Current Clinical Practice

FRANZ H. MESSERLI, M.D.
EDITOR

1987
W.B. SAUNDERS COMPANY
Philadelphia London Toronto
Sydney Tokyo Hong Kong

W. B. Saunders Company: West Washington Square
Philadelphia, PA 19105

Library of Congress Cataloging in Publication Data

Current clinical practice

1. Internal medicine.   2. Medicine, Clinical.
   I. Messerli, Franz H. [DNLM: 1. Medicine. WB 100 C976]

RC46.C95 1987   616   86–6512

ISBN 0–7216–1460–4

Editor: John Dyson
Developmental Editor: Carole Morrison
Designer: Terri Siegel
Production Manager: Bill Preston
Manuscript Editor: David Harvey
Illustration Coordinator: Walt Verbitski
Indexer: Ella Shapiro

Current Clinical Practice   ISBN   0–7216–1460–4

Last digit is the print number: 9   8   7   6   5   4   3   2   1

Contributors

CHARLES F. ABBOUD, M.B., B.Ch.

Associate Professor, Mayo Medical School; Consultant, Endocrinology and Internal Medicine, Mayo Clinic and Mayo Foundation, Rochester, MN

Hypopituitarism

MUZAFFAR AHMAD, M.D.

Chairman, Pulmonary Disease Department, Cleveland Clinic Foundation, Cleveland, OH

Pneumoconioses and Environmental Lung Disease

ROBERT E. ALBERTINI, M.D.

Clinical Professor of Medicine, Milton S. Hershey College of Medicine, Pennsylvania State University, Hershey, PA; Director, Department of Thoracic Medicine, and Assistant Chairman of Medicine, Geisinger Medical Center, Danville, PA

Dyspnea and Disability

GEORGE L. ALLEN, M.D.

Associate Professor of Medicine, Mayo Medical School; Consultant in Rheumatology, Mayo Clinic and Mayo Foundation, Rochester, MN

Osteoarthritis

JOHN ALBERT ANDERSON, M.D.

Clinical Professor of Pediatrics and Communicable Diseases, University of Michigan Medical School, Ann Arbor, MI; Chairman, Department of Pediatrics, and Head, Division of Allergy and Clinical Immunology (Department of Medicine), Henry Ford Hospital, Detroit, MI

Adverse Reactions to Foods

LYNN A. ANDERSON, M.D.

Resident, Department of Dermatology, Tulane University School of Medicine, New Orleans, LA

Atopic Dermatitis and Neurodermatitis

SANDRA L. ARGENIO, M.D.

Clinical Assistant Professor, Department of Family and Community Medicine, Milton S. Hershey College of Medicine, Pennsylvania State University, Hershey, PA; Attending Staff and Associate Physician, Geisinger Medical Center, Danville, PA

Immunizations in the Adult

ABDUL CADER ASMAL, M.D., Ph.D., M.R.C.P., F.C.P.

Assistant Professor of Medicine, Harvard Medical School; Attending Physician, New England Deaconess Hospital, Boston, MA. Formerly of the Joslin Clinic, Detroit, MI

Obesity; Disturbances in Electrolyte Metabolism, Diabetic Ketoacidosis, and Hyperosmolar Coma

RAYMOND G. AUGER, M.D.

Assistant Professor of Neurology, Mayo Medical School; Head, Section of Neurology, Mayo Clinic and Mayo Foundation, Rochester, MN

Treatment of Myopathies

RICHARD R. BABB, M.D.

Clinical Professor of Medicine, Stanford University School of Medicine; Staff, Gastroenterology Division, Palo Alto Medical Clinic, Palo Alto, CA

Peptic Ulcer Disease

LUIS A. BALART, M.D.

Staff, Department of Internal Medicine, Section on Gastroenterology, Ochsner Clinic and Alton Ochsner Medical Foundation, New Orleans, LA

Cirrhosis of the Liver

MARY C. BALDAUF, M.D.

Section Head, Blood Bank, St. Joseph's Hospital, Marshfield, WI; Pathologist, Marshfield Clinic, Marshfield, WI

Blood Transfusion

LAWRENCE V. BASSO, M.D., F.A.C.P.

Clinical Associate Professor of Medicine, Stanford University School of Medicine; Staff, Department of Endocrinology and Metabolics, Palo Alto Medical Clinic, Palo Alto, CA, and Stanford University Hospital, Stanford, CA

Acromegaly; Hirsutism

MARILYN BATEMAN, R.N., B.A.

Coordinator, Ochsner Foundation Community Clinical Oncology Program; Oncology Nurse Clinician, Ochsner Clinic and Alton Ochsner Medical Foundation, New Orleans, LA

Principles of Outpatient Chemotherapy

SURINDER K. BATRA, M.D., F.A.C.P., F.A.C.G.

Clinical Assistant Professor of Internal Medicine, University of Michigan Medical School, Ann Arbor, MI; Acting Division Head, Division of Gastroenterology, Henry Ford Hospital, Detroit, MI

Pancreatitis

JOHN F. BEAMIS, Jr., M.D.

Clinical Instructor in Medicine, Harvard Medical School, Boston, MA; Staff, Pulmonary Section, Lahey Clinic Medical Center, Burlington, MA

Common Fungal Diseases of the Lung

RICHARD S. BEASER, M.D.

Instructor in Medicine, Harvard Medical School; Senior Physician, Diabetes Treatment Unit, Joslin Clinic; Attending Physician, New England Deaconess Hospital, Boston, MA

Treatment of the Patient with Type I Diabetes

DAVID J. BECHTEL, M.D.

Clinical Instructor, Harvard Medical School; Staff Physician, Department of Emergency Medicine, Lahey Clinic Medical Center, Burlington, MA

Illness Caused by Cold

WILLIAM P. BEETHAM, Jr., M.D.

Assistant Professor of Medicine, Harvard Medical School, Boston, MA; Section of Rheumatology, Department of Internal Medicine, Lahey Clinic Medical Center, Burlington, MA

Crystal-Induced Arthritis: Calcium Pyrophosphate Deposition Disease and Pseudogout

STANLEY Z. BERMAN, M.D.

Clinical Assistant Professor, Department of Medicine, University of New Mexico School of Medicine; Chairman and Associate Staff, Department of Allergy and Immunology, Lovelace Medical Center; Attending Physician in Internal Medicine, Veterans Administration Hospital; Associate Medical Staff, University of New Mexico Hospital, Albuquerque, NM

Anaphylaxis

ERNEST BEUTLER, M.D.

Chairman, Department of Basic and Clinical Research, and Head, Division of Hematology/Oncology, Scripps Clinic and Research Foundation, La Jolla, CA

Hemolytic Anemia; Sickle Cell Disease and the Thalassemias

ANTHONY BILLAS, M.D.

Assistant Professor of Family and Community Medicine, Milton S. Hershey College of Medicine, Pennsylvania State University, Hershey, PA; Family Medicine Department, Geisinger Medical Center, Danville, PA

Viral Exanthems

WILLIAM L. BLACK, M.D., Sc.D.

Senior Staff, Diabetes Treatment Unit, Joslin Clinic, Boston, MA

Disturbances in Electrolyte Metabolism, Diabetic Ketoacidosis, and Hyperosmolar Coma

MICHAEL S. BLAISS, M.D.

Assistant Clinical Professor, Tulane University College of Medicine; Head, Department of Internal Medicine, Section of Allergy/Clinical Immunology, Ochsner Clinic and Alton Ochsner Medical Foundation, New Orleans, LA

Pruritus

CAREY A. BLIGARD, M.D.

Resident, Department of Dermatology, Tulane University School of Medicine; formerly affiliated with Ochsner Clinic and Alton Ochsner Medical Foundation, New Orleans, LA

Contact Dermatitis

MELVIN A. BLOCK, M.D., Ph.D.

Clinical Professor of Surgery and Consulting Staff, University of California School of Medicine and University Hospital, San Diego, CA; Chairman, Department of Surgery and Active Staff, Scripps Clinic and Research Foundation, La Jolla, CA; Courtesy Staff, Pomerado Hospital, Poway, CA

Parathyroid Disorders

LAWRENCE BLONDE, M.D.

Associate Director, Graduate Medical Education, Alton Ochsner Medical Foundation; Staff Physician, Department of Internal Medicine, Section of Endocrinology and Metabolic Diseases, Ochsner Clinic and Alton Ochsner Medical Foundation, New Orleans, LA

Cushing's Syndrome

JOSEPH B. BLOOD, Jr., M.D.

Assistant Clinical Professor of Medicine, Hahnemann University School of Medicine, Philadelphia, PA; Associate in Medicine, Guthrie Clinic and Robert Packer Hospital, Sayre, PA

Cough

FRANCIS BOUMPHREY, M.D.

Director, Center for the Spine, Cleveland Clinic Foundation, Cleveland, OH

Cervical and Lumbar Disc Disease

DONALD J. BRESLIN, M.D.

Assistant Clinical Professor of Medicine, Harvard Medical School, Boston, MA; Head, Section of Vascular Medicine and Hypertension, Lahey Clinic Medical Center, Burlington, MA; Staff, New England Deaconess Hospital, Boston, MA

Arteriosclerotic Occlusive Disease of the Aorta and Peripheral Arteries of the Lower Extremities; Venous Disorders and Pulmonary Embolism; Asymptomatic Carotid Disease; Hypertension in Acute Stroke and Hypertensive Encephalopathy

KAREN A. BRINGELSEN, M.D.

Instructor, Department of Pediatrics, Mayo Medical School; Associate Consultant in Pediatric Hematology and Oncology, Mayo Clinic and Mayo Foundation, Rochester, MN

The Inherited Disorders of Coagulation

G. THOMAS BUDD, M.D.

Attending Oncologist, Cleveland Clinic Foundation, Cleveland, OH

Soft Tissue and Bone Sarcomas

RONALD M. BUKOWSKI, M.D.

Staff Physician, Department of Medical Oncology and Hematology, Cleveland Clinic Foundation, Cleveland, OH

Tumors of the Intestinal Tract—Upper GI Tract, Carcinoid Syndrome, and Lower GI Tract

KEITH H. BURCH, M.D.

Assistant Clinical Professor of Internal Medicine, University of Michigan Medical School, Ann Arbor, MI; Medical Director, West Bloomfield Center, Henry Ford Hospital, Detroit, MI

Diagnosis and Treatment of Osteomyelitis

C. BRADDOCK BURNS, M.D.

Staff Physician, Department of Internal Medicine, Section on Pulmonary Diseases, Ochsner Clinic and Alton Ochsner Medical Foundation, New Orleans, LA

Bacterial, Viral, and Mycoplasmal Pneumonia

THEODORE W. BURNS, D.D.S., M.D.

Assistant Clinical Professor of Oral Medicine and Diagnosis, and Assistant Clinical Professor of Medicine, Louisiana State University Medical Center; Attending Gastroenterologist, Department of Internal Medicine, Section on Gastroenterology, Ochsner Clinic and Alton Ochsner Medical Foundation, New Orleans, LA

Esophageal Disorders and Disorders of Gastrointestinal Motility

ALAN L. BURSHELL, M.D.

Staff Physician, Section on Endocrinology and Metabolic Diseases, Ochsner Clinic and Alton Ochsner Medical Foundation, New Orleans, LA

Cushing's Syndrome

EDWARD J. BUSICK, M.D.

Instructor in Medicine, Harvard Medical School, Boston, MA; Physician, New England Deaconess Hospital, Boston, MA

Diagnosis and Management of Acid-Base Disturbances

RICHARD J. BUTCHER, M.D.

Clinical Associate Professor of Medicine, Milton S. Hershey College of Medicine, Pennsylvania State University, Hershey, PA; Associate in Cardiology, Geisinger Medical Center, Danville, PA

Pulmonary Hypertension and Cor Pulmonale

CAROL CAMP, M.S.

Microbiology Instructor, Robert Packer Hospital School of Medical Technology, Sayre, PA

Acute Bacterial Diarrhea and Food Poisoning

JULIO V. CARDENAS, M.D., F.A.C.P.

Clinical Assistant Professor, University of Michigan Medical School, Ann Arbor, MI; Division Head, Internal Medicine, Henry Ford Hospital, Detroit, MI

Malaria and Babesiosis

KEVIN V. CAREY, M.D.

Clinical Assistant Professor, State University of New York Upstate Medical Center, Syracuse, NY; Clinical Instructor, Hahnemann University School of Medicine, Philadelphia, PA; Staff Physician, Guthrie Clinic and Robert Packer Hospital, Sayre, PA

Diarrhea

WILLIAM D. CAREY, M.D.

Staff Physician, Co-Director, Liver Transplantation Section of Hepatology, Cleveland Clinic Foundation, Cleveland, OH

Cholecystitis and Cholelithiasis

JOHN H. CHAPMAN, M.D., F.A.C.P., F.A.C.C.

Clinical Professor of Medicine, Milton S. Hershey College of Medicine, Pennsylvania State University, Hershey, PA; Cardiology Associate, Geisinger Medical Center, Danville, PA

Coronary Artery Disease

A. RICHARD CHRISTLIEB, M.D.

Associate Professor of Medicine, Harvard Medical School; Physician, Joslin Clinic and New England Deaconess Hospital; Consultant in Medicine, Brigham and Women's Hospital, Boston, MA

Hypertension in the Diabetic Patient

HERBERT B. CHRISTIANSON, M.D.

Ochsner Clinic and Allan Ochsner Medical Foundation, Department of Dermatology, New Orleans, LA

Diseases of the Skin

BLAINE W. COBB, M.D.

Associate Staff, Department of Gastroenterology, Guthrie Clinic, Sayre, PA

Diverticulosis and Diverticulitis

GREGORY B. COLLINS, M.D.

Section Head, Alcohol and Drug Recovery Center, Department of Psychiatry, Cleveland Clinic Foundation, Cleveland, OH

Drug Abuse and Withdrawal

KENNETH H. COOPER, M.D., M.P.H.

Visiting lecturer, National Defense University, Washington, D.C.; President and founder, The Aerobics Center, Dallas, TX

Exercise in Health and Prevention of Disease

RAMACHANDIRAN COOPPAN, M.B.Ch.B., F.R.C.P.(C)

Instructor in Medicine, Harvard Medical School; Attending Physician, New England Deaconess Hospital; Attending Endocrinologist, Diabetes Treatment Unit, Joslin Clinic, Boston, MA

Trace Elements; Vitamins

EDWARD M. CORDASCO, M.D., F.C.C.P., F.A.C.P., F.A.C.A., F.A.O.M.

Head, Occupational Chest Clinic; Staff Physician, Pulmonary Disease Department, Cleveland Clinic Foundation, Cleveland, OH

Pneumoconioses and Environmental Lung Disease

JOSEPH C. CORKERY, M.D.

Clinical Instructor in Medicine, Harvard Medical School, Boston, MA; Head, Section of General Internal Medicine, Lahey Clinic Medical Center, Burlington, MA

Anxiety and Depression

LAURENCE M. CORTEZ, M.D.

Clinical Associate Professor of Medicine, Tulane University School of Medicine; Clinical Assistant Professor of Medicine, Louisiana State University School of Medicine; Epidemiologist; Associate Head, Section on Infectious Diseases, Department of Internal Medicine, Ochsner Clinic and Alton Ochsner Medical Foundation, New Orleans, LA

Medical Advice for Travelers

ROGER W. COUNTEE, M.D.

Staff, Department of Neurosurgery, Lahey Clinic Medical Center, Burlington, MA

Subarachnoid Hemorrhage

MICHAEL D. CRESSMAN, D.O.

Staff, Research Institute, Department of Hypertension and Nephrology, Cleveland Clinic Foundation, Cleveland, OH

Mild Essential Hypertension

GEORGE E. DAILEY III, M.D.

Assistant Clinical Professor of Medicine, University of California, San Diego, School of Medicine; Head, Division of Diabetes and Endocrinology, and Associate Member, Research Institute, Scripps Clinic and Research Foundation, La Jolla, CA; Courtesy Staff, Sharp Memorial Hospital and Alvarado Hospital, San Diego, CA, and at Pomerado Hospital, Poway, CA

Hormones and Cancer

DONALD J. DALESSIO, M.D.

Clinical Professor of Neurology, University of California, San Diego, School of Medicine; Chairman, Department of Medicine and Physician in Chief, Scripps Clinic and Research Foundation, La Jolla, CA

Giant Cell Arteritis and Polymyalgia Rheumatica

J. THOMAS DANZI, M.D., F.A.C.P.

Chief, Section of Gastroenterology, Guthrie Clinic and Robert Packer Hospital, Sayre, PA

Idiopathic Inflammatory Bowel Disease

RICHARD A. DART, M.D.

Associate Clinical Professor of Medicine, University of Wisconsin Medical School, Madison, WI; Marshfield Clinic and St. Joseph's Hospital, Marshfield, WI

Tubulointerstitial Nephropathy and Urinary Tract Infections

CHRISTOPHER J. DEGNEN, M.D.

Clinical Instructor in Emergency Medicine, Harvard Medical School, Boston, MA; Attending Physician, Emergency Department, Lahey Clinic Medical Center, Burlington, MA

Diseases due to Hypobaric and Hyperbaric Environments

JOHN A. D'ELIA, M.D.

Assistant Professor of Medicine, Harvard Medical School; Senior Physician, Joslin Clinic; Active Staff, New England Deaconess Hospital, Boston, MA

Chronic Renal Failure; The Kidney in Systemic Disease

RICHARD A. DeREMEE, M.D.

Professor of Medicine, Mayo Medical School; Attending Physician, St. Mary's Hospital and Methodist Hospital, Rochester, MN

Sarcoidosis

JAMES H. DIAZ, M.D.

Associate Professor of Anesthesiology (Clinical) Tulane University School of Medicine; Attending Anesthesiologist and Co-Director, Intensive Care Unit, Ochsner Clinic and Alton Ochsner Medical Foundation, New Orleans, LA

Diagnosis and Management of Acid-Base Disturbances

ROBERT P. DINAPOLI, M.D.

Assistant Professor, Mayo Medical School; Consultant in Neurology, Mayo Clinic and Mayo Foundation, Rochester Methodist Hospital, and St. Mary's Hospital, Rochester, MN

Acute Spinal Cord Disorders

MATTHEW B. DIVERTIE, M.D.

Consultant in Division of Thoracic Diseases, Consultant in Section of Critical Care—Respiratory; Professor of Medicine, Mayo Medical School, Rochester, MN

The Respiratory System

ANDREA DLESK, M.D., F.A.C.P.

Clinical Associate Professor, University of Wisconsin Medical School, Madison, WI; Staff Rheumatologist, Marshfield Clinic and St. Joseph's Hospital, Marshfield, WI

Reiter's Disease

DOUGLAS P. DUFFY, M.D.

Assistant Clinical Professor of Medicine, University of Wisconsin Medical School, Madison, WI; Staff Nephrologist, Marshfield Clinic and St. Joseph's Hospital, Marshfield, WI

Tubulointerstitial Nephropathy and Urinary Tract Infections

JOHN J. DUNCAN, Ph.D.

Research Associate, Department of Exercise Physiology, Institute for Aerobics Research, Dallas, TX

Exercise in Health and Prevention of Disease

PAUL G. DYMENT, M.D.

Clinical Professor of Pediatrics, Case Western Reserve University School of Medicine; Chairman, Department of Pediatric and Adolescent Medicine, and Head, Section of Adolescent Medicine, Cleveland Clinic Foundation, Cleveland, OH

Medical Care of the Adolescent Patient

NEIL M. ELLISON, M.D.

Clinical Assistant Professor of Medicine, Milton S. Hershey College of Medicine, Pennsylvania State University, Hershey, PA; Associate Physician, Department of Hematology/Oncology, Geisinger Medical Center, Danville, PA

Unproven Methods of Cancer Therapy

W. BROOKS EMORY, M.D.

Chief, Section on Pulmonary Diseases, Department of Internal Medicine, Ochsner Clinic and Alton Ochsner Medical Foundation, New Orleans, LA

Bacterial, Viral, and Mycoplasmal Pneumonia; Influenza

STEPHEN B. ERICKSON, M.D.

Assistant Professor of Medicine, Mayo Medical School; Consultant, Division of Nephrology and Internal Medicine, Mayo Clinic and Mayo Foundation, Rochester, MN

Nephrolithiasis

VIRGIL F. FAIRBANKS, M.D.

Professor of Laboratory Medicine and Internal Medicine, Mayo Medical School; Consultant in Hematology and Internal Medicine, Mayo Clinic and Mayo Foundation, Rochester Methodist Hospital, and St. Mary's Hospital, Rochester, MN

Iron Deficiency

PATRICIA K. FARRIS, M.D.

Assistant Professor, Department of Dermatology, Tulane University School of Medicine, New Orleans, LA; Private Practice–Dermatology

Atopic Dermatitis and Neurodermatitis

LUIS FERNANDEZ-HERLIHY, M.D.

Lecturer on Medicine, Harvard Medical School, Boston, MA; Head, Section of Rheumatology, Lahey Clinic Medical Center, Burlington, MA

Seronegative Spondyloarthropathies

WILLIAM A. FERRANTE, M.D.

Clinical Professor of Medicine, Tulane University School of Medicine and Louisiana State University School of Medicine; Staff, Department of Internal Medicine, Section on Gastroenterology, Ochsner Clinic and Alton Ochsner Medical Foundation; Senior Visiting Physician, Charity Hospital of Louisiana, New Orleans, LA

Nausea and Vomiting

BERNARD T. FERRARI, M.D.

Clinical Associate Professor, Department of Surgery, Tulane University School of Medicine; Vice Chairman, Department of Colon and Rectal Surgery, Ochsner Clinic and Alton Ochsner Medical Foundation, New Orleans, LA

Common Anorectal Problems in Internal Medicine

JULIO E. FIGUEROA, M.D.

Senior Active Staff, Department of Internal Medicine, Section on Nephrology, Ochsner Clinic and Alton Ochsner Medical Foundation, New Orleans, LA

Clinical Approach to the Patient with Renal Disease

RICHARD M. FINKEL, M.D.

Clinical Instructor in Medicine, Harvard Medical School, Boston, MA; Staff, Department of Internal Medicine, Section of Nephrology, Lahey Clinic Medical Center, Burlington, MA

Acute Renal Failure

EVELYN J. FISHER, M.D.

Clinical Associate Professor of Medicine, University of Michigan Medical School, Ann Arbor, MI; Staff Physician, Division of Infectious Diseases, Henry Ford Hospital, Detroit, MI

Pneumocystis carinii, Giardiasis, Cryptosporidiosis, Trichinosis, and Echinococcosis

MORRIS A. FLAUM, M.D.

Clinical Assistant Professor, Department of Medicine, Tulane University School of Medicine; Staff Physician, Department of Internal Medicine, Section on Hematology and Oncology, Ochsner Clinic and Alton Ochsner Medical Foundation, New Orleans, LA

Pain

W. NEATH FOLGER, M.D.

Assistant Professor, Mayo Medical School; Consultant, Neurology, Mayo Clinic and Mayo Foundation, Rochester Methodist Hospital, and St. Mary's Hospital, Rochester, MN

Ischemic Cerebrovascular Disease: Vertebrobasilar System

PIERRE FORGACS, M.D., F.R.C.P. (C)

Clinical Instructor in Medicine, Harvard Medical School, Boston, MA; Head, Section of Infectious Diseases, and Staff, Department of Internal Medicine, Lahey Clinic Medical Center, Burlington, MA

Infective Endocarditis: A Disease in Evolution; Common Otolaryngologic Problems; Brain Abscess and Subdural Empyema; Acute and Chronic Meningitis

MAURICE FOX, M.D.

Clinical Professor of Medicine, Stanford University School of Medicine; Staff, Department of Endocrinology and Metabolics; Codirector of Laboratory, Palo Alto Medical Clinic and Stanford University Hospital, Stanford, CA

Acromegaly

STEPHEN R. FREIDBERG, M.D.

Chairman, Department of Neurosurgery, Lahey Clinic Medical Center, Burlington, MA

Brain Abscess and Subdural Empyema; Management of Increased Intracranial Pressure

JEFFERY P. FREY, M.D.

Assistant Professor of Medicine, Tulane University School of Medicine and Louisiana State University School of Medicine; Staff, Department of Internal Medicine, Division of Primary Care, Section on Community Internal Medicine, Ochsner Clinic and Alton Ochsner Medical Foundation, New Orleans, LA

Perioperative Medical Management

WILLIAM R. FRIEDENBERG, M.D., F.A.C.P.

Clinical Associate Professor, University of Wisconsin Medical School, Madison, WI; Staff Hematologist/Oncologist, St. Joseph's Hospital, Marshfield, WI

Immunodeficiency; Neutropenia

NEAL M. FRIEDMAN, M.D.

Chairman, Department of Endocrinology, Lovelace Medical Center; Clinical Assistant Professor of Medicine, Department of Internal Medicine, University of New Mexico School of Medicine; Chairman, Department of Endocrinology, Lovelace Medical Center, Albuquerque, NM

Goiter and the Single Thyroid Nodule

EDWARD D. FROHLICH, M.D.

Alton Ochsner Distinguished Scientist and Vice President for Academic Affairs, Alton Ochsner Medical Foundation; Member, Section on Hypertensive Diseases, Ochsner Clinic; Professor, Departments of Medicine and Physiology, Louisiana State University; Clinical Professor of Medicine and Adjunct Professor of Pharmacology, Tulane University, New Orleans, LA

The Cardiovascular System

ANTHONY J. FURLAN, M.D.

Director, Cerebrovascular Program, Cleveland Clinic Foundation, Cleveland, OH

Cardioembolic Stroke

HAROLD A. FUSELIER, Jr., M.D.

Clinical Assistant Professor, Department of Urology, Tulane University School of Medicine; Head, Department of Urology, Ochsner Clinic and Alton Ochsner Medical Foundation; Director, Mims Gage Ochsner Lithotripsy Center; Consultant in Urology, Charity Hospital of Louisiana, New Orleans, LA, and Southeast Louisiana Medical Center, Houma, LA

Common Urologic Problems in Internal Medicine

LEONARD E. GATELY III, M.D.

Assistant Professor of Dermatology, Tulane University School of Medicine; Staff Physician, Tulane Medical Center; Visiting Physician, Charity Hospital of Louisiana; Consultant in Dermatology, Ochsner Clinic and Alton Ochsner Medical Foundation, New Orleans, LA

Psoriasis

J. BYRON GATHRIGHT, Jr., M.D.

Chairman, Department of Colon and Rectal Surgery, Ochsner Clinic and Alton Ochsner Medical Foundation, New Orleans, LA

Common Anorectal Problems in Internal Medicine

GERALD T. GAU, M.D.

Assistant Professor of Medicine, Mayo Medical School; Consultant in Cardiovascular Disease, Mayo Clinic and Mayo Foundation, Rochester Methodist Hospital, and St. Mary's Hospital, Rochester, MN; Floyd County Memorial Hospital, Charles City, IA; St. Francis Hospital, New Hampton, IA

Rehabilitation After Myocardial Infarction and Cardiac Surgery

JANE A. GEHLSEN, M.D.

Private practice, Hilton Head Island, SC; formerly affiliated with Marshfield Clinic, Marshfield, WI

Tumor Lysis Syndrome

EDWARD GENTON, M.D.

Attending Cardiologist, Department of Internal Medicine, Section on Cardiology, Ochsner Clinic and Alton Ochsner Medical Foundation, New Orleans, LA

Anticoagulants and Platelet Inhibitors

BERNARD J. GERSH, M.B., Ch.B., D. Phil.

Associate Professor of Medicine, Mayo Medical School; Consultant, Division of Cardiovascular Diseases and Internal Medicine, Mayo Clinic and Mayo Foundation, Rochester, MN

Heart Block

RAY W. GIFFORD, Jr., M.D.

Staff, Department of Hypertension and Nephrology, Cleveland Clinic Foundation, Cleveland, OH

Mild Essential Hypertension

GERALD S. GILCHRIST, M.D.

Professor and Chairman, Department of Pediatrics, Mayo Medical School; Consultant in Pediatric Hematology and Oncology, Mayo Clinic and Mayo Foundation; Director, Mayo Comprehensive Hemophilia Center, Rochester, MN

The Inherited Disorders of Coagulation

PAUL F. GILLILAND, M.D.

Professor of Internal Medicine, Texas A&M University College of Medicine, College Station, TX; Director, Division of Endocrinology and Metabolism, Scott and White Clinic; Consultant in Endocrinology and Metabolism, Olin E. Teague Veterans Administration Hospital, Temple, TX

Hypothyroidism

JOSEPH A. GOLISH, M.D.

Professional Staff, Department of Pulmonary Medicine, Cleveland Clinic Foundation, Cleveland, OH

The Common Cold

LILIAN GONSALVES-EBRAHIM, M.D.

Section Liaison—Psychiatry, Department of Psychiatry, Cleveland Clinic Foundation, Cleveland, OH

Psychological Aspects (Chronic Renal Failure)

CAROL E. GOODMAN, M.D.

Head, Department of Physical Medicine and Rehabilitation (Retired), Ochsner Clinic and Alton Ochsner Medical Foundation, New Orleans, LA

Pain

GERALD GORDON, M.D.

Clinical Associate Professor, Milton S. Hershey College of Medicine, Pennsylvania State University, Hershey, PA; Associate in Infectious Diseases, Geisinger Medical Center, Danville, PA

Anaerobic Infections: Tetanus and the Gangrenes; Chlamydia

RALPH GREEN, M.D.

Chairman, Laboratory Hematology, Cleveland Clinic Foundation, Cleveland, OH

Hemochromatosis

MEIR GROSS, M.D., F.A.P.A.

Faculty, Cleveland Clinic Educational Foundation; Head, Section of Eating Disorders, Cleveland Clinic Foundation, Cleveland, OH

Anorexia

PAUL T. GROSS, M.D.

Assistant Professor of Neurology, University of Massachusetts Medical School, Worcester, MA; Clinical Instructor in Neurology, Harvard Medical School, Boston, MA; Staff Neurologist, Department of Neurology, Lahey Clinic Medical Center, Burlington, MA, and Department of Neurology, Children's Hospital, Boston, MA

Sleep Disorders

A. DALE GULLEDGE, M.D.

Head Liaison—Psychiatry, Department of Psychiatry, Cleveland Clinic Cancer Center, Cleveland, OH

Nonmedical Support for Cancer Patients and Their Families; Psychological Aspects (Chronic Renal Failure)

JOSÉ A. GUTRECHT, M.D., M.Sc.

Staff Neurologist, Department of Neurology, Lahey Clinic Medical Center, Burlington, MA

Acute and Chronic Viral Encephalitis

STEPHEN C. HAMMILL, M.D.

Assistant Professor of Medicine, Mayo Medical School; Consultant, Division of Cardiovascular Diseases and Internal Medicine, Mayo Clinic and Mayo Foundation, Rochester, MN

Syncope

MAURICE R. HANSON, M.D.

Assistant Clinical Professor, Department of Neurology, Case Western Reserve University; Staff Neurologist, Cleveland Clinic Foundation, Cleveland, OH

Coma and Confusional States

RUSSELL W. HARDY, Jr., M.D.

Director, Center for the Spine, Cleveland Clinic Foundation, Cleveland, OH

Cervical and Lumbar Disc Disease

JOHN W. HARE, M.D.

Assistant Professor of Medicine, Harvard Medical School; Senior Physician, Joslin Clinic; Attending Physician, New England Deaconess Hospital; Consultant (Obstetrics), Brigham and Women's Hospital, Boston, MA

Treatment of the Patient with Type 1 Diabetes

EDWARD W. HEIN, M.D.

Assistant Professor of Pediatrics, Temple University School of Medicine; Chief, Section of Allergy, St. Christopher's Hospital for Children, Philadelphia, PA; Formerly of the Cleveland Clinic Foundation, Cleveland, OH

Allergic Reaction to Insect Sting

FREDERICK W. HEISS, M.D.

Staff, Department of Gastroenterology, Lahey Clinic Medical Center, Burlington, MA

Parasites of the Gastrointestinal Tract

PAUL E. HERMANS, M.D.

Professor of Medicine, Mayo Medical School; Consultant in Infectious Diseases, Methodist Hospital and St. Mary's Hospital, Rochester, MN

Outpatient Antibiotic Therapy; Toxic Shock Syndrome and Pelvic Inflammatory Disease

ROGER H. HERZIG, M.D.

Associate Clinical Professor of Medicine, Case Western Reserve University; Director, Bone Marrow Transplantation, Cleveland Clinic Foundation, Cleveland, OH

Tumors of the Skin: Malignant Melanoma

TERRY C. HICKS, M.D.

Staff Surgeon, Department of Colon and Rectal Surgery, Ochsner Clinic and Alton Ochsner Medical Foundation; Clinical Instructor in Surgery, Department of Surgery, Tulane University School of Medicine; Surgical Staff, Tulane University Hospital, and Charity Hospital of Louisiana, New Orleans, LA

Common Anorectal Problems in Internal Medicine

CHESLEY HINES, Jr., M.D.

Clinical Associate Professor, Tulane University School of Medicine; Staff, Department of Internal Medicine, Section on Gastroenterology, Ochsner Clinic and Alton Ochsner Medical Foundation, New Orleans, LA

Malabsorption and Maldigestion

ELEANOR T. HOBBS, M.D.

Clinical Instructor in Medicine, Harvard Medical School, Boston, MA; Chairman, Department of Emergency Medicine, Lahey Clinic Medical Center, Burlington, MA

Approach to the Poisoned Patient

WILLIAM GRAY HOCKING, M.D.

Assistant Clinical Professor, University of Wisconsin Medical School, Madison, WI; Staff, Department of Hematology and Oncology, Marshfield Clinic, Marshfield, WI

Polycythemia: Primary and Secondary Erythrocytosis

WENDELL W. HOFFMAN, M.D.

Clinical Instructor of Medicine, Harvard Medical School, Boston, MA; Consultant in Infectious Diseases, Lahey Clinic Medical Center, Burlington, MA

Brain Abscess and Subdural Empyema; Acute and Chronic Meningitis

DAVID R. HOLMES, Jr., M.D.

Associate Professor of Medicine, Mayo Medical School; Consultant, Division of Cardiovascular Diseases and Internal Medicine, Mayo Clinic and Mayo Foundation, Rochester, MN

Syncope

HENRY A. HOMBURGER, M.D.

Associate Professor of Laboratory Medicine, Mayo Medical School and Mayo Graduate School of Medicine; Consultant in Clinical Immunology, Mayo Clinic and Mayo Foundation, Rochester, MN

Laboratory Testing in Evaluation and Management of Allergic Diseases

FRANK M. HOWARD, Jr., M.D.

Professor of Neurology, Mayo Medical School; Consultant, St. Mary's Hospital, Methodist Hospital, and Mayo Clinic and Mayo Foundation, Rochester, MN

Treatment of Diseases Affecting Neuromuscular Transmission

RICHARD D. HURT, M.D.

Assistant Professor of Medicine, Mayo Medical School; Consultant in Internal Medicine, Division of Community Internal Medicine, Mayo Clinic and Mayo Foundation, Rochester, MN

Alcoholism

FRED E. HUSSERL, M.D.

Staff, Department of Internal Medicine, Section on Nephrology, Ochsner Clinic and Alton Ochsner Medical Foundation, New Orleans, LA

Leg Cramps and Restless Legs; Toxic Nephropathies and Drug Use in Patients with Renal Impairment

JEFFREY C. HUTZLER, M.D.

Section Liaison—Psychiatry, Department of Psychiatry, Cleveland Clinic Foundation, Cleveland, OH

Psychological Aspects (Chronic Renal Failure)

ROGER L. HYBELS, M.D.

Clinical Assistant Professor of Otolaryngology, Boston University School of Medicine, Boston, MA; Senior Staff, Department of Otolaryngology–Head and Neck Surgery, Lahey Clinic Medical Center, Burlington, MA

Common Otolaryngologic Problems

EDWARD R. JEWELL, M.D.

Staff, Section of Peripheral Vascular Surgery, Lahey Clinic Medical Center, Burlington, MA

Arteriosclerotic Occlusive Disease of the Aorta and Peripheral Arteries of the Lower Extremities

VICTOR E. JIMENEZ-LUCHO, M.D., M.S., D.T.M. & H. (Lond.)

Assistant Professor of Tropical Medicine, San Marcos University, Lima, Peru; Research Fellow, National Institutes of Health, Bethesda, MD; Former Infectious Diseases Fellow, Henry Ford Hospital, Detroit, MI

Malaria and Babesiosis

H. ROYDEN JONES, Jr., M.D.

Neurologist, Lahey Clinic Medical Center, Burlington, MA

Current Perspectives of Cerebrovascular Disease; Uncommon Causes of Stroke; Intracerebral Hemorrhage

JOHN F. JOVANOVICH, M.D.

Senior Staff Physician, Department of Internal Medicine (Infectious Disease), Henry Ford Hospital, Detroit, MI

Rickettsiosis and Pasteurella Infections; Genital Herpes

DOROTHY M. KAHKONEN, M.D.

Clinical Assistant Professor of Internal Medicine, University of Michigan, Ann Arbor, MI; Attending Physician, Department of Metabolism, Henry Ford Hospital, Detroit, MI

Non-Insulin–Dependent Diabetes Mellitus

ANTOINE KALDANY, M.D.

Assistant Professor of Medicine, Harvard Medical School; Senior Physician, Joslin Clinic; Investigator, E. P. Joslin Research Laboratories; Active Staff Physician, New England Deaconess Hospital; Associate in Medicine, Brigham and Women's Hospital, Boston, MA

Chronic Renal Failure; The Kidney in Systemic Disease

CARL G. KARDINAL, M.D.

Associate Professor of Clinical Medicine, Louisiana State University School of Medicine; Principal Investigator, Ochsner Foundation Community Oncology Program; Medical Oncologist, Department of Internal Medicine, Section on Hematology and Oncology, Ochsner Clinic and Alton Ochsner Medical Foundation, New Orleans, LA

Principles of Outpatient Chemotherapy

HAROLD P. KATNER, M.D.

Assistant Professor, Department of Internal Medicine, and Chief, Section on Infectious Diseases, Mercer University School of Medicine; Teaching and Consulting Staff, Medical Center of Central Georgia, Macon, GA; Consulting Staff, Veterans Administration Hospital, Dublin, GA. Formerly of Ochsner Clinic and Alton Ochsner Medical Foundation, New Orleans, LA

Sexually Transmitted Infections

NORMAN KATTWINKEL, M.D.

Clinical Instructor in Medicine, Harvard Medical School, Boston, MA; Senior Staff Physician, Department of Internal Medicine Section of Rheumatology, Lahey Clinic Medical Center, Burlington, MA

Lyme Disease

RONALD L. KAYE, M.D., F.A.C.P.

Clinical Professor of Medicine, Stanford University School of Medicine; Attending Physician, Stanford University Hospital, Veterans Administration Hospital, and Children's Hospital at Stanford; Staff Physician, Department of Metabolics, Palo Alto Medical Clinic, Palo Alto, CA

Rheumatoid Arthritis

JOSEPH E. KELLEHER, Jr., M.D.

Senior Staff Physician, Department of Allergy and Dermatology, Lahey Clinic Medical Center, Burlington, MA

Allergen Immunotherapy

JOSEPH F. KELLEY, M.D.

Senior Clinical Instructor, Department of Medicine, Case Western Reserve University; Chairman and Staff Physician, Department of Allergy and Immunology, Cleveland Clinic Foundation, Cleveland, OH

Urticaria and Angioedema

MICHAEL H. KESLIN, M.D.

Associate Clinical Professor, University of New Mexico School of Medicine; Associate Staff, Department of Allergy and Immunology, Lovelace Medical Center, Albuquerque, NM

Anaphylaxis

H. STEPHEN KOTT, M.D.

Clinical Instructor in Neurology, Harvard Medical School, Boston, MA; Chairman, Department of Neurology, Lahey Clinic Medical Center, Burlington, MA

Multiple Sclerosis

ROBERT S. KUNKEL, M.D.

Staff Physician; Head, Section of Headache, Department of Internal Medicine, Cleveland Clinic Foundation, Cleveland, OH

Headache

CHARLES A. LAUBACH, Jr., M.D.

Clinical Professor of Medicine and Adjunct Professor of Applied Physiology, Milton S. Hershey College of Medicine, Pennsylvania State University, Hershey, PA; Director Emeritus and Senior Consultant, Department of Cardiology, Geisinger Medical Center, Danville, PA

Diseases of the Pericardium and Myocardium

FERROL J. LEE, M.D.

Associate in Endocrinology, Guthrie Clinic and Robert Packer Hospital, Sayre, PA

Thyroiditis; Thyroid Cancer

ROBERT LENOX, M.D.

Staff, Department of Pulmonary Diseases, Guthrie Clinic and Robert Packer Hospital, Sayre, PA

Pleural Effusion

KERRY H. LEVIN, M.D.

Staff Neurologist, Cleveland Clinic Foundation, Cleveland, OH

Peripheral Neuropathy

NATHAN W. LEVIN, M.D.

Clinical Professor of Internal Medicine, University of Michigan Medical School, Ann Arbor, MI; Head, Division of Nephrology and Hypertension, Henry Ford Hospital, Detroit, MI

Chronic Renal Failure; Dialysis and Transplantation

RANDY LINDE, M.D., F.A.C.P.

Assistant Clinical Professor of Medicine, Stanford University School of Medicine, Staff, Department of Endocrinology, Stanford University Hospital, Stanford, CA and Palo Alto Medical Clinic, Palo Alto, CA

Hirsutism; Infertility

ROBERT L. LONGMIRE, M.D.

Staff Physician, Department of Hematology, and Adjunct Associate Member, Department of Basic and Clinical Research; Staff physician, Scripps Clinic and Research Foundation, La Jolla, CA

Multiple Myeloma and Related Disorders

WALLACE E. LOWRY, Jr., M.D.

Associate Professor, Texas A&M University College of Medicine, College Station, TX; Staff, Department of Orthopedics, Scott and White Clinic, Temple, TX

Common Orthopedic Problems in Internal Medicine

DENNIS J. LYNCH, M.D.

Professor, Department of Surgery, Texas A&M University College of Medicine, College Station, TX; Staff, Division of Plastic Surgery, Scott and White Clinic, Temple, TX

Snakebites, Spider Bites, and Fire Ant Stings

BRUCE R. MacKAY, M.D.

Associate Professor of Medicine, Hahnemann University School of Medicine, Philadelphia, PA; Clinical Associate Professor of Medicine, Syracuse University School of Medicine, Syracuse, NY; Chairman, Department of Medicine and Chief of Endocrinology, Guthrie Clinic and Robert Packer Hospital, Sayre, PA

Thyroiditis; Thyroid Cancer

HUGH L. N. MacKECHNIE, M.D.

Clinical Assistant Professor, University of Michigan Medical School, Ann Arbor, MI; Director, Adult Allergy, Henry Ford Hospital, Detroit, MI

Allergic and Nonallergic Rhinitis

JAMES W. MANIER, M.D.

Clinical Professor of Medicine, University of New Mexico School of Medicine; Chief of Gastroenterology, Lovelace Medical Center, Albuquerque, NM

Constipation; Tumors of the Intestinal Tract—Upper GI Tract, Carcinoid Syndrome, and Lower GI Tract

NIRMAL S. MANN, M.D., M.S. (Gastro), F.A.C.N., F.A.C.G., F.R.C.P.(C), F.A.C.P.

Professor of Medicine, Texas A&M University College of Medicine, College Station, TX; Chief, Gastroenterology–Hepatology–Nutrition Section, Olin Teague VA Center (affiliated with Scott and White Clinic), Temple, TX

Gastrointestinal Bleeding

SURINDER K. MANN, M.D., F.A.C.N.

Assistant Professor of Medicine, Texas A&M University College of Medicine, College Station, TX; Staff Physician, Geriatric Gastroenterology Section, Olin Teague VA Center (affiliated with Scott and White Clinic), Temple, TX

Gastrointestinal Bleeding

ALICE MAROSI, M.D.

Assistant Clinical Professor of Pediatrics, University of New Mexico School of Medicine; Associate Staff, Department of Allergy and Immunology, Lovelace Medical Center; Active Medical Staff, University of New Mexico Hospital, Albuquerque, NM

Anaphylaxis

DAVID A. MATHISON, M.D.

Clinic Senior Consultant and Adjunct Member, Division of Allergy and Immunology, Scripps Clinic and Research Foundation, La Jolla, CA

Adverse Reactions to Drugs

JOSEPH J. MAZZA, M.D.

Associate Professor of Clinical Medicine, University of Wisconsin Medical School, Madison, WI; Associate Staff Physician and Consultant in Hematology and Internal Medicine, Marshfield Clinic, St. Joseph's Hospital, Marshfield, WI

Chronic Lymphocytic Leukemia; Chronic Myelogenous Leukemia

ELIZABETH I. McBURNEY, M.D., F.A.C.P.

Clinical Associate Professor of Dermatology, Louisiana State University School of Medicine; Clinical Assistant Professor of Dermatology, Tulane University School of Medicine; Consulting Staff, Charity Hospital of Louisiana, New Orleans, LA; Staff Physician, Slidell Memorial Hospital, and Active Staff, Northshore Regional Medical Center; Private practice, Slidell, LA (formerly affiliated with Ochsner Clinic and Alton Ochsner Medical Foundation, New Orleans, LA)

Herpes Zoster

A. MARY McCARROLL, M.D.

Attending Endocrinologist, Scripps Clinic and Research Foundation, La Jolla, CA, and Sharp Memorial Hospital, San Diego, CA

Multiple Endocrine Neoplasia (MEN); Pluriglandular Autoimmune Syndrome

RICHARD Y. McCONNELL, M.D.

Chairman, Department of Emergency Medicine, Ochsner Clinic and Alton Ochsner Medical Foundation, New Orleans, LA

Heat-Related Illnesses

JAMES M. McCULLOUGH, M.A., M.D.

Private Practice, General Pulmonary Medicine and ICU Medicine, Metairie, LA. Formerly affiliated with Ochsner Clinic and Alton Ochsner Medical Foundation, New Orleans, LA

Perioperative Medical Management

DOUGLAS B. McGILL, M.D.

Professor of Medicine, Mayo Medical School; Consultant in Internal Medicine and Gastroenterology, Mayo Clinic and Mayo Foundation, Rochester, MN

Hepatitis

URSULA G. McKENNA, M.D.

Assistant Professor of Medicine, Mayo Medical School; Consultant, Emergency Medical Services, St. Mary's Hospital and Methodist Hospital, Rochester, MN

Toxic Shock Syndrome and Pelvic Inflammatory Disease

ROBERT McMILLAN, M.D.

Director, Weingart Center for Bone Marrow Transplantation, Division of Hematology/Oncology, Scripps Clinic and Research Foundation, La Jolla, CA

Platelet Disorders

RAYMOND C. MELLINGER, M.D.

Clinical Professor of Medicine, University of Michigan Medical School, Ann Arbor, MI; Head, Division of Endocrinology, Department of Internal Medicine, Henry Ford Hospital, Detroit, MI

Prolactinoma

JOHN W. MELSKI, M.D.

Pediatric Dermatologist, Marshfield Clinic; Staff, St. Joseph's Hospital, Marshfield, WI

Common Skin and Soft Tissue Infections; Acne Vulgaris

F. J. MENAPACE, M.D., F.A.C.C.

Clinical Professor of Medicine, Milton S. Hershey College of Medicine, Pennsylvania State University, Hershey, PA; Staff, Geisinger Medical Center, Danville, PA, and Temple University Hospital, Philadelphia, PA

Valvular Heart Disease

DONALD J. MIECH, M.D.

Associate Clinical Professor of Medicine (Dermatology), University of Wisconsin Medical School, Madison, WI; Assistant Clinical Professor of Dermatology, University of Minnesota, Minneapolis, MN; Attending Dermatologist, Department of Dermatology, Marshfield Clinic and St. Joseph's Hospital, Marshfield, WI

Management of Decubitus and Leg Ulcers

DONALD G. MILLER, M.D.

Clinical Instructor in Medicine, Harvard Medical School; Active Staff, New England Deaconess Hospital, Renal Department, Joslin Clinic, Boston, MA

Parenteral Nutrition

O. FRED MILLER III, M.D.

Director, Dermatology Department, Geisinger Medical Center, Danville, PA

Cutaneous Manifestations of Rheumatoid Arthritis

FERNANDO G. MIRANDA, M.D.

Clinical Assistant Professor (Neurology), University of New Mexico School of Medicine, Albuquerque, NM; Staff Neurologist, St. Rose Hospital, Hayward, CA, and Eden Hospital, Castro Valley, CA. Formerly at Lovelace Medical Center, Albuquerque, NM

Insomnia

HIROSHI MITSUMOTO, M.D., D.M.Sc.

Staff Neurologist and Director, Neuromuscular Disease Program, Department of Neurology, Cleveland Clinic Foundation, Cleveland, OH

Motor Neuron Disease

MONICA L. MONICA, M.D., Ph.D.

Staff, Eye, Ear, Nose and Throat Hospital, New Orleans, LA; Private Practice, Metairie, LA. Formerly at Ochsner Clinic and Alton Ochsner Medical Foundation, New Orleans, LA

Common Eye Problems in Internal Medicine

RONALD P. MONSAERT, M.D.

Clinical Professor of Medicine, Milton S. Hershey College of Medicine, Pennsylvania State University, Hershey, PA; Director, Department of Endocrinology and Metabolism, Geisinger Medical Center, Danville, PA

Hypothalamic Disorders; Hypoglycemia

ANTHONY P. MOORE, M.D.

Clinical Instructor, University of California, San Diego, School of Medicine; Head, Division of Community Medicine, and Member, Board of Governors and Board of Directors, Scripps Clinic Medical Group; Staff Physician, Department of Internal Medicine, Scripps Clinic and Research Foundation, La Jolla, CA

Fatigue

TOMASZ MROCZKOWSKI, M.D.

Visiting Assistant Professor, Department of Dermatology, Tulane University School of Medicine, New Orleans, LA

Atopic Dermatitis and Neurodermatitis

DOUGLAS B. MUCHMORE, M.D.

Assistant Adjunct Member, Research Institute of Scripps Clinic; Staff Physician, Scripps Clinic and Research Foundation, La Jolla, CA

Osteomalacia and Osteoporosis

JANE MUELLER, B.A.

Affiliated with Ochsner Clinic and Alton Ochsner Medical Foundation, New Orleans, LA

Ideals in the Physician-Patient Relationship

CHARLES Z. NAGGAR, M.D., F.A.C.C.

Assistant Clinical Professor of Medicine, Harvard Medical School, Boston, MA; Director, Non-Invasive Laboratory; and Staff, Section of Cardiology, Lahey Clinic Medical Center, Burlington, MA

Infective Endocarditis: A Disease in Evolution

THOMAS F. NIKOLAI, M.D., F.A.C.P.

Clinical Assistant Professor of Medicine, University of Wisconsin Medical School, Madison, WI; Staff Physician and Consultant, Section of Endocrinology, Department of Internal Medicine, Marshfield Clinic; Consultant and Attending Physician (Internal Medicine and Endocrinology), St. Joseph's Hospital, Marshfield, WI

Hyperthyroidism

ROBERT G. NORFLEET, M.D., F.A.C.P.

Associate Clinical Professor of Medicine, University of Wisconsin Medical School, Madison, WI; Attending Gastroenterologist, Marshfield Clinic and St. Joseph's Hospital, Marshfield, WI

Premalignant Lesions of the Gastrointestinal Tract

DONALD G. NORRIS, M.D.

Head, Section of Pediatric Oncology/Hematology, Cleveland Clinic Foundation, Cleveland, OH

Infectious Mononucleosis

PETER OLIVER, M.D.

Staff Otolaryngologist, Lahey Clinic Medical Center, Burlington, MA

Dizziness and Vertigo

JOHN M. O'LOUGHLIN, M.D.

Clinical Instructor in Medicine, Harvard Medical School, Boston, MA; Chairman, Department of Allergy and Dermatology, Lahey Clinic Medical Center, Burlington, MA

Allergen Immunotherapy

DENNIS R. OWNBY, M.D.

Clinical Assistant Professor of Pediatrics, University of Michigan Medical School, Ann Arbor, MI; Head, Division of Pediatric Allergy, Henry Ford Hospital, Detroit, MI

The Hyper-IgE Recurrent Infection Syndrome

E. PRATHER PALMER, M.D.

Staff Physician, Department of Neurology, Lahey Clinic Medical Center, Burlington, MA; Instructor in Neurology, Boston University School of Medicine; Consultant in Neurology, Boston VA Hospital, Boston, MA

Dementia Syndrome

GEORGE A. PANKEY, M.D.

Clinical Professor of Medicine, Department of Medicine, Division of Infectious Diseases, Tulane University School of Medicine; Clinical Professor, Louisiana State University School of Medicine; Clinical Professor of Oral Diagnosis, Medicine and Radiology, Louisiana State University School of Dentistry; Head, Section on Infectious Diseases, Ochsner Clinic and Alton Ochsner Medical Foundation; Senior Visiting Physician, Charity Hospital of Louisiana, New Orleans, LA; Consultant, Department of Medicine, VA Medical Center, Biloxi, MS

Sexually Transmitted Infections

JOHN P. PARKER, M.D.

Assistant Clinical Professor of Medicine, University of Wisconsin Medical School, Madison, WI; Staff, Department of Nephrology, Marshfield Clinic and St. Joseph's Hospital, Marshfield, WI

Tubulointerstitial Nephropathy and Urinary Tract Infections

STEVEN I. PFEIFFER, Ph.D.

Adjunct Professor of Psychology, Tulane University; Staff Psychologist, Ochsner Clinic and Alton Ochsner Medical Foundation, New Orleans, LA

The Practice of Brief Psychotherapy

ROBERT V. PIERRE, M.D.

Professor of Internal Medicine and Laboratory Medicine, Mayo Medical School; Staff, Mayo Clinic and Mayo Foundation, Rochester, MN

The Preleukemic or Myelodysplastic Syndromes (PL/MDS)

V. K. PIZIAK, M.D., Ph.D.

Associate Professor of Internal Medicine, Texas A&M University College of Medicine, College Station, TX; Senior Staff, Scott and White Clinic, Temple, TX

Menopause

JOHN POPOVICH, Jr., M.D.

Clinical Assistant Professor of Medicine, University of Michigan Medical School, Ann Arbor, MI; Senior Staff Physician, Division of Pulmonary and Critical Care Medicine, Henry Ford Hospital, Detroit, MI

Respiratory Failure

JOSEPH D. PURVIS, M.D.

Attending Physician, Department of Hematology and Medical Oncology, Cleveland Clinic Foundation, Cleveland, OH

Breast Cancer

ROBERT J. QUINET, M.D.

Staff, Department of Medicine, Section on Rheumatology, Ochsner Clinic and Alton Ochsner Medical Foundation; Clinical Assistant Professor of Medicine, Division of Rheumatology, School of Medicine, Louisiana State University, New Orleans, LA

Osteoarthritis

EDWARD L. QUINN, M.D., F.A.C.P.

Clinical Professor of Medicine, University of Michigan Medical School, Ann Arbor, MI; Emeritus Chairman, Division of Infectious Disease, Department of Medicine, Henry Ford Hospital, Detroit, MI

Infectious Diseases

JORGE RAKELA, M.D.

Assistant Professor of Medicine, Mayo Medical School; Consultant in Internal Medicine and Gastroenterology, Mayo Clinic and Mayo Foundation, Rochester, MN

Hepatitis

HENRY W. RANDLE, M.D., Ph.D.

Associate Professor of Medicine (Dermatology), Texas A&M University College of Medicine, College Station, TX; Private Practice, Austin, TX. Formerly affiliated with Scott and White Clinic, Temple, TX

Erythema Multiforme

JOHN E. RAY, M.D.

Clinical Professor of Surgery, Tulane University School of Medicine; Chairman Emeritus, Staff Surgeon, Department of Colon and Rectal Surgery, Ochsner Clinic and Alton Ochsner Medical Foundation, New Orleans, LA

Common Anorectal Problems in Internal Medicine

MARILYN C. RAY, M.D.

Clinical Instructor, Tulane University School of Medicine and Louisiana State University School of Medicine; Staff, Department of Dermatology, Ochsner Clinic and Alton Ochsner Medical Foundation, New Orleans, LA

Contact Dermatitis; Pemphigus and Pemphigoid

RICHARD RE, M.D.

Vice-President, Director of Research, Alton Ochsner Medical Foundation; Head, Department of Internal Medicine, Section on Hypertensive Diseases, Ochsner Clinic and Alton Ochsner Medical Foundation; Associate Professor of Medicine, Louisiana State University School of Medicine; Associate Clinical Professor of Medicine, Tulane University School of Medicine, New Orleans, LA

Medical Management of Secondary Hypertension

RICHARD A. REINHART, M.D., F.A.C.P., F.A.C.C.

Clinical Assistant Professor, University of Wisconsin Medical School, Madison, WI; Attending Cardiologist, St. Joseph's Hospital and Marshfield Clinic, Marshfield, WI

Acute Pulmonary Edema

FRANK A. RIDDICK, Jr.

Clinical Professor of Medicine, Tulane University School of Medicine; Medical Director and Chairman, Board of Management, Ochsner Clinic and Alton Ochsner Medical Foundation; Emeritus Head, Department of Internal Medicine, Section on Endocrinology and Metabolic Diseases, Ochsner Clinic and Alton Ochsner Medical Foundation, New Orleans, LA

Ideals in the Physician-Patient Relationship

ALFRED G. ROBICHAUX III, M.D.

Staff Physician, Department of Obstetrics and Gynecology, Ochsner Clinic and Alton Ochsner Medical Foundation, New Orleans, LA

HELLP syndrome

FREDERICK B. ROSE, M.D., F.A.C.P.

Clinical Assistant Professor of Medicine (Infectious Diseases), Hahnemann University School of Medicine, Philadelphia, PA; Clinical Assistant Professor, Upstate Medical Center, Syracuse, NY; Director of Medical Education, Robert Packer Hospital, and Chief, Infectious Disease Section, Guthrie Clinic, Sayre, PA

Acute Bacterial Diarrhea and Food Poisoning

A. DAVID ROTHNER, M.D.

Chief, Pediatric Neurology, Cleveland Clinic Foundation, Cleveland, OH

Seizure Disorders

STEVEN BRYAN ROUSE, M.D., F.R.C.S. (C)

Clinical Instructor, State University of New York at Stony Brook; Staff, Department of Obstetrics and Gynecology, Guthrie Clinic and Robert Packer Hospital, Sayre, PA

Medical Treatment During Pregnancy

WILMER M. RUTT, M.D.

Director, Primary Care Medicine, Henry Ford Hospital, Detroit, MI

Medical Care of the Healthy Adult

M. SAEED-UZ-ZAFAR, M.D.

Clinical Assistant Professor of Medicine, University of Michigan Medical School, Ann Arbor, MI; Staff Physician, Department of Endocrinology, Henry Ford Hospital, Detroit, MI

Prolactinoma

JOHN A. SARYAN, M.D.

Instructor in Pediatrics, Tufts University School of Medicine, Boston, MA; Senior Staff Physician, Department of Allergy and Dermatology, Lahey Clinic Medical Center, Burlington, MA

Allergen Immunotherapy

ROBERT F. SAUL, M.D.

Clinical Assistant Professor of Medicine (Neurology) and Surgery (Ophthalmology), Milton S. Hershey College of Medicine, Pennsylvania State University, Hershey, PA; Associate in Neurology and Ophthalmology, Geisinger Medical Center, Danville, PA

Brain Tumors

DAVID J. SCHEINHORN, M.D.

Clinical Associate Professor of Internal Medicine, Louisiana State University School of Medicine and Tulane University School of Medicine; Associate Head, Section on Pulmonary Diseases, Department of Internal Medicine, Ochsner Clinic and Alton Ochsner Medical Foundation, New Orleans, LA

Chronic Obstructive Pulmonary Disease and Bronchiectasis; Legionnaires' Disease

ALEXANDER SCHIRGER, M.D.

Professor of Medicine, Department of Cardiovascular Diseases, Mayo Medical School; Consultant in Medicine, Division of Cardiovascular Diseases, Hypertension and Internal Medicine, Mayo Clinic and Mayo Foundation, Rochester, MN

Edema

GEORGE T. SCHNEIDER, M.D., F.A.C.S., F.A.C.O.G.

Clinical Professor, Department of Obstetrics and Gynecology, Louisiana State University School of Medicine; Senior Surgeon (Ob/Gyn), Charity Hospital of Louisiana; Senior Consultant, Department of Obstetrics and Gynecology, Ochsner Clinic and Alton Ochsner Medical Foundation, New Orleans, LA

Oral Contraception; Common Gynecologic Problems in Internal Medicine

JOSEPH E. SEBER, M.D.

Private Practice and Staff Physician, Parkway Regional Medical Center and Southeastern Medical Center, N. Miami Beach, FL

Sunburn

LEONARD H. SEREBRO, M.D.

Clinical Instructor, Louisiana State University School of Medicine; Staff Physician, Department of Internal Medicine, Section on Rheumatology, Ochsner Clinic and Alton Ochsner Medical Foundation, New Orleans, LA

Hyperuricemia and Gout

JOHN A. SHEA, M.D.

Clinical Instructor, Harvard Medical School, Boston, MA; Staff, Department of Gastroenterology, New England Deaconess Hospital, Boston, MA, and Lahey Clinic Medical Center, Burlington, MA

Parasites of the Gastrointestinal Tract

KIRK V. SHEPARD, M.D.

Staff, Department of Hematology and Oncology, Cleveland Clinic Foundation, Cleveland, OH

Tumors of the Intestinal Tract—Upper GI Tract, Carcinoid Syndrome, and Lower GI Tract

MURRAY N. SILVERSTEIN, M.D., Ph.D.

Professor of Medicine, Mayo Medical School; Staff, Division of Hematology, Mayo Clinic and Mayo Foundation, Rochester, MN

Chronic Myeloproliferative Diseases

ROBERT T. SIMKINS, D.O.

Senior Staff Neurologist, Director of EEG, Department of Neurology, Henry Ford Hospital, Detroit, MI

Lacunar Stroke

ROBERT E. SMITH, M.D.

Fellow, Department of Gastroenterology, Dartmouth-Hitchcock Medical Center; Instructor in Internal Medicine, Dartmouth Medical School, Hanover, NH. Formerly at Geisinger Medical Center, Danville, PA

Chlamydia

DAVID W. SNYDER, M.D.

Attending Cardiologist, Department of Internal Medicine, Section on Cardiology, Ochsner Clinic and Alton Ochsner Medical Foundation, New Orleans, LA

Arrhythmias

JOHN A. SPITTELL, Jr., M.D.

Mary Lowell Leary Professor of Medicine, Mayo Medical School; Consultant in Medicine, Division of Cardiovascular Diseases, Hypertension and Internal Medicine, Mayo Clinic and Mayo Foundation, Rochester, MN

Edema

WAYNE E. SPRUCE, M.D.

Assistant Clinical Professor, University of California, San Diego, School of Medicine, La Jolla, CA; Director, Bone Marrow Transplantation Program, and Co-Director, Hematology/Oncology Division, Children's Hospital, San Diego, CA; Assistant Adjunct Member, Scripps Clinic and Research Foundation, La Jolla, CA

Bone Marrow Transplantation in the Treatment of Severe Aplastic Anemia

RAY W. SQUIRES, Ph.D.

Director, Cardiovascular Health Clinic, Mayo Clinic and Mayo Foundation, Rochester, MN

Rehabilitation After Myocardial Infarction and Cardiac Surgery

A. DEAN STEELE, M.D.

Professor of Medicine, Texas A&M University School of Medicine, College Station, TX; Director, Division of Rheumatology, Scott and White Clinic, Temple, TX

Fibrositis

DAVID STEINBERG, M.D.

Clinical Assistant Professor of Medicine, Harvard Medical School, Boston, MA; Head, Section of Hematology, Lahey Clinic Medical Center, Burlington, MA

Megaloblastic Anemia

W. PERRY STOKES, M.D.

Former Fellow in Gastroenterology, Ochsner Clinic and Alton Ochsner Medical Foundation, New Orleans, LA; Currently Staff Gastroenterologist, Iberia General Hospital and Medical Center, and Dauterive Hospital, New Iberia, LA; and Franklin Foundation Hospital, Franklin, LA

Nausea and Vomiting

BRADLEY J. SULLIVAN, Ph.D., M.D.

Pediatric Infectious Disease Specialist, Marshfield Clinic and St. Joseph's Hospital, Marshfield, WI

Common Skin and Soft Tissue Infections; Deep Fungal Infections

FREDERICK S. SUNDERLIN, M.D.

Clinical Associate Professor of Medicine, Milton S. Hershey College of Medicine, Pennsylvania State University, Hershey, PA; Associate, Department of Endocrinology, and Vice-President, Director of Medical Education, Geisinger Medical Center, Danville, PA

Adrenocortical Insufficiency

ERIC G. TANGALOS, M.D.

Assistant Professor of Medicine, Mayo Medical School; Consultant, Division of Community Internal Medicine, Mayo Clinic and Mayo Foundation, Rochester, MN

Medical Treatment of the Elderly

EDWARD TARLOV, M.D.

Neurosurgeon, Lahey Clinic Medical Center, Burlington, MA

Intracerebral Hemorrhage

STUART J. TIPPING, M.D.

Section Chief, Medical Oncology, Marshfield Clinic; Attending Oncologist, St. Joseph's Hospital, Marshfield, WI

Genitourinary Tumors; Gynecologic Tumors

DENNIS TORETTI, M.D.

Clinical Professor of Medicine, Milton S. Hershey College of Medicine, Pennsylvania State University, Hershey, PA; Associate, Department of Rheumatology, Geisinger Medical Center, Danville, PA; Consultant, Williamsport Hospital, Williamsport, PA

Polyarteritis Nodosa

GREGORY S. UHL, M.D.

Clinical Associate Professor of Medicine, University of New Mexico School of Medicine; Director of Nuclear Cardiology, Lovelace Medical Center, Albuquerque, NM

Congestive Heart Failure

GREGORY T. VALAINIS, M.D.

Fellow, Department of Internal Medicine, Section on Infectious Disease, Ochsner Clinic and Alton Ochsner Medical Foundation, New Orleans, LA

Kawasaki Syndrome

RICHARD G. VAN DELLEN, M.D.

Associate Professor of Medicine, Mayo Medical School; Consultant, Division of Allergic Diseases and Internal Medicine, Mayo Clinic and Mayo Foundation, Rochester, MN

Asthma

ELLIS J. VAN SLYCK, M.D.

Clinical Associate Professor of Medicine, University of Michigan Medical School, Ann Arbor, MI; Head, Division of Hematology, Henry Ford Hospital, Detroit, MI

Acute Leukemia

JORGE A. VELOSA, M.D.

Associate Professor of Medicine, Mayo Medical School; Consultant, Division of Nephrology and Internal Medicine, Mayo Clinic and Mayo Foundation, Rochester, MN

Primary Glomerular Diseases

K. K. VENKAT, M.D.

Clinical Assistant Professor of Internal Medicine, University of Michigan Medical School, Ann Arbor, MI; Senior Staff Physician, Division of Nephrology and Hypertension, Department of Medicine, Henry Ford Hospital, Detroit, MI

Chronic Renal Failure; Dialysis and Transplantation

HECTOR O. VENTURA, M.D.

Fellow, Department of Internal Medicine, Section on Cardiology, Ochsner Clinic and Alton Ochsner Medical Foundation, New Orleans, LA

Fever; Leg Cramps and Restless Legs

CARLOS A. VERDONK, M.D.

Associate Professor of Medicine, Texas A&M University College of Medicine, College Station, TX; Senior Staff, Division of Endocrinology, Scott and White Clinic, Temple, TX

Hypercalcemia and Hypocalcemia

CHARLES N. VERHEYDEN, M.D., Ph.D.

Associate Professor, Department of Surgery, Texas A&M University College of Medicine, College Station, TX; Staff, Division of Plastic Surgery, Scott and White Clinic, Temple, TX

Snakebites, Spider Bites, and Fire Ant Stings

DONALD G. VIDT, M.D.

Chairman, Department of Hypertension and Nephrology, Cleveland Clinic Foundation, Cleveland, OH

Accelerated Hypertension, Malignant Hypertension, and Hypertensive Emergencies

FRANCIS J. VIOZZI, M.D.

Clinical Professor of Medicine, Milton S. Hershey College of Medicine, Pennsylvania State University, Hershey, PA; Director, Department of Rheumatology, Geisinger Medical Center, Danville, PA

Cutaneous Manifestations of Rheumatoid Arthritis

RANDALL S. VOLLERTSEN, M.D.

Assistant Professor of Medicine, Mayo Graduate School of Medicine, Rochester, MN

Systemic Lupus Erythematosus

PETER C. WALTHER, M.D.

Associate Clinical Professor of Urology, University of California, San Diego, School of Medicine; Attending Urologist, Scripps Clinic and Research Foundation, La Jolla, CA, and at Sharp Cabrillo Hospital and University Hospital, San Diego, CA

Male Hypogonadism and Impotence

JOHN L. WANAMAKER, M.D.

Associate Clinical Professor of Medicine (Cardiology), Hahnemann University School of Medicine, Philadelphia, PA; Chief of Cardiology, Guthrie Clinic and Robert Packer Hospital, Sayre, PA

Common Congenital Heart Disease in the Adult

STEPHEN L. WANGER, M.D.

Clinical Instructor in Neurology, Harvard Medical School, Boston, MA; Staff, Department of Neurology, Lahey Clinic Medical Center, Burlington, MA

Parkinson's Disease and Other Movement Disorders

JACK WAXMAN, M.D.

Associate Professor of Medicine, Louisiana State University School of Medicine; Chief, Section on Rheumatology, Department of Internal Medicine, Ochsner Clinic and Alton Ochsner Medical Foundation, New Orleans, LA

Tendinitis and Bursitis

DAVID C. WEBB-JOHNSON, M.A., M.B. (B.Chir.), M.R.C.P.

Clinical Instructor in Medicine, Harvard Medical School, Boston, MA; Staff Physician, Department of Pulmonary Medicine, Division of Internal Medicine, Lahey Clinic Medical Center, Burlington, MA

Interstitial Lung Disease

JAMES K. WEICK, M.D.

Chairman, Department of Hematology and Medical Oncology, Cleveland Clinic Foundation, Cleveland, OH

Cancer of the Lung

THOMAS E. WEISS, M.D.

Emeritus Head and Honorary Staff, Department of Internal Medicine, Section on Rheumatology, Ochsner Clinic and Alton Ochsner Medical Foundation; Emeritus Clinical Professor of Medicine, Tulane University School of Medicine, New Orleans, LA

Hyperuricemia and Gout

K. M. A. WELCH, M.D.

Professor of Clinical Neurology, University of Michigan Medical School, Ann Arbor, MI; Chairman, Department of Neurology, Henry Ford Hospital, Detroit, MI

Lacunar Stroke

RALEIGH R. WHITE IV, M.D.

Professor, Department of Surgery, Texas A&M University College of Medicine, College Station, TX; Staff, Division of Plastic Surgery, Scott and White Clinic, Temple, TX

Snakebites, Spider Bites, and Fire Ant Stings

WILLIAM L. WHITE, M.D.

Assistant Professor of Medicine, Mayo Medical School; Consultant in Hematology, Mayo Clinic and Mayo Foundation, Rochester, MN

Hodgkin's Disease; Non-Hodgkin's Lymphomas

FRED W. WHITEHOUSE, M.D.

Clinical Professor of Internal Medicine, University of Michigan Medical School, Ann Arbor, MI; Attending Physician, Department of Metabolism, Henry Ford Hospital, Detroit, MI

Non–Insulin-Dependent Diabetes Mellitus

DAVID O. WIEBERS, M.D.

Consultant in Neurology, Mayo Clinic and Mayo Foundation, Rochester, MN

Ischemic Cerebrovascular Disease: Carotid System

HERBERT P. WIEDEMANN, M.D.

Pulmonary Staff and Head, Section of Respiratory Therapy, Cleveland Clinic Foundation, Cleveland, OH

The Common Cold

ASA J. WILBOURN, M.D.

Assistant Clinical Professor, Case Western Reserve University School of Medicine; Staff Neurologist and Head, EMG Lab, Cleveland Clinic Foundation, Cleveland, OH

Peripheral Neuropathy

DAVID E. WILLIAMS, M.S., M.D.

Assistant Professor of Medicine, Mayo Graduate School of Medicine and Mayo Medical School; Consultant, Division of Thoracic Diseases and Internal Medicine, Mayo Clinic and Mayo Foundation, Rochester, MN

Tuberculosis and Tuberculoidoses

GARY W. WILLIAMS, M.D., Ph.D.

Executive Officer, Department of Medicine; Staff, Department of Rheumatology, Scripps Clinic and Research Foundation, La Jolla, CA

Giant Cell Arteritis and Polymyalgia Rheumatica

R. K. WINKELMANN, M.D., Ph.D.

Professor of Dermatology, Mayo Medical School; Consultant in Dermatology, Mayo Clinic and Mayo Foundation, Rochester, MN

Scleroderma and Mixed Connective Tissue Syndrome

JOSEPH I. WOLFSDORF, M.D.

Assistant Professor of Pediatrics, Harvard Medical School; Associate in Endocrinology, Children's Hospital; Associate Physician, New England Deaconess, Hospital; Chief, Pediatric and Adolescent Unit, Joslin Clinic, Boston, MA

Inborn Errors of Carbohydrate Metabolism

DOUGLAS L. WOOD, M.D.

Assistant Professor of Medicine, Mayo Medical School; Consultant, Division of Cardiovascular Diseases and Internal Medicine, Mayo Clinic and Mayo Foundation, Rochester, MN

Heart Block

LINDA YAZVAC, M.D.

Assistant Clinical Professor, Department of Medicine, Louisiana State University School of Medicine; Instructor in Physical Diagnosis, Tulane University School of Medicine; Assistant Section Head, General Internal Medicine, Ochsner Clinic and Alton Ochsner Medical Foundation, New Orleans, LA

Fever

JESS R. YOUNG, M.D.

Chairman, Department of Peripheral Vascular Diseases, Cleveland Clinic Foundation, Cleveland, OH

Systemic Embolism

BRUCE R. ZIMMERMAN, M.D.

Associate Professor of Medicine, Mayo Graduate School of Medicine; Vice Chairman, Division of Endocrinology, Mayo Clinic and Mayo Foundation, Rochester, MN

Hyperlipidemia

THOM J. ZIMMERMAN, M.D.

Professor and Chairman, Department of Ophthalmology, Professor of Pharmacology and Toxicology, University of Louisville School of Medicine; Staff Physician, Humana Hospital University, Louisville, KY. Formerly with Ochsner Clinic and Alton Ochsner Medical Foundation, New Orleans, LA

Preface

Even in medicine though it's easy to know what wine, honey, hellebore, cautery, and surgery are, to know to *whom, when,* and *how* to apply them so as to effect a cure is not less an undertaking than to be a physician.

Aristotle, Nicomachean Ethics, Vol. 9

Although those words were written more than 2000 years ago, they still make crystal clear the dilemma modern physicians face throughout their careers. We learn in medical school and in our postgraduate training how to arrive at a working diagnosis by applying clinical facts gained from the history, physical examination, and appropriate laboratory tests. We gain an acquaintance with the "real-life" applications of the basic sciences we have been taught and become familiar with the biochemistry, pharmacology, and pharmacokinetics of a myriad of therapeutic agents. But medical school cannot provide us with the experience that tells us how, when, and to whom such agents should be given.

During our years as interns and residents, the facilities and the superspecialists of a teaching hospital are reassuringly at our disposal. Those of us who then choose to enter private practice are abruptly torn from this setting, finding ourselves remote, both physically and spiritually, from our mentors. Worse, we are ill prepared to face the common ailments of the general patient population. Instead of managing gravely ill patients in a controlled environment, the physician must deal with chronic complaints that range from mild constipation to headaches to low back pain. Instead of having the option to discharge a patient from the hospital after a few days, the physician now deals with the same patient and the same disease, day in, day out for many years.

This is why *Current Clinical Practice* was written. It is intended to show the physician, whether tyro or seasoned, how the tools of modern internal medicine are used by the specialists and superspecialists of the major private clinics in the United States. The clinics represented here are totally committed to excellence in medical practice, providing referral centers for patients from the United States and Europe, the Middle East, South America, and elsewhere who seek the highest standards of medical care.

The editors and authors of *Current Clinical Practice* do not attempt to teach what wine, honey, hellebore, cautery, and surgery are. They have not written another textbook of medicine. Although diagnostic criteria and pathophysiologic processes are presented in brief, these authors assume that the physician has made the diagnosis and that he or she has mastered the basic skills and tools of our profession. This book's focus is on patient management in a broad range of diseases and disorders. It tells its physician-reader how patients are managed at the *clinics*— how Ernest Beutler treats hemolytic anemia at the Scripps Clinic; how Ray Gifford lowers high blood pressure at the Cleveland Clinic; how Royden Jones manages stroke patients at the Lahey Clinic. However, the clinics are not only committed to excellence in medical care. As private institutions they are compelled to practice medicine in the most cost-efficient way. Thus, socioeconomic considerations and cost-benefit ratios, which have become progressively important aspects of medicine over the past few years, are an integral part of each chapter of *Current Clinical Practice*.

Our book is organized into thirteen specialty areas, with a fourteenth section concerning the problems of general patient care. Although these authors have been careful to deal with the common complaints and diseases physicians see daily, they have not neglected more esoteric entities. Thus, leg cramps are here, but so is Lyme arthritis. No claim is made or implied that what we offer is complete; however, we did try to be thorough. Our goal, put simply, is to be the physician's faithful adviser in the clinical practice of medicine.

Acknowledgements

I am deeply indebted to many talented and dedicated persons for their contributions to this product. *Current Clinical Practice* would not have been possible were it not for the invaluable help of Carole Morrison and Susan Barker who served as assistant editors in this project. Without the thorough work of Juanita Shipman, Marion Stafford, and the Medical Editing staff at Alton Ochsner Medical Foundation, this book would not have become a reality.

Clearly, however, my special gratitude goes to the editorial departments of various clinics, in particular to Pauline Zarolow at the Lahey Clinic Foundation, Connie Cryar at Henry Ford Hospital, Shannon Henry at Cleveland Clinic Foundation, Phyllis Minick at Scripps Clinic and Research Foundation, and Rosemary Perry and Dr. Bernard Forsher at the Mayo Clinic Publications Office. All of the science editors and clinic editors who spontaneously were willing to embark on a task of these dimensions, despite an already crowded professional life, deserve a special word of appreciation.

Finally, my very special thanks go to the W. B. Saunders Company and its staff, who provided us with excellent advice and support throughout this complex endeavor. I particularly appreciated the help of John Dyson who was exceedingly helpful at various crossroads in the planning and execution of *Current Clinical Practice*. We were fortunate enough to have the collaboration of David Harvey, who established the style of the book, and Bill Preston, who oversaw the technical details of production.

Finally, I thank my wife Veronica and my children Adrian, Franziska, and Alexander, who provided the understanding and emotional support which made my own commitment to this endeavor easier and more enjoyable.

Franz H. Messerli

Contents

SECTION VI
THE DIGESTIVE SYSTEM

SECTION XIII
DISEASES OF THE JOINTS AND CONNECTIVE TISSUE

SECTION **1**

GENERAL PATIENT CARE

FRANK A. RIDDICK, JR.

1 · IDEALS IN THE PHYSICIAN-PATIENT RELATIONSHIP

Frank A. Riddick, Jr.
Jane Mueller
OCHSNER CLINIC AND ALTON OCHSNER MEDICAL
FOUNDATION

THE PHYSICIAN

The ideal physician is, we think, the one who combines knowledge and skill with the attitude exemplified in Francis Peabody's wonderfully ambiguous observation, "The secret of the care of the patient is in caring for the patient."

The physician who spoke those words practiced medicine from 1907 until 1927. In his short but intense career, he was researcher, clinician, professor of medicine, member of illustrious scientific bodies, and chief of the clinic at a large public hospital. But he is remembered today not for the breadth and intensity of his activities but for those qualities that, Zinsser says, "brought him distinction as a human being." Peabody had "a rare blending of learning and humanity, incisiveness of intellect and sensitiveness of the spirit, which occasionally come together in an individual who chooses the calling Medicine; and then we have the great physician."

The physician who cares for the patient in Peabody's sense knows the patient as a person, not simply as an instance of disease; that is, the physician knows the relevant details of the patient's emotional, domestic, work, and financial lives, and the details of his medical past and present. And the physician considers all aspects of the patient as he bends his efforts to treat the whole person, not just his illness. "The care of the patient must be completely personal," Peabody warned, "because in an extraordinarily large number of cases both diagnosis and treatment depend on an intimate personal relationship between physician and patient."

In Peabody's era, impelled by the application to patient care of discoveries from physics, chemistry, and bacteriology, medicine was entering its scientific age. Peabody feared that as medicine became more scientific it would become less humanistic. The threats that scientific advances pose to humanistic medicine are even more challenging today than in Peabody's time. The challenge of seeing the patient as a human being has already been mentioned. The hospital experience still is often a dehumanizing one as the patient is stripped of his "accustomed environment," even of his clothes. The stripping robs the physician also—of the chance to see the patient in his own circumstances, the circumstances to which the physician seeks to restore the patient.

The patient who has a functional illness is still at some risk of being dismissed by his doctor as having nothing the matter with him or, more likely, nothing that interests or involves the physician. Ironically, although society in general has become keenly aware of the prevalence and importance of emotional disorders, that awareness is not fully reflected in medical practice. Too many physicians do not consider either the emotional components of illness or illnesses that have emotional causes to be valid objects of their concern. Whatever the reasons (perhaps one reason is that the pressures of medical training and practice have led the physician to neglect his own, and his patient's, emotional life), the attitude is unfortunate and unscientific. As Peabody says, "Disease in man is never the same as disease in an experimental animal, for in man the disease at once affects and is affected by what we call the emotional life. Thus the physician who attempts to take care of the patient while he neglects this factor is as unscientific as the investigator who neglects to control all the conditions that may affect his experiment."

William Locke, an endocrinologist at the Ochsner Clinic, addresses the same issue with compelling succinctness: "Every patient is his own disease."

THE PATIENT

What of the ideal *patient*? How might he be described? Peabody would perhaps be taken aback by the questions and consider them irrelevant. Peabody asked nothing of the patient except, by implication, that he be the recipient of the physician's caring. Peabody was—to use an adjective less pejorative in his medical circles than in our own—paternalistic. But Peabody's paternalism was so benign and so founded on respect for the patient and his sensitivities that, we dare to say, even a modern patient who values independence highly would be tempted to succumb to it.

Although we cannot know what Peabody would have said about patients, we do know that patients are changing, at least significant numbers of them. Most notably, patients are changing the way they look at

1

their role and the physician's role. A survey made in 1985 under the auspices of the American Board of Family Practice noted that Americans were assuming more responsibility for decisions about their health, life, and death. Both physicians and laymen responding to the survey said that laymen should educate themselves about preventing disease and maintaining health and that they should do so by reading about health, by listening to and watching broadcasts about health issues, and by taking courses.

We see the trend toward responsible patienthood as a logical and ideal extension of Peabody's equation, "The secret of the care of the patient is in caring for the patient"—*and* in helping the patient engage his physical, emotional, and intellectual resources as fully as possible in his own care.

THE RELATIONSHIP

In the best of all possible worlds, the ideal physician and the ideal patient have an ideal relationship. The 1984 *Cumulated Index Medicus* lists five columns of articles under the heading "Physician-Patient Relations." Drawing on the thoughts expressed in those articles, but chiefly on reflections upon our own experiences as doctor and patient, we have arrived at the following list of characteristics of the ideal physician-patient relationship:

1. Mutual respect. Both physician and patient regard each other as adults who have equal worth as persons despite their unequal medical skills and knowledge.

2. Mutual openness. Both physician and patient tell each other the whole story. The physician tells the patient the whole story about the diagnosis, possible treatments, and possible outcomes, and the patient tells the physician the whole story of his illness, including any embarrassing parts that are relevant to the illness, such as alcoholism or an emotional disorder.

3. Mutual trust. Not the blind trust in the physician that has characterized too many physician-patient interactions of the past, in which both parties saw the physician as an all-knowing parent and the patient as an unquestioningly obedient child. Rather, the two-way trust that can arise when physician and patient talk to each other about the patient's hopes, fears, values, goals, and priorities.

4. Mutual decision-making. The physician and patient who trust each other decide together which of the possible treatments is most suitable for the patient.

THE OBSTACLES

The obstacles to forming the ideal physician-patient relationship are many and severe. Some of the most serious ones did not exist in Peabody's time. Perhaps the most stringent today is that the relationship necessarily involves more than two persons. And those other persons are often decision-makers whose first concern is how to cut costs or how to use medical facilities more efficiently, rather than how to best treat the individual patient. Those other persons may be agents of the government or of insurance companies, or they may be gatekeepers for health maintenance organizations or health programs subsidized by employers.

A look at the way in which outside agents have shaped medical care in other countries indicates what might happen in our own. It is sobering for one of us, who is now 55, to realize that if he had renal failure in Great Britain he would be considered too old for renal dialysis, because, in the British view, "we all get a bit crumbly at that age."

It is also disturbing that despite the general agreement that medical care should be tailored to the overall needs of the individual patient, the appropriateness of the physician's care is now evaluated by "norms of care," average lengths of hospital stay, and payments based on the patient's disease, rather than on how simple or how complicated its treatment is or the physiologic and emotional setting in which it occurs. Locke's "every patient is his own disease" gets short shrift in an era of cost containment.

Such constraints on diagnosis and treatment are repugnant to the physician who is trying to care for the patient in Peabody's sense. Levinsky says that the physician *cannot* be the agent of society in the rationing of health care; he must be an advocate for the patient, not for the economic interests of others.

Certain other obstacles also keep the modern physician and patient from working together as well as they might. Too much of the medical information aimed at the layman is unfocused and inappropriately emotional, and sometimes it is dangerously inaccurate. Not all patients want to be responsible for their own health, and not all doctors want patients to be responsible. Also, some doctors and patients, by temperament or from habit, are probably incapable of the partnership that that responsibility implies. Robb writes about an English woman who thought that American physicians gave the patient too much information. "In England," she said, "we trust our doctors to tell us what we ought to know." Katz, a psychoanalyst who advocates shared decision-making between physicians and patients, would both understand and be distressed by the woman's attitude.

The last obstacle to be mentioned is also a serious one—the tremendous increase in the number of medical malpractice suits that makes even the most caring doctor pause, willy-nilly, to wonder whether a new patient is a potential adversary.

THE OUTLOOK

However, there are also bright sides to the physician-patient relationship today. Patients are increasingly well informed about health, and willing and able to participate in the choices they face. Much medical information written for the layman is excellent, easily available, and inexpensive. Physicians would do well to acquaint themselves with this literature and to encourage their patients to read it. The liability penalties for the physician are far less severe than those imposed by the Code of Hammurabi. Economic limitations on medical care have always existed, but overall the limitations today are fewer than ever before.

The ideal physician, the ideal patient, and the ideal physician-patient relationship do not exist and never will exist. They are abstractions. But they are important, even necessary, abstractions, because they give physicians and patients goals at which to aim. All thinking physicians and patients are idealists; they are also realists, because they know that without goals they are apt to go astray. Whatever one's stage of becoming the great physician (another useful ideal), whether neophyte or veteran, it is not too early or too late to consider Peabody's observation that good medical care necessarily involves paying attention to the patient's humanity.

REFERENCES

Aaron HJ, Schwartz WB: The Painful Prescription: Rationing Hospital Care. Brookings Institute, Washington DC, 1984.

Burros M: Poll finds public is assertive on health. New York Times, May 2, 1985.

Katz J: The Silent World of Doctor and Patient. Free Press, New York, 1984.

Levinsky NG: The doctor's master. N Engl J Med 311:1573–1575, 1984.

Peabody FW: Doctor and Patient. Macmillan Co, New York, 1930.

Robb, JW: The British choice in health care: a report from London. Pharos 48:33–37, 1985.

Zinsser H: Introduction. In Peabody FW: Doctor and Patient. Macmillan Co, New York, 1930, pp. ix–xi.

2 · FEVER

Linda Yazvac
Hector O. Ventura
OCHSNER CLINIC AND ALTON OCHSNER MEDICAL
FOUNDATION

Humanity has but three great enemies; fever, famine and war; of these by far the greatest, by far the most terrible, is fever.

Sir William Osler

Fever is a ubiquitous response that occurs not only in mammalian species but also in crustaceans, fish, amphibians, and reptiles. The association between fever and disease was recognized centuries ago, yet it was not until the latter half of the 19th century that regular measurement of body temperature as a means of monitoring disease became common.

In man, thermoregulation is centered in the preoptic area of the anterior hypothalamus, where heat-producing and heat-conserving activity is balanced to maintain body temperature at $37 \pm 1°C$. Diurnal variation normally occurs, even when fever is present. Temperature is lowest in the early morning hours and peaks in the late afternoon. In fever, the hypothalamic thermostat is reset at a higher level and the body responds by increasing internal temperature to meet the new setting.

PYROGENS

Although fever can be produced in a myriad of ways, a common mediator is endogenous pyrogen, a protein (first described by Beeson in 1948) that has the ability to reset the hypothalamic thermostat upward. Exogenous pyrogens such as antigen-antibody complexes, viruses, fungi, bacteria, and their products are capable of inducing production of endogenous pyrogen, now recognized as interleukin 1, by bone marrow–derived phagocytes. Some human tumor cells have been found capable of producing a substance antigenically identical to endogenous pyrogen, which explains in part the pathogenesis of fever in some neoplastic disease.

The precise mechanism of action of endogenous pyrogen at the hypothalamic level remains unclear, but monoamines and prostaglandins, particularly prostaglandin E_2, are thought to play an important role. Inhibition of prostaglandin synthesis in the hypothalamus is believed responsible for the antipyretic effects of aspirin and nonsteroidal anti-inflammatory drugs, while corticosteroids exert their effect by decreasing chemotaxis and production of interleukin 1 by phagocytes.

HYPERTHERMIA

Hyperthermia is a condition distinct to fever. Diurnal variation disappears and hypothalamic control is lost: although the thermostat remains at the correct setting, pathologic increases in both heat production and conservation mechanisms result in a progressive rise in internal temperature. Since hypothalamic function is set at normothermic levels, antipyretics are ineffective in treatment. A very small percentage of patients suffer from disorders of thermoregulation rather than fever. Heat stroke, malignant hyperthermia, hyperthyroidism, and pheochromocytomas can cause elevation of body temperature, but diurnal variation is lost. Pharmacologic agents that affect the body's ability to produce or dissipate heat can also result in hyperthermia. In infiltrative, vascular, or infectious processes directly involving the hypothalamus, hypothermia is more common than hyperthermia. If hyperthermia does occur, body temperature may become extremely high, exceeding even 106°F, the apparent thermal maximum allowed by the hypothalamus in response to endogeneous pyrogen stimulation.

MANAGEMENT

Fever is one of the most common signs confronting the physician and may be provoked by a wide assortment of disease processes. Interview and physical examination performed in the physician's office will frequently permit diagnosis of the condition producing fever. Therapy may then be instituted promptly. The short-term goal of treatment is to alleviate the patient's discomfort by:

1. Reducing fever through the use of antipyretics such as aspirin or acetaminophen.

2. Maintaining hydration by enteral or parenteral administration of fluids.

3. Meeting metabolic requirements through appropriate rest and nutritional intake.

4. Limiting pain through judicious use of analgesics and other therapy.

The ultimate goal, of course, is to reverse or eradicate the disease process responsible for the production of fever. In many cases, particularly in many viral illnesses, the physician can only provide supportive care while allowing time for the patient's own immune system to respond appropriately to the challenge. In other cases, antibiotics, antineoplastics, anti-inflammatory agents, incision and drainage, or other surgical intervention may be required. The treatment chosen is predicated by the specific disease entity being treated. Since success or failure of treatment is thus largely dependent on the accuracy of diagnosis of the underlying condition producing fever, a careful assessment is mandatory.

Every form of therapy is fraught with the potential for complications, and the treatment of fever is no exception. Empiric methods should be avoided. The physician must be alert to the possibility of electrolyte or fluid imbalance, adverse medication effects, or failure of the prescribed treatment to control the underlying disease. Patients should be instructed about signs and symptoms to be reported immediately, and in the use of pharmacologic and nonpharmacologic measures prescribed to treat them. Potential adverse effects and interactions of these measures should be discussed and follow-up arrangements made.

FEVER OF UNKNOWN ORIGIN

Fortunately for the physician as well as the patient, the cause of fever is clear and the process self-limiting most of the time. Nevertheless, in a significant number of cases, the duration of fever is prolonged and the etiology elusive. This subset of febrile patients is classified under the heading "fever of unknown origin (FUO)," which constitutes both dilemma and delight for the clinician.

The criteria for entry into this elite group were first outlined by Petersdorf and Beeson:

1. Illness of more than three weeks' duration.
2. Fever higher than 101°F on several occasions.
3. Diagnosis uncertain after one week of study in the hospital.

Because fever has so many potential etiologies (see Table 1), diagnostic possibilities are numerous, and the relative incidence of a disorder varies depending on age, geographic location, and the socioeconomic characteristics of the patient population studied. Effective evaluation of the patient with fever of unknown origin requires that certain basic principles be applied. There is no substitute for meticulous history-taking and physical examination. Recent or remote travel to foreign or even domestic locales, toxin exposure, contact with wild or domestic animals, use of current or antecedent medications, sexual preference, and a host of other questions must be explored in detail with the patient. Physical examination must be exhaustive, with close attention to the eyes, skin, heart, and reticuloendothelial structures. Examination must be repeated on a daily basis to detect such findings as an evanescent skin rash or fundal exudate. A thorough dental examination should be made with appropriate x-rays to exclude occult dental abscesses. If the illness appears progressive, severe, or unremitting, the patient should be hospitalized. Loss of circadian variation of temperature should alert the physician to potential factitious or hypothalamic disorders. Characterization of fever patterns may even be helpful in a few disorders, such as cyclic neutropenia, malaria, and some cases of Hodgkin's disease.

Factitious illness is being recognized with increasing frequency and has been found in 3% to 9% of patients complaining of prolonged fever. Some patients attempt to misrepresent true body temperature curves, while others induce disease by self-inoculation with a variety of contaminated substances. Most of these patients are female and a large percentage are employed in allied health fields. A history of previous psychiatric problems is unusual. Many respond well to psychiatric intervention.

In spite of exhaustive and meticulous evaluation

Table 1. PRINCIPAL CAUSES OF FEVER OF UNKNOWN ORIGIN IN ADULT PATIENTS LIVING IN THE UNITED STATES

Infections (40%)	**Miscellaneous Causes (25%)**
Tuberculosis	Drug therapy
Subacute bacterial endocarditis	Penicillin
Parasitic infection (e.g., malaria)	Sulfonamides
Viral infection	Phenytoin
Systemic fungal infection	Quinidine
Localized infections	Allopurinol
Pelvic abscess or inflammatory disease	Procainamide
Intra-abdominal abscess following surgery or leakage from GI tract	Methyldopa
Osteomyelitis	Propylthiouracil
Genitourinary infection	Iodides
Hepatobiliary infection	Phenobarbital
	Salicylates
Neoplasms (20%)	
Lymphomas, Hodgkin's, and non-Hodgkin's	Granulomatous Disease
Hypernephroma	Regional enteritis
Atrial myxoma	Temporal arteritis
Leukemia	Polymyalgia rheumatica
Gastrointestinal tumors	Sarcoidosis
Pancreatic tumors	Granulomatous hepatitis
Disseminated carcinomatosis	
	Factitious Fever
Autoimmune or Collagen Vascular (15%)	Others
Rheumatic fever	Familial Mediterranean fever
Systemic lupus erythematosus	Fabry's disease
Polyarteritis nodosa	Cyclic neutropenia
Mixed connective tissue disease	Pulmonary embolism
Still's disease	Cause undetermined
Allergic vasculitis	

using an extensive arsenal of laboratory and radiologic tests, 5% to 8% of patients with fever of unknown origin defy diagnosis. In some, future reevaluation proves more productive. In most of the others, however, fever remits spontaneously and the patient recovers.

REFERENCES

Aduan RP, et al: Factitious fever and self-induced infection. A report of 32 cases and review of the literature. Ann Intern Med 90:230–242, 1979.

Beeson PB: Temperature-elevating effect of a substance obtained from polymorphonuclear leukocytes. J Clin Invest 27:524, 1948.

Bernheim HA, Block LH, Atkin E: Fever: pathogenesis, pathophysiology, and purpose. Ann Intern Med 91:261, 1979.

Dinarello CA: Pathogenesis of fever. In Wyngaarden JB, Smith LH (eds): Cecil Textbook of Medicine, 17th ed. W.B. Saunders Co, Philadelphia, 1985, pp 1471–1473.

Dinarello CA, Wolff SM: Pathogenesis of fever in man. N Engl J Med 298:607, 1978.

Dinarello CA, Wolff SM: Fever of unknown origin. In Mandell G, Bennett JE, Douglas RG (eds): Principles and Practices of Infectious Diseases, Vol 1. John Wiley & Sons, New York, 1979, pp 407–428.

Dinarello CA, Wolff SM: Molecular basis of fever in humans. Am J Med 72:799–819, 1982.

Jacoby GA, Swartz MN: Fever of undetermined origin. N Engl J Med 289:1407–1409, 1973.

Osler W: The study of the fevers of the South. JAMA 26:999–1004, 1896.

Petersdorf RG, Beeson PB: Fever of unexplained origin. Report on 100 cases. Medicine 40:1–30, 1961.

Wolff SM: The febrile patient. In Wyngaarden JB, Smith LH (eds): Cecil Textbook of Medicine, 17th ed. W.B. Saunders Co, Philadelphia, 1985, pp 1470–1471.

Wolff SM, Fauci AS, Dale DC: Unusual etiologies of fever and their evaluation. Annu Rev Med 26:277–281, 1975.

3 · PAIN

Morris A. Flaum
Carol E. Goodman
OCHSNER CLINIC AND ALTON OCHSNER MEDICAL FOUNDATION

DEFINITION AND DIAGNOSTIC CRITERIA

"An emotional experience due to the perception of unpleasant sensations carried to the central nervous system by a complex nociceptive (pain-receptive) system of afferent pathways" defines pain as both a physiologic and psychologic experience. Many times, pain can be alleviated only when the patient's anxiety is assuaged as well as the discomfort.

Acute pain lasts for a few days up to six months and results from tissue irritation, inflammation, or damage. Medical or surgical treatment and healing usually relieve the acute pain with no residual symptoms or functional impairment. Chronic pain lasts for more than six months, often accompanies ongoing pathologic processes such as cancer and degenerative arthritis, and frequently is associated with emotional distress.

Unfortunately, in many patients with chronic pain the cause of continuing symptoms cannot be found. Evidence of suffering is exaggerated by pain behavior such as limping, grimacing, and preoccupation, and can often disrupt employment and family relationships.

Persistent intractable pain, known as "chronic benign pain syndrome," is a major burden of health care systems today. Treatment of benign pain focuses on relief of acute symptoms to prevent chronic pain syndromes. Treatment of malignant pain should help decrease both physical and mental debility, allowing the patient to maintain function with minimal emotional distress and suffering.

PATHOPHYSIOLOGY

Pain sensations are initiated by strong mechanical, thermal, electrical, or chemical (e.g., bradykinin, prostaglandin) stimuli acting upon free nerve endings in almost all tissues of the body. Impulses propagate along small myelinated and unmyelinated pain fibers (A delta and C fibers) of the primary afferent nociceptor neurons, pass through dorsal root ganglia, and synapse with second-order neurons in the dorsal horn gray matter by the action of chemical neurotransmitters (e.g., substance P). Large myelinated mechanoreceptor fibers (carrying sensations of pressure, vibration, and so forth) have lower thresholds for stimulation, and synapse with the same second-order neurons. Sensory input of this type can prevent propagation of pain sensation from the nociceptors. Linking interneurons containing enkephalin, one of the body's natural opioid peptides, can also block the pain message. Axons ascend to several supraspinal sites, including the brain stem reticular nuclei, thalamus, and cortex. The brain interprets a stimulus applied anywhere along the nerve as pain coming from the origin of that pathway (e.g., "phantom" pain). In "referred" pain, visceral sensations are perceived as coming from the periphery because visceral and somatic axons ascend along the same pathways (Fig. 1).

For therapeutic purposes, pain may be suppressed at four levels: at the tissue level by removing noxious stimuli; at the spinal cord level by applying different sensory impulses; at the brain stem level by stimulating the production of opioids and activating descending pain modulation systems; and at the cortical level by modifying the emotional consequences of the pain experience. Many forms of treatment are effective because the body's natural pain modulation systems are activated.

CLINICAL ASPECTS

Treatment of pain includes establishing rapport with the patient, gathering pertinent historical details, conducting the appropriate examination, and educating the patient. For a motivated patient, accurate diagnosis and effective treatment by an interested physician can prevent the development of chronic pain syndromes. Patients are asked not only to complete questionnaires about the history and nature of the pain, but also to describe the mode of onset and associated factors.

Physical examination begins at the pain site, which should guide investigation of the disease process, whether it be mechanical, inflammatory, metabolic, degenerative, or malignant. Tenderness of ligaments at the cervicothoracic or lumbosacral junction differentiates ligamentous from muscular strain. Tapping over irritated nerves elicits Tinel's sign. Passive stretching

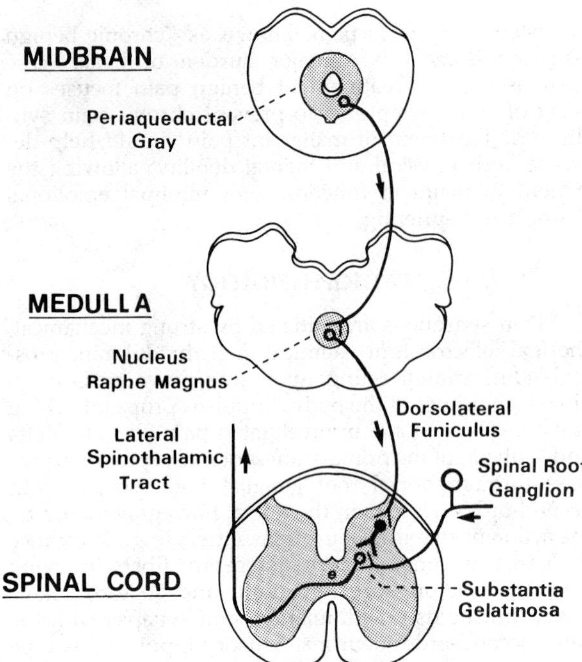

Figure 1. Excitatory stimuli ascend via afferent neurons and spinothalamic tracts. Inhibitory pathways originate in periaqueductal gray and nucleus raphe magnus (and other nuclei), descend in spinal funiculi, and synapse with enkephalin-containing interneurons (*black*) in substantia gelatinosa that exert presynaptic inhibition on nociceptive neurons. (From Goodman CE: Pathophysiology of pain. Arch Intern Med 143:529, 1983. By permission.)

causes discomfort in muscle spasm and fibrositis; active contraction against resistance produces pain at the tendinous origin or insertion (e.g., tennis elbow or supraspinatus tendinitis). Observation of posture, muscle development, and alignment of extremities can reveal lumbar lordosis, scoliosis, and leg length discrepancy, which cause back and neck pain. The neurologic examination should pay particular attention to reflex asymmetry, minimal muscle weakness, and sensory abnormalities, and should include nerve stretching and compression tests for assessment of pain origin (e.g., root vs. peripheral nerve). Pulses, skin temperature and texture, and edema should be noted.

Once the diagnosis is made, educating the patient may be time-consuming but is equally important. Patients appreciate a clear explanation of the cause, organ involvement, and rationale of treatment.

MANAGEMENT

The initial aim of treatment of acute benign pain is to remove the cause. A combination of nonpharmacologic therapies is appropriate, including rest and physical modalities, as well as drug therapy with anti-inflammatory, antispasmodic, and analgesic medications. The goal is adequate relief of symptoms with minimal side effects and little danger of habitual use. Goals of rehabilitation to prevent prolongation of acute into chronic pain are (1) relief of pain, (2) reduction of spasm and swelling, (3) restoration of mobility, (4)

muscle strengthening and support, (5) recovery of normal agility and endurance, and (6) reestablishment of a healthy self-image. In chronic diseases, additional aims include (1) directing the patient's attention away from the pain (behavior modification, psychotherapy), (2) participation in group exercises, (3) balancing relaxation and activity (biofeedback, relaxation techniques), (4) planning for vocational or productive participation, and (5) changing to more self-directed treatment.

Benign pain can usually be treated at home or with outpatient physical and occupational therapy. Instructions for home treatment specify frequency and duration of heat or cold applications and exercises. Prescriptions for physical therapy should include diagnoses, goals, precautions, and modalities. Close communication is maintained with therapists. Patients are reevaluated after two to four weeks of treatment and, if possible, placed on a home program. Prolonged periods of outpatient therapy often reinforce the "sickness role" and may have a negative influence on rehabilitation. When benign pain develops into a syndrome of chronic pain and disability, the teamwork of a specialized stress or pain clinic is needed.

Therapy for acute malignant pain begins with thorough and complete history-taking and physical examination, with appropriate diagnostic studies to define the cause and determine the most appropriate treatment. This may consist of symptomatic relief, radiation therapy, or surgery. Although the pain may be responsive to other measures, analgesics must be prescribed early to allow important diagnostic procedures and to assure the patient that the pain will be alleviated.

NONPHARMACOLOGIC MEASURES

Physical modalities (cold, heat, electricity, water, and mechanical agents) have been used for centuries. Many sophisticated devices have been developed, but the rationale for each remains quite simple. These agents produce analgesic effects at two sites of pain suppression: (1) at the tissue level where increased circulation removes noxious chemical by-products of inflammation, trauma, and anoxia; and (2) at the spinal level where intense sensory input by thermal and mechanoreceptors blocks transmission of painful stimuli.

Cold reduces edema, hematoma formation, inflammatory reaction, and (in some instances) acute muscle spasm. Cold is contraindicated in peripheral vascular disease, ischemia, or Raynaud's syndrome.

Heat relieves pain, produces relaxation, increases local circulation, and promotes healing. Range-of-motion exercises are preceded by heat application. Moist heat is especially effective for muscle spasm and arthritic joints. Paraffin bath units provide comfortable, superficial heat to extremities in arthritis and joint contractures. Heat can be applied to multiple joints with hydrotherapy in a tank for 20 to 30 minutes. Duration should be short and temperatures lower for elderly patients with cardiovascular disease.

Ultrasound, short wave, and microwave diathermy produce deeper heating. These modalities are contraindicated in areas of hemorrhage or malignancy, and over metallic implants. Ultrasound should be used for bursitis, tendinitis, neuritis, contractures, and muscle spasm, sometimes in combination with pulsed electrical stimulation.

Massage is added in cases of muscle spasm, tension, and fibrositis, but should be avoided in patients with hemostatic disorders or infection.

Transcutaneous electrical nerve stimulation (TENS) provides intense sensory input and may enhance endorphin production in the midbrain. It is an adjunct to other therapy for pain when pain is intractable or severe enough to warrant the expense. The dosage of narcotic drugs should be reduced to allow endorphin production and enhance patient alertness. Comfortable, pulsed electrical current, produced by a battery-operated device, is applied by surface electrodes. Electrodes are placed proximally and distally on the nerve in peripheral nerve injury, along the spine and dermatome in cervical and lumbosacral radiculopathy, and over trigger points in myofascial syndromes. Alternative locations are acupuncture points in proximal and distal regions. In painful dysesthesias (e.g., diabetic neuropathy and postherpetic neuralgia), electrodes to "bridge" the involved nerve provide greater benefit. A trial of three to four weeks is necessary to evaluate effectiveness. Electrode placement and stimulus settings may be changed to provide optimal relief. A TENS unit should not be used near a demand-type cardiac pacemaker or over the carotid sinus area. Skin hygiene and proper use of contact gel can prevent skin irritation.

Acute pain is often relieved by general body rest and local joint rest with use of splints, collars, and supports. The proportion of rest versus exercise is determined for individual cases. Weight reduction is a form of rest that reduces load on weight-bearing joints. Bed rest for at least four days can abort prolonged back pain. Mobility is preserved by slow stretching of the paraspinal muscles in a knee-to-chest flexion exercise. Later, walking and other exercises are allowed, with follow-up visits to monitor any neurologic consequences. Almost all patients tolerate swimming. After acute neck injuries, slow stretching exercises are performed during or after the application of heat, with intermittent use of a cervical collar to position the neck in slight flexion (never extension). Traction is not used in an acute cervical or low back condition until muscle spasm is relaxed and the ligamentous sprain is healed. However, traction is essential for relief of impingement on nerve roots from spondylosis or herniated disc.

Lumbosacral or thoracolumbar supports with shaped steel stays or plastic inserts are useful in obesity, extensive degenerative spine disease, and osteoporosis. Strengthening exercises supplement these supports to avoid further decompensation. Brief repetitive exercises help maintain joint range of motion. Flexion and rotation exercises early in the course of acute inflammation can prevent frozen shoulder syndromes.

Recurrent pain may be prevented if the patient can detect and change daily activities that perpetuate symptoms. Faulty posture, work positions, hobbies (needlework, reading in bed), and inadequate rest all contribute to chronic musculoskeletal strain. Small bifocal lenses and high-foam pillows can aggravate cervical problems. "Bucket" automobile seats and low-backed sofas can cause thoracic pain. Patients who are alerted to these situations can take the responsibility for remedying them and thus preventing onset of chronicity.

PHARMACOLOGIC THERAPY

Non-Narcotic Analgesics. Nonsteroidal anti-inflammatory agents inhibit the production of prostaglandins and thus decrease pain perception. Aspirin is the prototype and the most widely utilized of these drugs. It is effective in a number of painful disorders in the adult analgesic dose of 650 mg PO every four hours. While short-term therapy with aspirin has relatively few side effects, long-term use may result in gastrointestinal blood loss and renal dysfunction. Aspirin also inhibits platelet aggregation and may result in gastrointestinal upset.

Acetaminophen is an effective analgesic although it has little anti-inflammatory activity. It is effective in the relief of mild to moderate pain, the usual adult dose being 650 to 1000 mg PO every four hours. Acetaminophen is free of antiplatelet and gastrointestinal side effects. Overdoses, however, are extremely toxic to the liver. Aspirin and acetaminophen are commonly used in combination with other analgesics.

Numerous nonsteroidal anti-inflammatory agents are available to treat pain. Diflunisal is a derivative of aspirin, can be administered less frequently, and has a comparable analgesic effect. Ibuprofen, fenoprofen calcium, naproxen, and mefenamic acid are also used for mild to moderate pain. These agents have similar but variable GI, hepatic, renal, and CNS side effects. They are highly protein-bound and therefore may result in adverse drug interactions. Sulindac, tolmetin sodium, and indomethacin produce analgesia in conditions associated with inflammation. The commonly utilized non-narcotic oral agents for mild to moderate pain are summarized in Table 1.

Narcotic Analgesics. Morphine-like agonists, such as codeine and oxycodone, and mixed agonists-antag-

Table 1. NON-NARCOTIC ANALGESICS AND ANTI-INFLAMMATORY AGENTS

Analgesic	Dosage Schedule (Oral)	Comments
Acetaminophen	650–1000 mg every 4 hrs	Little GI or hematologic side effects
Aspirin	650 mg every 4 hrs	
Choline magnesium trisalicylate (Trilisate)	1000–1500 mg every 12 hrs	Does not affect platelet aggregation
Diflunisal (Dolobid)	500 mg every 8–12 hrs (maximum dose = 1500 mg/d)	Derivative of salicylate
Fenoprofen (Nalfon)	200 mg every 4–6 hrs	
Ibuprofen	400 mg every 6 hrs	
Indomethacin (Indocin)	25–50 mg three times daily	High incidence of CNS side effects
Mefenamic acid (Ponstel)	Initial dose 500 mg, then 250 mg every 6 hrs	Short-term use only
Naproxen (Naprosyn)	Initial dose 500 mg, then 250 mg every 6–8 hrs (maximum dose = 1250 mg/d)	May be given on twice-daily schedule
Naproxen sodium (Anaprox)	Initial dose 550 mg, then 275 mg every 6 hrs (maximum dose = 1375 mg/d)	
Sulindac (Clinoril)	150–200 mg every 12 hrs	
Tolmetin (Tolectin)	400 mg three times daily	

Table 2. NARCOTICS FOR MILD TO MODERATE PAIN

Analgesic	Dosage Schedule (Oral)	Comments
Codeine	30–60 mg every 4–6 hrs	Commonly utilized in combination Biotransformed to morphine
Meperidine	50–150 mg every 4 hrs	Metabolite is toxic and may result in CNS excitation
Oxycodone	5 mg every 4–6 hrs	Commonly utilized in combination
Pentazocine	30 mg every 4 hrs	Mixed agonist-antagonist
Propoxyphene napsylate	100 mg every 4 hrs	Cumulative toxicity May result in CNS depression
Propoxyphene HCl	65 mg every 4 hrs	Cumulative toxicity May result in CNS depression

onists, such as pentazocine, may be used either alone or in combination with non-narcotic analgesics to treat mild to moderate pain (Table 2). Administration and dosage must be individualized. These agents are addictive with long-term use.

Narcotics used for severe pain are morphine-like agonists and mixed agonist-antagonists (Table 3). These bind to the CNS opiate receptors. It is vital to individualize therapy for the patient and the severity of pain. For severe pain of acute onset, parenteral analgesia is the preferred mode of therapy, whereas oral therapy is preferred for chronic pain. Narcotics should be used in a stepwise fashion unless the severity of the pain dictates that the most potent agent is chosen initially. The agent elected should be given on a routine and regular schedule, since this will decrease the recurrence of severe pain and may allow a reduction in the total amount of analgesic given. In this way, the pain can be controlled while the incidence of adverse effects is lowered. If adverse effects do occur, they should be treated appropriately but the patient must not be allowed to lapse into severe pain. The addictive potential of these agents must be considered, especially in patients with nonmalignant diseases.

Several new techniques have recently been introduced to manage pain. These include continuous IV or SC infusion of analgesics with a patient-controlled programmable device. Intrathecal and epidural administration of narcotics, typically morphine, have proved useful to treat postoperative and chronic pain. This technique reduces the dose of narcotic required for effectiveness and results in prolonged analgesia without systemic side effects. The rapid development of tolerance may limit this approach.

Adjuvant Analgesics. Phenothiazines, tricyclic antidepressants, and other agents are useful for selected patients with pain. The phenothiazines, such as promethazine, and the butyrophenones, such as haloperidol, can be used to potentiate analgesia and enhance the sedative effect of other agents. Hydroxyzine, an antihistaminic and antiemetic, has similar effects.

Tricyclic antidepressants are also useful in adjuvant therapy for chronic pain, especially when there is concomitant depression. They may be effective in treating postherpetic neuralgia. Amitriptyline, 50 to 100 mg at bedtime, can be given with fluphenazine, 1 to 3 mg in divided doses, in the multi-agent management of chronic pain.

Cyclobenzaprine hydrochloride (Flexeril), 10 mg every eight hours, or diazepam (Valium), 5 mg three times per day, is effective in treating muscular spasm and relieving local pain. Diazepam is also useful in the patient with anxiety. These agents should be used cautiously in combination with other drugs. L-Tryptophan, an amino acid, may help to treat insomnia and depression in a dose of 500 to 3000 mg at bedtime. The anticonvulsants phenytoin and carbamazepine are effective for neuritic pain and trigeminal neuralgia.

Table 3. NARCOTICS FOR SEVERE PAIN

Analgesic	Analgesic Dose* (mg)	Duration of Action (hrs)	Comments
Butorphanol (Stadol)	IM 2	4–6	Agonist-antagonist
Codeine	IM 130	4–6	See Table 2 for initial dosage
	PO 200	4–6	
Hydromorphone (Dilaudid)	IM 1.5	4–5	
	PO 7.5	4–6	
Levorphanol (Levo-Dromoran)	IM 2	4–6	May accumulate with repeated administration
	PO 4	4–7	Excellent oral potency
Meperidine (Demerol)	IM 75	4–5	
	PO 300	4–6	Poor oral potency
Methadone (Dolophine)	IM 10	4–6	Accumulation with repeated administration
	PO 20	4–7	
Morphine	IM 10	4–6	
	PO 60	4–7	
Nalbuphine (Nubain)	IM 10	4–6	Agonist-antagonist
Pentazocine (Talwin)	IM 60	4–6	Agonist-antagonist
	PO 180	4–7	

*These doses are equivalent to 10 mg of intramuscular morphine.

Adapted from Inturrisi CE: Role of opioid analgesics. Beaver WT (ed.) Proceedings of a symposium: appropriate management of pain in primary care practice. Am J Med 77:29, 1984.

Surgery for Pain. Some neurosurgical procedures are effective in treating pain. These include neuroablative procedures such as radio frequency ablation of neural ganglia (i.e., the trigeminal ganglion), dorsal rhizotomy, spinal cordotomy, and transsphenoidal hypophysectomy. Microsurgical decompression of the trigeminal root helps some patients with trigeminal neuralgia.

Behavior Modification. Biofeedback, hypnosis, cognitive training, and relaxation training are increasingly used to treat chronic pain and are effective for patients with the chronic pain syndrome. Such patients should be considered for evaluation and therapy in a pain treatment center where a multidisciplinary approach can be used for this chronic disabling disorder.

REFERENCES

Beaver WT (ed): Appropriate management of pain in primary care practice. Am J Med (Symposium) 77(3a), Sept. 10, 1984.

Cailliet R: Soft Tissue Pain and Disability. F.A. Davis Co, Philadelphia, 1977.

Goodman C: Pathophysiology of pain. Arch Intern Med 143:527–530, 1983.

Swerdlow M (ed): The Therapy of Pain. J.B. Lippincott Co, Philadelphia, 1981.

4 · DIARRHEA

Kevin V. Carey
GUTHRIE CLINIC

ACUTE DIARRHEA

Diarrhea is one of the most common maladies of man. Fortunately, in the "developed nations" it is usually self-limited and mild. A physician generally is not required for a brief illness (under ten days). When a patient's diarrhea is acute and mild, diagnostic testing and medications should be avoided. Even when an exhaustive work-up is performed, a cause for the diarrhea cannot be found in about 40% of cases.

EVALUATION: SPECIAL GROUPS

Evaluation is necessary for the very young, the elderly, patients with serious chronic illness (all of which groups are particularly likely to become dehydrated), and those who report bleeding or toxicity. Evidence of dehydration indicates a need for hospitalization and intravenous fluid support. A person of any age who reports bleeding, fever, or chills should be seen urgently. When there is bleeding, hospitalization to monitor blood count and severity of diarrhea is necessary. A stool culture for invasive bacteria and an examination for parasites is required. Toxicity is indicated by fever, prostration, or tachycardia. With toxicity, one needs to be aware of the possibilities of bacterial sepsis or toxic megacolon. Blood cultures should be obtained. If abdominal distention occurs, plain x-ray examinations should be done initially and daily until toxicity resolves. Megacolon often presents with the sudden cessation of diarrhea while bloating and fever continue. Toxic patients should be treated with vigorous hydration and intravenous antibiotics.

All diarrhea patients should be questioned about recent travel, which may have caused an infection. Following trips to tropical climes, diarrhea is usually due to toxin-producing noninvasive bacteria. Patients with traveler's diarrhea require stool examination for ova and parasites and bacterial culture, followed by antibiotic treatment. I recommend trimethoprim and sulfa (Bactrim DS or Septra DS-1 b.i.d. for five days).

Giardiasis may be acquired during travel, often in cool mountainous areas. It is characterized by abdominal cramps, which are frequently epigastric.

Two other groups carry a high risk of intestinal infection. Homosexual males have a high incidence of multiple infectious organisms and parasites (e.g., *Giardia* and *Cryptosporidium*.) Children who attend day care centers where there are infants or toddlers, their families, and workers in such centers have an increased risk of bacterial and parasitic infection.

MANAGEMENT

Nonpharmacologic Measures. The vast majority of diarrhea patients do not need testing or treatment, but should first be reassured about the usually benign course of such illness. They should be advised to drink large amounts of water and juices, and to eat salty foods such as saltine crackers and bouillon, and sugar as in hard candies, gelatins, or flat soda. Beverages that are advertised to contain large amounts of electrolytes (e.g., Gatorade) are helpful but are not as effective as salty foods. Patients need to know that although efforts to increase their intake will often increase the amount of diarrheal flow, the absorption of fluid and electrolytes will increase.

I discourage the use of several "home remedies." I am amazed how often milk and dairy products are thought to be helpful as "binders" and stomach coating. This is ironic because enteritis can actually lower intestinal lactase levels. Gas, cramps, and worsened diarrhea result when dairy products are ingested; they should be introduced only after recovery, and even then may not be well tolerated for weeks or months. Magnesium-containing antacids and alcoholic beverages have a laxative effect even in normal individuals and are particularly undesirable in diarrhea patients.

Drug Therapy. I do not usually prescribe strong antidiarrheal drugs such as opioids, paregoric, diphenoxylate and atropine, and loperamide or narcotics such as codeine. Patients require an explanation for this, since many seek help only in order to obtain such a prescription. These drugs are not of proven benefit in acute diarrhea because they may impair the body's ability to rid itself of infectious agents and also increase the risk of megacolon in patients with toxic colitis. Antibiotics usually are not helpful and sometimes can lead to prolonged carriage of infectious agents. If patients insist on some form of drug therapy, I recommend bismuth subsalicylate (Pepto-Bismol). This drug has proven efficacy in traveler's diarrhea and seems to provide some symptomatic relief in other acute diarrheas. The usual dosage is 1 or 2 oz every 30 minutes for four hours. Patients should be warned that it may turn the stools black.

CHRONIC DIARRHEA

Chronic diarrhea presents a much more difficult problem, chiefly because there are so many possible causes. In evaluating chronic diarrhea, it is very important to determine exactly what the patient means by diarrhea: whether increased frequency, liquidity, or volume of stool, or all three.

EVALUATION

History. One should try to identify those patients who do not have true diarrhea but rather have incontinence. These patients usually have anal sphincter dysfunction or incontinence due to chronic severe constipation or impaction. They report frequent small bowel movements with soiling of underwear or uncontrollable oozing of liquid fecal material. This is best managed by bowel training programs, which attempt to induce bowel movements at an appropriate time rather than constantly trying to retard bowel function. Antidiarrhea medications do not help and may worsen incontinence.

Next, the patient should be questioned for the characteristic history of irritable bowel syndrome (IBS), the most common cause of chronic diarrhea. In IBS, there are frequent small bowel movements, often with mucus. Frequently, there is pain and bloating relieved by flatus or a bowel movement. Patients report longstanding bowel irregularities involving either diarrhea or constipation, or sometimes alternating diarrhea and constipation. There should not be weight loss, nocturnal diarrhea, episodes of incontinence, or bleeding. Answers to questions about IBS will help determine the severity of the illness.

Further pursuing the history, it is important to ask about drugs. The drugs often associated with diarrhea include antacids containing magnesium, antibiotics, antihypertensives (propranolol, guanethidine), cimetidine, colchicine, digitalis, lactulose, laxatives, quinidine, and thryoxine. The complete list of the patient's medications should be closely scrutinized. Occasionally, hyperosmotic nutritional supplements or dietetic foods that contain sorbitol and other nonabsorbable sugars cause diarrhea. Always questions should be asked about alcohol intake.

Surgical history should be reviewed. Resection of the ileum frequently causes bile salt malabsorption. This can be controlled with loperamide hydrochloride (Imodium) or cholestyramine (Questran). Gastric resection can cause diarrhea by several different mechanisms.

In chronic diarrhea, as in acute diarrhea, it is important to remember the various infections seen in homosexual male patients.

The history of flushing of the skin is highly suggestive of carcinoid syndrome. Finally, a history of Raynaud's phenomenon should lead to consideration of bacterial overgrowth due to altered bowel motility.

Sigmoidoscopy. Examination of the patient with chronic diarrhea should include sigmoidoscopy. This should be done without enema preparation. The finding of an impaction indicates a diagnosis of anal incontinence. A formed stool raises the question whether there is diarrhea at all. Finally, minor changes of inflammatory bowel disease—edema and erythema—are normal after an enema. Sigmoidoscopy can confirm a diagnosis of carcinoma, colitis, pseudomembranous colitis, or melanosis coli (suggesting laxative abuse).

Often a stool specimen can be obtained at sigmoidoscopy. In all patients, the stool should be examined for occult blood and fecal leukocytes. A positive test suggests carcinoma or colitis (pseudomembranous, infectious, ischemic, or inflammatory). Alkalinizing a sample of stool with a few drops of sodium hydroxide may reveal the purple stain of phenolphthalein, indicating surreptitious use of that laxative. A Sudan stain for fat can indicate malabsorption.

Laboratory Tests. Routine laboratory analysis (CBC, chemistry profile) can help categorize the diarrhea and guide further testing. For example, anemia indicates malabsorption or blood loss due to cancer or inflammatory diseases. Low potassium suggests secretory diarrhea.

Thyroid hormone and immunoglobulin levels should be measured. Other tests that can be done on an outpatient basis include xylose absorption, urinary 5-HIAA, and the Schilling test.

MANAGEMENT

Nonspecific Drug Therapy. If IBS seems likely, treatment for that condition should be given. If one is uncertain, it is useful to try antidiarrheal therapy to see if the diarrhea can be controlled by simple measures. This may include antidiarrheal drugs such as loperamide, two capsules after the first bowel movement in the morning and one after each subsequent bowel movement up to a maximum of eight per day. Other drugs such as diphenoxylate and atropine (Lomotil), two tablets up to four times a day or codeine, 30 to 60 mg up to four times a day may be substituted. Codeine should be avoided in patients who may abuse it. I do not use codeine in patients with IBS. However, codeine does offer significantly decreased cost.

Hospitalization. If there is weight loss or disability, or if symptoms are severe, hospitalization is recommended. In cases of doubt, a stool volume quantitation, which can be done on an outpatient basis, may help to decide. A normal stool volume is less than 250 gm per day. Stool volumes are usually normal in cases of incontinence and in IBS. In secretory diarrhea, volumes often exceed 1000 gm per day. A collection can be measured for 48 or 72 hours. Patients with higher than normal stool volumes warrant hospitalization.

Upon hospitalization, the outpatient work-up should be reviewed. Then, a stool collection for 48 hours while the patient is kept fasting (with IV fluid and electrolyte support) is helpful. Continued diarrhea while fasting indicates a secretory diarrhea. If the fast stops the diarrhea, food intolerance or malabsorption is suggested.

The causes of secretory diarrhea include surreptitious laxative abuse, carcinoid tumor, medullary carcinoma of the thyroid, gastrinoma, pancreatic cholera, ganglioneuroma, and villous tumors. Therefore, if not already done, colonoscopy and small bowel follow-through x-ray examinations should be performed. Detailed evaluation for secretory diarrhea includes serum hormone measurements, celiac angiography, CT scan of the abdomen, and exploratory laparotomy. Since this is expensive and potentially dangerous, and since surreptitious laxative use is a common cause of secretory diarrhea, a search of the patient's room in his absence is mandatory prior to further evaluation.

Table 1. EVALUATION OF CHRONIC DIARRHEA

History
1. IBS
2. Drugs, alcohol
3. Previous surgery
4. Life style (travel, day care, homosexuality)
5. Skin flushing
6. Raynaud's syndrome

Sigmoidoscopy

Stool Analysis
1. Blood cells, leukocytes
2. Alkalinize
3. Sudan stain for fat

Laboratory Tests
1. CBC, chemistry profile
2. Thyroid function
3. Immunoglobulin assay
4. Xylose absorption
5. Urinary 5-HIAA
6. Schilling test

X-Ray Examination
1. Small bowel follow-through
2. Barium enema

Stool Weight Measurement and Stool Weight Measurement While Fasting

---

If the diarrhea ceases with fasting, work-up for malabsorption should be pursued. Malabsorption may be due to liver failure, pancreatic failure, or small intestinal disease. Liver evaluation should include a liver spleen scan. Pancreatic evaluation includes plain film of the abdomen for pancreatic calcification and, if available, pancreatic function tests. A trial of pancreatic enzyme replacement can be given. Evaluation for small intestinal disease includes a small bowel biopsy and aspirate for *Giardia*. A trial for possible bacterial overgrowth should be considered: metronidazole (500 mg q.i.d. for seven days) or another antibiotic such as ampicillin, tetracycline, or trimethoprim and sulfa.

If the entire work-up to this point is negative, a check list such as suggested in Table 1 should be reviewed. Other therapeutic trials of steroids, indomethacin, or cholestyramine can be given, but these are not likely to be successful if a diagnosis cannot be made.

REFERENCES

Bond JH: Office-based management of diarrhea. Geriatrics 37:52–55, 61–64, 1982.

Fordtran JS: Diarrhea. *In* Wyngaarden JB, Smith LH, Jr. (eds): Cecil Textbook of Medicine, 17th ed. W.B. Saunders Co, Philadelphia, 1982, pp 712–719.

Goldfinger S, Phillips S, Rogers A: Diarrhea: A Practical Guide to Diagnosis and Management. Projects in Health, New York, 1976.

Read NW, Kiejs GJ, Read MG, et al: Chronic diarrhea of unknown origin. Gastroenterology 78:264–271, 1980.

5 · CONSTIPATION

James W. Manier
LOVELACE MEDICAL CENTER

DEFINITION AND DIAGNOSTIC CRITERIA

Constipation has been defined variously as excessive hardness of the stools, small stools, incomplete emptying of the rectum, and infrequent stooling. All of these have been found unreliable except stool frequency. Four studies in Western nations have shown a stool frequency of at least three times a week.

PATHOPHYSIOLOGY AND DIAGNOSIS

Constipation is a symptom, not a disease. Successful management depends on correct identification of cause (Table 1), which is most commonly apparent after a carefully performed history-taking and physical examination. When these are not definitive or when symptoms are not quickly responsive to a trial treatment with a high-fiber diet and bulk laxatives, an extensive laboratory investigation may be necessary.

Proctosigmoidoscopy is very helpful and may reproduce symptoms of the irritable bowel. Dark pigmentation of the bowel wall (melanosis coli) is seen with long-term use of anthracene cathartics. A flexible sigmoidoscope can reveal 60% to 70% of rectosigmoid cancers.

A helpful determination of colonic transit can be obtained by administering 20 rings cut from a radiopaque nasogastric tube and placed into gelatin capsules. The progress of these markers is then followed through the bowel with daily abdominal x-rays for seven days or until defecation of all of them, if this occurs earlier. This study allows separation of causes of colonic constipation into outlet obstruction (clustering of markers in the rectum), colonic inertia (markers throughout the colon), and hindgut inertia (markers in the left colon).

Anorectal manometry is useful to document anal sphincter function. It consists of insertion of a two-balloon assembly into the rectum and between the anal sphincter. Rectal distention with one balloon normally causes relaxation of the internal sphincter, which is recorded by the second balloon. Conditions such as Hirschsprung's disease and idiopathic constipation fail to show this response.

Full-thickness biopsies can be obtained from the

Table 1. ETIOLOGY OF CONSTIPATION

Metabolic Diseases		
Diabetes mellitus	Porphyria	
Panhypopituitarism	Pregnancy	
Hypothyroidism	Pheochromocytoma	
Hypercalcemia	Enteric glucogen excess	
Hypokalemia		
Central Nervous System		
Peripheral	*Peripheral (Continued)*	Cerebral
Aganglionosis	Multiple sclerosis	Parkinsonism
Ganglioneuromatosis	Tabes dorsalis	Tumors
Autonomic neuropathy	Shy-Drager syndrome	Vascular accident
Chagas' disease	Trauma	
Pseudo-obstruction	Cauda tumors	
Meningocele		
Drugs		
Analgesics	Antihypertensives	Psychotropic agents
Anesthetics	Bismuth salts	Parkinson drugs
Antacids	Barium	
Anticholinergics	Diuretics	
Anticonvulsants	Heavy metal poisoning	
Antidepressants	Iron	
	Ganglionic blockers	
Diet Habits		
Change in environment	Laxative abuse	
Ignoring call to stool	Low bulk diet	
Lack of exericse	Lack of water intake (?)	
Large Bowel Constipation		
Obstruction	*Motor Abnormalities*	*Rectal disease*
1. Extraluminal:	Irritable bowel	Tumors
Tumors	Diverticulosis	Ulcerative proctitis
Volvulus	Myotonic dystrophy	Proctocele
Hernias	Collagen vascular disease	*Anal Disease*
2. Intraluminal:	Idiopathic slow transit	Fissure
Tumors	Idiopathic megacolon	Hemorrhoids
Strictures		Prolapse
		Stricture

rectum with a suction biopsy instrument. These are of little value in adults, but may be diagnostic in infants and young children with one of the aganglionotic diseases such as Hirschsprung's.

Psychologic evaluation should be carried out by the managing physician, but a Minnesota Multiphasic Personality Inventory (MMPI) can uncover significant additional data such as underlying depression or psychosis.

MANAGEMENT

GOALS

Constipation is a common problem usually handled by patients without calling in a physician. It is thus important to heed those who do seek medical attention. Short-term goals should be to provide as rapid relief of the acute episode of constipation as possible. In the long term it is necessary to define the cause so that permanent control can be obtained. Evaluation and treatment usually can be handled in the office.

NONPHARMACOLOGIC MEASURES

Once the diagnosis of idiopathic constipation has been established, all possible offending drugs should be discontinued. Drug trials have shown that normal bowel function is reestablished in half the patients when laxatives are stopped. Unfortunately, some patients continue laxatives surreptitiously. Dietary fiber should be increased by adding high-fiber foods such as whole-grain baked foods, fresh fruits, and vegetables. Peanuts, popcorn, wheat, and corn bran are good sources of extra fiber. Corn bran seems to make patients less gassy (perhaps through lack of colonic digestion by bacteria). Patients should be taught to heed the call to stool in order to avoid extinction of the defecation reflex. Learning to use the toilet after eating (particularly the dinner meal) takes advantage of the gastrocolic reflex. Sitting exercises will strengthen weak abdominal muscles important in accomplishing the voluntary act of defecation. A small step stool under the feet when sitting on the toilet will make abdominal muscles more effective. Ingestion of large amounts of fluid and laxative foods such as figs and prunes may help. Daily exercise is important.

DRUG THERAPY

Laxatives, except bulk cathartics, should be used on a long-term basis only when all other therapy fails and when all specific diseases have been excluded. The choice of a specific laxative is dictated by cost, availability, and side effects (Table 2).

Bulking Agents. These agents are preparations of natural and semisynthetic polysaccharides and cellulose derivatives (Table 2). These compounds form emollients and gels when mixed with water. This action holds water in the stool. Although indigestible by the human bowel, some of them represent a major food source to colonic bacteria, which results in proliferation of these organisms and a resultant increase in stool bulk. The

Table 2. LAXATIVES

Bulk Agents

Product	Manufacturer	Active Agent	Dose
Konsyl	Lafayette	Psyllium	1 tsp with glass water 1–3 × daily
Konsyl-D	Lafayette	Psyllium + 50% dextrose	1 tsp with glass water 1–3 × daily
Metamucil	Searle	Psyllium	1 tsp with glass water 1–3 × daily
Modane Bulk	Adria	Psyllium	1 tsp with glass water 1–3 × daily
Serutan Toasted Granules	Williams	Plantago	1 tsp with glass water 1–3 × daily
Serutan Powder	Williams	Plantago	
Syllact	Wallace	Psyllium husks	1 tsp in water 1–3 × daily
Perdiem Plain	Rorer	Psyllium	1–2 tsp with glass liquid 1–5 × daily
Effersyllium	Stuart	Psyllium	1 tsp or packet with glass liquid 1–3 × daily
Fiberall	Rydelle	Psyllium	1 tsp + glass liquid 1–3 × daily
Lyoroeil	Powell	Psyllium	1 tsp + glass water 1–3 × daily
Mitrolan	Robins	Calcium polycarbopyl	Chew tablets 4 × daily
Movicol	Norgine	Gum karaya	1–2 tsp with water 1–2 × daily
Nuggets	Jayco	Psyllium	1 tsp with water 1–3 × daily

Osmotic Agents

Product	Manufacturer	Active Agent	Dose
Phosphosoda	Fleet	Sodium phosphate	4 tsp glass water + 2nd glass water
Phillips' Milk of Magnesia	Glenbrook	Magnesium hydroxide	2–4 tbsp with water
Chronulac Syrup	Merrell Dow	Lactulose	1–2 tsp daily

Surface-Active Agents

Product	Manufacturer	Active Agent	Dose
Argoral	Parke-Davis	Phenolphthalein + oil	½–1 tbsp
Cholase	Mead Johnson	Docusate sodium	1–3 tsp. 3 × daily
Correctol	Plough	Phenolphthalein	1–2 tablets daily
Decholin	Miles Pharm.	Bile salts	1–2 tablets 3 × daily
Dialose	Stuart	Decusate potassium	1 tablet 1–2 × daily
Dulcolax	Boehringer	Bisacodyl	2–3 tablets daily
Exlax	Exlax Pharm.	Phenolphthalein	1–2 tablets daily
Evac-U-Gen	Walker	Phenolphthalein	1–2 tablets 2 × daily
Doxidan	Hoechlst-Roussel	Danthron + docusate	1–2 capsules daily
Modane	Adria	Danthron	1 tablet at bedtime
Perdiem	Rorer	Senna + psyllium	1–2 tsp with water 2 × daily
Carter's Pills	Carter	Bisacodyl	1–3 pills at bedtime
Senokot	Purdue Fredrick	Senna	1–2 tsp daily
Fleet Castor Oil	Fleet	Castor oil	3 tbsp daily

Lubricants

Product	Manufacturer	Active Agent	Dose
Agoral, Plain	Parke-Davis	Agar, tracacanth, acacia	1–2 tbsp daily
Haley's M-O	Winthrop	Mineral oil + milk of magnesia	2 tbsp 2 × daily
Fleet Mineral Oil	Fleet	Mineral oil	1–2 tbsp daily
Milkinol	Kremers-Urban	Liquid petroleum	1–2 tbsp daily

overall effect of administration of these laxatives is to increase stool bulk, speed intestinal transit, and ease stool evacuation. Side effects are minimal and consist of increased colonic gas secondary to the digestive activities of colonic bacteria. These agents may interfere with magnesium, iron, zinc, and calcium absorption. Calcium supplements should be added to the diets of patients at risk of osteoporosis. Rarely, bulking agents have been implicated as a cause of intestinal obstruction in patients with strictures from such conditions as inflammatory bowel disease, neoplasia, and diverticulitis.

Osmotic Agents. These cathartics act by drawing fluid into the bowel lumen through the semipermeable membrane of the gut wall via osmosis (Table 2). The distention of the bowel thus produced reflexly stimulates propulsive bowel contractions. Members of this group include the sulfate and phosphate salts of sodium and magnesium (the saline cathartics) and lactulose, a synthetic disaccharide of galactose and fructose for which the bowel has no disaccharidase. The action of lactulose is enhanced by its colonic bacterial digestion, which increases the number of osmotically active molecules present. Phosphate cathartics with long use can decrease serum calcium levels by binding calcium in the bowel lumen, preventing absorption. In renal insufficiency, magnesium and phosphate levels may rise precipitately because of inability of the kidney to excrete them.

Surface-Active Agents. In this group are the most potent laxatives including castor oil, the anthracene cathartics, phenolphthalein, and the various diphenyl methane derivatives (Table 2). Current evidence, unfortunately incomplete for some members of this group, implicates the intestinal epithelium as the primary site of action of these drugs. The mode of action varies among the different members of the group; several have more than one mode operational. Some work through a second messenger system present in the enterocyte, most commonly adenyl cyclase and cyclic adenosine monophosphate to stimulate intestinal secretion of fluid and electrolytes into the lumen. Some inhibit sodium potassium adenosine triphosphatase–mediated sodium absorption, thus limiting sodium-assisted solvent drag of water from the lumen. Others alter mucosal permeability by damaging the enterocyte so that a concentration gradient across the epithelium is lost that normally prevents secretion into the lumen. Others stimulate cyclo-oxidase, which produces more prostaglandin E, which in turn increases intestinal secretion into the gut lumen. Some stimulate intestinal motility, and some damage the intestinal mucosa itself.

Long-term administration of anthracene cathartics in animals has led to myenteric plexus degeneration, and resultant interference with intestinal motility. Docusate sodium, a compound of many laxatives (Table 2), has a detergent effect that increases the absorption of certain drugs, leading to toxic levels. The large losses of fluid and electrolytes induced by these agents can be harmful, particularly in very young and elderly patients. Long-term use of these drugs can produce a featureless colonic mucosa radiologically (the laxative colon). Melanosis coli, a dark pigmentation of the bowel mucosa from an increase in macrophages containing a brownish-black melanotic pigment in the lamina propria, is seen with long-term use of anthracene cathartics.

Lubricants. This group is composed of the various mineral oils that are nonabsorbable hydrocarbons (Table 2). These compounds act by lubricating the colonic contents and by coating the surface of the stool, preventing colonic absorption of fecal fluid and thus increasing stool bulk to stimulate defecation. Side effects include impairment of fat-soluble vitamin absorption, inducement of chronic perianal inflammation, and lipid pneumonia secondary to accidental pulmonary aspiration. Lubricants can interfere with absorption of lipid-soluble drugs, thus lowering effective blood levels.

Rectal Administration. Some laxatives are available in a suppository form. Prolonged use can produce perirectal inflammation. Castile soapsuds enemas have led to acute colitis. No evidence exists to support the contention that they restore rectal sensation. Their use should be restricted to preparation for radiologic and endoscopic procedures, and removal of fecal impaction.

PATIENT EDUCATION AND INFORMATION

One publisher has prepared a written sheet on care of constipation, which can be distributed to patients.* A film strip prepared by a commercial company has proved helpful in my office.† If available, a dietary consultant can be beneficial, particularly when a high-fiber diet must be combined with other dietary restrictions. Printed handouts on high-fiber diets have helped my patients.

PERIODIC REEVALUATION

Follow-up visits allow patients to know the physician is concerned and allow the physician to determine that the prescribed program is being followed and is effective, or if not to immediately reexamine the patient. The initial follow-up visit should be within two to three weeks of prescribing treatment. The patient should be invited to call earlier if unanticipated problems arise. If everything is well at the return visit, the time should be used to reinforce the plan of treatment and answer questions.

PATIENT COMPLIANCE

Compliance varies widely. It may be nonexistent in the laxative abuser. One group of laxative abusers may present an interesting clinical picture of watery diarrhea, weight loss, and weakness. These patients are often medical personnel and more often female than male. They usually have had multiple previous negative medical examinations for their "diarrhea." They may exhibit hypokalemia, metabolic alkalosis, evidence of malabsorption, and secretory diarrhea. Ten per cent show a cathartic colon on x-ray film. Proctoscopy may show melanosis coli if patients have been taking anthracene cathartics. Addition of sodium hydroxide to a stool specimen will demonstrate a red color if phenolphthalein cathartics are being used. Stool osmolality may demonstrate an anion gap if osmotic laxatives are being ingested. Search of the patient's room for concealed laxatives is important, since this is a potentially fatal disease if not diagnosed.

PREVENTIVE MEASURES

Chronic constipation, although basically a benign condition, does carry some risks. The disappearance of myriads of complaints after correction indicates that constipation is uncomfortable. In chronic fecal impaction, pressure on the mucosa by inspissated feces can produce mucosal ulcers. Some urinary infections are associated with constipation. Diarrhea can result from the ball valve effect of impacted stool, and in children is a cause of encopresis. Four studies suggest an association with rectal cancer. Constipation can be secondary to serious organic diseases that are a threat to the patient. These risks can be modified by correct diagnosis and appropriate treatment.

Some individuals resort to laxatives even when asymptomatic. Fewer laxatives are being used today in older people, and the long-held misconception that constipation produces toxic symptoms is being corrected. The best preventive is to educate patients regarding normal stooling, the importance of a high-fiber diet, and the need to avoid laxatives if bowel function is normal.

SOCIOECONOMIC ASPECTS OF MANAGEMENT

The economic aspects of constipation are high. In 1976, laxative consumption in the United States was estimated to cost 225 million dollars annually. Laxatives are of themselves not without danger. More important is the risk that injudicious use of laxatives without establishing a cause for the constipation may prevent the diagnosis of a correctable disease or of colon cancer and inflammatory diseases, some of which are potentially fatal. The problem of constipation is serious. It should not be ignored by the physician, and requires careful and diligent efforts on the part of both physician and patient to correct.

REFERENCES

Clayden GS, Lawson JO: Investigation and management of long-standing chronic constipation in childhood. Arch Dis Child 51:918–923, 1976.

Elliot DL, Watts WJ, Girard DE: Constipation. Mechanisms and management of a common clinical problem. Postgrad Med 74:143–149, 1983.

Kazzman H: Constipation in the elderly. AFP 27:179–184, 1983.

Poisson J, Devroede G: Severe chronic constipation as a surgical problem. Surg Clin North Am 63:193–212, 1983.

Stratton JW, Mackeigan JM: Treating constipation. AFP 25:139–142, 1982.

---

*Patient Care Communications, Inc., 16 Thorndal Circle, Daren, CT 06820.

†Milner Fenwick, Inc., 2125 Green Spring Drive, Timonium, MD 21093.

6 · COUGH

Joseph B. Blood, Jr.
GUTHRIE CLINIC

DEFINITION AND DIAGNOSTIC CRITERIA

The successful treatment of cough is dependent on accurate diagnosis. The more specific the cause, the more successful is the treatment. When the cough is associated with other systemic signs and symptoms, a specific disease state may be readily apparent and the treatment of this disease state will alleviate the cough. This discussion will deal with those diseases in which cough is the most prominent or perhaps the only symptom.

One must decide whether a cough is due to excessive mucus production by the tracheobronchial tree and nasal passages, or to excessive irritation of the cough receptors. If none of these is present, a diagnosis of nonspecific cough can be made.

About 75% of patients present with chronic bronchitis, postnasal drip, asthma, or some combination of these as a cause of the chronic cough. The next most common causes are postviral tracheitis (a dry cough following a viral bronchitis some weeks later), congestive heart failure, or reflux esophagitis, which are found in about 15% of patients. The remaining 5 to 10% make up a group of rare presentations such as diffuse interstitial fibrosis, bronchial tumors, and pneumoconiosis.

MANAGEMENT

NONPHARMACOLOGIC MEASURES

Pulmonary Toilet. If a cough is due to excessive secretions, good pulmonary toilet is needed, which takes precedence over the empiric pharmacologic suppression of a cough. It is well to remember that smokers may not have a productive cough at first owing to suppression of normal tracheobronchial clearance mechanisms and the presence of thick viscid sputum, but with proper pulmonary toilet the true amount of secretions may be cleared from the lung.

Pulmonary toilet has three important components. First, proper humidification of the airway. This is essential in patients who are chronic bronchitics and who have mucoid impactions in the lower airways from heavy smoking. A hand-held nebulizer such as the Handivent is inexpensive and easy to use. The more complicated and expensive IPPB machines offer no advantage over nebulizers except when severe lung disease makes it impossible for patients to take deep breaths without assistance from a positive-pressure source. Oral hydration with 2 to 3 liters of extra water per day is helpful in patients who appear to be clinically dehydrated. A helpful guide is to have patients observe their urine color: it should be water clear.

The second important component includes postural drainage with percussion and vibration to the chest wall. Because the aerosol is effective in humidifying only the upper tracheobronchial tree, inspissated sputum in the lower smaller airways must be loosened and moved proximally to the larger air passages. This can be done in a 20° Trendelenburg position and can be taught by a well-trained physical therapist to the patient or relative for home therapy.

The third important factor is the double-cough technique. This is used to clear the upper passages and then the lower passages sequentially. Many patients are unable to perform this technique effectively without being taught.

When patients need pulmonary toilet, I have them use a good steam vaporizer or a Handivent nebulizer four times a day followed by 10 to 20 minutes of good postural drainage if tolerated. Instructional sheets are available.

PHARMACOLOGIC MEASURES

Oral Expectorants. In order to increase secretions, I recommend oral expectorants. The object of this class of agents is to increase the volume and decrease the viscosity of sputum. The following agents are very helpful. First, mucolytic agents such as acetylcysteine (Mucomyst), which is best given by nebulization in a 10% to 20% solution mixed with normal saline: 3 to 5 ml of 20% solution; 6 to 10 ml of 10% solution every six hours. More frequent nebulization is associated with a bronchial irritation or even bronchospasm, especially in asthmatic patients.

Second, organic iodides (Organidin and its preparations) are effective in loosening secretions and promoting drainage in the lower airways. I find them particularly effective when used in patients with chronic lung disease who are also bronchitics. Organic iodides stimulate gastric mucosal receptors by a reflex mechanism, increasing the volume of low-viscosity sputum and making it easier for patients to clear secretions. Nausea and abdominal bloating are the most common side effects. Organidin comes in three forms: a solution in which 20 drops in juice or water three times a day are used; an elixir, 5 cc three times a day; or in tablet form, one tablet three to four times a day. I prefer the solution since dosage allows larger quantities to be given for hydration.

An alternative medication for the patient who cannot take the organic iodides is guaifenesin (Robitussin), which has an action similar to that of the organic iodides. The dosage is 30 ml three times a day and there are very few side effects. However, in my experience this preparation is of doubtful efficacy.

Decongestion. A cough accompanied by excessive nasopharyngeal and nasal secretions requires a suppression of the secretory output by the upper passages. One possible exception would be in those patients with acute purulent sinusitis in whom the treatment of choice would be to stimulate the sinus secretions and promote drainage with organic iodides.

The suppression of excessive upper respiratory tract secretions can be best accomplished with the use of vasoconstrictor medications. If an allergic component is detected by the observation of bluish boggy nasal mucosa, an antihistamine can be added.

Topical Decongestants. Topical decongestants work very nicely, but have several drawbacks. Most of these agents are short-acting; provide only temporary relief for a few hours; may not reach all the effective areas of the nasal mucosa, particularly in the posterior pharyngeal areas; and produce a rebound phenomenon known as rhinitis medicamentosa, particularly after long and indiscriminate use. Since little of the topical decongestant is absorbed, the main advantage is that cardiac stimulation, tremulousness, and hypertensive effects are not seen. If the above effects are observed, one should suspect that the patient is using the medication indiscriminately.

Oxymetazoline hydrochloride (Afrin) can be used in adults and older children: two sprays or two to four drops in each nostril of a 0.5% solution every 12 hours for four to five days maximum. Rhinitis medicamentosa may develop with longer use. Another alternative, xylometazoline hydrochloride (Otrivin) should be used as one to two drops of a 0.1% solution every eight to ten hours. Burning of the nasal mucosa for a brief period is the main side effect.

Oral Decongestants. Oral decongestants can be more effective than topical decongestants for several reasons. They have a long duration of action, they can be given every 12 hours or even once daily with good effect, and they cover the areas of the nasopharynx usually inaccessible to the topical sprays. They therefore do not cause rhinitis medicamentosa with prolonged use. In the treatment of cough due to excessive nasal or upper respiratory secretions, a pure vasoconstrictor agent, or one with a small amount of antihistamine, is the drug of choice. This is particularly true in that segment of the population whose work involves running of heavy machinery or driving motor vehicles. The following preparations are useful:

1. Those with no antihistamine:
   a. Pseudoephedrine hydrochloride (Sudafed), 60-mg or 30-mg tablets. One tablet every six to eight hours, usually for three to four days. The 30-mg tablets can be used if the 60-mg tablets are not tolerated.
   b. Phenylephrine hydrochloride plus phenylpropanolamine (Entex LA), one tablet every 10 to 12 hours.
2. Those with very little antihistamine:
   a. Actifed tablets (pseudoephedrine 60 mg plus triprolidine 2.5 mg), one tablet every eight hours.
   b. CoTylenol OTC preparation and Teldrin, both containing pseudoephedrine 30 mg and chlorpheniramine 2 mg, two tablets or capsules every six hours.

Topical Steroid Sprays. Topical steroid sprays are very effective in treating cough due to allergic rhinitis and postnasal drip, particularly if polyposis is present. Some of the corticosteroid is absorbed, but suppression of the adrenopituitary axis and development of cushingoid signs are not a problem unless the medication is used in excessive quantities. In general, after a week of continuous usage there is a marked decrease in drainage of the upper respiratory tracts, and thus a lessening of the cough.

Beclomethasone dipropionate (Beconase, Vancenase), dexamethasone sodium phosphate (Decadron, Turbinaire), and flunisolide (Nasalide) are all available and equally effective. One to two sprays in each nostril two to four times a day are appropriate, depending on the severity of the symptoms. Beconase spray gives the least nasal burning and may be easiest to use. After one week of therapy, maximal effect should be obtained and efforts should be made to decrease the dosage to once a day or as needed.

Oral corticosteroid preparations such as prednisone should be used only in short courses of 10 to 14 days' maximum duration, and only as a last resort if the above sprays do not work.

Special Problems. The dry cough with excessive stimulation of cough receptors such as seen after a viral infection, the so-called postviral tracheitis, responds to two medications. First, Tessalon Perles is a peripherally acting medication that acts as a local anesthetic, and its main action is to suppress peripheral cough receptors: 100 mg three to four times a day. Side effects include rash, nasal congestion, constipation, headache, nausea, and drowsiness, which are quite rare. A short course of high doses of oral prednisone is also effective. A typical schedule would be 40 mg prednisone per day on a once daily dosage for two to three days, and then tapering rapidly by 10-mg decrements every two to three days until a dosage of 10 mg can be reached. The medication then can be discontinued entirely, thus completing the cycle in no more than 14 days. There have been no reported side effects with this regimen since there is no suppression of the adrenopituitary axis or development of other forms of hypercortisolism. Osteoporotic patients tolerate this regimen well without any ill effects, but it should not be used in insulin-dependent diabetics or patients on antimetabolite chemotherapy.

For patients with a background of atopy, the dry hacking cough may be associated with an early asthmatic state. This type of cough responds well to long-acting theophylline preparations or selective beta$_2$-adrenergic agents. Theo-Dur or a similar agent, 300 mg every 12 hours, is the preparation I prefer. The new long-acting preparations appear also to be effective for 24 hours. Dosage must be modified for children, who often require a relatively larger dosage of theophylline preparation on a per weight basis owing to increased drug metabolism; for older individuals the dosage must be lowered because of decreased drug metabolism. Monitoring theophylline levels is useful in adjusting dosage to the usual therapeutic range of 10 to 20 μg/ml.

The beta$_2$-adrenergic selective agents are better than nonselective agents because of the decreased incidence of tremulousness and tachycardia with the former. The tablets appear to be more effective in older patients, who seem to adapt to them better and have fewer problems than with the sprays. Individuals in their teens and twenties appear to find sprays more to their liking. Oral preparations such as albuterol (Ventolin, Proventil), a 4-mg tablet three times a day, are usually effective in suppressing asthmatic cough. This also comes in a spray preparation. The usual dosage is one to two sprays three times a day. A new preparation, terbutaline (Brethine), also appears to be effective.

Cough Suppressants. A cough not due to excessive secretions or irritation of the receptors in the tracheobronchial tree may be treated with a general antitussive agent if a cause cannot be identified. The antitussives used to suppress a nonspecific cough can be classified as centrally acting (i.e., suppression of the cough at the medullary center) or peripherally acting (i.e., suppression of the submucosal receptors in the tracheobronchial tree. The former group of medications includes the opiates such as codeine, hydrocodone, and hydromorphone, which have a similar mode of action; the latter group includes dextromethorphan and caramiphen.

The narcotic preparations, in my opinion, should be used only for a cough that is associated with severe pain and anxiety, such as from fractured ribs and abdominal trauma, or for a severe, aggressive, *nonproductive* cough. Use of these agents to suppress a *productive* cough may lead to sputum retention and its attendant complications. Codeine phosphate or codeine sulfate (all forms are generic) can be used in the 15- or 30-mg tablets every six hours, depending on the size of the adult patient. For an adult weighing less than 150 lb I use 15 mg; for an adult weighing more than 150 lb I use 30-mg tablets. The side effects are nausea, vomiting, dizziness, constipation, and drowsiness. The potential for drug abuse is low and respiratory depression occurs only with overdoses.

The centrally acting nonopiates are dextromethorphan and caramiphen. Dextromethorphan is the most widely prescribed cough preparation in the United States. It is available in OTC preparations as well as in prescription medications. Although its efficacy has never been unequivocally confirmed in a controlled study, it seems to work well clinically. The dosage form is a generic liquid of 10 mg dextromethorphan per 5 ml, or Benylin DM, 10 mg per 5 ml in 5% alcohol. The recommended dosage is 15 ml every six to eight hours, not to exceed 60 ml in 24 hours. The drug is essentially free of narcotic addiction and other side effects associated with codeine and its derivatives. Caramiphen is the other centrally active non-narcotic antitussive, available only in combination with other cold remedies—usually a vasoconstrictor. Tuss-Ornade, one capsule every 12 hours, is particularly useful.

REFERENCES

American Medical Association Drug Evaluations, 5th ed. AMA, Chicago, 1983, pp 549–600.

Irwin RS, Rosen MJ, Braman SS: Cough. A comprehensive review. Arch Intern Med 137:1186–1191, 1977.

Pierce JA: Cough. *In* MacBryde CM, Blacklow RS (eds): Signs & Symptoms, 6th ed. J.B. Lippincott Co, Philadelphia, 1977.

Zanjanian MH: Expectorant and antitussive agents. Ann Allergy 44:290, 1980.

7 · INSOMNIA

Fernando G. Miranda
LOVELACE MEDICAL CENTER

DEFINITION AND DIAGNOSTIC CRITERIA

Sleep disturbance and inadequate wakefulness are among the most usual subjective symptoms of patients referred to physicians. If the physician is unable to diagnose or even suspect sleep pathology, the treatment of such patients cannot be suitable. This in turn affects patients' social functioning and work performance, and often their personal life. Research in the field of sleep physiology in the 1950s and early 1960s has focused more attention on an objective understanding of the pathophysiologic mechanisms of sleep disturbances and the neurophysiologic mechanisms involved in normal sleep and wakefulness.

Most physicians are clearly surprised to discover that the traditional approach to diagnosis and treatment is both frustrating and inconclusive. With a sleep disturbance, patients' complaints often are not verified, and a diagnostic protocol cannot be strictly followed. Many times, physicians tend to prescribe medication that often may not be necessary at all.

Those of us involved in this field believe that if the general practitioner or specialist understands a classification of the sleep pathology, these disorders will be "demystified" and he will be able to use findings of abnormal sleep patterns and symptoms to detect medical and psychiatric illnesses in his patients.

GLOSSARY OF TERMS USED IN THE CLASSIFICATION OF SLEEP DISORDERS

Circadian rhythm: An innate, daily fluctuation of physiologic and behavioral functions, including sleep-waking. Generally tied to the 24-hour day-night cycle but sometimes to a measurably different periodicity when light/dark and other time cues are removed.

Conditioned insomnia: An easily overlooked form of chronic insomnia (sometimes a component of psychophysiologic DIMS) caused by the development, during an earlier experience of sleeplessness, of a negative association between characteristics of the customary sleep environment and sleeping.

"Deep" sleep stage: Common term for NREM sleep stages 3 and 4.

Delta sleep stage(s): Stage(s) of sleep in which EEG delta waves are prevalent or predominant (sleep stages 3 and 4, respectively).

Early AM *arousal:* Premature morning awakening.

Insomnia: Difficulty in sleeping. A confusing term, though ubiquitously employed, because it is used to indicate any and all gradations and types of sleep loss.

"Light" sleep stage: Common term for NREM sleep stage 1 and sometimes stage 2.

Myoclonus: Muscle contractions in the form of "jerks" or twitches. In sleep-related (nocturnal) myoclonus, the jerks are primarily of the flexor groups in the lower extremities, and have a characteristic frequency of 20 to 40 seconds.

NREMS period: The NREMS portion of NREMS-REMS cycle; such a period consists primarily of sleep stages 3 and 4 early in the night, and sleep stage 2 later.

Polysomnogram: The continuous and simultaneous recording of physiologic variables during sleep: EEG, EOG, EMG, EKG, respiratory air flow, respiratory excursions, lower limb movements, and other electrophysiologic variables.

Sleep stages:

Sleep stage NREM: The other major sleep stage apart from REMS. Consists of sleep stages 1 to 4, which constitute areas in the spectrum of NREMS.

Sleep stage REM: The stage of sleep found in all mammals studied, including humans, in which brain activity is extensive, brain metabolism is increased, and vivid hallucinatory imagery or dreaming occurs (in humans). It is also called "paradoxical sleep" because, in the face of this intense excitation of the CNS and the presence of spontaneous rapid eye movements, resting muscle activity is suppressed. The EEG is a low-voltage, fast-frequency non-alpha record. Stage REM sleep usually takes up 20% to 25% of total sleep time.

CLINICAL ASPECTS

The physician must elicit from the patient a significant amount of data in terms of quality as well as quantity of the insomnia complaint. A depressed individual may be able to fall asleep fairly quickly, but unable to maintain the continuity of sleep with premature morning arousal. In contrast, inability to fall asleep is quite frequent in patients who are anxious, worried, or guilty, whether they are essentially normal or in a psychotic state.

Probably the most important and powerful disrupter of the sleep process is internal arousal related to conscious and excessive "trying" to fall asleep, opposed to early night inability to sleep in delayed sleep phase, which represents a sleep-wake cycle shift, and not a true abnormality of the sleeping process. In addition, periodic awakenings through the night might represent interruption of rapid eye movement (REM) sleep. Also, some insomniacs may be totally relaxed and still sleep poorly because of weakness in their sleep system.

When a practitioner encounters a patient with a sleep disturbance (either insomnia, hypersomnia, or the parasomnias—abnormal behavior during the night) that is important enough to disrupt functioning at work or family life, the patient should be referred to a sleep disturbance center. Here, he can be evaluated by the proper diagnostic criteria (discussed below). Polysomnography may or may not be indicated. However, the patient is evaluated by a physician or a psychologist keenly familiar with sleep disorders.

In many instances, I have used the original visit to reassure the patient that the difficulty is a transient one. In many cases, this is all that is needed.

PSYCHOPHYSIOLOGIC DIMS (DISORDER OF INITIATING OR MAINTAINING SLEEP)

Transient and Situational. This represents a brief period of sleep disturbance usually provoked by an acute emotional arousal or conflict caused by a loss or perceived threat. Normally, the patient presents with difficulty in falling asleep, intermittent awakenings, and premature morning arousal. In order to be classified as a transient DIMS, this disturbance may not last longer than three weeks following termination of the precipitating event.

These emotions are usually triggered by experiences such as a marriage proposal or an unfamiliar sleep environment. Individuals who are insecure and have a low threshold for emotional arousal are most vulnerable.

Differential diagnoses include temporary periods of insomnia that have origins in medical, toxic, and environmental conditions.

Persistent Psychophysiologic DIMS. This is a sleep-onset and intermediary-sleep-maintenance insomnia that develops as a result of the mutually reinforcing factors of chronic, somatized tension, anxiety, and negative conditioning to sleep. It usually starts with a prolonged episode of stress in a person who sleeps adequately but not well before the stress. The maladaptive behavioral habits learned during the stress episode are not extinguished because of the occasional spontaneous nights of poor sleep. Somatized tension, anxiety, and some depression are often evident in such insomnias, but they are not serious enough to warrant a psychiatric diagnosis.

These are best treated with behavioral techniques and relaxation training. This works most of the time, since a conditional internal factor is the apprehension about falling asleep that builds up in connection with unsuccessful and excessive efforts to sleep.

DIMS ASSOCIATED WITH PSYCHIATRIC DISORDERS

Emotional and psychiatric problems are in many cases the underlying factor of many insomnias. Psychotherapy for these patients differs from therapy for those who know that they are emotionally distressed. It has been suggested that these types of insomniacs may need a very firm, direct approach similar to the one used for other psychosomatic conditions.

Symptoms and Personality Disorders. This is a sleep-onset and intermediary-sleep-maintenance insomnia that is clearly related to the psychologic and behavioral symptoms of the clinically well-known and classified nonaffective and nonpsychotic psychiatric disorders. These distinctive conditions include generalized anxiety, panic, and phobic disorders; hypochondriasis; obsessive–compulsive disorders; various personality disorders; and other conditions usually designated "neurotic." Many of these represent disorders that are the expression of an incompletely successful personality and of behavioral attempts to control anxiety.

Depression and abnormalities in sleep have been studied extensively. They are characterized by a short REM latency of less than 50 minutes, by long and intensive REM periods early at night, and by poor sleep efficiency (long sleep latencies, many awakenings during the night, and early morning awakenings). Delta sleep is decreased. It is not unusual for younger patients to show hypersomnia associated with their depression.

In patients with manic depressive illness, the manic phase is characterized by short sleep, and the depressive phase is often associated with hypersomnia. However, the typical features of short REM latency and reduced delta sleep are still present.

Some authors recommend that sleep-inducing antidepressants be given only at bedtime, making maximal use of their sedating side effects.

DIMS And Other Functional Psychoses. These usually consist of severe sleep-onset insomnia and often sleep continuity difficulties, which develop with acute psychotic decompensations or exacerbations. The components that usually underlie the sleep disturbance are anxiety, fear, suspiciousness, urgency of thought, and extreme guilt. Also, DIMS often remains a significant problem in chronic psychosis. Chronic schizophrenics show decreased delta sleep but normal amounts of REM. Dream-content schizophrenia fluctuates with the clinical status.

DIMS ASSOCIATED WITH USE OF DRUGS AND ALCOHOL

With sustained use of such agents, usually undertaken to fight DIMS arising from a different source, tolerance increases and the depressants lose their sleep-inducing effects. This often leads to an increase in dosage. In addition, unrecognized periods of partial and relative withdrawal occur, which contribute to the development of secondary, drug-related DIMS. After discontinuance of some drugs, severe sleeplessness occurs. This is sometimes accompanied by features of a drug withdrawal syndrome.

During chronic use of a hypnotic agent, nocturnal sleep is marked by frequent awakenings, lasting for more than five minutes, occasionally including periods out of bed. Progressive prolongation of sleep latency also occurs as the ingestion of the drug lengthens in time. Chronic alcoholic patients show sleep manifested by many awakenings, many stage changes, little or no delta sleep, and decreased REM sleep. Total time in bed is often increased and the sleep-wake rhythm is blurred.

It has been noted that after one or two years of abstinence, the sleep of many alcoholics remains disturbed. Delta sleep remains low, sleep is excessively fragmented, and there are difficulties in falling asleep.

DIMS ASSOCIATED WITH SLEEP-INDUCED RESPIRATORY IMPAIRMENT

Sleep Apnea DIMS Syndrome. Sleep apneic patients who complain of insomnia usually show predominantly central sleep apneas (diaphragmatic paralysis).

Nocturnal Myoclonus. This is DIMS associated with sleep-related (nocturnal) "myoclonus and restless legs." It is a condition in which insomnia is associated with the occurrence during sleep of periodic and repetitive episodes of highly stereotyped muscle jerks. In some individuals, excessive daytime sleepiness rather than insomnia is the chief complaint. The leg twitches repeat every 20 to 40 seconds, occasionally unilaterally, sometimes bilaterally. The episodes last anywhere from five minutes to two hours and they alternate with periods of normal sleep. These are not related to the "hypnic jerks" that occasionally startle many of us when we are falling asleep. The incidence of sleep-related myoclonus increases with age.

This type of disorder is responsive to treatment with clonazepam, starting at 0.5 mg q.h.s.

"Restless Leg Syndrome." In contrast to nocturnal myoclonus, this occurs while patients are awake and relaxing. In some cases the syndrome is related to peripheral neuropathies, circulatory insufficiencies, carcinoma, and vitamin deficiencies.

DIMS ASSOCIATED WITH MEDICAL, TOXIC, AND ENVIRONMENTAL CONDITIONS

This category covers those medical, toxic, and environmental conditions that are invariably associated with DIMS: CNS disorders, renal failure, infections, arthritis, endocrine and metabolic disorders, and poisoning (e.g., with mercury, arsenic, and alcohol). Environmental conditions such as noise, heat, and humidity may directly disturb sleep. Treatment must be directed toward the conditions that cause poor sleep.

CHILDHOOD-ONSET DIMS

This is a sleep-onset and sleep-maintenance insomnia, resulting in daytime symptoms of inadequate sleep. It is characterized by a distinctive history of unexplained development before puberty and persistence into adulthood.

These patients take significantly longer to fall asleep than adult-onset insomniacs, sleep less, and show excessive amounts of ill-defined REM sleep. They also show evidence of soft neurologic impairments such as hyperkinesis, dyslexia, or attention deficit disorders. Many show atypical EEG waves of unknown significance. The diagnosis is usually made retrospectively in adults.

Many of these insomniacs are exquisitely sensitive to noise and stimulants. A cup of tea or a chocolate drink hours before bedtime may seriously interfere with their sleep.

REPEATED REM SLEEP INTERRUPTIONS

This condition is diagnosed only if the patient presents with a sleep-maintenance insomnia having a characteristic pattern of awakenings starting in the first REM sleep period, about 90 minutes after sleep onset, and recurring in almost every subsequent REM sleep period.

ATYPICAL POLYSOMNOGRAPHIC FEATURES

This condition is diagnosed when there is a mixing of EEG waves from different sleep-awake stages or very many arousals. Clinically, patients displaying these features often do not feel restored after apparently adequate sleep. They may also complain of morning stiffness, aches, and increased sensitivity to pain. Most patients with fibrositis display an excessive intrusion of alpha EEG waves in their sleep. This condition seems to improve with chlorpromazine, which helps to decrease alpha intrusions and increase delta sleep.

NO DIMS ABNORMALITY

Some patients who complain of insomnia have no diagnosable sleep problem when evaluated at the sleep disturbance center. These may be "short sleepers" who need little sleep. They also may have "subjective" DIMS complaints without objective findings.

REFERENCES

Current Concepts, The Sleep Disorders. Peter Hauri, PhD, October, 1982.
Sleep, Vol 2, No 1, 1979. Raven Press, New York.

8 · ANXIETY AND DEPRESSION

Joseph C. Corkery
LAHEY CLINIC MEDICAL CENTER

Anxiety

DEFINITION AND DIAGNOSTIC CRITERIA*

Anxiety is the subjective feeling of fear, worry, or dread, often in association with an outpouring of sympathetic nervous system response. Four signs of a generalized anxiety disorder are enumerated in DSM-III: *motor tension*, such as shakiness, trembling, inability to relax, facial strain, and sighing; *autonomic hyperactivity*, including sweating, palpitations, tachycardia, lightheadedness, polyuria, or a sense of a lump in the throat; *apprehensive expectation* manifested by worry, rumination, or anticipation of misfortune; and *vigilance and scanning* evidenced by hyperattentiveness, insomnia, impatience, irritability, or feelings of being on edge. The specific criteria detailed in DSM-III require that symptoms from three of these four categories be present and that the anxious mood be of more than one month's duration and be unrelated to some other psychiatric disorder, such as depression or schizophrenia.

PANIC DISORDER

In addition to the previously described generalized anxiety disorder, DSM-III includes the distinct entity of panic disorder with its own clinical features and response to therapy. Panic disorder is manifested by spontaneous, sudden, intense attacks of overwhelming outpouring of sympathetic nervous system response associated with a feeling of impending doom.

The criteria for panic attacks as presented in DSM-III require that at least four of the following symptoms appear during each attack: dyspnea, palpitations, chest pain, choking, dizziness, feelings of unreality, paresthesias, feelings of hot or cold, sweating, faintness, trembling, and fear of dying or of becoming insane.

Episodes usually last approximately ten minutes. They are often so severe that patients go to the emergency room, where an unsatisfying diagnosis of hyperventilation syndrome is made. These attacks may be so terrorizing that phobias of objects, places, persons, or situations associated with such attacks may develop. Typical phobias include fear of crowds, shopping malls, heights, bridges, traffic, or closed-in places. These patients may become so polyphobic that they are comfortable only at home or with familiar persons. This ad-

---

*The diagnostic criteria for anxiety and depression are based on guidelines of the Diagnostic and Statistical Manual of Mental Disorders (DSM-III).

vanced condition is known as *agoraphobia* (fear of the marketplace).

Agoraphobia. The diagnosis according to DSM-III depends on a marked fear and avoidance of being alone or in a public place, and constriction of normal activities. In some patients a progression seems to take place from panic attacks to phobias to crippling agoraphobia. For other patients, this progression does not occur, but some element of a mild, generalized state of anxiety may be present between panic attacks.

CLINICAL RECOGNITION

Any clinician can immediately recognize the large area of overlap between the symptoms of anxiety and many medical illnesses. Because these varied physical symptoms often lead patients to believe that they have disease of the heart, lung, or brain, the internist is challenged with not only making a diagnosis but also convincing the patient of the presence of a psychiatric disorder in the face of distressing physical symptoms.

How then does the physician recognize the patient who is experiencing anxiety? This can be difficult, but a few guiding principles are useful. First, the physician should observe the feelings evoked in himself or herself by the patient. Anxiety is a contagious disease, and an anxious patient creates an anxious physician. An anxious person describing palpitations, chest tightness, and smothering sensations of choking evokes more unease in the physician than a patient describing angina pectoris or orthopnea. Second, the symptoms are never typical of any classic physical illness, and they leave the physician groping with such vague diagnoses as migraine equivalent, hypoglycemia, near-syncope, or costochondritis. This inability to explain the myriad of symptoms in terms of any single organic illness should alert the physician to the possibility of an anxiety disorder. The physician usually must then choose a balanced approach to these atypical complaints and must order tests and radiography to rule out important medical illnesses such as hyperthyroidism, mitral valve prolapse, pheochromocytoma, or seizure disorder. With attention to these guidelines, the diagnostic criteria in DSM-III, and follow-up office visits, the diagnosis of anxiety can be made.

MANAGEMENT

The benzodiazepines, antihistamines, β-blockers, barbiturates, tricyclic antidepressants, monoamine oxidase (MAO) inhibitors, and antipsychotic drugs have antianxiety activity. For generalized anxiety states the benzodiazepines are probably the most useful. The choice from several benzodiazepines often depends on the half-life of the drug and the status of the patient's liver function. Oxazepam (Serax) has a brief half-life of five to 15 hours and may be given to patients with liver impairment, whereas diazepam (Valium) has a half-life of 20 to 200 hours and will accumulate when disease of the liver is present. Alprazolam (Xanax) is a new benzodiazepine that has a brief to intermediate half-life and a tenfold greater potency than diazepam on a milligram for milligram basis. Like the other drugs in its class, alprazolam is effective in the treatment of generalized anxiety. Also, unlike all the other benzodiazepines, it is effective for panic disorder and agitated depression.

I usually choose alprazolam to treat anxiety states because it bridges both generalized anxiety disorder and panic disorder. In addition, it has a rapid onset of action and relatively mild side effects. The initial dose is 0.25 mg PO three times per day. If the patient's condition does not improve, the dose may be increased to 0.5 mg three times per day with subsequent increases up to 6 mg per day in three divided doses. Relief from anxiety and panic attacks is often dramatic. In addition, the phobias and even agoraphobia may gradually resolve as a patient regains control and loses fear of panic attacks. These benefits usually outweigh the side effects of sedation. Unfortunately, the potential for habituation associated with other benzodiazepines is also present. The substitution of diazepam or supplementation with a bedtime dose of a tricyclic antidepressant often facilitates tapering the dose.

Panic disorder also may be controlled with the MAO inhibitors, such as phenelzine sulfate (Nardil), or tricyclic antidepressants. If a patient with panic disorder does not respond to alprazolam, I either substitute a tricyclic antidepressant or refer the patient to a psychiatrist for therapy with an MAO inhibitor or to a behavioral psychologist for nonpharmacologic therapy such as relaxation training, biofeedback, or systematic desensitization.

Depression

DEFINITION AND DIAGNOSTIC CRITERIA

Depression is easily recognized in patients who complain of sadness, cry easily, and have suicidal thoughts. However, many depressed patients report physical complaints such as fatigue, weight loss, headache, or constipation, rather than complaints about mood. Therefore, the internist must be alert to these varied presentations and should directly question patients about mood.

Two major depressive disorders, unipolar and bipolar depression, must be considered. The unipolar disorder is a pure depression, whereas the bipolar illness has two components, depression and mania. The diagnostic criteria established in DSM-III for a major depressive episode include two main features, a dysphoric mood and neurovegetative symptoms. The dysphoric mood is manifested by gloominess, crying readily, sadness, hopelessness, and helplessness. The neurovegetative symptoms (four of eight must be present) include weight loss or gain, altered sleep pattern, psychomotor agitation or retardation, loss of pleasure in usually enjoyable activities, loss of energy, guilt or worthlessness, poor ability to concentrate, and recurrent thoughts of death and suicide. Patients with unipolar depression meet these criteria, and those with bipolar disorder have the additional features of mania.

The diagnostic criteria posed in DSM-III for a manic episode are an elevated expansive mood and three of the following: increase in activity, talkativeness, flight of ideas, inflated self-esteem, decreased need for sleep, distractibility, and involvement in risky ventures with the possibility of harmful consequences. The intensity of these manic episodes varies greatly. Some manic patients may be productive and successful because of extra energy during manic phases. Identification of mania may be difficult for the physician because many patients disguise it well and actually enjoy their high level of energy. The physician may have to contact a patient's friends or family to secure a diagnosis of mania. This extra effort is worthwhile because treatment of bipolar disorder differs from that of unipolar depression.

CLINICAL ASPECTS

Suicide may be a consequence of either type of depression, and the physician should directly question a patient about thoughts and plans to take his or her own life. Patients at high risk of committing suicide often have concrete detailed plans, whereas those at lower risk have suicidal thoughts but no specific plan. High-risk patients should be referred immediately to a psychiatrist for further evaluation.

The physician must be aware of the differential diagnosis of depression. Physically ill patients, much like depressed patients, may become lethargic, lose interest in activities, have multiple physical complaints, and appear sad. Therefore, the internist should thoroughly evaluate apparently depressed patients for evidence of occult malignant disease, hypothyroidism, dementia, or depressive side effects of antihypertensive drugs such as clonidine, methyldopa, propranolol, and reserpine, as well as of cimetidine (Tagamet) or steroids.

MANAGEMENT

The physician's first decision is to determine whether to refer a patient to a psychiatrist or to treat a patient himself. I refer patients with concrete plans for suicide, manic depressive illness, or major depression. However, such individuals constitute a minority of the depressed patients seen by internists. Fortunately, several valuable antidepressant medications are available to the internist for the treatment of depression.

Several tricyclic antidepressants are approximately equivalent in their ability to treat depression but differ somewhat in their side effects. Selection of a particular drug depends on the major side effects of sedation: postural hypotension, cardiac conduction disturbances, and such anticholinergic reactions as dry mouth, constipation, and retention of urine.

Doxepin (Sinequan), trazodone (Desyrel), and amitriptyline hydrochloride (Elavil) have greater sedative effects than other tricyclic antidepressants and may be particularly useful in depression with considerable insomnia or agitation, whereas imipramine (Tofranil), desipramine (Norpramin), and protriptyline (Vivactil) have fewer sedative effects and are useful in depression with motor retardation and hypersomnia. Postural hypotension, which occurs most often with imipramine, may be predicted by a postural drop in a patient's blood pressure before medication is administered. The potential for cardiac arrhythmia, which probably has been overstated, is associated with all these medications but seems to be less pronounced with doxepin and trazodone. The anticholinergic effects of dry mouth, urinary retention, constipation, and blurred vision are intolerable to many patients, particularly the elderly. Trazodone, which appears unique in that it is unassociated with any anticholinergic reactions, may be useful for such patients.

The nonpsychiatrist, who need not be familiar with all the details of the many tricyclic antidepressants currently available, should choose one or two drugs and use them appropriately. I use trazodone as my first-line antidepressant because of its high potency in sedation and its freedom from associated anticholinergic side effects. For other patients, I select desipramine because of its low potential for sedative effects and its moderately low anticholinergic effects. The starting dose (trazodone or desipramine) is 50 mg given at bedtime. This is increased by 50-mg increments every three days until a target dose of 200 mg is reached. A patient may note improvement in a sleep disorder almost immediately, whereas the antidepressant effects may not appear for one month. If no benefit is observed after one month, the dose should be increased gradually. The therapeutic range of dosage is 50 to 600 mg for trazodone and 50 to 300 mg for desipramine. If the medication is effective, it should be continued for six months and gradually tapered by 25 mg per week until it is discontinued. Patients who do not tolerate tapering should be evaluated by a psychiatrist.

An exciting new development in the treatment of depression is the availability of alprazolam, the only member of the benzodiazepine group with antidepressant effects. This drug seems to be most useful in depressed patients with agitation and features of anxiety and insomnia. Treatment plans were noted previously for alprazolam in management of panic disorder and anxiety, and the same dose and schedule (0.75 to 6 mg per day in divided doses) are applicable in depression as well. The antidepressant effects are seen within a matter of days, in contrast to the delayed benefits of tricyclic medications. An additional benefit of alprazolam is the absence of postural hypotension and the anticholinergic or cardiac side effects associated with tricyclic drugs. However, like the other benzodiazepines, alprazolam carries the associated risk of habituation and possible difficulty in withdrawal.

REFERENCES

American Psychiatric Association: Diagnostic and Statistical Manual of Mental Disorders (DSM-III). American Psychiatric Association, Washington, DC, 1980.

Judd LL: Current concepts in pharmacology. *In* Petersdorf RG, Adams RD, Braunwald E, et al (eds): Harrison's Principles of Internal Medicine, Update VI. McGraw-Hill Book Co, New York, 1985, pp 229–250.

Sheehan DV: Panic attacks and phobias. N Engl J Med 307:156–158, 1982.

9 · NAUSEA AND VOMITING

W. Perry Stokes
William A. Ferrante
OCHSNER CLINIC AND ALTON OCHSNER MEDICAL FOUNDATION

DEFINITION

Nausea is the sensation of impending emesis. Vomiting occurs when a complex set of contractions and relaxations result in retrograde movement of gastric contents into the esophagus. This process is under the control of a vomiting center located in the medulla oblongata. The vomiting center receives vagal afferent fibers from the gastrointestinal tract, from higher cortical centers, from the vestibular apparatus, and from the chemoreceptor trigger zone. Dopaminergic receptors are stimulated by emetic agents induced by metabolic disorders, pregnancy, drugs, or radiation therapy. Efferent fibers from the vomiting center innervate the diaphragm, the abdominal musculature, the stomach, and the esophagus.

DIFFERENTIAL DIAGNOSIS

Separation of nausea and vomiting into acute and chronic forms helps the physician make a specific diagnosis (Table 1). The contents and odor of the vomitus and its temporal relationship to meals are important historical features. A thorough physical examination complements the history and may lend support to specific diagnostic possibilities.

Relevant features of the history and physical dictate which diagnostic investigations need to be performed. Tables 2 and 3 outline evaluation for both acute and chronic cases.

In the absence of demonstrative lesions, abdominal exploration for symptoms of nausea and vomiting is usually unrewarding. However, the physician may occasionally find himself in a situation in which operation is necessary to rule out surgically correctable lesions. If none are found, full-thickness biopsy of the bowel should be performed to help rule out bowel neuropathy or myopathy.

Psychogenic disorders are one of the more common causes of chronic nausea and vomiting. These are di-

Table 1. CAUSES OF VOMITING

Acute	Hepatobiliary
Gastroenteritis	Pancreatic
Intra-abdominal inflammation or obstruction	Peritoneal
Drugs	Vascular
Systemic febrile illness	Pseudo-obstruction
Myocardial infarction	Parasitic infestation
Metabolic derangements	Metabolic and endocrine
	Acidosis
Chronic	Hypothyroidism and hyperthyroidism
Psychogenic	Uremia
Central nervous system	Hyponatremia
Intracranial hypertension	Hypercalcemia
Trauma	Hyperkalemia
Anoxia	Addison's disease
Hypertensive encephalopathy	Pregnancy
Hydrocephalus	Miscellaneous
Space-occupying lesion	Cardiopulmonary disease
Vestibular disorders	Sinusitis rhinitis
Glaucoma	Radiation sickness
Migraine headache	Chronic smoking
Gastrointestinal	General anesthesia
Obstructive	
Nonobstructive	

agnoses of exclusion, and psychiatric testing should be undertaken when the history or physical and laboratory tests are suggestive. It is important to remember that patients with psychiatric disorders also develop organic illnesses. Thus, any complaint of nausea and vomiting associated with psychiatric illness should be investigated.

MANAGEMENT

DRUG THERAPY

Treatment of nausea and vomiting should be directed at the cause, symptoms, and metabolic consequences. Every reasonable effort should be made to arrive at an accurate diagnosis, so that treatment can be

Table 2. EVALUATION OF THE PATIENT WITH ACUTE NAUSEA AND VOMITING

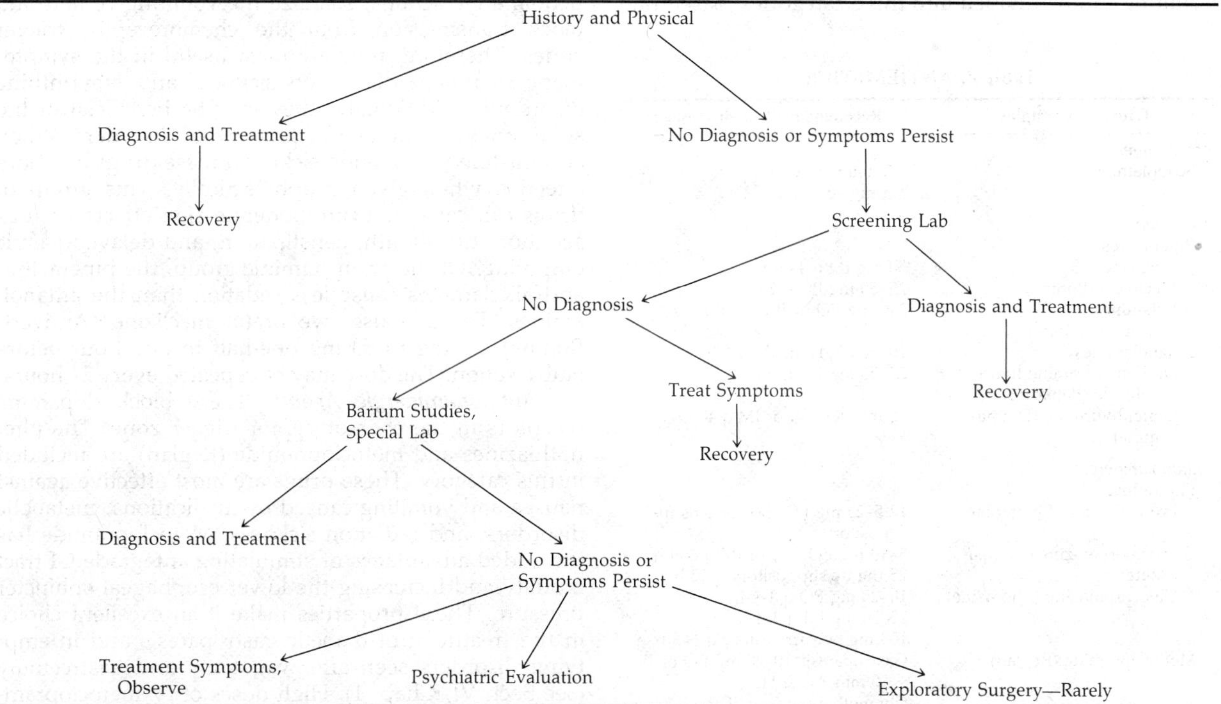

Table 3. EVALUATION OF THE PATIENT WITH CHRONIC NAUSEA AND VOMITING

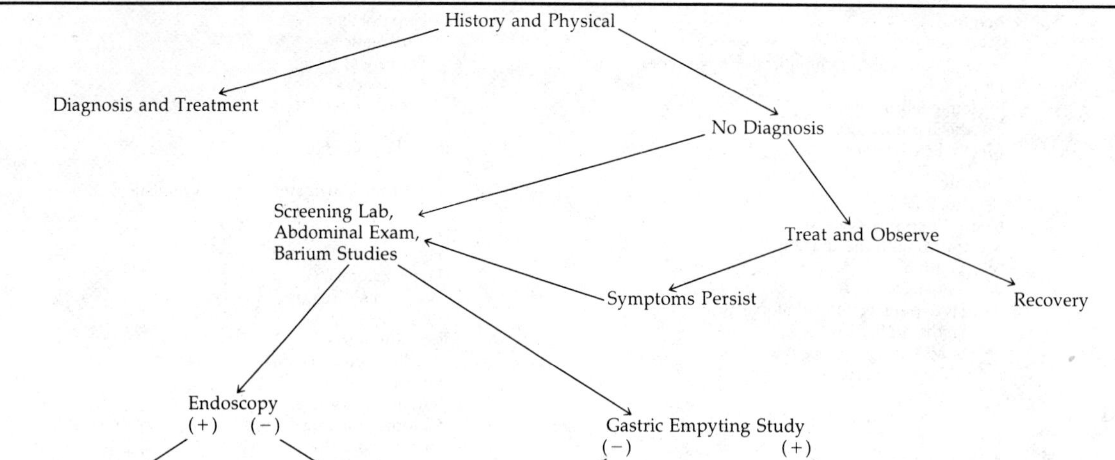

targeted. However, symptomatic treatment may be adjunctive in these patients or primary in patients in whom the diagnosis is not readily apparent.

Drugs used in symptomatic relief of nausea and vomiting can be divided into three categories, based on their mechanisms of action: (1) anticholinergics and antihistaminics, (2) antidopaminergics, and (3) a miscellaneous category (Table 4).

Anticholinergics and Antihistaminics. These have anticholinergic actions, stabilize the vomiting center, and block transmission from the chemoreceptor trigger zones. Therefore, they are most useful in the symptomatic treatment of motion sickness and labyrinthine disorders. Additionally, they may be beneficial in the symptomatic treatment of primary GI disorders. When administered for motion sickness, these drugs are more effective when given prophylactically. This group of drugs can cause mild to moderate side effects such as sedation, dry mouth, constipation, and delayed gastric emptying. Of the antihistaminic group, the piperazines and alkylamines cause less sedation than the ethanolamines. For oral use, we prefer meclizine (Antivert, Bonine), 25 mg to 50 mg one-half to one hour before embarkation. The dose may be repeated every 24 hours.

Antidopaminergic Agents. These block dopamine receptors in the chemoreceptor trigger zone. The phenothiazines and metoclopramide (Reglan) are included in this category. These drugs are most effective against nausea and vomiting caused by medications, metabolic disorders, and radiation sickness. Metoclopramide has the added advantages of stimulating antegrade GI tract motility and increasing the lower esophageal sphincter pressure. These properties make it an excellent choice in the treatment of diabetic gastroparesis and in emptying disorders seen after vagotomy and gastrectomy (see Sect. VI, Chap. 1). High doses of IV metoclopramide, given prophylactically, have been shown to be

Table 4. ANTIEMETICS

Category/Examples	Recommended Adult Dosage
Anticholinergics	
Scopolamine	0.3–0.6 mg PO q.d.
	1.5 mg adhesive q 3 d
Antihistamines	
•Piperazines	
Cyclizine (Marezine)	50 mg IM q 4–6 h
Meclizine (Bonine)	25–50 mg PO q 24 h
Alkylamines	2–4 mg PO or IM q 4–6 h
Chlorpheniramine	
Ethanolamines	10–50 mg IV or IM q 6 h
Diphenhydramine hydrochloride (Benadryl)	25–50 mg PO q 6 h
Dimenhydrinate (Dramamine)	50 mg PO, IV, or IM q 4–6 h
Antidopaminergics	
Phenothiazines	
Promethazine (Phenergan)	12.5–25 mg PO, IM, or by suppository
Prochlorperazine (Compazine)	5–10 mg PO, IV, or IM q 6–8 h
	25 mg by suppository q 12 h
Chlorpromazine (Thorazine)	10–25 mg PO q 4–6 h
	25–50 mg IM q 3–4 h
	100 mg by suppository q 6–8 h
Metoclopramide (Reglan)	Gastroparesis 10–20 mg PO or IV 30 min AC & HS
	Chemotherapy (see PDR)

effective in treating emesis secondary to some chemo-therapeutic agents. Restlessness, drowsiness, fatigue, and extrapyramidal reactions are side effects of these preparations. Although the phenothiazines are excellent short-term antiemetics, they should be used with caution when prescribed for long periods of time because of their tendency to cause extrapyramidal reactions, galactorrhea, cholestatic jaundice, and bone marrow suppression. Since these agents are antidopaminergic, they should not be given concomitantly, as side effects may be additive. Additionally, anticholinergics block the actions of metoclopramide, and use of these medications together should be avoided.

The miscellaneous category includes dexamethasone, methylprednisolone, and cannabinoids. The mechanism of action of these drugs is unknown. They are most effective for chemotherapy-induced emesis.

NONPHARMACOLOGIC MEASURES

In the more severe cases of nausea and vomiting, loss of potassium, hydrogen, and chloride in the vomitus leads to hypokalemic metabolic alkalosis. Nasogastric suction frequently compounds the electrolyte losses. Replacement should be instituted with IV normal saline and potassium chloride or potassium phosphate supplementation.

In the obtunded patient, the clinician should watch for aspiration pneumonia or its subsequent chemical pneumonitis. In this group of individuals, the prescribed regimen should include small-volume liquid meals, the reverse Trendelenburg position, and antiemetic medication.

COMPLICATIONS

Two complications of nausea and vomiting deserve special mention: bleeding from esophageal tears and esophageal perforation. Bleeding from Mallory-Weiss esophagogastric junction tears is characterized by bloody vomitus, usually occurring after vigorous retching, and endoscopy is necessary for diagnosis. Treatment consists of replacement of blood loss and observation. Bleeding is usually self-limiting, but if it persists or recurs, electrocautery with a heater probe, arterial embolization therapy, or surgery may be indicated. Balloon tamponade is contraindicated for this lesion. Esophageal perforation (Boerhaave's Syndrome) is a catastrophic event in which the patient experiences excruciating pain and shows signs and symptoms of sepsis. Treatment requires antibiotic administration and emergency surgery.

REFERENCES

Feldman M: Nausea and vomiting. *In* Sleisenger MH, Fordtran JS (eds): Gastrointestinal Disease: Pathophysiology, Diagnosis, and Management. W.B. Saunders Co, Philadelphia, 1983, pp 160–177.
Hanson JS, McCallum RW: The diagnosis and management of nausea and vomiting: a review. Am J Gastroenterol 80:210–218, 1985.
Malgelado JR, Camilleri M: Unexplained vomiting: a diagnostic challenge. Ann Intern Med 101:211–218, 1984.

10 · DIZZINESS AND VERTIGO

Peter Oliver
LAHEY CLINIC MEDICAL CENTER

Management of the patient with dizziness or vertigo depends primarily on a thorough multidisciplinary evaluation. Dizziness is a lay person's term for a constellation of symptoms ranging from the vague lightheadedness of hyperventilation, as evidenced in 23% of patients seen in one dizziness clinic, to the violent whirling or pulsion attacks of Meniere's disease. Vertigo is a medical term used narrowly by some physicians to describe exclusively a sense of rotation and applied broadly by others to include all the symptoms of vestibular dysfunction. This discussion is confined to vestibular dysfunction, which produces an illusory or distorted sensation of motion, such as rotation, rocking, tilting, and bouncing, and my use of *vertigo* includes all of these symptoms.

A peripheral vestibular disorder, the most common diagnosis, was found in 38% of patients at a dizziness clinic. Such disorders may be classified according to frequency as benign positional vertigo, acute vestibulopathy (e.g., post-traumatic, vestibular neuritis, or perilymphatic fistula), Meniere's disease, and chronic vestibulopathy (e.g., postlabyrinthectomy or the result of aminoglycoside ototoxicity). These conditions may overlap, but can be differentiated largely by descriptive and temporal criteria.

Benign Positional Vertigo

DEFINITION AND DIAGNOSTIC CRITERIA

Benign positional vertigo is characterized by brief (seconds to one minute) episodes of a sense of motion when a patient assumes a specific position or moves in a particular way. Episodes are recurrent but diminish in intensity and severity with repetition, i.e., fatigue. Nausea is uncommon and associated cochlear symptoms are rare. Benign positional vertigo is common in older persons on a degenerative basis and after an acute vestibulopathy. It is episodic in the former and is usually self-limited in the latter. The pathophysiologic mechanism is irritation of the cupula of the posterior semicircular canal by fragmentation or displacement of otoconia of the macula utriculi. Diagnosis is confirmed by a positive response to a Nylen-Bárány maneuver. With the patient seated on the edge of the examining table, he is moved quickly to a supine position with his head hanging 45° backward and rotated 45° to one side while he is observed for development of nystagmus and vertigo. The test is then repeated with the head turned the opposite way.

MANAGEMENT

Benign positional vertigo is treated with exercises to induce habituation. These consist of a patient's repetitive induction of vertigo several times a day until the vertigo fatigues; failure to do so is a sign of disease of the central nervous system. Over a period of one to four weeks, positional dizziness usually disappears. If vertigo recurs, the exercises should be repeated. Singular neurectomy (denervation of the posterior semicircular canal) is necessary in rare instances.

DRUG THERAPY

Drug therapy is seldom necessary for benign positional vertigo; it suppresses the reaction that is necessary for habituation to occur.

Acute Vestibulopathy

DEFINITION AND DIAGNOSTIC CRITERIA

Acute vestibulopathies produce severe vertigo that lasts from hours to days with gradual recovery. Nausea and vomiting are common, and auditory symptoms are variable. Vestibular neuritis may accompany or be the only manifestation of viral illness. Vertigo associated with acute or chronic otitis media is rare. It should be treated vigorously and the patient should be observed closely for signs of intracranial infection. Injury to the head sometimes produces vestibular symptoms by shaking (commotio labyrinthus) or a fracture through the labyrinth; by stretching the eighth nerve as the brain torques within the skull; or by creating a perilymphatic fistula (leakage from the oval or round window). The latter may also result from barotrauma caused by aerotitis or scuba diving. Findings on electronystagmography of semicircular canal paresis and positive results of positional and fistula test, respectively, support the previous diagnoses.

MANAGEMENT

Immediate treatment of acute vertigo addresses the anxiety of and provides reassurance for the patient who wonders, "Am I having a stroke or seizure?" Positional exacerbations respond to bed rest, usually with the affected ear down, and limitation of head motion. The vomiting patient is rehydrated with intravenously administered fluids, which usually are necessary only in acute vestibulopathies. Prolonged hospitalization for several days may be necessary to treat vertigo due to suppurative otitis media with parenteral administration of antibiotics. Operation for acute otitis media that does

not respond to antibiotic therapy ranges from myringotomy to mastoidectomy. Chronic suppurative otitis media (often present with cholesteatoma) that produces vertigo requires mastoidectomy unless the patient is a poor operative risk.

DRUG THERAPY

Regardless of its etiologic basis, an acute and prolonged attack of vertigo is best treated by parenterally administered diazepam (Valium), 5 to 10 mg every three to four hours, or droperidol (Inapsine, Innovar), 2.5 to 5 mg every six to eight hours. Potentiation of the analgesic and respiratory depressant effects of narcotics occurs particularly with the latter. For use at home, promethazine hydrochloride (12.5, 25, or 50 mg every four to six hours) or prochlorperazine (2.5, 5, or 25 mg every eight to 12 hours) suppositories help to control vomiting. I have found diazepam, 2 to 5 mg every four to six hours, to be the most effective orally administered vestibular suppressant. For patients who are young, elderly, or depressed, however, I prefer meclizine hydrochloride, 12.5 to 25 mg every four to six hours.

Meniere's Disease

DEFINITION AND DIAGNOSTIC CRITERIA

Meniere's disease is characterized by episodic attacks of vertigo with nausea and vomiting, fluctuations in hearing, and roaring tinnitus in one ear. Episodes occur one to two times a week, month, or year and last from one-half hour to several hours. The cochlear symptoms are more likely than the vestibular symptoms to precede the complete triad. The pathophysiologic condition is defective absorption of endolymph, which results in dilation (hydrops) and periodic rupture of the membranous labyrinth. The diagnosis of Meniere's disease is best supported by the patient's pathognomonic history and by a perceptive hearing loss at low tones; results of vestibular tests are extremely variable.

MANAGEMENT

Treatment of Meniere's disease is controversial and varies with frequency and severity of vertigo attacks, response to medication, unilateral or bilateral (20% to 30%) occurrence of disease, and age and general health of the patient. Because attacks are brief (hours), hospitalization is rare.

Medical therapy for Meniere's disease is as controversial as the surgical. I routinely prescribe a diet without added salt, i.e., approximately 4 gm of salt per day, and Dyazide—a combination of triamterene, 50 mg, and hydrochlorothiazide, 25 mg—each morning. If such symptoms as vertigo, hearing loss, or both are not controlled, I supplement or replace the diuretic with furosemide (Lasix), 20 to 80 mg per day. Supplemental potassium is usually necessary only with the latter. Vertigo is controlled within three to six months in 70% to 80% of patients. The effect on hearing is less predictable. If vertigo is uncontrollable or if hearing loss is the patient's major complaint, drainage of the endolymphatic sac is my next step. Vestibular nerve section or labyrinthectomy are last resorts.

Patients with Meniere's disease require a thorough explanation of the chronicity of their problem. Reduction of stress, often including a change in job or life style, can be more beneficial than all the previously mentioned medical and surgical measures. Follow-up visits after initial evaluation take place at three months, six months, and annually. Audiologic evaluation and determination of serum potassium levels are obtained at these times. Compliance of patients is usually excellent.

SURGICAL THERAPY

Operation, which is reserved for disease that is intractable to medical treatment, includes procedures that preserve hearing: drainage of the endolymphatic system or vestibular nerve section and, when hearing loss has become severe, destructive labyrinthectomy. Endolymphatic drainage is less effective in long-term relief of vertigo (60% to 70%) but is associated with minimal rates of morbidity. Vestibular nerve section is associated with a small but noteworthy risk of operative morbidity and even mortality, as is any intracranial procedure.

Like destructive labyrinthectomy, vestibular nerve section is associated with a prolonged postoperative ataxia that lasts from one month to permanently, especially in older patients.

The vast majority of patients under age 60 years who undergo labyrinthectomy or vestibular nerve section achieve satisfactory balance within one to three months. Occasional ataxia in the dark or on uneven ground is not uncommon. Elderly patients with intractable Meniere's disease must be warned before such an operation that they may have to trade violent attacks of vertigo for continuous imbalance that requires use of a cane when outside the home.

Chronic Vestibulopathy

Chronic vestibulopathies most commonly produce ataxia rather than vertigo. Oscillopsia (unusual bouncing of the environment when walking) and difficulty in reading are typical symptoms. Bilateral vestibular paresis may be found on caloric testing after ototoxic drug therapy; loss of hearing may be variable or absent. A patient who has had a labyrinthectomy has, of course, unilateral paresis and complete loss of hearing.

Vertigo is rarely seen as an isolated phenomenon in neurologic disease but may be the presenting symptom in ischemia of the brain stem or multiple sclerosis. An acoustic neuroma rarely causes vertigo or dizziness except when it is large; ataxia is more common.

OTOTOXICITY

The most lamentable situation occurs when a patient undergoes bilateral vestibular ablation as a result of the administration of ototoxic drugs. This occurs most commonly in bedridden patients who receive aminoglycoside antibiotics for life-threatening infections. Prevention is the only satisfactory treatment for this therapeutic disaster, and daily inquiries as to whether a patient has noted any disequilibrium on motion are essential. A history of previous treatment with an aminoglycoside (and exposure to noise that may lead to further hearing loss) warn the physician that brief courses of aminoglycoside therapy may have an additive effect on a previously affected vestibular or auditory system. Renal disease and the concomitant administration of diuretics, especially furosemide and ethacrynic acid (Edecrin), increase the risk of aminoglycoside ototoxicity. Frequent monitoring of renal function, serum levels of antibiotics, and vestibular and auditory function are mandatory. If vestibular ablation occurs, little can be done to rehabilitate the patient except instruction in the use of a walker, advice to move always in an adequate light, and encouragement to be as active as the disability permits. Administration of a vestibular suppressant is obviously counterproductive.

REFERENCES

Drachman DA, Hart CW: An approach to the dizzy patient. Neurology 22:323–334, 1972.

Jackson CG, Glasscock ME 3rd, Davis WE, et al: Medical management of Meniere's disease. Ann Otol Rhinol Laryngol 90:142–147, 1981.

Norre ME, De Weerdt W: Treatment of vertigo based on habituation: 1. Physiopathological basis. 2. Technique and results of habituation training. J Laryngol Otol 94:689–696, 971–977, 1980.

Oliver P: Evaluation of the patient with dizziness. Lahey Clin Found Bull 26:172–174, 1977.

Snow JB, Kimmelman CP: Assessment of surgical procedures for Meniere's disease. Laryngoscope 89:737–747, 1979.

11 · FATIGUE

Anthony P. Moore
SCRIPPS CLINIC AND RESEARCH FOUNDATION

DEFINITION AND DIAGNOSTIC CRITERIA

Fatigue is one of the most common of patient complaints to primary care physicians. In the laboratory, fatigue consists of the inability of muscle to respond to repetitive, specific stimuli. Fatigue in the clinical setting is far more difficult to quantitate. This is the tired patient, the one with lack of energy, pep, or stamina. Synonyms include weariness, listlessness, lassitude, exhaustion, and ennui. Fatigue is a symptom and, as such, is totally subjective. Although the patient may "look tired," fatigue is not a physical sign and certainly not a diagnosis. It is important to understand exactly what patients mean by fatigue, and to distinguish it from weakness, lack of muscular strength, sleepiness, and dyspnea. Its nature often remains vague and ill defined.

PATHOPHYSIOLOGY

Fatigue is the "final common pathway" of a number of physiologic states and emotional or physical disorders. No *one* mechanism accounts for all the features of fatigue. After vigorous physical exertion, we all experience fatigue eventually. We recall from physiology that with repetitive physical activity, ATP molecules are depleted and the muscle fatigues. If exertion proceeds further without oxygen (anaerobic glycolysis), there is build-up of lactic acid. The muscles are tired and sore; we have to stop to "catch our breath." With rest there is repletion of oxygen, glucose, nutrients, and ATP. The muscle is ready to contract again.

Pathologic states include the anemias in which there is decreased oxygen-carrying capacity of the blood. In heart failure or chronic lung disease, there is inadequate perfusion of the skeletal muscle and vital organs with blood and oxygen. Metabolic disorders may disturb the delicate balance between sodium, potassium, and calcium required for normal muscle contraction. In diabetes, insulin deficiency or resistance leaves the muscles and tissues starved of glucose. In neurologic diseases, fatigue may relate to a "lesion" preventing conduction between the central nervous system, the peripheral nerve, and the muscle. Other disorders such as hypothyroidism, alcoholism, and carcinomatosis may lead to a myopathy with muscle tissue wasting. In major depression, there are changes in the biogenic amines and neurotransmitters in the brain. In other cases the precise pathophysiology remains obscure: e.g., the inexplicable fatigue that can occur early in patients with malignancy. Another current controversy is the exact mechanism and extent of fatigue from deficiencies of iron, trace minerals, and vitamins. In any individual, there may be multiple reasons for fatigue.

CLINICAL ASPECTS

As a diagnostic predictor, the symptom of fatigue is high in sensitivity but low in specificity. In other words, it can be an *early* sign of almost *any* disorder. The evaluation of fatigue presents a real challenge for the primary care physician.

The three general categories of fatigue relate to physiologic, physical, and psychogenic disorders. The classification is useful for diagnostic purposes, but the functions of the mind and body are inseparable. The patient's perception of the symptoms of fatigue, or of any illness, depends on a complex interaction of psychosocial, biologic, and environmental factors.

PHYSIOLOGIC FATIGUE

Fatigue is the biologic signal in the healthy body that rest is needed. All of us have experienced physiologic fatigue from overexertion, boredom, or lack of sleep. The physically deconditioned (i.e., "out of shape") or overweight may lack energy. Women at certain times during their menstrual cycle or pregnancy may feel drained of energy. These conditions are "normal," not pathologic. People rarely bring these complaints to their doctors.

ORGANIC FATIGUE/PHYSICAL DISORDER

In organic or physical disorders, the fatigue is more likely to be acute or progressive. The patient will be specific about complaints and limitations. Physical activity or exercise exacerbates organic fatigue. It is worse in the afternoon or evening. In diagnosing the underlying physical disorder, the review of systems is a key factor. Other accompanying symptoms may often be clues: fever or weight loss increase the chances of an organic disorder; fatigue and weight loss may implicate diabetes, apathetic hyperthyroidism, malabsorption, or malignancy; and weight gain may signal hypothyroidism.

There are scant data showing the relative frequencies of various physical disorders in patients presenting with generalized fatigue. Reviews in family practice journals reveal the most frequent physical cause to be a "viral syndrome." Patients may have lingering fatigue long after a "cold" or "flu." Recent data show that a "viral syndrome," the Epstein-Barr virus, may cause chronic, recurrent, fatiguing illness. Hematologic illnesses, particularly anemia, often present with fatigue. Up to 5% of all women have iron deficiency anemia.

Fatigue caused by endocrine or metabolic disorders is relatively frequent and eminently treatable. Previously undiagnosed diabetes mellitus may present as a "flu" with dehydration and polyuria. The diagnosis of hypoglycemia is currently in vogue, and its incidence therefore overestimated. Don't overinterpret the glucose tolerance test. Up to 50% of all normal women drop their glucose to a level of 50 mg/dl sometime during the test, and achieve blood glucose values in this range on a prolonged fast.

Hypothyroidism is a relatively common cause of chronic fatigue. The fatigue may long antedate the other classic symptoms of weight gain, constipation, cold intolerance, and so forth. Incipient hypothyroidism presents with an elevated TSH before the T_4 begins to fall. One study shows that L-thyroxine may be useful even for patients with subclinical hypothyroidism. Addison's disease, on the other hand, is rare: early in this century its cause almost always was tuberculosis, but now an autoimmune etiology is more common. There is an association with other autoimmune disorders, e.g., Hashimoto's thyroiditis, pernicious anemia, and vitiligo. In a busy internal medicine practice you may detect a new case every few years if you are alert and lucky. The odds are that the diagnosis will have been missed by several other physicians. Consider Addison's disease when the patient is relatively hypotensive with pigmented scars or creases or vitiligo, and (as Thomas Addison pointed out) "general languor and debility"; and in a patient with hypothyroidism who is on adequate thyroid hormone but continues to complain of fatigue.

Cardiopulmonary disorders presenting with fatigue usually have associated dyspnea or chest discomfort. However, patients who have congestive heart failure with "low-output" cardiomyopathies may simply complain of fatigue. Some reports indicate that patients with mitral valve prolapse have an increased incidence of fatigue due to autonomic nervous system dysfunction. Most neurologic diseases have focal deficits, depending on the site of the "lesions." Because of the characteristic "lesions scattered in time and space," symptomatic fatigue can be a prominent feature of multiple sclerosis. This fatigue is often induced by warm temperatures, in addition to physical exertion. Easy fatigability that responds promptly to rest, particularly if associated with ptosis, diplopia, or facial weakness, should raise the possibility of myasthenia gravis. Fatigue can be the initial symptom of connective tissue disorders, especially rheumatoid arthritis and systemic lupus erythematosus. The severity of the fatigue generally parallels the activity of these diseases. However, other criteria should be met before these diagnoses are seriously considered. A positive low-titer ANA can be overinterpreted to the detriment of the patient. It becomes, in fact, a lab abnormality in search of a disease.

Almost any drug can potentially cause fatigue. Look for the temporal relationship of symptoms to the initiation of drug therapy. Common offenders are antihypertensive drugs, e.g., reserpine, beta-blockers, and diuretics (hypokalemias). Sedative hypnotics and tranquilizers are obvious suspects. With daily use they may accumulate in the blood. Antidepressants, especially at the initiation of therapy, may create an overly tired sedated patient. Birth control pills and corticosteroids can cause depression and fatigue. Alcohol exerts a potentially toxic effect on all organ systems. Alcohol-induced fatigue may be the result of malnutrition, hypoglycemia, neuropathy, myopathy, or liver, kidney, or heart damage. Caffeine may give patients a boost, but when the effect wears off they feel drained. Amphetamines and "diet pills," particularly when taken on a chronic basis, have a similar effect.

Fatigue may also be associated with true sleepiness. Patients may be sleep deprived from insomnia related to anxiety or caffeine excess. Early morning awakening (e.g., 2 AM) is typical of depression and alcohol excess. Consider obstructive sleep apnea when snoring is followed by arousals from sleep. The patient may be overweight, with thick neck and redundant pharyngeal tissue, high blood pressure, and polycythemia. In this case both the patient and his or her mate will be tired and sleepy. The patient with narcolepsy has an uncontrollable urge to doze off during the day when not stimulated. He may have learned chemical (amphetamine, caffeine) and physical means of keeping himself awake. The public is way ahead of us in its concern about sleep problems and snoring, as evidenced by the more than 300 antisnoring devices registered with the U.S. Patent Office. Sleep disorder medicine is emerging as a new specialty currently with 30 such centers around the country.

Any form of malnutrition, from malabsorption to malignancy, can cause fatigue. Any trauma, whether it follows surgery, concussion, or myocardial infarction, can cause fatigue.

Any infection may cause fatigue. We have noted the common diagnosis of "viral" etiology. In the young adult, consider hepatitis or mononucleosis if there are prolonged or severe symptoms. In bacterial infection, there generally is fever. Tuberculosis is a classic cause of fatigue but is now on the wane; however, consider it especially in a patient from Mexico or Southeast Asia.

PSYCHOGENIC FATIGUE

Fatigue in the clinical setting is usually psychogenic. A 1944 study from Lahey Clinic analyzed 300 consecutive patients who presented with fatigue. After a complete work-up, 80% were found to be suffering from psychogenic or "nervous" disorders, and only 20% had "organic" or physical disorders. Since 1944 we have developed sophisticated CT scanners and immunologic and serologic tests, but studies continue to show that in 50% to 80% of patients there is a predominantly psychogenic cause of fatigue. In psychogenic fatigue the history is vague, inconsistent, or even bizarre. Symptoms are usually chronic, and previous medical evaluations may be negative. Such patients may make *the physician* feel anxious, depressed, frustrated, or helpless.

Depression, in some form, is the most common form of fatigue. This diagnosis is not simply one of exclusion. The depressed patient's chief complaint is usually "I'm tired," rather than "I'm depressed." With a major depression there may be other "vegetative" symptoms: loss of appetite, loss of libido, and sleep disturbance. Patients may wake up in the morning "too tired to get out of bed." They may say that they lack motivation, "can't concentrate," or have a "poor memory." They lack interest in daily activities. To their families they may seem preoccupied and withdrawn from personal relationships. The depression may be "masked," with patients showing little insight into their emotional problems, and instead attributing their symptoms to physical illness.

Other forms of depression presenting as fatigue may be related to life stresses. As a chronic relapsing problem fatigue may be associated with personality disorders, including dependent, histrionic or manipulative behavior. Fatigue may provide a patient with secondary gain, e.g., it may be part of a disability syndrome. Fatigue may be one of multiple physical symptoms in a somatization disorder.

Other psychosocial factors may be the root of the symptoms. Persistent anxiety will leave the patient enervated and sleepless. There is often stress at home or at work: perhaps the transient stress related to moving or divorce, or something as irrevocable as dealing with death or taxes. On closer questioning the patient may reveal dissatisfaction, agitation, or tearfulness.

After history-taking and physical examination, the cause is usually obvious. However, a reasonable data base for most patients with significant chronic fatigue may include CBC, sedimentation rate, chemistry panel including electrolytes, fasting blood glucose, liver function tests, BUN, creatinine, calcium, T_4, TSH, urinalysis, and chest x-ray. Depending on the clinical picture, other tests may include a monospot, B_{12}, serum iron levels, ACTH stimulation test, PPD, urine, blood, and stool cultures, plus exam for ova and parasites, ANA, RF, CPK, EKG, treadmill, cardiac echo, arterial blood gas, gastrointestinal series, EMG, and various CT scans. Judgment is required to arrive at a diagnosis while containing costs and avoiding potentially hazardous tests. An MMPI can provide invaluable objective documentation of suspected depression, somatization, and hysteria.

MANAGEMENT

A holistic approach demands that a treatment program be aimed not only toward the symptoms or a disease, but toward the patient as a whole. The chief concern in most of these patients is the possibility of organic illness. Specific therapy, depending on the underlying physical disorder, should be instituted. General measures can also be helpful. The patient who is not feeling well is optimally receptive to advice about life style modifications. Adverse health habits, including smoking, drug and alcohol excess, poor sleep habits, sedentary life style, improper diet, and obesity, all aggravate fatigue. Make the patient an active participant in the healing process. Implicit in the therapeutic relationship are rapport with and trust and confidence in the physician. Support and empathy facilitate recovery.

EXERCISE

Patients in the grip of an organic illness require more rest. However, at some point the inactivity becomes counterproductive. Paradoxically, patients with chronic fatigue and a sedentary life style benefit from exercise. They may be looking for "permission" or encouragement from their physician. An exercise prescription must be individualized, but most patients benefit from a structured aerobic exercise program, beginning with a 30-minute brisk daily walk for those who are ambulatory.

Patients who are overweight and fatigued may need some additional incentive. Most know that obesity is a risk factor for multiple diseases and they look better when they are thinner. They should also realize they will be *feeling better* with weight loss when they don't have to tote around the excess baggage all day.

DRUG-INDUCED FATIGUE

Drug regimens causing fatigue should be modified to minimize this side effect. For example, an antihistamine prescription can be changed to a bedtime dose only. Unnecessary drugs can be tapered and stopped. Consider always whether the disease being treated justifies the untoward drug side effects.

STIMULANTS

Despite increasing public awareness, many patients still don't understand that caffeine and diet pills, when used in the long term, can overstimulate and thereby tire them out. Likewise, most patients do not make the connection between alcohol, sleep disorder, and fatigue. Patient education may suffice; if not, referral to an alcohol and chemical dependency program is indicated.

REASSURANCE

For patients with a benign disease, reassurance is a major part of therapy. Whether they are the "worried well" or overtly hypochondriacal, they will benefit. Although you may quickly suspect that the fatigue is functional, finish the history-taking and physical exam before you attempt reassurance. Premature attempts leave the patient feeling "dismissed" or not taken seriously. They need to know that you fully understand their symptoms. You need to know their underlying concern (or "self-diagnosis"), be it anemia, hypoglycemia, thyroid or vitamin deficiency, or cancer. Be open to their "hidden agenda." When the symptoms are explained, patients are receptive to reassurance.

DEPRESSION

Concomitant assessment of psychologic status often reveals "functional overlay" if not overt depression. Anxiety and depression may be an appropriate reaction to organic illness. Certain physical disorders (e.g., hypothyroidism, multiple sclerosis, systemic lupus erythematosus, and pancreatic cancer) have an increased incidence of depression. Conversely, some studies reveal that patients with psychiatric illness have an increased incidence of physical disorders. From a holistic standpoint, a healthy mind helps to maintain a healthy body.

Patients with major depression respond to pharmacotherapy in 60% to 70% of cases when tricyclic antidepressants are used. The choice of specific drug is partly empirical. However, amitriptyline hydrochloride (Elavil) is useful for patients with depression and insomnia. Dosage should begin with 25 mg PO q.h.s. and slowly advance by increments to 150 mg daily. Occasionally, some patients may require as much as 300 mg daily. Early in therapy, patients may complain of side effects such as dry mouth and sedation. It may take one month for depression to lift and fatigue to improve. A newer drug, trazodone hydrochloride (Desyrel), a triazolopyridine, may be better tolerated. Relative contraindications include benign prostatic hypertrophy, glaucoma, and cardiac arrhythmia. Ask about suicidal ideation in patients with major depression.

Patients whose fatigue is related to psychophysiologic, somatization, or personality disorders may prove more difficult to handle. As a rule they are reluctant to accept a psychologic interpretation for their symptoms; the symptoms may provide a means of getting attention. When one symptom is removed, it is replaced by another. Drug therapy should be limited, since these patients increasingly complain of side effects. Likewise, invasive tests and procedures should be kept to a minimum. These patients may be manipulative and disability prone, and it is important to set limits. They have difficulty with compliance because they don't always have motivation to lose their symptoms. A regular appointment is helpful for "somatizers" so that they don't need to come up with new symptoms to justify an appointment. The above measures will help to manage the patient who is seen as a "crock" and to limit "doctor shopping."

ANXIETY

Many patients with mild anxiety respond to reassurance and the general measures noted above. For those with more serious anxiety, specific treatment is indicated. Counseling and support for the underlying stress is helpful. Those with "pacing" problems need to set limits on work and responsibility. Severe anxiety interferes with functional states and with sleep, and leads to more anxiety. In the short term during a situational stress or adjustment reaction, benzodiazapines may be helpful if used judiciously. Alprazolam (Xanax), one to two 0.25-mg tablets two to three times a day, may help to break that vicious cycle by reducing the anxiety without causing too much sedation. Judicious use of triazolam (Halcion) as a short-acting sedative hypnotic, 0.25 mg at night, may be helpful. Patients with persistent anxiety need behavioral modification or psychotherapy.

REFERENCES

Allan FN: Differential diagnosis of weakness and fatigue. N Engl J Med 231:414–418, 1944.
Cooper DS, Halpern R, Wood LC, et al: L-Thyroxine therapy in subclinical hypothyroidism. Ann Intern Med 101:18–24, 1984.

Crosby WH: Current concepts in nutrition: who needs iron? N Engl J Med 297:543–545, 1977.

Hollister LE: Drug therapy: tricyclic antidepressants (two parts). N Engl J Med 299:1106–1172, 1978.

Solberg LT: Lassitude, a primary care evaluation. JAMA 251:3275–3276, 1984.

Straus SE, Giovanna T, Armstrong G, et al: Persistent fatigue and illness in adults with evidence of Epstein-Barr virus infection. Ann Intern Med 102:7–16, 1985.

12 · HEADACHE

Robert S. Kunkel
CLEVELAND CLINIC FOUNDATION

The overwhelming majority of headache complaints are not due to any serious organic or structural disease and are classified as either vascular, muscle contraction, or mixed headache pattern. Muscle contraction headache is the most common type afflicting man. Migraine, which occurs in 12% to 15% of the U.S. population, undoubtedly accounts for the most disability in the common headache syndromes. Cluster headache, like migraine, is also vascular, occurs mostly in men, and can be very disabling, although the attacks are usually short and there are periods of remission. Mixed headache syndromes are commonly seen in headache clinics and are often associated with drug dependency.

It is of course most important to recognize headaches that may be due to disease. Headaches of recent onset, those associated with neurologic or visual symptoms, or a change in the headache pattern in a person who has had chronic headaches all warrant diagnostic evaluation. Inflammatory conditions and infections of the eyes, ears, nose, and throat may cause headache. Mass lesions or bleeding within the cranium may also cause headache but are usually associated with neurologic signs and symptoms. Temporal arteritis is an inflammatory condition of the cranial vessels and should be considered in anyone over 55 who begins to have headache for the first time. A sedimentation rate is very suggestive of this condition, and the diagnosis is confirmed by a temporal artery biopsy. Treatment is with corticosteroids in an initial dosage of 60 mg a day. This may be gradually tapered but will probably have to be used for many months. The activity of the disease should be followed by periodic measurements of sedimentation rate.

Muscle Contraction (Tension) Headache

Muscle contraction (tension) headache is the most common one. Acute episodic muscle contraction headache usually does not bring the patient to the doctor and is readily treated by over-the-counter analgesics and sleep. Chronic muscle contraction headache or frequent episodic muscle contraction headache, on the other hand, is very commonly seen in the doctor's office and needs treatment, since this type of patient seems particularly prone to dependency on analgesics or tranquilizers.

PATHOPHYSIOLOGY

In most patients with muscle contraction headache, there is a sustained chronic contraction of scalp and neck muscles, which may cause diminished blood flow through the muscular arterioles, leading to ischemia and metabolic acidosis in the muscles. This acidosis can cause further muscle contraction and pain. Although anxiety and depression are the most common causes of this headache, any inflammatory or infectious condition of the head and neck organs may cause muscle spasm. Cervical spine disorders and postural abnormalities can also cause muscle spasm and subsequent muscle contraction headache.

CLINICAL ASPECTS

The pain is usually described as a dull, tight, aching pressure sensation and is rarely localized. It is usually global, over the entire head, and the neck often feels stiff and tight. Decreased range of motion of the neck frequently can be demonstrated. There may be rounding of the shoulders with poor posture. On examination, it is often possible to find tender areas of the scalp. The neck muscles may be very tender and in a state of spasm. Diseases of the head and neck causing secondary spasm should be excluded by examination and diagnostic x-rays. Sleep disturbances are common and the patient often is unaware of any specific emotional factors.

MANAGEMENT

Treatment begins with explaining the cause of the discomfort to the patient. Tense, tight muscles do cause pain, and the pain is not imaginary. The physician should help the patient to identify any stresses or emotional factors that may play a role. Necessary diagnostic studies should be made to exclude any underlying condition.

NONPHARMACOLOGIC MEASURES

Nonpharmacologic measures include relaxation techniques, physical therapy, and biofeedback. The last-named may be helpful in teaching relaxation techniques, but many people can learn these without more formal biofeedback training. I have found physical therapy and exercises quite helpful in people with poor posture and a lot of tightness in the neck muscles. Patients must be instructed and encouraged to follow a home exercise program. Without it, little progress can be made with only one or two weekly visits to the therapist.

DRUG THERAPY

If drugs are deemed necessary to reduce the discomfort, the choice must be made between daily prophylactic medication or medication only at the time of the discomfort. Chronic muscle contraction headache, which is usually present most of the time, should be treated with a daily prophylactic medical program. The drug of choice is one of the tricyclics, such as amitriptyline or doxepin, 25 to 100 mg once a day in the evening. Antidepressants are preferred to anxiolytics because they are more effective and less likely to produce dependency. Antidepressant side effects such as constipation, dryness of the mouth, and weight gain are occasionally intolerable to the patient.

Nonsteroidal anti-inflammatory agents may be useful in chronic muscle contraction headache and are usually quite safe. They may be used prophylactically or as analgesics. For prophylactic use, I prefer naproxen, 200 to 375 mg twice daily; fenoprofen calcium, 300 to 600 mg three times daily; or indomethacin, 25 to 50 mg q.i.d. Common side effects include gastrointestinal disturbances and edema. For the relief of pain, if simple aspirin or acetaminophen are not beneficial, choose one of the milder muscle relaxants or short-acting, nonsteroidal, anti-inflammatory drugs. Norgesic, Equagesic, Soma Compound, or Parafon Forte may be helpful. Meclofenamate sodium, 50 to 100 mg every six hours or ibuprofen, 400 to 600 mg every six hours are short-acting anti-inflammatory drugs that are often helpful as analgesic agents.

Since this group of patients is very likely to become dependent on tranquilizers, barbiturates, and analgesics, do not prescribe such agents on a regular daily basis. Combination drugs such as Fiorinal, Esgic, Axotal, and Phrenilin all contain barbiturates along with analgesics and/or caffeine. These work very well to relieve head pain but should be used only sporadically. Daily use of analgesics can actually perpetuate the chronic discomfort, probably by altering output of endorphins from the central nervous system.

As with any chronic condition, follow-up examination is important and the medication should be changed if necessary. Referral for counseling or psychotherapy may be necessary.

Migraine Headache

Migraine headache probably accounts for the most disability and time lost from work. It is a vascular headache in that the pain arises from the vessels and the structures supporting the vessels. Classic migraine headache is preceded by a specific 20- to 30-minute warning, usually of a visual nature. Common migraine accounts for some 80% to 85% of all migraine headaches and there are no specific warning symptoms.

PATHOPHYSIOLOGY

The pathophysiology of migraine is not well understood. Several biochemical and hormonal abnormalities have been demonstrated, but these are not universally present. Platelet agglutination often occurs at onset. Most recent researchers consider the initiating event of each attack to be neurogenic in nature and to arise from a midbrain dysfunction. Undoubtedly, there is a very complex series of triggering events.

CLINICAL ASPECTS

Migraine is a familial disorder of altered sensitivity of vessels, three times more common in women than in men. It usually begins in the late teens or early 20s and often eases after menopause. Many women note their worst headaches occur around the time of the menstrual period.

Typically, migraine is a pounding, pulsatile pain on one side of the head, although it may be a generalized headache. Accompanying this throbbing headache is usually nausea and vomiting; anorexia; sensitivity to light, noise, and odors; chills and sweats; and problems with cognition. The attack lasts 12 to 48 hours and sleep is often beneficial.

MANAGEMENT

NONPHARMACOLOGIC MEASURES

The short-term goal of treating migraine is to bring relief to the patient. The long-term goal should be control of the number of attacks and prompt relief for those that do occur. If there are more than three attacks a month, daily prophylactic medical treatment is indicated. If the attacks are less frequent, treatment is aimed at their prompt abortion and cessation. Nonpharmacologic measures such as biofeedback training may be helpful in the motivated patient, but biofeedback does not seem as useful in migraine as in chronic muscle contraction headache. One should help the patient identify triggering events such as stress, environmental factors, and fatigue. A few migraineurs note that their attacks are triggered by the ingestion of certain foods. Although specific food allergies are not thought to trigger migraine, certain chemical substances in food such as tyramine may bring on an attack owing to their vasomotor activity.

DRUG THERAPY

The mainstay of treatment for the migraine patient consists of drug therapy (Table 1). For prophylaxis, the beta-blockers, specifically propranolol, 80 to 320 mg a day, nadolol, 40 to 160 mg a day, or atenolol, 50 to 100 mg a day, are the drugs of choice if not contraindicated. All these agents may cause fatigue and should be used with caution in a patient with allergic pulmonary disorders. The calcium channel blocker verapamil, 320 to 480 mg a day, may be quite helpful in prevention of migraine. It may take six to eight weeks before much effect is seen. Many other calcium channel antagonists currently on the horizon may prove more effective in controlling migraine than is verapamil. The nonsteroidal anti-inflammatory agents also help to control the number of attacks. Methysergide maleate is one of the better prophylactic agents, but must be used with caution, and the patient should take a drug holiday of four to six weeks every four months if taking this medication. It has occasionally been shown to cause fibrotic reactions when taken for a prolonged period. This possible risk is greatly reduced by intermittent use.

Other less effective preventive agents that may at times be useful include clonidine, 0.2 to 0.4 mg daily, cyproheptadine, 12 to 16 mg daily, Bellergal-S b.i.d., and amitriptyline, 25 to 100 mg daily at bedtime.

Table 1. PROPHYLACTIC AGENTS FOR MIGRAINE

Preparation	Daily Dose
Beta-blockers	
Propranolol (Inderal)	80–320 mg
Nadolol (Corgard)	40–160 mg
Atenolol (Tenormin)	50–100 mg
Timolol (Blocadren)	20–40 mg
Metoprolol (Lopressor)	100–200 mg
Calcium channel blockers	
Verapamil (Calan, Isoptin)	320–480 mg
Nifedipine (Procardia)	40 mg
Nimodipine*	
Flunarizine	
Methysergide (Sansert)	6–8 mg
Anti-inflammatory agents	
Naproxen (Naprosyn)	500–1000 mg
Ibuprofen (Motrin, Rufen)	1200–1600 mg
Indomethacin (Indocin)	75–200 mg
Fenoprofen calcium (Nalfon)	900–1800 mg
Antidepressants	
Amitriptyline (Elavil, Endep, Amitid)	25–100 mg
Phenelzine (Nardil)	45 mg
Doxepin (Sinequan, Adapin)	25–100 mg
Bellergal-S	2 daily
Clonidine (Catapres)	0.2–0.4 mg
Guanabenz (Wytensin)	8–16 mg
Cyproheptadine (Periactin)	12–16 mg

*Miles Laboratories. Expected for release in the U.S. soon; currently being studied.

DRUG THERAPY FOR ACUTE MIGRAINE ATTACK

The acute attack of migraine is best treated with one of the ergotamine preparations either by tablet, sublingual tablet, inhaler, or suppository (Table 2). Ergotamine tartrate should not be used in a patient with peripheral vascular disease. It causes nausea in perhaps 50% of people. The tablet form should be taken two tablets at once followed by one tablet every half-hour for two or three more doses if needed. The suppository is used at the onset of a headache and repeated in one hour if necessary. The only other vasoconstrictive agent available at this time is Midrin, which contains the vasoconstrictive agent isometheptene mucate. Midrin should be taken two capsules at once and one or two

Table 2. ABORTIVE THERAPY FOR MIGRAINE

Vasoconstrictive Agents
Ergotamine tartrate
  Oral: Cafergot, Cafergot PB, Wigraine
  Rectal: Cafergot, Cafergot PB, Wigraine
  Sublingual: Ergostat, Ergomar, Wigrettes
  Inhalant: Medihaler Ergotamine
  Intramuscular: Dihydroergotamine
Isometheptene mucate
  Oral: Midrin, Migralam

Anti-inflammatory Agents
Nonsteroidal
  Ibuprofen (Motrin, Rufen Advil, Nuprin), 400–600 mg q 6 h
  Naproxen sodium (Anaprox), 275 mg q 6 h
  Meclofenamate sodium (Meclomen), 50–100 mg q 6 h
  Diflunisal (Dolobid), 500 mg b.i.d.
Steroids
  Methylprednisolone acetate (Depo-Medrol), 40–80 mg IM
  Dexamethasone acetate (Decadron-LA), 8–12 mg IM
  Dexamethasone (Decadron), 5–12 PAK, PO

Antiemetics
  Metoclopramide (Reglan), 20 mg
  Hydroxyzine HCl (Atarax, Vistaril), 25–50 mg
  Promethazine HCl (Phenergan), 50 mg

Analgesics
  PO or IM

capsules in an hour if needed. Some of the shorter-acting nonsteroidal anti-inflammatory agents such as ibuprofen or meclofenamate may work quite well in aborting a migraine attack. Sometimes none of these oral agents work and an injection of a narcotic, sedative, and antinauseant may be necessary. At times one of the long-acting steroid preparations such as Depo-Medrol, 40 to 80 mg, or Decadron-LA, 8–12 mg, may be taken IM after an attack has lasted a few days without relief.

Recently, IV dihydroergotamine has been found helpful in aborting an attack of migraine if initial measures have been to no avail: 1 mg added to 30 to 50 ml of saline is run in IV over 15 to 20 minutes. This often stops a migraine attack even if it has been present for many hours or several days. This may have to be repeated in six or eight hours for two or three doses before the attack is terminated. It is quite well tolerated and has been shown to be very useful. As an adjunct to the treatment of migraine, metoclopramide hydrochloride, 20 mg at onset, may help to control the nausea and enhance absorption of orally ingested medications. This is usually prescribed in the oral form but can be given IV if desired.

SUPPORTIVE MEASURES

It is important to discuss medications and their actions with the patient. Pamphlets on migraine are available from pharmaceutical companies and at my institution we show a slide presentation to patients followed by a discussion with a patient educator.

Patients should be told that not every medication works for everyone and a change may be necessary. Follow-up visits are important so that dosage may be altered or medication changed. Many patients whose migraine attacks are well suppressed by medication may be able to greatly reduce or even eliminate the dosage after several months of good control. However, we stress that migraine is a familial disorder for which there is no present cure. Our goal is to reduce the frequency and severity of attacks as well as to provide good prompt relief at onset.

Cluster Headache

Cluster headache is a headache of a vascular etiology due to dilation of branches of the external and internal carotid artery. Diagnosis is made from the history and as yet there are no specific diagnostic tests to confirm the diagnosis.

PATHOPHYSIOLOGY

Like migraine, this vascular headache is not well understood so far as the pathophysiologic events are concerned. It is known that up to one third more blood flows through the orbital vessels on the side of the headache during the attack than on the noninvolved side. Many workers feel that this headache is somehow triggered by a hypothalamic dysfunction since it does occur in a cyclic pattern. Histamine, serotonin, and other vasoactive substances may be involved in producing the dilation of the arteries and the pain.

CLINICAL ASPECTS

This condition is about ten times more common in men than in women. It is almost always unilateral, and the pain centers around the orbit, temple, and face. The pain is steady and constant as opposed to the throbbing, pulsating pain of migraine. The attacks of pain are short, lasting less than two hours. They may occur several times a day and typically recur daily for several weeks or months, only to be followed by complete remission with pain-free intervals lasting months or years. Accompanying the severe pain are often symptoms of parasympathetic stimulation, such as tearing of the eye, conjunctival infection, and ipsilateral nasal congestion.

Many men with cluster headache seem to have an excessive alcohol intake and smoke excessively. Other conditions associated with stress, smoking, and alcohol ingestion (such as ulcer disease, ruddy complexion, and elevated hemoglobin levels) all occur more commonly in patients with cluster headache.

MANAGEMENT

The treatment of cluster headache should concentrate on prevention. Attacks usually hit abruptly and are of short duration, making the use of analgesics for each attack impractical. Each cluster is treated with daily prophylactic medication until the attacks are suppressed. Daily prophylactic medication does not usually prevent the cluster from recurring, and so medication should be stopped once the cluster is over. Very few nonpharmacologic measures are useful in cluster headache. Most patients greatly curtail or cease the ingestion of alcoholic beverages, since alcohol triggers an attack. Occasionally, patients believe that vigorous exercise and the use of ice on the side of the head involved may make the attacks less severe.

Methysergide four times daily or prednisone, 5 to 10 mg four times daily, are the two most widely used preventive medications for cluster headache. They may be used together or separately. Ergotamine tartrate three to four times a day on a regular basis may also control the attacks; unlike migraine there is usually no problem with ergotamine rebound even though it is used daily. Lithium carbonate, 300 mg three to four times daily, is also a good preventive medication. The calcium channel antagonists hold great promise in prevention of cluster attacks, but they tend to be slow-acting and may not show much effect before the cluster is over. Their place will probably be in the management of chronic cluster headache, a rare condition in which the patient has no sustained periods of remission. Other occasionally helpful medications include cyproheptadine and the nonsteroidal noninflammatory agents.

Medications used to control cluster headache have numerous side effects. Methysergide should be used for a maximum of four months at a time; it can be restarted after a four- to six-week drug holiday. Fortunately, it is rarely needed for more than a few weeks or a few months. Likewise, long-term use of prednisone can have deleterious side effects. Both these medications are usually effective fairly quickly, and need not be tried for long periods if they are not effective within a few days.

For the acute cluster headache attack, narcotic medications are often necessary. Ergotamine in any one of its available forms may help shorten the attack. Oxygen in pure form, when breathed at a rate of 7 liters a minute, may effectively control an attack of pain within five to ten minutes. It seems to be effective in about 60% to 70% of patients. Of course, oxygen therapy is inconvenient when the headache attacks occur away from home.

Patients need to be followed and observed for complications of the medications rather than for any long-term side effects of the condition itself.

Mixed Headache

Mixed headache by definition implies that the patient has several varieties of headache at the same time. Mixed headaches are very commonly seen in headache centers. Usually they occur in people who have had migraine in the past and now have a superimposed daily muscle contraction–type headache. Since many of these patients have daily pain, they become dependent on analgesics or tranquilizers; the main goal of therapy often is to reduce the intake of these. Drug therapy consists of the use of antidepressant medications and nonaddicting analgesics. These patients usually need some psychologic counseling, and biofeedback may also be helpful.

REFERENCES

Diamond S, Dalessio DJ: The Practicing Physician's Approach to Headache, 3rd ed. Williams & Wilkins Co, Baltimore, 1982.

Diamond S, Medina JL: New drug therapies for headache. Postgrad Med 68:125–140, 1980.

Edmeads J: Headache. *In* Rakel RE (ed): Conn's Current Therapy. W.B. Saunders Co, Philadelphia, 1986, pp 717–722.

13 · PRURITUS

Michael S. Blaiss
OCHSNER CLINIC AND ALTON OCHSNER MEDICAL FOUNDATION

DEFINITION AND DIAGNOSTIC CRITERIA

Pruritus, or itching, can be defined simply as a sensation of the skin that evokes scratching. This condition can occur in many disorders with or without dermatologic manifestations.

PATHOPHYSIOLOGY

The pathophysiology is not completely understood because of the lack of an animal model to study itching and a true objective measurement for itching in man.

Many different stimuli have been noted to provoke itching such as temperature change, trauma, touch, and emotional stress. It is believed that these and other stimuli cause the release of chemical mediators in the skin. The most studied mediator is histamine, which is liberated from mast cells. Intradermal injection of histamine elicits itching and a wheal, which can be blocked by antihistamines. Other studies have shown that endopeptidase, another mediator, can produce itching when injected into the skin. Peptides such as kinin and leukotrienes probably play a role in itching, although the mechanisms are not clear.

These mediators of itching appear to stimulate nerve endings in the epidermal junction of the skin. The sensation of itch is then carried by two sets of nerve fibers, the nonmyelinated, slow-conducting C fibers and the myelinated, rapidly conducting delta A fibers. Poorly localized itch is probably conducted by C fibers, while highly localized areas of itch travel by delta A fibers. Pain is also carried in these same fibers but is recognized as a completely different sensation from itching. Itch is then transmitted through these fibers by the anteriolateral spinothalamic tracts to the thalamus, and lastly to the sensory cortex.

CLINICAL ASPECTS

Pruritus can be divided into two large classifications for ease of diagnosis: that with skin manifestations and that without skin manifestations (Table 1). This classification can help in diagnosis and formulation of a rational plan of management.

Pruritus with skin manifestations is much easier to diagnose. This group includes many different dermatoses such as atopic dermatitis, scabies, allergic contact dermatitis, dermatitis herpetiformis, urticaria, pruritus ani and vulvae, and lichen simplex chronicus.

Pruritus without skin lesions is usually more difficult to assess. Dry skin or xerosis is a common cause of itching in the elderly and is due to dehydration in the stratum corneum.

Many conditions of pruritus without skin manifestations are associated with systemic disorders. Pruritus secondary to obstructive biliary disease is seen with primary biliary cirrhosis, drug-induced cholestasis, and cholestasis in pregnancy. These conditions cause itch secondary to high levels of bile salts in the skin. The reason for this is not clear. Generalized pruritus also occurs in certain malignancies, especially Hodgkin's disease and leukemia. Endocrine disorders with generalized pruritus are hyperthyroidism, hypothyroidism, and carcinoid syndrome. There is no convincing evidence that diabetes mellitus itself is a condition associated with pruritus. The itching seen with hypothyroidism appears to be due to the accompanying xerosis in this condition. Chronic renal failure is commonly associated with generalized pruritus. The cause is unknown but may be due to the hypercalcemia that occurs with this condition. Iron deficiency anemia, systemic mastocytosis, and polycythemia vera are implicated as hematologic causes of generalized itching. Drug abuse, parasitic infestation, and psychogenic disorders can also have pruritus as a major symptom.

MANAGEMENT

PLAN

Because of the many different etiologies for pruritus, there is no single treatment that will work for all patients. Management depends on being able to diagnose the particular cause, and thus choose the appropriate treatment of the itching.

The work-up for pruritus can usually be done on an outpatient basis. If skin manifestations are present, recognition of the disorder should lead to specific therapy. When no skin manifestations are present, a careful physical examination and appropriate laboratory tests to check for the above systemic diseases should be undertaken (Table 2).

NONPHARMACOLOGIC MEASURES

Many nonpharmacologic measures can help relieve pruritus and in certain conditions completely alleviate the problem. Scratching helps control itching, probably by replacing itch with another sensation, pain. In many dermatoses, especially atopic dermatitis, scratching may worsen the condition and increase the likelihood of secondary infection.

Cold can be helpful in general management of pruritus. Cool baths can temporarily relieve itching, and maintenance of a cool environment around the patient can decrease symptoms.

Hydration of the skin in patients with xerosis will help lessen itching. After a cool bath, an emollient such as Lubriderm should be applied to the body before drying off. This keeps moisture in the stratum corneum, which lessens the dryness and decreases the pruritus.

Itching can be made worse by several different conditions which should be avoided. Emotional stimuli such as stress and anxiety can worsen itching. Tight clothing and rough material such as wool can irritate the skin and increase pruritus. Alcohol, coffee, tea, and colas can contribute to itching in some patients and should be avoided.

DRUG THERAPY

Several different groups of drugs have been shown to be effective in controlling pruritus. Obviously, the appropriate drug therapy depends on the etiology.

Table 1. PRURITUS WITHOUT SKIN MANIFESTATIONS

Liver disorders	Kidney disorders
Primary biliary cirrhosis	Chronic renal failure
Drug-induced cholestasis	Blood disorders
Cholestasis in pregnancy	Iron deficiency anemia
Malignancies	Systemic mastocytosis
Hodgkin's disease	Polycythemia vera
Leukemia	Miscellaneous conditions
Endocrine disorders	Xerosis
Hyperthyroidism	Drug abuse
Hypothyroidism	Parasitic infestation
Carcinoid syndrome	Psychogenic disorders

Table 2. LABORATORY WORK-UP OF PRURITUS

1. CBC	6. Thyroid screen
2. Sedimentation rate	7. Chest x-ray
3. Urinalysis	8. Stool for blood, ova, and parasites
4. Liver function studies	9. Serum glucose
5. Kidney function studies	10. Serum calcium and phosphate

H_1-antihistamines help control pruritus in many patients by acting as competitive inhibitors of histamine at the target organ. These drugs are very effective in most cases of pruritus associated with dermatoses, especially urticaria and atopic dermatitis, but are of limited value in pruritus of systemic disorders such as biliary cirrhosis, Hodgkin's disease, and uremia. Several families of antihistamines are available, but hydroxyzine HCl (Atarax) has been shown to be the most effective in controlling pruritus induced by histamine in the skin. Because almost all available antihistamines can cross into the central nervous system and cause sedation, I usually start with a single nightly dose of hydroxyzine (e.g., 25 mg) and slowly increase the dose as needed to control itching. After several days of continued use of the antihistamine, most of the sedation problem resolves. Patients need to be warned of this potential side effect and cautioned about using alcohol while taking these drugs, as it can add to the sedation problem.

A new H_1-antihistamine, terfenadine (Seldane), has been released in the United States. This drug has been shown to be highly effective in controlling pruritus and does not cause sedation because it does not cross into the central nervous system. Other nonsedating H_1-antihistamines are awaiting FDA approval.

Another drug, doxepin (Sinequan), an antidepressant, acts like an H_1-antihistamine when given in low doses, e.g., as 25 to 50 mg a day. It is also effective in controlling pruritus but is not approved by the FDA for this use.

H_2-antihistamines, cimetidine (Tagamet) and ranitidine (Zantac), are rarely effective by themselves in decreasing itching. In some studies, H_2- and H_1-antihistamines together were effective in controlling chronic urticaria when H_1-antihistamines alone were not. So far the use of H_2-antihistamines for other causes of pruritus has not been rewarding.

Topical antihistamines such as diphenhydramine cream (Benadryl) should not be used to treat pruritus. They are not very effective and can produce contact sensitization.

Corticosteroids, both topical and systemic, are valuable agents in relieving many causes of pruritus. They are extremely important in pruritus of inflammatory skin disorders such as allergic contact dermatitis, atopic dermatitis, and lichen simplex chronicus. Like the antihistamines, they are less effective in controlling pruritus in systemic diseases. The weakest-strength topical agent should be tried first: e.g., 1% hydrocortisone cream. If needed I next try stronger, fluoronated steroid creams or ointments, and lastly oral corticosteroids. The fluoronated steroids should not be used on the face or on intertriginous areas because they can produce dermal atrophy, stria, and telangiectasia. Also chronic use of fluoronated steroids, especially if placed over large areas of the body or with occlusive dressings, can lead to adrenal suppression and the other numerous side effects associated with chronic oral corticosteroid use. There are fewer side effects when the patient takes oral steroids on alternate days rather than on a daily regimen. Caution needs to be observed with these drugs because adverse side effects can often be worse than the disease being treated.

Pruritus associated with many systemic disorders can be treated specially. In patients with pruritus due to hepatitis or extrahepatic cholestasis and jaundice, cholestyramine, the nonabsorbable anion exchange agent, has been effective in relieving itching. This agent decreases itching by reducing the level of bile salts in the skin and serum. It appears that the bile salts are the cause of the pruritus. Plasma exchange and extracorporeal charcoal perfusion are other effective treatments but also have the potential for more side effects. In women with pruritus due to cholestasis during pregnancy, cholestyramine has been shown to be safe and useful.

Several treatments have been tried in patients with uremic pruritus. Antihistamines and corticosteroids are not usually helpful in this condition. In some patients dialysis decreases the itching, but in most patients the itching is worsened. Both cholestyramine and oral charcoal have been used with minimal results. There is a subset of uremic patients with secondary hyperthyroidism who have a marked decrease in itching after a subtotal parathyroidectomy. Ultraviolet light, especially UV-B (290 to 320 nm), has also been reported to reduce itching in this disorder.

PATIENT INFORMATION AND EDUCATION

On initial evaluation the patient must understand that there are numerous causes of pruritus. The work-up to find the underlying disorder can be extensive, especially in patients with no skin manifestations or chronic urticaria. In most of these conditions it is important for the patient to know that the treatments prescribed are simply attempts to control the itching, not cures for the underlying disorder, and therefore the itching may not be completely relieved. It is necessary to explain the possible side effects. When corticosteroids are used, detailed instructions are given and the patient cautioned about complications with long-term use. A patient who is well informed during the first visit will help the work-up proceed smoothly and be more compliant. The physician managing the patient who has pruritus with no skin manifestations must not too quickly categorize the condition as psychogenic. As with any disease of unknown cause, the patient will show signs of stress and anxiety. Patients often believe family and friends who tell them the itching is due to "nerves." Before the condition is labeled psychogenic, the physician must thoroughly evaluate and reevaluate all possible organic causes.

SOCIOECONOMIC ASPECTS OF MANAGEMENT

The physician caring for these patients must be their strongest advocate. The patient often receives "advice" from family and friends about unproven and possibly harmful treatments for the itching. The physician should consult the patient about this possibility and be prepared to explain the condition to family members. When everyone concerned with the patient understands the problem, the patient's stress is often reduced, and this can lessen itching.

Fortunately, itching can be controlled. If an underlying cause is found, treatment usually relieves the itching. If no cause is found, the nonpharmacologic and pharmacologic measures outlined should give significant relief.

REFERENCES

Gilchrest BA: Pruritus: pathogenesis, therapy, and significance in systemic disease states. Arch Intern Med 142:101–105, 1982.

Greaves MW: The nature and management of pruritus. The Practitioner 226:1223–1225, 1982.

Tonnesen MG: Pruritus. *In*: Fitzpatrick TB, Eisen AZ, Wolff K, Freedberg IM, Austen KF (eds): Dermatology in General Medicine. New York, McGraw-Hill Book Co., 1979, pp 32–34.

Winkelman RK: Pharmacologic control of pruritus. Med Clinics North Am 66:1119–1133, 1982.

14 · EDEMA

Alexander Schirger
John A. Spittell, Jr
MAYO CLINIC AND MAYO FOUNDATION

Edema, or swelling of the limbs and dependent portions of the body, has been recognized as a serious symptom of illness by physicians since ancient times. Accumulation of fluid in the peripheral tissues, whether in the limbs or in the dependent parts of the torso, suggests to both laymen and physicians a severe physiologic disturbance, the cause residing in the heart, kidneys, or liver. Less commonly, swelling or edema may be due to local circulatory disturbances in the affected extremity or organ.

Systemic Edema

Systemic edema occurs in the course of cardiac failure, advanced liver disease, severe nutritional disease, or renal failure. What are the features that indicate or point to a systemic cause of swelling of the extremities? Bilaterality, extension above the knees and into the presacral areas, and associated symptoms and signs of cardiac, hepatic, renal or nutritional disease indicate a systemic type of edema rather than one with a local cause. The alert clinician seeks other physical clues when confronted with bilateral edema of the extremities. Particularly in edema of recent onset, softness of the edematous tissues and easy pitting with pressure suggests systemic edema. With lymphatic obstruction, the edema is firm because tissue reaction has proceeded to the point of fibrous induration.

CARDIAC EDEMA

Associated symptoms of dyspnea, oppressive sensations in the chest, palpitations, or historical evidence of an irregular heartbeat in association with the onset of edema may suggest atrial fibrillation and point to the heart as a cause. Estimation of jugular venous pressure and careful evaluation of jugular venous pulse waves often provide useful confirmatory evidence of cardiac failure. An important type of cardiac edema, which may be difficult to distinguish from localized edema, is that due to chronic constrictive pericarditis. When this is suspected, the clinician must seek other clues such as the characteristic X and Y descent of the jugular venous pulse. In patients with other forms of cardiac disease, careful auscultation for murmurs, evidence of rheumatic heart disease, left-to-right shunts, or a gallop rhythm frequently identify the edema as cardiac in origin.

HEPATIC EDEMA

In the patient whose systemic edema is due to liver dysfunction, there usually is historical support in the form of excessive alcohol intake or a viral infection affecting the liver. Other characteristic signs of advanced hepatic disease may include spider angiomata, palmar erythema, gynecomastia, loss of axillary hair, or evidence of collateral venous circulation of the abdominal wall. An important clinical point is that when peripheral edema is due to hepatic dysfunction, ascites is almost always present and splenomegaly is not uncommon.

RENAL EDEMA

In patients suspected of having renal dysfunction, a history of acute streptococcal pharyngitis, acute glomerular nephritis, or symptoms suggestive of recurrent urinary tract infections will direct attention to the kidneys. Characteristic changes of the ocular fundi, hemorrhages, and exudates may be seen in individuals who have long-standing, severe renal disease. A rare form of systemic edema due to renal dysfunction is seen in the patient with renal vein thrombosis characterized by acute onset, accompanied by abdominal or flank pain with or without hematuria, but with fairly massive edema of the lower extremities. Patients with renal vein thrombosis may have systemic edema owing on one hand to kidney dysfunction and on the other hand to extension of thrombus into the vena cava, which results in venous obstruction, presenting the striking clinical picture of combined acute renal vein thrombosis and acute iliofemoral thrombophlebitis. We have seen such a patient in whom the iliac vein thrombosis became so massive that it was mistaken for a tumor on CT scan of the abdomen.

NUTRITIONAL EDEMA

Edema of nutritional causes is rare. However, one must be aware of it in our culture where undernutrition may be due to economic factors but more commonly to emotional factors associated with chronic alcoholism, chronic drug abuse, intestinal malabsorption, or diet faddism combined with anorexia nervosa. In the last-named condition, physical signs of cheilosis, redness of the tongue, and evidence of weight loss will call attention to the diagnosis.

IDIOPATHIC EDEMA

A form with features of both systemic and local edema is "idiopathic edema," which at times can tax both the clinician's acumen and the patient's endurance. Idiopathic edema is seen most often in women and is characteristically cyclic or periodic. The degree of fluid retention may result in a weight gain of 10 lb or more in the course of a day. The extremities bear the major brunt of fluid retention, but there may also be increased abdominal girth and engorgement of the breasts, as well as an uncomfortable sensation due to a puffiness of the face. The edema occurs when the patient is in an erect posture and is ameliorated when lying down; nocturia then is a frequent complaint.

Edema Due to Local Causes

Edema of systemic cause falls within the purview of several disciplines, but edema of local causes is in the domain of the internist with a special interest in cardiovascular disease. Local edema may be due to venous obstruction, lymphatic obstruction, or a particular type of lipodystrophy.

EDEMA OF VENOUS OBSTRUCTION

Edema due to venous obstruction can result from: (1) external venous compression or thrombosis, as in acute thrombophlebitis; (2) localized venous hypertension from chronic deep venous insufficiency; or (3) arteriovenous fistula. Swelling due to acute thrombophlebitis characteristically involves the foot and leg and, depending on the location of the thrombotic process, may involve the thigh and extend up to the inguinal ligament. The swelling is firm, but it pits in the initial stages and is commonly unilateral. If this occurs in the postoperative period, following prolonged immobilization, or in the patient with an underlying malignancy, and if the swelling is unilateral, one should assume that the problem is due to venous obstruction. Usually the diagnosis of venous edema is supported by other signs of venous obstruction such as increased venous pattern. Also, in the patient with acute thrombophlebitis, careful palpation along the course of the deep venous channels of the calf and thigh will demonstrate tenderness over the deep veins. Swelling of massive degree with minimal tenderness in Scarpa's triangle and little or no calf and lower thigh tenderness indicates thrombophlebitis involving the iliofemoral system. Pain in the calf evoked on dorsiflexion of the foot is, in our opinion, nonspecific and the least reliable sign of deep venous thrombosis. Thrombophlebitis most commonly is unilateral but on rare occasions affects both legs, when confirmatory evidence of deep venous thrombosis is provided by noninvasive means with venous Doppler studies (Fig. 1) and impedance plethysmography (Fig. 2). Currently, venography remains the best means to provide the diagnosis when clinical evidence and laboratory findings are inconclusive or contradictory.

LYMPHEDEMA

Lymphedema is swelling due to impaired flow of lymph. It may be due to a primary disorder of the lymphatic vessels (idiopathic lymphedema) or may have an extrinsic cause such as lymphatic obstruction or inflammatory changes (secondary lymphedema). Characteristically, lymphedema is firmer and less pitting than systemic edema or venous edema, is not associated with

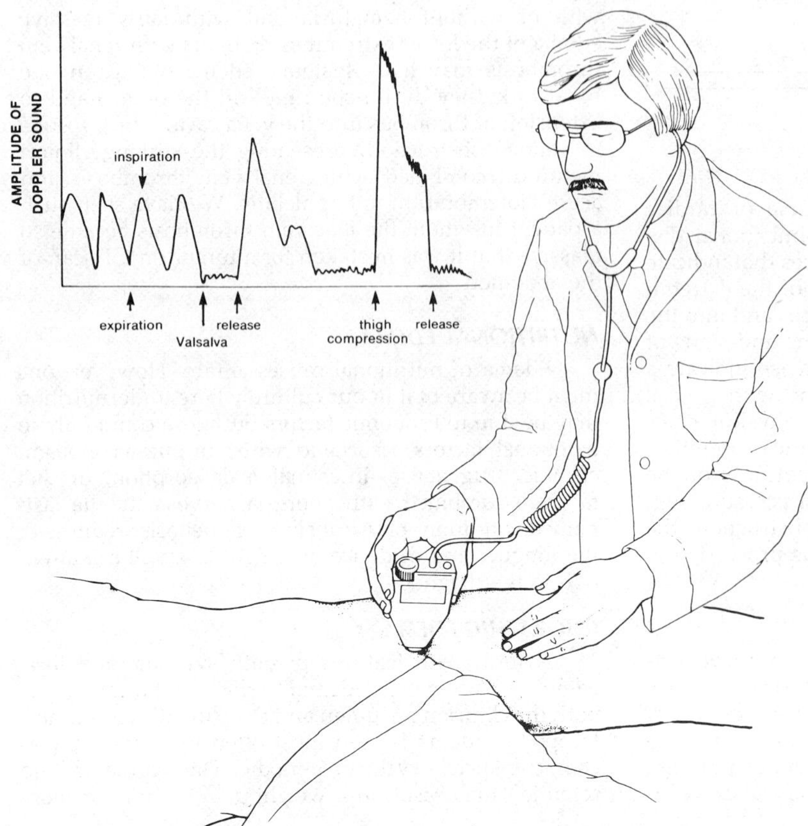

Figure 1. Doppler flowmeter positioned over femoral vein permits examiner to hear sounds reflecting velocity of blood flow. Graph shows a condensed record of sound amplitudes normally heard during respiration, Valsalva maneuver, and distal compression of vein. The presence of a thrombus diminishes or obliterates these flow sounds. The compression and release test can also be used on superficial femoral, popliteal, and posterior tibial veins. (From Wheeler HB: A modern approach to diagnosing deep venous thrombosis. J Cardiovasc Med 5:217–231, 1980. By permission, Group Medicine Publications, New York.)

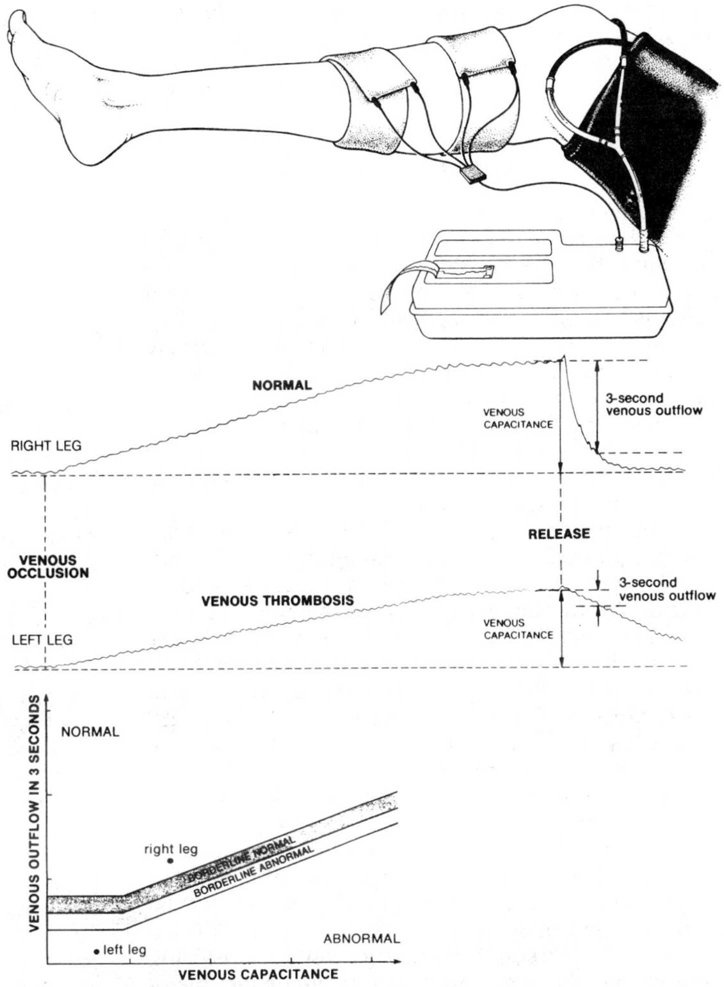

Figure 2. An inflated pneumatic cuff around the thigh traps blood in the lower leg, causing a rise in venous capacitance. Upon deflation, the normally rapid venous outflow is reduced if a thrombus obstructs any major vein draining the leg, as is shown in the paired graphs of a normal right leg and an obstructed left leg. Electrodes around the calf detect resistance changes reflecting venous outflow in the first three seconds after cuff release. Diagnostic results are plotted on the bottom graph in which a diagnonal line separates normal and abnormal findings. Results that fall in the shaded areas on either side of the line are considered slightly less reliable than those in the clearly normal and abnormal ranges. (From Wheeler HB: A modern approach to diagnosing deep venous thrombosis. J Cardiovasc Med 5:217–231, 1980. By permission, Group Medicine Publications, New York.)

an increased venous pattern or stasis pigmentation, and (in contrast to venous edema) has no associated tenderness along the deep veins of the calf or thigh. In patients with lymphedema of longer duration, there may be a peculiar deformity characterized as squaring of the toes, and in some patients with idiopathic lymphedema there is the peculiar yellowish discoloration of the nails, the yellow nail syndrome. In about half the patients with idiopathic lymphedema, the swelling is bilateral.

Onset during the early decades of life strongly suggests that the edema is idiopathic. In the patient in whom swelling first appears in the fifth decade of life or later, a secondary cause is more likely. Idiopathic lymphedema developing in infancy has been referred to as congenital; when the swelling begins at puberty or later, it is called lymphedema praecox. Idiopathic lymphedema that appears later in life is referred to as "forme tardive" of idiopathic lymphedema.

The abnormality in idiopathic lymphedema resides in the lymphatic vessels, but in secondary lymphedema the swelling is due to an inflammatory reaction or other obstructive process involving the lymphatics. Of the neoplastic diseases causing obstructive lymphadema, carcinoma of the prostate is the most common in men and lymphoma the most common in women. Diagnosis is made on the basis of careful physical examination of the prostate in men, and careful palpation of the inguinal nodes and a bimanual pelvic examination in search of lymphoma in women. CT scan of the abdomen is valuable in diagnosis of obstructive lymphedema.

In patients with a characteristic clinical picture of recurrent lymphangitis and cellulitis, lymphedema is due to repeated infection of the lymphatic system by streptococci. It has been postulated that streptococci enter the macerated skin at sites of active fungal infection or trichophytic fissures between the toes. The clinical picture is that of an acute inflammatory episode characterized by temperature elevation to 104°F, shaking chills, headaches, and generalized malaise accompanied by local tenderness in the affected limb. Redness either involves the entire circumference of the limb or appears as reddish streaks, which are in fact the inflamed lymphatic vessels. Recurrent streptococcal lymphangitis and cellulitis is the most common form of inflammatory lymphedema in North America, but in other cultures filariasis is more common.

LIPEDEMA

The last form of local edema is lipedema, which is due to a peculiar accumulation of fatty tissues in the legs but may involve the entire lower extremity, sparing the feet and toes. Lipedema is symmetric and most often occurs in women. In addition to being aware of large legs, these patients complain of orthostatic edema, tenderness, and easy bruising, all readily explained by the excess of fatty tissue. Why some patients are more prone to develop lipedema than others is not clear. The clinical picture is so typical that the diagnosis is readily made by examination alone.

MANAGEMENT

Treatment of edema must be directed toward correcting the basic cause, or if that is not possible, to controlling the edema. Judicious administration of diuretics helps mobilize fluid, but one should be mindful of the risk of potassium depletion. Elevation of the legs by raising the foot of the bed or by a specifically designed sling is useful in chronic forms of edema. After maximal reduction of the edema, the patient is measured for a fitted elastic stocking. In an attempt to ensure a maximal fluid-free state, a thiazide diuretic may be administered on an intermittent basis following discharge from the hospital.

If the patient has swelling due to recurrent lymphangitis and cellulitis, any fungal infection of the toes must be treated vigorously by local measures and, if refractory, with systemic antifungal therapy. We have found intermittently administered long-term antibiotic prophylactic therapy effective in preventing bacterial infection. We customarily use phenoxymethyl penicillin V or erythromycin in patients allergic to penicillin, 250 mg four times daily, for the first seven to ten days of each month for at least one year.

Surgical treatment of lymphedema should be considered for patients who do not respond to medical management, including elastic compression in the form of stockings, physical therapy, and intermittent pneumatic compression treatment. Excisional surgery such as the modified Homans operation or the Thompson "buried dermal flap" procedure is indicated only in disabling forms of lymphedema. Advances in lymphatic microsurgery (lymphovenous anastomoses, lymphatic transplantation) give hope to patients with secondary lymphedema. Early clinical reports are encouraging but long-term results are still necessary to confirm the value of these procedures.

Patients with lipedema are best managed by a sympathetic explanation of the nature of the problem plus weight control measures and the avoidance of extra sodium in the diet. The occasional use of diuretics for special occasions may help to control orthostatic edema, but the regular use of diuretics is discouraged. Because of tenderness, patients seldom tolerate any support more than supportive hose. Management of patients with idiopathic edema is challenging. We have found restriction of sodium, weight control, and fluid restriction to be the most helpful measures.

REFERENCES

Allen EV: Lymphedema of the extremities: classification, etiology and differential diagnosis: a study of 300 cases. Arch Intern Med 54:606–624, 1934.

Edwards OM, Bayliss RIS: Idiopathic edema of women. Q J Med 177:124–144, 1976.

Smith RD, Spittell JA, Schirger A: Secondary lymphedema of the leg: its characteristics and diagnostic implications. JAMA 185:80–82, 1963.

Streeten DHP: Understanding and treating idiopathic edema. Consultant 20:82–88. 1980.

Wheeler HB: A modern approach to diagnosing deep venous thrombosis. J Cardiovasc Med 5:217–231, 1980.

15 · MEDICAL CARE OF THE ADOLESCENT PATIENT

Paul G. Dyment
CLEVELAND CLINIC FOUNDATION

Adolescent medicine has been defined as "that body of knowledge and set of skills necessary to meet the health care needs of young people from the onset of puberty to the acquisition of autonomous adulthood, or approximately . . . 10–21 years of age." Puberty refers to the physiologic changes accompanying sexual maturation, but does not include the psychosocial dimensions implicit in our definition of adolescence—the period of life during which these physical and psychologic changes are occurring.

This chapter will focus on the adolescent office visit and how it should differ from the routine adult history-taking and physical examination. Clearly, adolescents are a unique group with a special set of physical and emotional concerns. The enlightened physician will certainly approach them as such. Since many office visits by adolescents are prompted by physical examination requirements for school or college or for routine health maintenance reasons, these are excellent opportunities for the physician to question them about physical and psychologic growth and development, or to elicit any concerns that might trigger detection of occult disease. The much maligned "sports physical" could be expanded for this same purpose, especially if this is conducted in the physician's office instead of the school locker room.

THE OFFICE VISIT

Most teenagers are more comfortable if there are others of their own age group in the waiting room, or at least evidence that adolescents are welcome by the presence of teen-oriented magazines, or possibly a "rock" poster on the wall. It is frequently possible to set aside time exclusively for teenagers—after school, or a certain time on Saturday—to show your concern for them and your understanding of their life style. The pamphlet rack in the waiting room should contain adolescent-oriented pamphlets on topics such as sexually transmitted disease, breast and testicular self-examination, and harmful practices such as cigarette smoking and drunk driving.

ATTITUDE OF PHYSICIAN

There is little purpose in deploring the generation gap between physicians and adolescents. It is a biologic fact of life, and we must accept that teenagers' life styles and perceptions of the world may differ from ours. They are trying to find a sense of identity, and often trying to cast off adult domination, so physicians must be careful not to adopt a rigid position that might engender a defensive and uncooperative reaction. Tolerance and patience are probably the most important virtues of the successful physician in adolescent medicine practice. Unfortunately, the friendliest physician can still be sabotaged by a receptionist or nurse who clearly has trouble relating to adolescents. "Programming" employees in this regard is an important part of practice management.

ROLE OF PARENTS

The parent generally makes the first appointment only. Parents have a role in giving the history of the young adolescent; they should be present at the beginning of the office visit, but should be asked to leave during the examination. When the examination is complete I confer with the teenager about what will be discussed with the parents, and they are then brought back in to review the clinical situation. The patient is encouraged to initiate all subsequent phone calls to the office.

MEDICAL HISTORY

I introduce myself to the patient and parents when entering the office and ask the adolescent to sit in the chair beside my desk. All questions are directed to the patient. Occasionally I put a question also to the parents to make sure this becomes a joint history, and I carefully observe the interaction between patient and parents (frequently the most valuable part of the entire process). A questionnaire is often more rewarding than a person-to-person traditional Review of Systems, and I use the one developed by Johnson and Tanner (Table 1). The patient completes this in the waiting room beforehand. The rest of the medical history-taking is much the same as for adults, but the psychosocial history is taken from the patient alone and after the parents have gone, either before or after the actual physical examination. If done after the examination, patients are frequently more comfortable: they are dressed, their anxieties about the physical examination have been allayed, and they may then be more likely to reveal what is really bothering them.

Many experienced physicians prefer to continue the medical history during the physical examination, believing this helps to distract the patient. When the psychosocial history is taken I make sure that at least one question is asked about each of the following subjects: sex, drugs, home, and school. Sometimes a facial reaction to the question is more rewarding than the actual reply. It is often necessary to reassure patients that I am their doctor, not their parents' doctor, and that the things we talk about are confidential. A nonjudgmental stance is extremely important, although it is arguable that remaining nonjudgmental when the patient is describing an unwise life style (e.g., taking androgens for body building, practicing unprotected intercourse) could be interpreted by the patient as evidence of my acceptance of that particular behavior. The medical and social reasons why that particular behavior is of concern must be clearly expressed by the physician, albeit nonjudgmentally.

PHYSICAL EXAMINATION

If parents are present at this stage, they are now asked to sit in the waiting room. The young patient should be given privacy in the examining room while undressing, so I leave the room with the parents, which provides an opportunity to elicit from them whether there are further problems they would like me to know about their adolescent. The common practice of having the adolescent already undressed and wearing a gown while giving the initial medical history is undesirable and somewhat dehumanizing, and does not help the patient feel at ease.

The physical examination is carried on as if the patients were adults, with due respect for adolescents' frequently heightened sense of modesty. It is a good idea not only to keep the door shut, but to use a second curtain-barrier in case someone comes in unexpectedly during a rectal or pelvic examination. During the physical examination, teenagers can benefit from reassurance that everything seems to be normal. It is important to reassure young people about their physical development. Sexual development should always be recorded with the standard Tanner rating system. There is no real purpose in doing a "routine" rectal examination on adolescents unless there is abdominal pain or some rectal symptomatology. Similarly, pelvic examinations in girls should be considered routine only if they are sexually active or have gynecologic symptoms. If older adolescent males have little or no knowledge of testicular self-examination, this is a good time to teach the technique and provide a pamphlet on the subject. Breast self-examination by the older adolescent girl should be approached in an identical fashion.

CONCLUDING INTERVIEW

The conclusion of the visit is frequently the most important part. Adolescents may need to be reassured that you will be honest with them. Teenagers are very concerned about physical problems, and it is not wrong to reassure them more often than may be strictly necessary. Nonconfidential matters can be discussed when the parents rejoin you, and this helps to clarify your instructions. Adolescents should be in charge of their own therapy as far as possible.

HEALTH MAINTENANCE

The goals of the health maintenance examination are multiple: detection of occult physical and emotional abnormalities; reassurance of adolescents and parents regarding physical development; education about preventive health matters such as testicular and breast self-examination, the risks of alcohol and cigarette smoking, and so forth; and counseling if the patient or the family is suffering from significant stress.

SCREENING TESTS

The American Academy of Pediatrics has recommended the following schedule for adolescents. A physical examination should be performed every two years from 12 to 21 years of age, with screening for visual acuity at 16 years, and for hearing at 14, 16, and 20 years. Routine tuberculin skin tests should be done every one to two years in areas of high endemicity of that disease; in areas of low occurrence the physician may elect not to test routinely, or to test at longer intervals. Both urinalyses and hemoglobin or hematocrit determinations are being reevaluated in regard to the frequency and timing of routine performance. Until these issues are settled, the Academy suggests doing at least one urinalysis and one determination of either hemoglobin or hematocrit at some time during adoles-

Table 1. HEALTH QUESTIONNAIRE

This questionnaire will help us to better know you.
Sometimes it is easier to raise questions you have on your mind this way. Check "YES" or "NO" to the questions on page 1; check the appropriate column for the problems listed on page 2. Hand this paper directly to your physician. You may have it back if you wish.

1. What do you like to be called? _______________________

2. Why are you coming to the doctor today? _______________________

	YES	NO
3. Do you have any other things needing medical attention?	☐	☐
4. Do you think you are a healthy person in general?	☐	☐
5. Have you been seriously ill, had an operation, or been in the hospital overnight?	☐	☐
6. Do you think you have heart trouble?	☐	☐
7. Do you think you have cancer?	☐	☐
8. Have you ever had low blood or anemia?	☐	☐
9. Are there any foods you can't eat or medicines you can't take because you are allergic to them?	☐	☐
10. Have you ever had a discharge or other problems with your sex organs?	☐	☐
11. Do you have any questions about pregnancy or birth control?	☐	☐
12. Do you have any questions about drinking or drug use?	☐	☐
13. Do you have any questions about smoking cigarettes?	☐	☐
14. Do you have any questions about venereal disease?	☐	☐
15. Do you have any worries about how your body is developing?	☐	☐
16. Are you happy with your weight?	☐	☐
17. Are you happy with your height?	☐	☐
18. Are you absent from school (or job) a lot?	☐	☐
19. Are you having any trouble passing your courses at school?	☐	☐
20. Does anything bother you about school (or job)?	☐	☐
21. Can you talk to your parents about important things or worries?	☐	☐
22. Do you get along with your brothers and sisters?	☐	☐
23. Are there any big problems at home?	☐	☐
24. Do you have any problem making friends?	☐	☐
25. Do you date?	☐	☐
26. Do you go steady?	☐	☐
27. Do you have any worries about your sex feelings?	☐	☐

This is a list of conditions and problems that sometimes give young people trouble. Check each one as to whether you are troubled by it a lot, once in a while, or never.

	A LOT	ONCE IN A WHILE	NEVER
Skin problems; rashes, pimples	☐	☐	☐
Headaches	☐	☐	☐
Dizzy spells, fainting, blackouts	☐	☐	☐
Eye or vision problems	☐	☐	☐
Do you wear glasses?	☐	☐	☐
Ear or hearing problems	☐	☐	☐
Stuffy, runny, or bleeding nose	☐	☐	☐
Colds or sore throats	☐	☐	☐
Trouble with teeth or gums	☐	☐	☐
Coughing or wheezing	☐	☐	☐
Get out of breath more than friends	☐	☐	☐
Pain or aches in stomach	☐	☐	☐
Vomiting (throwing up)	☐	☐	☐
Diarrhea (loose bowels)	☐	☐	☐
Constipation	☐	☐	☐
Problems with urination (passing water); pain, burning, blood, urinate too often	☐	☐	☐
Pain or aches in back, arms, legs, muscles, or joints	☐	☐	☐
Hay fever, hives, or asthma	☐	☐	☐
Feel upset or nervous	☐	☐	☐
Feel angry	☐	☐	☐
Feel lonely, sad, or depressed	☐	☐	☐
Feel tired all day; no energy	☐	☐	☐
Have problems sleeping	☐	☐	☐
Eat too much or too little	☐	☐	☐
Don't eat right foods	☐	☐	☐
Girls: problems with your period (menstruation)	☐	☐	☐

	YES	NO
Is there anything else your doctor should know about you?	☐	☐
Do you have any other health questions?	☐	☐

Do you wish to make any comments about your health, have concerns about seeing the doctor, being examined, or about this questionnaire? If, so, write it here. _______________________

____

____

____

From Johnson RL, Tanner NM: Approaching the adolescent patient. *In* Hofmann AD, Greydanus DE (ed): Adolescent Medicine. Copyright 1983, Addison-Wesley Publishing Company, Inc.

cence, leaving the timing of further tests up to individual practice experience. Screening for sickle cell disease in black patients should be done primarily to initiate a discussion of its genetic implications, rather than to discover a previously undetected disorder. Most physicians do not believe it necessary to screen patients of Mediterranean heritage for glucose-6-phosphate dehydrogenase (G6PD) deficiency, as the frequency of clinically significant hemolytic reactions in these patients is exceedingly small.

BLOOD PRESSURE ASSESSMENT AND IMMUNIZATION STATUS

Careful measurement of blood pressure, with the cuff covering two thirds of the right arm, when the patient is seated, is an important part of the health maintenance examination. Normal BP measurements, particularly the systolic, increase during adolescence. Levels suggesting hypertension and those warranting follow-up are indicated in Table 2.

Patients who have received the customary childhood immunizations need only a booster tetanus-diphtheria immunization at 14 years of age. Those with an incomplete or an unknown immunization history require "catch-up" immunizations, following guidelines of the American College of Physicians.

SPORTS PHYSICAL

One study showed that only 1% of youth had abnormalities detected by physicians in the standard medical examination that disqualified them from high school and college athletics. Perhaps this low statistic perpetuates the typical cursory approach and attitude of both physicians and school officials toward the sports physical. Ideally, the examination should take place in the private office of the physician and should include all the features of a complete health maintenance visit, as described above. Unfortunately, this is not often the case and such exams are often conducted en masse in the school locker room.

Most physical abnormalities that affect the adolescent's participation in athletics are the result of previous injuries, so the focus of the physical examination should be on the musculoskeletal system. A thorough "orthopedic" examination, which can take less than two minutes, should be made in addition to the standard medical examination. Table 3 outlines the format; if this

is followed, about 10% of athletes prove to have a musculoskeletal abnormality that may need rehabilitative treatment such as specific exercises or weight training. If there is a certified trainer at the school, he can be helpful in supervising the rehabilitation process. If the disability is severe, referral to an orthopedic surgeon, preferably one experienced in sports injuries, should be considered.

If the preparticipation physical examination is done in the privacy of the office, the physician should add to the customary subjects discussed at the time of the health maintenance examination (sex, drugs, home, and school) some sports-specific advice. This should cover ill-advised practices such as androgen use by football players and weight lifters, inappropriate "making weight" techniques of wrestlers attempting to lose weight, and fasting by gymnasts (who need supplemental vitamins).

Proper medical care for adolescents requires a physician sensitive to the emotional expressions and needs of young people, with a considerable degree of tolerance for their life styles and behaviors, a willingness to alter the traditional adult approach and thus win acceptance by them, and a sincere desire to help them through this most difficult decade. Adolescents can readily discern whether you display all, some, or none of the above characteristics. If you pass muster, they can make this part of your practice the most personally rewarding of all.

REFERENCES

Dyment PG: Drugs and the adolescent athlete. Pediatr Ann 13:602–604, 1984.

Guide for Adult Immunizations. American College of Physicians, Philadelphia, 1985.

Guidelines for Health Supervision. Committee on Practice and Ambulatory Medicine, American Academy of Pediatrics, 1981.

Table 3. MUSCULOSKELETAL SCREENING EXAMINATION

Instructions	Observation
Stand facing examiner	Acromioclavicular joints; general habitus
Look at ceiling; over both shoulders; touch ears to shoulders	Cervical spine motion
Shrug shoulders (examiner resists)	Trapezius strength
Abduct shoulders 90° (examiner resists at 90°)	Deltoid strength
Full external rotation of arms	Shoulder motion
Flex and extend elbows	Elbow motion
Arms at sides, elbows 90° flexed; pronate and supinate wrists	Elbow and wrist motion
Spread fingers; make fist	Hand or finger motion and deformities
Tighten (contract) quadriceps; relax quadriceps	Symmetry and knee effusion; ankle effusion
"Duck walk" four steps (away from examiner with buttocks on heels)	Hip, knee, and ankle motion
Back to examiner	Shoulder symmetry; scoliosis
Knees straight, touch toes	Scoliosis, hip motion, hamstring tightness
Raise up on toes, raise heels	Calf symmetry, leg strength

From Preparticipation health evaluation. *In* Sports Medicine: Health Care For Young Adults. American Academy of Pediatrics, Evanston, IL, 1983, p 87. Reprinted by permission.

Table 2. ADOLESCENT BLOOD PRESSURE LEVELS

Blood Pressure (mm Hg)	Normal Average Male	Normal Average Female
Systolic	119 ± 13*	111 ± 12
Diastolic	75 ± 10	72 ± 10
Persistent levels suggesting hypertension = ≥ 2 S.D. above mean		
Systolic	≥ 145	≥ 135
Diastolic	≥ 95	≥ 92
Persistent levels warranting follow-up = ≥ 1 S.D. above mean		
Systolic	≥ 132	≥ 123
Diastolic	≥ 85	≥ 82

*Mean ± 1 S.D.

Reprinted by permission of the New York State Journal of Medicine, copyright by the Medical Society of the State of New York. From Kilcoyne MM: Adolescent hypertension. NY State J Med 76:2002–2006, 1976.

Hofmann AD: Foreword. *In* Hofmann AD, Greydanus DE (eds): Adolescent Medicine. Addison-Wesley, Menlo Park, CA, 1983.

Hofmann AD, Becker RD, Gabriel HP: The Hospitalized Adolescent: A Guide to Managing the Ill and Injured Youth. Free Press, New York, 1976.

Johnson RL, Tanner NM: Approaching the adolescent patient. *In* Hofmann AD, Greydanus DE (eds): Adolescent Medicine. Addison-Wesley, Menlo Park, CA, 1983, pp 10–11.

Linder CW, Durant R, Seklecki RM, et al: Preparticipation health screening of young athletes. Am J Sports Med 9:187–193, 1981.

Tanner JM: Growth at Adolescence. Blackwell, Oxford, 1962.

Thompson TR, Andrish JT, Bergfeld JA: A prospective study of preparticipation sports examinations of 2670 young athletes: method and results. Cleve Clin Q 49:225–233, 1982.

16 · MEDICAL TREATMENT OF THE ELDERLY

Eric G. Tangalos
MAYO CLINIC AND MAYO FOUNDATION

DEFINING THE PROBLEM

People never think they are old until their body starts to tell them so. Whether at age 65, 75, or 85, the definition of who is elderly is based more on functional criteria than on chronologic age. The definition of aging is even more obscure and in the clinical sense is a relative one.

Depending on one's perspective, an individual is both young and old at the same time. Visual and auditory acuity reach their peak by 10 years of age. Most athletes are at their prime between the ages of 20 and 30. Neuronal loss from our brains may begin at age 35, and by age 40 all of us are starting to lose bone and muscle mass. Physicians are said to be most productive between 40 and 50.

The aging process seems to be random and unorganized and varies from individual to individual. Unlike childhood, which can be marked by the calendar and gauged by growth and development charts, there is nothing to tell us how the average 65-year-old should look or feel. Clinical experience has taught us that an 85-year-old may look 20 years younger and that a 65-year-old may have the equivalent of 85 years of wear and tear on his frame.

The gerontologist (i.e., scientist) finds it relatively easy to categorize age-related change on the cellular and structural level. The geriatrician (i.e., clinician) has the more difficult job of anticipating and treating the maladies of an entire species. If we are to categorize the elderly, we could say that this is the population at high relative risk for such disorders as Alzheimer's dementia, hip fractures, cataracts, and drug toxicity.

CLINICAL IMPLICATIONS

The aging of America is as important a development in our nation's history as our western migration and the exploration of space. Each day our "aged" population increases by some 1400 as 5000 Americans reach age 65 and 3600 of the elderly die. The texture of society will change as significantly as it did with the European immigration of the late 19th and early 20th centuries.

American demographers may well conclude that the most striking difference between the late 20th century and the world of our grandchildren will be the presence of so many elderly in the population. Today the United States has 24 million persons age 65 or older, and this number is increasing twice as fast as the rest of the population. Since 1950 the number of people over age 65 has doubled, and since the 1970s it has increased by one fourth (Fig. 1). The first postwar "baby-boomers" turn 65 in the year 2011, causing a sexagenarian explosion at an increase of 1 million persons per year for the ensuing 20 years (59%). By the year 2030, our elderly population will go from 24 million to 51.5 million, from 11% to almost 17% of the total population.

The impact on medical care will be immense as we experience a demand on resources never before encountered. Given just the nursing home population, expenditures in the last 10 years have gone from 7 billion to over 30 billion dollars annually. Each year the public burden for nursing home support increases and now accounts for 60% of these payments.

The major factors that have allowed a greater portion of our population to reach senior citizen status in this century include the development of chlorinated public water supplies, sanitary sewage systems, widespread application of childhood immunizations, and the introduction of antibiotics into medical practice. The big change in life expectancy has occurred because of reduced infant and childhood mortality rates. In 1841 a newborn female could expect to live 42 years and a male 41 years, whereas in 1973 a newborn female could expect 76 years of life and a newborn male 72 years of life. In contrast, a 65-year-old in 1841 could expect to live about 11 more years while his 1983 counterpart could improve on that very little.

Little has been done to alter longevity beyond age 65, and the biologic clock of unmodified human survival

U.S. POPULATION 65 AND OLDER

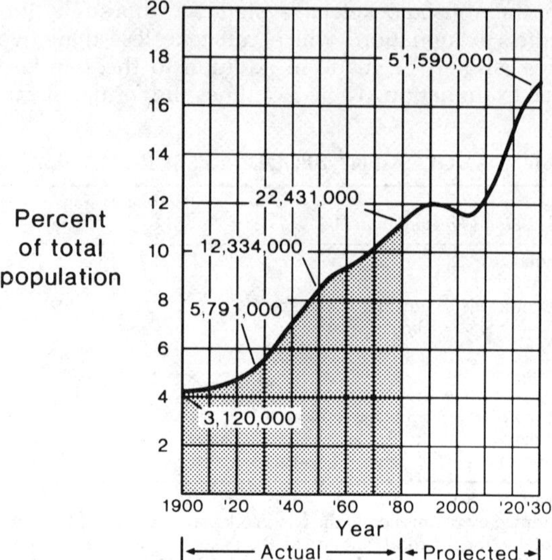

Figure 1. From U.S. Bureau of Census.

appears to run down close to age 100. Despite reports from Soviet Georgia and Ecuador, the oldest human is probably a female close to 115 years of age. As life expectancy approaches the biologic limits of life span, physicians must attend to an enlarging older population with problems that are multifaceted and interwoven.

The field of geriatrics has grown rapidly in the last ten years as medicine and government prepare for increasing demands on services. Geriatric fellowships are now common across the country, the Association of American Medical Colleges recognizes the need for geriatric curriculum development, and the National Institute on Aging's expanding budget funds research on questions this population poses to science and medicine. The organ-specific approach to medical problems must blend in a synthesis of the physiologic, sociologic, and psychologic parameters that determine overall health. In a more frail and unforgiving body, the elderly will require more gentle care and ultimately redefine what is meant by "quality of life."

MEDICAL MANAGEMENT

GENERAL PRINCIPLES

In dealing with the elderly, physicians already have the advantage that the patient is a survivor. Physician interaction may have done little to influence the course of the lives of many of them thus far, and our goal should be to perpetuate good health habits and intervene only when necessary.

Medical care of the elderly is predominantly an outpatient practice—a trend that is likely to continue as a government thrust in the next decade for continuing care of even the "frail elderly" is to keep costs down and allow these people to remain at home as long as possible. For the elderly, the doctor-patient relationship and continuity of care become crucial. The primary care physician is the one most likely to provide this. He must play an active role as patient advocate and intermediary, often having to decide when treatment should be initiated and when not. We have all witnessed the unfortunate episode that develops when a 90-year-old confused patient with pneumonia is brought into the emergency room. The primary care physician can often avert such situations, discussing with patients the possibility of hospitalization, continuing care options, socalled "living wills," and patients' intentions regarding resuscitative efforts, long before these become a reality.

Elderly patients need easy access to their physician, and time set aside to answer telephone calls is one of the best ways for a physician to provide this. The aging process makes many patients introspective and distrusting while at the same time increasingly reliant on others. The physician needs to move into a role of increasing responsibility, sharing his expertise and advice and providing support and reassurance to a population whose lives may be as unsteady as their gait.

For the management of elderly patients with chronic diseases, routine office visits may prove very worthwhile. It is usually best to make a definitive follow-up arrangement while patients are still in your office, and to remind them by phone or mail.

NONPHARMACOLOGIC MEASURES

The physician's ability to maintain good health in the elderly patient goes beyond knowing which drugs are appropriate. Understanding the environment of the elderly, how they perceive it, and how they move around in it are hallmarks of geriatric care. Environmental modification can be a shared responsibility with occupational therapy.

Sensory deprivation is an important determinant in the health and well-being of elderly patients. Bright colors and adequate lighting can help counter any loss of depth perception. Hearing aids may put a dull, withdrawn individual back in touch with family and environment. Poor vision and cloudy mental images may both clear after cataract surgery. For the patient with poor position sense, poor balance, or a peripheral neuropathy, a cane provides both support and the reassurance of additional sensory input.

Protecting brittle bones from injury should be a consideration at all times. Hand rails on stairways and in the bathroom may prevent falls. Removal of throw rugs and use of night lights may also prevent accidents.

Demented patients present a particular challenge, since as yet no pharmacologic agents are available to correct the disorder. Home care may be feasible if the environment is stable and certain needs are met. Care givers should not disrupt familiar routines and habits. For example, brushing teeth in the safety of one's own bathroom requires almost no cognition or memory function, yet the same task during a visit to relatives may unmask severe intellectual deficits. Encourage these patients to keep lists and have paper and pen close to the telephone.

DRUG THERAPY

With advancing age, the incidence of chronic disease increases (Fig. 2), and the complexity of patient care becomes more challenging as the physician encounters numerous interrelated medical problems and a wide variety of pharmacologic agents.

The elderly account for more than 25% of all prescription drugs. It is estimated that they receive about 50% of all hypnotics produced, and some studies show that up to 90% of all nursing home patients receive a sedative on at least a p.r.n. basis. According to the 1977 National Health Care Expenditure Study, persons 65 and older average 10.8 prescriptions annually.

With aging the absorption, distribution, metabolism, and excretion of most drugs is altered. Rational drug therapy requires an understanding of the agent, the clinical situation, and the specific patient.

Factors that contribute to differing drug response in the elderly are described below.

Absorption. In most situations, drug absorption should be considered slower and less efficient in the elderly. This may be due to decreased intestinal blood flow, a decreased absorptive surface along the GI tract, or altered GI motility. In addition, lowered gastric acidity alters the ionization and solubility of certain drugs.

Distribution. Reduced lean body mass, a decrease in total body water, and an increase in fat:protein ratio all affect drug distribution. Changes in serum albumin with age alter protein binding. Two drugs that competitively bind for the same receptor sites may cause toxicity by displacing more free (unbound) drug than if each drug were used alone.

Metabolism. Factors influencing the rate and extent of drug metabolism include cardiac output and hepatic

INCIDENCE OF CHRONIC DISEASE
WITH ADVANCING AGE

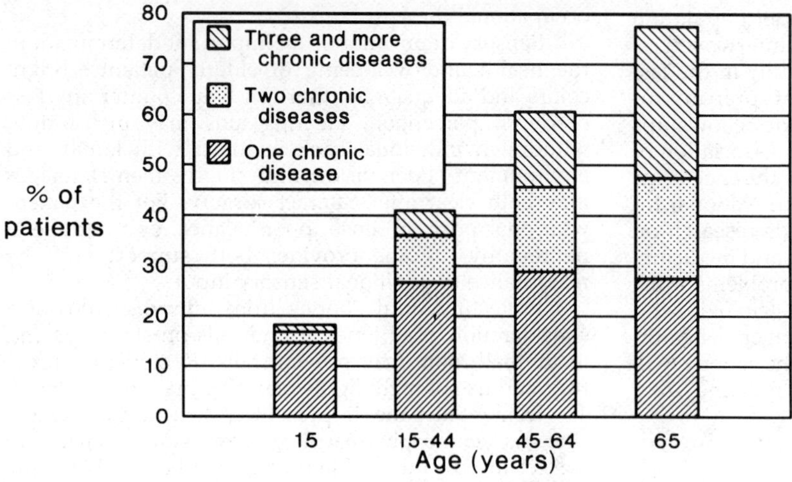

Figure 2. Adapted from Covington TR, Walker JI: Current Geriatric Therapy. W.B. Saunders Co, Philadelphia, 1984, p 36.

blood flow. With age there is a decrease in cardiac output, liver mass, and hepatocyte efficiency.

Excretion. Renal function is probably the single factor most responsible for altered drug levels in the aging population. The body most often converts a drug to a more water-soluble product for elimination by the kidneys. Some drugs are simply filtered while others are actively excreted by the kidney. Studies of water diuresis show that with aging there is reduced maximal rate of urine flow and formation of solute-free water. Renal concentrating ability is also significantly reduced. The kidneys are estimated to lose function at a rate of 1% per year after age 35.

As Vestal advises, we must:

1. Strive for a diagnosis before starting treatment.
2. Take a careful drug history.
3. Know the pharmacology of drugs prescribed.
4. Titrate drug dosage with patient response.
5. Use smaller doses for the elderly.
6. Simplify the therapeutic regimen.
7. Regularly review drugs and treatment plan and stop those not needed.
8. Remember that drugs may cause illness.

When contemplating a new prescription, ask yourself:

1. Does the condition warrant a new treatment modality?
2. Should the new therapy be additive or can it replace some other medication?
3. Will this medication fit into the treatment regimen comfortably?
4. Will the therapeutic schedule confuse the patient?

It is best to start or add only one drug at a time and to begin with a small dose. Newer agents with simpler pharmacokinetics are often easier to use. The triazolobenzodiazepines, for example, have eliminated worry over long-lasting active metabolites as the triazolo ring prevents hepatic metabolism and allows the kid-

neys to excrete these drugs unchanged. Frequent visits with the patient may still be necessary as you gradually increase the dose to an optimal level.

Changing drug therapy for elderly patients is not always easy. They are often resistant to change and may attribute to the medication some mystical properties never described in your PDR. They are often on a fixed income and are understandably displeased when large quantities of medications from an old regimen are discarded, but this is better than allowing them to stockpile and practice self-treatment with outdated and inappropriate drugs.

Patients should be supplied with economical quantities of a medication but should not be allowed indefinite refills. Question your patients about their prescriptions and encourage them to call drugs by their proper names. When a question of drug misuse arises, either accidental or intentional, encourage patients to bring all their medications to the office. This should be a mandatory requirement during posthospital check-up; it is amazing how often some unexpected drugs have crept into the regimen!

An elegant dosing schedule may be sacrificed for a simple one that patients can understand. The newer, more expensive, once-a-day drugs may also be more appropriate for these patients, despite the costs. A significant improvement is the change that has occurred with beta-blockers, allowing once-daily medication for hypertension. If drug expense is a particular concern, breaking scored tablets in half can save some money: production costs are related more to the pill itself than to how much drug it contains.

Pillboxes that can accommodate seven days of therapy are useful for the patient who is mildly confused but can follow a program when medications are laid out a week in advance. The box should have a clear cover with multiple partitions for each day, so that one can easily check how many pills have been taken. It is estimated that up to 25% of hospitalizations of the elderly are caused by medication difficulties. A patient who has been doing poorly at home on his own is often much improved after admission to a hospital or long-

---

Vestal RE: White House Conference on Aging, 1981.

term care facility where a medication routine can be established.

COMMUNITY RESOURCES

Senior Citizen Centers across the country, funded through the Older Americans Act, serve as county-wide resources and focal points for federal programs. Congregate dining, meals on wheels, legal services, and a wide variety of social services for the elderly are also available at these sites.

Public health departments now provide many services to keep patients functioning in their own homes, and alternate-care grants help to finance these activities. Private nursing services may also contract with Medicare for home health aides, physical therapy, and visiting nurse services.

Support groups for seniors and their families are also available in urban areas. The Alzheimer's Disease and Related Disorders Society is the most notable of these. Any physician caring for the elderly should be able to provide names and addresses to assist in arranging additional help for patient and family.

PREVENTIVE MEASURES

Environmental modification and adequate sensory input have already been alluded to and are truly preventive measures. Exercise to preserve mobility and improve cardiovascular tone should be encouraged. Weight loss should be accomplished by dieting and efforts should continue to get patients to stop smoking and maintain control of their blood pressure.

Hypertension in the elderly exists as a disease as well as a physiologic process. What constitutes "normal" can be debated, but evidence suggests that at some point untreated patients have increased mortality and morbidity risks. Kannel estimates that the incidence of congestive heart failure is 8.5 times higher in the elderly male hypertensive patient than in one who is normotensive. The extended Framingham Study has also shown that overall mortality due to cardiovascular disease is higher among hypertensive elderly than among their normotensive counterparts.

Pneumococcal vaccine should be offered to your patients and needs to be given only once. Influenza vaccination should be offered yearly and some attempt should be made to determine tetanus immunization.

THE NURSING HOME

More than 1 million Americans over age 65 are in nursing homes. This group represents only 5% of the elderly population but accounts for more than 25% of their health care expenditures. The primary care physician should be comfortable in the nursing home and cooperative with its staff. Routine nursing home visits enable the physician to keep in touch with the patient, the family and the problems of long-term care.

Although the presence of health care extenders may not be as dominant as predicted in the 1970s, the geriatric nurse practitioner's role in the nursing home is a major development in providing efficient comprehensive care to these patients. For practices with large numbers of long-term care patients, the geriatric nurse practitioner is a logical extension of the office practice. Clinical skills are highly refined and these practitioners provide accurate information and excellent assessments. Their routine rounds at the nursing home reassure the staff, satisfy the family, and prevent unnecessary calls. Hospitalizations are more appropriate and occur when problems are at an early stage of development. Most "teams" using this system work because of the close relationship and trust between the geriatric nurse practitioner and the supervising physician.

SOCIOECONOMIC IMPACT

The elderly represent the most rapidly expanding and demanding group on whom the health care dollar is spent. Medical schools throughout the country are devoting more curriculum time to the aging process and offering senior electives in geriatric medicine, so that partly by selection and partly by training, attitudes toward the care of the elderly are changing. Practicing physicians must take heed of this movement.

The elderly will not go away and will not be disenfranchised. Their demands upon society and medicine must always be met. Whether your patient is a 70-year-old grandmother confined to a wheelchair or an 80-year-old just in from nine holes of golf, the care needs of these people are as varied as their personalities and their backgrounds. As time progresses, the vitality of this group will have an even more dominant effect upon American society.

THEORETICAL CONSIDERATIONS

Man has always been fascinated with youth and survival. Aging is a part of our being and up to now has been an anticipated consequence of our existence. Molecular biologists with their studies on DNA transcription and repair are continuing to wage an assault on the premise that when you get old enough, you can expect to die.

Rat experiments from the 1930s showed that by limiting food intake in early life the animal would live longer. Other studies have yet to conclude that human life span can be modified in this way. A tremendous improvement in infant mortality and childhood deaths has "rectangularized" the human survival curve in developed countries, but this only leaves more individuals vulnerable to chronic disease later in life.

Fries and Crapo have advanced the concept of the "compression of morbidity" to distinguish the morbidity of patients with prototypical lingering chronic illness from that seen in patients with delayed-onset chronic disease. They argue that the ability to postpone chronic disease, taken together with the biologic limits represented by the life span, results in a shortened period between the clinical onset of chronic disease and the end of life. Should this be true, physicians will find healthier older patients who for a relatively short time will require significant supportive and terminal care.

REFERENCES

Covington TR, Walker JI: Current Geriatric Therapy. W.B. Saunders Co, 1984.

Cowley M: The View From 80. Penguin Books, New York, 1980.

Fries JF, Crapo LM: Vitality and Aging. W. H. Freeman & Co, San Francisco, 1981.

Kannel WB: Blood pressure and development of cardiovascular disease in the aged. *In* Caird FI, Dall JL, Kennedy RD (eds): Cardiology in Old Age. Plenum Press, New York, 1976.

Reichel W: Clinical Aspects of Aging. Williams & Wilkins Co, Baltimore, 1983.

Stegner W: The Spectator Bird. Doubleday & Co, Garden City, NY, 1976.

Williams TF: Rehabilitation in the Aging. Raven Press, New York, 1984.

17 · MEDICAL TREATMENT DURING PREGNANCY

Steven Bryan Rouse
GUTHRIE CLINIC

The delivery of a normal, healthy infant is one of the great miracles of nature. Modern obstetrics attempts to provide every newborn with the highest probability of normal physical and mental development. Pregnant women with concurrent diseases are often subject to medical therapy that may have significant bearing on the ultimate outlook of their infants. The use of drugs in pregnancy is an area of specific concern to all physicians.

GENERAL COMMENTS ON DRUGS IN PREGNANCY

The concept of the placental barrier should be abandoned. All drugs known to cross biologic membranes will enter the fetal circulation. Drugs may influence the fetus directly on entering its circulation or indirectly through their effects on placental function. The pharmacodynamics of pregnant women are markedly different from those of nonpregnant patients with respect to many drugs. During pregnancy, mean arterial blood pressure falls, cardiac output rises, intravascular and extravascular fluid (IVF, EVF) volume markedly increases, glomerular filtration rate (GFR) increases, and the hepatic production of many binding proteins is also increased. Standard dosage regimens are inadequate for many drugs such as penicillins, aminoglycosides, and anticonvulsants.

Approximately two thirds of patients take medication at some time during their pregnancies. Often, these are over-the-counter preparations that have been poorly evaluated in pregnant patients and for which the therapeutic indication often is dubious. Little information, at best, is available on most drugs, and there are virtually no data on drug combinations. We all recall the thalidomide experience and should remember that gross abnormalities are probably only the extreme manifestation of drug effect. It took years to associate the marked effects of thalidomide with the drug itself, and the more subtle changes in obstetric outlook related to drug usage may never be recognized. All physicians should try to minimize the use of drugs in pregnancy. A clear indication must be present beforehand, and the risks of not using a drug must be clearly established as greater than those associated with its use. The routine use of over-the-counter preparations by pregnant patients should be discouraged. When drugs *are* prescribed, the dosage must be sufficient for patients' needs. It is essential that all physicians prescribing drugs for pregnant patients have a reference text providing current information on drugs in pregnancy.

ANTIBIOTIC USAGE

As many as 30% to 50% of pregnant women receive antibiotics. Before prescribing the drug, it is necessary to understand the tissue distribution, protein binding and plasma clearance, and potential fetal effects. The GFR markedly increases in pregnancy, clearing the plasma of drugs normally excreted by the kidneys. IVF and EVF volumes increase 30% to 50% in pregnancy, producing a much larger volume for drug distribution. The liver produces a significant increase in drug-binding proteins, thereby decreasing the concentration of free drugs available. Often, because of the physiologic changes in pregnancy, antibiotic dosage recommendations for nongravid patients do not apply. Penicillins, cephalosporins, and aminoglycosides, given orally or parenterally, achieve lower plasma concentrations than in nongravid patients. Plasma levels of drugs, when available, are of tremendous value. In a failed response in a clinical situation, when experience and drug sensitivities indicate that improvement is in order, an increase in dosage may be appropriate.

Virtually all antibiotics readily enter the fetal circulation. The pharmacodynamics of antimicrobials in the fetus is poorly understood because direct measurement of fetal blood levels is not possible. Umbilical cord measurements do not accurately reflect either blood or tissue concentrations in the infant. The half-life of antibiotics is usually longer in the infant than in the mother. Table 1 illustrates commonly used antibiotics and relevant facts about their application in pregnancy.

ANTIHYPERTENSIVE DRUGS

There are physiologic changes in pregnant women that affect the course of hypertensive disease. These women develop a relative insensitivity to angiotensin I and II, and therefore are less sensitive to the endogenous pressor agents. They also experience a significant decrease in peripheral vascular resistance, sufficient to produce a falling mean arterial pressure in the first and second trimester despite the marked increase in cardiac output. This occurs in both hypertensive and normal patients. There is a significant increase in IVF volume throughout pregnancy. Because of the fall in mean arterial pressure, previously hypertensive women are usually normotensive on their first prenatal visit. On subsequent evaluations, blood pressures rise progressively during the third trimester. Previously unrecognized hypertension is not obvious until patients approach term. This allows room for diagnostic errors so that careful, frequent monitoring of the BP, even in routine patients, is essential in the third trimester. Patients on chronic antihypertensive therapy may need dose readjustment as term approaches. Because of the increase in IVF volume, clinical signs such as edema, which would be alarming in normotensive patients, may have little or no significance in gravid women.

Concern for fetal well-being justifies increased monitoring and intervention if diastolic BP is consistently above 85 mm Hg in the second trimester and 90 mm Hg in the third trimester. Many women with mild to moderate chronic hypertension demonstrate normal BP in the first and second trimesters. There is no justification for continuing antihypertensive therapy in patients

Table 1. ANTIBIOTICS IN PREGNANCY

Antibiotic	Dosage Adjustment	Safety	Comments
Penicillins	Increased dosage usually required	Safe No evidence of harm to fetus	For ampicillin and amoxicillin, double standard dosage at usual frequency is appropriate
Erythromycin	Increased dosage usually required	Safe for fetus Do not use estolate salt of erythromycin because of potential hepatotoxicity	Does not appear to prevent congenital syphilis; therefore, if mother is treated with erythromycin, infant should be treated postnatally with penicillin
Nitrofurantoin	Standard doses used	Not teratogenic May cause hemolysis in G6PD-deficient babies	Avoid use in last month of gestation
Aminoglycosides	Usually must give highest recommended dosage per kg to achieve therapeutic blood levels	Only streptomycin is associated with fetal ototoxicity, but caution with all members of this group is warranted	Blood levels are very useful in monitoring dosage
Sulfonamides	No alteration in dosage required	Theoretically increases risk of kernicterus because of displacement of bilirubin from albumin No teratogenicity documented	Do not use in third trimester
Metronidazole	No alteration in dosage required	Mutagenic in rodents Although not clearly teratogenic, caution is advised Do not use in first trimester	Clotrimazole cream often gives relief from *Trichomonas* infection in pregnancy
Trimethoprim-sulfamethoxazole	No alteration in dosage required	Teratogenicity of other folate antagonists has led to avoidance of this drug combination in pregnancy	Used widely in other countries in pregnancy
Chloramphenicol	No alteration in dosage required	Contraindicated No congenital defects associated with drug's use, but lethal "gray baby" syndrome from neonatal exposure	Most workers consider that drug is not indicated in pregnancy
Tetracyclines	No alteration in dosage required	Not safe owing to teratogenicity, neonatal dental discoloration, and maternal hepatotoxicity	Alternative drugs are almost always more suitable

whose BP is normal on presentation for prenatal care. If diastolic BP is less than 85 mm Hg, I prefer to stop all antihypertensive drugs at the first prenatal visit. Patients are then carefully instructed in techniques of BP measurement, and requested to record lateral recumbent BP twice daily. Office visits are set at two-week intervals. Patients are told to call if diastolic BP remains above 90 mm Hg on two occasions more than six hours apart.

PREECLAMPSIA

The risk of superimposed preeclampsia is very high in patients with a history of essential hypertension, especially if combined with evidence of renal impairment. A 24-hour protein excretion and creatinine clearance is measured in the first trimester and repeated at eight-week intervals for recognition of any compromise in renal function. If BP remains consistently below 140/90 mm Hg on home monitoring, patients are carefully followed at home. If BP rises above this level or if there is significant proteinuria (1+ or over on routine urinalysis), patients are admitted to the hospital for strict bed rest. A baseline 24-hour urine protein check is repeated; this should be less than 300 mg/L for 24 hours. Proteinuria exceeding 300 mg/L for 24 hours usually suggests preeclampsia superimposed on chronic hypertension, justifying careful observation and aggressive management. If BP stabilizes at normal on rest in the hospital, patients may be discharged on continued rest at home to record blood BP three times daily. They are seen at least twice a week in the office to review the BP log, assess fetal well-being, and evaluate for albuminuria. If

BP rises further they are readmitted, often for the remainder of the pregnancy.

DRUG THERAPY

BP above 100 mm Hg diastolic on bed rest justifies antihypertensives in chronic hypertensive patients. Methyldopa is started at 750 to 1000 mg per day in divided doses. This usually suffices, although 1500 mg per day is not unusual. If higher doses of methyldopa are insufficient, 25 mg of hydralazine is added three times daily. These two agents are chosen because we have the greatest experience in treating hypertension in pregnancy with these. They enter the fetal circulation but are not known to produce fetal anomalies.

There is virtually no place for diuretics in the management of hypertension in pregnancy. They reduce edema, but this is of little or no benefit. They are reserved for the treatment of serious cardiac disease in pregnancy. There is very little evidence that antihypertensive therapy prevents the superimposition of preeclampsia on hypertensive vascular disease. Careful monitoring for the early manifestation of this dreaded complication is absolutely essential.

Although the safety of beta-blocking agents has not been established in pregnancy, I sometimes discontinue hydralazine and substitute propranolol, 40 to 80 mg twice a day. Labetalol, an agent with both alpha- and beta-blocking properties, has been extensively used in Europe in pregnancy hypertension (200 to 400 mg twice a day). In the severe, chronic hypertensive group, perinatal mortality is high and careful fetal monitoring is justified. Clinical and ultrasound assessment of fetal growth is essential. Serum estriol levels are taken and weekly stress tests are made in the third trimester. If severe preeclampsia occurs, the infant must be delivered regardless of the gestational age. If maternal BP status is stable but critical, time of delivery is dictated by amniocentesis to establish the degree of fetal lung maturity.

ANTICOAGULANT THERAPY

Pregnancy is relatively thrombogenic, and thrombotic phenomena are a major cause of maternal morbidity and mortality. Because of venous stasis and a relatively increased coagulability associated with pregnancy, the gravid woman at risk of thromboembolic disease must be treated prophylactically. Candidates for therapy are those with a prosthetic heart valve, atrial fibrillation, a history of documented iliofemoral thrombosis, or pulmonary emboli. If there is a possibility of deep venous thrombosis, Doppler and impedance plethysmography are used to assess the iliofemoral veins (see Chap. 14, Figs. 1 and 2). If abnormality is detected, the patient is treated prophylactically; if not, she is followed with repeat vascular examinations but no therapy.

I prefer to avoid oral anticoagulants. Bishydroxycoumarin (Dicumarol) crosses the placenta and is associated with fetal anomalies when used in the first trimester. It also exerts an anticoagulant effect on the fetus and markedly increases the risk of intracranial bleeding if vaginal delivery is allowed in the third trimester. Heparin does not cross the placenta because of its large molecular size and negative charge; it is fairly simple to use and is easily monitored. Hemorrhage is the most important risk of heparin use, but thrombocytopenia and osteoporosis, although uncommon, are also encountered. Patients with acute thrombotic events are heparinized therapeutically in the hospital via standard, continuous infusions for approximately seven days. Over a two- to three-day period, the patient is then switched to subcutaneous heparin on a twelve-hourly regimen. For prophylaxis and long-term therapy, 150 to 250 units per kg every 12 hours SQ usually keep the partial thromboplastin time (PTT) at 1½ times control. One week after discharge a PTT and platelet count are performed and repeated twice monthly after stabilization. The usual warnings and instructions should be given while the patient is on anticoagulants, especially regarding the avoidance of aspirin and acetaminophen. The required dose of heparin increases for many patients as the pregnancy progresses.

DELIVERY

Anticoagulant therapy at the time of delivery in patients on long-term SQ heparin is straightforward. For planned cesarean sections, the patient is admitted 48 hours in advance and switched to a continuous IV infusion, which is discontinued two to three hours before the procedure. Forty-eight hours after the cesarean section, continuous heparin therapy is reinstituted for approximately seven days. The patient is then discharged on an SQ program identical to the prenatal dose-adjusted heparin protocol for the next six weeks.

For planned vaginal delivery, a similar protocol is used except that the infusion is discontinued at onset of induction of labor.

ANTICONVULSANTS

Seizure disorders are probably the most common neurologic problem encountered in everyday practice by the obstetrician. Congenital anomalies occur at an increased rate in patients with seizure disorders who are on anticonvulsants. The relationship to specific drug use has been difficult to clarify in the past because of the multiple drugs often taken by these patients.

Phenytoin is associated with the fetal hydantoin syndrome: intrauterine growth retardation, craniofacial anomalies, hypoplasia and ossification of the distal phalanges, optic nerve hypoplasia, and mental retardation. The teratogenic potential of phenobarbital is less certain. Barbiturate withdrawal is possible in the newborn and the attending pediatrician should be aware of the antepartum use of phenobarbital.

Higher doses of anticonvulsants are required to prevent seizures. Measurement of drug levels and dosage adjustment may be required throughout pregnancy.

No woman should receive anticonvulsants in pregnancy unless there are clear indications. A patient who has been free of seizures for years should be taken off the drugs before she conceives, if at all possible. Women with seizure disorders should be fully informed of the reproductive consequences of anticonvulsants before they conceive. Pregnant women on phenytoin may experience a depletion of vitamin K factors, and are usually given 10 mg parenteral vitamin K (phytonadione) weekly for the last month of gestation and when admitted to the labor suite. The newborn is also treated after delivery.

DIABETES

Insulin is the only agent useful for maintaining normal blood sugar levels in a pregnant patient. Oral hypoglycemics should not be used. Recognition and management of the so-called gestational diabetic is controversial and is not discussed here. My colleagues and I prescribe an appropriate diet for all women who have a documented glucose intolerance in pregnancy with fasting blood sugar levels over 100 mg/dL and/or two-hour postprandial blood sugar levels over 150 mg/dL.

For the insulin-dependent diabetic, euglycemia is essential. Patients should be euglycemic at the time of conception, an important consideration in the family planning of diabetic women. The risks of diabetes, including congenital anomalies, are markedly reduced by maintaining strict euglycemia.

Careful home monitoring of blood sugar is important, and a reflectance colorimeter is far more accurate than urine testing. The patient is carefully taught all aspects of management of diabetes in pregnancy, and actively participates in dosage decisions. Blood sugar measurements are performed before breakfast and two hours postprandially throughout the day, several times weekly, and recorded in a log book for examination by the physician on prenatal visits. Fasting morning blood sugar levels are kept below 100 mg/dL and two-hour postprandial levels below 150 to 160 mg/dL. Twice daily dosage of insulin, using regular and NPH, is given before breakfast and before the evening meal: roughly two thirds in the morning. Approximately twice as much NPH as regular insulin is usually required. Patients are seen twice monthly for assessment of fetal growth and examination of the blood sugar log book, and are encouraged to call for advice if questions about dosage arise.

Fetal hyperinsulinemia related to maternal hyperglycemia is the source of fetal and neonatal complications. Patients are usually reassured that transient hypoglycemia has little effect on the infant. Hyperglycemia is the condition to be avoided. Symptomatic hypoglycemia may be effectively treated by 6 or 8 oz of skimmed milk, which corrects the problem without the large swings in blood sugar often associated with orange juice or soft drinks.

All patients with long-standing diabetes, especially those with retinal or renal disease, are assessed by an ophthalmologist within the first trimester and then at appropriate intervals if retinal disease is encountered. Proliferative retinopathy developing during the pregnancy is treated by laser therapy. A 24-hour urinalysis for protein determination and creatinine clearance is made at eight to 12 weeks' gestation, and repeated at four- to six-week intervals to detect any renal involvement. Patients with any evidence of renal disease are instructed on twice daily BP measurement.

Any complication such as pyelonephritis, more than 1+ proteinuria, hypertension, or unsatisfactory fetal growth is an indication for hospitalization. Noncompliant patients are often admitted for regulation by the medical staff.

Assessment of fetal well-being in a diabetic patient is essential. Gestational dates are confirmed by ultrasound at 16 weeks, and repeated at four- to six-week intervals. In the last trimester, ultrasound examinations and serial determination of the symphysis fundal height are essential to rule out intrauterine growth retardation or fetal macrosomia. Daily estriol determinations have been found of value in predicting impending fetal problems, but are expensive and subject to great variation; I generally obtain them only for poorly controlled patients with clearly increased fetal risk. Nonstress and oxytocin challenge tests are extremely important in establishing fetal well-being, on a weekly basis in the last six to eight weeks before delivery.

DELIVERY

The timing and method of delivery of infants of diabetic mothers are highly individualized. Delivery takes place at 36 to 38 weeks' gestation if both maternal and fetal well-being is established. Fetal lung maturity is first confirmed by amniocentesis. If the cervix is unripe, some physicians perform a cesarean section. However, 5 mg of prostaglandin in gel applied directly to the cervix the night before induction is very effective and safe, provided that the infant is carefully monitored during the ensuing uterine contractions. If concern for fetal or maternal well-being is the reason for hospitalization, delivery is usually effected without regard to lung maturity at any time after 34 weeks. Cesarean section is often the safest course in these patients.

Intrapartum insulin management is greatly simplified by a constant insulin infusion. A 5% dextrose solution in normal saline is administered at 125 cc per hour during induction of labor. All other solutions, used in infusing other medications, should be free of dextrose or other sugars. One unit of regular insulin per hour is infused, and blood sugars are initially obtained at hourly intervals. Maternal blood sugar is kept between 70 and 90 mm/dL. After delivery of the placenta, a 10% dextrose solution at 100 cc per hour for approximately eight hours is given to prevent maternal hypoglycemia. If preoperative blood sugar is normal, no insulin is given before planned cesarean section. Avoidance of sugar-containing solutions is important until the cord is clamped, to prevent neonatal hypoglycemia. In the recovery room, blood sugar is immediately measured and constant insulin infusion is initiated.

The above recommendations for insulin management are simple and usually highly effective, but dietary instructions to the diabetic, pregnant woman are critical. I prefer not to make recommendations on the basis of ideal body weight. Usually 1800 to 2400 calories are required for sustained weight gain in pregnancy. An American Diabetic Association diet is used. The higher caloric intakes are used for larger women, dietary intake being individualized on the basis of daily activity, maternal body size, and weight gain in pregnancy. At present, I do not recommend the use of aspartame in pregnancy, pending further clarification of its safety.

REFERENCES

Briggs GG: Drugs in Pregnancy and Lactation: A Reference Guide to Fetal and Neonatal Risk. Williams & Wilkins Co, Baltimore, 1983.
Rayburn W, Suspan FP: Drug Therapy in Obstetrics and Gynecology. Appleton-Century-Crofts, New York, 1982.

HELLP Syndrome

Alfred G. Robichaux III

OCHSNER CLINIC AND ALTON OCHSNER MEDICAL FOUNDATION

DEFINITION AND DIAGNOSTIC CRITERIA

The HELLP syndrome was first described in 1982 as a complication in pregnant patients. The acronym "HELLP" signifies the characteristic abnormalities of the syndrome: "H" for hemolysis, "EL" for elevated liver function, and "LP" for low platelet counts. This acronym was designed to call attention to this variant of preeclampsia, which is frequently confused with GI diseases and which, if misdiagnosed, may prove fatal for mother and baby. Preeclampsia is a well-known entity in obstetrics, occurring most commonly during a first pregnancy. Severe preeclampsia is defined as (1) BP of 160/110 on two occasions more than six hours apart, (2) proteinuria greater than 5 gm in 24 hours, (3) oliguria, (4) cerebral or visual disturbances, and (5) pulmonary edema or cyanosis. "Eclampsia is the occurrence of convulsions, not caused by coincidental neurologic disease such as epilepsy, in a woman whose condition also fulfills the criteria for preeclampsia" (Pritchard et al, 1980).

The diagnosis of HELLP syndrome should be suspected in any pregnant patient complaining of malaise or epigastric pain.

PATHOPHYSIOLOGY

The exact underlying pathophysiology is not well understood but is thought to be within the spectrum of severe, pregnancy-induced hypertension. It is a state of vasospasm probably mediated by a defect in the prostaglandin pathways.

CLINICAL ASPECTS

The HELLP syndrome represents a medical emergency. Primigravid women are affected slightly more often than multigravid women. The syndrome may occur from 24 weeks of pregnancy on. Patients usually present with specific complaints of "not feeling well" (aside from the usual discomforts of pregnancy) and of epigastric or right upper quadrant pain. Elevated BP is not a reliable finding. The most frequent differential diagnosis is (1) pancreatitis, (2) acute cholecystitis, (3) acute fatty liver of pregnancy, or (4) hemolytic uremic syndrome. All too often, precious time is lost in the work-up of these other diagnoses.

MANAGEMENT

Confirmation of the HELLP syndrome is an indication for immediate hospitalization to perform baseline laboratory assessment, with the ultimate goal of terminating the pregnancy as soon as the patient has been stabilized.

Bed rest, with the patient lying in the left lateral recumbent position, has been a cornerstone of therapy to prolong pregnancies complicated by pregnancy-induced hypertension. The same treatment applies for HELLP syndrome while the patient is being stabilized.

LABORATORY EVALUATION

A quick dipstick test of the urine usually detects proteinuria, 2+ or greater. The patient should be directly admitted to the labor and delivery area. Intravenous infusion is started and complete blood count, including platelet count, and biochemical screening profile obtained. A peripheral smear should be examined immediately for evidence of hemolysis. The CBC usually indicates a state of hemoconcentration unless there is severe hemolysis. A hemoglobin level below 10 gm/dL is an indication for transfusion with packed red cells. There will be abnormally elevated liver function study results and, if the disease has reached an advanced stage, elevated BUN and creatinine. Hypoglycemia is a very ominous finding as it reflects impending liver failure and coma. Platelet counts of less than 100,000 per cu mm are an indication for immediate delivery.

DRUG THERAPY

Magnesium sulfate should be administered initially as a bolus of 2 to 4 gm in 250 ml of 5% glucose in water over 20 minutes, and then a continuous drip of 1 to 2 gm per hour. Hydralazine (Apresoline) should be the initial drug of choice for severe hypertension.

We use magnesium sulfate to prevent seizures and Apresoline to control BP in efforts to stabilize the patient while preparing for delivery. Therapeutic levels of magnesium sulfate are 5 to 7 mEq/ml. As magnesium sulfate levels in the blood increase over 8 mEq/ml, deep tendon reflexes decrease. Above 10 to 12 mEq/ml, respirations decrease; above 12 to 14 mEq/ml, respiratory and cardiac arrest may occur. Apresoline may result in hypotension and reflexive tachycardia. It is still the best antihypertensive agent because of the ease of titration with BP and because it does not decrease uterine blood flow.

Since magnesium sulfate is metabolized by the kidneys, we insert a Foley catheter to monitor urine output when administering this drug. If urine output falls, the dose of magnesium sulfate should be decreased.

TERMINATING PREGNANCY

The pregnancy should be terminated by the most technically feasible method. A period of short inductions should be attempted if the cervix is favorable, but if it is unfavorable or induction is prolonged, cesarean section is indicated. The rate of perinatal mortality is surprisingly low for the degree of prematurity encountered. It is unwise to delay delivery in an attempt to accelerate the degree of fetal maturity by corticosteroid therapy.

The postpartum period is managed by Pritchard's 30/30 rule, "Keep the hematocrit above 30% and the urine output above 30 cc/hr." Fresh-frozen plasma should be used for any clotting problems. Platelet transfusions are not usually indicated unless the platelet count is less than 50,000 per cubic millimeter. The blood count will probably be much lower than anticipated from the estimated blood loss at delivery because of hemolysis. Appropriate replacement with packed red blood cells is indicated. The magnesium infusion should be continued for 24 hours. Accurate assessment of urinary input and output is necessary. It usually takes 24 to 72 hours for the patient to reach stable clinical conditions. Abnormal liver function studies and platelet counts usually return to normal rapidly.

PATIENT INFORMATION AND EDUCATION

The HELLP syndrome appears to affect women from all socioeconomic backgrounds. A patient thought to be a candidate for pregnancy-induced hypertension should be instructed to begin a bed rest program and to report any rapid increase in weight gain, headache, or epigastric distress. She should be seen more often than is laid down in the traditional schedule of obstetric visits.

There is no known preventive measure for pregnancy-induced hypertension or its variant, HELLP syndrome, and at present there is no known evidence of predisposition for this disease in subsequent pregnancies.

REFERENCES

Goodlin RC: Severe pre-eclampsia: another great imitator. Am J Obstet Gynecol 125:747–753, 1976.

Pritchard JA, Cunningham FG, Mason RA: Coagulation changes in eclampsia: their frequency and pathogenesis. Am J Obstet Gynecol 124:855–864, 1976.

Pritchard JA, MacDonald PC, Gant NF: Williams' Obstetrics, 16th ed. Appleton-Century-Crofts, New York, 1980, p 665.

Weinstein L: Syndrome of hemolysis, elevated liver enzymes, and low platelet count: a severe consequence of hypertension in pregnancy. Am J Obstet Gynecol 142:159–167, 1982.

18 · THE PRACTICE OF BRIEF PSYCHOTHERAPY

Steven I. Pfeiffer
OCHSNER CLINIC AND ALTON OCHSNER MEDICAL FOUNDATION

Many patients seeking medical attention suffer from underlying emotional problems. Often a socioemotional problem masquerades as a physical complaint, and it is not uncommon for patients to turn to their physician for help with their mental health.

It is estimated that the prevalence of mental illness in primary care settings is as high as 14% to 22%, and that more than 50% of patients seeking medical consultation present both functional and organic dysfunction. Primary care physicians can expect many of their patients to complain of anxiety, depression, work-related stress, drug and alcohol abuse, obesity, marital discord, family dysfunction, child management problems, or vague somatic problems.

Brief psychotherapy affords a supportive and accepting atmosphere in which the physician can help patients find more effective ways of mastering their problems and life circumstances. The primary care physician who incorporates brief psychotherapy into his medical practice can assist many patients with transient or mild psychologic disorders.

There are well over 200 different schools of psychotherapy, each with its own, albeit overlapping, conceptualization of health and mental illness, therapeutic techniques, and treatment goals. Brief psychotherapy encompasses many divergent approaches, all of which share three basic attributes. First, therapy focuses primarily on the conscious and here-and-now, rather than probing the unconscious or past. Second, treatment goals are limited to the relief of symptoms, in conjunction with modification of patients' attitudes and behavior. No attempt is made to change basic character structure. Third, the physician's posture and techniques are of necessity action oriented, with an emphasis on promoting experimentation with new and more adaptive behavior. No deliberate attempt is made to search for underlying psychic trauma or conflict. Physicians who practice brief psychotherapy utilize little or no dream material, transference manifestations, or free associations. Treatment generally is limited to no more than six to eight 30- to 45-minute sessions. Successful outcome is defined as modifying or eliminating existing symptomatology, furnishing new and more extended perspectives, and providing support and direction to alternative patterns of interpersonal behavior.

Wolberg views all schools of psychotherapy as forms of personal influence in which emotional problems are treated by trained persons who establish professional relationships with their patients. Strupp argues that ''. . . good psychotherapy of whatever description results in an emotional and cognitive restructuring of the patients' view of themselves, others, and reality.'' Whether one perceives psychotherapy as an exercise in advising, educating, guiding, coaching, influencing, or treating, a successful outcome should provide patients with a corrective emotional experience that reorganizes their attitudes and assumptions about themselves and their world, and affords them alternative means for engaging in constructive behavior change.

The physician who adheres to a biopsychosocial model of illness and is interested, comfortable, and skilled in providing counseling services in his practice will find brief psychotherapy useful. It is cost effective and requires considerably less psychiatric training or technical skill than the more intensive, depth-oriented reconstructive approaches. Also, brief psychotherapy consists of a circumscribed, structured series of sessions that avoids iatrogenic complications such as negative therapeutic responses, secondary gain, and unmanageable patient transference.

THE PROCESS OF BRIEF PSYCHOTHERAPY

In my view, brief psychotherapy consists of five interrelated, dynamic stages or phases of treatment. The first entails an *initial assessment* of the problem, including an appraisal of personality variables, family and environmental factors, and possible contraindications (i.e., patients not ideally suited for short-term psychotherapy). The second stage reflects an evolving emphasis on the development of a *working therapeutic relationship* and formation of a *therapeutic contract.* During this second stage, which can occur as early as the first session, the physician seeks to arouse positive patient expectations and motivation, gain the patient's confidence and commitment to the conditions of therapy, and clarify misconceptions. The physician also enters into developing, in collaboration with the patient, a behavioral contract that specifies the projected number of sessions, the procedures and their rationale, expected benefits, and possible discomfort and risks the patient may reasonably be expected to experience, and the limits of confidentiality.

The third stage of treatment, generally considered the grist of psychotherapy, begins with *planned change efforts.* The physician actively employs psychotherapeutic tasks, techniques, and assignments to create incentives for behavioral change. Patients are helped to understand their perceptions, feelings, and actions and are simultaneously prompted to give up maladaptive responses while experimenting with more adaptive behavior. Commonly used techniques particularly well suited for brief psychotherapy include biofeedback, homework assignments, hypnosis, relaxation training, role rehearsal, and systematic desensitization. Wolberg's excellent compendium describes a variety of technical procedures.

Psychotherapeutic techniques do not exist either in isolation from the person of the therapist or apart from the complex interpersonal features of the therapeutic encounter. Strupp aptly states that any psychotherapy, including behavior therapy, is always a very human endeavor and can never be a purely technical enterprise.

As brief psychotherapy progresses, the physician quite often encounters resistance to change. The fourth stage entails *identifying patient resistance* and *monitoring the relative success of the planned interventions.* The fourth stage can occur as soon as planned change efforts are initiated, and serves an important feedback function in keeping patient and physician on task. The physician continually examines whether the patient is meeting the agreed objectives and expectations for meaningful change.

Like the preceding four stages, the fifth and final stage, *termination,* should occur in a planned and deliberate fashion. Patients should be afforded the opportunity to survey progress, explore the degree to which they have attained the goals specified during development of the therapeutic contract, and evaluate how they plan to maintain improvement after therapy ends. Termination should be viewed by the patient not as an end point, but as the springboard for more independent intra- and interpersonal growth.

ASSESSMENT OF THE PATIENT

Systematic and thorough assessment is crucial to successful outcome in brief psychotherapy. Unfortunately, the greatest obstacle to a comprehensive clinical picture of the patient's psychosocial, emotional, and mental status is the physician's reluctance to ask questions that may elicit highly personal and potentially embarrassing material.

The initial assessment needs to include a careful delineation of symptomatic and functional problems; possible environmental, family, and occupational factors contributing to the referral problem; the presence of apparent secondary gain (see below); the degree of distress and anxiety; and personal assets and resources available to the patient. Early in the initial session the physician should determine the degree of emergency, whether psychotropic medication should be combined with psychotherapy, and whether brief psychotherapy is preferable to no treatment or to an alternative (and possibly less expensive) social intervention.

Ansteh and Hipskind and Frank both provide descriptions of patient qualities that predispose to a favorable response to brief psychotherapy. They include the following questions: Can the patient benefit from four to eight sessions? Is the patient reasonably intelligent and verbally adroit? Does the patient appear dependable, nonimpulsive, and trusting? Does the patient present a high degree of motivation to change, and accept that his problem is psychologic in nature? Does the patient bring to the session a history of previous, meaningful interpersonal relationships and successes in other endeavors? Is the presenting problem of relatively brief duration, and is there one or more identifiable acute precipitants? Is the patient experiencing enough distress to want to change, and can he tolerate a moderate degree of anxiety?

To this list I would add the following five criteria: Is the patient self-observant and psychologically minded? Does the patient share the same values as the physician? Is the patient capable of separation from the physician and therapy at termination? Can the patient be expected to benefit enough from short-term psychotherapy not to require long-term or maintenance treatment? And finally, what is the physician's internal response to the patient and his presenting problem (including whether the patient evokes obvious countertransference feelings in the physician such as hostility, sympathy, revulsion, pity, or sexual attraction).

It is equally important during the first contact to consider patients who are poor candidates or high risks for a negative response to brief psychotherapy. Those who strongly suggest an unfavorable outcome include:

1. Patients presenting organic brain syndromes, acute psychoses (manic depression and schizophrenia), or severe personality disorders (the antisocial, avoidant, borderline, histrionic, hypochondriacal, narcissistic, paranoid, and sociopathic).

2. Patients with alcohol and drug dependence.

3. Patients displaying only marginal to weak ego strength and with a history of poor personal and occupational involvements.

4. Depressed patients with family histories of suicide or who have experienced a recent suicide by a friend or acquaintance.

5. Patients presenting primarily somatic complaints or factitious illness.

6. Patients who enter treatment primarily for secondary gain (i.e., secondary advantages accruing from an illness, such as gratification of dependency yearnings).

7. Patients with a poor response to previous psychotherapy.

8. Patients who enter psychotherapy under duress or threat (from school authorities, occupation, etc.).

These types of patients are poor candidates for short-term counseling because they are either too disorganized, debilitated, distrustful, or impulse ridden or anxious to develop a working therapeutic alliance in a few brief sessions. Their emotional problems generally reflect chronic and deeply entrenched conditions that are more responsive to long-term psychiatric treatment.

Assessment should also include an appraisal of patients' expectations. Patients enter counseling anticipating that psychotherapy will help them accept their troublesome feelings and behavior, remold their personalities, exorcise evil thoughts and actions, provide instruction in more righteous or moral living, and afford a friend, lover, or surrogate parent. One of the physician's early tasks is to clarify patients' expectations and bring them in line with what can be reasonably expected given the evolving therapeutic contract.

CREATION OF A FACILITATIVE THERAPEUTIC CLIMATE

Brief psychotherapy shares with most other schools of therapy the need for the physician to establish a secure, permissive, and confidential atmosphere in which patients can feel comfortable while freely discussing their innermost thoughts and feelings. It is very important for patients to be able to express themselves candidly and unreservedly without worrying whether their ideas, actions, or emotions are perceived as banal, comical, offensive, or bizarre.

An accumulating body of research has consistently found a number of nonspecific or extratherapeutic facilitative conditions that create a positive climate for change. The physician must convey acceptance and reassurance, concern, understanding, respect, kindness, an accurate empathy and nonpossessive warmth, and an ability to guide and instruct without moralizing. The physician must also be attuned to the nonverbal communications and multi-level messages of his patient and be acutely aware of his own values, biases, and predilections so that they don't intrude into his therapeutic work. He must be able to comfortably tolerate divergent ideas that may conflict with his own belief system. Finally, the physician needs to possess a compassion for human suffering, misery, and interpersonal failings.

Strupp, a prominent researcher in the field of psychotherapeutic outcome, contends that facilitative conditions are absolutely indispensable for good therapeutic outcome. He has found that successful therapists possess a gentleness and proclivity to comfort and not hurt, a deep desire to help the patient become more autonomous and competent, and the ability to listen actively and immerse themselves in their patient's inner world, life experiences, and current conflict.

If brief psychotherapy is to be successful, the nonspecific facilitative ingredients common to all forms of psychotherapy—hope; trust; freedom to express oneself; a view of the therapist as an empathic, compassionate, and nonjudgmental helping professional; and an emotional catharsis—must all be operative. The efficacy of brief psychotherapy relies in large part on the quality of the therapeutic climate that serves as the context in which technical interventions can be introduced.

ROLE REHEARSAL: AN ILLUSTRATIVE THERAPEUTIC TECHNIQUE

Role rehearsal is one of the many techniques ideally suited to brief psychotherapy. Space permits a discussion of only this one procedure, but the physician should not rely on only one technique. Maslow's warning should be heeded: if the only tool you have is a hammer, you tend to treat everything as if it were a nail. One further precautionary note bears mentioning: that for any technical intervention to succeed, both the timing and the therapist-patient relationship must be right.

Role play or role rehearsal can be used with individuals, couples, or families and combines behavioral, gestalt, family systems, and transactional analysis principles. The enactments are structured by the physician to give patients the opportunity to try out new behaviors, resolve internal conflicts, and gain greater insight into how they think, feel, and behave in situations that have created problems for them in the past.

Top Dog-Underdog Dialogue. This type of role simulation is best applied with patients embroiled in neurotic conflicts involving opposing impulses or feelings. The physician can suggest to the patient that he enact each part of the conflict in turn by means of a dialogue. During the role play, the physician encourages the patient to emphasize, exaggerate, or even repeat a particular aspect of the enactment to help clarify or bring into focus a significant dynamic. This type of drama often evolves into a "top dog-underdog" dialogue that allows the patient to express an unresolved conflict. These typically reflect harsh, parent/superego demands at variance with infantile, child/id impulses. Enactments should be brief, without extensive preliminary preparation, and the patient should be prompted to exchange roles.

The Empty Chair. A related role simulation procedure, the empty chair, is appropriate when patients are experiencing conflict with or ambivalent feelings toward an important person in their lives. Patients are urged to sit facing the empty chair and express, in the security of the therapy setting, their innermost feelings toward the figure that the chair represents. The physician provides feedback, recommends alternative tactful and assertive ways of expressing communications, and allows for reinforced practice of these new skills.

Sculpting. One final variant of role rehearsal, sculpting, is best applied with couples and families. The physician structures the actual physical positions of each participant in relation to the underlying theme being dealt with in therapy. During the sculpting activity, individuals enact their assigned roles, such as bossy, meek, clingy, demanding, distant, rebellious, or scapegoat. The physician provides feedback, direction, and encouragement much as a drama director. The benefits of these three interventions include providing expanded awareness, insight, catharsis, and simulated practice with new interpersonal behaviors.

ETHICS, CONFIDENTIALITY, AND PROFESSIONAL OBJECTIVITY

The establishment of a positive, therapeutic climate for change requires a *relationship of trust* between patient and physician, and this alliance must be carefully protected through the course of the therapeutic experience. The American Psychiatric Association is sensitive to the special ethical problems inherent in psychotherapy and has appended an annotation to the AMA *Principles of Medical Ethics.*

INFORMED CONSENT

The concept of informed consent for psychotherapy is particularly relevant to the establishment of a relationship of trust with the patient. For consent to be informed, patients must possess relevant information regarding the procedures to be performed, the physician's qualifications as a psychotherapist, the discomforts or risks reasonably to be expected, the benefits reasonably to be expected, alternatives to brief psychotherapy that might provide similar benefits, and a freedom to withdraw consent and discontinue participation in treatment. For patients considered legally incompetent, such as minors, substitute informed consent from parents should be obtained.

CONFIDENTIALITY

Confidentiality refers to the uses of information obtained during psychotherapy. The Hippocratic oath requires a clear and unmistakable "duty of silence," which in most instances of brief psychotherapy practiced in the physician's office is a reasonable ethical standard. However, the seemingly straightforward confidentiality principle can become somewhat more ambiguous and complex when the physician works with couples and families. Additionally, the physician should be expected to divulge confidential material under the following four conditions: (1) if a criminal action is (potentially) involved, (2) if the information is made an issue in a court action, (3) if the information is obtained for the purpose of rendering an expert opinion to a lawyer, and (4) if the physician is acting in a court-appointed capacity.

COUNTERTRANSFERENCE

The physician experiences a range of emotions and reactions toward his patients, some more realistic than others. The physician-as-therapist must examine his feelings critically to ensure that a countertransference response is not developing. I have found it useful to ask myself the following questions before and after each therapy session: How do I feel about the patient? Am I obtaining pleasure out of seeing the patient? Do I overidentify with, feel sorry for, or become angry with the patient? Do I want to protect, reject, punish, or control the patient?

The physician needs to appreciate when he may be reacting to the patient on the basis of intensely personal feelings that may interfere with his helping the patient. For example, a physician who has recently divorced and is finding it hard to handle his own sexual feelings may unconsciously inhibit the patient's expression of sexual material brought up during the session. The physician may unwittingly change the topic, appear disinterested, underreact to the patient's communication, and reinforce less personally sensitive material with differential attention and interest.

In some instances, the physician may simply not be the "right" therapist for a particular patient. At other times, the physician may find that a patient is not suited to brief psychotherapy and requires more intensive, long-term treatment. Finally, some patients are simply not ready for psychotherapy when first seen by the physician. These three types of patients all require the physician's support, with the assurance that he will refer the first two groups of patients to an alternative therapist and that he will be available to the third group when they are ready to enter into therapy.

SUMMARY

Brief psychotherapy is an action-oriented intervention system. It requires that the therapist develop a working therapeutic relationship and behavioral contract with the patient and establish a facilitative therapeutic climate in which planned interventions can be introduced. Careful initial assessment and ongoing monitoring of patient resistance and the relative success of the planned change effects reinforce the short-term, goal-oriented nature of this approach.

Brief psychotherapy can provide patients with strategies for abandoning unrealistic fears and troubling impulses, techniques for getting along better with themselves and others, and procedures for enhancing feelings of self-acceptance and efficacy.

REFERENCES

American Medical Association: The Principles of Medical Ethics: With Annotations Especially Applicable to Psychiatry. American Psychiatric Association, Washington, DC, 1978.

Ansteh R, Hipskind M: Selecting patients for brief office counseling. J Fam Pract 13:195–199, 1981.

Arnold JF, Chapman RJ: The primary care physician and psychotherapy. In Rakel RE (ed): Textbook of Family Practice, 3rd ed. W.B. Saunders Co, Philadelphia, 1984, pp 1330–1347.

Frank JD: Persuasion and Healing: A Comparative Study of Psychotherapy. Johns Hopkins Press, Baltimore, 1973.

Maslow AH: Toward a Psychology of Being, 2nd ed. Van Nostrand, Princeton, NJ, 1968.

Strupp HS: A psychodynamicist looks at modern behavior therapy. Psychother: Ther Res Pract 16:124–131, 1979.

Wolberg LR: The Technique of Psychotherapy (2 vols), 3rd ed. Grune & Stratton, New York, 1977.

19 · PERIOPERATIVE MEDICAL MANAGEMENT

Jeffery P. Frey
James McCullough
OCHSNER CLINIC AND ALTON OCHSNER MEDICAL FOUNDATION

The role of the physician in the care of surgical patients is not readily apparent. Skill in identifying disease at an early stage and in managing nonsurgical problems in the perioperative period makes the physician a valuable asset. The physician can also help surgeon and patient weigh the relative risks versus benefits of a surgical procedure by providing a comprehensive view of the patient's total health.

INCIDENCE OF PERIOPERATIVE COMPLICATIONS

The incidence of operative and postoperative death is approximately 0.3% and has shown continuous decline. Of these deaths, 10% occur with induction of anesthesia, 35% during the actual operative procedure, and 55% in the 48 hours following surgery. The leading causes are respiratory failure, aspiration of gastric contents, sudden cardiac difficulty (due either to pump failure or to arrhythmia), and hypovolemic shock (usually secondary to hemorrhage). The relative incidence of each of these has remained between 10% and 15% despite the decline in overall mortality. Hypoxia has been estimated to play a role in about 50% of anesthetic deaths.

Death in the postoperative period has not been well studied: studies are anecdotal, retrospective, and sometimes contradictory. Several studies have been skewed because of the inclusion of high-risk and elderly populations. Clearly, the overall death rate has also declined. The principal cause of postoperative death is myocardial infarction, often painless, which may present as congestive heart failure or malignant arrhythmia. The combined mortality from pulmonary emboli, pneumonias, sepsis, and other causes contributes less to the total than does death from cardiogenic causes.

EVALUATION OF THE HEALTHY PATIENT

In a study of cost effectiveness, the only procedure found to be of value in evaluating the healthy preoperative patient was the internist's history-taking and physical examination. Tradition, the demands of our institutions, and our colleagues dictate what other testing is done. Ideally, tests ordered should be based on the findings of the history and physical examination.

PATIENTS WITH NUTRITIONAL DISORDERS

Obesity is the most common nutritional disease in the Western world. It increases the risk of postoperative complications such as infection, thromboembolic disease, respiratory failure, and wound dehiscence. If the surgical procedure is not urgent, the recommendation of weight reduction might be reasonable. The potential benefit in decreased surgical mortality and morbidity must be weighed against the potential harm in delaying surgical therapy.

The patient in negative nitrogen balance is at greater risk of infection and poor wound healing. Survival can be improved by establishing positive nitrogen balance through enteral, and if necessary parenteral, hyperalimentation. Negative nitrogen balance should be considered in patients with chronic infections, chronic inflammatory diseases, or malignancy. Gastrointestinal operative procedures increase the postoperative risk of negative nitrogen balance.

PATIENTS WITH CARDIAC DISEASE

Perioperative myocardial infarction is a complication of preexisting coronary artery disease. The great success of coronary artery bypass surgery has demonstrated that these patients can safely undergo surgery. The presence of congestive heart failure, a history of myocardial infarction within the previous six months, or angina pectoris in an unstable pattern were most predictive of a poor outcome in a large retrospective study of cardiac death occurring with noncardiac surgery. The risk was low in the following conditions: chronic stable angina, cardiac risk factors but without known coronary disease, previous successful coronary artery bypass surgery, peripheral vascular disease, asymptomatic carotid bruits, and previous infarction longer than six months before surgery.

Goldman has developed a statistical point system

Table 1. COMPUTATION OF CARDIAC RISK INDEX FOR NONCARDIAC SURGERY

Risk Factors	Points
History	
Age > 70 yr	5
MI in previous 6 mo	10
Physical examination	
S_3 gallop or JVD	11
Important valvular aortic stenosis	3
Electrocardiogram:	
Rhythm other than sinus or PACs on last preoperative EKG	7
> 5 PVCs/min documented at any time before operation	7
General status:	
$Po_2 < 60$ or $Pco_2 > 50$ mm Hg, K < 3.0 or $HCO_3 <$ 20 mEq/liter, BUN > 50 or Cr > 3.0 mg/dl, abnormal SGOT, signs of chronic liver disease, or patient bedridden from noncardiac causes	3
Surgery:	3
Intraperitoneal, intrathoracic, or aortic	
Emergency	4
Total possible	53 points

Point Total	No or Only Minor Complications	Life-Threatening Complications	Cardiac Deaths
0–5	99%	0.7%	0.2%
6–12	93%	5%	2%
13–25	86%	11%	2%
≥ 26	22%	22%	56%

Modified from Goldman L, et al: Multifactorial index of cardiac risk in noncardiac surgical procedures. N Engl J Med 297:848, 1977. Reprinted by permission of The New England Journal of Medicine.

for assessing the potential risk of noncardiac surgery to cardiac patients (Table 1). It highlights the importance of a simple, noninvasive preoperative evaluation in identifying potential risk factors. The same factors are useful in following patients postoperatively. The degree of hydration must be closely monitored, and if doubt exists, pulmonary artery pressure monitoring may become necessary. Postoperative EKGs, cardiac enzyme measurement, and continuous EKG monitoring are indicated in those patients at highest risk of intraoperative infarction or who have had an arrhythmia during surgery or recovery.

PATIENTS WITH PULMONARY DISEASE

Anesthesia in normal subjects causes ventilation-perfusion mismatching, impaired oxygenation, altered chest wall mechanics, and mucociliary activity. Postsurgical pain, particularly after abdominal procedures, may inhibit effective respiration and cough reflex. Narcotic analgesics may inhibit respiratory drive and alter the ventilatory pattern. In patients with lung disease, such alterations can be catastrophic. Such individuals should be identified at the preoperative examination, and appropriate treatment should be prescribed to try to reduce the perioperative morbidity and mortality.

Preoperative pulmonary testing (spirometry and arterial blood gases) is indicated in patients who have known pulmonary disease (regardless of age), are older than age 70, are obese, have a significant smoking history, or are scheduled for upper abdominal or thoracic surgery. One or more of the following results should alert the physician to a high risk of pulmonary complications: MVV less than 50% of predicted, FEV_1 less than 2 liters, Pco_2 greater than 45 mm Hg, or Po_2 less than 50 mm Hg. Such high-risk patients require close follow-up and aggressive pulmonary management both before and after surgery. Incentive spirometry, cessation of smoking, infection control, and bronchodilators are useful in this management. Early ambulation, pulmonary toilet, and pain control, including epidural narcotics if feasible, are highly desirable in the postoperative period.

The effects of loss of a lung must be assessed in the patient who is being considered for a pulmonary resection. Bronchospirometry is an invasive means of measuring the pulmonary functions of each lung. A less invasive method involves quantitative ventilation-perfusion scanning: multiplying the fraction of perfusion to the nonoperative lung by the MVV and FEV_1 gives a reasonable prediction of postoperative pulmonary function. If the FEV_1 is anticipated to be greater than 800 cc, or the MVV is greater than 50% of that predicted by BSA, the patient can be expected to come off ventilatory assistance postoperatively. A third means of evaluating these patients is with a pulmonary artery catheter: if mean pulmonary artery pressure is greater than 25 to 30 mm Hg at rest, the patient should not be considered a candidate for pneumonectomy.

The risk of postoperative pneumonia is more difficult to predict. Patients who smoke, are obese, or have secretions in the large airways (detected with the "loose cough test") are at greater risk. This risk can be reduced by preoperative respiratory therapy.

PATIENTS WITH HEPATIC AND GASTROINTESTINAL DISEASE

The patient with hepatic abnormalities poses a frequent dilemma to the physician and the surgical team. The patient with frank jaundice and hepatomegaly, as well as asymptomatic abnormalities in hepatic enzymes, requires further evaluation with serologic markers for hepatitis B to protect health care personnel who may come into contact with the patient's blood. If there is evidence of hepatic dysfunction—depressed albumin production, prolonged prothrombin time, or elevated bilirubin—special care should be taken (1) to minimize the risk of bleeding through the use of fresh-frozen plasma, (2) to observe for postoperative blood loss, (3) to maintain normal fluid and electrolyte balance, and (4) to identify and treat hepatic encephalopathy in the intraoperative period. Anesthetic agents that are hepatotoxic or require hepatic metabolism should be avoided. The patient with portal hypertension or ascites presents the additional challenge of the necessity of maintaining renal perfusion while minimizing excessive fluid retention. All patients with advanced liver disease should also be evaluated as candidates for possible parenteral nutritional support.

Surgical patients with GI disease frequently present with anorexia, nausea, vomiting, malabsorption, obstruction, or chronic diarrhea. Hence, they frequently have underlying fluid and electrolyte abnormalities or are chronically malnourished. Preoperative evaluation of these patients should assess the degree of abnormality with the goal of returning them to as near normal as possible before surgery. Patients with inflammatory bowel disease are often treated with corticosteroids, and the physician must be vigilant to prevent adrenal insufficiency.

PATIENTS WITH ENDOCRINE ABNORMALITIES

The physician most frequently is called on to evaluate and treat patients who have diabetes or thyroid disease or have been treated with steroids. Endocrine abnormalities also can be insidious in their presentation and unknown to patient and surgeon. Therefore, signs and symptoms of diabetes, hyperthyroidism, hypothyroidism, and adrenal insufficiency must be carefully sought preoperatively.

Intraoperatively, when caloric intake is uncertain, the diabetic on insulin is best treated by halving the usual dose of intermediate-acting insulin and using fluids that contain glucose. During surgery, the patient should have glucose measurement every two to four hours and coverage with regular insulin. If the patient is on an insulin pump, the basal infusion rate should be maintained and insulin coverage can be given through the infusion system. The type II diabetic treated with oral hypoglycemic agents or diet alone should have regular glucose determinations and regular insulin coverage for hyperglycemia greater than 200 mg/dl. Ideally, diabetes should be well controlled before surgery.

One third of all cases of thyroid storm are precipitated by surgery. Even minor procedures such as dental extraction and forceps delivery have been implicated. The physician needs to be alert for the signs and symptoms of thyrotoxicosis in the preoperative evaluation. Elderly patients may not exhibit the typical findings, and tachycardia, atrial fibrillation, or other arrhythmias may be the only clues to hyperthyroidism. Measurement of serum thyroxine level is usually sufficient to establish the diagnosis of significant hyperthyroidism. If surgery can be delayed for one to three months, the patient should be made euthyroid with propylthiouracil or methimazole. If surgery is more urgent, the patient may be prepared with a beta-adrenergic blocking agent and iodides, in addition to 300 to 450 mg PTU and 20 to 30 mg methimazole. These patients must be followed closely postoperatively, since the effect of iodides is short-lived and beta-antagonists may be insufficient to prevent thyroid storm.

Patients who have myxedema are prone to prolonged sedation and unconsciousness from anesthetics and sedatives. They have abnormalities in respiratory and myocardial function, which can be reversed by thyroid hormone replacement. They also have electrolyte abnormalities associated with an impairment in free water clearance. Nevertheless, studies involving a limited number of patients have shown that those with hypothyroidism can undergo major surgery without mishap. Considering the contradictory data, it would be best to delay elective surgery while full replacement is established, and allow emergency surgery with ample warning to the anesthesiologist about the presence of hypothyroidism. The patient with frank myxedema should be treated with IV triiodothyronine, 100 to 300 mg, before administration of an anesthetic agent. After emergency surgery, replacement can be begun slowly postoperatively. Adrenal insufficiency sometimes occurs in the same patient, either because of accompanying Addison's disease or (less often) because the hypothyroidism is secondary to pituitary disease.

The physiologic stress of surgery demands full use of the adrenal gland's hormonal reserves. In normal patients, plasma cortisol levels have been seen to increase as much as sevenfold in response to surgery. In one study of intraoperative hypotension, a large percentage of patients were found to have an abnormally small response to cosyntropin (Cortrosyn) stimulation. Because steroids are widely used in the appropriate treatment of allergic and inflammatory diseases, this diminished reserve is seen most commonly in asymptomatic and apparently normal patients. Naturally the stigmata of Addison's disease should be sought preoperatively, but it is more important to obtain a careful history of steroid use. Steroid preparation is necessary preoperatively for patients who have Addison's disease, are on steroids at the time of surgery, have been on steroids for one month in the previous six months, or have had a total steroid dose equivalent to 1 gm of cortisol in the preceding six months. In elective surgery, the steroid preparation consists of 100 to 200 mg hydrocortisone IM the day before surgery; 100 mg IV immediately before induction of anesthesia; 100 to 200 mg IV during surgery; and 100 mg IM immediately postoperatively. In emergency surgery, an additional 100 mg should be given with induction of anesthesia to replace the dose usually given the day before elective procedures. Postoperatively the patient needs a tapering schedule beginning at 200 mg IM or IV hydrocortisone (or equivalent).

ANTIMICROBIAL PROPHYLAXIS

The prophylactic use of antibiotics continues to stir controversy. Their use in the prevention of endocarditis and infection in prostheses and vascular shunts is not as controversial. Patients undergoing a procedure with a high risk of significant bacteremia, and who have an area of turbulent blood flow where blood moves from an area of high pressure to one of low pressure, are at greatest risk. These include patients with prosthetic heart valves; rheumatic valvular disease; and congenital lesions such as a small VSD, tetralogy of Fallot, patent ductus arteriosus, and coarctation of the aorta. Patients who have mitral valve prolapse need prophylaxis if they have a persistent late systolic murmur or midsystolic click. The need for antibiotic prophylaxis in patients with intermittent murmurs and clicks is not uniformly accepted. Any patient with a history of endocarditis is considered to be at risk and should be given prophylaxis. The following procedures have been identified as carrying a high risk of bacteremia: prostatectomy (when the urine is infected), esophageal dilation (with a non-

Table 2. SUMMARY OF RECOMMENDED ANTIBIOTIC REGIMENS FOR DENTAL/RESPIRATORY TRACT PROCEDURES

Standard Regimen	
For dental procedures that cause gingival bleeding, and oral/respiratory tract surgery	Pencillin V 2.0 gm PO 1 hr before, then 1.0 gm 6 hr later; for patients unable to take oral medications, 2 million units of aqueous penicillin G IV or IM 30–60 min before a procedure and 1 million units 6 hr later may be substituted
Special Regimens	
Parenteral regimen for use when maximal protection desired; e.g., for patients with prosthetic valves	Ampicillin 1.0–2.0 gm IM or IV plus gentamicin 1.5 mg/kg IM or IV, ½-hr before procedure, then 1.0 gm penicillin V 6 hr later; alternatively, parenteral regimen may be repeated once 8 hr later
Oral regimen for penicillin-allergic patients	Erythromycin 1.0 gm PO 1 hr before, then 500 mg 6 hr later
Parenteral regimen for penicillin-allergic patients	Vancomycin 1.0 gm IV *slowly* over 1 hr, starting 1 hr before; no repeat dose is necessary

SUMMARY OF RECOMMENDED REGIMENS FOR GASTROINTESTINAL/GENITOURINARY PROCEDURES

Standard Regimen	
For genitourinary/gastrointestinal tract procedures listed in text	Ampicillin 2.0 gm IM or IV plus gentamicin 1.5 mg/kg IM or IV, given ½–1 hr before procedure; one follow-up dose may be given 8 hr later
Special Regimens	
Oral regimen for minor or repetitive procedures in low-risk patients	Amoxicillin 3.0 gm PO 1 hr before procedure, then 1.5 gm 6 hr later
Penicillin-allergic patients	Vancomycin 1.0 gm IV *slowly* over 1 hr plus gentamicin 1.5 mg/kg IM or IV 1 hr before procedure; may be repeated once 8–12 hr later

From Shulman ST, et al: Prevention of bacterial endocarditis. Circulation 70:1124A–1125A, 1984. By permission of the American Heart Association, Inc.

sterilized instrument), tonsillectomy, dental extraction, periodontal surgery, burn surgery, or surgery on infected tissue. The American Heart Association's recommendations for antimicrobial prophylaxis are listed in Table 2.

PATIENTS WITH DISORDERS OF HEMOSTASIS

Abnormal hemostasis from all causes occurs in about 0.02% of the population. Of these, 10% to 20% have no history of abnormal bleeding. One should seek a history of abnormal bleeding following surgery, dental extraction, or trauma; a history of unexplained hematuria; or a family history of bleeding disorders or of abnormal bleeding. Of less use is a history of easy bruising or epistaxis. The examiner should look for petechiae, large and unexplained hematomata, or evidence of hemarthrosis. Any patient in whom there is a suspicion of abnormal hemostasis should be evaluated for prothrombin time, partial thromboplastin time, platelet count, and bleeding time. If a bleeding abnormality is confirmed, further evaluation is needed to pinpoint the exact cause.

Disseminated intravascular coagulation (DIC), immune thrombocytopenic purpura (ITP), isolated deficiencies of factor VIII or factor IX, and von Willebrand's disease are the most commonly encountered abnormalities. DIC is best treated by therapy for the underlying disease. ITP often resolves spontaneously within six months; if possible, surgery should be delayed until the platelet count rises over 100,000. If surgery is urgent, the patient can be treated with prednisone; if this is unsuccessful, the physician should consider splenectomy. The factor deficiencies should be treated with their specific factor cryoprecipitates. Replacement factor should be given one hour before surgery, approximately 40 units per kg to raise the level of assayed factor to about 80% of normal. This level is maintained for 48 hours following surgery with hourly infusions of the factor. For ten more days this level should be maintained with infusions every eight hours to maintain levels at about 40% of normal.

Von Willebrand's disease can be identified by demonstrating prolonged bleeding time, abnormal ristocetin-induced platelet aggregation, and a deficiency of factor VIII. Factor VIII should be replaced continuously as in patients with hemophilia A; however, replacement must continue even when suitable levels are detected since the bleeding time will become prolonged within 12 hours if the cryoprecipitate is not given on a regular basis. For dental surgery, the hemophiliac patient can be managed with epsilon-aminocaproic acid (EACA) which inhibits salivary fibrinolysis; 0.5 mg per kg per 24 hours (up to a maximum of 24 gm) is given in divided doses every four hours. The EACA should be started 12 hours before the procedure, and a single dose of factor cryoprecipitate should be given immediately before the procedure. The EACA should be continued for ten days following dental surgery.

The use of anticoagulants in surgical patients presents a relatively common problem. The physician should be concerned not only about reversal of the anticoagulant effect, but also whether and when the anticoagulants need to be restarted after surgery. Heparin should be withheld for six hours before surgery, and surgical hemostasis should be given extra attention. Heparin can be restarted at half the presurgical dose after surgery, and full doses can be resumed four days postoperatively. Protamine sulfate can be used to reverse the heparin effect in emergency situations. Ideally, warfarin therapy should be stopped two to four days before surgery. Vitamin K, IV, can be used to reverse the abnormal prothrombin time when there is not time to wait for reversal of the warfarin effect. Aspirin affects platelet aggregation for the life of the platelet, abnormal bleeding being seen up to five days after a dose. Abnormal bleeding from aspirin can be reversed in about 12 hours with the transfusion of platelet concentrates, one unit per 10 kg of body weight.

PATIENTS WITH OTHER HEMATOLOGIC ABNORMALITIES

Anemia detected preoperatively requires the usual evaluation. If the surgery is elective, appropriate therapy to correct the abnormal hemoglobin levels is the preferred course. In more urgent situations (particularly in patients who are elderly, are symptomatic, or have a history of ischemic cardiovascular disease or when the anticipated blood loss from surgery is potentially great), the patient should be transfused, ideally with saline-washed packed RBCs. Patients with sickle cell anemia have an increased risk of vasoocclusive crises during and after surgery. The risk can be lessened with adequate hydration, oxygenation, and maintenance of normal body temperature. Exchange transfusions with washed packed cells in the 24 hours before and two weeks after surgery, maintaining a hemoglobin of 10 gm %, reduce the risk further.

Leukopenia by itself is not a contraindication for surgery. Again, its cause should be sought. Thrombocytopenia requires not only such evaluation but also appropriate transfusions to maintain a platelet count ideally over 100,000 (if the problem is inadequate platelet production).

HYPERTENSIVE PATIENTS

Surgery on hypertensive patients is a common event. The anesthesiologist needs to know which antihypertensive medications his patient is taking so that attention can be given to drug interactions and electrolyte abnormalities. Only for patients with malignant or accelerated hypertension should surgery be postponed pending control of blood pressure. Greater importance is placed on history suggestive of encephalopathy, on eye ground changes, on evidence of congestive heart failure, and on proteinuria than on absolute BP levels. Severe elevations can be controlled with IV nitroprusside, IV labetalol, or sublingual nifedipine. If the hypertension is caused by volume overload, IV loop diuretics can be used.

PATIENTS WITH ARTHRITIS

The principal goal in caring for the patient with inflammatory arthritis who also needs surgery is to maintain joint mobility during the intraoperative period. Minimal interruption of anti-inflammatory therapy, regular physical therapy, and early ambulation need to be encouraged. Particular care should be taken in intubation of patients with rheumatoid arthritis or ankylosing spondylitis with cervical involvement, to prevent serious injury. Since many of these patients have been treated with corticoids, the physician should take steps to prevent adrenal insufficiency. Steroid use in this group of patients should be investigated and appropriate preparation given.

PATIENTS WITH RENAL FAILURE

Patients who have renal failure are particularly challenging. They may be malnourished and require nutritional support; frequently have fluid and electrolyte abnormalities; may have myocardial dysfunction or ischemic disease; may have abnormalities in gastrointestinal motility; are often on steroids or are diabetic; have a potential site for infection if they have an AV shunt used for access in hemodialysis; have abnormal platelet aggregation and bleeding tendencies; and have severe hypertension. Appropriate perioperative care requires diligent attention to all organ systems.

CONCLUSION

This review is far from comprehensive. Every medical disease has a potential for creating problems in the perioperative period. The physician must be compulsively concerned about the adequacy of nutritional support, including normal balance of electrolytes and fluid; gas exchange; circulation and tissue perfusion; elimination of wastes; and metabolism of drugs. The patient must be observed by both physician and surgical team for blood loss and infection. Present trends suggest that we can expect to care for older and sicker patients and to employ more complex and hazardous surgical procedures. As physicians, our role can only expand in preoperative evaluation and postoperative care of these patients.

REFERENCES

Committee on Prevention of Rheumatic Fever and Bacterial Endocarditis. Circulation 56:139A, 1977.

Corman L, Bolt R: Medical evaluation of the preoperative patient. Med Clin North Am 63, 1979.

Goldman L, Caldera DL, Nussbaum SR: Multifactorial index of cardiac risk in noncardiac surgical procedures. N Engl J Med 297:845–850, 1977.

Tisi GM: Preoperative evaluation of pulmonary function. Am Rev Respir Dis 119:293–310, 1979.

20 · MEDICAL CARE OF THE HEALTHY ADULT

Wilmer M. Rutt
HENRY FORD HOSPITAL

Prevention of disease is the ultimate goal of medicine. In daily practice, however, urgent symptoms and signs, time pressures, and the lack of third party payment for preventive services have forced physicians to accord prevention a low priority.

Prevention occurs at several levels. An intervention that reduces the likelihood of a disease developing, such as immunization against influenza, is called primary prevention. Identification and treatment of streptococcal sore throat, which interrupts or minimizes the progress of a disease or irreversible damage from a disease by early detection and treatment, is called secondary prevention. Tertiary prevention, such as identification and treatment of hypertensive heart disease, slows the progress of the disease and reduces the disability arising from it.

To speak of caring for asymptomatic or even healthy patients distorts the truth. Measures to enhance health, prevent disease, and slow its progress apply to all patients, including those with major disorders. Attention is often given to major disease at the expense of maintaining the health of other systems of the body.

The office patient most likely to receive good advice is the one who initially requests advice and examinations to promote his or her health. This type of patient is now more prevalent. Most people who feel well, however, still do not go to physicians. In some health care systems, free comprehensive health maintenance packages have been offered. Only about 40% of people participate when ordinary methods of informing them of available services are used. Additional supportive phone calls and repeat mailing of letters can increase this number to about 60%. Thus, about 40% probably do *not* participate in screening programs.

A plethora of so-called screening programs are sponsored by service clubs, hospitals, insurance companies and industry. Many of these attend to only one risk factor, such as glaucoma, hypertension, or diabetes. I have been unable to find any screening program that addresses other health issues thought to be cost effective by such conservative groups as the Canadian Task Force (Table 1). Many programs also offer procedures that provide extensive biochemical profiles, which are not likely to be helpful in a general population.

Most screening programs do not segment the population in terms of the indicated procedures for age and sex or increased risk. This is usually justified in the name of efficiency. However, simple protocols could make this possible. Most programs also do not spend time on really significant risk factors related to life style: stress, cigarette smoking, inappropriate alcohol and

Table 1. CHECKLIST TO IDENTIFY AND REDUCE RISK FACTORS (REVIEW ON FIRST VISIT AND EVERY FIVE YEARS)

Condition	Technique
Syphilis, gonorrhea and other venereal disease*	In persons with multiple sexual partners, screening tests at least every 2 years, VDRL and GC Screen in first trimester of pregnancy. Consider immunization against hepatitis B in selected patients. Disease avoidance counseling.
Congenital toxoplasmosis*	Identify and counsel pregnant women who have pet cats and who eat raw meat.
Carcinoma of cervix*	In persons with multiple sexual partners and those with previous abnormal Pap smears, reinforce necessity of annual Pap smear.
Breast cancer*	In persons whose immediate relatives have breast cancer, nulliparous persons, and persons with previous breast cancer, mammography every 1–3 years from age 35 to 50. Teach all women self-examination.
Hearing loss*	Inquire about listening to loud music more than 2 hours a week or working in noisy areas. Counsel when appropriate.
Smokers‡	Counseling, literature, consider referral to smoking cessation group. Spirometry every 5 years in persons smoking more than 10 years. Consider urine cytology in heavy smokers over 50.
Automotive accidents‡	Counsel persons who drive after using alcohol, cannabis, or sedative drugs. Encourage use of seat belt and shoulder harness. Look for mental impairments, expecially in older patients.
Unwanted pregnancy*	Counseling to prevent second pregnancy.
Diseases of occupational exposure*	Identify work and leisure exposures, check against known toxic agents, and counsel.
Stressed life style	Counseling and possible referral to stress reduction program.
Diseases of international travel*	Identify high-risk travel destinations anticipated and follow recommendations in Chapter 21.
Skin cancer†	While examining skin, counsel patients (especially those with fair skin) about risk of high-intensity solar exposure and appropriate methods of avoidance (e.g., use of sunscreens and reporting of changing skin lesions).
Malnutrition‡	Analyze diet for prudence every 5 years. Identify persons more than 20% over or 10% under ideal weight. Offer counseling, especially groups using behavior modification techniques.
Thyroid cancer	If there is history of radiation treatment to head and neck, perform physical examination of thyroid gland annually.
Vaginal cancer	Reinforce need for annual pelvic examination in daughters whose mothers have received high-dose estrogens during pregnancy.
Dental disease†	Refer all patients who have not seen a dentist in previous year.
Cancer of testes†	Teach young men self-examination.
Sickle cell trait,† Thalassemia trait,† Tay-Sachs disease†	Identify trait in appropriate population groups and refer for genetic counseling.
Muscular dystrophy†	Female relatives of persons with muscular dystrophy should have several CPKs to identify carrier state.
Tuberculosis*	Tuberculin skin test for persons who have had contact with disease recently, live in high-risk area, are part of a high-risk group, or are poorly nourished.
Osteoporosis	In women, discuss calcium intake and option of estrogen replacement beginning at menopause.
Substance abuse‡	Ask key questions about amounts and type of alcohol and other drugs. Appropriate counseling and referral.
Poor physical conditioning	Ask if person gets at least three periods of vigorous exercise for at least 20 minutes each week. If not, counsel.
Retirement distress‡	Final counseling examination before retirement.

*Good evidence; † fair evidence; ‡ poor evidence (Canadian Task Force on Periodic Health Examination—CTFPHE).

drug consumption, excessive body weight, and unbalanced diet. Professionals should use all the power they have to influence organizations that provide health screening and maintenance programs in the community to emphasize high-priority items.

Tables 1 and 2 present a personalized approach based on studies and current literature, and a bias that promoting life style changes is worthwhile. The checklist in Table 1 should be thoroughly reviewed at the first visit and every five years thereafter. Self-administered or assisted checklists, in either paper or electronic format, simplify the process. Tickler messages to physicians, office staff, or patients improve compliance.

THE ANNUAL PHYSICAL

The annual physical was promoted by the American Medical Association 50 years ago and has been a sacred part of physician behavior. Patients frequently demand a "physical examination" and are convinced of its importance.

What is considered a "physical examination" varies widely. Many patients do not believe it necessary to remove their clothes for a physical. Others consider that BP determination, several blood tests, and urinalysis constitute a physical. I most often find that physicals do not include significant attention to behaviors that are known to be important to health. Think of your patients who come for periodic health examinations. Try to divide the time you spend with them into four segments: (1) symptoms, (2) signs, (3) identification and discussion of risk factors, and (4) detection of occult disease. You may be surprised at the percentages. Most of us could improve our balance by devoting more attention to (3) and (4), and less but more focused attention to (1) and (2).

Table 2. ROUTINE EXAMINATION TECHNIQUES

Technique	Frequency	
	To Age 50	*After Age 50*
Blood pressure*	Every visit	Every visit
Breast examination and reinforcement of self–breast-examination technique*	Annual	Annual
Mammography*	Baseline 35	Every 1–2 years
Periodic health examination*	Every 5 years	Every 2 years
Tonometry and refraction†	Every 5 years	Every 2 years
Occult blood in stool†	Every 5 years	Annually
Sigmoidoscopy	No	Every 5 years
Pap smear†	Annual—may decrease if several normal	Every 2 years
CBC (not including differential)‡	Every 5 years	Every 5 years
Cholesterol‡	Every 5 years	Every 5 years
Glucose	Every 5 years	Every 2 years
Rubella hemagglutination inhibition test*	All nonimmunized women of child-bearing age at first visit and immunization of seronegative women if pregnancy can be avoided for 3 months.	
Influenza immunization*		Annual after 65
Pneumonia immunization*		Once after 65
Diphtheria/tetanus* immunization	Every 10 years	Every 10 years

*Good evidence; † fair evidence; ‡ minimal evidence (Canadian Task Force on Periodic Health Examination—CTFPHE).

GENERALLY NONINDICATED PROCEDURES

Except for specific indications, tests such as chest radiography, automated biochemical profiles (SMA-12, SMAC), thyroid function testing, resting EKGs under age 40, and treadmill EKGs in low-risk persons have not been found generally useful.

EXERCISE

More than 50% of my patients have fewer than three sustained periods of exercise per week. Many who do not exercise regularly do so only during certain seasons and expose themselves to the risk of initiating vigorous exercise without a proper conditioning program. Many patients select activities that do not have aerobic qualities, such as golf, baseball, bowling, and other activities with only brief bursts of exercise. I counsel selection of lifetime exercises that produce minimal aggravation of the normal degenerative processes in the muscles and joints. Favorites are brisk walking, swimming, cross-country skiing, jogging, and dancing.

I teach my patients that regular, vigorous exercise programs over long periods produce a trend toward decreased cardiopulmonary morbidity and mortality. I also emphasize the benefits of enhanced neuromuscular coordination and efficiency, maintenance of bone strength, metabolic effects such as weight control and enhancement of high-density lipoproteins. Many patients with a tendency to anxiety and depression benefit from a carefully supervised program of progressively more vigorous regular exercise. A referral to an exercise physiologist is beneficial for some.

DIETARY HABITS

Approximately one third of people over age 30 are more than 20% over ideal weight. Increased morbidity and mortality associated with conditions such as diabetes, osteoarthritis, hypertension, hyperlipidemia, and gout have been demonstrated.

Each patient should have an optimal weight established, based on standard charts. This weight should be placed on the Problem List at the first visit, and the percentage deviation from ideal weight calculated. This should be repeated at five-year intervals. Many persons who are at ideal weight at age 25 show gradual increases in their early 30s. It is at this time, rather than when the weight has become more pronounced and clearly medically important, that intervention in dietary habits should be made.

Cynicism about weight reduction programs is no longer appropriate. Through in-depth education about food, self-help groups, professionally directed groups with carefully formulated behavior modification, and exercise programs, significant long-term adjustments in body weight have been made by many persons.

Patients who needlessly spend much time and money on fad diets should be warned of the dangers of extreme unsupervised diets, which cause unnecessary morbidity.

There are several dozen computer programs, many adapted for home personal computers, that can assist patients. Based on a several-day diet diary, programs such as the DINE Program suggest to the patient which portions of the diet are optimal and which need improvement.

Much education regarding diet should be given in schools, both during formal schooling years and in community education programs. Many community education programs include courses in diet that are faddish and have poor scientific basis. As physicians, we need to use our influence so that state-of-the-art school curriculums are developed and offered in an attractive format.

STRESS REDUCTION

Stress from a host of sources is a common cause of lack of well-being, and consequently is not understood. It is essential to find some means of gently assessing whether the patient has problems relating to marriage, sexual adjustment, family, finances, drugs, employment, and the like. Many people have severe, unidentified problems in these areas and do not consider them to be related to health.

Young persons who are developing their careers frequently adopt a pattern of sustained work that includes long hours and weekend work. These should be counseled early and perhaps referred to one of the increasing number of quality stress reduction programs.

SMOKING

Smoking, one of the most common self-inflicted injuries, has been well documented in the past decade by both retrospective and prospective epidemiologic and experimental studies to be a significant cause of disability and death.

Despite the cynics who say that smoking habits cannot be altered, the percentage of the population that smokes has progressively decreased over the last two decades. However, approximately one third of adults are still regular smokers and should be educated systematically and intensively regarding the medical aspects of smoking.

Without question, smoking is the primary cause of chronic obstructive lung disease and lung cancer. It is a significant cause of cancers in the oral cavity, larynx, esophagus, and bladder. It is an important independent risk factor for coronary artery disease and is thought by some experts to be the most important risk factor for men under age 50.

Women who smoke and become pregnant have smaller babies and an increased rate of spontaneous abortion and perinatal mortality. Thousands of deaths each year can be attributed to smoking during pregnancy. Each woman of reproductive age should be fully apprised of these facts and given access to literature, proven group therapies, and repeated assessment.

For people who have smoked for more than 10 years, simple spirometry demonstrates early emphysematous changes. A careful explanation of the irreversible nature of obstructive lung disease is important. This should be done by creative use of paramedical personnel, audiovisual devices, group teaching, and literature.

The declining risk of the development of lung cancer after smoking cessation should be emphasized to patients as a positive health promotion tactic.

ALCOHOL AND OTHER DRUG USE

Aside from considerations of alcoholism, one should check patients' irrational use of alcohol. Nearly one half of young drivers in a recent Michigan survey indicated that they had driven after moderate to heavy alcohol consumption within the past year. This documents what we already know from newspapers. The intermittent, heavy use of alcohol results in much morbidity and mortality from vehicular accidents and domestic violence.

The identification of persons with heavy alcohol use, who may or may not be defined as alcoholic, is also of importance. Three questions I use on my health questionaire are: (1) How much alcohol do you drink?, (2) Do you have a drinking problem?, and (3) Has anyone in your family complained about your drinking? Other sets of questions have been supported by various authorities. I have been surprised with the honesty with which people answer these questions in writing. I believe they answer them more honestly in writing than they do in oral conversation.

Other nonalcoholic drugs have assumed major importance in all portions of our culture. When I ask about medication usage, I also ask in a nonjudgmental fashion about over-the-counter and street drugs. As part of the medication history, many people are ready to discuss these matters and to listen to advice. The caring physician will do this on a regular basis.

PEOPLE ARE GENERALLY WELL

LaRouchefoucauld, a 17th century French essayist, said that "devoting one's life to keeping well is one of the most tedious of ailments." A perusal of popular literature could lead to the conclusion that everyone is sick. The overemphasis on detection of hidden disease in physician offices can also convince patients that they are sick although the precise illness has not yet been found! Some patients are more susceptible than others to this and develop a dependency relationship, reporting the slightest symptoms.

One should generally avoid tests in patients without indication, because of the frequency of false-positive results. The worried well will find these false positives even more reason to search further for occult disease, which usually is not there. I try to remember when confronted with results in an asymptomatic patient that a large dose of clinical judgment is indicated and a wider range of normal values is probably indicated. In patients at low risk, the predictive value of a positive result is low.

Self-help books such as Vickery's *Take Care of Yourself* are useful in emphasizing the positive aspects of health care. In my group, we have placed a copy of this book in each examination room. Approaches such as this produce a positive feeling about wellness and create independence rather than dependence.

REFERENCES

Breslow L, Somers AR: The Lifetime Health Monitoring Program—a practical approach to preventive medicine. NEJM 296:601–608, 1977.
Council on Scientific Affairs: Medical evaluation of healthy persons. JAMA 249:1626–1633, 1983.

Medical Practice Committee, American College of Physicians: Periodic health care in the asymptomatic patient. Ann Intern Med 95:729–732, 1981.

Spitzer WO, Battista RN, Bayne RD, et al: The Periodic Health Examination, 1984 Update, Canadian Task Force on the Periodic Health Examination. CMAJ, 130:1278–1285, 1984.

Spitzer WO, Bayne JR, Charron KE, et al: The Periodic Health Examination, Canadian Task Force on the Periodic Health Examination. CMAJ 121:1193–1250, 1979.

21 · MEDICAL ADVICE FOR TRAVELERS

Laurence M. Cortez
OCHSNER CLINIC AND ALTON OCHSNER MEDICAL FOUNDATION

As the numbers of Americans traveling abroad continue to increase, physicians in all practice settings are continually consulted regarding health concerns abroad. In 1983, 12½ million citizens departed for overseas destinations, and 5 million new passports were issued. During the first nine months of 1984, 9½ million U.S. citizens departed our international borders. Some concern on the part of the traveler is natural and justified and the physician is the appropriate source for information. The physician's responsibilities include (1) ensuring that medical requirements for overseas travel are fulfilled, (2) prescribing the appropriate immunizations and chemoprophylaxis specific to particular regions of travel and to each individual, and (3) advising the traveler on common sense precautions and additional helpful measures to prevent injury or illness.

The chance of an American contracting a serious illness in developed countries is rather slim, and the risk of travel in continental Europe, Canada, Australia, and New Zealand is about the same as in the U.S. Even in developing countries, travelers are relatively safe if they confine their activities to tourist areas. Nonetheless, the physician should take this opportunity to update routine immunizations such as diphtheria/tetanus, measles, and polio. The risk of measles, mumps, and polio is greater for travelers. The risk of contracting malaria, a disease seldom considered by American physicians, is real and the results can be fatal.

GENERAL ADVICE*

All travelers should have both physical and dental examination at least four weeks, if not more, before travel in order to allow for vaccinations that may be necessary. Either the physician or the patient should contact the appropriate yellow fever vaccination center. Immunization certificates and passports should be validated well in advance of departure. Travel agencies and airlines can usually be relied on for help in such matters.

*See Table 1.

Table 1. DRUGS AND SUPPLIES CHECKLIST FOR TRAVELERS

1. Copy of brief history and pertinent physical findings, and description of therapeutic regimen (patients with medical problems)
2. Extra prescription drugs, properly labeled, with copies of each prescription
3. Supply of aspirin, Tylenol, antidiarrhea medication, antacids (buying over-the counter medications is strongly discouraged)
4. Bacitracin or Neosporin ointment for treatment of superficial skin infections
5. Caladryl lotion for mild sunburn, heat rash, and pruritus
6. First-aid kit with Band-Aids of several sizes, 3-inch Ace wrap, Betadine solution
7. Insect repellent
8. An extra pair of sunglasses, eyeglasses, lens prescriptions, suntan lotion and sunscreen
9. Soap, tampons, toothpaste, sunscreen, moisturizing lotion, etc.

Patients with marked allergy to ragweed pollen are warned that they may react to the pyrethrum-containing insecticides used on airplanes. They should ask the flight attendant for a damp cloth with which to cover their faces during spraying.

REQUIRED VACCINATIONS

YELLOW FEVER

Some countries require an international certificate of vaccination against yellow fever. This vaccine is recommended for those traveling to areas reporting infection or to known endemic zones (in equatorial Africa and many areas of South America), even if infection is not currently reported. The vaccine is a live virus grown in chick embryos and is approved for individuals over the age of six months, with a booster every ten years. As with any live virus vaccine, administration is contraindicated in certain patients (see "Special Considerations" below). Administration may be associated with fever, pain at the injection site, headache, and malaise for 24 to 48 hours (another good reason for obtaining it well before departure). Yellow fever vaccine can be obtained only from designated centers that receive weekly updates on yellow fever activity. A list of designated centers is available from local or state health departments or from the Centers for Disease Control (see "Where to Call or Write" below).

CHOLERA

Few countries require vaccination against cholera. Travelers who follow the usual tourist routes, stay in hotels catering to tourists, and avoid roadside food and drink are at little risk of contracting cholera even in endemic areas. This is fortunate since cholera vaccine (a killed vaccine) is only about 50% effective. A single dose within six months before travel will satisfy international health requirements. Cholera vaccine has side effects similar to those of yellow fever vaccine.

RECOMMENDED VACCINATIONS*

TYPHOID

Vaccine for typhoid is recommended for those traveling to rural areas where typhoid is endemic or where

*Must be individualized.

infection is being reported. The vaccine often causes pain at the injection site and constitutional symptoms for one or two days, and does not confer complete protection. Primary immunization consists of two doses at four-week intervals; if time is lacking, three doses may be given at weekly intervals. Booster doses are necessary every three years.

MEASLES, MUMPS, AND RUBELLA

All three of these viral diseases present significant hazards and are uncontrolled in both developed and developing countries of the world. Most individuals born before 1957 are immune to measles because of naturally acquired antibody. Neither they nor persons born later who received measles immunization are at further risk. Adults, especially women of childbearing age, should be immune to rubella. Evidence of immunity consists of proof of immunization after the age of 15 months or serologic evidence of immunity. These three vaccines are live virus preparations, and therefore contraindicated in certain patients (see "Special Considerations" below).

POLIOMYELITIS

In general the risk of acquiring polio in Canada, continental Europe, Australia, New Zealand, and Japan is no greater than in the U.S. Outbreaks can occur, however, as evidenced by the 1984 occurrence of many cases in Finland. Polio should be considered endemic in all developing countries of the world, and travelers to these lands should be immune. Those previously immunized should receive one dose of oral polio vaccine (OPV), except immunosuppressed hosts, who should receive one dose of inactivated polio vaccine (IPV). OPV is the vaccine of choice for children requiring primary immunization. IPV is preferred for patients over the age of 18 years. For nonimmunized adults without sufficient time to complete more than one dose of the three-dose series, a single dose of OPV is recommended.

DIPHTHERIA-TETANUS

The diphtheria-tetanus booster should be administered every ten years.

HEPATITIS A

Immune globulin should be administered to nonimmune individuals traveling to developing nations if they are traveling away from usual tourist routes. Dosage varies with the person's weight: for those traveling for less than three months, 0.5 cc for less than 50 lb, 1 cc for 50 to 100 lb, and 2 cc for more than 100 lb. For stays of longer than three months, immune globulin should be given in a dose of 1 cc for less than 50 lb, 2.5 cc for 50 to 100 lb, and 5 cc for more than 100 lb. For prolonged stays, the latter schedule should be repeated every six months (see "Special Considerations" below).

HEPATITIS B

Vaccine for hepatitis B is recommended for all travelers who are negative for hepatitis B serologic markers if they are traveling for more than six months to an area of high endemicity (eastern and southeastern Asia, sub-Sahara Africa and the Pacific Basin), or even for short stays if they anticipate sexual contact or contact with blood from within the local population. The vaccine is administered in three doses over a six-month period.

Optimal protection is not conferred until all three have been administered, but ample protection of questionable duration may be realized in some people after only one or two doses, so it is worthwhile starting this program at any time.

SPECIAL CONSIDERATIONS AND CONTRAINDICATIONS FOR VACCINATIONS

Live virus vaccines (measles, mumps, rubella, yellow fever, oral polio) should not be given to pregnant women or to persons with known or potential immune deficiency states caused by disease or therapy (such as hematologic or lymphoproliferative disorders, malignancies, and conditions caused by immunosuppressive therapy). Oral polio vaccine should not be administered to a patient living with an immunodeficient person.

Immunoglobulins may mute the host response to live virus vaccines (yellow fever and oral polio vaccines being the exceptions) if given less than three months before or two weeks after the vaccines.

Several vaccines may be given at once but typhoid, cholera, and yellow fever vaccines are best given separately, since each can cause unpleasant side effects.

Package inserts of the vaccines should be reviewed and patients questioned thoroughly regarding any allergies to components such as egg protein and neomycin. If allergy history is positive and time permits, evaluation by an allergist is recommended. If there is a medical reason for a traveler not to take a vaccine, the physician must provide such information and reasons on a dated, signed statement for the traveler to carry.

MALARIA

Chemoprophylaxis for malaria is the most important preventive measure taken on behalf of the traveler. Acquisition of malaria by travelers is not rare, and *Plasmodium falciparum* malaria may be fatal. Only the United States, Canada, Europe, and Japan are free of vector-related malaria. The risk of malaria in other areas varies on the basis of weather, elevation, mosquito activity, time of year, and so forth. If there is any doubt, give prophylaxis, even if your patient is only stopping over in an endemic area. It only takes one mosquito bite to get malaria.

Chloroquine phosphate is the drug of choice for malaria prevention and is given as a 500-mg (300-mg chloroquine base) tablet once weekly beginning two weeks before entering an endemic area, while residing there, and for six weeks after leaving. Chloroquine should be used with caution in the presence of liver disease, alcoholism, or blood disease. It can also aggravate porphyria and psoriasis.

Unfortunately, the areas of the world with chloroquine-resistant *P. falciparum* malaria (CRFM) are increasing. Since its release in 1982, Fansidar (pyrimethamine-sulfadoxine) has been used in addition to chloroquine for people traveling to known risk areas for CRFM, and has obviated the problem of chloroquine resistance. Both drugs must be administered and the dosage schedule is the same. Fansidar has been generally well tolerated. However, severe adverse reactions have been seen, similar to those associated with other sulfonamides. The CDC (advisory memo No. 75 dated 12/24/84) reported ten cases (four fatal) of skin reactions attributable to Fansidar in American travelers during the preceding two years. These cases are being investigated by the CDC. Until this relationship and risk are more completely defined, the CDC recommends: (1) careful questioning of travelers regarding any previous sulfonamide intolerance, and withholding of the drug if there is a positive history; (2) addition of Fansidar to chloroquine in regimens of travelers to CRFM areas in Asia or South America only if they are staying overnight; (3) continued use of the combination of Fansidar and chloroquine in travelers to east and central Africa where transmission of CRFM has been documented, and discontinuation of Fansidar if any skin or mucous membrane lesions or symptoms develop. Continuous updates on the CRFM/Fansidar situation can be expected, and the CDC may be contacted if there is a question. In black patients the G6PD level should be checked in order to warn of possible hemolysis. In a sulfa-allergic individual who must go to a CRFM region, doxycycline, 100 mg once a day, may be of benefit since some activity against *Plasmodia* is present.

Travelers can also take precautions to avoid mosquitoes, which are attracted by perfumes and dark colors. Light-colored clothing should be worn and it should cover the arms and legs. Advise travelers to remain inside from dusk to dawn, the insects' main feeding time. Unless they are staying in a hotel with tight-fitting windows and central air conditioning, they should sleep under mosquito netting. Insect repellent may be applied to thin clothing as well as to exposed skin. The most effective is *N*,*N*-diethylmetatoluamide (deet), an ingredient in many commercially available insect repellents such as Off.

Prophylaxis can fail, so malaria must be considered in the differential diagnosis for any traveler.

TRAVELER'S DIARRHEA

Traveler's diarrhea (also known as Montezuma's revenge, Aztec two-step, Delhi belly, Tokyo trot, and others, depending on geographic area) is usually defined as four or more loose stools in a 24-hour period. It may be associated with nausea, vomiting, abdominal cramps or pain, bloody stools and fever.

The incidence of traveler's diarrhea depends on the area of travel, the duration of stay, and whether the stay is confined to tourist-oriented areas. Up to 50% of visitors to some areas are affected, making diarrhea responsible for more lost time than any other hazard to the traveler. Enteropathogenic *E. coli* has been isolated in 40% to 70% of travelers with diarrhea, *Shigella* in 5% to 20%. Many other agents have been implicated, including *Campylobacter*, but about one third of cases remain undiagnosed and approximately one fifth are mixed infections, so the exact cause is frequently undetermined.

PREVENTIVE MEASURES

Avoidance of contaminated food and drink is the best preventive for traveler's diarrhea. Water in hotels and restaurants that cater to American tourists may be safe. If there is any doubt as to adequate chlorination, the water should be avoided. Chlorination does not kill parasites such as *Giardia* and *Amoeba*, and pepper sauces do not kill microbes. Only bottled or purified water is safe for drinking and tooth brushing. Carbonated beverages are usually safe. Caution should be taken to avoid drinking alcoholic beverages mixed with contaminated water, local beers containing unpurified water, and contaminated ice cubes. Water may be purified by iodinating with tetraglycine hydroperiodide tablets, available at pharmacies and sporting goods stores. The best method of purification is by boiling vigorously for several minutes.

Most diseases acquired from contaminated water can also be acquired from foods. Any foods thoroughly cooked are generally safe, as are canned foods. Products considered unsafe to eat are raw vegetables, salads, and fresh fruit (except fruit that is easily peeled, such as bananas). Caution tourists against buying food from street vendors. Milk is safe only if boiled or in canned evaporated form (diluted with uncontaminated water). Ice cream or cheese are considered unsafe as they may be made with contaminated milk.

TREATMENT

Most cases of traveler's diarrhea are mild and self-limiting, lasting less than four days, and can be managed with the above-mentioned modalities and with adequate fluid and electrolyte replacement (see Table 2).

Bismuth subsalicylate (Pepto-Bismol) is effective in a prophylactic adult dose of 2 oz four times a day; for mild cases, 1 to 2 oz every 30 minutes for eight doses. However, it is often impractical to carry Pepto-Bismol in large supplies. Travelers should be warned that Pepto-Bismol contains salicylate and will turn the stool black.

For mild diarrhea and cramps, diphenoxylate (Lomotil), loperamide (Imodium), codeine, and opiates can be used, but may be dangerous in patients with significant dysentery and fever.

Prophylactic antibiotics usually are not wise because of the risk of untoward side effects and development of resistant organisms. If patients insist on taking these, the physician can only warn about the complications. There is no hard-and-fast rule. For a businessman making a short but important visit, prophylaxis may be reasonable since even a very brief illness may be detrimental. Long-term prophylaxis (for more than a week) is hard to justify.

Doxycycline, 100 mg once a day, is effective against susceptible strains of enteropathogenic *E. coli*, but resistant strains occur in many parts of the world. Side

Table 2. FORMULA FOR TREATMENT OF DIARRHEAL DISEASE (Replacement of Fluid and Electrolytes)

Prepare two separate glasses of the following:	
Glass No. 1	
Orange, apple, or other fruit juice	8 oz
Honey or corn syrup	½ tsp
Salt, table	1 pinch
Glass No. 2	
Water (carbonated or boiled)	8 oz
Soda, baking	¼ tsp

Drink alternately from each glass until thirst is quenched. Supplement as desired with carbonated beverages, water, or tea made with boiled or carbonated water.

From Health Information for International Travelers, 1984. Centers for Disease Control, Quarantine Division, 1600 Clinton Road, Atlanta, GA 30333.

effects include photosensitivity, GI upsets, or diarrhea due to overgrowth of resistant organisms.

The combination of sulfamethoxazole and trimethoprim (Bactrim, Septra), one double-strength tablet twice a day, is also an effective preventive. Sulfa drugs are also associated with significant adverse reactions, especially rash and anemia. Enteric pathogens are already resistant in some areas. If prophylactics are used, they should not replace good hygienic practices and caution in selecting food and drink. Even if the most common pathogens are susceptible to the prophylactic agent employed, the traveler is not protected from helminthic, parasitic, viral, or other bacterial causes of diarrheal illness.

Sulfamethoxazole-trimethoprim or doxycycline therapy are both effective in treating diarrhea caused by susceptible organisms, in the same doses as for prophylaxis. The traveler can be given a five-day supply in case of severe diarrhea, although there is considerable variation in individual definition of "severe." Most patients with significant diarrhea realize benefit within 24 to 48 hours. If symptoms persist longer than 48 hours, medical attention should be sought.

Recommended diet for those suffering from traveler's diarrhea includes dry toast, crackers, bouillon, gelatin, and broiled or baked chicken. Patients with traveler's diarrhea may develop a transient lactase deficiency, so that milk and dairy products should be avoided. Raw fruit and foods that are greasy, highly seasoned, or fried can provoke recurrent symptoms.

WHERE TO CALL OR WRITE FOR INFORMATION

Advice for the physician and traveler may be obtained from local and state health authorities. Specific concerns can also be addressed by contacting the embassy or local consulate general office of countries to be visited. Several publications are available at all yellow fever vaccination centers or from the CDC (Centers for Disease Control, Quarantine Division, 1600 Clinton Road, Atlanta, GA 30333). Publications include *Health Information for International Travel* (yearly publication); *Blue Sheet* (a bi-weekly summary of health information for international travel); and *Advisory Memoranda* (periodically updated as needed).

A summary of cruise ship sanitation inspections or a copy of the last inspection report of a specific vessel may be obtained from the office of the Chief, Sanitation and Vector Control Activity, Division of Quarantine, 1015 North America Way, Room 107, Miami, FL 33132.

Quality medical care in the tropics and developing countries varies greatly. In developing countries, such care is provided at most missionary hospitals. The names of well-trained physicians who speak English may be obtained from:

1. International Association for Medical Assistance to Travelers (IAMET), 736 Center Street, Lewiston, NY 14092 (716-754-4883).
2. Intermedic, 777 Third Avenue, New York, NY 10017 (212-486-8974).
3. Health Care Abroad, 923 Investment Building, 1511 K Street NW, Washington, DC 20006 (800-336-3310).
4. American residents of the country.
5. Managers of larger hotels, especially those catering to tourists.
6. Travel services: American Express, Cook's, etc.
7. The airlines.
8. The American embassy or consulate.

Handicapped travelers may write to Access America, Washington, DC 20202-2101 for *A Guide to Accessibility of Terminals.*

The American Diabetes Association Inc., 2 Park Avenue, New York, NY 10016 (800-227-6776) provides a list of affiliated organizations throughout the world.

Travelers or physicians with questions regarding travel are welcome to contact a member of the Infectious Diseases Section, Ochsner Clinic Yellow Fever Vaccination Center, 1514 Jefferson Highway, New Orleans, LA 70121 (504-838-4000), Telex 810-951-6183 OCHS.

REFERENCES

Advisory Memorandum No. 75, Department of Health and Human Resources, 12/24/84.

Dupont HL, Reves RR, Galindo E, et al: Treatment of traveler's diarrhea with trimethoprim/sulfamethoxazole and with trimethoprim alone. N Engl J Med 307:841–844, 1982.

Health Information for International Travel. MMWR 33 (Suppl):1, 1984.

Steffen R, van der Linde F, Gyr K, et al: Epidemiology of diarrhea in travelers. JAMA 249:1176–1180, 1983.

22 · LEG CRAMPS AND RESTLESS LEGS

Franz H. Messerli
Fred E. Husserl
Hector O. Ventura
OCHSNER CLINIC AND ALTON OCHSNER MEDICAL FOUNDATION

Spontaneous leg cramps (charley horses) are a common complaint heard by physicians of all specialties. A distinction between nocturnal leg cramps and so-called restless legs is not always possible since both disorders overlap and can be found in the same patient. Cramps occur in all age groups but are somewhat more common in the elderly. Most often the calf muscles (gastrocnemius or soleus) or the intrinsic muscles of the sole are involved. However, other muscle groups of the foot, as well as in the upper extremity, may be the site of muscle cramps. These usually awaken the patient after a few hours of sleep and are precipitated by a muscular contraction producing an intensely painful spasm of the affected muscle. Patients describe them as excruciating and they may cause much insomnia, anxiety, and distress.

PATHOPHYSIOLOGIC CONSIDERATIONS

The cause of leg cramps and "restless legs" is unknown. However, certain physiologic and pathologic states such as pregnancy, dehydration, denervation, alcohol abuse, diabetes, electrolyte disturbances, uremia and gout, as well as certain medications (diuretics), have been shown to be associated with the painful syndrome. An entity known as "benign fasciculation syndrome" seems to predispose to muscle cramps, and calcium deficiency, hyponatremia, hypokalemia, and hypomagnesemia seem to produce them consistently. Although repletion of a deficient ion most often cures the disorder, treatment with calcium, sodium, potassium, or magnesium in patients who have no documented deficiency has usually little, if any, beneficial effect.

Contraction is the only possible response of muscle tissue to whatever stimulus. Therefore, the passive plantar flexion of the foot that occurs when patients lie down seems to predispose them to leg cramps. Spontaneous neural stimulation of a flaccid and tensionless gastrocnemius and soleus muscle beyond a physiologic limit results in a painful spasm.

MANAGEMENT

NONPHARMACOLOGIC MEASURES

A variety of drugs and maneuvers have been suggested in relieving cramps and restless legs. Stretching exercises of the calf muscles seem to bring relief in about half of all instances. Even in patients who show little response, stretching maximizes any pharmacologic effect sought from medical therapy. The patient is instructed to stand with shoes off in front of a wall 3 to 4 ft away and to lean forward, keeping the heels on the floor, for about ten seconds. During that time, the patient should detect a feeling of pulling in the calf without experiencing any pain. The excercise can be done with both legs at the same time, or alternately with first one then the other. Approximately half of the patients seem to be cured within a week if the stretching exercise is done at least three times a day.

The application of heat in the form of a heating pad or hot compresses may also help some patients.

DRUG TREATMENT

Calcium supplements seem to be particularly effective for leg cramps that occur during pregnancy. The dose we recommend is 1 gm calcium PO twice a day in the form of calcium carbonate. Patients with achlorhydria may have to take gluconate or lactate salt of calcium. Calcium seems to be less effective in the absence of any other disorder.

Quinine and quinidine sulfate have been used to treat leg cramps for several decades. An increase in the refractory period and a decrease in the excitability of the motor end plate occur, and calcium influx is also affected. Quinidine is very effective in uremia or in patients who are on hemodialysis and suffer from excruciatingly painful cramps. The concomitant use of a high sodium dialysate (140 mEq) seems to have an additional beneficial effect. Patients with idiopathic leg

Table 1. PROVED AND UNPROVED MEASURES FOR LEG CRAMPS AND RESTLESS LEGS

Proved Measures	Unproved Measures
Stretching exercises	Magnet between mattress and lower sheet
Quinine and quinidine sulfate	
Vitamin E (tocopherol)	Novocain infiltration
Phenytoin	Injections of vitamin B_{12}
	Disopyramide phosphate (Norpace)
	Sodium fluoride
	Prophylactic hydration
	Vasopressin spray
	Vasodilators (calcium entry blockers, hydralazine [Apresoline])

cramps often show an excellent response to quinidine. The usual dose is 200 to 300 mg PO at bedtime or before dialysis.

Ayres and Mihan reported a series of patients whose leg cramps improved considerably or disappeared completely when *vitamin E*, 100 IU, was given three times a day before meals. In our experience, vitamin E is effective in certain patients and the response is usually seen within a day or two. Many patients, however, do not respond to it.

Occasionally, *phenytoin*, 200 to 400 mg a day, reverses recurrent cramps. A brief course of three to four weeks may be effective and afford long-lasting benefits.

Side effects from calcium, quinidine, and vitamin E in the doses cited are virtually nil. Vitamin E may improve glycogen storage in the muscles and thereby decrease insulin requirements in diabetics. Since leg cramps are common in diabetic patients, this adverse effect should be kept in mind, although it rarely becomes clinically important. Quinidine sulfate may give rise to hemolysis in patients with G6PD deficiency. Acute intravascular hemolysis with tubular necrosis and renal failure have been reported even in otherwise healthy subjects. Quinidine sulfate also can elevate the plasma level of digoxin and prolong the effects of warfarin.

OTHER ANECDOTAL AND UNPROVED MEASURES

A variety of agents mentioned in the literature supposedly bring relief for leg cramps (Table 1). Most of these measures and drugs are anecdotal; however, they seem to help dramatically in a few patients. Since most of these are relatively harmless, they may be tried if the above measures fail.

REFERENCES

Ayres S Jr, Mihan R: Leg cramps (systremma) and "restless legs" syndrome. Calif Med lll:87–91, 1969.
Daniell HW: Simple cure for nocturnal leg cramps (letter to the editor). N Engl J Med 300:1115, 1979.
Hammar M, Larsson L, Tegler L: Calcium treatment of leg cramps in pregnancy. Acta Obstet Gynaecol Scand 60:345–347, 1981.
Parrow A, Samuelsson SM: Use of chloroquine phosphate—a new treatment for spontaneous leg cramps. Acta Med Scand 181:237–244, 1967.
Weiner IH, Weiner HL: Nocturnal leg muscle cramps. JAMA 244:2332–2333, 1980.

23 · EXERCISE IN HEALTH AND PREVENTION OF DISEASE

John J. Duncan
Kenneth H. Cooper
*INSTITUTE FOR AEROBICS RESEARCH
AND THE COOPER CLINIC, DALLAS, TX*

EXERCISE AS PROSPECTIVE MEDICINE

The number of drug prescriptions far exceed the number of exercise prescriptions written annually. This may be paradoxical since the prevalence of sedentary life style is greater than that of any single disease entity. There may be several reasons why exercise is not widely prescribed as prospective medicine: (1) physicians are skeptical of the value of exercise in preventing or altering the natural course of disease, (2) there is no evidence that exercise prolongs life, and (3) exercise is often thought of as difficult in implementation and adherence. However, these three points are not unique to exercise therapy; there is no known treatment to prevent coronary heart disease or prolong life.

Several consistent findings are common to the epidemiologic studies reviewed in this chapter: (1) physical activity status is inversely related to the risk of cardiovascular mortality and morbidity, (2) coronary risk can be reduced by relatively low levels of activity, (3) any protection from coronary heart disease conferred by exercise can be maintained only by lifelong commitment to an exercise program, and (4) reduction of coronary risk through increased exercise occurs independent of concomitant changes in other risk factors. Participation in activities reported to confer protection from coronary disease (walking, cycling, swimming, jogging, tennis, or cross-country skiing) is within the capacity of almost everyone.

EXERCISE AND CORONARY RISK FACTORS

Epidemiologic studies have provided strong evidence linking physical inactivity to greater incidence of coronary heart disease. However, this information does not adequately explain the mechanism(s) by which exercise may confer a protective effect from the development of coronary heart disease. This section will focus on alterations of plasma lipids, blood pressure, glucose intolerance, obesity, and fibrinolysis associated with exercise.

EXERCISE AND LIPIDS

Both epidemiologic and longitudinal evidence indicate that regular aerobic exercise favorably alters lipid concentrations. Such alterations may be one means of explaining a reduction of coronary risk. Improvements of lipid profile after exercise are clinically and statistically significant, with a reduction in coronary risk ascribed

to exercise. HDL-cholesterol and triglyceride levels are the lipid components most often affected by exercise regimens. HDL-cholesterol levels may not change until a "threshold" of exercise has been attained and then increase in a dose-related manner depending on the intensity, frequency, and length of time (in weeks) of exercise.

EXERCISE AND BLOOD PRESSURE

Epidemiologic studies indicate that individuals in better cardiovascular fitness have lower resting blood pressures (both systolic and diastolic) than people in the low-fitness categories. Exercise intervention studies show that BP response is dependent on initial level of BP, those having the highest baseline values experiencing the greatest increase. Significant reductions of resting systolic and diastolic BP attributed to exercise are usually found in individuals with baseline resting BP at the upper end of the normotensive range. The magnitude of changes in systolic BP is generally 3 to 10 mm Hg, while diastolic BP is generally lowered by 3 to 6 mm Hg. These changes are as great as those found after pharmacologic therapy in normotensive patients. Blood pressure reductions found in these studies could be of therapeutic value in individuals with "high normal" BP (diastolic 85 to 89) and those with diastolic BP of 90 to 95 mm Hg.

GLUCOSE INTOLERANCE AND EXERCISE TRAINING

Improved glucose tolerance and increased insulin sensitivity are associated with higher levels of physical activity. Alterations in glucose metabolism generally occur after three months of exercise training. However, studies are needed to investigate the independent effects of exercise on glucose metabolism that are independent of adiposity, diet, and aging and the interrelationships between muscle fiber types, exercise, and glucose metabolism. In view of the current state of knowledge regarding exercise and glucose homeostasis, recommendation of an exercise program with weight control seems warranted for the prevention of adult-onset diabetes.

OBESITY

Obesity has become so prevalent in our society that many regard this condition as a "normal" and inevitable by-product of existence. However, the increase of body weight with age clearly is not inevitable. Dietary and exercise interventions lower the percentage of body fat while preserving lean body mass. Exercise that elicits an increase in heart rate to 70% to 85% of maximal capacity for a minimum of 20 minutes at least three days per week, combined with dietary restriction, appears to be the most effective means of altering body composition. Reversing obesity may lower the risk of coronary heart disease.

EXERCISE AND HEMATOLOGIC ALTERATIONS

Exercise may be effective in preventing intravascular thrombus formation and coronary heart disease by increasing fibrinolysis. Exercise training has also been shown to lower platelet adhesiveness and aggregation, both of which have been implicated in the development of atherosclerosis. By this mechanism, exercise may lessen the potential for deleterious thrombosis formation

Table 1. GUIDELINES IN WRITING AN INDIVIDUAL EXERCISE PRESCRIPTION

Components	Activities	Approximate Time
Baseline medical evaluation:	Suggested for all individuals over 35 years of age or symptomatic individuals under 35 years of age	
Mode of exercise:	Continuous movements utilizing large muscle groups: walking, swimming, cycling, jogging	
Warm-up period:	Stretching, low level calisthenics, etc.	5–10 min
Aerobic phase:		20–30 min
Intensity	Beginning exercisers start at 50%–60% of maximal heart rate, gradually progressing to 70%–85%	
Frequency	3–5 days per week	
Duration	Beginning exercisers should initially exercise for 5–10 min, gradually increasing duration 15–20 sec per session until exercise is performed for 20–30 min	
Cool-down	Calisthenics and/or brisk walking	5–10 min

and resultant clinical manifestations—sudden death, myocardial infarction, or angina.

WRITING AN EXERCISE PRESCRIPTION

Proper prescription of exercise is similar to prescription of medication. One should have an understanding of the physiologic responses of exercise, and the dosage should be titrated to meet individual needs. Writing an exercise prescription entails several sequential steps, including: (1) baseline medical evaluation; (2) determination of the mode of exercise; (3) initial and follow-up calculation of intensity, duration, and frequency; and (4) detailed instructions regarding warm-up and cool-down periods (Table 1). Periodic follow-up consultations are necessary to reassess progress, revise the prescription, and improve patient compliance. The patient should be taught the values of exercise, how to establish goals, and what is expected of him or her.

BASELINE MEDICAL EVALUATION

Baseline medical evaluations are necessary to assess the presence or absence of disease and the functional capacity of each participant. Before an exercise program is begun, a thorough medical screening consisting of medical history, physical examination, and resting and exercise EKGs should be administered. These evaluations help to identify individuals who should not participate in an exercise program or who need special adjustments. Data collected from the exercise stress test also help to determine the intensity, duration, and frequency of exercise required to improve cardiovascular fitness, and lessen the potential for deleterious effects.

MODE OF EXERCISE

Aerobic exercise involves activities that emphasize continuous movement of large muscle groups for extended periods. Activities such as weight lifting increase muscle mass but do little to improve cardiovascular fitness. Thus, activities such as walking, jogging, cycling, and swimming provide optimal cardiovascular benefit. Other activities, such as basketball, can be adapted to aerobic exercise provided the rules are changed to incorporate continuous movements for sufficient time periods. Almost any activity can be aerobic if it elicits the proper heart rate response for the specified duration.

INTENSITY

Several methods can be used to prescribe proper intensity levels of each exercise session. Heart rate is perhaps the most frequently employed method of calculating exercise intensity. A percentage of the maximal heart rate obtained during a multi-stage exercise test is used in an equation to calculate the target heart rate zone. With this method, maximal heart rate, resting heart rate, and intensity level are entered into an equation that computes target heart rate zone. Maximal heart rate should preferably be obtained from a multi-stage exercise test, but can be estimated by subtracting the patient's age from 220. The following example illustrates the steps needed to calculate proper target exercise level serving to enhance cardiovascular fitness for a 20-year-old:

$$
\begin{aligned}
\text{Maximal heart rate} &= 200 \\
\text{Resting heart rate} &= \underline{-65} \\
& \ \ 135 \\
\text{Intensity level (70\%)} &= \underline{\times .70} \\
& \ \ 94.50 \\
\text{Resting heart rate} & \underline{+65.00} \\
\text{Minimal heart rate} &= 159.50
\end{aligned}
$$

This value represents the minimal heart rate for the target zone. The maximal training level would be calculated in a similar manner but with a different intensity level (i.e., 85%). In this example, this maximal training level is calculated as approximately 180 beats per minute. Previous research has shown that optimal cardiovascular benefits are derived with exercise intensities between 70% and 85% (in this example, between 159.50 and 180 beats per minute). However, beginning exercisers should probably start at between 60% and 70%. Exercise heart rates can be measured during the activity by stopping, counting the number of beats in ten seconds, and multiplying by six to obtain a heart rate per minute. It is important not to stop for more than ten seconds during vigorous exercise because this results in a precipitous decrease in heart rate. Carotid or brachial pulse may be used to compute heart rate, but massaging or depressing the carotid bodies may precipitate dangerous arrhythmia.

Metabolic equivalents (METS) are used as an estimate for intensity of various exercises. Since some individuals have difficulty recording or obtaining an accurate heart rate, there are tables that estimate energy requirements of each activity (i.e., running 10 mph). One MET is equivalent to 3.5 ml/kg/min of oxygen. Similar procedures used to calculate target heart rate levels are employed with METS: (1) calculate the maximal MET level obtained during a multi-stage exercise test (i.e., 6 METS); (2) add the maximal MET level to

60% (i.e., 6 + 60 = 66%); (3) multiply the value in the second step by the maximal MET level (66% × 6 = 3.96 METS); and (4) choose the activities that correspond to this intensity level (3.96 METS). MET levels for a wide variety of occupational and recreational activities are provided by the American Heart Association. Exercise based on these levels has been shown to improve cardiovascular fitness.

DURATION

Each exercise session should consist of a 5- to 10-minute warm-up, a 20- to 30-minute aerobic phase, followed by a 10- to 15-minute cool-down period. The warm-up phase serves to stretch the muscles and gradually increase heart rate. Stretching exercises should concentrate on trunk and leg muscle groups (i.e., hamstring, quadriceps, and gastrocnemius).

Optimal cardiovascular health is achieved with 20 to 30 minutes per session. Many of the beneficial effects of exercise, such as higher HDL, improved glucose tolerance, and decreased BP, generally require 20 to 30 minutes of exercise three to five days per week. However, for beginning exercisers it is important to start at minimal durations (10 to 15 minutes) and gradually increase over a period of weeks. There is a higher incidence of musculoskeletal injuries in individuals who begin exercising at too high an intensity or for too long. A good rule-of-thumb to prevent musculoskeletal injuries is not to change exercise intensity, duration, or frequency abruptly or simultaneously.

The third phase of the exercise session is the cool-down period. This serves to lower heart rate gradually and prevent peripheral pooling of blood in the lower extremities. Motionless activity after strenuous exercise can precipitate syncope or dangerous arrhythmia due to inadequate venous return to the myocardium. Thus, it is important to remain in motion after the aerobic phase is over, but at a slower level. Recovery heart rates can be checked after five minutes of cool-down; rates below 120 beats per minute generally indicate a cardiovascular training effect.

FREQUENCY

Optimal health benefits are obtained from participating in exercise programs three to five days per week. The beginning exerciser should start at three days per week, with each exercise day separated by one day of rest. Increasing the frequency to four to five days per week provides additional cardiovascular improvement, but risks an increased incidence of musculoskeletal injuries. Maintenance of any cardiovascular health benefit derived from exercise training requires that exercise be adopted as a lifelong habit. Regression of health benefits may occur in as little as five weeks after discontinuation of exercise. Thus, it is recommended that exercise become an integral part of daily routine.

AEROBIC POINT SYSTEM

The "aerobic point system" of Cooper accurately quantitates the cardiovascular value of various activities. Each aerobic point reflects the intensity and duration of an activity. This system allows novices and experienced exercisers alike an opportunity to understand and compare the aerobic benefits of various types of activities. Cooper recommends earning a minimum of 30 aerobic points per week. This value corresponds to a "good" category of cardiovascular fitness obtained on a maximal exercise tolerance test (VO_2 max = 42.0 mg/kg/min).

Cooper's program includes "field tests" to measure cardiovascular fitness, and chart packs that calculate the aerobic benefits derived from various activities. The 12-minute walk-run test involves covering the greatest distance in 12 minutes; the 1.5-mile test involves the amount of time needed to cover 1.5 miles. Norms for both tests are based on maximal aerobic capacity (maximal VO_2 ml/kg/min). Individuals over the age of 35 or who have any cardiovascular risk factors should not participate in field testing.

CONCLUSIONS

Sedentary life styles predominate in our society despite an abundance of evidence indicating that exercise may be a versatile medicine to prevent deleterious health consequences. Exercise of adequate intensity, frequency, and duration has many salutary effects including increased fibrinolysis and HDL levels, and lowered BP, plasma insulin level, glucose levels, LDL level, platelet adhesiveness, and adiposity. Sufficient experimental and epidemiologic evidence exists to indicate that the relationship between exercise and good health is more than circumstantial. Most people can participate in some form of exercise program. However, physicians have a role in persuading, educating, and motivating their patients.

EXERCISE AND SECONDARY PREVENTION OF CORONARY DISEASE

Secondary prevention of coronary heart disease involves modification of coronary risk factors after an event has occurred. Modification of risk factors at this point serves to alter the normal course of coronary disease and prevent recurrence of coronary events (i.e., myocardial infarction).

EXERCISE AND HYPERTENSION

Aerobic exercise training has consistently been shown to lower systolic and diastolic BP of hypertensive patients. Interpretation of the findings is often difficult because of concomitant weight reductions, changes in diet, or lack of control groups. However, a recent well-controlled study demonstrated that exercise significantly lowered systolic and diastolic BP in mildly hypertensive patients, without concomitant changes of body weight or diet. BP reductions after training were statistically significant. Diastolic BP is often lowered 5 to 12 mm Hg immediately after exercise training.

EXERCISE PRESCRIPTION FOR HYPERTENSIVE PATIENTS

All hypertensive patients should undergo maximal exercise tolerance testing with EKG and BP monitoring. Repeat testing should occur at specified intervals during the exercise program. Maximal tolerance testing is conducted to evaluate the presence of underlying coronary disease and to record BP response to acute exercise. Patients with resting diastolic BP between 90 and 104 mm Hg safely participate in an exercise program of adequate intensity (70% to 85%), duration (20 to 30 minutes), and frequency (three to five days per week).

Activities such as walking, jogging, swimming, and cycling are recommended as the aerobic activities from which hypertensive patients will derive optimal health dividends. Exercise may be used as primary therapy for the first six months in asymptomatic patients with diastolic BP of 90 to 104 mm Hg. If diastolic BP is not below 90 mm Hg after six months, pharmacologic treatment should be administered along with exercise.

EXERCISE AND ANTIHYPERTENSIVE MEDICATIONS

Diuretics generally do not attenuate cardiovascular responses to exercise, but do lower BP. Thus, exercise prescription based on heart rate may be utilized in a routine manner. However, special precautions should be taken to prevent hypokalemia, especially during the summer months. Individuals experiencing difficulty regulating potassium levels should be switched to a potassium-sparing diuretic or another medication. Exercise may also precipitate nocturnal leg cramps in patients taking diuretics, possibly because of extensive dehydration and/or electrolyte (potassium, magnesium) depletion.

Beta-blockade attenuates heart rates, and cardiac output at rest, during submaximal exercise and at maximal levels of exercise. Lower cardiovascular hemodynamics occur with both selective and nonselective beta-blockers, but the effects are dose dependent, higher doses being associated with greater attenuation of cardiac function. Studies with low-dose beta-blockade generally are able to improve exercise capacity, while the effects of higher dose are inconsistent. In any event, exercise heart rates need to be adjusted since a patient may not be able to attain the same training heart rate that was achieved before receiving beta-blocker therapy. Exercise heart rates should be recalculated to values of 70% to 85% from the maximal heart rate the patient achieved while receiving beta-blockers.

Sympatholytic drugs either produce relatively minor reductions of resting and exercise heart rate or no change. Likewise, resting and exercise cardiac output is generally lowered to a small extent. These drugs also lower exercise BP without compromising exercise capacity. Improvement in maximal oxygen uptake occurs following an adequate aerobic exercise program. However, special consideration should be given to the cool-down period to prevent hypotension. Stress testing should also be conducted to provide a basis for prescribing proper heart rate intensity.

Vasodilators and alpha-blockade generally do not interfere with cardiovascular response to exercise. Increases in maximal oxygen uptake occur in hypertensive patients receiving treatment with prazosin. From a physiologic standpoint, prazosin may be one of the drugs of choice in hypertensive patients who desire to participate in an exercise program, because it does not interfere with normal cardiac responses to exercise. However, the cool-down period after exercise is very important to prevent postexercise hypotension. Patients should walk slowly for five to ten minutes after cessation from activity. Similarly, patients taking calcium entry blockers and angiotensin converting enzyme inhibitors can expect to have a normal hemodynamic response to exercise.

In summary, hypertensive patients receiving anti-hypertensive medication may safely engage in exercise programs provided there are no other conditions contraindicating participation. With the exception of beta-blockers, most antihypertensive medication does not significantly affect cardiovascular hemodynamics during exercise. Improvements in maximal oxygen uptake generally occur with concomitant pharmacotherapy. However, depending on the dose, beta-blockers may attenuate the rise in maximal oxygen uptake associated with exercise training. Exercise prescriptions based on heart rates are written in a usual manner for all patients except those receiving beta-blocker therapy. Exercise heart rates in these individuals should be adjusted to reflect a percentage of the maximal heart rate obtained while they are receiving beta-blocker therapy.

DIABETES

Exercise provides an excellent adjunctive means of controlling glucose levels in both non–insulin-dependent and insulin-dependent diabetes. There are at least five favorable effects of exercise on glucose homeostasis: (1) increased insulin sensitivity, (2) decreased body weight, (3) decrease in cardiovascular risk factors, (4) acute and carry-over improvement of glucose tolerance, and (5) increased metabolism of ketone bodies.

EXERCISE PRESCRIPTION FOR DIABETES

Several important considerations for the non–insulin-dependent diabetic, including hypoglycemia and dehydration during or following exercise, have been stressed by Devlin. These situations can be overcome by carrying a rapidly absorbable source of carbohydrate, and by ingestion of an adequate amount of water. Hypoglycemia may be precipitated by the combination of exercise and sulfonylurea drugs, while other drugs such as phenylbutazone, sulfonamides, and monoamine oxidase inhibitors may further exaggerate the action of sulfonylureas. Exercise programs also should not be started in poorly controlled diabetes owing to the risk of ketosis.

Exercise alters insulin and glucose kinetics. Exercise performed immediately after an injection of insulin causes an increased absorption of insulin, which in turn inhibits glucose production, finally culminating in lower availability of blood glucose for skeletal muscle uptake and hypoglycemia. To reduce the possibility of exercise-induced hypoglycemia, Devlin recommends injection into the abdomen or nonexercising limb (if exercise is performed within 30 minutes of injection; otherwise, the patient should wait to exercise for 30 to 60 minutes following injection). Insulin injections may be made anywhere if exercise is not performed for at least 60 minutes.

Insulin doses have to be retitrated for each patient. Devlin recommends decreasing the dose by one third in patients receiving only one injection of intermediate-acting insulin per day, omitting the short-acting injection and reducing the intermediate by one third in patients who normally use a combination of intermediate- and short-acting injections. Also, if insulin is delivered via a continuous subcutaneous pump, reduce the rate by one third.

Exercise intensity, duration, and frequency can be prescribed in a usual manner: intensity, 70% to 85%;

duration, 20 to 30 minutes; frequency, three to five days per week. Like other patients, diabetics should have a thorough physical examination, including maximal EKG tolerance testing. These tests are necessary to rule out any underlying coronary disease, a common clinical manifestation in this population.

PERIPHERAL VASCULAR DISEASE

EXERCISE PRESCRIPTION FOR PERIPHERAL VASCULAR DISEASE

All patients with peripheral vascular disease should undergo a complete physical examination including a symptom-limited exercise tolerance test. Exercise may be contraindicated in patients whose disease is severe. Walking may be the best form of exercise for patients with peripheral vascular disease because of the principle of specificity of training. This means that oxidative and morphologic changes occur in specific muscles in response to specific exercises. Since claudication generally occurs while the patient is walking, conditioning of these muscles and vasculature to this specific form of activity should provide optimal improvements. Each patient should exercise just below the threshold of claudication, but not to levels that precipitate pain. This threshold will change following several months of a walking program, so that the intensity may be increased while exercise is still kept below the pain threshold.

CHRONIC OBSTRUCTIVE PULMONARY DISEASE (COPD)

EXERCISE PRESCRIPTION FOR COPD

Activities that utilize small muscle groups should be avoided (e.g., arm ergometry) owing to substantial increases of lactate and increased ventilatory response compared with similar workloads utilizing large muscle groups (e.g., leg muscles). Exercise should be conducted in an environment with relatively low levels of atmosphere pollutants. If pollution is high enough to impair pulmonary function, exercising should be performed either early in the morning, when environmental pollution may be lower, or indoors.

Psychologic benefits derived from exercise may explain any improvements in physiologic status induced by exercise training. Exercise can exaggerate dyspnea in COPD patients, which creates anxiety and a fearful state, thus limiting the amount of exercise. Lack or total avoidance of exercise owing to psychologic perception of physiologic effects leads to absenteeism, which in turn contributes to a further deterioration of pulmonary function and general health. Thus, it is important to incorporate exercise slowly, motivate and reassure patients, and explain to them the type of physiologic response that may be elicited by exercise. Improvements in maximal ventilation, maximal exercise time, and cardiac function are often found in individuals who are able to attain higher levels of exercise.

Initially, COPD patients should participate in several short periods of walking, each lasting one to two minutes. Duration should be increased by one to two minutes every two weeks until the patient is able to exercise continuously for 20 to 25 minutes. The intensity of each exercise session should be below the threshold of dyspnea. The frequency should be three to five days per week.

Hypoxia and pulmonary hypertension may occur in COPD patients during exercise. Supplemental oxygen often corrects these symptoms. Bronchodilators also are effective in prophylaxis during exercise.

SUMMARY

Exercise can have an important beneficial influence on many disease states. There are many other applications of exercise to disease states such as osteoporosis, arthritis, and some psychologic disorders. Exercise in these contexts may not be curative but may lessen symptoms, improve capacity, and decrease the possibility of secondary events. Exercise is not a panacea or cure-all, but approached rationally may serve as valuable adjunctive therapy. Perhaps contemplation of the benefits of exercise led to these inspired words:

> Better to hunt in Fields, for Health unbought,
> Than fee the Doctor for a nauseous Draught.
> The Wise, for Cure, on Exercise depend;
> God never made his Work, for Man to mend.
>
> JOHN DRYDEN

REFERENCES

American College of Sports Medicine: Guidelines for Graded Exercise Testing in Exercise Prescription, 2nd ed. Lea & Febiger, Philadelphia, 1980.

American Heart Association: The committee on exercise. Exercise testing and training in individuals with heart disease are at high risk for its development. American Heart Association, Dallas, 1972.

Blair SN, Goodyear NN, Gibbons LW, et al: Physical fitness and incidence of hypertension in healthy normotensive men and women. JAMA 252:487, 1984.

Braun SR, Fregosi, R, Reddan WG: Exercise training in patients with COPD. Postgrad Med 71:163, 1982.

Cooper KH: The Aerobics Program for Total Well-being. M. Evans Co, New York, 1982.

Devlin JT, Horton ES: An exercise regimen for diabetics. Cardiovasc Med 10:65, 1985.

Duncan JJ, Hagan RD, Upton S, et al: The effects of an aerobic exercise program on plasma catecholamines and blood pressure in patients with mild essential hypertension. JAMA 254:2609, 1985.

Pollock ML: The quantification of endurance training program. In Wilmore J (ed): Exercise and Sports Science Review. Academic Press, New York, 1973.

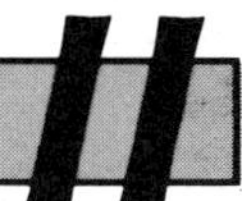

THE CARDIOVASCULAR SYSTEM

EDWARD D. FROHLICH
EDWARD GENTON

1 · CORONARY ARTERY DISEASE

John H. Chapman
GEISINGER MEDICAL CENTER

DEFINITION

The coronary arteries are commonly involved by obstructive atherosclerosis, resulting in myocardial ischemia. Angina pectoris and myocardial infarction (MI) with its complications are the clinical manifestations that constitute the major epidemic of our time: coronary heart disease.

PATHOPHYSIOLOGY

The symptom angina is usually an oppressive chest discomfort precipitated by stress and relieved by rest after two to ten minutes. This discomfort is caused by an imbalance between the oxygen (O_2) demands of the myocardium and O_2 supply by the coronary blood flow. Assuming an adequate perfusion pressure, blood flow depends on the resistance of both large arteries and distal arterioles. Flow is normally controlled by arteriolar responsiveness to metabolic demands, but with large vessel disease this capacity becomes limited because of proximal resistance, which dominates. This resistance may be reversible in coronary spasm (Prinzmetal angina), but more often is fixed owing to atherosclerotic narrowing of the vessel. A decrease in the O_2 content of blood, as with anemia or hypoxemia, also limits O_2 supply.

With fixed disease, then, we must understand the determinants of myocardial O_2 demand that govern the clinical syndrome. These are (1) heart rate, (2) contractility, and (3) ventricular wall stress during systole. Wall stress depends on both left ventricular (LV) systolic pressure and LV volume (law of Laplace). Accordingly, hypertension aggravates angina by increasing wall stress. Digitalis in a nonfailing heart may aggravate angina because of its effect on contractility, but would help if it controlled the heart rate in atrial fibrillation.

In a failing heart, digitalis, diuretics, or nitrates may help angina by shrinking a dilated heart.

Several factors are involved in the initiating sequence leading to infarction: intimal damage, platelet aggregation, and vasospasm with modulating influence by circulating thromboxane A_2 and local production of prostacyclins, histamine, and serotonin. Although the sequence is unclear, thrombosis does appear to be the final common pathway in most patients evolving transmural (Q-wave) infarctions. The incidence of thrombosis is lower in nontransmural (non–Q-wave) infarctions, suggesting that in these patients a severe imbalance between myocardial O_2 supply and demand may be the predominant factor. By definition, infarction implies myocardial necrosis; however, the process of cell death is not at all instantaneous. In any patient, there is a given amount of ischemic myocardium at risk, the fate of which is dependent on the delicate balance between O_2 demand and supply.

CLINICAL ASPECTS: DIAGNOSIS

Fear of heart disease is prevalent in our society, and accompanying anxiety leads to a loss of life quality as great as or greater than the disease itself. We must, therefore, be absolutely certain and confident in diagnosis. It is better to go as far as cardiac catheterization to be certain than to treat tentatively as "possible" angina.

Chest pain can be classified by history into three categories: (1) typical angina, (2) noncardiac chest pain, and (3) atypical chest pain of undetermined origin. The patient with *typical exertional pain* should be treated as such. Exercise testing is unnecessary for diagnosis, though you may wish to assess functional capacity in a stable patient for management planning. Remember, however, that many patients with a typical history have come to the physician only after the symptoms have become unstable. These individuals should never be put on a treadmill; they need medical stabilization, which often involves hospitalization. Patients with obvious *noncardiac pain* should be reassured completely. They should *not* be given nitroglycerin "just in case." This approach reflects uncertainty on the part of the physician, which is sensed immediately by patients, continuing the cycle of fear. If you cannot confidently reassure people, a diagnostic test should reaffirm your diagnosis. Patients with *atypical pain* should undergo diagnostic testing before any treatment program is started. Remember that a 12-lead EKG *during* pain can be as useful as any of the more expensive diagnostic procedures.

Treadmill exercise electrocardiography is an important diagnostic tool and, as long as its limitations are understood beforehand, can serve as a sound basis for clinical judgment. For functional assessment of a patient with known disease, it is unparalleled. In patients with hypertension, valvular heart disease, LV hypertrophy, QRS prolongation, or resting ST-T abnormality or who are on digitalis, there is a high chance of false-positive EKG changes. If diagnosis is the goal, these individuals should have a concomitant radionuclide study whenever feasible. In the absence of these factors, ST segment depression (≥ 1.0 mm) that is either horizontal or downsloping can be considered abnormal. Under ideal circumstances, the exercise EKG has a sensitivity of 70% and a specificity of 90%. In expert hands, concomitant radionuclide testing may improve the sensitivity to 90%. Keep in mind that a "positive" exercise test is just as much based on the reproduction of pain as it is on the appearance of the EKG or scan.

The diagnosis of MI is based on history, EKG changes, transitory cardiac enzyme elevation, and (occasionally) cardiac imaging with technetium-99m stannous pyrophosphate (TcPYP). At least two of these diagnostic procedures should be positive before a diagnosis is made. In transmural MI, there is typical EKG evolution with development of new 0.04 second Q waves. In nontransmural MI, there are usually persistent new ST- and T-wave abnormalities without Q waves. The creatine kinase (CK) isoenzymes are not perfect, but are remarkably specific and should be available in all institutions. In our laboratory, an elevation of the CK-MB fraction to $\geq 2.5\%$ of the total CK is considered abnormal. Most of the rare conditions that could give false-positive CK-MB, such as dermatomyositis or Duchenne's muscular dystrophy, should be clinically obvious. The lack of specificity of other cardiac enzymes has led us away from their routine use, though lactic dehydrogenase (LDH) isoenzymes may be useful in late diagnosis. The TcPYP is needed only when (1) bundle branch block or pacemaker rhythm obscures the EKG diagnosis or (2) the patient arrives 36 or more hours after onset of pain, when enzymes might be missed.

The EKG may still be normal early in the course of MI. A decision to admit should be based on the history. Chronic atypical, nonexertional chest pain should be treated as noncardiac pain until proved otherwise. This approach allays fear, but when a patient is frightened enough by a new prolonged episode to come to the emergency room, it is wise to have a high index of suspicion. The classic presentation with crushing pain, nausea, and diaphoresis does occur, but atypical presentations such as those mimicking gastrointestinal distress are very common. If you are concerned enough to do enzyme tests, the patient should be observed in the hospital. We do, however, tend to practice a little too carefully (and expensively); some patients with low-probability episodes do not need admission to the Coronary Care Unit (CCU) to be "ruled out."

MANAGEMENT OF ANGINA

APPROACH TO THE PATIENT

The angina patient is experiencing physical symptoms he does not understand that interfere with usual activity. More than that, he is fearful. *Initial goals* in therapy should be to (1) stabilize symptoms with a good medical regimen; (2) educate the patient, avoiding any confusion or uncertainty; (3) establish a plan the patient has confidence in, including optimistic goals tempered with realistic expectations; and (4) take "control" of an unsettled situation with confident reassurance. *Long-term goals* include (1) regular adjustments of the program in order to achieve a high-quality life, (2) willingness to change the plan if goals are not achieved or to help change to more realistic ones if necessary, (3) long-term behavior modification regarding risk factors, and (4) ongoing reassurance and support.

Taking the time to educate early will pay big dividends later. A diagram can be used to demonstrate the three major coronary arteries, explaining angina and heart attack in very simplified terms: angina as a "warning" and heart attack as "permanent damage." Risk factors are reviewed but it should be made clear that the cause of atherosclerosis is unknown and there is therefore no "cure." The three approaches to treatment (medicine, surgery, angioplasty) are reviewed optimistically with the patient, but the limitations of our knowledge and capabilities should be made clear so that goals are realistic. The role of catheterization should be explained. Keep it simple. Fancy words like "revascularization" may impress your patient but won't mean a thing; "detour or bypass so blood has a new way to get to the heart muscle" will make it clear. This education session takes only 20 to 30 minutes, but whenever I have "not had the time," it has always come back to haunt me.

Patients do better in the long run if from the very beginning they work on learning to live with the disease rather than struggling to be rid of it. It is human nature to fight something threatening in order to get it solved and over with. So often after surgery patients psychologically consider it "over with," but when angina recurs a year later, or a bypass graft closes, they feel shattered. They fight back by blaming the surgeon or stresses at work, and frantically ask "what do we do now?" Eventually, this attitude may lead to misery and failure to cope, even in patients whose disease is relatively mild.

This dilemma is caused by unrealistic expectations about coronary artery bypass surgery and angioplasty, and we physicians are partly responsible. We recommend the procedure as a way to "fix" the patient because we are human and we want it to be so. But this unrealistic attitude must be avoided by honest discussion *beforehand*. Patients need to know that after successful surgery there may be some recurrent angina that will require medication, that not all grafts stay open forever, that angioplasty may have to be repeated, and that the disease itself may progress. This can be explained in an optimistic and soothing manner.

We can be both realistic about the limitations of current therapy and positive in setting goals: to maintain for each patient as full, active, productive, and enjoyable a life style as possible. To accomplish this, our objectives should be not only control of pain, but also control of fear and preservation of self-confidence.

The phrase "surgery only if refractory to medical therapy" is inadequate. Patients may be symptom free on $50.00 a month worth of medications, but unhappy because they have also given up the things they find meaningful. You must know your patients, what makes them the happiest and what gives them the most sense of self-worth; these are the activities to set as goals. It may be golf, tennis, hunting, or farming. It may be the job. Forced early retirement can be a severe blow to an already battered ego. If a long awaited vacation trip was planned, the goal should be to make that trip. If these positive goals cannot be achieved with medical therapy, catheterization and either surgery or angioplasty should be considered. Your initial interview should include discussion of these positive goals with both patient and spouse, because patients' natural tendency is to give up the things they love out of fear. They need to know that these activities do not cause heart attacks. Your encouragement and support will allow for a better quality of life than patients would allow themselves.

Because of their coronary anatomy, not all patients are good candidates for surgery or angioplasty. Knowledge of that anatomy is a major factor in setting realistic goals of therapy. *Catheterization is not a commitment to surgery or angioplasty*; it is the acquisition of information to allow more meaningful planning. The patient with unfavorable anatomy is likely to be continued on medical therapy with more restricted goals, whereas the patient with favorable anatomy is likely to be nudged toward surgery in order to preserve higher goals. We must not make the mistake of "operating on an anatomy," but the procedure is necessary to establish the options.

Indications for catheterization are (1) uncertainty as to diagnosis, (2) unacceptable quality of life due to angina despite optimal medical therapy, (3) markedly abnormal stress test at low workload, (4) recurrent angina after MI, and (5) new-onset angina in a young, active patient. Age is relative. Many 70-year-olds are "younger" than others at 55 because of their active life style; the goal should be to preserve it. No patient should ever be pushed into invasive procedures, but all patients should be educated on their level as to the risks and benefits.

The mortality risk from diagnostic catheterization in experienced hands is less than one in 1000 (<0.1%). An unstable patient with class IV angina has a higher risk, one in 150 (0.67%). Life-threatening complications are more likely in patients with advanced disease (particularly left main coronary stenosis), but these are also the individuals most likely to benefit from surgery, making the risk well worth the benefit. The decision to recommend catheterization should never be undertaken lightly. As long as you and your patient set goals together, the decision will come naturally.

Percutaneous transluminal coronary angioplasty (PTCA) has expanded our capabilities and found a definite role in management. It provides an intermediate step to apply in earlier stages of the natural history, primarily single-vessel disease, reserving surgery for a later stage when multiple vessels are involved. I do not think of PTCA as a substitute for surgery, but rather as an adjunct. Before PTCA we were in an all-or-none therapeutic situation, surgery or no surgery, and for good reasons refrained from definitive treatment for patients with single-vessel disease unless they really were "refractory." Now we can avoid premature surgery and at the same time maintain a high quality of life. The procedure is economical both in the hospital and in terms of days lost from work. In experienced hands, PTCA is 80% to 90% successful.

The risk of the procedure, however, is quite real. Approximately 5% of patients develop a complication that necessitates emergency surgery, so there must be a surgical team available. There is approximately a 20% clinical recurrence rate after successful angioplasty, which may require a second procedure. Thus, PTCA has many advantages but is not a cure-all, and it carries a mortality risk (1.0%) not dissimilar to that from surgery. A candidate for angioplasty should also be a candidate for surgery.

As with any new procedure, the indications for PTCA are still in a state of flux and vary somewhat, depending on the experience of the operator. Our indications are (1) single-vessel disease, (2) "second"-vessel disease with previous infarction from first-vessel occlusion, (3) bypass graft stenosis at distal anastomotic site, (4) new-vessel stenosis in previously operated patients, and (5) selected multi-vessel disease cases with favorable anatomy.

The randomized coronary artery surgery study (CASS) has demonstrated that coronary artery bypass surgery (CABG) does not improve survival rate or subsequent infarction rate in patients who either are asymptomatic after MI or have mild stable angina. Further analysis of the data, however, suggests that a subset of patients with poor LV function (ejection fraction <50%) may fare better with surgery. Because they were not included in the study, nothing can be said about patients with severe angina. Three definite statements can be made: (1) surgery does improve prognosis in patients with left main coronary disease, (2) patients with poor LV function and multi-vessel disease are more likely to benefit from surgery, and (3) surgery can improve the quality of life in patients whose symptoms are not adequately controlled medically. Our decision-making should be based on each patient's own assessment of life quality rather than strictly on anatomy. I am very aggressive about treatment in patients who are significantly symptomatic, because I am convinced of the positive effect of surgery, not only on symptoms but also on a sense of well-being and self-confidence.

Unstable Angina. Mild changes in frequency of angina can be dealt with on an outpatient basis, but whenever there is a dramatic change in pain pattern, particularly pain at rest, the situation is dangerous and hospitalization is indicated. An EKG is helpful for diagnosis when there is pain. Intravenous nitroglycerin generally controls symptoms while other adjustments are made. Often, bed rest and sedation suffice. Avoid rushing an unstable patient off to the catheterization laboratory; the risk is high. Whenever possible, the patient should first be stabilized and observed for several days. If urgent catheterization is necessary, it is best to insert an intra-aortic balloon counterpulsation unit, which may by itself stabilize the situation and allow for catheterization and surgery under safer conditions.

Prinzmetal's Angina. Variant angina (Prinzmetal's) is diagnosed by an EKG during pain demonstrating ST-segment elevation that disappears after pain relief. Documentation is essential. The pain itself is usually rather typical in character but occurs at rest, often in a cyclical pattern. If your suspicion is high, hospitalize the patient without medications and wait for the opportunity to document with an EKG during pain. On occasion, an outpatient Holter monitor study picks up an obvious case, but this is a less reliable method of diagnosis. Catheterization should be done in documented cases because severe fixed disease is so often present. If suspicion is very high but documentation lacking, an ergonovine provocation test can be performed at catheterization, but my own experience is that spending the time and effort to get an EKG during pain is far more productive. Once a diagnosis is made, calcium antagonist therapy is quite specific and effective.

NONPHARMACOLOGIC THERAPY

When managing coronary disease, look for any correctable factors that are adversely affecting myocardial O_2 supply and demand. *Oxygen supply* may be diminished by (1) hypoxemia due to asthma or pneumonia; (2) anemia due to occult GI bleeding; (3) hypotension due to overdiuresis or drug intolerance; and (4) severe bradycardia due to sinus node disease, heart block, or drug overdose. *Oxygen demand* may be increased by (1) increased wall tension due to hypertension, LV outflow tract obstruction, or congestive failure (CHF); (2) increased heart rate due to fever, hyperthyroidism, hypovolemia, anxiety, pain, drug toxicity, or primary tachyarrhythmia; and (3) increased contractility due to inotropic agents in a nonfailing heart.

This should be an automatic checklist on every encounter. Patients whose angina is out of control may not need medication changes or immediate catheterization; rather, they may have dropped hemoglobin to 9 gm, slipped into CHF, or developed pneumonia. Patients with BP of 180/100 should not be labeled "refractory" until the BP is controlled.

There comes a point in the natural history when disabling angina demands a reduction in stress and a significant decrease in normal activities despite continued attempts to adjust the medical program. Optimistic goals should be stressed early in the natural history because it is possible to maintain an almost full life style for many years. Aside from teaching patients to "pace" and avoid extremes such as shoveling snow or lifting heavy weights, it is unfair to restrict them unnecessarily. But a time does come that we are often slow to recognize, when expectations have to change and no more "fixing" can or should be done. This realization should be gentle and gradual. Once both patient and doctor accept it, we learn to stop fighting the angina and start adapting to it. I am continually amazed at how beautifully people do once they make that psychologic adjustment of "acceptance."

The physician's role is to encourage and suggest, not to dictate changes. Patients usually make their own adjustments and simply ask for your advice. Even sensitive problems such as sexual activity generally work themselves out; it is not usually necessary to discuss "positions" of intercourse, but you should be prepared to do so. Driving a car is often a basic necessity and, except for discouraging long trips, I try not to restrict this unless syncope or recurrent arrhythmia require it.

Patients recuperating from surgery need special support. There is almost always incisional chest pain, which frightens patients and must be differentiated from pericarditis; all that's required is analgesics and reassurance. Families and friends tend to "baby" patients, slowing their progress. This requires family counseling and frequent support, best supplied by a trained cardiac rehabilitation team. *Patients must be constantly reminded of the goals you set out in the beginning.* Particularly in men, a postoperative depression often occurs and may be accompanied by temporary sexual dysfunction. Open discussion, reassurance, and frequent encouragement to get back to normal activities (including work) almost always solves these problems.

Later in the course, real angina may recur, particularly in those whose revascularization was incomplete or whose graft flows were poor owing to diffuse disease. This is where your preoperative discussion regarding expectations will pay off; the problem may be easily managed by reinstitution of a good medical program. I try to avoid any discussion of repeat catheterization, which only starts the fear cycle over again. *Many patients need both surgery and medical therapy to achieve their goals, and should be told so from the beginning.*

DRUG THERAPY

Just as there is no evidence that surgery prolongs life in most situations, so there is no evidence that drug therapy prolongs life, with the exception of beta-blockers in the first three years following MI. It is not mandatory for coronary patients to take a lot of medicine. The goal of drug therapy is the same as for other therapies: quality of life. Sometimes the drugs we prescribe do more to lessen the enjoyment of life than to enhance it. Frequent reassessment and flexibility are crucial to good management (Table 1).

There is no cookbook treatment plan for angina. Each patient is different and may respond differently to medication. I generally start off with a combination of oral isosorbide dinitrate and propranolol, adjusting the doses upward as required. If beta-blockers are contraindicated because of CHF or bronchospasm, calcium antagonists may be needed early; otherwise, they probably should be held in reserve because of their cost.

Nitrates. Nitrates remain the cornerstone of angina therapy. Their mechanism of action is not completely understood, but involves an indirect effect through systemic vasodilation and the direct effect of coronary vasodilation. Some patients are exquisitely sensitive when therapy is begun and develop headache due to meningeal vessel dilation. All patients should be warned about headache, given low dosage to start, and urged

Table 1. SIDE EFFECTS OF ANTIANGINAL DRUGS*

	Hypotension, Flushing, Headache	Left Ventricular Dysfunction	Decreased Heart Rate Atrioventricular Block†	Gastrointestinal Symptoms	Bronchoconstriction‡
Betablockers	0	+ +	+ + +	+	+ + +
Nitrates	+ + +	0	0	0	0
Diltiazem	+	+	+	0	0
Nifedipine	+ + +	0	0	0	0
Verapamil	+	+	+ +	+ +	0

*0 = absent; + = mild; + + = moderate; + + + sometimes severe.

†In patients with sick sinus node syndrome or conduction system disease.

‡In patients with obstructive lung disease.

From Braunwald, E: Mechanisms of action of calcium-channel-blocking agents. N Engl J Med 307:1624, 1982. Reprinted by permission of The New England Journal of Medicine.

to use acetaminophen (Tylenol) if it occurs. Most patients adapt after a week and can then tolerate full doses, but they need to be gently coaxed through this initial period. Occasional patients can never tolerate nitrates, but in my experience these are rare. Given patience and experimentation with different dosage forms, a tolerable and effective program can be found. More than one dosage form can be used to tailor a program to fit the patient's needs. Most patients with significant angina need medication three or four times a day and may as well get used to it early.

Sublingual nitroglycerin (TNG), 0.4 mg normally or 0.3 mg in a sensitive individual, should be carried by most patients. Onset of action is two to three minutes and duration 15 to 20 minutes. I prefer patients to use TNG sparingly and learn to "pace" themselves, but they should be encouraged to use it if pain does not let up immediately on rest. If a patient is using more than one or two doses a week, the other medication should be adjusted. However, if the patient is already on maximal medication, prophylactic TNG before an activity known to produce angina is one of the tricks of learning how to live with the disease. If pain persists, the patient should take up to three TNG five minutes apart before coming to the hospital. However, there is a very fine balance between adequate education of the patient and unnecessary raising of fears.

Sublingual isosorbide dinitrate (2.5 to 10 mg) acts in five minutes and lasts up to two hours, making it a good form to use prophylactically before a specific activity such as sexual intercourse or a shopping trip. If used for day-long prophylaxis, however, it should be taken every three or four hours to be fully effective. This frequency is too cumbersome for most patients, but for active individuals working outside it may be preferred because it does not require a glass of water.

Oral isosorbide dinitrate (10 to 60 mg) has a duration of up to six hours and is probably the form of choice for daily anginal prophylaxis taken q.i.d. The dose required varies widely; many patients require and tolerate 40 mg or more q.i.d. I have also had success with the sustained release form (Isordil Tembids, 40 mg), which extends the duration slightly and can be taken t.i.d. or once at night as a supplement.

Nitroglycerin ointment (½ to 3 inches) has a duration of up to eight hours and can be used t.i.d. or q.i.d. or as a supplement at night. Most patients find it messy and inconvenient, but this may well be the best tolerated form of nitrate in terms of side effects. Elderly patients in particular may not tolerate any other dosage form, but do well on ointment q.i.d. The transdermal discs probably do not give 24-hour protection, often cause skin irritation, and are outrageously expensive.

Beta-blockers. The Beta-adrenergic receptor blocking agents are very effective in managing exertional angina but are ineffective or even detrimental in coronary spasm. These drugs reduce myocardial O_2 demands, particularly during exercise, by limiting the effect of sympathetic nerve stimulation; this results in a reduced heart rate, contractility, and cardiac output for any given level of exercise. The antihypertensive and antiarrhythmic effects are added benefits in many patients. In the doses required for angina control, minor differences in cardioselectivity and intrinsic sympathomimetic effect among the many products are of very little concern.

I use propranolol (Inderal) in almost all patients and have become comfortable with its use. When initiating therapy it is easiest to prescribe 40-mg size tablets, start with one half tablet q.i.d. for a week, and then increase to 40 mg q.i.d. Most patients with angina need at least 160 mg per day and many require 320 mg per day. Don't be over-concerned with heart rate. Many physicians are afraid to increase the dosage when the pulse is <60 per minute and do not reach therapeutic levels because of this. Most patients do well with a resting pulse of 45 to 50 per minute. After an effective dose is established, the total daily amount can be given once daily (q.d.), using the long-acting form (Inderal LA) if practical. For example, a construction worker may do well with Inderal LA in the morning and sublingual isosorbide dinitrate during the day. On the other hand, a patient taking oral nitrates q.i.d. might as well stay with propranolol q.i.d. taken at the same time.

Patients with CHF who are dependent on basal adrenergic tone usually do not tolerate beta-blockers. In borderline cases, addition of digitalis may allow continued use, but switching to a calcium antagonist such as nifedipine is usually best. Patients with bronchospasm do not tolerate beta-blockers well and often need a change to calcium antagonists. Switching to a cardioselective beta-blocker such as metoprolol (Lopressor) may help, but in my experience is unlikely to improve the situation. If atrioventricular (AV) block or symptomatic sinus bradycardia occur, you will have to back off the dose, but always watch for drug interaction with digitalis, verapamil, or diltiazem. All these drugs must be used with caution, particularly in patients with known conduction system disease or sick sinus syndrome. I have had to recommend permanent pacing in this situation, not because of syncope, but in order to give adequate doses of antianginal drugs to control symptoms.

Other side effects such as aggravation of claudication, depression, vivid dreams, and GI upset are often dose dependent and can be acceptable if the dose is kept below a certain level. Beta-blockers with less lipid solubility possibly cause fewer CNS problems. If these are bothersome, it is worth trying atenolol (Tenormin) or nadolol (Corgard). In a brittle diabetic, nonselective agents may mask the warning symptoms of hypoglycemia, and a cardioselective agent such as metoprolol or atenolol is recommended. I have not seen this problem in diabetics under reasonable control. Most cases of impotence are not related to propranolol, so do not discontinue this drug in sick patients for this reason only.

Calcium Antagonists. Calcium antagonists increase myocardial O_2 supply by direct coronary vasodilation, and are therefore ideally suited for management of variant angina and cases of unstable angina with rest pain where vasospasm may be a factor. However, they are also remarkably effective in patients with chronic exertional angina, as a result of improved O_2 supply and decreased demand related to peripheral vasodilation.

The three currently available calcium antagonists (verapamil, nifedipine, and diltiazem) have significant differences that must be recognized to avoid complications but may also be utilized to optimize a medical program. All three lower peripheral vascular resistance, but this is much more evident with nifedipine (Procardia), which not infrequently causes side effects of reflex tachycardia, dizziness, flushing, and edema. In patients with CHF, however, this afterload-reducing property of nifedipine can be used to advantage. All three drugs also have negative inotropic effects, but verapamil (Calan or Isoptin) is more prominent in this regard and should be avoided in CHF, particularly in combination with beta-blockers.

In a nonfailing heart, nifedipine causes significant reflex tachycardia owing to its vasodilator effect; this may even cause angina in sensitive patients, and for this reason nifedipine should be used in conjunction with beta-blockers in the absence of failure. Conversely, this property makes nifedipine the best choice in a patient with AV block or sick sinus syndrome. Diltiazem (Cardizem), and to a lesser extent verapamil, cause sinus bradycardia owing to a direct effect on the sinus node and should be avoided in sick sinus syndrome. Verapamil exerts a potent effect on the AV node, slowing conduction; this property also makes it an important antiarrhythmic agent. However, verapamil should be avoided in any patient with known AV node disease, particularly if beta-blockers are being used.

Nifedipine is most likely to cause side effects but is the best choice in the presence of CHF or sinus node dysfunction. *Verapamil* is better tolerated but causes constipation in 10% to 20% of patients. It should be avoided in patients with CHF or AV node or sinus node disease, and should be used with extreme caution in conjunction with beta-blockers. *Diltiazem* is very well tolerated in most patients; I tend to use it in most situations and have found it remarkably effective in patients who are poorly controlled on other medications.

Diltiazem can be started with 60-mg tablets, having the patient test dose ½-tablet q.i.d. for a few days, increasing up to 60 mg q.i.d., which is generally effective. Some patients require 90 mg q.i.d. for full benefit. I have had very few problems adding full-dose diltiazem to a patient already on maintenance propranolol. If there is definite evidence of sinus node disease, nifedipine is a better choice. Equivalent dosages are (1) nifedipine, 20 mg q.i.d.; (2) verapamil, 120 mg q.i.d.; and (3) diltiazem, 60 mg q.i.d.

Indications for salicylates (aspirin) and dipyridamole (Persantine) are somewhat controversial and we do not use them routinely in the management of angina. We use them after CABG because of data suggesting an improvement in long-term graft patency rate.

PATIENT INFORMATION

Patient education has been stressed because it is an integral part of management. "Failures" in therapy can usually be traced back to misunderstanding and unrealistic expectations. The patient must be involved in decision-making from step one. Usual side effects of drugs should be explained when writing a prescription, but common sense dictates that rare side effects not be mentioned. The mere suggestion that propranolol may cause impotence is more likely to cause it than the drug itself. Even a simple treadmill test can be terrifying; all it takes is an explanation and reassurance *before* the test.

Cardiac catheterization goes easily if patients know exactly what to expect at the laboratory. The worst fear is that of the unknown. Reporting results to the patient requires time, sensitivity, and a positive attitude. If either PTCA or CABG is indicated, the procedure should be recommended with enthusiasm. Patients who are poor surgical candidates need to know that the test was worthwhile and that information was gained to direct a new emphasis in therapy. That emphasis may mean acceptance of a more limited life style, but if this is put over gently and optimistically, the results will be positive. Above all, it is critical to maintain an attitude of hope.

PERIODIC EVALUATION

Good follow-up makes the plan work. Very few management decisions are unchangeable. The goal of each visit is to reassess life quality as the patient sees it and to review treatment options. Medications may need to be changed or adjusted, depending on their side effects and efficacy. The risks of CABG or PTCA should be considered in relation to the severity of symptoms. The more limited the life style, the more reasonable those risks become. As the natural history progresses, goals and expectations may have to change.

Surgical options change as the disease progresses. All too often patients are managed over-conservatively on the basis of an "old" catheterization study in which CABG was not considered. A patient told not to have CABG two years ago when he had double-vessel disease may very well now have triple-vessel disease and be a definite surgical candidate. This progression can occur rapidly; I have very often seen "40%" lesions become "90%" lesions in less than a year.

"Routine" tests are not often indicated. Most stable patients should have an EKG yearly so that for future events there will be a legitimate comparison study. The stable patient with a known "50%" lesion and previous good functional capacity should have a treadmill test for objective follow-up on approximately a yearly basis. Management of angina patients with a history of previous infarction and clinical evidence of LV dysfunction may be assisted by a noninvasive assessment of LV function with either echocardiography or radionuclide angiography. Demonstration of LV dilation or evidence of elevated end-diastolic pressure may suggest the need for digitalis or diuretics. An ejection fraction less than 30% suggests caution in recommending catheterization because of increased risk of intervention. However, catheterization should still be considered if a patient has severe angina without gross evidence of congestive failure.

PATIENT COMPLIANCE

Compliance problems usually reflect inadequate communication between patient and physician. The overall plan, goals, and options should be reviewed at each visit to avoid confusion. Noncompliance with medications may simply require careful review of instructions, or may necessitate dose modification or drug change because of side effects. More often, however, the medication schedule simply does not fit in well with the individual's life style. Here it is important to be flexible. Remember that the goal is life quality, not obedience. Fit the program to the patient, not the patient to the program.

In some patients, angina is controlled on a long-acting beta-blocker q.d. and Isordil Tembids b.i.d. But if q.i.d. medication is necessary to control symptoms, try to keep it as simple as possible. If a drug such as nifedipine causes so many immediate side effects that the patient has to "stagger" the dose at times different from those of the other medications, try switching to diltiazem so that all pills can be taken at once. Or, if q.i.d. doesn't work, try using the same drugs t.i.d., perhaps with a higher dosage. Work with the patient to find an acceptable combination.

PREVENTIVE MEASURES

Behavior modification to take into account risk factors is essential and should be readdressed on every encounter, but should not be pushed to the point where quality of life is seriously affected, marital discord occurs, or the doctor-patient relationship is threatened. Hypertension should be carefully controlled. I am very strict on smoking but have been known to suggest a pipe to the recalcitrant patient. There is no magic formula for stopping smoking, but group therapy such as in a cardiac rehabilitation program, combined with a lot of exercise, probably has the best chance of success. Patients need to find enjoyable ways to start and maintain an exercise program.

A low-cholesterol diet should be stressed for all patients. The emphasis is on basic eating habits we must all struggle with, such as red meat once or twice instead of six times a week, and margarine instead of butter. A fasting lipid profile is done early on, and at least one good session with a dietitian is arranged for both patient and spouse. I try to avoid lipid-lowering drugs such as cholestyramine unless cholesterol levels remain >250 mg per 100 ml after conscientious diet therapy. Checking blood cholesterol too frequently, though, can be counterproductive by producing a cholesterol obsession that really does more harm than good. People need to live their lives and not spend every moment worrying about their health.

SOCIOECONOMIC ASPECTS

It is important to be aware of the family dynamics and marital stresses involved with every coronary patient. Individuals' egos are battered and their family role is often altered. Spouses are threatened and may harbor more fear than the patients do. There is a tendency for family, friends, and employers to overprotect patients, which only pushes the ego further down; they reject this and in so doing come into conflict with loved ones whose motivation is good but whose methods are counterproductive. This is why optimistic goals must be stressed from the beginning, to try and keep patients' life roles as close to normal as possible. Aim to get patients back to work as soon as possible and avoid prolonged periods of unnecessary inactivity from which many never recover. Families need counseling and reassurance to allay their own fears that the patient's future depends on what they do; it doesn't. They must come to understand the patient's need to be himself, to get back to living rather than stop living because of the illness. *Remember that preservation of self-confidence and a sense of self-worth are every bit as important goals as control of the symptoms themselves.*

The management of coronary disease has come to be dominated by "high technology." The major diagnostic and therapeutic advances of the past decade, when ordered wisely for a specific purpose and when performed by a highly trained person with strict quality control, have clearly improved our ability to deal with this disease. Cardiac "testing," however, is very expensive, and it is my impression that we do far too many tests and far too little communicating. The patient with known coronary disease who just played 18 holes of golf without symptoms does not need a thallium exercise test to decide that he's stable. He probably doesn't even need a treadmill. The patient whose typical angina can no longer be controlled acceptably despite medical adjustments does not need an exercise MUGA to decide that a catheterization is indicated. Most of what we need to know to make decisions is learned by talking to the patient.

MANAGEMENT OF MYOCARDIAL INFARCTION

PLAN

Primary goals in management of MI include (1) stabilization of rhythm and prevention of arrhythmic death; (2) limitation of the extent of injury; (3) treatment of acute complications; (4) rehabilitation, including education and emotional support; and (5) long-range planning for management of coronary disease. We now keep a patient hospitalized for seven to ten days in an uncomplicated MI, with graduated activity starting early under the guidance of an organized cardiac rehabilitation team. Management of specific complications such as arrhythmias, pericarditis, CHF, cardiogenic shock, and heart block are discussed in other sections of this text.

INDICATIONS FOR INVASIVE MONITORING

There is no substitute for *frequent*, careful bedside observations of BP, pulse, mental status, skin color and temperature, neck veins, cardiac sounds, and urine output. The physical examination not only answers most questions about therapy; the "laying on of hands" serves to relax and reassure the patient. Invasive hemodynamic monitoring is not a replacement but is an adjunct to clinical evaluation. It should be reserved for these very specific indications: (1) signs of low cardiac output when LV filling pressure cannot be determined adequately on clinical grounds, (2) CHF complicated by low output for monitoring response to positive inotropic and/or vasodilator agents, and (3) appearance of a new murmur for differential diagnosis of mitral regurgitation versus ruptured interventricular septum. Data obtained are not always accurate, owing to many technical pitfalls, and quality control is essential. As with any of our diagnostic tests, it must be correlated with all the clinical parameters.

DYSAUTONOMIA

Many patients present with an acute dysautonomia accompanying the MI, which may need treatment. With severe pain and overwhelming fear, there is a tremendous discharge of both the parasympathetic and sympathetic nervous systems. In inferior wall MI, the parasympathetic discharge often dominates, causing sinus bradycardia, AV block with junctional escape, and associated hypotension. The physician should not overtreat in this situation for fear of unmasking the overactive sympathetic system, causing tachycardia and hypertension, which increase myocardial O_2 requirements and extend the injury. Bradycardia alone is not harmful as long as BP is adequate; in fact, it is protective. Atropine should be given only if *both* bradycardia and hypotension are present, and in small increments (0.3 to 0.5 mg, repeated twice if necessary every five to ten minutes) so as to correct the hypotension but not overshoot the mark. Even those with AV block and an adequate junctional escape rhythm with narrow QRS should be left alone if BP is adequate; the block usually reverses itself. Remember that these patients may also be relatively hypovolemic and need volume replacement.They may be particularly vulnerable to nitrates, which should be avoided until BP is stable.

Other patients present with sympathetic dominance, sinus tachycardia, and hypertension. In addition to pain relievers, these patients should be given IV beta-blockers followed by oral treatment. This reduces myocardial O_2 demands, protects against ventricular fibrillation, and may reduce myocardial injury. For this purpose I use propranolol (1 mg IV every three minutes up to 10 mg) or metoprolol (5 mg IV every two minutes for three doses).

PROPHYLACTIC LIDOCAINE

Unless contraindicated by severe hypotension, CHF, hepatic dysfunction or advanced age, I use prophylactic lidocaine infusions in most patients, starting with a bolus of 1 mg/kg followed by an infusion of two to three mg per minute. The infusion may be discontinued after 24 hours unless otherwise indicated. In patients receiving beta-blockers, the infusion rate should be lowered because of the known effect on lidocaine clearance rates.

LIMITATION OF INJURY

Although no specific treatment regimens can be recommended as proved, a clinical approach to MI aimed at "preservation of myocardium" is both theoretically sensible and clinically practical. Rather than simply observing for complications, we actively work to prevent them by limiting the extent of injury. Many of the most practical considerations in this regard are often totally ignored in a busy CCU.

REST, SEDATION, PAIN RELIEF

Modern CCUs have become machine- rather than patient-oriented. The atmosphere is noisy, exciting, and therefore terrifying. Patients need to be isolated from this excitement as much as possible, and we should use more sedatives such as diazepam (Valium). Morphine sulfate (2- to 8-mg increments) should be used in adequate doses to control pain. If the drug causes hypotension, the patient probably needs volume replacement. For persistent or recurrent pain, we use IV nitroglycerin (Tridil, 25 mg in 500 cc D5W = 50 μg/cc). This should be started at 5 μg/min, with the dose doubled at ten-minute intervals until the pain is controlled. We have had very little trouble using the drug without invasive monitoring, utilizing an automated BP device (Critikon Dinamap).

CORRECTABLE FACTORS

Fever, anemia, and hypoxemia must be treated and all tachyarrhythmias addressed immediately. Digitalis should be avoided if possible but is still the drug of choice for rapid atrial fibrillation. Hypertension, persistent despite pain relief, sedation, and beta-blockers, should be brought under control starting with IV nitroglycerin, reserving nitroprusside for the most malignant cases. CHF is managed initially with diuretics and nitrates. An adequate perfusion pressure between 90 and 120 mm Hg systolic must be maintained. Many patients are relatively hypovolemic owing to diaphoresis, vomiting, and lack of intake; volume replacement is all that is required. Persistent hypotension in an inferior wall MI with distended neck veins but clear lungs should always raise the possibility of right ventricular infarction. These individuals require very large amounts of fluid and may require hemodynamic monitoring. Positive inotropic agents should be avoided if possible because of their cost in O_2 requirement. Before any such drug is used, hemodynamic monitoring should be done to ensure an optimal filling pressure of between 18 and 20 mm Hg. If necessary, dobutamine (250 mg in 500 cc = 500 μg/cc, starting dose 2.5 μg/kg/min) is probably the most protective of the myocardium.

ADDITIONAL MEASURES

We generally maintain patients on *nitrate therapy* in the CCU, nitroglycerin ointment (½ to 2 inches q.6 h.). *Beta-blockers* are started in all patients without contraindications before discharge because of evidence from several good randomized trials (timolol, propranolol) showing a reduction in mortality for three years following MI. Their use in the acute period is not as well established but is certainly advised for patients with tachycardia or hypertension, as discussed. *Calcium antagonists* are being used more and more frequently in MI. Coronary spasm may play an initiating role in the pathophysiology of the event and these drugs also have an important "protective" action at the cellular level, which may delay the process of cell death. These agents should be used in patients having persistent pain, but cannot yet be recommended as standard care. Active research continues at our institution and others to define the role of calcium antagonists in myocardial preservation.

THROMBOLYTIC THERAPY

It has been demonstrated that it is possible to reperfuse an acutely occluded coronary artery in the setting of MI by administration of a fibrinolytic agent such as streptokinase, either directly into the coronary artery at catheterization or by systemic IV infusion. If a safe, clot-selective activator of fibrinolysis (such as tissue plasminogen activator) could be developed that would not cause a generalized lytic state when given systemically, patients could be treated early without the need for catheterization. The role of immediate PTCA or CABG after clot lysis remains controversial. Much more research is needed before a safe agent can be made widely available and any specific recommendations made for standard treatment of MI. In my opinion, clinical application has moved too fast with this therapy, and its use should be restricted to centers directly involved in carefully designed clinical trials.

DISCHARGE PLANNING

Patients with postinfarction angina should be stabilized and considered for early catheterization, preferably after two to three weeks of convalescence, particularly after nontransmural MI. Asymptomatic patients should have *low-level treadmill testing*, symptom limited to no more than 5 METS, unless otherwise contraindicated by significant CHF, advanced age, or inability to ambulate. Those who have an abnormal response, with ST-segment depression ($\geq$ 2 mm) or hypotension, are at high risk and should be considered for an aggressive approach with early catheterization. *Ambulatory EKG monitoring (Holter)* is desirable in most patients, but should be done after good beta-blockade. If paroxysmal ventricular tachycardia is seen despite this therapy, additional antiarrhythmics are indicated. Noninvasive assessment of LV function by *radionuclide ventriculography or echocardiography* is very useful in determining prognosis. Patients with an ejection fraction <50% are at higher risk and should be considered for aggressive management. However, the cost effectiveness of these tests is questionable. I do not recommend their routine use but advise selective use when decisions cannot be made on the basis of other studies.

FAMILY CONCERNS

Finally, there must be frequent sensitive communication with both patient and family as to the clinical course. It is important to remain optimistic with the patient while at the same time realistic about expectations following discharge. Definite plans for further evaluation and long-term management must be made so that the family is not left confused and excessively fearful of the future.

REFERENCES

Hoekenga D, Abrams J: Rational medical therapy for stable angina pectoris. Am J Med 76:309–314, 1984.

Lipid Research Clinics Coronary Primary Prevention Trial Results II: The relationship of reduction in incidence of coronary heart disease to cholesterol lowering. JAMA 251:365–374, 1984.

Principal Investigators of CASS and Their Associates: Myocardial infarction and mortality in the Coronary Artery Surgery Study (CASS) randomized trial. N Engl J Med 310:750–758, 1984.

Silverman KJ, Grossman W: Angina pectoris: natural history and strategies for evaluation and management. N Engl J Med 310:1712–1717, 1984.

Spann JF: Changing concepts of pathophysiology, prognosis, and therapy in acute myocardial infarction. Am J Med 74:877–886, 1983.

2 · CONGESTIVE HEART FAILURE

Gregory S. Uhl
LOVELACE MEDICAL CENTER

DEFINITION

A state of congestive heart failure (CHF) exists when cardiac function is insufficient to meet all the body's physiologic needs. The cardiovascular system can be challenged by a variety of cardiac and extracardiac disorders, eventually resulting in a common group of symptoms and signs that the clinician recognizes as CHF. These cardiovascular burdens can be categorized as one of the following. First, there is a volume or preload abnormality characterized by conditions that increase blood volume, such as mitral or aortic valvular insufficiency, left-to-right shunts, or chronic severe increases in cardiac output such as anemia or hyperthyroidism. Second, there may be a pressure or afterload mismatch accompanying conditions (hypertension, aortic or pulmonic valvular stenosis, or coarctation of the aorta) that increase the resistance to which the heart must pump blood. Third and most common are primary ventricular muscle problems, either segmental due to coronary artery disease or diffuse, with subsequent fibrosis and hypertrophy such as cardiomyopathic states.

PATHOPHYSIOLOGY

An understanding of the Frank-Starling mechanism of myocardial contractility as the operational and compensatory mechanism to enhance cardiac contractility is important to an understanding of CHF therapy. This is best depicted as a ventricular function curve (Fig. 1) that plots cardiac output against some measure of ventricular volume or stretch (usually filling pressure). Nonischemic or nonfibrous myocardium will compensate for a decrease in stroke output with greater myocardial stretch to increase the force of contraction and attempt to return stroke volume toward normal. In CHF, for any given filling pressure the ventricular stroke volume is decreased, and for any given stroke volume the filling pressure is increased. When cardiac and stroke outputs are reduced because of a loss of contractility, ventricular end-diastolic volume enlarges, which increases wall stress, a major determinant of myocardial oxygen consumption. In an attempt to restore wall stress to normal, myocardial hypertrophy develops, further

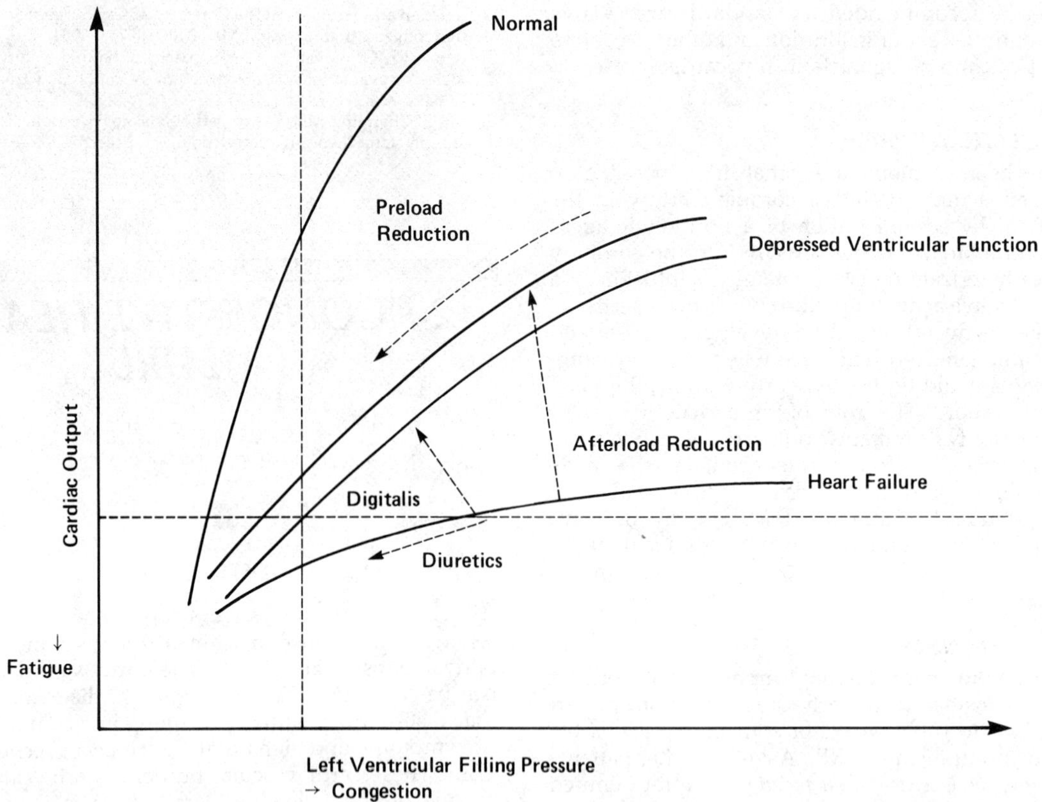

Figure 1. Ventricular function curve relating cardiac function to ventricular volume and the effects of therapeutic interventions.

increasing wall thickness. If blood supply to the remaining hypertrophied myocardium is adequate, a stable compensated state results despite extensive loss of functional myocardium from fibrosis or scar. However, if there is diffuse coronary artery disease, chronic ischemia may hamper myocardial compensatory mechanisms.

The progressive impairment of pump function results in increased systemic vascular resistance and sympathetic tone in an attempt to maintain arterial pressure. Plasma renin activity is considerably higher than normal, owing to decreased renal perfusion pressure and decreased renal sodium load. As depicted in Figure 2, the renin-angiotensin-aldosterone cycle begins with $alpha_2$ globulin in the liver which enhances further renin release from the kidneys and releases angiotensin I. Increased aldosterone promotes salt and water retention and loss of potassium, which may predispose to arrhythmias, and usually results in the clinician adding a diuretic to further stimulate renin release. Angiotensin I circulates to the lung and is converted to angiotensin II, a potent vasoconstrictor. This results in further sodium retention, contributing to the vicious cycle depicted in Figure 2.

CLINICAL ASPECTS

The symptoms and signs of CHF are well known and will not be dealt with in great detail here. Dilated or congestive cardiomyopathy is usually a biventricular dilatation so that right ventricular failure often accompanies, rather than follows, left ventricular failure. Signs of pulmonary congestion, which appear early in isolated left ventricular failure owing to hypertensive or ischemic heart disease, may be absent or delayed.

Elevated venous pressure may be seen as distended neck veins, hepatojugular reflux, and hepatic congestion. Eventually peripheral edema may develop, especially after the right ventricle is dilated to a point of functional tricuspid insufficiency. Other physical findings could include low blood pressure, a narrow pulse pressure, sinus tachycardia, and cardiac arrhythmias. Ventricular ectopy may be the first and only manifestation of CHF, and as the atria dilate, atrial fibrillation tends to be a late finding.

GOALS OF THERAPY

The course of the patient with CHF is that of a chronic and progressive limitation of exercise tolerance due to declining left ventricular performance. Aside from treatment of hypertension and surgical intervention for valvular or coronary artery disease when appropriate, all treatment strategies are directed at improving the quality of life. This is a rather nebulous term, differing in application from one individual to another, and involving interplay between patients' expectations, their mood, their satisfaction with life style, and their coping mechanisms. Therapeutic interventions that can affect functional capacity can determine patients' mobility, independence, and participation in hobbies, rec-

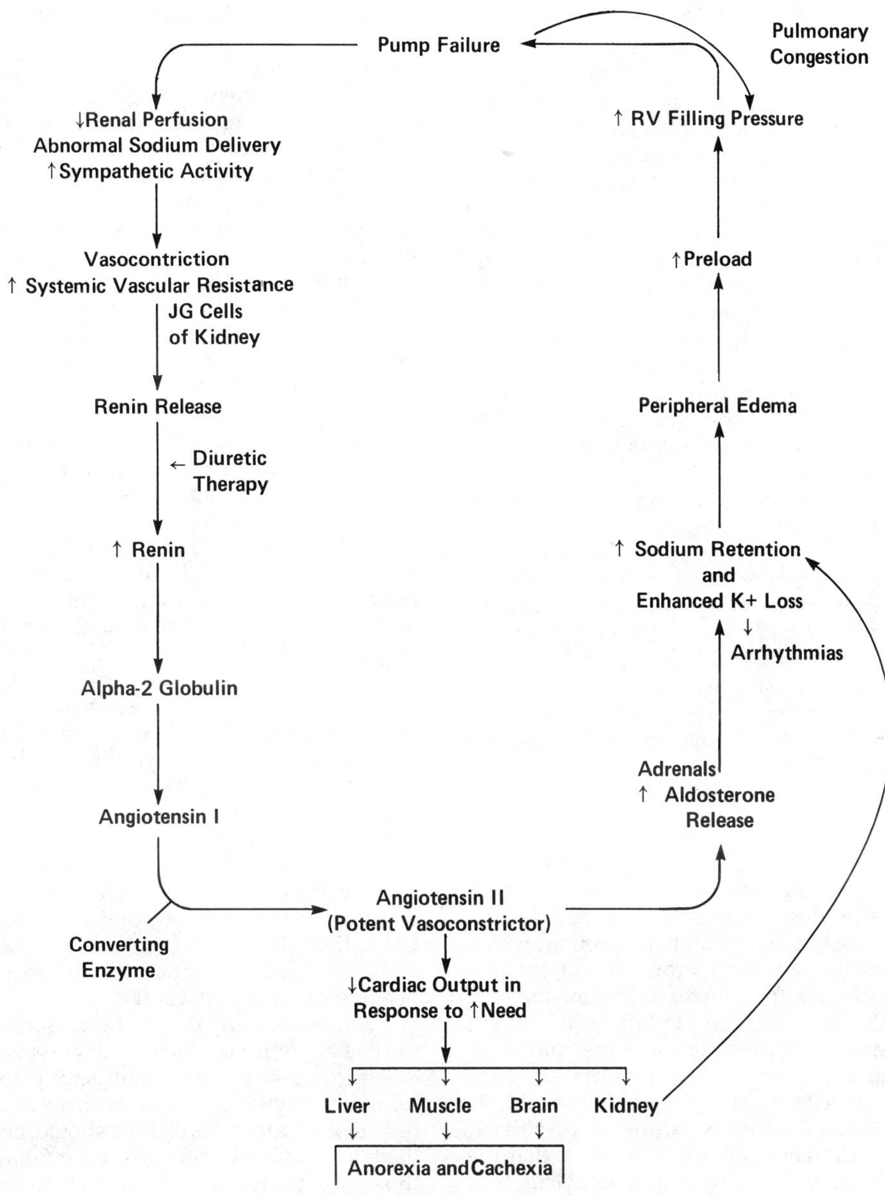

Figure 2. Physiology of heart failure.

reation, and sexual activity. Adding to the stress of CHF symptoms are ineligibility for insurance, discrimination against employment even if recovery is made to a reasonable level of activity, and possible premature retirement. Patients may experience a slight improvement in the quality of life but not see it as worth the trade-off in price of medications or side effects, or even the need for intermittent hospitalization. Thus, the physician and patient may occasionally be adversaries when considering changes in treatment or rehospitalization.

HOSPITALIZATION

Hospitalization of CHF patients is occasionally warranted. Some beneficial medications can only be given parenterally. An afterload mismatch can be reduced by valvular replacement in aortic stenosis or by aggressive therapy for hypertension. Diastolic volumes can be reduced by medications, or surgical correction can be considered before major decompensation and irreversible dilatation occur, such as in aortic insufficiency. Ischemia can be treated with medication or surgical intervention before the loss of a significant myocardial mass, which would result in irreversible CHF. Hospitalization should be considered when symptoms worsen and medications may be needed that require measurements of left ventricular filling pressure with invasive monitoring. In general, however, home health care and ambulatory treatment is the ideal, since the prognosis is so poor and maintenance of quality of life is supreme.

NONPHARMACOLOGIC MEASURES

Bed Rest. In the treatment of mild to moderate CHF, and even during an acute exacerbation of pump failure, the prescription of rest, both physical and emotional, can reduce demand for cardiac output considerably. Bed rest for a limited time frequently precipitates diuresis, lowering left ventricular filling pressure and decreasing heart size, which in turn reduces wall tension and possibly reverses the vicious cycle of CHF symptoms.

Sodium Restriction. This remains a valuable therapeutic intervention, especially in patients accustomed to a greater than normal sodium intake. Sodium restriction to less than 2 gm of sodium per day is difficult to achieve, unpalatable, and probably unnecessary with today's potent diuretics. However, dietary sodium restriction allows us to reduce the dose of various medications and, in addition, slows the loss of renal potassium or magnesium wasting.

Oxygen Therapy. Oxygen is a mainstay in therapy for worsening CHF symptoms. Hypoxia of the myocardial cell enhances tissue damage. Hypoxemia results from pulmonary congestion and resultant ventilation/perfusion mismatches, as well as widened arterial venous oxygen differences from depressed cardiac output. Oxygen therapy may be of hemodynamic benefit, and may reduce ventricular irritability and protect the myocardium from further damage by fibrosis if the hypoxia is severe. Low-flow home oxygen is beneficial in the later stages of CHF.

DRUG THERAPY

Diuretics. Diuretics are among the principal therapeutic agents in CHF, but care must be taken in their judicious use. Large doses may result not only in loss of electrolytes, but in excessive volume depletion, which may lower ventricular filling pressure without enhancing cardiac output, and may increase symptoms such as fatigue (Fig. 1). The relief of tissue congestion caused by increased capillary hydrostatic pressure and fluid accumulation in the tissues is the goal of diuretic therapy. If severe pulmonary edema does not exist, simple agents such as thiazide diuretics can be used initially. Administration of diuretics should be timed so that the effects are largely confined to waking hours. The peak action of most diuretics is usually two to four hours after oral administration. With furosemide and other potent loop diuretics that work in the proximal tubule where 65% to 70% of the glomerular filtrate is absorbed, the onset of action is after about one hour. Excessive use of these powerful diuretics may result in hypochloremic alkalosis, dehydration, hypotension, prerenal azotemia, and digitalis intoxication, especially if the patient becomes hypokalemic. Potassium supplements may be required, and care must be taken if potassium-sparing agents such as triamterene or spironolactone are used, since these may produce hyperkalemia. Potassium chloride is the supplement of choice to replace body potassium. Perhaps the best way to avoid hypokalemia is to give diuretics intermittently (two to three times a week), guided by daily weights. Any sudden weight increase of more than 1 kg in one day can be treated with additional diuretics.

As heart failure worsens, even large doses (160 mg furosemide) may not be effective to maintain an adequate diuresis. The addition of metolazone, 2.5 to 10 mg per day, to the loop diuretic may markedly enhance the diuretic effect.

Inotropic Drugs. The use of inotropic agents is based on the physiologic fact that the normal heart is only partially activated and that in CHF there may be stimulation of residual contractile reserve sufficient to improve cardiac performance. Digitalis glycosides remain the principal positive inotropic agents and should be used, with rare exceptions. There is much disagreement concerning the efficacy of digitalis, and some experts consider the medication ineffective in CHF if normal sinus rhythm is present. In acute studies, digitalis is most effective in patients with recent-onset CHF and in patients with atrial fibrillation in which the ventricular response is controlled by digitalis. The advantage of digitalis is that the patient's congestive failure can conceivably be improved on a once-a-day medication—a fact that markedly improves compliance. Initial therapy with digoxin is 0.5 mg PO or IV if the patient is critically ill or has atrial fibrillation with a rapid ventricular response. This is followed by 0.25 mg PO every six hours for 24 hours and a maintenance daily dose (0.125 to 0.375 mg) adjusted to clinical response, side effects, or drug levels.

The main limitation of the clinical effectiveness of digitalis is the low toxic/therapeutic ratio, which often results in conduction defects and arrhythmias as more drug is given to control symptoms of heart failure. Little can be expected from digitalis when the problem is primarily a severe mechanical obstruction such as an aortic stenosis or an end-stage cardiac disease in which there is severe pump failure due to myocardial infarction. In these settings, toxicity occurs frequently since dosages are increased to combat the advancing signs of CHF. Digitalis therapy in CHF may actually shift the entire ventricular function curve upward because of its positive inotropic effects (Fig. 1).

Antiarrhythmic Drugs. Indications for therapy for cardiac arrhythmias include disturbing symptoms, undesirable hemodynamic effects, and the prevention of serious arrhythmias such as heart block. Ventricular response to atrial fibrillation should be controlled with digitalis to allow better ventricular filling in diastole and thus improve cardiac output. Tachycardia per se increases myocardial oxygen requirements and decreases ventricular filling time. High-grade ventricular irritability generally is associated with a more guarded prognosis. However, almost all available antiarrhythmic agents have a negative inotropic effect, especially disopyramide, so should be used sparingly and with caution in CHF patients. The physician should search carefully for precipitating causes that may respond to therapy other than antiarrhythmic agents. Examples include electrolyte imbalance, anemia, digitalis toxicity, and hypoxia.

Preload and Afterload Reducing Drugs. Systemic vasodilators represent an important addition to therapy for heart failure. Patients with reduced function operate on the flat portion of the depressed function curve, which is less affected by changes in preload but very afterload dependent (Fig. 1). The rationale for using afterload reduction is that the compensatory mechanisms of increased sympathetic tone and vasoconstriction have gone beyond the point necessary to maintain perfusion pressure, and result in an impediment to cardiac output (Fig. 2). Preload reduction is obtained by an increase of capacitance of the atria and the systemic and pulmonary veins.

Currently used drugs have vasodilating effects on both the venous and arteriolar capacitance beds to differing degrees. They can be classified according to their predominant effects: (1) primarily arteriolar dilatation, from hydralazine and minoxidil; (2) venous capacitance dilatation, from isosorbide dinitrate and nitroglycerin; and (3) mixed arteriolar and venous dilatation, from prazosin and angiotensin converting enzyme (ACE) inhibitors.

The selection of nonparenteral vasodilators for long-term management of CHF patients should be based on the primary hemodynamic abnormalities. Nitrates and nitroglycerin are most useful for patients with elevated pulmonary venous pressure and adequate cardiac output. If cardiac output is low but pulmonary venous pressure is not markedly elevated, hydralazine or minoxidil may be sufficient. Since most patients have elevated pulmonary venous pressure, prazosin or ACE inhibitors may be more appropriate. Alternatively, minoxidil or hydralazine combined with nitrates offer similar results and may actually be tried if tolerance develops to the other medications. Prazosin or ACE inhibitors should be avoided in relatively hypotensive patients because further hypotension can precipitate renal failure. When an agent that is less likely to produce hypotension, such as hydralazine, is combined with digitalis the combination is more effective than one would expect from either one alone.

If nitrates are used, they should be titrated to decrease filling pressure and reduce shortness of breath. If filling pressure is reduced too much there may be a fall in stroke volume (Fig. 1). In addition, tolerance to long-acting nitrates often develops early, so that their effects may be modest and short-lived. Isosorbide dinitrate, 20 to 80 mg PO, can have a sustained effect for up to four hours and may improve exercise tolerance. Nitroglycerin paste, 1 to 2 inches every six hours, is also effective. The acute response may not always be equal to the chronic response and there are often clinical improvements without objective changes in ejection fraction, chest x-rays, or echocardiograms. Certain patients demonstrate less tolerance or attenuation of the effect of nitrates with the addition of spironolactone.

Prazosin has a theoretical advantage over other arteriolar and venodilators and has shown beneficial effects in chronic double-blind trials. Nearly every patient develops hypotension after the first several doses and should therefore be started on a low dose (i.e., 1 mg). The maintenance dosage of prazosin is 3 to 5 mg every six hours. Troublesome side effects include dizziness, nausea, vomiting, diarrhea, palpitations, drowsiness, and nervousness. The major clinical disadvantage of long-term prazosin therapy is an attenuation of the hemodynamic and clinical effects; this can often be blunted or prevented by the addition of spironolactone.

Hydralazine sometimes requires very large doses (200 to 400 mg per day) to be effective in CHF patients. The incidence of side effects from these relatively large doses is considerable, including gastrointestinal symptoms, fluid retention, weight gain, systemic lupus erythematosus, and a peripheral neuropathy. A sustained clinical improvement is sometimes seen, but tolerance to the medication can occur.

Minoxidil is a potent vasodilator whose effects are similar to those of hydralazine. In dosages of 20 to 40 mg per day it often produces beneficial hemodynamic and clinical effects, the major side effects being fluid retention, weight gain, and hypertrichosis. Some patients develop a negative inotropic effect from minoxidil and may actually have a worsening of CHF. However, an increase in diuretics or the addition of an antialdosterone agent may prevent fluid retention in long-term minoxidil therapy.

The calcium antagonists, especially nifedipine, can cause significant vasodilatation and a drop in systemic vascular resistance. The major limitations of these medications lie in the development of peripheral edema and significant orthostatic hypotension. However, their great advantage is that they may be titrated rather closely to an ideal effect.

Captopril and other ACE inhibitors are extremely effective arteriolar vasodilators. Because of their effect on the renin-angiotensin system, they may cause marked BP reduction. For this reason, when therapy is begun the patient must be closely observed and is often hospitalized. A relatively small dose equivalent to 6.25 mg of captopril every eight hours often has beneficial effects. The dose can be increased gradually, but 20% of all patients with chronic CHF develop hypotension. Care must be taken to avoid proteinuria, especially if there is preexisting renal disease, but this usually disappears after stopping the drug. Azotemia is most likely to occur in sodium-depleted patients. Careful titration of dosage with close supervision can be accomplished on an outpatient basis. Major side effects include anemia, neutropenia, and dermatitis.

Complications of Drug Therapy

Most complications in CHF patients occur in those who develop hepatic dysfunction. This is common because of a decrease in hepatic blood flow compromising oxygen delivery to the parenchyma, as well as a rise in systemic venous pressure, which causes edema and atrophy of hepatocytes. The major effect of hepatic dysfunction is on the pharmacokinetics of drugs. Lidocaine has a high extraction rate in the liver and the clearance is influenced by hepatic blood flow. Thus, overdosages of lidocaine must be guarded against. Quinidine is eliminated as an intact drug by the kidney and transformed to its active metabolites in the liver; therefore, the clearance of these by-products may be reduced and dosage change may be required. This obviously has significant effects on the digoxin-quinidine interaction, which can result in digitalis intoxication. Prazosin is metabolized in the liver and its use requires close monitoring. This does not account for tachyphylaxis to the drug. Digitalis is excreted unchanged via the kidney, but with GI distress it may be difficult to differentiate between right heart failure and digitalis toxicity. Diuretics can induce alkalosis and hypokalemia, especially when their metabolism in the liver is poor. Anticoagulants interfere with hepatic synthesis of vitamin K–dependent clotting factors, so that frequent adjustments in the dosage of these medications may be required in CHF patients.

PERIODIC EVALUATION

Despite being severely ill with end-stage cardiomyopathy or arteriosclerotic heart disease, a number of fortunate patients can improve with therapy and enhance their functional capacity. Some can even return to work, although the socioeconomic impact of CHF is often quite remarkable. Unfortunately, the ultimate prognosis depends on the severity of the underlying cardiac lesions, and most patients who reach the stage of severe failure at any point usually succumb within six months to one year. It has been pointed out by numerous investigators that all our therapeutic interventions may produce subjective clinical improvement without actually prolonging life. Routine follow-up should consist of evaluation of exercise performance, since indices of left ventricular function are expensive and not consistently useful for following left ventricular performance and assessing treatment. Since exercise capacity is a major determinant of quality of life, the serial performance of a relatively inexpensive and reproducible exercise test is most valuable in assessing therapy and clinical decision-making.

REFERENCES

Abelmann WH: Classification and natural history of primary myocardial disease. Prog Cardiovasc Dis 27:73–94, 1984.

Chatterjee K: Congestive cardiomyopathy: therapeutic approach. Compr Ther 8:25–34, 1982.

Franciosa JA: Effectiveness of long-term vasodilator administration in the treatment of chronic left ventricular failure. Prog Cardiovasc Dis 24:319–330, 1982.

Johnson RA, Palacios I: Dilated cardiomyopathies of the adult. N Engl J Med 307:1051–1058, 1119–1126, 1982.

Pantley GA, Bristow JD: Ischemic cardiomyopathy. Prog Cardiovasc Dis 27:95–114, 1984.

3 · ACUTE PULMONARY EDEMA

Richard A. Reinhart
MARSHFIELD CLINIC

If I'm asked why the heart pumps, I have to say because it likes to. It feels more comfortable in pumping.

E. A. STEAD, JR.*

DEFINITION

Acute cardiogenic pulmonary edema is an excess of lung water in the interstitial and/or intra-alveolar spaces. This usually results from an abrupt increase in pulmonary venous and capillary pressure due to the inability of the left ventricle to eject the blood delivered to it from the right heart.

CLINICAL ASPECTS

Clinically, the patient presents with dyspnea, cough, wheezing, and usually inability to lie down. The patient often is unable to talk effectively because of the

*From Schoonmaker F, Metz E: Just Say For Me. World Press, Denver, 1968.

dyspnea. His or her appearance may vary from calmness to extreme anxiety and agitation. The integument may be clammy. Respirations are labored. Examination of the lungs usually reveals wheezing, rales, or rhonchi but they may be clear to auscultation. Detailed cardiovascular examination may be difficult because of the patient's agitation and the noises coming from the lungs. Careful inspection of the neck veins is important since venous distention is most often present; however, the neck veins may be flat since acute left ventricular dysfunction may result in pulmonary vascular congestion without changes in systemic venous volume. The pulse is usually rapid.

LABORATORY DATA

Laboratory tests are used to confirm the diagnosis of acute pulmonary edema. Chest x-ray usually shows interstitial or intra-alveolar fluid as the hallmark of this condition, and is also most useful to differentiate acute asthma with bronchospasm from acute pulmonary edema, which clinically is often difficult. However, there may be atypical radiologic features of pulmonary edema, and clinical assessment remains the primary mode of diagnosis. Arterial blood gases are useful for determining the severity of the condition rather than for diagnosis. If metabolic acidosis and respiratory acidosis are associated with CO_2 retention, respiratory muscle exhaustion is likely. The chest x-ray and arterial blood gases are therefore the most useful and readily available confirmatory tests in the initial stages of evaluation and treatment.

PATHOPHYSIOLOGY

The causes of pulmonary edema are many (Table 1), but the end result is elevated pulmonary venous pressure produced by left ventricular or mitral valve dysfunction.

MANAGEMENT

The short-term goal in the treatment of acute pulmonary edema is to reduce pulmonary venous pressure.

Table 1. CAUSES OF ACUTE PULMONARY EDEMA

Hypertensive cardiac disease
Acute myocardial infarction
Acute myocardial ischemia without infarction
Congestive cardiomyopathy with added stress of:
  Atrial fibrillation with rapid ventricular response
  Acute volume expansion
  Pulmonary embolism
  Acute blood pressure rise
Acute mitral regurgitation secondary to ruptured chord or papillary muscle
Aortic stenosis
Aortic regurgitation
Mitral stenosis with onset of atrial fibrillation
Noncardiogenic pulmonary edema secondary to:
  Shock
  Trauma
  High altitude
  Near-drowning
  Acute pancreatitis
  Smoke inhalation
  Exposure to high concentrations of inspired oxygen

The long-term goal is to determine the cause of this increased pressure and to prevent recurrence.

Most patients with acute pulmonary edema present as an emergency. Initial therapy is in the emergency room and stabilization is generally achieved within hours. Because there is usually a severe underlying cause, hospitalization is almost always indicated. Admission to a general floor has been advocated after initial stabilization, but in most instances an intensive care unit is preferred because the underlying cause usually warrants this.

NONPHARMACOLOGIC MEASURES

Nonpharmacologic therapy when immediately applied can often be life-saving. Placing the patient in a sitting position decreases venous return and reduces pulmonary congestion; it also increases vital capacity and decreases the work of breathing. Administering oxygen by nasal prongs at 6 liters per minute will sufficiently improve oxygenation yet not give the smothering sensation of a mask, thereby being more acceptable to the patient. Rotating tourniquets are of limited use since peripheral venous pressure is likely to be high and systemic veins are constricted. Likewise, phlebotomy is usually unnecessary, particularly since venous pressure can be rapidly reduced by pharmacologic measures.

DRUG THERAPY

Drug therapy is directed at arteriolar and venous dilatation, diuresis, and increasing myocardial contractility. Vasodilatation increases the size of the large systemic capacitance veins, reducing venous return to the heart, and reduces systemic arteriolar resistance, enhancing ventricular function without a concomitant increase in myocardial oxygen consumption.

Morphine sulfate remains the mainstay of drug therapy for acute cardiogenic pulmonary edema: 2 to 4 mg IV, repeated every several minutes until the desired effect is achieved or until adverse effects preclude additional doses. Pulmonary capillary wedge pressure and left ventricular filling pressures fall after IV morphine administration (preload reduction). Morphine also decreases systemic vascular resistance by dilating peripheral arterioles (afterload reduction). It also reduces anxiety and thereby may reduce the oxygen requirements of the peripheral tissues by preventing unnecessary skeletal muscle movement. Adverse effects of morphine include excessive respiratory depression, nausea and vomiting. Increase in vagal tone caused by morphine may lead to bradycardia and atrioventricular block. Hypotension is more likely to be a problem in the hypovolemic patient. By using smaller, repeated IV boluses, some unwanted effects can be avoided.

Nitroglycerin, administered sublingually, topically, or IV, can produce rapid clinical improvement in pulmonary edema. The main action of nitroglycerin is dilatation of the venous system and decrease in left ventricular filling pressure (preload reduction). Arteriolar dilatation also occurs with the use of nitroglycerin and may also reduce systemic vascular resistance (afterload reduction). A single 0.6 mg tablet of sublingual nitroglycerin can be given immediately, and hemodynamic effects occur within five to ten minutes. A constant infusion of IV nitroglycerin, beginning at 10 µg per minute, can be titrated to achieve the desired effect of symptomatic improvement. Topical nitrates may be less useful because of the arteriolar and venous constriction that commonly occurs in acute pulmonary edema, inhibiting transcutaneous absorption. Nitroglycerin is a safe drug in this setting; its adverse effect of hypotension disappears within minutes when the drug is discontinued or the dosage reduced.

Furosemide given IV has been shown to have both renal and extrarenal hemodynamic effects. Clinical relief of symptoms of pulmonary congestion frequently precedes any demonstrable diuretic effect because of an increase in venous capacitance which, in turn, reduces venous return to the heart. The initial IV dose depends on the size of the patient, whether he has previously been treated with a diuretic, and the severity of the condition. If no diuretic has been previously used, 0.5 to 1 mg per kg body weight is the initial IV dose for moderate to severe pulmonary edema. Previous chronic use of a diuretic usually requires a larger dose (1 to 2 mg/kg/body weight). Subsequent doses are tailored to the patient's needs, depending on the clinical response to the initial dose. The major adverse effect of IV furosemide is hypotension secondary to either excessive venodilatation or excessive diuresis.

Inotropic Drugs

Drugs that can be used to increase myocardial contractility include digoxin and sympathomimetic amines. Digoxin, although its positive inotropic effect is delayed by hours, has an immediate effect of venodilatation in congestive heart failure, rapidly reducing ventricular preload. It is given initially as 0.5 mg IV followed in two to four hours by an additional 0.5 mg. This schedule is used as a loading dose if the drug has not been previously taken by the patient. If the patient is already taking a digitalis preparation, additional doses may be of benefit, particularly in the setting of atrial fibrillation with an uncontrolled ventricular response. Digoxin is particularly useful if atrial fibrillation with a rapid ventricular response is a precipitating or contributing factor to acute pulmonary edema. Digoxin usually slows the ventricular response of atrial fibrillation within one to two hours.

Dobutamine is a useful sympathomimetic amine to treat CHF. It is usually reserved for patients who do not respond to other measures. It is started as a continuous infusion at 2 to 3 µg/kg/body weight per min, with 2 to 3 µg/kg/body weight per min increments every 10 to 30 minutes until the desired hemodynamic effects are obtained or undesirable effects appear. Optimal maintenance doses usually range between 7.5 and 15 µg/kg/body weight per min; doses above this frequently elicit undesirable side effects, including tachycardia, arrhythmias, and excessive rise in BP. Dobutamine is a positive inotropic agent with mild vasodilating properties, and results in improved ventricular function while reducing elevated ventricular filling pressures and vascular resistance. In CHF, dobutamine tends to improve renal blood flow by increasing cardiac output rather than activating renal dopaminergic receptors. Another sympathomimetic amine used in this setting is dopamine. This has a similar effect to that of dobutamine, but the undesirable effects of greater positive chronotropy and peripheral vasoconstriction make it a less desirable drug.

INTUBATION

Inadequate ventilation and oxygenation, as evidenced by arterial $P_{O_2} < 50$ mm Hg or $P_{CO_2} > 50$ mm Hg, deserve special attention. Interstitial lung fluid can increase lung stiffness or decrease the caliber of small airways, both of which increase the work of breathing and interfere with gas exchange in the lungs. If there is marked fatigue of the patient, as evidenced clinically or by arterial blood gases showing CO_2 retention and respiratory acidosis combined with metabolic acidosis, intubation and assisted ventilation with a respirator may become necessary. This decision is based both on observation of the patient showing clinical deterioration and on arterial blood gases showing progressive acidosis and CO_2 retention despite initial therapy. Initial stabilization is usually attempted, however, with the non-pharmacologic and pharmacologic measures described above. Only when the patient continues to deteriorate clinically are intubation and assisted ventilation indicated. Applying positive end-expiratory pressure (PEEP) while the patient is on the ventilator has become a useful clinical tool to treat pulmonary edema. PEEP has a dual beneficial effect by increasing arterial P_{O_2} and lung compliance.

OTHER DRUG THERAPY

Aminophylline and *sodium bicarbonate* are used in extreme circumstances only. An initial loading dose of aminophylline, 3 to 5 mg/kg/body weight IV over a 20-min period followed by a constant infusion of 0.5 mg/kg lean body weight per hr, is used to alleviate extreme bronchospasm. Monitoring of theophylline blood levels is recommended, however, since reliance on weight-derived formulas to determine constant infusion dose can be inaccurate and can lead to toxicity. Adverse effects are atrial and ventricular arrhythmias, nausea and vomiting. Sodium bicarbonate is reserved for correction of extreme acidosis (metabolic and respiratory when arterial pH is < 7.0). The initial dose of sodium bicarbonate is 0.5 to 1 mEq/kg/body weight. Its use, however, should be limited because it presents a large sodium and volume load to the system and may further exacerbate pulmonary edema. In this context, it must be remembered that, as the patient improves, lactic acid is metabolized to bicarbonate, thereby often giving rise to metabolic alkalosis.

FOLLOW-UP

Follow-up of the patient after initial stabilization includes an attempt to delineate the precise cause of the acute pulmonary edema. Therapy directed at these specific causes is instituted to prevent recurrence. More detailed diagnostic procedures, however, generally follow this initial stabilizing period. Continued assessment may include insertion of a flow-directed pulmonary artery catheter to more closely follow left ventricular filling pressures over the subsequent days. This is best done following transfer of the patient to the intensive care unit. To follow systemic arterial pressure more closely and to facilitate frequent arterial blood gas determinations, insertion of a catheter into a peripheral artery may also be useful.

Sodium nitroprusside, a potent and rapidly acting arteriolar and venous dilator, may be indicated in continued care if hemodynamic and symptomatic improvement does not occur in the first few hours of treatment. Careful monitoring of pulmonary artery pressures and systemic arterial pressures is needed when this drug is applied. A continuous IV infusion of nitroprusside is begun, 0.1 to 0.2 µg/kg/body weight. This drug is titrated to obtain a reduction in pulmonary artery diastolic pressure to 15 to 18 mm Hg. This may occur rapidly and with small doses. Systemic arterial pressure has to be monitored since this drug is a potent arteriolar as well as venous dilator that may produce rapid reduction in BP to a hypotensive range. Hypotension can readily be reversed by stopping the infusion; reversal usually occurs within minutes.

Noncardiogenic Pulmonary Edema

DEFINITION

Noncardiogenic pulmonary edema can present a clinical picture similar to that of acute cardiogenic pulmonary edema. Diffuse injury of the pulmonary capillary membrane leads to exudation of proteinaceous material into the lung interstitium despite normal pulmonary venous pressure. This exudation of fluid in turn leads to decreased lung compliance and impaired gas exchange.

Differentiation of this entity from acute cardiogenic pulmonary edema is made on clinical grounds, and can be confirmed by demonstrating normal left ventricular filling pressure with a flow-directed pulmonary artery catheter. The causes of noncardiogenic pulmonary edema are many (Table 1).

THERAPEUTIC GOALS

Therapeutic goals are respiratory support and specific therapy for the precipitating disease process. Since maintenance of adequate oxygenation is often difficult, intubation and assisted ventilation with a respirator are often needed. Utilizing the lowest necessary inspired oxygen concentration to maintain adequate oxygenation is important since higher inspired concentrations of oxygen may exacerbate lung injury. PEEP is helpful in this setting. It is important to prevent the complication of intercurrent pulmonary infection, and appropriate sputum and blood cultures should be obtained when infection is suspected. Pulmonary embolism is another common complication in noncardiogenic pulmonary edema, and specific measures such as low-dose subcutaneous heparin, at 5000 units every 12 hours, should be considered. Acute pulmonary embolism should also be suspected if acute clinical deterioration occurs. Since noncardiogenic pulmonary edema can be a long-term illness, it is important to support nutrition of the patient with either enteral or parenteral supplement.

REFERENCES

Chatterjee K, Parmley WW: The role of vasodilator therapy in heart failure. Prog Cardiovasc Dis 19:301–325, 1977.

Leier CV, Unverferth DV: Drugs five years later. Dobutamine. Ann Intern Med 99:490–496, 1983.

Rizk NW, Murray JF: PEEP and pulmonary edema. Am J Med 72:381–383, 1982.

Schoonmaker F, Metz E: Just Say for Me. World Press, Denver, 1968.

Shanies HM: Noncardiogenic pulmonary edema. Med Clin North Am 61:1319–1337, 1977.

Staub NC: The pathogenesis of pulmonary edema. Prog Cardiovasc Dis 23:53–80, 1980.

Staub NC: Role of the endothelium in lung fluid balance. *In* Crandall ED, moderator: Recent developments in pulmonary edema. Ann Intern Med 99:808–822, 1983.

Zelis R, et al: Morphine: its use in pulmonary edema. Cardiovasc Rev Rep 2:257–267, 1981.

4 · REHABILITATION AFTER MYOCARDIAL INFARCTION AND CARDIAC SURGERY

Ray W. Squires
Gerald T. Gau
MAYO CLINIC AND MAYO FOUNDATION

Cardiac rehabilitation is a longitudinal form of care designed to develop and maintain a desirable level of physical, social, and psychologic ability in patients with cardiovascular disease. Education, counseling, and exercise are combined to help patients return to a near-normal existence as soon as possible after the clinical event, or adapt to the limitations imposed by the disease. Acknowledged goals of rehabilitation include restoration of function, surveillance and feedback regarding convalescence and treatment, and risk factor modification for secondary prevention.

BRIEF HISTORICAL PERSPECTIVE

Until the 1950s, prolonged bed rest was part of the customary treatment after acute myocardial infarction. In 1951, Levine and Lown advocated early mobilization and noted that in patients who were allowed progressive periods of sitting upright in an armchair, morbidity and mortality rates were lower than in those given the standard treatment. Formalized physical activity programs for inpatients described by Wenger, Hellerstein, and others followed, and the concept of cardiac rehabilitation emerged. Exercise training dominated the field during the early years, but the concept of multidisciplinary rehabilitation and risk factor modification became more prominent during the late 1970s.

CARDIAC REHABILITATION PROGRAM SPECIFICS

THE PATIENTS

Candidates for cardiac rehabilitation include patients with acute myocardial infarction, angina pectoris, peripheral vascular disease, hypertension, cardiomy-opathy, and angiographically demonstrated but asymptomatic disease, and those who have undergone cardiac surgery (coronary artery bypass grafting, valve repair or replacement, congenital abnormalities, percutaneous transluminal coronary angioplasty, cardiac transplantation, and so on). Patients considered at high risk of developing cardiovascular disease, e.g., renal dialysis and transplant patients, are also candidates. Advanced age is not necessarily a contraindication for participation, and we have seen several active octogenarians benefit from rehabilitation efforts.

Depressed left ventricular function is not by itself a contraindication to participation in a cardiac rehabilitation program. Exercise capacity and the potential to improve exercise tolerance with exercise training is not necessarily related to resting left ventricular ejection fraction (LVEF). Many patients with depressed left ventricular function may return to active life styles. We recently reviewed our experience with 20 patients with resting LVEFs of less than 25% who entered the rehabilitation program. Mean age was 55 years, with a follow-up interval of 11 to 30 months. Fourteen of the patients (70%) were employed full-time. One patient was retired but fully active. Three experienced recurrent symptoms of congestive heart failure and were restricted to limited activity. Two (10%) had experienced sudden cardiac death, far below the expected mortality for this patient group.

Almost all patients have the potential to benefit from the education and counseling aspects of rehabilitation. The exercise portion of the program should be restricted to patients who do not exhibit the following contraindications to exercise training: unstable angina pectoris, overt cardiac failure, severe left ventricular outflow tract obstruction, life-threatening arrhythmias, dissecting aneurysm, acute myocarditis, serious systemic disease, thrombophlebitis, recent systemic or pulmonary embolus, severe hypertension, overt psychoneurotic disturbances, uncontrolled diabetes mellitus, and severe orthopedic limitation.

THE TEAM

A team approach has been adopted at the Mayo Clinic and is headed by a cardiologist. Team members include nurses, physical therapists, occupational therapist, dietician, psychiatrist, psychologist, social worker, exercise physiologist, pharmacist, physiatrist, chaplain, and vocational rehabilitation counselor. The team approach allows diverse patient problems to be approached and solved in a logical manner. Utilization of the collective skills and experience of the team can be effective in attaining individual patient rehabilitation goals. Current practice addresses multiple aspects of a patient's life: risk factor modification, nutrition, exercise, psychosocial status, stress management, family relationships, vocational adjustment, and understanding of heart disease. The primary physician retains control of and responsibility for care of the patient. The program provides patient surveillance to help the primary physician to determine the effectiveness of the treatment plan, and communication between the team and the primary physician is maintained.

The rehabilitation process is arbitrarily divided into four phases (Table 1). Patients may enter the program at any phase depending upon their clinical situation.

Table 1. CARDIAC REHABILITATION PROGRAM PHASES

Phase	Characteristics	Duration
I	Inpatient program: education, counseling, early mobilization with progressive physical activity, group meetings, predischarge or soon after discharge low-level graded exercise test	Period of hospitalization
II	Immediate posthospital outpatient program (medical center based): education, counseling, risk factor modification, close medical supervision, progressive physical activity, availability of continuous EKG monitoring during exercise sessions, symptom-limited graded exercise test near program completion	4 to 8 weeks after hospital dismissal
III	Late recovery outpatient program (YMCA or home exercise): continued regular exercise training, education, risk factor modification, evaluations (dietary, blood lipids, exercise program, occupation, weight, etc.) at 3, 6, and 9 months, symptom-limited graded exercise test at 6 months	9 months beyond end of Phase II
IV	Maintenance outpatient program (YMCA or home exercise): continued regular exercise training and risk factor modification, yearly general medical evaluation with symptom-limited graded exercise test	Continued indefinitely

INPATIENT PROGRAM: PHASE I

For hospitalized patients, Phase I begins with admission and continues until dismissal. Typical patients involved in Phase I include those with acute myocardial infarction, angina pectoris, and percutaneous transluminal coronary angioplasty, and those who have undergone cardiac surgery. Program components include patient and family education, group and individual counseling, group discussion sessions, and low-level exercise. The objectives are to:

1. Hasten adjustment to the hospital environment and the acute event.

2. Prevent potential deleterious effects of prolonged bed rest.

3. Facilitate return to physical activity and reduce the feelings of invalidism.

4. Begin risk factor assessment and modification.

A multimedia presentation of information (verbal, written, and audiovisual) is coordinated by the cardiac rehabilitation nurse. Topics include diet, smoking cessation, physical activity, normal psychologic responses, medications, cardiovascular pathology, and other risk factor concepts. However, the current trend toward shorter hospital stays, and the inherent anxiety and depression that commonly affect patients after an acute event, indicate that the period of hospitalization is not an ideal time for patient learning. Phase I physical activity follows a gradual progression scheme beginning with passive range-of-motion exercise and early mobilization and advancing to ambulation, stair climbing, and cycle ergometry. For cardiac surgery patients, specific upper extremity exercises are used to maintain range of motion and to facilitate sternal wound healing by increasing local blood flow. Detailed exercise programs for inpatients have been published. The safety of low-level inpatient exercise for cardiac patients has been established. Hemodynamic responses are moderate and acceptable.

Most patients undergo submaximal graded exercise testing before or very soon after hospital dismissal. A Naughton treadmill protocol or a rest and exercise (cycle ergometer) radionuclide angiogram with an end point of an energy expenditure of 4 to 6 METs (METs = multiples of resting metabolism) is employed. Valuable prognostic factors such as symptoms, EKG signs of ischemia, arrhythmias, blood pressure response, ventricular function during exercise, and exercise tolerance are gleaned from the exercise test. The test serves to instill confidence into the patient and family and is useful in determining a safe home exercise prescription.

OUTPATIENT PROGRAM: PHASE II

In many respects, Phase II (the immediate posthospitalization period) is the most critical stage of rehabilitation in that patients are most receptive to changes in life style and are motivated by clear recollections of the acute event. Phase II rehabilitation takes place at the medical center in a special clinic and generally begins within one week of hospital dismissal. Phase II objectives are to:

1. Instruct patients in proper exercise principles and restore them to a desirable exercise capacity.

2. Provide understanding for patient and family regarding cardiovascular disease and to continue appropriate risk factor modification steps—smoking cessation, attainment of ideal weight, decreased saturated fat and cholesterol in the diet, control of blood pressure, stress management, and regular exercise.

3. Meet psychosocial needs, restore confidence, and reduce anxiety and depression.

4. Assist the primary physician in identifying medical problems.

5. Assist the patient in gradual return to occupational and avocational activities.

Educational needs are assessed by interview and a pencil and paper knowledge test. Individual and group discussions and lectures are held. All patients and spouses are encouraged to meet individually with the dietician. Return to previous activities such as sex, hobbies, and vocation is planned. Medications are reviewed by the nurse to ensure compliance with the treatment plan. A standard Phase II program consists of frequent visits to the outpatient rehabilitation center (three per week) for supervised exercise and education. Additional home exercise sessions are usually prescribed. For patients who live some distance from the medical center, less frequent visits are scheduled. The average Phase II program duration is six to eight weeks. Low-risk patients (i.e., those with no signs of CHF or severely depressed left ventricular function, no ischemic signs or symptoms during graded exercise testing with exercise capacity of 4 METs or greater, normal systolic BP response to exercise, no recurrent angina pectoris, and no history of life-threatening ventricular arrhythmias) may safely perform most of the exercise program at home. In our opinion, high-risk patients are best served by close supervision in a monitored exercise program.

Exercise Sessions

The exercise sessions at the medical center are supervised by cardiac rehabilitation nurses and therapists. Continuous EKG monitoring and periodic BP measurements are routine. Aerobic activities such as treadmill walking and cycle ergometry (forms of exercise that are quantifiable and easily reproducible) form the core of the physical activity program, but flexibility, upper extremity muscle strengthening, and relaxation exercises are included. Warm-up and cool-down activities are always performed. Initial aerobic exercise is prescribed conservatively, i.e., 10 to 15 minutes per session at an energy cost of 1.5 to 2.5 METs. A safe upper limit heart rate is derived from the low-level graded exercise test. The perceived exertion scale developed by Borg is used to adjust exercise intensity to a comfortable level for the patient. Patient signs and symptoms are also used to adjust exercise intensity. During the first two to three weeks, aerobic exercise duration is increased to approximately 40 minutes while exercise intensity is maintained in the moderate range. In general, uncomplicated post–cardiac surgery patients are progressed more rapidly than post–myocardial infarction patients. Exercise frequency is set at five to seven sessions per week (three or fewer at the clinic) for the average patient. Properly designed exercise programs for outpatients are safe, and untoward events rarely occur.

Beta-adrenergic receptor blocking agents are commonly prescribed for cardiac patients. Because these drugs lower both resting and exercise heart rate, concern has been expressed that these patients would not exhibit an exercise training effect. However, our experience and that of others indicate substantial training effects in patients taking beta-blockers.

Continuous EKG monitoring during exercise sessions in Phase II serves to document heart rate, ischemia, and arrhythmias precisely. In our experience, most patients can be safely weaned from EKG monitoring after six weeks of Phase II. Patients with a history of either dangerous arrhythmias or extremely poor left ventricular function receive a longer period of monitoring.

Near the end of Phase II, a symptom-limited (maximal) graded exercise test is performed. Results are used to determine readiness for return to work and to update the exercise prescription. Most patients return to work six to eight weeks after hospital dismissal. Exercise intensity is set at approximately 60% to 70% of functional capacity and at a level below signs and symptoms of ischemia. Exercise duration continues indefinitely at 30 to 45 minutes, with a frequency of at least three sessions per week. Exit criteria from the Phase II program include a functional capacity of at least 5 METs, control of BP and arrhythmias, and an absence of angina pectoris at a desirable level of activity for the patient's life style.

PHASE III

Phase III of rehabilitation continues for at least nine months after Phase II. The exercise program either is medically supervised at the YMCA or is purely a home exercise program. The YMCA exercise program does not include EKG monitoring. The objectives of the program are a further increase in exercise capacity and a continuation of risk factor modification steps. A formal evaluation occurs at three, six, and nine months; this includes progress made in exercise, diet, smoking cessation, blood lipids, body weight, medications, and previously unsolved problems. At six months, a symptom-limited graded exercise test is performed.

As with all longitudinal forms of treatment, compliance with rehabilitation recommendations is of concern. Life style changes are not easily accomplished by most patients. Although dropouts cannot be accurately predicted, certain factors do increase the chance of noncompliance: continued cigarette smoking, depressed mood, blue collar occupation, poor left ventricular function, and obesity. Compliance is improved by ensuring quality staff/patient interaction, precise and consistent giving of information, periodic follow-up, and physician/patient interaction. The three-, six-, and nine-month follow-up visits have enhanced patient compliance with life style changes, in our experience, and represent a very important component of the atherosclerosis secondary prevention program. In addition, coronary clubs or other patient organizations serve as support groups for patients and families.

PHASE IV

In Phase IV, patients are encouraged to continue indefinitely with risk factor modification steps and to maintain a regular exercise program. Yearly evaluations, including graded exercise testing, are recommended, beginning one year after the six-month Phase III evaluation.

BENEFITS AND LIMITATIONS OF CARDIAC REHABILITATION

Table 2 lists benefits that may result from comprehensive cardiac rehabilitation. Physical work capacity is improved by regular exercise training. The product of heart rate and systolic BP is lower for a given amount of exercise, indicating a reduction in myocardial oxygen

Table 2. BENEFITS RESULTING FROM LONG-TERM OUTPATIENT CARDIAC REHABILITATION

Physiologic*	Psychologic
↑ $\dot{V}O_2$ max	↓ Anxiety and depression
↓ $M\dot{V}O_2$ for given workload	↑ Confidence and self-esteem
↑ Muscle strength and endurance	↑ Knowledge
↑ Blood fibrinolytic activity	Epidemiologic
↓ Catecholamines	↓ Morbidity[†]
	↓ Mortality[†]
Symptomatic	
↓ Angina pectoris	Risk factors
↓ Dyspnea	↓ Smoking
↓ Claudication	↓ Total cholesterol and triglycerides
↓ Fatigue	↑ High-density lipoprotein cholesterol
Anatomic	↓ Obesity
↓ Progression of disease[†]	↓ Hypertension
Regression of disease[†]	↑ Carbohydrate metabolism

Economic
↑ Patient productivity[†]
↓ Disability cases[†]
↓ Physician office visits[†]
↓ Medications

*$\dot{V}O_2$ max = maximal oxygen uptake; $M\dot{V}O_2$ = myocardial oxygen demand.

[†]Potential benefits.

requirement. Much of the improvement in exercise capacity is the result of peripheral changes in the exercise-trained skeletal muscle. There is some evidence that central circulatory function, i.e., stroke volume, may be improved in selected cardiac patients after exercise training.

The major limitation of cardiac rehabilitation is the lack of definitive evidence that future morbidity and mortality can be improved by efforts at secondary prevention. Randomized clinical trials have been undertaken to determine the effects of rehabilitation on future clinical events, but to date have yielded inconsistent results. Kallio and colleagues provided evidence that multidimensional rehabilitation programs (exercise, diet change, smoking cessation, and so forth) may favorably impact on mortality. Other studies have been less encouraging notwithstanding the monumental problems associated with clinical trials.

There is little question that cessation of cigarette smoking after myocardial infarction or coronary artery bypass graft surgery improves survival and the myocardial infarction recurrence rate. Data from the Mayo Clinic indicate that adequate treatment of hypertension after acute myocardial infarction improves chances of survival. There is evidence that control of hyperlipidemia by either dietary manipulation or drug therapy retards progression of coronary atherosclerosis in patients with symptomatic coronary disease. In addition, progression of disease either in the native coronary arteries or in saphenous vein grafts has been shown to be related to adverse plasma lipid levels.

In our experience, cardiac rehabilitation is a useful form of therapy for most patients. Those who participate in rehabilitation appear to work more effectively, have fewer symptoms and limitations, comply more closely with treatment plans, have more positive self-perception and confidence, and lead more active life styles with more physical and sexual activity than patients who are left to fend for themselves.

REFERENCES

Connolly DC, Elveback LR, Oxman HA: Coronary heart disease in residents of Rochester, Minnesota, 1950–1974. III. Effect of hypertension and its treatment on survival of patients with coronary artery disease. Mayo Clin Proc 58:249–254, 1983.

Kallio V, Hamalainen H, Hakkila J, et al: Reduction in sudden deaths by a multifactorial intervention programme after acute myocardial infarction. Lancet 2:1091–1094, 1979.

Kellerman JJ: Cardiac rehabilitation: reminiscences, international variations, experiences. J Cardiac Rehab 1:43–50, 1981.

Pollock ML, Wilmore JH, Fox SM: Exercise in Health and Disease: Evaluation and Prescription for Prevention and Rehabilitation. W. B. Saunders Co., Philadelphia, 1984, pp 298–373.

Squires RW, Gau GT: Cardiac rehabilitation and cardiovascular health enhancement. *In* Brandenburg RO, Fuster V, McGoon DC, et al (eds): Mayo Clinic Textbook of Cardiology, in press.

Wenger NK, Hellerstein HK (eds): Rehabilitation of the Coronary Patient. John Wiley & Sons, New York, 1978.

5 · MILD ESSENTIAL HYPERTENSION

Michael D. Cressman
Ray W. Gifford, Jr.
CLEVELAND CLINIC FOUNDATION

DEFINITION AND DIAGNOSTIC CRITERIA

Many controversial issues are encountered when discussing recommendations about the care of hypertensive patients. A prime example is the definition of hypertension. There are theoretical difficulties in ascribing any number to constitute a diagnosis of mild hypertension, since there is no clear numerical level at which blood pressure can be considered "safe." Insurance actuarial studies have found that diastolic blood pressures (DBPs) ranging from 83 to 87 mm Hg are associated with an increased incidence of cardiovascular mortality when compared with the population at large. The mortality experience (actual to predicted mortality) in men is increased by another 18% when DBPs range from 88 to 92 mm Hg and by 51% when DBPs range from 93 to 97 mm Hg. This increment in risk is also apparent in women, but the actual mortality experience for any given range of DBP is lower in women than it is in men. It is also important to keep in mind that the absolute cardiovascular risk of any given BP level depends on the presence or absence of a variety of associated cardiovascular risk factors. In other words, the cardiovascular risk of a 35-year-old woman with a DBP of 95 mm Hg and no other risk factors is quite different from the risk of a similar DBP in a man who has hypercholesterolemia, glucose intolerance, a family history of premature cardiovascular disease, and a habit of heavy cigarette smoking.

RECOMMENDATIONS OF THE THIRD JOINT NATIONAL COMMITTEE

Despite these theoretical problems, some simple guidelines are required for physicians who treat hypertensive patients. We feel that the recommendations of the Third Joint National Committee (JNC III) on Detection, Evaluation, and Treatment of High Blood Pressure are useful for practicing physicians. Simply stated, patients with DBPs that are repeatedly demonstrated to range from 90 to 104 mm Hg are considered to have mild hypertension. Because of the social and psychologic implications of labeling a patient "hypertensive," considerable care should be taken in establishing this diagnosis. The fact that BP levels may vary considerably in certain patients, and the clear demonstration that exercise and environmental stress can transiently increase BP, have prompted the JNC III to make several recommendations in reference to the confirmation of hypertension.

Recordings of BP should not be obtained until the patient has been seated quietly for several minutes. Clothing that constricts the arm should be removed. A mercury sphygmomanometer or a recently calibrated aneroid device is used to record BP while the patient is seated. At least two measurements are obtained at each visit, and the average of these is recorded. If DBP ranges from 90 to 104 mm Hg at the initial visit, BP should be rechecked within two months. If it is still high at the second visit, the patient should be evaluated or referred within two weeks. If DBP remains in the 90 to 104 mm Hg range at the third visit, a diagnosis of mild diastolic hypertension can be made. Patients with DBPs ranging from 85 to 89 mm Hg are said to have "high-normal" pressures, and should have BP rechecked within one year.

SYSTOLIC BLOOD PRESSURE AND CARDIOVASCULAR RISK

Epidemiologic evidence clearly shows that systolic blood pressure (SBP) is as predictive of long-term cardiovascular mortality as DBP. In general, SBP and DBP rise proportionally in patients with essential hypertension. However, some young patients and many elderly individuals have "isolated systolic hypertension." The JNC III Report contains recommendations for managing this group of patients. The current chapter will deal only with the management of mild diastolic hypertension (DBP, 90 to 104 mm Hg).

PATHOPHYSIOLOGY

The cause of essential hypertension is unknown. The familial clustering observed suggests a genetic influence; the association between the level of salt intake and the prevalence of hypertension in different societies is a prime example of a potential environmental factor that could unmask hypertension in a susceptible person.

Hemodynamically, chronic essential hypertension is usually characterized by high peripheral vascular resistance, normal or reduced cardiac output, and reduced circulating blood volume. However, the chronic phase may represent evolution from a state of salt and water excess with an increase in cardiac output. It has been postulated that a circulating natriuretic substance that inhibits Na/K ATPase is released when blood volume is expanded. The sodium transport inhibitor produces natriuresis but leads to vasoconstriction via a calcium-mediated enhancement of smooth muscle contraction. This series of events could explain the "low-renin" hypertension observed in certain subsets of the hypertensive population. Other investigators have questioned the role of baroreceptor dysfunction or other neurogenic factors, cardiac abnormalities (particularly abnormalities in diastolic filling of the heart), overactivity of the renin-angiotensin system, or an intrinsic abnormality of sodium handling by the kidney. It is safe to say that a variety of factors are involved and any single explanation for the genesis of essential hypertension is probably inadequate. The pathophysiology is multifactorial, and different mechanisms are operative in individual hypertensive patients.

CLINICAL ASPECTS

It is estimated that approximately 60 million people in the United States are hypertensive. Roughly two thirds of these patients have mild diastolic hypertension. The massive effort to educate the community about the risks of high BP has undoubtedly increased detection of mild hypertension in its asymptomatic phase. These efforts must continue since the long-term goal of antihypertensive therapy is to *prevent* complications of unrecognized and untreated hypertension. However, many patients have already developed target organ damage (e.g., stroke, left ventricular hypertrophy or failure, myocardial infarction, renal insufficiency) at the time of presentation. The location and extent of this involvement influences the choice of drug treatment or the goal level and rate of BP reduction.

The physician must be concerned with several aspects of the health care of the hypertensive patient. Adequate care requires not only a program of BP reduction by nonpharmacologic or pharmacologic means. Attention must also be given to other factors that place patients at risk of subsequent cardiovascular disease. Measures to improve glucose tolerance, reduce blood lipid levels, and decrease cigarette consumption may be required. Recognition and management of preexisting atherosclerotic cardiovascular disease by surgical means can drastically alter subsequent clinical course. For this reason, a careful history and physical examination must be performed with particular reference to the cardiovascular system. The impact of an aggressive approach to treatment of asymptomatic aortic aneurysms, severe extracranial carotid artery disease, or coronary artery disease is difficult to define for the population at large, but in individual cases appropriate surgical intervention can prevent a catastrophic cardiovascular event.

MANAGEMENT

EVALUATION OF THE HYPERTENSIVE PATIENT

The initial evaluation of the hypertensive patient is designed to assess the presence of associated cardiovascular risk factors (smoking, family history, hypercholesterolemia, hyperglycemia), detect the presence of target organ involvement, and determine if a secondary cause of hypertension is present. This investigation does not require hospitalization. The physician must perform a detailed history and physical examination with emphasis on the cardiovascular system. A limited number of laboratory tests are required, including urinalysis with careful examination of the urine sediment, serum creatinine, potassium, and uric acid, hemoglobin and hematocrit, total and high-density lipoprotein (HDL) cholesterol level, and fasting venous plasma glucose. In addition, a resting EKG should be obtained, to identify patients with left ventricular hypertrophy or evidence of ischemic heart disease.

The results of the initial investigation are discussed with the patient before any specific treatment program begins. It is helpful to teach the patient to record BP at home; the technique is easily learned and a variety of relatively inexpensive sphygmomanometers are available. Home BP monitoring aids the detection of "office hypertension" and reduces the need for repeated BP checks in the physician's office. Home recordings are especially helpful in long-term follow-up when decisions must be made to increase or decrease dosages of antihypertensive medications.

As stated, the long-term objectives of antihypertensive therapy (the chronic reduction of BP to normotensive levels and the modification of correctable associated risk factors) must be emphasized to the patient. This may require some life style changes, e.g., smoking, drinking, or dietary habits. The success of the program depends to a large degree on the ability to gain compliance.

NONPHARMACOLOGIC MEASURES

Concern about long-term risks of pharmacologic therapy has led to increased interest in nonpharmacologic antihypertensive therapy. Obese patients may become normotensive if they lose weight. Patients who ingest more than 2 oz. of ethanol per day may respond to a reduction in alcohol intake. Reduction of saturated fat intake has been reported to lower BP. There have also been reports of modest BP reduction when calcium, potassium, or magnesium intake is increased. Finally, isotonic exercise, biofeedback, and various relaxation techniques may reduce BP in certain patients.

Curtailment of heavy alcohol intake, reduction in saturated fat consumption, the use of dietary supplements (calcium, potassium, magnesium), or a reasonable exercise program are obviously appealing therapeutic measures, but their ability to reduce BP chronically has not been rigidly tested. If these measures are employed, BP should be followed as closely as it is in patients receiving drug treatment. In our opinion, weight reduction in obese patients and moderate sodium restriction are the most useful and effective nonpharmacologic methods of treatment. However, not every patient will comply with the diet and not all patients who comply will respond. For this reason, patients treated by salt restriction or weight reduction should also be carefully followed. If an adequate response has not been observed after approximately six months of any nonpharmacologic therapy, drug treatment should begin. It is reasonable to begin drugs earlier if the patient simply is not interested in following a low salt diet or any other nonpharmacologic measure.

Physicians who choose to treat hypertensive patients with a low-sodium diet should recognize that the success of the dietary manipulation depends to a large degree on the effort given to instruct the patient. For this reason, the help of a dietician should be enlisted whenever possible. We recommend a diet containing approximately 2 gm sodium (5 gm salt). It is important to emphasize the difference between "salt" (NaCl) and sodium (Na). Salt is approximately 40% Na; thus, a 5-gm salt diet contains 2 gm sodium. A 2-gm sodium diet contains roughly 87 mEq Na. Thus, 5 gm NaCl = 2 gm Na = 87 mEq Na. The average American diet contains 10 to 20 gm salt per day, and approximately 30% to 40% of this salt is added to food during its preparation or at the table. Another 30% is contained in various processed foods ("fast" foods, canned foods, lunch meat, etc.).

Thus, if these two salt sources are eliminated or significantly reduced, the diet will contain approximately 5 gm salt, a restriction considered moderate.

It is helpful to reduce the salt intake gradually rather than abruptly. The taste for salt is acquired and clearly diminishes with time as salt intake is reduced. We have our patients eliminate salt first during the preparation of food, and remove it from the table later. Lists of foods containing high salt levels should be given since many patients are not aware that items such as canned tomatoes or tomato juice, dill pickles, milk and cheese, monosodium glutamate, sodium monophosphate, ketchup, soy sauce, and certain "salt substitutes" all contain sodium. It is helpful to have the patient or food preparer learn to read labels, but this may require much time and patience.

It should be reemphasized that some patients cannot or will not follow a low salt diet. Others who do comply will not respond. Compliance is difficult to determine solely by speaking with the patient, but a reasonable estimate of sodium intake can be obtained by measuring the sodium content of a 24-hour urine specimen. The physician should recognize that patients have difficulty remembering to save all the urine excreted in a 24-hour period. Adequacy of the collection can be assessed by measuring the creatinine content of the specimen. Women excrete approximately 15 mg creatinine/kg/day; men excrete 20 mg creatinine/kg/day.

We monitor sodium excretion (1) in patients who have not responded to the sodium-restricted diet, if they wish to continue the diet; and (2) in patients who have not had an appropriate response to drug therapy. The results of the collection should be used to identify hidden sodium sources of which the patient is unaware, not to chastise the patient for not complying. This would only place a barrier between the patient and the physician, and ultimately reduce subsequent compliance with any dietary or drug treatment.

Some physicians feel that salt restriction plays little if any role in the management of hypertensive patients. Recognizing that salt restriction is not always possible and not universally effective in lowering BP, we advocate a moderately restricted diet in the vast majority of our hypertensive patients because:

1. Moderate salt restriction is unlikely to do any harm (since a 5-gm salt diet contains 40 times more salt than is physiologically needed).

2. Many patients have a moderate antihypertensive response if compliance is achieved.

3. There is no good way to separate responders from nonresponders.

4. Salt restriction may obviate the need for drugs, enhances the efficacy of antihypertensive agents, and reduces the hypokalemic response to diuretic treatment.

DRUG THERAPY

The pattern of drug treatment has changed in the last decade. Comparison of the 1980 and 1984 JNC reports reflects some of these changes. In 1980, diuretics at a dosage of 50 to 100 mg per day hydrochlorothiazide or its equivalent were recommended as the only first step in drug treatment. In 1984, diuretics or beta-blockers were recommended as the first step and the recommended diuretic dosage was reduced by 50%. Diuretics and beta-blockers are not the only agents that have been successful as monotherapy. Some patients do well with centrally acting sympatholytic agents (clonidine, guanabenz, methyldopa), peripherally acting alpha-receptor antagonists (prazosin), combined alpha/beta-blockers (labetalol), converting enzyme inhibitors (captopril, enalapril), or calcium channel blockers (diltiazem, nifedipine, verapamil). The clinician is now faced with a seemingly endless list of antihypertensive agents and information from the pharmaceutical industry and medical literature supporting the widespread use of many of these as the first step in drug therapy. However, information concerning the long-term safety and efficacy of monotherapy with agents other than diuretics or beta-blockers is incomplete, and we continue to use either a diuretic or a beta-blocker as the first step in the vast majority of our hypertensive patients.

Several factors influence the choice of drug treatment for mild hypertension, including age, race, and the presence or absence of conditions that may be associated with hypertension. Many patients with mild hypertension are asymptomatic and will not tolerate a treatment program that is inordinately expensive, inconvenient, or associated with symptomatic side effects. There is a need for individualization of treatment, but this should not involve a haphazard approach to drug selection. It can be argued that any "stepped-care" approach ignores the variability in the mechanism of each individual patient's hypertension. Although this criticism may be valid, no one can argue that (1) the stepped-care approach successfully reduces BP for prolonged periods; and (2) diuretic-based, stepped-care antihypertensive therapy decreased cardiovascular mortality in patients with mild hypertension in the Hypertension Detection and Follow-Up Program (HDFP), even in those with DBPs ranging from 90 to 94 mm Hg.

Diuretics As Initial Drug Treatment. Since thiazide diuretics are inexpensive, convenient to administer, and well tolerated, a strong argument can be made for choosing these agents initially in patients with mild hypertension. They are effective in both young and elderly individuals and reduce BP in white and black hypertensives. However, a number of biochemical abnormalities (hypokalemia, hyperuricemia, hyperglycemia, hyperlipidemia, hypomagnesemia, and hypochloremic metabolic alkalosis) may develop during long-term treatment. It has been suggested that these abnormalities offset the benefit of their antihypertensive effect and minimize their ability to reduce long-term cardiovascular morbidity and mortality. The increased coronary mortality in hypertensive patients with abnormal resting EKGs in the special intervention group of the Multiple Risk Factor Intervention Trial (MRFIT) has led to a reassessment of their use in the treatment of hypertension. A clear role for thiazide-induced hypokalemia in the increased incidence of sudden death in hypertensive patients with abnormal EKGs in MRFIT has not been proved, but is of great concern. Because of this concern, we consider it reasonable to (1) reduce the dosage range of hydrochlorothiazide (or its equivalent) to 25 to 50 mg per day, (2) maintain serum potassium above 3.5 mEq/L in any patient with clinical or EKG evidence of organic heart disease, and (3) consider using a beta-blocker initially in patients with ischemic heart disease. Doses of hydrochlorothiazide in excess of 50 mg produce more side effects and do not often induce a more profound antihypertensive response.

Beta-Blockers As First Step in Drug Treatment. Many physicians advocate a more widespread initial use of beta-blockers, chiefly because of concern about the aforementioned biochemical effects of the thiazides. However, beta-blockers can increase serum triglycerides, reduce high density lipoprotein (HDL) levels, and alter glucose metabolism. In addition, there is currently no firm evidence that beta-blockers reduce the incidence of primary (as opposed to recurrent) myocardial infarction in hypertensive patients. The recently reported Medical Research Council trial of the diuretic bendrofluazide versus propranolol showed no difference in coronary events in these treatment groups, but there was a reduction in coronary events in nonsmokers receiving propranolol. Beta-blockers can reduce BP for prolonged periods in certain hypertensive patients, but are not as versatile as the thiazides. For example, patients with bronchial asthma, congestive heart failure, severe sinus bradycardia, or heart block greater than first degree should not receive beta-blockers. Patients with Raynaud's phenomenon or severe occlusive peripheral vascular disease have a relative contraindication to beta-blocker treatment. Black patients as a group respond more favorably to thiazide diuretics than to beta-blockers. Elderly individuals have more side effects and a less favorable antihypertensive response to beta-blockers than do younger patients. Finally, patients with chronic renal failure generally have a volume-dependent form of hypertension that is difficult to control without a diuretic.

Many patients do very well with beta-blocker monotherapy, and some have associated medical conditions that also respond to beta-blockers. A subset of young hypertensive patients have evidence of a hyperkinetic circulation characterized by resting tachycardia, hyperdynamic precordium, systolic flow murmur, or symptoms of vasomotor lability (sweating, palpitations, or labile BP). Hemodynamically, these patients have an increased cardiac output, which distinguishes them from most hypertensive patients whose hypertension is characterized by high peripheral vascular resistance and normal or decreased cardiac output. This may explain the favorable response to beta-blockade in the former group of patients.

We use beta-blockers initially in these patients and in patients with the associated medical conditions listed in Table 1. Thus, our initial choice of diuretics or beta-blockers is dictated by clinical characteristics of individual hypertensive patients. Some physicians advocate further individualization of treatment based on an anal-

Table 1. INDICATIONS FOR BETA-BLOCKERS (OTHER THAN HYPERTENSION)

Cardiovascular	Noncardiovascular
1. Angina pectoris	1. Migraine headache
2. Supraventricular tachyarrhythmias	2. Essential tremor
3. Postmyocardial infarction prophylaxis	3. Anxiety
4. Aortic dissection	4. Glaucoma
5. Hypertrophic cardiomyopathy	
6. Mitral valve prolapse	
7. Mitral stenosis	

ysis of the relative importance of volume and pressor mechanisms. One analysis is based on "renin profiling," and requires collection of a 24-hour urine specimen for determination of sodium intake and measurement of plasma renin activity (PRA) in a peripheral venous blood sample. Patients with "low-renin" hypertension are treated with diuretics; those with "high-renin" hypertension are treated with beta-blockers. Although this approach has theoretical appeal, it is quite costly and has never really been shown to be any more effective than one that relies on clinical criteria to select initial drug treatment.

Diuretic and Beta-Blocker Dosages. The JNC III recommends diuretic treatment as the first step in "patients over 50 years of age, in black patients, and in patients with peripheral vascular disease, asthma, or other forms of chronic pulmonary disease." We usually initiate treatment with 25 mg hydrochlorothiazide or its equivalent as a single morning dose. If DBP is not reduced to less than 90 mm Hg after one to three months of treatment, the dose is increased to 50 mg once a day. Serum potassium should be checked when the maintenance dose of the diuretic is reached. Oral potassium supplements or potassium-sparing diuretics (amiloride, spironolactone, triamterene) are added if serum potassium is below 3.5 mEq/L in elderly patients, patients receiving digitalis, and patients who have clinical evidence of organic heart disease. The value of potassium supplements in young asymptomatic patients with mild hypokalemia (serum potassium ranging from 3.0 to 3.5 mEq/L) is not defined. Several thiazide/potassium-sparing combinations (Dyazide, Aldactazide, Maxzide, Moduretic) are also available and convenient to use.

Table 2 provides a list of currently available diuretics and beta-blockers. The pharmacologic properties of the various beta-blockers are the subject of several recent reviews and will not be reiterated here. Our choice of a beta-blocker is dictated largely by the ability of the individual drug to reduce BP for a 24-hour period when given once a day. Atenolol, metoprolol, nadolol, acebutolol, and a long-acting preparation of propranolol can all be given on a q.d. basis. The other beta-blockers must be given twice a day. The water-soluble drugs (atenolol, nadolol, acebutolol) should be avoided in patients with chronic renal failure (because they are excreted by the kidney) but are preferred in patients with chronic liver disease. Atenolol, a long-acting, water-soluble, "cardioselective" beta-blocker, differs from the other beta-blockers in that its dose-response relationship (dose to antihypertensive response) is relatively flat. Doses in excess of 100 mg rarely produce an additional antihypertensive response. This negates the need to titrate the dose frequently and eliminates the cost and inconvenience of these titration visits.

The maximal response to either diuretic or beta-blocker monotherapy may not be achieved for several weeks and a second drug should not be added prematurely. In general, a two- to three-month trial is reasonable since the risk of mild hypertension over this interval of time is minimal. We usually add a beta-blocker to the diuretic (if no contraindications exist) or add a diuretic to the beta-blocker if beta-blocker monotherapy was used initially. Beta-blockers are much more effective when used with a diuretic in black hypertensive patients than when they are used as monotherapy in blacks.

Other Antihypertensive Agents. As previously stated, centrally acting alpha$_2$ agonists (clonidine, guanabenz, methyldopa), alpha$_1$ antagonists (prazosin), combined alpha and beta antagonists (labetalol), ACE inhibitors (captopril, enalapril), and calcium channel blockers (diltiazem, nifedipine, verapamil) are effective as monotherapy in certain patients. The efficacy of these drugs is enhanced by diuretics. Clonidine, guanabenz, and methyldopa are particularly useful in the elderly and in young patients with symptoms of adrenergic excess who do not tolerate beta-blockers. Hydralazine can be used alone in elderly patients provided that a marked reflex tachycardia does not occur; this tends to be less of a problem in the elderly because of their decreased baroreceptor sensitivity. Prazosin and the centrally acting alpha$_2$ agonists cause few biochemical side effects. The occurrence of orthostatic hypotension (particularly early in treatment) makes prazosin less desirable in elderly patients, particularly if they have severe cerebrovascular disease.

Low-dose captopril therapy (12.5 to 25 mg two or three times daily) is associated with a low incidence of symptomatic and biochemical side effects. It tends to be less effective as monotherapy in blacks. Diuretics increase the efficacy of captopril and negate the racial difference in response to the drug. In addition, captopril blunts the hypokalemic effect of diuretics. The use of potassium supplements and potassium-sparing agents in conjunction with captopril may cause hyperkalemia (especially in patients with abnormal renal function) and should be used only if hypokalemia occurs. Captopril has proved useful to treat patients with chronic CHF and is particularly indicated for patients with heart failure who remain hypertensive on diuretics. However, a profound hypotensive response can occur with the first few doses (particularly in patients with high pretreatment plasma renin levels) and can jeopardize cerebral, coronary, or renal perfusion. It is reasonable to begin therapy with captopril at 6.25 to 12.5 mg b.i.d. in patients with heart failure or with known or suspected renal artery disease. Particular caution should be exercised in patients with bilateral renal artery disease since captopril has caused acute renal failure in this setting. Enalapril is a newer ACE inhibitor differing from captopril in that it (1) is more potent, (2) has a longer duration of action, and (3) lacks the sulfhydryl group, which is felt to produce some of the serious but uncommon side effects of captopril.

The calcium channel blockers have not yet been approved for use in hypertension but produce a moderate antihypertensive response even when used alone. They share the important advantage of beta-blockers inasmuch as they are useful for angina pectoris, migraine headache, and atrial tachyarrhythmias (where verapamil may be the drug of choice). In contrast to the beta-blockers, these agents lower BP by reducing peripheral vascular resistance, and seem to be particularly effective in elderly patients. Since the elderly have a high incidence of coronary artery disease, it is likely that these agents will enjoy increased use in these patients. Caution should be exercised with nifedipine since a significant first-dose hypotensive response

Table 2. ANTIHYPERTENSIVE AGENTS

	Daily Dose (mg)		
	Initial	Maximal	Frequency/Day
DIURETICS			
Thiazide and Related Sulfonamide Diuretics			
Bendroflumethiazide (Naturetin)	2.5	5	1
Benzthiazide (Aquatag, ExNa, Hydrex)	25.0	50	1
Chlorothiazide sodium (Diuril)	250.0	500	1
Chlorthalidone (Hygroton, Thalitone)	25.0	50	1
Cyclothiazide (Anhydron, Fluidal)	1.0	2	1
Hydrochlorothiazide (Esidrex, Hydro-Diuril, Oretic)	25.0	50	1
Hydroflumethiazide (Diucardin, Saluron)	25.0	50	1
Indapamide (Lozol)	2.5	5	1
Methyclothiazide (Aquatensen, Enduron)	2.5	5	1
Metolazone (Diulo, Zaroxolyn)	2.5	5	1
Polythiazide (Renese)	2.0	4	1
Quinethazone (Hydromox)	50.0	100	1
Trichlormethiazide (Metahydrin, Naqua)	2.0	4	1
Loop Diuretics			
Bumetanide (Bumex)	0.5	10	2
Ethacrynic acid (Edecrin)	50.0	200	2
Furosemide (Lasix)	80.0	480	2
Potassium-Sparing Agents			
Amiloride hydrochloride (Midamor)	5.0	10	1
Spironolactone (Aldactone)	50.0	100	1
Triamterene (Dyrenium)	50.0	100	1
ADRENERGIC INHIBITORS			
Beta-Adrenergic Blockers			
Acebutolol	200.0	800	1
Atenolol (Tenormin)	25.0	100	1
Metoprolol tartrate (Lopressor)	50.0	300	1
Nadolol (Corgard)	20.0	240	1
Pindolol (Visken)	20.0	60	1
Propranolol hydrochloride	40.0	480	2
Propranolol long-acting (Inderal LA)	80.0	480	2
Timolol maleate (Blocadren)	20.0	60	1 2
Central Adrenergic Inhibitors			
Clonidine hydrochloride (Catapres)	0.2	1.2	2
Guanabenz acetate (Wytensin)	8.0	32	2
Methyldopa (Aldomet)	500.0	2000	2
Peripheral Adrenergic Antagonists			
Guanadrel sulfate (Hylorel)	10.0	150	2
Guanethidine monosulfate (Ismelin)	10.0	300	1
Rauwolfia alkaloids			
Rauwolfia whole root (Raudixin)	50.0	100	1
Reserpine (Sandril, Serpasil, Rau-sed, Reserpoid)	0.05	0.25 (additional derivatives available)	1
Alpha$_1$ Adrenergic Blocker			
Prazosin hydrochloride (Minipress)	1.0	20	2
Combined Alpha- and Beta-Blocking Agents			
Labetalol hydrochloride (Normodyne, Trandate)	200.0	1200	2
VASODILATORS			
Hydralazine (Apresoline)	50.0	300	2
Minoxidil (Loniten)	2.5	50	2
ANGIOTENSIN CONVERTING ENZYME (ACE) INHIBITORS			
Captopril (Capoten)	37.5	150	2
Enalapril maleate (Vasotec)	10.0	40	1
SLOW CHANNEL CALCIUM ENTRY BLOCKING AGENTS			
Diltiazem hydrochloride (Cardizem)	60	240	2
Nifedipine (Procardia)	30	180	3
Verapamil hydrochloride (Calan, Isoptin)	240	480	3

associated with a reflex tachycardia may occur. Many patients require a beta-blocker or centrally acting alpha$_2$ agonist during nifedipine treatment because of the reflex tachycardia observed with this vasodilator. Reflex tachycardia generally does not occur with diltiazem or verapamil because these drugs have negative chronotropic effects. Diltiazem and verapamil should be avoided in patients with severe sinus bradycardia or significant AV nodal conduction disturbances, a consideration that must be observed if one of these agents is used to treat the elderly hypertensive. Dosing schedules for these antihypertensive drugs are in Table 2.

PATIENT INFORMATION AND EDUCATION

The importance of patient education can hardly be overstated. The key elements of this process include:

1. Emphasis on the risks of long-standing, untreated hypertension.

2. Recognition and modification of associated cardiovascular risk factors.

3. Instruction in home BP monitoring.

4. Emphasis on the role of dietary sodium restriction. A dietician should assist in the prescription of a low salt diet. Caloric restriction and reduction in saturated fat intake may also be required.

5. Recognition by the patient that adherence to the prescribed therapeutic regimen is critical for success of the treatment program.

PERIODIC EVALUATION

The frequency of follow-up visits to reexamine the patient and monitor various laboratory parameters must be individualized. Frequency depends on the clinical condition of the patient, adequacy of BP control, compliance, and choice of drug treatment. As previously stated, diuretic treatment especially requires laboratory surveillance because these agents produce hypokalemia and other metabolic disturbances. It is reasonable to check the serum potassium shortly (within one month) after the maintenance diuretic dose is reached. Hyponatremia can also develop, particularly in elderly patients, and should also be monitored. Monitoring of blood glucose and blood lipids should be performed annually and perhaps more often in patients with diabetes or hyperlipidemia. Office BPs should be recorded in both supine (or seated) and standing positions, to detect the presence of orthostatic hypotension. This is particularly true in elderly patients who are prone to this side effect.

In patients who are truly resistant to a regimen of moderate sodium restriction and adequate doses of standard triple drug therapy (diuretic plus antiadrenergic agent plus vasodilator), there may be a secondary cause of hypertension. However, resistance is more often due to noncompliance, or inappropriate combinations or inadequate dosage of the various pharmacologic agents. Inadequate diuretic dosages have frequently been the cause of resistance to treatment in the past, and this should be kept in mind when approaching the patient with resistant hypertension, notwithstanding the recent trend to reduce diuretic dosages. If noncompliance does not seem to be an issue and the secondary causes are reasonably excluded, the physician may (1) further restrict sodium and alcohol intake, (2) reemphasize weight reduction in obese patients, (3) substitute or add a second antiadrenergic agent, (4) increase the dose of the previously prescribed antiadrenergic agent (except for reserpine), (5) substitute minoxidil for hydralazine, or (6) refer the patient for further evaluation.

PATIENT COMPLIANCE

The success of the antihypertensive treatment program is directly related to the patient's ability to maintain compliance, which is best achieved by:

1. Educating the patient about the risks of hypertension and the need for continuous treatment and follow-up.

2. Involving the patient and possibly the spouse in the treatment program. Home BP monitoring increases this involvement.

3. Avoiding repeated office visits and long delays in the physician's waiting room.

4. Prescribing a treatment regimen that is convenient, well tolerated, and not unduly expensive.

5. Providing positive reinforcement to the patient.

Noncompliance should always be considered when treatment is ineffective. Patients who do not know the names of their medications or when they take them, who frequently miss visits, or who complain of multiple side effects are often noncompliant. Certain patients may not cooperate because their medications are too expensive. When beta-blockers are used, failure to demonstrate a decrease in the resting heart rate should suggest noncompliance since the antihypertensive dose of a beta-blocker (except for pindolol and possibly acebutolol) is much greater than the dose required to reduce heart rate. The lack of change in serum potassium, uric acid, or chloride suggests noncompliance in diuretic-treated patients.

Pill counts can be used to detect noncompliance. Sometimes it is helpful to administer the drugs and observe the antihypertensive response in the office. Patients who do not appear to be responding but whose BP normalizes after the drugs are given in the office may not be taking their medications. A transdermal preparation of clonidine, applied on a weekly basis, may improve compliance in patients who have an aversion for or difficulty in remembering to take their BP medications. The fatigue and dry mouth frequently encountered early in oral clonidine treatment appear to be less prominent with the transdermal form of the drug.

PREVENTIVE MEASURES

No known measures have been proved to prevent the development of hypertension. However, some nonpharmacologic measures (sodium restriction, potassium feeding, and calcium supplementation) appear to delay the onset and decrease the severity of hypertension in certain animal models. For this reason, some physicians advocate the use of these nonpharmacologic measures in patients at risk of developing hypertension. Prevention of the atherosclerotic complications of hypertension requires a multifaceted approach that includes (1) control of hypertension; (2) dietary modification in patients with obesity, glucose intolerance, or hypercholesterolemia; (3) stopping cigarette smoking; and (4) maintenance of adequate physical conditioning with a reasonable exercise program.

SOCIOECONOMIC IMPACT

Critics of an aggressive approach to management of mild hypertension often use an economic argument for withholding treatment. It is true that many patients with mild hypertension must be treated to affect overall mortality since the risk is small, especially in the young. However, the economic impact of treatment cannot be measured solely by the cost of therapy. Cardiovascular disease continues to be the number one cause of mortality in the U.S. In addition, the expense of treating complications once they have occurred, coupled with the cost of lost work time in previously productive members of society, must be considered. This is not to deny the need for establishing a treatment program that adequately considers cost. In our opinion, the approach outlined by the JNC III has the best chance of providing cost-effective treatment of mild hypertension.

REFERENCES

Hypertension Detection and Follow-Up Program Cooperative Group: Five-year findings of the hypertension detection and follow-up program. I. Reduction in mortality of persons with high blood pressure, including mild hypertension. JAMA 242:2562–2571, 1979.

Hypertension Detection and Follow-Up Program Cooperative Group: The effect of treatment and mortality in "mild" hypertension. Results of the hypertension detection and follow-up program. N Engl J Med 307:976–980, 1982.

Joint National Committee on Detection, Evaluation, and Treatment of High Blood Pressure: 1984 Report of the Joint National Committee on Detection, Evaluation, and Treatment of High Blood Pressure. Arch Intern Med 144:1045–1057, 1984.

Multiple Risk Factor Intervention Trial Research Group: Multiple Risk Factor Intervention Trial. Risk factor changes and mortality rates. JAMA 248:1465–1477, 1982.

Society of Actuaries and Association of Life Insurance Medical Directors of America: Build and Blood Pressure Study 1979. Recording and Statistical Corp. USA, 1980.

6 · ACCELERATED HYPERTENSION, MALIGNANT HYPERTENSION, AND HYPERTENSIVE EMERGENCIES

Donald G. Vidt
CLEVELAND CLINIC FOUNDATION

Sustained arterial hypertension results in progressive vascular damage and progression to accelerated or malignant hypertension, and considerably shortens life. The presence of cerebral, cardiac, or renal complications influences both prognosis and therapy. The continuing development of effective antihypertensive drugs over the past three decades has been associated with a progressive decline in hypertension resistant to therapy. Truly refractory hypertension is rare today. Major clinical trials have demonstrated the effectiveness of drug therapy in preventing stroke, congestive heart failure, aortic dissection, progressive renal failure, and progression to more severe or accelerated hypertension.

DEFINITIONS

It is desirable to define the various terms used and to recognize that they may all represent phases in the course of this chronic disease if it is inadequately treated. *Resistant hypertension* represents failure to control blood pressure adequately (<150/100 mm Hg) despite compliance with an appropriate three-drug regimen. *Accelerated hypertension* represents severe hypertension (≥180/120 mm Hg) with evidence of CNS, cardiac, and renal damage, with Grade III hypertensive retinopathy characterized by hemorrhages and exudates, but without papilledema. *Malignant hypertension* presents the features of accelerated hypertension and is associated with necrotizing arteriolitis, retinal hemorrhages, exudates, and papilledema (Grade IV funduscopic changes). With progression of target organ damage, the risk of encephalopathy, intracranial hemorrhage, left ventricular failure, and renal failure is significant. In untreated patients, mortality from malignant hypertension approaches 100% within one year.

A number of disease conditions of varied etiologies may be complicated by accelerated or malignant hypertension. This severity of hypertension is most commonly seen in the course of untreated or inadequately controlled essential hypertension, but may occur as a complication of renovascular hypertension, acute or chronic glomerulonephritis, preeclampsia of pregnancy, and pheochromocytoma. Accelerated or malignant hypertension may also be observed in association with collagen vascular illnesses such as scleroderma, polyarteritis, or systemic lupus erythematosus. Although it is less common, it may also present a management problem in association with the hemolytic-uremic syndrome, atheroembolic renal disease, primary aldosteronism, or Cushing's disease. Any form of secondary hypertension, inadequately controlled, carries the risk of progression.

Any of these situations may be considered a matter of *hypertensive urgency* or *emergency* if target organ complications supervene to impose an immediate threat to the integrity of the cardiovascular system. For convenience, hypertensive urgencies are defined as situations in which BP should be reduced within 24 hours; in a hypertensive emergency, BP reduction within one hour is considered desirable. A hypertensive emergency depends more on the patient's clinical state than on the absolute level of BP. A patient with accelerated or malignant hypertension and sustained BP of ≥230/130 mm Hg, but with no evidence of acute target organ compromise, does not necessarily require immediate reduction of BP by administration of parenteral agents. Prompt and aggressive therapy with oral agents, in combination, may suffice. In contrast, even moderate elevation of BP, if complicated by acute CHF or aortic dissection, represents a true emergency requiring aggressive treatment with parenteral agents and immediate reduction of BP. Whether the condition is encountered in the office, clinic, or emergency room, the clinician must be prepared to judge whether the patient can be appropriately and safely managed on an ambulatory basis, or whether hospitalization is desirable for initial treatment and control of BP.

MANAGEMENT OF RESISTANT HYPERTENSION

Hypertension resistant to a suitable regimen should stimulate a search for other causes of resistance. In most cases, patient noncompliance, failure to restrict sodium intake, or an inadequate drug regimen can be identified. Potential drug interactions must be expected, e.g., when giving tricyclic antidepressants to a patient taking guanethidine or clonidine. Concurrent administration of indirectly acting sympathomimetic agents in many over-the-counter preparations, or the use of oral contraceptives, may interfere with antihypertensive drug effects. If these issues have been addressed and a secondary cause of hypertension is ruled out, further study may be appropriate to identify the underlying hemodynamic and humoral mechanisms responsible for the resistance. The regimen may then be changed appropriately.

A discussion of the clinical pharmacology of available antihypertensive agents is beyond the scope of this chapter, but suitable reviews are available. I have reviewed briefly the clinical pharmacology of three newer families of antihypertensive agents that have demonstrated particular efficacy in the treatment of accelerated or malignant hypertension and in hypertensive urgencies or emergencies.

CALCIUM ENTRY BLOCKERS*

Three calcium entry blockers (nifedipine, diltiazem, and verapamil) have been approved for treatment of angina pectoris and cardiac arrhythmias. These agents are potent vascular smooth muscle dilators and possess a hemodynamic profile that makes them potentially useful in management of severe hypertension and hypertensive emergencies. Calcium entry blockers inhibit the passage of extracellular calcium across cell membranes and the release of calcium ions from binding sites in sarcoplasmic reticulum. This effect lowers calcium-dependent splitting of adenosine triphosphate and results in the uncoupling of excitation-contraction. Furthermore, contractile activity of the heart is reduced, resulting in coronary and systemic vasodilatation. Negative inotropic effects are offset by vasodilatation and reflex sympathetic cardiac stimulation preventing adverse effects on left ventricular function. Since these drugs are also potent coronary vasodilators, they are particularly useful for reducing blood pressure in ischemic heart disease.

The most extensive experience has been reported with oral or sublingual nifedipine. Maximal reduction in BP has been observed within 15 to 30 minutes following 10 to 20 mg of sublingual nifedipine and within one hour after oral administration. The degree of BP decrease appears related to baseline BP. Hypoten-

sion has rarely been observed when nifedipine is administered alone, but appropriate caution is warranted in patients on concurrent therapy with other agents, particularly diuretics. Cerebral blood flow is maintained or increased after nifedipine intake, thus providing potential protection to the cerebral circulation in association with rapid BP reduction. Nifedipine has also been administered safely in patients with hypertensive crises complicated by left ventricular failure. Acute reductions in systemic and pulmonary arterial pressures are associated with improvement in CHF. Concomitant administration of other adrenergic inhibitors such as beta-blockers, clonidine, guanabenz, or methyldopa can effectively suppress the reflex tachycardia seen with nifedipine alone.

Intravenous verapamil has also been effective in hypertensive crises: 5 to 10 mg is followed by a maximal BP reduction within five minutes. A continuous infusion of 3 to 25 mg per hour can maintain hypotensive effects for longer periods. Unlike nifedipine, verapamil interferes with AV conduction, resulting in various degrees of heart block. The combination of verapamil with a beta-blocker is therefore relatively contraindicated. Experience with diltiazem in the treatment of severe hypertension is somewhat limited. A moderate response has been noted following IV diltiazem in incremental doses of 5 to 20 mg.

With all three agents, hypotensive effects may persist for one to several hours after initial dosing, allowing conversion to maintenance oral doses of these same agents or conversion to other drug combinations. An important advantage of calcium entry blockers is the potential preservation of left ventricular and cerebral function in treating hypertensive emergencies associated with left ventricular failure and coronary or cerebral insufficiency.

ANGIOTENSIN CONVERTING ENZYME (ACE) INHIBITORS

Captopril, the prototype of the ACE inhibitors, was approved initially to treat severe or refractory hypertension. This agent blocks the conversion of angiotensin I to angiotensin II and secondarily suppresses aldosterone secretion. Following oral administration, onset of action is seen within 15 to 30 minutes, and maximal effects are observed in 60 to 90 minutes. Although dosage titration increases the magnitude of the hypotensive response, the major effect observed is prolongation of the duration of response. Recommended dosage ranges from 75 to 450 mg daily, divided and administered every eight to 12 hours. A precipitous first-dose response may occur in patients with high angiotensin II levels. An initial test dose of 12.5 mg is useful to determine the initial response before proceeding with dose titration. The correlation between pretreatment plasma renin activity and response to captopril has been variable, and even patients with low plasma renin activity can exhibit a marked fall in BP.

Particular caution must be exercised in considering captopril for patients with accelerated or malignant hypertension in whom renal artery stenosis and angiotensin II–dependent hypertension exist. A marked first-dose response may be accompanied by acute renal failure in susceptible patients, particularly those with preexistent renal impairment, bilateral renal artery ste-

---

*Not approved by the F.D.A. for hypertension.

nosis, or renal artery stenosis in a solitary functioning kidney. Loss of renal autoregulation appears to play a role in renal failure. Rash and dysgeusia are common, but more serious adverse effects include heavy proteinuria with nephrotic syndrome, neutropenia, or agranulocytosis. The sulfhydryl group in the captopril molecule has been incriminated as a possible contributor to the agent's toxicity. Recent experience with small doses of captopril suggests that the toxicity is dose related. In treatment of mild to moderate hypertension, doses of 25 to 150 mg per day have been associated with few serious side effects.

Enalapril maleate, a nonsulfhydryl ACE inhibitor, has also proved effective and safe in all degrees of hypertension and in some cases of renovascular hypertension. A longer duration of activity suggests that once-a-day dosing may be appropriate. Extensive studies in mild to moderate hypertension have shown enalapril to be safe and effective, but more studies are required to clarify its role in the management of accelerated or malignant hypertension.

COMBINED ALPHA- AND BETA-BLOCKERS

Labetalol is a unique, new antihypertensive agent with both alpha- and beta-adrenergic receptor blocking properties. Systemic vascular resistance and BP are reduced within minutes following IV injection, while the heart rate is unchanged or slightly reduced. The alpha-blockade is selective for postsynaptic receptors, whereas the beta-blocking properties are noncardioselective. Labetalol undergoes extensive first-pass hepatic metabolism, and its plasma half-life is a relatively short 1.5 to 2 hours. Elimination kinetics are not altered in patients with renal failure and no dose adjustments are required. Peak effects are seen within two hours of oral administration, and despite rapid clearance a prolonged antihypertensive effect is observed and maintained with twice-daily dosing. Orthostatic hypotension is the most common side effect due to the drug's alpha-blocking properties, whereas side effects relating to beta-blocking properties are similar to those seen with beta-blocking agents. Labetalol may be combined with a diuretic and other agents in treating hypertension of all degrees of severity.

Table 1 outlines the current consensus on step-care

Table 1. PHARMACOLOGIC MANAGEMENT OF ACCELERATED AND MALIGNANT HYPERTENSION

Initial therapy:	Thiazide or loop diuretic*
(Step 1 and 2)	plus
	Adrenergic inhibitor†
Proceed to full doses as needed.	
Add vasodilator:	Hydralazine
(Step 3)	Prazosin‡
Additional drugs:§	Minoxidil
	Captopril
	Nifedipine
	Guanethidine

*If creatinine >3.0 mg/dl, substitute furosemide, 40–240 mg b.i.d., or bumetanide, 1–10 mg b.i.d.

†These include beta-adrenergic blockers, central adrenergic inhibitors, peripheral adrenergic antagonists, alpha₁ adrenergic blocker, combined alpha- and beta-adrenergic blocker.

‡If not utilized in Steps 1 and 2, prazosin may be added as a Step 3 agent.

§These agents may be substituted for other drugs (captopril, minoxidil, nifedipine) or added as Step 4 (guanethidine). Use guanethidine with caution, if at all, in patients with impaired renal function.

management of moderate to severe hypertension based on the report of the Joint National Committee. Patients with severe or resistant hypertension require two or often three drugs for adequate control. For BP not controlled with optimal doses of a diuretic plus an adrenergic inhibitor, small doses of a vasodilator may be added to the regimen. Hydralazine is an effective vasodilator when administered with an adrenergic inhibitor in the regimen to prevent headache, palpitations, or anginal chest pain. Minoxidil is more potent than hydralazine but causes hypertrichosis and significant fluid retention. If adequate BP control is not achieved with three drugs and if secondary hypertension as well as the causes of unresponsiveness have been excluded, the addition or substitution of guanethidine or another adrenergic inhibitor may be considered. Captopril has been used in place of second-line adrenergic inhibitors or may be added as a third- or fourth-line drug. Similarly, calcium channel blockers are being used increasingly as add-on drugs for patients with resistant hypertension. Recommended daily dosages of currently used agents are listed in Table 2, Chapter 5.

This program of step-care therapy controls BP in most patients but may not provide optimal control in others. For patients in whom high diastolic BP persists despite maximally tolerated doses of medication, several additional steps may be considered. Further restriction of dietary sodium intake to less than 2 gm daily may be tried and the addition or substitution of a loop diuretic may be considered. Further weight reduction efforts in obese patients may be particularly helpful at this point and an additional second-line drug may be substituted or added to the regimen. There is little pharmacologic advantage in combining two agents of the same class, e.g., two beta-blockers or two central alpha-agonists. In selected cases, increasing the dose of a second-line agent beyond recommended levels may be effective and may require toleration of more adverse effects to achieve and maintain a goal BP. Such increases are not recommended in the case of reserpine.

MANAGEMENT OF ACCELERATED AND MALIGNANT HYPERTENSION

Accelerated and malignant hypertension are indistinguishable in course and prognosis, and are considered together here. In most cases, the constellation of symptoms and progressive target organ dysfunction warrant hospital admission for initial management, including diagnostic studies and aggressive drug therapy to ensure adequate control of BP. Sudden deterioration in target organ function may precipitate a hypertensive urgency or emergency requiring immediate BP reduction with parenteral drug administration. The decision to manage on an outpatient basis demands that the clinician have suitable knowledge of the patient's history, including associated diseases and secondary causes, if likely, and meticulous follow-up and supervision is necessary until BP is adequately controlled.

Accelerated or malignant hypertension is more commonly seen in patients not receiving therapy, or in those treated inadequately or intermittently for established hypertension. On occasion, a patient may present with malignant hypertension who has no awareness of previous high BP. Progression to a malignant phase in a known medically compliant hypertensive patient strongly suggests a secondary cause, such as renovascular hypertension.

For accelerated or malignant hypertension uncomplicated by renal failure, left ventricular failure, or encephalopathic symptoms, there is no need for parenteral administration of drugs such as diazoxide, nitroprusside, labetalol, or trimethaphan. Therapy, however, requires optimal doses of at least two, and often three, effective agents. A regimen consisting of an oral diuretic plus a beta-blocker or another adrenergic inhibitor may be complemented by the addition of a vasodilating agent, such as hydralazine (Table 1). The presence of significant renal insufficiency (serum creatinine >3.0 mg/dl) necessitates substitution of a loop diuretic such as furosemide or bumetanide, and the potent vasodilator minoxidil may be substituted for hydralazine in refractory cases. The ACE inhibitor captopril has proved a suitable substitute for second- or third-line agents in selected cases, and response to this agent does not appear dependent on plasma renin activity. The calcium channel blocking agents, while not yet approved in the United States for the treatment of hypertension, have also been tried mainly as third-line agents. Nifedipine has proved efficacious for oral or sublingual administration in initial therapy for severe hypertension and in hypertensive urgencies or emergencies. A new alpha- and beta-blocker, labetalol, available in both parenteral and oral forms, has also proved useful for initial and long-term treatment of accelerated or malignant hypertension.

In light of current knowledge of disordered autoregulation of cerebral blood flow in hypertension, it seems more appropriate to achieve gradual control of BP during the first week of therapy. Blood pressure should be reduced to about 160/110 mm Hg during the first 48 to 72 hours, with gradual titration of drugs to achieve a goal diastolic BP below 90 mm Hg over the succeeding three to five days. Close attention should be paid to renal function during the first seven to ten days of treatment. If this is impaired at the initiation of therapy, early worsening of renal function is commonly noted, but stabilization followed by improvement can be expected to occur in most individuals with sustained, optimal control of BP.

With some agents, effects may be enhanced by alternative dosing methods. Clonidine, a central alpha-agonist, acts by stimulating central alpha-receptors to decrease sympathetic outflow and lower BP. Rapid absorption occurs with oral administration, the peak effect occurring in two to four hours. Clonidine loading is obtained by administering 0.1 to 0.2 mg hourly for several hours. The most common side effects are drowsiness and dry mouth. A newer alpha-agonist, guanabenz, has very similar pharmacokinetic properties and should provide similar results. Ten to 20 mg of nifedipine orally or sublingually brings about a rapid reduction in BP (within 15 minutes when sublingual nifedipine is used, and after a slightly longer time following oral administration). Blood pressure is lowered as a result of peripheral vasodilatation, while the cardiac index and heart rate are increased. Nifedipine may offer the added advantage of selectively increasing cerebral and coronary blood flow in patients with associated ischemia of the cerebral or coronary vasculature. Concomitant administration of a diuretic and a beta-blocker will minimize fluid retention, suppress reflex tachycardia, and enhance the antihypertensive effects of nifedipine. Since plasma renin activity is elevated in most patients with malignant hypertension, the ACE inhibitor captopril has been suggested as a particularly appropriate therapeutic agent: 25 to 50 mg may reduce BP to normal within 60 to 90 minutes. The onset of effect will be seen within 15 minutes and may be enhanced by concomitant administration of oral furosemide. Further clinical trials of labetalol appear warranted in the initial management of accelerated or malignant hypertension. Unlike traditional beta-adrenergic blockers, a hypotensive response to the combined alpha- and beta-blocking effects of labetalol is seen within two hours and is maximal at three hours. The fall in BP appears dose related and may persist for eight hours or longer. Although extensive data are available on the efficacy of labetalol for mild to moderate hypertension, more information is needed to assess its role in initial oral therapy of accelerated or malignant hypertension. Each of these agents offers the potential of providing initial control of severe to malignant hypertension with variable loading regimens, and allows sustained control with subsequent b.i.d. or t.i.d. dosing. Concomitant

Table 2. AGENTS FOR TREATMENT OF HYPERTENSIVE EMERGENCIES*

	IM	Intermittent IV	Continuous[+]
Direct Vasodilating Drugs			
Sodium nitroprusside			0.5–10 µg/kg/ml
Nitroglycerin			5–100 µg/min
Diazoxide		50–100 mg bolus inj. (within 30 sec) every 15 min	15–30 mg/min
Hydralazine	5–10 mg	5–10 mg bolus inj.	200 mg/L
Verapamil		5–10 mg/20 ml	5–25 mg/hr
Nifedipine	10–20 mg PO or sublingual		
Sympathetic Inhibition Drugs			
Labetalol		20–80 mg by intermittent inj. every 10–15 min	0.5–2.0 mg/min
Trimethaphan			1000 mg/L
Phentolamine	5–10 mg	5–10 mg bolus inj.	200 mg/L
Reserpine	1–5 mg	1–5 mg from syringe over 3–5 min	
Methyldopa		250–500 mg in 100 ml over 30–60 min	

*Concomitant administration of a rapidly acting diuretic (furosemide or bumetanide) IV is desirable in most cases. May repeat at appropriate intervals.

[+]Infusion rate will be titrated under continuous supervision until desired effect obtained.

therapy with a suitable diuretic is needed to avoid early resistance or "pseudotolerance," and other agents may be added to the regimen when appropriate.

MANAGEMENT OF HYPERTENSIVE EMERGENCIES

When hypertension poses an immediate threat to the integrity of the cardiovascular system, immediate parenteral administration of an appropriate agent should be initiated. The rate and degree of BP reduction will be determined by the agent selected and the mode of administration. In most cases, initial reduction of diastolic BP to the range of 100 to 110 mm Hg is sufficient to reduce the immediate risk of an acute event. Care must be taken with initial therapy to avoid compromising the cerebral or coronary circulation.

Table 2 lists agents currently available for parenteral use, with dosage and recommended means of administration. Although nitroprusside remains the gold standard among parenteral agents, this drug is safely administered only in the intensive care unit where continuous supervision of the infusion can be maintained. Agents such as labetalol and diazoxide are more cost effective. Intermittent pulse administration, a maximal observed effect from each pulse within five minutes, obviates the need for continuous monitoring and allows many patients to be managed with close supervision on a medical/surgical floor. This can add significantly to the cost effectiveness of caring for patients with a hypertensive emergency.

Conditions that often require management as a hypertensive emergency are listed in Table 3. Appropriate caution cannot be overemphasized in the selection of an appropriate parenteral agent in these conditions, and necessitates an understanding of the clinical pharmacology and adverse effects of available drugs. Labetalol must be used with caution or avoided in any hypertensive emergency complicated by left ventricular failure, since the beta-adrenergic effects of this agent may further impair cardiac function. Direct vasodilators such as diazoxide or hydralazine should be avoided in hypertensive emergencies in association with acute in-

Table 3. HYPERTENSIVE EMERGENCIES

Cerebrovascular Emergencies:
Hypertensive encephalopathy
Hypertensive intracerebral hemorrhage
Subarachnoid hemorrhage
Acute atherothrombotic brain infarction with severe hypertension
Malignant hypertension (some cases)

Cardiac Emergencies:
Acute congestive heart failure
Acute coronary insufficiency
Postcoronary artery bypass hypertension
Acute aortic dissection

Other Conditions:
Pheochromocytoma
Rebound hypertension following sudden withdrawal of antihypertensive agents (clonidine, guanabenz in some cases)
Food or drug interactions with monoamine oxidase inhibitors
Severe preeclampsia and eclampsia
Acute glomerulonephritis
Postoperative hypertension (particularly vascular procedures)
Head injury
Severe body burns

tracerebral events, coronary insufficiency, or dissecting aneurysm, conditions in which a precipitous reduction in BP or associated reflex tachycardia may pose a hazard. The ganglion blocker trimethaphan should be avoided in management of eclampsia of pregnancy (particularly before delivery) and in acute postoperative hypertension, in view of associated parasympatholytic side effects. Somnolence, often obfuscating neurologic evaluation, limits the use of reserpine or methyldopa ester in cerebrovascular emergencies, including hypertensive encephalopathy.

REFERENCES

Cressman MD, Vidt DG, Gifford RW Jr, et al: Intravenous labetalol in the management of severe hypertension and hypertensive emergencies. Am Heart J 107:980–985, 1984.
Frishman WH, Weinberg P, Peled HB, et al: Calcium entry blockers for the treatment of severe hypertension and hypertensive crisis. Am J Med 77:35–44, 1984.
Gifford RW Jr: Management and treatment of essential hypertension, including malignant hypertension and emergencies. *In* Genest J, Kuchel O, Hamet P, et al (eds): Hypertension. McGraw-Hill Book Co., New York, 1983, pp. 1127–1170.
Gifford RW Jr, Tarazi RC: Resistant hypertension: diagnosis and management. Ann Intern Med 88:661–665, 1978.
Vidt DG: Accelerated hypertension, malignant hypertension and hypertensive emergencies. *In* Glassock RJ (ed): Current Therapy in Nephrology and Hypertension 1984–1985. C.V. Mosby Co., St. Louis, 1984, pp. 324–333.
Vidt DG, Gifford RW Jr: A compendium for the treatment of hypertensive emergencies. Cleve Clin Q 51:421–430, 1984.

7 · HYPERTENSION IN THE DIABETIC PATIENT

A. Richard Christlieb
JOSLIN CLINIC

DEFINITION AND DIAGNOSTIC CRITERIA

The generally accepted definition of hypertension as blood pressure of 140/90 mm Hg or greater may be too liberal for the patient with diabetes mellitus. Cardiovascular risk and renal deterioration are compounded when elevated BP complicates the diabetes, and "acceptable BP" should be lower, preferably near 120/80 mm Hg, especially in younger patients.

PATHOPHYSIOLOGY AND CLINICAL ASPECTS

Diabetics are prone to the various types of hypertension encountered in the general population plus some forms peculiar to the diabetic state:

1. Hypertension secondary to diabetic nephropathy occurs in insulin-dependent diabetes (IDDM) with juvenile onset, and in many patients with a later onset of diabetes. It is characterized by hypervolemia, hyporeninemia, increased peripheral vascular resistance, and increased cardiac output. Hyporeninemic hypoaldosteronism with hyperkalemia is present in many of these patients.

2. Fluid retention causing hypertension can occur

in diabetics without nephropathy. Here, hyperglycemia causing an increased extracellular fluid osmolality can increase blood volume. Recent data suggest that hyperinsulinemia in obese patients with early non–insulin-dependent diabetes (NIDDM) may cause sodium retention and increased sympathetic activity, resulting in hypertension.

3. Systolic hypertension is most frequently seen in older diabetics and results from a combination of mechanisms, including increased peripheral vascular resistance, increased cardiac output, and decreased compliance in major arteries.

4. Supine hypertension with orthostatic hypotension is most common in patients with autonomic neuropathy who may also have nephropathy and hyporeninemic hypoaldosteronism.

MANAGEMENT

PLAN

Blood pressure should be recorded both supine and standing, the goal of treatment in most patients being a standing BP of 120–130/70–80 mm Hg. In patients with renal failure or systolic hypertension, such a reduction may not be tolerated and higher BP will be acceptable. Home BP monitoring is advisable for many patients. Hospitalization should be considered whenever the hypertension becomes accelerated or cannot be adequately controlled in the presence of renal failure.

NONPHARMACOLOGIC MEASURES

Achievement of ideal body weight, sodium restriction, and individualized physical activity are always indicated. These measures alone may achieve the desired goal in those with mild hypertension.

DRUG THERAPY

Drug selection should be individualized for the various types of hypertension (Table 1). Treatment for each type can be initiated with a long-acting thiazide

Table 1. ANTIHYPERTENSIVE DRUGS FREQUENTLY PRESCRIBED IN DIABETICS AT THE JOSLIN CLINIC

| Drugs* | Dose | |
	Initial (mg)	Maximum (mg)
Diuretics		
Thiazide		
Loop	*	*
Potassium-sparing		
Vasodilators		
Hydralazine (Apresoline)	10–25 q.i.d.	75 q.i.d.
Minoxidil (Loniten)	5 q.d.	40 q.d.
Beta-adrenergic blockers		
Metoprolol (Lopressor)†	50 q.d. or b.i.d.	100 q.i.d.
Atenolol (Tenormin)†	50 q.d.	100 q.d.
Propranolol (Inderal)	40 b.i.d.	120 q.i.d.
Alpha-adrenergic blockers		
Prazosin (Minipress)	1 b.i.d.	5 q.i.d.
Sympathetic inhibitors		
Methylodopa (Aldomet)	250 b.i.d.	500 q.i.d.
Clonidine (Catapres)	0.1 b.i.d.	0.6 q.i.d.
Reserpine	0.1 q.d.	0.25 q.d.
Converting enzyme inhibitor		
Captopril (Capoten)	25 t.i.d.	150 q.i.d.

*See PDR or appropriate texts for complete information.
†Cardioselective.

Table 2. SOME POTENTIAL COMPLICATIONS OF ANTIHYPERTENSIVE DRUGS TO MONITOR IN PATIENTS WITH DIABETES MELLITUS

Drug	Possible Complications
Diuretics	
Potassium-losing	Decreased glucose tolerance in non–insulin-dependent diabetics, hypercholesterolemia, impotence
Potassium-sparing	Hyperkalemia, impotence
Vasodilators	Precipitate or aggravate symptomatic coronary heart disease
Beta-adrenergic blockers	Impaired insulin release with hyperglycemia, delayed recovery from hypoglycemia, blunted symptoms of hypoglycemia (palpitations, tremor, anxiety), cardiac failure, hypertension during hypoglycemia
Alpha-adrenergic blockers	Orthostatic hypotension
Sympathetic inhibitors	Orthostatic hypotension, impotence
Converting enzyme inhibitors	Proteinuria, renal failure, hyperkalemia

diuretic. In patients *with nephropathy* in which serum creatinine levels approach 3.0 mg/dl, a loop diuretic should be used in divided doses. Metolazone, which acts synergistically with loop diuretics, can be added. Hypovolemia is avoided by maintaining a trace of peripheral edema. A vasodilator (hydralazine, or if needed, minoxidil, which is more potent) or an alpha-adrenergic blocker (prazosin) can be added. The associated autonomic neuropathy generally prevents the tachycardia induced by vasodilatation. Beta-adrenergic blockers (e.g., metoprolol), which have a relatively short half life and are metabolized in part by the liver, or sympathetic agents can be added as third-line drugs. In patients *without nephropathy*, a beta-adrenergic blocker, prazosin, a sympatholytic agent, or captopril can be added to the diuretic, followed by the addition of a vasodilator if necessary. Patients with *systolic hypertension* generally do best with drugs decreasing cardiac output, such as beta-blockers or methyldopa, added to the diuretic. *Supine hypertension with orthostatic hypotension* presents a most difficult therapeutic challenge. To decrease supine BP, hydralazine (25 to 75 mg), which has a relatively short duration of action, is prescribed before retiring, and 9-alpha-fludrocortisone in the morning. This drug replaces mineralocorticoids and, contrary to common belief, is not contraindicated in this form of hypertension. Ephedrine can be added in divided doses. If edema is present, a diuretic may be needed. Raising the head of the bed 10 inches allows gravity to decrease the supine BP, and use of effective elastic hose counteracts gravity to increase BP when upright.

The potential for adverse effects of antihypertensive drugs in the diabetic is enormous (Table 2). Diuretics that waste potassium (e.g., thiazides and loop diuretics) can decrease glucose tolerance in NIDDM because of the decreased insulin release associated with hypokalemia. Adequate potassium replacement or the use of potassium-sparing diuretics can reverse this effect. Control of diabetes in patients dependent on exogenous insulin should not be affected. An increased cholesterol, which is of questionable significance, can also occur with these drugs. Potassium-sparing diuretics (spironolactone, triamterene, amiloride) should not be used in patients with nephropathy or hyporeninemic hypoaldosteronism (which is common in diabetic patients), because lethal hyperkalemia may ensue. Orthostatic hypotension and impotence in males, so commonly present in diabetics, can be precipitated or aggravated, especially by the sympathetic inhibiting drugs, but also by other classes of drugs (Type II). Increased cardiac work associated with vasodilator therapy can aggravate symptomatic coronary heart disease. The effect is minimized when diuretic and beta-adrenergic blocking drugs are prescribed concomitantly. The potential complications of beta-blockers occur most frequently with the nonselective variety but can also occur with cardioselective beta-blockers, especially with increasing dosages wherein cardioselectivity can be lost. Delayed recovery from hypoglycemia, aggravation of peripheral vascular disease, severe hypertension during hypoglycemia, and blunting of the symptoms of hypoglycemia may occur. There are many symptoms of hypoglycemia, but only palpitations, anxiety, and tremor are minimized with beta-blockade. Sweating is enhanced by these drugs. Converting enzyme inhibitors can cause proteinuria, accelerate renal failure, and (because they block angiotensin II formation) decrease the stimulation of aldosterone release, causing hyperkalemia.

Should complications of an antihypertensive drug occur in the diabetic patient, a drug in another class that does not produce this complication can be substituted. For instance, a patient who develops orthostatic hypotension or a man who becomes impotent while on methyldopa may reverse these symptoms and have well-controlled BP after substituting hydralazine, prazosin, or metoprolol. There are no contraindications to the use of antihypertensive drugs concomitantly with insulin or with first- or second-generation oral glucose–lowering agents.

PATIENT INFORMATION AND EDUCATION

Diabetic patients with hypertension must be educated regarding the possible complications of both conditions, the need for treatment in avoiding such complications, their own role in the treatment program, and the complications of treatment itself. Instructions should be given for a diabetic meal plan using appropriate sodium and lipid restriction. A program for monitoring BP and glucose and for adjusting insulin- or oral glucose–lowering agents should be designed to make these activities a part of everyday living. Patients should be advised of potential serious complications of antihypertensive drugs, especially orthostatic hypotension and those associated with beta-blockade. Although the latter do occur, they have rarely been a problem in our experience. We use beta-blockers freely, always discussing the potential side effects before beginning treatment.

PERIODIC EVALUATION

Diabetic patients routinely are seen often, at least every six months. Once the desired BP level is achieved, the hypertension can be followed adequately during these routine visits. During the initial phases of therapy, more frequent visits, e.g., every three to 12 weeks, may be necessary. During these visits, it is important to question the patient regarding side effects of therapy such as lightheadedness, impotence, or the loss of hypoglycemia symptoms, and then alter the antihypertensive program as necessary. In addition to determinations of blood glucose, glucosuria, and glycosylated hemoglobin, patients with hypertension should have periodic checks for serum potassium, renal function, and proteinuria.

PATIENT COMPLIANCE

Compliance of patients is best achieved through education and their active participation in the treatment program. Many patients master not only insulin adjustment, using home glucose monitoring, but also antihypertensive drug adjustment, using home BP monitoring. The personal interest of physicians in their patients goes a long way toward achieving such goals. Physicians should take the initiative in ferreting out problems. As an example, BP in a patient with nephropathy and blindness was poorly controlled on what appeared to be an adequate drug regimen. After repeated visits and discussion with the patient, he finally related that his wife, who dispensed his medications daily, was distressed by his impotence and, hearing that this was caused by antihypertensive medications, refused to give him these. A change of medications and appropiate education of the wife remedied this situation, and BP control was achieved.

PREVENTIVE MEASURES

Education is an integral part of therapy for the diabetic patient. From the onset of diabetes, the patient should be counseled regarding the various risk factors leading to hypertension and other complications. Control of diabetes, appropriate exercise, achievement of ideal body weight, avoidance of excess salt intake, and cessation of smoking are all recommended. Unfortunately, human nature being what it is, they cannot be achieved universally.

SOCIOECONOMIC AND PSYCHOLOGICAL ASPECTS

Just having diabetes places an emotional and economic burden on patients and their families. This is especially noticeable in younger patients. Adding hypertension to the diabetes compounds these burdens. In addition to family support, it is often of great benefit for patients with similar problems to meet in peer groups to share their problems and experiences under the supervision of qualified medical personnel. A better understanding of one's own problems and the knowledge that one is not alone generally cultivate improved compliance with treatment programs, and improved longevity.

REFERENCES

Christlieb AR: The hypertensions of diabetes. Diabetes Care 5:50–58, 1982.
Drury PL: Diabetes and arterial hypertension. Diabetologia 24:1–9, 1983.

8 · MEDICAL MANAGEMENT OF SECONDARY HYPERTENSION

Richard Re
OCHSNER CLINIC AND ALTON OCHSNER MEDICAL FOUNDATION

Medical treatment of the secondary forms of hypertension should be considered in certain well-defined circumstances. *First,* medical therapy can be undertaken as a temporizing measure permitting the physician to assess the patient without fear of hypertensive crisis. *Second,* it is appropriate when a definitive surgical cure is impossible because of either the nature of the lesion or the patient's overall medical condition. *Finally,* there are those few forms of secondary hypertension that are optimally treated medically. The challenge to the physician is to determine for each individual the best strategy for providing control of hypertension with the least overall risk. How medical versus definitive surgical therapy enters into the equation is determined in the final analysis by the physician's judgment.

The more common secondary forms of hypertension (excluding oral contraceptive–induced hypertension, which is optimally treated by withdrawal of these agents) are renal artery stenosis secondary to either fibrodysplastic disease or atherosclerotic disease, the different forms of hyperaldosteronism, and pheochromocytoma. Each presents unique challenges and opportunities, and the therapy for each is continuously evolving. In addition, strategies based on outcome probabilities from today's treatment figures may be inapplicable tomorrow with the advent of improved technology for definitive cure. Thus, the decision to use medical therapy must be constantly reevaluated for each form of hypertension.

RENOVASCULAR HYPERTENSION

Renovascular hypertension is the most common form of secondary hypertension in man. It can occur as fibrodysplastic disease and present as medial fibromuscular dysplasia, intimal fibroplasia, or adventitial and periarterial fibroplasia. The most common of these, medial fibrodysplasia, produces the well-known beads-on-a-string pattern on arteriography, and although it can lead to significant renovascular hypertension, it generally is not a progressive disease. When hypertension ensues or when renal failure is (rarely) threatened in any of these disease categories, surgical correction can be undertaken. More recently, renal artery angioplasty has been found to be a safe, effective therapy for these disorders with reported long-term remissions. In the patient with atherosclerotic renal artery stenosis angioplasty can be effective, but the lesions often recur relatively quickly, requiring either repeat angioplasty or definitive surgery. Additionally, because in the older patient with atherosclerotic disease there is a predilection for coexisting carotid or coronary artery disease, the risk involved with either angioplasty or definitive surgery is considerably greater than that confronted by the patient with fibromuscular disease. Thus, for the most part, the medical treatment of renovascular hypertension is a problem to be confronted in the elderly patient with atheromatous disease.

PATHOPHYSIOLOGY

The pathophysiology of renovascular hypertension in man can be considered roughly akin to the one-kidney, one-clip Goldblatt animal model. That is to say, in the early stages of the disease plasma renin activity probably rises, causing elevation in pressure and a hypersecretion of aldosterone. This in turn causes fluid retention, with intravascular volume expansion and renin suppression. Thus, when the patient presents in the chronic phase, the renin, although not low, need not be abnormally high, and he in fact presents in a state of mixed vasoconstriction and hypervolemia. Therefore, the medical treatment of this disorder is designed to lower renin secretion to the extent possible and to treat any residual hypertension with volume-reducing agents. This strategy can serve to control blood pressure in many patients, but it in no way influences the long-term progression of the disease and does nothing to preserve renal function other than the preservation of the contralateral kidney that might be derived from the BP-lowering effects. The vascular lesion per se is unaffected by such medical treatment and may go on to complete occlusion. Follow-up of these patients under medical treatment requires detailed evaluation of both BP and renal function.

SPECIFIC DRUG THERAPY

Plasma renin activities can be lowered by a large number of drugs, particularly the beta-blockers and the alpha$_2$ agonist clonidine. In our experience, clonidine is probably the most potent renin suppressor currently available. Of course, the converting enzyme inhibitors are more effective in interrupting the renin system, not by suppressing renin but by uncoupling it from the angiotensin II–producing cascade. Thus, even though renin levels remain high and angiotensin I levels actually rise in the face of converting enzyme inhibition, plasma angiotensin II levels fall and pressure tends to decrease. In view of this, it would appear reasonable to begin treating renovascular hypertension with a converting enzyme inhibitor such as captopril or enalapril. The addition of a diuretic or clonidine to those patients who are refractory often provides the added margin needed for BP control. Should this fail, additional drugs such as minoxidil can be used, but these are rarely required.

There is, however, one caveat to be applied to this strategy. It has been well established that captopril, and probably other converting enzyme inhibitors, can result in a marked rise in creatinine (i.e., a marked decline in renal function) in patients with bilateral renal artery stenosis or patients with one kidney and renal artery stenosis. This phenomenon probably occurs because during states of decreased blood flow to the kidney, local generation of angiotensin II causes increased efferent renal arteriolar tone and therefore permits the maintenance of glomerular filtration pressure. Once converting enzyme inhibition is applied, angiotensin II levels fall and glomerular filtration fraction declines, leading to a worsening of renal function. Therefore, the drug must be used with caution in patients with renal vascular hypertension if unacceptable rises in creatinine are not to be produced. Also, because many patients with renovascular hypertension have prodigiously elevated renin levels and because captopril, for example, acutely lowers angiotensin II levels, there is a risk of dramatic falls in BP. In these high-risk patients, captopril should be given in a ¼ tablet test dose (6.25 mg PO), and they should be observed for approximately two hours. If precipitous falls in pressure are noticed, the patient should lie down and, if pressure is not immediately restored, IV saline should be administered. Rarely is anything more, such as pressor administration, required. Many of the newer converting enzyme inhibitors may have a more gradual onset of action and thus may be potentially easier to use. Finally, because captopril can produce renal damage in high-risk patients, careful follow-up testing of urine for protein and of renal function by creatinine clearance is recommended. Because changes in white cell count have also been noted, this parameter should also be followed. Patients suffering from collagen vascular disease are extremely susceptible to the severe side effects of captopril therapy.

Thanks to the modern pharmaceutical armamentarium, the BP of almost any patient with renovascular hypertension can be acceptably controlled by currently available medications. This greatly enhances the physician's range of opportunities for dealing effectively with these patients.

HYPERALDOSTERONISM

Although hyperaldosteronism is a less common cause of secondary hypertension than is renovascular stenosis, it is nonetheless a disorder the physician is often compelled to treat medically. Of the three common forms (adenomatous hyperaldosteronism, hyperaldosteronism associated with bilateral idiopathic adrenal hyperplasia, and glucocorticoid-remediable hyperaldosteronism), all but adenomatous hyperaldosteronism must currently be treated medically. In general, medical treatment of all three forms is similar. Although glucocorticoid-remediable aldosteronism can in theory be treated with low doses of glucocorticoids (i.e., dexamethasone), this treatment is often associated with some tendency toward Cushing's syndrome, as is the case in congenital hyperplasia. Therefore, many of these patients are treated somewhat unphysiologically, but effectively, with aldosterone-blocking agents and diuretics. However, if a case of glucocorticoid-sensitive hyperaldosteronism is discovered, we recommend that a trial of low-dose dexamethasone (0.75 to 1.0 mg per day) be given to assess the efficacy of this treatment. Occasionally, glucocorticoid supplementation at night can help reduce side effects, and other strategies can be undertaken in this regard just as in congenital adrenal hyperplasia. Thus, a patient with a familial history of hyperaldosteronism and bilateral adrenal hyperplasia can benefit from a trial of dexamethasone to see if he falls into this category (glucocorticoid-remediable hypertension is often familial.) If he does, trial-and-error manipulations of glucocorticoid replacement should be undertaken to see if the patient can be effectively treated. One risk is that dexamethasone can raise BP in any patient with hyperaldosteronism, so that patients must be followed carefully during this trial period.

Spironolactone. The twin aims of medical treatment of hyperaldosteronism are to lower BP and raise potassium levels. This can be accomplished by either aldosterone antagonists, such as spironolactone, or antagonists of non–aldosterone-sensitive sodium-potassium exchange in the distal tubule, such as amiloride or triamterene. Because high doses of spironolactone are often associated with breast tenderness, it is sometimes impossible to use this agent conveniently at full therapeutic doses. Diuretics, of course, can be used in conjunction with spironolactone to offset sodium retention and help lower BP. Thus, the combination of a thiazide diuretic and spironolactone, or a thiazide diuretic and a triamterene or amiloride, can be quite effective in these patients.

Additionally, routine antihypertensive medications such as alpha-adrenergic blocking agents can be added to control BP in resistant patients with idiopathic hyperplasia. Most patients with adenomatous hyperaldosteronism undergo surgery and are not really candidates for long-term medical therapy because in this group the surgical cure of both BP and potassium abnormalities is often achieved. In patients with bilateral adrenal hyperplasia, surgical cure is uncommon; therefore medical therapy is the therapeutic mode of choice.

Calcium Channel Blockers. A relatively new form of therapy for these patients consists of calcium channel blockers. These tend to lower pressure in low renin states, and we have used them successfully to treat hyperaldosteronism. Some reports have also suggested that converting enzyme inhibitors can be useful for idiopathic hyperaldosteronism (as contrasted with adenomatous hyperaldosteronism). At first this may seem paradoxical, but one must remember that the renin-angiotensin system exists not only in the blood, but also in the arterial wall and the adrenal gland. It may be that although idiopathic hyperaldosteronism is associated with low plasma renin activity, there is adequate renin activity in the walls of vessels and in the adrenal gland for these converting enzyme inhibitors to be useful. In any event, calcium channel blockers and even converting enzyme inhibitors can be of use in selected patients with hyperaldosteronism.

PHEOCHROMOCYTOMA

The greatest challenge to the physician undertaking medical treatment of secondary forms of hypertension is presented by the patient with pheochromocytoma. Virtually all these patients require therapy prior to definitive diagnostic testing, such as angiography, and prior to surgery. Failure to treat a patient adequately before operative removal of a pheochromocytoma can lead to disaster. There are also patients with either inoperable pheochromocytomas or malignant pheochromocytomas in whom medical therapy must be undertaken.

Phenoxybenzamine. A patient can generally be prepared for surgery or invasive diagnostic testing with phenoxybenzamine, 10 mg PO every 12 hours, the dose being gradually increased at one- to two-day intervals until nasal stuffiness and some postural hypotension are noted. This recommendation must be tempered by the condition of the patient. Extremely ill patients might best be served by IV phentolamine or IV nitroprusside until oral blockade can be undertaken.

Beta-Blockers. It is our policy not to begin beta-blockers in these patients unless cardiac arrhythmias intervene and require beta-blocker treatment. It is an old nostrum that using beta-blockers in the absence of full alpha-blockade can be dangerous, since pressures can rise by virtue of the blockade of vasodilatory beta-receptors in the muscle beds. Therefore, beta-blockers such as propranolol are used sparingly, if at all, and only after alpha-blockade has been established.

Alpha-Methyltyrosine. This agent, an inhibitor of catecholamine biosynthesis, can be similarly used to prepare patients for surgery or diagnostic testing. We usually prefer the tried and true phenoxybenzamine. It is true that alpha-methyltyrosine inhibits the activity of tyrosine hydroxylase, the enzyme that catalyzes the rate-limiting step in the biosynthesis of catecholamines, and therefore gradually lowers plasma epinephrine and norepinephrine levels. However, this drug is associated with crystalluria, so that patients on this medication must maintain urine volumes of about 2 L per day. Also, the dosage should be kept under 3 gm per day in order to reduce the risk of crystalluria. It can be started at 250 mg twice daily and gradually increased up to 2 or 2.5 gm. Its use is associated with transient drowsiness and with extrapyramidal side effects such as drooling and tremor, as well as anxiety. Phenothiazines should probably be avoided in patients on this medication, since they can potentially exacerbate extrapyramidal signs.

In general, patients should be alpha-blocked for about one week before any surgical procedure. This gives blood volume a chance to reaccumulate, and a declining hematocrit is a good sign that this is taking place. Acute crisis can be managed with phentolamine or nitroprusside, and we have successfully controlled intraoperative BP with nitroprusside, its rapidity of onset and offset being very helpful.

Prazosin. Prazosin, a selective alpha$_2$-receptor blocker, has been used in isolated cases of pheochromocytoma. However, this drug alone is unlikely to provide adequate blockade in these patients, although it may serve an ancillary role. For the most part, we have not used it for pheochromocytoma.

In conclusion, there are multiple forms of secondary hypertension that require medical treatment by virtue of the nature of the disease or the status of the patient's overall health. Fortunately, we now have an armamentarium adequate to deal with virtually all these situations. Although no absolute rules can be applied to the medical treatment of secondary forms of hypertension, good judgment and consideration of the medical status, coupled with a knowledge of the wide variety of drugs now available, make successful management possible in most cases.

REFERENCES

Atuk NO: Pheochromocytoma: diagnosis, localization, and treatment. Hosp Pract 18:187–202, 1983.
Bravo EL, Tarazi RC, Dustan HP, et al: The changing clinical spectrum of primary aldosteronism. Am J Med 74:641–651, 1983.
Edwards CRW, Padfield PL: Angiotensin-converting enzyme inhibitors: past, present, and bright future. Lancet 1:30–34, 1985.
Modlinger RS, Ertel NH, Hauptman JB: Adrenergic blockade in pheochromocytoma. Arch Intern Med 143:2245–2246, 1983.
Treadway KK, Slater EE: Renovascular hypertension. Annu Rev Med 35:665–692, 1984.
Weinberger MH: Primary aldosteronism. In Genest J, Kuchel O, Hamet O, et al (eds): Hypertension: Pathophysiology and Treatment, 2nd ed. McGraw-Hill Book Co., New York, 1983, pp 922–947.

9 · ARTERIOSCLEROTIC OCCLUSIVE DISEASE OF THE AORTA AND PERIPHERAL ARTERIES OF THE LOWER EXTREMITIES

Edward R. Jewell,
Donald J. Breslin
LAHEY CLINIC MEDICAL CENTER

Arteriosclerotic occlusive disease of the aorta and peripheral arteries of the lower extremities is a common clinical problem. At first, patients are asymptomatic, but as disease progresses they present with claudication and eventually with limb-threatening ischemia. The presentation depends on the severity of disease and to a lesser extent on activity level. Recommended treatment is directly related to clinical status.

MANAGEMENT OF ASYMPTOMATIC PATIENTS

Some elderly patients with peripheral vascular disease are asymptomatic because a sedentary life style prevents development of symptoms. When subtle clinical findings in these patients are ignored, a limb-threatening situation may develop that might have been avoided had the proper measures been taken. In asymptomatic patients, risk factors should be identified and reduced if possible. The importance of excellent foot care should be stressed, and follow-up evaluation should be carried out at appropriate intervals.

Tobacco Abuse. This is one of the most important risk factors associated with the progression of arteriosclerosis. Despite intensive efforts, few of these patients are able to refrain from cigarette smoking for any prolonged period. Methods that can help patients stop smoking include hypnosis, acupuncture, and behavior modification therapy. In addition, nicotine polacrilex (Nicorettes) may be used as adjunct therapy with a behavior modification program. The usefulness of nicotine gum alone is unproved. When patients have the urge to smoke, a piece of gum is chewed slowly. They are instructed to wean themselves gradually from nicotine gum, and length of treatment should not exceed six months. Even the most successful of these therapies has only about a 20% long-term success rate. Although it is difficult to motivate a patient to stop smoking, the effort is worthwhile.

Other Reversible Risk Factors. Factors that play a role in the progression of arteriosclerosis include diabetes, hyperlipoproteinemia, and hypertension. An effort should be made to control these problems in the hope of retarding the progression of peripheral vascular disease.

Foot Care. Asymptomatic patients should be taught the importance of good foot care. A minor trauma can lead to a foot lesion that may eventually become limb-threatening and necessitate surgical intervention. Patients with peripheral vascular disease, especially those who have diabetes and may be neuropathic, should avoid placing their feet in hot water. Hot water burns not uncommonly precipitate a limb-threatening condition. Patients with peripheral vascular disease should make sure new shoes fit properly and wear them only for short periods until broken in. Walking barefoot should be avoided because stepping on a sharp object may result in trauma and infection. Care should be taken when cutting toenails because even a slight injury may cause toe ulcer and limb-threatening infection.

Asymptomatic patients should be evaluated at intervals of three to 12 months depending on the severity of ischemia. At follow-up visits the lower extremities are reexamined, and patients are reminded to contact their physician in case of ischemic rest pain, nonhealing ulcer, or other symptoms of limb-threatening ischemia.

CLAUDICATION

In active patients with peripheral vascular disease the presenting symptom is often intermittent claudication. The term claudication, from the Latin word *claudico,* "to limp," refers to pain or severe fatigue produced by exertional ischemia. The characteristic clinical presentation is an aching or cramplike pain brought on by a specific amount of exercise and relieved within one or two minutes by standing and resting. After resting the pain is again precipitated by the same specific amount of exercise. Most patients with lower extremity claudication can accurately describe the distance they can walk before the onset of symptoms. Symptoms occur sooner when walking up an incline or at a faster pace. The location of the symptoms is determined by the site of the arterial disease. Patients with symptomatic aortoiliac occlusive disease often present with hip and thigh claudication, and sometimes with claudication in the calf. Superficial femoral artery disease is associated with calf claudication, and severe tibial disease with foot claudication. However, foot claudication is extraordinarily rare and usually a manifestation of thromboangiitis obliterans.

Although claudication has a characteristic pattern and ordinarily is easy to identify, its symptoms can be confused with those of other common problems, such as degenerative joint disease, lumbar disc disease, and spinal stenosis.

NEUROSPINAL COMPRESSION SYNDROME

Neurospinal compression syndrome is probably the clinical entity most easily confused with claudication. It is secondary to spinal stenosis, which may be either acquired or congenital, and results in lower extremity discomfort with exercise. The discomfort associated with this syndrome usually has the character of numbness or weakness, similar to that sometimes present with atypical claudication. Although symptoms of spinal stenosis may be precipitated by exercise, the amount of exercise varies, and the symptoms may be relieved better by sitting for prolonged periods than by standing. Symptoms of spinal stenosis are usually aggravated by any activity that increases lumbar lordosis and are decreased by flexion of the lumbar spine. Differentiation between claudication and spinal stenosis can be difficult because many patients with spinal stenosis are elderly and may also have decreased pulsations in the lower extremities due to peripheral vascular disease. Although a good history and physical examination can identify some of these patients, others require further evaluation of the lumbar spine by either myelography or computed tomography.

CLINICAL ASPECTS

Physical examination of patients with claudication usually reveals decreased pulsation below the level of the identifiable lesion. Doppler examination can be used to document the presence of peripheral vascular disease, to follow its progression, and to help assess its severity and clinical importance in complex problems. The examinations can be performed in a vascular laboratory or a physician's office. Doppler pressures are obtained with a blood pressure cuff at the calf and the Doppler probe over the posterior tibial and dorsalis pedis arteries. These pressures together with brachial pressures can be used to create an ankle-to-brachial index. In a normal patient, this index is slightly greater than 1. As a rule of thumb, each flow-reducing arterial lesion results in a 0.3 decrease in the index. For example, a patient with hemodynamically significant aortoiliac occlusive disease may present with an index of 0.6 to 0.7; a patient with both stenotic aortoiliac disease and superficial femoral artery disease may present with an index around 0.4. In patients with claudication alone the presenting index may be 0.5 to 0.6, and in patients with limb-threatening ischemia, usually less than 0.35. Because of calcified noncompliant arteries, pressures in diabetic patients may be artificially high and unreliable.

MANAGEMENT

In patients with claudication, as in asymptomatic patients with arteriosclerotic peripheral vascular disease, risk factors should be identified and if possible controlled. Patients should be taught the importance of excellent foot care and placed on an exercise program. Exercise has been shown to be of benefit in patients with claudication and may bring 100% improvement by six months. We suggest that our patients walk once or twice a day for 30 to 60 minutes, exerting themselves to the limits imposed by their pain, and then resting. Patients who are able to stop smoking and be faithful to an exercise program can have very gratifying results.

DRUG THERAPY

Until recently, effective medical therapy for claudication did not exist. However, the introduction of pentoxifylline (Trental) has provided a method for increasing walking distance. In a double-blind randomized trial, patients treated with pentoxifylline could walk about 50% farther without symptoms after 24 weeks than patients treated by placebo. This difference was statistically significant. Pentoxifylline is not primarily a vasodilator but a hemorrheologic agent that increases malleability of red blood cells and allows them to squeeze through capillary beds more easily. Although the primary effect of pentoxifylline is on malleability of red blood cells, it may also have some effect on vascular smooth muscle and platelet functions. This agent is easily absorbed when taken orally. It is metabolized by red blood cells and the liver and excreted by the kidney. The usual dose is 400 mg PO three times a day with meals. It usually is effective within two to four weeks, but the recommended therapeutic trial period is eight weeks. Side effects are mild and include headache, dizziness, and nausea. If these occur, the dose of pentoxifylline can be reduced until the patient becomes tachyphylactic to them. The dose can subsequently be increased to the recommended amount as tolerated. Few patients have symptoms severe enough to prevent them from taking this medication. Ketanserine, a new serotonin antagonist available in Europe, seems to be another promising agent to bring symptomatic relief in patients with claudication. Patients must be told, however, that these agents provide only relief of a symptom and that control of risk factors plays a more vital role in the treatment. It should be explained to them that such measures may inhibit the progression of both lower extremity arteriosclerosis and disease in coronary arteries, extracranial vasculature, and renal arteries.

We should realize and stress to patients that claudication is a benign symptom. In studies of the natural history of arteriosclerosis before the advent of surgical intervention, only about 7% of patients with claudication progressed to tissue loss in five years and about 12% in ten years. The condition of most patients with claudication remained stable, and a small percentage improved. Because claudication is benign and may be helped medically, surgery should be offered to only a selected group of patients with this symptom. If patients represent an acceptable medical risk, have trouble performing their job or some other desired activity, and understand the risks and benefits of surgery, angiography may be performed. If this study shows a lesion that can be easily bypassed, surgery is considered. However, claudication alone is rarely an indication for operation.

LIMB-THREATENING ISCHEMIA

Patients with ischemic rest pain, ischemic nonhealing ulcers, or limited gangrene are considered to have limb-threatening ischemia. Without invasive therapy a large percentage of these patients will require major amputation.

Ischemic Rest Pain. This is characteristically a severe pain that occurs at night when the patient lies in bed with legs elevated. It usually occurs in the toes or across the metatarsal head and is relieved by placing the foot in a dependent position. Rest pain can be confused with pain associated with diabetic neuropathy, which is usually bilateral. It is neither precipitated nor relieved by changes of position, and physical examination usually shows decrease in sensation to light touch and vibration in the lower extremities. Differentiation between ischemic rest pain and neuropathic pain in a patient who has both diabetic neuropathy and severe ischemia is difficult, and taxes the judgment of even the most sophisticated clinician.

Nonhealing Ischemic Ulcers. These ulcers are a serious problem because they can become infected at any time and can result in a limb- or life-threatening condition. Ischemic ulcers and gangrene usually involve the distal part of the foot or sometimes a more proximal area that has been traumatized. These ulcers usually have well-defined edges without granulation tissue. They may have a shaggy gray or yellow base or be covered with an eschar. Such ulcers are often painful and tender to the touch. In patients with diabetic neuropathy, on the other hand, there may be no pain or tenderness.

Physical examination in these patients reveals many signs of distal ischemia, such as absence of palpable pedal pulses, thin and atrophic skin over the distal leg and foot, considerable loss of hair, sparse subcutaneous tissue, and rubor in the dependent position. With the patient in the supine position the feet blanch when elevated, and when legs are placed in a dependent position the capillary filling may be delayed noticeably. In our experience, the amount of blanching with elevation and the increase in capillary filling time provide an estimation of the degree of ischemia. Venous filling time is also a valuable indicator (except when venous insufficiency leads to premature filling). This is the time required for superficial veins in the feet to fill when the legs are returned to the dependent position after elevation. In normal patients the venous filling time is usually less than 10 to 15 seconds; in patients with mild to moderate ischemia, 15 to 25 seconds; and in patients with limb-threatening ischemia, more than 25 seconds. In patients with severe ischemia and venous filling times of more than 25 seconds, the ankle-to-brachial index is usually less than 0.35.

Percutaneous Angioplasty and Surgery. These present definite risks and are recommended only to patients with limb-threatening conditions. However, with careful patient selection these methods can provide long-term benefit and reasonable safety (Table 1). Angioplasty is most useful for short, isolated areas of stenosis. Unfortunately, patients with isolated stenosis are usually asymptomatic or present with claudication, and are not ordinarily considered candidates for invasive therapy. Patients with limb-threatening ischemia usually

Table 1. RESULTS OF INVASIVE THERAPY

Procedure	Mortality (%)	Five-year Patency (%)	Five-year Limb Salvage (%)
Aortoiliac reconstruction	3	95	
Iliac angioplasty	0.5	70*	
Femoropopliteal reconstruction	0.3	75	85†
Superficial femoral angioplasty	0.5	55*	

*Two-year patency.

†With distal bypass surgery the five-year limb salvage rate is commonly 10% to 15% higher than the five-year graft patency rate, because some grafts that fail remain patent long enough to heal an ulcer and convert a limb-threatening condition into one less serious.

have extensive disease that can be treated only by surgery. In some patients with multiple lesions, a combination of percutaneous angioplasty and surgery offers the best solution.

REFERENCES

Boyd AM: The natural course of arteriosclerosis of the lower extremities. Angiology 11:10–14, 1960.

Fielding JE: Smoking: Health effects and control. N Engl J Med 313:491–498, 555–561, 1985.

Jonason T, Jonzon B, Ringqvist I, et al.: Effect of physical training on different categories of patients with intermittent claudication. Acta Med Scand 206:253–258, 1979.

Porter JM, Cutler BS, Lee BY, et al: Pentoxifylline efficacy in the treatment of intermittent claudication: multicenter controlled double-blind trial with objective assessment of chronic occlusive arterial disease patients. Am Heart J 104:66–72, 1982.

Rutherford RB: Vascular Surgery, 2nd ed. W. B. Saunders Co, Philadelphia, 1984.

10 · INFECTIVE ENDOCARDITIS: A DISEASE IN EVOLUTION

Charles Z. Naggar
Pierre Forgacs
LAHEY CLINIC MEDICAL CENTER

Infective endocarditis is best characterized as a changing disease. Increasingly, its complications rather than the infection itself pose the major therapeutic challenge. New antimicrobial agents and echocardiographic visualization of bacterial vegetations, along with improved surgical skills, have favorably altered the natural history of infective endocarditis. Because of the existing numerous excellent and exhaustive reviews, we elected not to add yet another. Instead we discuss the changing nature of infective endocarditis, emphasize the newer diagnostic tools, and highlight recent therapeutic modalities.

DEFINITION AND PATHOGENESIS

Defined as an intravascular infection, endocarditis results from colonization of the endothelium by microorganisms. Infective endocarditis usually refers to microbial, bacterial, or fungal infection within the heart.

Bacteremia may follow dental extraction; periodontal procedures; urethral instrumentation; curettage; incision of abscesses; gastrointestinal surgery; septorhinoplasty; or the use of contaminated hypodermic needles for parenteral use, ear piercing, or acupuncture. Bacteremia is the principal insult that initiates the process of endocarditis.

THE DIAGNOSTIC CHALLENGE

Infective endocarditis, which is preponderant in men, rarely occurs in the first decade of life. Currently,

drug abusers without structural heart disease, patients with prosthetic valves, older patients with degenerative aortic valves, and patients with mitral valve prolapse account for a large percentage of all those with infective endocarditis. Often disguised, infective endocarditis can run a protracted course masquerading as a disease of the lung, eyes, central nervous system, bones, kidneys, or joints or as an anemia.

HISTORY: THE FIRST CLUE

Correct diagnosis requires a high degree of suspicion. A detailed history may afford the physician the first clue to the presence of structural heart disease predisposing a patient to infective endocarditis.

In addition, when a characteristically acute, short-lived infection assumes an evanescent recurrent course, the physician should consider a more chronic disease, such as infective endocarditis.

Recurrent fever and malaise subsequent to a recent three- to six-month gynecologic or urologic instrumentation, dental or periodontal procedure, ear or nose piercing, self-treated skin abscess, or bowel, kidney, or pelvic surgery should alert the physician to the possibility of infective endocarditis. A history compatible with multiple systemic or pulmonary emboli, unexplained congestive heart failure, or joint pain associated with anemia is the common presentation of infective endocarditis in today's clinical practice.

PHYSICAL EXAMINATION: THE CAREFUL SEARCH

Because patients with infective endocarditis rarely present with symptoms of heart disease, extracardiac manifestations of infective endocarditis are often more helpful than cardiac signs. Conjunctival petechiae in the palpebral conjunctivae and Roth's spots are characteristic of the disease. Subungual splinter hemorrhages and clubbing are less specific signs of infective endocarditis, but they occur frequently enough to be important clues. Osler's nodes and Janeway's subcutaneous lesions are rare findings. Splenomegaly, seldom documented in the early stages of infective endocarditis, is an important but inconsistent finding in the chronic stages.

Intracardiac manifestations of infective endocarditis result from destruction of normal valves or further aggravation of preexisting lesions. The changing acoustic characteristics of regurgitant murmurs are a hallmark of infective endocarditis that we have rarely encountered. Much less specific are the systolic flow murmurs that are commonly present because of anemia, fever, and systemic infection. Severe perivalvular leaks commonly lead to CHF. Occasionally fungal endocarditis, *Staphylococcus* endocarditis on heterograft porcine valves, and endocarditis on mitral valve prolapse cause exuberant vegetations that obstruct the flow of blood and result in functional valvular stenoses. Septic pericarditis is extremely rare, and coronary artery emboli occur less frequently than systemic arterial emboli.

LABORATORY TESTS: THE CONFIRMATORY EVIDENCE

Our initial outpatient evaluation includes three blood cultures obtained at 20-minute intervals, hematocrit, hemoglobin, total and differential WBC, Westergren erythrocyte sedimentation rate, serum urea nitrogen and creatinine, rheumatoid factor, and urinalysis. A resting EKG, two-dimensional echocardiogram, and routine chest radiograph provide all the diagnostic confirmation required. We then instruct the patient to keep an accurate temperature diary. At least 80% of patients with infective endocarditis have mild anemia, i.e., hemoglobin between 10.5 and 12.9 gm/dL. The anemia is rarely severe or hemolytic unless the patient has malfunction of a prosthetic valve, with or without perivalvular leakage. Total WBC count is usually within the normal range but the differential WBC count shows a leftward shift. The ESR is elevated in 90% of patients to a level above 40 mm/h. Assessment of serum urea nitrogen and creatinine serves to rule out any noteworthy azotemia. Urinalysis may show microscopic hematuria and proteinuria.

Two-dimensional echocardiography is currently the most complete anatomic study of the beating heart. It visualizes cardiac valves with a high degree of resolution and is capable of demonstrating intracardiac vegetations. Noninvasive visualization of bacterial and fungal vegetations in vivo represents a definite diagnostic advantage. In our series of 35 consecutive patients with infective endocarditis at Lahey Clinic Medical Center, routine diagnostic echocardiography demonstrated 24 vegetations on native valves of 19 patients. In addition to its ability to image bacterial vegetations on valvular surfaces, echocardiography defines the size, mobility, and natural history of these vegetations; the degree of valvular destruction; and the hemodynamic derangements caused by infective endocarditis.

CLINICAL MANAGEMENT

BACTERIOLOGIC CURE

Proper identification of the microbial organism is the most important step in controlling the infection. Clinical microbiology laboratories are increasingly skilled in detection of the organisms that cause endocarditis and in precise elucidation of antimicrobial susceptibility. Table 1 contrasts the variety and frequency of microbial organisms encountered in various groups of patients with infective endocarditis. Better understanding of the bacteriologic properties of antibiotics, the synergistic drug interaction, and the mechanisms by which organisms resist antibiotics has led to the development of highly effective antibiotic regimens for most types of infective endocarditis (Table 2). As a result, patients rarely die of uncontrolled infection; more often they die of CHF, arrhythmia, or embolization. For selection of optimal antibiotic therapy, the causative organism and a profile of its antibiotic susceptibility are needed. In hemodynamically stable patients with indolent infective endocarditis, a few days' wait for such information is preferred. In contrast, empiric antibiotic therapy must be used in urgent situations. We use detailed microbiologic tests to choose antibiotic regimens for infective endocarditis caused by organisms other than *Streptococcus viridans*. Minimal bactericidal concentration, serum bactericidal titer, and synergy studies help to characterize the microorganism. The causative organism must remain in the laboratory until therapy has been completed because adverse reactions to a drug may necessitate a revision in antibiotic therapy.

Although increasingly less prevalent, culture-negative endocarditis usually presents as unexplained fever and heart murmur in patients with structural heart disease. In such patients, echocardiography may demonstrate vegetations. Immunologic clues, such as an elevated rheumatoid factor and a high ESR, are corroborative evidence of infective endocarditis. In indolent infective endocarditis, the rheumatoid factor may be as high as 1:2560 or greater dilution of serum. Levels in this range are usually encountered in patients with severe seropositive rheumatoid arthritis or with systemic lupus erythematosus. In the absence of either of

Table 1. MICROBIOLOGY OF INFECTIVE ENDOCARDITIS

Organism	Native Valve Endocarditis*		Endocarditis in Narcotic Addicts†		Prosthetic Valve Endocarditis‡	
	No.	%	No.	%	No.	%
Staphylococcus aureus	72	18	208	55	65	14
Staphylococcus epidermidis	16	4	9	2	130	20
Streptococcus	228	58	73	19	116	25
S. viridans	149			28	64	
S. pneumoniae	0			1	5	
Group D	79			27§	32	
Other	0			17	15	
Gram-negative and gram-positive bacilli	35	9	30	8	99	21
Diphtheroids	NS			2	30	
Pseudomonas aeruginosa	NS			16	0	
Enteric and other gram-negative bacilli	NS			12	69	
Fungi	0	0	16	4	43	9
Candida	0			16	30	
Other	0			0	13	
Other organisms	29		0		9	
Multiple organisms in culture	0		17		0	
Negative blood cultures	13	3	27	7	0	0
Total	393		380		462	

*Modified from Wilson WR, Giuliano ER, Danielson GK, et al: General considerations in the diagnosis and treatment of infective endocarditis. Mayo Clin Proc 57:81–114, 1982.

†Modified from Reisberg BE: Infective endocarditis in the narcotic addict. Prog Cardiovasc Dis 22:193–204, 1979.

‡Modified from Mayer KH, Schoenbaum SC: Evaluation and management of prosthetic valve endocarditis. Prog Cardiovasc Dis 25:43–54, 1982.

§Includes enterococci only.

NS = Not specified.

Table 2. ANTIBIOTIC DRUG THERAPY FOR ADULTS WITH ENDOCARDITIS

Infection	Most Effective Regimen		Alternative Regimen†		Weeks of Treatment	
	Drug	Dosage*	Drug	Dosage*	Native Valve	Prosthetic Valve
Streptococcal						
Penicillin-susceptible nonenterococcal streptococci (*S. viridans* and *S. bovis*, MIC <0.2 and minimal bactericidal concentration <20)	Aqueous penicillin G	20 million U/d IV in divided doses every 4 h	Vancomycin	30 mg/kg/d IV in divided doses every 6 or 12 h	4	4–6
			or			
			Cephalothin	2 mg IV every 4 h	4	4–6
	Aqueous penicillin G plus	As above for 4 wk	Cephalothin	In above doses	4	4–6
			or			
	Streptomycin	500 mg IM every 12 h during initial 2 wk	Vancomycin	In above doses	4	4–6
			or			
			Clindamycin plus	1.2 gm every 8h		
			Streptomycin	As noted		
	Penicillin plus	20 million U/d IV	Clindamycin plus	1.2 gm IV every 8 h	2	NA
	Streptomycin	In above doses	Streptomycin	500 mg IM every 12 h		
Enterococci	Aqueous penicillin G	20 million U/d IV in divided doses every 4 h	Vancomycin	1 gm IV every 12 h	4–6	6
	plus		plus			
	Gentamicin	1 mg/kg IV every 8 h	Gentamicin	1 mg/kg IV every 8 h		
	or		or			
	Streptomycin‡	In above doses	Streptomycin‡	In above doses		
Staphylococcal						
S. aureus (methicillin-susceptible, penicillin-resistant)	Nafcillin	2.0 gm IV every 4 h	Cephalothin	2 gm IV every 4 h	4–6	6
	or		or			
S. epidermidis (methicillin-susceptible)	Oxacillin		Vancomycin	1 gm IV every 12 h		
S. aureus (methicillin-resistant)	Vancomycin	1 gm IV every 12 h			4–6	6
S. epidermidis (methicillin-resistant)	Vancomycin	1 gm IV every 12 h	Design according to special susceptibility studies		4–6	6
	plus					
	Rifampin	300 mg orally every 8 h				
	or					
	Vancomycin and Rifampin	In above doses			4–6	6
	plus					
	Gentamicin	1 mg/kg IV every 8 h during initial 2 wk				
	or				4–6	NA
	Vancomycin	1 gm IV every 12 h				
Gram-negative						
Fastidious gram-negative coccobacilli (*Haemophilus; Cardiobacter*)	Ampicillin	12 gm/d IV in divided doses every 4 h			4–6	4–6
	plus					
	Streptomycin	500 mg IM every 12 h				
	or					
	Ampicillin	12 gm/d in divided doses			4–6	6
Pseudomonas aeruginosa	Ticarcillin	18 gm/d IV			6	6
	or					
	Carbenicillin	30 gm/d IV in divided doses every 4 h				
	plus					
	Tobramycin	2.5 mg/kg IV every 8 h				
	or					
	Gentamicin	2.5 mg/kg IV every 8 h				
Corynebacterium sp.	Vancomycin	1 gm IV every 12 h	Penicillin	20 million U/d IV in divided doses	4–6	6
			plus			
			Streptomycin	500 mg IM every 12 h		

*Dosages given are for 70-kg adult with normal renal function. Appropriate adjustment must be made for renal insufficiency (especially with vancomycin, streptomycin, gentamicin) and for patients allergic to penicillin.

†For patients allergic to drugs suggested in "Most Effective Regimen" column.

‡If enterococcus is susceptible to 2000-µg disc of streptomycin or penicillin-streptomycin synergism is demonstrated.

NA = Not applicable.

these, such high levels of the rheumatoid factor strongly suggest infective endocarditis. The level of rheumatoid factor and ESR both decrease to normal levels following successful antibiotic therapy.

Patients are hospitalized just before initiation of antibiotic therapy. To reduce hospital costs, IV antibiotic therapy in an outpatient setting is occasionally advocated, but we do not recommend it. Patients with infective endocarditis associated with mild CHF, ventricular ectopic activity, or considerable mitral regurgitation require cardiac monitoring. Diuretic therapy with its inevitable shifts in electrolytes may aggravate ventricular arrhythmias. An EKG is usually obtained every 48 to 72 hours during the first two weeks of antibiotic therapy, and weekly thereafter, to search specifically for any abnormalities in conduction. Serum urea nitrogen and creatinine are determined every 48 hours to monitor aminoglycoside-related renal toxicity. Audiometry is performed periodically in such patients.

RECURRENT EMBOLIZATION

Echocardiography has been used recently in infective endocarditis, not only for its diagnostic capabilities but also for follow-up study of patients with vegetative endocarditis. We recommend that it be repeated every eight to ten days during antibiotic therapy in patients with initially demonstrable vegetations. In our series of 35 consecutive patients with infective endocarditis, 20 patients had 25 vegetations. Within the first 12 weeks of antibiotic therapy, 12 of 25 vegetations increased in size, three of 25 became more mobile, and five of 18 extended to the chordae tendineae. However, in the late follow-up period, an average of 160 weeks after antibiotic therapy, 18 of 23 vegetations remained unchanged in size, one decreased, and one increased. In two patients, exuberant vegetations were documented by echocardiography. The first patient with mitral valve prolapse and infective endocarditis experienced repeated systemic embolization to the brain. In a second patient who had endocarditis of a porcine prosthetic mitral valve, a large obstructing vegetation attached to

the mitral porcine cusps was associated with hemolytic anemia, intravascular coagulation, and low cardiac output. In both of these patients, echocardiography contributed to decisions for early surgical intervention. In two other patients, echocardiography documented enlarging vegetations, the first on the atrial side of the posterior mitral leaflet and the second on the atrial side of the septal leaflet of the tricuspid valve. Recurrent embolization in both patients was successfully treated with chronic anticoagulation with warfarin (Coumadin) for nine and 18 months, respectively, and no recurrences of emboli were evident after a year of follow-up. We recommend anticoagulation until two echocardiograms three months apart demonstrate stability.

Anticoagulation, although complicated, is not always contraindicated in infective endocarditis. Chronic anticoagulation in patients with prosthetic valve endocarditis is usually continued without interruption during and after antibiotic therapy. Anticoagulant therapy does not appreciably increase the rate of morbidity or mortality in patients with prosthetic valve endocarditis. Careful monitoring of prothrombin time is essential during administration of broad-spectrum antibiotics.

INDICATIONS FOR CARDIAC SURGERY

The hemodynamic state of the patient dictates the necessity for valve replacement. Progressive or severe CHF in patients with aortic valve endocarditis carries a high mortality rate if treated medically. Early valve replacement in such patients is advised despite the risk of prosthetic valve endocarditis and valve dehiscence. Any patient who has more than one major embolus, especially if a large mobile vegetation is demonstrated on echocardiography, deserves serious consideration for valve replacement. Patients with perivalvular or interventricular septal abscesses unresponsive to medical therapy, patients with relapsing endocarditis caused by *Staphylococcus aureus* without identifiable metastatic foci, and patients with fungal endocarditis require valve replacement. Purulent pericarditis mandates surgical drainage.

Table 3. RECOMMENDED DOSES FOR ANTIBIOTIC PROPHYLAXIS*†

Procedure	Routine Prophylaxis	High-Risk Prophylaxis (Valve Prostheses)
Dental, otorhinolaryngologic, or bronchoscopic	Penicillin V, 2 gm PO 1 h before and 1 gm 6 h later	Ampicillin, 1–2 gm IV or IM plus Gentamicin, 1.5 mg/kg IV or IM ½ h before procedure then penicillin V, 1 gm PO 6 h later
	or (for penicillin-allergic patient)	
	Erythromycin, 1 gm PO 1 h before and 500 mg 6 h later	Vancomycin, 1 gm IV 1 h before (slowly, 1 dose only)
Urologic	Ampicillin, 2 gm IM or IV 1 h before and 6–8 h later plus Gentamicin, 1.5 mg/kg IM or IV 1 h before and 6–8 h later	Same as for routine prophylaxis
	or (for penicillin-allergic patient)	
	Vancomycin, 1 gm IV 1 h before and 12 h later plus Gentamicin, 1.5 mg/kg IM or IV 1 h before and 8–12 h later	Same as for routine prophylaxis

*For adults with normal renal function. Reduce dosage in children weighing less than 60 lb but do not exceed adult dosage as follows: penicillin V, one half adult dose; erythromycin, 20 mg/kg initially, then 10 mg/kg; gentamicin, 2 mg/k per dose; vancomycin, 20 mg/kg; ampicillin, 50 mg/kg.
†Modified from American Heart Association: Prevention of bacterial endocarditis. Circulation 70:1123A–1127A, 1984.

RECURRENT FEVER AND RELAPSES

During the course of antibiotic therapy for infective endocarditis, the portal of entry of the infection must be identified and eliminated. We recommend a complete dental evaluation and sinus radiography for patients with infective endocarditis caused by *S. viridans*, and proctosigmoidoscopic and barium enema studies for patients with infective endocarditis caused by *S. bovis*. However, certain types of endocarditis, such as that caused by enterococcus and *S. aureus*, can relapse. Such relapses are treated medically. Metastatic infections, such as septic arthritis and purulent pericarditis, and large CNS abscesses require surgical drainage and can be the source of recurrent fevers. In the absence of such metastatic infections, the possibility of a drug-related fever should be considered.

In our experience, drug-related fevers may lack the diurnal variation common to septicemia. Drug-related fever, which is not usually associated with chills and rigor, may be associated with skin eruptions and an elevated eosinophil count.

FOLLOW-UP AFTER DISCHARGE

After a full course of antibiotic therapy for infective endocarditis, antibiotics are discontinued and patients are observed by us for 24 to 48 hours before being discharged. During hospitalization we and the nursing staff undertake an educational program to inform patients and their families of the nature of structural heart disease that predisposes them to infective endocarditis. All portals of entry for bacteremia are discussed in detail, as well as the use of prophylactic antibiotics.

Optimal antimicrobial prophylaxis for all known procedures associated with endocarditis can be expected to prevent only a few cases. This lack of effectiveness prevails because no apparent portal of entry for bacteremia is recognized in most patients with infective endocarditis. With certain procedures associated with substantial risk for bacteremia, however, antibiotic prophylaxis should be prescribed. Such prophylaxis is recommended for patients with rheumatic valvular heart disease, congenital heart disease excluding secundum atrial septal defects, acquired valvular heart disease, idiopathic hypertrophic subaortic stenosis, mitral valve prolapse (particularly with associated mitral regurgitation), prosthetic heart valves, or previous infective endocarditis and for patients with any form of aortic regurgitation. These procedures include dental and periodontal procedures, tonsillectomy, adenoidectomy, bronchoscopy, urologic procedures, and operative procedures involving infected tissue, such as incision and drainage of an abscess. Our recommendations for prophylactic antibiotics are outlined in Table 3.

Patients return to the clinic for a follow-up visit two to four weeks after discharge and at three-month intervals for the first year after completion of antibiotic therapy. Within four weeks after discharge, blood cultures are obtained, and hematocrit, total WBC count, and ESR are evaluated. In patients with vegetative endocarditis, echocardiography is repeated within three months. An adequate diet with or without supplemental vitamins usually restores hematocrit and hemoglobin to normal levels within eight to 12 weeks after discharge.

In our experience, cardiac medications require frequent adjustment in the outpatient setting. The prothrombin time is measured monthly in every patient undergoing chronic anticoagulant therapy.

Acknowledgment

We greatly appreciate the secretarial help of Ms. Diane Gallagher, CMT, and the collation of echocardiographic data by Ms. Debra A. Dumont, RDMS.

REFERENCES

Johnson CM, Rhodes KH: Pediatric endocarditis. Mayo Clin Proc 57:86–94, 1982.

Naggar CZ, Pippin JP, Forgacs P: Infective endocarditis, a changing disease, abstracted. Chest 86:316, 1984.

Poretz DM, Eron LJ, Goldenberg RI, et al: Intravenous antibiotic therapy in an outpatient setting. JAMA 248:336–339, 1982.

Rahimtoola SH (ed): Infective Endocarditis. Grune & Stratton, New York, 1977.

Wilson WR: Symposium on infective endocarditis. Mayo Clin Proc 57:3–32, 81–114, 145–175, 1982.

Wilson WR, Geraci JE, Danielson GK, et al: Anticoagulant therapy and central nervous system complications in patients with prosthetic valve endocarditis. Circulation 57:1004–1007, 1978.

11 · HEART BLOCK

Douglas L. Wood
Bernard J. Gersh
MAYO CLINIC AND MAYO FOUNDATION

Disturbances of atrioventricular (AV) conduction, often collectively referred to as heart block, are common causes of syncope and presyncope. Our understanding of the causes of heart block and the ability to diagnose disorders of transmission of cardiac impulses within the conduction system have improved dramatically within the last few years by virtue of intracardiac electrophysiologic studies. These diagnostic advances and increasing knowledge of the natural history of conduction disturbances, coupled with rapid advances in design, manufacture, and application of pacing devices, require a more specific definition of the generic term "heart block" so that available therapy may be better understood and more precisely applied.

In general, "heart block" refers to conduction disturbances presenting as a bradycardia and dropped beats because of a failure of impulse conduction from the atria to the ventricles. However, other patients with conduction disorders (e.g., bifascicular block) who may or may not have symptoms referable to intermittent bradycardia caused by intermittent heart block often come to a physician's attention with an electrocardiographic abnormality. In the choice of therapeutic approach, the acute or chronic nature of the conduction disturbance and the natural history of the disorder are important. This chapter emphasizes the diagnosis and treatment of chronic heart block and conduction disturbances.

DEFINITION AND DIAGNOSTIC CRITERIA

ATRIOVENTRICULAR BLOCK

Clinically, AV block can be classified according to degree and/or site. Decisions regarding treatment, usually the need for a pacemaker, are influenced primarily by the presence of symptoms that are directly attributable to the development of heart block and the site at which it occurs. Heart block can be classified as first-degree, second-degree, or third-degree (also called complete) heart block.

First-degree AV block is defined as fixed prolongation of the P-R interval exceeding 210 msec. In second-degree heart block, not every sinus impulse reaches the ventricles. Second-degree AV block is subdivided into Mobitz Type I or Wenckebach block, where there is a progressive increase in the P-R interval prior to the dropped beat, and Mobitz Type II block, in which the P-R intervals are constant. Third-degree, or complete, AV block occurs when there is no relationship between atrial activity and ventricular activity. This diagnosis requires the atrial rate to be faster than the ventricular rate, which is controlled by a subsidiary pacemaker in the His-Purkinje system.

Invasive electrophysiologic studies have demonstrated that the EKG descriptions of heart block do not have distinct anatomic correlations. The P-R interval is the sum of conduction times in several parts of the heart. The P-A interval is the time from impulse formation in the sinoatrial node in the high right atrium to the atrium; the A-H interval is the conduction time from the atrium through the AV node; and the H-V interval is the conduction time through the His-Purkinje to the beginning of ventricular activation. The P-A interval corresponds to conduction in the atrium, the A-H interval to conduction in the AV node, and the H-V interval to conduction in the bundle of His. First-degree heart block generally results from a delay in conduction within the AV node, but may be related to an increase in the time necessary to conduct from the AV node to the ventricles over the His-Purkinje system. Second-degree heart block of the Wenckebach variety is most often a reflection of an abnormality within the AV node, but in rare circumstances Wenckebach periodicity may occur in the His-Purkinje system. Generally, Mobitz Type II block or complete heart block reflects significant disease in the bundle of His or the bundle branches. The QRS complex in such patients is frequently widened and the rate of ventricular escape rhythm is slow.

BIFASCICULAR BLOCK

Bifascicular block includes several EKG patterns: right bundle branch block and left anterior fascicular block; right bundle branch block and left posterior fascicular block; and, more debatably, left bundle branch block with left or right axis deviation. Trifascicular block is defined as any pattern of bifascicular block associated with a prolonged P-R interval.

PATHOPHYSIOLOGY

Several pathologic processes may affect the specialized conduction system resulting in heart block.

Table 1. CAUSES OF COMPLETE HEART BLOCK

Acute
  Myocardial infarction
  Cardiac surgery
  Drugs—Beta adrenergic blocking agents, calcium antagonists, digoxin, antiarrhythmic agents (quinidine, procainamide, disopyramide, amiodarone)
  Electrolyte disorders
  Hypercalcemia
  Myocarditis (e.g., coxsackievirus), diphtheria (now uncommon)

Chronic
  Idiopathic fibrosis or sclerosis (Lev's disease, Lenegre's disease)
  Cardiac surgery (valve replacement, VSD repair)
  Coronary artery disease and previous myocardial infarction
  Congenital heart disease (e.g., corrected transposition of the great vessels)
  Calcific aortic valve disease
  Rheumatic heart disease
  Congenital heart block (maternal heart block)
  Connective tissue disease—scleroderma, systemic lupus erythematosus
  Calcific mitral annulus
  Parasitic coronary artery disease (including Chagas' disease)
  Myocardial infiltration—amyloid, sarcoid, hemochromatosis
  Neoplasms—metastatic, leukemia
  Familial

Idiopathic fibrosis or degeneration of the specialized conducting tissues is the most common pathologic finding in patients with chronic heart block. Other causes of heart block are listed in Table 1. Heart block is a common complication of acute myocardial infarction, but since many patients with acute heart block after myocardial infarction die, chronic heart block is only rarely related to myocardial infarction. Acute and chronic complete heart block may follow valve replacement surgery. Connective tissue disease may be an important cause of complete heart block; in young or middle-aged women with complete heart block, connective tissue disorders should always be considered.

CLINICAL ASPECTS

Acquired complete heart block, either fixed or intermittent, was for many years the arrhythmia for which pacing was most frequently utilized. In most circumstances, syncope or presyncope has been the indication for pacing. Although some patients with heart block are asymptomatic, many report symptoms of presyncope, syncope, and dyspnea. Some report feelings of fatigue, some have intermittent confusion, and others may suffer ventricular tachyarrhythmias as a result of the bradycardia.

The advent of the permanent pacemaker dramatically altered the prognosis for patients with symptomatic heart block. Recent and continuing technologic advances in pacemaker design, and increasing knowledge of the natural history of conduction disturbances derived from invasive electrophysiologic studies, have expanded the indications for permanent pacemaker implantation to patients with conduction disturbances other than second- or third-degree heart block (Table 2). In expert hands, the morbidity rate of permanent pacing is low and the benefits significant. However, the ease of pacemaker implantation and the costs behoove the physician to have a clear idea of the indications for pacing.

Table 2. GUIDELINES FOR PERMANENT PACING

I. Pacing in Acquired Atrioventricular Block in Adults
  A. Conditions for which permanent pacemakers should be implanted:
    1. Complete heart block, permanent or intermittent, regardless of site associated with any of the following:
      Symptomatic bradycardia
      Congestive heart failure
      Tachyarrhythmias requiring therapy that would suppress escape foci
      Asystolic pauses of ≥ 3 seconds or escape rate of <40 b.p.m. in asymptomatic patients
      Confusion or other CNS symptoms that clear with temporary pacing
    2. Second-degree heart block associated with symptomatic bradycardia
    3. Atrial fibrillation or flutter associated with symptomatic complete heart block
  B. Conditions for which permanent pacemaker may be implanted but for which controversy exists regarding its use:
    1. Asymptomatic complete heart block with escape rate ≤ 40
    2. Asymptomatic Mobitz Type II second-degree heart block
    3. Asymptomatic Mobitz Type I second-degree heart block localized to His bundle or below
II. Pacing in Atrioventricular Block Associated with Myocardial Infarction
  A. Conditions for which permanent pacemakers should be implanted:
    1. Persistent complete heart block or Mobitz II second-degree block
    2. Transient complete heart block and associated bundle branch block (except in inferior wall infarction)
  B. Conditions for which permanent pacemakers may be implanted:
    1. Persistent first-degree AV block with new bundle branch block
III. Pacing in Chronic Bi- or Trifascicular Block
  A. Conditions for which permanent pacemakers should be implanted:
    1. Bifascicular block with symptomatic intermittent Mobitz Type II second-degree or complete heart block
  B. Conditions for which permanent pacemakers may be implanted:
    1. Bi- or trifascicular heart block with asymptomatic Type II second-degree block
    2. Bi- or trifascicular block and syncope without an identifiable cause
    3. Significant His-Purkinje disease identified by electrophysiologic study in patients who will require antiarrhythmic therapy that would aggravate His-Purkinje dysfunction

Adapted from Special Report: Guidelines for permanent cardiac pacemaker implantation. A report of the Joint American College of Cardiology/American Heart Association Task Force on Assessment of Cardiovascular Procedures. JACC 4:434–442, 1984.

MANAGEMENT

GENERAL APPROACH

In evaluating a patient for a permanent pacemaker in the treatment of heart block, several factors must be considered. Pacing may be *therapeutic* in patients with symptomatic heart block and other symptomatic conduction disturbances. Pacing may be *prophylactic* in patients with asymptomatic heart block or certain other conduction disturbances. In some patients, the decision for permanent pacing can be made on assessment of the EKG symptoms and associated pathologic states and, in other circumstances, on the results of EKG monitoring, the results of electrophysiologic studies, or (in those with associated tachyarrhythmias) the continuing need for therapy with drugs that would impair cardiac conduction. Patients with sustained ventricular tachycardia associated with syncope who require therapy with antiarrhythmic drugs may require prophylactic pacing based on electrophysiologic testing of the conduction system after administration of specific antiarrhythmic drugs.

There are few contraindications to permanent pacing in the treatment of heart block. Age alone is not a contraindication, but the presence of debilitating general diseases that in and of themselves would limit a patient's prognosis may influence the decision for pacing. However, when such relative contraindications exist, pacing may still be indicated if the management of other medical problems could be facilitated by permanent pacing.

There continue to be circumstances in which a small group of patients will have had serious injury associated with cardiogenic syncope where no cause for their symptoms is found in spite of extensive investigations, including invasive electrophysiologic studies. In this group of patients, if the syncope is regarded as being more life-threatening or potentially harmful than the morbidity risks of the pacemaker implantation, permanent pacing may be indicated.

TREATMENT OF SPECIFIC TYPES OF CHRONIC HEART BLOCK

First-Degree AV Block. This is an electrocardiographic entity without hemodynamic sequelae or symptoms. Permanent pacing is unnecessary in patients with asymptomatic first-degree AV block localized to the AV node. The decision to pace patients with asymptomatic first-degree AV block in the His bundle or infra-His structures is less clear and depends in part on the results of invasive electrophysiologic tests. In patients who have first-degree AV block in association with new bundle branch block following myocardial infarction, the decision to pace is controversial (discussed later).

Second-Degree Heart Block. Second-degree heart block of the Wenckebach variety may occur in 5% to 9% of asymptomatic individuals who undergo 24-hour ambulatory EKG monitoring. Type I second-degree heart block is more likely to occur during sleep or in athletic or well-trained individuals, suggesting that increased vagal tone is an important determinant of the development of Type I AV block. However, when the heart rate is sufficiently low, symptoms of presyncope or syncope may occur. Permanent pacing is indicated for all patients with symptomatic permanent or intermittent second-degree Wenckebach block unless this is due to heightened vagal tone when drugs such as propantheline, scopolamine, or theophylline may be used. The approach to an asymptomatic patient with Type I second-degree block using an invasive electrophysiologic study is illustrated in Figure 1. If the site of

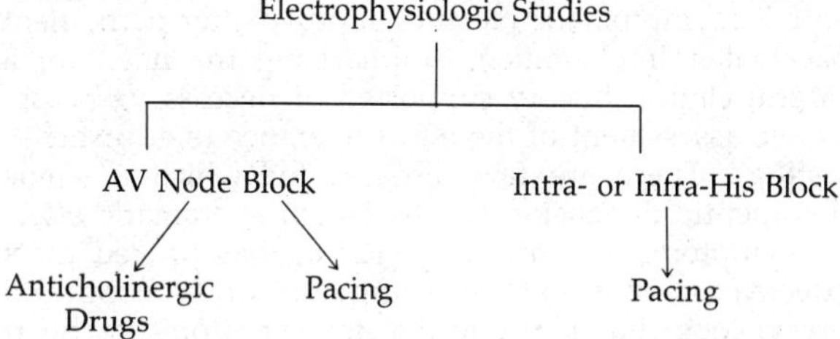

Figure 1. Approach to symptomatic Type I second-degree heart block.

block is in the AV node or proximal to the His bundle, a reasonable first step would be a trial of anticholinergic drugs or theophylline. If this fails, permanent pacing is indicated. On the other hand, if block is localized to the His bundle or distal to His, the likelihood of eventual complete heart block with an unstable escape pacemaker warrants permanent pacing, as initial therapy. A further determination of the potential utility of pacing in these circumstances can be gained from the administration of IV procainamide during the electrophysiologic study, with determination of its effect on AV node and His-Purkinje system function.

Type II Second-Degree AV Block. The prevalence of Type II second-degree AV block in normal patients is extremely low. The site of block in patients with Type II AV block is confined to the His bundle or below. The prognosis for these patients is determined by the presence not only of heart block but more significantly of associated cardiac disease. There is a high incidence of progression to complete AV block in patients with intra-His and infra-His disease.

Any patient with asymptomatic Type II heart block deserves electrophysiologic study unless EKG monitoring shows a strong correlation between symptoms and bradycardia. Patients who develop infra-His block with atrial pacing at low rates, and who develop complete heart block or marked prolongation of the H-V interval after administration of procainamide are better served by prophylactic pacing.

Chronic Complete AV Block. This is detected infrequently in the general population and is more related either to degenerative changes in the conduction system or to underlying heart disease. In certain groups of patients, such as those with recent myocardial infarction or who have undergone cardiac surgery, especially valve replacement, the incidence of complete heart block is considerably higher.

A diagnosis of complete AV block is straightforward in patients in whom the complete heart block is persistent. However, in many patients with presyncope or syncope, the rhythm disturbance is intermittent. If the diagnosis of complete heart block is suspected on clinical grounds, ambulatory EKG recordings, exercise testing, and occasionally telephone transmitters or patient-activated recorders may provide the diagnosis. In most circumstances, invasive electrophysiologic studies in patients with recurrent presyncope or syncope in whom a diagnosis of complete heart block is suspected can define the diagnosis and guide the treatment.

In symptomatic adult patients with intermittent or persistent complete heart block at any anatomic level, permanent pacing is indicated. The issue in asymptomatic patients is more complex, but even many "apparently" asymptomatic patients improve after permanent pacemaker implantation, emphasizing the need for a careful clinical history supported, if necessary, by objective assessment of the effort tolerance (e,g., exercise testing). There are few diseases for which a single therapeutic dimension has had such a dramatic effect on symptoms and mortality. Pacing has proved most effective in relieving the symptoms of syncope and presyncope, but less effective for symptoms of heart failure.

Thus, permanent pacing is indicated in all patients with presyncope or syncope associated with permanent or intermittent complete heart block. Patients who have CHF and heart block may benefit from permanent pacing, possibly by utilizing techniques of physiologic pacing (in which AV synchrony is maintained) or by simply increasing the rate of ventricular demand pacing. Permanent pacing is also indicated in patients with ventricular tachyarrhythmias requiring therapy with antiarrhythmic drugs which would exacerbate a conduction disturbance or suppress an escape focus. Permanent pacing is also indicated for treatment of asymptomatic patients with intermittent or permanent complete heart block when there are documented periods of asystole exceeding 3 seconds, when the escape rate is less than 40 beats per minute, or when the morphology of the escape focus suggests that this arises distal to the AV node. Permanent pacing is also indicated in patients with confusion or other CNS symptoms that appear related to bradycardia and have been shown to improve with temporary pacing.

In the prepacemaker era, the one-year mortality rate with complete heart block ranged from 30% to 80%. Since the introduction of permanent pacing, the long-term prognosis has changed considerably. In the absence of severe associated heart disease and impaired left ventricular function, prognosis after pacing in patients with complete AV block becomes similar to that for the general population.

Congenital AV Block. A subgroup of patients with complete AV block are those in whom it is congenital. Although antenatal diagnosis may be possible, the diagnosis is frequently delayed. Most patients with congenital complete heart block may have few symptoms until they reach their second or third decade.

The prognosis for congenital complete AV block varies according to age. The highest mortality in congenital heart block occurs in infancy and may be related to the presence of other congenital defects. For adolescents and adults, the prognosis is not entirely benign, and when ventricular rates begin to slow, ventricular ectopy may become a more prominent clinical finding. Patients with congenital complete heart block who are symptomatic with syncope or presyncope should be permanently paced. Patients who develop moderate to marked exercise intolerance associated with congenital heart block should also be permanently paced. The role of pacing in *asymptomatic* patients with congenital complete heart block and frequent ventricular ectopy has not been clarified, but permanent pacing in this situation is reasonable. In asymptomatic patients, permanent pacing is indicated when the site of block can be localized to the bundle of His or infra-His structures at the time of invasive electrophysiologic studies. In children and adolescents with congenital complete heart block, there is a high association of syncope and death with ventricular rates of less than 45 beats per minute in the awake state. In these circumstances, permanent pacing is controversial but may help to reduce the potential for syncope or death.

INDICATIONS FOR PERMANENT PACING IN ATRIOVENTRICULAR BLOCK FOLLOWING MYOCARDIAL INFARCTION

Patients who survive myocardial infarction with evidence of transient high-grade second-degree heart block or complete heart block are candidates for permanent pacing but this has been controversial. Results of multicenter studies have helped to clarify the indications for prophylactic permanent pacing in survivors of myocardial infarction. With transient reversible complete heart block accompanying acute inferior myocardial infarction, the role of prophylactic permanent pacing is small, since patient prognosis is dependent on the extent of coronary artery disease and not the conduction abnormality. However, the development of high-degree AV block, even if transient, after anterior myocardial infarction is a particularly lethal complication. The conduction disturbance is a marker of extensive necrosis, and many of the *late* deaths are due to pump failure and *ventricular tachycardia/fibrillation*. The impact of permanent pacing in this situation is difficult to evaluate, but a multicenter trial showed that although complete heart block occurs in less than 10% of patients who survive anterior myocardial infarction, the acute mortality rate in this group of patients is approximately 75%. Prophylactic permanent pacing is indicated in most patients who survive anterior myocardial infarctions complicated by *transient* complete heart block during the course of the acute infarction. The results of a multicenter trial of pacing in patients who survived myocardial infarction demonstrated that in patients with anterior infarction there was an overall 28% incidence of sudden death or recurrent heart block in the first year of follow-up; however, the incidence of sudden death or recurrent heart block was highest in patients who were not paced, of whom approximately three-fourths died or had recurrent heart block. In patients who survived anterior myocardial infarction and who had transient complete heart block or high-grade second-degree heart block, the incidence of sudden death or recurrent heart block was only 10% when permanent pacing was utilized.

Patients who have persistent high-degree AV block after inferior myocardial infarction should have permanent pacing. Transient advanced AV block after inferior infarction is not an indication for pacing.

Controversy remains over the utility of permanent pacing in patients who develop associated bundle branch block and advanced AV block after myocardial infarction. In general, we recommend permanent pacing in patients who survive myocardial infarction with bifascicular block and evidence of transient high-grade AV block. In patients who develop bifascicular block without evidence of high-grade AV block, electrophysiologic studies should be undertaken to determine the potential for development of complete heart block as well as for sustained ventricular arrhythmias. Patients with markedly prolonged H-V intervals at rest, an H-V interval ≥ 100 msec after procainamide, or pacing-induced infra-His block should be permanently paced. It should be emphasized that most of these patients have significant underlying left ventricular dysfunction, and death is often related to ventricular tachyarrhythmias.

PACING IN BIFASCICULAR AND TRIFASCICULAR BLOCK

Patients with bi- or trifascicular block usually have advanced disease of the conduction system and may experience symptoms related to intermittent complete heart block. When complete heart block occurs either transiently or permanently in patients with bi- or trifas-

cicular block, there is an increased incidence of sudden death. Because many such patients have transient complete heart block that goes undetected, it is not unreasonable to assume that syncope in such patients may be due to complete heart block. However, since many of these die as a result of ventricular tachyarrhythmias probably as a manifestation of severe underlying cardiac disease, we routinely carry out electrophysiologic studies in these patients to guide therapy. Some investigators have proposed that prophylactic permanent pacing is indicated in all patients with transient syncope and bifascicular block. However, although complete heart block is often preceded by bifascicular block, a considerable body of evidence suggests that the rate of progression of bifascicular heart block to complete heart block is low. Unfortunately, there are no reliable clinical or laboratory findings that identify patients at high risk of developing complete heart block. The invasive electrophysiologic study is useful in patients with syncope and bifascicular block.

Because some patients with bifascicular block and advanced heart disease may have a transient ventricular tachyarrhythmia as a cause of their syncope, we generally recommend electrophysiologic studies to evaluate patients with bi- or trifascicular block who experience syncope. At the time of the electrophysiologic study, most of these patients have H-V intervals that are long, but a prolonged H-V interval per se is not an independent predictor of progression to complete heart block, except in patients with an H-V interval ≥ 80 to 100 msec. In the absence of inducible ventricular tachyarrhythmias or in the absence of identifiable significant sinus node or AV node disease in such patients, or another cause of syncope such as carotid sinus hypersensitivity, we infuse procainamide to evaluate the response of the His-Purkinje system to the pharmacologic stress. If the H-V interval lengthens to 80 to 100 msec or more, or if infra-His block develops, pacing is recommended in patients who have cardiogenic syncope or other symptoms referable to heart block.

Patients who have bi- or trifascicular block without symptoms of presyncope or syncope are not treated with permanent pacing and do not require further investigation. Such patients likewise are not subjected to temporary pacing in preparation for surgery or other procedures.

CLINICAL SELECTION OF VARIOUS PACING MODES

Available pulse generators are capable of pacing either in a single chamber or in both chambers with back-up programming available to allow pacing in a single chamber. Virtually all available pulse generators are multiprogrammable, which provides extreme adaptability to changing clinical situations. The increasing complexity of pacemaker pulse generator design has been accompanied by escalating cost, an issue of increasing importance.

Several factors are important in the choice of pacing mode. In general, patients with heart block are treated with single-chamber pacemakers and function in a ventricular inhibited mode. The exceptions to this rule are patients who have intact retrograde VA conduction and are potential candidates for the pacemaker syndrome. Other exceptions to ventricular pacing alone include patients who have had known "pacemaker syndrome" or symptoms produced by temporary ventricular pacing before or at the time of initial pacemaker implantation, and patients who require maximal atrial contribution because of hemodynamic impairment, increased left ventricular compliance, or a special need for rate responsiveness. These patients are all better served by dual-chamber pacing.

The pacemaker syndrome initially was defined simply as lightheadedness or syncope related to long cycles of ventriculoatrial association, with 1:1 VA conduction that occurred during VVI or VOO pacing. The definition of the pacemaker syndrome has been expanded to include episodic weakness or syncope associated with periods of AV association, probably due to a reflex response mediated by atrial receptors.

LONG-TERM MANAGEMENT

Patients treated with permanent pacing for manifestations of heart block or who undergo prophylactic permanent pacing because of a concomitant need for drug therapy should be followed at regular intervals. We currently examine patients one month after pacemaker implantation and then evaluate pacemaker performance utilizing transtelephonic transmissions on a quarterly basis.

Asymptomatic patients with first-degree heart block, Mobitz Type I second-degree heart block, or bi- or trifascicular heart block require routine follow-up and education regarding the need to report symptoms possibly related to bradycardia. No special precautions are necessary for these patients, but if symptoms potentially referable to transient heart block develop they should be considered for permanent pacing. When there is still clinical uncertainty regarding the need for permanent pacing in relation to symptoms not easily referable to transient heart block, invasive electrophysiologic studies may help provide information necessary to make a decision. Unfortunately, there are no reliable noninvasive studies available today to help answer this question unless an episode is documented during a period of ambulatory EKG monitoring. New recording systems are being developed that allow continuous EKG monitoring for prolonged periods in which a microprocessor continuously stores several minutes of information. At the time when patients feel an unusual event, or if they have syncope that is witnessed and the device can be signaled by a bystander, these microprocessors record enough information to document the rhythm at the time of the symptom. In between times when patients are asymptomatic, the memory of this microprocessor can be cleared continuously by one of several methods. It remains questionable whether these devices will be available in large numbers and will be reliable enough to use in these clinical circumstances.

REFERENCES

Mond HG: The bradyarrhythmias: current indications for permanent pacing (I and II). PACE 4:432–442, 538–547, 1981.

Nishimura RA, Gersh BJ, Holmes DR, et al.: Outcome of dual-chamber pacing for the pacemaker syndrome. Mayo Clin Proc 58:452–456, 1983.

Rossi L: Anatomopathology of the normal and abnormal AV conduction system. PACE 7:1101–1107, 1984.

Special Report: Guidelines for permanent cardiac pacemaker implantation. A report of the Joint American College of Cardiology/American Heart Association Task Force on Assessment of Cardiovascular Procedures. JACC 4:434–442, 1984.

12 · ARRHYTHMIAS

David W. Snyder
OCHSNER CLINIC AND ALTON OCHSNER MEDICAL FOUNDATION

The various cardiac arrhythmias differ in underlying electrophysiology, site of origin within the heart, hemodynamic consequence, prognosis, and response to therapy. Furthermore, a given arrhythmia will vary in clinical impact among different patients owing to differences in arrhythmia frequency and duration, heart rate, and underlying cardiac pathology. When an individual presents with arrhythmia, the first goal is to document its type and mechanism. The second is to decide whether or not (and how urgently) it must be treated. Drug therapy can then be rationally prescribed, with subsequent methodical assessment of the effectiveness of the treatment. This chapter explores management problems and strategies as they apply to three commonly encountered rhythm disorders.

Atrial Fibrillation

DEFINITION

Atrial fibrillation is a common arrhythmia characterized by completely disordered depolarizations of the atria and "wavelets" of activation fronts bombarding the AV node. These wavefronts may collide with each other and cancel or they may conduct into the AV junction. Many impulses block in the AV node owing to refractoriness following an earlier depolarization, but others conduct to the ventricles. The resultant rhythm is rapid (100 to 160 per minute) and irregular.

CLINICAL ASSESSMENT

Atrial fibrillation is suggested clinically by the irregularity of the tachycardia. Marked variability in cycle length results in variable diastolic filling of the ventricles. Following short cycles, little blood is ejected and no peripheral pulse is palpable. Thus, the true pulse rate exceeds the palpated radial pulse. Variable diastolic filling time also explains the changing intensity of the first heart sound. The electrocardiogram shows atrial fibrillatory waves of varying amplitude and rate (350 to 600 per minute) but no discrete P waves. The QRS morphology is usually normal, though aberrant intraventricular conduction occurs with early beats, especially if they follow a preceding long cycle length (Ashman's phenomenon).

Atrial fibrillation may occur in the absence of predisposing cardiovascular disorder and is then referred to as lone atrial fibrillation. However, in 70% of cases the arrhythmia results from preexisting metabolic disturbance or pulmonary or cardiac pathology. Patients with rheumatic mitral valve disease are at highest risk but, because of its prevalence, hypertension is the most common factor producing atrial fibrillation in the U.S. Chronic atrial fibrillation is usually due to underlying heart disease, whereas paroxysmal atrial fibrillation is often seen in the absence of other problems. Atrial fibrillation with a slow ventricular response in the absence of drug therapy implies impaired AV nodal conduction and is commonly associated with concomitant sinus node dysfunction. Very rapid atrial fibrillation should suggest hyperthyroidism or one of the ventricular preexcitation syndromes.

PATHOPHYSIOLOGY

Hemodynamic consequences of atrial fibrillation relate both to the rapid heart rate and to the loss of atrial systole. As the heart rate accelerates, myocardial oxygen demand increases and diastolic coronary perfusion time is reduced, precipitating angina in individuals with coronary artery disease or left ventricular hypertrophy. The loss of atrial contraction reduces left ventricular filling, particularly in patients with poor left ventricular compliance (as in coronary heart disease, hypertension, or hypertrophic cardiomyopathy). Cardiac output declines by 15% to 30%, and systemic and pulmonary venous pressures rise. Drugs that slow the heart rate allow more time for passive ventricular filling, but cardiac output will remain low until effective atrial systole can be restored.

An additional consequence of atrial fibrillation is enlargement of the atria and stasis of blood within the noncontracting chambers. This predisposes to intra-atrial thrombosis and systemic embolization. Thrombosis is most common in patients with markedly dilated atria (as in mitral valve disease and hypertrophic cardiomyopathy) or those with a very low cardiac output. Even patients with structurally normal hearts face a fivefold increased risk of stroke due to embolization; there is a 17-fold increased risk in patients with rheumatic heart disease.

MANAGEMENT

Management of patients with atrial fibrillation should include an evaluation of the predisposing cause and judicious treatment of the rhythm disorder. Hyperthyroidism may present with atrial fibrillation in the absence of other clinical manifestations, especially in the elderly. In patients with chronic lung disease or heart disease, optimal treatment of the underlying disorder may greatly facilitate restoration and maintenance of sinus rhythm. Electrolyte imbalance, particularly hypokalemia, must be corrected.

The specific treatment of atrial fibrillation differs according to the urgency of the situation. In sick sinus syndrome, atrial fibrillation may represent a welcome change from symptomatic bradyarrhythmias and, unless the ventricular rate is excessive, may require no therapy. The patient with mitral stenosis tolerates atrial fibrillation poorly and can present with pulmonary edema requiring immediate electrical cardioversion. In most instances, however, the primary goal is rate control, achieved by suppressing conduction through the AV node. This can often be accomplished on an outpatient basis, with follow-up adjustment of drug doses according to rate response.

Digoxin may be given PO or IV. A loading dose is required to achieve prompt effects, with a total loading dose of 1.0 to 1.5 mg over the first 24 hours. Thereafter, the usual daily dose is 0.125 to 0.5 mg, depending on rate response, body size, and renal function. Doses should be lower in the elderly, regardless of serum creatinine levels.

An exception to the use of digoxin is the patient with paroxysmal atrial fibrillation without structural heart disease. Fibrillation often occurs at times of augmented vagal tone, such as after meals or during sleep. Digoxin has profibrillatory effects in these patients; this is probably partly due to its vagotonic properties. Digoxin should usually be avoided in lone atrial fibrillation.

Digoxin slows the resting heart rate but is less effective when sympathetic tone is high, such as with exercise or during an acute illness. High doses of digoxin in the acutely ill patient are unlikely to provide adequate rate control but are more likely to cause serious toxicity. The addition of a beta-adrenergic blocking drug offers better rate control in this setting. A beta-blocker may be given PO, beginning at low doses, and titrated against the heart rate response. In an acute condition, propranolol (up to 0.1 mg/kg) or metoprolol (up to 0.2 mg/kg) can be given IV with cautious monitoring of BP and heart rate.

If there is coexistent lung disease, peripheral vascular disease, or heart failure, beta-blocking drugs may be contraindicated. A rate-lowering calcium channel blocker such as verapamil or diltiazem should then be considered. Verapamil may be given IV over 10 to 15 minutes to a total dose of 0.15 mg/kg, to acutely lower the rate. If atrial fibrillation is of recent onset, this restores sinus rhythm in about 15% of patients. Since verapamil is a vasodilator, BP should be monitored closely and hypotension treated by withholding verapamil, volume expansion, and (if needed) administration of vasopressors or calcium. Verapamil (80 to 120 mg t.i.d.) or diltiazem (30 to 90 mg q.i.d.) may be given PO to maintain control of AV conduction. Verapamil, but not diltiazem, has significant negative inotropic effects and may aggravate or precipitate congestive heart failure in predisposed individuals. Verapamil reduces the clearance of digoxin as well as its volume of distribution. The digoxin dose should be halved when verapamil is added, and blood levels of digoxin should be measured.

RESTORATION OF SINUS RHYTHM

Rate control generally is easily achieved and maintained in the outpatient setting. When atrial fibrillation is of recent onset, digoxin, with or without a betablocker or calcium channel blocker, may also restore sinus rhythm in a significant number of patients. However, atrial fibrillation that is long-standing or that occurs in the digitalized patient is less likely to resolve. Cardioversion may then be considered, based on such important factors as the potential hemodynamic benefit from sinus rhythm, the likelihood of maintaining sinus rhythm in the long term, the toxicity of drugs required to preserve sinus rhythm, and the chance of systemic embolization at the time of cardioversion (Table 1). When atrial fibrillation is poorly tolerated, cardioversion should be attempted even if the chance of persistent sinus rhythm is remote. Type Ia antiarrhythmic drugs

Table 1. ATRIAL FIBRILLATION: FACTORS PREDISPOSING TO THROMBOEMBOLISM AND RECURRENT FIBRILLATION

Thromboembolism	Recurrent Fibrillation
Mitral valve disease	Mitral valve disease
Recent-onset fibrillation	Long-standing fibrillation
Prior emboli	Prior recurrence
Very large left atrium	Very large left atrium
Prosthetic mitral valve	Persistent thyrotoxicosis
Congestive heart failure	Intolerance to antiarrhythmics

such as quinidine, procainamide, or disopyramide phosphate should be used in preparation for cardioversion, and in 20% of patients brings about "chemical" conversion to sinus rhythm.

Certain cautions should be noted in the use of these drugs. All antiarrhythmic drugs can exacerbate arrhythmia, and quinidine produces torsade de pointes pleomorphic ventricular tachycardia in 5% of patients with atrial fibrillation. This life-threatening arrhythmia is more likely in patients with a prolonged EKG QT interval prior to therapy, those with hypokalemia or hypomagnesemia, and those using other drugs that may prolong the QT interval. If such predisposing factors exist, hospital admission for treatment should be considered.

Quinidine reduces the clearance of digoxin as well as its volume of distribution, so that digitalis intoxication may be precipitated by the addition of quinidine. In this event, the digoxin dose should be reduced by half and plasma digoxin levels monitored. Procainamide and disopyramide also may cause torsade de pointes ventricular tachycardia, but they do not alter digoxin pharmacokinetics.

ANTICOAGULATION

Anticoagulation lowers the risk of peripheral embolization in patients with chronic atrial fibrillation and in those undergoing cardioversion. High-risk patients (see Table 1) should be anticoagulated with heparin and/or warfarin for two weeks before chemical or electrical cardioversion. If atrial fibrillation is chronic, patients should continue taking warfarin indefinitely. Antiplatelet drugs have not been shown to prevent intracardiac thrombosis and are not recommended.

Once antiarrhythmic therapy has been initiated, adequate plasma drug levels attained, and anticoagulation maintained for two weeks in high-risk patients, electrical cardioversion is attempted. Over 90% of patients convert to sinus rhythm with DC shock, although only 30% to 50% remain in sinus rhythm for 12 months. Those who revert to atrial fibrillation can generally be managed best by controlling the heart rate with digoxin and providing chronic anticoagulation if embolic risks are high. However, repeated cardioversions may be justified if fibrillation is poorly tolerated. Amiodarone, an investigational antiarrhythmic drug, may succeed in preserving sinus rhythm when other drugs have failed.

Paroxysmal Atrial Tachycardia

DEFINITION

Paroxysmal atrial tachycardia (PAT) is a descriptive term that encompasses several different types of supraventricular arrhythmias. These arrhythmias are rapid and regular, and begin and end abruptly. The patient with PAT notes a sudden onset of fluttering in the chest that may be associated with shortness of breath, lightheadedness, or chest tightness. Typical anginal pains may occur even in the absence of coronary artery disease. Rest and recumbency may alleviate the tachycardia, and some patients learn to use cough or Valsalva maneuvers to terminate the arrhythmia.

The history often suggests the correct diagnosis, although paroxysmal atrial fibrillation or episodes of sustained ventricular tachycardia can present similarly. A definitive diagnosis is based on EKG findings during an episode of tachycardia. The patient should be instructed to report for an EKG when sustained tachycardia occurs. If this is not feasible, a device for transmitting the EKG by telephone is invaluable (e.g., a Cardiobeeper). The EKG shows a regular tachycardia, generally with a normal QRS configuration. Occasionally, aberrant intraventricular conduction produces a wide-complex tachycardia difficult to distinguish from ventricular tachycardia. The demonstration of AV dissociation by routine EKG or by esophageal or intracardiac recordings makes ventricular tachycardia likely; a typical right or left bundle branch block pattern favors PAT. A very wide QRS complex (more than 140 msec) is uncommon with PAT, as is a frontal plane QRS axis in the superior, leftward quadrant (−90 to −180 degrees). Termination of the arrhythmia by vagal maneuvers is more likely in PAT than in ventricular tachycardia.

ELECTROPHYSIOLOGY

PAT may be due to enhanced automaticity of the atria or AV node, but more often is due to reentry. The most common site of reentry is within the AV node and depends on slow conduction in a circular pattern through dual AV nodal pathways. The AV nodal pathways differ in their conduction velocity, refractoriness, and response to antiarrhythmic drugs. Typically, AV nodal reentry is initiated by an atrial premature depolarization that conducts down the slow-conducting pathway to excite the ventricles and returns via the faster pathway to reexcite the atria as well as the proximal portion of the slow AV pathway.

The second common form of PAT is due to reentry via an anomalous AV bypass tract. In most instances, this tract is capable of only retrograde conduction from ventricle to atrium and is termed a "concealed" bypass tract. Other bypass tracts conduct antegrade during sinus rhythm and preexcite the ventricles, giving rise to the characteristic EKG delta wave in Wolff-Parkinson-

White syndrome. In either case, the bypass tract generally conducts in a retrograde fashion during PAT, antegrade conduction being mediated by the AV node and His-Purkinje system. The rhythm is rapid, usually >200 beats per minute, and the QRS is followed by an inverted P wave with a short R-P interval.

Uncommon causes of reentrant PAT involve reentry within the sinoatrial node or within the atria themselves. Other uncommon types of PAT are due to enhanced automaticity. In contrast to reentrant tachycardias, automatic tachycardias generally reflect some underlying disease process or drug effect. Thus, automatic atrial tachycardia is seen with sick sinus syndrome, chronic lung disease, myocarditis, myocardial infarction, acute ethanol ingestion, or digitalis intoxication. Management of automatic tachycardias centers on appropriate therapy for the underlying condition, antiarrhythmic therapy being reserved for arrhythmia that persists afterward.

MANAGEMENT

Since in 90% of cases PAT is due to a reentrant circuit utilizing the AV node, vagal maneuvers that slow conduction within the AV node may terminate the reentry cycle. Initial management should include calm reassurance, and placement of the patient in the supine position to reduce sympathetic tone. The Valsalva maneuver, followed by cautious carotid sinus massage, may be effective. If not, vagal effects can be potentiated by IV administration of edrophonium chloride (Tensilon). A test dose of 2 to 5 mg is followed by the remainder of a 10-mg dose, and carotid massage is repeated. Verapamil, however, has largely replaced other drugs in the initial therapy for reentrant PAT. When given IV in a total dose of 0.15 mg/kg (as outlined in the section on atrial fibrillation), this calcium channel blocker is effective in 90% of patients. However, because verapamil is a vasodilator, it should be given cautiously to hypotensive individuals. Instead, phenylephrine given as a slow bolus dose of 0.5 to 1.0 mg will increase BP and, through baroreceptor-mediated vagal stimulation, may terminate the arrhythmia. If the arrhythmia persists, verapamil can then be used with less concern for hypotension.

Other drugs that have been utilized acutely are now rarely needed because of the predictable efficacy of verapamil. Propranolol and digoxin in full loading IV doses have been effective in the past. The combined use of IV propranolol and verapamil is contraindicated, since cases of asystole and severe hypotension have followed this combination. The unstable patient who does not respond promptly to therapy should have cardioversion with low-energy DC shock, and further pharmacologic manipulations should not be risked.

Long-term management of PAT depends on the frequency and severity of attacks. Infrequent episodes can be treated as they arise with vagal maneuvers or a cocktail of drugs known to be effective. Verapamil alone (160 to 240 mg PO) or in combination with a beta-blocker and/or sedative may be rapidly effective and avert expensive visits to the emergency department. If attacks are frequent or very severe, maintenance therapy is needed to prevent recurrence. Digoxin alone is the initial drug of choice as it is easily taken and tolerated. When digoxin alone is ineffective and adequate plasma levels have been attained (1.5 to 2.0 ng/ml), a second drug may be added to further suppress the AV node. Any of the beta-blocking agents (except perhaps pindolol, which has little beta-blocking effect at rest) can be added and the dose titrated to reduce the resting and exercise heart rate. Alternatively, either verapamil (80 to 120 mg three times daily) or diltiazem (60 to 120 mg three or four times daily) can be used. When given PO, these agents are not as universally effective as when given IV, and high doses are often required. Nifedipine has no effect on the AV node or on arrhythmia.

Combinations of drugs that slow AV nodal conduction are sometimes ineffective. However, the retrograde fast AV nodal pathway as well as the AV bypass tract can be suppressed with membrane-active antiarrhythmic agents. When other measures fail, one may add or substitute quinidine, procainamide, or disopyramide phosphate in standard doses. Amiodarone blocks both antegrade and retrograde limbs of these reentrant circuits and is highly effective in controlling otherwise refractory PAT.

ELECTROPHYSIOLOGIC TESTING

Since episodes of PAT are sporadic, it is difficult to be sure whether a drug regimen is effective. In problematic cases, the induction of PAT with programmed atrial stimulation can permit rapid assessment of treatment efficacy. Drugs that terminate and prevent induction of PAT in the laboratory are generally effective long term. If no effective drug is found, pacing modalities can be tested to terminate the arrhythmia electrically. A permanently implanted pacemaker can then be programmed to interrupt spontaneous PAT. When PAT is mediated by reentry through an anomalous pathway, that pathway can be localized by mapping techniques and then surgically divided or destroyed by electrical catheter ablation, thus removing the substrate for reentry.

The Wolff-Parkinson-White syndrome requires special precautions. Since the AV bypass tract can conduct antegrade to the ventricles, it may transmit atrial activity rapidly during atrial fibrillation. A drug that shortens the refractory period of the bypass tract will accelerate the ventricular rate in atrial fibrillation, which explains episodes of circulatory collapse and death in this setting. Digoxin should not be used unless its effects on refractoriness in the bypass tract have been established. Membrane-active drugs, on the other hand, prolong refractoriness and are particularly effective in patients with the Wolff-Parkinson-White syndrome. Surgical interruption of the bypass tract should be considered in patients known to have a short antegrade refractory period.

Ventricular Arrhythmias

CLINICAL ASSESSMENT

Ventricular ectopic activity (VEA) occurs in most healthy adults and in most patients with intrinsic heart disease. Some degree of VEA is therefore normal and expected. On the other hand, complex VEA in patients with advanced heart disease has been associated with a high risk of sudden death due to ventricular fibrillation. The principal task when evaluating the patient with VEA is therefore a careful assessment of risk and the likelihood of modifying that risk through suppression of ventricular arrhythmias.

Advanced left ventricular dysfunction, whether due to coronary artery disease, cardiomyopathy, or other processes, is the strongest factor predisposing to sudden cardiac death. However, when left ventricular failure is the result of ischemic heart disease, particularly in the face of left ventricular aneurysm or recent myocardial infarction, it becomes even more ominous. Additional risk factors include the extent of occlusive coronary disease, the presence of inducible myocardial ischemia, and the complexity of VEA. This last-named factor has received a great deal of attention, especially in survivors of acute myocardial infarction. Increasing frequency of ventricular ectopy, especially when associated with ventricular couplets and salvoes of ventricular tachycardia, has been associated with progressively higher rates of sudden death. Whether this association is causal, and whether suppression of high-grade VEA can modify the sudden death risk, have been debated. However, evidence now supports arrhythmia suppression in patients at high risk because of the demonstrated reduction in mortality in treated patients.

MANAGEMENT

When approaching the patient with VEA, an assessment of left ventricular function, underlying heart disease, coronary anatomy, and the frequency and complexity of ventricular arrhythmia should precede any decision regarding therapy. The patient with a structurally normal heart rarely requires treatment unless the observed ventricular arrhythmia is itself directly life-threatening. The patient with recent infarction and left ventricular failure may merit treatment for frequent VEA, even if ventricular tachycardia has not been observed. Occasionally, a patient will be at intermediate risk, and the decision to treat may be quite difficult. In this instance, treatment may be considered optional and therapy continued only if an effective regimen can be found easily that is well tolerated by the patient.

Effective treatment of VEA is a demanding process that requires the use of potentially toxic drugs that have no predictable effect on the arrhythmia. Any given drug may suppress the arrhythmia, have no effect, or in 5% to 15% of cases actually worsen the arrhythmia. A careful strategy is needed to document treatment efficacy and to screen for pro-arrhythmic effects. The two most widely used approaches have been based either on suppression of spontaneous arrhythmia as documented by ambulatory monitoring or on the ability to prevent ventricular tachycardia induced by invasive programmed stimulation of the ventricles.

The noninvasive approach requires that arrhythmia documented by ambulatory monitoring and exercise stress testing be reproducible from one day to another. Spontaneous fluctuation in arrhythmia frequency and complexity can give the false impression of drug efficacy. However, as pointed out by Lown and collaborators, patients with frequent and high-grade arrhythmia usually have little significant variability in ambient arrhythmia. Their group has established criteria for adequate arrhythmia suppression and documented a dramatic improvement in long-term prognosis when a drug regimen providing this suppression can be found. Complete elimination of ventricular tachycardia, 90% suppression of couplets, and 50% reduction in total ventricular premature beats during ambulatory monitoring and exercise testing must be achieved for satisfactory rhythm control.

In at least one third of patients with documented, life-threatening ventricular arrhythmia, ambulatory monitoring shows infrequent or low-grade VEA. In these cases, arrhythmia reproducibility is low and the noninvasive approach has no reliable end point by which to gauge treatment. Invasive ventricular stimulation should be performed for these patients in an attempt to reproducibly induce ventricular tachycardia. A drug regimen that subsequently eliminates inducibility of ventricular tachycardia is generally effective in preventing the spontaneous arrhythmia.

ANTIARRHYTHMIC AGENTS

Regardless of which method is used, the goal is to find a drug or combination of drugs that is effective and can be tolerated by the patient. Until recently, this goal has been extremely difficult to reach with only the Type Ia drugs quinidine, procainamide, and disopyramide phosphate, all three of which have common side effects and serious potential toxicity (Table 2). All share similar electrophysiologic effects, and thus an arrhythmia refractory to one agent is somewhat less likely to respond to the other related drugs. Newer agents are now being approved for use in the U.S. that have very different electrophysiologic effects and are better tolerated by patients. Tocainide is a Type Ib drug similar to lidocaine, but it can be taken orally. It can be given two or three times daily, is cleared predominantly by the kidneys, and has side effects that are usually minor and dose dependent. In contrast to Type Ia drugs, tocainide has little effect on contractility, sinus node function, or intraventricular conduction. A trial of IV lidocaine may predict the effect of tocainide, as most patients who respond to one drug will respond to the other.

An antiarrhythmic drug recently marketed in this country, flecainide, has the advantages of unique electrophysiology, high rate of efficacy, and relatively few side effects. However, flecainide does have negative inotropic effects as well as a depressant effect on the AV node and intraventricular conduction. It should be used with caution in patients with left ventricular dysfunction or preexisting intraventricular conduction defects. The drug has a long half-life and can be administered twice daily. Proarrhythmic effects with flecainide appear less commonly than with quinidine.

Amiodarone is a Type III antiarrhythmic agent that

Table 2. ORALLY ACTIVE ANTIARRHYTHMIC DRUGS

Class	Drug	Dose (mg)	Clearance	Adverse Effects
Ia	Quinidine	200–400 q.i.d.	Hepatic	GI intolerance, fever, cinchonism, thrombocytopenia, hemolytic anemia, elevation of digoxin levels.
	Procainamide	500–1500 q.i.d. (sustained release)	Renal/hepatic	GI intolerance, fever, rash, CNS effects (confusion, hallucination), agranulocytosis, lupus syndrome.
	Disopyramide	100–200 q.i.d.	Renal	Anticholinergic effects, negative inotropic effects.
Ib	Phenytoin	300–400 q.d.	Hepatic	Cerebellar dysfunction, megaloblastic anemia, neuropathy, lupus syndrome, lower quinidine levels.
	Tocainide	400–600 t.i.d.	Renal/hepatic	GI intolerance, CNS effects (dizziness, tremor, confusion), hypotension, ?pulmonary fibrosis.
Ic	Flecainide	100–300 b.i.d.	Hepatic	Dizziness, visual disturbance, negative inotropic effect, impaired AV and intraventricular conduction.
II	Beta-blockers	Variable	Variable	Negative inotropic and chronotropic effects, bronchoconstriction, vasoconstriction, depression.
III	Amiodarone	200–600 q.d.	Unknown	Corneal microdeposits, constipation, photosensitivity, thyroid dysfunction, pulmonry fibrosis, hepatitis, elevated digoxin levels.
IV	Verapamil	80–120 t.i.d.	Hepatic	Negative inotropic and chronotropic effects, constipation, elevated digoxin levels.
	Diltiazem	30–120 q.i.d.	Hepatic	Negative chronotropic effects, edema.

markedly prolongs the action potential and refractory period in all cardiac tissues. The drug has complex pharmacokinetics including poor bioavailability, a very large volume of distribution, and a low rate of clearance. These result in a plasma half-life measured in weeks rather than hours, a prolonged period required for loading before a steady state is reached, and variability in required maintenance dose among individuals. This agent will soon be available in the U.S. and has been used extensively as an investigational drug. It is remarkably effective in the treatment of atrial, ventricular, and AV reentrant arrhythmias. Amiodarone has been effective in 75% of patients with recurrent ventricular tachycardia refractory to standard drugs. Although it generally is well tolerated, constipation, photosensitivity, and asymptomatic corneal microdeposits are very common. Serious toxicity, including thyroid dysfunction, reversible liver function abnormalities, and life-threatening pulmonary fibrosis, are being increasingly recognized.

The availability of these newer drugs should increase our ability to control dangerous ventricular arrhythmias without causing intolerable side effects. Certain important principles may help in the selection of a proper drug regimen. First, a "therapeutic" plasma level is that which controls arrhythmia without toxicity, regardless of what value returns from a laboratory assay. One should not discard a drug as ineffective unless the dose has been pressed to maximally tolerated levels, nor should one increase the dose of an already effective drug just because of low measured plasma levels. Nonetheless, plasma levels are useful to document patient compliance, to assess drug absorption and elimination, and to ensure that high levels have been attained before abandoning the drug. When arrhythmia recurs despite apparent initial control, measurement of the plasma drug level is essential in order to judge dosing adequacy.

Another important consideration is that electrolyte imbalance may dramatically affect the response to therapy. Hypomagnesemia and particularly hypokalemia must be corrected. Similarly, concomitant drug therapy must be examined. Digoxin has been shown to suppress arrhythmia in about one half of patients, but can aggravate arrhythmia in one third. Concomitant use of quinidine, verapamil, or amiodarone significantly reduces digoxin clearance and elevates plasma levels. Phenytoin,

a rather weak antiarrhythmic agent, has been used in combination regimens but markedly accelerates the clearance of quinidine and disopyramide, thus requiring that these drugs be given in higher doses and more frequently. Drugs with negative inotropic effects, such as beta-blockers, disopyramide, flecainide, amiodarone, or verapamil, have additive effects and should not be combined in patients with left ventricular dysfunction.

On the other hand, certain drug combinations have been found effective in treating otherwise refractory arrhythmia. Many of the electrophysiologic effects of membrane-active drugs are reversed by catecholamine stimulation. This can be avoided by the addition of a beta-blocking drug with resultant improved efficacy. The combination of a Type Ia and Type Ib drug may be effective when either alone is not. This has been best documented with the combination of mexiletine (a lidocaine-like drug) and quinidine or procainamide. When no effective regimen can be found, referral for the use of investigational drugs or for surgical arrhythmia ablation might be considered.

Regardless of which therapeutic avenue is ultimately chosen, initial arrhythmia suppression must be documented. However, the realities of a clinical practice are such that no regimen is guaranteed long term. Side effects prompt dosage changes, companion drugs are altered, electrolytes may vary, and the underlying heart condition may progress. Follow-up evaluation is mandatory. Ambulatory monitoring must be repeated on a regular basis, the frequency depending on the severity of the initial arrhythmia. Reevaluation is also appropriate after any change in cardiac status, such as following myocardial infarction, revascularization, or left ventricular aneurysm repair.

REFERENCES

Benditt DG, Benson DW Jr, Dunningan A, et al: Atrial flutter, atrial fibrillation, and other primary atrial tachycardias. Med Clin N Am 68:895–918, 1984.

Benditt DG, Benson DW Jr, Klein GJ, et al: Prevention of recurrent sudden cardiac arrest: role of provocative electropharmacologic testing. J Am Coll Cardiol 2:418–425, 1983.

Graboys TB, Lown B, Podrid PJ, et al: Long-term survival of patients with malignant ventricular arrhythmia treated with antiarrhythmic drugs. Am J Cardiol 50:437–443, 1982.

Josephson ME, Kastor JA: Supraventricular tachycardia: mechanisms and management. Ann Intern Med 87:346–358, 1977.

Torres V, Flowers D, Somberg JC: The arrhythmogenicity of antiarrhythmic agents. Am Heart J 109:1090–1097, 1985.

13 · DISEASES OF THE PERICARDIUM AND MYOCARDIUM

Charles A. Laubach, Jr.
GEISINGER MEDICAL CENTER

The incidence of cardiomyopathies seen in the ambulatory clinic has increased in the past decade. Depending on the demographics of the population served, estimates of current incidence range from 5% to 15%.

PATHOPHYSIOLOGY

Myocardial systolic function is concerned with contractility. Myocardial diastolic function is concerned with relaxation. When contractility is normal, stroke volume and cardiac output vary directly with preload and inversely with afterload. With abnormal contractile function the modification of preload, afterload, or both allows the physician to improve cardiac output. Ventricular filling is dependent, at least to some extent, on myocardial relaxation. Impaired relaxation affects diastolic function. Normal pericardium has both systolic and diastolic functions: it (1) prevents heart chamber dilatation, (2) prevents ventricular hypertrophy in response to strenuous exercise, (3) limits right ventricular stroke work with left ventricular outflow resistance, and (4) prevents ventriculoatrial regurgitation in the presence of increased ventricular end-diastolic pressure.

An abnormal amount of fluid in the pericardial space or constrictive disease of the pericardium impairs diastolic function—relaxation of the myocardium. *Systolic* dysfunction is commonly associated with increased chamber volume—a dilated cardiomyopathy. *Diastolic* dysfunction, due to infiltrative myocardial disease or constrictive pericardial disease, usually has a nondilated chamber or only mildly dilated chambers—a restrictive cardiomyopathy. *Combined* systolic and diastolic dysfunction is associated with hypertrophic cardiomyopathy. Early in the natural history of hypertrophic cardiomyopathy there may be normal or supernormal systolic function; later it becomes depressed and chamber dilatation may develop. This pathophysiologic approach to myopericardial diseases provides a convenient clinical scheme to classify them physiologically and anatomically.

Pathophysiology	*Pathoanatomy*
Systolic dysfunction	→ *Dilated cardiomyopathy*
	→ *Hypertrophic cardiomyopathy*
Diastolic dysfunction	→ *Restrictive cardiomyopathy*

Dilated cardiomyopathy, the most frequently encountered, generally has multiple chamber involvement with near-normal wall thickness. Systolic function impairment is present because of a generalized decrease in contractility. By contrast, in ischemic cardiomyopathy the left ventricle is predominantly involved with segmental contractile defects and segmental wall thinning where there is scar formation due to infarction.

Hypertrophic cardiomyopathy may be generalized or focal, such as septal or apical hypertrophy. Septal involvement can result in obstruction to one or both ventricular outflow tracts. Most commonly the left ventricle is involved. The left ventricular cavity is not dilated, although dilatation may occur late in the natural history of the obstructive type. The anterior leaflet of the mitral valve moves anteriorly in systole, contributing to the obstruction of the left ventricular outflow tract. There is premature closure of the aortic valve.

Restrictive myocardial disease is usually due to an infiltrative myocardial disease, such as amyloidosis. However, it can be caused by constrictive pericardial disease or, rarely, endomyocardial fibrosis. Generally, an increase in wall thickness can be documented by echocardiography. The ventricles are not dilated. With pericardial or endocardial disease, ventricular filling is impaired but contractile function is fairly well preserved. With infiltrative myocardial disease, both systolic and diastolic function may be impaired. Good-quality echocardiography can demonstrate abnormal endocardial or pericardial thickening and a hyperrefractile granular and sparkling appearance of the myocardium in infiltrative disease, such as amyloidosis.

CLINICAL ASPECTS

The most frequent symptomatic presentation for the dilated and restrictive cardiomyopathies is dyspnea or some degree of congestive heart failure. A few patients with dilated cardiomyopathy present with a rhythm disorder. In contrast, most patients with hypertrophic cardiomyopathies are asymptomatic when initially seen, having been referred because of a heart murmur or an abnormal EKG. Only a small number present because of dyspnea on effort or arrhythmia. All patients with dilated cardiomyopathies have evidence of cardiac enlargement on physical examination. An S_3 gallop sound can be heard in three fourths of the patients, and an apical systolic murmur consistent with mitral regurgitation in more than one third.

In most cases of obstructive cardiomyopathies a systolic ejection murmur is heard along the left sternal border and in the apical region, modified in intensity by physiologic maneuvers—handgrip or squatting.

DIAGNOSTIC STUDIES

Echocardiography is the most useful laboratory study in the diagnosis of myopericardial disease because it provides both anatomic and physiologic information. Doppler flow studies expand the physiologic parameters. In obstructive hypertrophic cardiomyopathy the systolic gradient across the obstruction in the ventricular outflow tract can be estimated. With echocardiography, serial examinations can be used to follow the clinical course and the response to treatment.

Used selectively, endomyocardial biopsy represents another useful diagnostic tool. It can be performed safely during one-day hospitalization. It is helpful in documenting the type of restrictive disorder (infiltrative myocardial process, constrictive pericardial disease, or, rarely, endomyocardial disease), and when dilated cardiomyopathy is caused by acute inflammatory myocarditis.

The EKG frequently shows a pattern of left ventricular hypertrophy in hypertrophic cardiomyopathy, particularly if there is outflow tract obstruction. Septal hypertrophy may be associated with Q waves in the right precordial leads, a pseudoinfarction pattern. The dilated and restrictive cardiomyopathies have a broad spectrum of nonspecific EKG findings: low voltage, conduction defects, and nonspecific ST–T wave abnormalities.

Finally, ambulatory electrocardiography (Holter) has had selective usefulness in identifying patients with cardiomyopathy who are at increased risk owing to the random occurrence of complex ventricular ectopy including ventricular tachycardia.

MANAGEMENT

DILATED CARDIOMYOPATHY

Since most of the dilated cardiomyopathies are of unknown etiology, treatment is directed toward improving contractile function. A digitalis preparation, digoxin, continues to be the principal inotropic agent for outpatient management. If edema is present, preload reduction with a diuretic, such as furosemide in initial dosage of 20 to 40 mg daily, is the next pharmacologic intervention. If there is no edema, a nondiuretic preload reducing agent, such as a nitrate, in combination with digoxin may further improve systolic function.

Excessive diuresis should be avoided to prevent volume depletion. Excessive volume depletion can result in below-optimal preload and paradoxic reversal of clinical improvement.

Periodic determinations of serum digoxin and potassium levels should be performed to minimize the risk of deleterious rhythm disorders due to digitalis toxicity and/or hypokalemia. If preload reduction alone is not sufficient, gradual afterload reduction must be achieved in order to decrease left ventricular work. A number of agents have been demonstrated to be of value: nitrates alone, hydralazine, hydralazine in combination with nitrates, prazosin, angiotensin inhibitors (e.g., captopril) with a calcium blocking agent (e.g., nifedipine).

Table 1. DRUGS IN THE TREATMENT OF MYOCARDIAL DISEASE

Cardiotonic	
Digoxin	0.25 mg once
Venous pooling	
Nitroglycerin	2.5–6.5 mg b.i.d.
Nitrates (Peritrate, Isorbide)	20–30 mg q.i.d.
Arterial dilatation	
Hydralazine (Apresoline)	25–50 mg q.i.d.
Nifedipine (Procardia)	10–20 mg t.i.d.
Venous and arterial pooling	
Prazosin (Minipress)	1–5 mg q.i.d.
Captopril (Capoten)	12.5–25 mg t.i.d.
Diuretics	
Furosemide (Lasix)	20–40 mg b.i.d.
Ethacrynic acid (Edecrin)	50 mg b.i.d.
Others	
Prednisone	1.0–1.5 mg/kg/day
Hydroxyurea (Hydrea)	500 mg/day
Melphalan (Alkeran)	0.25 mg/kg/day
Azathioprine (Imuran)	1.0–1.25 mg/kg/day

As with excessive diuresis, too vigorous afterload reduction with a vasodilator may cause orthostatic hypotension resulting in cerebral ischemic symptoms and a paradoxic change in the clinical course of CHF.

Beta-blocking agents have been used cautiously to improve hemodynamics when resting heart rate is inappropriately elevated. The decrease in heart rate permits more optimal ventricular filling. Generally a modest dosage of propranolol, not in excess of 1 mg/kg/24 hr, will produce this negative chronotropic effect. If antiarrhythmic agents are needed, quinidine or procainamide is preferred because each has considerably less negative inotropic effect than disopyramide.

Thromboembolism, particularly in the presence of atrial fibrillation and/or chronic CHF, is another risk in the clinical course of dilated cardiomyopathy. Chronic anticoagulation can decrease this risk.

There is a group of dilated cardiomyopathies having a more specific etiology. In addition to the supportive measures discussed for the idiopathic group, certain specific measures in the treatment program are to be considered. Anthracycline antibiotics, specifically doxorubicin (Adriamycin), are frequently used in cancer chemotherapy. Repetitive administration is associated with dose-related myocardial injury and may be complicated by heart failure. The use of endomyocardial biopsy to follow patients receiving this agent permits early identification of cardiac toxicity and discontinuation of the drug before clinical signs of heart failure develop. Several biopsies are done at one- to two-month intervals, when the total accumulated dose is $\geq$ 100 mg/m².

Acute inflammatory myocarditis is a cardiomyopathy that may respond to immunosuppressive treatment. Treatment should be undertaken only in biopsy-proven cases. Mason and colleagues have reported a favorable experience using a combination of steroid and azathioprine (azathioprine [Imuran], 1.00 to 1.25 mg/kg/day). Steroids alone may be effective in myocarditis associated with hypereosinophilic syndrome.

Alcoholic cardiomyopathy may be improved by abstention from alcohol. Complete reversal of severe congestive cardiomyopathy after one-year abstinence has been reported.

HYPERTROPHIC CARDIOMYOPATHY

Beta-blockers are useful in the management of obstructive hypertrophic cardiomyopathy. Large doses of propranolol such as 180 to 320 mg/day have been recommended and seem to lower the risk of sudden death. Calcium channel blockers have added another pharmacologic tool. Verapamil is effective in relief of obstructive symptoms. However, because adverse effects such as syncope and atrial fibrillation have occurred during the administration of these agents, some caution is required.

Arrhythmias are a part of the natural history of hypertrophic cardiomyopathy. Type I antiarrhythmic agents alone or in combination with digoxin are effective in controlling supraventricular tachydysrhythmias. Propranolol or a Type I agent are useful to treat ventricular ectopic activity.

Since infective endocarditis may be a complication of obstructive hypertrophic cardiomyopathy, bacterial endocarditis prophylaxis should be practiced. Finally, surgical intervention should be considered for those patients with high-grade outflow tract obstruction who have a decline in functional capacity despite maximal medical treatment.

RESTRICTIVE AND CONSTRICTIVE MYOPERICARDIOPATHY

Restrictive cardiomyopathy and constrictive pericardial disease have a similar pathophysiology and frequently the same clinical presentation. Differentiation of restrictive from constrictive disease may be difficult but is important, since pericardiectomy often allows complete reversal of the pathophysiology due to constrictive disease. The management of restrictive disease is discouraging. A diuretic will reduce preload and the associated congestive symptoms, but must be used with caution to avoid excessive volume depletion. As the disease progresses and systolic dysfunction develops, digoxin may provide some clinical improvement.

Identification of the infiltrative pathologic processes by biopsy often allows selection of specific therapies that may reverse or control progression of the disorder. Corticosteroids may be helpful in sarcoidosis or hypereosinophilic myocardial disease. The use of steroids in combination with hydroxyurea may be effective when steroids alone have resulted in only limited improvement (steroids [prednisone], 1.00 to 1.5 mg/kg/day for one week, then every other day; and hydroxyurea [Hydrea], 500 mg/day). An alkylating agent, such as melphalan (Alkeran), 0.25 mg/kg/day, in combination with corticosteroids for four days per month, has been reported to be helpful in primary amyloidosis. Finally, deferoxamine mesylate, which has been used to control iron overloading in hemochromatosis, may be tried when there is cardiac involvement.

REFERENCES

Child JS: Echocardiographic evaluation of cardiomyopathies. Appl Cardiol 2:15–20, 1985.

Fenoglio JJ Jr, Ursel PC, Kellog CF, et al: Diagnosis and classification of myocarditis by endomyocardial biopsy. N Engl J Med 308:12–18, 1983.

Mason JW, Billingham ME, Ricci DR: Treatment of acute inflammatory myocarditis assisted by endomyocardial biopsy. Am J Cardiol 45:1032–1044, 1980.

Miller DH, Borer JS: The cardiomyopathies. A pathologic approach to therapeutic management. Arch Intern Med 143:2157–2162, 1983.

14 · VALVULAR HEART DISEASE

F. J. Menapace
GEISINGER MEDICAL CENTER

The long-term outpatient management of patients with valvular heart disease is dependent on (1) the physician's recognition that a patient's symptoms or, just as important, the abnormal physical or laboratory findings may be due to valvular problems; (2) the precise anatomic and physiologic definition of the valve or valves involved; (3) the natural history of a particular valve pathology, treated medically, surgically, or with a combination; and (4) strict attention to modification of coronary risk factors such as hypercholesterolemia, smoking, and so forth. Patients should be taught about dietary restriction of fats, cholesterol, and sodium. They should be encouraged to exercise within their limits unless this is absolutely contraindicated (e.g., in tight aortic stenosis). Also, despite great advances in cardiovascular surgery and edifying long-term results, an artificial valve substitutes a whole new set of problems, and to date the ideal prosthesis is not available.

Noninvasive studies, especially echocardiography, have revolutionized our approach to suspected or documented valvular disease. Echocardiography allows us to determine the etiology of a specific valvular problem or document the anatomic sequelae (e.g., degree of ventricular hypertrophy). In addition, the physiologic significance of valve lesions is being deduced by Doppler echocardiography. Most important, echocardiography allows easy follow-up to aid clinical decision-making. Every physician caring for patients with valvular heart disease should have access to an echocardiography lab offering M-mode, two-dimensional, and Doppler echocardiography.

Aortic Stenosis

DEFINITION AND PATHOPHYSIOLOGY

Aortic stenosis is created by rheumatic damage to the leaflets, degenerative deposition of calcium, or the gradual fibrosis and calcification of a congenitally malformed and often bicuspid valve. All lead to a progressive decrease in orifice size. Most workers consider critical aortic stenosis to be present when the valve area is 0.6 cm^2 or less. This usually corresponds to a 50 mm Hg or greater left ventricular outflow gradient in patients with normal cardiac output. The obstruction leads to a progressive increase in left ventricular systolic pressure to maintain cardiac output. This pressure overload on the left ventricle is a stimulus for the development of concentric left ventricular hypertrophy. There is a concomitant decrease in left ventricular compliance and therefore an increase in left atrial work. This compensatory hypertrophy allows for maintenance of cardiac output for long periods until, for as yet unknown reasons, myocardial failure ensues.

CLINICAL ASPECTS

Patients with significant aortic stenosis present with angina, syncope, or symptoms of congestive heart failure. Examination reveals a carotid pulse that is decreased both in overall amplitude and in speed of upstroke (parvus et tardus). Jugular venous distention is not remarkable unless CHF has intervened. The apical impulse is usually minimally displaced and forceful, often with a prominent presystolic movement. A thrill should be carefully sought anywhere from the second intercostal space to the carotids. Its presence is usually indicative of at least a 50 mm Hg outflow gradient. A harsh systolic ejection murmur heard best at the base is the auscultatory hallmark. It does not change its intensity with bedside hemodynamic maneuvers.

The murmur of aortic stenosis in the elderly may actually be best heard in the apical region. Other physical findings may not be as striking as in younger patients. The quality of the aortic component of the second heart sound thus becomes important. A significantly calcified valve will lead to diminution or absence of the aortic component of S_2 where nonhemodynamic flow murmurs (aortic sclerosis) do not diminish this sound. Also, one must remember that in patients with low cardiac output there is a marked decrease in the murmur, and the possibility of aortic stenosis as a cause of CHF in the older age group must always be kept in mind.

Two-dimensional echocardiography is used to confirm the site of left ventricular outflow obstruction (excludes subvalvular, muscular, and supravalvular obstruction). It can reliably measure the compensatory mechanisms such as left ventricular hypertrophy, left atrial size, and (most important) left ventricular systolic function. Prediction of transaortic gradients by Doppler echocardiography is useful in clinical decision-making and in screening patients for cardiac catheterization.

MANAGEMENT

Management of patients with aortic stenosis is primarily dependent on the presence of symptoms. The natural history is well known. The survival of patients with isolated aortic stenosis and angina is generally about five years; syncope, three years; and CHF patients, two years. There is a long latent period between initial damage or deformity and these symptoms. What becomes of paramount importance is the identification of patients with congenital aortic stenosis. All patients with an early systolic ejection click and murmur should have two-dimensional echocardiography in an attempt to identify this abnormality. During adolescence and early adult life, subacute bacterial endocarditis prophylaxis may be the only therapy required. For dental procedures, patients should be given penicillin V, 2 gm PO one hour beforehand, then 1 gm five hours after the procedure. For upper respiratory tract surgery and gastrointestinal or genitourinary procedures, administer ampicillin, 1 to 2 gm IM or IV plus gentamicin, 1.5 mg/kg IM or IV one hour beforehand followed by 1.0 gm of oral penicillin V six hours later. For penicillin-allergic patients, give erythromycin, 1 gm PO one hour before, then 500 mg five hours after the procedure. Exercise is proscribed only in patients with marked obstruction. Symptoms should herald a consideration of surgery since medical treatment of this disease is unsatisfactory and nitrates, diuretics, and vasodilators are potentially dangerous for this group. Cardiac catheterization is generally needed to exclude concomitant significant coronary artery disease. Valve replacement is usually recommended for patients with gradients greater than 50 mm Hg. Decision-making becomes difficult once the patient has slipped into failure and has poor left ventricular function. In this setting of de-

creased cardiac output, a 30 to 35 mm Hg gradient may be significant and valve replacement recommended. Fortunately, many of these patients, although at increased risk for valvular surgery, do remarkably well owing to postoperative increase in ejection fraction.

Aortic Insufficiency

PATHOPHYSIOLOGY

Incompetence of the aortic valve may occur from (1) diseases that affect the cusps, such as rheumatic fever (scarring and retraction lead to inadequate coaptation; (2) dilatation of the ascending aorta (Marfan's syndrome); or (3) an inflammatory process involving the root at valve level (ankylosing spondylitis). The first two mechanisms can give rise to aortic insufficiency with acute dissecting thoracic aneurysm, and the combination of chest pain and the murmur of aortic insufficiency should always bring this up as a possible cause. Congenitally bicuspid valves are being recognized with increasing frequency as an etiology, but in many cases the exact cause of aortic insufficiency is not readily discernible.

The basic compensatory mechanism in chronic aortic insufficiency is left ventricular dilatation. Owing to the increased wall tension from this dilatation, there is a stimulus for development of hypertrophy, but not to the degree occurring in the pure pressure overload of aortic stenosis. This "eccentric" left ventricular hypertrophy (dilatation and hypertrophy) occurs with only minimal elevation of left ventricular end-diastolic pressure. In acute aortic insufficiency there is little time for development of ventricular dilatation, and a rapid rise in left ventricular end-diastolic pressure ensues. This leads to distinct clinical presentation, findings, and course.

CLINICAL ASPECTS

Clinical features of chronic aortic insufficiency include a widened pulse pressure (increased systolic and decreased diastolic) and a diastolic murmur usually best appreciated along the left sternal border. The pulses are characterized by a very rapid rise as well as a rapid fall. The apical impulse is usually displaced laterally and inferiorly and may be more diffuse in nature. An apical diastolic rumble due to the aortic insufficiency (the so-called Austin Flint murmur) may also be noted. The first heart sound is usually normal in intensity. A systolic ejection murmur is usually appreciated owing to the increased forward flow. Tall stature, arachnodactyly, dolichostenomelia, ocular problems, and high arched palate should raise the possibility of Marfan's syndrome.

M-mode and two-dimensional echocardiography are indicated in all patients. It may reveal the etiology, confirm the diagnosis, and provide an estimate of left ventricular size and performance. Echocardiography is also a much more sensitive means of measuring ascending aortic root dilatation than chest x-ray. If an adequate echo cannot be obtained, radionuclide angiography with reporting of left ventricular volumes and ejection fraction should be obtained.

MANAGEMENT

The volume overload imposed by chronic aortic insufficiency is tolerated well by most patients for considerable periods. There is, however, a subgroup of patients with aortic insufficiency who are symptomatic, have left ventricular dysfunction, do not benefit from aortic valve replacement, and eventually die, usually of progressive left ventricular dysfunction. Some authors have suggested aortic valve replacement in patients with impaired left ventricular function who are asymptomatic or mildly symptomatic. Some also suggested aortic valve replacement to "preserve left ventricular function" in all patients with significant aortic insufficiency. At present, we know that the prognosis of patients with aortic insufficiency and normal left ventricular function is generally good. These individuals may remain symptom free for a considerable time. Patients with chronic aortic insufficiency should be followed with yearly echocardiographic studies. If these reveal an increase in end-systolic volume or end-systolic dimension, more frequent follow-up is warranted, at four- to six-month intervals. Surgery should be considered when patients develop symptoms of CHF or when there are signs of progressive left ventricular dysfunction (decreased fractional shortening on echocardiogram or decreased ejection fraction by radioangiography). Excellent surgical results can be expected in most patients following this approach.

Management of patients with Marfan's syndrome should also include beta-adrenoreceptor blocker therapy to decrease the "shear" forces on the aorta, in the hope of delaying the rate of root dilatation. Aortic root replacement should be considered when aortic root dilatation has reached 6.0 cm or more. The rationale for this is that the development of a dissecting aneurysm is common once this amount of dilatation has occurred and that elective replacement carries a lower mortality risk than emergency surgical repair. Contact sports should be proscribed, and swimming substituted, in this subset of patients with aortic insufficiency.

Acute Aortic Insufficiency

The syndrome of acute aortic insufficiency may occur in patients with bacterial endocarditis, trauma, or a dissecting aneurysm involving the ascending aorta. The acute regurgitation leads to a rapid rise in left ventricular diastolic pressure. The patient experiences symptoms of heart failure, usually in the form of acute pulmonary edema. This sequence of events should be considered in a patient with acute pulmonary edema and a normal- or near–normal-sized cardiac contour on chest x-ray. One of the key points on physical examination is a soft or absent first heart sound, due to a marked early rise in left ventricular end-diastolic pressure that prematurely closes the mitral valve. The murmur of aortic insufficiency may also be short and difficult to appreciate owing to the rapid equilibration of left ventricular end-diastolic and aortic diastolic pressure as a result of the torrential aortic insufficiency. Echocardiography may aid in the diagnosis by demonstrating the premature closure of the mitral valve and evidence of aortic insufficiency. Identifiable vegetations or root pathology may also give a clue to the etiology. Management consists of treatment of failure with the addition of parenteral vasodilators such as sodium nitroprusside (Nipride), 40 to 60 μg/min. Urgent surgery is needed for the great majority of these patients.

Mitral Stenosis

PATHOPHYSIOLOGY

Mitral stenosis is usually caused by rheumatic fever; the congenital variety is rare. The rheumatic inflammatory process leads to fusion, thickening, and fibrosis of the mitral valve cusps and chordae tendineae. This causes a progressive decrease in mitral valve orifice area: the normal adult size is 4 to 6 cm^2. When the orifice has been reduced to 2 cm^2, mild mitral stenosis results. It is at this point that left atrial pressure must elevate to sustain cardiac output. Elevation of left atrial pressure leads to pulmonary venous and capillary hypertension. This mechanism is responsible for the common patient complaint of dyspnea with exertion. Reactive pulmonary hypertension initially occurs, and some fixed element ensues as changes occur in the pulmonary vascular bed. This eventually leads to right ventricular hypertrophy. Critical mitral stenosis is felt to be present when valve area is reduced to 1.0 cm^2 or less.

CLINICAL ASPECTS

This disease entity should be suspected in patients with symptoms of CHF, atrial arrhythmias, embolic phenomenon, hemoptysis, or low cardiac output. This is seen most typically today in native American women in their sixth or seventh decade. The hallmarks are an accentuated first heart sound, an opening snap (the timing of which may indicate severity), and diastolic rumble. Exercise is often a helpful technique in accentuating these findings. Chest x-ray often reveals left atrial enlargement and an increased pulmonary venous pattern. Electrocardiography is most likely to show left atrial abnormality, atrial arrhythmias, right axis deviation, or right ventricular hypertrophy. Echocardiography is the procedure of choice to confirm the diagnosis.

MANAGEMENT

Long-term management of these patients is predicated upon both symptomatology and objective, noninvasive data. Most patients with a mitral valve orifice of less than 1.0 cm² require surgical treatment, either mitral commissurotomy (for the relatively young patient with a valve that is not calcified) or mitral valve replacement. The classification (isolated vs. nonisolated mitral disease) and severity can be accurately estimated by a combination of M-mode, two-dimensional, and Doppler echocardiography.

Pharmacologic treatment consists of loop diuretics such as furosemide (Lasix), 40 mg PO daily, with potassium supplementation (dietary or pharmacologic) in those with dyspnea on effort or other congestive symptoms. Vasodilators are usually contraindicated in patients with fixed valvular obstruction. Patients in normal sinus rhythm usually do not benefit from digitalis glycosides since neither the increased pulmonary capillary pressure nor cardiac output is positively affected owing to the mechanical obstruction. Atrial fibrillation, either intermittent or fixed, usually leads to a marked decline in functional capacity. This is due to loss of the atrial contribution to cardiac output, increase in pulmonary capillary wedge pressure, and decrease in cardiac output when diastole is shortened. Digitalis should be utilized under these circumstances.

Attempts at pharmacologic conversion and maintenance are warranted with Type I antiarrhythmic drugs. Quinidine sulfate is the preferred agent. Hospitalization is usually required for this conversion, since if fibrillation persists after an adequate trial, electrical cardioversion after anticoagulation is indicated.

All patients who cannot be maintained in normal sinus rhythm require a coumarin type of anticoagulant unless there is a strong contraindication. The ventricular response to atrial fibrillation should be monitored, rather than drug levels. A ventricular rate of approximately 80 beats per minute after mild exercise is a reasonable response. A beta-blocker such as propranolol (Inderal), 20 to 40 mg every six hours, or verapamil (Isoptin), 30 to 180 mg every six hours, may be added to the digoxin to decrease conduction through the AV node and better control the rate.

Follow-up visits, usually at yearly intervals, are warranted. Periodic reexamination of valve orifice size can be obtained with echocardiography. Progressive symptomatology (Class III or IV New York Heart Association classification) or critical orifice size should prompt consideration of surgical treatment. Whether cardiac catheterization is needed or adds any additional information in patients not suspected of having concomitant associated valve or coronary disease is debatable and usually is an institutional preference.

Mitral Insufficiency

PATHOPHYSIOLOGY

The mitral valve is the most complex of the four cardiac valves and itself has several components. These consist of leaflets, chordae tendineae, mitral annulus, and papillary muscles with their underlying myocardium. Mitral insufficiency can result from damage to or dysfunction of any of these structures. With the decreasing incidence of rheumatic fever, mxyomatous degeneration of the valve is becoming one of the most common causes. In chronic mitral regurgitation, the volume overload is ejected into the low-resistance left atrium. The left ventricular systolic pressure is normal or low, and there is therefore a decreased afterload on the left ventricle. The basic problem is that since there is a low pressure reservoir into the left atrium, decreased myocardial function can occur without causing striking alterations in clinical symptoms. Many patients with chronic mitral regurgitation have a fall in ejection fraction following valve replacement, since the left ventricle can now pump only into the relatively high-pressure aorta. This probably explains the poor postoperative survival curves in patients with chronic mitral regurgitation as compared to those with chronic aortic insufficiency.

CLINICAL ASPECTS

Symptomatically, patients with chronic mitral regurgitation usually complain of symptoms of CHF or of a low cardiac output with fatigue, especially late in the day (as opposed to the early morning fatigue of depressed individuals). Pulmonary hypertension is usually a late manifestation, generally accompanied by signs of "right heart failure." Atrial fibrillation results from progressive left atrial dilatation. Embolic events are relatively uncommon, unlike the situation in mitral stenosis.

On examination, the arterial pulse is generally normal in contour and amplitude; venous distention occurs late in the course. (The apical impulse is usually displaced laterally and may be more diffuse.) The hallmark on auscultation is a holosystolic murmur best heard at the apex. The aortic component of the second heart sound is normal and the pulmonic component is accentuated late in the course. A third heart sound is common.

Two-dimensional echocardiography reveals the cause of the mitral regurgitation in many cases. More important, it reveals the degree of left atrial and left ventricular enlargement and global as well as segmental left ventricular function.

MANAGEMENT

Management of patients with chronic mitral regurgitation is probably the most difficult of all, since definite left ventricular dysfunction may be present despite an asymptomatic patient. In patients who are asymptomatic yet have cardiomegaly, yearly clinical and noninvasive follow-up are needed, either echocardiography or radionuclide studies. If the left ventricular end-diastolic dimension is 80 mm or greater, the end-systolic dimension 50 mm or greater, the fractional shortening less than 35%, or the ejection fraction less than 55%, cardiac catheterization is warranted. Mitral valve replacement should be considered for this group as well as for symptomatic patients.

Acute Mitral Regurgitation

This syndrome, which can be seen in patients with bacterial endocarditis, trauma, acute myocardial infarction, or spontaneous rupture of a myxomatous chord, results in a sudden high degree of mitral regurgitation. The high pressure of the left ventricle is transmitted to a normal or near-normal left atrium that cannot dilate rapidly. The high pressures are therefore transmitted into the pulmonary veins and capillaries. Acute pulmonary edema occurs along with pulmonary hypertension. Again, this is a cause of acute pulmonary edema with a normal or near-normal heart size on chest x-ray. On examination, there is a marked contrast to chronic mitral regurgitation. The patient is generally in sinus rhythm, a forceful atrial contraction is noted as a fourth heart sound, the systolic murmur may actually be shorter and not holosystolic (rapid rise in left atrial pressure leads to equalization and decreased flow), and a third heart sound and accentuation of the pulmonic component of the second heart sound are appreciated. Therapy, in addition to digitalis and loop diuretics, should include vasodilators such as sodium nitroprusside (Nipride), 40 to 60 µg/min, to increase flow and output. Unless rapid improvement results, surgical therapy will be needed.

Mitral Valve Prolapse

PATHOPHYSIOLOGY

The mitral valve prolapse syndrome is thought to be one of the most common cardiac problems, estimates suggesting that 5% to 10% of the population is affected. In many cases examined, myxomatous proliferation of leaflets, chordae, and annulus can result in a redundant valve that prolapses into the left atrium in systole. The degree of prolapse determines the degree of mitral regurgitation. Some authors have also hypothesized that localized myocardial abnormalities allow inadequate tethering and subsequent prolapse. Mitral valve prolapse has been associated with a wide variety of diseases such as Marfan's syndrome, Ehlers-Danlos disease, and Duchenne's muscular dystrophy. There is a high incidence in patients with atrial septal defects and thoracic chest wall deformities, suggesting a possible genetic defect at the time when these structures are developing.

CLINICAL ASPECTS

Most patients with mitral valve prolapse are asymptomatic. Atypical chest pain and palpitations (with poor correlation to documented arrhythmia) are common.

Symptoms of classic anxiety neurosis are usual and probably represent two common disorders in the same patient. Recent attention has been focused on patients with a variety of neurologic symptoms (e.g., transient cerebral ischemia, amaurosis fugax, or retinal infarcts), which may be the presenting manifestation, especially in a younger patient population. Sudden death is an extremely rare complication of the disease.

Examination typically reveals an asthenic individual, often with chest wall deformity such as pectus excavatum. Lax joints are common with positive wrist and thumb signs. The hallmark on auscultation is a systolic click that occurs after the beginning of the carotid upstroke. A late systolic (at times holosystolic) murmur, often high-pitched and honking, is noted best at the apex. The murmur changes in intensity with maneuvers that affect left ventricular volume. A smaller left ventricular volume, such as seen with the patient upright, causes earlier prolapse, and the click and murmur occur earlier in systole.

Echocardiography has become the procedure of choice in documenting the diagnosis and excluding associated abnormalities. It also provides left atrial size and left ventricular size and performance. Patients should not be labeled unnecessarily with this diagnosis, since they are prorated by insurance companies at the same rate as patients with chronic rheumatic mitral valve disease.

MANAGEMENT

Management of most patients need involve only subacute bacterial endocarditis prophylaxis. Patients should have a baseline echocardiogram to determine left atrial and left ventricular size. Yearly follow-up is indicated, since a subset of patients with the prolapse syndrome will develop progressive, hemodynamically significant mitral regurgitation. These patients are handled in the same way as those with any other form of chronic mitral regurgitation. Patients who develop neurologic symptoms should initially be treated with a combination of dipyrimadole (Persantine), 75 mg b.i.d., and aspirin, 500 to 1300 mg daily. A beta-blocker, propranolol, 40 mg every six hours, can be prescribed for patients with symptomatic palpitations. These may also be beneficial in some patients with chest pain. Nitrates are essentially of little help and may actually make the prolapse more severe by causing smaller left ventricular volume.

REFERENCES

Bonow RG, Rosing DR, McIntosh CL, et al: The natural history of asymptomatic patients with aortic regurgitation and normal left ventricular function. Circulation 68:509–517, 1983.

Council on Cardiovascular Disease in the Young: Committee on Rheumatic Fever and Infective Endocarditis. Statement for health professionals. Circulation 70:1123A–1127A, 1984.

Roberts WC, Perloff JK: Mitral valve disease: a clinicopathologic survey of conditions causing the mitral valve to function abnormally. Ann Intern Med 77:939–975, 1972.

Ross J Jr, Baumwald E: The influence of corrective operations on the natural history of aortic stenosis. Circulation 37(Suppl V):61, 1968.

Waith DC, Stewart WJ, Block PC, et al: A new method to calculate aortic valve area without left heart catheterization. Circulation 70:978–983, 1984.

15 · VENOUS DISORDERS AND PULMONARY EMBOLISM

Donald J. Breslin
LAHEY CLINIC MEDICAL CENTER

Chronic Venous Insufficiency

CLINICAL ASPECTS

Prolonged venous stasis can produce firm, thickened, painful, tender, dull red skin, which gradually becomes "bound down" as the underlying tissues contract. Deposition of brown pigment and coarsening and scaling of the skin follow. Ulceration can occur, particularly on the ankle, commonly on its medial aspect.

MANAGEMENT

MECHANICAL COMPRESSION

Deep venous insufficiency of the lower extremity affects the skin of the leg and spares the thigh. Consequently, elastic supports need not extend higher than just below the knee unless swelling of the thigh bothers the patient. The best support is provided by Ace bandages, 4 inches in width, but graduated compression stockings, heavy in weight and usually knee length, provide an alternative approach. Jobst stockings (Jobst Institute Inc., Toledo, OH), which are custom fit, and Sigvaris (Camp International Inc., Jackson, MS) stockings, which are available in a variety of sizes, are satisfactory. The pressure exerted by the supporting stockings should be designated by prescription. For deep venous insufficiency, 30 mm Hg usually suffices. Stasis also tends to recur even with conscientious use of supporting stockings. In such instances, elastic bandages are preferable.

BOOT DRESSINGS

Dome-Paste (Dome-Paste, Miles Pharmaceuticals, West Haven, CT) or Gelocast boots (Beiersdorf Inc., South Norwalk, CT) are useful once stasis dermatitis has occurred. They are applied from the base of the toes to below the knee, covered with an elastic paper bandage (Coban, Medical Products Division/3M, St. Paul, MN), and reinforced with two or three longitudinal strips of ½-inch adhesive tape. The boots should be replaced after ten days and should not be applied over infected areas or if associated arterial insufficiency is present.

LOCAL TREATMENT

When fever is absent and an area of redness is localized, an antibiotic is usually unnecessary. If the skin of the leg is thickened and red, fluocinolone acetonide (Synalar), 0.025% cream or ointment, is applied to the involved area of skin three or four times during the day, covered with Saran Wrap, and wrapped with an Ace bandage during the day.

An antibiotic is given when stasis ulcers are associated with fever or discharge. The patient with diabetes mellitus is more susceptible than others to associated cellulitis. Treatment for the patient with draining stasis ulcer is bed rest and topical applications of moist cotton soaked in 0.9% saline solution, or half-strength Burow's solution applied for 15 minutes five times a day. When the moist compresses are removed, neomycin sulfate (Neo-Synalar) cream can be applied to the skin surrounding the stasis ulcer.

Treatment for ambulatory patients with nondraining stasis ulcers is neomycin sulfate cream applied to the ulcer and surrounding skin covered with Telfa, a ½-inch-thick foam rubber pad that extends well beyond the ulcerated area, and the Gelocast or Dome-Paste boot. When the ulcer is draining and the patient must remain ambulatory, Ace bandages are used instead of a boot. The leg is unwrapped intermittently for application of moist compresses, as previously outlined. The leg is elevated four times a day for 30 minutes and at night. Large stasis ulcers will heal with ambulatory treatment in two to three months. An ulcer 3 cm or more in diameter will require split-thickness skin grafting. Once a stasis ulcer has healed, the measures previously described for stasis dermatitis must be continued. A generalized pruritic dermatitis resulting from a hypersensitivity ("id") reaction is treated with topical steroid cream and systemic steroids if necessary.

Varicose Veins

Varicose veins, abnormally dilated superficial veins commonly found in the lower extremities, result from weakness in vein walls or venous hypertension. Most varicosities can be treated with elastic supports. Some women want varicose veins removed surgically for cosmetic reasons, but they must recognize that adequate surgery leaves extensive scarring. Operation usually should be deferred until no future pregnancies are planned. Although varicose veins are incompetent, removal can further impair venous outflow from the limb if proximal deep venous occlusion is present. Sclerosing injections are rarely used.

A congenital venous malformation must be suspected in the young patient with varicose veins. This can be associated with hypertrophy of the involved limb and cutaneous hemangioma. Arteriography will demonstrate arteriovenous connections. Elastic supports are usually sufficient treatment. Superficial venous malformations are sometimes excised.

Superficial Thrombophlebitis

Superficial thrombophlebitis, usually a self-limited disorder that resolves in two to three weeks, may suggest an underlying systemic disease causing hypercoagulability. Pain and inflammation are helped by phenylbutazone (Butazolidin), 100 mg four times a day, or indomethacin (Indocin), 25 mg four times a day for four to six days, and applications of hot packs. Anticoagulants are not indicated unless the long saphenous vein is involved above the knee and inflammation seems to be extending proximally. Recurrence in a varicosity may indicate the need for venous stripping and ligation.

Acute Obstruction of Deep Veins

CLINICAL ASPECTS

To help allay anxiety in patients fearful of the consequences of a pulmonary embolism, use of the word "clot" should be avoided. A clear explanation helps to prevent the patient's misunderstanding of the illness.

In chronic venous insufficiency, pain and swelling in the leg that occur after prolonged dependency and subside in less than 24 hours with elevation do not usually represent new thrombophlebitis. Occasionally a swollen leg becomes hot, red, and tender with associated fever of 101° to 106°F and chills. These findings are sometimes mistaken for thrombophlebitis when they may be caused by cellulitis in a previously lymphedematous leg. When severe pain and a swollen lower extremity are unrelieved by elevation, pelvic tumor must be suspected with pain due to nerve root compression.

A thrombus limited to the calf is an uncommon source of pulmonary emboli unless it extends proximally. Accuracy in diagnosis of proximal deep vein thrombosis has been improved greatly by the use of noninvasive venous studies. Noninvasive monitoring with serial impedance plethysmography or phleborheography is an effective approach for suspected thrombophlebitis of the calf. A change from negative to positive result indicates proximal extension and need for anticoagulants. In the absence of monitoring, deep calf thrombophlebitis should be treated like other deep vein thrombosis with anticoagulants in standard doses.

MANAGEMENT

The standard treatment of deep vein thrombosis includes elevation of the limb to 30° above the horizontal, application of hot packs, and use of nonsalicylate analgesics. Pillows should not be placed behind the legs because this can cause local venous compression.

HEPARIN

Heparin is given by continuous IV infusion with a pump. Initially a bolus of 5000 units of heparin is given, followed by a dose of 1000 to 1500 units per hour depending on partial thromboplastin time (PTT), which should be about 1.5 to two times the patient's control value. Administration of intermittent boluses of IV heparin, 5000 to 7500 units every four hours, is an alternative to continuous infusion. Repeated determination of PTT is unnecessary with intermittent bolus treatment, but PTT is checked at least once between the third and fourth hour to ensure the presence of an anticoagulant effect. Treatment with intermittent bolus may carry a higher risk of bleeding than continuous infusions of heparin. Subcutaneous low-dose heparin (5000 units every 12 hours) is reserved for prophylaxis. Moderate doses of subcutaneous heparin can be used for outpatient treatment if sodium warfarin (Coumadin) is contraindicated. If therapeutic doses of subcutaneous heparin are given every 12 hours, PTT should be 1.5 to two times normal six hours after SQ administration, and some anticoagulant effect should still be present one to two hours before the next dose. The total 24-hour dose is usually 20,000 to 40,000 units by this route. Doses of more than 40,000 units in 24 hours by any route are rarely needed. Hirsh and colleagues advise exceeding this dose only if the serum level of heparin is less than 0.3 unit per ml. Larger doses of heparin can be used, but no controlled studies support this at present. To avoid hematoma, no IM heparin injections of any kind are given.

A rare complication of heparin therapy consists of life-threatening thromboembolism involving arteries and veins related to platelet aggregation, heralded by increasing heparin resistance and thrombocytopenia. Platelet counts are monitored during heparin therapy on the fifth day of therapy and every three days thereafter.

SODIUM WARFARIN (COUMADIN)

Treatment with Coumadin is initiated at the same time as heparin treatment because four to six days are required before adequate Coumadin effect is achieved. After the prothrombin time (PT) has been in the therapeutic range for 48 hours, heparin is stopped and Coumadin is continued. The PTT is maintained with heparin in a range of 1.5 to two times control during the first six to ten days of treatment, after which a PT of 1.5 times control is effective. Higher levels are unnecessary and cause an increased risk of bleeding. Elderly frail patients who may require extremely small doses of Coumadin must be treated cautiously. During initial Coumadin therapy, the PT must be checked just before the next dose of heparin is due, to avoid a misleading prolongation of PT, which heparin can induce. In the absence of continued known risk factors for venous thromboembolism, Coumadin is discontinued after three months. Recurrences are rare with this treatment schedule. No "rebound" effect causing recurring venous thrombosis after discontinuance of Coumadin has been evidenced clinically.

If bleeding occurs or surgery is contemplated, three or four units of fresh-frozen plasma is usually enough to revert the PT to an acceptable level. In addition, if bleeding is severe, orally administered vitamin K_1, 2.5 to 10 mg, may be sufficient to decrease the PT to an acceptable range. Much of the effect will be seen in six to eight hours. The IV route should be avoided because of hypotension and rare anaphylaxis.

Moderate doses of heparin are as effective as standard doses of Coumadin, and cause less bleeding. After an initial two weeks of large IV doses of heparin to produce a PTT of 1.5 to two times normal, heparin is given SQ for three months in lower doses. Heparin is injected SQ every 12 hours and is adjusted to keep the PTT at 1.5 times control value (when measured six hours after injection). Once the dose is fixed, no further anticoagulant monitoring is needed. The average dose is 10,000 units of heparin every 12 hours. This is a useful technique, particularly for pregnant women in whom Coumadin is associated with a risk of fetal deformity or for patients who cannot be monitored regularly.

COMPLICATIONS

Recurrence of thrombophlebitis during adequate Coumadin therapy is rare; if it does recur, heparin in therapeutic doses should be resumed for three or four weeks followed by 12 months of treatment with Coumadin. For further recurrences or an underlying coagulopathy, such as antithrombin III or protein C deficiency, Coumadin must be continued indefinitely. Recurrent venous thrombosis when a patient is receiving adequate therapeutic doses of orally administered anticoagulants should always raise the suspicion of underlying malignant disease.

The rare combination of extensive venous obstruction complicated by secondary decrease in arterial perfusion produces gangrene. Circulating blood volume depletion because of venous pooling can be fatal. Experimentally, lumbar sympathectomy has not proved useful. Fibrinolytic agents are prescribed unless contraindicated; alternatively, standard heparin therapy is used. Elevation of the legs to 60° and replenishment of blood volume are important. Venous thrombectomy is performed if patients are unresponsive to medical treatment.

FIBRINOLYSIS

Agents that activate the body's proteolytic system include urokinase and streptokinase. Both activate plasminogen to form plasmin. Urokinase is much more expensive and is reserved for patients with resistance or allergy to streptokinase. Fibrinolytic treatment of thrombophlebitis should be started within five days of onset of symptoms and continued for four to six days. The earlier treatment is initiated, the more likely it is to achieve complete lysis of clot. Postphlebitic valve damage can be prevented by successful fibrinolytic therapy. Most hospitalized patients have underlying conditions that contraindicate fibrinolytic treatment because of the unacceptable risk of bleeding.

If anticoagulant therapy is contraindicated in the patient with deep vein thrombosis or if anticoagulants fail to prevent recurrences, an inferior vena caval filter or clip is inserted surgically. Venography, including inferior venacavography, should be performed first to establish the extent of the clot.

Antibiotics are not needed for thrombophlebitis, with the rare exception of septic thrombophlebitis, which may be associated with septic abortion or IV injections by addicts. Antibiotics and anticoagulants are effective without the need for ligation of the inferior vena cava and ovarian veins.

Pulmonary Embolism

Normal levels of arterial Po_2 or negative noninvasive venous studies or venography do not exclude pulmonary embolism. If results of ventilation-perfusion lung scans with multiple views are negative, clinically significant pulmonary emboli are excluded. When pulmonary embolism is suspected clinically but results of lung scans are indeterminate, pulmonary angiography is required.

Pulmonary emboli are treated by standard anticoagulation with heparin and Coumadin, as previously described. Initial requirements for heparin may be high: an initial IV bolus of 10,000 units is usually given.

The mortality rate of patients with massive pulmonary embolism complicated by systemic hypotension is about 50%, and the rate for those who undergo pulmonary embolectomy with cardiopulmonary bypass is often 40% to 50%. Fibrinolytic treatment promptly decreases pulmonary hypertension and improves hemodynamics in patients with massive pulmonary embolism. It is our treatment of choice and is continued for 24 to 48 hours.

PROPHYLAXIS

Most patients who die of pulmonary embolism do so within the first two hours, before standard treatment can help them. Prophylactic methods will prevent many of these deaths.

Heparin administered SQ in low doses of 5000 units is effective in preventing venous thromboembolism. It is started two hours before operation and is administered at 12-hour intervals until the patient is fully ambulatory. Recent evidence suggests that adding dihydroergotamine mesylate (DHE 45), 0.5 mg with each heparin dose, gives added protection. Low-dose heparin is not adequate in the patient who has had bone trauma or who is undergoing prostate surgery or pelvic surgery for extensive carcinoma. Although the overall risk of bleeding is low, heparin should be avoided even in small doses in neurosurgical patients.

Intermittent compression boots are an alternative method of prevention and are particularly useful when all risk of bleeding must be avoided. They are applied preoperatively and continued while the patient is in bed for the postoperative period. The value of aspirin prophylaxis in patients undergoing hip surgery has not been determined.

High-risk patients with a past history of thrombophlebitis who are undergoing hip surgery, or those with extensive carcinoma having pelvic surgery, should receive therapeutic doses of Coumadin despite the increased risk of bleeding. We usually start with 10 mg of Coumadin commencing 24 hours after operation.

Noninvasive venous monitoring in high-risk patients has been helpful in conjunction with other methods. Baseline noninvasive testing is followed by monitoring every three days. Any change from the baseline study indicates a need for venography and standard anticoagulant treatment if thrombosis is found. No prophylactic approach will entirely eliminate venous thromboembolism. Noninvasive venous monitoring provides additional protection by detecting patients who need aggressive treatment with anticoagulation.

REFERENCES

Hirsh J, Genton E, Hull R: A Practical Approach to the Diagnosis, Prevention and Treatment of Venous Thromboembolism. Grune & Stratton, New York, 1981.

Hull R, Delmore T, Carter C, et al: Adjusted subcutaneous heparin versus warfarin sodium in the long-term treatment of venous thrombosis. N Engl J Med 306:189–194, 1982.

Hull R, Hirsh J, Jay R, et al: Different intensities of oral anticoagulant therapy in the treatment of proximal-vein thrombosis. N Engl J Med 307:1676–1681, 1982.

Moser KM, LeMoine JR: Is embolic risk conditioned by location of deep venous thrombosis? Ann Intern Med 94:439–444, 1981.

Sasahara AA, DiSerio FJ, Singer JM, et al: Dihydroergotamine-heparin prophylaxis of postoperative deep vein thrombosis: a multicenter trial. JAMA 251:2960–2986, 1984.

16 · SYNCOPE

Stephen C. Hammill
David R. Holmes, Jr.
MAYO CLINIC AND MAYO FOUNDATION

INTRODUCTION

A brief disturbance in normal consciousness is a common ailment. When it is an isolated occurrence that is easily explained, the physician is seldom consulted. However, if the disturbance recurs, it may become a matter of concern and prompt the physician to search for evidence of an underlying disease and to distinguish among syncope, epilepsy, vertigo, hyperventilation, and a number of other conditions. Patients with syncope often present diagnostic and therapeutic challenges because of the etiologic diversity that includes benign, self-limited causes and life-threatening arrhythmias (Table 1). The spells are often sporadic and unpredictable in their occurrence, but the patient usually is extremely anxious and strongly desires to prevent recurrence.

DEFINITION

Syncope is defined as a transient loss of consciousness associated with a loss of ability to maintain postural tone. The subjective feeling of an impending loss of consciousness, along with an onset of generalized weakness, is described as "presyncope" or "near-syncope."

Table 1. SPECIFIC DISORDERS ASSOCIATED WITH SYNCOPE

Vasodepressor (vasovagal) syncope
Orthostatic syncope
  Poor postural adjustment
  Orthostatic hypotension
Cardiac syncope
  Arrhythmias
  Ischemic heart disease
  Valvular heart disease
  Congenital heart disease
Carotid sinus syncope
Syncope due to pulmonary disease
Cough syncope
Micturition syncope
Neurovascular syncope
  Cerebrovascular syncope
  Cerebral artery spasm
  Subclavian steal
  Glossopharyngeal syncope

Both syncope and near-syncope may exist in the same patient, with near-syncope preceding syncope or as an isolated event.

INCIDENCE AND PROGNOSIS

Syncope is a relatively common clinical problem that is probably underreported. There is little information on its specific frequency in patient populations but surveys of young people and healthy adults have demonstrated it to be present in 10% to 50% of persons interviewed.

The long-term prognosis of patients presenting with syncope depends on the cause and the presence of associated medical problems. Vasodepressor syncope (vasovagal syncope or a simple faint) in an otherwise healthy person has little, if any, negative long-term prognosis. In contrast, syncope due to ventricular tachycardia occurring in the setting of cardiomyopathy or coronary artery disease identifies a patient at high risk of subsequent cardiac events. The incidence of sudden death during follow-up in patients with a cardiovascular cause for syncope is between 20% and 25%, compared with 5% in patients with a noncardiac cause and 3% in patients with syncope of unknown cause.

MECHANISM

Syncope results from cerebral hypoxia secondary to a global impairment in cerebral perfusion. If the cardiac output decreases, cerebral resistance decreases to allow an increase in flow; however, for this compensatory mechanism to occur, the perfusion pressure must remain adequate.

An important hemodynamic relationship is the relative distribution of blood flow between the venous and arterial circulations. Approximately two thirds of blood volume is in the venous circulation, and when a person is in an upright position, the blood shifts into the deep venous system of the pelvis and lower extremities. Blood pressure and cerebral perfusion are maintained by several physiologic reactions that occur as a person assumes the upright posture. These include (1) reflex acceleration of heart rate, with a transient increase of 5 to 25 beats/min; (2) reflex arteriolar constriction to maintain arterial pressure; (3) reflex vasoconstriction and an increase in muscular tone and tissue pressure in the legs and abdominal muscles, to decrease the pooling of blood in the venous capacitance vessels and to facilitate venous return; and (4) increase in plasma catecholamine levels. Failure of one or more of these compensatory reflexes may result in syncope.

SPECIFIC SYNCOPE-ASSOCIATED DISORDERS AND THEIR TREATMENT

VASODEPRESSOR (VASOVAGAL) SYNCOPE

Vasodepressor syncope is the classic benign faint and may be the most common cause of syncope. The precipitating events vary widely from unaccustomed physical and mental exhaustion to anxiety, emotional shock, and systemic or visceral pain.

Vasodepressor syncope results from a decrease in peripheral vascular resistance and an inability to maintain an adequate systemic pressure. Vasodepressor syncope, as with other forms of syncope, can result in an anoxic convulsion if loss of consciousness is sufficiently abrupt and prolonged. Occasionally, persons may have a typical history of vasodepressor syncope with the typical prodrome and, in addition, have occasional episodes of syncope without warning.

In most patients with classic vasodepressor syncope and known precipitating factors, avoidance of the event, recognition of the prodrome, and early resumption of the recumbent position may successfully prevent syncope. Treatment with an anticholinergic (propantheline, 7.5 to 15 mg three times daily), theophylline, or permanent cardiac pacing may be required in selected patients.

ORTHOSTATIC SYNCOPE

As discussed previously, reflex cardiovascular mechanisms are needed to maintain cerebral perfusion when the upright position is assumed. Inappropriate postural responses to BP change can be divided into (1) poor autonomic adjustment to the upright posture and (2) orthostatic hypotension. Both conditions are associated with syncope.

Poor Autonomic Adjustment to Upright Posture. This is most commonly observed among the elderly, in whom postural adaptation reflexes are slowed by physiologic aging. Other conditions include physical exhaustion, prolonged recumbency, hot weather, pregnancy, and gastrectomy. Cardiovascular alterations consist of an exaggerated pooling of blood in the distended capillary beds, an inadequate cardiac venous return, and an increase in peripheral vascular resistance. The net result is an abnormal decrease in systolic pressure, an abnormal increase in diastolic pressure, and an excessive acceleration in heart rate. It is usually a harmless condition and can be aided by having the patient assume the upright posture more gradually and by use of support stockings to help maintain venous tone.

Orthostatic Hypotension. Secondary orthostatic hypotension may be seen in patients with endocrinologic and metabolic disorders (Table 2). Secondary orthostatic hypotension also may be seen in central and peripheral nervous system and other miscellaneous disorders (Table 2). One of the most commonly observed causes of secondary orthostatic hypotension is the excessive use of diuretics for the treatment of hypertension, heart failure, or peripheral edema.

Primary or idiopathic orthostatic hypotension is a disease of the autonomic nervous system and is associated with other signs of autonomic dysfunction, including impairment of sweating, impotence, and bowel-bladder disregulation.

On assuming the upright position, the patient may lose consciousness at the height of the decrease in postural BP, and syncope usually lasts no longer than seconds. The postural symptoms are often worse in the morning and are aggravated by heat, humidity, a heavy meal, and exercise. Treatment of orthostatic hypotension is often complex, but progress continues to be made (Table 3).

Table 2. ORTHOSTATIC SYNCOPE

Poor postural adjustment
  Prolonged recumbency
  Physical exhaustion
  Advanced age
  Pregnancy
  Gastrectomy
  Young persons with tall asthenic habitus
Orthostatic hypotension
  Primary (idiopathic) orthostatic hypotension
    Idiopathic orthostatic hypotension
    Shy-Drager syndrome (idiopathic orthostatic hypotension with neurologic deficit)
  Secondary orthostatic hypotension
    Central and peripheral nervous system disorders
      Peripheral neuropathies
      Guillain-Barré syndrome
      Brain stem lesions
      Traumatic, inflammatory myelopathies
      Intracranial tumors
    Endocrinologic-metabolic disorders
      Primary and secondary adrenal insufficiency
      Primary amyloidosis
      Pheochromocytoma
      Diabetes mellitus
    Miscellaneous disorders
      Extensive surgical sympathectomy
      Hypovolemia (including drug-induced)
      Anorexia nervosa

Table 3. THERAPY OF ORTHOSTATIC HYPOTENSION

Correct volume depletion and electrolyte disturbance
  Discontinue hypotension-inducing drugs
  Treat identifiable disorders: adrenal insufficiency, hypothyroidism, anemia
Mechanical methods
  Mild exercise if tolerated
  Head-up position of bed
  Elasticized body garment
Plasma and extracellular fluid expanders
  High salt diet
  Fluorocortisone
Vasoconstrictor drugs
  Ephedrine
  Phenylephrine
  Midodrine
  Phenylpropanolamine
  Clonidine
  Amphetamine
  Methylphenidate
  Dihydroergotamine
Other drugs
  Indomethacin
  Propranolol
  Pindolol

CARDIOVASCULAR SYNCOPE

Syncope due to cardiac abnormalities is caused by a transiently diminished cardiac output as a result of a cardiac arrhythmia or reduced stroke volume. Cardiac syncope usually has a more rapid onset and recovery than do the other types of syncope, and often there are no premonitory symptoms. The patient can exhibit an anoxic convulsion during an episode. Cardiac syncope may occur with the patient in either the recumbent or upright position.

Cardiac Arrhythmias. In this group belong the excessively slow and fast heart rates that may result in syncope from severely reduced cardiac output. Any of these disturbances in rhythm may be transitory and are not necessarily found at a subsequent examination. Use of a telephone transmitter, prolonged ambulatory monitoring, or invasive electrophysiologic testing may be required to identify the mechanism of the rhythm disturbance.

Sinus Node Dysfunction. "Sick sinus syndrome" is a general term used to describe disorders of sinus function that result in failure of the sinus node impulse to activate the atrium, or failure of the sinus node to perform its pacemaking function adequately (Fig. 1). A major subset of the sick sinus syndrome is the tachycardia-bradycardia syndrome, which is characterized by episodes of paroxysmal supraventricular tachycardia and sinus bradycardia. At the termination of supraventricular tachycardia, there is often prolonged delay before sinus rhythm returns. The patient may experience syncope during this transitional phase. Generally, sinus node dysfunction is found in association with abnormalities of the subsidiary pacemakers in the atrioventricular node and His-Purkinje system, such that adequate cardiac rhythm is not maintained during the absence of sinus node activity.

Paroxysmal Supraventricular Tachycardia. Patients with episodes of paroxysmal atrial fibrillation, atrial flutter, and atrial tachycardia may have a history of syncope. Heart rates in excess of 180 to 200 beats/min are generally necessary before consciousness becomes clouded or lost. However, most patients can tolerate such accelerated heart rates without a significant alteration in consciousness. In patients with impaired cerebral perfusion or associated cardiac diseases, a supraventricular arrhythmia may be associated with a profound decrease in cerebral perfusion during heart rates that would be tolerated in a normal heart. Accelerated AV conduction resulting in a rapid ventricular rate and syncope during episodes of supraventricular tachycardia can occur in patients with the Wolff-Parkinson-White syndrome.

Atrioventricular Block. Syncope in patients with AV block can result from superimposed tachyarrhythmias or a failure of subsidiary pacemakers to maintain cardiac rhythm.

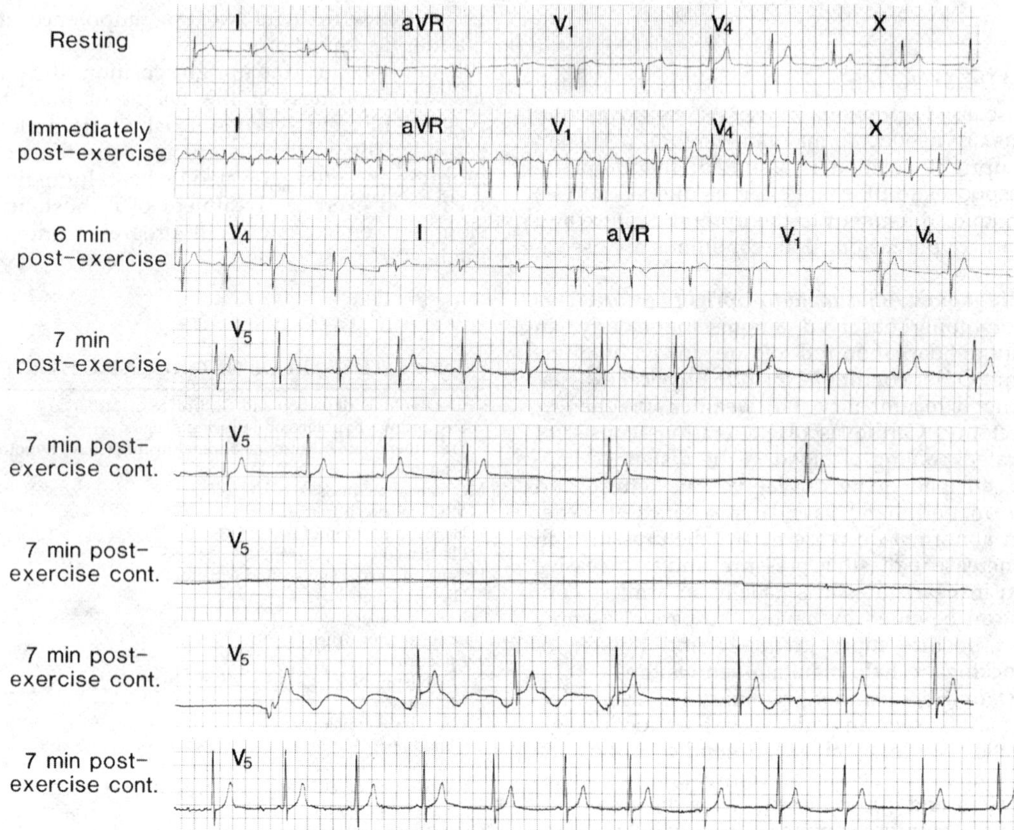

Figure 1. Sinus pause followed by sinus arrest after exercise stress testing. (From Hammill SC, Holmes DR Jr, Wood DL: Cardiac arrhythmias. *In* Conn RB (ed): Current Diagnosis, 7th ed. W.B. Saunders Co, Philadelphia, 1985, pp 405–433. By permission.)

Ventricular Arrhythmias. Paroxysmal ventricular tachycardia or ventricular fibrillation can occur not only in patients with heart disease but also in those who appear to have otherwise normal cardiac function. Patients with paroxysmal ventricular tachycardia and otherwise normal cardiac function generally do not experience syncope. However, syncope may be experienced by individuals whose ventricular tachycardia results in an excessively rapid ventricular rate or who have an associated cardiac condition such as ischemic, myopathic, valvular, or congenital heart disease.

A long Q-T interval is associated with rapid paroxysmal ventricular arrhythmias (torsades de pointes) and syncope. It can be a familial abnormality or may result from drugs, including quinidine, procainamide, disopyramide, and the phenothiazines, and from electrolyte imbalance, including hypokalemia, hypomagnesemia, and hypocalcemia.

Asystole. Asystole can develop in the presence of complete heart block or atrial standstill when junctional or ventricular pacemakers fail to pace the heart.

Treatment of patients with symptomatic bradycardia, AV block, and asystole requires permanent cardiac pacing. Prevention of syncope due to tachycardia requires antiarrhythmic medication, as discussed in Chapters 11 and 12, Section II.

Ischemic Heart Disease. During cardiac ischemia, syncope can result from ventricular arrhythmias or conduction disturbance, increases in parasympathetic activity with consequent bradycardia and hypotension, and severely impaired left ventricular function.

Valvular Heart Disease. Patients who have valvular heart disease that results in a relatively fixed cardiac output (aortic and pulmonary stenoses) can experience syncope. Characteristically, their syncope is associated with exertion and does not occur at rest. Syncope during exertion results from an increase in peripheral vasodilatation and a failure to increase cardiac output commensurately. Syncope occurs in 20% to 25% of patients with aortic stenosis and is almost always induced by physical activity. Rarely, mitral stenosis can cause syncope by a greatly decreased cardiac output after exercise, by the development of a ball-valve type of thrombus, or by the onset of a rapid supraventricular tachycardia. Myxomas also can cause syncope as a result of ball-valve obstruction of cardiac outflow. Patients with prosthetic cardiac valves who have syncope should be evaluated aggressively, because the syncope may be secondary to mechanical malfunction or obstruction caused by damage to the valve or by thrombus formation on the valve structures. Finally, syncope may be associated with dynamic left ventricular outflow obstruction, as seen in hypertrophic cardiomyopathy. In the latter, syncope is associated with events that result in a decrease in diameter of the left ventricular cavity during systole, such as increased contractility, or a decrease in afterload and thus in left ventricular distending pressure. Syncope may occur during exertion or after administration of drugs that have a positive inotropic effect, such as digitalis or isoproterenol, or drugs that cause peripheral vasodilatation. Also, arrhythmia due to valvular heart disease may cause syncope.

Congenital Heart Disease. In patients with congenital heart disease, the transient loss of consciousness has been most commonly observed in those with tetral-ogy of Fallot, but it also can occur in patients with truncus arteriosus, Eisenmenger complex, aortic stenosis, pulmonary stenosis, transposition of the great vessels, or ventricular septal defect. Syncope usually becomes manifest in early childhood and is precipitated by physical activity. It may be secondary to a decrease in cardiac output, to cardiac arrhythmias, or to a decrease in arterial oxygen saturation.

CAROTID SINUS SYNCOPE

Stimulation of the carotid sinus elicits the carotid reflex because of activation of baroreceptors within the wall of the sinus itself, the vagal efferents producing cardiac slowing. This is a physiologic reflex; however, some individuals have an exaggerated or even pathologic response, with spontaneous activation of the reflex or activation of the reflex from only slight pressure on the carotid sinus. The carotid sinus reflex is composed of a cardioinhibitory response and a vasodepressor response. The cardioinhibitory response is present in most patients with carotid sinus hypersensitivity, but 5% to 10% of patients exhibit a pure vasodepressor response. A mixed cardioinhibitory and vasodepressor response is observed in 30% of patients. The definition of a normal response to carotid sinus stimulation is arbitrary; ventricular asystole of 3 seconds or more (cardioinhibitory response) and a decrease in BP of 50 mm Hg or more (vasodepressor response) are definitely abnormal.

Approximately 30% of patients over 50 years of age have an abnormal response to carotid sinus massage yet remain asymptomatic. In selected patients with recurrent syncope, the typical spell can be reproduced by carotid sinus stimulation.

In the patient whose syncope is primarily due to the cardioinhibitory response, a permanent pacemaker will eliminate the spells. Unfortunately, a pacemaker is not as effective in eliminating syncope in the patient with a predominantly vasodepressor response, and treatment of such a patient is often similar to that of one with primary orthostatic hypotension.

PULMONARY DISEASE

Syncope due to primary pulmonary hypertension is characteristically related to effort and occurs in 20% of patients with this abnormality. Patients with pulmonary hypertension are often unable to increase cardiac output to compensate for the vasodilatation of exercise, and thus experience a decrease in arterial pressure. If the decrease is sufficient, syncope results. A second mechanism of syncope in such patients is cardiac arrhythmia associated with the abnormal right ventricular function.

Syncope also may be an early manifestation of a massive pulmonary embolism. Although syncope is usually preceded by typical pleuritic chest pain and dyspnea, these symptoms may be absent. The pulmonary embolism results in an acute decrease in cardiac output and decrease in the cerebral circulation.

COUGH SYNCOPE

Cough syncope, or tussive syncope, is a faint that accompanies an attack of coughing. The mechanism of fainting is similar to that associated with other strenuous activity, such as laughing, straining at stool, sneezing, and lifting. This abnormality generally affects males 40 years of age or older, and chronic obstructive pulmonary disease is often a predisposing factor.

MICTURITION SYNCOPE

Micturition syncope usually occurs after a patient has been recumbent for some time and then assumes the upright position while urinating. Micturition syncope results from a lack of the normal postural adaptive mechanisms, which are impaired because of the previous prolonged recumbency in a warm bed and the absence of a period of adjustment. In addition, visceral afferent stimulation from a full bladder probably contributes to the syncope, as a similar type of syncope has been observed during catheterization of a distended bladder and rapid drainage.

NEUROVASCULAR SYNCOPE

Cerebrovascular Disease. Syncope is uncommon in patients with cerebrovascular disease. When it occurs, it implies a partial or complete occlusion of at least one of the carotid or vertebral arteries. Syncope generally occurs while the patient is in the upright position, although those with vertebral artery disease may experience syncope with a change in head position.

Cerebral Artery Spasm. Patients with migraine or hypertensive encephalopathy can experience syncope, but this is not common.

Subclavian Steal Syndrome. Patients with the subclavian steal syndrome may present with an occlusion or high-grade stenosis of the subclavian artery proximal to the origin of the vertebral vessel. During exercise of the upper extremity, blood may be shunted away from the vertebral system, resulting in symptoms of cerebrovascular insufficiency and occasionally syncope.

Glossopharyngeal Syncope. Patients with glossopharyngeal neuralgia may experience syncope during stimulation of the pharynx, tonsillar area, base of the tongue, or ear. An electrocardiogram recorded during the syncopal spell usually demonstrates bradycardia or asystole. Such syncope may be eliminated by sectioning of the glossopharyngeal nerve. Some patients with this mechanism of syncope may have associated malignancy involving the neck.

REFERENCES

Day SC, Cook EF, Funkenstein H, et al: Evaluation and outcome of emergency room patients with transient loss of consciousness. Am J Med 73:15–23, 1982.

Kapoor WN, Karpf M, Wieand S, et al: A prospective evaluation and follow-up of patients with syncope. N Engl J Med 309:197–204, 1983.

Lipsitz LA: Syncope in the elderly. Ann Intern Med 99:92–105, 1983.

Morley CA, Perrins EJ, Grant P, et al: Carotid sinus syncope treated by pacing: analysis of persistent symptoms and role of atrioventricular sequential pacing. Br Heart J 47:411–418, 1982.

Robertson D, Robertson RM: Orthostatic hypotension—diagnosis and therapy. Mod Concepts Cardiovasc Dis 54:7–12, 1985.

Thomas JE, Hammill SC: Syncopal disorders. In Brandenburg RO, Fuster V, Giuliani ER, et al (eds): Cardiology: Fundamentals and Practice. Year Book Medical Publishers, Chicago, in press.

17 · SYSTEMIC EMBOLISM

Jess R. Young
CLEVELAND CLINIC FOUNDATION

DEFINITION AND DIAGNOSTIC CRITERIA

Virchow's definition of an arterial embolus as "the sudden blocking of an artery . . . by a clot or obstruction which has been brought to its place by the blood current" seems as appropriate today as it was 100 years ago. Although an embolus may consist of cholesterol plaque, tumor, fat, air, or foreign body, the clinical picture most commonly results from a thrombus formed in the heart or in an aortic or peripheral aneurysm that has migrated to an arterial bifurcation, where it lodges and obstructs flow.

Acute arterial embolism is a dramatic event that requires quick action and decisive judgment. Arterial spasm and propagating thrombus increase the urgency of prompt diagnosis and treatment if amputation and death are to be prevented. To avoid incorrect diagnosis and procrastination, the physician must understand the causes of acute ischemia, the clinical picture presented, and the indicated treatment.

Arterial embolism should be suspected in any patient who experiences sudden onset of pain, pallor, coldness, and numbness of an extremity. This suspicion is greatly strengthened by the presence of cardiac disease, especially when associated with atrial fibrillation or recent myocardial infarction. The diagnosis of systemic embolism should also be considered in a patient with cardiac disease who develops signs or symptoms of arterial insufficiency to the brain, spleen, kidneys, or intestines.

PATHOPHYSIOLOGY

SOURCES

About 90% of systemic emboli originate in the heart (Table 1). Over the past 40 years, the cardiac source of emboli has shifted. Previously, most patients were in

Table 1. ETIOLOGY OF ARTERIAL EMBOLI

Etiology	Incidence (%)
Arteriosclerotic heart disease	60
Rheumatic heart disease	20
Prosthetic heart valves, atrial myomas, myocarditis, and other cardiac sources	10
Proximal aneurysms, parodoxic embolus	5
Undetermined	5

their fourth decade of life and had emboli as a result of rheumatic heart disease. Antibiotic therapy has reduced the incidence and complications of rheumatic heart disease. Today, most patients are in their sixth and seventh decades and have emboli caused by the complications of arteriosclerotic heart disease.

Atrial fibrillation enhances the likelihood of formation of mural thrombus, but is not an essential prerequisite for embolization. Cardiac surgical procedures such as excision of a ventricular aneurysm, valve replacement, and (occasionally) coronary bypass surgery may be complicated by systemic embolism. Embolism may occur as a late complication of prosthetic valve replacement, although the incidence has dropped markedly in recent years as a result of the introduction of less thrombogenic valves and the use of anticoagulants. Other causes of mural thrombi and embolization include myocarditis, cardiomyopathies, myxomas, ventricular aneurysms, and chronic congestive failure.

Intriguing but rare is the parodoxic embolus that arises from a venous thrombus and is transported to the systemic arterial circulation through a septal defect with a right-to-left shunt. Usually, one or more previous pulmonary emboli have set the stage for the parodoxic embolus by increasing blood pressure in the pulmonary arteries and right side of the heart, thereby creating a right-to-left shunt through an otherwise asymptomatic atrial septal defect.

Atheromatous debris from a diseased aorta or more distal artery may be responsible for the sudden appearance of cutaneous gangrene of the feet and toes.

SITES OF SYSTEMIC EMBOLI

An arterial embolus usually progresses distally until it reaches an arterial bifurcation whose diameter is smaller than that of the occluding embolus. The most common sites are listed in Table 2. Most carotid emboli progress intracranially, but an occasional large embolus lodges at the bifurcation of the common carotid artery. Most emboli of the legs involve the common femoral artery bifurcation, followed by the aortoiliac and the popliteal artery bifurcations. About 15% of emboli involve the arm and another 10% either the mesenteric circulation or the renal arteries.

EFFECTS OF EMBOLISM

When a major arterial trunk suddenly becomes occluded with an embolus, the distal tissues must be nourished by collateral vessels. The adequacy of the collateral circulation is the biggest factor in the eventual outcome. Initially, there is usually reflex arterial spasm involving the main trunk proximal and distal to the site of occlusion as well as the small collateral channels. If the spasm is prolonged, endothelial damage occurs in

the arterial tree, favoring deposition of thrombus in the collateral channels and thus diminishing the prospects for recovery. However, when the collateral channels remain patent and are reasonably adequate, it is unlikely that irreversible ischemia will occur.

Spontaneous improvement with return of pulsations in major arteries occurs when spasm abates or when endogenous fibrinolysin permits lysis and fragmentation of a large embolus. The resulting fragments are swept by the bloodstream to more distal sites, with a diminishing of the extent and severity of ischemia.

CLINICAL ASPECTS

The diagnosis of sudden arterial occlusion usually is correctly made in the presence of the typical clinical picture of acute onset of pain, coldness, numbness, and hypoesthesia of the involved extremity. The two most common causes of sudden arterial occlusion are embolization and thrombosis in situ. Sudden local thrombosis of an artery usually occurs at the site of an atherosclerotic plaque. Sometimes, sudden arterial thrombosis is the first clinical manifestation of atherosclerosis, but more often it occurs as an unexpected complication of preexisting symptomatic arteriosclerosis obliterans.

Typically, the patient with thrombosis is older, has a history of claudication, evidence of occlusive disease in the contralateral limb, no obvious source for an embolus, and a more gradual onset of symptoms.

Other entities to consider in a patient with acute arterial occlusion include traumatic thrombosis, dissecting aneurysm, ergot toxicity, blood dyscrasias, arteritis, and septicemia. Venous gangrene (phlegmasia cerulea dolens) may also present clinically with a picture difficult to differentiate from an acute arterial occlusion.

It is very important to differentiate embolism from thrombosis. The treatment of choice for embolism is embolectomy since it is a limited procedure, can be done under local anesthesia if necessary, and is usually successful. Thrombectomy for thrombosis, on the other hand, is often unsuccessful. It may aggravate the ischemia, necessitating a major arterial reconstruction on an emergency basis in an often poorly prepared patient. For these reasons, the indications for surgery are more strict for thrombosis than for embolism.

Arteriograms are not necessary when the diagnosis is obvious. When there is doubt as to the etiology of the ischemia, arteriography can be done. The usual arteriographic pattern in embolism is that of an abrupt cut-off of arterial continuity, with minimal or no collateral circulation. Occasionally, the outline of the embolus itself can be seen as a filling defect.

In half the patients with arterial embolism, pain is not the initial symptom and the onset is not acute. In 25% of cases, pain is entirely absent and the only symptoms may be numbness and coldness. Sometimes, the only clinical manifestation of sudden arterial occlusion may be the abrupt appearance or worsening of intermittent claudication. Paresis is almost never the presenting complaint. If it occurs, it usually appears several hours after other symptoms of ischemia have been present. Sudden onset of ischemic symptoms simultaneously in both legs implies either that an embolus has lodged at the bifurcation of the aorta (saddle embolus) or that acute aortic thrombosis has occurred.

Table 2. SITES OF SYSTEMIC ARTERIAL EMBOLI

Site	Incidence (%)
Carotid	20
Femoral	20
Aortoiliac	15
Popliteal	15
Upper extremity	15
Mesenteric	5
Renal	5
Other (splenic, coronary, tibial, etc.)	5

The most important physical sign in establishing the diagnosis of sudden arterial occlusion is the absence or severe impairment of pulsations in arteries that were known previously to have had palpable pulses. The acutely ischemic extremity appears pale or cyanotic and is cold and hypoesthetic or anesthetic, and the superficial veins have collapsed. In the later stages, muscular weakness can sometimes be demonstrated.

MANAGEMENT

PLAN

The short-term goal of management is to make a correct diagnosis of embolism, try to determine the cause, and attempt to give specific treatment as soon after onset of ischemia as possible. The patient should be hospitalized for close observation. When CHF, recent massive myocardial infarction, life-threatening arrhythmias, hemorrhage, severe electrolyte disturbances, shock, or diabetic coma is present, the primary measures must be directed toward saving the life of the patient.

If conservative measures do not produce rapid improvement in circulation within two to three hours, surgical removal of the clot must be considered. Although it is wise to avoid an unnecessary operation, the patient must be referred to the surgeon while treatment can still be effective. There is no arbitrary time limit beyond which a limb is unsalvageable. As long as irreversible gangrene is not present, the limb can be restored if the embolus can be removed. The best indications of viability are the preservation of light touch, motion of the digits, and the presence of capillary blanching on pressure. If these are not present, the limb is severely ischemic and irreversible gangrene will result if circulation cannot be restored within eight to 12 hours. The decision to operate must take into consideration not only the general condition of the patient, but also the fact that the leg will probably progress to gangrene and subsequently require amputation if severe ischemia is not relieved.

The actual surgical technique of embolectomy has been so simplified that it is much less hazardous, even in the very ill, to restore blood flow under local anesthesia than to wait and then perform amputation under general anesthesia. Since the introduction of the intra-arterial catheter technique by Fogarty and Cranley, all embolectomies can be performed under local anesthesia, and total restoration of blood flow can be expected in most instances. The procedure in itself has low rates of morbidity and mortality and, at present, embolectomy for moderately to severely ischemic limbs should not be withheld without good reason.

Long-term goals should include removing the source of the embolus whenever possible. Mitral valve surgery and atrial appendectomy should be considered if rheumatic heart disease with mitral stenosis is the source of the embolus. Aneurysmectomy should be done when an aneurysm is the source. Stricter control or elimination of arrhythmias should be attempted if arrhythmia is the cause of embolus. When the cause cannot be eliminated, permanent anticoagulation should be recommended.

NONPHARMACOLOGIC MEASURES

A warm environment is one of the best measures for relieving arterial spasm; thus, the patient should be placed in a room where the temperature can be kept between 80° and 85°F. It is also advisable to wrap the involved extremity loosely in a blanket to preserve body heat and protect the limb from trauma. The head of the bed should be elevated on blocks 8 to 10 inches high so that the patient's arms and legs are in a dependent position and the effect of gravity augments the flow of blood to the involved extremity. A foot cradle is helpful in protecting the leg, and a foam rubber boot will help protect the foot and heel. It is worth emphasizing that elevation of an acutely ischemic extremity and the application of heat to it are contraindicated and may hasten the onset of gangrene.

The blocking of appropriate sympathetic ganglia has been advocated by some for the treatment of sudden arterial occlusion. This should be done before heparin is administered and should not be repeated while effective anticoagulation is being maintained, because of the danger of bleeding at the injection sites. Anticoagulation is more important in the management of acute ischemia than is regional sympathetic denervation, and therefore heparin should not be withheld for the purpose of blocking sympathetic ganglia safely.

DRUG THERAPY

Selection of Drugs. Severe pain, which aggravates arterial spasm, usually requires the use of narcotics. They should be given in adequate doses as often as necessary. Clinicians differ regarding other methods of attempting vasodilation. Vasodilators are not effective when given orally, but intra-arterial administration may be beneficial. Papaverine hydrochloride, 30 to 60 mg, or tolazoline hydrochloride (Priscoline), 25 to 50 mg, injected intra-arterially will improve flow within a few minutes, if they are effective at all. In the absence of contraindications to anticoagulant therapy, the patient should be given a bolus of heparin IV, 4000 to 7000 units. An IV drip should also be started, giving about 10 units of heparin hourly for each pound of body weight to maintain coagulation time or partial thromboplastin time at twice normal. Administration of an anticoagulant is important because it prevents propagation of thrombus and decreases the possibility of recurrent emboli. This immediate anticoagulation can provide time for transfer of the patient to a hospital if not already there, and permit a more thorough preoperative evaluation if surgery is necessary.

Low-molecular-weight dextran has been shown to be of value in the treatment of acute arterial embolism. By preventing erythrocyte aggregation and capillary stagnation, dextran decreases blood viscosity and increases blood flow and tissue perfusion. Best results are obtained when treatment is started within four to eight hours of onset of symptoms. The usual dosage is 500 ml of a 10% solution every six hours. It should be given cautiously in patients with limited cardiac reserve because of the danger of overloading the heart and precipitating CHF. Dextran should not be given to patients with borderline renal function because renal failure has been reported after its use in this situation. A rare patient may experience an anaphylactic reaction with dextran.

The place of thrombolytic therapy in the management of embolic occlusions remains unsettled. The embolic material may be well organized and resistant to lysis. Local delivery of thrombolytic agents by way of an arteriographic catheter left at the site of occlusion seems to have a better chance of success. However, a major concern is that the lytic agent may also cause lysis and fragmentation of the thrombus at the site of origin of the embolus, resulting in a new shower of emboli. Hence, an embolus, if accessible to a surgical approach, is best removed operatively. Most cerebral emboli are intracranial and not accessible to surgical embolectomy. However, a large embolus can be accessible at the common carotid artery bifurcation. Mesenteric, renal, and splenic emboli still require laparotomy and surgical embolectomy.

Management of Complications. If an embolus involves the terminal aorta, severe shock may be present, necessitating rapid fluid infusion.

In some patients with prolonged severe limb ischemia, renal failure with acidosis and hyperkalemia may follow the release of toxic products from ischemic muscles. The incidence of this complication is minimized by adequate hydration, alkalinization of the urine, and use of dextran. If it does occur, dialysis may be necessary.

There is a frequent association of deep venous thrombosis with acute arterial occlusion. Pulmonary embolism has also been noted as a complication or a cause of death in many patients with acutely ischemic limbs. This risk should be minimized by anticoagulant therapy.

Recurrent arterial embolism is common if the source of the embolus is not eliminated and the patient is not given adequate anticoagulant therapy. Inadequate therapy can result from either insufficient dosage of medication or poor patient compliance. This emphasizes the need for full and careful anticoagulation. The prothrombin time should be checked at no longer than weekly intervals for the first four to six weeks to make sure that the amount of coumarin needed to keep the PT at about 1½ to two times the control does not vary much from week to week. Following this trial period, the interval between blood checks can be lengthened to every two to four weeks. Lifelong anticoagulation is generally indicated unless the source of the embolus can be eliminated. Examples of such eradication are resection of an aneurysm responsible for a peripheral embolus, or conversion of atrial fibrillation to normal sinus rhythm. Patients with an acute myocardial infarction complicated by mural thrombi, but uncomplicated by ventricular aneurysm or atrial fibrillation, rarely have emboli after four months, and anticoagulants can be discontinued at that time.

PATIENT INFORMATION AND EDUCATION

Patients must be well informed regarding their condition and treatment in order to improve compliance. The importance of antiarrhythmic agents, if needed, should be stressed. If anticoagulant therapy is necessary, the dangers of either too little or too much therapy must be explained clearly. It must be emphasized that an inadequate dose of anticoagulants can result in recurrent embolism, and too great a dose can produce dangerous bleeding complications. Written material regarding coumarin therapy should be given so that patients can learn about side effects, drug interactions, the use of alcohol, and what to do when bleeding occurs. Patient compliance is usually excellent as long as the risks of noncompliance are well outlined.

PERIODIC EVALUATION

Patients should be seen in the office four to six weeks after discharge. All pulses should be checked and compared with those found at the time of discharge. If a Doppler or Pulse Volume Recorder is available, this should also be used to check and compare with the hospital findings. Basic information regarding the patients' condition and treatment should be reviewed with them. Following this, visits can be at three- to six-month intervals if all is going well. Consultations regarding PT determinations every one to four weeks and coumarin dose adjustments can be handled by telephone.

PREVENTIVE MEASURES

Patients with arteriosclerotic heart disease should be counseled regarding risk factor modification. Tobacco in any form should be forbidden. The diet should be tailored to get rid of excess weight and to restrict saturated fats and cholesterol. If dietary measures fail to reduce the concentration of cholesterol to reasonably normal levels, lipid-lowering agents should be added. If the patient has markedly elevated cholesterol, other family members should be checked. Diabetes mellitus and hypertension should be adequately controlled.

Systemic embolization can result from bacterial endocarditis. Patients with valvular heart disease should be instructed regarding antibiotic prophylaxis for dental manipulations or tooth extractions, urethral catheterization, surgery on the urogenital or gastrointestinal tracts, and several other clinical situations.

SOCIOECONOMIC ASPECTS OF MANAGEMENT

The cost of supervising a prophylactic program for a patient who has had a systemic embolus is not great. The average dose of coumarin costs about $20.00 a month. The laboratory charge for a prothrombin determination, which must be done one to four times a month, is about $10 to $15. There will also be an office charge for visits every three to six months. These expenses are minimal compared with the economic and medical consequences of a poorly supervised prophylactic program.

REFERENCES

Fogarty TJ: Management of arterial emboli. Surg Clin North Am 59:749–753, 1979.

Hight DW, Tilney NL, Couch NP: Changing clinical trends in patients with peripheral arterial emboli. Surgery 79:172–176, 1976.

Hollier LH: Acute arterial occlusion. *In* Spittell JA Jr (ed): Clinical Vascular Disease. F. A. Davis Co, Philadelphia, 1983, pp 49–57.

Young JR: Sudden arterial occlusion: medical aspects. *In* Gifford RW Jr (ed): Peripheral Vascular Disease. F. A. Davis Co, Philadelphia, 1971, pp 159–172.

18 · ANTICOAGULANTS AND PLATELET INHIBITORS

Edward Genton
OCHSNER CLINIC AND ALTON OCHSNER MEDICAL FOUNDATION

Thrombosis is the principal event in the pathogenesis of many cardiac or vascular diseases, and complicates the course of patients with conditions of varied etiologies. In the management of these patients, it is important that the clinician have a thorough understanding of thrombosis to identify predisposing factors, anticipate prognosis, and select the optimal approach to antithrombotic therapy.

THROMBOGENESIS

The sequence by which blood is transformed from its fluid state to a hemostatic plug or intravascular thrombus is a multi-stage process involving the endothelial cell, blood platelet, coagulation and fibrinolytic systems, and various inhibitory mechanisms. In most instances the initiating event is damage to the endothelial cells, which stimulates the adhesion of platelets at the site of damage, followed rapidly by aggregation of additional platelets to form a primary hemostatic plug. Simultaneously the coagulation system is activated through the extrinsic and/or intrinsic thromboplastin pathways. This activation of the coagulation system results in formation of thrombin that converts fibrinogen to a fibrin gel, which stabilizes the platelet plug and forms a permanent hemostatic plug or thrombus. Thrombi are of several types, depending on predominating constituents, and their internal organization may consist of primarily platelets, primarily fibrin, or a mixed variety. Thrombi that form in the arterial circulation with rapid flow consist predominantly of platelets, while those forming in low-pressure or slow-flow areas (as in veins or partially occluded arteries) consist predominantly of red cells within a fibrin latticework, with platelets dispersed irregularly throughout. In the region of thrombosis, the fibrinolytic system is activated by release of tissue plasminogen activator from damaged endothelial cells. This degrades plasminogen adherent to fibrin within the thrombus or in the circulation to plasmin, which leads to proteolytic digestion of fibrin within the thrombus.

MANAGEMENT

Antithrombotic therapy may be variable, depending on the clinical situation, and may alter one or a combination of the thrombogenic components. Treatment may (1) prevent damage or inhibit response to endothelial cells, (2) prevent stasis of blood flow, (3) inhibit platelet reactivity, (4) inhibit the coagulation pathway, or (5) stimulate the fibrinolytic system. Methods for each of these approaches are currently available. The choice of

Table 1. EFFECTIVENESS OF ANTITHROMBOTIC THERAPY

	Heparin Dosage			War-farin	Aspirin	Dipyrid-amole
	High	*Moderate*	*Low*			
DVT/PE						
Treatment	+	±	−	−	−	−
Prophylaxis						
Primary	+	+	+	+	±	−
Secondary	+	+	−	+	−	−
Acute MI						
Venous thrombi	+	+	+	+	−	−
Systemic emboli	+	±	−	+	−	−
Prosthetic heart valve	+	+	−	+	−	−

approach requires consideration of several factors including whether the therapeutic objective is primarily prophylaxis of a thrombotic event, inhibition of an established thrombosis, or "secondary prophylaxis." Further, the approaches vary for the high-flow arterial system or the low-pressure venous circulation. For the former, a method to alter platelet reactivity is most rational, while for venous thrombosis inhibition of the coagulation system or prevention of stasis of blood flow is more appropriate. Once thrombosis exists, prophylactic methods are inappropriate, and treatment requires a method to arrest the thrombotic process and prevent further fibrin formation. In selected cases, optimal therapeutic outcome involves not just arresting the thrombotic process but accelerating resolution of the occlusive thrombus, using agents that activate the fibrinolytic system. The techniques currently used most frequently are those that modify the coagulation mechanism or platelet reactivity.

ANTICOAGULANT DRUGS

Basically, the coagulation system may be altered to prevent thrombosis by (1) creating a deficiency in the level or potency of one or several of the clotting factors; or (2) preventing the activation of, or inhibiting the effect of, activated clotting factors to interrupt the sequential reaction that leads to thrombin formation and fibrinogen conversion to fibrin. Heparin is an example of a drug that inhibits activated clotting factors, whereas oral anticoagulants alter the synthesis of several clotting factors.

Heparin

Heparin is a sulfated mucopolysaccharide extracted commercially from mast cells in the mucosa of hog intestine or beef lung. During preparation the native molecule undergoes cleavage, which results in widely varying molecular weights in the final material. It is likely that the numerous effects on coagulation produced by heparin reside in different-sized molecules. Most of the heparin molecules in commercial heparin are biologically inactive, and evidence suggests that the anticoagulant effect resides in low-molecular-weight molecules (below 5000 angstroms). Heparin from the different animal and organ sources has identical effects on coagulation assay.

The action of heparin as an anticoagulant when added to plasma results from its complexing with antithrombin III, which is a naturally occurring globulin. The complexing with heparin greatly enhances the inhibitory activity of the protein. This enhancement probably is caused by a conformational change in the AT-3 molecule, which increases the inhibitory activity by exposing more reactive sites. AT-3 is a naturally occurring inhibitor of enzymes with a serine protease residue at their enzymatically active center. Several clotting factors, when activated, are serine protease inhibitors, including Factors IX, X, XI, and XII and thrombin, or Factor IIa. The reaction between inhibitor and enzyme is stoichiometric and irreversible, and greatly accelerated by the presence of heparin. Once the clotting factor complex reaction occurs, which is irreversible, heparin may separate and return to the circulation to react with other AT-3 molecules. The amount of heparin needed to accelerate the rate of interaction between thrombin and AT-3 is minute. Some evidence suggests that the rate of reaction of the heparin antithrombin III complex differs for the various activated clotting factors. The more sensitive factors, such as Factor Xa, require lesser concentrations to be inhibited. This may explain the effectiveness of thrombosis prophylaxis when heparin is administered in low doses, which inhibit Factor Xa and thereby prevent formation of thrombin; once thrombin has formed, however, a larger concentration of heparin is necessary to arrest the thrombotic process.

Heparin is effective only when administered parenterally because the molecule is inactivated by gastric acidity. It may be injected subcutaneously or by the intravenous route as a bolus injection or sustained infusion. The clearance of heparin from the circulation has two phases: approximately 40% of the dose disappears in five to ten minutes, some because it enters the extravascular space, and most because it binds to the membrane of endothelial cells. Heparin remaining in the circulation is removed with a half-life of 60 to 90 minutes. It is thought that most of the drug is cleared by the reticuloendothelial system, with small amounts cleared by hepatocytes and excreted into the bile. With customary doses, most of the drug is desulfated and excreted in the urine within 24 hours as an inorganic sulfate. With larger doses there is a longer half-life and slower excretion. For parenteral use a number of concentrations of the drug are available, ranging from 1000 to 40,000 units per ml. For SQ use the more concentrated aqueous preparations are best to keep the injected volume at 0.5 ml or less. For IV bolus or continuous infusion, the drug can be diluted to the desired volume in either dextrose or saline. The dose of heparin used depends on whether it is being given for prophylaxis or for treatment of active thrombosis. Because of variation in specific activity of heparin preparations, the drug should always be prescribed in units rather than milligrams.

For *prophylaxis of venous thrombosis,* a dose of 10,000 to 15,000 units per 24 hours is usually sufficient and produces a blood level of 0.05 to 0.1 units per ml of plasma. The most convenient approach is to administer the drug SQ in low dosage of 5000 units every eight to 12 hours. For least discomfort and hematoma formation, the injection should be given by a 26-gauge, ½-inch needle in a volume of 0.25 to 0.5 ml, injected into the subcutaneous fat of the anterior abdominal wall or anterior thigh. Care must be taken to avoid disruption of capillaries or injection into muscles.

For "low-dose heparin," monitoring is unnecessary in most patients, but it may be useful to document the effect on partial thromboplastin time (PTT) in patients at high risk of thrombosis or bleeding. In most patients the PTT is not prolonged significantly; however, in 5% to 10% of patients it will be, and a lesser dose is required. A similar number of patients will have no measurable blood level of heparin with the low dose and require increased amounts. This can be determined by adjusting the dosage to prolong the PTT by three to five seconds. Once proper dosage is established, further monitoring is unnecessary. The drug must be continued for as long as the provocation to thrombosis persists.

To treat *active thrombosis,* "full-dose heparin" is required. Both experimentally and in clinical practice, heparin in an amount that prolongs the PTT 1½ to two times control and produces heparin plasma concentration of 0.3 units per ml achieves this objective. In practice, this translates into a daily dose of 20,000 to 30,000 units in most patients. Treatment is begun with a priming dose of 5000 to 10,000 units, which achieves anticoagulation in approximately 85% of patients. To confirm that anticoagulation has been achieved, a PTT should be obtained 15 to 30 minutes following the IV bolus. If the desired effect has been accomplished, treatment can be continued with intermittent bolus of heparin at four- to six-hour intervals in a dose of 5000 to 10,000 units or as a continuous infusion averaging 20,000 to 30,000 units per 24 hours. The dose required varies considerably from 10,000 to occasionally as much as 100,000 units per day. Where in the therapeutic range an individual patient is kept depends on several factors. For massive pulmonary embolism, it is recommended that treatment be initiated with a higher dose of heparin than required to prolong the PTT to "therapeutic range," whereas patients considered at high risk of bleeding might well be kept near the lower limits of the therapeutic range.

Heparin Monitoring. Whether monitoring of heparin therapy with coagulation episodes is necessary is a matter of controversy. In most cases it is probably possible to predict a dose that will achieve anticoagulation and make monitoring unnecessary; however, it is desirable to document that anticoagulation has been achieved. Further, excessive amounts of the drug should be avoided, to reduce the risk of hemorrhage. Thus, routine monitoring is recommended, the first assay being obtained within 30 minutes after the heparin bolus has been given to confirm the achievement of anticoagulation. Monitoring should be done subsequently with intermittent bolus administration to obtain a clotting time before a dose, to establish that anticoagulation extends throughout the time period but is not excessive. Adjustment in dosage may be made on the basis of coagulation tests and is required in many cases after 36 or 48 hours, possibly because the heparin clearance is altered as the thrombotic process is arrested.

Complications of Heparin Therapy. The most important complications of heparin therapy are thrombocytopenia and hemorrhage. The reported frequency of *thrombocytopenia* varies widely, but it probably occurs in less than 2% of patients treated with IV heparin and in a smaller number treated with low-dose heparin. The mechanism of the thrombocytopenia is uncertain and may be multiple. Evidence suggests that platelet aggregation may be induced by the drug. Later reactions up to 20 days after initiation of therapy are probably on the basis of antiplatelet antibody formation.

Bleeding constitutes the most important complication of heparin therapy because of its frequency and significance. Hemorrhage occurs in 5% to 10% of patients and is of major consequence in about one half of the cases because of the severity or location of the bleeding. Patients at particular risk are (1) those with underlying hemostatic defect; (2) those being treated with other drugs that compromise hemostasis, such as aspirin; (3) those who have been exposed to recent surgery or vascular trauma; or (4) especially the elderly. Patients with compromised hemostatic capability are prone to bleed even with moderate levels of heparin, and the risk of bleeding increases with intensity of heparin in such cases. Patients considered at high risk of bleeding should have heparinization adjusted to the lower side of the therapeutic range, with the PTT kept near 1½ times control value. These patients should also receive a continuous infusion of heparin rather than intermittent boluses, to avoid the peaks of activity unavoidable with intermittent injections. To reduce bleeding complications, trauma should be avoided, including vascular or intramuscular injection. If serious bleeding begins, heparin should be terminated for 24 hours, during which time hemostasis is usually accomplished. If the indication for heparin remains strong, it may be resumed by continuous infusion and a lower dosage. When rapid reversal of heparin is required, protamine sulfate, a strong basic substance that combines with and inhibits heparin, may be used: 1 mg of protamine inhibits 1 mg (approximately 100 units) of heparin. It is seldom necessary to give more than 50 to 100 mg of protamine sulfate, but the drug is rapidly cleared from the circulation and may have to be repeated as determined by coagulation tests.

Other side effects of heparin include transient alopecia or osteoporosis. Osteoporosis occurs only after heparin administration in excess of three months and in patients receiving more than 15,000 units per day. The mechanism for this complication is uncertain.

Oral Anticoagulants

Mechanism of Action. Oral anticoagulants are organic compounds with molecular structure similar to vitamin K. Two groups used clinically are coumarin or indanedione derivatives. The differences between the various compounds relate to their potency, duration of action, rapidity of onset, and toxicity. All the oral anticoagulants have the common action of blocking membrane transport of vitamin K in hepatocytes and thereby inhibiting the effect of vitamin K on a postribosomal step in the synthesis of several clotting factors, including Factors II, VII, IX, and X. Vitamin K modifies the final structure of these clotting factors with a step that is essential for their normal biologic activity. With vitamin K deficiency or in the presence of oral anticoagulants, an immunologically detectable but biologically inactive protein results. The rate of activation of the clotting factor is accelerated several thousandfold when complexed with phospholipid, but this reaction is prevented with the abnormal clotting factor.

Oral anticoagulants are well absorbed from the GI tract or may be injected parenterally. In the circulation the drugs are more than 90% bound to albumin, and only the unbound fraction is pharmacologically active upon hepatocytes. Most of the drugs are metabolized in the hepatic endoplasmic reticulum and excreted in urine or stool. Metabolites may have slight but insignificant biologic activity.

Drug Regimen. Treatment is begun by oral or parenteral administration of the drug. The effect on hepatocytes is dose dependent and due to drug unbound to plasma proteins. Thus, small changes in the non–protein-bound fraction may lead to large changes in the anticoagulant activity produced. After treatment is begun, the development of anticoagulation is dependent on the clearance of normal circulating clotting factors present at the start of treatment. This clearance in turn is dependent on the half-life of clotting factors, which varies considerably from about six hours for Factor VII to 24 to 40 hours for Factors IX and X and 60 hours for Factor II. It therefore takes four or five days following the initiation of anticoagulant therapy before there is necessary depression of all four coagulation factors. Treatment should be initiated with doses of the oral anticoagulant approximately twice the anticipated maintenance dose. This reduces clotting factors gradually over three or four days. Thereafter, maintenance doses are given to maintain the desired level of anticoagulation.

Although the response to anticoagulants is reasonably predictable, there may be considerable variation in individual patients and in relation to a variety of clinical circumstances. In particular, the effects of clinical conditions that affect the intake and absorption of vitamin K and diseases of the hepatobiliary and renal systems result in varied response to the oral anticoagulants. In addition, many other drugs alter the anticoagulant effects through a variety of mechanisms. It is prudent to consider a drug interaction at any time that a medication is to be terminated or begun, and the prothrombin time (PT) should be checked frequently as a safeguard.

Monitoring. Anticoagulant therapy should always be monitored by appropriate coagulation tests, most often the one-stage PT. The tests should be obtained prior to treatment to exclude a hypocoagulable state, then after 48 hours, and thereafter at appropriate intervals, to document the level of anticoagulation achieved. In practice this usually requires PT checks three times weekly for two or three weeks and then less frequently, but never to exceed three or four weeks. Even when patients have been stabilized for months or years, fluctuations may occur for reasons that are often uncertain.

The optimal range of anticoagulation to achieve antithrombotic effect is difficult to define and may vary for different circumstances based on intensity of the stimulus for thrombosis. It is recommended that the PT be prolonged to 1.3 to two times the control value. The lower level is adequate for venous thrombosis prophylaxis. The higher levels are possibly necessary for prophylaxis of arterial thromboembolism, such as in patients with substitute heart valves.

Complications and Special Considerations. Complications of oral anticoagulants include hypersensitivity reactions and hemorrhagic complications. *Hypersensitivity* is uncommon with coumarin derivatives but more frequent with the indanedione derivatives; reactions include dermatitis, fever, hepatitis, and renal failure. Rarely, after one or two weeks of treatment with the coumarin derivatives, skin necrosis occurs in areas containing large deposits of subcutaneous fat such as breasts, thighs, and buttocks. This complication is most likely due to vasculitis and requires prompt termination of treatment.

The major complication of anticoagulation is *hemorrhage*, which occurs in 2% to 10% of patients during a course of treatment lasting several months. Bleeding is of major proportion in about half of these cases and fatal bleeding occurs in 0.01% to 1% of anticoagulated patients. In most instances, bleeding occurs with excessive anticoagulation. When it occurs with therapeutic levels, a local lesion such as peptic ulcer or malignant disease is usually present. Death from bleeding is most often due to intracerebral hemorrhage, but may result from bleeding into the GI tract.

Pregnancy presents a particular difficulty because oral anticoagulants cross the placenta and anticoagulate the fetus. This may lead to hemorrhage, especially during delivery. Additionally, oral anticoagulants have teratogenic effects, and "coumarin embryopathy" consisting of chondrodysplasia of the face and long bones may occur in more than 10% of infants exposed to the drug during the first trimester of the pregnancy.

Reversal of Oral Anticoagulant Effect. This can be accomplished with small doses of vitamin K given either orally or by parenteral injection. If the PT is excessively prolonged to levels more than three times control, a dose of 3 mg of parenteral vitamin K_1 oxide will return the PT to therapeutic range within six to eight hours without completely reversing the effect. If sufficient hemorrhagic complication occurs, a dose of 10 to 20 mg of K_1 oxide will completely reverse the drug effect. If bleeding is severe and life-threatening, the anticoagulation can be rapidly reversed by IV infusion of concentrates of coagulation Factors II, VII, IX, and X derived from two or three units of frozen plasma.

PLATELET-SUPPRESSANT DRUGS

The concept of pharmacologic inhibition of platelet reactivity as an approach to prophylactic antithrombotic therapy has gained considerable support with the recognition of the important role of platelets in thrombosis formation, especially in the arterial circulation, and the identification of drugs that suppress platelet function and retard thrombus formation in experimental animals. Although many drugs inhibit platelet function in vitro, only a few have demonstrated antithrombotic effects in vivo and are suitable for clinical use. Most of these agents have pharmacologic actions other than platelet effect and have been used in therapeutics for other purposes. Of these drugs, only acetylsalicylic acid and dipyridamole have been documented to have beneficial effects and are being widely used clinically.

Aspirin

The analgesic, anti-inflammatory and antipyretic actions of aspirin have long been known. More recently, it has been appreciated that bleeding time was prolonged in many patients following administration of this drug. Aspirin seems to inhibit the platelet release reaction induced by a number of stimuli, including collagen,

epinephrine, and thrombin in low concentrations. It probably inhibits platelet reactivity by several pathways. The one best elucidated has been the effect of the drug on the prostaglandin pathway: aspirin has been shown to inhibit the synthesis of cyclic endoperoxides and thromboxane A_2 from platelet membrane arachidonic acid by inhibiting the enzyme cyclo-oxygenase in the platelet. This effect is thought to result from acetylation of the cyclo-oxygenase, which irreversibly inhibits its action. Aspirin acetylates numerous platelet membrane proteins and inhibits platelet membrane enzymes that may contribute to its inhibitory effect on platelet function. The clearance of aspirin from the circulation is rapid and occurs within 15 to 30 minutes, but its effect on platelet proteins is permanent for the life of the platelet since the acetylation is irreversible and the platelet, being a non-nucleated cell, cannot regenerate enzymes. The dose of aspirin necessary to produce maximal cyclo-oxygenase inhibition is small, probably less than 150 mg for an adult, and the effect of even this small dose persists for several days.

Aspirin also inhibits prostaglandin synthesis by the endothelial cells of blood platelets and, in particular, the synthesis of prostacyclin (PGI_2), which is a potent inhibitor of platelet aggregation and a vasodilator. The dose of aspirin necessary for prostacyclin inhibition is considerably larger than for cyclo-oxygenase inhibition and may require dosages greater than are used clinically. The optimal dose of aspirin for platelet-inhibiting effect is currently uncertain; as little as 60 mg daily inhibits both thromboxane A_2 and PGI_2 formation, and as much as 2600 mg allows continued synthesis of some PGI_2. For the antithrombotic effect, no aspirin dosage tested is more or less effective than another, and presently no thrombogenic dosage has been found.

Dipyridamole

Dipyridamole is a vasodilator that weakly inhibits platelet aggregation induced by adenosine diphosphate, and in larger concentration inhibits platelet release reaction induced by collagen, epinephrine, or thrombin. In adults the drug (400 mg daily) shortens platelet survival time, and a similar effect is produced with as little as 100 mg of dipyridamole daily in combination with 1 gm of aspirin. This augmentation effect by aspirin has not been fully explained, but may relate to the ability of aspirin to inhibit cyclo-oxygenase and thereby potentiate the antithrombotic effect of dipyridamole. The drug is administered to adults in dosages of 50 to 75 mg, two or three times daily, and is generally well tolerated. No bleeding diathesis or other adverse platelet effects have been demonstrated.

REFERENCES

Bertele V, Salzman EW: Antithrombotic therapy in coronary artery disease. Arteriosclerosis 5:119–134, 1985.

Genton E, Turpie AG: Anticoagulant therapy following acute MI. Mod Concepts Cardiovasc Dis 52:45–51, 1983.

Hersh J, Genton E, Hull R: Venous Thromboembolism. Grune & Stratton, Orlando, 1981.

Hull R, Delmore T, Carter C, et al: Adjusted subcutaneous heparin vs. warfarin sodium on the long-term treatment of venous thrombosis. N Engl J Med 306:1985, 1982.

19 · PULMONARY HYPERTENSION AND COR PULMONALE

Richard J. Butcher
GEISINGER MEDICAL CENTER

DEFINITION AND DIAGNOSTIC CRITERIA

Pulmonary hypertension exists when mean pulmonary artery pressure exceeds 20 mm Hg. It may occur in response to left heart disease or increased pulmonary blood flow due to left-to-right shunting; these entities are discussed elsewhere in this book. *Cor pulmonale* consists of some combination of hypertrophy and dilatation of the right ventricle resulting from pulmonary hypertension not caused by left heart disease or intracardiac shunt. Cor pulmonale may be caused by disorders of the lung or the pulmonary vessels, or by extrapulmonary disorders of ventilation. When no underlying disease can be found, *primary pulmonary hypertension* exists. *Right heart failure* may result from cor pulmonale but need not always be present.

PATHOPHYSIOLOGY

The various disorders that may result in pulmonary hypertension (see Table 1) do so through just a few

Table 1. DISEASES TO BE CONSIDERED IN DIFFERENTIAL DIAGNOSIS OF PULMONARY HYPERTENSION

Diseases causing pulmonary venous hypertension
  Left ventricular systolic or diastolic failure
  Constrictive pericarditis
  Left atrial hypertension due to mitral stenosis, left atrial myxoma, or cor triatriatum
  Pulmonary veno-occlusive disease
  Fibrosing mediastinitis
Left-to-right shunt (intracardic or involving great vessels)
Diseases causing hypoxia
  Chronic obstructive lung disease
  Bronchiectasis, cystic fibrosis
  Chest wall deformities
  Lymphangitic spread of tumor
  Hypoventilation in presence of normal lungs
    Central hypoventilation
    Obstructive sleep apnea
    Neuromuscular disease
    Cord lesion or bilateral diaphragmatic paralysis
    Chronic mountain sickness
Mechanical occlusion of pulmonary vessels
  Pulmonary thromboembolism
  In situ thrombus (as from hemoglobinopathy)
  Nonthrombotic pulmonary emboli (tumor, fat, marrow, right atrial myxoma, vegetation, abscess, Gaucher's cells)
Pulmonary vascular involvement in collagen vascular diseases (systemic sclerosis, CREST, SLE, rheumatoid arthritis) or sarcoidosis
Lung diseases causing variable degrees of hypoxia and obliteration of pulmonary vessels
  Pulmonary fibrosis and other parenchymal lung diseases
  Lung resection; congenital absence of one pulmonary artery
Pulmonic stenosis - valvar or supravalvar.
  Congenital
  Acquired (usually extrinsic compression by mediastinal mass)
Drug-induced disease (anorexics)
Idiopathic disease

basic mechanisms. *Hypoxia* of any cause results in reflex pulmonary vasoconstriction; over time it may lead to irreversible hypertrophy of the pulmonary arteriolar walls and resultant hypertension. *Loss of functioning pulmonary arterial bed* can result in hypertension of the remaining arteries; thromboembolism, occlusion by in situ thrombosis (as by sickling in hemoglobinopathy), or destruction of vessels by pulmonary fibrosis all can cause pulmonary hypertension in this manner. *Intimal proliferation* of pulmonary arteries may lead to pulmonary hypertension in collagen vascular disorders, especially the CREST syndrome variant of systemic sclerosis. Some diseases act through multiple mechanisms: parenchymal lung disease may cause both hypoxia and direct destruction of vessels; in schistosomiasis, ova embolize the lungs and also provoke intense inflammation of pulmonary arteriolar walls.

Primary pulmonary hypertension appears to result from hyperreactivity of muscular pulmonary arteries and arterioles, leading eventually to hypertrophy of the arteriolar walls and the histologic findings of a necrotizing arteritis and characteristic plexiform lesions. The cause of primary pulmonary hypertension is unknown. Its predilection for women of childbearing age; its occasional familial occurrence; its known association with portal hypertension and with Raynaud's phenomenon; and its occurrence in the small percentage of patients exposed to the drug Aminorex (an appetite suppressant, since banned) or certain plant substances, all seem to suggest that multiple mechanisms, each as yet unidentified, may produce the increase in local vascular reactivity. To complicate the picture further, patients with the clinical syndrome of primary pulmonary hypertension may on occasion demonstrate two other distinct histopathologic pictures. One is that of widespread deposition of thrombi in small and medium-sized pulmonary arteries; these may occur in situ or represent occult thromboemboli. The other is that of *pulmonary veno-occlusive disease* with thickening ("arteriolization") of normally thin-walled venules.

Persistent pulmonary hypertension at first results in hypertrophy of the right ventricle; later, dilatation and systolic impairment occur and increased right heart filling pressures develop. The left ventricle is essentially spared.

CLINICAL ASPECTS

Cor pulmonale is at times difficult to distinguish from other causes of right heart failure; dyspnea may erroneously be taken to indicate left heart failure when it is actually due to the underlying lung or pulmonary vascular disease.

Almost all patients have dyspnea and fatigue. Chest pain, palpitations, or syncope may occur with exercise. Before right heart failure develops, physical examination usually shows a right parasternal lift and a loud pulmonic component of the second heart sound, which is often palpable. A right-sided fourth heart sound and jugular venous A wave, a pulmonic ejection sound, and the Graham Steell diastolic murmur of secondary pulmonic insufficiency (heard at the left upper sternal border) may all be present.

As right heart failure develops, the second heart sound becomes widely split. Tricuspid insufficiency, when present, may produce a systolic murmur at the fourth interspace increasing during inspiration, as well as jugular venous V waves and hepatic pulsation. Peripheral edema and ascites are late signs. Cyanosis may result from right-to-left shunting within the lung or through a patent foramen ovale.

The *chest x-ray* may show prominent pulmonary arteries and at times peripheral oligemia. *Electrocardiographic* signs are those of right ventricular hypertrophy, right axis deviation, P pulmonale, right bundle branch block (complete or incomplete), or loss of anterior precordial forces. The *echocardiogram*, often technically difficult if lung disease is present, may show right ventricular hypertrophy or dilatation, straightening of the interventricular septum, and a pulmonic valve with an absent A wave and partial midsystolic closure. *Radionuclide ventriculography* often shows right ventricular enlargement or hypokinesis, a prominent pulmonary artery, or reflux of isotope into the inferior vena cava during a first-pass study. A dilated or thick-walled right ventricle is occasionally noted on *thallium perfusion imaging*.

Right heart catheterization provides definitive hemodynamic data but carries a slight risk, which is lower if pulmonary angiography is avoided.

Patients with pulmonary hypertension are also at unusual risk from general anesthesia, even for minor surgical procedures. Deaths may also occur during venous cut-down procedures and arterial cannulations, as well as after perfusion lung scanning. The clinical course of cor pulmonale, irrespective of cause, consists of periods of stability punctuated by abrupt deterioration; improvement tends to occur only with successful therapy for an underlying process. Survival varies from months to a few years. Periods of stabilization lasting several years may occasionally occur.

MANAGEMENT

Because of the poor prognosis for patients with pulmonary hypertension of unknown or untreatable cause, they must be meticulously evaluated for treatable causes of pulmonary hypertension or diseases that mimic it (Table 1). If a careful history and physical examination does not provide specific diagnostic clues, the following data base should be obtained to identify remediable causes: chest x-ray, EKG, two-dimensional echocardiogram, arterial blood gases, spirometry, lung volumes, diffusing capacity, antinuclear antibody, perfusion lung scan, and impedance plethysmography or radionuclide venography of the lower extremities. In the absence of correctable factors, the treatment plan outlined below is designed to provide relief and to prevent or delay deterioration.

Right heart catheterization, requiring hospitalization, should be performed if no cause of pulmonary hypertension is evident. This will confirm the diagnosis, gauge its severity, and exclude the rare correctable cause that cannot be diagnosed noninvasively. Hospitalization (generally with right heart pressure monitoring) is mandatory if vasodilator therapy is begun. Hospital care is also necessary for the episodic acute or subacute deteriorations that occur in virtually all patients. Patients with cor pulmonale due to obstructive lung disease often benefit from follow-up by a pulmonary nurse clinician who can help them cope with the complex treatment plan and can identify clinical deterioration before it reaches a crisis.

NONPHARMACOLOGIC MEASURES

Chronic low-flow oxygen therapy is indicated when cor pulmonale is present and PaO_2 <55 mm Hg. Flow rates should be adjusted to produce a PaO_2 >60 mm Hg; initially, patients must be observed for progressive hypercapnia. Patients with chronic bronchitis, bronchiectasis, and cystic fibrosis may benefit from percussion and postural drainage. Phlebotomy to control secondary polycythemia should be considered when the hematocrit exceeds 60%. No further benefit can be demonstrated from decreasing the hematocrit below 55%. Salt and fluid restriction and bed rest benefit patients with right heart failure.

DRUG THERAPY

Since patients with severe pulmonary hypertension of any cause are prone to pulmonary embolism once right heart failure and a state of low cardiac output develop, I believe that long-term anticoagulation is indicated irrespective of the underlying etiology unless there is a definite contraindication. Warfarin should be used to maintain a prothrombin time (PT) of 1.5 to 1.8 times the control value. A PT determination should be performed every two to four weeks, depending on the patient's stability. Hemoglobin and stool must be monitored for occult blood loss.

Digoxin should be used if associated left ventricular failure or atrial arrhythmias are present, despite its risk of toxicity in the presence of hypoxia. Often a dose of 0.125 mg/day, keeping the digoxin level well below 1.5 ng/dl, is safest. Digoxin may be useful in treating acute exacerbations of cor pulmonale. Surveillance for the arrhythmias of digitalis toxicity (high-grade ventricular ectopy, AV junctional tachycardia, and atrial tachycardia with AV exit block) should be maintained; once the patient is stable, the drug may often be safely omitted. Multifocal atrial tachycardia and sinus tachycardia do not respond to digoxin.

Diuretics should be used to control edema and ascites, recognizing that decreasing intravascular volume may further decrease an already low cardiac output and that diuretic-induced hypokalemia may potentiate serious arrhythmias. Usually loop diuretics (furosemide, 20 to 80 mg/day and up) are required. Potassium replacement or potassium-sparing diuretics (triamterene, 25 to 100 mg/day, amiloride, 5 to 10 mg/day, or spironolactone, 25 to 100 mg/day) may be needed.

Theophylline has been shown to produce chronic improvement of hemodynamics in patients with cor pulmonale; thus, a long-acting theophylline preparation (e.g., Theo-Dur), starting at 200 mg PO every 12 hours and adjusting dosage to a serum level of 10 to 20 μg/ml should be given to patients with obstructive lung disease causing cor pulmonale. Theophylline toxicity, presenting as nausea, restlessness and irritability, insomnia, arrhythmia, and occasionally seizures, may be minimized by attention to serum levels. In the absence of immediate life-threatening manifestations, theophylline toxicity is best managed by monitored withdrawal of the drug. I have seen overzealous treatment of mild theophylline toxicity with cathartics result in osmotic diarrhea leading to hypovolemia, renal failure, and death in this setting.

Sympathomimetic bronchodilators may be used as needed for bronchospasm. Arrhythmias have not been a major problem, particularly with the cardioselective agents (albuterol, two metered doses every four to six hours).

Vasodilator drugs, including hydralazine, calcium channel antagonists, captopril, and nitrates among others, have produced beneficial hemodynamic or clinical responses in individuals or small groups of patients with primary or secondary pulmonary hypertension. However, none of these drugs is consistently effective, and all are capable of producing life-threatening systemic hypotension in this setting. Thus, these agents cannot be initiated in outpatients; their risk-to-benefit ratio does not justify their inclusion as standard therapy.

PATIENT INFORMATION AND EDUCATION

Prognostic information to the patient and family should convey the generally progressive nature of the disorder without communicating hopelessness (since occasional long periods of stabilization and rare remissions occur). Patients using warfarin need explicit instructions concerning mandatory follow-up and signs of bleeding. No patient with pulmonary hypertension should smoke. Because hypoxia may worsen pulmonary hypertension, commercial air travel poses an inherent risk.

Abstinence from smoking, prevention and treatment of deep venous thrombosis, and avoidance of skin exposure to water infested with schistosomes will significantly reduce the incidence of the three major causes of cor pulmonale.

A minority of cases of primary pulmonary hypertension are transmitted as an autosomal dominant trait. Presence of the disease in two family members establishes this pattern; presence of disease in a male suggests it.

PERIODIC EVALUATION

Reevaluation of patients with primary pulmonary hypertension at six to 12 months after diagnosis should include reconsideration of potentially treatable causes. Occasionally, pulmonary hypertension turns out to have been the first manifestation of a generalized collagen vascular disease.

Follow-up visits are required from time to time to evaluate increasing symptoms. Intercurrent pulmonary embolism, left ventricular failure, arrhythmia, and cardiac tamponade may need to be excluded before symptoms can be attributed to progression of the original process. Routine laboratory tests may include hemoglobin for blood loss or polycythemia, stool Hemoccult in anticoagulated patients, arterial blood gases, potassium, and digoxin and theophylline levels.

If complete compliance with continuous home oxygen therapy cannot be obtained, hypoxemic patients derive partial benefit from nocturnal oxygen therapy (at least 12 hours per day). Noncompliance with warfarin follow-up requires discontinuation of the drug. Inferior vena caval interruption should be considered if pulmonary emboli have been demonstrated.

Heart/lung transplantation has become technically feasible for patients terminally ill with pulmonary hypertension. Whether society should support this treatment, and if so, under what clinical circumstances, remains controversial.

REFERENCES

Fuster V, Steele PM, Edwards WD, et al: Primary pulmonary hypertension: natural history and the importance of thrombosis. Circulation 70:580–587, 1984.
Green LH, Smith TW: The use of digitalis in patients with pulmonary disease. Ann Intern Med 87:459–465, 1977.
Matthay RA, Berger HJ: Cardiovascular function in cor pulmonale. Clin Chest Med 4:269–295, 1983.
Peter RH, Rubin L: The pharmacologic control of the pulmonary circulation in pulmonary hypertension. Adv Intern Med 29:495–520, 1984.
Weir EK, Reeves JT (eds): Pulmonary Hypertension. Futura Publishing Co., Mt. Kisco, NY, 1984.

20 · COMMON CONGENITAL HEART DISEASE IN THE ADULT

John L. Wanamaker
GUTHRIE CLINIC

The spectrum of patients with congenital heart disease presenting for management as adults has broadened greatly in recent years. The physician responsible for their care must broaden his knowledge accordingly. In addition to recognizing and understanding the simpler and milder forms of congenital defects, he must appreciate the more complex and severe malformations that are now survivable because of the remarkable accomplishments of cardiac surgery in the past few decades.

A few congenital lesions are truly corrected by surgery, such as ligation and division of a patent ductus arteriosus with normal pulmonary resistance and primary closure of a secundum atrial septal defect in early childhood. Repair of other lesions may leave residual defects of varying severity requiring careful follow-up. Procedures to improve reduced pulmonary flow require careful observation to provide optimal timing for second-stage procedures. Knowledge of the details of previous surgery is crucial to the care of these patients. By focusing on the characteristics and behavior of the patches, conduits, and prosthetic valves used, one can anticipate problems. Distortion of natural structures by patch insertions or incisions for access may explain the electrocardiographic abnormalities and arrhythmias that appear later.

Treatment approaches to congestive heart failure and preventive measures for infective endocarditis are common to all forms of heart disease. However, the problem of pulmonary hypertension and increased pulmonary vascular resistance is especially prevalent among congenital heart patients. Once established, pulmonary hypertension is generally refractory to therapeutic measures that prove effective in acquired heart disease.

Pregnancy is well tolerated by women with mild to moderate defects who have reasonable effort tolerance. However, exceptions occur in those with pulmonary hypertension or cyanotic lesions, in whom maternal risk is significantly higher and fetal mortality is high.

Finally, couples with congenital heart disease may need counseling about family planning. No cause has been established for the great majority of congenital defects. The presence of congenital heart disease in a first-degree relative increases the risk four to eight times above that of the general population, in which there are eight cases per 1000 live births.

MANAGEMENT

LEFT-TO-RIGHT SHUNTS

Atrial Septal Defect. Atrial septal defect is the most common shunt lesion in the adult population. The systolic murmur is often inconspicuous and its true significance not appreciated until a pre-employment chest film displays cardiac enlargement and pulmonary plethora, or a preoperative EKG suggests right ventricular volume overload, calling attention to the underlying defect. The murmur, fixed split of the second heart sound, and prominent right ventricular impulse form a constellation of physical findings that allow accurate diagnosis in combination with the above findings.

As a rule of thumb, when a secundum atrial septal defect is recognized clinically, it is large enough to warrant surgical closure. The size of the defect may be confirmed by cardiac catheterization. Surgical repair is recommended for all uncomplicated defects with pulmonary flows equal to or greater than 1.5 times systemic flows. An aggressive approach is justified because of the low mortality rate (less than 1% of surgical repair) and the benefit of successful closure.

Unoperated, patients with significant defect show a small but progressive increase in pulmonary vascular resistance with advancing age. Increasing heart size is to be expected and associated atrial arrhythmias may occur. Successful surgery will arrest or reverse these trends. The longer surgery is delayed, the less likely are salutary results to be anticipated. Nonetheless, closure of large atrial septal defect has provided increased effort tolerance and decrease in congestive symptoms when performed in patients in the sixth and seventh decades of life.

Ventricular Septal Defect. The clinical manifestations of ventricular septal defect are dependent on the size of the defect and the response of the pulmonary vascular bed. In small defects, those whose diameter is less than the diameter of the aortic valve, shunt flow is restricted and pulmonary arterial pressure is normal to slightly increased. These defects generally cause no significant clinical problems unless complications develop. Defects larger than the aortic diameter allow excessive shunt flows and are often associated with pulmonary hypertension. If pulmonary resistance rises, shunt reversal with cyanosis may appear. Many of these large defects will have caused heart failure in childhood, so that the behavior may have been modified by previous medical or surgical treatment.

The hallmark of ventricular septal defect is the systolic regurgitant murmur heard along the lower left sternal border with transmission to the right side of the sternum. Large defects are associated with hyperdynamic and large left ventricles, ventricular gallops, and diastolic mitral flow rumbles. Elevated pulmonary pressure may be recognized by accentuation of pulmonic closure. The chest x-ray may be virtually normal in small defects, but in significant ones cardiac enlargement is displayed along with an increase in pulmonary vascularity.

When patients with ventricular septal defect have symptoms or objective signs to suggest significant shunts, cardiac catheterization should be performed to assess the magnitude of the shunt and to measure pulmonary vascular resistance. In uncomplicated cases, a pulmonic-to-systemic flow ratio greater than 2:1 is an indication for surgical repair. The mortality rate in these cases should be less than 5%. When pulmonary vascular resistance is calculated to be greater than 70% of systemic, the mortality rate is prohibitive and surgery is contraindicated.

Patients with nonsurgical defects are followed annually to observe for the development of complications. Infective endocarditis is an important threat. An appropriate antibiotic prophylactic program must be emphasized at each follow-up visit. American Heart Association guidelines call for penicillin at the time of dental procedures, and combined penicillin or ampicillin with aminoglycosides in genitourinary or gastrointestinal procedures. Effective blood levels to combat the anticipated bacteremia are achieved by dosing one hour before the procedure and at regular intervals for 48 hours after the procedure.

Aortic regurgitation may develop in ventricular septal defects, even small ones, if the defect is placed strategically below the aortic valve. Lacking support, an aortic cusp may prolapse through the defect and produce significant regurgitation.

Abnormal hypertrophy in the pulmonary outflow tract may occur and produce infundibular pulmonic stenosis. While this may limit the magnitude of the left-to-right shunt, it does so at the expense of development of right ventricular hypertrophy and, at times, right ventricular failure. These complications may be recognized during periodic follow-up; if symptoms accompany them, further study is warranted.

Patients with small, uncomplicated ventricular defects who are asymptomatic need not be restricted. They have excellent prognoses and may be allowed to participate in vigorous life styles. Pregnancy may be undertaken with confidence, but antibiotic prophylaxis at the time of delivery is a necessary precaution.

EISENMENGER REACTION

Excessive pulmonary flow may result in anatomic changes in the small pulmonary arteries. Medial hypertrophy, intimal thickening, and development of plexiform lesions occur with time. In situ thromboses may develop. These changes reduce the pulmonary vascular bed and lead to progressive elevations in pulmonary arterial pressure and resistance. Ultimately, the left-to-right shunt is reduced and bidirectional or predominant right-to-left shunting develops. This sequence may occur with a large shunt at any level, but is most likely with those at the great vessel or ventricular level, as they expose the pulmonary vascular bed to systemic systolic pressure as well as large volume flow. As these changes occur, the clinical findings of the specific defect are replaced by those of pulmonary hypertension. Pulmonic closure is accentuated and may be felt in the second left interspace. A right ventricular impulse becomes prominent. Pulmonic ejection sounds and short systolic ejection murmurs in the pulmonic region; the atrial gallop of right ventricular hypertrophy; and the systolic regurgitant murmur of tricuspid regurgitation may all be detected. The magnitude of right-to-left shunting determines the depth of cyanosis and the extent of digital clubbing. At this stage, the chest x-ray displays prominent central pulmonary arteries with decreased vascular markings in the periphery. Right ventricular hypertrophy of systolic overload will be noted on the EKG. Cardiac catheterization demonstrates the underlying lesion and allows assessment of pulmonary vascular resistance, as well as the major direction and magnitude of shunt flow. When pulmonary vascular resistance exceeds 70% of systemic resistance, surgery is contraindicated.

Survival is limited in this group of patients; the average age at death is 35 years. There are unique complications. Paradoxic systemic emboli may arise from venous sources. Patients with known venous disease must be followed carefully and treated aggressively when phlebitis occurs. Brain abscess is a relatively frequent complication and must be suspected when unexplained neurologic symptoms are noted. Appropriate evaluation and treatment may then be carried out.

Pregnancy is ill advised in these patients, being associated with increased maternal mortality as well as a high incidence of abortion and neonatal mortality. The increased risk appears due, at least in part, to the fall in systemic vascular resistance that occurs normally in the third trimester of pregnancy. This is attended by an increase in the right-to-left shunt and further hypoxia. Pregnancy therefore should be avoided when pulmonic vascular resistance has reached the inoperative level.

Oral contraceptives containing estrogen have been suspected of increasing thromboembolic complications and intensifying pulmonary hypertension, and are contraindicated. Intrauterine devices have been used successfully, but carry a risk of bleeding and infective endocarditis. Laparoscopic surgical sterilization is preferred by most authorities but may be complicated by bleeding or infection.

The secondary polycythemia of the Eisenmenger reaction is associated with both thrombotic and bleeding complications. Antiplatelet agents may be used to prevent thromboembolic episodes, but their value has not been proved conclusively. Headaches not associated with other neurologic symptoms or signs prove troublesome in many patients with polycythemia. The increased blood viscosity that accompanies the polycythemia may interfere with circulatory dynamics when the hematocrit reaches 70%. Phlebotomy and volume replacement with plasma to maintain the hematocrit at less than 65% may be useful in some patients, and should be given a trial when the hematocrit exceeds 70%; the troublesome headaches may subside and effort tolerance may improve substantially. Reducing the hematocrit by 10% usually proves adequate to produce a beneficial effect.

Hemoptysis may occur and become a distressing symptom. It appears usually in older patients with the Eisenmenger reaction. Treatment is symptomatic and consists of sedation and the use of cough suppressants. Syncope may occur when a sudden fall in systemic vascular resistance allows an increase in the right-to-left shunt and hypoxia. Drugs that reduce systemic vascular resistance selectively must be used with great caution. Vigorous exercise may produce the same hemodynamic effect and should be curtailed.

Sudden death may occur in up to one third of these patients, presumably owing to an arrhythmia. Holter monitoring should be performed on patients who complain of palpitations or syncopal episodes. Appropriate antiarrhythmics may be selected on the basis of identification of the abnormal rhythm.

VALVULAR LESIONS

The most common congenital heart defects are those that may go unrecognized until adulthood. Mitral valve prolapse is discovered most frequently in adolescence and early adulthood.

The bicuspid aortic valve may not declare its presence until the fourth or fifth decade. Some patients seen have undergone surgical repair of significant aortic stenosis in childhood. Residual aortic regurgitation of varying degrees is the rule, and restenosis is likely. Prophylaxis for infective endocarditis is necessary, along with careful follow-up for further valve deterioration. These topics are covered in detail in Chapter 12.

COARCTATION OF AORTA

In adults, coarctation is most likely to be discovered during investigation for systemic hypertension. The complaints are related to hypertension or reduced arterial flow to the legs. Occasionally, the presenting manifestation may be one of the complications of coarctation such as CHF, aortic rupture, or rupture of a Berry aneurysm with intracranial hemorrhage.

The pathognomonic clinical finding is a discrepancy between the rapid-rising, large-volume arterial pulses in the neck and arms and the slow-rising, low-volume pulses in the legs. Blood pressure differences between the upper and lower extremities will confirm the findings on palpation. The systolic ejection murmur is heard best in the back in the interscapular region.

The classic figure 3 seen on chest x-ray is produced by the dilated aortic knob and poststenotic descending thoracic aorta separated by the segments of coarctation. Rib notching is due to erosion by the enlarged intercostal collateral vessels. Catheterization is required to identify the level, length, and severity of the obstruction, as well as associated defects and the extent of arterial collateral development.

Survival is adversely affected by the presence of the coarctation, so that surgery is indicated when the diagnosis is confirmed. A peculiar syndrome may arise two to ten days after repair, consisting of acceleration of hypertension associated with abdominal pain, nausea, and fever. The abdominal complaints have been attributed to mesenteric vasculitis. Vigorous treatment with parenteral antihypertensives, such as nitroprusside beta-blockers, and vasodilators usually is effective and brings BP under control.

Annual follow-up is required following surgery for

several reasons. Obstruction may recur; residual hypertension at rest may be present despite successful surgery; and hypertension may recur after a period of normal levels and need not be related to recurrent coarctation. In these situations, antihypertensive treatment should be continued or resumed and monitored. In a small percentage of patients, BP may be normal at rest but increased significantly with exercise. For this reason, careful BP monitoring during a stress test should be carried out in the first year after successful surgery. If exercise hypertension of this type is present and cannot be controlled adequately with antihypertensives, activities should be restricted.

The annual reevaluation allows the detection of associated lesions, especially a bicuspid aortic valve, which is felt to be present in at least 50% of patients with aortic coarctation. Until the aortic valve lesion becomes important in its own right, the annual revisit allows reindoctrination in the importance and techniques of antibiotic use to prevent infective endocarditis.

Since complications arise more frequently in patients over 20 years old when the repair was carried out, these should be seen every six months to detect early signs of left ventricular hypertrophy or CHF.

TETRALOGY OF FALLOT

The most common of the cyanotic congenital lesions, tetralogy of Fallot, consists of pulmonic stenosis, ventricular septal defect, overriding aorta, and right ventricular hypertrophy. The ventricular septal defect is usually large and located high in the septum. Pulmonic stenosis may be valvular, infundibular, or supravalvular, either alone or in combination and of variable severity. The anatomic circumstances dictate the clinical presentation. If the pulmonic stenosis is mild or moderate, the manifestations are those of a large ventricular septal defect with predominant left-to-right shunt. If pulmonic stenosis is severe, a right-to-left shunt predominates, resulting in cyanosis and hypercyanotic spells. Chest x-ray findings suggestive of tetralogy include right ventricular hypertrophy and a right-sided aortic arch.

The natural survival with this combination is poor. Less than 5% of patients survive to age 25; therefore, it is unlikely that a cardiologist will encounter an untreated adult patient with tetralogy. Initial surgical palliative procedures and more recent intracardiac repair have improved life expectancy, so that current estimates suggest that 75% of surgical patients will achieve age 40. These are the patients whose ongoing care will be provided.

Many of these patients have no symptoms and normal heart size. Nearly all have a residual pulmonic ejection murmur. Most have an early diastolic murmur of pulmonic regurgitation. Some 80% display right bundle branch block on EKG. In this asymptomatic group with normal cardiac silhouette on chest x-ray, full activities and a normal life style may be allowed. Antibiotic prophylaxis for infective endocarditis should be stressed. Annual follow-up is in order, since the long-term effect of ventriculotomy on the right ventricle is not known.

Residual right ventricular outflow obstruction and residual shunt are factors that lead to shortened survival. If clinical improvement seems less than anticipated, repeat cardiac catheterization should be carried out. If right ventricular systolic pressure exceeds 60 mm Hg or if the residual intracardiac shunt is greater than 1.5 to 1, repeat surgery to correct the abnormal hemodynamics should be seriously considered.

CONGENITAL HEART BLOCK

Failure of development of normal communications between supraventricular and junctional components of the conduction system may result in complete AV block. This condition is suggested by inappropriately slow heart rate in infancy and childhood. It is easily confirmed by the EKG. The frequent association of corrected transposition of the great arteries should arouse suspicion of this entity or some other structural cardiac disease, but in about 50% of cases the heart block is an independent anomaly. When there is no associated structural heart disease, these patients nearly always survive to adulthood.

The escape focus is generally stable and often exhibits the ability to accelerate when circulatory demands increase. The condition is therefore well tolerated for long periods, although fatigue or syncope may develop gradually, and survival may be shortened somewhat. Some patients may remain active and comfortable into their sixth decade, with heart rate in the mid-40s. If the QRS complexes are narrow, the ventricular rate is above 40, and there is some acceleration with exercise, observation should continue every four months. When symptoms develop or if the ventricular rate falls below 40, permanent pacemaker implant is recommended.

REFERENCES

Borow KM, Alpert JS, Braunwald E: Congenital heart disease in the adult. *In* Braunwald E (ed): Heart Disease: A Textbook of Cardiovascular Medicine, 2nd ed. W. B. Saunders Co, Philadelphia, 1984, pp 1024–1046.
Engle MA, Perloff JK (eds): Symposium on postoperative congenital heart disease in adults. Parts I and II. Am J Cardiol 50:541–657, 1982.
Perloff JK: The Clinical Recognition of Congenital Heart Disease, 2nd ed. W. B. Saunders Co, Philadelphia, 1978.
Roberts WC: Congenital Heart Disease in Adults. F. A. Davis Co, Philadelphia, 1979.

1 · CHRONIC OBSTRUCTIVE PULMONARY DISEASE AND BRONCHIECTASIS

David J. Scheinhorn
OCHSNER CLINIC AND ALTON OCHSNER MEDICAL
FOUNDATION

Chronic Obstructive Pulmonary Disease

DEFINITION AND DIAGNOSTIC CRITERIA

Chronic obstructive pulmonary disease (COPD) encompasses the clinical entities chronic bronchitis and emphysema. Chronic bronchitis is characterized by a daily cough and sputum production of long duration, and is diagnosed by a history of such symptoms. Emphysema is dilatation of alveolar spaces with rupture of alveolar walls throughout the lung. It is diagnosed by a history of chronic progressive breathlessness, with physical examination and roentgenographic evidence of hyperinflation, confirmed by pulmonary function testing that also demonstrates a decreased diffusing capacity.

PATHOPHYSIOLOGY

Cigarette smoking is associated with an inflammatory reaction in both the conducting airways and alveoli, and paralysis of normal mucociliary clearance. In chronic bronchitis the bronchi are then narrowed by inflammatory cell infiltrates, edema, mucous gland hypertrophy, smooth muscle hypertrophy, and spasm mediated by irritant reflexes and humoral factors. The

**Dr. Divertie passed away while this book was in progress. We regret the loss of our respected colleague. FRANZ H. MESSERLI*

bronchial lumen is further compromised by excessive mucus secretion, which may be infected.

In emphysema, when there is influx and breakdown of inflammatory cells, the polymorphonuclear leukocyte proteases that are released overwhelm local antiproteases, causing degradation of elastin and collagen. Alveolar walls are weakened by this process and rupture, leading to collapse of small airways normally "tethered" open by those walls.

Because of differences between intraluminal and pleural pressure, normal airways narrow during expiration. The airway narrowing becomes more pronounced as lung volume decreases because of decreased tethering forces. This and the pathologic changes described above result in the severe respiratory air flow obstruction that characterizes COPD.

CLINICAL ASPECTS

Patients with COPD usually have both chronic bronchitis and emphysema. They seek medical attention with the complaint of shortness of breath. Frequently, patients with more chronic bronchitis than emphysema regard their morning cough with sputum production as a natural consequence of smoking, and notice dyspnea only when it interferes with important daily activities. Patients with more emphysema than bronchitis often have no chronic cough, only breathlessness. Patients with advanced COPD are tachycardic, have a hyperresonant barrel chest with distended neck veins, and on auscultation have decreased breath sounds or wheezing, the loud rattling of large airway mucus, and a prolonged expiratory note. A point of maximal cardiac impulse in the epigastrium, a right ventricular heave or gallop, and peripheral edema are frequently found. Chest roentgenograms show enlarged central pulmonary vessels along with the hyperinflation, and peripheral paucity of bronchovascular markings. Spirometry reveals obstruction to air flow, increased lung volumes, and decreased diffusing capacity. Arterial blood gases reveal hypoxemia of varying degree and hypercapnia in those with chronic bronchitis who have lost normal CO_2 control of ventilation. Hypoxemia with secondary pulmonary hypertension and right ventricular failure occurs early in patients with predominantly chronic bronchitis and can last for many years because, with treatment, the causes of bronchial obstruction can be reversed. In contrast, when patients with emphysema progress to cor pulmonale, they are at the end of the natural history of the illness.

MANAGEMENT

The short-term goal of treatment in stable patients with COPD is relief of dyspnea and other daily symptoms. Long-term goals begin with educating patients to understand the symptoms and how to alter them. They should be instructed to stop personal pollution (smoking) and to remove themselves from environmental pollution. Other important goals of therapy are to decrease the frequency of infections and hospitalizations, increase activities (which may include employment), and improve psychologic well-being.

Acute respiratory failure with life-threatening hypoxemia and acidosis mandates hospitalization. Other conditions or agents that may necessitate hospitalization to avert respiratory failure include infection, congestive heart failure, bronchospasm, drugs that depress respiratory function, and pulmonary emboli. Surgical intervention is indicated only in a small subset of emphysema patients with "giant bullous disease," not in usual COPD. Home health care is indicated for patients whose advanced disease has caused breathlessness that interferes with activities of daily living. Ambulatory treatment is desirable for all patients with COPD, including use of portable oxygen therapy when necessary, as patients who become bedridden suffer the complications of pulmonary embolism, loss of muscle mass, and emotional collapse.

NONPHARMACOLOGIC MEASURES

Cessation of cigarette smoking is essential to successful COPD treatment. Debilitating symptoms such as cough with sputum production improve or cease in three to six months following cessation. Dyspnea may lessen and pulmonary functions improve. Importantly, the progressive yearly decline in pulmonary function seen in COPD is less (by 11% to 13%) after smoking cessation. Oxygen transport is improved when 5% to 15% of hemoglobin is no longer saturated with carbon monoxide, and hypoxemia is lessened. Most patients who succeed in quitting smoking do so on a physician's advice. The success rate for all smokers is only 10% to 15% in one year, but is probably higher for symptomatic patients with COPD. Several studies indicate that aids such as nicotine gum double the success rate. A "smoking clinic," if available, may be helpful.

Follow patients closely at first to support smoking cessation. Both negative and positive reinforcement can play an important role. Carboxyhemoglobin levels will confirm the patient's progress in quitting, and a radioimmunoassay for nicotine metabolites (in less than 1 ml of saliva) is a reliable, less invasive test to document and encourage cessation.

Remove patients from environments with provocative levels of dust and fumes. These pollutants trigger the nonspecific bronchial hyperactivity of COPD. Before giving patients a physician's note to take to their employer, it is important to discuss their job security. Patients must understand that they may risk losing their job if no position with decreased dust or fume exposure is available.

Encourage regular exercise, such as brisk walking, within the confines of the dyspnea, with a goal of gradual increase in distance or time. In more severe climates I recommend the use of a stationary exercising bicycle with supplemental oxygen available if needed.

In some areas, comprehensive exercise programs, including graded treadmill exercise with oxygen, may be available. Gains in exercise capacity have been documented with such programs, but are of short duration unless a home program follows.

Adequate nutrition is important, employing dietary supplements when necessary. The skilled dietician can evaluate and improve a patient's diet to ensure the maintenance of muscular mass sufficient for ventilation. Avoidance of dehydration has a beneficial effect on mucociliary clearance, but excessive hydration has not been shown to be useful.

Mechanical clearance of airway secretions with outpatient or home respiratory therapy maneuvers is necessary in some ambulatory patients with copious secretions (discussed later).

DRUG THERAPY

Theophylline. Initial bronchodilator therapy for patients with COPD is treatment with an oral theophylline preparation and an inhaled beta-2 agonist. Spirometric air flow improvement need not be demonstrated, as improved respiratory muscle contractility or central effects can lead to symptomatic improvement. A trial of therapy is justified after weighing benefits against side effects in the individual patient. Preparations taken once a day are gaining in popularity over those taken twice a day. I start patients with Theo-Dur, 300 mg twice a day, or Theo-24, 600 mg every day, and instruct the patient to call if nervousness, insomnia, or nausea are bothersome. I draw a theophylline level in one to two weeks (although steady levels are achieved in three days) and instruct patients to call the office for their dosage adjustment; 50% changes in dose are used. The 10 µg/ml to 20 µg/ml serum level is well tolerated by most. A six-week trial is sufficient to assess the benefit. If bronchospasm is prominent, there is no concomitant disease, including recent myocardial infarction, that will be worsened by theophylline therapy. Several reviews have stressed the need for increased dosage in children and smokers, and decreased dosage in the elderly and those with CHF or liver disease. The most frequently encountered drug that decreases metabolism of theophylline is cimetidine (Tagamet), which reliably raises serum levels by one third. Erythromycin may also raise serum levels.

Because gastrointestinal toxicity usually precedes cardiac arrhythmias or seizures, patients can usually avoid these more serious problems. If accidental or intentional overdosage with oral (or intravenous) theophylline occurs, treatment with oral-activated charcoal (Arm-A-Char), 30 gm every two hours for four doses, significantly speeds decline in blood levels. In such cases, patients should be hospitalized with cardiac monitoring.

Beta-Receptor Stimulation. Albuterol (Proventil, Ventolin), administered by metered dose inhaler, two puffs three to four times a day, is good initial therapy to use with oral theophylline, particularly in patients with chronic bronchitis. Enhanced mucociliary clearance is an important adjunct to prolonged (more than six hours) bronchodilatation. Patients can use two puffs twice during hours of sleep if breakthrough wheezing occurs. A spacer or inhalation chamber (Aerochamber) provides more reliable drug delivery, but patients may not readily accept these cumbersome additions to the inhaler. It is essential to demonstrate the correct use of the metered dose inhaler. Patients should be warned to expect five to ten minutes of tachycardia and one hour of nervousness and tremor. The beta-2 specificity of these drugs is relative and dose dependent. However, since there is little systemic absorption, and supraventricular tachyarrhythmias may be the result of lung disease, withholding such treatment should be considered only in patients with serious ventricular arrhythmias. Beta-blockade, even with selective blockers (atenolol, metoprolol) should be avoided in patients with bronchospasm, but if these agents must be used they probably do not block the local effects of inhaled beta-agonists, which should be continued. Overuse of inhaled beta-agonists is usually limited by their side effects. With worsening dyspnea, patients may overuse inhalers without serious complications, perhaps because bronchospasm limits drug deposition.

Antibiotics. Treatment of acute bronchitis with increased sputum and change in sputum color is a seven- to ten-day course of doxycycline, 100 mg twice a day, or amoxicillin, 250 mg three times a day. These drugs are first choice because of their antibacterial spectra, their demonstrated efficacy, and the infrequent dosages needed. (In fact, placebo performs as well as a wide variety of antibiotics in the treatment of purulent bronchitis.) Tetracycline, trimethoprim-sulfamethoxazole, and cefaclor are also used with success. Secretions of patients with COPD are most often colonized with *Haemophilus influenzae* and *Streptococcus pneumoniae*. However, Gram stains and cultures of sputum, along with any attempt to treat specific organisms, are unnecessary unless there are signs and symptoms of pneumonia.

Corticosteroids. These have always been used in patients with end-stage disease. A one-month trial contributes to a sense of well-being and increases exercise ability without objective improvements in pulmonary function or arterial blood gases. Prednisone is used, 10 to 15 mg per day. Recently, 20% of COPD patients have been shown to respond with significant increased air flow when given 32 mg of medrol every day for a two-week trial. After such a response, they were tapered to low-dose steroid every other day or inhaled beclomethasone or triamcinolone, two to four puffs four times a day. Such a trial should be considered in patients with severe obstruction.

Unestablished Drugs. Chromolyn sodium has no place in COPD therapy, and oral beta-agonists generally have stimulant side effects that outweigh their benefits. Calcium channel blockers such as nifedipine and inhaled anticholinergics such as Robinul block exercise-induced bronchospasm, but as yet have no defined role in COPD treatment; neither do central respiratory stimulants.

Ipratropium Bromide and Newer Agents. A new drug soon to be released in the U.S. that shows promise for the future is inhaled ipratropium bromide, an atropine-like inhaled agent. It is an effective bronchodilator when added to the basic regimen of theophylline and inhaled beta-agonists. Watch for urinary obstruction in the elderly. Alpha-blockers and ketotifen, an oral bronchodilator used in Europe, may be useful in the future. Drugs that change ventilation-perfusion relationships in the lung, such as almitrine, look good experimentally and may have an important role in treating COPD patients if multicenter trials prove them safe.

Oxygen. One of the most important drugs in the treatment of advanced COPD is oxygen. Acute home O_2 therapy is prescribed during the month following an exacerbation of disease that requires hospitalization. Chronic O_2 therapy begins after one month of a stable comprehensive treatment regimen. Low-flow treatment, 1 to 2 liters per minute by nasal cannula for 24 hours, is best, and at least 16 hours of 24 hours is better than none to prevent or slow down advancing cor pulmonale. A few patients with severe documented desaturation during sleep will benefit from therapy during hours of sleep; p.r.n. therapy is of no value. We favor an O_2 extractor for the mainly homebound patient and a liquid system for the more ambulatory.

Whenever a patient has a resting PO_2 less than 55 mm Hg or higher PO_2 that drops below 55 mm Hg with steady-state exercise testing or when measured while the patient sleeps, supplemental oxygen is indicated. There are good data to support the benefit of supplemental oxygen for patients whose PO_2 is below 60 mm Hg at rest if they have cor pulmonale, left ventricular dysfunction, angina, arrhythmias, or significant secondary polycythemia. Third-party payers require a physician's letter to justify supplemental oxygen supply to these patients.

Serious adverse effects of chronic oxygen administration, such as low grade oxygen toxicity, have been investigated but not demonstrated convincingly. Oxygen therapy should not be used if patients continue to smoke. Ignition of nasal cannulae may occur with third-degree nasal flash burns. There is little to no danger of home fires.

CONTINUING EDUCATION

There is no substitute for the physician's time spent in the office talking to patients about their illness and medications. For patients eager to learn more, I recommend the excellent and comprehensive book by Petty and Nett, which will help COPD patients develop realistic goals and expectations. The local branch of the American Lung Association provides excellent literature about smoking cessation, and the AMA supplies informational flyers about some theophylline and inhaled beta-agonist preparations. The manufacturer of the metered dose inhaler provides a tear sheet of illustrated instructions as a helpful office handout to supplement a *demonstration* of correct inhaler use. The physician's availability by telephone to discuss symptoms, medication problems, and psychologic questions and crises is essential.

New symptoms in the patient with COPD should alert you to related disease processes that share the common risk factor of a history of smoking (i.e., coronary artery disease, other vascular disease, and lung cancer). Incomplete response to therapy may prompt an allergy evaluation, especially in patients who have chronic bronchitis with prominent bronchospasm or sinus problems.

FOLLOW-UP

The first few visits should be four to six weeks apart to adjust medication dosages, add and subtract medicines, reinforce compliance and smoking cessation, and answer questions. I usually follow the patient who is doing well every three to four months, but emphasize that they should call if specific problems develop, such as changes in sputum color and amount, ankle edema, or even daily weight change in more advanced disease. I usually let patients initiate their own course of doxycycline for acute bronchitic flares, and instruct them to call only if they do not respond and progressive shortness of breath or fever develops.

There are no routine laboratory tests that are absolutely necessary. Theophylline levels should be measured to adjust dosage and check compliance at first. Office spirometry is an excellent way to follow the progress of COPD and to assess objective response to therapy.

Patients generally seek medical attention when their COPD interferes with activities they expect to perform (though they often do not realize that their activity level has declined). This makes compliance with the medical program better than average. Compliance is better with an unremitting illness such as COPD than with an episodic one such as asthma. Try to use tolerable medicines in the simplest form and most infrequent dosage schedules. Once-a-day theophylline preparations and twice-a-day inhaled steroids are attractive now, and twice-a-day inhaled beta-agonists will be perfected in the future to help simplify programs.

PREVENTIVE MEASURES

A yearly influenza vaccination is important for those patients with COPD, as they are at high risk. Side effects are rare and do not cause decompensation. Pneumonia vaccine (Pneumovax 23) should be administered at least once and essentially has no side effects. Repetition is unnecessary. Patients who have received the 14-valent vaccine should not receive the 23-valent vaccine because severe local and sometimes systemic reactions have been reported. Some infectious disease specialists circumvent this problem in high-risk patients by administering one tenth the recommended dose of the 23-valent vaccine.

Family counseling will help relatives know what to expect from the COPD patient's abilities, capabilities, limitations, fears, goals, and prognosis. The family can be very helpful in daily home care, such as in mechanical sputum dislodgment in some instances of chronic bronchitis (and bronchiectasis, see below).

Marital or genetic counseling may be needed for those younger patients with emphysema associated with homozygous levels of alpha$_1$-antitrypsin deficiency; relatives of these individuals should be screened for levels less than 50 mg%. Cigarette and other fume inhalation may cause onset of severe symptomatic disease ten years earlier in these individuals.

SOCIOECONOMIC CONSIDERATIONS

COPD ranks fifth as a cause of death in the U.S., and 200,000 persons will be disabled with it in 1986. The costs of care and loss of productivity to society amount to millions of dollars. Individual treatment costs can be kept down by using generic preparations in quantities that the pharmacist can dispense without counting (tabs 100). Home oxygen is particularly expensive, at $300 to $800 per month. One should choose an oxygen system closely tailored to the patient's individual needs; for example, the more expensive portable system is not appropriate for a housebound individual. Intensive care unit treatment is very expensive and should be discussed with patients and their close relatives before it is needed. In patients of whom you know nothing, and in those familiar to you who have reversible decompensating factors, one episode of assisted ventilation is justified. There are very few patients who cannot be weaned from assisted ventilation and who require home mechanical ventilation.

Bronchiectasis

Bronchiectasis is saccular dilatation of bronchial walls caused by a destructive process. A bronchogram demonstrating the saccular dilatation is necessary to prove the diagnosis. Bronchiectasis can be caused by remote disease processes such as tuberculosis or bacterial pneumonia, or can be the result of an ongoing disease process (usually interstitial pneumonitis, vasculitis, or sarcoidosis).

Patients usually complain of cough with sputum production, often mucopurulent, sometimes in large quantity, and commonly with episodes of hemoptysis. Associated sinusitis is common. Progression of the disease is characterized by fever, increase in amount and purulence of sputum, and increased dyspnea in advanced disease. On physical examination, crackles and wheezes are heard over the involved areas, and clubbing of the nails is seen (unlike COPD). Recurrent pneumonias are characterized by organisms increasingly resistant to antibiotics, finally by mucoid strains of *Pseudomonas* and multiple drug-resistant *Staphylococcus aureus*. The chest x-ray film is usually normal between pneumonias, although honeycombing is the final common result of lung destruction, both radiographically and pathologically.

MANAGEMENT

Short-term goals of therapy are treatment of bronchospasm (prominent in at least one half of the patients), antibiotics for increased infection, and mechanical clearance of infected airway secretions. Long-term goals include slowing the course of lung destruction and helping the patient maintain an active and productive lifestyle. When pneumonia is present, hospitalization is usually needed for IV antibiotic therapy and intensive respiratory therapy.

Mechanical clearance of airway secretions can be accomplished with a daily home program of inhaled bronchodilator, inhalation of mist (the best thinner of mucus), and postural expulsive coughing, with or without percussion. After morning and night dosages of albuterol, two puffs by metered dose inhaler, patients are instructed to wait 10 to 20 minutes to let bronchodilatation commence and to prevent bronchospasm induced by the next step. They spend 10 minutes under a mist mini-tent formed by a towel over their heads as they lean over a sink with hot running water. They should then lie on a bed with hands resting on the floor, inclining the head and trunk downward. In this position they perform expulsive forceful coughing for 10 to 15 seconds, rest on the bed, and repeat this procedure for a total time of 10 minutes. Percussion with cupped hands may be added to this by another person. Patients may find positional variations to elicit the most mucus.

Bronchodilatation therapy as described for COPD is used. Antibiotic therapy is the same as in COPD for repeated infection, using ambulatory doxycycline or amoxicillin over many years for resurgence of purulent bronchitis without signs of pneumonia. In following a given patient over years, it becomes clear when these antibiotics will partially succeed or fail (immediate flare of signs and symptoms of infections after discontinuation of medication).

Therefore, in more advanced disease and recurrent pneumonia, antibiotics with antipseudomonal and antistaphylococcal spectra must be started immediately on hospitalization, and coverage narrowed when sputum bacteriology provides drug susceptibility. A Gram stain may show a marked predominance of either organism to help narrow coverage from the start. If not, IV gentamicin, 1 mg/kg every eight hours, is combined with oxacillin, 2 gm every four to six hours. Other aminoglycosides can be used, but in every instance the dosage interval must be lengthened proportionately to serum creatinine levels if renal insufficiency is present, and peak and trough levels should be used for final dose adjustment. Cefazolin, 1 gm IV every four to six hours, may be substituted for oxacillin to provide even stronger gram-negative coverage in patients known to have recurrent gram-negative infection.

If *Pseudomonas* is strongly suspected from the history or implicated by culture, IV carbenicillin, 5 gm every four hours, or IV ticarcillin, 3 gm every four hours, is added to the other antibiotics.

Susceptibility testing usually allows the drug regimen to be narrowed to two IV antibiotics for a 10- to 14-day course in these serious infections. I do not use nebulized antibiotics or nebulized mucolytics; the latter are poorly tolerated and questionably effective. Anaerobic organisms less commonly cause pneumonias in these patients, but if they are the only organisms cultured, they should be treated with high-dose IV penicillin, 5 million units every six hours. Because of the saccular abscess-like pathology in patients with bronchiectasis, the choice of drugs is not as important as the need for intensive respiratory treatment for mechanical drainage. For a discussion of complications and side effects of antibiotic treatment, see Chapter 6.

We treat massive hemoptysis, such as a half-cupful of blood expectorated with each cough over hours to days, with bed rest. The patient is positioned with the affected side down, and mild cough suppression is obtained with oral codeine, 32 to 64 mg every four to six hours. However, we carefully monitor by physical examination (breath sounds), chest roentgenogram (alveolarization of blood, blood ''bronchograms''), and arterial blood gases (PO_2, A-a gradient) to make sure that blood is being adequately cleared. If these parameters steadily worsen, surgery may be needed after intraoperative bronchoscopy, using a rigid ventilating bronchoscope to localize the bleeding lobe if possible. A previous *selective* bronchogram is the procedure of choice for diagnosis of bronchiectasis, but this does not guarantee that the abnormal area is the site of hemorrhage.

In exsanguinating hemoptysis, placement of an endotracheal tube in the main bronchus of the nonbleeding side may be life-saving. Bronchial artery embolization requires a skilled angiographer not only to perform it, but to recognize and avoid a significant branch of the anterior spinal artery that may arise from the target bronchial artery. Vasopressin (Pitressin), 0.3 units per minute IV, has been used by some authors to control hemorrhage.

Other aspects of therapy for bronchiectasis are the same as for COPD. Patient compliance with the mechanical drainage program is most important. I often emphasize the importance of treatment compliance by describing how it is a life-or-death matter in cystic fibrosis patients, who have similar problems with mucopurulent airway infection and obstruction. Those who continue their mechanical drainage programs can live nearly normal life spans, but those who rebel (as teenagers will) and stop their drainage may die at an early age.

REFERENCES

Bukowsky M, Nakatsu K, Mundt PW: Theophylline reassessed. Ann Intern Med 101:63–73, 1984.
Flenley DC: Long-term home oxygen therapy. Chest 87:99–103, 1985.
Petty TL, Nett LM: Enjoying Life with Emphysema. Lea & Febiger, Philadelphia, 1983.
Scheinhorn DJ, Emory WB: Putting spirometry to use in your practice. J Respir Dis 2:8–18, 1981.
Weg JG: Bronchiectasis. *In* Cherniack RM (ed): Current Therapy of Respiratory Diseases. B. C. Decker, Philadelphia, 1984, pp 154–158.

2 · ASTHMA

Richard G. Van Dellen
MAYO CLINIC AND MAYO FOUNDATION

DEFINITION AND DIAGNOSTIC CRITERIA

Asthma is generally easy to diagnose. The typical episodic symptoms of cough, wheezing, and dyspnea; wheezing on examination of the lungs; and evidence of obstructive airway disease reversed, either spontaneously or with therapy, make the diagnosis. However, cough or dyspnea alone without the typical wheezing can occur with asthma, and wheezing can occur from causes that mimic asthma, including high airway obstruction, congestive heart failure, pulmonary embolism, and infiltrative processes in the bronchi. Patients with severe asthma may not show immediate improvement in pulmonary function after bronchodilator therapy, and evidence of reversibility becomes apparent only after treatment with corticosteroids. In the patient who presents with normal pulmonary function and a history compatible with asthma, reversible airway obstruction can be documented by (1) a bronchial challenge with methacholine or (2) measurement of peak expiratory flow during and after an attack. The first can be done at most medical centers; the second can be done at home with a mini-Wright Peak Flow Meter (Armstrong Industries, Northbrook, IL). Although not helpful in asthma, a roentgenogram of the chest should be taken to rule out other diseases.

How Severe Is the Asthma? Once asthma has been diagnosed, assessment of its severity is critical in planning therapy. Patients with mild asthma do not need the vigorous and urgent therapy required by those with severe asthma. Several sources are helpful in assessing the severity of asthma.

History. Suggestive of severe asthma are increased frequency and severity of wheezing; attacks occurring at night, awakening the patient; and the more frequent use and abuse of aerosolized bronchodilators. Obvious clues, such as previous hospitalizations or ventilatory failure and previous need for steroid therapy, should alert the physician to the possibility of severe asthma.

Physical Examination. Dyspnea and use of accessory muscle are suggestive of severe airway obstruction, although this is not uniformly true, since hyperventilation can produce similar findings. Wheezing on examination, the sine qua non of asthma, is notoriously misleading, and absence of wheezing may be an ominous sign, indicating severe airway obstruction. The amount of wheezing on examination does not correlate with the degree of functional impairment. In acute asthma, the presence of paradoxical pulse—a greater decrease in arterial pressure than the normal decrease of 10 mm Hg during inspiration—correlates somewhat with the severity of airway obstruction. Its absence, however, does not rule out severe airway obstruction. An assessment of the degree of airway obstruction is unreliable if based solely on the physical examination.

Arterial Blood Gases. The Pa_{O_2} correlates reasonably well with the degree of severity of asthma: the lower the Pa_{O_2}, the worse the airway obstruction. The Pa_{CO_2} is usually low in the typical acute asthma attack and does not become elevated until the expiratory flow is less than 20% of predicted. However, many patients with airway obstruction of less than 20% do not have an elevated Pa_{CO_2}. Patients with CO_2 retention and acidemia have severe asthma and need immediate treatment.

Measurement of Pulmonary Function. The objective measurement of pulmonary function is usually an accurate method for assessing the degree of airway obstruction in asthma. Pulmonary function should be measured periodically in all asthma patients. Either a Wright Peak Flow Meter or a mini-Wright Peak Flow Meter may be used. Both measure the peak expiratory flow and both are inexpensive, easy to use, and adequate for following and assessing airway obstruction in asthma patients. The peak expiratory flow correlates well with the FEV_1; however, one must remember that the peak expiratory flow is effort dependent. Other measurements of expiratory flow, such as the FEV_1, maximal midexpiratory flow rate, and flow at 50% of vital capacity, are also helpful. Because of its small size, the mini-Wright Peak Flow Meter can be used at home to follow the course of the asthma. The peak expiratory

flow can be falsely elevated at high lung volumes and the flow rate can be falsely low with poor effort.

Summary. None of the above four sources can be independently or consistently relied on to assess accurately the severity of asthma; all must be considered together. Some authors have tried to stage the asthma or to use either a scoring system or a predictor index, but it is doubtful whether these help. Judgment must be used in deciding on the severity of the asthma, and the initial treatment is based on this first assessment.

PATHOPHYSIOLOGY

Common findings in most patients with asthma include hyperreactive airways and sputum eosinophilia. Despite this, the myriad causes with different mechanisms and the variable patterns of this disease make a unifying pathogenesis enigmatic. Pathologic material is found mostly in patients with severe asthma. Pathologic findings include mucous plugging, a sometimes dense eosinophilic infiltrate, hypertrophy of the smooth muscle of the bronchial wall, increased numbers of goblet cells, and mucosal damage that includes denuding or stripping of the mucosal cells from the basal cell layer. These findings are not those of bronchospasm alone and require days or weeks to reverse. On the basis of these pathologic findings in severe asthma, one may think that bronchodilators alone will not suffice and that steroids are needed.

MANAGEMENT

PLAN

Goals of treatment include reversing the obstructive airway disease and decreasing the symptoms. Any plan relies on an assessment of the severity of the asthma.

Which Patients Should Be Hospitalized? Only a small percentage of asthma patients require or should be considered for hospitalization: (1) those with respiratory failure; (2) those who do not respond to therapy in the emergency room or the office; (3) those with complications that either aggravate the asthma, such as pneumonia or a respiratory infection, or result from it, such as pneumothorax; (4) those with recent repeated attacks of increasing severity and frequency, particularly if there is abuse of bronchodilator aerosols; (5) those who have peak expiratory flow rates (or some other measure of pulmonary function) less than 20% of predicted, despite appropriate initial therapy; and (6) those who are noncompliant or living alone and unable to provide self-care.

Treatment in the Hospital. Patients who are hospitalized should receive bronchodilator therapy, intravenous fluids, oxygen therapy, and corticosteroids. (Drug therapy will be discussed later.) Sedation should be avoided. Sodium cromolyn and inhaled steroids have no role in severe asthma. Once the asthma is controlled, inhaled steroid therapy can be started as the dose of systemic steroids is decreased.

Death From Asthma. Although death is uncommon, it can occur during a severe attack. Many such deaths are preventable. Studies of patients who died from asthma indicate that some had not received steroid therapy and some had received sedation. In severe asthma, sedation should not be given, whereas the use of corticosteroids is very important. Other factors that contribute to death from asthma are abuse of aerosolized bronchodilators and failure by both patient and physician to recognize the severity of an attack.

Is There a Cause? Consideration should be given to allergic or occupational causes of asthma or the possibility that aspirin ingestion or sulfite exposure could be the cause of a severe exacerbation. A careful history is important when allergic and occupational causes are considered. In addition, most patients with asthma should undergo a screening series of allergy skin tests (immediate wheal and flare skin tests). An alternative to skin testing is the radioallergosorbent test (RAST), also called the "allergen-specific IgE antibody" test. The RAST is more expensive but is a blood test available to physicians who do not do allergy skin testing. The results of both skin tests and RAST need to be correlated with the history. Most cases of adult-onset asthma do not have an allergic cause, although this is a possibility. One should not be concerned with the cause of the asthma until the diagnosis is made and the asthma, if severe, is treated. Avoidance of allergic causes, such as pets, occasionally effects a cure, and the use of cromolyn is particularly applicable in patients with allergic asthma. Occupational causes of asthma sometimes require bronchial challenges for confirmation.

NONPHARMACOLOGIC MEASURES IN TREATMENT

General Measures. Patients with asthma should avoid respiratory irritants such as dust, smoke, fumes, allergens when appropriate, and occupational causes if present. Patients with asthma should not smoke. Hobbies and avocations that aggravate asthma need to be considered. A common situation that worsens stable asthma and sometimes leads to hospital admission is exposure to dust and fumes, such as in remodeling a home. Common sense avoidance measures should be used by asthma patients. Dust and cold air masks are helpful. Air conditioning helps some patients, as do dust precipitators mounted in central ducts on furnaces. An atmosphere that is too humid or too dry should be avoided. A new space-age mask, although expensive, is useful for some patients with temporary, unavoidable exposure to irritants or allergens (Airstream by Racal Airstream, Rockville, MD). This mask has been particularly helpful for patients who are allergic to laboratory animals and have only intermittent, temporary exposure. Sulfites, aspirin, and nonsteroidal anti-inflammatory drugs should be avoided when appropriate. Influenza often aggravates asthma, and immunization is advisable if the patient is not allergic to eggs or the vaccine.

Avoidance of Aspirin. Between 8% and 20% of adult patients with asthma have an adverse reaction to aspirin ingestion, consisting of nasal symptoms or an asthmatic attack (or both), sometimes severe and life-threatening; rarely, these patients have hives. The incidence of this adverse reaction is around 40% in patients who have nasal polyps and asthma; its mechanism is unknown. All asthma patients should be questioned regarding possible allergy to aspirin, and if the history is suggestive, aspirin should be avoided. A challenge to aspirin is possible but dangerous and needs to be done cautiously, starting with very low doses and gradually increasing them. One must be prepared to treat a severe asthma attack when a challenge is undertaken.

Patients with sensitivity to aspirin experience a similar adverse reaction to the ingestion of nonsteroidal anti-inflammatory drugs, all of which inhibit the cyclooxygenase pathway of arachidonic acid metabolism. These drugs should be avoided. Patients usually can safely take acetaminophen, propoxyphene, choline salicylate, and sodium salicylate. Patients with nasal polyps and asthma should be warned about the possibility of reactions to aspirin, because the incidence in that group is so high.

Avoidance of Sulfites. A small group of patients have been found to experience severe asthma attacks, some life-threatening, after the ingestion of sulfites. Sulfites in the form of metabisulfite or bisulfite are employed widely as antioxidants, whitening agents, and food preservatives. They are used to prevent spoilage by bacteria and to prevent the browning of lettuce, fruits, potatoes, and other vegetables. In restaurants, sulfite solutions are commonly sprayed on lettuce, salads, and fruits to keep them looking fresh and to avoid browning. Sulfites are used in some dehydrated fruits, dehydrated and frozen potatoes, dehydrated soups, maraschino cherries, wines, some beers, some shrimp, guacamole dip, and some soft drinks.

Patients who have had severe asthma after the ingestion of sulfites should carry injectable epinephrine in case of accidental ingestion.

Of concern is the sulfite found in some medications used by this subset of patients with asthma. Some intravenous medications contain sulfites. Local anesthetics and epinephrine also contain small quantities, but subcutaneous injection does not provoke asthma in these patients. Asthma can occur, however, after the inhalation of sulfites found in some bronchodilator solutions. There are no sulfites in the metered-dose inhalers commonly used for the treatment of asthma patients.

DRUG THERAPY

Medication is the mainstay of therapy for many asthma patients. Asthma medications can be grouped into three large categories: bronchodilators, cromolyn, and corticosteroids.

Bronchodilators

Adrenergic Agonists. Beta-adrenergic agonists are rapid and potent bronchodilators that are widely used. Epinephrine, 0.2 to 0.5 ml of a 1:1000 solution, and terbutaline, 0.25 mg, are available for SQ injection. For patients with severe asthma, the dose can be repeated every 30 minutes for several doses. Caution is needed in patients with coronary artery disease and hypertension.

Inhaled adrenergic agonists are commonly used for asthma. For mild asthma, these agents are sometimes sufficient and can be used intermittently as needed. They are excellent in preventing exercise-induced asthma. Aerosolized epinephrine was historically the first one available, followed by isoproterenol. The newer agents, which are $beta_2$-adrenergic agonists, include isoetharine, metaproterenol, albuterol, and terbutaline; the last-named three are also available for oral use and have replaced ephedrine. Tremor can occur when these agents are used PO. The tremor lessens with time but is a limiting factor in the treatment of many patients. Isoproterenol has a rapid onset and is short-acting, whereas the newer agents are longer-acting. Recent evidence that the heart contains beta$_2$-adrenergic receptors makes the selectivity of these new agents less of an advantage.

Does refractory bronchoconstriction result from long-term chronic use of adrenergic agents? The answer remains unknown. Evidence shows that abuse of isoproterenol and probably other aerosols can worsen the asthma. Whether this occurs with the recommended doses of adrenergic agents is also unknown, but the severe unresponsive bronchoconstriction in patients on chronic therapy is more likely due to worsening of the asthma itself, with inflammation of the airways, which requires corticosteroid therapy.

Another concern is possible cardiac damage when adrenergic agents are used with theophylline. Despite long-term clinical experience with this combination, animal studies and anecdotal information have only recently raised this question. Further studies are needed to resolve this issue.

Theophylline. Theophylline is a widely used bronchodilator. In addition to dilating bronchial smooth muscle, it enhances relaxation of the lower esophageal sphincter, the uterus, and the ureters; enhances contractility of the diaphragm; causes mild diuresis; stimulates the respiratory center; has both a chronotropic and an inotropic effect on the heart; and is a stimulant of the central nervous system.

Theophylline is available for PO, IV, and rectal administration. It is well absorbed when given PO. Rectal suppositories are erratically absorbed and should be avoided. Solutions, however, are well absorbed when given rectally. Theophylline is degraded by the liver. Renal clearance of theophylline is low, ranging from 2.7 to 8.5 ml/min/m^2. Available for oral administration are anhydrous theophylline and several salts of theophylline, including aminophylline (the ethylenediamine salt), oxtriphylline, and dyphylline. These come in various forms: short-acting tablets and solutions, and long-acting or delayed-release tablets and capsules. The commonly used IV form is aminophylline, although IV theophylline is available. Rectal forms are not used often. Aminophylline is equivalent to 80% to 85% anhydrous theophylline; oxtriphylline is equivalent to 64% anhydrous theophylline.

The half-life of theophylline varies widely among patients (Table 1). Disease states and drugs affect the clearance, and the half-life in asthmatic adults who are otherwise healthy ranges from 2.9 to 12.8 hours. Erythromycin, troleandomycin, and cimetidine prolong the half-life, as do fever, obesity, and viral upper respiratory infections. Smoking, phenobarbital ingestion, and some dietary factors can shorten the half-life.

No one dosage for maintenance therapy can be used for all patients because of the wide variability in theophylline pharmacokinetics among patients. Methods to determine the serum level of theophylline are available and should be used in guiding both PO and IV therapy. The loading dose for IV aminophylline is 5.6 mg/kg, given slowly during a 20- to 30-minute period. This dose will increase the serum theophylline level approximately 10 μg/ml. For patients who have been taking regular theophylline, a loading dose should

Table 1. HALF-LIFE OF THEOPHYLLINE

Patient	Age Range	Half-life (hr)	
		Mean	Range
Normal or asthmatic adults	19–79 yr	8.7	2.9–12.8
Smokers	19–47 yr	4.9	4.0–7.7
Liver disease (cirrhosis)	43–72 yr	25.6	7.1–59.1
Congestive heart failure	53–87 yr	22.9	3.1–82.0
Asthmatic children	6–16 yr	3.96	1.4–7.9
Premature babies	3–15 days	30.2	14.4–57.7

not be given unless the baseline level of serum theophylline is known. For maintenance therapy, the most important, helpful information when deciding on dosage is the patient's previous experience with theophylline preparations. If the history is not helpful, IV aminophylline can be started at 0.5 mg/kg/hr, and the dose adjusted according to the theophylline level. A widely recommended maintenance dosage schedule of 0.9 mg/kg/hr for IV aminophylline is too much for many patients and can result in serious toxicity. Patients' previous experience should be a guide. If, when initially hospitalized, a patient is on a maintenance program of 1 gm of anhydrous theophylline daily, has no side effects, and has a serum theophylline level in the therapeutic range, a similar maintenance schedule of IV aminophylline, of 1200 mg/24 hr (50 mg/hr), should be started. If a dose of several hundred milligrams of oral theophylline has caused toxicity, aminophylline should be given cautiously and at a lower dose than the recommended maintenance schedule formula. For patients with congestive heart failure or liver disease, therapy should be started with 0.2 mg/kg/hr of IV aminophylline.

For oral therapy in adults, a 12-hour anhydrous theophylline preparation can be used, starting with 200 mg twice daily and gradually increasing the dose, if needed, guided by serum theophylline levels. The relationship of the theophylline level and the dose is not linear at high serum theophylline levels. Thus, the serum theophylline level may increase more than expected with small dosage increases, particularly at high serum levels. The mild nausea and upset stomach so common with theophylline is lessened by increasing the dose gradually. Since food may increase the absorption of 24-hour preparations, these should be given on an empty stomach.

The usual therapeutic serum theophylline level is between 10 and 20 μg/ml. However, bronchodilatation can occur with levels as low as 5 μg/ml. In mild to moderate asthma, bronchodilatation increases as the theophylline level is increased. Toxicity—usually nausea, vomiting, and headache—can be seen at levels of 13 μg/ml or lower, and increases in incidence with higher levels of theophylline. Thus, toxicity can occur even when the level is within the therapeutic range, although the incidence is low. At higher theophylline levels, usually above 35 μg/ml, seizures, serious cardiac dysrhythmias, and death can occur. Seizures have occurred at lower levels. Tachycardia is common. Recent reports of minimal toxicity despite very high levels of serum theophylline do not lessen the need to be aware of the potential seriousness of theophylline toxicity.

Patients with serious toxicity and dangerously high levels of serum theophylline can be treated with charcoal hemoperfusion or oral-activated charcoal, 30 gm every two hours, to a total of 120 gm. Oral charcoal increases the clearance rates of theophylline but not quite to the same level as does charcoal hemoperfusion; however, the former is easier to administer and has fewer side effects. Oral charcoal increases the clearance whether the previous theophylline has been given PO or IV.

Cromolyn. Cromolyn is most helpful for patients with allergic asthma. It is not a bronchodilator and is poorly absorbed after oral administration. The drug is given by inhalation as either a powder or an aerosol. Cromolyn should not be used for acute asthma attacks and is most effective in patients with allergic asthma, i.e., seasonal asthma with positive skin tests corresponding to the season in which the asthma occurs. Cromolyn also helps some patients with exercise-induced asthma when it is inhaled before exercising. It is excellent for asthma patients who have allergy as a result of periodic, unavoidable exposure to animals, such as during occasional visits to a relative, or who have occasional occupational exposure. The dose is 20 mg inhaled before exposure or every four to six hours.

Corticosteroids. Corticosteroids remain a necessary and helpful medication for patients with severe asthma, although the mechanism of action remains unknown. Patients with severe asthma need systemic steroids. Unfortunately, only a few studies have compared the efficacy of various doses. One study comparing doses of methylprednisolone found that 125 mg IV every six hours resulted in more improvement in pulmonary function at 24 hours than did 40 mg. At 48 and 72 hours there was no difference in effect between the two doses, but both the 125-mg and the 40-mg doses gave statistically significant improvement in pulmonary function, compared with a 15-mg dose. Actual differences, however, were not great. In the low-dose (15-mg) group, the FEV_1 improved from 25% to approximately 55% of the predicted value, whereas with the other two dosage schedules, the FEV_1 improved from 25% to 65% of the predicted value. For patients with respiratory failure, the steroid should be given IV, 40 to 125 mg of methylprednisolone every six hours, or its equivalent if another steroid is used. Once the asthma has improved, a change to oral medication should be made and the dosage reduced. For patients who do not need IV steroids or hospitalization, the usual daily starting dose is 40 to 60 mg of prednisone or its equivalent in divided doses. When the asthma is improved, a change to a single morning dose should be made. Patients who have never been on steroid therapy may need only a short course. For these, 40 mg of prednisone daily can be given until the asthma is controlled, after which the dosage should be reduced by 5 mg each day, resulting in a one- to two-week course of systemic steroids. Nonsteroid medication should be carefully evaluated to ensure that treatment is optimal.

If the patient needs long-term steroid therapy, attempts should be made to control the asthma by inhaled steroids such as beclomethasone, triamcinolone acetonide, or flunisolide. The inhaled steroid medications have enabled many patients who previously required low-dose, long-term systemic steroids to stop using systemic steroids. Patients who had required 10 to 15 mg of prednisone daily (or its equivalent) have been able to stop using systemic steroids and change to one of the inhaled steroids. For patients who have never received systemic steroids and who need something in addition to bronchodilators or cromolyn to control the asthma, a short course of prednisone (as discussed above) can be given and an inhaled steroid can be started. The steroid aerosols require approximately seven to ten days to have their full effect, so the peak effect can be expected during the time when the dose of prednisone is reduced. For patients with mild asthma who do not require systemic steroids yet whose asthma is not controlled by nonsteroid medication, the steroid aerosols may be helpful.

The usual dose of beclomethasone is two inhalations, 42 μg per inhalation four times daily, to a total of 336 μg daily. The dose can be increased to 800 μg daily. Patient compliance and the expense become problems with high doses. The usual dose of triamcinolone is similar, two inhalations four times daily. Each inhalation gives approximately 100 μg of triamcinolone. The usual dose of flunisolide is two inhalations twice daily, each delivering 250 μg.

Although short-term studies of inhaled steroids indicate no suppression of the hypothalamic-pituitary-adrenal axis at the usual doses, several have suggested that adrenal suppression occurs with long-term use. Thus, when these patients encounter unusual stress, such as surgery, additional systemic steroids should be given.

The main side effect from inhaled steroids is candidiasis of the pharynx and mouth. This is often asymptomatic, infrequent, and easily treated with nystatin. Some patients have hoarseness and throat irritation without candidiasis.

Patients who require long-term systemic steroids should be treated when possible with alternate-morning (every-other-day) prednisone or methylprednisolone. Once the asthma is controlled by daily steroids, a change to alternate-morning prednisone should be made, either gradually over several weeks or all at once, depending on the patient's previous experience with systemic steroids. If the patient's asthma had previously been controlled by alternate-morning prednisone therapy and requires, for example, 40 mg of prednisone daily for five days to achieve control, the dose could be changed to 40 mg on alternate mornings. An alternative approach would be to continue taking 40 mg on the even days and gradually reduce the dose on the odd days, until after several weeks the dose is 40 mg taken on alternate mornings. If the asthma is well controlled, the dose could be reduced by 5 mg every two to four doses to the lowest possible dose that will give reasonable control of the asthma. Some patients require daily steroids to control their asthma. Attempts should constantly be made to reduce the dose gradually to the lowest possible dose. In patients receiving systemic corticosteroids over a long period, the serum glucose and potassium levels should be monitored periodically and a calcium supplement given if there is no contraindication.

IMMUNOTHERAPY

Immunotherapy, also called "desensitization" or "hyposensitization," is used to treat patients with allergic asthma. Double-blind, placebo-controlled studies have demonstrated the efficacy of immunotherapy in patients with seasonal rhinitis for several allergens. The value of immunotherapy for asthma patients is not as well documented, although a few studies indicate that immunotherapy reduced the severity of asthma when the asthma was due to specific allergens. Other carefully controlled, well-designed studies are needed. Many allergists believe that immunotherapy is helpful in patients with seasonal asthma due to mold or pollen allergy. Several reports have shown that bacterial vaccine is ineffective in the treatment of asthma, and its use, common 20 years ago, has diminished today.

PATIENT INFORMATION AND EDUCATION

General Information. Educational information for asthma patients is available through several organizations, including the Asthma and Allergy Foundation of America and the American Lung Association. Both groups have newsletters and resource material, and there are local chapters. The Mayo Clinic has prepared a small booklet on asthma and encourages attendance at a patient education session, where a videotape is shown and nurses are available to answer questions. Several videotapes are available. At these sessions, we use "Living With Your Asthma" from Instructional Media Services, Medical Sciences Building, University of Toronto, Toronto, Ontario, Canada. Our pharmacists have prepared handouts on drugs used in the treatment of asthma—a single sheet for each drug. Informational sheets are also available on the avoidance of sulfites and the use of epinephrine.

Use of Aerosols. Proper technique is crucial in the use of aerosolized medications for asthma, both bronchodilator and corticosteroid aerosols. Recent evidence suggests that inhaling these aerosols through a spacer or tube increases their efficacy, although they are efficacious without this if inhaled properly. When metered-dose inhalers are placed directly in the mouth, much of the spray hits the back of the oral pharynx and is swallowed. A spacer or tube between the mouth and the inhaler results in more medication entering the trachea and bronchi.

Although several commercial products are available, my colleagues and I have found that a simple rolled tube, 8 to 12 inches long, is helpful. The most important aspect is to observe the patient to be certain that aerosolized medication is used properly. The spacer tubes have helped some patients to time the use of these sprays correctly so that the metered-dose aerosol is triggered at the onset of inspiration.

PERIODIC EVALUATION

The frequency of follow-up for asthma patients depends on the severity. Those with mild, intermittent asthma that is readily reversed or controlled by aerosolized bronchodilators need not be seen as long as their disease is stable. Patients requiring long-term systemic steroids should be seen frequently, probably every one to three months when possible and more often when the steroid dosage is changed. A Wright Peak Flow Meter can be used as an office procedure for flow measurements. A helpful tool in chronic asthma is the mini-Wright Peak Flow Meter. Patients can purchase one of these and follow the course of their asthma at home by measuring their own peak expiratory flows.

PATIENT COMPLIANCE

Compliance in patients with daily wheezing is ordinarily not a major problem. However, many patients dislike the tremor that occurs from the use of oral adrenergic agents, and so prefer not to take this medication. Also, because corticosteroid aerosol medications do not produce an immediate bronchodilator effect, some patients assume they do not work. The physician must reemphasize the need for regular use of this medication for it to be effective.

ALLERGIC BRONCHOPULMONARY ASPERGILLOSIS

Allergic bronchopulmonary aspergillosis (ABPA) is a complication of asthma in patients who are allergic to the *Aspergillus* molds, mainly *A. fumigatus*. In addition to having typical asthma, these patients have attacks associated with malaise, low-grade fever, and pulmonary infiltrates noted on the chest roentgenogram. Sometimes they cough up brown plugs.

ABPA is diagnosed when the following criteria are satisfied: evidence of asthma, peripheral blood eosinophilia, a positive immediate skin test to *Aspergillus*, the presence of serum precipitating antibodies to *Aspergillus*, an elevated level of total serum IgE, an elevated allergen-specific IgE (or RAST) to *Aspergillus*, pulmonary infiltrates, and proximal or central bronchiectasis. These patients also can have a positive sputum culture for, and a dual skin test response to, *A. fumigatus*, with a positive immediate skin test at 15 to 20 minutes and a late reaction usually peaking at eight to 12 hours and resolving by 24 hours.

A positive skin test to *Aspergillus* alone is not diagnostic because *Aspergillus* can cause allergic asthma unassociated with ABPA. The presence of *Aspergillus* in the sputum is common, particularly during the summer and fall months, and cannot be considered diagnostic. The *Aspergillus* mold also can cause hypersensitivity pneumonitis, as well as a saprophytic aspergilloma, both of which give precipitating antibodies to *Aspergillus*. The bronchiectasis can sometimes be demonstrated by tomography; thus, bronchography, which entails some risk, is often not necessary.

One long-term follow-up study of patients with untreated ABPA suggests that the course is chronic and that some have severe lung destruction. Because most of these patients are young and the treatment involves systemic steroids, an accurate diagnosis is very important.

Corticosteroids must be given in large enough doses for a sufficient period to control the disease. Therapy with prednisone, 0.5 mg/kg/day, has been recommended until the chest roentgenogram shows clearing, or for two weeks. The dose of prednisone can then be changed to 0.5 mg/kg every other day for three months, and slowly reduced during a second three-month period. Recent evidence suggests that monitoring the total IgE antibody level is useful in the management of these patients, and an increasing IgE level may be predictive of a clinical flare. Antifungal drugs have not been helpful. Remissions do occur and can last for years.

REFERENCES

Bernstein IL, Johnson CL, Ted Tse CS: Therapy with cromolyn sodium. Ann Intern Med 89:228–233, 1978.

Greenberger PA: Allergic bronchopulmonary aspergillosis. J Allergy Clin Immunol 74:645–653, 1984.

Hendeles L, Weinberger M: Theophylline. *In* Middleton E Jr, Reed CE, Ellis EF (eds): Allergy: Principles and Practice, 2nd ed. C. V. Mosby Co, St. Louis, 1983, pp 535–574.

Stevenson DD: Diagnosis, prevention, and treatment of adverse reactions to aspirin and nonsteroidal anti-inflammatory drugs. J Allergy Clin Immunol 74:617–622, 1984.

Stevenson DD, Simon RA: Sulfites and asthma (editorial). J Allergy Clin Immunol 74:469–472, 1984.

3 · *RESPIRATORY FAILURE*

John Popovich, Jr.
HENRY FORD HOSPITAL

DEFINITIONS AND DIAGNOSTIC CRITERIA

The primary function of the lung is to exchange gas between the inspired air and blood within the pulmonary capillaries. Disturbances in this gas exchange result in abnormalities of respiratory gases within the arterial blood. Thus, respiratory failure is defined as a condition in which arterial P_{O_2} is below the predicted normal range for the patient's age at the prevalent barometric pressure (excluding hypoxemia from intracardiac right-to-left shunting), or arterial P_{CO_2} is above the normal range (excluding respiratory compensation for metabolic alkalosis). This definition implies that the diagnosis of respiratory failure is made by the laboratory analysis of arterial blood and represents the consequences of impaired lung function.

As respiratory failure is a disorder of function and not a disease, it may be caused by a variety of conditions that affect lung function (see Table 1). These include abnormalities of ventilation where the lung is entirely normal (e.g., neuromuscular disease).

Respiratory failure may be subclassified into types based on the physiologic derangements: (1) hypoxemic respiratory failure without hypercapnia and (2) hypoxemic, hypercapnic respiratory failure. Respiratory failure also is often classified into acute and chronic forms, as well as acute exacerbations of chronic respiratory failure. These distinctions are helpful in determining both etiologic diagnosis and therapy.

PATHOPHYSIOLOGY

Respiration can be subdivided into four functional processes: ventilation, perfusion, gaseous diffusion, and control of breathing. The interplay of each of these processes keeps oxygen and carbon dioxide tensions normal in the arterial blood. Abnormalities in these processes, either singly or together, may result in respiratory failure.

Values of arterial oxygen tension (PaO_2) below normal or $PaCO_2$ above normal indicate the presence of respiratory failure, if intracardiac right-to-left shunt and respiratory compensation for metabolic alkalosis are excluded.

HYPOXEMIA

Pathophysiologically, there are four major causes of hypoxemia: (1) ventilation-perfusion inequality; (2) hypoventilation; (3) diffusion impairment; and (4) shunt. The most common cause of these is ventilation-perfusion inequality. Calculation of the alveolar-arterial gradient ($A\text{-}aD_{O_2}$) helps to determine the physiologic cause of hypoxemia, in that pure hypoventilation as a cause of hypoxemia has a normal calculated $A\text{-}aD_{O_2}$, whereas other causes of hypoxemia have an increased $A\text{-}aD_{O_2}$. Further differentiation can be made by determining the response of the PaO_2 to increasing inspired oxygen tensions: PaO_2 increases to normal values when a hypoxemic patient breathes 100% oxygen if the hypoxemia is due to ventilation-perfusion inequality or diffusion impairment; hypoxemia persists despite 100% oxygen if its cause is shunt.

HYPERCAPNIA

The two major causes of hypercapnia are ventilation-perfusion inequality, which causes alveolar ventilation ($\dot{V}_A$) to decrease as dead-space ventilation increases, and hypoventilation. Excessive carbon dioxide production, as may occur during fat deposition states and excessive carbohydrate feeding, may also cause hypercapnia.

ACID-BASE DISTURBANCES

An increase or decrease in Pa_{CO_2} in the blood has a direct effect on hydrogen ion concentration (through

Table 1. PARTIAL LIST OF CAUSES OF RESPIRATORY FAILURE

Airway disease
  Chronic obstructive airway disease
  Upper airway obstruction (inflammatory, foreign body)

Chest wall disease
  Fibrothorax
  Flail chest
  Kyphoscoliosis
  Massive pleural effusion
  Pneumothorax

Neuromuscular disease
  Central nervous system disease
  Cervical or thoracic spine injury
  Drug overdoses
  Muscle disease (myasthenia gravis, muscular dystrophy)
  Peripheral nerve disorders (motor neuron disease, Guillain-Barré syndrome)
  Sleep apnea (central, obstructive mixed)

Pulmonary parenchymal disease
  Pulmonary edema (cardiogenic, noncardiogenic, adult respiratory distress syndrome)
  Pulmonary infiltration (pneumonia fibrosis)

Pulmonary vascular disease
  Pulmonary emboli (thromboemboli, fat emboli)
  Pulmonary vasculitis

the amount of carbonic acid produced) and a reciprocal effect on pH. Acute changes in Pa_{CO_2} have a more profound effect on pH than chronic changes because of the lower amount of bicarbonate present to buffer pH. Hypoxemia and inadequate blood flow to meet the needs of aerobically metabolizing respiratory muscles may also produce a metabolic acidosis through lactic acid production.

CARDIOVASCULAR DISTURBANCES

Hypoxemia, hypercapnia, and acidosis produce vasoconstriction of the pulmonary vasculature. Pulmonary arterial pressure increases and, if sufficiently high, causes right heart failure. Hypoxemia and hypercapnia induce increased sympathetic nervous system activity, leading to tachycardia, systolic hypertension, and arrhythmias.

CLINICAL ASPECTS

The clinical aspects of respiratory failure are usually overshadowed by the symptoms and signs of the disease that results in the respiratory failure. Dyspnea often accompanies respiratory failure, although in many hypoventilating patients even this most basic symptom may be absent. Most other manifestations result from hypercapnia, hypoxemia, and right heart failure. The most common associated symptom with hypercapnia is headache. It is often more severe in the morning owing to worsening of hypoventilation during sleep. Alterations in mental function, such as short-term memory loss, cognitive diminishment, and eventually obtundation, occur as hypercapnia worsens. Physical findings are of tachycardia, systolic hypertension, bounding pulses, sweating, and constricted pupils, as well as orbital hyperemia and chemosis.

The symptoms of hypoxemia are similar to those of intoxication. Mental status abnormalities of personality changes, cognitive dysfunction, and inappropriateness are frequent. Alveolar hypoxemia is the most potent pulmonary vasoconstrictor and may result in pulmonary hypertension and cor pulmonale with attendant findings. Renal hypoxemia (if present for weeks or months) results in polycythemia.

MANAGEMENT

Management of respiratory failure can be divided into (1) management of the underlying disease precipitating respiratory failure; (2) treatment of hypoxemia; and (3) treatment of hypercapnia.

Differentiation of respiratory failure into acute or chronic variants is extremely helpful for clinical management. As the management strategies differ for each, they will be discussed separately.

MANAGEMENT OF ACUTE RESPIRATORY FAILURE
Plan

The major management questions in cases of suspected acute respiratory failure are: (1) What is the degree of physiologic derangement in oxygenation and acid-base balance caused by the acute respiratory failure? (2) What is the underlying precipitating cause? (3) What is the natural history of the underlying cause and is the cause readily reversible?

Most patients with acute respiratory failure caused by conditions that are not readily and totally reversible require hospitalization for treatment of the underlying disease and the physiologic derangements. Some cases, such as acute asthma or narcotic overdose, can be reversed entirely. Others, such as severe pneumonia or the adult respiratory distress syndrome, require significant time for improvement. Often the most pressing question is whether the failure is severe enough to require intensive care placement for observation and tracheal intubation and mechanical ventilation for support. This usually requires sound clinical judgment and careful assessment of the severity of the blood gas derangements. Ensuring adequate oxygenation is paramount. Oxygen therapy is indicated to sustain life until other therapeutic measures effect a reversal of the acute cause of respiratory failure. Reversal of hypoxemia by administering supplemental oxygen to achieve a Po_2 of 60 to 70 mm Hg (with resultant hemoglobin saturations of 90% to 94%) should be the first therapeutic goal. Sedative medications should be avoided. Left heart failure should be treated with careful diuresis. If progressive hypercapnia occurs and/or if pH is below 7.25, immediate intubation should be performed and mechanical ventilation initiated. Severe hypoxemia with Pa_{O_2} less than 60 mm Hg on a high-flow non-rebreather oxygen mask also often requires intubation and positive pressure therapy.

Nonpharmacologic Measures

An assessment of upper airway patency is essential in the patient presenting with respiratory failure. Tracheal intubation (oral or nasal) serves to relieve upper airway obstruction and provide access for tracheal suctioning and mechanical ventilation, if needed.

Significant secretions that cannot be expectorated by cough may require nasotracheal suctioning. Mobilization of secretions by chest percussion and postural drainage is often effective, but does not speed the rate of resolution of processes such as uncomplicated pneumonia or produce sputum that is not present ("thumping on an empty ketchup bottle"). Optimal hydration reduces sputum tenacity and allows easier sputum removal. Mucolytic agents and ultrasonic nebulization of saline are generally ineffective.

Mechanical aids to assist lung inflation, such as intermittent positive pressure breathing (IPPB), incentive spirometry, or continuous positive airway pressure (CPAP) by face mask, may be of benefit in patients who cannot or will not take periodic deep breaths, or who have chronically decreased compliance of the respiratory system.

Mechanical ventilation is indicated to provide work of breathing and return pH to normal range (7.35 to 7.42). Initial tidal volumes of 10 to 15 ml/kg, ideal weight, are recommended; flow rates should be adjusted to allow adequate time for expiration. Owing to tenuous respiratory status and cardiovascular instability, patients in acute respiratory failure often require invasive monitoring with arterial, central venous, or thermodilution pulmonary artery catheters. These provide vascular access for arterial and/or mixed venous blood samples, central vascular pressures, and cardiac output determinations. Newer fiberoptic pulmonary artery catheters allow continuous monitoring of mixed venous oxygen saturation, providing a measure of the adequacy of oxygenation and cardiac output. Noninvasive respiratory gas monitoring can be provided by transcutaneous oxygen and carbon dioxide tension electrodes, oximeters (ear, finger, pulse), and expired carbon dioxide analyzers.

Drug Therapy

Drug therapy for respiratory failure is aimed at treatment of the underlying disease, treatment of respiratory infections, reversal of airway obstruction, and treatment of concomitant heart failure.

For a few diseases causing respiratory failure, there is specific treatment. Hypersensitivity pneumonitis, desquamative interstitial pneumonitis, Goodpasture's syndrome, and Wegener's granulomatosis require treatment with corticosteroids or other immunosuppressive drugs and techniques (e.g., plasmapheresis). Myasthenia gravis and narcotic overdose are neuromuscular disorders that may result in respiratory failure and are treated with specific therapy. Nevertheless, these disorders constitute a minority of cases of both acute and chronic respiratory failure, which are more frequently caused by respiratory infections and chronic obstructive lung disease.

Respiratory infection as a primary or exacerbating cause of respiratory failure must be suspected and aggressively treated with broad-spectrum antibiotics, guided by sputum Gram stain and cultures. Increasingly, atypical pneumonias may play significant pathogenic roles, requiring specific diagnostic tests beyond routine Gram stain and culture.

Bronchodilators

Airway obstruction caused by smooth muscle contraction and airway inflammation is treated by bronchodilator medications and corticosteroids. The principal bronchodilators in clinical practice are methylxanthine drugs (aminophylline, theophylline) and beta-adrenergic stimulants. Theophylline compounds provide bronchodilation by preventing the phosphodiesterase degradation of cylic AMP; increased cyclic-AMP levels produce bronchodilation. These compounds also probably increase diaphragmatic muscle strength and central respiratory drive. Therapeutic levels of 12 to 16 μg/ml are usually adequate to achieve maximal benefit; higher levels, especially those greater than 20 μg/ml, are associated with greater gastrointestinal, cardiovascular, and CNS toxicity. During acute respiratory failure, IV aminophylline is used to rapidly produce steady serum levels. Titration of these levels and frequent monitoring of serum levels are necessary both to avoid undertreatment and, more important, to prevent toxic levels. Toxicity is frequent not only because of the narrow therapeutic window, but also because of the variability of drug volume of distribution and metabolism noted in acutely ill patients due to organ system dysfunction and concomitant drug therapy (e.g., cimetidine, propranolol, and erythromycin).

The preferred beta-adrenergic stimulant is a beta-2 receptor selective drug (e.g., albuterol, metaproterenol) given by inhalation. Application by properly used metered dose inhaler or aerosol generator achieves greatest bronchodilation with the least systemic adrenergic effects. Infrequently, these drugs may need to be given PO or SQ. Combined therapy of airway obstruction with methylxanthine and beta-adrenergic drugs has additive and, possibly, synergistic bronchodilator effects.

More recently, aerosolized atropinic agents (e.g., atropine sulfate, 0.01 to 0.05 mg/kg, q 6 hr), which affect bronchodilation by parasympathetic blockade, have been investigated for use in obstructive airway disease. Use of these agents in acute respiratory failure appears most helpful as an adjunct to conventional methylxanthine and beta-adrenergic therapy, especially in patients with chronic bronchitis or predominantly central airway obstruction. Caution in their use is important: currently available atropinic agents can be significantly absorbed systemically, causing ocular, CNS, cardiovascular, and urinary tract problems, and can also significantly dry tracheobronchial secretions, potentially worsening airway obstruction on a structural basis. Future atropinic agents, such as ipratropium bromide and atropine methonitrate, may have far fewer side effects.

Corticosteroids frequently act adjunctively with bronchodilator medications by enhancing responsiveness to beta-adrenergic drugs and by general antiinflammatory actions on airways. Corticosteroids appear most beneficial in patients with demonstrable reduction of airway obstruction in response to beta-adrenergic stimulants and in patients with markers of atopic disease. In acute respiratory failure secondary to obstructive airway disease, an initial IV dose of 1 mg/kg methylprednisolone every six hours appears most appropriate, with subsequent tapering and conversion to oral preparations determined by clinical course.

When present, left ventricular failure should be treated by improvement in oxygenation and normalization of acid-base status, diuretics, afterload reducing agents, and (possibly) digitalis. The overaggressive use of diuretics in misdiagnosed left ventricular failure may result in significant cardiac output reductions and concomitant worsening of hypoxemia and tissue oxygenation in respiratory failure patients. A reduction of blood flow to the respiratory muscles may occur, thereby precipitating acute respiratory muscle fatigue and respiratory arrest. Afterload reducing agents may also act as pulmonary vasodilators; worsening of hypoxemia by lowering ventilation-perfusion ratios may occur. These agents must be given under careful clinical and, possibly, invasive cardiorespiratory monitoring. Cor pulmonale, or pure right heart failure, is best treated by relief of hypoxemia, normalization of pH, bed rest, and mild diuresis. There is no role for digitalis in treating cor pulmonale.

MANAGEMENT OF CHRONIC RESPIRATORY FAILURE

The management of chronic respiratory failure entails treatment of the underlying disease and its attendant complications and alleviation of the physiologic derangements caused by hypoxemia and hypercapnia. Major goals of such treatment include the return of the patient to as normal a functional life style as possible, minimizing complications and the need for hospital admission.

Hospitalizations are frequently required during so-called acute exacerbations of chronic respiratory failure. These are usually due to worsening of the primary disease, the development of cardiovascular complications, or infection. The need for admission should be determined by whether the cause of the exacerbation is reversible, by the severity of blood gas derangements, and by the ability of the patient to meet her or his needs in the home setting. Home health care professionals can help provide monitoring and treatment (e.g., chest physiotherapy) previously available only in the inpatient setting.

Surgical Correction

Certain patients with sleep apnea and chronic respiratory failure who require ventilatory assistance can be managed surgically. Patients with obstructive sleep apnea and either life-threatening cardiac arrhythmias or significant disability may be candidates for tracheotomy. Structural abnormalities causing sleep-related obstruction (tonsillar hypertrophy, mandibular malformations) should be surgically corrected. Recently, removal of obstructive oropharyngeal tissues by uvulopalatopharyngoplasty has shown promise as a treatment for the patient with obese obstructive sleep apnea. An alternative to surgical intervention in these patients is nocturnal nasal CPAP, which presumably acts as a pressure "splint" of the upper airway. It is paramount that the rules for patient selection be rigid, requiring detailed general and sleep-related history and physical examination, nocturnal polysomnography, and direct nasopharyngolaryngoscopy. These patients are best managed by multidisciplinary teams in tertiary referral settings. Patients with central sleep apnea plus marked hypoventilation and cardiorespiratory failure may require mechanical support of ventilation during sleep. Techniques such as electrophrenic diaphragmatic pacing or nocturnal positive pressure ventilation can be employed in carefully selected patients.

Continuous Ventilatory Assistance

Some patients with chronic respiratory failure cannot be weaned from ventilatory assistance and remain on chronic ventilatory support. Ideally, such patients should be discharged to a home setting. An organized team of physicians, nurses, and respiratory therapists is required for home mechanical ventilation. As patients with restrictive chest wall disease or central sleep apnea often require mechanical ventilatory assistance only at night, they may assume reasonably normal life styles and often return to employment.

Nocturnal ventilation may be provided by positive pressure ventilation via tracheotomy or by noninvasive negative pressure means, such as cuirass ("chest shell"), whole body shell, or caisson ("iron-lung") ventilators. Patients not requiring full ventilatory support but who have sleep-worsened hypoventilation may benefit from assistance devices such as oscillating or rocking beds; individuals with diaphragmatic paralysis or neuromuscular diaphragmatic impairment are included in this group.

Drug Therapy

Aside from agents used to treat the primary disorder causing respiratory failure, the most important drug used in chronic respiratory failure is oxygen. Supplemental oxygen is employed in patients with chronic hypoxemia of sufficient magnitude to cause organ dysfunction. Indications for oxygen therapy are as follows: (1) resting chronic PaO_2 less than 56 mm Hg and/or (2) signs of hypoxia-induced organ system dysfunction or complications, including polycythemia, cor pulmonale, impaired sleep pattern, and impaired mentation.

More controversial indications are exercise-induced hypoxemia and nocturnal desaturation. The former is often recognized in patients with severe restrictive lung disease, pulmonary vascular disease, or obstructive lung disease with diffusion reduction. Graded exercise testing with monitoring of oxygen saturation by continuous oximetry can identify such patients when activity is limited by hypoxemia. This allows quantitation of the dose requirements of oxygen. Ordinarily, exercise-induced desaturation does not occur in obstructive lung disease patients with resting PaO_2 greater than 60 mm Hg unless both severe obstruction and diffusion reductions are present. Nocturnal oxygen desaturation appears to occur frequently in chronic bronchitic patients and should be treated if secondary organ effects (cor pulmonale, secondary polycythemia, nocturnal dysrhythmias, or nocturnal cardiac ischemia) are present.

Oxygen is generally delivered by nasal cannula. PaO_2 should be increased to 65 mm Hg. Patients should be routinely advised to increase nasal cannula flow rate by 1 L/min during exercise or sleep.

To be most effective in reducing mortality risks, patients should use oxygen continuously for at least 18 hours per day or during the period (e.g., sleep, exertion) when desaturation occurs. Oxygen requirements should be frequently reassessed by measurement of arterial oxygen tension and saturation. In stable patients, arterial blood gases should be checked at least every three months or after signs of clinical deterioration.

Occasionally, drugs used as respiratory stimulants, such as medroxyprogesterone (20 mg q 6 hr) and acetazolamide (250 mg q 8 hr), are effective in some forms of chronic hypoventilatory respiratory failure. Drug therapy for obstructive sleep apnea (e.g., protriptyline) has been generally ineffective.

Patient Information and Education

Patients with chronic respiratory failure and their families need to recognize symptoms and signs of respiratory, cardiovascular, and infectious complications. Education regarding disease pathophysiology, optimal breathing patterns, relaxation techniques, and exertional tasks helps to optimize life style and maintain close patient-clinician ties. Counseling related to general health considerations, such as nutrition, is also important.

Rehabilitation programs, including exercise training, are effective means of improving muscular efficiency to perform the training tasks. To be effective, patients must be able to perform some exertional tasks and be willing to apply themselves to the training program and to continue maintenance training programs. These must be tailored to improve general cardiovascular performance and muscular performance of certain tasks. For example, swimming programs may improve cardiovascular performance but may not necessarily help a patient walk further.

Periodic Evaluation

The frequency of evaluation is highly dependent on the stability of the patient. Generally, patients should be seen every two to six months. Routine laboratory tests should include arterial blood gases and hemoglobin concentrations. Spirometric tests may be helpful periodically in patients with obstructive lung disease but are generally employed only if clinical deterioration occurs, or yearly as general prognostic monitors. Electrocardiogram and chest radiographs should be obtained at the time of suspected deterioration in clinical status. Determination of oxygen requirements should be done at intervals dependent on arterial blood gas results and changes in the patient's condition.

Patient Compliance

Compliance with prescribed drug, nonpharmocologic, and oxygen therapy regimens should be checked at each clinic visit. Home health personnel can reinforce the therapeutic program at times. Most important, patients requiring oxygen need reminding about the appropriate daily duration of use, as they often use oxygen only when short of breath or otherwise symptomatic.

Preventive Measures

General and respiratory health must be emphasized. Obviously, the patient should stop smoking and try to eliminate passive inhalation of family members' smoke. Preventive vaccination with pneumococcal vaccine and yearly influenza vaccine are indicated. Treatment of early influenza or prophylaxis during epidemics with amantadine should be considered.

Patients and family members need to be counseled regarding the use of artificial ventilation. Patients who are terminally and irreversibly ill from respiratory failure should be helped to accept their disease and imminent death. Forestalling measures that merely prolong life without offering recovery, such as mechanical ventilation, are not indicated in such patients. Multi-professional counseling helps patients and families to deal with chronic illness, and should be instituted as early as possible in the course.

REFERENCES

Anthonisen NR: Hypoxemia and O_2 therapy. Am Rev Respir Dis 126:729–733, 1983.

Aubier M, Murciano D, Milic-Emili J, et al: Effects of the administration of O_2 on ventilation and blood gases in patients with chronic obstructive pulmonary disease during acute respiratory failure. Am Rev Respir Dis 122:747–754, 1980.

Bone RC: Treatment of respiratory failure due to advanced chronic obstructive lung disease. Arch Intern Med 140:1018–1021, 1980.

Lertzman MM, Cherniak RM: Rehabilitation of patients with chronic obstructive pulmonary disease. Am Rev Respir Dis 114:1145–1165, 1976.

Nocturnal Oxygen Therapy Trial Group: Continuous or nocturnal oxygen therapy in hypoxemic chronic obstructive lung disease. A clinical trial. Ann Intern Med 93:391–398, 1980.

4 · COMMON FUNGAL DISEASES OF THE LUNG

John F. Beamis, Jr.
LAHEY CLINIC MEDICAL CENTER

Fungal infections of the lung represent an increasingly important group of diseases in our society. The fungi that produce these infections are grouped into two broad, occasionally overlapping categories: endemic fungi and opportunistic fungi. As the population of the United States shifts to sunbelt areas for recreation or permanent residence, more people will be exposed to the endemic fungi—*Coccidioides immitis*, *Histoplasma capsulatum*, and *Blastomyces dermatitidis*. Modern transportation permits these organisms to produce disease far from their areas of endemicity. For example, *C. immitis* infections have been described in every continent except Antarctica.

With the increasing use of chemotherapy for malignant neoplasms, the number of patients at risk of development of infections by *Aspergillus* sp., *Cryptococcus neoformans*, and *Candida* sp., the opportunistic fungi, is also increasing. A new disease, the acquired immune deficiency syndrome (AIDS), is producing a rapidly expanding group of patients at risk of diseases caused by opportunistic fungi.

Fungi are capable of producing several different interactions with lung tissues: allergic, invasive, or saprophytic. The interaction is determined by the immunologic status of the patient. Since treatment may vary from mere observation to amphotericin B to corticosteroids, the clinician must not only isolate the organism but also define the reaction it is producing in the host.

A fungal etiology should be considered in the evaluation of every pulmonary infiltrate. This requires an awareness of fungi common to a local area as well as detailed knowledge of the patient's travel history and current immunologic status.

Aspergillus Lung Diseases

Six separate pulmonary syndromes are caused by the interaction between the lung and the ubiquitous *Aspergillus* sp. of fungi (Table 1). These fungi, usually *A. fumigatus*, *A. niger*, or *A. flavus*, are continually aerosolized into the lung from the ambient air and are

Table 1. *ASPERGILLUS* PULMONARY SYNDROMES

	Predisposition	Presence of Organism	Laboratory		Chest Radiography	Treatment
Aspergillus asthma	Reactive airway disease	Intermittent exposure	Eosinophilia IgE PPTNS* Skin test	+ + + + + − I†	Normal or hyperinflation	Avoid exposure; bronchodilators (immunotherapy), corticosteroids
Aspergillus hypersensitivity pneumonitis	Occupational setting (malt workers, farmers)	Intermittent exposure	Eosinophilia IgE PPTNS Skin test	− Normal + + + D‡	Interstitial or alveolar infiltrates originally transient; may progress to fibrosis	Avoid exposure; corticosteroids
Allergic bronchopulmonary aspergillosis	Reactive airway disease	Chronic colonization; intra-airway	Eosinophilia IgE PPTNS Skin test	+ + + + + + + + + I†, D‡	Fleeting infiltrates; bronchial shadows; ring shadows; fibrosis	Corticosteroids
Invasive pulmonary aspergillosis	Malignancy; chemotherapy; corticosteroid therapy	Invading tissue (may be extrapulmonary)	Eosinophilia IgE PPTNS Skin test Antigen§	− Normal + − − +	Progressive infiltration; round pneumonia; hemorrhagic infarct	Amphotericin B
Aspergilloma	Cavitary lung disease	Chronic colonization; intracavitary	Eosinophilia IgE PPTNS Skin test	+ − Normal + + + + D‡	Cavity with intracavitary mass; crescent sign	Observation; operation if complications arise; ? intracavitary amphotericin B
Chronic necrotizing pulmonary aspergillosis (semi-invasive aspergillosis)	Mild alteration in host defenses	Local invasion; mycetoma	Eosinophilia IgE PPTNS Skin test	− ? + + + ?	Infiltrate with development of cavity and mycetoma	Amphotericin B; surgical drainage

*Serum precipitating antibodies; I† = immediate skin test (wheal and flare); D‡ = delayed skin test (Arthus reaction); § antigen occasionally found in serum or bronchoalveolar lavage fluid.

capable of initiating allergic reactions, establishing a saprophytic infestation, or producing local and disseminated tissue invasion. One or all of these reactions may occur in the same patient, which emphasizes the need for proper diagnosis. Immediate life-threatening *Aspergillus* infections occur in hospitalized individuals, but chronic infections and allergic reactions are more common in outpatients.

leukocytosis, and interstitial pulmonary infiltrates shortly after exposure. The organism may be cultured from the environment and occasionally from sputum, but this mainly serves to confirm exposure. Precipitating serum antibodies to *Aspergillus* sp. are always present, but again this only indicates past exposure. From 30% to 50% of similarly exposed but asymptomatic individuals also demonstrate precipitating antibodies. Treatment is the same for other hypersensitivity pneumonitis described under *Chronic Berylliosis* (see Chap. 9).

Aspergillus Asthma

On rare occasions typical bronchial asthma develops from exposure to *Aspergillus* sp. Diagnosis is based on the history of specific exposure followed by asthmatic symptoms. Baker's asthma has at times been attributed to the inhalation of *Aspergillus* spores. Management is similar to that for bronchial asthma (see Chapter 2).

Aspergillus Hypersensitivity Pneumonitis

Malt worker's lung is the classic *Aspergillus* hypersensitivity pneumonitis. Hypersensitivity pneumonitis may also occur after inhalation of the fungus during exposure to moldy fertilizer. Diagnosis of this condition is primarily based on history of exposure and development of classic symptoms of fever, chills, dyspnea,

Allergic Bronchopulmonary Aspergillosis

DEFINITION AND DIAGNOSTIC CRITERIA

This complex pulmonary immunologic condition results from chronic colonization of airways of patients with chronic air flow obstruction by organisms of the *Aspergillus* sp. Major diagnostic criteria are bronchospasm, peripheral blood eosinophilia, immediate skin reactivity to *Aspergillus* antigen, precipitating antibodies against *Aspergillus* antigen, elevated serum levels of IgE, transient or fixed pulmonary infiltrates, central bronchiectasis, and specific IgE or IgG antibodies to *Aspergillus* sp. The minor criteria are isolation of *A. fumigatus* in sputum, history or expectoration of plugs, and delayed (Arthus) skin reaction to *Aspergillus* antigen. Of these criteria, only central bronchiectasis and the presence of specific IgE or IgG antibodies to *A. fumigatus* can be considered pathognomonic of allergic bronchopulmonary aspergillosis.

PATHOPHYSIOLOGY

Chronic colonization of the airways of patients with air flow obstruction results in the development of IgE and precipitating antibodies to *Aspergillus* sp. An immunologic reaction takes place within the bronchial wall, producing granulomatous inflammation and mild invasion of the walls of the airway by fungus. Central airways are involved most often. This chronic inflammation will eventually lead to central bronchiectasis. Delayed clearance of secretions in the airway results in plugging of mucus and obstruction of the large airways, leading to pulmonary infiltrates.

CLINICAL ASPECTS

Allergic bronchopulmonary aspergillosis should be considered in any patient whose asthma is difficult to manage, any patient with asthma who has an abnormal result on chest radiography, and any cystic fibrosis patient with eosinophilia. Patients may present with acute symptoms of fever, pleuritic chest pain, malaise, and pulmonary infiltrates. Eosinophilia is often found. The presentation can be more subacute with prolonged pulmonary infiltrates and refractory bronchospasm. Many patients are asymptomatic despite the presence of pulmonary infiltration.

The most cost-effective screening test used to rule out allergic bronchopulmonary aspergillosis is the immediate skin test with *Aspergillus* antigen; a negative result effectively rules out allergic bronchopulmonary aspergillosis, while an immediate wheal-and-flare reaction warrants further testing, such as serum levels of IgE and precipitating antibody tests. Plain x-ray films of the chest demonstrating ring shadows and pulmonary densities representing impaction of mucus in dilated bronchi (gloved finger sign) can suggest central bronchiectasis. Bronchography is rarely indicated to demonstrate central bronchiectasis and carries some risk in these patients with reactive airway disease. Whole lung tomography or computed tomography may demonstrate the dilated central bronchi without risk to the patient.

MANAGEMENT

The only effective treatment for allergic bronchopulmonary aspergillosis has been corticosteroid agents, and prednisone is the drug of choice. The drug works by controlling the immunologic reaction, which occurs within airway walls. The goal of immediate therapy is to relieve bronchospasm and to open plugged airways by reducing the inflammatory reaction in the airway walls. Long-term therapy is usually indicated to prevent further development of bronchiectasis and progressive damage to the lung. Hospitalization is indicated only for treatment of severe bronchospasm.

Patients are initially treated with prednisone, 40 to 60 mg daily until they show clinical improvement and the pulmonary infiltrates clear, usually in one to two weeks. The medication is then slowly tapered by 5 mg/wk until a level of 15 mg/day is achieved. At this point, alternate-day therapy is instituted. Radiography of the chest and serum levels of IgE are monitored monthly for two to three months to ensure stability. Extremely high levels of IgE are associated with acute flare-ups of allergic bronchopulmonary aspergillosis. With effective therapy the level of IgE should return toward normal. In a patient with confirmed allergic bronchopulmonary aspergillosis, levels of IgE should be obtained periodically even when the patient is asymptomatic, as a rise in the level of IgE may be a forewarning of an impending acute exacerbation. Occasionally a patient will have good control of bronchospasms taking prednisone in a low dose, but continue to demonstrate activity of allergic bronchopulmonary aspergillosis by the presence of pulmonary infiltrates or by a persistently elevated IgE. In this event the dose of corticosteroid agents should be increased until the allergic bronchopulmonary aspergillosis is controlled despite the increased risk of side effects from the corticosteroids. Continued progress of the disease can result in end-stage pulmonary fibrosis. Inhaled corticosteroids do not control allergic bronchopulmonary aspergillosis, nor does local or systemic antifungal therapy.

Patients should be informed that they have a chronic allergic pulmonary condition that can result in persistent and progressive pulmonary disability if not effectively treated. They should also know that symptoms suggestive of acute pneumonia—fever, chills, cough, and purulent sputum—may well represent a flare of the allergic bronchopulmonary aspergillosis and not a pulmonary infectious process. All patients should be told of the potential ill effects of chronic use of corticosteroid agents, and methods to reduce these should be employed such as the use of vitamin D, calcium supplements, and measures to prevent weight gain and fluid retention.

This condition is also discussed in Section III, Chapter 2.

Invasive Pulmonary Aspergillosis

DEFINITION AND DIAGNOSTIC CRITERIA

This highly fatal pulmonary *Aspergillus* syndrome results from direct invasion of the lung parenchyma by *Aspergillus* organisms. It is often associated with dissemination to extrapulmonary sites such as the brain, heart, bone marrow, and liver. This condition usually occurs in patients with well-defined immunocompromised states; e.g., patients receiving therapy for hematologic malignancies, taking immunosuppressive agents after renal transplantation, or taking corticosteroid agents. Therapy with corticosteroid agents and prolonged neutropenia have been implicated as the major risk factors for invasive aspergillosis. Occasionally, it has developed in patients with other *Aspergillus* syndromes such as allergic bronchopulmonary aspergillosis and mycetoma, without their being obviously immunocompromised. Invasive *Aspergillus* pneumonia has rarely developed in immunocompetent patients without obvious risk factors.

PATHOPHYSIOLOGY

Loss of cellular and immune pulmonary and systemic host defense mechanisms allows invasion of lung tissue by the *Aspergillus* organisms delivered to the lung in inhaled air, producing a necrotizing pneumonia. The organism has the propensity to grow in and around pulmonary blood vessels, and damage to these vessels may lead to distal pulmonary infarction. The organism is often spread to remote tissues by the bloodstream. Because most of these patients are immunocompromised, the development of antibodies to the organism is unpredictable. Detection of an *Aspergillus* antigen in the serum or in bronchoalveolar lavage fluid offers promise as a diagnostic tool, but this test is currently available only in a few research centers.

CLINICAL ASPECTS

The clinical presentation is varied, but a common scenario is that of unremitting fevers, pulmonary infiltrates, and lack of response to antibiotic therapy in a known immunocompromised patient. Patients may also present with pleuritic chest pain, fever, tachypnea, and pleural rub—all reminiscent of pulmonary embolism. Minor or massive hemoptysis may also be the presenting symptom. Radiographic findings are nonspecific, varying from diffuse interstitial infiltrates to a dense localized, round pneumonia resembling a pulmonary infarct. Cultures of sputum or bronchial washings are occasionally positive but cannot separate colonization from tissue invasion by the organism. However, positive results from culture should raise the index of suspicion and suggest further diagnostic evaluation. Transbronchial lung biopsy through a fiberoptic bronchoscope produces notoriously inaccurate results in this condition, and open lung biopsy is usually required for a definitive diagnosis. Detection of tissue invasion by the organism in a nonpulmonary site also establishes a diagnosis.

MANAGEMENT

Invasive *Aspergillus* pneumonia was initially considered to be a universally fatal condition. Some case reports have now demonstrated that therapy can be successful. The main determinant of success is early diagnosis. Intravenously administered amphotericin B (Fungizone) is the treatment of choice. Patients should be given the standard 1-mg test dose IV followed within six hours by the first therapeutic dose of amphotericin B, 10 mg in 500 ml of D5W given over two to four hours. Larger doses are given on subsequent days to achieve a maximal daily dose of 30 to 50 mg. The addition of flucytosine (Ancobon) may improve the outcome, but the potential bone marrow toxicity from this medication may contraindicate its use in patients with hematologic malignancies or bone marrow suppression from chemotherapy. Prognosis depends as much on the behavior of the underlying disease as on the invasive *Aspergillus* syndrome.

Patients are usually given a total dose of 1 to 2 gm of amphotericin B over several weeks. Patients who recover from the *Aspergillus* pneumonia may be left with chronic pulmonary cavitation, aspergilloma, or both at the site of the necrotizing pneumonia.

Preventive measures against the development of this condition are unavailable. Serial determination of serum antigen or antibody to *Aspergillus* and serial surveillance nasal swab cultures for the fungus may permit earlier diagnosis once an opportunistic infection has developed.

Aspergilloma

DEFINITION AND DIAGNOSTIC CRITERIA

Solid masses of the mycelial form of the *Aspergillus* fungus are prone to develop within the cavities of patients with long-standing cavitary lung disease of any cause (previous tuberculosis, remote fungal or necrotizing pneumonia, cystic lung disease, or long-standing sarcoidosis). This is called a mycetoma or an *Aspergillus* fungus ball. These usually occur within cavities in the upper lobes of the lung and are described as spherical masses within a cavity often surrounded by a rim of free air, i.e., the crescent sign.

PATHOPHYSIOLOGY

The delayed clearance of bronchopulmonary secretions from any chronic cavity permits the residence of the *Aspergillus* fungus. The mycelial form of the organism multiplies and forms a large conglomerate mass of fungus. In surgical or autopsy specimens, organisms may be seen within the wall of the cavity, but no further tissue is invaded. Because of chronic inflammation, the wall of the cavity often develops squamous metaplasia and granulation tissue, which is friable and can lead to frequent hemoptysis. Massive hemoptysis is usually the result of bleeding from a bronchial artery supplying the wall of the cavity.

CLINICAL ASPECTS

Patients may present with hemoptysis, usually mild but occasionally massive. Many patients are asymptomatic until a mass lesion is found within an old cavity on routine chest films. Tomography may be helpful to define the intracavitary location of the mass. Movement of the fungus ball within the cavity on decubitus films confirms the diagnosis of an intracavitary mass. Culture of sputum or bronchial washings frequently grows *Aspergillus* sp. Precipitating antibodies to the *Aspergillus* fungus are almost always present in high titers. Some patients have systemic symptoms such as fever, malaise, and weight loss.

MANAGEMENT

Treatment of aspergilloma remains controversial and must be individualized, taking into account the overall pulmonary status and the severity of symptoms. Patients who are asymptomatic or who have minimal hemoptysis should be observed. Mild hemoptysis, especially when accompanied by purulent sputum, may clear with a brief course of broad-spectrum antibiotics, as in the treatment of bacterial bronchitis (ampicillin, 500 mg four times a day; tetracycline, 500 mg four times a day; or trimethoprim-sulfa, two tablets twice a day for 10 to 14 days). Mild persistent hemoptysis occasionally responds to a brief course of prednisone, such as 20 mg/day for 10 to 14 days. This seems to reduce some of the inflammation within the cavity wall. With this conservative approach, the aspergilloma may resolve spontaneously in up to 30% of patients.

Patients with massive hemoptysis should be hospitalized and undergo fiberoptic bronchoscopy to localize the site of bleeding. Surgical resection of the cavity and fungus ball should then be considered. Frequently these individuals have such severe diffuse fibrotic or cystic lung disease that they may not be surgical candidates owing to poor pulmonary function. In this event, bronchial arteriography and embolization occlusion therapy for the bleeding vessel could be considered. This technique requires considerable expertise on the part of the angiographer and may not be readily available in most hospitals. The prognosis for patients with massive hemoptysis who cannot be treated with surgical resection is poor.

Chronic Necrotizing Pulmonary Aspergillosis

DEFINITION AND DIAGNOSTIC CRITERIA

The most recently described pulmonary *Aspergillus* syndrome has been termed chronic necrotizing pulmonary aspergillosis or semi-invasive aspergillosis. In this condition, pulmonary cavitation, limited tissue invasion, and mycetoma develop over a matter of weeks in a previously normal area of the lung.

PATHOPHYSIOLOGY

This condition usually occurs in patients with mild defects in systemic or pulmonary defense mechanisms, which predispose them to a chronic low-grade pulmonary infection with *Aspergillus*. Certain conditions, such as diabetes mellitus, chronic obstructive pulmonary disease, radiation fibrosis, sarcoidosis, and malnutrition, have been considered risk factors for chronic necrotizing pulmonary aspergillosis.

CLINICAL ASPECTS

Patients are usually found to have a pneumonic pulmonary infiltrate. Over a period of days to weeks cavitation develops within the infiltrate, and a mycetoma may develop within the cavity. Usually there is a long history of cough, production of sputum, weight loss, and low-grade fever. In patients who have been treated with surgical resection for this condition, the fungus has been seen within the wall of the cavity and to a mild degree within the surrounding lung parenchyma, indicating tissue invasion. The organism does not disseminate systemically.

MANAGEMENT

Chronic necrotizing pulmonary aspergillosis is difficult to treat. Systemically administered amphotericin B has proved successful in several reported cases. It is also evident that it is most important to drain the cavity. Amphotericin B frequently does not sterilize the cavity, and a chronic external drainage procedure is required either by a closed thoracostomy tube or by open drainage with a limited rib resection. Secondary infections with bacteria should be treated with antibiotics appropriate for the culture and sensitivities.

The long-term prognosis is unknown. Patients often are chronically disabled with cough and sputum production, and are malnourished.

Blastomycosis

DEFINITION AND DIAGNOSTIC CRITERIA

Blastomycosis is a pulmonary infection caused by the inhalation of the fungus *B. dermatitidis*. This may appear as an acute pneumonia, or pulmonary manifestations may be entirely asymptomatic and be recognized only when a patient presents with evidence of extrapulmonary dissemination. Diagnosis of blastomycosis is established by culturing the organism from sputum, bronchial washings, or biopsied tissue. The characteristic yeast form of the organism can be demonstrated by smears of sputum using potassium hydroxide, by sputum cytologic samples prepared by Papanicolaou's technique, or by periodic acid–Schiff staining of fixed tissue.

PATHOPHYSIOLOGY

Our knowledge of the epidemiology of this disease has many gaps. Blastomycosis is confined to the North American continent, most infections occurring in the southwest or midwestern states, especially Minnesota and Wisconsin. Culture of the organism from soil has been difficult. One study associated the fungus with bird droppings. Dogs are particularly susceptible to pulmonary infection with *B. dermatitidis*.

CLINICAL ASPECTS

Patients may present with acute symptomatic pneumonia manifesting as cough, high fever, and myalgias. At times the presentation may be more subacute with cough, hemoptysis, and weight loss being the most frequent symptoms. Another group of patients presents with extrathoracic dissemination (e.g., osteomyelitis, skin papules, or ulcers), an asymptomatic pulmonary infiltrate being noted on chest radiography.

The chest radiographic findings in pulmonary blastomycosis are nonspecific and range from localized consolidation to a patchy, diffuse, alveolar filling process. As in other fungal pneumonias, hilar adenopathy may be seen; cavitation seems less common. Pleural effusions may be present. Skin tests and complement fixation and immunodiffusion serologic tests are available but usually do not help to establish a diagnosis or predict the prognosis. Demonstration of the fungus in sputum or tissue by culture or smear is required to establish a definite diagnosis. Occasionally, small epidemics of blastomycosis occur. The diagnosis of blastomycosis in a dog often helps explain a respiratory illness in its owner.

MANAGEMENT

Intravenously administered amphotericin B is the treatment of choice for blastomycosis. All patients with disseminated disease and most of those with progressive or chronic blastomycosis (longer than three weeks of illness) should receive therapy. Usually a total dose of amphotericin B, 2 gm, is given over a number of weeks. Many people can be treated as outpatients.

Some patients with pulmonary blastomycosis are now recognized to have an acute self-limited pneumonia requiring no therapy. Patients who show evidence of improvement at the time of diagnosis or within two weeks of illness should be observed closely. Serial chest radiographs and erythrocyte sedimentation rates (ESR) should be obtained monthly for three months, and then every three months for the first year to confirm continued resolution.

Extrathoracic recurrence has been described years after the initial infection. Patients should be advised to have any new cutaneous ulceration or soft tissue swelling examined carefully by a physician. Immunosuppression in the future from cytotoxic therapy or treatment with corticosteroid agents may lead to recurrence or dissemination of a previously well-healed infection.

Coccidioidomycosis

DEFINITION AND DIAGNOSTIC CRITERIA

Both pulmonary and disseminated forms of coccidioidomycosis result from the inhalation of the arthrospore form of the dimorphic fungus *Coccidioides immitis*. Diagnosis is established by culturing the organism from sputum or tissue or by demonstrating the characteristic spherule form of the fungus within human tissue. In the appropriate clinical setting, a fourfold rise in the coccidioidal complement fixation titer or conversion of the coccidioidin skin test from negative to positive can be considered diagnostic.

PATHOPHYSIOLOGY

The fungus resides in the soil of the Lower Sonoran Life Zone, which is noted for its semi-arid climate and short, intense rainy season. These areas include much of the southwestern United States, certain areas of northern Mexico, and several South and Central American countries. In soil, the organism is seen in its mycelial form; in human tissue, the spherule form of the fungus is demonstrated.

Unlike other common fungal diseases, laboratory evaluation of coccidioidomycosis is helpful in establishing diagnosis and predicting prognosis. The intradermal coccidioidin or spherulin skin tests usually turn positive within three to four weeks after acute infection. Conversion of the skin test from negative to positive in the setting of an acute respiratory illness is diagnostic of a recent coccidioidal infection. A positive skin test in an individual from an endemic area indicates either a past or present infection. Skin testing does not alter serologic titers.

Serologic studies for coccidioidomycosis are also helpful for diagnosis and prognosis, although in nonendemic areas they may be available only from reference laboratories. The latex particle agglutination test measures IgM antibodies, which develop within four weeks of acute infection and disappear by 12 weeks; thus, a positive result on this test is usually diagnostic of an acute coccidioidomycosis infection. Specific IgG antibodies are measured by the quantitative complement fixation or agar-gel immunodiffusion assays. The complement fixation test may not show positive results for six to eight weeks after infection, but findings remain positive for from months to years. A complement fixation titer of 1:16 dilution or less usually indicates a well-controlled infection, while a titer of 1:32 or greater often accompanies progression of the initial infection, development of chronic pulmonary coccidioidomycosis, or extrapulmonary dissemination. When therapy is effective, the complement fixation titer will return to low levels.

CLINICAL ASPECTS

Several pulmonary coccidioidal syndromes exist. The initial pulmonary reaction resulting from inhalation of *C. immitis* spores is termed primary pulmonary coccidioidomycosis and is asymptomatic in more than 60% of patients. The asymptomatic infection is evidenced only by a positive skin test during epidemiologic studies or radiographic findings of previous granulomatous disease. The 40% of patients who become symptomatic usually present with typical symptoms of acute pneumonia—cough, fever, malaise, and pleuritic chest pain. In 10% to 20% of patients, erythema nodosum, erythema multiforme, and polyserositis are present (acute valley fever). Routine laboratory studies are usually nonspecific but often demonstrate eosinophilia and elevated ESR. Chest radiography shows a patchy segmental infiltration, which may be single or multiple, and occasionally is fleeting. Either unilateral or bilateral hilar adenopathy is a hallmark of acute coccidioidomycosis. Acute cavitation and pleural effusion can occur but are uncommon.

Most primary coccidioidal pneumonias resolve clinically and radiographically within six to eight weeks. Occasionally patients are persistently fatigued, but as long as the complement fixation titer remains below 1:32 and skin reactivity is maintained, no therapy is indicated. Although primary pulmonary coccidioidomycosis has no racial predilection, Filipinos and blacks are at higher risk of developing extrapulmonary dissemination from the acute infection. During the acute pneumonia, these patients should be observed carefully for signs of dissemination to skin, meninges, bone, or liver. A complement fixation titer that continues to rise or remains persistently elevated is a poor prognostic sign even without obvious evidence of dissemination.

Although most patients with acute coccidioidomycosis either never realize their illness or improve spontaneously, progressive coccidioidal pneumonia, which carries with it a high mortality, occasionally develops. This syndrome is manifested by persistent fever, prostration, copious sputum production, and radiographic progression of the pneumonia often associated with cavity formation. Patients usually have some defect in systemic or pulmonary immune defenses, such as diabetes mellitus, or underlying malignancy.

Miliary pulmonary coccidioidomycosis is a highly fatal acute coccidioidal syndrome. This infection results from diffuse hematogenous spread of fungus throughout the lung, often with extensive extrapulmonary dissemination.

Chronic pulmonary coccidioidomycosis is an indolent pulmonary infection produced by *C. immitis*. This condition occasionally follows an episode of primary coccidioidal pneumonia, but more often the initial infection cannot be dated. Chronic pulmonary coccidioidomycosis resembles chronic pulmonary tuberculosis in that biapical fibronodular lesions and multiple cavities with retraction and surrounding infiltration are the most common radiographic findings. Sputum and bronchial washings are almost always positive for *C. immitis*, and the complement fixation titer is usually elevated.

The two most common forms of remote pulmonary coccidioidomycosis are the coccidioidoma and the coccidioidal cavity. In endemic areas, single nodular parenchymal lesions resulting from previous primary coccidioidal pneumonia, a coccidioidoma, make up a large percentage of resected solitary pulmonary nodules, i.e., coin lesions. Unlike solitary nodules from remote tuberculosis or histoplasmosis, coccidioidomas rarely calcify, which makes their differentiation from cancer difficult without benefit of thoracotomy. Late coccidioidal cavities are classically thin-walled and may represent the shelling out of a granulomatous nodule. Most patients, although asymptomatic, have positive sputum cultures for *C. immitis*. These cavities are usually small, less than 4 cm, and most resolve spontaneously within two years. Complications of coccidioidal cavities include hemoptysis, pneumothorax, bronchopleural fistula, and secondary infection with the development of a mycetoma from *Aspergillus* sp.

MANAGEMENT

More than 95% of primary coccidioidal pneumonias resolve clinically and radiographically within six to eight weeks without therapy. General supportive measures, such as rest, adequate fluids and nutrition, and aspirin or acetaminophen for fever, are recommended. Most people with acute coccidioidomycosis can be managed as outpatients. Hospitalization is indicated if dehydration, severe toxicity, or signs of respiratory insufficiency are present. Results of the skin test are initially negative; tests should be repeated at weekly intervals to demonstrate conversion. A complement fixation titer should also be repeated at weekly intervals until evidence proves that it has peaked and returned to levels below 1:32. Once improvement has taken place, the complement fixation titer should be repeated every three months for the next year.

Patients in high-risk groups, e.g., blacks, Filipinos, diabetics, or individuals with immune deficiencies, should be observed closely for evidence of dissemination. Even when disease is limited to the thorax and is resolving, some patients tend to have prolonged malaise and may complain of fatigue for months. When the complement fixation titer remains above 1:64, evaluation for systemic dissemination should be carried out. This includes a lumbar puncture and measurement of the complement fixation titer in CSF, a technetium 99m bone scan, and a total body gallium-67 nucleotide scan.

The persistence of a high complement fixation titer without obvious dissemination would be an indication to treat a high-risk patient who has primary coccidioidomycosis. Other indications for treatment of primary coccidioidal pneumonia include coexistent diabetes mellitus, concurrent therapy with immunosuppressive agents, and the development of primary coccidioidomycosis in the third trimester of pregnancy. Amphotericin B remains the agent of choice for these infections: usually a total of 2 gm given in 50-mg increments three times per week controls the disease, in contrast to disseminated coccidioidomycosis, which usually requires more than 2 gm of amphotericin B. Ketoconazole (Nizoral) has been used to treat acute coccidioidomycosis, but the exact indications for this drug have yet to be defined. Ketoconazole offers the advantages of oral administration and produces minimal toxicity compared with amphotericin B. In patients with disseminated disease, however, the drug is unable to eradicate the organism, and the disease often flares when the drug is discontinued. At present, amphotericin B is preferred; ketoconazole should be saved for patients who demonstrate toxicity to the first-line drug.

Patients with progressive coccidioidal pneumonia and miliary pulmonary coccidioidomycosis should be admitted to the hospital for IV administration of amphotericin B. They may have extreme toxicity, and respiratory failure occasionally may develop. Amphotericin B should be given daily until toxicity has improved; once clinical improvement occurs, the drug may be given three times per week to reduce toxicity.

Amphotericin B is also the treatment of choice for chronic pulmonary coccidioidomycosis. However, many patients with this condition may be asymptomatic, have stable pulmonary infiltrates, and not need treatment. If symptoms are severe or progression of disease is seen radiographically, therapy is indicated. Amphotericin B, totaling about 30 mg/kg, usually produces radiographic evidence of improvement and eradication of *C. immitis* from the sputum. In one large study using ketoconazole, 400 mg/day for up to 18 months, subjective symptoms improved, but this drug failed to change findings in the sputum, alter serologic titers, or produce appreciable radiographic evidence of improvement. Again, ketoconazole should be reserved for the patient in whom toxicity to amphotericin B develops.

When a coccidioidal pneumonia resolves into a small pulmonary nodule, the diagnosis of coccidioidoma can easily be made and the patient observed. Most coccidioidal nodules, however, are found without a previous history of pneumonia, and if noncalcified they must be removed surgically to rule out cancer. Coccidioidal cavities less than 4 cm in diameter should be observed because they usually resolve spontaneously. Large cavities, especially if subpleural, should be considered for surgical resection, as the chance for rupture is high.

Cryptococcosis

DEFINITION AND DIAGNOSTIC CRITERIA

Cryptococcosis is a pulmonary infection produced by the fungus *Cryptococcus neoformans*. The diagnosis of pulmonary cryptococcosis requires cultures or fungal stains to demonstrate that the fungus has invaded lung tissue.

PATHOPHYSIOLOGY

C. neoformans enters the body by inhalation. This fungus, an encapsulated yeast distributed widely in nature, is usually associated with soil containing pigeon droppings. Alterations in host defenses result in pulmonary infection or systemic dissemination by the fungus.

CLINICAL ASPECTS

Although cryptococcal meningitis is the most common disease produced by *C. neoformans*, three forms of cryptococcosis are limited to the respiratory system. In the immunocompromised host, pulmonary cryptococcosis is a major risk factor for dissemination to the central nervous system or other extrathoracic sites, such as skin, bone marrow, or the genitourinary tract. The immunocompetent host seems to be able to limit this infection to the lung and often requires no treatment.

Simple colonization of the airways by the organism is the most benign of the three pulmonary cryptococcal syndromes. A sputum culture positive for *C. neoformans* is occasionally found in patients with normal results on chest radiography or whose chest films show abnormal findings because of other pulmonary conditions such as lung cancer.

A second form of pulmonary cryptococcosis presents as a well-defined pulmonary mass lesion 2 to 5 cm in diameter. Biopsy reveals a glistening, gelatinous ball sharply delineated from surrounding lung tissue. This fungus ball is composed of a uniform collection of *C. neoformans* organisms without surrounding inflammation. The lesion is often completely resected at the time of open biopsy and no further therapy is needed. A thorough search for common sites of extrapulmonary dissemination should be performed in the immunocompromised patient.

The third or pneumonic type of pulmonary cryptococcosis presents with nonspecific respiratory complaints. Radiographic findings are those of segmental consolidation, poorly defined masses, and irregular masslike infiltrates. The organism is seen on biopsy to be surrounded by granulomatous inflammation. Hilar adenopathy, cavitation, and pleural effusion can occur. The diagnosis of cryptococcal pneumonitis requires either open or transbronchial lung biopsy or transthoracic needle aspiration for confirmation. A positive result on sputum culture and compatible findings on chest radiography are only presumptive evidence of cryptococcal pneumonitis, especially in an immunosuppressed host.

Serologic measurement of cryptococcal antigen and cryptococcal antibodies can be helpful in establishing the diagnosis but not in determining the prognosis.

MANAGEMENT

The patient with normal findings on chest film, no evidence of extrathoracic dissemination, and positive results on sputum culture for *C. neoformans* should be observed. Patients with *C. neoformans* in the sputum and apparent noncryptococcal abnormalities seen on chest films need not be treated for cryptococcosis unless the organism is seen within biopsied lung tissue or cultured from some extrapulmonary site.

The pneumonic form of pulmonary cryptococcosis resolves without therapy in most immunocompetent patients. Therapy is indicated when chest radiographs show progression of the infection during a period of observation or when the patient remains symptomatic. Symptoms usually include malaise, fatigue, and low-grade fever.

When the decision to treat pulmonary cryptococcosis is made, amphotericin B and flucytosine in combination should be given. The addition of flucytosine enables amphotericin B to be used in a lower daily and total dose with resulting lower toxicity. Usually the maximal daily dose of amphotericin B is 20 to 30 mg. Flucytosine should not be taken alone because it causes rapid development of resistant organisms. Amphotericin B can be prescribed singly when the patient is sensitive to flucytosine. Duration of the combination therapy should be four to six weeks, determined by clinical response. Any immunocompromised patient in whom pulmonary cryptococcosis develops should be treated immediately, because the incidence of dissemination is high.

Histoplasmosis

DEFINITION AND DIAGNOSTIC CRITERIA

Inhalation of spores of the fungus *Histoplasma capsulatum* results in the pulmonary infection known as histoplasmosis. Several syndromes have been described (Table 2). Acute pulmonary histoplasmosis, a pneumonic illness, develops 10 to 15 days after inhalation of the fungus. This is usually a benign, self-limited illness but it can lead to extrapulmonary dissemination in the susceptible host. Chronic pulmonary histoplasmosis is a low-grade chronic pulmonary infection produced by *H. capsulatum* in patients with bullous emphysema. Past (remote) histoplasmosis is usually an asymptomatic condition.

The diagnosis of acute pulmonary histoplasmosis requires the clinical picture of acute pneumonia along with a history of exposure to the fungus, a fourfold rise in the histoplasmosis complement fixation titer, or a titer of greater than 1:32 dilutions. Unlike acute pulmonary histoplasmosis in which the organism is rarely cultured, the diagnosis of chronic pulmonary histoplasmosis requires culturing of the organism from sputum

Table 2. CLASSIFICATION OF HISTOPLASMOSIS

Histoplasmosis in normal hosts (acute pulmonary histoplasmosis)
   Usual asymptomatic infection
   Occasional symptomatic infection
   Rare complications
     Pericarditis
     Mediastinal granuloma
     Mediastinal fibrosis
     Histoplasmomas
Opportunistic infections
   Disseminated histoplasmosis (immune defect)
   Chronic pulmonary histoplasmosis (structural defect)

From Goodwin RA, Lloyd JE, Des Prez RM: Histoplasmosis in normal hosts. Medicine 60:231–266, 1981. © 1981, The Williams & Wilkins Company, Baltimore.

on multiple occasions along with evidence of progressive pulmonary infiltration in a patient with bullous disease. Remote histoplasmosis is usually a diagnosis established in an asymptomatic patient. It presents with one of many radiographic patterns of previous granulomatous lung disease and a history of travel to or residence in an endemic area.

PATHOPHYSIOLOGY

H. capsulatum, a dimorphic fungus, is highly endemic in the central United States and in some Central and South American countries. The mycelial form resides in the soil and grows best in soil fertilized with bird droppings. Within living tissue, the organism is found in the yeast stage.

The organism is inhaled into the alveoli and small airways of the lung, where it is phagocytized by pulmonary macrophages. More macrophages and lymphocytes are brought to the area, resulting in a zone of inflammatory cells, which eventually is recognized radiographically as a pulmonary infiltrate. Delayed hypersensitivity develops in approximately two weeks and produces further inflammatory reaction in the lung parenchyma and in the regional lymph nodes, which may also contain organisms. As the lesion enlarges, areas of necrosis develop, and healing gradually occurs. The necrotic areas become walled off by fibrous tissue and eventually calcify. Repeated exposure to the fungus (reinfection) results in a more rapid and exuberant inflammatory reaction as the host's previous immunity leads to a greater mobilization of sensitized lymphocytes and macrophages. Extrapulmonary dissemination of histoplasmosis usually occurs in immunocompromised patients. Patients with AIDS have recently been found to be at high risk for dissemination.

CLINICAL ASPECTS

The majority (more than 90%) of patients with histoplasmosis infections have no referable symptoms. Patients symptomatic from acute pulmonary histoplasmosis have had a moderate to heavy exposure to the organism or have been sensitized by past exposures. Epidemics of acute symptomatic histoplasmosis have been linked to exposures, such as cleaning a chicken coop, archaeologic digging, bulldozing a bird or a bat roost, urban excavating, or chopping decayed wood. Headaches and fever are the most common features of acute symptomatic histoplasmosis, followed by cough, chills, and substernal chest pain. Erythema nodosum can also occur. Chest radiography shows a patchy infiltrate with hilar adenopathy. Very heavy exposures are associated with diffuse patchy infiltrates, which at times resemble a miliary pattern, or the diffuse ground-glass pattern commonly seen with the adult respiratory distress syndrome. The WBC count is normal or mildly elevated and the ESR is usually increased. A skin test for histoplasmosis is not helpful for diagnosis of an acute infection, but serial skin tests may demonstrate conversion in a patient with an initial negative result. A histoplasmin complement fixation titer of 1:32 or more or a fourfold rise in the titer confirms the diagnosis in the appropriate clinical setting.

Chronic pulmonary histoplasmosis occurs almost exclusively in patients with underlying emphysematous changes. In this condition, the large air spaces produced by centrilobular or panacinar emphysema become infected with *H. capsulatum*. Male sex, age over 40 years, and immune deficiency are other risk factors. Findings on chest radiographs mimic pulmonary tuberculosis, cavitation and infiltration in the upper lobes of the lungs being the most common findings. Complement fixation titers are usually positive. Diagnosis is made by sputum culture or culture of bronchial washings. Symptoms are nonspecific, cough and weight loss being common.

Remote histoplasmosis presents with a variety of radiographic findings of old pulmonary granulomatous disease. Patients are usually asymptomatic and most often cannot date the primary infection. The fungus is presumed to be dead or dormant and walled off within healed granulomas. Although not totally distinguishable from the granulomatous changes of tuberculosis, the calcified granulomas of histoplasmosis have certain radiographic characteristics, in that they tend to be multiple, small (2 to 3 mm), and heavily calcified. Within the granuloma the calcifications may be central, scattered, circumferential, or lamellar. The hilar calcifications in remote histoplasmosis are larger than those seen in tuberculosis and may be 1 to 2 cm in size. Splenic calcifications may also be seen radiographically. Because some patients may lose skin reactivity unless repeatedly reinfected, skin tests for histoplasmin may reveal either positive or negative findings in previous granulomatous disease. Results of complement fixation serologic testing are usually negative in remote histoplasmosis.

Complications of remote histoplasmosis include broncholithiasis, which occurs when calcified peribronchial lymph nodes erode into and through a bronchial wall. This condition may cause hemoptysis, large airway obstruction and lithoptysis (spitting of calculi). Mediastinal fibrosis, a rare but potentially fatal complication, is stimulated by chronic inflammation surrounding mediastinal lymph nodes infected with *H. capsulatum*. Any of the mediastinal structures may be incorporated within the fibrosis. Patients may present with large airway obstruction, superior vena caval syndrome, or underperfusion of a lung from obstruction of a pulmonary artery or pulmonary vein.

MANAGEMENT

Acute symptomatic pulmonary histoplasmosis in a healthy individual usually requires no therapy. Symptoms should resolve in one to two weeks except for a feeling of fatigue, which may be prolonged. Chest radiographs should be obtained weekly for comparison until definite improvement is seen. A lowering of the ESR is a promising sign. Patients should be encouraged to rest and not return to work until the infiltrate and the fatigue have almost completely cleared; relapse may occur if they return prematurely to their usual activities.

Patients who are immune deficient from other diseases or therapies and patients with symptomatic illness of more than three weeks' duration should be considered for treatment of acute pulmonary histoplasmosis. Some experts have advocated a short course of amphotericin B, a total dose of 500 mg over a period of several weeks. However, a total dose of 1 gm is more appropriate for most patients. This can usually be accomplished by giving 30 to 50 mg/day three times a week on an outpatient basis for those who are not acutely ill. Patients (1) with diabetes, (2) with hematologic malignancies, (3) receiving chemotherapy or immunosuppressive therapy after transplantation, and (4) with AIDS should be considered for treatment of acute pulmonary histoplasmosis. The role of ketoconazole in therapy for acute histoplasmosis is undefined. This orally administered agent has been shown to be effective in anecdotal cases and, as in acute pulmonary coccidioidomycosis, can be given when amphotericin B cannot be tolerated.

The course of chronic pulmonary histoplasmosis is uncertain and may depend as much on the underlying bullous disease as on the histoplasmosis infection. Up to 30% of patients improve spontaneously. Thus, those who are stable or clinically improving should be observed. A three-month period of observation and rest are probably warranted in every patient in whom this condition is diagnosed, as long as systemic symptoms are not severe. Amphotericin B is the standard treatment for chronic pulmonary histoplasmosis. Again, the role of ketoconazole in treatment of this condition is undefined: 200 to 400 mg/day might be indicated during the period of observation.

Patients with symptomatic broncholithiasis should be considered for surgical resection of the involved area when the calcification is localized in an airway that can be resected without removing a critical mass of functioning lung. Bleeding from broncholithiasis, as in other hemoptysis syndromes, often stops with bed rest, and suppression of cough with codeine, 30 mg every four to six hours. Patients presenting with more than 100 ml of hemoptysis are best treated in the hospital. The hemoptysis occasionally responds to antibiotics, such as ampicillin, tetracycline, and trimethoprim-sulfa because this condition is often associated with bronchitis. Prednisone, 20 mg/day for 10 to 14 days, may reduce some of the inflammation surrounding the broncholith, with a corresponding reduction in bleeding.

No specific treatment exists for mediastinal fibrosis from past histoplasmosis. Patients should be informed that they have a chronic, slowly progressive condition that may produce serious untreatable symptoms if the trachea or one of the great vessels becomes obstructed. Surgical bypass of the blocked superior vena cava has occasionally been successful. The progressive fibrosis does not respond to therapy with corticosteroid agents.

Patients with pulmonary granulomas from remote histoplasmosis require no therapy. Tuberculin skin tests are performed to rule out tuberculosis as the cause of the granulomas. Occasionally, a solitary granuloma, the histoplasmoma, may be confused with lung cancer if calcium is not present within the lesion. Fortunately, most histoplasmomas are calcified and often show the characteristic pattern of central or lamellar calcifications. Some histoplasmomas may grow in size, which further confuses the diagnosis. When the growth is asymmetric or if tomography demonstrates asymmetric calcification within the granuloma, cancer cannot be ruled out and surgical resection should be recommended.

REFERENCES

Drutz DJ, Catanzaro A: Coccidioidomycosis: Parts I and II. Am Rev Respir Dis 117:559–585, 727–771, 1978.
Goodwin RA Jr, Des Prez RM: Histoplasmosis. Am Rev Respir Dis 117:929–956, 1978.
Goodwin RA, Lloyd JE, Des Prez RM: Histoplasmosis in normal hosts. Medicine 60:231–266, 1981.
Pennington JE: Aspergillus lung disease. Med Clin North Am 64:475–490, 1980.
Sarosi GA, Davies SF: Blastomycosis. Am Rev Respir Dis 120:911–938, 1979.

5 · PLEURAL EFFUSION

Robert Lenox
GUTHRIE CLINIC

DEFINITION

A pleural effusion is a collection of fluid in the pleural space detectable by clinical or roentgenographic means. Fluid accumulation occurs when the dynamic balance between the hydrostatic pressures pushing fluid out of the circulatory system and oncotic pressure pulling fluid back into blood vessels is upset. Factors that increase hydrostatic pressure or decrease oncotic pressure, as well as blockage of lymphatics or inflammation of the pleural space, all lead to fluid accumulation.

CLINICAL ASPECTS

Patients with effusions present with symptoms of the underlying disease, or with complaints of dyspnea or a feeling of fullness in the chest. In most instances, stimulation of mechanical receptors is thought to be the cause of dyspnea. On examination the findings are dullness to percussion, decreased tactile and vocal fremitus, and decreased or absent breath sounds. Effusion with less than 200 to 300 cc of fluid may have no abnormal physical findings.

Findings on chest x-ray vary. Increased density within the chest and a meniscus sign are usually present. With a small or subpulmonic effusion the costophrenic angle will be blunted. In reviewing lateral chest roentgenograms, identification of both diaphragms is helpful. Inability to see both diaphragms indicates lung consolidation or pleural disease. Effusions can be separated from massive atelectasis by looking for mediastinal shifts away from effusions or toward the side with massive atelectasis. A lateral decubitus view with the involved side down is the standard means of confirming free fluid within the pleural space. Ultrasound can help differentiate loculated fluid from pleural fibrosis.

DIAGNOSTIC CRITERIA

The discovery of a pleural effusion requires a systematic approach. Looking at the whole patient may provide all the information needed to both diagnose and treat (e.g., in a case of congestive heart failure). Likewise, risk-benefit ratios are important. An abortive tap of a minuscule effusion may harm the patient. Tapping a very small effusion increases the risk of pulmonary, hepatic, or splenic laceration. Care should be taken in doing the tap: enter over the top of the rib one interspace below the physical findings. Nevertheless, a thoracentesis can provide a safe means to obtain material leading to correct diagnosis and treatment.

Closed pleural biopsy, using either the Abrams or Cope needle, can provide useful information. This closed procedure is safest when there is ample fluid, and should be considered before the space is tapped dry. It is most useful in diagnosing tuberculosis effusion (65% diagnostic). Carcinoma can be proved by closed needle biopsy, but this is not as sensitive as cytologic examination. Closed pleural biopsy is a relatively safe procedure with only a 4% complication rate.

Pleuroscopy or visualization of the pleural space by an appropriate flexible endoscopy while the involved lung is collapsed is sometimes helpful. Adequate visualization is possible only when there are no pleural adhesions and it is used mainly to exclude malignancy.

Open pleural biopsy has been done less often in recent years. Unless there is a strong possibility of mesothelioma or other malignancy, open biopsy often adds little to less invasive procedures (and most idiopathic pleural effusions have a benign outcome). However, open pleural biopsy is appropriate in the presence of progressive pleural disease of unknown etiology.

In reaching a correct diagnosis a review of the differential diagnosis is essential (Table 1). A useful practice is to separate the fluid into a transudate or an exudate. This can be done by comparing pleural LDH and protein with that found in blood serum. Three factors are useful: an effusion protein-to-serum-protein ratio greater than 0.5; effusion LDH-to-serum-LDH greater than 0.6; and LDH greater than 250 milliunits/ml. If two of these factors are found, there is a 90% chance of the effusion being an exudate.

Historical and physical findings aid interpretation. Exposure to asbestosis raises the possibility of mesothelioma as well as bronchogenic carcinoma. A history of tobacco abuse with findings of clubbing or a localized wheeze suggests bronchogenic carcinoma. A septic patient suggests infection or other inflammatory processes.

Laboratory studies done on fluid contribute to a correct diagnosis. Pleural fluid cytology positive for malignancy is diagnostic. A low glucose level is seen in rheumatoid arthritis, bacterial and tuberculous infections, and cancer. An elevated amylase level raises the possibility of pancreatic disease or esophageal rupture. A positive culture or stain is also diagnostic. Nevertheless, most diagnoses are reached by interpreting the data in light of the clinical setting.

Table 1. CAUSES OF PLEURAL EFFUSIONS

Transudates
  Cardiovascular
    Congestive heart failure
    Constrictive pericarditis
    Superior vena cava obstruction
  Low oncotic pressure
    Cirrhosis with ascites
    Malabsorption
    Nephrotic syndrome
    Peritoneal dialysis
Exudates
  Neoplasm
    Bronchogenic carcinoma
    Metastatic carcinoma
    Mesothelioma
    Intra-abdominal tumors (Meigs' syndrome)
    Lymphomas
    Chest-wall neoplasms
  Infections
    Bacterial empyema
    Parapneumonic
    Tuberculosis
    Fungi
    Parasites
    Viruses and mycoplasma
    Legionella, Chlamydia, Rickettsia
  Collagen vascular disease
    Lupus erythematosus
    Rheumatoid arthritis
  Trauma
    Hemothorax
    Chylothorax
    Esophageal rupture
  Intra-abdominal disorders
    Pancreatitis
    Subphrenic hepatic and splenic abscesses
  Drugs
    Drug-induced lupus erythematosus
    Nitrofurantoin
    Methylsergide
  Other causes
    Pulmonary embolism
    Myxedema
    Familial Mediterranean fever
    Post myocardial infarction

MANAGEMENT

Treatment of pleural effusions depends on the underlying cause. If the cause is removed, the effusion will resolve. There are instances when this cannot be done and when the patient will benefit from manipulation within the pleural space.

Hemothorax refers to frank bleeding within the pleural space. It occurs spontaneously in rare cases associated with hematologic disorders, but most commonly is associated with trauma. If the pleural effusion is small, thoracentesis and careful observation may be adequate, but most cases require thoracostomy tube drainage. Large tubes to ensure adequate drainage are recommended. If brisk bleeding continues, thoracotomy is warranted. In the presence of a left-sided hemothorax, rupture of the aorta should be considered, since a ruptured aorta requires immediate surgery.

Malignant pleural effusions cannot be cured. Significant palliation can be obtained by pleurodesis. Before proceeding with pleurodesis, the effusion should be symptomatic and a pattern of reaccumulation requiring repeated thoracenteses should be established. The lung must also fully expand following removal of fluid. A thick protein pleural coating can prevent reexpansion, and unless the clinical situation warrants thoracotomy with removal of this coating, there is no possible way to achieve pleurodesis.

The most successful nonoperative methods of pleurodesis combine thoracostomy tube drainage with the installation of a sclerosing agent. Agents used for sclerosis include tetracycline, bleomycin, nitrogen mustard, talc, and radioisotopes of gold, phosphorus, and yttrium. The technique of installation is as important as the agent used. There has been more clinical experience with tetracycline than with other agents. A thoracostomy tube should be inserted and all pleural fluid drained. The patient should be premedicated with narcotic analgesics. If tetracycline is used, 15 mg/kg of ideal body weight or 500 mg has been advocated. The tube is clamped and the patient is rotated for the next hour to ensure contact of the sclerosing agent with all pleural surfaces. The tube is then unclamped until drainage is less than 250 cc in 24 hours. A success rate of about 80% to 85% can be achieved with this method.

Another condition that requires drainage of the pleural space is empyema, which literally means pus in the pleural space but has grown to connote infection in the pleural space. Features of pleural fluid suggesting infection are loculation, pus, pH of pleural fluid less than 7.3, rapid accumulation of pleural fluid following removal, a low glucose level, and positive cultures or Gram stain of pleural fluid.

Proper treatment of empyema requires appropriate antibiotics combined with adequate drainage of the pleural space. Adequate drainage is usually achieved with a closed thoracostomy tube. If the fluid is loculated, more than one tube may be needed. Fluoroscopy can be helpful in placing tubes into loculated effusions. The tube is left in place until defervescence, cessation of drainage, and clinical improvement occurs.

If the patient does not respond to closed tube drainage, a limited thoracotomy with rib resection and manual lysis of adhesions may be helpful. If this fails, radical thoracotomy with decortication of the pleural space is indicated.

Parapneumonic effusions are effusions resulting from the accompanying inflammation of the pleural space as a consequence of a nearby pneumonia. They are not the result of direct pleural space infection. Parapneumonic effusions that do not show criteria found in empyema should be followed. They initially should be drained by thoracentesis. The underlying pneumonia is treated with appropriate antibiotics, and thoracentesis is repeated as fluid reaccumulates.

Tuberculous effusion can be the result of spread of the organism into the pleural space, or can follow primary tuberculosis. Post primary tuberculous effusion tends to resolve spontaneously, but such patients should be treated with standard double drug regimens, otherwise a high percentage (65%) will develop apical tuberculosis.

Chylothorax is the accumulation of chyle within the pleural space, as a result of thoracic duct rupture or blockage. Usually it follows trauma or lymphoma, but idiopathic cases do occur. Diagnosis is based on the milky color of the pleural fluid at thoracentesis; a creamy layer forms on top when the fluid is left to stand. The pleural fluid is predominantly lymphocytic. Total cholesterol is 65 to 220 mg/dl with a total fat of 0.4 to 6.0 gm/dl. Chylothorax should be differentiated from a pseudochylous effusion found in some patients with long-standing pleural effusion; this also is a high-fat-content effusion, but the principal fat is cholesterol. Pseudochylous effusion is found in cases of tuberculosis and rheumatoid arthritis. Cholesterol levels vary from 140 to 4500 mg/dl. Lipid protein electrophoresis can help differentiate these effusions. A Type I pattern is seen in chylothorax. Therapy for pseudochylous effusion consists of treating the underlying disease.

Chylothorax usually reaccumulates rapidly following thoracentesis. Repeated thoracentesis or chest thoracostomy will lead to rapid loss of fat, protein, and lymphocytes. Treatment is begun by stopping oral feeding and maintaining the patient on IV fluids or parenteral hyperalimentation. If the patient is not responding by a drop in the thoracic drainage within a week or two, surgical repair is recommended. If the chylothorax is caused by lymphoma, chemotherapy or radiation therapy often remedy the problem; if these fail, surgery can be considered.

Mesotheliomas are primary neoplasms of the pleura or peritoneum, and are either benign or malignant. Benign mesotheliomas present as a pleural mass and are best treated by surgical removal.

Malignant mesotheliomas are usually associated with asbestos exposure. There is an exudative effusion in most instances. The tumor spreads widely within the pleural space. Histologically the tumor can appear as an adenocarcinoma, fibrosarcoma, or fibroma, or there may be a mixture of the above microscopic findings. The gross appearance of the chest cavity is characteristic and the surgeon can help the pathologist by conveying this information. There is no effective means of treating malignant mesotheliomas at present. The patient usually dies of respiratory insufficiency, often resulting from local spread. Supplemental oxygen and narcotics should be used when needed. Surgical resection followed by radiation and chemotherapy has provided the most prolonged survivals.

Putrid Lung Abscess

A lung abscess is an area of necrotic lung containing pus. It appears as a cavity with an air fluid level on a chest roentgenogram. Abscess cavities can result from obstruction of a bronchus (tumor or foreign body), pulmonary infarct, or infection with necrosis (gram-negative bacilli, *Staphylococcus aureus*, *Mycobacterium*, fungi, *Nocardia*, and actinomycetes). These entities are discussed elsewhere.

Putrid lung abscesses are believed to be caused by aspiration. They have a marked tendency to occur in patients with gingival disease or impaired consciousness: e.g., alcoholics, drug addicts, victims of seizures, and people undergoing general anesthesia. Putrid lung abscesses are usually located in dependent portions of the lung; it is unusual to find them in the anterior segments of the upper lobes.

The organisms involved are those found in the gingival crevice. There is a mixture of different anaerobic organisms.

Patients present with a one- to three-week history of illness. Symptoms include fever, chills, and productive cough. There is copious, foul-smelling purulent sputum. Physical examination reveals intermittent fever with localized findings of consolidation. Chest x-ray shows a single thin-walled cavity with an air fluid level. A thick-walled cavity suggests carcinoma with necrosis.

MANAGEMENT

Following history-taking, physical examination, and chest roentgenogram, therapy may be started after sputum cultures have been obtained. If there is suspicion of endobronchial obstruction, bronchoscopy is indicated. If no obstructive lesion is found during bronchoscopy, a double-sheathed brush can be used to obtain cultures to rule out other infectious causes of a lung cavity.

Once the diagnosis is established, treatment with antibiotics is started. Penicillin, cefoxitin, clindamycin, chloramphenicol, and metronidazole are agents of established efficacy. Penicillin has been the treatment of choice for many years in patients with anaerobic lung abscesses. Even though *Bacteroides fragilis* is often present, these abscesses respond well to penicillin; the usual dose is 4 to 8 million units per day IV. When the patient is afebrile and clinically improved, oral penicillin VK is used, 500 to 750 mg q.i.d. for four weeks.

There is little information comparing other antimicrobials to penicillin in therapy for putrid lung abscess. Evidence shows clindamycin to be somewhat more effective than penicillin; in a comparative study, clindamycin was 100% effective and penicillin 60% effective. The dose of clindamycin most often used for putrid lung abscess is 600 mg IV q.i.d. until the patient is clinically improved, followed by 300 mg q.i.d. P.O. for four weeks.

Adjuvants to antimicrobial therapy include bronchodilators, postural drainage, hydration, chest physiotherapy, and oxygen. These measures usually are only necessary for a short time.

Surgical intervention is required in a few cases but should be avoided if possible. Indications for surgery include massive hemoptysis, bronchopleural fistula, failure of medical therapy, and empyema unresponsive to closed chest thoracostomy.

The outcome of putrid lung abscess is dependent on host factors, but prognosis is usually good in otherwise healthy young patients. Concurrent disease often determines the outcome. Chronic debilitating diseases, alcoholism, or esophageal disease adversely affect results; lung abscesses in such patients carry a 15% to 20% mortality rate.

Following successful treatment of a putrid lung abscess, it is important to try to eliminate predisposing factors such as gingival disease or poor seizure control. Follow-up chest x-rays usually show some fibrotic strands or pleural thickening. Lung function generally returns to near baseline.

REFERENCES

Abrams LD: A pleural-biopsy punch. Lancet 1:30–31, 1958.
Cope C: New pleural biopsy needle. JAMA 167:1107–1108, 1958.
Guenter CA, Welch MH: Pleural disease. *In* Pulmonary Medicine, 2nd ed. J.B. Lippincott Co, Philadelphia, 1982, pp 567–605.
Hausbeer FH, Yarbo JW: Diagnosis and treatment of malignant pleural effusion. Semin Oncol 12:54–75, 1985.
Hinshaw HC, Murray JF: Lung Abscess. *In* Diseases of the Chest, 4th ed. W.B. Saunders Co, Philadelphia, 1980, pp 287–297.
Levison ME, Mangura CT, Lorber B, et al.: Clindamycin compared with penicillin for the treatment of anaerobic lung abscess. Ann Intern Med 98:466–491, 1983.
Light RW, MacGregor MI, Luchsinger PC, et al.: Pleural effusions: the diagnostic separation of transudates from exudates. Ann Intern Med 77:507–513, 1972.
Prakash UBS, Reiman HM: Comparison of needle biopsy with cytologic analysis for evaluation of pleural effusion; analysis of 414 cases. Mayo Clin Proc 60:158–164, 1985.
Rumbaugh IF, Prior JA: Lung abscess: a review of 41 cases. Ann Intern Med 55:223–234, 1961.

6 · *THE COMMON COLD*

Herbert P. Wiedemann
Joseph A. Golish
CLEVELAND CLINIC FOUNDATION

DEFINITION AND DIAGNOSTIC CRITERIA

The common cold is a self-limited viral infection of the upper respiratory passages. Since everyone suffers an average of two to five episodes per year, the symptom complex is universally recognized. The hallmarks are nasal congestion, nasal discharge, and sneezing. In addition, the common cold is characterized by nonsuppurative inflammation and the relative absence of high fever or significant constitutional symptoms. These points are useful in differentiating the common cold from other, sometimes more serious infections of the respiratory tract, including pneumonia, sinusitis, otitis, and pharyngitis. The typical presence of mild myalgias, malaise, headache, chilly sensation, and a dry scratchy throat usually makes it easy to distinguish the common cold from hay fever or vasomotor rhinitis.

The economic impact of the common cold is immense. It accounts for approximately 60 million lost days of work or school annually. Sales of proprietary cold remedies and analgesics in the United States total over $2 billion per year.

PATHOPHYSIOLOGY

Several different viruses are capable of producing the common cold (Table 1). About 25% to 50% are caused by rhinovirus, of which there are more than 100 known serotypes. Rhinoviruses grow best in tissue cultures maintained at 33°C, similar to the temperature in the nose of man. Members of the rhinovirus family

Table 1. VIRUSES THAT CAUSE THE COMMON COLD SYNDROME

Frequent	Infrequent
Rhinovirus	Coxsackievirus
Adenovirus	Enterovirus
Influenza virus	Rubeola
Parainfluenza virus	Rubella
Respiratory syncytial virus	Varicella
Coronavirus	

rarely cause illness other than the common cold, whereas many of the other viruses associated with mild upper respiratory infection also produce more serious illness such as pneumonia (influenza virus), exudative pharyngitis (adenovirus, coxsackievirus), conjunctivitis (adenovirus), and in young children croup (parainfluenza virus) or bronchiolitis (respiratory syncytial virus).

The nasopharynx and conjunctivae are the portals of infection. Transmission is either by direct exposure to airborne droplets emitted by infected persons during sneezing or coughing, or by hand contact with contaminated surfaces and subsequent placement of a contaminated finger near the nasal or conjunctival mucosa. Experimental studies with rhinovirus indicate that infection is most efficient by the latter mechanism, although airborne transmission may be more important for other viruses. Experimental studies do not support the notion that damp feet or exposure to chilling air makes an individual more susceptible to rhinovirus infection.

The pathologic changes in the nasal mucosal membranes are hyperemia, edema, and transudation. Marked cytopathic changes are rare, in contrast to the effect of influenza virus on the lower respiratory tract. Repair is usually rapid and without any known residual changes. The local production of interferon, which protects uninfected cells, probably accounts for the rapid termination of infection before the development of specific antibody.

Complications of the common cold are rare, although bacterial infections such as otitis or sinusitis sometimes occur. Viral infection does not appreciably alter the bacterial flora of the nasopharynx. Bacterial complications are probably caused more by ostial obstruction or damage to the mucociliary clearing mechanism than by the emergence of superinfecting or virulent bacteria.

CLINICAL ASPECTS

Signs and symptoms that develop in volunteers challenged with rhinovirus are similar to those seen in the naturally occurring illness. Initial symptoms are a burning sensation of the eyes and nose, a dry scratchy throat, and mild headache, malaise, and chilly sensation. Sneezing, nasal discharge, and nasal congestion soon follow and reach a peak on the second or third day of illness. Fever is usually mild and transient. A severe sore throat is rare and no pharyngeal exudate is observed. Mild or moderate cervical adenopathy may occur. Cough is absent or mild in most patients and usually nonproductive, although a small amount of mucoid sputum may be seen. When it does occur, cough tends to be a persistent symptom, often lingering after the nasal discharge and congestion have subsided. Coughing may be particularly marked and prolonged in cigarette smokers and asthmatics; the latter may also experience an exacerbation of wheezing during the common cold. The mean duration of rhinovirus illness is about seven days, although up to 25% of patients are symptomatic for two weeks.

Physical examination may reveal mild erythema of the pharynx and tympanic membranes. The nasal turbinates are swollen and boggy. Laboratory investigation may show mild leukocytosis and elevation of the erythrocyte sedimentation rate. Physical and laboratory examination are primarily important for the diagnosis or exclusion of more severe illnesses that patients may designate a "cold."

MANAGEMENT

Throughout history, numerous cures for the common cold have been advocated. Perhaps none are more curious (nor, unfortunately, more effective) than the suggestion of Pliny the younger in the first century to "kiss the hairy muzzle of a mouse." To date, there remains no specific therapy against infection by the rhinovirus or other cold viruses. Research currently in progress may lead to effective and practical application of interferon, antiviral drugs, or vaccination. However, until such time, no compelling argument can be advanced that anything more than simple bed rest and warm clothing is prudent or necessary.

PHARMACOLOGIC THERAPY

Many patients feel better with symptomatic treatment of their systemic, nasal, or pharyngeal complaints. Aspirin (0.6 gm for an adult) helps relieve headache, fever, and myalgias. However, aspirin has no apparent worth for other cold symptoms, and may actually prolong the duration of viral shedding.

Temporary relief of nasal congestion can be achieved with oral pseudoephedrine (Sudafed) or oxymetazoline nasal spray (Afrin). Decongestants should not be used for more than a few days, in view of the rebound effect from prolonged use. Cough can often be controlled by over-the-counter medications containing dextromethorphan (Robitussin-DM cough syrup and Mediquell chewing gum); more severe coughs may require codeine or related derivatives (Hycodan) for suppression. Warm saline gargles or throat lozenges are appropriate for mild pharyngitis.

Routine use of antibiotics is discouraged. Suppurative complications of the common cold are rare and are not prevented by antibiotic prophylaxis. Antibiotic therapy should be reserved for documented or suspected purulent otitis, sinusitis, bronchitis, or pharyngitis. Pneumococci, *Haemophilus influenzae*, group A streptococci, and *Mycoplasma* are common causes of these complications and usually respond well to appropriate antimicrobial agents.

Large doses of vitamin C (ascorbic acid) are not recommended. Although some controlled studies demonstrate an apparent modest benefit from vitamin C, a placebo effect may have been involved since volunteers were able to taste the vitamin C capsules. Several other controlled studies show no ability of vitamin C to prevent, ameliorate, or shorten cold symptoms.

Nasal interferon drops or sprays have been tested. Although some efficacy in preventing or treating the common cold is seen, effective doses are associated with side effects such as bloody mucus, nasal stuffiness, nasal mucosal erosions, and submucosal infiltration by mononuclear cells. Thus, interferon is not currently suitable for prevention or treatment of common colds.

Drugs that have direct antiviral activity or that stimulate interferon release (interferon inducers) are not yet effective or practical against rhinovirus infection. However, the efficacy of amantadine against influenza and of ribavirin aerosol against respiratory syncytial virus suggests that future research into this topic may provide dividends in treating the common cold.

ENVIRONMENTAL CONTROL AND PREVENTION

Since contact transmission appears to be a major feature of rhinovirus infection, environmental control would seem to be a practical means of prevention. Patients with active infection frequently have virus on their hands (40% to 90%), and environmental objects such as door knobs and counter tops are often contaminated (6% to 15%). The susceptible individual contaminates his finger and then transmits the virus to his nasal or conjunctival surface. Thus, frequent handwashing is a sensible admonition.

Rhinovirus is relatively resistant to many disinfectants. Tincture of iodine and a phenol/alcohol agent (Lysol) are most effective. Experimental studies indicate that treating contaminated surfaces with phenol/alcohol, or fingers with 2% aqueous iodine, is helpful. Unfortunately, the phenol/alcohol disinfectant has no residual activity, which limits its benefit.

There is no vaccine available for rhinovirus infection. The large number of different serotypes of rhinovirus makes this approach unattractive. Furthermore, there is some evidence that rhinovirus exhibits antigenic variation, similar to that exhibited by influenza. It should not be forgotten that rhinoviruses account for at most about 50% of common colds. Nevertheless, interest in the vaccine approach has been stimulated by recent studies suggesting that relatively few rhinovirus serotypes account for the vast majority of clinical infections. A final stumbling block in the path of vaccines against the common cold is the fact that systemically administered antigen, which stimulates specific serum antibodies, may not provide protection against infection at mucosal surfaces. Thus, the most effective vaccine against the common cold may ultimately prove to be an aerosol.

Two recent reports* indicate the effectiveness of alpha-interferon nasal spray for short-term prophylaxis of rhinovirus infection in high-risk individuals. Side effects of this medication included a 10% incidence of minor nasal bleeding.

---

*N Engl J Med 314:65–70, 71–75, 1986.

REFERENCES

Couch RB: The common cold: control? J Infect Dis *150*:167–173, 1984.
Gwaltney JM: The common cold. *In* Mandell GL, Douglas RG Jr, Bennett JE (eds): Principles and Practice of Infectious Disease. John Wiley & Sons, New York, 1985, pp 351–355.
Hall CB, McBride JT: Upper respiratory tract infections. *In* Pennington JE (ed): Respiratory Infections: Diagnosis and Management. Raven Press, New York, 1983, pp 79–95.
Kapikian AZ: The common cold: *In* Wyngaarden JB, Smith LH Jr (eds): Textbook of Medicine, 17th ed. W.B. Saunders Co., Philadelphia, 1985, pp 1691–1695.

7 · BACTERIAL, VIRAL, AND MYCOPLASMAL PNEUMONIA

C. Braddock Burns
W. Brooks Emory
OCHSNER CLINIC AND ALTON OCHSNER
MEDICAL FOUNDATION

DEFINITION, DIAGNOSIS, AND CLINICAL ASPECTS

Despite the dramatic improvement in our ability to treat bacterial infections with antimicrobial agents, pneumonia remains an important cause of morbidity and mortality in the general population. The primary challenge to the clinician is to determine the specific organism responsible for the infection, and thus ensure the most effective therapy.

Pneumonia is, by definition, an infection of the lower respiratory tract and lung parenchyma. The most common modes of transmission of organisms to these sites are inhalation of small, airborne, infectious particles or aspiration of secretions containing resident naso-oropharyngeal flora. Since lung defense mechanisms are well suited to defend against infection, factors that impair the normal host defenses are usually present at the time of infection.

In the setting of an acute illness characterized by fever, cough, dyspnea, pleuritic pain, and general malaise, the diagnosis of pneumonia is readily suggested. An abnormality on chest radiograph consistent with pneumonia is essential for the diagnosis. Atypical and less dramatic presentations of pneumonia are common in elderly persons and patients with concurrent illnesses. A definitive diagnosis requires isolation of the specific organism from material obtained directly from the lower respiratory tract, the pleural space, or the bloodstream; or by documentation of specific serologic changes indicative of an acute infection. Infections from organisms outside the classes of agents considered here, pulmonary edema, pulmonary embolism with infarction, drug reactions, pulmonary hemorrhage, primary or metastatic neoplasms, radiation pneumonitis, nonspecific interstitial pneumonitis, and vasculitic processes may all produce radiographic changes mimicking pneumonia. A specific diagnosis is made in less than 50% of cases.

Clearly, initial therapy must be based on a presumptive diagnosis or chosen empirically. The list of probable organisms can be narrowed by considering the setting and host in which the infection arises. In general, cases can be divided into three categories: community-acquired pneumonia, nosocomial or hospital-acquired pneumonia, and pneumonia occurring in the immuno-compromised host. We are concerned with community-acquired pneumonias. Here, a few organisms cause the majority of infections among otherwise normal persons. Patients with concurrent illnesses that may alter their defense mechanisms (e.g., diabetes mellitus, chronic lung disease, congestive heart failure, or alcoholism) can acquire bacterial pneumonias from additional organisms. We will refer to this latter group of patients as "complicated hosts." These additional bacteria overlap with those frequently encountered in nosocomial pneumonias. Pneumonias in persons with severe impairment of their defense mechanisms (e.g., hematologic malignancies, immunosuppressive agents, or acquired immune deficiency syndrome) make up the final category, but are not discussed here.

INITIAL EVALUATION

Because it is often impossible to know the clinical course of each infection at the time of presentation, it is necessary to evaluate thoroughly every suspected case of pneumonia. It is very important to pay attention to the patient's life style, occupation, recent activities, and current and past medical problems, as well as to the dominant features of the present illness. Physical examination provides information about the extent of infection and the possibility of complicating problems, but only rarely establishes the specific diagnosis.

Abnormalities of routine laboratory studies are usually nonspecific. Leukocytosis is expected in bacterial pneumonias, is often present in *Mycoplasma* pneumonia, and may be seen initially in viral infections. Leukopenia in the presence of infection is an ominous sign, and leukocyte counts above 35,000 to 40,000 per cu mm indicate response to a severe infection. Blood cultures and arterial blood gases are appropriate tests for all patients being hospitalized.

A chest radiograph should be obtained in every patient suspected of having pneumonia, since physical findings correlate with radiographic abnormalities in no more than half of the cases. The radiograph helps define the extent of involvement. Broad overlap in the radiographic patterns that result from infections with different organisms precludes making a specific diagnosis from the radiograph alone. Lobar pneumonia begins in the alveolar spaces and spreads centrifugally to produce an infiltrate that abuts the pleural surface. A pattern of bronchopneumonia results from segmental involvement due to infections that spread along airways to the surrounding parenchyma. Finally, a pattern of patchy involvement dominated by accentuation of interstitial markings typically results from nonbacterial infections.

The most readily available source of information to help determine a specific diagnosis is the Gram stain of expectorated sputum. Microscopic features indicating that the specimen comes from the lower respiratory tract are the presence of alveolar macrophages and the absence of squamous epithelial cells. The presence of more than 20 to 25 squamous epithelial cells per low-power field, even when many neutrophils are present, indicates that the specimen is unsuitable for examination and culture. Isolation of a pathogen from sputum culture that is consistent with the predominant organism seen on Gram stain supports the presumptive diagnosis.

Despite best efforts, the patient may be unable to produce an adequate sputum sample. In the setting of community-acquired pneumonia, invasive procedures to obtain secretions from the lower respiratory tract are rarely indicated. When concurrent illnesses produce a difficult diagnostic problem, or the severity of the infection makes the most accurate initial therapy essential, an invasive procedure may be justified. Methods employed are transtracheal aspiration, bronchoscopy with a protected brush catheter, or transthoracic needle aspiration. All have some associated risk of morbidity or mortality, and all require a cooperative patient and a skilled operator. Quantitative cultures of the specimens obtained by transtracheal aspiration or bronchoscopy are necessary. These two procedures should be done before administration of any antibiotics. Open lung biopsy is the most definitive method of establishing a diagnosis, but its use should be limited primarily to pneumonias occurring in the immunocompromised host.

TREATMENT

GENERAL ASPECTS

Community-acquired pneumonias range in severity from mild, self-limited infections to fulminating infections that are rapidly fatal despite appropriate therapy. Mortality rates in recently reported series remain as high as 10% to 15% among hospitalized patients. This makes careful follow-up of all patients mandatory regardless of their symptoms at presentation. Reliable, young or middle-aged patients without coexisting medical problems are often treated outside the hospital.

Initial therapy includes attention to several general problems. Maintenance of adequate hydration is probably as helpful in mobilization of secretions as any other form of therapy. Expectorants, aerosols with bronchodilators or mucolytic agents, and humidifiers or nebulizers are of no proven value in uncomplicated pneumonia. Bronchodilators and chest physical therapy are indicated when conditions associated with increased bronchial secretions, such as chronic bronchitis or bronchiectasis, are present and in the treatment of lung abscess.

Supplemental oxygen should be given as needed to maintain an arterial oxygen tension of approximately 60 mm Hg. Raising the Pa_{O_2} above this level produces little increase in arterial oxygen content and may expose the patient to toxic concentrations of oxygen. It is important to maintain the hemoglobin concentration above 10 gm/dl to ensure adequate oxygen delivery. Adequate Pa_{O_2} can often be achieved with nasal oxygen delivered at a rate between 2 to 4 L/min. When higher concentrations of oxygen are required, delivery by mask will help avoid drying of the upper respiratory mucosa.

Tachypnea is often the result of decreased lung compliance and pleuritic pain rather than of hypoxemia. Relief of pain with codeine (30 mg PO every six to eight hours), a nonsteroidal anti-inflammatory agent such as indomethacin (25 mg q.i.d. PO with meals), or parenteral meperidine (25 to 75 mg IM every four to six hours) is often helpful.

Finally, in the presence of pneumonia, patients with marginal spontaneous ventilation are better managed by early intubation and support with mechanical ventilation. The long course of the illness eventually makes this necessary in most cases.

SPECIFIC THERAPY

Normal Host. Up to 90% of community-acquired pneumonias occurring in adults without an underlying illness result from a virus, *Streptococcus pneumoniae* or *Mycoplasma pneumoniae*. Many of the remaining cases are due to *Legionella* spp., discussed in Section IV, Chapter 10.

Pneumococcal Pneumonia. *S. pneumoniae* remains the cause of infection in most patients hospitalized with community-acquired pneumonia. The organism is found in the normal oral flora in a small percentage of healthy adults and in a greater percentage of persons with an upper respiratory illness. Aspiration of secretions containing the organism is the usual sequence leading to infection. The typical history is of a preceding upper respiratory illness punctuated by an abrupt rigor and high fever spike, followed by pleuritic pain and a cough productive of rust-colored sputum. The chest radiography shows a bronchopneumonia or lobar pattern with a pleural effusion in approximately one third of cases. Sputum culture is positive in roughly 50% of cases and blood cultures in up to 30%.

For patients hospitalized with suspected pneumococcal pneumonia, standard antibiotic therapy is 600,000 units of procaine penicillin G, IM every 12 hours. For patients with penicillin allergy we usually give erythromycin, 500 mg IV every six hours. Cephalothin and vancomycin are also effective alternatives. We continue parenteral therapy until the patient has been afebrile for 48 hours, then give antibiotics PO to complete a total of 10 to 14 days of therapy. Those who have mild symptoms may be treated as outpatients with phenoxymethyl penicillin, 250 mg PO every six hours, after an initial IM injection of procaine penicillin. Infections with *S. pneumoniae* resistant to penicillin continue to be reported, and to date have remained sensitive to vancomycin.

If extrapulmonary sites of infection such as empyema, arthritis, meningitis, or endocarditis are suspected, diagnostic procedures should be done before antibiotic therapy is started. In these cases, initial treatment should be with aqueous penicillin G, 20 million units daily by constant infusion.

Response to antibiotics is often dramatic, but some patients remain febrile for several days. Persistent fever during the initial three or four days should not be taken alone as an indication for changing or adding antibiotics.

Mycoplasmal Pneumonia. The spectrum of infections produced by *M. pneumoniae* ranges from mild upper respiratory infections to severe, life-threatening pneumonias. Infection is spread to close contacts by inhalation of aerosols containing the organism. The settings of classrooms, college dormitories, and military bases favor spread to large numbers of persons. Mycoplasmal pneumonia is uncommon in those over the age of 50.

Onset of illness is usually insidious, with prominent symptoms of headache, cough, pharyngitis, and fever. Radiographic changes typically are patchy bronchopneumonia in a single site or multiple sites. Only patients with abrupt onset of illness, lobar infiltrates, and signs of consolidation are likely to require hospitalization.

Diagnosis is generally based on documentation of a fourfold rise in complement-fixing antibody titer. Cold agglutinins appear in approximately 50% of cases and usually peak in the second or third week of illness, but are nonspecific since they also occur with some viral infections and in noninfectious disorders.

Erythromycin is the antibiotic of choice, 500 mg every six hours. Tetracycline in similar dosage is a suitable alternative. Antibiotics shorten the duration of symptoms and hasten clearing of the abnormalities seen on chest x-ray films, but they do not eradicate the organism from the respiratory tract. Antibiotics should be given for three weeks in an effort to prevent relapse of symptoms.

Hemolytic anemia, myocarditis, myringitis, polyarthritis, rash, erythema multiforme, and neurologic symptoms are among the most common extrapulmonary manifestations and can be severe.

Viral Pneumonia. Influenza (types A and B) and adenovirus are the only viruses that regularly cause pneumonia in adults. The exact incidence and clinical spectrum of these infections in the general population are uncertain.

Influenza A usually occurs in epidemics and is the topic of Chapter 12, Section IV. Adenovirus causes sporadic cases of pneumonia in the general population, but may be responsible for outbreaks of pneumonia among military recruits. The disease is characterized by fever, pharyngitis, bronchitis, and a cough productive of mucoid sputum. Chest x-ray changes range from patchy accentuation of interstitial markings to bilateral infiltrates characteristic of the adult respiratory distress syndrome. This is the virus that most commonly produces life-threatening respiratory failure in the general population.

Isolation of viruses from respiratory secretions requires special handling and culture techniques and is time-consuming. More often the diagnosis is based on documentation of specific serologic changes. Treatment of adenovirus infection is supportive. Full recovery of pulmonary function can be expected in most cases, even when severe respiratory failure is initially present.

Complicated Host. When pneumonia occurs in a debilitated or institutionalized person, as a complication of advanced chronic lung disease or recent influenza, or as a result of aspiration, additional organisms must be considered. These include *Staphylococcus aureus*; the gram-negative bacilli *E. coli*, *Klebsiella pneumoniae*, and *Haemophilus influenzae*; and anaerobic organisms.

Staphylococcal Pneumonia. *S. aureus* is responsible for only a small percentage of pneumonias acquired outside the hospital. Along with *Streptococcus pneumoniae* and *H. influenzae*, it is an important cause of post-influenza pneumonia and should be considered in this specific situation. Retirement homes commingle elderly people and are the sites for pandemics of influenza. The typical picture of staphylococcal pneumonia in a patient from such a setting is a pneumonic infiltrate with areas of cystic hi-light (cavitation), an associated pleural effusion, and leukocytosis in the range of 15,000 to 25,000 per cu mm. Primary staphylococcal pneumonia has a mortality rate of 20% to 30%. Treatment of choice is a penicillinase-resistant penicillin (oxacillin or nafcillin), 2 gm every four hours IV for 14 days. Therapy should be extended for four to six weeks in cases with associated bacteremia. In penicillin-allergic patients, and in cases where methicillin-resistant organisms are isolated, vancomycin (1 gm every six hours) is a reliable alternative.

Gram-negative Bacillary Pneumonia. In persons with chronic debilitating illnesses there is an increased incidence of colonization of the respiratory tract by gram-negative bacilli. Acute decompensation due to a complicating pneumonia occurs commonly in this setting, and identification of the causative organism may be difficult. Expectorated sputum often yields "mixed flora." Initial coverage with broad-spectrum antibiotics is prudent in these instances and usually successful. Reasonable empiric combinations include an aminoglycoside (gentamycin or tobramycin) with either an extended-spectrum penicillin (ticarcillin or mezlocillin) or a second-generation cephalosporin (cefamandole or cefoxitin). Dosages following the first 24 hours of treatment must be tailored for patients with altered renal function. Peak and trough serum levels of the aminoglycoside should be measured in all patients to ensure that therapeutic levels are obtained and to help avoid renal toxicity.

Klebsiella pneumoniae infections should be suspected in middle-aged and elderly male patients with a history of chronic alcohol abuse. Typically, the onset of illness is acute with prostration, dyspnea, severe hypoxemia, chest pain, and hemoptysis (a picture not dissimilar to pneumococcal pneumonia). Sputum may be gelatinous and red (currant jelly). Classically, this is a lobar pneumonia involving the upper lobe. Treatment of choice is with an aminoglycoside, as noted, and cephalothin or cefazolin (4 to 6 gm daily).

Haemophilus influenzae pneumonia is a more frequently recognized condition in patients with underlying chronic obstructive lung disease or alcoholism. These small, pleomorphic, gram-negative coccobacilli may be overlooked or misinterpreted on Gram stain. Parenchymal necrosis and empyemas often occur. Treatment of choice has been ampicillin (2 gm every four hours IV); however, increasing isolation of beta-lactamase–producing organisms makes the combination of an aminoglycoside plus either mezlocillin or a second-generation cephalosporin more reasonable initial therapy. When an ampicillin-resistant organism is suspected or proved, chloramphenicol (1 gm every six hours) remains a reliable alternative.

E. coli infection should be suspected in patients who develop pneumonia in the setting of concurrent urinary infection or a recent urologic procedure. The typical patient is one with diabetes mellitus and pyelonephritis. The primary mode of spread of infection to the lung is hematogenous; therefore, blood and urine cultures may be positive when sputum cultures are nondiagnostic. Treatment of choice is with a combination of an aminoglycoside with a cephalosporin or ampicillin, on the basis of sensitivity results. Recent studies document a growing incidence of ampicillin resistance among *E. coli* isolates, including organisms acquired outside the hospital.

Anaerobic Lung Infection. Infections due to anaerobic organisms should be considered in patients presenting with pneumonia and a history of altered consciousness or dysphagia that suggests possible aspiration. Predisposing factors include alcoholism, seizure disorders, cerebral vascular accidents, drug addiction, or esophageal disorders. The presence of periodontal disease is an important contributing condition since this greatly increases the concentration of bacteria in the oral cavity and secretions. If treatment is delayed, aspiration pneumonia is usually followed by formation of a lung abscess. This is heralded by production of putrid sputum in at least 50% of cases. Location of the process in a dependent area of the lung (when supine, the posterior segment of the upper lobes and the superior segment of the lower lobes) is an important clue to diagnosis. Indeed, occurrence of a lung abscess in an atypical location or in an edentulous patient should raise the suspicion of endobronchial obstruction.

Anaerobic organisms are found in 90% of abscesses following aspiration pneumonia. Treatment of choice in most cases is with penicillin (12 to 20 million units daily, IV). Critically ill patients should be treated with a combination of penicillin and either clindamycin or metronidazole; or, if penicillin allergic, with chloramphenicol. Patients who fail to respond to penicillin usually respond to clindamycin or metronidazole. Antibiotic treatment for an extended period is often needed when an abscess cavity is present.

Unusual Pneumonias. Pneumonia caused by an unusual organism should be considered when the patient's recent activity suggests possible exposure. For example, chlamydial infection (psittacosis) occurs in persons having close contact with birds. The history of a recent tick bite or exposure to squirrels or rabbits suggests possible infection from *Francisella tularensis* (tularemia). Pneumonia in a veterinarian or livestock worker may be due to the *Rickettsial* organism *Coxiella burnetii* (Q fever). These infections merit consideration in the proper setting; otherwise, pneumonia in a few patients will go undiagnosed and possibly be mistreated.

STRATEGY FOR EMPIRIC THERAPY

When initial assessment provides a presumptive diagnosis, initial therapy should be directed at that cause of infection. Many times, however, therapy must be chosen empirically and must be broad enough to encompass several common pathogens. Table 1 lists suitable regimens for presumed nonviral pneumonias based on the clinical setting. These have been our choices for moderately ill patients. In the face of an apparent overwhelming illness, additional antibiotics may be indicated to ensure coverage of less common organisms or drug-resistant species, as detailed in the discussion of specific infections above. Newer, third-generation cephalosporins and clavulanic acid–penicillin combination antibiotics are currently under intense evaluation and may supersede current choices for empiric treatment of pneumonias in the complicated host.

COMPLICATIONS

Antibiotic therapy has decreased dramatically the incidence of complications with bacterial pneumonias. Secondary infections such as septic arthritis, meningitis, and endocarditis are now unusual. Empyema remains a common complication and the likelihood of occurrence varies with the infecting organism. The chance that a parapneumonic effusion will prove to be infected ranges from as many as 80% to 90% of effusions associated with pneumonias due to anaerobic organisms or *E. coli*, to 20% to 25% of those associated with *K. pneumoniae* and *S. aureus*, to only 1% to 2% of effusions occurring with pneumococcal pneumonia.

It is important to recognize effusions that are in-

Table 1. EMPIRIC THERAPY FOR PRESUMPTIVE BACTERIAL PNEUMONIA

Clinical Setting	Common Pathogen*	Initial Therapy
Normal Host		
Acute onset	Pneumococcus,† *Mycoplasma*	Procaine penicillin, 600,000 units/12 hrs IM. Alternate: erythromycin, 500 mg/6 hrs IV.
Atypical onset	*Mycoplasma,*† virus, pneumococcus	Erythromycin, 500 mg/6 hrs PO or IV. Alternate: doxycycline, 100 mg/12 hrs PO or IV.
Complicated Host		
Institutionalized or debilitated	Pneumococcus, gram-negative bacillus	Gentamycin or tobramycin, 3–5 mg/kg/day IV, plus mezlocillin, 3 gm/4 hrs IV or cefamandole, 2 gm/6 hrs IV.
Alcoholic or COPD	Pneumococcus, *Klebsiella pneumoniae,*	
Urologic infection	*Haemophilus influenzae*	
	E. coli,† other gram-negative bacilli	
Postinfluenza	Pneumococcus, *Staph. aureus,*† *H. influenzae*	Oxacillin or nafcillin, 2 gm/4 hrs IV, plus cefamandole, 2 gm/6 hrs IV.
Aspiration	Anaerobic organisms	Penicillin G, 12–20 million units/day IV. Alternate: clindamycin, 600 mg/6 hrs IV.

**Legionella* pneumonia may occur in either normal or complicated hosts. If *Legionella* pneumonia is suspected, erythromycin, 1 gm/6 hrs IV, should be added to the regimens listed above.

†Major organism.

fected since successful treatment usually requires chest tube drainage. Any of the following four criteria is an indication for chest tube drainage of a *parapneumonic effusion*: (1) organisms seen on Gram stain or cultured from the pleural fluid, (2) fluid with the appearance of gross pus, (3) fluid with a pH <7.00, or (4) fluid with a glucose <40 mg%. If the fluid has a pH between 7.00 and 7.20 or an LDH above 1000 IU, the decision for tube drainage should be individualized. If tube drainage is not instituted, a repeat thoracentesis should be done in 24 to 48 hours.

Lung abscess is another complication resulting from necrotizing infections. As with empyemas, most abscesses are associated with anaerobic infections. Necrotizing pneumonias due to *S. aureus* and gram-negative bacilli are important other causes of cavitary lesions. Standard therapy with prolonged antibiotics and vigorous postural drainage is usually successful. The therapeutic role of bronchoscopy is unproved. It should be performed to evaluate abscesses that fail to respond to medical management, to exclude an obstructing or cavitating neoplasm. Surgery is rarely necessary to manage a lung abscess.

FOLLOW-UP CARE

The ideal duration of antibiotic treatment of pneumonia is unproved. It is not necessary to continue therapy until all radiographic changes have resolved. This may occur within two to three weeks, but can require up to six to eight weeks with extensive infiltrates. Abnormalities persisting beyond this time suggest endobronchial obstruction, and bronchoscopy to exclude this possibility is indicated.

Lasting impairment in pulmonary function is unusual following bacterial pneumonia, even when multiple lobes were involved. Cavitary lesions usually close, leaving surprisingly little residual radiographically visible change.

PREVENTIVE MEASURES

Immunizations against influenza A and *S. pneumoniae* are currently available for general use. Indications for administration of the vaccine for influenza are discussed in Section IV, Chapter 12. Immunization has been proved effective in preventing pneumococcal infections in high-risk patient groups. It is reasonable to expect that immunization is also beneficial for patients in the general population who are at increased risk of infection. These include (1) any patient over the age of 2 years with splenic dysfunction; (2) persons with chronic respiratory, cardiac, renal, or hepatic disease; and (3) anyone over the age of 65 years or with diabetes mellitus. The currently available vaccine (Pneumovax) is given at a dose of 0.5 ml IM or SQ, and should be a one-time treatment only. Local soreness and mild fever are the most common adverse effects.

REFERENCES

Bartlett JG, Finegold SM: Anaerobic infections of the lung and pleural space. Am Rev Respir Dis 110:56–77, 1974.

Fraser RG, Paré JAP: Infectious diseases of the lungs. *In* Diagnosis of Diseases of the Chest, 2nd ed. W. B. Saunders Co, Philadelphia, 1978, pp 657–731.

Levison ME: The Pneumonias. John Wright PSG, Boston, 1984.

Light RW, Girard WM, Jenkinson SG, et al: Parapneumonic effusions. Am J Med 69:507–511, 1980.

Pennington JE: Respiratory Infections: Diagnosis and Management. Raven Press, New York, 1983.

8 · SARCOIDOSIS

Richard A. DeRemee
MAYO CLINIC AND MAYO FOUNDATION

DEFINITION AND DIAGNOSTIC CRITERIA

There is no simple definition of sarcoidosis. Because no specific etiologic agent or agents have been discovered, a definition must necessarily be descriptive and syndromic in character. Definitions may vary widely from authority to authority, but all should include a few critical criteria. First, the disease should be considered systemic as opposed to local: i.e., virtually every organ system may be involved at the same time. Second, the pathology is characterized by a sequence of inflammatory events, beginning with thymus-dependent lymphocytes that lead to the formation of noncaseous granuloma, which, by a process of hyalinization and fibrosis, may distort the architecture of vital organs and impair their function. Third, specific causes of the non-caseous granuloma, such as fungal or mycobacterial infections or berylliosis, must be excluded. Finally, the disease observed should behave in a manner clinically consistent with sarcoidosis. It is this concept of clinical consistency that is most difficult to convey, requiring a degree of clinical expertise and familiarity.

In more than 90% of cases, sarcoidosis has a major intrathoracic manifestation, with involvement of the lungs and/or hilar lymph nodes. Other key organ involvement includes the liver, spleen, skin, eyes, heart, central nervous system, joints, and bones. Thus, to make the diagnosis it is necessary to biopsy an involved organ (usually lung, lymph node, or skin) and demonstrate noncaseous granuloma. Next, a specific cause of the granuloma should be excluded. The information obtained must then be evaluated in the context of the patient in whom there is evidence of a systemic disease that acts like sarcoidosis.

PATHOPHYSIOLOGY

Recent studies with bronchoalveolar lavage have helped to clarify the pathogenesis. An unknown agent or agents stimulates a cascade of inflammatory events that appears to begin with thymus-dependent lymphocytes (T cells). These T cells elaborate kinins that promote the ingress of lymphocytes and mononuclear cells into the alveolar spaces and walls. Monocytes are then stimulated to form the noncaseous granuloma. Persistence of the granuloma may be associated with hyalinization and fibrosis, which leads to irreversible damage. Although studies of the T-cell inflammation that leads to granuloma have been done chiefly on the lung, it is thought that a similar process occurs in other organs such as the liver, spleen, or skin, or wherever the granuloma is found. In the case of the lung, both granuloma and fibrosis disturb the function of the alveolar capillary membrane, reducing the surface area for diffusion of gases, thereby leading to hypoxemia. The granuloma is potentially reversible, but fibrosis is not. An understanding of the dichotomous elements of reversible inflammation and irreversible fibrosis is important in order to form an approach to treatment. Hypercalcemia is associated with and due to sarcoidosis in 10% to 20% of cases. Recent investigations point to the activated monocyte as the probable source of increased production of $1,25(OH)_2$ vitamin D, which causes altered calcium metabolism. Although altered calcium metabolism is probably present in all patients with sarcoidosis, it is unknown why only a few develop frank hypercalcemia and hypercalciuria. Persistent hypercalcemia can lead to impaired renal function due to nephrocalcinosis. Renal damage due primarily to granulomatous infiltration is rare. An interesting feature of sarcoidosis is its propensity to undergo spontaneous remission and leave the patient with no detectable damage. It is a challenge to try to predict such remissions, aided by the plain chest roentgenogram.

CLINICAL ASPECTS

Pulmonary sarcoidosis is, at least in its early development, an asymptomatic disease. Thus, it is often discovered by chance on routine screening chest roentgenogram or in the course of evaluating symptoms unrelated to sarcoidosis. An understanding of the roentgenographic staging system is essential. Stage I is represented by bilateral, symmetric hilar lymphadenopathy, often with a right paratracheal lymph node enlargement without parenchymal infiltration. Stage II is bilateral hilar lymphadenopathy plus parenchymal infiltration, and stage III is parenchymal infiltration in the absence of hilar lymphadenopathy. This staging scheme not only conveys visual information, but is closely connected with prognosis, the approximate degree and kind of pulmonary function abnormality to be anticipated, and the frequency of breathlessness. Breathlessness is a prime symptom of pulmonary disease. In a personal series of 165 patients, only 29 (18%) complained of breathlessness when first seen for evaluation; most of these were in stage III. Cough was the initial complaint in about 30% of patients. About 10% complained of arthralgias. Most were unaware of sarcoidosis at its discovery. Occasionally, patients present with ocular symptoms related to uveitis, or with skin lesions. In these situations, a chest roentgenogram should be obtained and may uncover unsuspected pulmonary disease. Involvement of the heart may be manifested by arrhythmias and conduction disturbances on electrocardiogram. Sudden death due to involvement of the heart has been reported, presumably caused by arrhythmia. The prognosis for spontaneous remission is 60% or better for stage I, 50% for stage II, and 30% for stage III. Pulmonary function measurements are usually normal in stage I, although slight decreases in the diffusing capacity for carbon monoxide may be seen, and rarely an obstructive airway component. In stages II and III, almost half the patients still have pulmonary function within normal limits. Others show a decrease in static lung volumes (restriction). In very late stages, severe airway obstruction may be superimposed; this strongly correlates with the symptom of breathlessness.

MANAGEMENT

This discussion relates primarily to pulmonary sarcoidosis, but the principles elaborated apply also to involvement of other critical organs.

The treatment of pulmonary sarcoidosis is controversial. Although agents such as oxyphenbutazone, chloroquine, alkylators, and other immunosuppressants have been reported to be effective, glucocorticoids, and particularly prednisone, or prednisolone, have been the most widely used and most effective in current practice. Whereas there is little or no disagreement about the prompt use of glucocorticoids in the treatment of uveitis, CNS involvement, myocardial sarcoidosis, or hypercalcemia, the use of these agents for pulmonary sarcoidosis remains controversial. There appear to be two opposing viewpoints. One contends that glucocorticoids do not affect the natural course of the disease, i.e., do not prevent the evolution to fibrosis and irreversible pulmonary damage. Adherents to this view tend to recommend glucocorticoids only if the patient develops symptoms, such as breathlessness or cough. The other view is that glucocorticoids can reverse the inflammatory phase and prevent irreversible fibrosis if dosage and duration are sufficient. The definitive scientific study to resolve this controversy has not yet been properly carried out. Nonetheless, a physician caring for a patient with sarcoidosis must decide either to treat with glucocorticoids, or not to treat and simply observe the natural course of the disease. However inconclusive the scientific data, I feel the evidence weighs on the side of early intervention with glucocorticoids, particularly for patients in stages II and III.

Once the proper diagnosis has been made, a number of questions arise: (1) Is the disease active or inactive? (2) If active, what is the prognosis for spontaneous remission? (3) Does the patient have symptoms such as breathlessness, cough, or arthralgias that call for relief? (4) What is the degree of pulmonary function change, if any? (5) Is there critical involvement of organs other than the lung, such as the eye, CNS, or heart? (6) Is there hypercalcemia?

PLAN

Patients are first classified according to the roentgenographic staging scheme described earlier. All have baseline pulmonary function studies and basic blood tests, such as hemogram, creatinine, calcium, and serum angiotensin converting enzyme (SACE). A detailed examination of the ocular fundus should also be made even in asymptomatic patients, as uveitis may be subclinical. Patients in stage I are not treated unless they have uncomfortable erythema nodosum with arthritis, or an unusual complication of obstructive airway disease due to granulomatous bronchitis. The prognosis for stage I is excellent and there is usually no or little derangement of pulmonary function. These patients can be observed with chest roentgenogram at three- to six-month intervals until the disease resolves, usually within the first one to two years. If the chest reoentgenogram shows evolution into stages II or III, the patient is considered for treatment.

All patients in stages II or III are potential candidates for glucocorticoid treatment if, after a period of observation of three to six months following diagnosis, their disease is not spontaneously regressing or has progressed. The basic principles underlying early treatment of these patients have to do with the elements of inflammation (T-cell alveolitis leading to granuloma) and fibrosis, the presumed result of such inflammation. It has been clearly demonstrated that glucocorticoids readily suppress the inflammation, and it is reasoned that thereby fibrosis will not ensue, or, if it has already occurred, will not recur. Hence, the short-term goals are to identify patients at risk of developing fibrosis and to introduce glucocorticoid to suppress inflammation and prevent or minimize fibrosis. The long-term goals are to decide in which treated patients the underlying cause of the inflammation is no longer present and treatment can be withdrawn, leaving minimal, if any, residual pulmonary damage.

Most of these individuals will be ambulatory and outpatients. Hospitalization for sarcoidosis is infrequently indicated, usually for respiratory failure, found in those with far-advanced, irreversible fibrosis. Rarely, massive hemoptysis from a fungus ball inhabiting a fibrotic cavity may require hospitalization, as this may be life-threatening. For these patients, control of hemorrhage may be attempted with embolization of the affected bronchial artery, or resection of lung tissue may be required. Resection of fungus balls generally carries a high morbidity and mortality rate.

DRUG THERAPY

Glucocorticoids, especially prednisone or prednisolone, are the current drugs of choice. I advocate alternate-day regimens, with rare exceptions. Such regimens require glucocorticoids of intermediate biologic half-life (12 to 36 hours), of which prednisone and prednisolone are examples. Glucocorticoids of long biologic half-life (36 to 72 hours), such as paramethasone, dexamethasone, or betamethasone, should not be used on an alternate-day basis or they will cause pituitary adrenal axis suppression, the avoidance of which is the intention of such regimens. With alternate-day administration, long courses (many months to years) can be given with few, if any, side effects, and withdrawal from glucocorticoids can be effected more rapidly and safely than with daily regimens.

There is no preference between prednisone and prednisolone. In the liver, prednisone is converted to prednisolone by hydroxylation at the eleventh carbon atom. Theoretically, prednisolone might be preferred in patients having severe liver damage, to avoid the necessity of hydroxylation by the liver, but I have never encountered a patient in whom this consideration was important.

Other drugs used include chloroquine, oxyphenbutazone, alkylating agents, and other immunosuppressants. When the patient is entirely unable to tolerate glucocorticoids or there are contraindications to their use, the other agents may be considered, although these all have significant side effects also. Indomethacin, 25 mg three times daily, is effective in relieving pain from erythema nodosum and arthritis or suppressing fever.

Patients treated with glucocorticoids are started on prednisone, 40 mg PO on alternate days; it is not necessary to begin with daily doses and then taper to alternate days. In fact, by such practice the patient may undergo a reactivation when changing to alternate days, probably owing to a relative adrenal insufficiency on the off day. Periodic evaluation and modification of dosage are described later. Occasionally, a patient does not respond to the 40-mg dose, and the dose may then be increased to 60 mg on alternate days. If the disease still does not respond, it is likely that irreversible fibrosis has already occurred and the patient is unlikely to improve on higher doses. Even hypercalcemia responds within seven to 14 days on alternate-day regimens. Ocular sarcoidosis can often be treated with topical glucocorticoids, particularly if found in stage I. An ophthalmologist should advise on the form of administration.

Black patients tend to experience a more aggressive prolonged course. They are handled in the same way, but prednisone therapy may need to last longer than for whites.

The adverse effects of glucocorticoids are well known. Among the most frequently encountered are central obesity, impaired glucose metabolism or frank diabetes mellitus, hypertension, osteoporosis, proximal myopathy, and cataracts. It is difficult to treat these side effects short of discontinuance of the drug, but their frequency and severity are mitigated by alternate-day regimens. A patient should be warned of, but not alarmed about, the possible side effects. Diets can be prescribed to avoid weight gain. If frank diabetes occurs, diet, oral hypoglycemic agents, or even insulin may be necessary as long as glucocorticoids are in use. Similarly, if hypertension occurs it should be treated with whatever is required. Some physicians have advocated the concomitant use of calcium and vitamin D, especially for women, in an effort to prevent osteoporosis. As long as supraphysiologic levels of glucocorticoids are present, such prophylactic measures are unlikely to be effective.

If a patient has any of the conditions mentioned above, the addition of glucocorticoids will obviously aggravate them. Therefore, the physician must be circumspect about beginning treatment if the potential adverse effects outweigh the prospect of improving the patient's overall status. Opportunistic infections are more likely in patients treated with more than 40 mg of prednisone (or equivalent in another congener) on a daily basis. Patients on alternate-day regimens seem to be less vulnerable to such infection. Obstructive airway disease or frank asthma may complicate sarcoidosis. Glucocorticoids can ameliorate these conditions, but bronchodilators, both inhaled and systemic, may often be indicated.

PATIENT INFORMATION AND EDUCATION

As sarcoidosis occurs relatively infrequently, there is very little information concerning it in lay publications and the general public are mostly ignorant of it. Hence, a patient having sarcoidosis may be fearful on hearing the diagnosis. The physician should attempt to explain the nature of the disease in lay terms. It is important to allay fear and reassure the patient that the disease is not a malignancy, but an inflammation affecting many different organs, especially the lungs and lymph nodes in the chest. Emphasis is placed on the usually benign course of the disease, particularly when discovered in stage I. However, it should be pointed out that glucocorticoid treatment may be necessary in stages II and III to reduce the possibility of fibrosis. The side effects of glucocorticoids should be reviewed, especially those pertaining to increased appetite with possible weight gain, osteoporosis (especially in women), hypertension, and cataract development. However, it should be emphasized that alternate-day regimens greatly reduce the possibility of these. Until the disease is arrested, regularity of follow-up should be firmly impressed on the patient. As in most unfamiliar situations, thorough and understandable explanations can help rid the patient of fear and improve cooperation with management.

A satisfactory outcome cannot be guaranteed. Factors influencing outcome include the degree of fibrosis present at detection and patients' diligence in following a program of management. Patients obviously vary in their motivation and some cannot be motivated at all. To ensure the best possible compliance, the physician must educate patients fully concerning the nature of their disease.

PERIODIC EVALUATION

Regular periodic follow-up is mandatory. Intervals will vary according to the patient's roentgenographic stage and whether or not treatment is being used.

Patients in stage I are usually not treated unless they have involvement of the eyes, CNS, or heart, or have hypercalcemia. It is my custom to advise a repeat chest roentgenogram in six months. Spontaneous remission, if it occurs, usually happens in the first one to two years. It may occur after only one month, but I have also observed patients who have persistent, stable stage I disease for over 15 years, while remaining entirely asymptomatic. Once spontaneous resolution occurs, it is unlikely the disease will ever recur and the patient may be released from follow-up. Baseline pulmonary function studies and SACE activity are obtained at the time of diagnosis. Pulmonary function studies are repeated only if the patient becomes breathless or progresses to stages II or III. SACE is measured at each visit, since this is an inexpensive and easily performed blood test that gives real-time information concerning the activity of the granulomatous inflammation.

Patients in stages II or III are seen at three-month intervals. All who show no spontaneous improvement or progress during a three- to six-month period of observation are considered as candidates for prednisone treatment, usually beginning at 40 mg on alternate days or increased to 60 mg on alternate days if there is no improvement. Pulmonary function studies, including diffusing capacity for carbon monoxide and SACE activity, are obtained at time of diagnosis and each follow-up visit. Hemoglobin and WBC counts are also taken. If the patient has hypercalcemia or hyperglycemia, one should obviously measure serum calcium and fasting plasma glucose. If the composite clinical and laboratory picture shows improvement and if the SACE has been suppressed within the normal range or significantly below baseline levels, the dose of prednisone can be progressively reduced by 10 mg at each three-month follow-up visit. Evidence of reactivation is met by an increase in the dose to the previously effective level, and the follow-up sequence is repeated. While three fourths of patients become inactive with one standard course (approximately 15 months), others may require extended treatment for up to many years. It is important to individualize treatment based on the activity of the inflammatory component. In my view, SACE activity measurements provide the least expensive, most easily obtained method of assessing such activity. Much recent publicity has been given to bronchoalveolar lavage and gallium-67 citrate lung scanning as tools to assess inflammatory activity, but in my opinion these should at present be considered research tools and not a part of the routine management of patients with sarcoidosis.

After completion of a course of prednisone treatment, follow-up is conducted at increasingly extended intervals, e.g., every six months. If the patient is stable one year after stopping prednisone, it is likely the disease has been arrested. Nevertheless, yearly examinations for up to five years after treatment are reasonable to detect cases with very subtle, smoldering inflammatory activity.

PREVENTIVE MEASURES

As there is no known cause of sarcoidosis, there are no known specific preventive measures, but some measures related to pulmonary disease in general can be helpful. Patients should be warned not to smoke. The use of antipneumococcal and influenza vaccines is reasonable, particularly for patients having significant irreversible fibrosis and chronic breathlessness or cough. For such patients, antimicrobial agents such as tetracycline, amoxicillin, or trimethoprim/sulfamethoxazole should also be prescribed for intercurrent lower respiratory tract infections. Familial occurrences of sarcoidosis are recorded, but are rare. Families should be informed of the noncontagious nature of the disease and the unlikelihood of coincident occurrence among blood relatives.

SOCIOECONOMIC ASPECTS OF MANAGEMENT

Individuals with sarcoidosis can usually be managed in an outpatient setting. The relative economic costs should therefore be small compared with those for patients with chronic obstructive airway disease and emphysema, who may require more frequent hospitalizations. Because of low incidence of sarcoidosis (11 to 71 cases per 100,000 in the United States), the total treatment bill nationally should be quite small. Nevertheless, if patients are not properly diagnosed, evaluated, and treated, there is the potential for irreversible fibrosis with consequent respiratory impairment, leading to increased hospital and human costs. The early investment of expertise with appropriate laboratory aids can lead to overall savings.

REFERENCES

DeRemee RA: The present status of treatment of pulmonary sarcoidosis: a house divided. Chest 71:388–393, 1977.

DeRemee RA, Rohrbach MS: Serum angiotensin-converting enzyme activity in evaluating the clinical course of sarcoidosis. Ann Intern Med 92:361–365, 1980.

James DG, Williams WJ: Sarcoidosis and Other Granulomatous Disorders. W. B. Saunders Co, Philadelphia, 1985.

Sharma OP: Sarcoidosis: Clinical Management. Butterworths, London, 1984.

9 · PNEUMOCONIOSES AND ENVIRONMENTAL LUNG DISEASE

Edward M. Cordasco
Muzaffar Ahmad
CLEVELAND CLINIC FOUNDATION

DEFINITION AND DIAGNOSTIC CRITERIA

PNEUMOCONIOSIS

Inhalation of inorganic dust of respirable size results in pneumoconiosis. The inorganic dust may be fibrogenic, which is capable of causing a tissue reaction. Examples are silicosis, coalworker's pneumoconiosis, and asbestosis. Nonfibrogenic responses following inhalation of nonreactive dusts such as iron, tin, and barium result in benign pneumoconiosis and do not cause disability. High-risk jobs responsible for various pneumoconioses are summarized in Table 1.

Table 1. PNEUMOCONIOSES AND HIGH-RISK JOBS

Pneumoconiosis	Occupations at Risk
Silicosis	Tunneling, mining, quarrying, gold mining, foundry work, sandblasting, ceramics, granite mining
Coalworker's pneumoconiosis	Coal mining (at face of mine and transportation)
Asbestosis	Asbestos mining, insulation, textile manufacturing, construction and ship building, repair of gaskets, brake linings and clutches
Berylliosis	Processing and handling of beryllium compounds, aerospace industry, manufacture of gyroscopes and nuclear reactors

HYPERSENSITIVITY PNEUMONITIS

Disorders produced by inhalation of organic material are classified as allergic alveolitis or hypersensitivity pneumonitis and have an immunologic mechanism. These include farmer's lung (from *Thermoactinomyces* and *Micropolyspora faeni*), and bagassosis (from *Thermoactinomyces sacchari*). Hypersensitivity pneumonitis also results from exposure to contaminated mushrooms, grain, cheese, and hay, all of which are common in farm communities. Individuals living adjacent to or just visiting farms can acquire these illnesses.

OCCUPATIONAL ASTHMA

Occupational asthma results from inhalation of organic materials, even though some varieties, such as toluene diisocyanate–related asthma, may have potent pharmacologic mechanisms.

Environmental and occupational asthmas are associated with urban areas and primarily originate from the chemical and plastic industries, but can also be of domestic origin. This problem has multiplied enormously in the past few years. Some agents presently used in industry capable of evoking this type of asthma include detergent enzymes, urea formaldehyde, cotton dust, and paint solvents and thinners such as epoxy resins and toluene diisocyanate. The last-named substance is used in the manufacture of rubber compounds and foam materials. City dwellers living near plastic and chemical plants may become ill through exposure to high concentrations of these agents coupled with the direction and velocity of wind flow. Individuals may also become ill at home while using plastic and paint compounds in hobbycrafts.

ACUTE INTERSTITIAL PNEUMONITIS

Acute interstitial pneumonitis is a serious occupational lung disease that also has environmental causes. The most common causes of industrial interstitial pneumonitis are hafnium, niobium, tungsten (cobalt carbide), polyvinyl chloride (plasticizers), and polypropylene. Polyvinyl chloride (PVC) is one of the major plastics used in the auto industry and in hospitals, as a main component in various kinds of tubing. Plastic wrap films and photocopying films are also made from PVC. It is an outstanding component of many finished products and as such is a superb chemical compound. These agents may cause toxicity or adverse hypersensitivity in persons exposed to PVC dust, fumes, or decomposition products of PVC plasticizers that result from thermal decomposition of these materials. Such products can disseminate into the ambient atmosphere and endanger community health.

To produce lung disease of environmental origin, a potentially toxic inhalant must be capable of reaching the lower respiratory tract in the range of 1 to 10 μ in size (maximal 0.5 to 5 μ), be deposited or absorbed by the bronchial or alveolar epithelial surface membranes, and be retained long enough to produce specific injury. Irritant gases, fumes, and smoke are also causes of environmental lung disease and are likely to result in direct alveolar and endothelial cell damage.

New environmental lung diseases are turning up at the rate of several per year, primarily owing to the introduction of a vast number of new industrial processes and to the increased necessity of chemical dump sites (landfills). With the advent of prominent government agencies exhibiting a regulatory effect on industrial health in the past few years, labor force, management, and the public itself are now conspicuously aware of occupational and community health hazards. Moreover, newer chemical compounds, particularly of the hydrocarbon group, are having a major national impact on community health, as exemplified by crises in New York, North Carolina, Michigan, and Missouri involving massive toxic chemical landspills.

Community-acquired toxic gas from massive gas tank explosions or leaks in industrial cities may involve several hundred people near the specific industrial complex. This has been reported as acute chlorine gas intoxication from spontaneous or accidental explosions in some cities. One such explosion in New York State in 1975 resulted in three deaths, and approximately 150 individuals had acute toxic reactions.

Accidental spread of potentially toxic gas and solid chemicals has been reported in various cities throughout the U.S., particularly in Michigan, North Carolina, and Ohio. Agents involved included nitrogen dioxide, phosphene, hydrogen sulfide, hydrochloric acid, phosphorus pentoxide, and polychlorinated biphenyls. Horrendous chemical disasters occurred in Mexico and India in 1984; the accident in India caused over 2000 deaths, many victims being urban dwellers living adjacent to the industrial complex. Petrochemicals and hydrogen cyanide gas were the offending agents in these two catastrophes. The list of occupational lung diseases should also include lung cancer (Section V, Chap. 21).

CLINICAL ASPECTS

The most important factor in the evaluation of an occupation-related lung disease is getting a thorough work history. This must be detailed and specific and usually requires that the physician invest a significant amount of time with the patient. All jobs, beginning with the very first one, should be chronologically listed. There should be a precise description of the job activity and a listing of all materials the patient habitually handles or is exposed to at work. Duration and intensity of exposure to every material and the protective measures taken must be documented. Information should be obtained about any examination (if offered by the industry) including lung function testing and x-rays. It is also very important to document the relationship between severity of symptoms and absence from work, especially during weekends and vacations. The exact identification of the suspected hazardous material and

information about its toxicity are of paramount importance to a diagnosis of occupational pulmonary disease.

There are no classical symptoms or signs in pneumoconiosis. Early silicosis, for example, may produce no symptoms except for recurrent respiratory infections. Symptoms may range from those of chronic bronchitis (cough and sputum) to severe dyspnea on exertion, depending on the extent of involvement. Cor pulmonale may develop in patients with far-advanced silicosis and may be manifested by weight gain, peripheral edema, and a congested liver. The usual exposure ranges from three to six years in acute silicosis, to 20 to 40 years in chronic silicosis. Coalworker's pneumoconiosis, on the other hand, usually requires 10 to 12 years of exposure. Cough with expectoration is a common symptom, especially among smokers. In asbestosis, the characteristic symptom is dyspnea on exertion, usually accompanied by a nonproductive cough. Radiographic appearance in pneumoconiosis is one of rounded regular opacities varying from 1 to 10 mm with predominant distribution in the upper and mid-lung fields. Silica and coal dust produce this characteristic appearance. These nodules can coalesce and produce large, rounded opacities, especially when complicated by tuberculosis. The phenomenon is observed in conglomerate silicosis and in progressive massive fibrosis. Lower lobe irregular linear opacities due to pulmonary fibrosis are characteristic of asbestosis. In asbestosis, pleural disease may be present and is an extremely useful aid to diagnosis. Pleural plaques with calcification may be quite marked and effusions may occasionally be observed even in the absence of mesotheliomas. The radiographic findings in chronic berylliosis usually consist of regularly distributed, diffuse, fine granularity in both lungs. Hilar nodes may be slightly enlarged and linear patterns may develop that proceed to contraction of involved lung tissue and hyperlucency of adjacent areas. Pneumothorax as a result of cyst formation is not uncommon.

Pulmonary function studies can vary greatly, depending on the degree of involvement and smoking history, from normal lung function in a nonsmoker with simple silicosis to a severe obstructive and restrictive ventilatory defect. The extent of obstructive changes usually depends on other factors, especially smoking in relation to silica exposure. Conglomerate silicosis is usually associated with severe airway obstruction. The same statements are generally true of other pneumoconioses with the exception of berylliosis, in which the characteristic finding is a reduction in diffusing capacity and a restrictive ventilatory defect resulting from extensive distribution of granuloma in the interstitium.

MANAGEMENT

There is no specific treatment for most pneumoconioses. Management involves prevention and control of exposure to noxious substances. In the case of silicosis, high exposures must be avoided by use of respiratory protection (e.g. respirator mask or self-contained breathing apparatus [SCBA]), improved ventilation (improved air circulation with fans, window vents, etc.), and wet techniques for dust suppression. Once silicosis is established, further exposure must be avoided. The effects of exposure should be monitored by serial chest x-rays; when the disease is simple, no further measures may be required. Aluminum dust has been inhaled in the past to prevent progression of silicosis, but its value has not been established. Specific therapy in silicosis is directed at complications. In patients with conglomerate silicosis, prophylactic treatment with antituberculosis chemotherapy, i.e., isoniazid, is indicated if tests are tuberculin positive in a daily dose of 100 to 300 mg. The proper duration of prophylactic treatment has not been determined, but one year is adequate in most cases. In severe conglomerate silicosis, life-long prophylaxis may be indicated at the same dosage. Clinically active tuberculosis requires a multiple drug regimen based on established principles of therapy, which may have to be modified by antibiotic sensitivity studies if acid-fast bacilli are recovered on culture. Treatment should include at least two drugs for 18 to 24 months; however, concomitant use of rifampin and isoniazid may shorten this period.

In smokers, airway obstruction may be the prominent symptomatic feature of the disease. Smoking should be completely discontinued and bronchodilator therapy instituted. We prefer a theophylline compound, preferably long-acting, to maintain a therapeutic level. Bronchodilatation is supplemented with a beta-agonist. A selective beta-agonist is most appropriate and albuterol (Proventil or Ventolin), two inhalations every four to six hours through a metered dose device, should suffice. Patients should be instructed how to use the device; those having trouble with coordination should be given a spacer device. Respiratory infections should be treated aggressively. Sputum cultures are not necessary in most cases unless a new infiltrate is visualized on chest x-ray. Ampicillin, tetracycline, or erythromycin in a seven- or ten-day course is an effective treatment for an infectious exacerbation. Patients with cor pulmonale should be treated with diuretics, salt restriction, and continuous low-flow oxygen. Arterial blood gas measurements are necessary for assessment of hypoxemia and we recommend use of oxygen when the PaO_2 is 60 mm Hg or below. A level of oxygen in the mid-60's is adequate and can be provided conveniently with supplemental oxygen at home via nasal prongs with an FiO_2 of 24% to 28%. Gaseous oxygen, liquid oxygen, or a membrane oxygenator may be used as the source. Continuous oxygen, defined as use of oxygen for at least 18 out of 24 hours, has been shown to affect both morbidity and mortality favorably in hypoxemic chronic obstructive lung disease. The same beneficial effect can also be expected in patients with silicosis and air flow limitation leading to significant hypoxemia. Prevention of infection is also important and is accomplished via influenza vaccination every fall and a one-time administration of pneumococcal vaccine.

As with silicosis, there is no specific treatment for coalworker's pneumoconiosis. Patients should be advised to cease exposure either through transfer to the outside or by leaving the industry. Just as in silicosis, one treats only complications. Patients who are positive reactors and those with established tuberculosis should have the same treatment as silicosis patients. Air flow obstruction and cor pulmonale need the same measures, with emphasis on continuous low-flow oxygen in the presence of resting hypoxemia.

ASBESTOSIS

Asbestosis has no specific treatment. The most important complication is the development of lung cancer, since 50% of patients with asbestosis die from lung cancer. Asbestos exposure should be eliminated or reduced to the lowest level technically achievable. Periodic surveillance of asbestos exposure should include a respiratory questionnaire, a chest x-ray, and lung function studies. Any new roentgenographic density should be pursued and a neoplasm ruled out whenever possible. It is extremely important for asbestos workers to completely discontinue smoking since cigarettes greatly increase the risk of lung cancer. As in other pneumoconioses, air flow obstruction should be handled via bronchodilators, and hypoxemia, when present, with continuous low-flow oxygen to optimize the cardiopulmonary status.

CHRONIC BERYLLIOSIS

Chronic berylliosis is thought to be a hypersensitivity phenomenon and is treated with corticosteroids. The idea is to diminish inflammatory exudations and edema and to limit the progression of the granulomatous process. The rationale for the use of steroids is based on the clinical impression of improvement following steroid therapy. We treat these patients in the same manner as those with sarcoidosis. An initial dose of prednisone in an adult of average weight is a single 60-mg dose daily, maintained for six to eight weeks and gradually tapered, depending on radiographic and clinical pulmonary function response. In four to six months, the drug is usually tapered and maintained at a daily single dose of 10 mg. Respiratory infections are treated aggressively; cor pulmonale is treated in the usual manner, along with administration of continuous oxygen in the hypoxemic patient.

Treatment of the hypersensitivity pneumonitis group consists primarily of removal of the offending material, use of corticosteroids, and administration of oxygen when varying degrees of hypoxia are manifest. The more modernized ventilated silos have markedly reduced the incidence of silo-filler's disease, a nitrogen dioxide pneumonitis. General improvement in public health education has also reduced the incidence of farm-acquired problems.

ENVIRONMENTAL ASTHMA

Environmental asthma is treated primarily with bronchodilators and cromolyn sodium inhalation. The latter therapy is used primarily as a prophylactic taken before entering the work environment, thereby preventing recurrence of symptoms. Corticosteroids are employed in more severely ill patients. Beta$_2$-agonists (such as metaproterenol, salbutamol, and fenoterol) play a major role in therapy. In our opinion, theophylline alone is not quite as effective, but adequate data for a comparison of these two types of bronchodilators are still not available. The monitoring of industrial hygiene in and around the occupation site and analysis of atmospheric pollution by public health personnel are of paramount importance to maintain a safe community. Periodic monitoring of the workplace is essential, and when a substance known to be hazardous is used, all efforts must be directed toward keeping atmospheric concentrations below the threshold limit (TLV) level, to prevent adverse health effects upon the general public. When noxious gases or fumes are present, appropriate dust masks or respirators at work are usually beneficial. Adequate ventilation in and around the industrial complex is of utmost importance. Conversion to a different chemical or mechanical process may be necessary.

Management of severe toxic pulmonary edema requires urgent treatment, consisting of high-flow oxygen, usually with positive end-expiratory pressure; endotracheal intubation in most cases with ventilatory therapy (assist-control ventilation); the addition of corticosteroids in the most overwhelming cases; broad-spectrum antibiotics to combat secondary bronchitis and bronchiolitis; and, in specific instances, blocking agents such as has hexamethylenetetramine (HMT), which has been efficacious in phosgene intoxication.

PREVENTIVE MEASURES

Since there is no specific therapy, preventive measures in pneumoconiosis are of extreme importance. Environmental standards for silica exposure are regulated by the Department of Labor for both mining and general industry. Carborundum shot or substitute materials obtained from coal slag can be used and should markedly reduce the risk of respiratory disease. Exhaust ventilation can reduce exposure, and properly fitted and maintained air supply respirators are of utmost importance in protecting exposed individuals. Annual surveillance of high-risk jobs is essential and there should be a cooperative program of prevention by industry, labor, and government in all areas of major occupational exposure.

The Coal Mine Health and Safety Act of 1969 was the landmark legislation that provided the means to control and prevent coalworker's pneumoconiosis. The act mandated a respirable dust standard of 3 mg/m^3, to be reduced in two years to 2 mg/m^3. Compliance with the new dust standard was quickly accomplished in a high proportion of mining sections. The only opportunity for intervention in coalworker's pneumoconiosis exists before the disease has progressed to a severe or complicated state. Therefore, whenever simple pneumoconiosis is diagnosed, further exposure must be avoided. The current OSHA standard for asbestos exposure is 2 fibers/cubic foot/hr. The National Institute for Occupational Safety and Health has recently recommended reducing this exposure to an eight-hour exposure limit of 0.1 fiber/cubic foot/hr and elimination of all but essential use of asbestos. Processing of asbestos in a wet form has been effective in many plants, and exhaust ventilation is another valuable control technology during exposure from cutting and weaving asbestos. High-efficiency vacuum cleaners and proper disposal of asbestos waste are also vital factors.

An important aspect of management of patients with pneumoconiosis and environmental lung disease is proper counseling and education. Time spent with the patient discussing the pathogenesis and mechanisms of the disease and possible complications go a long way to ensure patient compliance and ease of follow-up. A strong effort should be made to help the patient discontinue smoking, to improve air flow obstruction and reduce the risk of cancer, especially in asbestosis. Disability evaluation for the purpose of compensation is important and should be carried out under optimal laboratory and radiographic conditions within Federal guidelines.

All hospitals, university centers, and clinics should

Table 2. PROPHYLACTIC MEASURES FOR TOXIC CHEMICALS

1. Stringent Federal control acts regarding toxic substance review and surveillance should be initiated and rigorously enforced. Enforcement should include periodic review by Federal inspectors without prior announcement.
2. Toxic chemical drums, tanks, and other containers should be labeled appropriately.
3. Adequate preparatory evacuation plans should be drawn up between the community and industry in each heavily industrialized city.
4. Good communications with city fire departments should be mandatory.
5. The work force should be educated on a continuous basis by industrial safety and health personnel regarding appropriate handling, bagging, transporting, and discharge of toxic substances.
6. The occupational environment should be monitored frequently by diligent, capable industrial hygienists.
7. Ambient air pollutants should be monitored on a daily basis by public health–pollution control engineers and physicians.

have occupational and/or environmental departments as specific medical units to initiate and conduct many of the programs listed in Table 2. These units should work closely with county and city health departments and private occupational health centers to assist in the management of serious emergency public health problems.

REFERENCES

Council on Scientific Affairs: A physician's guide to asbestos-related diseases. JAMA 252:2593–2597, 1984.

Fraser RG, Pare JAP: The pneumoconioses and chemically-induced lung diseases. *In* Diagnosis of Diseases of the Chest, 2nd ed. W. B. Saunders Co, Philadelphia, 1979, pp 1475–1570.

White RP, Cordasco EM: Occupational asthma: a frequently overlooked entity. IM—Internal Medicine for the Specialist 3:90–100, 1982.

Ziskind M, Jones RN, Weill H: State of the art: silicosis. Am Rev Respir Dis 113:643–665, 1976.

10 · INTERSTITIAL LUNG DISEASE

David C. Webb-Johnson
LAHEY CLINIC MEDICAL CENTER

DEFINITION AND DIAGNOSTIC CRITERIA

The interstitial lung diseases are a group of different and often fatal disorders that diffusely affect the lung parenchyma. They are termed interstitial because thickening and inflammatory cell infiltration of the alveolar wall occur, but the small airways, blood vessels, and (as in alveolar proteinosis and desquamative interstitial pneumonia) alveolar spaces themselves may also be affected.

PATHOPHYSIOLOGY

The common denominator of interstitial lung diseases is eventual fibrosis of the interstitium. More than 140 different types have been identified. The cause is known in about 35% of these, including inorganic (silicosis, asbestosis, talcosis, berylliosis) and organic (farmer's lung, bagassosis, sequoiosis) dust diseases. Interstitial lung disease can be caused by exposure to gases (sulfur dioxide, chlorine); drugs; poisons, such as paraquat; radiation; viral, bacterial, and fungal infections; uremia; and pulmonary edema. Approximately 65% of interstitial lung diseases have no known cause.

CLINICAL ASPECTS

Patients present with breathlessness and often with nonproductive cough. On physical examination they usually have bibasilar end-inspiratory dry crackles and may have cyanosis and clubbing of the fingers and toes. Chest radiography shows a wide variety of patterns but usually demonstrates a diffuse reticulonodular infiltrate throughout both lung fields, progressing eventually to diffuse fibrosis and honeycomb lung. Mediastinal adenopathy is common only in sarcoidosis, silicosis, tuberculosis, and fungal infection. Sarcoidosis often affects the upper lobes, whereas idiopathic interstitial pneumonitis and asbestosis usually affect the lower zones. Spontaneous pneumothorax is most often seen with eosinophilic granuloma.

Pulmonary function tests show a purely restrictive pattern (although sarcoidosis often has a coexistent obstructive defect). In early restriction the only abnormality is a reduced diffusing capacity on exercise. As the disease progresses the resting diffusion becomes abnormal, and hypoxemia develops on exercise. With further progression, lung volumes (total lung capacity, vital capacity) are reduced, followed by hypoxemia at rest with mild alveolar hyperventilation and chronic respiratory alkalosis. With further fibrosis, lung volumes become severely reduced. Next, severe hypoxemia leads to the development of pulmonary hypertension and eventual cor pulmonale. Finally, hypercapnia and respiratory failure supervene.

A careful and comprehensive history is essential. This should include all past and present occupations, all environmental exposures, all drugs taken, any history of previous malignant or collagen disease, any exposure to radiation, and any relevant family history.

Laboratory tests include a complete blood count; urinalysis to determine the presence of vasculitis or Goodpasture's syndrome; protein electrophoresis and immunoelectrophoresis; tests for rheumatoid factor and antinuclear antibody; measurement of muscle enzymes to rule out myositis; fungal complement fixation titer determination; tuberculin skin test with tests for anergy and serum and urine calcium; and perhaps a measurement of angiotensin-converting enzyme. If organic dust disease is suspected, hypersensitivity precipitins should be ordered. Sputum cytology may show malignant cells in lymphangitic carcinoma, ferruginous bodies in asbestosis, or occasionally a causal organism in infection.

MANAGEMENT

To treat interstitial lung disease, a specific diagnosis must be made. Most patients respond to prednisone, but tuberculosis, fungal infections, and alveolar proteinosis are worsened by steroid agents, whereas amyloidosis and most pneumoconioses are unaffected.

Idiopathic Interstitial Pneumonitis (Cryptogenic Fibrosing Alveolitis)

DEFINITION AND DIAGNOSTIC CRITERIA

First described as a rapidly fatal condition in the 1930s by Hamman and Rich, idiopathic interstitial pneumonitis (cryptogenic fibrosing alveolitis) is now known to range from a chronic process that may remain stable over years to one that progresses rapidly to irreversible pulmonary fibrosis. For interstitial pneumonitis to qualify as truly "idiopathic" or "cryptogenic," known causes, such as asbestosis, radiation treatment, drug reactions, exposure to toxic fumes, and collagen vascular disease, must be excluded. The diagnosis can rarely be made on transbronchial biopsy, but open lung biopsy is almost always needed.

In 1965, Liebow and others described desquamative interstitial pneumonia (DIP), in which the alveolar wall or interstitium was relatively normal but prominent desquamation of alveolar cells into the alveolar space occurred. Usual interstitial pneumonitis (UIP) may also show desquamated cells, but the principal pathologic finding is a chronic inflammatory cell infiltrate (lymphocytes, plasma cells, histiocytes) in the alveolar walls with varying degrees of fibrosis.

More recently, idiopathic interstitial pneumonitis has been further divided, depending on the predominant inflammatory cell or the site of inflammation. In a few patients a component of bronchiolitis obliterans occurs in conjunction with UIP, which is termed bronchiolitic interstitial pneumonitis or bronchiolitis obliterans organizing pneumonia. This appears to carry a better prognosis than UIP alone. In giant cell interstitial pneumonia, numerous large, multinucleate giant cells appear, mainly in the alveolar spaces. The disease responds poorly to steroids and leads to death from progressive interstitial fibrosis. Lymphocytic interstitial pneumonia affects principally the lower lobes, with an interstitial infiltrate consisting mainly of mature lymphocytes plus a few plasma cells and histiocytes. It must be distinguished from pseudolymphoma, a more localized condition, and lymphoma of the lung, in which invasion of pleura or blood vessels may occur. Dysproteinemia with an increase or decrease in gamma globulin occurs in up to two thirds of patients. Sjögren's syndrome and the eventual development of lymphoma are often seen. The prognosis for lymphocytic interstitial pneumonia is better than that for UIP because it responds more favorably to corticosteroids.

PATHOPHYSIOLOGY

The cause of idiopathic interstitial pneumonitis is unknown but available evidence points to an immune basis. Low titers of rheumatoid factor in the serum are found in 10% to 20% of patients, and antinuclear antibodies are detected in up to 40%. The histologic picture is indistinguishable from that of lungs involved by collagen vascular disease. Circulating immune complexes and the deposition of immunoglobulins in alveolar walls have been shown in some patients with DIP.

Bronchoalveolar lavage fluid contains an increased number of neutrophils, contrasted with the increase in lymphocytes in patients with sarcoidosis and chronic hypersensitivity pneumonitis, both granulomatous forms of alveolitis. More than 10% of neutrophils in lavage fluid of patients with interstitial infiltrates suggests a diagnosis of idiopathic pulmonary fibrosis or asbestosis.

CLINICAL ASPECTS

Idiopathic interstitial pneumonitis occurs in either sex at any age but is most common in patients between 40 and 70 years old. In early disease, findings on physical examination may be normal, but later dry "Velcro" crackles are heard at first over the lower lung fields and increasingly higher as the disease progresses. Clubbing of the fingers and occasionally of the toes is seen in 60% to 70% of patients, whereas this is uncommon in other forms of pulmonary fibrosis, except asbestosis. Symptoms are typical of any interstitial disease, with increasing dyspnea, dry cough, and eventual fatigue, anorexia, weight loss, and sometimes arthralgia. In up to 10% of patients with biopsy-proved interstitial lung disease, there are normal findings on chest radiography. Most of these have a positive gallium scan, but a negative finding on gallium scan does not exclude disease. Pulmonary function testing shows classic restrictive changes, with exercise hypoxemia and a reduced diffusing capacity preceding reductions in lung volumes.

MANAGEMENT

Any previous chest radiographs must be obtained. Chronic findings that remain unchanged over several years suggest stable fibrosis and make further diagnostic work-up unnecessary. A tuberculin skin test is helpful, and any sputum produced should be smeared and cultured for acid-fast and fungal organisms. Patients with active disease as shown by gallium scan, bronchoalveolar lavage, progression on chest radiography, or worsening symptomatology require a tissue diagnosis. Lung biopsy is the most important diagnostic and prognostic procedure in the management of idiopathic pulmonary fibrosis. Open biopsies are taken ideally from two sites away from the lingula, which frequently shows nonspecific changes. An area that appears macroscopically normal and one that is minimally involved are chosen because many different interstitial diseases look the same once the advanced fibrotic stage is reached.

The short-term goal of treatment is to improve dyspnea and cough; the long-term goal is to suppress alveolitis and therefore prevent pulmonary fibrosis. A favorable overall response occurs in only about one third of patients with UIP. Steroids appear to decrease production of immune complexes, depress infiltration of neutrophils and lymphocytes into the lung tissue, inhibit secretion of chemotactic factors and enzymes from macrophages, and reduce adhesion of neutrophils

to endothelial surfaces. Hospitalization is usually indicated only for open lung biopsy. Diffusing capacities, vital capacity, chest radiographs, arterial blood gases, gallium scans, and even bronchoalveolar lavage can all be obtained on an outpatient basis. Corticosteroid treatment is with oral agents, usually prednisone, in a single daily dose because alternate-day therapy is probably not as effective. We use prednisone, 1 mg/kg (60 to 80 mg) daily for six weeks, and then reduce this slowly (2.5 to 5 mg each week) until a daily maintenance dose of 0.25 mg/kg (around 15 to 20 mg) is reached. Others would use up to 1.5 mg/kg per day (not exceeding 120 mg/day) initially. If the alveolitis clears on gallium scan or bronchoalveolar lavage, the dose of prednisone can be tapered and stopped; if the alveolitis remains stable, the maintenance dose is continued. If lung disease progresses with the patient receiving low doses of prednisone, a high-dose trial of prednisone for six weeks can be attempted, or cyclophosphamide (Cytoxan) or azathioprine (Imuran) can be added. Patients receiving prednisone therapy should be reevaluated after six to eight weeks and subsequently at three-month intervals.

Serious side effects from steroid therapy are common. These include increased appetite and weight gain, which may affect vital capacity or blood oxygen tension. Fluid retention, hyperglycemia or frank diabetes, depression, hyperexcitability or actual psychosis, osteoporosis with compression fractures, peptic ulcer disease, and ischemic necrosis of hip joints are all possible side effects. Immunosuppression can lead to opportunistic infection, and any severe worsening observed on chest radiography may require repeat biopsy. Other side effects include hypertension, hypokalemia, poor wound healing, cataracts, glaucoma, phlebitis, hirsutism, ecchymosis, pancreatitis, pseudotumor cerebri, and myopathy. Informed consent must be obtained from the patient before treatment with steroids is initiated.

Cyclophosphamide is given in a dose of 2 mg/kg per day and controlled by blood counts. Azathioprine, 3 mg/kg per day, can be used but can give rise to fever, diarrhea, and skin rash. When the patient does not respond to prednisone alone, either drug can be added in a single daily dose, preferably with prednisone, 15 to 20 mg daily, and treatment continued for six to nine months.

The possibility of secondary malignancies arising after treatment with cyclophosphamide must be considered. Leukopenia is an expected effect of the drug and is used as a guide to therapy. The WBC count is monitored twice weekly for the first month, then weekly until stable, and thereafter every two weeks. The dose of cyclophosphamide is adjusted to keep the total WBC count above 3500/mm³ and the total neutrophil count above 1500/mm³. Sterile hemorrhagic cystitis can also result from cyclophosphamide administration and can be severe and even fatal. Ample fluid intake and frequent voiding help to prevent this, but urinalysis should be performed weekly. If microscopic hematuria develops, the drug should be stopped and only restarted at a lower dose after the urine has cleared. Gonadal suppression with amenorrhea or azoospermia and impotence can be expected, and alopecia is common. Hypersensitivity pneumonitis and interstitial pulmonary fibrosis have been reported.

Interstitial Lung Disease and Rheumatoid Arthritis

DEFINITION AND DIAGNOSTIC CRITERIA

Rheumatoid arthritis may be complicated by a variety of pulmonary lesions, the classic syndromes being pleurisy with or without effusion, diffuse interstitial pneumonitis, necrobiotic or rheumatoid nodules, Caplan's syndrome (rheumatoid nodules associated with pneumoconiosis), and pulmonary vasculitis with or without pulmonary hypertension. Bronchiolitis obliterans has now been added to the list. These pulmonary syndromes may appear up to ten years before the arthritis.

CLINICAL ASPECTS

About 2% of patients with rheumatoid arthritis show an interstitial pattern on chest radiography, but 30% to 40% have a reduced diffusing capacity for carbon monoxide despite normal chest radiographs. Biopsy shows mild fibrosis. The degree of fibrosis bears no relationship to the activity of the arthritis. Clinically, dyspnea, dry cough, weakness, fever, and weight loss are the most common symptoms, and dry "Velcro" crackles may be heard. The lung disease tends to progress slowly over years and the ability of steroids to alter this downhill progression remains unproved. A presumptive clinical diagnosis can be made by a highly positive test for rheumatoid factor together with a compatible chest radiograph, which most often shows a reticulonodular infiltrate in the lower and middle lung zones. However, many different histologic patterns have been described, and open lung biopsy is preferable, both to confirm the diagnosis and to gauge prognosis. As we would expect, patients in whom biopsy shows rheumatoid nodules have the best prognosis. Patients with cellular interstitial pneumonia without much fibrosis, lymphoid hyperplasia, and bronchiolitis obliterans organizing pneumonia have a better prognosis than those with the pattern of UIP.

MANAGEMENT

In patients with dyspnea or progressively deteriorating lung function, we advise a trial of steroids. We give prednisone, 1 mg/kg per day for four weeks, and then reassess the patient. An increase in vital capacity of 10% or more, in arterial oxygen tension of 10 mm Hg or more, or in diffusing capacity of 20% or more over baseline studies constitutes a positive response. Unfortunately this is seen in less than 20% of all patients. If treatment is successful, prednisone should be decreased by 5 to 10 mg every two weeks to the minimal dose required to maintain improvement, usually 20 to 30 mg/day. Administration of steroids on alternate days is usually not helpful. If steroids are not successful, a trial of cyclophosphamide, 2 mg/kg per day, together with a low dose of prednisone, can be attempted, with scant hope of success. Because of the immunosuppressive effect of this combination of drugs, treatment should be interrupted or the dose modified if bacterial, fungal, or viral infections develop. Penicillamine therapy has been tried in rheumatoid lung disease but may itself be associated with an increased incidence of bronchiolitis obliterans.

Pulmonary vasculitis is rare and usually occurs in the setting of general systemic vasculitis. This should be more responsive to steroids, with or without cyclophosphamide, but response may still take up to three months. Treatment should continue for about one year after the vasculitis becomes inactive. If chest radiography, electrocardiography, or clinical evaluation suggests pulmonary hypertension, a trial of oxygen in patients who have hypoxemia has more chance of success than vasodilator therapy with agents such as hydralazine, nifedipine (Procardia), and phentolamine (Regitine).

Gold salts used to treat rheumatoid arthritis can produce a hypersensitivity pneumonitis with a histologic picture of UIP, diffuse alveolar damage, lymphoid hyperplasia, or bronchiolitis obliterans. One half of patients also have a fever or skin rash, and eosinophilia is often seen. Most patients recover slowly when the drug is stopped, but deaths have been reported. Prednisone, 1 mg/kg per day, should give improvement within two to four weeks, but should be continued at a minimal dose of 15 to 20 mg/day for at least four months and possibly longer because gold is retained in body tissues. Diagnosis is made from the temporal relationship of injections of gold to development of interstitial lung disease. Bronchoalveolar lavage shows an increase in the percentage of lymphocytes, whereas neutrophils are increased in rheumatoid lung disease. Methotrexate, also used to treat rheumatoid arthritis, produces a similar hypersensitivity pneumonitis, which responds more rapidly and requires a course of prednisone in a tapered dosage, starting at 1 mg/kg per day, over a three- to four-week period. Repeat challenge with the drug may not reproduce the disease.

Systemic Lupus Erythematosus

Involvement of the lungs or pleura occurs in 50% to 70% of patients with systemic lupus erythematosus, more frequently than in any other collagen vascular disease and with a female predominance of about 10:1. Pleuritis with or without effusion is the most common abnormality. The incidence of interstitial pneumonitis is controversial and depends on definition, because horizontal, bibasilar "line shadows" or platelike atelectasis are common, but progressive pulmonary fibrosis is rare.

Acute lupus pneumonitis may be a variant of interstitial pneumonitis and have a fulminant course, characterized by severe dyspnea, a cough with scant sputum, a fever up to 100° to 104°F, hypoxia, and bilateral alveolar filling patterns on chest radiography, typically radiating from the hila toward the lower lobes. Cultures of blood and sputum are negative, and biopsy shows a mononuclear cell infiltration with hyaline membranes and hemorrhagic pulmonary edema. Vasculitis is often present. Treatment is with prednisone, 1 mg/kg per day, and usually cyclophosphamide, 1.5 to 2 mg/kg per day, or azathioprine for about six weeks; the dose is then reduced to the minimum necessary to control the disease.

Linear fibrosis or platelike atelectasis requires no treatment. Diffuse interstitial fibrosis, which may progress to honeycomb lung, is seen in 2% to 3% of patients; management is principally supportive, but steroids may be needed. Death is usually the result of renal or CNS disease and not lung disease, unless pulmonary superinfection occurs. Drug-induced lupus affects the lung in up to 50% of patients, causing pleuritis, effusion, or pulmonary infiltration. These may improve spontaneously if the offending drug is stopped, but again a course of steroids may be required.

Polymyositis-Dermatomyositis

In 5% of patients with polymyositis-dermatomyositis, interstitial lung disease develops, which may precede the skin and muscle disease by up to 24 months. Response to corticosteroids is good if treatment is started early, especially in young patients and those with a cellular biopsy. Weakness of the pharyngeal muscles can cause aspiration pneumonia, and respiratory muscle weakness may produce hypoventilatory respiratory failure; pleural involvement has not been reported. Diagnosis rests on recognition of typical clinical features, presence of diffuse lung disease, and characteristic changes on electromyography and muscle biopsy, together with elevated levels of serum creatine kinase and serum aldolase.

Scleroderma (Progressive Systemic Sclerosis)

Interstitial lung disease is found eventually in more than 90% of patients with scleroderma. Recurrent aspiration pneumonitis from abnormal esophageal motility may complicate the picture. Scleroderma lung disease has the worst prognosis of all the collagen vascular diseases, the four- to five-year survival rate being only around 50%. Pulmonary hypertension may develop, independent of the degree of pulmonary fibrosis, from a vasculitis of the arterioles and capillaries of the lung. The incidence of lung cancer, especially alveolar cell carcinoma, is increased. Cystic lesions may occur. These are often subpleural and may give rise to pneumothorax if they rupture. A variable degree of pleuritis is seen in up to 30% of patients.

The diagnosis of scleroderma lung disease is made by typical skin changes. The antinuclear antibody test is positive in 30% to 80% of patients and typically is in a speckled pattern; rheumatoid factor may be present in 25% to 35%. Because patients with mixed connective tissue disease respond better to steroids, as do those with a so-called overlap syndrome, a blood test for extractable nuclear antigen should be obtained. An appreciable vasculitis is almost always present and can occur independently of pneumonitis or fibrosis. The gallium scan has been reported to be positive in as many as 70% of patients, suggesting active inflammation, but response to steroids remains poor. No evidence has shown any of the traditional therapies for interstitial lung disease to be of help in classic scleroderma lung disease.

Eosinophilic Granuloma

DEFINITION AND DIAGNOSTIC CRITERIA

First described in 1940 in bone and then associated with lung lesions, eosinophilic granuloma affects men more than women and occurs especially in the third and fourth decades of life. Chest radiography shows discrete, small pulmonary densities, especially in the upper lobe, or a reticulonodular pattern. Hilar adenopathy may be found, and a pneumothorax, uncommon in other interstitial lung diseases, may occur in 25% of patients. Definitive diagnosis is made by open lung biopsy. End-stage disease results in a typical honeycomb lung with fibrosis and cyst formation. On electron microscopy, intracytoplasmic rodlike structures or X bodies are seen; thus, bronchoalveolar lavage can provide a firm diagnosis and the need for open lung biopsy may be avoided in the future.

PATHOPHYSIOLOGY

Eosinophilic granuloma represents a relatively benign disease of bone, lung, and occasionally oropharynx, thyroid, hypothalamus, prostate, GI tract, or vulva. Hand-Schüller-Christian disease (a more severe multisystem disease in which diabetes insipidus and even panhypopituitarism are frequent) and Letterer-Siwe disease in infants share a similar histology. These three diseases together are called histiocytosis X. The pathogenesis is unknown, but immune complexes have been found in the serum of some patients with active disease.

CLINICAL ASPECTS

About one quarter of all patients present solely with an abnormal chest radiograph. Others may have a nonproductive cough, breathlessness, and less frequently chest pain, fatigue, malaise, weight loss, or fever. Eosinophilic granuloma is usually a mild disease in which spontaneous resolution is common, but it can progress to honeycomb lung, cor pulmonale, and eventual respiratory failure. Spontaneous regression may develop in 10% to 25% of patients within months of diagnosis.

MANAGEMENT

Corticosteroids are not particularly effective in suppressing the disease, but their use may improve the appearance of the chest radiograph and suppress inflammation until the disease stabilizes and burns out. All patients should be monitored with regular chest radiography and pulmonary function tests. Treatment should be started only if progression occurs, if vital capacity or diffusing capacity is less than 70% of predicted or the alveolar arterial oxygen gradient more than 35 mm Hg, or if symptoms are moderate or severe. Bone scans should be performed because bone lesions will eventually develop in 20% of patients; these are treated by curettage and local radiotherapy. Steroids may be tried in advanced fibrosis but with little hope of success. The dose of prednisone is around 1 mg/kg per day to a maximum of 80 mg for six to eight weeks, which in our experience may be adequate. The drug can either be tapered rapidly or reduced over three months to 15 mg on alternate days, this dose being maintained for six to nine months and then discontinued. If prednisone brings no response or if side effects are intolerable, second-line drugs such as penicillamine, 750 to 1000 mg/day, or antimetabolite agents such as vinblastine (Velban), can be tried.

Pulmonary Hemorrhagic Syndromes

Diffuse alveolar hemorrhage with hemoptysis (sometimes severe), anemia, and bilateral diffuse infiltrates on chest radiographs (often air bronchograms) can be seen in a number of diseases (Table 1). After repeated hemorrhages a reticular pattern can develop. Hemosiderin-loaded macrophages are seen in the sputum, bronchoalveolar lavage secretions, or gastric washings. Microscopic examination of lung tissue shows blood in the alveolar spaces and hemosiderin both in macrophages and in the extracellular space. On bronchoscopy no major bleeding site, but rather a diffuse "ooze," is seen. Pulmonary function tests show hypoxemia and decreased lung volumes. Diffusing capacity may be reduced or actually increased because of the presence of hemoglobin in the alveoli taking up carbon monoxide.

IDIOPATHIC PULMONARY HEMOSIDEROSIS

Idiopathic pulmonary hemosiderosis is a disease of children and young adults. It presents with occasional hemoptysis, which persists over many years, producing iron deficiency anemia and finally interstitial pulmonary

Table 1. DISEASES CAUSING DIFFUSE ALVEOLAR HEMORRHAGE

Goodpasture's syndrome
Idiopathic pulmonary hemosiderosis
Immune complex glomerulonephritis
Wegener's granulomatosis
Uremic pneumonitis
Acute necrotizing pneumonia
Acute lupus pneumonia
Mitral stenosis
Pulmonary veno-occlusive disease

fibrosis and cor pulmonale. Hepatosplenomegaly or adenopathy is found in 20% to 25% of patients. Diagnosis is by open lung biopsy to rule out Goodpasture's syndrome, which can at first be limited to the lung without renal involvement. Immunofluorescent stains in patients with idiopathic pulmonary hemosiderosis are negative.

Length of survival from onset of idiopathic pulmonary hemosiderosis is from 2½ to 20 years, but spontaneous remission is possible. In prospective controlled trials, no treatment altered the outcome of the disease. In patients with massive hemorrhage, hypoxemia should be relieved by oxygen administration through a mask. An endotracheal tube may be needed for suction, mechanical ventilation, or both. The anemia requires iron replacement and sometimes blood transfusion with a 40-μm filter in the line to remove any WBC aggregates. If respiratory failure occurs, the customary indications for mechanical ventilation apply.

The use of steroids is empiric, but in theory they can inhibit complement (C5a)-mediated intravascular granulocyte aggregation and the release of toxic oxygen radicals that damage endothelial cells. They also reduce inflammation and decrease vascular permeability. Methylprednisolone, 30 mg/kg, is given intravenously, as in the prevention of adult respiratory distress syndrome, and is changed to a maintenance dose of approximately 60 mg of prednisone per day when the crisis is over. This is continued for four weeks and then reduced to a dose sufficient to prevent relapse or fibrosis, usually 5 to 15 mg/day or 10 to 30 mg every other day for 18 months to two years. Young patients with active alveolitis probably respond best. Plasmapheresis can be tried in acute idiopathic pulmonary hemosiderosis but is less successful than in Goodpasture's syndrome. Cytotoxic drugs, such as azathioprine and 6-mercaptopurine (Purinethol), are reserved for patients with massive hemorrhage not responding to large doses of steroids.

GOODPASTURE'S SYNDROME

DEFINITION AND DIAGNOSTIC CRITERIA

Goodpasture's syndrome is characterized by pulmonary hemorrhage with hemoptysis, diffuse alveolar infiltrates, anemia, and glomerulonephritis, the last-named often rapidly progressive. In most patients, antiglomerular basement membrane antibodies are detected. The disease is most common in young, particularly white, men. Initially described as occurring after influenza, it may follow a minor respiratory infection or heavy exposure to hydrocarbons and clinically presents with cough, hemoptysis, and dyspnea, followed weeks to years later by proteinuria, hematuria, and renal failure. Some patients actually present with renal failure.

CLINICAL ASPECTS

The causes are unknown, but the syndrome is thought to be related to infectious or chemical injury to the capillary basement membranes in the lung and then in the kidney, which apparently share common basement membrane antigens. More than 80% of patients present with proteinuria, microscopic hematuria, and rarely pyuria. Renal failure requiring dialysis usually occurs within 12 to 14 months after onset, and iron deficiency anemia is present. The differential diagnosis includes vasculitis (Wegener's granulomatosis and polyarteritis nodosa), pulmonary edema, uremic lung, immune complex disease (systemic lupus erythematosus), and occult systemic mitral stenosis, which should be excluded by echocardiogram. A test for circulating antiglomerular basement membrane antibody in the blood is perhaps the best and least invasive method to obtain a diagnosis, but it may take several days before results are received.

MANAGEMENT

The prognosis is poor, with a median survival time of 15 weeks in several large series, about one half the patients dying of lung hemorrhage and one half of uremia. Reports of spontaneous remission and long-term survival are scattered. Emergency stabilization of diffuse pulmonary hemorrhage should be performed in a critical care unit with available ventilatory support. Anemia should be corrected by transfusion of packed red blood cells, using fresh-frozen plasma if clotting defects are demonstrated. Oxygen is given to raise arterial oxygen tension above 60 to 70 mm Hg, and emergency rigid bronchoscopy and lavage may be required. Corticosteroids may temporarily suppress pulmonary hemorrhage, and one dose of 100 to 150 mg of methylprednisolone should be given. Plasmapheresis to remove the circulating antiglomerular basement membrane antibody is the definitive treatment of choice; it may be life-saving if continued daily until pulmonary hemorrhage decreases and then given every other day to a minimum of six exchanges, but continuing until renal function has stabilized and antiglomerular basement membrane antibody levels in the blood are no longer detectable. Dangers of plasmapheresis include infection, loss of plasma proteins, and hypotension.

Fresh-frozen plasma, salt-free albumin, and saline are required to keep clotting parameters normal and albumin levels above 2.5 gm/dl. At the same time, daily administration of prednisone, 1 mg/kg, and cyclophosphamide, 3 mg/kg, or azathioprine, 1 to 2 mg/kg, is started to suppress further production of antiglomerular basement membrane antibody. Initial response to this treatment is good and relapse does not usually occur if prednisone and cyclophosphamide are continued. Treatment with bilateral nephrectomy, which was used in earlier years to control massive hemoptysis, should no longer be needed. The alveolar infiltrates clear slowly after hemorrhage stops and pulmonary fibrosis does not usually develop. When the disease is stable or after administration of a high dose of prednisone for six weeks, the dose can be reduced slowly to 15 to 20 mg/day and the cyclophosphamide dose kept between 2 and 5 mg/kg per day, using a WBC count of 3000 to 4000/mm³ and a neutrophil count of around 1500/mm³ to monitor the dose. Any flare-up of pulmonary or renal disease may require further plasmapheresis and full doses of immunosuppressants. Chronic renal failure develops in some patients despite this treatment.

Drug-Induced Lung Disease

Drug-induced lung disease is increasing as a major cause of morbidity and death, while the list of drugs

Table 2. DRUG-INDUCED PULMONARY DISEASE SYNDROMES

Aspiration
Hilar adenopathy and mediastinal widening
Hypoventilation and respiratory failure
Predisposition to pulmonary thromboembolism
Bronchospasm
Vasculitis
Pulmonary infiltrates with eosinophilia
Drug-induced lupus
Pulmonary edema
Interstitial fibrosis
Bronchiolitis obliterans

known to cause diffuse pulmonary damage grows longer. Several distinct syndromes have been described (Table 2).

Pulmonary edema has been attributed to the use of heroin, methadone, codeine, propoxyphene (Darvon), hydrochlorothiazide, chlordiazepoxide (Librium), ethchlorvynol (Placidyl), aspirin, phenylbutazone, nitrofurantoin, some chemotherapeutic agents, and blood transfusion (leukoagglutinins). This may produce an interstitial pattern on chest radiography, as may drug-induced lupus, which has been associated with at least 25 drugs, pulmonary manifestations occurring in 40% to 80% of patients. We are concerned here with drugs giving rise to diffuse interstitial pneumonitis and fibrosis. These include ganglion-blocking agents, methysergide (Sansert), gold salts, bleomycin (Blenoxane), chlorambucil, methotrexate, melphalan (Alkeran), cyclophosphamide, busulfan (Myleran), sulfasalazine, mitomycin (Mutamycin), and amiodarone (Cordarone). Nitrofurantoin can produce an acute pleuropulmonary reaction two hours to ten days after the drug is started, with fever, chills, dry cough, and dyspnea or pleuritic chest pain or both. One third of patients may have eosinophilia, and the reaction usually clears within two to four days after the drug is stopped. Steroids are helpful and should be used if symptoms are severe. The chronic reaction occurs after six months to six years of therapy and presents with insidious dry cough and dyspnea. Lung biopsy shows fibrosing alveolitis; reversibility is variable, steroids sometimes proving beneficial.

Busulfan causes pulmonary fibrosis after an average of 3½ years of therapy. Biopsy shows organizing interstitial infiltrates with bizarre type II pneumonocytes. Changes are usually irreversible, but discontinuation of the drug and the use of steroids can produce improvement. Bleomycin is the most common chemotherapeutic agent to result in pulmonary fibrosis, with an incidence of 3% when the total dose is less than 400 mg of bleomycin and up to 20% when the total dose is greater than 500 mg. Even a total dose of 60 mg has been reported to cause changes. Previous lung irradiation predisposes a patient to pulmonary involvement, as does administration of oxygen. Older patients are more susceptible to pulmonary fibrosis. The treatment is to stop the drug and, if necessary, to use steroids in a high dose, but the mortality rate is nevertheless around 10%. Early diagnosis improves the prognosis, and patients treated with this potentially toxic drug should be monitored with regular measurement of diffusing capacity.

Radiation Pneumonitis

DEFINITION AND DIAGNOSTIC CRITERIA

Patients vary greatly in the amount of pulmonary radiation they can withstand. When a dose of 200 rad daily is given five days a week, pneumonitis can occur after 2000 rad, is rare with less than 3000 rad, is common after 3500 rad, and always occurs with 4000 rad or more. With radiotherapy for carcinoma of breast, for example, radiographic manifestations of radiation pneumonitis occur in about 40% of patients and clinical manifestations in 11%.

CLINICAL ASPECTS

Symptoms of radiation pneumonitis usually begin gradually six to 12 weeks after completion of therapy, and occasionally are seen as early as four weeks after treatment. In general, the earlier the onset, the more severe is the disease. Symptoms include dry cough, dyspnea usually on exertion, limitation of full inspiration, and often fever. Infiltrates tend to have sharp margins that relate to the borders of the radiation port, so review of the treatment portal films is helpful in making the diagnosis. Pleural effusion sometimes occurs. The clinical course of radiation pneumonitis varies from days to weeks, clinical resolution usually taking place within a month. The radiographic picture may take longer to clear.

The late, chronic phase of radiation fibrosis may follow the acute pneumonitis or may develop insidiously in patients who have not had the acute reaction. Correlation between clinical symptoms of dyspnea and radiographic findings is poor. The process usually is completely stable after 12 to 18 months. Rarely, pneumonitis or fibrosis can occur outside the irradiated field, possibly from lymphatic obstruction, hypersensitivity reaction, previous use of chemotherapeutic agents, or coexisting opportunistic infection. Both the pneumonitis and fibrosis are aggravated by preexisting interstitial lung disease and by administration of oxygen and bleomycin. Steroids markedly increase tolerance to radiation, but the pneumonitis may occur four to eight weeks after steroids are stopped.

MANAGEMENT

Treatment of acute radiation pneumonitis is usually supportive and expectant. If symptoms are severe or the extent of lung involvement is extensive on radiographic examination, a trial of steroids is warranted, as these often dramatically improve radiation pneumonitis. Prednisone, 40 to 60 mg/day, is given PO each morning; this is reduced slowly by about 5 mg weekly or biweekly, because relapse is seen if steroids are withdrawn too rapidly. The typical patient requires treatment for 10 to 12 weeks, usually with not less than 15 to 20 mg/day of prednisone. If the pneumonitis flares up during withdrawal of steroids, the dose is increased again to 40 to 60 mg/day. Radiation fibrosis is unresponsive to treatment, and these patients usually require cough suppressants and oxygen for hypoxemia.

REFERENCES

Carrington CB, Gaensler EA, Coutu RE, et al: Natural history and treated course of usual and desquamative interstitial pneumonia. N Engl J Med 298:801–809, 1978.

Cherniack RM: Current Therapy in Respiratory Medicine 1984–1985. C.V. Mosby Co, St. Louis, 1984.

Crystal RG, Gadek JE, Ferrans VJ, et al: Interstitial lung disease: current concepts of pathogenesis, staging and therapy. Am J Med 70:542–568, 1981.

Hamman L, Rich AR: Fulminating diffuse interstitial fibrosis of lungs. Trans Am Clin Climatol Assoc 51:154–163, 1935.

Liebow AA, Steer A, Billingsley JG: Desquamative interstitial pneumonia. Am J Med 39:369–404, 1965.

Weinberger SE, Kelman JA, Elson NA, et al: Bronchoalveolar lavage in interstitial lung disease. Ann Intern Med 89:459–466, 1978.

11 · *TUBERCULOSIS AND TUBERCULOIDOSES*

David E. Williams
MAYO CLINIC AND MAYO FOUNDATION

DEFINITION AND DIAGNOSTIC CRITERIA

The term "tuberculosis" is now generally restricted to mean the infectious disease caused by the mammalian tubercle bacilli *Mycobacterium tuberculosis* and *M. bovis*. These two mycobacteria cause a contagious disease with public health implications. They can be isolated from the diseased animal, using laboratory culture media with similar techniques, and then can be reintroduced into animals to reproduce the disease (Koch's postulate). Since infections of *M. bovis* have become very rare in the North American continent in recent years, and disseminated disease from the attenuated strain of *M. bovis*, the bacillus of Calmette and Guérin (BCG), is also very rare, the term tuberculosis is used in the discussion that follows to refer to infections caused by *M. tuberculosis*.

Division of mycobacteria into the four groups tubercle bacilli, tuberculoid bacilli, saprophytic mycobacteria, and *M. leprae* appears more relevant for *clinical* use than the Runyon system, which divides tuberculoid bacilli and saprophytic mycobacteria into four groups based on *cultural* characteristics. The term "tuberculoidosis" suggested by Francis and Abrahams (1982) will be used to refer to infections caused by the "tuberculoid" bacilli in preference to earlier terms such as "atypical mycobacterial infections," "nontuberculosis mycobacterial infections," or "myocobacteria other than tuberculosis" (MOTT).

Tuberculosis

PATHOPHYSIOLOGY

INITIAL INFECTION

Following inhalation of tiny "droplet nuclei" containing mycobacteria, those reaching the alveolar level may be ingested by nonactivated macrophages, newly migrating into the area. The rate of multiplication of tubercle bacilli in macrophages is relatively slow and the earliest clinical manifestations of their presence are not evident for several weeks. Early dissemination occurs by means of lymphatics to regional lymph nodes and into the bloodstream.

The inhaled bacilli usually locate in the lower lung fields; if the site heals, it may undergo calcification, and the roentgenographic appearance is called a primary Ghon lesion. Calcification of this initial focus along with the involved regional (hilar) lymph nodes is referred to as the Ranke complex. Within the first few weeks, the tubercle bacilli may be seeded in many organs and tissues of the body. The bacilli replicate more readily in those tissues with higher oxygen levels, such as the metaphyseal ends of long bones, vertebral column, renal cortex, and lung (particularly the apex). Impaired clearance mechanisms related to decreased lymphatic flow in the lung apices may also explain the predilection of tubercular foci in the apical posterior segments of both lungs.

TUBERCULOUS DISEASE

Primary Infection. Up to 15% of infected persons are unable to contain tubercle bacilli in a dormant fashion. The bacilli replicate in the lungs or foci in other organs, and manifestations of active disease are noted. This may occur as the result of a large inoculant of infecting bacilli, or it may be related to rapid growth in a host with incomplete or impaired immune response such as a young child or persons with the acquired immune deficiency syndrome (AIDS), or in patients with certain orders involving lowered resistance such as silicosis, diabetes mellitus, postoperative gastrectomy, or diseases associated with immunosuppression by corticosteroids or other immunosuppressive drugs.

Reactivation. Reactivation or postprimary tuberculosis refers to the disease that occurs when dormant bacilli in infected persons begin to actively multiply. The most common clinical form of postprimary tuberculosis in the United States is seen in the elderly patient.

CLINICAL ASPECTS

PULMONARY

Although cavitation of pulmonary lesions is an uncommon event in primary tuberculosis, it is a common feature of progressive postprimary disease. It develops in a small patch of pneumonia, usually in the posterior or apical segment of an upper lobe or an apical segment of a lower lobe following reactivation of previously seeded hematogenous foci (Simon foci). The onset of dyspnea suggests the complication of spontaneous pneumothorax (particularly if onset is abrupt), pleural effusion, or miliary disease. Another worrisome symptom, hoarseness, suggests the highly contagious form—laryngeal tuberculosis.

Death can eventually occur from untreated progressive tuberculous pneumonia, with loss of lung either through direct pneumonic involvement or indirectly through obstruction of bronchi with caseous material or involved lymph nodes. Life-threatening hemorrhage poses a continuing hazard in untreated or incompletely treated patients.

In primary tuberculous infection in children, the pulmonary parenchymal involvement is often rather insignificant on roentgenographic examination, while the regional lymph nodes are greatly enlarged.

MILIARY

Hematogenous dissemination results in many tubercles of uniform size. These miliary lesions, so named because at 2 mm in size they resemble millet seeds, may occur in both lungs. If untreated, an acute respiratory distress syndrome may develop and rapidly lead to death.

Presentation of miliary tuberculosis may vary from an acute febrile onset in a child or younger adult, with a typical uniformly stippled pattern in the chest roentgenogram, to a more cryptic form in the older patient. It is more common in males, non-Caucasians, persons with some compromise in their immune competence (alcoholism, malignancy, diabetes, AIDS), or patients placed on steroids or given other immunosuppressive treatment.

EXTRAPULMONARY

For some years the number of cases of extrapulmonary tuberculosis reported in the United States has remained constant at approximately 4000 per year in spite of the fact that the number of cases of pulmonary tuberculosis has progressively declined. Although most extrapulmonary disease follows lymphohematogenous dissemination (e.g., miliary tuberculosis), direct extension from an adjacent structure (e.g., pericarditis from an adjacent involved lymph node) and conduit spread (e.g., tuberculosis of the lower urinary tract) may also occur.

CLASSIFICATION OF TUBERCULOSIS

Table 1 is an abbreviated summary of the five classes of tuberculosis infection accepted in the official American Thoracic Society (ATS) statement of 1980.

MANAGEMENT

PLAN

Short-Term and Long-Term Goals. The immediate objective for the individual recently diagnosed as having active tuberculosis is to treat the disease so as to decrease morbidity and eliminate mortality. For the public the objectives are to interrupt and prevent the transmission of tubercle bacilli. The longer-term goal is the eradication of tuberculosis in the U.S. To accomplish these aims, tuberculosis control is based on the principles of surveillance and containment. The reader is referred to a joint statement of the ATS and the Centers for Disease Control (CDC) in 1983.

Two important principles regarding screening for tuberculosis are (1) screen only when services are available for appropriate follow-up management for detected

Table 1. CLASSIFICATION OF TUBERCULOSIS

0. No tuberculosis exposure, not infected (no history of exposure, negative tuberculin skin test)
I. Tuberculosis exposure; no evidence of infection (history of exposure, negative tuberculin skin test)
II. Tuberculous infection, without disease (positive Mantoux, negative bacteriologic studies [if done], no clinical or roentgenographic findings compatible with tuberculosis)
III. Tuberculosis: infected, with disease (specify location, bacteriology, and chemotherapy status)
IV. Tuberculosis: No current disease but history and/or clinical finding(s) of previous disease
V. Tuberculosis suspect (diagnosis pending)

cases and (2) screen only those subpopulations where infection is more likely than in the general U.S. population, or where the presence of an individual with disease would pose a particular hazard to others (e.g., in child care facilities and newborn nurseries). Mass radiography of the general population was once a generally accepted screening procedure, but more recently infection rates have become so low that the Mantoux skin test is accepted as the preferred initial method of screening.

A chest roentgenogram serves as a screening technique in persons who report a positive Mantoux test some time in the past. For those who have never had this test or had a previous negative reaction, the 5-TU tuberculin skin test is usually the preferred screening method. Persons without a significant reaction can be retested after one to two weeks to identify those who demonstrate "boosting," i.e., a considerable increase in the size of a reaction, representing an amnestic recall of a previously positive tuberculin reaction that has waned. This is particularly recommended for certain populations including older persons. Those with a significant tuberculin reaction should be evaluated for evidence of disease. Those with a negative Mantoux result should be retested at intervals that can be determined by their relative risk of acquiring new infection.

The most easily identified high-risk groups are contacts of newly diagnosed cases. Members of the immediate family or others who have shared accommodations with a known case are labeled "household contacts." Other high-risk contacts are those who have shared environmental air at work, leisure, or other similar settings.

When a fresh case of tuberculosis is discovered in our clinic (or hospital), we discuss the importance of contact screening with the patient and close relatives. We urge them to contact their local public health department to initiate these investigations even before routine notification has been completed via the state departments of health.

Indications for Hospitalization vs. Ambulatory Treatment. Isolation is not in itself a justification for hospitalization; indeed, the safest situation is keeping the patient at home, on chemotherapy, while contacts receive preventive treatment. Obviously, patients who are very sick or whose management is complicated by drug resistance or drug reactions may require hospitalization. A community general hospital usually suffices, but appropriate infection control practices should be followed to protect employees and other patients from infection. Ideally, the patient's room ventilation should be handled separately from that of the remainder of the hospital; more frequent air exchanges, ventilation to the outside, and the use of ultraviolet lights in the ventilation system are important factors in decreasing transmission of droplet nuclei.

Most infectious patients become noninfectious very rapidly after starting chemotherapy, e.g., within several days to a few weeks. The safe time for patients to resume normal activities depends on their response to treatment, the initial bacillary burden or infectivity (e.g., particularly high in cavitary disease and laryngeal disease), the nature of their activities, and the persons exposed to them in the course of those activities.

DRUG THERAPY

Principles of Drug Therapy. The *high rate of mutation* to drug-resistant forms is the reason for treatment with multiple drug combinations. The proportion of drug-resistant mutants in wild strains of tubercle bacilli are 10^{-5} to^{-6} for isoniazid, streptomycin, or ethambutol and 10^{-7} for rifampin. Since cavitary lesions may contain 10^{7} to 10^{9} bacilli, it follows that there may already be 100 to 10,000 mutants present within the cavity that are naturally resistant to any single drug. If only one bactericidal drug is used in the treatment, these resistant mutants may be permitted to multiply until eventually the total population is resistant. On the other hand, the chance of a naturally occurring mutant that is resistant to *both* isoniazid (10^{-6}) and rifampin (10^{-7}) is 10^{-13}. Thus, in previously untreated patients with tuberculosis, the occurrence of an organism naturally resistant to two antituberculosis drugs is extremely remote.

A second concept of chemotherapy acknowledges that there may be *four distinct populations* of tubercle bacilli in tuberculous lesions. Owing to variables in their environment within various tissues, these four populations differ in their metabolism and, therefore, in their susceptibility to antituberculosis drugs.

The largest population of organisms are those actively growing at neutral pH in a cavity wall. Appropriate doses of isoniazid, rifampin, and streptomycin are all bactericidal in this metabolically active population. Rapid control of this population not only avoids the selection of resistant mutants and eventual therapeutic failure because of acquired resistance, but also eliminates viable bacilli in the sputum of patients and, therefore, helps to control spread of the disease.

Three other slower growing populations are also present. One group (acidic environment, within macrophages) is particularly susceptible to pyrazinamide. Isoniazid and rifampin are effective to some degree against them; streptomycin is totally inactive. A third group of bacilli are extracellular (solid caseous areas) and may exhibit only "spurts" of metabolic activity during which rifampin appears to be the most effective drug. A fourth population of organisms (dormant) is difficult to eradicate with drugs, and thus largely dependent on the host defense mechanisms for destruction.

The organisms most susceptible to killing by drugs are those that are actively multiplying (mostly the first group), and these may be largely eliminated within two or three months. The other three populations are killed much more slowly, effective therapy for these slower growing or intermittently active populations being more dependent on the duration of the treatment as well as the drugs used. Failure to control these populations is quite unlikely to result in drug-resistant organisms because of the small size of the population. Nevertheless, such failures (e.g., through improper selection of drug, too short duration of therapy, or poor compliance) can show up later as "relapse" from persisting organisms. On the other hand, failure of a drug regimen to control the first group of metabolically active bacilli is evident within the first few months of chemotherapy when sputum conversion to culture-negative does not occur.

With the replication time of the tubercle bacillus between 15 and 20 hours, a once-daily dose of drugs is sufficient, particularly during the initial or "intensive" phase of therapy (approximately four to 12 weeks) while the population of actively multiplying organisms is being killed. As conversion to culture-negative occurs, the "continuation phase" of therapy begins, and the slower growing populations may be effectively treated with either daily or less frequent (but no less than twice-weekly) intervals.

Selection of Drugs and Adverse Reactions. Our concept of first-choice or first-line drugs in chemotherapy for tuberculosis includes the bactericidal drugs isoniazid, rifampin, streptomycin (neutral or alkaline pH), and pyrazinamide (acid pH) and the bacteriostatic drug ethambutol. Ethambutol is generally included because of its relative lack of serious side effects in comparison with other bacteriostatic drugs. The patient as well as the physician should be familiar with the major adverse effects of each drug and remain alert to their possible development throughout therapy. Some features regarding *first-line* drugs follow.

Isoniazid. Isonicotinic acid hydrazide (INH) is inexpensive, generally well tolerated, and readily absorbed from the gastrointestinal tract, and it diffuses into all tissues and body cavities.

Mild hepatic dysfunction occurs in 10% to 20% of patients taking this drug, but in most instances there is no need to discontinue treatment. Occasionally, however, progressive liver damage may occur, in which case the drug should be discontinued immediately. More careful monitoring of liver function is particularly important in patients with underlying liver disease, those who drink alcohol daily, or those also taking rifampin. None of these factors in itself constitutes a contraindication to trying the drug.

We emphasize to the patient the importance of contacting a physician immediately if symptoms or signs of possible liver disease develop, such as loss of appetite, low-grade fever, or discolored urine or sclerae. Since hepatotoxicity is so uncommon in younger patients, it is usually unnecessary to monitor liver function tests in individuals under 35 years of age unless they have a history of previous liver disease or alcoholism. In the older patient, we usually obtain pretreatment liver function tests, e.g., serum aspartate aminotransferase (AST) or glutamic-oxaloacetic transaminase (SGOT), serum bilirubin, and alkaline phosphatase, and then repeat them at appropriate intervals of one to three months. If any of the tests exceed three to five times laboratory normal, and if no intervening illness or associated drugs can be incriminated, it may be necessary to interrupt or completely discontinue INH.

Neurotoxicity for INH appears to be related to interference with pyridoxine metabolism. Peripheral neuritis may be prevented by administration of pyridoxine, 10 mg or more daily depending on the general nutrition of the patient. The usual dosage of INH is 300 mg per day for adults; for children, up to 15 mg/kg/day (not exceeding 300 mg) can be given because of its more rapid excretion. When used in intermittent therapy for adults, 15 mg/kg can be given twice weekly. INH inhibits hepatic metabolism of phenytoin, and may therefore result in toxic levels of phenytoin if the drug level is not carefully monitored and the dose adjusted accordingly.

Rifampin. Rifampin is a semisynthetic antibiotic derivative of rifamycin B, which is derived from *Streptomyces mediterranei*. It is well absorbed orally, penetrates tissue well, is not dialyzable, and is eliminated mainly through the bile. The patient should be alerted that rifampin and its metabolites may impart a reddish-orange color to saliva, sputum, sweat, tears, urine, and even feces.

Worrisome side effects include occasional hepatic toxicity, light-chain proteinuria, and occasional influenza-like syndrome with circulating antibodies. Thrombocytopenia, leukopenia, and hemolytic anemia have been seen, particularly with high-dose intermittent therapy, and renal failure may ensue.

Significant drug interactions include elevated serum levels when rifampin is used with probenecid, and delayed absorption when used with para-aminosalicylic acid (PAS); by way of liver enzyme induction it may reduce the anticoagulant effect of warfarin, reduce the reliability of oral contraceptives, or reduce the effects of corticosteroids, digitalis, hypoglycemic drugs, and methadone. The usual recommended adult dose is 600 mg once daily, preferably one hour or two before eating since the presence of food in the stomach delays absorption. The dose for children is 15 mg/kg/day (not exceeding 600 mg/day).

Streptomycin. This aminoglycoside was the first clinically successful chemotherapeutic agent against *M. tuberculosis*. It appears to be bactericidal against extracellular *M. tuberculosis*. It does not diffuse well into tissues and body cavities, but for reasons previously mentioned it may be particularly useful in cavitary tuberculosis. It shares three side effects with other aminoglycosides: renal toxicity, 8th nerve toxicity (both vestibular and auditory branches), and a curare-like neurotoxicity. It is best to check hearing acuity and vestibular function (caloric test) before undertaking therapy, and then to monitor periodically by whispering to the patient and asking him to execute a 180-degree turn quickly. Vestibular symptoms usually precede symptoms of auditory impairment, and the latter may be avoided if treatment is promptly discontinued when the patient complains of an unsteady gait or tinnitus. Avoid use in the elderly.

Other adverse reactions include drug fever, dermatitis, leukopenia or thrombocytopenia, optic neuritis, or even a peripheral neuritis. The usual dosage is given IM (approximately 15 mg/kg/day) as 1.0 gm per day for the average adult. The dosage may be reduced for persons over age 60 to 0.5 gm per day; it may be given five days of the week for the first one or two months and then decreased to two or three times per week for an additional period.

Pyrazinamide. Pyrazinamide appears to be bactericidal in an intracellular acid environment, and this should be kept in mind when drug sensitivities are performed. Its most serious adverse effect is hepatic toxicity, so liver enzyme determinations are also helpful in monitoring its use. Urate excretion may be somewhat inhibited by pyrazinamide, leading to hyperuricemia and acute gout in some patients. The dosage is 25 mg to 40 mg/kg/day, usually 2 to 3 gm daily for adults as a single dose. It has also been used in intermittent therapy, 50 mg/kg twice weekly.

Ethambutol. Ethambutol is excreted mainly by the kidneys and the dosage should be adjusted for patients with compromised renal function. It is bacteriostatic and finds its listing as a "first-line drug" primarily because of its minimal toxicity.

The only chief toxicity is retrobulbar neuritis, which may occur as two types: most commonly, the central fibers of the optic nerve are involved. The patient may complain of central scotomata and decreased visual acuity with loss of green and perhaps red color discrimination. The less common second type is constriction of peripheral visual fields due to involvement of peripheral nerve fibers. Toxicity is clearly dose related and occurs more frequently when the dose of 25 mg/kg is used. Nevertheless, use of ethambutol at this level for the first one or two months of therapy followed by the reduced 15 mg/kg dose seldom results in optic neuritis.

Table 2 lists adverse reactions and special precautions related to use of "second-line drugs."

Standard Course of Chemotherapy. As discussed, treatment of tuberculous disease should always include at least two drugs, preferably INH and rifampin. A third should be used in the initial regimen if primary drug resistance is suspected, e.g., in patients who come from an area where drug resistance is frequent. If a regimen fails to result in bacteriologic conversion and reasonable compliance can be assumed, at least two new drugs should be used with any change of therapy. A nine-month regimen consisting of INH and rifampin throughout, usually supplemented in the initial phase by ethambutol, streptomycin, or pyrazinamide, is well tolerated and cures virtually all patients with susceptible organisms.

Intermittent Supervised Course of Chemotherapy. A regimen used successfully in Arkansas consists of 300 mg INH and 600 mg rifampin daily for one month, followed by 900 mg INH and 600 mg rifampin twice weekly for another eight months. Results have been equal to those reported from use of daily medication for the entire period: bacteriologic conversion in 78% of patients within two months, failure of treatment in about 1%, and relapse after initial success in 1%. Major toxic effects of drug(s) that required withdrawal of one of them occurred in about 6% of patients. Not only does the shift to twice-weekly administration facilitate the opportunity for direct supervision, but the overall cost of the twice-weekly continuation phase is less than one half the cost of nine months of daily INH and rifampin. Medication taken once weekly is clearly less effective and unacceptable.

A third and even a fourth drug, streptomycin, pyrazinamide, or ethambutol, should be added if there is a likelihood of primary drug resistance, e.g., in an individual probably infected by another patient, who in turn came from a country in which drug resistance is common. In such cases, the practice should be to anticipate primary drug resistance so that the patient is on at least two, and preferably three, drugs to which the organisms are likely to be susceptible. Courses of treatment that do not contain both INH and rifampin throughout the full nine months should be lengthened to between 18 and 24 months, depending on how much the regimens rely on bacteriostatic drugs.

Some evidence suggests that a six-month regimen of therapy is effective if four drugs (INH, rifampin, pyrazinamide, and streptomycin or ethambutol) are given for two months, followed by an additional four months of INH and rifampin, all drugs being given under close supervision. Regimens less than six months in duration are not acceptable owing to high rates of treatment failure and relapse.

It is most important to obtain studies for drug susceptibility on the initial isolate whenever drug resistance is suspected. If the organism is resistant to more than one of the primary drugs, or if treatment has failed owing to drug-resistant disease, consultation with a physician experienced in the treatment of mycobacterial diseases is recommended. Subsequent options are beyond the scope of this chapter; the reader may find

Table 2. SECOND-LINE DRUGS USED IN TREATMENT OF TUBERCULOSIS

Drug	Usual Adult Dose and Method of Administration	Usual Adverse Reaction	Special Precautions	Remarks
Capreomycin	IM, 1.0 gm daily (15 mg/kg) 2–4 mo, then 3 times/week	Audiovestibular injury, renal damage, painful injections	Resembles aminoglycosides, hypokalemia	Cross-resistance with kanamycin
Cycloserine	PO 0.5–1.0 gm/day in divided doses	CNS toxic, seizures, psychosis	Contraindicated in epileptics and psychotics	Weakly effective, use 100 mg pyridoxine
Ethionamide	PO, 250 mg 3–4 times daily (after meals)	Nausea, vomiting, hepatitis, hypersensitivity, depression	May cause depression with cycloserine or isoniazid	Weakly effective, tolerated poorly, better if given at bedtime
Kanamycin	IM, 1.0 gm 3–5 times/week	8th nerve damage, curare effect, renal toxicity	Ototoxicity worse with furosemide, mercurial diuretics, mannitol	Injections painful
Para-aminosalicylic acid (PAS)	PO, 7–12 gm/day (200 mg/kg) in divided doses	GI irritation, hepatotoxicity, drug rash	Administer with meals, avoid sodium salt in the elderly	Poor patient compliance
Thiacetazone	PO, 150 mg/day, larger doses if intermittent	Nausea, vomiting, dizziness, hypersensitivity rash	Significant worldwide primary drug variation in sensitivities	Weakly effective, used widely in Asia and Africa, inexpensive
Viomycin	IM, 1 gm q. 12 hr, twice a week	Electrolyte disturbances, renal injury	Monitor electrolytes and renal function	No longer made in US

helpful information in several papers listed in the bibliography.

Special Treatment Situations. In patients with *renal failure*, INH and rifampin are satisfactory. Streptomycin, kanamycin, capreomycin, cycloserine, and ethambutol should be avoided if possible; if these *are* given, blood levels should be monitored carefully.

Unfortunately, hepatotoxicity of INH, rifampin, pyrazinamide, ethionamide, and PAS poses a problem in patients with *liver failure*. Nevertheless, mild hepatic dysfunction (as with alcoholism) should not eliminate one or even more of these drugs from consideration. For example, INH can be used along with streptomycin and ethambutol if liver function is carefully monitored.

Women of child-bearing age are advised to avoid pregnancy until they have completed treatment for tuberculosis. However, the physician may have to choose a drug regimen for the pregnant patient. Whenever possible, tuberculosis during pregnancy should be treated with at least two of the three drugs INH, ethambutol, and rifampin. Although these cross the placental barrier, they have not been shown to have teratogenic effects.

Prednisone, 1 mg/kg body weight for six to 12 weeks, has been used to supplement antituberculosis drugs in treating endobronchial disease, in the hope of reducing scar formation. Adjuvant steroids have also been used in certain manifestations of extrapulmonary tuberculosis (tuberculous meningitis, miliary and pericardial tuberculosis).

Patients who require total parenteral therapy can be given two or more of the following: INH, streptomycin, rifampin, kanamycin, and capreomycin.

MONITORING THERAPY AND PATIENT COMPLIANCE

More than 95% of patients undergoing initial treatment for tuberculosis can be cured upon completing their prescribed regimen. The major cause of treatment failure is patients who do not take their medications as advised. The single, inner city, unemployed, alcoholic patient is less likely to be compliant; however, it has been shown that physicians and other health care workers cannot accurately predict compliance, and indeed frequently overestimate it. The intermittent (twice-weekly) program facilitates direct observation of ingestion of medication and monitoring of side effects, and is particularly helpful for the noncompliant patient. Personnel who are not physicians or nurses should be permitted to supervise and observe drug administration. Limiting the prescription to one month's supply for those on daily therapy facilitates monitoring of side effects and patient compliance.

The private physician, having diagnosed a case of tuberculosis, is often inclined to follow patients through therapy. A mechanism must be set up, however, to alert the physician when patients do not appear on schedule for medication refill, so that they can be contacted promptly. In our mobile society, patients are too frequently lost from supervision. It is recommended that patients be provided with a brief summary of their status: i.e., bacteriologic and roentgenographic status (last positive culture); specific drugs received and duration; proposed date for discontinuing the drugs; and name, address, and telephone number of the physician

familiar with their chemotherapy program. Patients should also be told that, when away from home and out of medication, antituberculosis drugs are usually available at the nearest local health department. The public health department should be promptly notified following the diagnosis of tuberculosis not only for contact investigation, but to assume supervision of chemotherapy if the private practitioner is unwilling or unable to monitor or enforce it.

PREVENTIVE MEASURES

BCG. This preparation has been used to produce an artificial primary infection at an extrapulmonary site. BCG does not reduce the chance of infection with *M. tuberculosis*, but has been shown to provide up to 80% protection against the development of clinical disease. It is not routinely used in the U.S. or other countries with a low prevalence of tuberculosis. Nevertheless, it should be seriously considered for persons, especially children, who have negative reactions to tuberculin and who have repeated exposure to untreated or ineffectively treated patients with sputum-positive pulmonary tuberculosis. It might also be considered for individuals living in or working with a high-prevalence population: e.g., Peace Corps volunteers or medical personnel working in close contact with refugees, native Indian populations, migrants, or those who are chemically dependent.

Preventive Chemotherapy. The observation that, at any age, the risk of developing tuberculous disease is greatest shortly after infection, and that some risk persists for the total duration of an infected person's life, has prompted the concept of antituberculous chemoprophylaxis. This presumably acts by diminishing and possibly eliminating the bacterial population in the infected person. Several large-scale, well-designed clinical trials conducted by the Public Health Service in the 1950s and 1960s demonstrated that a one-year course of INH reduced the incidence of tuberculosis during the year of medication by 70% to 80%. A study by the International Union Against Tuberculosis (IUAT) revealed a 90% reduction in case rates for compliant patients who took 52 weeks of medication, a 70% reduction for those who received 24 weeks, and a 31% reduction for those receiving only 12 weeks of chemoprophylaxis.

Tuberculin reactors ($\geq$5-mm induration) have been shown to have a 1.6% incidence of tuberculosis during the first year after contact. Those in this group who have been identified as recent converters (within a two-year period) have a greater than 5% risk of developing clinical tuberculosis during several years of follow-up. Indeed, the cumulative lifetime risk for young infected contacts (under 35 years of age) may be over 10%.

All contacts with a positive skin test who are not subsequently found to have active disease should be strongly considered for chemoprophylaxis. Children who are contacts of patients with positive smears and cultures of sputum are at highest risk and should receive preventive treatment for three months even if the skin test is negative. At the end of three months, those with a negative skin test can have a repeat test. If this is negative and their exposure has ended, preventive therapy can be discontinued; otherwise (if their skin test has converted) they should receive continued INH prophylaxis for a total period of 12 months. Obviously, if evidence of disease has developed in the interim, multiple drug therapy is required. Many workers are inclined to follow the same guidelines for older children and young adults.

For older adults with significant tuberculin reactions, the risk of side effects from INH should be carefully considered before prescribing preventive therapy. The case rate for development of INH hepatitis has been virtually zero under age 20; 0.3%, ages 20 to 34; 1.2%, ages 35 to 49; and 2.3%, ages 50 to 64. It also ranges from 0.64% in nondrinkers to 2.65% in those who use alcohol daily.

A second group who should be strongly considered for preventive therapy are those who present with radiographic abnormalities suggestive of tuberculous parenchymal scarring (excluding calcified granulomas as the sole abnormality), and who have a positive tuberculin reaction. Long-term follow-up of persons in this category indicates a risk of disease ranging from 0.4% to 3.5% each year.

A third group is composed of tuberculin reactors in diverse clinical situations, e.g., patients with hematologic or reticuloendothelial neoplasms; those using systemic corticosteroids in doses of >15 mg/day of prednisone (or its equivalent) or other significantly immunosuppressive therapy for a prolonged time; those with silicosis; persons with chronic renal insufficiency; diabetes mellitus patients (particularly if it is poorly regulated); those who have conditions associated with nutritional deficiency; patients with substantial weight loss such as after gastrectomy and intestinal bypass; and heroin addicts. In none of these is the precise risk of tuberculosis well documented; the benefits of INH chemoprophylaxis are therefore less clear and the risk of drug toxicity more worrisome. Although chemoprophylaxis is generally recommended, the physician may feel that the risk of INH toxicity (particularly in older patients) outweighs the possible benefits, and prefer instead to monitor the patient carefully for any manifestation of disease.

Finally, patients found to have a positive tuberculin reaction without any of the above diseases, with no known recent contact, not known to be recent converters (during the past two years), and with no abnormality on the chest roentgenogram have an approximately 0.1% per year risk of developing active tuberculosis. We recommend chemoprophylaxis to those in this group who are 35 years of age or younger.

For patients who are intolerant of INH and have a strong indication for chemoprophylaxis, rifampin is an accepted alternative.

Tuberculoidoses

Tuberculoid bacilli have been defined by Francis and Abrahams as members of the genus *Mycobacterium* that generally grow relatively slowly on artificial media, do not spread from person to person, and yet have the capacity to cause lesions in humans that are usually indistinguishable from true tuberculosis. It is very im-

Table 3. MYCOBACTERIA: SOME CLINICALLY SIGNIFICANT SPECIES

Tubercle Bacilli
M. tuberculosis
M. bovis
M. africanum(?)

Tuberculoid Bacilli

Easy to Treat	*Difficult to Treat*
M. haemophilum	*M. avium intracellulare*
M. kansasii	*M. chelonei-fortuitum*
M. marinum (balnei)	*M. scrofulaceum*
M. szulgai	*M. simiae*
M. ulcerans	
M. xenopi	

Saprophytic

Rarely Pathogenic	*Nonpathogenic*
*M. asiaticum**	*M. flavescens*
M. gordonae	*M. gastri*
*M. malmoense**	*M. nonchromogenicum*, *M. triviale*
	M. parafortuitum
	M. phlei
	M. smegmatis
	M. terrae complex
	M. vaccae

M. leprae

**M. asiaticum* and *M. malmoense* might be classified with tuberculoid bacilli when more reports emerge regarding their pathogenicity in humans.

portant that laboratories should identify and report mycobacteria as species rather than some arbitrary classification or grouping. Nevertheless, with so many mycobacterial organisms to remember, the clinician needs a framework to refer to when considering the pathogenic significance of the organism isolated (Table 3).

RESERVOIR AND MODE OF INFECTION

Almost all mycobacteria, except *M. tuberculosis* complex, have been isolated from soils, and many from water. The one most commonly occurring is *M. fortuitum*.

Water is suitable for propagation and survival of most acid-fast microorganisms. The fresh water of lakes, rivers, ponds, and creeks may yield positive cultures for *M. gordonae*, *M. terrae*, *M. flavescens*, *M. fortuitum*, *M. vaccae*, and others. Home aquariums (both salt and fresh water) may serve as reservoirs for *M. marinum*. *M. kansasii*, *M. xenopi*, and the "tap water bacillus" *M. gordonae* itself can colonize water systems, hot water generators, shower outlets, and other parts of water pipes, and indeed contaminate the mycobacteria laboratory.

The observation that persons infected with mycobacteria other than tuberculosis may manifest a positive tuberculin skin test using PPD-S led to an attempt to develop other more specific tuberculins: e.g., PPD-B from *M. intracellulare* (Battey bacillus), PPD-G from *M. scrofulaceum* (Gause strain), and PPD-Y from *M. kansasii* (yellow bacillus). Useful in epidemiologic studies, these have been of limited help in clinical diagnosis because of their frequent cross-sensitivity to PPD-S.

UNDERLYING DISEASE

Although colonization with a mycobacterium may occasionally be found in patients with normal-appearing lungs, the development of disease is typically related to some underlying lung abnormality, including chronic bronchitis and emphysema, fibrosis, bronchiectasis, or even a previous infection with *M. tuberculosis*. Infection with tuberculoid bacilli can complicate mineral oil pneumonia; the mechanism by which oil enhances the pathogenicity of mycobacteria may relate in some way to mechanical protection of the organism. Contamination of penetrating injuries to the skin and soft tissues, joints, or bones as well as postoperative wound infections with tuberculoid bacilli, may occur. Use of prosthetic hip devices and heart valves, long-term intravenous catheters, and other prosthetic materials has been complicated by infection with tuberculoid bacilli. Other possible predisposing factors for infection are occupational exposure such as in silicosis, cancer, rheumatoid disease (ankylosing spondylitis and rheumatoid arthritis), gastrectomy, and diabetes. The immunosuppression associated with chronic hemodialysis and renal transplantation, leukemia and lymphoma, and AIDS predisposes patients not only to infection, but to dissemination with a number of mycobacteria.

CLINICAL ASPECTS

PULMONARY AND DIAGNOSTIC CRITERIA

The most common tuberculoid mycobacteria causing pulmonary disease are *M. kansasii* and *M. avium intracellulare*. *M. scrofulaceum* and *M. fortuitum* have been implicated much less frequently. *M. kansasii* lung disease most closely resembles classical tuberculosis with its apical posterior upper lobe predilection in fibronodular disease and/or cavitation, while *M. fortuitum* is least likely to simulate classical tuberculosis either roentgenographically or histopathologically. Although upper lobe cavitation with *M. fortuitum* may occur, the more frequent patchy lesions are less likely confined to the upper lobes and the histopathology is more frequently characterized by a dimorphic inflammatory response: microabscesses with acute inflammatory cells (polymorphonuclear leukocytes) rather than typical caseating granuloma.

Since various mycobacteria are known to colonize the respiratory tract without causing invasive disease, the isolation of tuberculoid mycobacteria in a patient with a pulmonary process poses a problem to the clinician: colonization versus disease? Generally accepted criteria for diagnosing significant pulmonary tuberculoidosis are:

1. The same organism should be repeatedly isolated from the same source, preferably over several weeks. This is particularly significant if the underlying pulmonary disease is being aggressively treated. A single instance of isolation is important if the source is a diseased but normally sterile site.

2. There should be clinical evidence of a disease compatible with a tuberculoid mycobacterial infection.

3. Other potential causes for this disease process should be excluded.

Cavities due to tuberculoid mycobacterial disease tend to be more thin-walled with less parenchymal infiltrate about them than those seen in *M. tuberculosis*. Serial roentgenograms and pulmonary function testing help to clarify the presence of underlying pulmonary disease and to document progression compatible with an active mycobacterial infection.

EXTRAPULMONARY AND DISSEMINATED DISEASE

Tuberculoid lymphadenitis most frequently involves the high cervical nodes and is usually unilateral. It is most often seen in otherwise healthy children and is much less likely than tuberculosis to be associated with evidence of pulmonary involvement. *M. scrofulaceum*, *M. kansasii*, and *M. avium intracellulare* are the three most common organisms isolated. Excision of the involved nodes is probably the treatment of choice and has often been accomplished in the process of diagnosis. However, if it is not possible to excise cleanly all involved nodes, progression of the disease is seldom enough to warrant an intensive three- or four-drug regimen. Cervical nodes infected with *M. tuberculosis* ("scrofula") are more apt to be in the posterior triangle of the neck or supraclavicular area.

MANAGEMENT

EASY TO TREAT

M. haemophilum. This organism requires the addition of ferric ammonium citrate or mycobactin to standard Lowenstein-Jensen media for culture. This is the most likely reason why this organism was not recognized until 1978. Of the few reported cases, most have presented with cutaneous nodules, abscesses, or ulcers associated with lymphoma or renal transplantation. Nevertheless, it is not confined to immunosuppressed patients and has been cultured from cervical lymph nodes. Rifampin and PAS have been reported to be effective, but experience with chemotherapy is too scant to suggest a specific successful regimen.

M. kansasii. Pulmonary disease from *M. kansasii* is the tuberculoidosis that most closely simulates typical tuberculosis. However, it is more often found in patients with chronic obstructive pulmonary disease. Although partial resistance to INH and one or more of the other usual antituberculosis drugs may occur in vitro, an excellent response usually occurs with a combination of INH, rifampin, and ethambutol for 18 to 24 months (preferably for six months following the last positive culture).

M. marinum. Infection with this organism occurs in cooler parts of the body, e.g., skin that has been injured and exposed to contaminated fresh or salt water. The infection is usually self-limited and generally resistant to INH, but susceptible to rifampin, ethambutol, ethionamide, cycloserine, pyrazinamide, viomycin, and kanamycin. Some strains have been sensitive to tetracycline, trimethoprim-sulfamethoxazole, and minicycline. However, one or more of the latter antibiotics may be used for several weeks or months, and if unsuccessful, a combination of ethambutol and rifampin may be tried, with or without surgical excision.

M. szulgai. *M. szulgai* has been isolated from olecranon bursae, but more commonly from pulmonary lesions. It has proved relatively drug susceptible; rifampin, ethambutol, and either streptomycin or ethionamide are recommended pending sensitivity results.

M. ulcerans. Chronic, nonhealing, cutaneous ulcers due to *M. ulcerans* are most commonly found in Africa or the South Pacific and Australia, where it was first described. Joints and adjacent bone may become infected, but disseminated or pulmonary disease does not occur. Surgical debridement of necrotic tissue is necessary, and occasionally complete excision including amputation. Local heat has been reportedly helpful, in addition to long-term treatment with streptomycin and rifampin.

M. xenopi. Some cases of pulmonary disease associated with *M. xenopi* have been reported in Europe, Australia, and the U.S. The organism is found rather commonly in water, including hospital water systems. Treatment with isoniazid, rifampin, and either streptomycin or pyrazinamide appears to be effective; the latter regimen was successful even in an AIDS patient.

DIFFICULT TO TREAT

M. avium intracellulare. *M. avium intracellulare* organisms are the most common mycobacteria other than tuberculosis isolated at the Mayo Clinic and many other laboratories reporting to the CDC. Its indolent course, association with underlying pulmonary disease, and nearly uniform in vitro resistance to the usual antituberculosis drugs present a major therapeutic challenge. The starting place is optimal therapy for the underlying disease, e.g., postural drainage when appropriate along with periodic antibiotic therapy for patients with bronchiectasis, those with bronchodilators, those with chronic obstructive pulmonary disease and significant bronchospasm, and so forth. Serial chest roentgenograms may demonstrate no evidence of progressive disease in a significant number of patients colonized with *M. avium*, and the clinician may simply elect to monitor the patient's drug therapy periodically.

Nevertheless, when the three criteria for establishing significant disease as previously described have been fulfilled, and there is clinical progression, multiple drug treatment may be undertaken. Despite the in vitro resistance to individual drugs, synergy has repeatedly been observed *clinically* by many physicians and also demonstrated in the laboratory. Indeed, in our laboratory 96% of the strains were susceptible to a combination of ethambutol and rifampin at concentrations obtainable clinically. The following recommendations have been made at a consensus conference on tuberculosis:

1. For patients with minimal disease, such as those found to have a solitary pulmonary nodule due to *M. avium intracellulare*, chemotherapy need not be given in the immunologically intact.

2. For the usually moderately severe case of pulmonary disease, initial therapy should consist of INH, rifampin, and ethambutol for 18 to 24 months; streptomycin may be used during the initial two or three months.

3. For patients with more severe progressive disease, the regimen should be expanded to five or six drugs, including the above plus ethionamide, cycloserine, or kanamycin (which may replace streptomycin). Duration of treatment depends on therapeutic response and is difficult to predict.

4. For patients with life-threatening disseminated disease such as AIDS, initial chemotherapy should include five or six drugs as above, plus ansamycin and clofazimine. Ansamycin is currently available only through CDC as an investigational new drug; and clofazimine may be obtained through the National Jewish Hospital, Denver, Colorado.

When multiple drug regimens are required, particularly in seriously ill patients, toxic side effects often pose serious challenges, and physicians experienced with these medications should be consulted. Transfer factor from PPD-positive donors may be helpful in disseminated disease. There is some evidence to suggest a favorable influence of indomethacin on the mononuclear cell dysfunction that may accompany *M. avium intracellulare* infections. Resectional surgery for patients with localized pulmonary disease and adequate cardiorespiratory reserve may be used in conjunction with chemotherapy.

M. chelonei *and* M. fortuitum. The two rapidly growing mycobacteria species *M. chelonei* and *M. fortuitum* are quite widely found in the environment, and both of the subspecies of *M. chelonei* (subspecies abscesses and subspecies chelonei) have been associated with infection in humans. *M. chelonei* infection has been reported in recipients of renal homografts and in patients undergoing cardiac surgery, particularly that involving implantation of porcine or prosthetic heart valves. *M. fortuitum* has been found in post-traumatic wound infections, lymphadenitis, and corneal ulcers and occasionally in progressive lung disease. There is an interesting association of *M. chelonei* and *M. fortuitum* with mineral oil aspiration pneumonitis, and these rapidly growing mycobacteria (Runyon group IV) may colonize patients with underlying pulmonary disease for years without evidence of invasion. Since most strains are highly resistant to most antituberculous and other antimicrobial drugs, careful study is indicated before subjecting the patient to an intensive drug regimen.

Isolates of *M. fortuitum* appear to be more susceptible to amikacin, doxycycline, and sulfonamides, while *M. chelonei* may exhibit susceptibility to cefoxitin, erythromycin, and tobramycin. Treatment of *M. chelonei* infection invariably entails parenteral therapy, but less severe infections with *M. fortuitum* may benefit from long-term treatment with oral agents, perhaps supplemented by an initial course of parenteral therapy. Surgical excision of infected wounds, prostheses, or localized pulmonary disease should always be seriously considered, and indeed may offer the only chance of "cure." Drug susceptibility studies should be performed, particularly in this mycobacteria complex. Since acquired resistance may develop during therapy even with multiple drugs, periodic drug sensitivity testing should continue and the treatment program altered appropriately.

One report of a patient with antigen-specific bactericidal defect for *M. fortuitum* organisms was corrected in vitro by the addition of a cholinergic agonist (bethanechol chloride) and a prostaglandin synthetase inhibitor (indomethacin); there was subsequent improvement.

M. scrofulaceum. The most common manifestation of disease with *M. scrofulaceum* is cervical adenitis in children. Usually the disease is unilateral and may be successfully managed by complete excision of the node. The organism may colonize patients with underlying chronic pulmonary disease, and its pathogenicity is very difficult to assess. The organism is resistant to almost all antituberculosis drugs, but on the basis of limited clinical experience a combination of four or five drugs has been suggested, as used with *M. avium intracellulare*.

M. simiae. Initially recovered from monkeys imported from India, *M. simiae* has rarely been associated with pulmonary disease in man. It is generally resistant to all antimycobacterial drugs except cycloserine and ethionamide. Nevertheless, four- and five-drug therapy programs have been suggested, as for *M. avium intracellulare* and *M. scrofulaceum*.

SAPROPHYTIC MYCOBACTERIA

These relatively common organisms in our environment are very rarely pathogenic in the nonimmunocompromised host, and even isolation of one from an immunocompromised host would be most unlikely to have pathologic significance (Table 3).

M. asiaticum. The first report of pulmonary disease from this organism in two patients in Australia in 1983 awaits confirmation from other cases. No satisfactory information is available regarding therapy.

M. gordonae. This rather ubiquitous mycobacterium is not infrequently found in tap water, and thus often signifies laboratory contamination. Indeed, disease in humans is rare. It has resulted in granulomatous infection of synovia and bursa as well as carpal tunnel syndrome. Even more rarely, it has been reportedly associated with pulmonary disease and AIDS. In vitro drug susceptibility studies may reveal *M. gordonae* susceptible to INH, rifampin, ethambutol, and streptomycin. Surgical excision of infected bursae has been proposed in the past; nevertheless, as might be predicted from its in vitro drug sensitivities, multiple drug chemotherapy alone has been successful.

M. malmoense. Pulmonary infections in coalminers and patients with cervical adenitis have been reported in England. Drug resistance patterns have been variable and no clear recommendations for therapy can be made yet.

REFERENCES

ACCP Consensus Conference on Tuberculosis: Standard therapy for tuberculosis. Chest (Suppl) 87:115S–139S, 1985.

ATS Statement: Control of tuberculosis. Am Rev Respir Dis 128:336–342, 1983.

Bailey WC: Treatment of atypical mycobacterial disease. Chest 84:626–628, 1983.

Dutt AK, Stead WW: Chemotherapy of tuberculosis for the 1980s. Clin Chest Med 2:243–252, 1980.

Francis J, Abrahams EW: The pathogenicity and nomenclature of the mycobacteria. Tubercle 62:309–310, 1982.

McDonald RJ, Memon AM, Reichman LB: Successful supervised ambulatory management of tuberculosis treatment failures. Ann Intern Med 96:297–301, 1982.

Standard therapy for tuberculosis 1985. Chest 87:117S–124S, 1985.

12 · DYSPNEA AND DISABILITY

Robert E. Albertini
GEISINGER MEDICAL CENTER

DEFINITION

Dyspnea is a sensation of breathlessness or respiratory distress experienced at levels of activity with which it is not normally associated. It is an awareness of the act of breathing, normally a subconscious process.

PATHOPHYSIOLOGY

The sensation of dyspnea—awareness of an altered relationship between functional respiratory output and central respiratory drive—results from multiple messages to the cerebral cortex. The afferent pathways from the thorax include both vagal and somatic nerves. Additionally, alterations in blood gas concentrations and acid-base balance, by their effects on respiratory drive, may contribute to the sensation of dyspnea by widening the gap between respiratory drive and the expected functional output.

Parenchymal pulmonary stretch receptors are stimulated by stiffness of the lung in restrictive disease, overinflation in obstructive disease, and vascular distention in pulmonary arterial or venous hypertension. Proprioceptor neurons terminating in chest wall muscles and the diaphragm sense alterations in muscle length–tension relationships that result from changes in lung compliance or resistance.

Hypercapnia and acidosis, sensed mostly in the brain stem, contribute to the sensation of dyspnea by widening the gap between respiratory drive and the mechanical ability to meet it. Hypoxemia is sensed primarily by chemoreceptors in the carotid and aortic bodies. Its perception and interpretation centrally are weaker in comparison with most other inputs; consequently, hypoxemia per se rarely contributes much to the overall sensation of dyspnea during rest. During exercise, however, the metabolic acidosis and muscle fatigue associated with hypoxemia enhance the sensation of dyspnea. The level of arterial oxyhemoglobin desaturation required to limit exercise, cause metabolic acidosis, and produce dyspnea is quite variable owing to the heart's ability to respond to tissue oxygen demand by increasing cardiac output. Anemia, by decreasing the oxygen content of the blood, can also reduce oxygen delivery. Administration of oxygen usually does not alleviate dyspnea at rest but may improve exercise performance by increasing oxygen delivery during maximal cardiac output.

CLINICAL ASPECTS

A comprehensive history and a thorough physical examination are the keys to a successful evaluation. Chronic cough and gradually worsening dyspnea in a smoker are the hallmarks of chronic airway obstruction. Episodic dyspnea with or without wheezing and/or cough, often precipitated by exercise, fumes, dust, or other inhaled irritants, makes bronchial asthma a strong consideration. A history of occupational exposure should be sought and may require detailed accounting of all previous jobs held by the patient. Often missed are short exposures to significant toxic substances such as asbestos. Increased cough and sputum production, chills, fever, or hemoptysis suggests infection or neoplasm as the cause of increased dyspnea in a patient with chronic obstructive pulmonary disease (COPD). Chest pain may accompany coronary heart disease, pleural disease (effusion, neoplasm), pulmonary embolism, or chest wall disease (rib fracture, ruptured diaphragm, unsuspected trauma). Orthopnea, paroxysmal nocturnal dyspnea, or edema suggests heart failure. Faintness, syncope, and palpitations, particularly with exertion, are often associated with a fixed or limited cardiac output, as seen in pulmonary vascular or heart disease. Symptoms of phlebitis or recent events (surgery, trauma, immobility) known to predispose to venous thromboembolism may be clues to the presence of occult recurrent pulmonary emboli.

As part of the examination, evidence of neuromuscular disease should be sought, including ptosis, diplopia, proximal muscle weakness or tenderness, fasciculations, and absent or decreased reflexes. A suggested approach to evaluation of dyspnea is illustrated in Figure 1.

DIAGNOSIS

A carefully conducted history and physical examination should narrow the differential diagnosis to a few specific entities. The chest roentgenogram can quickly exclude or at least make unlikely a host of possible causes of dyspnea. Signs suggestive of pulmonary vascular disease may be readily apparent (large proximal pulmonary arteries and peripheral oligemia). If parenchymal disease is present the investigation may be steered toward a specific diagnostic test, depending on the pattern of the abnormalities seen. A complete blood count, urinalysis, electrolytes, and biochemical panel should be used to look for primary or associated systemic disease. An electrocardiogram is indicated in most patients.

Pulmonary function tests (PFTs) may be done initially, particularly if there is an indication of airway or chronic parenchymal lung disease on the initial history

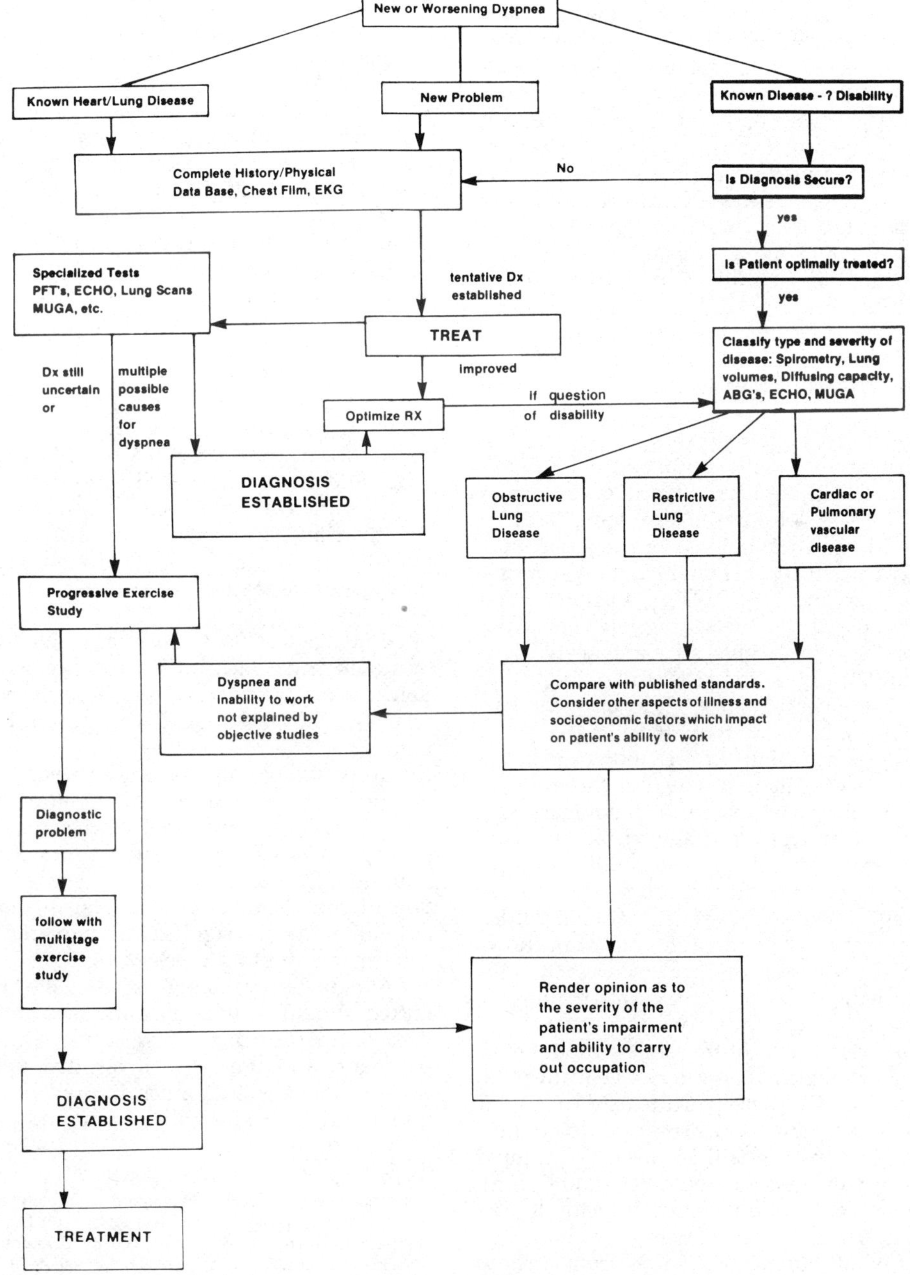

Figure 1. Approaches to dyspnea and disability.

and examination. However, patients with suspected infectious disease (especially tuberculosis), changing patterns of disease (e.g., heart failure under treatment), or unstable coronary disease should not undergo PFTs at this stage of the evaluation.

Further studies, in a cost-effective work-up, are indicated only if the initial evaluation is inconclusive or there is significant uncertainty regarding the cause of the dyspnea. Patients with easily documented disease such as emphysema or congestive heart failure need no further investigation; most will fall into this category. Those whose problem has not yet been clearly delineated require additional study beginning with spirometry and lung volumes. A repeat study after inhalation of an aerosolized bronchodilator is indicated if the baseline measurements of expiratory airflow (FEV_1, FEV_1/FVC, MMEF, or MVV) are reduced. Improvement (20% or greater) usually indicates bronchial asthma, a lesser-response chronic bronchitis, or no improvement emphysema. An increased lung volume when accompanied by reduced flow rates is suggestive of emphysema. When a patient with episodic dyspnea or cough has normal parameters of expiratory air flow, a challenge with aerosolized methacholine may uncover hyperreactive airways characteristic of asthma. Low lung volumes suggest interstitial, chest wall, or neuromuscular diseases. Measurement of maximal inspiratory and expiratory pressures is helpful in detecting muscle weakness as a cause of dyspnea. When airway disease is not suspected and spirometry and lung volumes are normal, the carbon monoxide diffusing capacity (DLCO) is the most sensitive study to detect early interstitial disease.

If primary or complicating heart disease is suspected, echocardiography with estimation of the ejection fraction can delineate the extent of ventricular dysfunction, if any, that is present. In some patients with COPD or a large chest, the echocardiogram may be technically poor; this problem is usually circumvented by gated radionuclide (MUGA) scanning. The MUGA scan, in addition to measuring left ventricular ejection fraction, may also give an estimate of right ventricular ejection fraction (first-pass study), indicating either primary right ventricular disease or secondary dysfunction due to pulmonary hypertension.

A radionuclide perfusion scan is indicated if the history or physical examination suggests thromboembolic disease (phlebitis; past history of pulmonary emboli; recent surgery, fracture, or immobilization; estrogen treatment; carcinoma) or if cardiac studies suggest right ventricular hypertrophy, particularly if no other cause is apparent. A normal perfusion scan excludes significant pulmonary emboli; an abnormal scan, however, has a 20% to 50% rate of error even when combined with ventilation scans. The indication for pulmonary angiography depends on the degree of suspicion and an assessment of the clinical situation.

A few patients remain a mystery even after the above sequence of study. These patients may have mild abnormalities that are, however, insufficient to account for the degree of dyspnea, or there may be multiple abnormalities with evidence of both heart and lung disease where the contribution of each factor to the symptoms is uncertain. Some patients may simply be deconditioned, while others may suffer from anxiety neurosis. A few may have occult, exercise-induced asthma, early primary pulmonary hypertension, or subtle coronary artery disease. It is here that exercise testing may allow the clinician to detect or rule out hidden disease and lead to either treatment or reassurance. The study is usually interpreted as indicating (1) exercise limitation due to cardiovascular or lung disease, (2) deconditioning, or (3) malingering, either alone or in combination with (1) or (2).

DISABILITY EVALUATION

Disability consists of inability to perform tasks. Because of the complex interaction among judicial, social, motivational, educational, and intellectual factors, physicians should not (and in most instances do not) make decisions concerning disability. This is an administrative function carried out by various judicial or compensation boards. However, physicians can and should make determinations concerning impairment.

Before evaluating patients, it is necessary to ensure that their condition has been properly diagnosed and maximally treated. Classification of the process and measurement of degree of impairment can usually be accomplished by appropriate use of PFTs and noninvasive cardiac studies. Results should be compared with published standards to determine if impairment is mild, moderate, or severe. Problems may occur when standards vary from one agency to another, and it is likely that the agency involved will apply its own criteria. Nonetheless, the physician should attempt to classify the degree of impairment independently. Generally accepted guidelines denote obstructive impairment as severe when values for FEV_1 or MVV compared with predicted normals or the FEV_1/FVC ratio are less than 40%. Restrictive impairment is severe when the FVC is less than 50% of predicted normal or the DLCO less than 40%. A resting PaO_2 of <55 mm Hg, regardless of the type of disease, indicates severe impairment of gas exchange.

Initial assessment of cardiac disability may be made by noninvasive measurements of resting ejection fraction. An ejection fraction significantly below normal at rest is usually associated with severe exercise impairment.

If preliminary PFTs and cardiac studies are not definitive, if less than severe impairment is present, or if the patient's complaints of dyspnea appear out of proportion to objective findings, an exercise study is indicated. The level of activity required by the occupation of the claimant must be taken into account. An individual may be significantly impaired for his job but still capable of other types of work.

When the evaluation is complete, the report submitted should include all data used in arriving at the decision, a statement of the cause and degree of impairment, and the reasons for that opinion. A well-written report will do much to prevent future administrative difficulties for both patient and physician.

REFERENCES

American Thoracic Society: Evaluation of impairment/disability secondary to respiratory disease. Am Rev Respir Dis 126:945–951, 1982.
Disability Evaluation Under Social Security: A handbook for physicians. HEW publication (SSA)79–10089, August, 1979.

Jones NL, Campbell EJM: Clinical Exercise Testing, 2nd ed. W. B. Saunders Co, Philadelphia, 1982.
Loke J, ed: Exercise: physiology and clinical application. Clin Chest Med 5:1–210, 1984.
Wasserman K, Whipp BJ: Exercise physiology in health and disease. Am Rev Respir Dis 112:219–249, 1975.

13 · COMMON OTOLARYNGOLOGIC PROBLEMS

Roger L. Hybels
Pierre Forgacs
LAHEY CLINIC MEDICAL CENTER

The physician who provides primary care sees many illnesses of the upper respiratory tract and diseases that secondarily affect this area. The emphasis in this chapter is on common conditions that make up the majority of complaints seen. In general, infections are unnecessarily blamed for a high percentage of head and neck symptoms. Most of these mistakes in diagnosis can be avoided by obtaining an adequate history from the patient and by working from an expanded differential diagnosis.

Nose and Sinus

DEFINITION AND DIAGNOSTIC CRITERIA

Most complaints and diagnoses of sinusitis represent some form of rhinitis. Many misconceptions about nasal and sinus disease are held by both the general public and the medical profession. Medical history is critical and usually is inadequately taken for these problems. A common tendency is to accept the patient's own diagnosis, usually expressed as "sinus problems." Much information can be obtained by simply asking patients what they mean by the term "sinus." In general, the three types of symptoms defined as a result of this question are obstruction, discharge, or pain. If physicians ask about each of these symptoms, they will go a long way toward making the proper diagnosis. Symptoms typically are a combination of these, but often one symptom can be identified as the primary complaint. Once this is determined, the factors that affect the symptoms, frequency, seasonal nature, and efficacy of past treatment can be determined.

PATHOPHYSIOLOGY

Obstruction. Obstruction of air flow through the nose results from mucosal swelling, polyps, or mechanical deformities. The latter two problems are identified by examination and the symptoms are more or less constant although their intensity may vary throughout the day or year. Mucosal edema is the sine qua non of rhinitis, of which the two major forms are allergic and vasomotor. Determination of the seasonal nature and environmental factors that affect the obstruction helps to distinguish between these two entities.

Drainage. Drainage is a common symptom of nasal mucosal disease. Unfortunately, mucus production is a constant physiologic process even in normal persons. The dilemma is to separate normal from abnormal, which depends a great deal on the subjective perception of the patient, and this varies greatly.

The immotile cilia syndrome is a genetic defect that leads to chronic rhinitis, sinusitis, otitis, and bronchitis, all of which are related to lack of ciliary motion and stasis of secretions. Diagnosis is made by electron microscopy of biopsied nasal mucosa.

CLINICAL ASPECTS

Most complaints of drainage deal with normal physiologic discharges or those secondary to rhinitis, and do not indicate infection. This distinction can be difficult even for the specialist, but some clues are helpful. Most complaints of postnasal drip, clearing of the throat, or chronic cough caused by nasal drainage can be assumed to be functional, yet these are the patients who complain the most vigorously. Anterior nasal discharge is more likely to indicate rhinitis or sinusitis. The white or clear mucus of vasomotor rhinitis can be differentiated from the yellow and greenish mucus of infection.

Pain occurs only in acute suppurative sinusitis and is usually localized to an area directly over the involved sinus. Chronic sinusitis refers to irreversible histologic changes in the mucosa, which have occurred from past infections, allergic influences, or both. These mucosal changes cause no pain. Pain results only when acute sinusitis occurs in these sinuses. All too often, headaches of varying location, frequency, and description are mistakenly diagnosed as "sinus headaches."

Acute Sinusitis. Acute sinusitis is distinguished by pain, pressure, or both in a consistent location and is more or less constant with pus visible in the nose and nasopharynx. If pus is not seen, the diagnosis of acute sinusitis is in doubt. Tenderness may be present over the involved sinus, and radiography shows either an opacified sinus or an air fluid level. Nasal obstruction is not a major part of this problem, but if pus is partially filling the nose on the ipsilateral side, some blockage occurs. Chronic sinusitis is characterized by recurrent acute infections in the same sinus.

Rhinitis Medicamentosa. One entity that should always be considered is the abuse of nasal sprays or drops (rhinitis medicamentosa), which is often missed because it is not considered. This is unfortunate because it is the most treatable form of rhinitis. The mucosal edema and inflammation resolve when the spray is stopped. When the patient lacks the willpower to abstain from these medications, corticosteroids given as a short tapering dose orally or injected into the inferior turbinates can be helpful.

MANAGEMENT

The organisms cultured from acutely infected sinuses are pneumococci or *Haemophilus influenzae* in 70% of patients. Cultures taken from the nose are of little use. To be accurate, material for culture must be taken by needle aspiration directly from the sinus. Anaerobes are present in 10% and *Staphylococcus aureus* in up to 10%. In patients with diabetes and in immunocompromised individuals, unusual microorganisms such as *Zygomycetes* and *Aspergillus* can cause sinusitis, and the clinician must constantly be on the alert for them. Ampicillin or amoxicillin has been used with good results as the first choice of antibiotic in treating acute sinusitis. In populations where *S. aureus* is considered a frequent cause of acute sinusitis, a combination of amoxicillin and dicloxacillin is a reasonable choice. In the penicillin-sensitive patient, trimethoprim-sulfamethoxazole can be used. In patients who do not respond to the initial choice of antibiotic, an attempt must be made to obtain a culture from within the sinus. The bacteria found in acute exacerbations of chronic sinusitis are different from those causing acute sinusitis. *S. aureus* and anaerobes, including *Bacteroides fragilis*, are involved. A good first choice of antibiotic for patients with chronic sinusitis is dicloxacillin alone or combined with metronidazole.

Rhinitis, both allergic and vasomotor, is not treated as easily as sinusitis, and an important aspect of therapy is to explain the chronic nature of the problem to patients. When allergies are suspected, patients should be evaluated and treated for them. Vasomotor rhinitis is the most resistant to therapy. It is not unreasonable to tell patients they have "to live with it" to a certain extent and that treatment will only help to control and not eliminate the rhinitis. Vasomotor rhinitis is essentially an exaggerated physiologic response to environmental stimuli. A good treatment for chronic rhinitis of either form is topical administration of beclomethasone diproprionate (Vancenase, Beconase), which is supplied in an inhaler. This medication must be applied daily to be effective, one to three sprays in each nostril one to three times per day. A newer topical medication is cromolyn sodium (Intal), one puff in each nostril four times per day.

Ear

DEFINITION AND DIAGNOSTIC CRITERIA

Pain in the ear can be an interesting diagnostic problem. Unfortunately, an infection is commonly presumed even when medical history and physical findings do not support this diagnosis. An important step is to determine the location of pain. The patient with "earache" often points to some other area on the side of the head. Presumably the ear is the only structure that patients can think of to blame for their discomfort. Other diagnoses to consider are temporomandibular joint syndrome; various headache syndromes; referred pain from the oral cavity, hypopharynx, or larynx; and musculoskeletal disorders of the neck. Some patients have difficulty only when they sleep on the ear or when cold air or water comes into contact with the involved ear. A simple history would expose these noninfectious situations and would avoid the multiple courses of antibiotics and ear drops these patients unnecessarily receive.

CLINICAL ASPECTS

Acute Otitis Media. Acute otits media is characterized by pain in the ear of relatively recent onset. Often a history of a preceding cold or nasal allergies is elicited. Hearing loss is associated with the discomfort since the middle ear is filled with pus, exudate, or both. Examination of the ear reveals the tympanic membrane to be dull, inflamed, and possibly bulging. If the drum has perforated, pus will be present in the ear canal. Pain that is chronic, recurs frequently, or is unremitting, should suggest another diagnosis, such as neoplasm.

External Otitis. External otitis and bullous myringitis are commonly confused with otitis media or lumped under the nonspecific heading of ear infections. External otitis is an infection of the skin of the ear canal; the middle ear is unaffected. Hearing may be diminished and discharge may be present, but the striking finding is that the skin of the ear canal is edematous, moist, and tender. The eardrum often is not visible, and traction on the external ear causes pain.

Bullous Myringitis. Bullous myringitis is a viral or mycoplasmal infection of the eardrum often associated with an infection of the upper respiratory tract. The rapidity with which pain develops and its severity are characteristic features with little if any effect on the hearing. The hallmark is a bullous, possibly hemorrhagic eruption over the tympanic membrane. Serosanguineous drainage may occur if a bulla ruptures, giving the impression of a perforated eardrum.

Chronic Suppurative Otitis Media. This is a difficult concept to understand. In most forms, the drum is perforated or retracted. These problems largely result from lifelong disease of the ear characterized by frequent infections. Dysfunction of the eustachian tube, severe enough to inhibit pneumatization of the mastoid bone in early childhood, is the underlying disorder explaining the radiographic findings of sclerosis of the mastoid bone typically noted in these patients. Mucoid drainage, one of the most common symptoms of chronic otitis media, originates from the mucosa of the middle ear and, because of the perforation, enters the ear canal; it is frequently treated with antibiotics unnecessarily. The drainage is exacerbated when the patient allows water in the ear, has an infection of the upper respiratory tract, or has a flare-up of allergic rhinitis.

Chronic Secretory Otitis Media. This is primarily a disease of childhood, resulting from inadequate function of an immature eustachian tube. An initial acute suppurative otitis media or chronic underlying allergic diathesis may play a contributing role.

Pruritus. Pruritus of the external auditory canal is common. It is either idiopathic with normal-appearing skin or is associated with dry, flaking skin. In either instance, the patient should be reassured that no appreciable problem exists, including infection, and that the symptoms can be controlled but not cured.

MANAGEMENT

The etiologic agents of otitis media have been established by aspiration and culture of the middle ear contents. Poor correlation is found between bacteria found in the nasopharynx or ear canal in patients with an intact tympanic membrane and bacteria isolated from the middle ear itself. Pneumococci, group A streptococcus, and *H. influenzae* account for 95% of isolates in children over 6 weeks of age. *H. influenzae*, although less common, is also found in adults. Viruses may also be the cause. A ten-day course of ampicillin or amoxicillin is considered the first line of treatment for children older than 6 weeks and adults with acute otitis media. Ampicillin-resistant *H. influenzae* may be the cause in 5% of episodes, since 25% of these bacteria are ampicillin resistant. Alternate regimens in patients allergic to penicillin or when initial treatment fails include trimethoprim-sulfamethoxazole, erythromycin, and sulfonamide or cefaclor (Ceclor). For children who experience recurrent attacks of acute otitis media, consideration should be given to insertion of ventilating tubes which are effective for this problem into the tympanic membranes.

External Otitis. It is important to recognize external otitis because treatment is topical and not systemic unless surrounding cellulitis is evident. Otic drops, such as neomycin sulfate (Cortisporin or Coly-Mycin), are placed directly into the ear canal four to six times per day. Ideal management also includes a wick placed carefully into the ear canal to absorb and hold the drops against the infected skin and to draw these solutions deeper into the canal. Wicks are commercially available, but a piece of twisted cotton works just as well.

Erythromycin can be used to treat bullous myringitis. Analgesics of codeine or oxycodone strength are necessary because of the severe pain.

Chronic Otitis Media. In chronic otitis media, topically applied otic drops are usually all that is necessary if the ear is draining, along with an explanation to patients of the recurring nature of the problem. Patients should also be advised to keep water out of the ear. Surgery is necessary for cholesteatoma but is elective in other situations, a discussion of which is beyond the scope of this chapter.

Serous Otitis Media. For serous otitis media, it is reasonable to initiate treatment with antihistamine decongestants and regular autoinflation of the ears; i.e., blowing against a closed mouth and nose, forcing air through the eustachian tube into the middle ear. When the fluid persists, when the loss of hearing is between 30 and 40 dB, or when the tympanic membrane is retracted or thinned or both, ventilation tubes should be inserted. This not only returns the child's hearing to normal during years critical to education, but minimizes the chance of development of future chronic ear disease. Serous otitis media becomes less frequent as the child matures.

Pruritus. Patients with pruritus should be encouraged to avoid scratching the canal since this perpetuates the problem. Instead, they should apply a topical steroid whenever the itching occurs. An over-the-counter preparation such as Cortaid can be tried; if this is unsuccessful, a stronger medication such as fluocinolone acetonide, 0.025%, may be prescribed.

Cerumen. Cerumen is a mundane but common problem. Patients should be reassured that most people never have to seek medical attention for it. Some worry that they never have wax; others are concerned that they seem to have it frequently even when it is not symptomatic. In patients in whom impactions occasionally develop, the best treatment is prophylaxis. One approach is to use a cotton-tipped applicator daily to wipe gently the entrance to the ear canal where the wax is produced by cerumen glands. Daily cleaning prevents collection of cerumen. The hazard with introduction of cotton applicators is that an existing collection of wax in the canal will be pushed in and impacted. Once wax occludes the canal, the safest approach is to remove it by irrigation after softening it first with a commercially available product or with 3% hydrogen peroxide, which works just as well.

Pharynx and Larynx

DEFINITION AND DIAGNOSTIC CRITERIA

Hoarseness is a frequent complaint and is fortunately a benign, self-limiting condition in most patients. In the nonsmoker, pharyngitis, laryngitis, or vocal abuse is the likely cause. As long as no airway problem or dysphagia exists, patients are advised to rest the voice. Bacterial laryngitis is rare and antibiotics are unnecessary. If the hoarseness persists for more than two weeks, patients should be referred to an otolaryngologist. Chronic change in voice is expected in the smoker, but progressive deterioration or severe abnormalities demand visualization of the vocal cords. The index of suspicion for neoplasm should be high in smokers of any age, especially if alcohol abuse is combined with the smoking habit. Hoarseness associated with pain is especially suspect. Cancer of the hypopharynx and larynx frequently causes pain on swallowing and referred otalgia on the ipsilateral side.

CLINICAL ASPECTS

Hoarseness. Of several benign lesions that can cause hoarseness, polyps, nodules, papillomas, and granulomas are the most common. Paralysis of the vocal cord is another entity seen in patients who are acutely hoarse. Unilateral paresis is commoner than bilateral paresis and creates a weak, breathy voice because the normally functioning cord cannot reach far enough laterally to contact the nonmoving cord during attempted phonation. The recurrent laryngeal nerve must be evaluated to determine where in its course it is affected. This nerve exits the skull in the jugular foramen with the vagus nerve, splits off in the neck, and approaches the larynx from an inferior direction posterior to the thyroid gland. On the left side, the nerve descends into the thorax and loops around the aorta, making it vulnerable to disease or operation in the chest; this therefore is the side most frequently paralyzed. The many functional disorders of the voice are difficult for the nonspecialist to diagnose. In these situations, the otolaryngologist relies heavily on the normal anatomic and functional appearance of the larynx on indirect laryngoscopy.

Pain in the Throat. Throat pain is typically assumed to be infectious. All too often, patients with cancer of the larynx or pharynx are treated initially with antibiotics, occasionally several times. Other causes should always be suspected and a careful history taken. Ideally the throat should be visualized by indirect laryngoscopy if the pain is persistent. The patient should describe the pain in detail. The physician may be surprised to discover that "pain" is actually pressure, tickling, dryness, or burning or cannot be verbalized, since nonorganic symptoms of the throat are extremely common. Infections tend to be infrequent and short-lived.

Epiglottitis. A potentially life-threatening infection of the supraglottic portion of the larynx, epiglottitis may develop in a short period. It is seen most commonly in children but is diagnosed with increasing frequency in adults, probably because of greater awareness. Throat pain is followed by difficulty in swallowing even normal secretions. As supraglottic edema increases, the airway is compromised. The smaller airway of children accounts for the overall increase in severity in their condition. The patient is febrile and appears acutely ill. If the patient can tolerate it, a lateral radiograph of the soft tissues of the neck can be obtained to show this edema. Typically, the diagnosis is strongly suggested by the clinical findings.

Tonsillectomy. Controversy has surrounded tonsillectomy for years. Discussion of adenoidectomy has been omitted from this chapter because indications for removal of adenoids should be considered separately from tonsillectomy and because severe nasal obstruction is the main, if not only, indication. Tonsillectomy has been an abused operation, providing a major source of income for some practitioners. On the other hand, many children and young persons who would benefit greatly from the operation suffer because of a commonly held belief, especially among pediatricians, that tonsillectomy is never necessary. Although studies have outlined specific criteria to be met before recommending tonsillectomy, it is difficult in practice to be precise. Medical history without good documentation is frequently given by a parent. When medical records accompany the patient, many episodes of sore throat treated without obtaining a culture or even examining the child may be described. As much as possible, objective evidence, including fever accompanying the sore thorat, several days of illness with each episode, palpable neck nodes, enlarged cryptic tonsils, and positive cultures for group A streptococcus, should provide the basis for the decision to operate. It may be necessary to withhold judgment until patients can be seen when they are acutely ill. In the end, the otolaryngologist must select patients for tonsillectomy who are having frequent episodes that disrupt their life style or education. Only under the most extreme conditions, e.g., chronic airway obstruction, is the size of the tonsil itself an indication for removal. Young adulthood is another period when recurrent tonsillitis can be a major problem.

Obstructive Sleep Apnea Syndrome. Described fairly recently, this syndrome is undoubtedly more common than previously thought. The cause is obstruction of the upper airway occurring during sleep, which causes apneic periods of variable duration. This involves frequent arousals to relieve the obstruction and consequently results in a poor quality of sleep. These patients experience sleepiness during the day and often fall asleep in the middle of activities, such as driving. They usually snore loudly, allowing family members to detect periods of apnea.

Neck Masses. Masses in the neck, especially in adults, should not be taken lightly. If each mass is assumed to be a neoplasm until proved otherwise, the proper respect will be paid to it. Medical history will detect recent disease in the areas draining into the cervical nodes, such as trauma, dental disease, infections, or neoplasms. Systemic signs and symptoms may accompany some illnesses. Important determinations are the date the mass was first noted and whether its onset was gradual or sudden. The rate and direction of growth should be elicited as well as any similar past episodes. Examination of the neck should be systematic to avoid concentrating only on the mass itself. All epithelial and mucosal surfaces of the head and neck should be examined.

Any nontender mass greater than 2 cm in diameter warrants further evaluation. A mass in the neck is the first sign of a tumor in 12% of patients with cancer in the head and neck. In patients under 20 years of age, inflammatory and congenital masses predominate. In patients between 20 and 40 years of age, inflammatory masses are frequent, but neoplasms of the lymphatic system and thyroid are important. In patients over 40, a mass should be considered malignant until proved otherwise.

MANAGEMENT

Any patient complaining of chronic or recurrent pain in the throat should see an otolaryngologist for definitive evaluation, and the irrational use of antibiotics should be stopped.

Epiglottitis. In epiglottitis, equipment for intubation and tracheotomy is kept at the bedside at all times and control of the airway is mandatory. If an intensive care facility with personnel experienced in endotracheal intubation is available, this procedure should be performed in place of tracheotomy. Young children should be treated at a pediatric facility, but the airway should be secured before transporting the patient. Little attempt should be made to examine the larynx in the office or emergency room because this may precipitate obstruction. The patient should be taken to the operating room, and with an anesthesiologist and otolaryngologist present, laryngoscopy can be followed by intubation. Tracheotomy can be performed if indicated. The usual organism is *H. influenzae* type B, which can be recovered in blood cultures in some patients. A combination of ampicillin and chloramphenicol or a third-generation cephalosporin is the initial treatment of choice.

Obstructive Sleep Apnea. The most effective treatment for obstructive sleep apnea is tracheotomy because it bypasses the site of obstruction in the upper airway. An alternative procedure is palatopharyngoplasty, in which the uvula and a margin of soft tissue are removed from the soft palate. In addition, the tonsillar pillars are sutured together, which requires tonsillectomy if not previously performed. This operation is not as successful (50%) for relief of apneas, but it is effective for elimination of snoring. Diagnosis is made by polysomnography, which is usually performed as an all-night study.

Neck Masses. At a minimum, the initial evaluation of a mass in the neck should include complete blood cell count with differential, serology for syphilis, and chest radiography. Fine needle aspiration cytologic study is rapidly becoming routine on the first office visit. The range of potential causes of neck masses is vast and beyond the scope of this chapter. The evaluating physician orders more specific studies on the basis of the history and physical examination to pinpoint the diagnosis. An important principle of surgery of the head and neck is that open biopsy is the last step in the evaluation of a mass in the neck since the possibility for ultimate cure is halved by indiscriminate biopsy of metastatic carcinoma. The first step is to search for the primary tumor on the epithelial mucosal surfaces of the head and neck by careful mirror examinations.

REFERENCES

Antimicrobial agents for acute otitis media. Med Letter 23:93–95, 1981.

Biedel CW: Modification of recurrent otitis media by short-term sulfonamide therapy. Am J Dis Child 132:681–683, 1978.

Evans FO, Sydnor JB, Moore WEC, et al: Sinusitis of the maxillary antrum. N Engl J Med 293:735–739, 1975.

Frederick J, Braude AI: Anaerobic infection of the paranasal sinuses. N Engl J Med 290:135–137, 1974.

Hamory BH, Sande MA, Sydnor A, et al: Etiology and antimicrobial therapy of acute maxillary sinusitis. J Infect Dis 139:197–202, 1979.

Haugsten P, Lorentzen P: The bacterial etiology of acute suppurative otitis media. J Laryngol Otol 94:169–176, 1980.

Schwartz R, Rodrigues WJ, Khan WN, et al: Acute purulent otitis media in children older than 5 years: incidence of *Haemophilus* as a causative organism. JAMA 238:1032–1033, 1977.

INFECTIOUS DISEASES

KEITH BURCH
EDWARD L. QUINN

1 · OUTPATIENT ANTIBIOTIC THERAPY

Paul E. Hermans
MAYO CLINIC AND MAYO FOUNDATION

There is nothing new about treating mild to moderately severe infections with orally administered antibiotics in an outpatient setting; for example, group A streptococcal pharyngitis, otitis, sinusitis, bronchitis, early community-acquired pneumonia, gastroenteritis, certain soft tissue infections, and uncomplicated urinary tract infections (UTI). What is new is the outpatient treatment of patients having *severe* infections with parenteral antibiotics after an initial period of hospitalization. This practice is gaining acceptance because of the large savings in treatment costs and the psychologic benefit to the patient, who can be dismissed earlier from the hospital to the home environment. Infections that otherwise require four or more weeks of hospital antibiotic therapy are especially interesting to consider for outpatient treatment: e.g., osteomyelitis, septic arthritis, endocarditis, and progressive pulmonary or disseminated fungal infections.

MANAGEMENT

SHORT- AND LONG-TERM GOALS

For patients with severe and moderately severe infections, hospitalization is initially required, during which parenteral antibiotics can be evaluated and patient tolerance and response measured. Surgical procedures such as sequestrectomy, wound packing, drainage of abscesses, and invasive diagnostic procedures are also performed before outpatient therapy is considered.

Only after the diagnosis is established, the patient's condition stabilized, and the infection controlled can one begin to assess the potential for outpatient continuation of parenteral antibiotic therapy (Table 1). We establish a working team approach. For moderately severe and severe infections, the team should include an infectious diseases specialist, the attending or referring physician, a pharmacist, a social worker, and spe-

cially trained nurses. The team approach should include a clinical evaluation, an estimate of the patient's ability to prepare and self-administer antibiotics, expected compliance, and an evaluation of home environment and insurance coverage. Unfortunately, not all patients have insurance coverage for treatment outside the hospital. In one series of 80 patients, the team rejected 49% because of various medical or psychosocial difficulties, physical disability, or financial problems stemming from lack of insurance.

If the individual is deemed acceptable for outpatient therapy, a training program begins to instruct him or her on the preparation and use of the same antibiotics used during the hospital stay.

Long-term objectives are the eradication of the infection and early diagnosis of complications or relapses. These necessitate follow-up examinations over periods ranging from four weeks for a UTI to two years for a disseminated fungal infection.

NONPHARMACOLOGIC MEASURES

For patients who are to be treated with intravenous antibiotics, access is usually provided with a heparin lock, occasionally a Hickman catheter. A system of inspection of the access route should be developed. On the average, a heparin lock needs replacement every three days.

Blood samples must be obtained to detect any side effects of antibiotic therapy. Serum creatinine must be measured every two or three days if aminoglycosides or amphotericin are used, or once a week if vancomycin is given. The prothrombin time is taken once a week if

Table 1. CRITERIA FOR OUTPATIENT PARENTERAL ANTIBIOTIC THERAPY

1. Non–life-threatening infection and no threat of serious complications that would be preventable or reversible with hospital care.
2. Completion of all necessary surgical procedures and consent of the attending surgeon.
3. The infection is considered curable with oral antimicrobial agents or parenteral agents that can be dosed at convenient intervals.
4. The prescribed antimicrobial agents do not pose a threat of serious side effects considering the patient's condition.
5. Communication among the responsible physician, the members of the outpatient treatment facility, the laboratory, and the patient are clearly established and understood.
6. No associated or underlying diseases exist that will make outpatient treatment difficult.
7. The patient can be expected to comply with the program of treatment.

broad-spectrum antibiotics are used, especially some of the third-generation cephalosporins, such as moxalactam. Regular follow-up visits with the responsible physician should be arranged, the frequency depending on the infection treated and the antibiotic used.

DRUG THERAPY

Selection of Antimicrobial Agent. A brief review of available antibiotics follows.

Penicillins

I. Natural penicillins: penicillin G, procaine penicillin G, penicillin V.
II. Extended-spectrum penicillins, with increased activity against gram-negative bacilli.
   A. Ampicillin, amoxacillin.
   B. Carbenicillin, ticarcillin.
   C. Azlocillin, mezlocillin, piperacillin.
III. Antistaphylococcal penicillins (penicillinase resistant).
   A. Orally: oxacillin, cloxacillin, dicloxacillin.
   B. Parenterally: nafcillin, oxacillin.

All the penicillins have a very short half-life, requiring dosage every four hours, in serious infections. Therefore, none is satisfactory for outpatient use, except procaine penicillin G, which should be given IM only. Penicillin V is the preferred penicillin for the oral route because of good absorption; amoxacillin gives higher blood levels than ampicillin; and dicloxacillin is the preferred agent, PO, for mild staphylococcal infections. There is no indication for ampicillin in acute pharyngitis, except when *Haemophilus influenzae* causes an upper respiratory infection in children.

Cephalosporins

I. *First generation*: cephalothin (Keflin), cephapirin (Cefadyl), cephradine (Velosef), and cefazolin (Ancef, Kefzol) for parenteral use; cephalexin (Keflex), cephradine (Velosef), cefadroxil (Duricef, Ultracef), cefaclor (Ceclor) for oral use.
II. *Second generation*: cefamandole (Mandol), cefoxitin (Mefoxin), cefonicid (Monocid), ceforanide (Precef), cefuroxime (Zinacef).
III. *Third generation:* cefoperazone (Cefobid), cefotaxime (Claforan), ceftazidime (Fortam), moxalactam (Moxam).

Several points should be emphasized. From the first to the third generation the cephalosporins show increased activity against enteric gram-negative bacilli, but in general decreased activity against gram-positive organisms, especially staphylococci. These agents should be used only for definitive treatment on the basis of in vitro susceptibility tests. I prefer cefazolin as a parenteral antistaphylococcal agent (or against other gram-positive cocci, except enterococci, which are never susceptible) because of high peak levels and prolonged half-life, allowing dosage every eight hours. Among second-generation cephalosporins I prefer cefonicid because its long half-life allows once- or twice-a-day dosage. Among third-generation cephalosporins I favor cefoperazone, which can be given every 12 hours, and moxalactam, every eight hours. Specific indications rest on in vitro susceptibility testing. Activity against *Pseudomonas aeruginosa, Serratia* sp. and *Bacteroides fragilis* is variable among third-generation cephalosporins and poor or absent among the first and second generations, except for cefoxitin, which has good activity against many strains of *B. fragilis*. None of the cephalosporins should be used against enterococci.

It should be clear that preference of agents with a long half-life is especially pertinent to the outpatient setting. For this reason, I prefer cefadroxil as an oral agent among first-generation agents because it may be given once or twice every 24 hours. It will be interesting to determine the role of ceftriaxone (Rocephin), a third-generation cephalosporin. It will require administration only once every 24 hours parenterally because of its unusually long half-life.

Aminoglycosides. Streptomycin is still used as an antituberculous agent and in combination with penicillin in endocarditis due to viridans streptococci and enterococci.

Kanamycin is no longer used much because of its lack of activity against *P. aeruginosa.*

Tobramycin, gentamicin, netilmicin, and amikacin are the most potent agents available against aerobic gram-negative bacilli, including *P. aeruginosa*. They must be given every eight hours parenterally. Although they have been used in the outpatient setting, one should consider their potential oto- and nephrotoxicity and problems of accurate dosage (requiring measurement of peak and trough serum levels). The following situations should preclude their use in outpatients: decreased renal function, patients over age 60, anticipated duration of treatment more than ten days, recent previous use of same or other aminoglycosides, concomitant use of other potential nephrotoxic agents, or inadequate supervision. When these agents are used, the serum creatinine should be measured daily.

Vancomycin. This agent has excellent antistaphylococcal activity and is also used in patients with endocarditis due to various streptococci and *Corynebacterium diphtheroides* (sometimes in combination with streptomycin).

Vancomycin is given IV every eight to 12 hours and is potentially ototoxic. The possible side effect of renal damage is still in doubt. Vancomycin is also used PO, although not absorbed, to treat antibiotic-induced enterocolitis (associated with *Clostridium difficile*).

Antifungal Agents. Treatment of deep-seated fungal infections, such as chronic progressive pulmonary or disseminated histoplasmosis, blastomycosis, coccidioidomycosis, and cryptococcosis, is expensive in hospitalized patients. We have had good experience continuing treatment on an ambulatory basis after initial stabilization in the hospital. During a period of two to three weeks it is possible to determine if there are more than the usual side effects of amphotericin B and if the infection can be brought under control. The febrile reaction during and soon after administration of amphotericin B diminishes or disappears in most patients in the first one to two weeks of therapy. The maximal tolerable dose with regard to renal toxicity given either daily (up to 0.6 mg/kg/body weight) or every other day (up to 1 mg/kg/body weight) can be determined for any given patient. It is also possible to determine during initial treatment if the patient tolerates rapid administration (e.g., about one hour).

As an example, a patient with disseminated histoplasmosis tolerates 40 mg of amphotericin B daily and the plan is to give a total of 2000 mg. If the entire course is given in the hospital, treatment will last at least 50 days. If the initial hospital treatment can be reduced to 14 days, the cost of at least 36 days of hospitalization will be saved.

Some patients with disseminated histoplasmosis exhibit only mild to moderate symptoms. We have treated successfully a small number of these with the oral antifungal agent ketaconazole on an outpatient basis. One should also consider bringing the infection under control in more severely ill patients in the hospital, giving amphotericin B and continuing treatment with ketoconazole thereafter on an outpatient basis. A few patients with disseminated candidiasis were similarly treated. Our initial experience with ketoconazole is promising, although more time is needed.

The treatment of choice for cryptococcal meningitis is with a combination of amphotericin B (20 mg IV daily) and 5-fluorocytosine (150 mg/kg/body weight PO daily divided over four equal doses) for a total of six weeks. Under careful supervision the better part of this course can be continued on an ambulatory basis.

The efficacy of outpatient treatment for dermatomycoses with griseofulvin and more recently with ketoconazole, and of monilial vaginitis with topical nystatin or miconazole, is well known.

Antimicrobial Agents That Can Be Given Orally. Penicillin and cephalosporins that can be given orally are listed above under their respective sections. Ketoconazole has been discussed under antifungal agents.

Well-known antibiotics used PO include erythromycins, tetracyclines, chloramphenicol, lincomycin, clindamycin, and agents used for UTI, such as nalidixic acid, nitrofurantoin, and sulfonamides. We shall not discuss these agents in any detail. Erythromycin remains the drug of choice to treat community-acquired pneumonias in the early stage in patients who are well enough to receive ambulatory treatment. Erythromycin is active against *Streptococcus pneumoniae, Legionella pneumophila,* and *Mycoplasma pneumoniae.* Erythromycin is also an important agent to treat enterocolitis due to *Campylobacter fetus* sp. *jejuni.* It is interesting that this microorganism is responsible for more cases of enterocolitis than are *Salmonella* and *Shigella* spp.

Tetracyclines should not be used in this setting because of resistant strains of *S. pneumoniae.* They may be employed as an alternative to treat mycoplasmal pneumonia in patients who do not tolerate erythromycin.

Patients with simple UTI can be treated as outpatients with standard regimen. The essential points here are (1) diagnostic work-up of men and women who have recurrent infections and (2) follow-up urine culture two to four weeks after completion of therapy to establish that the infection is eradicated. Because patients with a UTI, high fever, and chills have acute pyelonephritis and may have bacteremia, initial treatment in the hospital is preferred. Ambulatory treatment may be instituted, usually after three to four days of hospitalization. Sexually transmitted diseases are treated in the outpatient setting, unless there are complications such as pelvic inflammatory disease or disseminated gonococcal infection.

The value of acyclovir (Zovirax) PO has been established for primary or initial genital herpes, but it is not clear whether it is effective in recurrent genital herpes.

Clindamycin can be given PO or parenterally. Its main indication is for infections due to *B. fragilis.* It is also a good alternative in the treatment of infections due to *S. aureus* in patients who do not tolerate penicillins and cephalosporins. Co-trimoxazole (trimethoprim-sulfamethoxazole) has been used for many years for complicated UTI, including prostatitis. Co-trimoxazole has now also found application in the treatment of certain venereal infections (gonorrhea, lymphogranuloma venereum, and chancroid); gastroenteritis due to *Shigella, Salmonella,* and enteropathic *E. coli;* otitis media; sinusitis; and acute bronchitis; and for long-term treatment of infections due to *Nocardia asteroides* (nocardiosis). It is also used in the prophylaxis of UTI and traveler's diarrhea.

Interference with Concomitant Disorders. Potentially toxic agents should not be used on outpatients if an underlying illness other than the infection may lead to complications. For example, aminoglycosides should not be given to patients with impaired renal function, and moxalactam should be avoided in patients with coagulopathies.

PATIENT INFORMATION AND EDUCATION

Patients should be thoroughly informed as to the expected therapeutic response, symptoms of worsening infection, potential complications of the infection, and possible side effects of the antibiotics.

Patients who are accepted for and willing to participate in parenteral antibiotic self-administration need several training sessions to learn (1) the principles of aseptic technique, (2) how to prepare antibiotic solutions, and (3) how to care for the venous access system. Patients should also be counseled regarding possible adverse side effects of the antibiotics and the manifestations of worsening or nonresponse of the infection. The importance of communication with team members, including the referring physician, should be emphasized verbally and supplemented with written instructions. Patients should be encouraged to return to work.

PERIODIC EVALUATION

The frequency and type of evaluation depends on the patient, the infection, and the antibiotics used. Site inspection for evaluation of response and detection of complications or side effects is essential.

SOCIOECONOMIC ASPECTS OF MANAGEMENT

Cost analysis in one series of patients treated from 1979 to 1982 showed that the estimated average in-hospital treatment was $7,380 and the average outpatient cost $1,650, or an average saving of $5,728 per patient. This was equivalent to an average daily saving of $305. Owing to inflation, the average cost was lower in 1979 and higher in 1982.

REFERENCES

Antoniskis A, Anderson BC, Van Volkinburg EJ, et al: Feasibility of outpatient self-administration of parenteral antibiotics. West J Med 128:203–207, 1978.

Kind AC, Williams DN, Persons G, et al: Intravenous antibiotic therapy at home. Arch Intern Med 139:413–415, 1979.

Rehm SJ, Weinstein AJ: Home intravenous antibiotic therapy: a team approach. Ann Intern Med 99:388–392, 1983.

Stiver HG, Telford GO, Mossey JM et al: Intravenous antibiotic therapy at home. Ann Intern Med 89:690–693, 1978.

Symposium on Antimicrobial Agents (Hermans PE, ed): Mayo Clin Proc 58:6–32, 19–102, 147–168, 217–248, 1983.

2 · ACUTE BACTERIAL DIARRHEA AND FOOD POISONING

Frederick B. Rose
Carol Camp
GUTHRIE CLINIC

Man shares a world with large numbers of infectious agents capable of inducing acute diarrheal illness. It is not surprising, therefore, that gastroenteritis (superseded only by upper respiratory tract infections) is the second most common malady for which patients seek medical attention. The fact that these illnesses are not even more prominent is a tribute to the remarkable defense mechanisms and delicate ecologic balance maintained within the gastrointestinal tract. In treating gastroenteritis, which is very often minor and self-limiting, we must take care that our therapeutic agents do not compromise the patient in his struggle against these invaders. Such treatment, obviously, would be worse than none at all.

A few bacteria are responsible for almost all cases of bacterial gastroenteritis, dysentery, and food poisoning. Salmonellosis and shigellosis for years have been recognized as the primary bacterial pathogens involved in diarrheal illness. *Campylobacter jejuni* has now gained status as at least a coequal with these two organisms. *Yersinia enterocolitica*, a relatively infrequent isolate in the United States, is a common cause of acute GI disease in Scandinavian countries. *Escherichia coli* assumes an important role in a tourist who has traveled to Mexico or other foreign countries. A history of seafood consumption suggests both *Vibrio cholerae* and *V. parahaemolyticus*. *Staphylococcus aureus*, *Clostridium perfringens*, and *Bacillus cereus* are responsible for most cases of food poisoning. *Clostridium botulinum* is unique because of its life-threatening potential.

PATHOGENESIS

At the risk of oversimplification, the infectious diarrheal and vomiting agents can be divided between those that produce symptoms by the elaboration of toxins, some of which stimulate bowel secretions (enterotoxins), and those that do so by invasion of the bowel mucosa. These two mechanisms result in what are sometimes referred to as small bowel and large bowel (or dysentery) syndromes, respectively.

An enterotoxin-induced small bowel syndrome is best exemplified by cholera. The responsible organism, *V. cholerae*, manufactures an enterotoxin that results in the production of large amounts of fluid and electrolytes by the small bowel. The absorptive capacity of the large bowel is overwhelmed, resulting in voluminous amounts of watery diarrhea rich in electrolytes. The patient is usually afebrile and without tenesmus. Microscopic examination of stool is usually negative for leukocytes. Examples of other toxin-producing organisms are *S. aureus*, *C. perfringens*, *B. cereus*, toxigenic *E. coli*, and *C. botulinum*.

The *Shigella* family is the prototype for diarrheal illness induced by bacterial invasion. In this inflammatory diarrhea, patients have a dysentery illness consisting usually of fever, small-volume bloody stools, tenesmus, and leukocytes in the stool. Unlike toxin-producing organisms, these invasive bacteria are occasionally found in the bloodstream. *Salmonella, Campylobacter, Yersinia,* and sometimes *E. coli* and *V. parahaemolyticus* are other examples of bacteria considered to produce illness by invasion. However, even with these agents, many of the clinical manifestations are endotoxin induced.

BACTERIA PRODUCING ILLNESS BY TOXIN PRODUCTION

Four bacteria-producing toxins, usually grouped under the title "food poisoning," are *S. aureus*, *C. perfringens*, *C. botulinum*, and *B. cereus*. A common denominator in the diseases produced by all of these organisms is the absence of fever.

Because *S. aureus* manufactures its heat-stable toxin prior to consumption, a short incubation period of about four hours is usual. Warmed food, canned foods, cream fillings, frozen food, ice cream, salads, and meats are common food sources. The onset of illness is explosive, with continuous vomiting and sometimes diarrhea. Although severe prostration is common, the illness usually resolves within 12 hours after onset.

C. perfringens proliferates in warmed foods such as stews and gravies, which provide anaerobic growth conditions. Other sources include meats and poultry. Some toxin is preformed before ingestion, and further toxin is produced in the bowel after consumption. The average incubation period is 18 hours. The clostridial toxin induces diarrhea instead of vomiting. Abdominal pain and cramping may be severe.

The third organism of food poisoning group is *B. cereus*, responsible for two different syndromes. The emetic form resembles *S. aureus*, both clinically and in its incubation. The diarrheal form resembles *C. perfringens*. Fried rice is a common food source, especially for the form associated with vomiting. Chinese food, predominantly fried rice and raw vegetables, is a primary food source associated with this disease.

C. botulinum, primarily isolated from home preserved meats, fish, fruits, and vegetables, elaborates exotoxin that is detected in serum, food, and feces. The heat-labile neurotoxin is responsible for primarily neurologic manifestations including double and blurred vision, difficulty in speaking and swallowing, and paralysis of extremities. Occasionally weakness of respiratory muscles can proceed to the point where respiratory death may occur unless mechanical ventilation is initiated. *C. botulinum* generally does not produce major GI symptoms.

V. cholerae must be included in the differential diagnosis of bacterial-induced diarrheal illness. Emphasizing this fact is a recent isolation of *V. cholerae* from the coastal waters of the United States. Contaminated shellfish (crabs and shrimp) were the source of this disease. Cholera is characterized by voluminous amounts of watery diarrhea, often resulting in severe dehydration and electrolyte loss. This is an afebrile illness accompanied by chills, nausea, and abdominal pain with an incubation period of one to five days.

Traveler's diarrhea, a disease acquired by Americans or Europeans traveling to Mexico, Central and South America, or Asia, usually develops after ingestion of an enterotoxin-producing *E. coli*. This heat-labile toxin produces a small bowel syndrome in many ways similar to cholera.

BACTERIA PRODUCING ILLNESS BY INVASION

SALMONELLOSIS

Salmonellosis can be divided into two separate disease entities: typhoid (enteric) fever and nontyphoid salmonellosis. Typhoid fever, now extremely rare in the U.S., remains an important and severe illness in developing nations. It differs from the nontyphoid illnesses in a number of ways. The etiologic agent *S. typhi* is found only in humans, whereas nontyphoid salmonellae are ubiquitous. *S. typhi* is more apt to become systemic with enteric fever, consisting of severe prostration and fever. Other common clinical features are gastroenteritis, focal infection, and the development of the chronic carrier. Untreated typhoid fever is a prolonged illness of up to eight weeks' duration, whereas the nontyphoid varieties are milder diseases lasting usually four to seven days even when untreated.

Nontyphoid salmonellosis is primarily a summer illness found most commonly in young children. Of the more than 1500 serotypes of *Salmonella*, *S. typhimurium* is responsible for most human infections. Although the nontyphoid salmonellae can produce all the clinical symptoms of *S. typhi*, including an enteric fever–like illness (paratyphoid fever), they usually incite an acute enterocolitis accompanied by mild to moderate fever and resolution in less than a week. At high risk of this more benign disease are infants, the elderly, bacteremic patients, and those with underlying disease. Especially at risk are patients compromised by malignancy and hemoglobinopathies such as sickle cell disease.

Nontyphoid salmonellosis is almost always acquired through contaminated food prepared within the household. Poultry and other animals harbor these organisms in large numbers. Fortunately, 100,000 or more organisms are necessary to initiate illness. Salmonellosis is therefore less frequent than might be expected and is rarely transmitted from person to person.

SHIGELLOSIS

Shigellosis, or bacillary dysentery, needs very few organisms to induce infection (10 to 100) and spreads by person-to-person transmission throughout households and nursery schools. Unlike nontyphoid salmonellosis, man is the only host. *S. sonnei* accounts for 60% to 80% of the isolates in the industrial nations, whereas *S. flexneri* is more common in developing countries.

After an incubation period of 24 to 48 hours, patients present with varying symptoms. These range from mild afebrile gastroenteritis to frank dysentery with high fever. About one half of the patients have two to three days of crampy abdominal pain with watery diarrhea, which progresses to a dysentery syndrome. As a rule, fever abates in three days and dysentery resolves within a week. Bacteremia and extraintestinal complications occur infrequently.

CAMPYLOBACTER JEJUNI

C. jejuni has gained recognition as one of the leading causes of bacterial diarrhea. Although it cannot be distinguished from other bacterial diarrheas, there is evidence to suggest that this organism may elicit more abdominal pain, fever, tenesmus, and bloody diarrhea than the other infectious agents.

C. jejuni infections have an invariable incubation period (three to 11 days) and an apparent peak in summer months. There is a predilection for the 10- to 19-year-old age group. The most likely sources are contaminated poultry and meats, raw milk, and water. Infected dogs, cats, and farm animals are a source of this organism. Most illness resolves within a week, but up to 20% of patients relapse without therapy. Occasionally *C. jejuni* can produce illness indistinguishable from inflammatory bowel disease.

YERSINIA ENTEROCOLITICA

Of the bacterial diarrheal syndromes, *Y. enterocolitica* has the longest incubation (four to ten days) and one of the most insidious onsets. Many patients have a nonspecific febrile illness before developing acute GI disease ranging from acute gastroenteritis to pseudoappendicitis. The localization of right lower quadrant pain may be helpful in differentiating this illness from those caused by other bacterial agents. The development of erythema nodosum and arthritis in a patient with diarrhea is very suggestive of yersiniosis. In most cases the disease is mild and self-limiting, but the diarrhea usually lasts as long as one to two weeks; rarely, the diarrhea persists for months. Yersinia, like *C. jejuni*, can produce an illness that mimics inflammatory bowel disease.

VIBRIO PARAHAEMOLYTICUS

Although *V. parahaemolyticus* produces illness primarily in Japan, the organism is found in the coastal waters of the U.S. It produces illness in the U.S. mainly between June and October. Having an incubation period of approximately one day, this illness is associated with low-grade fever, explosive diarrhea, occasional vomiting, crampy abdominal pain, and headache. Resolution of all symptoms usually occurs within five days after the onset of illness.

DIAGNOSIS

HISTORY

Of all the diagnostic resources available to the outpatient physician, none is more cost effective in arriving at a diagnosis than the patient history. The answers to the following questions help to focus on the most likely etiologies: 1. Is fever present? 2. Is a similar illness afflicting family members? 3. What is the length of incubation? 4. Has there been a consumption of food notorious for causing infection? 5. Is there a recent travel history? 6. Is there a history of animal contact?

A febrile illness directs the physician away from toxin-mediated disease toward inflammatory invasive diseases such as shigellosis, salmonellosis, campylobacteriosis, or yersiniosis. A simultaneous onset of disease in different patients sharing the same meal or facilities points toward a common food source. A very short incubation period, especially in afebrile patients, is indicative of *S. aureus* or *B. cereus* food poisoning. A longer incubation period of up to 18 hours in afebrile patients suggests *C. perfringens* or the diarrheal form of *B. cereus* food poisoning. Gradual onset of neurologic symptoms without GI manifestations in patients consuming home-prepared alkaline food is compatible with botulism. Simultaneous onset of disease in febrile patients 20 to 30 hours after sharing a common food source is consistent with salmonellosis or campylobacteriosis infections, especially if the food source consisted of poultry or beef products. An insidious onset of disease with a prolonged incubation period is suggestive of yersiniosis. Spread of a dysentery illness sequentially through family members or children in a nursery school reflects person-to-person transmission associated with shigellosis or campylobacteriosis. A recent trip to Mexico greatly increases the likelihood of toxigenic *E. coli*. A patient having a diarrheal illness after close contact with animals (especially puppies or kittens) is a likely candidate for *C. jejuni* illness. A history of seafood consumption in a patient with a diarrheal illness should add the *Vibrio* organisms to the differential diagnosis.

PHYSICAL EXAMINATION

On physical examination, nearly all patients have diffusely tender abdomens and hyperactive bowel sounds. Tenderness in the right lower quadrant is consistent with yersiniosis or, occasionally, campylobacteriosis.

LABORATORY TESTS

Probably the most valuable diagnostic aid (and perhaps least used) is the stool analysis. The appearance of gross blood or pus is consistent with a bacterial dysentery syndrome. A drop of liquid stool stained with two drops of methylene blue can be examined microscopically in the office quickly and inexpensively. A specimen having more than 10 polymorphonuclear leukocytes (PMNs) per high-power field is indicative of most invasive bacterial infections. In typhoid fever, mononuclear cells are more common than PMNs. Other inflammatory processes such as ulcerative colitis, Crohn's disease, and antibiotic-induced colitis can create confusion because they all have fecal leukocytes. Stools from patients with early shigellosis may lack leukocytes.

Stool culture should be reserved for patients who are febrile and have severe diarrhea with fecal leukocytes present. In one study of febrile patients with diarrhea, almost one half of the stools that contained fecal leukocytes were culture positive for *Salmonella*, *Shigella*, or *Campylobacter*. Early specimen submission results in higher isolation rates. The laboratory should be notified by the physician submitting a stool specimen for *Campylobacter*, *Yersinia*, and *Vibrio* sp. when these organisms are suspected, so that appropriate culture techniques can be employed.

MANAGEMENT

The dictum "do no harm" is never truer than in the treatment of infectious diarrhea. Conservatism should be the guide in most of these diseases. Therapy can be broken into five areas: (1) fluid and electrolyte replacement, (2) nonspecific agents, (3) antispasmodics, (4) oral antibiotics, and (5) systemic antibiotics.

FLUID AND ELECTROLYTE REPLACEMENT

In the vast majority of patients with infectious diarrhea, oral fluids are sufficient to prevent dehydration until the diarrhea subsides. Broth with salted crackers, carbonated beverages, juices, or Gatorade are all acceptable. Diarrhea may increase with fluid intake but so will fluid absorption. Glucose potentiates the small bowel absorption of fluid and electrolytes. Milk should be avoided until diarrhea ceases, because temporary lactose intolerance may increase diarrhea and abdominal distress. Hospitalization may be necessary if there is a need for intravenous fluid replacement. This is particularly true in certain patient groups, mainly the very young, the elderly, and individuals with more than 15 to 20 bowel movements per day. Ringer's lactate or dextrose and normal saline with potassium chloride added are suitable choices.

NONSPECIFIC AGENTS

Kaopectate (kaolin + pectin) is a safe, common household remedy, our first line of defense after oral fluid replacement; 5 to 10 ml every four to six hours is the usual dose. Many patients seem satisfied and have subjective relief with this therapy. Control studies, however, show that this treatment fares no better than placebo therapy. Likewise, in controlled studies aluminum hydroxide has no proven efficacy in the reduction of diarrhea.

In experimental *Salmonella* animal infections, prostaglandin inhibitors such as indomethacin reduce the volume of diarrhea. The newer prostaglandin inhibitors may have a future role for some varieties of toxin-mediated diarrhea, but currently are not useful in human infection.

Bismuth subsalicylate (Pepto-Bismol) is effective in small bowel syndromes and especially traveler's diarrhea. The drug probably prevents the enterotoxin from reaching its target site in the small bowel. An effective dose is 30 ml every half-hour for eight doses, or an entire 8-oz bottle over four hours. We use this only in patients who are not obtaining relief from Kaopectate, who are afebrile, and who do not have fecal leukocytes as described above. The inconvenience of large doses is a major drawback. Furthermore, patients can develop salicylate poisoning, especially if they are on salicylate therapy for illness such as rheumatoid arthritis.

ANTIPERISTALTIC AGENTS

Diarrhea should be viewed as a mechanism for removing harmful toxins from the GI tract. It has been suggested that diarrhea is to infectious gastroenteritis what the cough is to bacterial pneumonia. Thus, with few exceptions the use of antiperistaltic agents such as codeine, loperamide (Imodium), and diphenoxylate with atropine (Lomotil) is to be avoided in the treatment of infectious diarrheal syndromes. In both salmonellosis and shigellosis a prolongation of the course and an increase in severity of disease have been observed with the use of these drugs. The same is probably true for campylobacteriosis. Antiperistaltic medicine can convert antibiotic pseudomembranous colitis into a severe, life-threatening megacolon.

Table 1. ANTIBIOTIC THERAPY FOR BACTERIAL DIARRHEA

Disease	Antibiotic	Dose Children	Dose Adults	Comments
Salmonella bacteremia, or typhoid fever	Chloramphenicol	50 to 75 mg/kg/day in four divided doses IV or PO for 2 wks	50 mg/kg/day in four divided doses preferably PO for 2 wks	Response to therapy may be slow. Chloramphenicol resistance when disease acquired in Mexico or Southeast Asia. Ampicillin resistance is also common and especially so with nontyphoid salmonellosis.
	Ampicillin	200 mg/kg/day in six divided doses IV for 2 wks	6–12 gm daily in four divided doses IV for 2 wks	
	TMP*/SMX† (Bactrim, Septra)	TMP 10 mg/kg/day and SMX 50 mg/kg/day PO in two divided doses for 2 wks	TMP 160 mg and SMX 800 mg (Bactrim DS, Septra DS) twice daily PO for 2 wks	
Shigellosis	TMP/SMX	TMP 10 mg/kg/day and SMX 50 mg/kg/day in two divided doses PO for 5 days	TMP 160 mg and SMX 800 mg (Bactrim DS, Septra DS) twice daily PO for 3–5 days	Ampicillin resistance common. Amoxicillin not to be used.
	Ampicillin	100 mg/kg/day in six divided doses IV or four divided doses PO for 5 days	2 gm/day in four divided doses PO for 3–5 days	
	Tetracycline	Not given to patients <10 yrs old	2 gm/day in four divided oral doses for 3–5 days	Tetracycline may be given in one 2.5-gm dose PO
Campylobacteriosis	Erythromycin	25 to 50 mg/kg/day in four divided doses PO for 7 days	2 gm daily in four oral doses for 7 days	In patients with systemic illness, gentamicin 3–5 mg/kg/day in three divided doses IV for 7–10 days.
Yersiniosis	Gentamicin	Gentamicin 5 mg/kg in three divided doses per day for 7–10 days	Same as for children	
Traveler's diarrhea	TMP/SMX		TMP 160 mg and SMX 800 mg once a day for 3–5 days	If no response, campylobacteriosis, giardiasis, vibriosis, and amebiasis must be considered.
	TMP (Trimpex)		200 mg once a day for 3–5 days	

*TMP = trimethoprim.
†SMX = sulfamethoxazole.

Occasionally an antiperistaltic agent may have a therapeutic role in an afebrile patient who has severe abdominal cramping with diarrhea without fecal leukocytes. We prefer loperamide, 4 mg initially followed by 2 mg (one capsule) after each unformed stool, not to exceed 16 mg per 24 hours. Remember, however, that even this type of patient may be in the early stage of shigellosis, and the absence of fecal leukocytes may be misleading.

ANTIBIOTICS

Antibiotics have a place in only a few cases of infectious diarrhea and should not be prescribed in the classical food poisoning syndromes (Table 1). In acute, nonbacteremic *Salmonella* gastroenteritis, even with high fever and multiple diarrheal stools, therapy is usually withheld.

Typhoid fever is always treated with antibiotics. Although ampicillin and trimethoprim-sulfamethoxazole (TMP/SMX) do not carry the risk of aplastic anemia that chloramphenicol does, the drug of choice for typhoid fever is still chloramphenicol. Even with this therapy, fever may persist for up to five days. Strains from Mexico and Southeast Asia are often resistant to chloramphenicol. If susceptibility patterns permit, ampicillin or TMP/SMX are suitable alternatives.

In bacteremic nontyphoid salmonellosis, the drug regimen is essentially the same as for typhoid fever. Perhaps for personal reasons, we prefer to use ampicillin or TMP/SMX before chloramphenicol. Since ampicillin resistance is being observed more frequently, care must be taken that the organism is susceptible.

Shigellosis is often a mild and self-limited disease, but because the organism is highly contagious and the carriage rate is shortened with antibiotics, we elect to treat all cases. Furthermore, there is a potential for severe dysentery syndrome in the untreated patient. When positive cultures are reported, we treat even those who appear to be improving.

TMP/SMX is recommended therapy for shigellosis. Ampicillin and tetracycline (in adults) are acceptable alternative antibiotics for susceptible strains. Amoxicillin, as compared with ampicillin, has superior absorption in the upper intestinal tract and does not reach the colon. Amoxicillin, therefore, should not be used to treat shigellosis because of inadequate concentration in the colon.

Since many cases of campylobacteriosis are mild, controversy exists over the necessity for the treatment of *C. jejuni* and the efficacy of erythromycin. In a controlled study the use of erythromycin did not shorten the natural course of this disease any more than a placebo. However, because 20% of untreated cases have recurrences and because we have been impressed with the severity of the illness in our untreated patients, we are currently treating all patients with diarrheal illness from which *C. jejuni* is isolated in stool specimens. Hospitalization with aminoglycoside therapy is necessary in the rare patient with bacteremia.

Systemic *Yersinia* infections necessitate hospitalization and aminoglycoside therapy. Oral chloramphenicol is an alternative but less acceptable therapy.

Single-dose, double-strength TMP/SMX per day has been shown to be effective in traveler's diarrhea. When there is a concern about sulfonamide allergy, trimethoprim alone has been used with favorable results. Failure to respond to these regimens suggests campylobacteriosis or giardiasis.

REFERENCES

Blaser MJ, Taylor DN, Feldman RA: Epidemiology of *Campylobacter jejuni* infections. Epidemiol Rev 5:157–176, 1983.

Blaser MJ, Wells JG, Feldman RA, et al: *Campylobacter* enteritis in the United States. Ann Intern Med 98:360–365, 1983.

Cohen ML, Gangarosa EJ: Nontyphoid salmonellosis. South Med J 71:1540–1545, 1978.

Kane JA, Blacklow NR: Infectious diarrhea. Primary Care 6:63–80, 1979.

Satterwhite TK, Dupont HL: Infectious diarrhea in office practice. Med Clin North Am 67:203–220, 1983.

3 · COMMON SKIN AND SOFT TISSUE INFECTIONS

Bradley J. Sullivan
John W. Melski
MARSHFIELD CLINIC

Impetigo

CLINICAL ASPECTS

Impetigo is classically associated with a honey-yellow, crusted lesion of children, usually about the nares or mouth in the winter and affecting legs or arms in the spring or summer. It may occur in the diapered area in infants. The earliest lesion is a pustule on an erythematous base, later evolving to irregular crusted erosions. Culture of the vesicopustules or removal of the crust and culture of the base yields group A streptococcus, *Staphylococcus aureus*, or both. Strep is believed to initiate the lesion with Staph invading secondarily. Very rarely other groups of streptococci are found.

MANAGEMENT

Local therapy includes soaking the crusts with a bacteriostatic soap (Hibiclens, pHisoHex) to remove them. Application of an iodine ointment (Betadine), bacitracin, or other antibiotic ointment may reduce local spread. Systemic therapy shortens healing time and more effectively reduces both contagiousness and local dissemination. Systemic therapy alone may be effective in children with eczema who might be irritated by bacteriostatic soaps. While penicillins are commonly recommended, our practice has been to consider erythromycin first. From a pediatrician's viewpoint, erythromycin is safe and inoffensive in taste and not more expensive than the usual penicillins. In some instances, it may be necessary to eliminate the cohabitating staphylococci in order to obtain resolution of the lesion, and erythromycin is a good drug for Staph. Usual dosage is 20 to 40 mg/kg/day divided by three or four for a duration of ten days. Cephalexin (Keflex) at 25 to 50 mg/kg/day divided by three or four is a more pleasant-tasting alternative. The newly introduced amoxicillin-clavulanate (Augmentin) is expensive but can be used as another alternative.

An occasional patient may develop poststreptococcal glomerulonephritis, which may not be prevented by the therapy for impetigo. All skin lesions should eventually resolve, including postinflammatory pigment changes.

Bullous Impetigo

CLINICAL ASPECTS

These patients are usually young, under 5 years. They have fragile blisters with little surrounding reaction. The blisters break easily, leaving circular, yellowish-brown crusted erosions. Culture and Gram stain of the vesicular fluid should confirm the presence of staphylococci. Bullous impetigo is one of several staphylococcal diseases attributed to toxins. In the scalded skin syndrome, there is extensive exfoliation of the skin.

MANAGEMENT

Lesions may be washed and treated locally as described under impetigo. Many authors recommend oral semisynthetic penicillinase-resistant penicillins (dicloxacillin or cloxacillin, 25 to 50 mg/kg/day divided by three or four, but they have obviously never tasted the liquid forms. Erythromycin (20 to 40 mg/kg/day divided by three or four) is much more palatable, with cephalexin (Keflex) at 25 to 50 mg/kg day divided by three or four a reasonable alternative.

With staphylococcal skin diseases other than bullous impetigo, the offending organism may be at a site remote from the skin, e.g., nares, abscesses, or, as with toxic shock syndrome, a tampon. The more serious illnesses deserve hospitalization.

Folliculitis

This is a pyoderma of terminal hairs (as opposed to vellus hairs), such as those in the male beard. *Staphylococcus aureus* can usually be cultured from expressed material. Rigorous hygiene is recommended, including shaving while in the shower under copious flow of water, discarding razor blades or soaking them in 70% alcohol (which may also be done with electric shaver heads). Bacteriostatic soaps such as chlorhexidine (Hibiclens) may be useful but can be irritating if used more than every other day. In areas other than the face, friction and occlusion may be significant and should be avoided. Chronic, recalcitrant infection (sycosis barbae) may respond to generous doses of oral erythromycin, dicloxacillin, or cephalexin (250 to 500 mg q.i.d.). Other antistaphylococcal antibiotics may occasionally be needed.

A modern era folliculitis is acquired in hot tubs or whirlpools. Within 48 hours of exposure, a pruritic folliculitis develops, usually demarcated by the level to which the person was submerged. *Pseudomonas aeruginosa* may be cultured from the lesions. They spontaneously regress in five to seven days without specific therapy. The cause is inadequate chlorination of the heated water.

Furuncles and Carbuncles

CLINICAL ASPECTS

Furunculosis is an extension of folliculitis in the abscess stage; carbuncles are abscesses that have invaded the subcutaneous fat. The most common causative organism is *Staphylococcus aureus*. Facial lesions near the upper lip, on the nose, cheeks, or forehead have some increased risk because of the venous drainage of these areas to the cavernous sinus. On the face they must be distinguished from inflammation acne nodules that are typically sterile. In the axillae and inguinal areas they must be distinguished from hidradenitis suppurativa, an acne-like disease of apocrine glands. Otherwise most occur on the nape of the neck, back, or thighs.

MANAGEMENT

Boils or carbuncles that are well localized at the time of presentation, not in the above-mentioned facial distribution, and causing no systemic reaction or local cellulitis can be conservatively managed with local moist heat, applied frequently until they point. Then they often drain spontaneously or can be cautiously incised and drained with the pus sent for bacterial culture.

Organisms other than *Staphylococcus aureus* may indicate immunodeficiency, e.g., chronic granulomatosis disease (as may recurrent staphylococcal infections). If systemic reaction, local cellulitis, or facial infection is present, antistaphylococcal antibiotics are recommended.

Recurrent furunculosis occasionally afflicts individuals or even small groups, usually a family. These are patients who relapse as soon as antibiotics are stopped or may have had boils for several months at the time of presentation. Unless they are immune deficient, e.g., chronic granulomatosis disease, Job's syndrome, hyper IgE syndrome, there is no proven cause for this phenomenon. However, the working hypothesis is that these patients harbor a virulent strain of *Staphylococcus aureus*. Seldom do these patients have bacteremia or systemic illness. Most of the time there are no predisposing factors to this illness.

Treatment of recurrent furunculosis addresses both the boils themselves and attempts to eradicate the carrier state. All of these patients are placed on adequate doses of antistaphylococcal drugs and maintained on the antibiotic until no more abscesses have occurred and the last lesions have resolved.

PREVENTIVE MEASURES

The organism is most often carried intranasally. Intranasal application of antibiotic ointments is one method to eradicate the carrier state. Our agents of choice are gentamicin or tobramycin applied in generous amounts on a Q-tip applicator, inserted as far up each nostril as is comfortable and rotated. Usually we advise nasal application twice or three times daily and to be continued for three months for all members of a family who are affected. While we have been very satisfied with intranasal aminoglycoside, Neosporin, Betadine, and bacitracin ointments are alternatives. Oral rifampin, 600 mg daily for five to ten days, may also eradicate nasal carriage of *Staphylococcus aureus*.

While the treatment just described may be sufficient, there are alternative therapies worth mentioning.

1. Thorough bathing and shampooing daily or even twice daily with a medicated soap such as chlorhexidine. Males may use the above-mentioned shaving precautions. Fingernails and toenails should be trimmed.

2. Personal linens and underclothing should be individualized, changed daily, and washed in soapy water. This precaution may extend beyond personal items such as towels to bedclothing and sheets. The purpose is to eliminate fomite carriage. Disposable garments and linens may achieve the same purpose.

3. All draining lesions should be well covered with sterile dressings; these should be disposed of promptly when removed and hands should be thoroughly washed afterward. Some authors even recommend disposable Kleenex tissues instead of cloth hankies for nasal discharge.

REFERENCES

Weinstein L, LeFrank J: Does antimicrobial therapy of streptococcal pharyngitis or pyoderma alter the risk of glomerulonephritis? J Infect Dis 124:229–231, 1971.

White A: The use of gentamicin as a nasal ointment. Am J Med Sci 248:52–55, 1964.

4 · BRAIN ABSCESS AND SUBDURAL EMPYEMA

Wendell W. Hoffman
Pierre Forgacs
Stephen R. Freidberg
LAHEY CLINIC MEDICAL CENTER

Brain Abscess

DEFINITION AND DIAGNOSTIC CRITERIA

A brain abscess is a focal, suppurative, intracranial space-occupying lesion that must be considered in the differential diagnosis of any expanding intracranial mass. The diagnosis is suggested when focal cerebral and/or cerebellar signs or evidence of increased intracranial pressure are present in the clinical setting of infection in the middle ear, mastoid, sinuses, lungs, or heart. A definitive diagnosis is made either through positive results of cultures and compatible histologic findings from surgically obtained specimens or through the clinical response to antimicrobial therapy (e.g., decrease in size of mass).

PATHOPHYSIOLOGY

Brain abscess most frequently arises from an adjacent infection, such as that involving the mastoid, middle ear, or paranasal sinuses. Less commonly it develops as a metastatic lesion from a distant primary site, such as the lung (e.g., bronchiectasis, lung abscess, empyema), heart (e.g., endocarditis, right-to-left shunts), or bone (e.g., osteomyelitis). Uncommonly brain abscess results from direct inoculation of organisms (e.g., neurosurgical procedures or compound skull fractures). In 20% of patients the source of infection cannot be determined.

The location of a brain abscess reflects the associated underlying source of infection. Otogenic and rhinogenic abscesses, which occur most often in the temporal and frontal lobes and less frequently in the parietal lobe, cerebellum, and occipital lobe, develop by direct extension through osteomyelitic foci or by spread along local venous pathways. Metastatic abscesses tend to arise in the distribution of the middle cerebral arteries and may be multiple in contrast to the more common single lesions of contiguous spread. In patients with cranial trauma, the site of penetration determines location of the abscess.

ETIOLOGIC AGENTS

The most common organisms causing brain abscess are anaerobic, microaerophilic, and aerobic streptococci; *Enterobacteriaceae*; and *Staphylococcus aureus*. Other caus-

ative organisms include *Bacteroides* sp., *Fusobacterium* sp., and *Actinomyces* sp.. The bacterial species vary with the site of abscess as well as with the underlying conditions. *Bacteroides fragilis*, *Enterobacteriaceae* (e.g., *Proteus* sp.), and streptococci predominate in otogenous abscesses of the temporal lobe. *Fusobacterium* sp., streptococci, and *Actinomyces* are most common in pulmonary-related brain abscesses. Staphylococcal abscesses are associated with bacteremia, endocarditis, and penetrating head trauma.

Organisms that cause brain abscess in the immunocompromised host include *Nocardia* sp., *Aspergillus* sp., *Mucor* sp., *Candida* sp., *Toxoplasma gondii*, and *Cryptococcus neoformans*. Although discussion of the management of these patients is beyond the scope of this chapter, the importance of early biopsy or aspiration to obtain a specific microbiologic diagnosis should be emphasized because empiric regimens are often inadequate.

In residents of developing countries, the most common organisms that cause brain infection include *Cysticercus* sp. and *Mycobacterium tuberculosis*.

CLINICAL ASPECTS

The symptoms of brain abscess are those of an intracranial mass. Severe headache, which is present in 70% of patients, is the most common symptom. Altered states of consciousness ranging from lethargy to coma occur in 50% to 70% of patients. Nausea and vomiting occur in about 50%, and either focal or generalized seizures are present in one third. In patients with chronic ear, sinus, or pulmonary infection, a reactivation of the infection often occurs before symptoms of central nervous system involvement.

Fever, which is usually low grade, is found in only 50% of patients and is most characteristic of the cerebritis stage. Focal neurologic deficits, with hemiparesis being the most common, also occur in 50%. Other clinical signs include nuchal rigidity (25%), papilledema (25%), and ataxia and nystagmus (in patients with cerebellar abscess).

When a brain abscess is suspected, a careful physical examination should be performed, searching specifically for otic, sinus, pulmonary, and cardiac disease.

A computed tomographic (CT) scan is the best diagnostic procedure for brain abscess and should be performed during the initial phases of evaluation. Even when clinically unsuspected, brain abscess is often diagnosed on CT. The use of a contrast agent enhances the selectivity of CT and permits visualization of even early abscess formation (i.e., focal cerebritis), and CT-guided stereotactic needle biopsy and aspiration have extended diagnostic and treatment abilities. Unfortunately, however, CT lacks specificity. Differentiation between abscess and tumor is at times impossible, necessitating surgical exploration.

The technetium-99m brain scan is sensitive in detection of intracranial suppuration and may be helpful in identification of early formation of abscess. A mass effect can be seen by cerebral angiography but its use has generally been obviated by CT. Electroencephalography may show a focus of delta-wave activity over the abscess and can be used to follow response to therapy.

Lumbar puncture is almost always contraindicated

because with increased intracranial pressure there is the danger of herniation. When studies of cerebrospinal fluid (CSF) are believed to be necessary to rule out meningitis, lumbar puncture should only be performed after CT. Findings on examination of CSF are nonspecific, with elevated level of protein, normal level of glucose (unless meningitis is present), and mild pleocytosis (i.e., several hundred cells/μL). Results of Gram stain and culture of CSF are negative unless the patient has meningitis or ventriculitis.

Many of the diagnostic tests can be performed on an outpatient basis, but hospitalization is absolutely necessary for proper treatment. When the typical clinical picture is present and a ring-enhancing lesion is demonstrated on CT, the diagnosis of brain abscess is made. However, the ring-enhancing lesion on CT is also seen with tumors, especially those that are metastatic. If no source of infection is found in the presence of signs and symptoms of an intracranial mass lesion, abscess must be differentiated from tumor, cerebral infarction, and hemorrhage. Another intracranial infection that may resemble brain abscess is herpes simplex encephalitis.

MANAGEMENT

Although the CT scan has greatly altered the management of brain abscess, general guidelines that guarantee optimal results in the individual patient are non-existent. Close cooperation between the internist and the neurosurgeon is of course mandatory.

ANTIBIOTICS

During the cerebritis stage, brain abscess can often be cured with adequate doses of parenterally administered antibiotics; an intracranial operation accomplishes little at this point and may cause neurologic deficit. Because the bacterial strain is presumptive, the choice of antimicrobial agents must be empiric. If cultures are believed to be necessary before starting antibiotic therapy, specimens can be obtained with CT-guided stereotactic biopsy. Traditionally the most common empiric regimen has been the combination of penicillin G, 20 to 30 million units administered intravenously per 24-hour period in divided doses, and chloramphenicol (Chloromycetin), 1 gm IV every six hours. Both drugs readily penetrate the blood-brain barrier, and penicillin G is active against all streptococci, anaerobes (except *B. fragilis*), and several strains of *Fusobacterium*. Chloramphenicol is active against virtually all anaerobes (including *B. fragilis*), aerobic streptococci, many *Enterobacteriaceae*, *Haemophilus* sp., and staphylococci. Metronidazole (Flagyl) has been advocated by some in place of chloramphenicol. If *S. aureus* is believed to be of primary importance as determined by positive results of blood cultures, either oxacillin or nafcillin (Nafcil, Unipen) should be administered IV in doses of 2 gm every four hours. In patients with allergy to penicillin, vancomycin hydrochloride (Vancocin), 500 mg IV every six hours, should be substituted for penicillin G, oxacillin, or nafcillin.

The optimal duration of antimicrobial treatment is unknown, but it probably should be continued for at least four to six weeks. Surgical therapy can be avoided if clinical improvement occurs. Multiple abscesses are usually not amenable to operation. During antibiotic

therapy a CT scan should probably be performed weekly. Cured abscesses may continue to appear as enhancing lesions on CT for up to ten weeks.

SURGICAL INTERVENTION

Surgical intervention is indicated when the abscess is large, when therapy with antibiotics alone is unsuccessful, or when the patient has increasing intracranial pressure. Total excision is possible when the abscess is in an accessible area and is encapsulated. Inaccessible abscesses may lend themselves to treatment by aspiration only, and the CT-guided needle has greatly improved this form of therapy. All surgical specimens should be submitted for Gram stain, aerobic and anaerobic bacterial cultures, acid-fast stains and cultures, and fungal stains and cultures. Appropriate changes in antibiotics should be made as dictated by results of culture.

Side effects of the most common antibiotics used in the treatment of brain abscess are relatively unusual. The most important toxic effects of chloramphenicol occur in the bone marrow and are of two types: a dose-related reversible bone marrow depression and an idiosyncratic aplastic anemia that occurs only rarely (one in 24,500 to 40,800 persons). Complete blood count should be performed twice weekly while chloramphenicol is being administered; if the WBC cell count decreases below 2500/μL, the antibiotic should be discontinued. Chloramphenicol prolongs the half-life of phenytoin (Dilantin) and phenobarbital, a factor that may be important in the management of abscess-related seizures.

COMPLICATIONS

The primary complications of brain abscess include elevated intracranial pressure and seizures. As noted previously, increased intracranial pressure is an indication for surgical intervention. Preoperative measures may include the use of mannitol (1 to 1.5 gm/kg of body weight IV over 10 to 15 minutes); hyperventilation (to a CO_2 of 30 torr); and dexamethasone (Decadron), 10 mg IV initially and 4 to 6 mg IV every six hours and continued postoperatively. Seizures should be treated with phenytoin or phenobarbital.

The mortality rate associated with brain abscess has decreased to 10% to 15% through the combined approach of surgery and antibiotics. Multiple abscesses, increased mental obtundation, ventricular rupture, and nonbacterial etiologic agents (e.g., fungi) are among the factors associated with mortality. Residual neurologic sequelae occur in approximately one third of patients, with focal seizures being of primary importance.

Subdural Empyema

DEFINITION AND DIAGNOSTIC CRITERIA

The term *subdural empyema* describes an intracranial suppurative collection in the preformed space between the inner dura and outer arachnoid surfaces. The diagnosis must be considered primarily in three groups:

patients who present with meningeal signs and a focal neurologic deficit, especially when the deficit suggests extensive involvement of one hemisphere; patients with a history of sinusitis who present with signs of meningitis; and patients in whom fever, subgaleal fluid collection, and a change in sensorium or focal neurologic signs or both develop after craniotomy.

PATHOPHYSIOLOGY

The frontal and ethmoidal sinuses provide the most common sources of infection, usually by direct extension through bone and dura as a result of thrombophlebitis of the emissary veins. Less often the focus is in the middle ear and mastoid. Infection only rarely occurs by hematogenous spread from the lung or other sources of sepsis, such as through abuse of intravenously administered drugs. Subdural empyema can also follow neurosurgical procedures or trauma to the skull, or it may extend from an earlier brain abscess. A previously sterile subdural hematoma can become infected. One or both hemispheres may be involved, and the empyema may be multiloculated. Focal osteomyelitis and epidural abscess can be seen in about 50% of these patients, but associated bacterial meningitis is uncommon.

The clinical picture in primary subdural empyema differs from that in patients with secondary infection of a chronic subdural hematoma. Pus in the subdural space, in contact with the cerebral cortex, is poorly tolerated. Cortical venous thrombosis can occur with irreversible massive cerebral infarction. In such patients no impediment exists to the rapid spread of pus, and it loculates in spaces where subdural hematoma is not seen, such as in the interhemispheric space. On the other hand, in the secondarily infected chronic subdural hematoma, the inner membrane protects the cortical veins from thrombosis and prevents the rapid dissemination of infection.

A variety of organisms are involved; aerobic streptococci and *S. aureus* are the most common, followed by anaerobic streptococci, *B. fragilis*, *Streptococcus pneumoniae*, *Haemophilus influenzae*, and other gram-negative organisms. As in brain abscess, the organisms that are isolated depend to a certain extent on the source of infection.

CLINICAL ASPECTS

The incidence of subdural empyema, which is highest in persons aged 20 to 40 years, reflects a 4:1 ratio of men to women. Fever, focal headaches, and malaise are present early in the development of the infection. As intracranial spread occurs, the headache becomes generalized with associated vomiting. Focal neurologic signs may progress rapidly within 24 hours or even develop suddenly. An entire hemisphere may show dysfunction with hemiparesis, hemianesthesia, hemianopsia, and aphasia. The patient with cerebral infarct may become comatose. Seizures occur in about one half of patients. Without surgical intervention, cerebral infarction and increased intracranial pressure with herniation will develop. In contrast to brain abscess, fever, leukocytosis, and stiffness of the neck are almost always present. The onset of symptoms may be more insidious than described previously, arising over several weeks. The clinical picture may also be masked somewhat by prior antibiotic therapy. As noted previously, subdural hematomas may become secondarily infected and present late in the course of disease (e.g., in the alcoholic patient).

MANAGEMENT

The single most useful diagnostic procedure is the CT scan. It usually shows a poorly circumscribed area of decreased density in the extra-axial region, surrounded by a thin rim of contrast enhancement. An interhemispheric collection of fluid is classically present. Associated edema, hemorrhage, and abscess formation are evident as well. Lumbar puncture is usually contraindicated because of the danger of transtentorial herniation.

Once the diagnosis is made, the neurosurgeon should be consulted immediately because treatment consists of prompt drainage. The best drainage procedure is one that facilitates both efficient removal of fluid and irrigation with antibiotics. In the infected chronic subdural hematoma, obliteration of the hematoma cavity is necessary, perhaps by removal of the skull bone and collapse of the scalp against the cortex. A postoperative continuous irrigation system should be used. The purulent drainage is submitted for aerobic and anaerobic bacterial cultures. Blood, sputum, and urine cultures should also be performed. Empiric antibiotic therapy includes nafcillin, 2 gm IV every four hours, combined with either metronidazole, 500 mg IV every six hours, or chloramphenicol, 1 gm IV every six hours. In the penicillin-allergic patient, vancomycin hydrochloride, 500 mg IV every six hours, can be substituted for nafcillin. These combinations may be changed as dictated by results of surgical cultures. Increased intracranial pressure and seizures should be treated as described previously for the patient with brain abscess. Prophylactic anticonvulsants are administered early in the course of therapy, and antibiotics should be continued for at least three to four weeks.

The longer therapy is delayed, the greater is the risk of permanent neurologic sequelae. Associated mortality ranges from 9% to 75%, depending on the degree of mental obtundation present initially, but the overall mortality is 14% to 18%. If cerebral infarction has developed as a result of venous thrombosis, the chance of survival is slight. Late onset of seizures after therapy may occur in up to 40% of patients.

REFERENCES

Bannister G, Williams B, Smith S: Treatment of subdural empyema. J Neurosurg 55:82–88, 1981.

Brewer NS, MacCarty CS, Wellman WE: Brain abscess: a review of recent experience. Ann Intern Med 82:571–576, 1975.

Britt RH, Enzmann DR: Clinical stages of human brain abscesses on serial CT scans after contrast infusion: computerized tomographic, neuropathological, and clinical correlations. J Neurosurg 59:972–989, 1983.

de Lourvois J: Antimicrobial chemotherapy in the treatment of brain abscess. J Antimicrob Chemother 12:205–207, 1983.

Gruszkiewicz J, Doron Y, Peyser E, et al: Brain abscess and its surgical management. Surg Neurol 18:7–17, 1982.

Kaufman DM, Miller MH, Steigbigel NH: Subdural empyema: analysis of 17 recent cases and review of the literature. Medicine 54:485–498, 1975.

Luken MG III, Whelan MA: Recent diagnostic experience with subdural empyema. J Neurosurg 52:764–771, 1980.

Yang S-H: Brain abscess: a review of 400 cases. J Neurosurg 55:794–799, 1981.

5 · ACUTE AND CHRONIC VIRAL ENCEPHALITIS

José A. Gutrecht
LAHEY CLINIC MEDICAL CENTER

Acute Viral Encephalitis

DEFINITION AND DIAGNOSTIC CRITERIA

Viral encephalitis describes a group of illnesses characterized by such symptoms as malaise, fever, myalgia, headache, alteration of consciousness, confusion, behavioral aberrations, seizures, and other focal or nonfocal neurologic deficits. These nonspecific symptoms and signs, which may occur in any combination, result from viral invasion of various tissues and organs in which the brain either is most involved or is the specific target organ.

Concomitant meningeal involvement and abnormal findings on examination of cerebrospinal fluid (CSF) are usually present. Initial CSF pressure may be normal or elevated. The CSF is clear and colorless. The white cell count in CSF is elevated (25 to 500 cells/μL) with a preponderance of mononuclear type cells. In the CSF the protein concentration is somewhat elevated while the glucose concentration is normal. Results of early studies of CSF may be normal or polymorphonuclear leukocytes may predominate.

PATHOPHYSIOLOGY

Invasion of the CNS usually occurs soon after the virus has entered and multiplied in other organs and tissues. Spread occurs by the neuronal or the hematogenous route. Pathologic changes in the brain include early infiltration by polymorphonuclear leukocytes followed by mononuclear cells, microglial hyperplasia, neuronal changes that may eventually lead to neuronal destruction, and in some types of encephalitis the presence of acidophilic inclusion bodies. Changes in the walls of blood vessels and invasion of white matter are more variable. The meninges are almost always involved. The extent and focus of these changes are responsible for variations in the severity and in the clinical manifestations of acute encephalitis.

CLINICAL ASPECTS

Acute viral encephalitis ranges from a brief, mild illness to severe illness leading to chronic neurologic sequelae or death. Focal neurologic deficits may appear superimposed on diffuse cerebral dysfunction. The clinical manifestations of viral encephalitis vary somewhat according to the type of causative virus, but the same virus may cause infections ranging in severity from subclinical to lethal.

Generalized metabolic, toxic, or anoxic encephalopathy, brain tumor, cerebrovascular disease, trauma, and nonviral infection may each produce a similar clinical picture. Thus the differential diagnosis is of paramount importance. The diagnosis of viral encephalitis should be made after careful exclusion of other causes of CNS dysfunction. Many processes that mimic acute encephalitis are often treatable and require prompt medical or surgical attention. Except for herpes simplex encephalitis, the diagnosis of viral encephalitis can usually wait because often only nonspecific supportive treatment is required.

VIRUSES COMMONLY IMPLICATED IN ACUTE ENCEPHALITIS

Herpes simplex virus (type I) is one of the commonest and most important causes of sporadic fatal encephalitis. The primary infection takes place by salivary or respiratory human-to-human contact. Neurologic disease occurs as a late reactivation secondary to nonspecific stimuli. Onset is marked by the sudden appearance of fever and headaches soon followed by focal seizures, impairment of consciousness, or both. During the next few hours or days, focal neurologic deficits arise in most patients.

Examination of CSF demonstrates the usual findings discussed previously, and red cells may also be found. In most patients single or multiple low-density abnormalities, usually in the temporal lobe, may be seen on CT scan. Radioisotope brain scan and angiography may also reveal focal lesions. Results of electroencephalography are almost invariably abnormal, and focal repetitive periodic complexes are found.

The diagnosis can be secured by examining brain tissue obtained by biopsy. Characteristic acidophilic intranuclear inclusions (Cowdry's type A) may be observed by light microscopy and virions by electron microscopy; positive fluorescent antigen staining may also be seen. The virus is rarely recovered from CSF. The illness is fatal in about three fourths of patients, and sequelae are usually found in survivors.

Equine encephalitis virus includes three types of togaviruses (formerly termed group A arboviruses) that are known to cause encephalitis, i.e., eastern equine, western equine, and Venezuelan equine. These viruses, which are transmitted by mosquitoes, tend to occur sporadically in summer and fall. Distribution is not confined to specific geographic regions. Infection tends to occur in children and older adults. Focal neurologic deficits are uncommon. The severity of the illness is variable.

St. Louis encephalitis virus, a togavirus (formerly a group B arbovirus) transmitted by mosquitoes, is responsible for outbreaks of encephalitis in the midwestern and southwestern United States, usually in summer and fall. Infection occurs in adults more often than in children. The associated mortality may be high, and sequelae often occur.

California encephalitis virus, a bunyavirus transmitted by mosquitoes, causes encephalitis almost exclusively in children. The associated mortality is usually low.

Enteroviruses (echoviruses and coxsackieviruses) rarely cause encephalitis, and the course of disease is usually benign.

Mumps (paramyxovirus) may cause encephalitis that develops before, during, or after parotitis. Encephalitis may be the only symptom of mumps infection. The illness rarely occurs in adults, and the course is usually benign.

Measles (paramyxovirus), which may cause encephalitis four to five days after the rash, occurs almost exclusively in children.

Varicella-zoster virus is an infrequent cause of encephalitis that usually develops two to eight days after the rash.

Epstein-Barr virus and *cytomegalovirus* produce encephalitis in rare instances.

Lymphocytic choriomeningitis virus (arenavirus) and *adenoviruses* rarely cause encephalitis.

MANAGEMENT

The short-term goal of treatment is entirely supportive whereas the long-range goal is to avoid neurologic sequelae and to return the patient to a normal life style. These objectives are best accomplished in a hospital setting because close nursing and medical supervision are usually required.

SUPPORTIVE CARE

Attention is first given to establishment of an adequate airway, including endotracheal intubation if necessary, and frequent checks of vital and neurologic signs. Symptomatic treatment is directed to relief of headache, fever, nausea, vomiting, and dehydration.

Headache may be treated with aspirin, acetaminophen, or codeine (30 to 60 mg every four hours intramuscularly); bed rest; and isolation from disturbing environments. Fever may be controlled with aspirin, cooling blankets, or alcohol sponge baths.

Dehydration is treated with 5% dextrose in isotonic saline solution or one half isotonic saline solution, and replacement of electrolytes as indicated by close monitoring of input and output of fluids and levels of electrolytes. Fluid overload must be avoided. Inappropriate secretion of antidiuretic hormone may occur, and restriction of fluids or hypertonic saline solutions may be needed.

Nausea and vomiting may be treated with prochlorperazine (Compazine), 10 to 20 mg, or trimethobenzamide hydrochloride (Tigan), 200 mg, parenterally or rectally every six to eight hours as needed.

Urinary catheterization is often necessary in the acute stages, and tube feedings may be needed later in the course of the illness.

NONSPECIFIC NEUROLOGIC TREATMENT

Status epilepticus or isolated major generalized seizures may occur, requiring prompt and vigorous treatment. In patients with status epilepticus, phenytoin (Dilantin), 500- to 1000-mg IV loading, is given at a rate of not more than 50 mg per minute in conjunction with electrocardiographic monitoring. The maintenance dose thereafter is approximately 5 mg/kg of body weight per day IV or through a nasogastric tube. Dilantin should never be administered intramuscularly.

Diazepam (Valium) may also be used alone as a first-choice drug or with phenytoin in more refractory cases. Diazepam is given IV in a 5-mg bolus over one to two minutes, repeated three to four times within a few minutes up to 20 mg, with close monitoring for respiratory depression. Use of diazepam alone is not indicated after initial treatment of seizure; other drugs, such as phenytoin, carbamazepine (Tegretol), or phenobarbital, must be used.

Phenobarbital may also be given either alone or with phenytoin, diazepam, or both for management of more refractory cases of status epilepticus. The initial dose is 100 mg IV over three to five minutes with loading continued up to a total dose of 500 to 800 mg. Monitoring of respiration is mandatory, and an immediate means of artificial ventilation must be available. Serum levels of drugs should be monitored frequently. Treatment is continued for one year or more if seizures persist.

Acute cerebral edema with increased intracranial pressure and herniation is frequently responsible for death in the acute stages of disease and for sequelae of varying degrees of severity in the chronic stages. Therapy must therefore be instituted promptly and aggressively. When herniation is imminent, 20% mannitol, 500 ml over 30 minutes, is administered IV. This is repeated every three to eight hours only when necessary because its effectiveness is diminished with repeated doses and a rebound increase of intracranial pressure may occur.

An IV bolus of dexamethasone, 10 to 20 mg, should be given early and continued in 4- to 8-mg doses every four to six hours thereafter. This drug may be continued for a few days as needed and then slowly tapered. Diuretics, such as IV furosemide (Lasix), 20 to 40 mg every six hours, may also be used. Replacement of fluids should be maintained to cover minimal needs.

SPECIFIC TREATMENT

Specific antiviral agents are available for the treatment of herpes simplex encephalitis. Vidarabine (Vira A) and acyclovir (Zovirax) reduce the associated mortality by more than one half and probably reduces the morbidity rate as well. Treatment must be initiated early in the course of the disease because a deteriorating level of consciousness is associated with a less favorable outcome. A high index of suspicion and a suggestive clinical picture should be followed quickly by electroencephalography, CT scan, and examination of CSF. Correct diagnosis depends on the study of brain tissue obtained at biopsy. Therapy should begin immediately after biopsy is performed.

The drug of choice is acyclovir, a selective inhibitor of the herpes simplex virus replication. Acyclovir, 30 mg/kg of body weight per day divided into three daily doses, is infused every eight hours in a minimum volume of 100 ml of standard IV fluid over a period of one hour for ten days.

Vidarabine is now considered a second therapeutic choice because of lesser effectiveness and more adverse reactions.

CHRONIC SUPPORTIVE CARE

Some patients recover incompletely from encephalitis, and late sequelae may develop that require continued treatment. From the medical standpoint, respiratory aids, enteral feeding, care of anal and urinary sphincters, and treatment of decubitus ulcers may be needed.

From the general neurologic standpoint, physical, occupational, and speech therapy with educational, social, and psychologic support are sometimes indicated. More specific pharmacologic treatment with anticonvulsant, psychotropic, sedative, hypnotic, or analgesic drugs may also be necessary.

Chronic Viral Encephalitis

Chronic or "slow" viral infections may involve the CNS. The infective agents may be conventional viruses, defective viruses, or unconventional transmissible agents of spongiform encephalopathy.

The pathologic changes may suggest a chronic inflammatory process (e.g., subacute sclerosing panencephalitis), but in other instances demyelination either coexists (e.g., progressive rubella panencephalitis) or is the dominant finding without inflammation (e.g., progressive multifocal leukoencephalitis). Unconventional transmissible agents cause noninflammatory degenerative changes (e.g., Creutzfeldt-Jakob disease).

SUBACUTE SCLEROSING PANENCEPHALITIS

Subacute sclerosing panencephalitis, which is caused by persistent infection with a defective measles virus, is characterized pathologically by perivascular infiltration by mononuclear and occasional plasma cells in the white and gray matter, patchy areas of demyelination and gliosis in the white matter and deep cortex with widespread degenerative neuronal changes. Intranuclear (Cowdry's type A) and ill-defined intracytoplasmic inclusion bodies are found in neurons and glial cells.

This disease affects children, more commonly boys, and is characterized by decline in schoolwork, intellectual deterioration, and personality changes. These signs are soon followed by ataxic gait, myoclonic jerks, and seizures leading to profound dementia, coma, and death.

Results of laboratory studies reveal elevated levels of measles antibodies in serum and CSF and a marked increase in IgG in CSF. Atrophy and focal or multifocal low-density lesions in white matter may be seen on CT scan. Repetitive periodic high-amplitude slow wave complexes at a rate of one every several seconds, which may coincide with the myoclonic jerks, and widespread abnormalities of background cortical activity are usually shown on electroencephalography. The illness is slowly progressive, leading almost invariably to death in one to five years. No specific treatment exists.

PROGRESSIVE RUBELLA PANENCEPHALITIS

Progressive rubella panencephalitis is an extremely rare disease that occurs in children and teenagers, primarily in those with congenital rubella syndrome. An inflammatory perivascular infiltration of lymphocytes and plasma cells takes place in the meninges and the white and gray matter. Extensive demyelination with atrophy and gliosis is usually found. The brunt of the illness is located in the cerebellum. Inclusion bodies have not been found.

Disease begins with intellectual deterioration and behavioral problems followed by progressive cerebellar ataxic gait and involvement of the corticospinal tracts, terminating eventually in coma and death in two to five years. Myoclonic jerks and seizures are not common. Examination of CSF may show lymphocytosis with increased concentration of total protein and markedly elevated IgG. The CT scan shows atrophy, particularly in the cerebellum. Electroencephalography demonstrates diffuse abnormalities without periodic or burst suppression patterns as seen in subacute sclerosing panencephalitis. Serum and CSF antibody titers against rubella virus are elevated.

PROGRESSIVE MULTIFOCAL LEUKOENCEPHALOPATHY

Progressive multifocal leukoencephalopathy is a rare demyelinating disease caused by an opportunistic papovavirus (most frequently JC strain) in immunocompromised adults. These patients most often have carcinoma, especially of the breast or lung; chronic leukemia; Hodgkin's disease; or other reticuloendothelial cell disease. Rarely, this disease has been found in patients without other underlying illness.

Clinical manifestations, which are usually insidious, include intellectual deterioration, hemiparesis, visual loss, and sensory deficits that appear up to several years after onset of the underlying chronic disease. Onset may sometimes be acute or subacute. The CSF is usually normal, electroencephalography reveals nonspecific focal or generalized abnormalities, and CT may show areas of low density. Death usually occurs within a year.

CREUTZFELDT-JAKOB DISEASE

Creutzfeldt-Jakob disease is rare and occurs late in middle age. Neuropathologic findings include neuronal destruction, astrocytosis, and status spongiosis (i.e., vacuolar changes in the cytoplasm of neurons and astrocytes). The cerebral cortex and basal ganglia are most prominently involved. The illness begins with vague symptoms of anxiety, asthenia, visual difficulties, disrupted sleep, impaired judgment, and mood changes. As the disease progresses, worsening intellectual impairment is accompanied by cerebellar gait ataxia, myoclonic jerks with prominent startle response, visual loss, and such signs of basal ganglia involvement as rigidity, tremors, and slowness. Electroencephalography usually shows a distinctive, periodic, generalized sharp wave pattern in patients with advanced disease. The course is usually rapidly progressive. No treatment is available, and death occurs within six months.

REFERENCES

Brown P: Acute viral encephalitis. *In* Conn RB (ed): Current Diagnosis. W. B. Saunders Co, Philadelphia, 1985, pp 918–923.

Johnson RT: Viral Infections of the Nervous System. Raven Press, New York, 1982.

Jubelt B, Harter DH: Viral infections. *In* Rowland LP, (ed): Merritt's Textbook of Neurology, 7th ed. Lea & Febiger, Philadelphia, 1984, pp 79–116.

Whitley RJ, Alford CA, et al: Vidarabine versus acyclovir therapy in herpes simplex encephalitis. N Engl J Med 314:144–149, 1986.

6 · ACUTE AND CHRONIC MENINGITIS

Wendell W. Hoffman
Pierre Forgacs
LAHEY CLINIC MEDICAL CENTER

Acute Meningitis

DEFINITION AND DIAGNOSTIC CRITERIA

Meningitis is an inflammation of the pia-arachnoid and the fluid in the intervening space. Infection extends throughout the subarachnoid space surrounding the brain, the spinal cord, and the optic nerves. Diagnosis is made by examination of cerebrospinal fluid (CSF). Separation of acute meningitis into two etiologic categories, bacterial meningitis and aseptic meninigitis syndrome, is clinically useful.

PATHOPHYSIOLOGY

The most common pathogens causing acute meningitis include *Streptococcus pneumoniae*, *Neisseria meningitidis*, and *Haemophilus influenzae*. These bacteria seem to possess a variety of mechanisms of pathogenicity. All three are colonizers of the nasopharynx and have definable antiphagocytic capsules that may confer tropism for the meninges.

Underlying factors in penetration of the mucosal barrier leading to bacteremia include defects in humoral immunity, complement-deficiency states, and antecedent viral infections of the upper respiratory tract. The most frequent mode of meningeal invasion appears to be bacteremia arising from pneumonia, endocarditis, gastroenteritis, urinary tract infection, or the nasopharynx. Entrance into the CSF from the blood is probably gained by way of the choroid plexuses. Other routes of infection include parameningeal foci and traumatic or congenital defects. Since the CSF is deficient in humoral factors and phagocytic cells, it is easy to see how initial invasion occurs.

Bacterial meningitis may lead to pathologic changes in adjacent structures, including cortical thrombophlebitis with infarction, cerebral edema, cranial nerve damage, ventriculitis, and hydrocephalus.

CLINICAL ASPECTS

ETIOLOGIC FACTORS

A wide variety of possible causes must be considered. In addition to bacterial pathogens the offending agent or condition may be fungal, mycobacterial, viral, parasitic, chemical, or neoplastic. Separation of acute

Table 1. MAJOR CAUSES OF MENINGITIS BY DIAGNOSTIC CATEGORY*

I. Acute and subacute bacterial meningitis (positive results of Gram stain or bacterial culture of CSF or both)
   Pneumococci
   Meningococci
   H. influenzae
   Gram-negative bacilli
   Group B streptococci
   L. monocytogenes
   Other (e.g., *S. aureus*, *S. epidermidis*)
II. Aseptic meningitis syndrome (negative results of Gram stain and bacterial culture of CSF)
   A. Antimicrobial therapy required
      Partially treated meningitis
      Parameningeal suppurative foci (e.g., brain abscess, paranasal sinusitis, cranial or spinal epidural abscess, subdural empyema, dermal sinus tract)
      M. tuberculosis
      Fungi
      Amebae
      Syphilis
      Herpes simplex, types 1 and 2
      Other (e.g., wall-defective bacteria, mycoplasma, bacterial endocarditis)
   B. Antimicrobial therapy not required
      Viruses (in general)
      Leptospirae
      Neoplastic
      Cyst related
      Chemical
      Other (e.g., Behçet's syndrome, Mollaret's meningitis, sarcoidosis, lupus erythematosus)

*Modified from McGee ZA, Kaiser AB: Acute meningitis. *In* Mandell GL, Douglas RG Jr, Bennett JE (eds): Principles and Practice of Infectious Diseases, 2nd ed. John Wiley & Sons, New York, 1979, p. 740.

meningitis into two categories based on results of Gram stain or culture of CSF is useful. When results of either of these are positive, a bacterial cause is defined (Table 1). Negative results of both indicate the presence of aseptic meningitis syndrome, which is further categorized into causes that require antimicrobial agents and those that do not (Table 1). As noted previously, aseptic meningitis does not automatically mean meningitis of viral origin, and therefore, a thorough evaluation for treatable causes should be performed.

PRESENTATION

Symptoms common to most types of meningitis include fever, generalized headache, stiffness of the neck, lethargy, confusion, and vomiting. The onset of symptoms may be acute (less than 24 hours) or subacute (one to seven days). This distinction is critical because the acute presentation almost always indicates a pyogenic bacterial cause and is associated with a much higher mortality rate. Subacute onset is much more common and its associated mortality rate is less than one half that for acute onset.

HISTORICAL CLUES AND CLINICAL SETTING

As in every medical emergency, a rapid and thorough history-taking and recognition of predisposing conditions are essential. Table 2 provides a clinical comparison of the most common causes of acute bacterial meningitis in adults.

Pneumococcal meningitis occurs in all age groups. It is associated with otitis media, mastoiditis, or both in 30% of patients; pneumonia in 25%; and sinusitis in an occasional few. A history of severe trauma to the head

Table 2. COMPARISON OF BACTERIAL MENINGITIS

Factor Compared	S. pneumoniae	N. meningitidis	H. influenzae	Gram-negative Organisms	S. aureus S. epidermidis	L. monocytogenes
Age	All ages	Children and young adults	Neonates to age 6 yr, elderly persons	Neonates, adults	Adults	All ages
Associated infections	Pneumonia, sinusitis, endocarditis, otitis media		Otitis media, pharyngitis	Gram-negative sepsis, ruptured brain abscess	Brain abscess, septicemia, endocarditis, sinusitis	
Predisposing conditions	CSF leakage, splenectomy, sickle cell disease, head trauma, alcoholism, bone marrow transplantation		CSF leak, humoral immune deficiency	Head trauma, neurosurgery, immunocompromised host, hospital acquired	CSF shunts	Immunocompromised hosts (especially renal transplant recipients), alcoholism
Clinical characteristics	Petechiae uncommon	Petechiae, purpura in 50%, disseminated intravascular coagulation common, most common in winter and spring, occurs in epidemics (serogroups A and C)	Petechiae rare, 10%–20% ampicillin resistant	*Klebsiella, E. coli, Pseudomonas* most common, Gram stain negative in 50%		Gram stain usually negative, occurs in neonates and elderly persons
Therapy of choice	Penicillin G	Penicillin G	Ampicillin and chloramphenicol	Third-generation cephalosporins +/− aminoglycosides	Oxacillin or nafcillin	Ampicillin, +/− aminoglycosides

is present in about 10% of patients, and CSF rhinorrhea occurs in 5%. Not infrequently, alcoholism is an underlying factor in pneumoccoal meningitis. Other factors such as sickle cell disease, postsplenectomy state, and bone marrow transplantation can also predispose patients to this infection.

Meningococcal meningitis primarily occurs in children and young adults, most cases arising in spring or winter. It has been responsible for major epidemics (serogroups A and C), such as those in military recruits.

H. influenzae is the most common cause of bacterial meningitis from the neonatal period to 6 years of age. Its occurrence in adults, which is rare, should prompt a search for a parameningeal focus, a CSF leakage, or an underlying immunodeficiency.

The incidence of meningitis caused by gram-negative organisms has increased appreciably over the past several years, probably reflecting the overall increase in hospital-acquired gram-negative infections. Possible clinical settings include previous neurosurgery, trauma to the head, and gram-negative sepsis. The specific organisms, which reflect the local hospital flora, most frequently include *Klebsiella* sp., *Escherichia coli*, and *Pseudomonas* sp. The presentation of meningitis in these patient populations may be more subtle and must be considered in the differential diagnosis of new fever or altered sensorium.

Staphylococcal meningitis must be considered in several settings. *Staphylococcus aureus* meningitis may occur in severe staphylococcal septicemia, endocarditis, sinusitis, and brain abscess. *S. aureus* and *S. epidermidis* cause infection of CSF shunts.

Listeria monocytogenes should be considered in the differential diagnosis of meningitis in immunocompromised patients, elderly persons, neonates, and especially renal transplant recipients. Results of Gram stain of CSF are often negative. Positive results may incorrectly be attributed to diphtheroid contaminants.

Other organisms, such as group A streptococci, are less common causes of meningitis. Group B streptococci are a major cause of neonatal meningitis.

When results of Gram stain and culture of CSF are negative, one is faced with aseptic meningitis syndrome. *Aseptic* implies for many a viral cause, and certainly viruses cause the majority of infections in this category. The differential diagnosis, however, must consider tuberculous, fungal (including *Cryptococcus* sp., *Coccidioides* sp., and *Candida* sp.), syphilitic, leptospiral, and amebic causes. Although the course of most of these infections is chronic, presentation may be subacute or acute. Noninfectious causes of aseptic meningitis syndrome include neoplasms, chemical agents, sarcoidosis, lupus erythematosus, and Behçet's syndrome.

The most common causes of viral meningitis are the enteroviruses that prevail in later summer and early fall. Other major causes include herpes simplex, mumps, and flavirviruses (e.g., St. Louis encephalitis). Less commonly, meningitis may occur secondary to such infections as measles, herpes zoster, cytomegalovirus, lymphocytic choriomeningitis, adenovirus, and Epstein-Barr virus.

PHYSICAL EXAMINATION

Signs of meningeal irritation include decreased mentation, stiffness of the neck, and positive Kernig's and Brudzinski's signs. These symptoms are similar despite the cause and may easily be overlooked, especially in neonates and elderly persons. Meningism with petechiae, purpura, or ecchymosis strongly suggests meningococcal infection. Similar skin lesions may rarely be associated with *S. aureus, S. pneumoniae,* and *H. influenzae*. Disseminated intravascular coagulation frequently accompanies meningococcemia and may result in adrenal infarction, renal cortical necrosis, shock, and acute respiratory distress syndrome. Neurologic signs, such as cranial nerve abnormalities, hearing loss, seizures, hemiparesis, and visual field defects, are relatively uncommon, occurring in 10% to 30% of patients. Increased intracranial pressure may develop, presenting as bradycardia, hypertension, and coma. There is no substitute for repeated examination, searching for changes in neurologic status. As noted previously, other associated infections must be sought on examination, including otitis media, sinusitis, pneumonia, and endocarditis. A clear nasal discharge suggests CSF rhinorrhea.

LABORATORY STUDIES

Examination of CSF should include total and differential cell counts, determinations of concentrations of protein and glucose, Gram stain, and bacterial cultures. Counterimmunoelectrophoresis for bacterial antigen is a valuable diagnostic tool that can be carried out within a few hours. The level of lactic dehydrogenase, which is consistently elevated in bacterial meningitis, is a nonspecific marker that may also be helpful when initial results of Gram stain are negative. If results of Gram stain, counterimmunoelectrophoresis, and culture are negative, a second CSF specimen can be obtained for additional studies, including cryptococcal antigen, acid-fast stain and fungal cultures, and cytologic examination.

A bacterial cause is suggested when the white cell count is greater than 1000/μL, the concentration of protein is more than 100 mg/dL, and the concentration of gluose is less than 40 mg/dL. The differential cell count usually shows a predominance of polymorphonuclear leukocytes (PMLs) in bacterial meningitis; however, in 10% of patients, more than 80% of lymphocytes is seen. Similarly, although lymphocytic pleocytosis usually suggests a nonbacterial cause, primarily PMLs are observed in up to 30% of patients with viral or tuberculous meningitis. Results of Gram stain are positive in 80% to 90% of those patients in whom subsequent results of bacterial cultures are positive.

A reduction of glucose concentration in CSF (hypoglycorrhachia) to less than 50% of a simultaneous blood level suggests a bacterial cause, but a normal concentration of CSF glucose does not exclude bacterial meningitis. Alternatively, hypoglycorrhachia can also be seen in mumps; lymphocytic choriomeningitis; and tuberculous, fungal, sarcoid, and carcinomatous meningitis. Initial CSF pressure usually is moderately elevated (200 to 300 mm). Pressures above 400 mm suggest brain swelling, whereas normal or low CSF pressures indicate the possibility of spinal needle occlusion or blockage in the subarachnoid space. As noted previously, concentrations of protein in CSF are often elevated above 100 mg/dL in bacterial meningitis. Pronounced elevations (greater than 1000 mg/dL) suggest blockage in the subarachnoid space.

Other laboratory tests should include complete blood count with differential, serum electrolytes, and creatinine. Blood cultures are essential and cultures of sputum and urine may be helpful. Radiographs of the chest, paranasal sinuses, and mastoids should be obtained in all patients with meningitis. When a mass lesion is suspected, computed tomography (CT) of the head should be performed.

MANAGEMENT

The approach in management of acute meningitis is largely dictated by the presentation. In the truly acute situation (i.e., symptoms for less than 24 hours), the immediate concern should be therapy. When the presentation is subacute, more time is often available to gather additional information before consideration of therapy.

In the patient with a fulminant presentation an abbreviated physical examination should be performed, searching for increased intracerebral pressure (i.e., papilledema) and focal neurologic deficits (excluding ophthalmoplegias). When either of these signs is present, blood cultures should be performed immediately, therapy with IV penicillin G and chloramphenicol (Chloromycetin) should be started, and arrangements should be made for a CT scan of the head. Lumbar puncture is contraindicated because of the risk of uncal herniation. If results of CT are negative for a mass lesion, lumbar puncture should be performed.

When physical examination does not reveal either papilledema or focal neurologic deficits, blood cultures and CSF studies are obtained, followed immediately by IV penicillin G or ampicillin (Polycillin). The goal is rapid initiation of therapy. Antibiotic therapy should be given immediately in bolus form. For example, penicillin G is given as a 5-million-unit bolus followed by continuous infusion of 1 million units/hr (24 million units/day). Ampicillin should be given as a 2- to 3-gm bolus followed by 2 gm every four hours (12 gm/day) IV. In penicillin-allergic patients, IV chloramphenicol is given, 1 gm immediately and 1 gm every four to six hours. If results of Gram stain of CSF or counterimmunoelectrophoresis are positive, therapy should be continued and altered as indicated by the findings. If results of Gram stain are negative but CSF WBC count is elevated, therapy should also be continued while further workup is initiated.

When the patient presents with a subacute course, a more complete initial history and examination may be possible. A search for papilledema, neurologic deficit, or both is performed as in the patient with acute onset, with the same requirement for a CT scan before lumbar puncture to exclude the presence of a mass lesion. Results of CSF examination determine whether immediate empiric antibiotic therapy is started. The approach for the patient with a depressed sensorium or who is comatose is similar to that described for acute presentation.

Patients with pneumococcal and meningococcal meningitis are treated with penicillin G, 20 to 24 million units/day IV. *H. influenzae* should be treated initially with ampicillin and chloramphenicol until beta-lactamase testing is completed. If results of such testing are positive, as occurs in 15% to 20% of patients, chloramphenicol alone should be continued; otherwise, ampicillin is the treatment of choice. Therapy for these three organisms should be continued for 10 to 14 days.

Chemoprophylaxis with rifampin (Rifadin) should be considered for contacts of patients with *H. influenzae* or meningococcal meningitis. If there are young children in the family other than the patient with *H. influenzae* infection, rifampin should be given to all members of the patient's household, both adults and children, and to contacts aged 4 years or under in day care centers. The patient should also receive prophylactic treatment because the carrier state may continue despite adequate therapy. In meningococcal meningitis, prophylaxis is indicated for contacts within the patient's household and in day care centers. Public health officials should be notified of these types of meningitis so that appropriate follow-up studies can be carried out. The dose of rifampin for contacts should be 20 mg/kg of body weight/day (not to exceed 600 mg) for four consecutive days in *H. influenzae*, and twice a day for two days in meningococcal infection.

Vaccines are available for use against certain strains of *S. pneumoniae*, *N. meningitidis*, and *H. influenzae*. The monovalent A or C meningococcal vaccine should be used in epidemics of either serogroup in conjunction with rifampin. The pneumococcal vaccine should be given to those groups of patients at higher risk as recommended by the Centers for Disease Control. A polysaccharide vaccine against invasive disease caused by *H. influenzae* type B was recently licensed in the United States. Administration is recommended at 18 months of age for children in known high-risk groups, and at age 24 months for all other children.

An optimal regimen for meningitis caused by gram-negative organisms has not been defined adequately, but the advent of third-generation cephalosporin antibiotics has altered the approach considerably. Initial therapy should include either cefotaxime (Claforan) or moxalactam disodium (Moxam), 2 gm every four hours IV in combination with an aminoglycoside, such as amikacin sulfate (Amikin), 5 mg/kg of body weight every eight hours IV. If the isolated organism is sensitive to the cephalosporin (e.g., *E. coli* or *Klebsiella* sp.), the aminoglycoside can be discontinued. In the presence of cephalosporin resistance, aminoglycosides should be given by both the systemic and intrathecal routes in combination with an extended-spectrum penicillin such as ticarcillin (Ticar) or piperacillin (Pipracil), both IV, 3 gm every four hours. Intrathecal aminoglycoside is given once every 24 hours (i.e., gentamicin [Garamycin], 4 to 8 mg). An intraventricular reservoir can be used at times to deliver the aminoglycoside. Total duration of therapy should extend 10 to 14 days after results of CSF cultures are negative. Prophylactic vitamin K should be given daily when moxalactam is used because of the tendency toward bleeding at high doses.

Meningitis resulting from *S. aureus* or *S. epidermidis* infection should be treated with nafcillin (Nafcil, Unipen), 2 gm every four hours IV. Vancomycin (Vancocin), 500 mg every six hours IV, is the drug of choice in penicillin-allergic patients or when the organism is nafcillin resistant. Duration of therapy should be at least four weeks.

L. monocytogenes meningitis is treated with ampicillin, 12 gm/day, and may require therapy of longer duration, i.e., more than three weeks.

When results of bacterial cultures of CSF are negative, aseptic meningitis syndrome is present and a systematic search should be undertaken for those causes that require antimicrobial therapy, e.g., partially treated bacterial meningitis or parameningeal infection.

Many patients with bacterial meningitis have received antibiotics before lumbar puncture. Results of CSF examination are not appreciably altered in the first few days by antimicrobial therapy and will continue to suggest a bacterial cause. Empiric antimicrobial therapy should be given, especially for the patient with a depressed sensorium. If a search for a bacterial cause yields negative results and antibiotic therapy is withheld, lumbar puncture may be repeated in eight to 12 hours. Brain abscess, tuberculous meningitis, and cryptococcal meningitis should be considered and appropriate studies ordered, including CT scan of the head.

Parameningeal foci can cause meningism and altered CSF parameters indistinguishable from those in bacterial or viral meningitis. Differential diagnosis includes brain abscess, subdural empyema, spinal epidural abscess, cranial osteomyelitis, mastoiditis, and infection of the middle ear and paranasal sinuses. A thorough examination usually indicates a parameningeal focus and prompt appropriate imaging studies, such as CT scan, radiography of the sinuses and mastoids, and myelography. Specific antibiotic therapy depends on the clinical situation.

Syphilis may present as acute meningitis months to years after primary infection, illustrating the need for serologic studies of serum and CSF in aseptic meningitis. The most effective therapy is aqueous penicillin G, 10 to 20 million units/day for ten days, followed by benzathine penicillin.

Herpes simplex (types 1 and 2) can cause meningoencephalitis. Type 1 infection usually presents as a progressive encephalitis. Type 2 can begin as aseptic meningitis and may progress to encephalitis, especially in the immunocompromised host. Both adenine arabinoside (Vira-A), 15 mg/kg of body weight/day for ten days IV and acyclovir sodium (Zovirax), 10 mg/kg of body weight every eight hours for ten days IV, have been shown to be effective in decreasing associated mortality rates and neurologic sequelae, especially in type 1 biopsy-proved encephalitis.

Amebic meningitis (*Naegleria* sp. and *Acanthamoeba* sp.) should be considered in the patient who presents with aseptic meningitis and a history of swimming in a fresh water lake or indoor pool. The organisms can be seen on a wet mount of CSF. Although infection is usually fatal, high doses of amphotericin B (Fungizone) given systemically and intraventricularly have been associated with clinical response and recovery in some patients.

Chronic Meningitis

DEFINITION AND DIAGNOSTIC CRITERIA

Chronic meningitis is marked by symptoms similar to those of acute meningitis. The syndrome applies if abnormalities of CSF persist for at least four weeks with clinical evidence of persistence or progression.

CLINICAL ASPECTS

PRESENTATION

In chronic meningitis the onset is insidious although there may be periods of acute deterioration with hydrocephalus, cerebral edema, or seizures. The usual presenting symptoms include headache, stiffness of the neck, fever, lethargy, confusion, nausea, and vomiting.

PHYSICAL EXAMINATION

Frequent findings include meningism and oculomotor palsies. Less often, focal neurologic signs and raised intracranial pressure may be evident. The syndrome of headache, nausea, vomiting, ataxia, incontinence, and papilledema suggests hydrocephalus, which may contraindicate lumbar puncture. Other findings, such as uveitis, skin lesions, and hepatomegaly, may suggest systemic disease.

ETIOLOGIC CATEGORIES

The differential diagnosis considers both infectious and noninfectious etiologic factors. Infectious causes may result from specific exposure in normal immune hosts or from the presence of opportunistic pathogens in a setting of disordered cellular immunity. Disease from noninfectious causes may be associated with extraneural involvement or may present exclusively in the central nervous system (Table 3).

INFECTIOUS CAUSES

Meningitis presents the most lethal form of tuberculosis. This diagnosis must be considered in the patient who has a history of notable exposure, positive results of tuberculin skin testing, or evidence of previous pulmonary tuberculosis or chest radiography. A careful history with respect to tuberculosis is imperative for every patient who presents with chronic meningitis. Overall, there is little about tuberculous meningitis to distinguish it from other causes of chronic meningitis.

Cryptococcal meningitis has several presentations ranging from subacute meningoencephalitis to the gradual onset of dementia. About one half of patients have an underlying cellular immune deficiency, such as in Hodgkin's disease, high-dose therapy with corticosteroids, and acquired immune deficiency syndrome.

When there is a history of travel to the southwestern United States, coccidioidomycosis must be considered. Coccidioidal meningitis may be part of generalized coccidioidomycosis or the only manifestation of active clinical disease.

Table 3. DIFFERENTIAL DIAGNOSIS OF CHRONIC MENINGITIS

Infectious Causes
1. Normal immune host, specific exposure
   Tuberculosis, coccidioidomycosis, histoplasmosis, brucellosis, syphilis, cysticercosis
2. Disordered cellular immunity, opportunistic infection
   Tuberculosis, coccidioidomycosis, histoplasmosis, cryptococcosis, nocardiosis, toxoplasmosis, candidiasis

Noninfectious Causes
1. Extraneural disease often present
   Lymphoma, leukemia, other neoplastic disease (e.g., breast, lung), Behçet's disease, lupus erythematosus, sarcoid
2. Extraneural disease usually absent
   Granulomatous angiitis, uveomeningoencephalitis, chronic benign lymphocytic meningitis, chronic meningitis of unknown cause

Most patients with *Candida* meningitis have notable underlying disease or predisposing factors, such as a prolonged course of antibiotic therapy, corticosteroid therapy, indwelling urinary or venous catheters, or previous abdominal surgery.

Syphilitic meningitis is a form of secondary or tertiary syphilis that is relatively rare but easily diagnosed and treated.

NONINFECTIOUS CAUSES

Primary and metastatic, hematologic, and solid tumors may spread to the meninges. Leukemia and lymphoma are usually apparent before meningeal involvement. In meningeal carcinomatosis the onset is subacute with rapid progression. The primary tumor in these patients may be occult, and sites include breast, lung, stomach, pancreas, and skin (i.e., melanoma). Diagnosis is usually made by cytologic studies of CSF.

Sarcoidosis, which characteristically involves the basilar meninges, most frequently occurs in the setting of systemic sarcoid and may be the sole manifestation of the disease. Diagnosis can be difficult, especially when only the CNS is involved.

Behçet's disease usually presents with orogenital ulcerations and iridocyclitis. The CNS may be involved in up to one fourth of patients. Granulomatous angiitis is a vasculitis that primarily involves the CNS. Diagnosis is made by brain biopsy, and the illness is invariably fatal.

LABORATORY EVALUATION

Examination of CSF usually shows a lymphocytic pleocytosis. A cell count of less than 50/μL is more characteristic of sarcoid, carcinoma, and chronic benign lymphocytic meningitis, whereas most patients with tuberculous and fungal meningitis have cell counts of 100 to 400/μL. Concentrations of total protein are most commonly greater than 100 mg/dL. Hypoglycorrhachia narrows the possibilities to primarily tuberculosis, fungal infection, carcinoma, and sarcoid.

Serologic studies of serum and CSF are critical in the diagnosis of syphilis, coccidioidomycosis, and cryptococcosis. In cryptococcal meningitis the direct antigen is measured. The value of serologic studies is less well established in histoplasmosis. High or rising serum antibodies may suggest *Brucella* sp. or toxoplasmosis.

The diagnostic gold standard for tuberculous and fungal meningitis is positive results of cultures. Multiple specimens or large amounts of CSF should be obtained; the associated rate of recovery is considerably increased when this is carried out. Ancillary urine, sputum, and gastric cultures should also be processed routinely.

In addition to previously mentioned studies, cytologic analysis of multiple specimens of CSF should be performed when necessary because initial negative results of studies do not exclude carcinomatous meningitis.

CT scan of the head, which should be performed in all patients with chronic meningitis, may show hydrocephalus or focal lesions. Chest radiography should also be performed routinely.

MANAGEMENT

As noted previously, certain initial positive results of CSF testing may call for specific therapy. These studies, which usually are rapidly available, include cryptococcal antigen, coccidioidal antibody, VDRL, acid-fast stain, and cytologic analysis. Specific treatments of the most common causes of chronic meningitis are listed in Table 4.

In the initial therapy for tuberculous meningitis, a three-drug regimen is usually recommended with isoniazid (INH), rifampin, and either streptomycin or ethambutol (Myambutol). The third drug may be discontinued once susceptibility testing confirms efficacy of the two ''mainline'' agents. Isoniazid and rifampin should probably be continued for 18 months.

Cryptococcal meningitis is treated with a combination of amphotericin B and flucytosine (Ancobon) for a duration of six weeks.

Amphotericin B remains the treatment of choice in coccidioidal, *Histoplasma*, and *Candida* meningitis. Both parenteral and intrathecal therapies are indicated in coccidioidal meningitis, the intrathecal dose administered three times a week for three months and then one to two times a week for several months, followed by a dose that is slowly tapered to one treatment every six weeks. Intrathecal therapy is discontinued after one year of normal results of CSF testing carried out once every six weeks. The total dose of parenterally administered amphotericin B varies somewhat depending on the fungus involved (e.g., *Coccidioides*, 2.5 gm; *Histoplasma*, 2.5 gm; *Candida*, 2 gm).

Syphilitic meningitis should be treated with high-dose penicillin G for ten days followed by benzathine penicillin.

If a specific cause is not identified and clinical deterioration ensues, empiric therapy must be considered. This is not an uncommon situation in therapy for tuberculous meningitis, and empiric therapy is certainly appropriate if historical or ancillary information is suggestive. Empiric use of amphotericin B is rarely indicated because of toxicity, but it may be considered for the patient with an indeterminate progressive chronic meningitis that is refractory to other forms of therapy. Empiric use of corticosteroids is primarily con-

traindicated. Steroid therapy has been advocated to treat tuberculous meningitis and may be important in therapy for sarcoidosis and conditions in which vasculitis is present.

Neurosurgical intervention may be important diagnostically when meningeal biopsy is believed to be indicated in indeterminate progressive meningitis. Shunting may become therapeutically necessary if hydrocephalus develops.

REFERENCES

Bennett JE, Dismukes WE, Duma RJ, et al: A comparison of amphotericin B alone and combined with flucytosine in the treatment of cryptococcal meningitis. N Engl J Med 301:126–131, 1979.

Bouza E, Dreyer JS, Hewitt WL, et al: Coccidioidal meningitis. An analysis of 31 cases and review of the literature. Medicine 60:139–172, 1981.

Carpenter RR, Petersdorf RG: The clinical spectrum of bacterial meningitis. Am J Med 33:262–275, 1962.

Cherubin CE, Corrado ML, Nair SR, et al: Treatment of gram-negative bacillary meningitis: role of the new cephalosporin antibiotics. Rev Infect Dis 4(suppl):S453–S464, 1982.

Ellner JJ, Bennett JE: Chronic meningitis. Medicine 55:341–369, 1976.

Hooper DC, Pruitt AA, Rubin RH: Central nervous system infection in the chronically immunosuppressed. Medicine 61:166–188, 1982.

Karandanis D, Shulman JA: Recent survery of infectious meningitis in adults: review of laboratory findings in bacterial, tuberculous, and aseptic meningitis. South Med J 69:449–457, 1976.

Lepow ML, Coyne N, Thompson LB, et al: A clinical epidemiologic and laboratory investigation of aseptic meningitis during the four-year period, 1955–1958: II. The clinical disease and its sequelae. N Engl J Med 266:1188–1193, 1962.

McGee ZA, Kaiser AB: Acute meningitis. *In* Mandell GL, Douglas RG Jr, Bennett JE (eds): Principles and Practice of Infectious Diseases, 2nd ed. John Wiley & Sons, New York, 1979, pp 738–760.

Stockstill MTG, Kauffman CA: Comparison of cryptococcal and tuberculous meningitis. Arch Neurol 40:81–85, 1983.

7 · ANAEROBIC INFECTIONS: TETANUS AND THE GANGRENES

Gerald Gordon
GEISINGER MEDICAL CENTER

Obligate anaerobic bacteria (bacteria that cannot multiply in the presence of oxygen) cause human illness by producing exotoxin (e.g., tetanus, botulism, pseudomembranous colitis, and gas gangrene) or by directly invading tissues (e.g., synergistic gangrenes, intra-abdominal abscesses, lung abscess, brain abscess, Vincent's angina, bacteremia). Anaerobic bacteria cause infections commonly attributed to their aerobic counterparts (e.g., endocarditis, urinary infections, osteomyelitis, septic arthritis, spontaneous peritonitis, empyema, and sinus infection). Complete characterization of each of these infections is beyond the scope of this chapter, which will discuss tetanus, synergistic and gas gangrene, and aspects of the role of anaerobes in various other disorders.

Table 4. TREATMENT CONSIDERATIONS IN CHRONIC MENINGITIS

Cause	Therapy
Tuberculosis	1. Isoniazid, 300 mg/day PO 2. Rifampin, 600 mg/day PO 3. Streptomycin, 500 mg IM every 12 h, or ethambutol, 15 mg/kg/day 4. Steroids?
Cryptococcal meningitis	1. Amphotericin B, 0.3 mg/kg/day IV 2. Flucytosine, 150 mg/kg/day in four divided doses
Coccidioidal, *Histoplasma*, *Candida*	1. Amphotericin B, 0.7–1.0 mg/kg/day IV 2. Amphotericin B, 0.25–1.0 mg intrathecally (in coccidioidal meningitis)
Syphilitic meningitis	1. Penicillin G, 10–20 million units/day IV for 10 days, followed by benzathine penicillin, 2.4 million units/wk for 3 wks
Sarcoidosis and CNS vasculitis	1. High-dose steroids
Lymphoma, leukemia	1. Chemotherapy, radiotherapy

Exotoxin Associated Diseases: Tetanus

Tetanus (lockjaw) is caused by an exotoxin (tetanospasmin) elaborated by *Clostridium tetani*, a gram-positive terminal spore-forming bacillus. *C. tetani* is found worldwide in soil, dust, water, animal and human feces, and other sources. Tetanus is a major problem in developing countries whereas in the United States only four cases per 10 million population occur yearly. Unimmunized individuals and those older than 60 years appear at greatest risk. Stab wounds, gunshot wounds, parenteral drug abuse, cutaneous burns, septic abortion, crush injuries, puncture wounds, or contaminated and devitalized wounds such as decubitus ulceration may predispose to tetanus. In 20% of cases a portal of entry is not identified. Neonatal tetanus is rare in this country but is a frequent cause of neonatal mortality in third-world countries.

PATHOPHYSIOLOGY

A wound contaminated with *C. tetani* spores that develops an anaerobic environment may favor sporulation. Vegetative *C. tetani* produces tetanospasmin, which then is bound in the spinal cord by transneuronal and/or hematogenous routes. Tetanospasmin acts to suppress GABA-ergic inhibitory influences without altering excitatory influences, resulting in the classical picture of involuntary muscle spasm.

CLINICAL FEATURES

Wounds infected with *C. tetani* are usually localized and may have minimal local reaction unless other microorganisms are present. The incubation period is two to more than 21 days. Initially, irritability, restlessness, headache, and low-grade fever may be present. Tetanus may occur uncommonly as a local phenomenon (localized tetanus) with muscle spasm in one muscle group or extremity or may be generalized with trismus, involuntary facial muscle spasm (*risus sardonicus*), and somatic muscle spasm resulting in opisthotonus. Involuntary muscle contraction (lasting seconds to minutes) may be stimulated by noise, light, eating, or drinking. Localized symptoms may be mild and occasionally self-resolving or become generalized and result in respiratory arrest and death.

The patient typically is alert and oriented. A hypermetabolic state exists. Hyperreflexia, the absence of sensory abnormalities, low-grade fever, and moderate to marked leukocytosis are noted. Cerebrospinal fluid chemistries and cell counts are normal, though CSF pressures may be elevated. The electroencephalogram and electromyogram are nonspecific.

Respiratory arrest from vocal cord spasm, myoglobinuria with or without acute renal failure, axial and peripheral bony fractures, muscle and/or tendon rupture, autonomic instability, decubitus ulceration, atelectasis, aspiration pneumonia, pulmonary embolism, gastric hyperacidity and peptic ulceration, traumatic glossitis, fecal impaction, and urinary retention may complicate the course of patients with tetanus. Mortality may approach 50%, but in centers treating tetanus more frequently, 90% survival occurs.

MANAGEMENT

Maintenance of an airway, ventilatory support, and special attention to the details of nursing care are important. Turning the patient frequently and removing pooled secretions are critical to minimize decubitus ulceration and hypostatic pneumonia. The patient's environment should be dark and quiet with a minimal amount of activity. Intermittent catheterization, adequate hydration, hyperalimentation, and the use of antacids and histamine (H_2) antagonist in doses to raise the gastric pH above 4.0 are all valuable. Use of laxatives and enemas may avoid complications of constipation.

Human tetanus immunoglobulin (Hyper-Tet), 500 to 3000 units, should be administered intramuscularly. The deltoid muscle group is preferred. While antibiotics do not initially alter the course of tetanus, penicillin G, 10 million to 20 million units per day, should be administered IV in divided doses to eradicate replicating *C. tetani* bacilli. Cefazolin, 1 gm IV every eight hours, or tetracycline, 500 mg PO four times a day, may be alternatives to penicillin. Therapy should be continued for 10 to 14 days.

Judicious use of muscle relaxants and sedatives allows adequate ventilation and minimizes complications of involuntary muscle contraction. Diazepam (Valium), 10 mg PO every four to six hours for mild cases or 120 mg over 24 hours as a constant IV infusion, may be helpful to diminish myoclonus. The sedative effect of these agents may also be useful. Curare-like agents are often needed to minimize intense muscle contraction. Since patients remain alert despite curarization, sedatives should be concomitantly administered. Tracheostomy should be performed in preference to oral or nasotracheal intubation when respiratory support is required, thereby preventing ulceration and scarring of the vocal cords from trauma due to vocal cord spasm.

Necrotic wounds should be debrided. Other antibiotics may need to be administered to treat coexisting infections. Complications of pneumonia, decubitus ulceration, duodenal or gastric ulceration with free perforation into the peritoneal cavity, fecal impaction, and urinary obstruction should all be vigorously attended. Diagnosis of peritonitis may be difficult, as peritoneal signs may be obscured by tetanic contraction of the abdominal musculature.

Alum adsorbed tetanus toxoid should be administered IM to patients who have tetanus, as the immunogenicity of tetanus toxin is poor. Recovery from tetanus does not ensure lasting immunity. A full series of immunizations of tetanus toxoid is required.

PREVENTION

Tetanus is clearly a disease for which the adage "an ounce of prevention is worth a pound of cure" holds true. Primary immunization of children and nonimmunized adults and reimmunization every ten years with tetanus-diphtheria (TD) booster injections should prevent most tetanus. The use of Hyper-Tet and booster doses of tetanus toxoid in patients who have severe wounds considered tetanus-prone is important. (See Chap. 20.)

Invasive Diseases: Gangrene and Clostridial Syndromes

DEFINITION AND DIAGNOSTIC CRITERIA

Gangrene represents avascular tissue death and may be dry (uninfected) or wet (infected). Wet gangrene has many causes, though anaerobic and mixed anaerobic/aerobic infection are usual; fungi and viruses (herpes zoster) may be etiologies. Diagnosis and subsequent treatment is pathogen specific, though a common approach is usually possible and involves vigorous debridement of devitalized tissues.

Cutaneous gangrenes can be caused by clostridia, by mixed anaerobic and aerobic bacteria, or by fungi (*Mucorales*), or they can be localized expressions of bacteremia (ecthyma gangrenosum).

CLINICAL FEATURES

Clostridium species cause a variety of superficial and deep structure (myonecrosis) gangrenes. Clostridial syndromes may present following trauma or surgery.

Superficial cellulitis due to clostridia may be localized and slowly progressive and may produce a small amount of gas in the soft tissues. Systemic symptoms are mild, though fever is present. Gangrene may not be present. Clostridia may be etiologic in diabetic foot ulcers, perirectal abscesses, and other devitalized infections. Gram stain of skin aspirates shows blunt-ended gram-positive rods, and cultures grow *C. perfringens* or occasionally other clostridial species.

Rapidly spreading superficial cellulitis with diffuse crepitus may be due to *C. perfringens* and occasionally other clostridial species. Typically, deep fascia and muscle are spared. Systemic manifestations may vary from none to overwhelming sepsis, diffuse intravascular coagulation (DIC), shock, and death. Cutaneous gangrene may occur.

Deeper involvement may occur with *clostridial myonecrosis*. Superficial hemorrhagic vesicle formation, wound edema and severe pain, low-grade temperature, profound toxemia, hemolysis, jaundice, and acute renal failure may occur. An unpleasant sweet odor may be noted. Gram stains of fluid from vesicles of subcutaneous tissues show gram-positive rods but few leukocytes. Typically, clostridial gas gangrene occurs six to 72 hours after traumatic injury or surgical procedure and should be considered in the differential diagnosis of wound infections in the immediate postoperative period. Patients usually remain alert despite hypotension and extreme toxemia, though delirium may be noted.

MANAGEMENT

When clostridial cellulitis with gangrene and/or clostridial myonecrosis is suspected, surgical confirmation and immediate aggressive debridement are mandatory. Incision into the subcutaneous tissue will define the degree of tissue involvement. Surgical exploration of infected areas may allow the physician to minimize the need for extensive mutilating surgery in some patients.

Patients with clostridial myonecrosis should have prompt and aggressive surgical excision of all nonviable tissue. Reexploration and further debridement of wounds within four to six hours after primary debridement are often necessary to remove retained nonviable infected tissues. It is important to remove all gangrenous tissue. Blood and tissue cultures for aerobic and anaerobic bacteria, Gram stains of tissue fluids, tissue histology, and fungal cultures should be performed, as multiorganism infection may occur. Superficial spreading cellulitis with subcutaneous gas may be caused by *B. fragilis*, *E. coli*, anaerobic streptococci, and other bacteria as well. In patients with pure clostridial infections, penicillin G, 20 to 30 million units IV, should be given in divided doses each day. The role of equine gas gangrene antitoxin is unclear and generally is not advocated. Hyperbaric oxygen may be a useful adjunct but should not delay aggressive surgical therapy.

Clostridial syndromes without myonecrosis require carefully coordinated medical and surgical therapy to remove all devitalized tissue. Superficial slowly spreading cellulitis may respond to penicillin G (12 to 20 million units IV daily in divided doses) therapy alone. Careful attention to hemodynamic and ventilatory stability and nutritional support are important.

Synergistic Cutaneous Gangrenes, Necrotizing Fasciitis, and Synergistic Necrotizing Cellulitis

PATHOPHYSIOLOGY

Mixed anaerobic and aerobic infection may occasionally cause a synergistic unrelenting spreading gangrene of skin and fascia. A hallmark of these infections is their progression despite appropriate antimicrobial therapy directed at individual bacteria. Anaerobic streptococci, anaerobic staphylococci, or anaerobic gram-negative bacilli may act synergistically with aerobic gram-negative bacilli or gram-positive cocci to cause synergistic gangrenes.

CLINICAL FEATURES

Synergistic cutaneous gangrene is uncommon but may occur as a complication of surgery or trauma. These infections may be seen in the extremities of diabetics, in parenteral drug abusers, or after trauma, or they may occur in the abdominal wall or perineum, complicating trauma or surgical procedures. The skin becomes indurated and initially quite tender; bullae may form in skin that is discolored dusky gray. Later in the course as cutaneous infarction occurs, the skin becomes anesthetic. Deeper structures (including muscle) are spared. The patient may be quite toxic or minimally so; fever may range from 101° to 105° F. Leukocytosis is moderate to marked. The spectrum of illness is broad, ranging from a relatively indolent process (Meleney's ulcer) to an aggressively progressing infection (synergistic necrotizing cellulitis).

Differentiating the degree of cutaneous and/or fascial involvement in patients with synergistic gangrenes is important therapeutically. Synergistic necrotizing cellulitis typically involves all dermal structures, fascia, and muscle. A foul-smelling "dishwater pus" is seen. Infection and necrosis of underlying fascia and muscle occurs with minimal cutaneous evidence of the degree of infection. Local pain and tenderness are marked and typically are more intense than one would expect for the amount of cutaneous involvement noted. Blood cultures grow pathogenic bacteria in about half the cases.

Synergistic necrotizing fasciitis involves dermal, subdermal, and fascial structures but not muscle. This process typically is acute. Diabetics appear to be at greatest risk. The affected area becomes indurated and initially quite painful. Bullae containing hemorrhagic fluid are seen overlying infarcted skin. Incision of affected areas demonstrates loss of integrity of the dermal layers. A probe can easily be passed through, demonstrating destruction of fascial planes.

MANAGEMENT

Surgical therapy is lifesaving in patients with synergistic necrotizing cellulitis and fasciitis. Extensive incisions should be made through the skin and subcutaneous tissue beyond the margins of involvement. Necrotic fascia, fat, and involved tissues should be resected. Wounds should be left open. While initial surgery involves incision and drainage, radical debridement may be necessary and may result in amputation or removal of large areas of gangrenous tissue.

Initial antimicrobial therapy should be directed by the results of Gram stain and culture and the sensitivity of excised material. Agents effective against *B. fragilis* (e.g., metronidazole, 500 mg IV every six hours; clindamycin, 600 mg IV every six hours; chloramphenicol, 1 gm IV every six hours; or cefoxitin, 2 gm IV every six hours) as well as against anaerobic streptococci (penicillin G, 20 million units per day) and the potential aerobic gram-negative organisms seen by Gram stain (an aminoglycoside and an acylamino penicillin or cephalosporin) may be valuable.

The role of hyperbaric oxygen in the management of these infections is undefined but may be valuable in centers in which providing this modality does not interfere with surgical therapy.

If synergistic gangrenes are not recognized and aggressively treated, infection will be unrelenting and will invariably result in death.

Head and Neck Infections

CLINICAL FEATURES

Anaerobic bacteria comprise the bulk of the bacteria colonizing the oropharynx. Aerobic bacteria cause acute superficial infections, such as pharyngitis due to group A streptococcus and epiglottitis due to *Haemophilus influenzae*. Anaerobic bacteria play a role more frequently in chronic infections, immediately postoperatively after dental or oropharyngeal surgical procedures, or in association with dental abscess (e.g., Ludwig's angina). Anaerobic bacteria (peptostreptococci, peptococci, *Bacteroides oralis* and *B. melaninogenicus*) may cause chronic sinus infections. Anaerobes rarely have been implicated in patients with acute and chronic otitis media. Recalcitrant cases of sinusitis or otitis media require a needle aspirate of the sinus or tympanocentesis with the culture for anaerobic bacteria as well as other pathogens. Swabs should be used only if mucosa can be avoided when cultures are obtained.

MANAGEMENT

Culture results may best dictate appropriate antimicrobial therapy, though penicillin VK, 500 mg PO every six hours or clindamycin, 300 mg PO every six hours for two to three weeks, may be effective choices in these situations. Susceptibility studies for gram-negative anaerobes recovered from head and neck infections should be requested; gram-positive anaerobic cocci are nearly always susceptible to penicillin and clindamycin.

Ludwig's Angina

CLINICAL FEATURES

Ludwig's angina is an uncommon but potentially lethal infection that should be recognized early and aggressively managed. Typically this infection presents as a submandibular space cellulitis progressing over 12 to 24 hours with bulging of the submaxillary space and elevation and posterior protrusion of the tongue against the palate, causing glottal obstruction. Infection may penetrate the mylohyoid muscle and spread downward toward mediastinal structures, resulting in mediastinitis.

Infection of the second or third molars appears to initiate Ludwig's angina. *Peptococcus, Peptostreptococcus, Bacteroides* species, fusobacteria, or aerobic streptococci usually appear to play an etiologic role. Occasionally, aerobic gram-negative rods are found.

MANAGEMENT

Recognition of signs of upper airway compromise and early tracheostomy may be lifesaving. Penicillin G, 20 million units parenterally in divided doses, is usually effective. Clindamycin, 450 to 600 mg IV every six hours, may be a satisfactory alternative. Agents effective against aerobic gram-negative rods are occasionally required (cefuroxime, 1.5 gm IV every eight hours; or carbenicillin, 5 gm every four hours, 30 gm/day IV; and gentamicin, 1.5 mg/kg IV every eight hours). Exploration of the submaxillary space may be necessary if abscess formation occurs.

General Overview of Anaerobic Infections

CLINICAL FEATURES AND DIAGNOSTIC FINDINGS

Anaerobic infections should be suspected in closed space, post-traumatic, or spontaneous infections in proximity to mucosal surfaces. Gram stain of purulent material may show multiple organism types, but aerobic cultures may show no bacterial growth or one organism type. A foul odor eminating from wounds may suggest the presence of an anaerobic bacterium (especially a peptostreptococcus), but the absence of pungent odors does not exclude the possibility that an anaerobe is present.

Anaerobic cultures should be obtained by aspiration of infected material into a sterile syringe; air should be excluded with the end of the syringe and needle sealed by a rubber stopper. Gram stains and appropriate aerobic and anaerobic cultures should then be performed.

MANAGEMENT

In most situations, preventing the spread of anaerobic bacteria into healthy tissue, making the environment of an infection as "aerobic" as possible to minimize the proliferation of anaerobic bacteria, drainage of abscesses, relief of obstruction, and removal of necrotic malignancies or foreign bodies are all important. The type, amount, and duration of antimicrobial agent are best defined by the disease one is treating and the bacteria involved. Unfortunately, because of delay in identification of anaerobic bacteria, presumptive therapy is often appropriate. Penicillin G (12 million to 20 million units/day IV), clindamycin (600 mg IV every six hours), cefoxitin (2 gm IV every six hours), and chloramphenicol (1 mg IV every six hours) are active against most gram-positive anaerobic bacteria. Metronidazole (7.5 mg/kg every six hours) appears to have the greatest in vitro activity against *B. fragilis* and other gram-negative anaerobic bacteria, though clindamycin, cefoxitin and chloramphenicol may be less active alternatives. Septic processes that originate below the diaphragm frequently involve *B. fragilis*, and initial therapy should be directed toward that organism as well as aerobic gram-negative bacilli. Penicillin-susceptible organisms continue to be frequent in supradiaphragmatic anaerobic infections, though as many as 20% of *B. melaninogenicus* and *B. oralis* are resistant to penicillin. Penicillin G, 12 million to 20 million units per day, remains a reasonable first agent in pleuropulmonary and oropharyngeal anaerobic infections. Clindamycin, 450 mg to 600 mg IV every six hours, is a reasonable alternative.

REFERENCES

Bartlett JG: Recent developments in the management of anaerobic infections. Rev Infect Dis 5:235–245, 1983.

Chow AW, Roser SM, Brady FA: Otofacial odontogenic infections. Ann Intern Med 88:392–402, 1978.

Finegold SM: Anaerobic Bacteria in Human Disease. Academic Press, New York, 1977.

Martin RR, Mandell GL, Douglas RG, Bennett JE: Clostridium tetani (Tetanus): Principles and Practice of Infectious Diseases, 2nd ed. John Wiley & Sons, New York, 1985, pp 1355–1359.

Stamenkovic L, Lew PD: Early recognition of potentially fatal necrotizing fasciitis. N Engl J Med 310:1689–1693, 1984.

8 · DIAGNOSIS AND TREATMENT OF OSTEOMYELITIS

Keith H. Burch
HENRY FORD HOSPITAL

In recent years changes have occurred in the clinical presentation of osteomyelitis and the associated etiologic agents. Factors contributing to these changes include more aggressive orthopedic procedures such as joint replacement and other reconstructive surgery, changes in the organisms responsible for hospital-acquired infections, and the abuse of intravenous drugs.

Osteomyelitis can be classified by the route through which the organism reaches bone and by the clinical manner of presentation. Infection may result from (1) hematogenous dissemination, (2) spread from a contiguous soft tissue infection or (3) direct inoculation secondary to trauma or surgery. Acute osteomyelitis relates to cases seen for the first time, whereas chronic cases have usually had prior admissions for the same infection.

Although not an uncommon infection, osteomyelitis can be difficult to diagnose and treat. Waldvogel in 1970 presented data on 247 patients at the Massachusetts General Hospital with osteomyelitis seen over a four-year period. Hematogenous infections were present in 19%, infection secondary to contiguous focus in 47%, and 34% of all cases were associated with vascular insufficiency. In this series 56% were acute and 44% were chronic.

Hematogenous Osteomyelitis

PATHOPHYSIOLOGY

Hematogenous osteomyelitis classically occurs in individuals less than 15 years of age although infections in adults are presently not uncommon. In children the infection occurs in the metaphysis of long bones, especially the femur, tibia, and humerus. Narrow capillaries enter the area of the epiphysis and make hair-pin turns, allowing infected emboli to lodge. Slow blood flow and the absence of phagocytic cells allow infection to progress. Necrosis secondary to vascular ischemia and the release of neutrophilic enzymes allows pressure to rise, and the inflammatory exudate pushes through the cortex and elevates the periosteum, which is not tightly bound to bone in children. In very young patients the joint space can also become involved, as capillaries still penetrate the epiphyseal growth plate.

Hematogenous osteomyelitis in adults, seen especially in the fifth and sixth decades, commonly involves the lumbar and thoracic vertebrae. Since the advent of intravenous drug abuse, such infections have been reported involving the vertebral column, pelvic girdle, sternum, and ribs. Heroin-related osteomyelitis is generally associated with a concomitant septic arthritis.

CLINICAL ASPECTS

Signs and symptoms of hematogenous osteomyelitis are diverse and may relate to the patient's age. Younger children and some adults present with fever, chills, pain, bone tenderness, and decreased motion. Others, particularly adults with vertebral osteomyelitis, have low-grade fever or pain alone. Heroin-related osteomyelitis usually presents with localized bone pain without leukocytosis or fever. The diagnosis must be suspected with a history of drug abuse.

LABORATORY FINDINGS

The sedimentation rate is usually elevated, but early x-rays may be negative, as at least ten days are required before bone changes occur. Technetium phosphate bone scans can be positive 10 to 14 days before radiographic changes can be seen. False-positive and rare false-negative scans are encountered, and differentiation by scans between cellulitis osteomyelitis and bone formation can be difficult. Gallium scans may also be helpful in conjunction with conventional bone scans.

Causative organisms of hematogenous osteomyelitis are variable. In neonates few systemic symptoms may be present. Joint effusion occurs in 60% to 70%, and at times decreased limb motion and edema may be the only signs of infection. Bacteria involved are usually *Staphylococcus aureus*, group B streptococcus, and *E. coli*, but other streptococci are now being more commonly encountered. In young children *S. aureus* accounts for 60% to 90% of cases. Group A streptococcus and gram-negative bacilli occur less frequently.

Pyogenic vertebral osteomyelitis of adults generally are secondary to *S. aureus* (50%), with gram-negative bacilli playing an increasing role. *E. coli* and other urinary tract pathogens are associated, and skin and respiratory tract infections may also lead to secondary bacterial seeding in bone. Heroin-related infections are usually due to *S. aureus, Pseudomonas aeruginosa,* or other gram-negative bacilli.

Salmonellae are uncommon causes of osteomyelitis unless the affected individual has sickle cell anemia or another hemoglobinopathy. *Salmonella choleraesuis, S. paratyphi,* and *S. typhimurium* account for two thirds of the cases of osteomyelitis in those with hemoglobinopathies. Long bone involvement may be well advanced before detection because bone infarction and osteomyelitis both have a similar clinical presentation.

Osteomyelitis Secondary to Contiguous Foci

Osteomyelitis due to contiguous spread comprises a large group of infections that commonly are encountered in patients over age 50. They may result from direct infection from sources outside the body or by progressive spread of infection from tissue adjacent to bone. Infection can be a result of penetrating wounds such as gunshots, open fractures, or surgical orthopedic procedures such as open reduction of closed fractures or internal fixation of a fracture involving the hip, femur, or tibia. Infections can occur after disc surgery, craniotomy, or repair of degenerative arthritis. Open fractures are particularly prone to infection as contamination occurs at the time of fracture.

Osteomyelitis of the mandible may occur in association with infected teeth, particularly after radiation therapy for carcinoma. Soft tissue infection of the fingers and toes may involve adjacent bones.

Frequently pain in the area of infection may be the only real complaint in osteomyelitis associated with a contiguous focus of infection, and localized tenderness with erythema and edema may indicate infection, with fever and leukocytosis only rarely associated.

S. aureus is the most common pathogen recovered, followed by gram-negative bacilli. Frequently, multiple causative organisms are encountered. There is an association of puncture wounds of the foot with gram-negative osteomyelitis, particularly *P. aeruginosa.*

Osteomyelitis Associated with Vascular Insufficiency

Contiguous spread of osteomyelitis associated with vascular insufficiency is a difficult clinical problem. Most of these patients have diabetes mellitus or severe vascular disease and are elderly. Infections frequently involve small bones of the feet and toes and are usually associated with an adjacent cellulitis in a pressure ulcer resulting from neuropathy. Many affected patients have concomitant diabetic gastropathy, retinopathy, and nephropathy. Infections are usually due to multiple organisms with combinations of *S. aureus* and *S. epidermidis*, streptococci excluding group A, and gram-negative bacilli frequently seen. Gram-negative bacilli are playing an increasingly important role, as are anaerobic organisms.

MEDICAL AND SURGICAL THERAPY

In all cases of osteomyelitis, attempts to identify the specific etiologic organism should be carried out. Blood cultures may be positive in 50% of cases of hematogenous osteomyelitis. If negative, percutaneous aspiration or open biopsy may be necessary. Cultures should be performed for aerobic and anaerobic bacteria, fungi, and mycobacteria. At times mycobacterium tuberculosis or systemic fungal infections (i.e., cryptococci) may present as isolated osteomyelitis. Sinus tract cultures do not correlate well with specimens cultured at the time of bone biopsy and cannot be relied on, but deep specimens taken at the time of surgical drainage are very valuable.

The cornerstone of therapy in acute osteomyelitis is high-dose parenteral antimicrobial therapy directed at the etiologic agent. Such early therapy may allow eradication of infection without surgery. However, if a young adult with acute hematogenous osteomyelitis in a long bone does not respond to therapy within 72 hours, surgical drainage is generally necessary. Heroin-related osteomyelitis usually requires aspiration or surgical drainage of the adjacent joint space, whereas vertebral osteomyelitis of older adults usually responds to antibiotics alone unless there is an associated paraspinal abscess.

ANTIMICROBIAL THERAPY

Antibiotics selected are given intravenously in high doses to ensure adequate drug concentrations in the infected area for protracted periods of time, usually four to six weeks. Eight to 12 gm of a penicillinase-resistant penicillin, ampicillin, cephalosporin, or a comparable dose of another appropriate antibiotic can be used. Vancomycin and parenteral sulfa-trimethoprim have been successfully utilized for osteomyelitis due to methicillin-resistant staphylococci. Resistant gram-negative osteomyelitis usually responds to a combination of agents that includes an appropriate broad-spectrum penicillin or a cephalosporin plus an aminoglycoside antibiotic.

Specific length of therapy is poorly defined but it appears that there is a high failure rate when parenteral antibiotics are given for less than three weeks. Although oral therapy is usually not given to adults with acute osteomyelitis, some studies in children with staphylococcal osteomyelitis have shown benefit, particularly when peak serum bactericidal titers achieved were $\geq$ 1:16 and trough titers were $\geq$ 1:2.

INDICATIONS FOR SURGERY

Surgery is needed at times for drainage and for removal of infected and compromised tissue. When osteomyelitis follows internal fixation of fractures, a stable implant is not immediately removed. If it is unstable, it should be removed and stability restored through external fixation, if possible. Once infection occurs early following total hip replacement, it may be possible to save the prosthesis with local surgery and antibiotics, but if it occurs several months post surgery, it may be necessary to remove the prosthesis.

Osteomyelitis associated with vascular insufficiency is very difficult to cure with antibiotics alone, and surgery may be necessary to remove devitalized infected tissue. Even with such an approach, cure rates are low and amputation may be necessary.

Chronic osteomyelitis is more difficult to deal with clinically than is acute osteomyelitis. Surgery is almost always necessary to remove sequestra and devitalized tissue in conjunction with specific antimicrobial therapy. After four to six weeks of parenteral therapy, oral antibiotics are generally given for protracted periods, even up to one year. Specific percentages are not available, but it is established that many patients with chronic osteomyelitis will respond to a combined medical surgical approach.

PREVENTION OF OSTEOMYELITIS

Osteomyelitis might be prevented in certain situations by prophylactic antibiotics. With open fractures, surgical debridement of the wound and prophylactic use of a first-generation cephalosporin have been useful to prevent *S. aureus* infections. Similar prophylactic use of cephalosporins has been of value in preventing staphylococcal infections following surgery for total hip and joint replacement.

CONCLUSION

Successful outcome of osteomyelitis depends on early diagnosis and therapy based on correct identification of the offending organism. Both proper antimicrobial agents and the appropriate use of surgery are necessary to achieve the best outcomes. Parenteral antibiotics should usually be given for four to six weeks, but children with acute osteomyelitis may respond to oral antibiotic programs if closely supervised. Long-term oral antibiotics may have value in treatment or suppression of chronic osteomyelitis of adults.

In our practice, parenteral home antibiotic programs have been very useful in treating such patients by allowing early discharge from the hospital and prompt return of the patent to the work place. Furthermore, home antibiotic programs are efficacious and cost effective for osteomyelitis.

REFERENCES

Armstrong EP, Rush DR: Treatment of osteomyelitis. Clin Pharm 2:213–222, May-June 1983.

Kind AC, Williams DN, et al: Intravenous antibiotic therapy at home. Arch Intern Med 139:413–415, 1979.

Waldvogel FA, Vasey H: Osteomyelitis: The past decade. N Engl J Med 303:360–370, 1980.

Waldvogel FA, et al: Osteomyelitis: a review of clinical features, therapeutic considerations and unusual aspects (first of three parts). N Engl J Med 282:198–206, 1970.

9 · TOXIC SHOCK SYNDROME AND PELVIC INFLAMMATORY DISEASE

Ursula G. McKenna
Paul E. Hermans
MAYO CLINIC AND MAYO FOUNDATION

Toxic Shock Syndrome

DEFINITION AND DIAGNOSTIC CRITERIA

Toxic shock syndrome (TSS) is defined as an acute illness characterized by high fever, diffuse erythematous rash followed by desquamation, hypotension, and multi-organ system dysfunction. The diagnostic criteria are listed in Table 1. Cases with less severe or even mild disease present with fewer criteria. Their recognition and treatment is equally important since they may progress to more severe illness or may recur if associated with menstruation. Until diagnostic laboratory tests exist, the diagnosis cannot be confirmed.

PATHOPHYSIOLOGY

There is strong evidence that the clinical and pathologic findings of TSS are mediated by toxins(s) released from a focus of staphylococcal infection, most often the

Table 1. CASE DEFINITION OF TOXIC SHOCK SYNDROME

1. Fever (temperature ≥ 38.9°C)
2. Rash (diffuse macular erythroderma)
3. Desquamation, 1–2 wk after onset of illness, particularly of palms and soles
4. Hypotension (systolic blood pressure ≤ 90 mm Hg, orthostatic hypotension, dizziness, or syncope)
5. Involvement of three or more of following organ systems:
   A. Gastrointestinal (vomiting or diarrhea at onset of illness)
   B. Muscular (severe myalgia or creatine kinase level ≥ 2 × ULN*)
   C. Mucous membrane (vaginal, oropharyngeal, or conjunctival) hyperemia
   D. Renal (BUN or creatinine level ≥ 2 × ULN or ≥ 5 WBC per high-power field in absence of urinary tract infection)
   E. Hepatic (total bilirubin, serum glutamic oxaloacetic transaminase, or serum glutamic pyruvic transaminase ≥ 2 × ULN)
   F. Hematologic (platelets ≤ 100,000/mm³)
   G. Central nervous system (disorientation or alterations in consciousness without focal neurologic signs when fever and hypotension are absent)
6. Negative results on following tests, if obtained:
   A. Blood, throat, or CSF fluid cultures; blood cultures positive for S. aureus, acceptable
   B. Serologic tests for Rocky Mountain spotted fever, leptospirosis, or measles

*Twice upper limits of normal for laboratory.

vagina. Most *S. aureus* isolates belong to phage group I, phage types 29 and 52.

Originally, two toxins were described: staphylococcal enterotoxin F and pyrogenic exotoxin C. These two toxins are identical proteins, now called TSS toxin-1. The major effect of the toxin is generalized vasodilatation with capillary leakage resulting in hypotension, hypoproteinemia, and hypoalbuminemia.

The pathologic findings in TSS are due to tissue hypoperfusion and direct effects of toxin such as microvesicular fatty changes and periportal inflammation of the liver, hemophagocytosis, vaginal and cervical ulcerations, and skin manifestations.

Most cases are menses associated. The majority involve users of tampons, particularly high-absorbency types. TSS also occurs in other settings: vaginal or pelvic infections, use of barrier contraceptives, post partum or post abortion, surgical wound infections, and other nonsurgical focal infection.

Recurrences are noted only in menses-associated cases. They may be related to lack of antibody formation to toxin. Recurrences diminish after treatment with antistaphylococcal antibiotics during an acute episode and if tampons are discontinued.

CLINICAL ASPECTS

Classical TSS is a multi-system disease with abrupt onset and rapid evolution. Prominent initial symptoms are fever, chills, nausea, vomiting, diarrhea, myalgias, muscle tenderness, arthralgias, headache, conjunctivitis, and sore throat. The erythematous rash is easily overlooked and is followed by a characteristic desquamation one to two weeks later. Vaginitis with malodorous discharge, labial swelling, and vaginal ulcers occurs in menses-associated TSS. The patient is often somnolent or confused. Nonpitting, periorbital, periarticular, or peripheral edema develops. Diffuse abdominal tenderness occurs, but signs of peritonitis are absent. Renal involvement is common, and acute oliguric and non-oliguric renal failure may ensue.

Orthostatic dizziness or syncope may rapidly progress to profound shock. Noncardiogenic pulmonary edema, disseminated intravascular coagulation (DIC), cardiac arrhythmias, and refractory shock may result in death.

Sequelae include transient loss of hair and nails, compromised renal function, impairment of higher mental functions, and neuromuscular abnormalities.

MANAGEMENT

PLAN

The short-term goal is treatment of the acute disease syndrome. The long-term goal is prevention of recurrence.

Patients who meet all criteria required for diagnosis must be hospitalized. Very ill patients with significant hypotension or in shock should be admitted to an Intensive Care Unit for careful monitoring of cardiac rhythm, arterial blood pressure, urinary output, respiratory rate, central venous pressure (or preferably capillary wedge pressure), pulmonary vascular resistance, arterial blood gases, chest x-ray findings, and serum electrolyte levels. This permits management of fluid replacement with large fluid volumes, and early recognition of life-threatening cardiac arrhythmias, noncardiogenic pulmonary edema, and renal failure.

Individuals with milder disease not meeting the case definition can often be successfully managed as outpatients if they are physiologically stable and can tolerate oral fluids. These will probably be menses-associated cases with recurrent milder episodes, which may precede or follow a severe one. Some patients do not even seek medical attention, and recover spontaneously.

Surgical intervention is often necessary in nonmenstrual TSS cases. Empyema, abscesses, and surgical wounds must be incised and/or drained.

NONPHARMACOLOGIC MEASURES

Offending foreign objects, such as tampons, sponges, barrier contraceptives, gauze packing in the nasal cavity, other surgical packing, or sutures, must be removed immediately. The vagina, cervix, or other foci must be cultured. A vaginal focus should be treated with saline irrigation.

Immediate aggressive treatment with normal saline or Ringer's lactate to restore intravascular volume is of crucial importance. Patients may require over 10 liters of crystalloid infusions per day. The use of colloid fluids is controversial. Hypoalbuminemia is significant, but administration of serum albumin may contribute to the development of noncardiogenic pulmonary edema.

Metabolic (lactic) acidosis resulting from hypotension is often significant. If the pH is under 7.1, bicarbonate may have to be given to prevent life-threatening cardiac arrhythmias. Hypokalemia is present in most patients and requires potassium replacement, usually for several days. Hypocalcemia is often pronounced, and out of proportion to the hypoalbuminemia. Elevated calcitonin levels have been found. In the presence of cardiac arrhythmias, parenteral calcium supplements should be given.

Hypotension and shock result in tissue hypoxia, requiring supplemental oxygen.

DRUG THERAPY

Antibiotics. A beta-lactamase–resistant antistaphylococcal antibiotic should be given, preferably oxacillin or nafcillin, 1.5 to 2 gm every four hours intravenously. If the patient is allergic to penicillin, a cephalosporin should be administered, e.g., cefazolin, 750 mg to 1.0 gm every six to eight hours. If the diagnosis is in doubt, an antibiotic coverage for gram-negative and anaerobic infections may be added until culture and laboratory reports are available. The optimal duration of therapy has not yet been established. Depending on the severity of the illness, we treat these patients with a parenteral antibiotic for seven to 14 days. Additional oral antistaphylococcal therapy (e.g., dicloxacillin, 500 mg every six hours) or a cephalosporin (e.g., cephalexin, 500 mg every six hours) for up to another two weeks is often appropriate.

Follow-up cultures are mandatory. Even after prolonged parenteral treatment with a beta-lactamase–resistant antibiotic, identical strains of *S. aureus* have been re-isolated. Treatment with an antistaphylococcal antibiotic during the acute episode reduces the risk of recurrent menstrual TSS and may prevent the rare bacteremia.

In patients who do not require hospitalization, we advise giving one of the above oral antibiotics for ten days.

Corticosteroids. The role of corticosteroids in treating the syndrome is unclear. A retrospective study suggested that corticosteroids, when started within two to three days after onset of the illness, reduce its severity. Thirty mg/kg of methylprednisolone should be given early and repeated in four to six hours. The optimal duration of the steroid treatment has not been established.

Pressor Agents. If hypotension is not corrected after rapid administration of 2 liters of crystalloid solution, pressor agents must be given. The preferred agent is dopamine, which at low doses (5 to 20 μg/kg/min), produces renal and mesenteric vasodilatation as well as increased cardiac output.

Management of Complications. Noncardiogenic pulmonary edema requires intubation and mechanical ventilation with positive end-expiratory pressure (PEEP). Hemorrhaging caused by DIC can be life-threatening and may require replacement of platelets and coagulation factors with fresh-frozen plasma. The use of heparin must be considered. Renal failure may necessitate hemodialysis.

PATIENT INFORMATION AND EDUCATION

Patients who have had menses-associated TSS are at risk of recurrences. We advise these patients to discontinue the use of tampons, and tell them to contact a physician immediately if fever, rash, nausea, vomiting and/or diarrhea, headache, myalgias, or dizziness occur during subsequent menstrual periods.

PERIODIC EVALUATION

Vaginal cultures in patients with menses-associated TSS should be performed during one to several subsequent menstrual cycles. If these are positive for *S. aureus*, we recommend a seven- to ten-day course of dicloxacillin during the menstrual cycle.

PREVENTIVE MEASURES

Menstruating women in general, in addition to patients with menses-associated TSS, need to be educated regarding prevention and early recognition of TSS. High-absorbency tampons should be avoided or used only at the time of heavy flow. If the symptoms described above are present during menstruation, the tampon should be removed immediately.

For non–menses-associated cases of TSS, early recognition is still the best way to prevent the full-blown syndrome. In postoperative or postpartum patients, watery diarrhea and erythroderma, especially if associated with hypotension, require a prompt search for a staphylococcal infection. The signs of a local infection may be minimal.

SOCIOECONOMIC ASPECTS OF MANAGEMENT

The cost of treatment of a case of TSS with many complications can be tremendous. Early recognition of symptoms and aggressive management is therefore extremely important.

Pelvic Inflammatory Disease

DEFINITION AND DIAGNOSTIC CRITERIA

Pelvic inflammatory disease is an infection of the fallopian tubes and the parametria with possible extension to the ovaries and peritoneum. Most cases develop as an ascending infection originating in the uterine cervix following a menstrual period, and are sexually transmitted. The diagnosis is primarily clinical and rests on the presence of pelvic and abdominal pain, severe tenderness on pelvic examination, malaise, and fever.

PATHOPHYSIOLOGY

In many cases in which cultures are obtained by culdocentesis or when a pelvic abscess is drained, multiple microorganisms are recovered. The etiologic agents include *Neisseria gonorrhoeae*; the anaerobes of the *Bacteroides* group (also non-*fragilis*, such as *B. bivius*, *B. disiens*, *B. melaninogenicus*), *Fusobacterium*, *Peptococcus*, and *Peptostreptococcus*; *Escherichia coli* and other enterobacteriaceae; group D streptococci; *Chlamydia trachomatis*; *Mycoplasma hominis*; and *Ureaplasma urealyticum*. *Actinomyces* species have been cultured from patients with an intrauterine device. Even when *N. gonorrhoeae* is clearly the causative organism (cultured from the cervix), cultures by culdocentesis may grow multiple microorganisms.

CLINICAL ASPECTS

The severity of the components of the clinical picture (abdominal and pelvic pain, tenderness on pelvic examination, malaise, fever, nausea, vomiting) varies from patient to patient. Leukocytosis and an increased erythrocyte sedimentation rate may not be present in the early stage.

Culture specimen for *N. gonorrhoeae* should always be obtained from the urethra, endocervix, and rectum. A Gram stain of a cervical specimen may show extra- and intracellular gram-negative cocci. Culdocentesis may be used to obtain material for aerobic and anaerobic cultures. It is usually not done because treatment is empiric anyway. One set of blood cultures should be taken in all febrile patients before antibiotic treatment is started.

Differential diagnoses include ectopic pregnancy, endometriosis, ruptured or twisted ovarian cyst, appendicitis, diverticulitis, and mittelschmerz. Laparoscopy may be required to establish a diagnosis in difficult cases.

The diagnosis of abscess formation is made easier by ultrasound and CT scanning. Rupture of an abscess is a life-threatening complication.

MANAGEMENT

PLAN

Short-term goals are to eradicate the infection, prevent abscess formation, and recognize and treat complications early, especially perforation of an abscess.

Long-term goals are to prevent infertility, relapse of the infection, and chronic pelvic pain.

Persons with fever of over 102°F, nausea and vomiting, and abdominal distention or who fail to improve after three days of outpatient treatment should be hospitalized. Pregnant women with pelvic inflammatory disease, suspected poor compliers, and patients who may not cooperate for follow-up examinations should also be hospitalized. Perforation of an abscess with generalized peritonitis is a surgical emergency requiring excision of infected tissue and drainage. A small abscess (less than 5 cm) may respond to conservative treatment, but most abscesses need to be drained. Poor response to medical treatment suggests an abscess. Patients who are mildly ill may receive ambulatory treatment and should be reevaluated in three days.

NONPHARMACOLOGIC MEASURES

In milder cases, bed rest and local heat using douches, sitz baths, or diathermy may suffice; in severe cases, bed rest, restriction of oral feeding, and intravenous fluids and electrolytes are appropriate. Nasogastric suction is used when abdominal distention is severe or bowel sounds are decreased or absent. Analgesics are prescribed for pain.

DRUG THERAPY

We follow the guidelines of the Centers for Disease Control (Table 2) with one exception. In the seriously ill patient with high fever, we add penicillin, 20 million units IV per 24 hours, to program B (clindamycin and gentamicin). This extends antimicrobial coverage to include group D streptococci. The CDC guidelines include recommendations for treatment of ambulatory and hospitalized patients.

In our opinion, single-drug programs using one of the new beta-lactamase agents such as moxalactam (Moxam), cefoperazone (Cefobid), cefotaxime (Cla-

Table 2. ANTIMICROBIAL THERAPY FOR PELVIC INFLAMMATORY DISEASE*

Parenteral Therapy

A. Doxycycline, 100 mg IV q 12 hr
   with
  cefoxitin, 2 gm IV q 6 hr
  for a minimum of 4 days and 48 hr after fever diminishes,
  followed by doxycycline, 100 mg q 12 hr PO approx. 10 more days

B. Clindamycin, 600 mg IV q 6 hr
   with
  gentamicin (or tobramycin), initial dose of 2.0 mg/kg IV, then 1.5 mg/kg IV q 8 hr (to be adjusted downward if renal function is impaired) for a minimum of 4 days and 48 hr after fever diminishes, followed by clindamycin, 300 mg q.i.d. PO for approx. 10 more days

C. Doxycycline, 100 mg IV q 12 hr
   with
  metronidazole, 1.0 gm IV q 12 hr for a minimum of 4 days and 48 hr after fever diminishes
  followed by same agents, same dosage PO for approx. 10 more days

Ambulatory Therapy

Cefoxitin 2.0 gm IV once or
amoxicillin, 3.0 gm PO once, or
ampicillin, 3.5 gm PO once, or
aqueous penicillin G, 4.8×10^6 units IM equally divided at two sites, once;
each of the above together with probenecid, 1.0 gm PO,
followed by doxycycline, 100 mg b.i.d. for approx. 14 days

*Centers for Disease Control Recommendations

foran), piperacillin (Pipracil), azlocillin (Azlin), or mezlocillin (Mezlin) have not been evaluated long enough in large enough numbers of patients. More information is needed before they can be recommended.

Adverse effects include allergic reactions to the antimicrobials used, potential nephrotoxicity of the aminoglycoside used, and antibiotic-induced ileocolitis (especially from clindamycin). Careful dosage of the aminoglycoside on the basis of patient weight, age, and renal function and dosage correction after actual measurement of peak and trough serum levels are mandatory.

Management of Complications. Early complications include abscess development and perforation. The latter is further complicated by peritonitis and requires immediate surgical intervention. Antibiotic treatment alone of a perforated abscess is associated with high mortality. Most abscesses require drainage. Antimicrobial treatment can be adjusted to the results of cultures obtained at surgery.

PATIENT INFORMATION AND EDUCATION

Patients receiving ambulatory treatment should be reminded of the importance of keeping regular appointments so that results can be evaluated. Hospitalized patients should be aware of the immediate and late goals of treatment. They all should know that their infection may have been sexually transmitted and that sterility may not be prevented by adequate treatment of the acute infection.

PERIODIC EVALUATION

A second look is required if there is a recurrence of symptoms or chronic pelvic pain. Follow-up visits one week and six weeks after discharge from the hospital are useful. At these times a WBC count, differential count, and ESR check should be done to ensure that the infection is under control.

PREVENTIVE MEASURES

Careful explanation of the mode of acquisition, the potential dangers of the infection, and the possibility of sterility are important. Too many people believe that a venereal infection is a minor problem that can readily be cured with penicillin. Contacts of patients with gonorrhea should be cultured and treated if positive.

SOCIOECONOMIC ASPECTS OF MANAGEMENT

Hospitalization lasts less than a week in most cases. However, IV administration of several antibiotics in separate solutions and the monitoring of aminoglycoside serum levels are expensive.

REFERENCES

Chesney PJ, Crass BA, Polyak MB, et al: Toxic shock syndrome: management and long-term sequelae. Ann Intern Med 96:847–874, 1982.

Eschenbach DA, Buchanan TM, Pollock HM, et al: Polymicrobial etiology of acute pelvic inflammatory disease. N Engl J Med 293:166–171, 1975.

McKenna UG, Meadows JA, Brewer NS, et al: Toxic shock syndrome: a newly recognized disease entity. Mayo Clin Proc 55:663–672, 1980.

Reingold AL, Hargrett NT, Dan BB, et al: Nonmenstrual toxic shock syndrome: a review of 130 cases. Ann Intern Med 96:871–874, 1982.

Sexually transmitted diseases: treatment guidelines, 1982. Rev Inf Dis 4:S729–746, 1982.

10 · LEGIONNAIRES' DISEASE

David J. Scheinhorn
OCHSNER CLINIC AND ALTON OCHSNER MEDICAL FOUNDATION

DEFINITION AND PATHOPHYSIOLOGY

Legionnaires' disease is the illness that results from pulmonary infection with *Legionella pneumophila*, an aerobic gram-negative bacillus. The diagnosis is made by demonstration of the organism by direct immunofluorescent antibody staining of infected secretions or tissue. Later confirmation of the diagnosis is possible by culturing the organism or finding a fourfold rise in complement-fixing antibody.

The organism can be isolated from indoor and outdoor sources of water, with a notorious predilection for the stagnant warm condensate of evaporative cooling towers. Infection occurs following inhalation with the establishment of a bronchopneumonia, leading to lobular and then lobar involvement. The inflammatory exudate may have fewer neutrophils than macrophages, and the organism readily multiplies within mononuclear cells. Hypoxemia is proportional to the extent of pulmonary involvement, but several endotoxins and exotoxins probably account for the toxic systemic symptoms and signs that serve as clues to the presence of infection with *L. pneumophila*.

CLINICAL ASPECTS

What aspects of the clinical presentation of legionnaires' disease differentiate it from other rapidly progressive bacterial or viral pneumonias? Patients with impaired cellular immunity form a group at highest risk. Antecedent upper respiratory symptoms are absent. Cough is often nonproductive during the first few days of illness, but when sputum is produced it is thin, nonpurulent, and blood streaked in one quarter to one third of patients. Headache, confusion, and disorientation (without localizing neurologic signs) are important clues to the diagnosis in our experience. Watery diarrhea without cramping should also heighten suspicion of infection with *L. pneumophila*. A disproportionately slow pulse is seen when compared to the height of fever.

The chest roentgenogram is nonspecific, but usually there is a nodular and lobular pattern with areas of coalescence to lobar involvement. Progression of infiltration after institution of therapy is also common. Hyponatremia (sodium less than 130 mEq/L) and hypophosphatemia with other clues just described should arouse suspicion of *Legionella* infection.

Expectorated sputum is the best material for diagnostic staining. Direct immunofluorescent staining requires three hours, is specific and moderately sensitive, and has only a 5% false-negative or false-positive result in experienced laboratories. This is an excellent test and the most useful one to guide therapy. This stain is also useful to identify organisms positively in histologic sections, again providing a rapid diagnosis. A Dieterle silver stain will confirm the presence of organisms but is not specific. The organism can be cultured on charcoal yeast extract media buffered with KOH. Smooth, gray, sticky colonies appear in two to four days. Saline and possibly lidocaine may inhibit bacterial growth and should not be used when specimens are transported or are obtained bronchoscopically. Blood culture and a variety of tissue sites have yielded positive cultures in patients with legionnaires' disease. Serologic confirmation of infection is by a fourfold rise in antibody titer that requires six to nine weeks.

MANAGEMENT

DRUG THERAPY

Early treatment with erythromycin results in probably a fourfold decrease in fatality rate. The most seriously ill patients with impaired host resistance have as high as an 80% fatality rate when untreated and often die with hemodynamic collapse in the first 48 hours following onset of symptoms.

Patients who have milder symptoms can be treated with oral erythromycin base, 500 mg every six hours; we have used the ethyl succinate (EES-400), 400 mg every six hours, with success. In most patients therapy should be initiated with erythromycin lactobionate or gluceptate, one gm IV every six hours. In the most seriously ill and immunocompromised patients, rifampin, 600 mg by mouth every 12 hours, should be used in addition to IV erythromycin. In patients who cannot take erythromycin, doxycycline, 200 mg loading dose, then 100 mg every 12 hours can be used PO or IV but may not be as effective as erythromycin.

After defervescence of clinical toxicity, most patients who have been given IV erythromycin can be changed to an oral preparation. If symptoms recur, several days of further IV therapy are indicated. We prescribe the ten days of oral therapy after IV therapy even in those who respond promptly to treatment. The overall fatality rate with treatment has been estimated at 5% to 20%.

Pyogenic complications of *L. pneumophila* pneumonia such as lung abscess or empyema are uncommon, but prolonged general debility is the rule. Most patients cannot return to work for a month after their illness, and lingering weakness, memory defect, and cough may persist for months. A follow-up visit is recommended in six weeks with a chest x-ray examination. The radiographic changes take longer to resolve than in most pyogenic pneumonias, more than six to eight weeks being usual.

HOSPITAL PRECAUTIONS

As the pathogenetic mechanisms become more clear, risk factor modification will become more specific. If a nosocomial outbreak is identified, susceptible hosts such as renal transplant patients may need to be transferred, and patients with positive sputum immunofluorescent smears may need to be placed in respiratory isolation even though person-to-person transmission has not been shown to occur. Hospital evaporative cooling tower reservoirs should be cultured when outbreaks occur and decontaminated with algicide and sodium hydroxide–containing preparations. Heating and additional chlorination have been used to control potable water sources in which organisms have been cultured in association with outbreaks.

REFERENCES

Davis GS, Winn WC, Beaty HN: Legionnaires' disease: infections caused by *L. pneumophila* and Legionella-like organisms. Clin Chest Med 2:145–166, 1981.

Edelstein PH, Meyer RD: Legionnaires' disease: a review. Chest 85:114–120, 1984.

Kugler JW, Armitage JO, Helms CM, et al: Nosocomial legionnaires' disease: occurrence in recipients of bone marrow transplants. Am J Med 74:281–288, 1983.

11 · VIRAL EXANTHEMS

Anthony Billas
GEISINGER MEDICAL CENTER

DEFINITION

Viral illnesses with cutaneous manifestations are common presenting complaints to primary care physicians, particularly those with large pediatric practices. Arriving at an accurate diagnosis can often be a frustrating experience for both the physician and the patient. Even though many times the treatment of viral exanthems is nonspecific, misdiagnosing these rashes can occasionally have disastrous results. This is particularly important when the differential diagnosis includes potentially lethal bacterial or rickettsial diseases or when pregnant or immunocompromised patients are involved. By taking a careful history and performing a thorough examination, the physician can often avoid expensive medical work-ups or potentially harmful procedures.

PATHOPHYSIOLOGY

Viruses can induce cutaneous lesions by directly infecting the epidermal or dermal structures or by various immunologic mechanisms. These manifestations are usually the result of hematogenous spread but can also occur by direct inoculation or even by migration along neurons (as in herpes zoster). Cutaneous lesions can vary from evanescent macules to crops of vesicles in various stages that can readily point to the diagnosis.

An attempt to describe the diagnosis and management of all known viral exanthems would be a formidable task. Several of these diseases, however, merit particular attention owing to the frequency with which they occur or to the seriousness of their complications if the diagnosis is missed.

Measles (Rubeola)

CLINICAL ASPECTS

Measles is an acute, highly contagious disease with significant morbidity and mortality. Its epidemiology has been drastically altered since the first measles vaccine was licensed in the United States in 1963. In fact, it has almost become a medical rarity, only 2813 cases being reported to the Centers for Disease Control (CDC) in 1985.

Typical measles affects the early school-age child (ages 5 to 9) and occurs principally in winter and spring. The incubation period is approximately five days and is followed by significant prodromal symptoms. These include malaise, cough, coryza, conjunctivitis with photophobia, and high fever. Pathognomonic Koplik's spots usually occur on the second or third day and consist of 1- to 2-mm white spots on an erythematous background (red halo). These typically occur on the buccal mucosa but can also be observed on lower labial, conjunctival, or vaginal mucosa. The rash usually appears on the fourth day, beginning behind the ears and on the forehead and spreading centrifugally to the extremities. It is erythematous and maculopapular, often becoming confluent on the face and upper trunk. The rash then clears over the next few days, also in a centrifugal pattern. Prominent lymphadenopathy, particularly cervical, is common. Leukopenia is a common laboratory finding, and x-rays show a nonspecific viral pneumonitis in approximately 70% of cases.

Since the introduction of measles vaccine, two new forms of measles have been described.

Mild Modified Measles. This occurs in partially immunized patients. This partial immunity can have a variety of causes, including administration of immune serum globulin on exposure to measles or in conjunction with measles vaccination. It can also occur in a patient who acquired measles or was immunized before one year of age. Mild modified measles is characterized by a prodrome of shorter duration and less intensity. Koplik's spots are less common and the rash seldom becomes confluent.

Atypical Measles. This is a more serious variant and occurs in previously immunized patients, particularly those who received the killed measles vaccine from 1963 to 1967. This disease is characterized by high fevers and an exanthem that progresses from peripheral to central areas. Petechiae and vesicles frequently occur, but Koplik's spots do not. Peripheral edema of the lower extremities and a typical nodular-appearing pneumonia are prominent features.

COMPLICATIONS

Complications of measles include otitis media, bacterial pneumonia, encephalitis (1 in 1000 cases), and rarely the late development of subacute sclerosing panencephalitis (SSPE).

Diagnosis can often be made on clinical grounds, but confirmation is important for epidemiologic reasons. Fourfold rises in measles hemagglutination inhibition (HAI) antibodies over two to four weeks, or similar rises in complement fixation (CF) or neutralizing antibodies, can be used. Viral cultures, when available, can also confirm the diagnosis.

MANAGEMENT

Prevention with vaccination is the best treatment, but supportive measures are needed for active disease. Antipyretics, bed rest, fluids, and antitussives can afford considerable relief. Close scrutiny for bacterial complications is vital, especially if fever persists beyond four days. Patients should be isolated until approximately five days after the onset of the exanthem. Follow-up chest x-rays are necessary before patients with atypical measles can resume full activities.

Exposed, susceptible, normal persons should receive a protective dose of gamma globulin (0.25 ml/kg) as soon as possible after exposure, followed by live vaccine after 12 weeks to induce lasting immunity. Exposed, susceptible, compromised hosts . . . should receive 0.5 ml/kg, up to 20 ml to 30 ml of gamma globulin. Live virus vaccine is contraindicated in such patients; indirect protection should be sought through immunizing all measles-susceptible close contacts of this group of patients.

MARCY AND KUBRICK

German Measles (Rubella)

CLINICAL ASPECTS

Rubella is a mild disease with minimal morbidity and mortality. Like rubeola, the incidence of rubella has been significantly decreased (604 cases in 1985) owing to the availability of rubella vaccine since 1969. The most important reason for accurate diagnosis of rubella today is to avoid the devastating development of congenital rubella syndrome (CRS), of which only two cases were reported in 1985.

In the prevaccine era, rubella typically struck young school-age children in winter and spring. Today the majority of cases occur in individuals over 15 years old. Incubation period is two to three weeks, and the prodromal phase varies from nonexistent in children to one to five days in adults. In adults it consists of eye pain, sore throat, headache, fever, chills, anorexia, and vomiting. These usually subside one day after the rash begins. The exanthem is variable but typically is an erythematous, discrete, and maculopapular rash that begins on the face and spreads to the extremities. It occasionally coalesces centrally and fades after about three days. It can be quite pruritic, which sometimes leads to a misdiagnosis of allergic reaction. Suboccipital and postauricular adenopathy are fairly specific findings. Owing to its variable and often mild presentation, the disease itself can be missed by both the patient and the doctor.

COMPLICATIONS

Complications are usually rare and consist of arthralgias and arthritis, thrombocytopenia (1 in 3000 cases), and encephalitis (1 in 6000 cases). The most dreaded complication occurs when a susceptible pregnant patient is exposed to rubella during the first trimester, with a 20% or greater incidence of CRS.

Diagnosis is suggested by history and clinical findings. A history of exposure is also helpful. Diagnosis can be confirmed by viral cultures (pharynx) or by a fourfold rise in either HAI, CF, or neutralizing antibodies.

MANAGEMENT

Treatment is often unnecessary since symptoms are usually mild. Aspirin can offer symptomatic relief with many of the minor complications. Bed rest is not usually necessary unless arthritis of the weight-bearing joints is involved. Strict avoidance of susceptible pregnant patients is a must.

Management of the pregnant patient exposed to rubella offers special problems. Obtaining HAI antibodies as soon as possible after exposure can rule out susceptibility if immunity is demonstrated (usually HAI $\geq$ 1:8 titer). If the antibody count is less than 1:8, a second specimen drawn two to four weeks later is indicated. A fourfold or greater rise in titer suggests infection in the mother with a risk of 20% or greater of CRS if exposure occurred in the first trimester. Detailed counseling is then needed, with the option of terminating the pregnancy. Postexposure immunoglobulin is not routinely recommended, but it has been used in women who absolutely ruled out termination of their pregnancies.

Chickenpox (Varicella)

CLINICAL ASPECTS

Chickenpox is a highly contagious disease with a relatively benign course. Unlike rubella and rubeola, this classic viral exanthem's epidemiologic picture has not yet been altered by immunizations. It typically occurs in children less than 9 years of age, especially in late winter or early spring. The incubation period is approximately 14 to 16 days after onset of the exanthem. Often the first symptom is the rash with a coincident fever. The lesions are initially more prominent centrally and begin as macules, progressing through various stages: papules, papulovesicles, crusting vesicles, and finally scab formation. Crops of lesions in various stages are a hallmark of varicella. The lesions are usually all crusted within ten days.

COMPLICATIONS

The most common complication is secondary skin bacterial infection though pneumonia can be prominent in adults. Encephalitis occurs in about 1 in 1000 cases and an association with Reye's syndrome has been noted in varicella patients receiving aspirin.

Laboratory studies are seldom necessary in this common and characteristic disease. Treatment is symptomatic, but aspirin should be avoided. Nails should be trimmed to reduce the risk of bacterial skin infections.

Table 1. CANDIDATES FOR WHOM VARICELLA-ZOSTER IMMUNE GLOBULIN (VZIG) IS INDICATED*

---

1. Susceptible to varicella-zoster
2. Significant exposure
3. Age of < 15 years, with administration to immunocompromised adolescents and adults and to other patients on an individual basis
4. One of the following underlying illnesses or conditions:
   a. Leukemia or lymphoma
   b. Congenital or acquired immunodeficiency
   c. Immunosuppressive treatment
   d. Newborn of mothers who had onset of chickenpox within five days before delivery or within 48 hours after delivery
   e. Premature infant ($\geq$ 28 weeks' gestation) whose mother lacks a prior history of chickenpox
   f. Premature infants (< 28 weeks' gestation or $\leq$ 1000 g) regardless of maternal history

---

From MMWR 33:89, 1984.
*Patients should meet the four criteria for VZIG candidates.

Polysporin ointment can be applied to excoriated lesions, and occasionally systemic antibiotics may be needed to control infections. Cool oatmeal baths (Aveeno) and antihistamines (diphenhydramine HCl 5 mg/kg/day) help to relieve the pruritus. The patient should be kept home for approximately one week following the eruption until all lesions are crusted. Contact with immunocompromised patients is strictly contraindicated.

Since 1978, varicella-zoster immune globulin (VZIG) has been available to prevent clinical varicella in susceptible immunocompromised patients. Table 1 gives a summary of candidates for whom VZIG is indicated.*

Exanthem Subitum (Roseola Infantum)

CLINICAL ASPECTS

Roseola is a benign disease of infancy (peak ages 7 to 13 months) that can lead to high anxiety in parents and doctors alike. It is the most common exanthem in children less than 2 years of age. Though no infectious agent has been isolated, it is thought to be of viral origin. Roseola typically begins with an abrupt fever (often up to 40.5°C) with few other signs or symptoms. Occasionally mild anorexia or irritability accompany the prodrome. Antipyretics cause a temporary decrease in temperature. After three to four days of high fever, the temperature suddenly plummets with the development of an exanthem. This rash usually begins on the trunk and spreads to the face and extremities. It consists of discrete erythematous macular or maculopapular lesions that last anywhere from two hours to two days. Laboratory results are generally unremarkable except for occasional leukocytosis early in the course, followed by leukopenia at the time of the exanthem.

---

*A complete discussion of this topic is included in the February 24, 1984 MMWR.

MANAGEMENT

Proper management begins with a careful history and particular emphasis on the child's general well-being. A thorough physical examination should rule out bacterial causes of hyperpyrexia such as otitis media, pneumonia, and especially meningitis. Close follow-up is essential, often on a daily basis with parental instructions to notify the physician if there is a change in the child's status. Loose-fitting clothes, antipyretics, and tepid baths can all be employed. Isolation is generally not indicated. Convulsions can often be the presenting complaint and should be treated as any other initial febrile seizure. This usually includes a diagnostic lumbar puncture to exclude a diagnosis of meningitis.

Erythema Infectiosum (Fifth Disease)

Fifth disease is a mildly contagious disease presumed to be of viral origin. It has very characteristic cutaneous manifestations with few constitutional signs. It often occurs in epidemics during the winter and spring and usually affects the 5- to 14-year-old age group. The incubation period is thought to be one to two weeks, and there is no associated prodrome. The exanthem is divided into three stages. It initially presents with characteristic fiery red "slapped" cheeks and circumoral pallor. The second stage (one to four days later) consists of an initially discrete, erythematous maculopapular rash on the proximal extremities that often takes on a reticular or "lacy" pattern. The final stage (approximately seven days after presentation) is similar to the second stage except that the rash waxes and wanes for one to three weeks. This can occur in response to temperature changes, sunlight, or trauma.

Laboratory results are seldom necessary and generally unremarkable. No treatment is needed except for support and reassurance and an occasional antihistamine if pruritus is present. Complications are very rare, but joint pain, myalgias, encephalitis, and hemolytic anemia have been reported.

Other Viral Exanthems

Many other viral agents are associated with exanthems that are either less common or have less significant implications. Adenoviruses are examples of common infectious agents in children and young adults with an approximately 2% to 5% occurrence of exanthems. Enteroviruses can be a leading cause of rashes, especially in summer and fall. Members of the herpes virus group, other than varicella, are well known for their cutaneous manifestations, such as herpes simplex or Epstein-Barr virus. Coxsackieviruses have been known to cause epidemics of hand-foot-and-mouth dis-

ease. Respiratory viral exanthems are important since they can result in a child being inappropriately labeled as allergic to an antibiotic.

REFERENCES

ACIP: Varicella-zoster immune globulin for the prevention of chicken-pox. MMWR 33:84–90, 1984.
ACIP: Rubella prevention. MMWR 33:301–317, 1984.
Cherry JD: Viral exanthems. DM 28(8):1–56, 1982.
Marcy SM, Kibrick S: Measles. *In* Hoeprich PD (ed): Infectious disease. Harper & Row, New York, 1983, pp 815–824.

12 · INFLUENZA

W. Brooks Emory
OCHSNER CLINIC AND ALTON OCHSNER MEDICAL FOUNDATION

ETIOLOGY

The influenza viruses (types A and B) are responsible for major morbidity and mortality affecting all ages worldwide. Three influenza viruses, types A, B, and C, are designated according to the antigenic character of their internal ribonucleoprotein. Serotypes A and B have two surface antigens (hemagglutinin and neuraminidase) in the viral envelope that are continually changing. Major antigenic changes, "shifts," occur in the surface antigens of type A at approximately ten-year intervals, while minor changes, "drifts," occur in A or B and are responsible for minor epidemics between the "shifts." Influenza C is associated with endemic outbreaks of upper respiratory infections but is not a clinically significant illness; hence it is not a component of the influenza vaccine.

PATHOPHYSIOLOGY

An influenza virus is labeled by its serotype (A, B, or C), the geographic area, the year it was first isolated, and the character of its surface antigens (e.g., type A has three hemagglutinin, H1, H2, and H3, and two neuraminidase, N1 and N2). Clinical illness occurs when the virus enters the upper respiratory tract as a result of inhalation of infected droplets. Incubation is usually 48 hours from exposure but ranges from one to four days. The viral hemagglutinin combines with a complementary molecular configuration of mucoprotein in the airway secretions. Then the viral neuraminidase lowers the viscosity of surface mucus, liquefying it and exposing cell surface receptors. Liquefaction of mucus retards removal of the virus by the mucociliary escalator and promotes spread of virus to the dependent portions of the tracheobronchial tree. Viral replication occurs within the cell after penetration of virus in vacuoles or by intake of RNA from particles disrupted at the surface. Release of the newly synthesized virus is enhanced by neuraminidase activity, and a new cycle of absorption, penetration, synthesis, and release is begun. A small percentage of patients develop a patchy viral pneumonia with capillary hemorrhage, viral inclusion bodies, and alveolar hyaline membranes. Necrosis and desquamation of the respiratory epithelium make the host vulnerable to secondary bacterial infections and are a significant source of mortality. The damage to the respiratory epithelium may explain the persistent nonproductive cough that lingers weeks after resolution of the acute infection.

CLINICAL ASPECTS

Major outbreaks of influenza A tend to occur at intervals of every two to four years from late autumn to early spring, and influenza B infections at intervals of every four to seven years. Epidemic behavior in a given locale is typical of the illness. The "flu" is characterized by symptoms of abrupt onset of chills, fever, headache, rhinorrhea, and myalgias of the legs and lower back, intensifying over the first 24 hours. The acute illness lasts four to seven days, but lassitude and persistent cough may linger for a much longer time. Viral serology and identification are more pertinent to confirming an outbreak in a specific locale but have little to no clinical benefit in management of an individual's illness.

The greatest threat from influenza occurs with the appearance of a new strain to which most of the population lacks immunity. In 1968 the Hong Kong influenza pandemic affected 25% of the U.S. population over a two- to three-month period because it was a new antigenic strain, with no native immunity in the U.S. population.

MANAGEMENT

Uncomplicated influenza infection is usually a self-limited outpatient illness. In children acute external otitis or pneumonia occurs in 25% of influenza A infections but in a much lower incidence with influenza B. Ampicillin would be appropriate treatment for otitis but patients (pediatric or adult) with pneumonia should be started on penicillinase-resistant penicillin (Nafcillin, 100 to 200 mg/kg IV per day at four- to six-hour intervals) while cultures are pending. Bacterial pathogens frequently causing pneumonia secondary to influenza infection are: *Staphylococcus aureus*, pneumococcus, and less commonly *Streptococcus* or *Haemophilus influenzae*.

REYE'S SYNDROME

Reye's syndrome in children is a serious complication of influenza B infection that may be associated with the administration of salicylates; hence acetaminophen preparations are advised for fevers and myalgias of viral illnesses in children. This syndrome of encephalopathy and fatty infiltration of the liver with hepatic failure occurs most frequently in children under age 16 and is fatal in 30% of patients. Recognition of encephalopathy early on is important, but therapy still remains supportive.

PRIMARY VIRAL PNEUMONIA

Primary viral pneumonia of influenza can progress rapidly to respiratory failure, necessitating intubation and mechanical ventilator support. Viral alveolar injury dictates the judicious use of positive end-expiratory pressure (PEEP) and the lowest inspired oxygen to maintain an arterial Po_2 of 65 mm Hg. Continuous positive airway pressure (CPAP) has been reported to be successful in nonintubated patients in maintaining viable Po_2. These ventilator-dependent patients are at risk for nosocomial infection, and intravenous mezlocillin (300 mg/kg per day at four- to six-hour intervals) and gentamicin (3–7.5 mg/kg per day at eight-hour intervals) should be started if such a problem occurs while cultures are pending.

The bacterial pneumonia that occurs four to seven days after a patient has the classic symptoms of flu should be treated with a penicillinase-resistant penicillin (nafcillin or methicillin) until cultures are positive.

Cardiac decompensation may complicate treatment of the elderly patient, and supportive care with oxygen, diuretics, and digitalis would be appropriate. Myocarditis may occur rarely as a feature of influenza and lead to a progressive cardiomyopathy.

The use of amantadine hydrochloride (Symmetrel) is 70% to 90% effective in preventing illness caused by type A influenza when administered within 24 to 48 hours of the onset of symptoms. It is not effective against influenza B. Amantadine can be used for short-term prophylaxis if there is an outbreak in one's community for selected high-risk patients, but it is expensive and therefore should not be used *carte blanche* through the "flu season." The dosage is 200 mg/day; splitting the dose to 100 mg/b.i.d. reduces the frequency of side effects of insomnia, lightheadedness, irritability, and difficulty in concentrating. Children should receive a lower dose (Tables 1 and 2), and those under age 1 year and persons with renal impairment should not take the drug.

Since 1963 the goal of management of influenza is to immunize annually the patient and medical population at greatest risk for disease. High-priority risk groups are nursing home residents, for whom attack rates are as high as 60%, with a fatality rate of 30%; persons with compromised immune function or metabolic diseases; and persons afflicted with chronic disorders of the cardiovascular, pulmonary, or renal systems. Medical personnel in contact with high-risk patients (i.e., ICU and PICU employees) and strategic service personnel (e.g., police and fire department members) are also strongly advised to have annual vaccinations.

IMMUNIZATION—PREVENTIVE MEASURES

The use of inactivated influenza vaccine is the single most important measure in preventing or attenuating infection. The vaccine for 1985–86 has 15 µg each of: A/Chile/83(H1N1), A/Philippines/82(H3N2), and B/USSR/100/83. It is considered safe for pregnant women, but it is better to wait until the second or third trimester to

Table 1. INFLUENZA VACCINE DOSAGE, BY AGE OF PATIENT (1984–1985 SEASON)

Age Group	Product	Dosage	No. of Doses
6–35 mo	Split virus only	0.25 ml	2
3–12 yr	Split virus only	0.5 ml	2
Over 12 yr	Whole or split virus	0.5 ml	1

From MMWR 34:256, 1984.

Table 2. AMANTADINE HYDROCHLORIDE DOSAGE BY AGE OF PATIENT AND LEVEL OF RENAL FUNCTION

Age Group	Dosage
Normal Renal Function	
1–9 yr	4.4–8.8 mg/kg/day once daily or divided twice daily; total dosages should not exceed 150 mg per day
10 yr	200 mg once daily or divided twice daily
Impaired renal function	Reduce to 100 mg daily

Modified from MMWR 33:259, 1984.

minimize any concern over the theoretical possibility of teratogenicity. Inactivated influenza vaccine should not be given to persons who have had anaphylactic reactions to eggs, and persons with a febrile illness should postpone vaccination until their acute illness has resolved. Side effects of the vaccine are mild. Local erythema and induration lasting one to two days occur in less than 30% of those vaccinated. Infrequently fever, malaise, and myalgias may affect those who have had no previous exposure to influenza virus, beginning six to 12 hours after vaccination and persisting for one to two days. This reaction is attributed to the influenza antigens. There has been no increased incidence of Guillain-Barré syndrome with the present vaccines. Pneumococcal vaccine can be given simultaneously.

REFERENCES

Centers for Disease Control: Provisional reports. MMWR 35:March, June, 1986.
Evans AS (ed): Viral Infections of Humans: Epidemiology and Control, 2nd ed. Plenum Medical Book Co, New York, 1982.

13 · KAWASAKI SYNDROME

Gregory T. Valainis
OCHSNER CLINIC AND ALTON OCHSNER MEDICAL FOUNDATION

DEFINITION AND DIAGNOSTIC CRITERIA

Kawasaki syndrome, otherwise known as *mucocutaneous lymph node syndrome*, was first described in 1967 by the Japanese investigator whose name the disease bears. It remains today a clinical diagnosis. Table 1 lists the six major diagnostic criteria, five of which must be met and for which no differential diagnosis can be made.

PATHOPHYSIOLOGY

Kawasaki syndrome is a multi-system disease of unknown etiology. It occurs worldwide in infants and young children of all ethnic groups. The primary pathologic changes are those of a vasculitis predominantly involving the proximal coronary arteries. Later aneurysmal dilatation is seen, which can lead to thrombus formation or rupture. Finally, scarring can occur with stenosis, which may lead to signs of myocardial ischemia.

CLINICAL ASPECTS

Kawasaki syndrome is characteristically a triphasic illness. The initial acute phase lasts approximately ten days, manifested by hectic fever, conjunctival injection, stomatitis, induration and reddening of the soles and palms, rash, and nonsuppurative cervical adenopathy. Aseptic meningitis, elevated hepatic transaminases, and diarrhea can also be seen. The subacute phase follows, lasting some 25 days, during which defervesence occurs. The other early manifestations resolve as well. Thrombocytosis peaks, and desquamation of the fingers and toes appears. Cardiac disease is most likely to occur in this phase, during which myocardial ischemia, arrhythmias, pericarditis, myocarditis, or heart failure can be seen. The convalescent phase occurs between the fifth and tenth weeks of illness. The return to normal of the erythrocyte sedimentation rate (ESR) marks the end of active disease.

No confirmatory laboratory tests are yet available. Some simple laboratory tests, such as a complete blood cell count (CBC), a platelet count, urinalysis, and ESR, can be helpful but are nonspecific.

MANAGEMENT

Since the etiology is unknown, specific rational therapy is unclear. The goals of therapy should be to mollify the acute phase symptoms and prevent the dreaded complications of vasculitis with aneurysm formation. In spite of therapy, approximately 20% of patients develop coronary aneurysms. The long-term prognosis has yet to be determined.

In general Kawasaki syndrome is a self-limiting illness, the only significant morbidity being cardiac damage. The mortality rate is less than 2%; thus, patients with mild cases who pose no diagnostic dilemma can be managed safely as outpatients with frequent clinic visits. Those patients with clinically severe disease (especially cardiac) or in whom the diagnosis is unclear should be monitored in a hospital setting.

Aspirin is the sole drug used for treatment in a three-pronged attack since it is (1) anti-inflammatory, (2) antipyretic, and (3) inhibitory of platelet aggregation. Initially high doses are used (80 to 100 mg/kg/day) in four divided doses. Salicylate levels must be monitored to maintain serum levels of 15 to 25 mg/dl. Parents should be made aware that although the acute-phase

Table 1. DIAGNOSIS OF MUCOCUTANEOUS LYMPH NODE SYNDROME

A. Fever for 5 or more days unresponsive to antibiotics
B. Conjunctival infection
C. Oral cavity changes: Strawberry tongue
                    Diffuse oropharyngeal erythema
                    Fissuring, erythema, and crusting of lips
D. Extremity changes: Erythema of soles and palms with induration
                    Late-onset desquamation of fingers and toes
E. Erythematous exanthem
F. Lymphadenopathy

manifestations may resolve more quickly with aspirin, the long-term morbidity and mortality may not be altered. We avoid glucocorticoid use because in one study a higher incidence of aneurysms was observed when compared with those patients treated with aspirin. Once the fever resolves, the aspirin dosage can be decreased to 10 mg/kg/day in two divided doses to inhibit platelet aggregation. A recent Japanese study in which high-dose IV gamma globulin reduced the incidence of coronary artery lesions when given within seven days of the onset of the illness holds great promise. It awaits multicenter testing in the United States for confirmation.

A real-time echocardiogram should be done initially to detect early coronary aneurysms. At first patients are seen at least twice weekly. Any abnormal studies should be repeated, and ESR and platelet counts should be obtained weekly. A careful cardiac examination is performed to detect any heart failure, a pericardial friction rub, mitral insufficiency, or irregular heart rhythms. The period from day 14 to day 35 marks the time of greatest risk of cardiac failure. A repeat echocardiogram is performed after 28 days of illness. Based on the clinician's accumulated data plus the repeat echocardiogram, clinic visits may then be decreased to once a week until the platelet count and ESR return to normal. Those patients with coronary aneurysms still present with inactive disease continue to receive aspirin indefinitely; those without can discontinue aspirin therapy.

Coronary angiography is reserved for equivocal cases or for patients who manifest coronary insufficiency. A rare patient will require coronary artery surgery for refractory disease. Balloon dilatation can also be used in very selected cases. The use of these adjuncts must be individualized.

Long-term follow-up is mandatory and should be reinforced with repeated statements to the parents. All patients should be seen every three to six months with repeat EKG and echocardiogram. Longer prospective studies are needed to determine the incidence of irreversible cardiac damage.

REFERENCES

Furusko K, Nakano H, Shinomiya K, et al: High-dose intravenous gammaglobulin for Kawasaki disease. Lancet 2:1055–1058, 1984.
Kato H, Koike S, Yokoyama J: Kawasaki disease: effect of treatment on coronary artery involvement. Pediatrics 63:175–179, 1979.
Kawasaki T: MCLS-clinical observation of 50 cases (in Japanese). Jpn J Allerg 16:178–222, 1967.
Kawasaki T, Kasaki F, Okuwa S, et al: A new infantile acute febrile mucocutaneous lymph node syndrome (MLNS) prevailing in Japan. Pediatrics 54:271–276, 1974.
Melish ME: Kawasaki syndrome (the mucocutaneous lymph node syndrome). Annu Rev Med 33:569–585, 1982.

14 · LYME DISEASE

Norman Kattwinkel
LAHEY CLINIC MEDICAL CENTER

DEFINITION AND DIAGNOSTIC CRITERIA

A form of arthritis first described in 1975 is now clearly defined as Lyme disease, which is heralded by a characteristic rash in most patients and is frequently accompanied by systemic symptoms including neurologic and cardiac changes. The rash is similar to one described previously in Scandinavian and European medical literature, and the arthritis is episodic and usually self-limited. The acute illness of Lyme disease may be mediated by immune complexes involving a spirochetal agent as demonstrated by low levels of serum complement, elevated cryoprecipitates, and antispirochetal antibodies. The disease usually carries a good prognosis but may cause appreciable morbidity.

PATHOPHYSIOLOGY

The vector of Lyme disease has been identified as a tiny (1- to 2-mm) tick, *Ixodes dammini*, first found in abundance in the region of Lyme, Connecticut, but now known to inhabit many states, primarily in southeastern New England. In the West another species, *I. pacificus*, has been incriminated. A similar tick, *Amblyomma americanum*, found especially in New Jersey, is probably another vector of Lyme disease. Natural hosts of these ticks are the white-footed mouse and the white-tailed deer. A causative agent isolated from midgut tissues of *I. dammini* ticks was first reported in 1982 and is identified as a spirochetal organism that has recently been classified and formally named *Borrelia burgdorferi*. This organism has been isolated from some although not all patients with Lyme disease, has been cultured, and has been used to induce the characteristic skin rash in rabbits. Elevated IgM specific antibody titer against the spirochete occurs early in the course of Lyme disease, whereas IgG antibody reaches a peak level several weeks later and may remain elevated for many months.

CLINICAL ASPECTS

A characteristic rash known as *erythema chronicum migrans* begins as a red macule or papule and expands in a circular fashion over several days, usually on the trunk. As the lesion grows, the outer ring becomes bright red while the center becomes clear, red, indurated, or (rarely) necrotic. The initial lesion may reach a diameter of 12 inches or more, and multiple smaller secondary lesions may appear. The rash is frequently asymptomatic and lasts about three weeks. Associated features at the time of the rash may include fever, stiff neck, backache, myalgias, sore throat, nausea, vomiting, headache, and Bell's palsy. Some patients have no associated symptoms.

Neurologic changes occurring with or after the rash include burning paresthesias, cranial nerve palsies, peripheral neuropathies, and aseptic meningitis. CSF analysis shows increased cellularity with lymphocytosis and a slight increase in protein.

Heart complications develop in approximately 10% of patients with Lyme disease. These consist of atrioventricular block or more diffuse cardiac involvement with electrocardiographic evidence of acute myocarditis, mild left ventricular dysfunction, or frank cardiomegaly. The duration of heart involvement is usually three days to six weeks.

Arthritis develops in 25% of patients with erythema chronicum migrans. It invades the large joints, particularly the knees, although the hands, feet, and elbows may be involved. The arthritis is usually monarticular, but some patients have several joints involved simultaneously or separately. The arthritis usually appears three to four weeks after the rash and may last from one week to six months. The attacks may be recurrent. Rarely a sustained, proliferative erosive synovitis similar to rheumatoid arthritis will develop.

LABORATORY TESTS

Serologic tests to detect elevated IgM and IgG specific antibodies against the spirochete are available and include an indirect immunofluorescent antibody test and an enzyme-linked immunosorbent assay (ELISA) test. These tests provide a high degree of specificity and sensitivity in the diagnosis of Lyme disease, especially if the disease progresses with heart, neurologic, or arthritic complications. The tests are relatively insensitive, however, for patients with the rash alone. Erythrocyte sedimentation rate and WBC count are usually within normal limits. Findings of latex fixation and antinuclear antibody tests are negative. Anemia and abnormalities of vital organs are usually absent.

MANAGEMENT

PLAN

To the unwary observer the frequently benign appearance and asymptomatic nature of erythema chronicum migrans might suggest that treatment is unnecessary. Indeed, since the rash is so mild and even absent in some patients, the decision to treat or not to treat may never arise. The alert physician, however, will recognize this rash and its infectious nature. The major late complications of arthritis, myocarditis, and neurologic changes require the persistence of a live spirochetal organism in the patient for some period beyond the early presence of the rash. In fact, if the infection is treated promptly with antibiotics at the time of the rash, these major late complications are unlikely to develop.

Minor late complications persist in nearly 50% of patients despite appropriate early treatment, and include headache, migratory myalgias, arthralgias, and lethargy. These minor complications tend to correlate with initial severity of the illness and may be caused by a small population of live spirochetes that fails to succumb to the antibiotic program. Despite a high dose of intravenously administered penicillin these minor complications may fail to improve, indicating that their development may not require persistent live organisms but may reflect the presence of retained antigen or some ongoing immune process. Therefore, the short- and long-term goals of management of Lyme disease include proper recognition of the characteristic erythema chronicum migrans and prompt institution of appropriate antibiotic treatment to eradicate the infection before complications develop.

Occasionally additional measures beyond antibiotic therapy become necessary. These include hospitalization for cardiac complications, such as complete heart block requiring implantation of a pacemaker; neurologic changes, such as meningoencephalitis; and arthritic problems when unusually painful and severe or when chronic and requiring synovectomy or other surgical intervention. Usually, however, people with Lyme disease are successfully treated as outpatients and respond promptly to oral administration of antibiotics and anti-inflammatory drugs.

NONPHARMACOLOGIC MEASURES

Although pharmacologic therapy is the mainstay of treatment of Lyme disease, other measures may be helpful and important. The rash, when pruritic or painful, may respond to cool compresses. The arthritis will be helped by splinting of particularly painful or swollen joints and bed rest in addition to anti-inflammatory agents. Both local heat and ice packs have been used with success in reducing pain.

DRUG THERAPY

Early experience between 1976 and 1980 showed that treatment with penicillin G, 250,000 units PO four times a day for ten days, as soon as the rash was seen shortened the duration of the rash and prevented later development of arthritis, but did not protect against later neurologic or cardiac complications. However, subsequent studies showed convincingly that use of tetracycline instead of penicillin definitely reduced the major late complications of myocarditis, meningoencephalitis, and recurrent attacks of arthritis. Therefore, the current recommended treatment program in adults is tetracycline PO, 250 mg four times a day for at least ten days, as soon as the rash is seen and again for another ten days if symptoms persist. Alternatively, phenoxymethyl penicillin, 500 mg four times a day for ten days, or benzathine penicillin, 2.4 million units IM, can be given.

Since tetracycline presents the danger of dental staining the recommended treatment for children is penicillin PO, 50 mg/kg of body weight per day (not less than 1 gm/day or more than 2 gm/day) in divided doses for ten days. In patients with sensitivity to penicillin, erythromycin, 30 mg/kg of body weight per day in divided doses for 15 to 20 days, is recommended.

Adverse Effects. One adverse effect of antibiotic treatment is that 10% to 14% of patients, usually those with severe disease, have higher fever, redder rash, and more severe joint pain during the first 24 hours of administration. This has been likened to a Jarisch-Herxheimer reaction caused by fast killing of large numbers of spirochetes during the early treatment period. The program should be continued in these patients, and subsequent improvement can be expected.

Cardiac Complications. As experience with Lyme disease has accumulated, the treatment of complications of the disease has evolved. With regard to cardiac complications, all patients with erythema chronicum migrans should have electrocardiography and if they have a slightly prolonged P-R interval should be followed as outpatients and advised to restrict their activities. Patients with a high degree of AV block or first-degree block with a P-R interval longer than 0.3 seconds should be hospitalized for monitoring, since these have a high risk of developing complete heart block. Patients with complete heart block will require implantation of a temporary pacemaker. If the complete AV block persists longer than a week, prednisone, 40 to 60 mg per day in divided doses, should be added with gradual tapering over the next week to ten days.

Neurologic Complications. Patients with neurologic complications usually have recurrent episodes of headache and stiff neck, and some have a peripheral neuropathy, such as facial palsy, and a convincing previous history of erythema chronicum migrans and exposure to ticks. A problem arises when the picture is incomplete and a patient presents only with signs and symptoms of meningitis. In such a patient, serologic testing is helpful, as discussed earlier. If Lyme meningitis is suspected, large doses of IV penicillin are now recommended, specifically penicillin G, 20 million units per day in divided doses for ten days. Adding prednisone to this program has not been shown to be helpful. In a patient with allergy to penicillin, tetracycline PO, 500 mg four times a day for 30 days, is reasonable.

Lyme Arthritis. Finally, the arthritis of Lyme disease is effectively treated with nonsteroidal anti-inflammatory medication, such as ibuprofen (Motrin), 600 mg four times daily, or indomethacin (Indocin), 25 to 50 mg three times daily. These drugs are necessary only if symptoms in the joints become troublesome despite previous use of antibiotic or corticosteroid medication. Occasionally chronic proliferative synovitis develops, in which case arthroscopic or open synovectomy is necessary.

PATIENT INFORMATION AND EDUCATION

Since the summer of 1975 when two mothers in Lyme, Connecticut first recognized a pattern of illness in their town's children, public awareness of the features of Lyme disease has grown at an unusually fast pace. Physicians working together with the lay press quickly appreciated the public health impact of this disease, and their efforts have done much to increase public education. Physicians and general populations in endemic regions of tick infestation are now acutely aware, particularly during summer months, of the implications of the typical rash and the need for early antibiotic treatment. Despite these advances, many physicians tend to forget that travel to endemic areas during the tick season may expose patients to the disease who otherwise would be safe from contact. Therefore, physicians and the public throughout the country should be aware of the features of Lyme disease. Physicians, in particular, should be alert to the rash and also be ready to consider the disease when complicating features, such as heart block, isolated arthritis, or neurologic changes, are present in the absence of the rash.

PERIODIC EVALUATION

In most patients, once the disease has been recognized and treated it will follow a smooth course with prompt resolution of symptoms. Complications will be minimized by early treatment. One or two follow-up visits usually are sufficient to ensure complete recovery. As mentioned earlier, IgM specific antibody titer becomes elevated as early as one week after symptoms begin, whereas the IgG antibody titer reaches a peak level several weeks later and may remain elevated for many months. The latter, in fact, is the only helpful laboratory test during the recovery phase. Once the nature of the disease and its possible serious complications are fully explained by the physician, patient compliance with the relatively innocuous and short course of antibiotic treatment is usually good. Sensitivity to antibiotics is easily managed by drug substitution in most patients.

PREVENTIVE MEASURES

Preventive measures against the disease have proved to be a more formidable challenge. During the winter months of indoor living no risk is present, but once summer arrives campers, backpackers, and vacationers are exposed to the potential risk of exposure to the tick environment—over which man has little control. Reducing the populations of white-tailed deer and white-footed mice is difficult and has political and environmental implications. Ultimately prevention depends on attention to avoidance of endemic areas known to harbor ticks, use of insect repellents (although these are only partially effective), and awareness of the characteristic erythema chronicum migrans and prompt treatment measures. In this way the considerable socioeconomic impact of Lyme disease on the general population can be controlled and minimized.

REFERENCES

Burgdorfer W, Barbour AG, Hayes SF, et al: Lyme disease—a tick-borne spirochetosis? Science 216:1317–1319, 1982.

Russell H, Sampson JS, Schmid GP, et al: Enzyme-linked immunosorbent assay and indirect immunofluorescence assay for Lyme disease. J Infect Dis 149:465–470, 1984.

Steere AC, Bartenhagen NH, Craft JE, et al: The early clinical manifestations of Lyme disease. Ann Intern Med 99:76–82, 1983.

Steere AC, Hutchinson GJ, Rahn DW, et al: Treatment of the early manifestations of Lyme disease. Ann Intern Med 99:22–26, 1983.

Steere AC, Pachner AR, Malawista SE: Neurologic abnormalities of Lyme disease: successful treatment with high-dose intravenous penicillin. Ann Intern Med 99:767–772, 1983.

15 · PNEUMOCYSTIS CARINII, *GIARDIASIS,* CRYPTOSPORIDIOSIS, TRICHINOSIS, AND ECHINOCOCCOSIS

Evelyn J. Fisher
HENRY FORD HOSPITAL

Pneumocystis Carinii *Pneumonia (PCP)*

DEFINITION, DIAGNOSTIC CRITERIA, AND CLINICAL ASPECTS

PCP is interstitial pneumonia due to the protozoan *Pneumocystis carinii.* Diagnosis is made by seeing the organism on special smear or histology from specimens obtained through bronchoscopy or open lung biopsy. *Pneumocystis carinii* is ubiquitous and exposure occurs in childhood. However, clinical disease is limited to severely immunodeficient persons and is particularly frequent in those with acquired immune deficiency syndrome (AIDS).

Usual symptoms are cough, fever, and dyspnea, the onset ranging from insidious to fulminant. Chest x-ray and arterial oxygen may be normal initially, and fever may be minimal. However, pulmonary diffusing capacity, arterial-alveolar oxygen gradient, and gallium scan are generally abnormal.

MANAGEMENT

All patients should be hospitalized until the disease is well controlled. Prompt invasive diagnostic procedures should be done. Oral therapy is possible with all of the drugs except pentamidine. Thus follow-up outpatient therapy is possible, provided that (1) oxygenation is adequate, (2) the patient is able to tolerate and adequately absorb oral drugs (AIDS patients often have malabsorption), (3) clinical status can be closely followed, (4) lab tests can be closely monitored for drug toxicity.

DRUG THERAPY

Four initial treatment regimens are available: sulfamethoxazole-trimethoprim (Bactrim, Septra), pentamidine (Pentam 300), the combination of dapsone plus trimethoprim, and an experimental drug, difluoromethylornithine (DFMO). Sulfamethoxazole-trimethoprim (SXT) and pentamidine are equally effective, and preliminary data suggest that dapsone plus trimethoprim is as effective also. Comparable efficacy data are not available for DFMO. SXT is less toxic than pentamidine, except in AIDS patients, 60% of whom get toxicity with either drug. DFMO and perhaps dapsone plus trimethoprim seem to be less toxic. I prefer to start with SXT since it is always available, and I use the other drugs as alternates. Experimental animal data suggest that it is not beneficial to combine SXT and pentamidine. (However, see *Management of Complications.*)

Full-dose treatment is for a minimum of two weeks in non-AIDS patients and three weeks in AIDS cases. Patients are then switched to long-term suppressive/prophylactic therapy for the duration of life in AIDS patients or duration of immune suppression in others. Four oral prophylactic regimens have been used. Pentamidine is not effective for prophylaxis of PCP in the rat model, and I am not aware of its use in man for prophylaxis. Instead, the combination drug Fansidar, which was developed for resistant falciparum malaria, has been successfully used for PCP prophylaxis.

Initial treatment doses are SXT, 20 mg/kg/d of trimethoprim component IV or PO divided into every-six-hour doses. (Note: this is *four* times the dose for urinary tract infection.) Pentamidine is administered 4 mg/kg/d as a single daily one-hour infusion (IV is better tolerated than IM). Dapsone is administered orally 50 mg b.i.d. plus trimethoprim, 20 mg/kg/d divided into four six-hour doses. For compassionate protocol for DFMO, call Merrell Dow in Cincinnati, Ohio (telephone 513-948-7868) for use and latest dosage recommendations. Long-term suppressive/prophylactic oral doses of SXT are 5 mg/kg/d divided into two doses. Dapsone is given 25 mg PO b.i.d. Fansidar (sulfadoxine 500 mg plus pyrimethamine 25 mg) is one tablet PO weekly. Leukovorin factor (folinic acid) can be used with the sulfa drugs in a dose of 10 to 25 mg/d PO, 9 mg/d IV or IM, to decrease potential bone marrow toxicity.

In pregnancy the choice is difficult: I prefer the use of SXT with leukovorin factor, except at term, when pentamidine may be preferable.

Major Adverse Effects. SXT frequently (especially in AIDS patients) results in blood dyscrasias, elevated liver enzymes, rash, nausea, vomiting, and drug fever and occasionally causes exfoliative dermatitis, Stevens-Johnson syndrome, or renal failure, especially in transplant patients. Pentamidine frequently results in elevated serum creatinine (24%), leukopenia (10%), elevated liver enzymes (9%), hypoglycemia (6%), hypotension (5%), thrombocytopenia (3%), GI disturbances, and sterile abscesses with or without pain if given IM. Side effects of dapsone plus trimethoprim and Fansidar are similar to those of SXT.

MANAGEMENT OF COMPLICATIONS

Drug failure is usually due to host factors, not drug resistance. Nevertheless, traditional therapy calls for switching to another agent if no response occurs in five to seven days. However, in AIDS patients the success rate of pentamidine or SXT when the other has failed is very low. It appears that in AIDS the critical treatment period is the first three to five days. If treatment is not successful, the patient generally experiences adult respiratory distress syndrome by that time. For this reason some clinicians have tried adding pentamidine to SXT at 72 hours if the patient has not started to improve on SXT alone. Pentamidine is then continued until improvement occurs. Preliminary data suggest that such short-term use of the combination of SXT and pentamidine is not harmful and might be helpful. Fluid overload is very common in AIDS patients. For this reason, if the patient appears to be going into respiratory failure, I give furosemide, 20 mg IV push, and repeat this dose once more if there is no response. If the patient does not wish to be put on a respirator, I have even tried corticosteroids for 24 hours with uncertain results. Symptoms of dyspnea can be greatly relieved, especially in terminal patients, with continuous morphine drip IV (usual initial dose 0.5 to 5 mg/h). One must remember that other concomitant infections are present in one third of AIDS patients, most frequently untreatable cytomegalovirus pneumonia.

Adverse drug effects are the rule. Before switching to another drug, I tolerate leukopenias to 1000/mm³; thrombocytopenia to 20,000/mm³; transaminase elevation to 150 IU or more; hypoglycemia to 25 mg/dl; hypotension to 60 mm Hg systolic; elevated levels of serum creatinine to 3 mg/dl (and even higher if pentamidine is the sole choice); rash, if not exfoliative, to patient tolerance; and vomiting, unless it significantly interferes with nutrition. If an AIDS patient is doing well otherwise on SXT but has problems with cytopenias or nausea and vomiting, I lower the dose to 75%, or even 50%, of the full dose in an attempt to achieve drug tolerance. Cross reactions between the sulfonamides SXT, dapsone, and Fansidar in AIDS patients appear low enough that it is justifiable in AIDS cases to try switching to another agent in this family if adverse reactions occur. It is not advisable to rechallenge patients with the same drug if life-threatening reactions have occurred.

PATIENT INFORMATION AND EDUCATION

Desires regarding ventilator or other extraordinary means should be discussed with patient and family at the beginning of treatment since respiratory failure can occur at any time.

PERIODIC EVALUATION

Outpatients on full-dose treatment are seen weekly; a chest x-ray is done weekly until clear or stable; and laboratory tests are done at least weekly. The patient should be seen one week after treatment, with further visits as necessary. Patients on full-dose therapy need a CBC and platelet estimate (count, if low), serum creatinine, and a transaminase at least every third day while inpatient and weekly afterward. In addition, those on pentamidine need serum creatinine and blood glucose at least three times per week and at least a weekly serum calcium and EKG. Patients on low-dose prophylactic/suppressive therapy should have blood count, transaminase, and creatinine monthly.

PREVENTIVE MEASURES

Immunosuppressive drugs should be reduced if possible. Immune-stimulating therapy so far has not been promising in AIDS. Patients with PCP should cover their mouths while coughing and not share a room with other immunosuppressed patients.

SOCIOECONOMIC ASPECTS OF MANAGEMENT

SXT and pentamidine are quite expensive. Leukovorin factor (folinic acid) is unbelievably expensive

(about \$1.00 per mg)! Dapsone plus trimethoprim is quite inexpensive; however, dapsone is not usually stocked in local pharmacies.

Giardiasis

DEFINITION, PATHOPHYSIOLOGY, AND CLINICAL ASPECTS

Giardiasis is an intestinal infection with the flagellate protozoan *Giardia lamblia*. Diagnosis is made by seeing *Giardia* organisms in a stool or small bowel sample.

Giardiasis is acquired by ingestion of the cyst through fecal-oral contamination of food or water or through sexual activity. Giardiasis should be suspected in any case of diarrhea that lasts over two weeks or is associated with any of the following seven factors: (1) foreign travel, (2) consumption of wilderness water, (3) custodial institutions or day care centers, (4) waterborne diarrhea outbreaks, (5) male homosexuality, (6) malabsorption, and (7) immune deficiency. *Giardia* can be difficult to eradicate in patients who have immune deficiencies or who are constantly being reinfected.

Giardia causes acute or chronic diarrhea in 20% to 50% of those infected and a further 5% to 15% remain chronic asymptomatic carriers. Because the incubation period is relatively long (at least one to two weeks), travelers often develop diarrhea after the trip is over. The diarrhea is usually chronic and intermittent, with a lot of malodorous gas. Malabsorption and lactose intolerance can occur, and failure to thrive is seen in children.

MANAGEMENT

DRUG THERAPY

There are three available drugs. Metronidazole (Flagyl) is the drug of choice owing to availability and tolerance. The other two drugs, quinacrine (Atabrine) and furazolidone (Furoxone), are seldom stocked in local pharmacies. Quinacrine may be slightly more effective in adults but is best avoided in children because of its side effects. Furazolidone is available as a suspension, but the volume required in children is quite large.

Metronidazole is taken 250 mg t.i.d. × 5d in adults or 5 mg/kg t.i.d. × 5d in children; quinacrine is in doses of 100 mg t.i.d. PO PC × 5d for adults; furazolidone is in doses of 100 mg q.i.d. × 7–10d in adults or 1.25 mg/kg q.i.d. × 7–10d in children.

Major Adverse Effects. Metronidazole frequently results in GI symptoms, disulfiram reaction with alcohol, and metallic taste; occasionally it causes stomatitis and rarely leukopenia, dizziness, ataxia, peripheral neuropathy with prolonged use, seizures, and red or brown urine. Metronidazole is mutagenic in vitro and carcinogenic in some animal models; short-term (ten-year) follow-up in man shows no evidence of carcinogenicity so far. Quinacrine frequently causes dizziness, headache, GI disturbance, and, occasionally, toxic psychosis, blood dyscrasias, and rashes. If treatment is absolutely necessary during pregnancy, I use metronidazole. Possible worsening of seizure disorder with metronidazole and of psychiatric disorders and psoriasis with quinacrine has been reported.

Quinacrine should not be used with the antimalarial primaquine or with alcohol, as it greatly increases their toxicity. Metronidazole potentiates the effects of warfarin.

Management of Complications. Postgiardial diarrhea is relatively frequent. The commonest causes are treatment failure (in 10% to 15%), reinfection, lactose intolerance, and psychogenic factors. One empiric retreatment course is reasonable, as is switching to quinacrine for one treatment course. When constant reinfection is occurring (three or more infections per year), it is best to treat only symptomatic cases. Such reinfection situations are common in day care centers, among some male homosexuals, and in areas with poor sanitation. In persons of limited means who clinically and epidemiologically are very likely to have giardiasis, one course of empiric therapy and one retreatment may be justified.

PERIODIC EVALUATION

If giardiasis is suspected and three stool exams are negative, a small bowel sample should be obtained. Three stools after treatment should be tested. The routine lab tests that are helpful are CBC and other tests for malabsorption if the case is chronic. Evaluation of immune function, particularly immunoglobulins, in refractory cases is important.

PREVENTIVE MEASURES

Improvement in sanitation and investigation of contacts (household, sexual, and food handlers) should be attempted. Travelers should be instructed in food and water precautions. Sexual precautions include the use of a condom and spermicidal jelly for vaginal or rectal sex, thorough washing before oral-genital sex, and avoidance of oral-anal sex. Persons should not share the same enema equipment. Chlorination or iodination of water may not kill all giardial cysts. Boiling water for one minute is effective.

Cryptosporidiosis

DEFINITION AND CLINICAL ASPECTS

Cryptosporidiosis is infection of the intestine with a newly recognized protozoan, *Cryptosporidium* sp. Diagnosis is made by finding the organism on stool parasite exam or in intestinal aspirates or biopsies. Exam for *Cryptosporidium* must be specially requested on stools because identification requires special techniques (e.g., modified acid-fast stain).

Cryptosporidium is a very common organism, perhaps even more common than *Giardia*. It is found in many animals and man, and transmission is fecal-oral, including anal-oral sexual contact. Several outbreaks in day care centers have occurred in the United States. Chronic cryptosporidiosis is an opportunistic infection. The diarrhea is generally similar to *Giardia* and malab-

sorption can occur. In normal hosts the diarrhea is self-limited, usually resolving within two weeks. In immunosuppressed patients, it is chronic and seldom cured. Cryptosporidial diarrhea of more than four weeks' duration may mean that the patient has AIDS if there is no other known cause of immune suppression. In AIDS patients, massive watery diarrhea of up to 17 liters per day has occurred.

MANAGEMENT

DRUG THERAPY

Treatment is attempted *only* in immunosuppressed patients and is *seldom* curative. The clinical response rate in AIDS is no more than 33%. The drugs currently being used are experimental: spiramycin (Rovamycin), a macrolide antibiotic that is on the market in Canada but not in the U.S., and difluoromethylornithine (DFMO). Spiramycin can be obtained in the U.S. from the FDA (telephone 301-443-4310), and DFMO can be obtained for compassionate use by calling Merrell Dow in Cincinnati, Ohio (telephone 513-948-7868). The dose for spiramycin is 0.5 to 1.0 gm PO t.i.d. × 7–14d or longer if chronic suppressive therapy is being attempted. Major adverse effects occurring with spiramycin are occasional GI disturbance (more frequent in AIDS patients) and rare allergic reaction. The preventive measures are the same as for giardiasis.

Trichinosis

DEFINITION, PATHOPHYSIOLOGY, AND CLINICAL ASPECTS

Trichinosis is muscle infection with the larval stage of a roundworm of carnivores, *Trichinella spiralis*. Diagnosis is presumptive based on clinical picture, serology, and eosinophilia. In some cases diagnosis may be confirmed by positive muscle biopsy.

The disease is acquired from consumption of undercooked carnivore meat. Pork is the commonest, but other carnivore meat may be the source, such as bear, rat, coyote, or dog. Larvae hatch in the intestine and end up encysted in voluntary muscle. Larvae also pass through other tissues, causing inflammatory reactions that are especially serious in myocardium or brain.

Initially abdominal symptoms and rash occur for one to two days after an incubation averaging nine days but ranging from two to 28 days. Then muscle pain occurs, often with edema of the eyelids and conjunctival and ungual hemorrhages. Fever is usual. Acute symptoms can last one to three weeks. Myocarditis and encephalitis can be fatal.

MANAGEMENT

Hospitalization is indicated for severe cases and any cardiac or CNS manifestations. Muscle biopsy may be indicated.

DRUG THERAPY

If the patient is suspected of having trichinosis at the abdominal symptom stage (this usually is only possible in cases that are part of an outbreak previously identified), PO thiabendazole or high-dose PO mebendazole is useful in killing larvae still in the intestine. In the later stages, the drug may kill adult worms in the intestine and keep them from producing more larvae, but drugs have no effect on larvae in muscle. The benefits of drug therapy have not been proved; it is therefore optional.

Drug doses recommended are thiabendazole (Mintezol): 25 mg/kg b.i.d. × 5d (maximum 3 gm/d); and mebendazole (Vermox): 200–400 mg t.i.d. × 3d, then 400–500 mg t.i.d. × 10d.

Corticosteroids are indicated for severe angioedema or urticaria and for myocardial and CNS inflammation.

Adverse Effects. Frequent side effects of thiabendazole are nausea, vomiting, anorexia, diarrhea, and dizziness. For adverse effects of mebendazole see under Echinococcosis, below.

Periodic Evaluation. Periodic checks include routine laboratory tests such as CBC and eosinophil count, creatinine and serologic tests. Serologic tests are positive in 85%, but not until three to four weeks after ingestion of meat; usually the test is not done locally. CBC, transaminase, and creatinine tests should be repeated weekly during drug therapy and one week after treatment.

Preventive Measures. Thorough cooking of carnivore meat, including wild game such as bear, prevents *Trichinella* infection. In the case of pork, cooking to an internal temperature of 66°C (150°F) provides a margin of safety. Freezing at −15°F for three weeks is also effective, but many home freezers do not reach this temperature. Garbage fed to hogs should be boiled for 30 minutes. Commercial pork in the U.S. is starting to be treated by gamma irradiation and should be *Trichinella*-free by 1987.

Echinococcosis

DEFINITION AND DIAGNOSTIC CRITERIA

Echinococcosis is infection of man with the larvae of an intestinal tapeworm of dogs and other canids (foxes, wolves, etc.). The result is potentially fatal larval cysts of internal organs, particularly the liver. Echinococcosis is only definitively diagnosable from surgical specimens. However, clinical suspicion may be high enough to treat when characteristic radiologic appearance, positive serology, and compatible epidemiologic history are obtained.

PATHOPHYSIOLOGY

When the eggs of *Echinococcus* found in dog or other canid feces are ingested, the larval stage can develop in man. Two species of *Echinococcus* infect man. *E. granulosus* causes one or more large cysts (*cystic hydatid disease*), and its normal intermediate (larval stage) host is an ungulate such as sheep, pig, reindeer, and camel. *E. multilocularis* causes a cancer-like lesion in the liver (*alveolar hydatid disease*) and its normal intermediate host is voles or mice. In the U.S. *E. granulosus* is endemic only in a few western states in sheepherders and in the northern woods of Canada and Alaska. Most cases of *E. granulosus* seen in the U.S. are in immigrants from the Mediterranean region, especially Italy, Greece, Yugoslavia, and the Middle East. *E. multilocularis* is seen in the extreme northern U.S., Canada, Alaska, Eastern Europe, and the U.S.S.R.

CLINICAL ASPECTS

The cysts of *E. granulosus* are most frequent in liver (65%) or lung (25%) and occasionally elsewhere, such as in bone or brain tissue. The cysts come to attention either because of their mass effect or incidental discovery on radiograph. The cysts grow 3 to 5 cm in the first year and very slowly, at 1 cm or less per year, after that. Cysts rupture, either spontaneously or at surgery, and can cause anaphylactic shock and disseminated infection, or cysts can become secondarily infected. The invasive mass of *E. multilocularis* can destroy the liver.

MANAGEMENT

One has to decide whether to attempt to cure or control the infection via surgery or drug therapy or simply to observe the patient. Both surgical and medical treatment are extremely expensive. Surgical resection usually is only possible with *E. granulosus*, not *E. multilocularis*. Surgical removal is treatment of choice for *E. granulosus*. Hypertonic saline (20%) is injected into the cysts during surgery to kill organisms prior to removal.

DRUG THERAPY

For *E. multilocularis* and unresectable *E. granulosus*, drug therapy has occasionally produced some benefits. This therapy is experimental and very expensive. One of two drugs can be used: mebendazole (Vermox) in very high doses of 12–14 gm/d PO or albendazole (Zentel, Smith Kline & French), which is experimental in the U.S., administered 800 mg/d in two divided doses. Treatment has been given for three to six months. For compassionate protocol for albendazole, call Smith Kline & French in Philadelphia (telephone 215-751-5231).

Adverse Effects. Although adverse effects are rare with low doses of mebendazole, as used to treat intestinal roundworms, they are common with high-dose regimens for echinococcosis. Problems include allergic reactions, alopecia, glomerulonephritis, leukopenia, drug fever, and elevated levels of liver enzymes. In the case of *E. multilocularis*, treatment must be continued for life. The mebendazole regimen is experimental and patient consent should be obtained. The drug is best given after meals and should be chewed well. Patients with preexisting liver disease are more likely to experience problems.

Anaphylactic shock is treated in the usual way. Secondarily infected cysts are treated with antibiotics.

Periodic evaluation should include monitoring cysts by liver echo or chest x-ray at three- to six-month intervals. Routine laboratory tests include serology, especially in cases where surgery is not done, and laboratory tests to monitor for drug toxicity. Preventive measures include washing hands before meals, deworming of dogs, and preventing dogs from eating infected carcasses.

REFERENCES

Drugs for parasitic infections: Med Letter Drugs Ther 26:27–34, 1984.

16 · MALARIA AND BABESIOSIS

Victor E. Jimenez-Lucho
Julio V. Cardenas
HENRY FORD HOSPITAL

Malaria

DEFINITION AND DIAGNOSTIC CRITERIA

Malaria is a febrile illness caused by four different species of the intracellular protozoa Plasmodium: *P. vivax, P. malariae, P. ovale*, and *P. falciparum*. It is widely distributed throughout the world and has a tremendous impact on the economy of infested areas. The last case of malaria acquired within the continental United States was reported in 1974, but the potential for transmission exists as long as the *Anopheles* mosquito populates the southern regions of the country.

Malaria should be considered in the differential diagnosis of any febrile illness in patients who have a history of travel to areas of the world where the disease is endemic.

PATHOPHYSIOLOGY

Man acquires the disease through the bite of an infected *Anopheles* mosquito, which is widely prevalent in tropical and subtropical areas of the world. Two stages develop after the inoculation of the parasites into the bloodstream. The first is an asymptomatic pre-erythrocytic stage with multiplication of the parasites within the liver parenchyma. This is followed by a symptomatic erythrocytic stage with alternating cycles of invasion and subsequent multiplication within the red blood cells, causing the classical periodic febrile attacks. A silent but persistent liver stage is responsible for the relapses commonly seen with *P. vivax* and *P. ovale* infection.

Man also may acquire the disease by transfusion of blood products from an infected donor.

CLINICAL MANIFESTATIONS

The incubation period is usually 10 to 20 days but in infections with *P. malariae* it may be longer. It is not unusual to see patients infected with *P. vivax* in whom onset of symptoms is more than six months after entering a nonendemic area such as the U.S. An important factor that contributes to these differences and that also produces some changes in the clinical picture is a semi-immune state often present in natives of endemic areas who have been exposed to repeated infections, and individuals who have been taking inadequate chemoprophylaxis with only partial parasite suppression.

The initial symptoms usually resemble an influenza-like illness with fever, chills, headache, myalgia, nausea, vomiting, and diarrhea. The classic malaria paroxysm is highly suggestive of this diagnosis. Within an hour or two the patient feels increasingly cold and shivery, and develops rigors. This is followed by the febrile phase with temperatures rising to 40°C or more for three or four hours, when the patient may develop vomiting, hypotension, and delirium. The defervescence that follows is associated with profuse sweating and exhaustion. Characteristically, the patient feels remarkably well between these paroxysms. The periodicity of the febrile attacks, every 72 hours for *P. malariae* (quartan malaria) and every 48 hours for the other three species (tertian malaria), may not be initially present or may never develop. This is especially true for infections with *P. falciparum* that commonly have daily febrile peaks.

The physical examination may be quite unremarkable during the periods between paroxysms, but after the second week of illness the spleen is usually palpable. The liver may be tender.

Basic laboratory studies are usually nonspecific and include a moderate leukopenia, mild to moderate anemia, and mild elevation of liver enzymes.

Life-threatening complications are more commonly seen in the patient heavily infested with *P. falciparum* malaria. Extensive intravascular hemolysis may lead to massive hemoglobinemia and hemoglobinuria (blackwater fever) with development of acute renal failure. Cerebral malaria is a fearful syndrome that includes seizures, meningism, and changes in mental status, apparently due to the lodging of parasitized erythrocytes within the cerebral blood vessels. Pulmonary edema, shock, and disseminated intravascular coagulation (DIC) may also occur. Less acute complications include immune complex–mediated glomerulonephritis, frequently seen in children with chronic *P. malariae* infection and the tropical splenomegaly syndrome.

Diagnosis must be made by identification of the parasite in a blood smear. It is easier to examine a thin smear stained with Leishman or Giemsa, but the thick smears have the advantage of concentrating more parasites. Thick smears, however, require considerably more expertise to read. Determining the species has both therapeutic and prognostic significance. The most important consideration is to decide whether the infection could be related to *P. falciparum* because of the high risk of lethal complications and drug resistance. The intraerythrocytic forms, which are more likely to be found in this case, are ring forms, usually small (1.2 µm) with a thin delicate cytoplasm, often in multiple numbers within each erythrocyte. Unfortunately, the characteristic large, banana-shaped gametocyte is seldom seen. In heavy, frequently fatal parasitemias, as many as 30% of the red blood cells may be parasitized. For more subtle distinctions of the parasite, several thin and thick blood smears should be obtained at different times and promptly submitted to a reference laboratory.

MANAGEMENT

If *P. falciparum* infection cannot be ruled out on the basis of blood smears or epidemiologic data, the patient should be hospitalized for further management; complications and rapid deterioration are possible even if the patient looks quite stable on the initial visit. If *P. falciparum* is excluded, the person may be managed in the outpatient setting.

In the acutely ill patient, it is critical to maintain adequate hydration and at the same time avoid fluid overload that could complicate pulmonary edema and renal failure. It is also essential to monitor the patient for CNS involvement and the development of DIC. It is not uncommon to have associated malnutrition in patients coming from underdeveloped areas of the world, and attention should be paid to this factor for ultimate recovery from the disease.

Chloroquine-Sensitive Malaria. Chloroquine is the drug of choice to treat malaria in areas where drug resistance has not been reported (Table 1). Chloroquine phosphate (Aralen) is given orally with a loading dose of 600 mg base (1 gm) followed in six hours by 300 mg base and then 300 mg base daily for two days. Total dose will be 1500 mg base. A rapid response is usual within 48 to 72 hours. Failure to respond may indicate resistance. In cases where oral treatment is not possible, chloroquine hydrochloride is available for intramuscular use, 200 mg base every 6 hours for a maximum of three days. Side effects with oral chloroquine are relatively unusual. Gastrointestinal discomfort can be prevented by taking the drug after meals. Occasionally, pruritus occurs and disappears after completion of treatment. Chloroquine retinopathy has been reported only with long-term use. Parenteral chloroquine, on the other hand, must be administered with caution, preferably in a hospitalized patient, owing to the risk of cardiovascular toxicity. It is not recommended for children.

Table 1. COUNTRIES WHERE CHLOROQUINE-RESISTANT *P. FALCIPARUM* HAS BEEN REPORTED

Angola	Malawi
Bangladesh	Malaysia
Bolivia	Mozambique
Brazil*	Namibia
Burma	Pakistan
Burundi	Panama*
Central African Republic	Papua New Guinea*
China, People's Republic	Peru
Colombia	Philippines
Comoros	Rwandapines
Democratic Kampuchea	Solomon Islands
(Cambodia)	Sudan
Ecuador	Surinam
French Guiana	Tanzania
Gabon	Thailand*
Guyana	Uganda
India	Vanuatua
Indonesia	Venezuela
Kampuchea	Vietnam*
Kenya	Zaire
Lao People's Democratic	Zambia
Republic	
Madagascar	

*Areas with reported Fansidar-resistant *P. falciparum* (as of February, 1985).

The relapsing forms of malaria, *P. vivax* and *P. ovale*, require additional treatment with primaquine to eradicate the persisting forms in the liver. Primaquine phosphate is given PO, 15 mg base daily for 14 days. Before primaquine is started, patients should be screened for G6PD deficiency, which would indicate that they are at risk for hemolysis. This drug is also contraindicated in pregnant women. If necessary, weekly doses of chloroquine will prevent relapses until delivery, after which primaquine can be given safely.

Chloroquine-Resistant* P. falciparum *Malaria. The therapy of choice for this form includes a combination of quinine, pyrimethamine, and a sulfonamide. In patients who have more than 5% of the red blood cells parasitized or who are suffering from one of the complications, quinine dihydrochloride should be given IV, 10 mg/kg diluted in 300 to 500 ml of saline administered slowly over at least four hours. This dose can be repeated in six to eight hours and again eight hours later. The total dose for the first 24 hours should not exceed 1950 mg. Close cardiovascular monitoring is required because of the potential cardiotoxicity. Besides cardiac toxicity, quinine may cause cinchonism characterized by tinnitus, headaches, nausea, and blurred vision. For the more stable patient, quinine sulfate, 650 mg PO t.i.d., can be given for seven to ten days.

Additionally, the patient should receive a combination of pyrimethamine, 25 mg. b.i.d. for three days and sulfadiazine, 500 mg q.i.d. for five days. A common alternative in the stable patient is the fixed combination of 25 mg of pyrimethamine and 500 mg of sulfadoxine (Fansidar) given as a single dose of three tablets. More recently the U.S. Army has reported the successful use of mefloquine to treat chloroquine-resistant *P. falciparum*. This was associated with mild and self-limited side effects. At present this drug is not commercially available. The fixed combinations of trimethoprim-sulfamethoxazole (Bactrim, Septra) have also been successfully used as alternatives to Fansidar when this is not readily available.

In the last few years, an increased number of cases have been reported from southeast Asia and the Amazon basin in South America, where Fansidar-resistant strains have been found. In these areas the treatment of choice includes a combination of quinine sulfate in the doses recommended above, plus tetracycline, 250 mg q.i.d. for seven to ten days.

All patients should be monitored with daily blood smears. There should be a decrease in the number of parasitized red blood cells, and by the fifth day after treatment no asexual forms of the parasite should be seen. Their presence suggests treatment has failed.

PREVENTION

All travelers to endemic regions should be warned about the possibility of contracting this infection and should be advised to use mosquito nets and insect repellents, especially between dusk and dawn when the likelihood of mosquitoes' biting is greater. More important, patients should be advised about chemoprophylaxis. Because of the changing pattern of drug resistance throughout the world, physicians should check the information published by the Centers for Disease Control: *Health Information for International Travel*, published annually, and periodic updates of the *Morbidity and Mortality Weekly Report*.

For travelers to areas without chloroquine resistance, the drug of choice is still chloroquine phosphate, 300 mg base once a week, starting two weeks before entering and continuing for six weeks after departure from the endemic area.

Travelers to areas with known chloroquine-resistant falciparum malariae should still use chloroquine in the same schedule as above, since chloroquine-resistant malaria can occasionally coexist with chloroquine-sensitive malaria. Until recently, weekly doses of Fansidar were also advised, but owing to the relatively high risk (1 in 18,000) of serious cutaneous reactions such as erythema multiforme, this is no longer indicated. Instead, it is advised that short-term travelers (for three weeks or less) to these areas be given three tablets of Fansidar to be taken as a single-dose treatment only in the event of a febrile illness during their travel when professional medical care is not readily available. The addition of Fansidar, one tablet weekly, is now restricted only to those long-term travelers who will have nighttime exposure in rural endemic areas in Africa, China, Southeast Asia, South America, and Oceania (Table 1). The traveler should be advised to discontinue the drug immediately if any mucocutaneous lesions appear.

Travelers should be warned that, even with adequate chemoprophylaxis, they can acquire malaria, and symptoms may appear months after they leave an endemic area. There is no adequate prophylaxis for Fansidar-resistant *P. falciparum* malaria.

Babesiosis

DEFINITION AND DIAGNOSTIC CRITERIA

Babesiosis is a less common protozoan disease caused by the intraerythrocytic organism called *Babesia*. This disease was well described in animals and only in 1957 was reported to cause human infection. Two species have been found to cause infections in humans, *B. microti* in North America and *B. divergens* in Europe. In the United States the disease is endemic along the northeastern coast, predominantly on Nantucket Island and Martha's Vineyard Island in Massachusetts, and on Long Island and Shelter Island in New York. Recently, a new focus in Wisconsin was reported. These areas are also endemic for Lyme disease as both pathogens have the same tick vector and animal reservoirs. The main vector is the northern deer tick, *Ixodes dammini*, and animal reservoirs are small mammals such as deer mice and meadow voles. Man is only an accidental host. Very occasionally the infection can be transmitted by blood transfusion.

The easiest and most practical means of diagnosis is examining a thin blood smear for the presence of intraerythrocytic inclusions that resemble the small ring shape of *P. falciparum* trophozoites. The erythrocyte parasitized by *Babesia* lacks the brownish pigment hemozoin, seen with older stages of *P. falciparum*. The rather unusual finding of intraerythrocytic dividing parasites consisting of two to four daughter cells held together by a thin strand of cytoplasm (tetrads or maltese cross forms) is regarded as highly characteristic of *Babesia*. The diagnosis can be confirmed by animal inoculation or by serologic testing through the CDC.

PATHOPHYSIOLOGY

The tick *Ixodes dammini* feeds during its larval and nymphal stage on the rodent population, and man becomes accidentally infected through the bite of the parasitized nymph. The tick may serve as both vector and reservoir, as it can pass the parasite to its next generation transovarially. After entering the bloodstream, the organism invades the red blood cells, where it further divides by budding. Thereafter, the erythrocyte ruptures and the new organisms invade other red blood cells, causing in some cases severe hemolytic anemia that can lead to acute renal failure. There is no exoerythrocytic or visceral stage as in malaria. A prolonged parasitemia for weeks to months may follow.

The spleen serves a very important role in resistance against this infection, since patients who are splenectomized have a more severe disease with a high mortality. The same is true for immunosuppressed patients and the elderly.

CLINICAL ASPECTS

As with other tick-related infections, there is increased incidence during the warmer months from May to September.

Most infections with *B. microti* are asymptomatic, and the disease in immunocompetent individuals is usually mild and self-limited. On the other hand, *B. divergens* has been reported to cause infections only in splenectomized persons with a high mortality rate.

In patients who develop symptoms the incubation period is usually one to two weeks but may take as long as nine weeks. The illness resembles a mild form of malaria with general malaise, fever, shaking, chills, diaphoresis, headaches, and myalgia. Unlike malaria, there is no periodicity and the characteristic febrile attack is not present. The physical examination is usually unrevealing but may show mild hepatosplenomegaly. The bite site is usually unrecognized.

A hallmark of the disease is hemolytic anemia of varying degree. The WBC count varies from low to elevated with an increase in the lymphocytes due to a larger number of B cells. There is a mild thrombocytopenia and in the most severe cases DIC. Mild elevation of liver enzymes and bilirubin may occur in half of the patients. Nonspecific polyclonal hypergammaglobulinemia as well as decreased complement levels during the acute phase have been described.

Regardless of the treatment, the recovery is often slow and symptoms such as fatigue and malaise may persist for several months. Parasitemia may also last for several weeks to months. Recovery is the rule for persons who are immunocompetent and have intact spleens.

Both splenectomized and immunosuppressed patients are at a higher risk of a more severe and protracted illness. Along with a hemolytic syndrome, marked liver dysfunction, hemoglobinuria, renal failure, and shock may occur. In one study the mortality rate in asplenic patients was 27%.

MANAGEMENT

Essential for the diagnosis is a high index of suspicion in any patient presenting with fever and constitutional symptoms who has come from a tick-infested area. The differential diagnosis should include other tick-borne diseases such as Lyme disease, Rocky Mountain spotted fever, and tularemia. The absence of rash or local inflammatory manifestations in babesiosis should help in making the distinction. Several thin blood smears with Giemsa or Wright stain should be done. It is also important to quantify the degree of parasitemia, as it usually involves 1% to 5% of the red blood cells but in splenectomized patients could involve more than 80% of them.

Once the diagnosis is made, most patients require only use of analgesics and antipyretics for symptomatic relief. Hospitalization is necessary for the high-risk group: splenectomized, immunosuppressed, or elderly patients. For patients with moderately severe hemolysis, close monitoring of blood count and renal and hepatic function are mandatory, and blood transfusions may be necessary.

There is no ideal drug therapy yet. Antimalarial drugs such as chloroquine, sulfadiazine, and pyrimethamine have little therapeutic effect. Antitrypanosomal drugs such as pentamidine or diminazene (Berenil) have improved some of the clinical manifestations but have failed to eradicate the parasite. Tetracycline and trimethoprim-sulfamethoxazole have been tested in clinical trials but proved unsuccessful. Quinine may be more effective. Recent clinical and experimental data show promising results with a combination of quinine, 650 mg and clindamycin, 600 mg t.i.d. for seven days.

Exchange transfusions have had some success as a heroic measure to decrease severe parasitemia in splenectomized patients.

PREVENTION

In general, persons entering an enzootic area, particularly during the summer, should try to avoid contact with the vector. In this regard the use of insect repellent containing diethyl toluamide may be helpful. The likelihood of infection seems to increase with the length of time that the vector feeds on the person. Because of the much higher risk of complications and death, splenectomized and immunosuppressed individuals should carefully reconsider their decision to enter these areas.

REFERENCES

CDC: Prevention of malaria in travelers. MMWR 31:1S–28S, 1982.
CDC: Health information for international travel. U.S. Public Health Service, Department of Health and Human Services. CDC Publication no. 84-8280:11–58, 1984.
CDC: Revised recommendations for preventing malaria in travelers to areas with chloroquine-resistant *Plasmodium falciparum*. MMWR 34:185–195, 1985.
Rosner F, Hosein Zarrabi M, Benach JL, et al: Babesiosis in splenectomized adults. Review of 22 reported cases. Am J Med 76:696, 1984.
Royal Society of Tropical Medicine and Hygiene: Symposium on human babesiosis. Trans R Soc Trop Med Hyg 74:143–158, 1980.
Stekettee RW, Eckman MR, Burgess EC, et al: Babesiosis in Wisconsin. JAMA 253:2675–2678, 1985.
WHO: Vaccination certificate requirements for international travel and health advice to travelers. World Health Organization, Geneva, 1983.
Wittner M, Rowin KS, Tanowitz HB, et al: Successful chemotherapy of transfusion babesiosis. Ann Intern Med 96:601–604, 1982.

17 · CHLAMYDIA

Robert E. Smith
Gerald Gordon
GEISINGER MEDICAL CENTER

Chlamydia psittaci and *C. trachomatis* are the two species of the genus *Chlamydia*. *C. psittaci* is an animal pathogen infecting avian and mammalian species. Human infection may be a zoonosis causing pneumonia and systemic illness. *C. trachomatis* is a human pathogen usually causing sexually transmitted diseases, inclusion conjunctivitis, and trachoma.

PATHOPHYSIOLOGY

Chlamydiae are incomplete bacteria and are dependent on animal cells for their energy source. They have a discrete cell wall and contain both RNA and DNA. Unlike bacteria, chlamydiae have a developmental cycle characterized by two morphologically distinct forms: the *elementary body* and the *initial body*. The elementary body is the infective chlamydial particle. It attaches to a susceptible host cell, enters the cell, and becomes the metabolically active initial body. Replication continues for 18 to 24 hours, at which time initial bodies condense into elementary bodies. Lysis of the host cell may occur, and newly formed elementary bodies may infect other nearby cells or another host. Laboratory diagnosis of chlamydial infections is outlined in Table 1.

Psittacosis (Ornithosis)

INTRODUCTION AND EPIDEMIOLOGY

C. psittaci typically causes pneumonia in humans by inhalation of infected aerosols from bird droppings, respiratory secretions, or infected avian tissues. Mammal-to-human and human-to-human transmission have occasionally occurred, though most human cases occur after exposure to infected birds of the psittacine species (parrots, parakeets, macaws, cockatiels, love birds, and cockatoos). Most infections have occurred in bird fanciers, pet store owners, bird importers, poultry processing plant workers, and others with frequent exposure to birds.

CLINICAL ASPECTS

The incubation period of psittacosis is seven to 14 days. Hematogenous spread occurs from the lungs to the liver, spleen, and hilar lymph nodes and less commonly to the brain, kidneys, endocardium, and myocardium. Clinical manifestations range from asymptomatic illness (25%) to a fulminant "toxic" illness resulting in death. Most symptomatic cases are characterized by an influenza-like illness with cough, fever, chills, and headache. Myalgias, arthralgias, weakness, weight loss, and anorexia are less commonly present. A dry cough is characteristic, but respiratory symptoms are usually less impressive than radiographic findings would suggest.

Patients' fever ranges from 38° to 41°C. An inappropriately slow pulse in relation to fever has been noted in as many as one third of cases. Pulmonary examination reveals localized end-inspiratory rales. Pleural friction rubs or signs of consolidation are rarely noted. Hepatosplenomegaly, rash (Horder's spots or erythema nodosum), and mental status changes are occasionally seen.

Chest x-ray demonstrates an infiltrate in 75% of cases and typically is a patchy unilateral perihilar or lower lobe infiltrate. Bilateral infiltrates, diffuse infiltrates, or lobar consolidation may occur. Pleural effusions and hilar adenopathy are uncommon.

Sputum is typically scant. Microscopic examination may reveal few polymorphonuclear leukocytes. Routine stains for bacteria, fungi, or other microorganisms including *Chlamydia* are negative. The white blood cell count and differential counts are usually normal, though leukocytosis and leukopenia may occur. Serum glutamate-oxalate transferase (SGOT), alkaline phosphatase, bilirubin, and creatine kinase (CPK) may be mildly elevated. Increased erythrocyte sedimentation rate (ESR), anemia, and mild proteinuria are nonspecific findings. Electrocardiography may demonstrate Q-T interval prolongation and ST-T wave changes.

Psittacosis is a rare cause of "culture-negative" endocarditis. Acute renal tubular necrosis, glomerulonephritis, pancreatitis, and diffuse intravascular coagulation may be seen in patients with severe psittacosis. A history of exposure to birds, an adequate sputum examination that shows no pathogens, and the presence of flu-like symptoms should strengthen the suspicion of psittacosis. Sick or dead birds should be examined by a qualified veterinarian, when zoonoses such as psittacosis are considered.

MANAGEMENT

Tetracycline, 250 mg PO every six hours, should be initiated when psittacosis is clinically suspected, since confirmation of this diagnosis is retrospective. Most patients become afebrile, with improvement in constitutional symptoms within 48 to 72 hours of initiating treatment. Slower rates of improvement are common and do not indicate treatment failure. Treatment should be continued for 21 days, otherwise relapse may occur. Erythromycin, 250 mg PO four times daily, has been used as an alternate therapy. One may give parenteral tetracycline HCl (500 mg IV every six hours) in critically ill patients. Side effects of treatment include those typical of tetracycline or erythromycin. Because of permanent discoloration of developing teeth, tetracycline is not recommended during pregnancy or in children under 8 years of age.

Supportive treatment is the same as for other pneumonias. Need for hospitalization is dictated by the severity of the illness. Most cases can be effectively treated on an outpatient basis. Follow-up visits are important as treatment failures may occur and require additional therapy. Less than 1% mortality occurs in properly treated patients. Long-term immunity to psittacosis does not develop after infection with *C. psittaci*, and reinfection may occur.

PREVENTION

Prevention of human psittacosis is directed toward eradication of *C. psittaci* in psittacine birds and avoidance of illegally imported psittacines. In the United States, all imported birds are required to undergo a 30-day quarantine in a USDA-supervised facility and receive a 30-day course of chlorotetracycline. Because human-to-human transmission can occur, patients with psittacosis who are hospitalized should be placed in respiratory isolation. Suspected or confirmed cases of psittacosis should be reported to the State Department of Health.

Genital Infections

INTRODUCTION AND EPIDEMIOLOGY

Genital infections with *C. trachomatis* may be the most prevalent form of sexually transmitted disease in the U.S. Clinical presentation depends on the patient's age, sex, sexual preference, and sexual practices.

C. trachomatis causes approximately 40% of nongonococcal urethritis in heterosexual males and may frequently be found as a copathogen with *Neisseria gonorrhoeae*. *C. trachomatis* has been implicated as a common cause of epididymitis in males under age 35 and is a possible etiology of Reiter's syndrome (oculogenital syndrome). Pharyngitis and/or proctitis due to *C. trachomatis* may also occur, depending on individual sexual practices.

C. trachomatis genital infections in females may be asymptomatic or cause low-grade salpingitis and be associated with infertility. Chlamydial urethritis in females is probably less common than in males and may account for some cases of the "dysuria–sterile pyuria" syndrome in young, sexually active women. Chlamydiae have been implicated in perihepatitis (Fitz-Hugh–Curtis syndrome). Neonates born vaginally to mothers infected with *C. trachomatis* may develop inclusion conjunctivitis and chlamydial pneumonia.

C. trachomatis causes nonepidemic adult inclusion conjunctivitis and is nearly always associated with genital tract infection in at least one sexual partner. It occasionally causes spontaneous bacterial peritonitis, meningoencephalitis, pneumonia with or without mediastinal lymphadenopathy in immunocompromised adults, and post–cesarean section sepsis.

PATHOGENESIS

Chlamydial genital and related infections are caused by the *C. trachomatis* serotypes D to K. Direct inoculation of a mucosal surface by infected genital secretions initiates infection by *C. trachomatis*.

CLINICAL ASPECTS

In males symptomatic chlamydial urethritis usually presents seven to 20 days after exposure as urethral pain with or without dysuria. A urethral discharge typically is present but may be minimal or grossly purulent. Inguinal adenopathy may be seen. Clinical characteristics alone cannot differentiate *C. trachomatis* urethritis from *Neisseria gonorrhoeae* urethritis. Microscopic examination of urethral discharge typically shows polymorphonuclear leukocytes but not bacteria.

Epididymitis due to *C. trachomatis* presents as an acute, intensely painful unilateral swelling in the scrotum, often associated with fever. Concomitant urethritis may be seen but often is absent.

Chlamydial proctitis in homosexual males and in women practicing anal intercourse may present with anorectal pain, hematochezia, anal discharge, and tenesmus. Proctoscopy reveals a nonspecific proctitis with mucosal erythema, friability, and edema. Smears of rectal secretions show leukocytes but no predominant bacterial types. Chlamydiae are not seen. Biopsy often demonstrates a mild, acute inflammatory infiltrate of the lamina propria. Asymptomatic anorectal infection occurs.

Many chlamydial infections in women are minimally symptomatic. Female sexual contacts of men with *C. trachomatis* urethritis may have cervical edema, erythema, friability, and mucopurulent discharge due to asymptomatic infection. Women with chlamydial urethritis (the pyuria-dysuria syndrome) may present with dysuria and urinary frequency. Urine cultures generally are sterile or show few bacteria. *C. trachomatis* salpingitis is usually subacute with low-grade fever, lower abdominal pain, moderate tenderness with cervical motion, and purulent cervical discharge. Development of pleuritic right upper quadrant pain with findings of a hepatic friction rub suggests perihepatitis. Laparoscopy may reveal fibrous plaque formation and friability of Glisson's capsule; rarely are the classically reported "violinstring" adhesions observed.

Neonates born to mothers infected with *Chlamydia* are at risk of developing conjunctivitis and pneumonia. Neonatal inclusion conjunctivitis usually presents five to 14 days after birth with acute onset of bilateral or unilateral conjunctival erythema and purulent discharge. Lymphoid follicular hyperplasia is not seen. Conjunctivitis may be mild or severe and may mimic bacterial conjunctivitis. Untreated, most cases spontaneously resolve over several weeks. Micropannus formation and corneal scarring have occasionally occurred. Within six months approximately 20% of infants with chlamydial conjunctivitis may develop chlamydial pneumonia. Progressive tachypnea, staccato cough, and absence of fever and constitutional symptoms are typical. Nasal obstruction and rhinorrhea occur. Physical ex-

amination usually reveals diffuse inspiratory rales; wheezes are absent. Chest x-ray shows diffuse interstitial infiltrates. Spontaneous resolution may occur over several weeks. Long-term sequelae are rare. Chlamydial pneumonia can occur without antecedent or concomitant conjunctivitis.

Adult inclusion conjunctivitis (oculogenital syndrome) presents sporadically as an acute follicular conjunctivitis in sexually active adults. As is the case in neonatal conjunctivitis, spontaneous resolution over a period of several weeks is the rule, and long-term sequelae are rare.

Adult inclusion conjunctivitis presenting as a follicular conjunctivitis is especially characteristic when the upper tarsal plate is involved. Conjunctival scrapings should be obtained and cultured for *Chlamydia* and should be stained with Giemsa stain for intracellular inclusions. Evaluation for synchronous genital tract infections should be performed in both the patient and identified sexual contacts.

MANAGEMENT

All patients with chlamydial infection and their sexual contacts should be treated with effective therapies (see Table 2).

Relapses may occur in 10% to 15% of patients treated with one week of therapy. Patients who relapse because of drug failure and not reinfection should receive three weeks of therapy. Penicillin G is ineffective against *Chlamydia*.

PREVENTION

Prevention of chlamydial genital infections is similar to prevention of most sexually transmitted diseases. General preventive methods can be recommended, such as use of condoms and washing of the genital area after sexual activity.

It is difficult to identify all sexually active persons with chlamydial infection. Until sensitive methods for diagnosis become less costly and routinely available, a large reservoir of asymptomatic carriers will likely remain undiscovered.

Prevention of neonatal infections is possible by identifying and treating asymptomatic maternal infections prenatally with an effective regimen that would also be safe to the fetus (e.g., erythromycin). Both parents of neonates with inclusion conjunctivitis or chlamydial pneumonia should be identified as infected with *C. trachomatis* and treated with tetracycline (or erythromycin if the neonate is breast fed).

Lymphogranuloma Venereum

INTRODUCTION AND EPIDEMIOLOGY

Lymphogranuloma venereum (LGV) is a distinct sexually transmitted disease caused by the L_1, L_2, and L_3 serotypes of *C. trachomatis*. LGV has a worldwide distribution but is more common in tropical regions.

Table 1. LABORATORY DIAGNOSIS OF CHLAMYDIAL INFECTIONS

Category	Test	Method Employed	Clinical Usefulness	Advantages	Disadvantages	Sensitivity
Delayed hypersensitivity	Frei antigen test	Intradermal injection of processed LGV antigen	LGV	Historical value	Prepared antigen not standardized Variable availability	Low
Serology	Complement fixation (CF)	Detects serum antibody to "group specific" antigen	LGV Psittacosis	Widely available Low cost	Does not differentiate between *C. trachomatis* and *C. psittaci*	High when used to diagnose LGV and psittacosis
	Micro-immunofluorescent antibody test (MIF)	Detects specific antibodies to *C. trachomatis* serotypes	Acute chlamydial urethritis Neonatal pneumonia Epidemiologic studies	Low cost High sensitivity (higher than CF)	High background titers in general population	High (80%) sensitivity in male urethritis
	ELISA antibody test	Detects anti–*C. trachomatis* antibodies utilizing an LGV antigen	Currently being investigated	Necessary equipment already available in most labs	Currently being investigated	Appears to have comparable sensitivity to MIF test
Cytology	Pap smear	Giemsa staining of routine Pap smear for chlamydial inclusion bodies	Genital tract infection in females	Technique already widely in use	Requires retraining of cytotechnicians Increases cost	Low (40%) sensitivity for cervical infection
	Conjunctival scrapings	Giemsa staining of conjunctival epithelial cells for inclusion bodies	Trachoma Adult and neonatal inclusion conjunctivitis	Rapid diagnosis Low cost	None	95% sensitivity in neonatal conjunctivitis; 45% sensitivity in trachoma and adult conjunctivitis
Immunologic detection of chlamydial antigens	Direct immunofluorescent staining of genital tract scrapings (DIF)	Both tests detect chlamydial antigens in scraped cells	Rapid diagnosis Low cost Requires little equipment investment	Currently being investigated	Genital tract infection Trachoma Adult and neonatal inclusion conjunctivitis	Sensitivities: 95% neonatal conjunctivitis 85% adult conjunctivitis 60% male urethra 66% female cervix

Few cases are acquired in the U.S.; most are contracted in Southeast Asia, South America, or the Caribbean Islands.

CLINICAL ASPECTS

LGV is transmitted sexually and has an incubation period of a few days to nearly a month. Three stages are generally described. In the first stage the initial lesion is usually painless and may appear as single or multiple ulcers, papules, or vesicles. In males these lesions may be found on the glans penis; in females the vaginal wall and cervix are the most common sites. In homosexual males and in some females, the primary lesion may be found in the perianal area of the rectum. The fingers, tongue, or perioral area may also be infected. Rarely the initial infection presents as a urethritis in males, probably reflecting a hidden urethral lesion. A primary lesion cannot be demonstrated either by examination or by history in as many as 60% of confirmed cases of LGV.

Table 2. TREATMENT OF CHLAMYDIAL SYNDROMES

	First-Line Agent	Alternative Agent
Urethritis Cervicitis Oculogenital syndrome	Tetracycline, 500 mg PO q.i.d. for 7–21 days	Erythromycin, 500 mg PO q.i.d. for 7–21 days Sulfisoxazole, 500 mg PO q.i.d. for 10 days
Pharyngitis Epididymitis Proctitis	Tetracycline, 500 mg PO q.i.d. for 7–21 days Therapy for this group of diseases is less clearly defined	Erythromycin, 500 mg PO q.i.d. for 7–21 days
Neonatal conjunctivitis	Oral erythromycin, 10 mg/kg q.i.d. for 14 days or in children older than 4 wk—sulfisoxazole 100 mg/kg/d oral or IV in four divided doses	
Lymphogranuloma venereum	Tetracycline, 250 mg PO q.i.d. for 21 days or more	Sulfisoxazole, 500 mg PO q.i.d. for 21 days or more
Psittacosis	Tetracycline, 250 mg PO q.i.d. for 21 days	Erythromycin, 250 mg PO q.i.d. for 21 days

The secondary stage is characterized by lymphadenopathy and follows the primary stage by one to six weeks. Adenopathy tends to be unilateral and occurs in the regional lymphatic tissue, draining the site of the primary lesion. Ileoinguinal adenopathy is noted when penile lesions occur. Retroperitoneal lymphadenopathy generally occurs in women. A single lymph node may be involved, but commonly contiguous nodes become enlarged and form a matted mass or *bubo*. Inguinal and femoral lymphadenopathy may occur unilaterally and be separated by an apparent groove caused by the inguinal ligament. This "groove sign," typical of LGV, is seen in less than 20% of cases. Adenopathy may spontaneously resolve over a few weeks, or enlargement and suppuration may occur. Chronic lymphadenopathy may persist for years.

Large fluctuant nodes may require percutaneous aspiration to forestall perforation. Spontaneously draining buboes may become secondarily infected. Histologically, lymph nodes demonstrate granulomas, and mononuclear cells may occasionally contain inclusion bodies.

The tertiary stage of LGV may present months or years after initial infection, usually as a nonspecific proctitis. Manifestations are rectovaginal fistulas and destructive vulvar lesions in females, and urethral fistulas in men; scrotal and vulvar elephantiasis secondary to lymphatic obstruction can occur.

MANAGEMENT

Patients with LGV should be treated with tetracycline (see Table 2). Response to therapy is variable and may be unsatisfactory if given late in the course. The earlier treatment is initiated, the better is the clinical response, as measured by diminution of lymphadenopathy and declining CF titers. Patients who fail treatment may respond to a second 21-day or longer course of therapy with tetracycline. Tertiary lesions usually show poor response to treatment, and even if the infection is resolved, residual permanent scarring may remain. Corrective surgery for rectal strictures is possible. Sulfisoxazole is an alternate therapy to tetracycline (see Table 2). The need for and efficacy of treatment of sexual contacts has not been studied, but it is prudent to treat sexual contacts as those with identified LGV.

PREVENTION

Confirmed cases of LGV should be reported to the State Board of Health. Sexual contacts should be identified and evaluated for presence of infection, and appropriate treatment instituted. General measures of public education concerning sexually transmitted diseases apply.

Trachoma

INTRODUCTION AND EPIDEMIOLOGY

Endemic trachoma is a chronic recurring follicular conjunctivitis due to *C. trachomatis* serotypes (A, B, B_1, and C). This infection is the leading cause of preventable blindness in the world. While *Chlamydia* conjunctivitis has a worldwide distribution, blinding trachoma usually occurs in areas that are economically underprivileged and are hyperendemic for *C. trachomatis* (regions of Africa, India, Asia, and the Middle East). In the U.S. a milder form of trachoma is seen in American Indians and emigrants from endemic areas (usually China, Japan, Samoa, and Pacific Micronesia). In these areas, infection usually occurs at an early age, followed by multiple reinfections throughout life. Children are thought to be the reservoir of infection, and human-to-human transmission appears to be the mode of spread, flies being an intermediate vector.

CLINICAL ASPECTS AND PATHOPHYSIOLOGY

Trachoma is characterized by formation of lymphoid follicular hyperplasia and papillary hypertrophy beginning in the upper tarsal plate. In the later stages the lower tarsal plate is involved. Chronic recurrent inflammation leads to conjunctival scarring and may lead to a characteristic inversion of the eyelashes known as *trichiasis* or *entropion*. Abrasion of the cornea by these inverted eyelashes leads to corneal scarring, corneal anesthesia, further scarring, micropannus formation, and ultimately corneal opacification. Secondary bacterial infection is common. Blindness occurs late in the course, usually 10 to 15 years after evidence that active infection has resolved.

DIAGNOSIS

The diagnosis of trachoma should be considered in any person who presents with a follicular conjunctivitis that has lasted for more than 15 days and who either lives in an area known to be endemic for trachoma or has emigrated from such an area. The diagnosis of trachoma can be confirmed by either Giemsa staining or fluorescent antibody staining of conjunctival scrapings, revealing characteristic cytoplasmic inclusion bodies. Culture may be helpful. Serologic testing is of epidemiologic interest but of little practical value.

TREATMENT

Oral and topical tetracycline, erythromycin, sulfonamides, and rifampin have all been found to be efficacious to varying degrees. However, treatment of patients with trachoma in the U.S. should be supervised by an ophthalmologist experienced in the care of trachoma and its complications.

Patients who have late manifestations such as lid distortion may benefit from corrective surgery. Blindness may be prevented if tarsorrhaphy is performed before permanent corneal damage has occurred.

PREVENTION

At the present time most treatment programs in endemic areas are directed toward control of infection in young children, and involve intermittent community-wide treatment with topical antimicrobials. Improvement of socioeconomic conditions in endemic areas would probably have a more significant and lasting impact on trachoma than any other single factor.

REFERENCES

Beem MO, Saxon EM: Respiratory tract colonization and a distinctive pneumonia syndrome in infants infected with *Chlamydia trachomatis*. N Engl J Med 296:306–310, 1977.

Hirschmann JV: Psittacosis. Medical Grand Rounds 2:57–66, 1982.

Holmes KK, Mardh PA, Sparling PF, et al: Sexually Transmitted Diseases. McGraw-Hill Book Co, New York, 1984, pp 243–290.

Schachter J, Dawson CR: Human Chlamydial Infections. PSG Publishing Co, Littleton, MA, 1978.

Stamm WE, Holmes KK: The expanding spectrum of *Chlamydia trachomatis* infections. *In* Isselbacher KJ (ed): Harrison's Principles of Internal Medicine Update IV. McGraw-Hill Book Co, New York, 1983, pp 9–24.

18 · RICKETTSIOSIS AND PASTEURELLA INFECTIONS

John F. Jovanovich
HENRY FORD HOSPITAL

DEFINITION AND DIAGNOSTIC CRITERIA

Rickettsiae are obligate intracellular organisms to which man is an incidental host. They are transmitted to man through the skin by appropriate tick vectors, with the exception of *Coxiella burnetii*. The disease state usually produced is a vasculitis caused by the proliferation of organisms in the endothelial lining of small blood vessels. The disease states produced by rickettsial organisms include Rocky Mountain spotted fever, rickettsialpox, Q fever, epidemic typhus, murine typhus, and scrub typhus. Not all the rickettsial infections are seen everywhere within the United States. Some are restricted to certain geographic locations such as the Rocky Mountain or southeastern states and some to certain environmental conditions such as poor urban housing.

Diagnosis of rickettsial disease occurs only when there is a strong suspicion. The presenting symptoms of fever, headache, and myalgias are very nonspecific and can be seen with any number of diseases. A rash is usually present in all rickettsial diseases with the exception of Q fever. However, this rash may not be present when the patient initially presents for evaluation. Serologic testing may be useful in confirming the diagnostic impression but often is of little value in the acute setting. Suspicion of a rickettsial disease and institution of antibiotic therapy may be crucial since a delay may be associated with disease complications and fatality.

Rocky Mountain Spotted Fever

CLINICAL ASPECTS

Rocky Mountain spotted fever is the most common rickettsial disease seen in the United States. The two vectors are *Dermacentor andersoni* and *D. variabilis*, the wood tick and dog tick, respectively. Seasonal variation is seen, the disease occurring primarily during the spring in the West and from May to September in the Southeast. This seasonal variation coincides with tick activity. A history of tick exposure may be elicited in up to 70% to 85% of patients with Rocky Mountain spotted fever. The incubation period is two to 14 days following the tick bite. Rickettsemia occurs early in the course of the disease and is followed by rickettsial invasion of the vascular endothelium.

The onset of clinical disease is often sudden and accompanied by fever, headache, chills, and myalgia. Temperatures of 41°C may be seen. Headache, usually frontal, is seen in approximately 90% of cases. Other nonspecific symptoms such as arthralgias, nonproductive cough, nausea, vomiting, diarrhea, and photophobia may be present.

The onset of the characteristic rash is generally in the third to fifth day of illness. The physician, however, must be careful not to exclude Rocky Mountain spotted fever from the differential diagnosis when a rash is not present. Less than 10% of all cases never experience the typical rash, and many fatal cases reported did not present with a rash when first seen by the physician. The rash itself consists of rose-colored blanching macules that appear peripherally on the hands, wrists, feet, and ankles, and it spreads in a centripetal fashion to involve the rest of the skin. If left untreated, the rash may become petechial and purpuric.

The generalized vasculitis produced by rickettsial organisms may result in widespread organ dysfunction if left untreated. A number of complications may develop including seizures, adult respiratory distress syndrome, myocarditis, and disseminated intravascular coagulation (DIC). Visceral and CNS dissemination may produce irreversible shock and death.

Serologic testing helps confirm the diagnosis. The most noted test is the Weil-Felix, which measures antibodies against *Proteus vulgaris* strains OX-19, OX-2, and OX-K. This test is of no value in the acute setting because of its poor sensitivity and specificity. Antibody titers may not be seen until after seven to ten days of illness and may not rise until later if antibiotic treatment has been started.

Complement fixation test is highly specific but has a low sensitivity. Other tests not widely available include microagglutination, microimmunofluorescence, and indirect hemoagglutination. A rapid diagnostic test utilizing skin biopsy material is the immunofluorescence of body tissues. It is very sensitive and highly specific. Skin specimens by biopsy may reveal rickettsial organisms as early as the third or fourth day of illness. The test can be performed within a few hours and may confirm the diagnosis. However, one problem encountered with this method is that a rash must be present clinically to determine the site of biopsy.

MANAGEMENT

Once the diagnosis of Rocky Mountain spotted fever has been entertained and other disease states have been excluded, antibiotic therapy is indicated. An adult who presents in one of the endemic areas and is seen with the symptoms of Rocky Mountain spotted fever deserves a therapeutic trial of tetracycline since a delay in diagnosis and treatment may lead to fatal complications.

Tetracycline, 25 to 50 mg/kg/day, and chloramphenicol, 50 mg/kg/day, are the two drugs used for treatment, administered for seven to ten days. It has been estimated that about one third of individuals with Rocky Mountain spotted fever have mild disease and may be treated as outpatients. Oral antibiotic therapy is appropriate on an outpatient basis as long as careful follow-up can be assured. Tetracycline and chloramphenicol are rickettsiostatic and should be continued for two to three days after the fever resolves. The average course of antibiotics is five to seven days. Relapses are uncommon, but if one occurs a second course of antibiotics should be given.

The remaining two thirds of patients who have more serious disease require hospital admission and careful monitoring. Complications that occur as a result of the disease need to be treated with appropriate supportive care.

Q Fever

CLINICAL ASPECTS

Q fever was first reported in 1937 following a series of outbreaks among slaughterhouse workers in Australia. Since then, it has been noted in many countries throughout the world. It is caused by *Coxiella burnetii*, an organism that is quite resistant to desiccation and to other environmental factors. Transmission is usually through inhalation, and the disease is more commonly encountered in areas where cows, sheep, and goats are raised. It is also possible that Q fever is transmitted to humans by milk.

The incubation period is usually 14 to 28 days. Q fever, like many other rickettsial diseases, usually presents as an acute febrile illness with symptoms of fever, headache, and myalgia. It may also present as prolonged fever, atypical pneumonia, and acute hepatitis. The chronic form may be seen as subacute endocarditis months or years after an acute attack.

The diagnosis and decision to treat are often made on clinical grounds. Serologic testing is available to aid in the diagnosis. A fourfold rise in antibody titer of paired sera is the most common method of establishing the diagnosis. The complement fixation test is the one most widely used.

MANAGEMENT

Tetracycline, 500 mg every six hours or doxycycline, 100 mg every 12 hours and chloramphenicol, 50 mg/kg/day, are the antibiotics used to treat Q fever. Some investigators, however, do not see any difference between treated and untreated persons in regard to the duration of the disease state. Q fever is not as responsive as other rickettsial diseases to antibiotics. In cases of Q fever endocarditis, mortality may be lowered by long-term antibiotic therapy, the drugs being administered for months or even years. Antibiotic regimens used to

treat endocarditis in the past have all included tetracycline. Valve replacement is carried out in individuals who have hemodynamic deterioration.

Other Rickettsial Diseases

The remaining rickettsial diseases include rickettsialpox, epidemic typhus, murine typhus, and scrub typhus. All present with the nonspecific symptoms of fever, headache, and myalgias. Each of these usually has an associated rash that occurs sometimes during the illness. Each has its own vector and environmental conditions that allow spread of the disease. Rickettsialpox and murine typhus usually require no specific therapy and have no associated mortality. However, tetracycline or chloramphenicol may speed recovery. Epidemic typhus and scrub typhus are not as benign in nature and may have a high mortality rate; antibiotic therapy is indicated for both.

Pasteurella

CLINICAL ASPECTS

Pasteurellae are known to cause infections in the animal kingdom. The organisms are carried in the nasopharynx or gastrointestinal tract of many animals such as cats, dogs, swine, and rats. *Pasteurella* infections can then be carried over to man simply through animal exposure or through animal contact by bite. They also are sometimes seen in individuals who have no history of animal exposure or contact.

Pasteurella infections that are the result of animal bite are probably the ones most commonly encountered in the outpatient setting. The patient may present with evidence of clinical infection a few hours after an animal bite. The bite wounds are usually located on the hands, arms, legs, or head-neck region. A low-grade fever may be present. Past history of animal exposure, particularly a bite with the onset of localized infection, should alert the physician to a possible *Pasteurella* infection. Antimicrobial therapy with penicillin (the drug of choice for *Pasteurella* infections), 500 mg every six hours, should be instituted, along with local care such as cleaning and debridement of the wound. In the case of penicillin allergy, tetracycline, 500 mg every six hours, may be used. Antibiotic treatment for seven to ten days is considered adequate.

The infections produced by animal bites are usually localized, but may become complicated because of the contiguous spread of organisms. Complications elsewhere in the body may also be seen as a result of bacteremia. *Pasteurella* infections usually present as respiratory tract disease in situations in which there is a history of animal exposure but none of bite. *Pasteurella* infections that occur when there is no history of animal exposure or bite comprise multiple clinical syndromes with no typical pattern.

REFERENCES

Mandell GL, Douglas RG, Bennett JE: Principles and Practice of Infectious Diseases, Vol 2. Ch 145–151 and Ch 185. John Wiley & Sons, New York, 1979.

Furie RA, Cohen RP, Hartman BJ, Roberts RB: *Pasteurella multocida* infection. Report in Urban Setting and Review of Spectrums in Human Disease. NY State J Med 80:1597–1602, 1980.

Marx RS: Rocky Mountain spotted fever. Compr Ther 9:43–48, 1983.

Spelman DW: Q fever. A study of 111 consecutive cases. Med J Aust 1:547–553, June 1982.

Walker DH, Burday MS, Folds JD: Laboratory diagnosis of Rocky Mountain spotted fever. South Med J 73:1443–1446, 1980.

19 · DEEP FUNGAL INFECTIONS

Bradley J. Sullivan
MARSHFIELD CLINIC

CLINICAL ASPECTS

Invasive fungal infections are rare diseases. There are endemic varieties—the well-known association of coccidioidomycosis with the arid, salty desert of the San Joaquin Valley, histoplasmosis in the Midwest, and blastomycosis in the Ohio River and eastern Mississippi watersheds. There are the sporadic illnesses affecting mainly immunocompromised individuals—*Candida* and *Cryptococcus*—among many others. With the exception of *Candida*, most of the above usually present as a pulmonary disease, unresponsive to antibacterial antibiotics. Dissemination to foci other than the lung is rare, but meningitis, osteomyelitis, pericarditis, skin infection, or a long list of other diseases actually may be the presenting problem.

In most cases the finding of the organism in sputum, cerebrospinal fluid (CSF), or blood or on biopsy confirms the diagnosis. Clinical suspicion is necessary to see that biopsy specimens are properly handled. Serology for histoplasmosis and coccidioidomycosis is most helpful. Skin tests are still useful in some situations (e.g., coccidioidomycosis) but may affect the serology. In blastomycosis we found neither to be helpful.

MANAGEMENT

With coccidioidomycosis, histoplasmosis, or blastomycosis the decision to treat rests on the impact of the disease on the patient. A good number of patients spontaneously resolve without medical intervention. Debilitated patients, those with seemingly overwhelming infection, and those "not getting better," however, deserve thorough work-up and treatment. Ketoconazole may be used for patients who are stable or not recovering satisfactorily. Blastomycosis, histoplasmosis, and occasionally coccidioidomycosis respond to the drug.

Other patients, including all immunocompromised individuals, should be treated with amphotericin B.

Candida infections, such as thrush or monilia, may develop in otherwise healthy patients. Traditional methods of treatment (mouthwash after eating, nystatin suspension, various creams) are sufficient in most instances. Ketoconazole may work in some recalcitrant infections but those will be seldom seen. The immunocompromised, on the other hand, can get candidal infections that can mimic any bacterial infection: fulminant candidemia, endocarditis, abscesses (particularly in the GI tract and liver), endophthalmitis (secondary to candidemia), esophagitis, oral thrush, pneumonia, urinary tract infection with fungus balls, and so on. These deserve aggressive management with amphotericin B, occasionally adding flucytosine for synergy. Oral prophylaxis with nystatin or ketoconazole has not worked.

Cryptococcus and *Aspergillus* afflict mainly the immunocompromised. The former can cause meningitis (best diagnosed by latex agglutination for the capsular antigen in the CSF), pneumonia, and disseminated disease. The latter causes pneumonia, sinusitis, meningitis, and other invasive disease. Amphotericin is the best drug for both, although there are some reports of the use of miconazole for *Cryptococcus*. *Aspergillus* is resistant to the imidazoles. *Cryptococcus* is sensitive to flucytosine but, because resistance can develop, it is used in combination with amphotericin, allowing a reduction in the dose of the latter.

AMPHOTERICIN B

Among the oldest and most reliable of antifungal agents is amphotericin B (Fungizone). Very few fungi are resistant to it. Failures are usually attributable to undertreatment—inadequate dose or duration. It is a drug, however, with a multitude of significant side effects, some immediate, some long term. Further, once committed to using it, the patient may require weeks to even months of therapy. Many patients require hospitalization for the entire course of therapy, but some may benefit from innovative approaches (mentioned below) that facilitate giving the drug in the outpatient setting.

A central venous line affords the best delivery system, both for inpatients and outpatients. Most clinics have teams well versed in the placement and care of such lines, and these should be consulted from the onset. Whoever administers the drug should pay due respect to aseptic technique since secondary sepsis from the line is a definite risk.

Preparation of amphotericin B is most often done by a pharmacist. While the final concentration in most instances is 0.1 mg/ml, increased concentrations may be advantageous, allowing less fluid delivery and perhaps more rapid administration. These variations should be individualized and are advised only when the catheter is in the vena cava in patients who are tolerating the medicine well.

Some important technical admonitions include:

1. Use 5% dextrose in water (D5W) for preparation and delivery of amphotericin. Salt solutions cause aggregation of the drug suspension. This means that the central line should be flushed with D5W before and after the infusion.

2. For optimal reconstitution of the drug, the man-

ufacturer recommends that the pH of the D5W should be greater than 4.2. In most instances, dextrose solutions have a pH measurement on the label, so the pharmacist seldom has to check the pH. The manufacturer also provides information on a buffer to lower the pH, if necessary. Sodium hydroxide should not be used.

3. Once prepared, the solution is stable for 24 hours. If it is not to be used immediately but transported to a distant site, heparin or hydrocortisone (both sodium salts) should be added and mixed just before infusion. Extremes of heat or cold should be avoided by transporting the solution in an insulated container.

4. There is no need to protect the amphotericin B solution from light, although this is commonly recommended. However, as a precaution, if transported, the solution should be protected from sunlight.

5. In-line millipore filters are not necessary but, if one is used, the pore size should be no less than 0.45 μm. Smaller pore size decreases the delivery of the drug.

The traditional method of administration of amphotericin suits most people. A test dose of 1 mg over one-half hour is given and the patient is monitored for febrile, pulmonary, and cardiovascular reactions. This is followed by a two- to six-hour infusion of 0.25 mg/kg. Maximal dosage (0.5 to 1.0 mg/kg/day for every-day therapy or 1.0 to 1.5 mg/kg/day for alternate-day therapy) is approached slowly, 5 to 10 mg at a time, for indolent diseases. In a rapidly deteriorating situation (e.g., candidemia in the septic, immunocompromised patient) the test dose may be skipped and dose increases made on an every-eight-hour basis, care being taken not to exceed the predetermined total daily dose in a 24-hour period. If the patient is already in renal failure or has marginal renal function, a loading dose should be given (cumulative 0.75 mg/kg) and the pharmacokinetic profile determined, with acceptable peak levels obtained right after delivery of the drug of 3 to 4 μg/ml as the goal.

Acute Reaction to Amphotericin. Reactions that initial administration of amphotericin B provokes are impressive: fever, chills, hypotension, headache, delirium, and occasionally wheezing and hypoxemia. These have prompted much advice about coadministration of "prophylactic" medications: (1) aspirin or acetaminophen at appropriate doses an hour before administration; (2) diphenhydramine (Benadryl), 25 to 50 mg PO (5 mg/kg/day divided by four for children) at the start of infusions; (3) meperidine (Demerol), occasionally recommended for sedation during infusion; (4) hydrocortisone, 25 to 50 mg (0.7 mg/kg for children) given concomitantly, either as a separate infusion or mixed with the amphotericin solution; or (5) heparin, 1 to 2 U/ml in the amphotericin solution to reduce phlebitis or clot formation.

Studies have not been done to determine whether any of the above recommendations have a definite impact on early, acute reactions to amphotericin B, but there are strong "clinical impressions" that they do. Steroids decrease the antifungal effect of amphotericin B in vitro, prompting some infectious disease consultants to advise against their use. In weakened patients who cannot tolerate the rigors of the side effects, the best approach is to increase the dose of amphotericin

very slowly. Most patients eventually become tolerant of it, at which time the ancillary medications are tapered.

Granulocyte Transfusions. A caveat was promulgated against simultaneous use of amphotericin B with granulocyte transfusions because of deaths due to acute respiratory decompensation. There are a number of alternative explanations for this phenomenon (and the original observation was not seen at other institutions), but caution is advised when treating neutropenic patients. Among precautionary measures advised are: (1) use fresh granulocytes prepared by centrifugation; (2) administer the granulocytes slowly; (3) observe patients carefully with frequent chest x-rays to look for developing infiltrates, and by performing blood gas studies to detect hypoxemia.

Long-term Adverse Effects. Once the hurdle of acute toxicity is passed, the cumulative renal and other toxicities become the focus of attention. The well-recognized renal toxicity and decreased glomerular filtration rate (GFR) deserve the most attention. No less intimidating are the other side effects: hematologic disorders (anemia, thrombocytopenia, leukopenia), headache, vomiting, cachexia, hypokalemia, hypomagnesemia, thrombophlebitis, anaphylaxis (which is rare), convulsions, generalized pain (one text describes burning sensations of the feet), and neurologic symptoms if intrathecal or intraventricular injections are given.

Nephrotoxicity. Although it may be a preliminary report to be refuted by later evidence, a study reporting decreased nephrotoxicity by salt repletion has attracted attention. Patients are given a high sodium diet or extra sodium in their IV fluids if there is evidence of sodium depletion (e.g., by history of diuretic use, dietary salt restriction, vomiting, or urine electrolytes with a low sodium). For the time being, I recommend this simple intervention at the onset of therapy as prophylaxis.

The nephrotoxicity is the main deterrent. Most authors recommend interruption of treatment when the serum creatinine reaches 3.0 to 3.5 mg/100 ml. Alternate-day therapy (Monday, Wednesday, and Friday) may reduce toxicity. In some institutions the MIC of amphotericin for the fungus can be determined and the peak serum level adjusted to twice that value, allowing for a lower dose. Synergy with other drugs may also allow reduction of the dosage of amphotericin.

Because of the complexities involved, I strongly advise consultation with an infectious disease specialist at the onset. However, a stable and trustworthy patient may even complete a course of therapy as an outpatient, attending a clinic or emergency room or even having house visits by a nurse.

KETOCONAZOLE

This oral antifungal agent (Nizoral) is relatively new but may have an impact on the management of fungal diseases. Already there are reports of the use of ketoconazole in blastomycotic osteomyelitis, mucocutaneous candidiasis and some other candidal infections, coccidioidomycosis, and occasionally in pulmonary histoplasmosis. In all instances of severe infection, certainly in meningitis, and (in my opinion) in all immunocompromised patients, amphotericin should be the first-choice drug. However, given relative clinical stability, therapy may be initiated with ketoconazole and the response determined. I suggest consultation with an infectious disease specialist to determine the appropriateness of this drug in any given situation since there is still much to be learned about the drug and its usefulness.

In order to be absorbed well, the drug needs an acid environment. It may be taken one-half hour before meals or even with a meal. Once-daily dosage is probably optimal, both in terms of achieving a high peak level and in probably decreasing some of the side effects. In my practice, I have the patients take a dose at breakfast. Once or twice weekly, I see them between 9 and 10 AM and obtain a serum level of the drug. This checks on patient compliance and absorption, and may correlate with outcome.

Dosage recommended by the manufacturer is ≤20 kg, 50 mg/d; 20–40 kg, 100 mg/d; >40 kg, 200 mg/d.

For the histoplasmosis and blastomycosis endemic to my upper Midwest region, I usually double the dose. This may be an appropriate maneuver in other settings.

Drug Interactions. Antacids or cimetidine decrease the absorption of ketoconazole dramatically. If the patient needs the antacid, the gastric acidity may be increased by ingesting the tablets with or dissolved in 4 ml of 0.2 N HCl. He should be advised to drink it with a straw and swallow quickly since the acid dissolves tooth enamel. A water chaser is advisable also.

Side Effects. Side effects are much fewer than those from amphotericin. Nausea and vomiting or abdominal pain may occur early in the course of therapy. This can be lessened in part by taking the medicine on a full stomach. Many patients eventually tolerate the drug with continued administration. Other side effects include gynecomastia, decreased adrenal steroidogenesis, chemical evidence of liver dysfunction, and (rarely) severe hepatotoxicity. The drug is excreted in breast milk, so lactating mothers should be warned. Also, since it may be teratogenic, pregnancy should be avoided during therapy.

FLUCYTOSINE (5-FLUOROCYTOSINE)

Flucytosine (Ancobon) acts synergistically with amphotericin against *Cryptococcus* and some *Candida* species. Although this means that lower doses of amphotericin may be used and that the duration of therapy may be shortened, particularly for cryptococcal meningitis, close attention must be paid to the risk of severe toxicity caused by flucytosine.

The usual oral dose is 150 mg/kg/d divided by four, but when in renal insufficiency (creatinine >1.7 mg/dl) the dose should be adjusted. Serum levels should be monitored and pharmocokinetics determined to best modify dosage. In combination with amphotericin, the amphotericin dose should be 0.3 mg/kg/d (or 0.6 mg/kg every other day) to gain the benefit of lowered renal toxicity.

Adverse Effects. Hematologic complications (anemia, leukopenia, and thrombocytopenia) may be reduced by maintaining peak levels of the drug below 100 μg/ml. Peak levels are obtained two hours after an oral dose. The incidence of GI dysfunction (including occasionally severe enterocolitis), rash, and reversible hepatotoxicity may also be reduced in this manner.

REFERENCES

Heidemann HT, Gerkens JF, Spickard WA, et al: Amphotericin B nephrotoxicity in humans decreased by salt repletion. Am J Med 75:476–481, 1983.
Hoeprich PD: Some aspects of the clinical use of amphotericin B. Infect Dis Newsletter 3:62–63, 1984.
Medoff G, Kobayaski GS: Strategies in the treatment of systemic fungal infections. N Engl J Med 302:145–155, 1980.

20 · IMMUNIZATIONS IN THE ADULT

Sandra L. Argenio
GEISINGER MEDICAL CENTER

DEFINITION

Routine immunization is considered basic practice in children and adolescents. It is an area of medicine that truly represents preventive care. Vaccinations against diphtheria, tetanus, pertussis, measles, mumps, rubella, and polio are routinely administered in the United States, usually in childhood. Immunization of adults is not generally routine, but it should be.

BASIC PRINCIPLES: ACTIVE AND PASSIVE IMMUNIZATION

Active immunization is a major tool of preventive practice. Active immunization mimics natural infection. With live vaccines, a mild infection is produced with little or no adverse reaction by the patient. An immunologic response is evoked to a dose of all or part of a microorganism or to a product of a microorganism such as a toxin. The body responds by producing antibodies that provide protection against the natural disease. A single dose of most live attenuated virus vaccines usually provides complete and lifelong protection. Inactivated vaccines and toxoids produce less complete responses after a single dose. Long-lasting immunity occurs with repeated doses of inactivated agents or toxoids, with periodic boosters given to maintain immunity.

Passive immunization involves the transfer of preformed concentrated antibody to provide temporary protection. Temporary protection can be provided against a disease for which there is no active immunizing agent. An example of this is protection of travelers against hepatitis A. When exposure to a disease has already occurred and time does not allow active protection, passive immunity provides antibodies until active immunity develops. Postexposure protection of rabies is a major example. Other uses of passive immunization include prophylactic therapy against hepatitis B and measles and replacement therapy in persons with immunodeficiency.

Recommendations for immunization are reviewed and updated periodically by the Advisory Committee on Immunization Practices (ACIP) of the United States Public Health Service. Two very useful sources are *The Morbidity and Mortality Weekly Reports* (MMWR), its yearly *Health Information for International Travel*, and the "Red Book" of the Infectious Disease Committee of the American Academy of Pediatrics.

Benefits and risks are associated with the use of all vaccines. Current recommendations represent a balancing of scientific evidence of benefits and risks to achieve optimal levels of protection against infectious diseases.

MANAGEMENT OF IMMUNIZATION

Immunization schedules must be individualized and must consider number and timing of doses, boosters, major precautions, and contraindications.

TIMING OF VACCINE SCHEDULES

Some vaccines require more than one dose for full protection. Others require booster doses to maintain protection. Most of the widely used vaccine antigens can safely and effectively be given at the same time. The following recommendations are summarized from MMWR's *Health Information for International Travel*.

Live Attenuated Vaccines. These include measles, mumps, rubella (MMR) vaccine, trivalent oral polio vaccine (TOPV), and yellow fever vaccine. Administration on the same day of the most widely used live virus vaccines (TOPV and MMR) has not resulted in impaired antibody response or increased rates of adverse effects.

There are theoretical concerns and data showing that the immune response to a live virus vaccine might be impaired if the vaccine is administered within the month following another live virus vaccine. Therefore, live virus vaccines should be administered either on the same day or at least one month apart.

Killed Inactivated Vaccines. Inactivated vaccines (cholera, typhoid, and plague) can be administered simultaneously at separate sites. However, local or systemic side effects may be increased. Generally, if practical, or if in persons known to experience side effects, inactivated vaccines should be given on separate occasions.

Toxoids. Field experience and antibody data suggest that simultaneous administration of DTP (diphtheria and tetanus toxoids and pertussis vaccine) and either TOPV or MMR provides adequate protection and does not increase the incidence of side effects. Simultaneous administration is especially recommended if it is doubtful that the patient will return to receive further doses of vaccine.

An inactivated vaccine and a live attenuated vaccine can be administered at separate sites. Decreased antibody levels have been observed when cholera (inactivated) and yellow fever (live attenuated) vaccines have been administered within three weeks of each other rather than at longer intervals. Therefore, the ACIP recommends that yellow fever and cholera vaccines can be administered simultaneously if necessary, but preferably at an interval longer than three weeks.

Immune Globulin. Inactivated vaccines can be given any time after immunoglobulin use. With live attenuated vaccines, passively acquired antibodies from the immunoglobulin may interfere with the replication of vaccine virus and thereby with the active antibody response of the patient. Live vaccines should not be given for at least six weeks, but preferably three months after the administration of immunoglobulin.

If it becomes necessary to administer immunoglobulin after a live vaccine, interference may occur. If the interval between vaccine and immunoglobulin is less than 14 days, the vaccine should be repeated about three months after immunoglobulin was given unless serologic testing indicates that antibodies were produced. If the interval was longer than 14 days, the vaccine need not be readministered.

SPECIAL CONSIDERATIONS

Hypersensitivity to Vaccine Compounds. Some vaccines are prepared from antigens derived from embryonated chicken eggs. Yellow fever, typhus, measles, mumps, and influenza are such vaccines. Rabies vaccine is now prepared in human diploid cell cultures, an improvement over the old vaccine prepared in embryonated duck eggs. Rubella vaccines are also prepared in human diploid cell cultures. Screening persons by history of ability to eat eggs without adverse effects is a reasonable way to identify those at risk of allergic reactions from receiving vaccines prepared in eggs. Patients who have had severe or anaphylactic reactions to eggs should not be given vaccines prepared in eggs. Live virus vaccines prepared in human tissue cell cultures are free of potentially allergenic substances. No severe hypersensitivity reactions have been reported to the live attenuated rubella vaccines prepared from virus grown in cell cultures. This vaccine can be given safely regardless of a history of egg allergy.

Some vaccines contain preservatives (mercurials or thimerosal) or traces of antibiotics (neomycin) and should not be given to patients allergic to these substances. Reactions are usually local rather than systemic. No currently recommended vaccine contains penicillin or its derivatives. Vaccine package inserts include information about preservatives or antibiotics used in preparation.

Patients with a Fever. In general, patients with a fever should not be given a vaccine until they have recovered, otherwise the vaccine may mask or superimpose adverse effects on the underlying illness. Mild upper respiratory infections, however, should not delay vaccination.

Patients with Immunodeficiency. Virus replication of live attenuated vaccines may be enhanced in patients with immunodeficiency diseases or malignancy or in those undergoing therapy with steroids or immunosuppressant agents. These patients should not be given live viruses. TOPV should not be given to a household member of an immunosuppressed patient because live TOPV vaccine viruses are excreted by the recipient and can be transmitted to other persons.

Pregnancy. The benefits to the mother must be balanced against the risk to the fetus. Live attenuated vaccines are generally not recommended for pregnant women or those likely to become pregnant within three months after vaccination because of the theoretical though low risk of teratogenic effects in the fetus. Measles, mumps, and rubella, all live vaccines, are contraindicated. Yellow fever and polio vaccines are relatively contraindicated but can be given if the woman is at high risk of exposure and infection with the natural disease. If possible, it is preferable to wait until the second or third trimester. Routine vaccination with MMR and TOPV does not have to be delayed in children of pregnant women.

There is no risk to the fetus from immunizing the mother with inactivated virus vaccines, bacterial vaccines, or toxoids or from passive immunization with immunoglobulin. Breast feeding is not a contraindication to immunization of the mother.

GUIDELINES AND SCHEDULES FOR IMMUNIZATIONS IN THE ADULT

Establishment and Updating of Basic Immunizations. Preventive medicine is the basic principle of pediatrics. The preventive emphasis is growing stronger in adult care as we urge patients to use seat belts, quit smoking, and modify life styles. However, many adults in the U.S. have inadequate basic immunization. The primary care physician must program his routine history to include an immunization history and must routinely update basic immunizations.

Diphtheria, Pertussis, and Tetanus (DPT). DPT involves a primary series of four doses in children under 7 years of age. In children over 7 and in adults, Td is used instead. Td consists of tetanus toxoid and a reduced dosage of diphtheria toxoid. It is not generally necessary to give pertussis vaccine to persons over 7 years old.

The primary series for patients over 7 is three doses of Td 0.5 cc IM initially, two months later, and six months later. A booster dose is required every ten years to maintain immunity. If the patient receives a dirty wound, a booster may be required after five years. Reactions are unusual and include local redness and swelling or moderate fever.

Polio. Polio is still endemic in large parts of the world. In children the primary series is two doses given six to eight weeks apart, with a third dose eight to twelve months after the second and a preschool booster. In adults over 18, routine immunization is not necessary because of the extreme unlikelihood of exposure to the disease. However, polio vaccination is recommended for travelers to endemic areas, members of populations with wild poliovirus disease, and lab and health care workers with viral contact.

For previously unimmunized adults, inactivated polio virus (IPV) is indicated because the risk of vaccine-associated paralysis following TOPV is slightly higher in adults than in children. The primary schedule for unvaccinated adults is three doses of IPV at one- to two-month intervals with a fourth dose six to twelve months after the third. If only four to eight weeks are available before exposure, two doses of IPV are given four weeks apart. If less than four weeks is available, give one dose of TOPV. Don't forget to complete the primary series later if exposure to polio continues.

If an adult has previously been partially immunized, the series should be completed with the remaining doses of either vaccine. An individual who remains at increased risk and who has previously received a complete primary series with TOPV should be given a single booster dose of TOPV. If the primary series was IPV, give one booster dose of either IPV or TOPV. If the primary series was exclusively IPV, a booster of IPV may be needed every five years if exposure continues.

Polio vaccine is very effective. Reactions are rare. There has been one case of vaccine-associated paralysis per 8.1 million doses given. As stated earlier, the live virus should not be given to immunodeficient individuals or their household contacts. Live virus is shed up to one month after vaccination with TOPV.

Smallpox. Smallpox has been essentially eradicated worldwide, an example of the success of preventive immunization programs. The vaccine is medically contraindicated and ineffective in the treatment of any disease (such as herpes or warts). At present the vaccine is no longer required by any country for entry.

Measles, Mumps and Rubella (MMR). MMR is given to children once at 15 months. Most adults born before 1957 were exposed to natural measles and are immune. Any adult born after 1957 who did not receive measles vaccine beyond the age of 1 year or who does not have a physician-documented history of disease should be vaccinated. Combined MMR vaccine is the agent of choice if the recipient is also susceptible to mumps and rubella. Certain individuals were given the killed form of measles vaccine between 1963 and 1967 and should be revaccinated with live measles vaccine because they can develop a severe atypical measles if exposed to the natural disease.

The incidence of mumps has decreased steadily since the vaccine became available in 1967. Mumps disease is a mild, self-limited infection, but meningeal signs or orchitis that can rarely lead to sterility may occur. Mumps vaccine is indicated for all adults, especially men, thought to be susceptible. In general, those born before 1957 are considered immune.

Rubella vaccine is indicated for all adults, especially women, who do not have proof of immunity—either documented rubella vaccination on or after the first birthday or documented serologic evidence of natural immunity. Because of the high incidence of congenital rubella syndrome and fetal wastage if rubella is contracted in the first trimester, it is advisable to immunize girls before the onset of puberty. Postpubertal girls should be warned of the teratogenic risks to the fetus and advised not to become pregnant for the next three months. They should not be vaccinated if pregnant.

Any contact with the health care system should be used as an opportunity to screen and vaccinate susceptible females. Prenatal or antepartum screening should be performed, and vaccine should be administered if indicated immediately postpartum before discharge.

These vaccines are very effective with a single subcutaneous dose of live attenuated vaccine. Reactions are rare and are usually a mild fever in two to three weeks or mild arthralgias. Contraindications include pregnancy, immunosuppression, and sensitivity to neomycin. Measles and mumps vaccine should not be given to patients sensitive to eggs. Rubella vaccine is prepared in human diploid cell culture and has not been associated with allergic reactions.

Influenza. Influenza vaccine is an inactivated virus vaccine. Annual vaccination is strongly recommended for all children and adults who are at increased risk of adverse consequences from lower respiratory tract infections.

The MMWR September 1984 supplement, *Adult*

Immunization, recommends vaccination of the following high-risk groups.

1. Adults at high risk of severe influenza who most warrant vaccinations, i.e., those with chronic cardiovascular or pulmonary disease severe enough to require regular follow-up or hospitalization in the previous year, and residents of nursing homes or chronic care facilities.

2. Physicians, nurses, and other personnel who have extensive contact with high-risk patients, to reduce the chance of nosocomial spread of influenza.

3. Other adults at moderately increased risk, i.e., healthy individuals over 65 years of age and persons with chronic metabolic disease, renal dysfunction, anemia, immunosuppression, or asthma.

The vaccine does not confer long-lasting immunity. Yearly vaccination is required. Reactions are mild and include local redness and induration or mild malaise and myalgia. Influenza vaccine should not be given to those with egg allergy. Pregnancy is not a contraindication, but public health authorities recommend waiting until the second trimester.

Pneumococcus. The pneumococcal vaccine is an inactivated vaccine that contains purified capsular material of 23 types of *Streptococcus pneumoniae* responsible for 87% of recent bacteremic pneumococcal infections. The duration of vaccine-induced immunity from a single 0.5-cc dose is unknown but appears to be long. It should be given to patients at special risk of pneumococcal infection: the elderly and persons with diabetes, chronic cardiovascular or pulmonary disease, and those who lack a spleen, have sickle cell disease, or are immunocompromised. Side effects are rare but appear to increase with subsequent doses. Therefore, boosters are not recommended. The safety of pneumococcal vaccine in pregnancy has not been evaluated.

Prophylaxis of Tetanus and Rabies in the Animal Bite Victim. Primary care physicians must be experts in the management of animal bites because of the increasing pet population in the U.S. and because of the increasing incidence of rabies in the wild animal population in certain regions of the country. Bite wound care demands consideration of four major problems: (1) care of lacerations and punctures, (2) assessment of the need for antibiotics, (3) tetanus prophylaxis, and (4) rabies prophylaxis. Only the last two topics will be discussed here as they relate to immunization in the adult.

Tetanus. Tetanus prophylaxis should be considered the standard of care in bite wounds. Primary immunization was discussed earlier. When providing tetanus prophylaxis, the immunization history is key (Table 1). If the primary series is incomplete, passive immunization with tetanus immune globulin (TIG) must also be considered.

For all wounds in patients with an incomplete primary series (zero, one, or two doses), a Td booster is required. If over ten years have elapsed since the last booster in a patient with a complete primary series, a booster is necessary. If the wound is small and clean, TIG is not necessary.

For large dirty wounds, TIG is not required if the primary series is complete and boosters are up to date. If the primary series is incomplete or uncertain or if more than five years have elapsed since the last booster, TIG is also indicated.

The dose of TIG is 250 to 500 IU given IM, the dose depending on the size of the wound. Td and TIG should be injected at separate sites, using different syringes because the two preparations can inactivate each other. Table 1 summarizes the recommendations.

Rabies. Human rabies is a preventable disease that, when contracted, is nearly always fatal. Preexposure prophylaxis should be offered to high-risk groups such as veterinarians and vet students, viral lab workers, forest rangers and explorers, taxidermists, trappers, and persons (adults and children) spending time in foreign countries in which rabies is a constant threat. Rabies human diploid cell vaccine (HDCV) is prepared in human diploid cell culture and therefore has a very low incidence of allergic or neurologic side effects. Preexposure prophylaxis consists of three 1-ml IM injections of HDCV on days 0, 7, and 28. Current studies suggest that preexposure prophylaxis with intradermal vaccine may also provide adequate antibody levels.

Preexposure vaccination does not eliminate the need for prompt postexposure prophylaxis. The latter includes active immunization with HDCV and passive protection with human rabies immune globulin (HRIG) if there has not been preexposure vaccination. In determining the need for protection, consider the species and vaccination status of the biting animal, the circumstances of the bite or exposure, and the incidence of rabies in the area. Wild animals such as skunks, raccoons, foxes, bats, coyotes, and other carnivores are at high risk for transmission of rabies. Rabies is rare in small rodents and rabbits.

Table 2 summarizes the Centers for Disease Control (CDC) recommendations for postexposure prophylaxis. Consider each case individually and consult public health officials when in doubt.

Postexposure prophylaxis consists of five doses of HDCV on days 0, 3, 7, 14, and 28. Passive protection should be provided to those who have not had preexposure prophylaxis with HRIG at 20 IU/kg. Half the dose is infiltrated into tissues around the wound and half is given IM. If the patient has been previously immunized, only HDCV is necessary, with doses on days 0 and 3.

Patient Education and Compliance. Most adults are aware of the need for immunization in children. However, physicians must also educate patients as to the need for immunization in adults, both basic and for special circumstances. A basic knowledge of the minimal risks and substantial benefits of immunization is important to both patient education and compliance. Patients should be told before vaccination of possible side effects.

Table 1. TETANUS PROPHYLAXIS RECOMMENDATIONS

Immunization History (Number of Doses)	Clean Wounds		Large Dirty Wounds	
	Td	TIG	Td	TIG
Uncertain	Yes	No	Yes	Yes
0–1	Yes	No	Yes	Yes
2	Yes	No	Yes	Yes, if wound over 24 hr old
3	Yes, if >10 yr since booster	No	Yes, if >5 yr since booster	No

Td = tetanus-diphtheria toxoid; TIG = tetanus immune globulin.

Table 2. RABIES POSTEXPOSURE IMMUNIZATION: WHEN TO TREAT (CDC RECOMMENDATIONS)

Animal	Condition of Animal	Treatment
Household pets	Healthy and vaccinated; can observe for ten days	None unless animal develops rabies
Household pets	Rabid or suspect	HRIG and HDCV; animal should be killed and tested
Household pets	Unknown (escaped)	Consult public health officials; HRIG and HDCV if indicated
Wild animals: skunks, bats, foxes, coyotes, raccoons, bobcats, other carnivores	Regard as rabid unless proven negative by laboratory test. If available, animal should be killed and tested.	HRIG and HDCV
Other animals: livestock, rodents, rabbits	CONSIDER INDIVIDUALLY—CONSULT PUBLIC HEALTH OFFICIALS. The following almost never require antirabies prophylaxis: squirrels, hamsters, guinea pigs, gerbils, chipmunks, rats, mice, rabbits.	

HRIG = human rabies immune globulin; HDCV = human diploid cell vaccine.

Some clinics require written informed consent. By talking with patients about the benefits in prevention of infectious diseases, the physician can minimize fears and doubts. This helps to ensure that patients will return to complete the primary series and to receive booster doses.

Patients need to know which immunizations they have received. In our highly mobile society, it is also important that they have written documentation of the vaccines and doses received. The physician should also keep a clear record of immunizations in an easily accessible area of the patient's chart.

Socioeconomic Aspects. Immunization is truly preventive medicine. The global eradication of smallpox is the best example of the socioeconomic possibilities of a well-organized worldwide vaccination program. The reductions in morbidity and mortality as well as financial savings from preventing many common infectious diseases are immeasurable. In the near future, an economic vaccine against hepatitis B may be available to help reduce the substantial incidence of hepatitis B in many nations of the world. As physicians, we must be alert to the continued need for immunization in the world.

REFERENCES

ACIP: Adult immunization. MMWR Supplement 33:12S–16S, 20S–22S, 24S, 30S, 1984.
ACIP: Rabies prevention—United States 1984. MMWR 33:393–408, 1984.
CDC: Health information for international travel 1984. MMWR Supplement 33:64–67, 70–71, 75, 1984.
Committee on Infectious Diseases of the American Academy of Pediatrics: Report of the Committee on Infectious Diseases. American Academy of Pediatrics, Evanston, IL, 1982, pp 29, 35.
Jackson RS: Immunization Practices for Adults. *In* Hook EW, Mandell GL, Gwaltney JM (eds): Current Concepts of Infectious Diseases. Wiley Medical Publications, New York, 1977, pp 135–138.

21 · GENITAL HERPES

John F. Jovanovich
HENRY FORD HOSPITAL

Genital herpetic infection is viewed as a disease of increasing incidence and importance. Following gonorrhea and nongonococcal urethritis in the male and gonorrhea and vaginitis in the female, genital herpes is now the third most common venereal problem. The occasional complications that are seen as a result of genital herpes are a matter of utmost concern. These complications include meningitis, radiculitis, and neonatal morbidity. In addition, the epidemiologic association of genital herpes with cervical cancer makes it a major health concern.

Herpes is not a new disease. Derived from a Greek word meaning "to creep," the term herpes was used in Greek medicine to include spreading cutaneous lesions of different etiologies. The herpetic eruptions that appear about the mouth at the crisis of fever were first noted around 100 AD by the Roman physician Herodotus. These are what we now refer to as herpes simplex virus type I (HSV-I) infections. These occur most commonly in children and on body sites above the waist. In 1600 AD, herpes of the genital tract in both men and women was reported by the French physician Astruc. Today these are referred to as herpes simplex virus II (HSV-II) infections. Most often these occur during adolescence and young adulthood (ages 15 to 30) and invade body sites below the waist. Seventy-five to 80% of all genital herpetic lesions are HSV-II in nature. Although HSV-I and HSV-II have distinct biologic and biochemical characteristics, there is some blending of their clinical and epidemiologic patterns. In addition, both these types of infections result in lifelong latent neural carriage of the virus. This carriage is in the trigeminal ganglion for HSV-I and in the sacral ganglia, S2 and S3, for HSV-II infections.

CLINICAL ASPECTS

Although the discussion in this chapter will center on the genital and oral lesions of herpes that are transmitted sexually, it is important to remember that not all herpetic infections are seen as cold sores or genital lesions. In medical and dental personnel, primary infection of the finger results from exposure to the virus in contaminated secretions. In this setting these infections are usually of the HSV-I type. When this same type of infection, or *herpetic whitlow* as it is known, is seen in the general population, it is usually of the HSV-II type. Herpes infections of the eye are also frequently encountered and are usually produced by HSV-I. These may present as unilateral follicular conjunctivitis or blepharitis.

Primary herpetic infection symptoms usually begin three to seven days after exposure and contact. Initially the patient complains of a burning sensation or paresthesia about the site of inoculation. Numerous small vesicles, bordered by an erythematous base, rupture and form shallow, moist ulcers. Pain and tenderness become very prominent with the appearance of the vesicles. Lmyph nodes may become enlarged and tender as the virus spreads to the lymphatics. Patients with primary HSV-II infections often have systemic symptoms including chills, low-grade fever, headache, or general malaise. Herpetic lesions may present for up to four weeks, and crusting will occur with epithelization.

In women infection has often been associated with dysuria, leukorrhea, and cervicitis. The cervicitis may be severe, with necrotic ulceration mimicking carcinoma on examination. Vulvar edema may also be seen secondary to the infectious process. Urinary retention is another problem encountered in the female patient with herpes. Anorectal herpes is becoming an increasingly recognized problem in the homosexual male. Symptoms that may be associated with anorectal herpetic lesions include rectal pain, itching, tenderness, and discharge.

AUTOINOCULATION

The question of autoinoculation of herpetic infections from one site, such as the genitals, to another, such as the eyes, is one often raised by patients. The concern is that the patient will transmit the herpes virus from an active lesion elsewhere on the body to the eyes. We know that transmission of HSV-II to other skin sites can occur, as, for example, with the passage of the virus from infected mothers to infants. Authorities also believe that autoinoculation to areas such as the hands, thighs, and buttocks is not uncommon. Although such autoinoculation from the skin to the eyes is theoretically possible, the chance circumstances under which this process would need to occur are rather unlikely. However, to avoid the possibility of autoinoculation from the genitals to other sites of the body, patients should be advised to practice principles of good hygiene, including thorough washing of the hands after contact with herpetic lesions, for example, after applying topical medications. This practice and general good hygiene help to reduce the risk of autoinoculation.

RECURRENCE

The major problem of herpetic infections is recurrence. Recurrent lesions are usually associated with less extensive involvement than the primary infection. Systemic symptoms usually are not present with recurrence. Approximately 75% of patients with herpetic infections have recurrences in the first year. The average number of recurrent episodes is four per year. It has been shown in some studies that persons infected with HSV-II are more likely to have recurrence than those infected with HSV-I. Some situations have also been said to be associated with, and perhaps to induce, recurrent episodes: e.g., emotional stress, sunburn, fever, menstrual periods, intercourse, surgery, and injury.

Diagnosis of herpetic infections is usually made on the basis of a careful history and examination. If there is any diagnostic doubt or confusion about the disease entity, a Tzanck smear can be taken. Definite confirmation is most reliably made with viral culture.

To perform a Tzanck smear, cells are scraped from the base of the vesicle and smeared onto a glass slide and then stained with Wright or Giemsa stain. The presence of multinucleated giant cells indicates a herpetic infection. Such cells as this can also be seen on Pap smear examination when taken from an infected patient. Unfortunately, the results from Pap smears are not as readily available as those from a Tzanck smear, which offers immediate results. However, most diagnoses of herpetic infections are made on clinical grounds alone. Definitive diagnosis can be made by viral culture of the suspected lesion.

MANAGEMENT

Treatment for the acute episode has, until recently, been only supportive. Sitz baths and cool water applications are usually advised. Drying agents such as calamine may also be applied. Narcotic analgesics often are also helpful in controlling the pain associated with herpetic infection.

There is a long list of previously used agents that are claimed to treat herpetic infections. This list includes such agents as L-lysine, BCG vaccination, lesion desiccation, topical salicylic acid, cryotherapy, photo inactivation, and dye. Most reports of success with these agents are anecdotal. Controlled investigation and studies do not support their claims. In addition, some of the agents listed above are thought to be possibly carcinogenic.

ACYCLOVIR

Only recently has medical therapy directed against the herpes virus been developed. A promising agent currently being marketed is acyclovir, which is believed to enter the virus infected cells more easily than normal noninfected cells. Once inside the cell, acyclovir is phosphorylated to a compound that interferes with viral DNA replication.

Topical acyclovir has been on the market and its application has been shown to be effective in decreasing the mean duration of viral shedding and the time needed to complete crusting of lesions in patients with primary herpes infections. These same type of effects, however, were not seen with recurrent infections, and the use of the topical agent has been promoted primarily for initial episodes of herpetic infection.

Recent investigations with oral acyclovir have been much more promising. It has been shown that the oral preparation is able to reduce viral shedding, formation of new lesions, and the duration of genital lesions in both primary and recurrent episodes. Systemic symptoms often associated with primary infection were also reduced with the oral compound. The dosage of oral acyclovir for treatment of primary and recurrent genital lesions is 200 mg five times daily for ten days. The dosage for recurrent episodes is 200 mg five times daily for five days.

Acute Episodes. A ten-day treatment regimen is recommended for the initial episode of herpes and a five-day treatment for recurrent lesions. Studies that were done to evaluate the effects of acyclovir on the episodes of recurrent herpetic lesions showed that patients did better when they themselves instituted the acyclovir treatment at the initial sign or symptom of a herpes outbreak than when they waited to see a physician. For this reason, it may be better for patients to have the medication on hand to begin treatment when the episodes recur.

Chronic Suppressive Therapy. In addition to treating individual episodes of herpes, work has also been done using acyclovir on a daily basis as chronic suppressive therapy. It has been shown that, when taken daily, acyclovir may prevent recurrent episodes of herpetic infections for as long as the medication is taken. However, once the medication is stopped, outbreaks recur. The recommended dosage of acyclovir for suppressive therapy is 200 mg three times daily for up to six months.

Side Effects. At the present time few side effects have been noted with acyclovir. Decreased spermatogenesis and mutagenesis have been reported with high doses of the drug in animal studies. Although not frequent, minor side effects such as nausea and vomiting have been seen with short-term administration of acyclovir for acute episodes of genital herpes. Headache and GI distress, although again not common, have been noted with patients in chronic suppressive treatment.

PSYCHOSOCIAL IMPLICATIONS

When treating sexually transmitted herpetic infections, the practitioner must not overlook the psychosocial issues raised. These issues appear greater in relation to herpetic infections because of the chronic, recurring nature of the infection. To the patient these issues may be just as important as the infectious process itself. Psychosocial support includes being able to provide the patient with information both about the infection and about the complications that may result. Two common areas often dealt with are neonatal infections and the risk of developing cancer as a result of herpetic infections.

Neonatal Infections. Most neonatal infections occur from a retrograde spread of the HSV-II infection from the genital tract of the mother or as a result of passage through the birth canal. The risk of infection is greater if the virus is present at the time of delivery and if the episode of infection is primary rather than recurrent. Patients need to be counseled about the possible alternative of cesarean section if infection is present at the time of delivery and if there is prolonged rupture of membranes. The possibility of transmitting infection to the child after birth also needs to be emphasized, along with the need for good practical hygiene to prevent spread of the virus.

Carcinoma of the Cervix. It has been suggested that genital herpetic infections may be a cause of carcinoma of the cervix. There seems to be a higher incidence of genital herpes and HSV-II antibodies in women with cervical carcinoma than in matched controls. It may be that these findings represent other variables, such as increased numbers of sexual partners or frequency of sexual activity, but this type of association has not been made between carcinoma and any other sexually transmitted disease.

At present it appears that we are able to offer patients with herpetic infections treatment not available in previous years. Because of the nature of the ongoing disease and the health threat it imposes, psychological support is considered a necessary part of this treatment. In spite of recent advances, herpes as a sexually transmitted disease continues to be a problem of increasing incidence and importance.

22 · SEXUALLY TRANSMITTED INFECTIONS

George A. Pankey
Harold P. Katner
OCHSNER CLINIC AND ALTON OCHSNER MEDICAL FOUNDATION

INTRODUCTION

An infectious disease that is sexually transmitted potentially affects all members of society. The long-term complications of sexually transmitted diseases, many of which may be undetected, have far-reaching ramifications for all members of society. Undetected infections in women can in many instances result in ectopic pregnancy, pelvic inflammatory disease, endometritis, salpingitis, and even sterility. In pregnant women, sexually transmitted infections can predispose to transplacental infection, premature labor, spontaneous abortion, or infection of the newborn during birth. There may be concomitant infections by a variety of pathogens, which makes accurate culture and diagnosis difficult. Fortunately, it is now becoming feasible to diagnose many potentially serious infections on the basis of clinical observation and laboratory testing.

In recent decades it has been recognized that certain segments of society have special needs regarding the management of their sexually transmitted diseases. This is the result not only of changing sexual orientations and sexual practices in our culture but also of the prevalence of various infecting organisms within subgroups of the population. Therefore, we have divided our chapter to discuss infections in homosexual or bisexual males as well as in the heterosexual population. (There is little evidence linking homosexuality in women to specific incidences of sexually transmitted infections). Specific chapters on some sexually transmitted diseases may be found elsewhere within the text.

Infections in Homosexual or Bisexual Males

During the past 15 years there has been a growing awareness of "gay-related diseases." Subsequent to the popularization of the Gay Rights Movement in the late 1960s, the homosexual minority became a vocal reality of Western culture. Long suppressed through nonacceptance, nonrecognition, and misunderstanding, this subculture began to identify itself as a community. Caught up in the sexual revolution that occurred in the late 1960s and 1970s, this group was plagued with a number of sexually transmitted diseases, as was society in general. It was recognized during this time that a number of diseases, such as hepatitis B and A, could be transmitted sexually and were highly prevalent in male homosexuals. The 1980s brought the AIDS epidemic, which chiefly hit the gay male community. It has since become apparent that many males are bisexual.

The significance of these events is that the effects are no longer restricted to male homosexuals but affect everyone. As physicians we are called on to treat and manage these problems. To do so without prejudice and with competency, we must understand homosexual practices as well as the emotional needs and medical problems of homosexuals.

SEXUAL PRACTICES

To evaluate the male homosexual adequately, a sexual history becomes imperative. The patient must be questioned as to whether he is orogenital active or passive, anogenital active or passive, and/or oral-anal active or passive; whether he has a single lover or multiple partners; and whether he participates in sadomasochistic practices such as fisting and piercing. It is beyond the scope of this chapter to discuss each of these in detail, but obviously if the patient is having anogenital intercourse, the rectum as well as the urethra should be evaluated adequately.

GONORRHEA

Infections with *Neisseria gonorrhoeae* may present in at least four different ways in male homosexuals; (1) genitourinary, (2) pharyngeal, (3) anorectal, and (4) disseminated. This is probably the most common sexually transmitted disease in the male homosexual community and has a two- to five-day incubation period.

GENITOURINARY INFECTION

Genitourinary infections may present asymptomatically, as urethritis with a purulent discharge and urethral discomfort, as epididymitis, as prostatitis, or as some combination of the above.

By far the most common presentation is uncomplicated urethritis. However, evaluation should include obtaining a history of painful or swollen testicles as well as of lower abdominal pain that worsens with urination, ejaculation, or defecation. Physical examination should include the urethra, testicles, epididymis, and prostate. An urethral swab often provides the answer on Gram stain alone, although culture is the gold standard. Culture becomes important if there is a high incidence of penicillin-resistant gonococci in the community, and as a test of cure after treatment.

PHARYNGEAL INFECTION

Pharyngeal infection is often asymptomatic and without physical findings, but may present with "sore throat" associated with pharyngeal erythema, with or without exudate. When this diagnosis is suspected, it can only be made definite with culture because the presence of nongonococcal *Neisseria* species in the throat makes a Gram stain useless.

ANORECTAL INFECTION

Anorectal infection may be asymptomatic or may present with tenesmus, mucopurulent discharge, rectal pain, or small amounts of blood in the stool. Symptomatic infections are present in less than 40% of patients and may be intermittently noted. Some of our patients have been misdiagnosed as having inflammatory bowel disease. Definitive diagnosis requires culture, but a positive Gram stain is sufficient to start therapy. Proctoscopic examination may be totally negative or show only nonspecific patchy mucosal lesions limited to the rectum.

DISSEMINATED INFECTION

Disseminated gonococcal infection in men is rare but may occur as a consequence of pharyngeal infection and possibly genitourinary involvement. The infection in this situation may involve the skin, joints, heart, and central nervous system. Fever, tenosynovitis, hemorrhagic pustules, and septic arthritis are the common features of this disease; endocarditis or meningitis are reported rarely. Diagnosis should be suspected from the history. Gram stain and culture of the skin lesions may be helpful but less so with joint fluid. In cases of endocarditis, gonococcus can be isolated from the blood, and with CNS involvement, spinal fluid may be positive.

Management of Genitourinary Infections

In uncomplicated urethral gonococcal infections, up to 40% of patients have been found to be coinfected with *Chlamydia trachomatis*. For this reason, in non–cephalosporin-allergic patients, we recommend ceftriaxone, 250 mg IM, followed by doxycycline (100 mg PO every 12 hours for seven days). In the cephalosporin-allergic patient, doxycycline alone is an alternative. When penicillin-resistant gonococci are documented or suspected, spectinomycin is recommended, 2 gm IM. Spectinomycin-resistant strains have also been documented. Nine trimethoprim-sulfamethoxazole 80/400-mg tablets, given as one dose daily for five days, may also be used.

Management of Pharyngeal Infections

Pharyngeal infections do not respond to ampicillin, amoxicillin, or spectinomycin. They do respond to ceftriaxone and to doxycycline. Pharyngitis due to penicillin-resistant gonococci can be treated with trimethoprim-sulfamethoxazole.

Management of Anorectal Infections

Anorectal infections respond to ceftriaxone and to spectinomycin, but not to ampicillin, amoxicillin, or tetracyclines.

If, for example, a patient is anal and oral receptive, with documented gonococcal infection, and is not cephalosporin allergic, treatment with ceftriaxone is recommended. If the same patient is cephalosporin allergic, a combination of doxycycline (for pharyngeal infection) plus spectinomycin (for rectal infection) is indicated.

Management of Disseminated Gonococcal Infections

In disseminated gonococcal infections, we recommend hospitalization and treatment with IV penicillin, 15 million units per day, until improvement occurs, followed by amoxicillin, 500 mg PO every eight hours for a total of seven days of treatment. Ceftriaxone, 2 gm daily IM, may be used for the patient who refuses hospitalization.

The homosexual male who is concerned about gonorrhea should have his urethra, posterior oropharynx, and rectum cultured even in the absence of signs and symptoms.

Management of these infections varies with the site, the incidence of penicillin- and tetracycline-resistant organisms in the community, and evidence or suspicion of coexistent infections (e.g., syphilis, *Chlamydia*).

An attempt should be made to treat all male and female sexual contacts, whether they are symptomatic or not. The likelihood of gonococcal infection may be decreased by the use of condoms.

CHLAMYDIA INFECTION

Chlamydia trachomatis is the major cause of nongonococcal urethritis in males. Its incidence varies among racial groups and it is thought to be most prevalent in heterosexual Caucasian males, but infection in homosexual males is not uncommon.

Patients who present with urethral discharge and dysuria and in whom gonorrhea has been ruled out should be evaluated for *Chlamydia*. Some authors feel that the quality of the discharge (mucoid with *Chlamydia*; purulent with gonorrhea) can help differentiate between the two infections but this is not always so. Because many laboratories cannot culture *Chlamydia* or have not yet obtained the rapid screening tests, empiric treatment is often prescribed.

Acute and chronic proctitis manifested by bloody, mucoid loose stools and rectal pain can occur in anal receptive patients. Diagnosis may require culture of a rectal biopsy.

Chlamydia has also been implicated as a cause of prostatitis, epididymitis, Reiter's syndrome (nongonococcal urethritis associated with arthritis, conjunctivitis, and dermal lesions occurring in HLA-B27 positive patients), and lymphogranuloma venereum (LGV). Some recent reports implicate *Chlamydia* as a cause of pharyngitis. We have also isolated it from the throats of asymptomatic males.

LGV is a systemic illness caused by certain strains of *C. trachomatis*. After a seven- to twelve-day incubation period following inoculation, a small, painless papule arises in an exposed area and is often missed by the patient. Subsequently, the infection spreads to the lymph nodes where swelling and matting of the nodes occur. Regression may take place, but often there is abscess formation with spontaneous drainage. Systemic manifestations may include fever, malaise, abdominal pain, nausea, vomiting, and urinary retention. If untreated, the infection may produce large, protruding swelling of the anal margin and rectal mucosa. Rectal strictures may develop. This remains a relatively uncommon disease but should be considered, especially if the patient gives a history of traveling to tropical or subtropical areas where this is more common.

Management

The treatment of uncomplicated chlamydial urethritis is doxycycline, 100 mg every 12 hours for seven days. If there is no response, treatment should be continued for another week. Erythromycin, 500 mg four times a day, or trimethoprim-sulfamethoxazole, 160/1600 mg twice daily for seven days, is also effective. Epididymitis and prostatitis may require longer therapy as judged by their clinical response. LGV requires three weeks of therapy.

As in gonorrhea, use of condoms decreases the chance of transmission of *Chlamydia*. Also, an attempt should be made to treat all male and female sexual contacts.

NONGONOCOCCAL, CHLAMYDIA-NEGATIVE URETHRITIS

In nongonococcal urethritis in homosexual males, only about 20% are positive for *Chlamydia*. Other etiologies of the syndrome have been looked for. *Ureaplasma urealyticum* has been implicated but not proved to be a cause. Enteric organisms that may have contaminated the urethra during rectal intercourse have also been implicated as a possible cause. Patients may present with a slightly to moderately clear, white, or gray morning discharge containing polymorphonuclear neutrophils (5 × 1000 × field). The incubation period is one to five weeks.

Management

Many of these infections respond to doxycycline, in regimens previously outlined. If no response is noted within seven days of therapy, some authors have recommended extending treatment to three weeks after noncompliance or reinfection has been ruled out.

The cause of the symptoms of a small percentage of patients may also be *Trichomonas vaginalis*, herpes simplex, *Candida*, or urethral condylomata acuminata (warts).

SYPHILIS

From 1970 to 1979 there was documented a more than 200% increase in the incidence of syphilis among homosexual men in the San Francisco area. Across the U.S. similar increases occurred.

Syphilis, caused by *Treponema pallidum*, presents in its primary form usually as a nontender, painless chancre. Chancres may be single or multiple and may be associated with regional lymphadenopathy. Again, evaluation in a homosexual male requires a thorough sexual history as well as physical examination. Chancres may be present in the oral cavity (e.g., tongue, lips, buccal mucosa); around or in the anus; on the rectal mucosa; and on the nipples, eyelids, fingers, wrists, and arms, as well as on the penis and scrotum. It is important to remember that secondarily infected chancres may be painful. Rectal chancres can be associated with rectal pain, diarrhea, constipation, rectal bleeding, and pain on defecation. Diagnosis can usually be made from the clinical evaluation and a dark-field evaluation (unless the lesion is within the mouth). Fluorescent treponema antibody absorption (FTA) is positive in over 95% of patients with primary syphilis.

Within a few weeks the disease enters the secondary stage. The manifestations of this form of syphilis are legion, including a variety of rashes, generalized lymphadenopathy, condylomata, noncicatricial alopecia, CNS involvement, and so on. Serologic diagnosis during this stage is invariably positive at high titers with the rapid plasma reagin test. Even if the disease is not treated, the titers will fall and the secondary manifestations spontaneously resolve.

If still left untreated, the patient goes into the latent stage where the spinal fluid serology remains negative. Early latent syphilis is defined as the first year following the secondary phase. Relapse with reappearance of "secondary lesions" can occur. If the patient still remains untreated, he may develop complications of late syphilis, which may include cardiovascular and neurologic involvement. Treatment and management are determined by the stage at time of diagnosis.

Management

Primary, secondary, or latent syphilis of less than one year's duration can be treated with benzathine penicillin G, 2.4 million units IM as a single dose. Patients allergic to penicillin can be treated orally with doxycycline, 100 mg every 12 hours for 15 days or erythromycin, 500 mg every six hours for 15 days. Latent syphilis of more than one year's duration without evidence of neurologic involvement (spinal tap for CSF and Venereal Disease Research Laboratory antibody and cell count required) should receive benzathine penicillin G, 2.4 million units IM every week for three successive weeks. Those allergic to penicillin can be treated orally with doxycycline, 100 mg every 12 hours for 30 days or erythromycin, 500 mg by mouth four times a day for 30 days, although there is no documentation of the adequacy of these regimens compared with penicillin. Some recommend the same regimens for tertiary syphilis with neurologic involvement or for those who have positive serology in CSF, but we use IV penicillin G, 15 million units per day for ten days followed by IM benzathine penicillin G, 2.4 million units weekly for three weeks. If patients are allergic to penicillin as determined by skin testing and have neurologic symptoms, we use doxycycline, 100 mg every eight hours for 42 days, or desensitize the patient to penicillin.

Procaine penicillin G, 4.8 million units IM and doxycycline, 100 mg every 12 hours for seven days are effective for incubating syphilis.

PROTOZOAL AND ENTERIC BACTERIAL PATHOGENS (GAY BOWEL SYNDROME)

In the late 1960s and early 1970s, infections with *Entamoeba histolytica* began to be recognized with increasing frequency in homosexual males. By the late 1970s the magnitude of this problem had reached epidemic proportions in some communities. Similar observations were made concerning the incidence of *Giardia lamblia* in this population. In the 1980s, *Cryptosporidia* became another related pathogen affecting this popu-

lation, but has been a major problem only among those with the acquired immune deficiency syndrome (AIDS).

The major reason for the spread of these pathogens is oral-anal contact (anilinction). Other possible mechanisms of spread include orogenital contact (fellatio) and, if the genitals have been contaminated previously with feces during anal intercourse and not washed, spread can occur from rectum to rectum with penises, fingers, contaminated colonic enema machines, or other shared foreign objects inserted into the rectum.

AMEBIASIS

The symptoms of amebiasis can range from none in carriers to diarrhea alternating with constipation, abdominal cramps, bloating, flatulence, and rarely systemic manifestations such as weight loss, fever, and prostration with amebic dysentery. More severe complications with hepatic, pulmonary, or brain abscesses are very rare with this form of the disease. Diagnosis can be made on stool examination, preferably a specimen obtained at proctosigmoidoscopy or a purged stool. Amebiasis should be strongly suspected if nonpathogenic protozoal cysts are also found, since up to two thirds of these patients have been found also to have *E. histolytica*.

Management

The simplest treatment of amebiasis, whether asymptomatic or not, is to use metronidazole, 750 mg PO three times a day for ten days. This dose will also eradicate *Giardia*. Patients should be warned to avoid ingestion of alcohol while taking metronidazole, to avoid a disulfiram (Antabuse) reaction.

GIARDIASIS

Giardiasis is usually asymptomatic but may present as explosive, foul-smelling diarrhea. A spectrum of symptoms may accompany the diarrhea including crampy abdominal pain, nausea, and flatulence. Anorexia and weight loss may occur with more chronic symptomatic infections, but usually the disease is self-limited. Patients with chronic infections tend to have episodic recurrence of symptoms.

Giardiasis is easy to diagnose when both purged and routine stools are examined.

Management

Treatment of giardiasis can be accomplished with seven days of quinacrine (Atabrine), 100 mg three times a day after meals or metronidazole, 250 mg three times a day.

The practice of anilinction, group anal sex, and oral sex with soiled penises has also predisposed the male homosexual community to *Shigella*, *Salmonella*, enteropathogenic *E. coli*, *Yersinia*, *Campylobacter*, and *Campylobacter*-like organisms. The management of these infections has been discussed in detail elsewhere. It must be remembered that if a male presents with severe diarrhea or dysentery secondary to one of these organisms, careful sexual history must be obtained so that proper patient education can be instituted.

SEXUALLY TRANSMITTED VIRAL INFECTIONS

The most common viral infections in homosexual males are due to cytomegalovirus and Epstein-Barr (EB)

Table 1. SEXUALLY TRANSMITTED PATHOGENS IN HOMOSEXUAL MALES

Pathogen	Disease or Syndrome
A. Bacteria	
1. *Neisseria gonorrhoeae*	Urethritis, epididymitis, proctitis, pharyngitis, prostatitis, disseminated gonococcal infection, sterility
2. *Chlamydia trachomatis*	Urethritis, epididymitis, proctitis, pharyngitis, lymphogranuloma venereum
B. Enteric Bacteria	
1. *Shigella* sp.	Diarrhea
2. *Campylobacter* sp. and related forms	Diarrhea
3. *Salmonella* sp.	Diarrhea
4. *Haemophilus ducreyi*	Chancroid (rare)
5. *Calymmatobacterium granulomatis*	Donovanosis (granuloma inguinale) (rare)
C. Virus	
1. Genital papilloma virus	Condyloma acuminatum, laryngeal or esophageal papilloma
2. Herpes simplex virus II	Initial and recurrent oral, genital, and anorectal herpes; aseptic meningitis
3. Hepatitis B virus	Acute hepatitis B, chronic active hepatitis, persistent (unresolved) hepatitis, polyarteritis nodosa, chronic membranous glomerulonephritis, mixed cryoglobulinemia, polymyalgia rheumatica, hepatocellular carcinoma
4. Cytomegalovirus	Heterophile-negative infectious mononucleosis, protean manifestations in immunosuppressed host (usually asymptomatic)
5. Hepatitis A virus	Acute hepatitis A
6. Molluscum contagiosum virus	Genital molluscum contagiosum, carcinoma of penis or anus
7. Hepatitis, non-A, non-B	Acute non-A, non-B hepatitis; persistent hepatitis; chronic active hepatitis
8. Human T-cell lymphotropic virus III	Acquired immune deficiency syndrome
9. Epstein-Barr virus	Mononucleosis (usually asymptomatic)
D. Spirochetes	
Treponema pallidum	Syphilis
E. Mycoplasma	
Ureaplasma urealyticum	Nongonococcal urethritis
F. Fungi	
Candida albicans	Balanitis
G. Protozoa	
1. *Trichomonas vaginalis*	Urethritis
2. *Entamoeba histolytica*	Diarrhea
3. *Giardia lamblia*	Diarrhea
H. Coccidia	
1. *Cryptosporidia*	Diarrhea
2. *Isospora belli*	Diarrhea
I. Metazoa	
1. *Phthirus pubis*	Pubic lice
2. *Sarcoptes scabiei*	Scabies

Table 2. BOWEL INFECTIONS IN HOMOSEXUAL MEN

	Proctitis	Proctocolitis	Enterocolitis	Enteritis
Anorectal pain	X	X		
Mucopurulent rectal discharge	X	X		
Bloody rectal discharge	X	X		
Tenesmus	X			
Constipation	X			
Diarrhea		X	X	X
Gonococcal infection, *C. trachomatis*, syphilis, herpes	X			
E. histolytica, Shigella, Campylobacter		X	X	
Giardia, Salmonella				X

virus, but these are usually asymptomatic and no treatment is recommended.

HERPES SIMPLEX

Herpes simplex infections are very common in the male homosexual community. The management of this problem is discussed elsewhere, but it is important to remember that herpes infections in gay males can have atypical presentations. Penile lesions may occasionally present within the urethra. Anorectal herpes usually causes severe rectal pain. If the infection extends or is present above the anal rings, severe inflammation and

induration may occur. Grossly these lesions may mimic anorectal carcinoma, requiring biopsy to make the diagnosis. Vesicular lesions of the hard palate are more likely to be herpetic rather than aphthous ulcers, which usually present on the buccal mucosa. Management of these infections, therefore, requires culture to confirm the diagnosis. Prevention includes avoiding sexual contact when active lesions are present. However, asymptomatic individuals can excrete the virus. Oral acyclovir is useful to treat active lesions and prevent frequent recurrences. Condoms decrease transmission of penile herpes.

HEPATITIS

In the early 1970s observations were made, and later confirmed, that various forms of hepatitis were sexually transmitted. Hepatitis A, shown to be transmitted via the fecal-oral route, has become epidemic in some male homosexual communities. The practice of anilinction places the patient at risk. As no vaccine against this virus exists, education remains the only means of preventing its spread.

A more significant problem has been the increasing prevalence of hepatitis B. The transmission of this infection has been correlated with passive anogenital intercourse, active oral-anal intercourse, rectal douching prior to passive anogenital intercourse, and passive manual anal intercourse (fist insertion into the rectum).

Management

With the development of the hepatitis B vaccine, we now have a way of preventing further spread of this potentially serious disease. The problem remains that many gay males are not aware of this risk nor of the vaccine. Education again must be our primary concern, especially when there are increasing numbers of carriers and patients with chronic active hepatitis B. Hepatitis B vaccine is indicated for all bisexual or homosexual males who do not have a hepatitis B antibody or antigen in the blood.

CONDYLOMATA ACUMINATA

Condylomata acuminata (venereal warts), caused by the human papillomavirus, are commonly found in the anorectal or urogenital area, but oral, vocal cord, and pharyngeal lesions also occur.

Management

Management depends on the extent of the warts and their responsiveness to topical therapy. Podophyllin in a 10% to 25% solution, the most successful of topical therapies, is applied to the lesions directly. Following the first application, it should be removed by washing with soap and water two hours later to avoid potential idiosyncratic reactions. Subsequent once-or-twice weekly applications are indicated until destruction of the wart is complete or for four weeks. Podophyllin should not be dispensed for home application, ulcerated warts, or very extensive warts and should never be injected into warts. Prolonged contact with podophyllin can cause second-degree burns.

Cryotherapy with liquid carbon dioxide (dry ice) or liquid nitrogen may be successful if podophyllin fails, especially in extensive warts. Occasionally, surgical excision and/or electrocautery is required. With extensive warts, general anesthesia may be required for adequate surgical removal. Recurrence following surgery is high, as it is with other methods. Laser therapy has been shown to be very effective and leaves few or no scars. The problem is that this form of therapy is not yet widely available.

MOLLUSCUM CONTAGIOSUM

Molluscum contagiosum, caused by a pox virus, is transmitted by close contact. Characteristically manifested by umbilicated papules in the pubic area, it is easily treated by curettage with a sharp dermal curet. Another approach involves expressing the content of the lesion with a curved forceps and destroying its base by touching it with phenol or silver nitrate.

INFECTED TRAUMATIC LESIONS ASSOCIATED WITH SEXUAL ACTIVITY

Infected anal fissures are common in males who participate in passive anal sex. The lesions are usually located posteriorly in the midline.

Management

Treatment is with a broad-spectrum antibiotic such as doxycycline plus cauterization with a 10% solution using silver nitrate on a cotton-tipped applicator, in conjunction with sitz baths and stool softeners. Healing usually occurs in three to four weeks. If the lesions are recurrent or unresponsive, surgical correction may be indicated. Anal intercourse and other forms of rectal trauma should be avoided during therapy.

Patients with retained foreign bodies in the rectum should be referred to a colorectal surgeon. Another increasingly recognized form of rectal trauma is associated with anal manual insertion (inserting the hands into the rectum for sexual stimulation), commonly known as fisting. Again, a colorectal surgeon should be consulted for careful evaluation if complications arising from this activity are suspected. Anal and rectal abrasions, perforation, and pelvic cellulitis have been reported. Broad-spectrum antibiotics as well as surgery are important in the management of these problems.

ACQUIRED IMMUNE DEFICIENCY SYNDROME

Of all the sexually transmitted diseases recognized in the homosexual male community, the most devastating has been the acquired immune deficiency syndrome (AIDS), caused by human T-cell lymphotropic virus type III infection (HTLV-III). It is beyond the scope of this chapter to discuss this in detail. If a patient is suspected of having AIDS, he should be sent to a tertiary care center, where appropriate evaluation can be performed. He should be referred to a person trained in infectious disease, preferably one who has had experience with AIDS.

REFERENCES

Centers for Disease Control: Sexually Transmitted Diseases Control Manual. DHHR 1985.

Centers for Disease Control: 1985 STD treatment guidelines. MMWR (Suppl), 34(4s), Oct 18, 1985.

Holmes KK, Mardh P, Sparling PF, et al: Sexually Transmitted Diseases. McGraw-Hill Book Co, New York, 1984.

Ostrow DG, Sandholzer TA, Felman YM (eds): Sexually Transmitted Diseases in Homosexual Men: Diagnosis, Treatment, and Research. Plenum Medical Book Co, New York, 1983.

Sexually Transmitted Diseases in Heterosexuals

Harold P. Katner
George A. Pankey
OCHSNER CLINIC AND ALTON OCHSNER MEDICAL FOUNDATION

GONORRHEA

The presentation of *Neisseria gonorrhoeae* in the heterosexual male is most often genitourinary, but pharyngeal and disseminated forms occur. In females, the spectrum of disease includes pharyngeal, anorectal, and disseminated infection, with a broad range of genitourinary manifestations. The clinical manifestations of pharyngeal and disseminated *gonorrhea* are no different from those in males (see p. 284).

Genitourinary Infection in the Female

Gonorrhea may cause dysuria, vaginal discharge, cervicitis, Bartholin's gland abscess, pelvic inflammatory disease, or any combination of these, but many if not most cases are asymptomatic.

Urethritis or urethral colonization usually accompanies endocervical infections, unless the patient has had a hysterectomy. The endocervix is the most common site of infection, which may present as an increase in vaginal discharge. Physical examination may be entirely normal or may reveal a mucopurulent endocervical discharge, friable endocervical mucosa, and/or erythema. With urethral involvement, a mucopurulent urethral discharge may be present. Bartholin's gland involvement presents as tender enlargement of the gland and swelling of the ipsilateral labia with abscess formation.

Pelvic Inflammatory Disease (PID)

One of the most serious complications of gonococcal infection in the female is pelvic inflammatory disease

(PID). It is estimated to occur in up to 15% of females infected with gonorrhea. Menstrual irregularities, lower abdominal pain, fever, chills, nausea, and vomiting may all be part of the presenting complaints. Physical findings range from significant tenderness with movement of the cervix or peritoneal findings to adnexal tenderness and masses. Tubo-ovarian abscess may result from salpingitis in PID. Rupture of such an abscess may result in peritonitis. Salpingitis may also lead directly to peritonitis or perihepatitis. Diagnosis of PID is supported by culture of endocervical and anorectal secretions or, if necessary, culdocentesis fluid, laparoscopically obtained fallopian tube exudate, or specimens obtained at surgery. Other bacteria, including *Chlamydia,* may be cultured. (For further discussion of PID, see Sect. IV, Chap. 9.)

Anorectal Infection

Anorectal gonorrhea occurs in females with or without a history of anal intercourse. A history of anal intercourse in a male suggests that he is bisexual. The presence of anorectal infection has been related to the duration of the endocervical infection, suggesting contamination from infected vaginal secretions. A significant percentage of infected individuals are asymptomatic. When symptoms do occur, pruritus, bleeding, a purulent discharge, or manifestations of proctitis can be expected. Routine culture of the anus in females suspected of having gonorrhea is carried out in many institutions and occasionally may be the only positive culture.

All male sexual partners of females with gonorrhea in any form should be treated with ceftriaxone and doxycycline, as outlined above.

SYPHILIS

The manifestations of syphilis are no different from those described for homosexual males (p. 285). A careful sexual history will help direct a more careful physical examination looking for "atypical" sites of primary lesions. A history of anal intercourse in a female with or without symptoms warrants examination by anoscopy or proctosigmoidoscopy.

Management

Management is no different for heterosexual males or nonpregnant females from that outlined for homosexual males. Pregnant females should be screened at their first prenatal visit with a rapid plasma reagent serology (RPR). If the test is negative but the patient is at high risk of contracting syphilis, the RPR should be repeated during the third trimester.

If syphilis is documented in a pregnant, nonallergic patient with a history of recent sexual exposure to an infected individual, benzathine penicillin G should be administered, in accordance with recommendations outlined for homosexual males.

In penicillin-allergic pregnant patients, the recommended treatment is erythromycin, 500 mg PO every six hours for 15 (for early and latent syphilis) to 30 days (for neurosyphilis).

TRICHOMONIASIS

Trichomonas vaginalis is a flagellated protozoan. Nonvenereal transmission probably occurs, but the most common means of transmission is believed to be sexual. It is predominantly an infection of the lower genitourinary tract in both men and women. Most women infected with *Trichomonas* are asymptomatic. Symptoms range from vaginal discharge, dyspareunia, dysuria, and urinary frequency to lower abdominal pain in rare instances. Physical examination may reveal a profuse vaginal discharge that is frothy and white.

Most men with *Trichomonas* are asymptomatic, but mild urethral itching or burning may be present.

Management

Metronidazole, 2 gm PO in a single dose, for the patient and the sexual partner(s) is the regimen of choice. Where treatment has failed, retreatment is recommended.

Because metronidazole is not recommended throughout pregnancy and contraindicated in the first trimester, clotrimazole, a 100-mg suppository intravaginally at bedtime for seven days, has been used with some success.

VAGINITIS

It is estimated that approximately 28% of women who attend clinics specializing in sexually transmitted infections exhibit the symptoms of vaginitis. Undoubtedly this is a common complaint of women in the clinical patient population as a whole. In postmenopausal women, the usual forms of infection should be distinguished from vaginal atrophy accompanying hormonal change.

Common forms of vaginitis include bacterial vaginosis, vulvovaginal candidiasis, *Gardnerella vaginalis,* and *Ureaplasma urealyticum.* (For further discussion, see Sect. VII, Chap. 21.)

REFERENCES

Centers for Disease Control: 1985 STD treatment guidelines. MMWR, 34(4S), Oct 18, 1985.
Holmes KK, Mardh PA, Sparling PF, et al (eds): Sexually Transmitted Diseases. McGraw-Hill Book Co, New York, 1984.
Medical Letter on Drugs and Therapeutics: Treatment of sexually transmitted diseases. 28:23–28, 1986.
Pritchard JA, MacDonald PC, Gant NF. Williams Obstetrics, 17th ed. Appleton-Century-Crofts, Norwalk, CT, 1985.

BLOOD AND NEOPLASTIC DISORDERS

ERNEST BEUTLER
JAMES K. WEICK

1 • BONE MARROW TRANSPLANTATION IN THE TREATMENT OF SEVERE APLASTIC ANEMIA

Wayne Spruce
SCRIPPS CLINIC AND RESEARCH FOUNDATION

ETIOLOGIC CONSIDERATIONS

Until the advent of bone marrow transplantation, severe aplastic anemia was associated with a high mortality rate. Most patients would succumb within the first six months of the onset of their disease. Treatment with anabolic steroids and corticosteroids had, in most cases, been disappointing and most patients died of hemorrhagic or infectious complications. The presenting symptoms of marrow aplasia are a result of the marrow failure and are usually easy bruising, spontaneous bleeding, and/or infection.

Severe aplastic anemia is a relatively uncommon disorder with an incidence of about 65 per million in adults over 65 years of age and 4 per million in children. Approximately 25% of cases occur in individuals under the age of 20 years and 30% in patients over the age of 60 years. Males and females are equally affected. While there are well-described congenital forms of marrow aplasia including Fanconi's anemia, the majority of the cases are acquired. A variety of etiologic agents including chemicals, drugs, ionizing radiation, and infections has been implicated. Occasionally pregnancy and thymomas have been associated with marrow failure, and paroxysmal nocturnal hemoglobinurea may occasionally present with pancytopenia. The best known drug association is the rare but often fatal association with chloramphenicol. Benzine and insecticides are chemical agents that have been implicated in cases of aplastic anemia. In spite of the multitude of possible etiologic agents, the majority of patients present with no clear-cut cause of their marrow failure.

DIAGNOSTIC CRITERIA

The criteria for severe marrow aplasia include a markedly hypocellular marrow and peripheral blood with any two of the three following findings: a neutrophil count of less than 500/dl, a platelet count of less than 20,000/dl, and a corrected reticulocyte count of less than 1%. Bone marrow aspirations are not adequate to make the diagnosis and a bone marrow biopsy is mandatory.

PATHOPHYSIOLOGY

Since aplastic anemia is not a single disease, the pathophysiology cannot be explained with a single concept. Theoretically, marrow failure could be explained as failure of the pleuripotential stem cell, or a failure of its microenvironment. Until recently it was felt that most cases of marrow failure resulted from an isolated failure of the stem cell. However, clinical experience in human marrow transplantation indicates that at least in some cases the cause may reside in the immune system. There are many well-documented cases of spontaneous autologous marrow recovery after unsuccessful attempts at marrow grafting. In addition, at least half of identical twin transplants have failed when no immunosuppression was used. Also, a growing number of individuals have been successfully treated with antithymocyte globulin (ATG). These observations implicate an immune mechanism in at least some patients.

PHARMACOLOGIC AND IMMUNOLOGIC THERAPY

Most of this chapter will deal with bone marrow transplantation as the treatment for severe aplastic anemia; however, a brief description of other forms of therapy will also be presented.

STEROIDS

Treatment with androgens such as testosterone and oxymetholone was reported to result in remission of severe marrow aplasia in small numbers of patients in the early 1960s. These reports were not confirmed in larger numbers of patients, and more recent studies in the 1970s showed that they provided no advantage over modern supportive care. Likewise, corticosteroids in conventional doses (1 to 2 mg/kg) and immunosuppressive drugs such as cyclophosphamide have been reported to be effective in small numbers of patients. Confirmation in larger numbers of patients is lacking.

ANTITHYMOCYTE GLOBULIN

Since Mathe's original report on autologous marrow recovery in three out of seven patients treated with antithymocyte globulin (ATG) in 1970, there have been many other studies confirming its efficacy used alone, with haplo-identical marrow, or with androgens. The doses of ATG and the source of the material have varied greatly from study to study. However, the response rate in most series is between 40% and 70%. Many patients do not respond completely; however, the majority of them are transfusion free. The role of haplo-identical marrow and androgens remains unclear. The use of large doses of methylpredisolone (20 mg/kg) along with ATG by the Swiss group has shown responses in 15 of 16 patients so treated. In most series of patients, the time to response has varied from a few weeks to several months and relapses have been seen in up to 10% of patients.

The toxic effect of ATG is considerable and includes fever, chills, urticaria, and hypotension. In addition, platelet counts usually drop and may be difficult to support. Many of these side effects can be modified with the use of antihistamines and corticosteroids. Many patients will develop serum sickness, which can usually be prevented or treated with corticosteroids.

Bone Marrow Transplantation

HISTOCOMPATIBILITY

HLA System. Early clinical work, primarily in murine systems, showed that marrow could be successfully transplanted in lethally irradiated animals only when they were histocompatible as determined by the H2 complex. The human equivalent is called the human leukocyte antigen (HLA) system. There is a series of closely related loci on the number six chromosome designated HLA-A, B, C, and D, which make up the human histocompatibility complex. Because of their close proximity on the chromosome, they are inherited as a unit in a mendelian codominant manner. Thus siblings have a 25% chance of being HLA identical. The A, B, C, and DR (D-related) loci are determined by anti-HLA antisera, and the D loci by the mixed lymphocyte culture. HLA testing can be done at all transplant centers and by most major blood banks. By and large, the majority of successful transplants have been performed between individuals who are HLA identical. At present, a patient must have siblings to have a marrow transplant for aplastic anemia. There have been occasional reports of successful transplants using parental or unrelated donors who are phenotypically identical to the patient, but these are rare.

PATIENT EVALUATION PRIOR TO TRANSPLANTATION

Once the diagnosis has been established, a decision needs to be made as to whether the patient is a candidate for transplantation. HLA typing of the patient and family should be done as soon as possible. The results of the HLA typing and mixed lymphocyte culture can usually be available within a week. Transplantation in patients over the age of 40 years is not usually successful, and these individuals should be considered for other forms of treatment.

During the evaluation period, blood product transfusions should be given very judiciously to avoid exposure of the patient to foreign antigens that might lead to graft rejection. Donors who are family members should be especially avoided. However, if the patient is extremely anemic or bleeding, transfusions should be given. The use of washed or frozen red cells and single donor, unrelated platelets may help to minimize sensitization. Infections should be treated vigorously; however, it may be necessary to go ahead with the transplant even in the face of active infections.

PREPARATIVE REGIMENS

Work done in animal systems showed that some form of immunosuppression was necessary in order for a marrow transplant to be successful. This has proved to be true in the human situation as well. Currently most centers, including our own, employ cyclophosphamide as the backbone of the preparative regimen. The dose is 50 mg/kg of lean body weight given intravenously over one hour daily for four days (total dose is 200 mg/kg). Most patients experience intense nausea and vomiting with the drug that lasts from several hours to several days. Other prominent side effects of the drug include an antidiuretic effect, hemorrhagic cystitis, and very rarely cardiac toxicity. Because of the antidiuretic effect and risk of hemorrhagic cystitis, a high urine flow must be maintained. A balanced electrolyte solution containing sodium bicarbonate, potassium, and furosemide (10 mg/L) is infused at a rate of 3000 ml/24 hours/m². In addition, we use continuous bladder irrigation with urologic saline at 1 liter per hour beginning at the time of the first cyclophosphamide infusion and continuing for 24 to 48 hours after the last dose of the drug.

In patients who have not been sensitized by prior blood product transfusions, this preparative regimen is usually adequate to allow engraftment. However, the majority of patients with aplastic anemia have required some blood component support either with packed cells or with platelets prior to coming to transplant. In these patients there is a definite risk of graft rejection, which may be as high as 30%, and additional immunosuppression appears to be necessary. Several methods have been used to provide additional immunosuppression. Our group currently employs total lymph node irradiation as suggested by the transplant group at the University of Minnesota. It involves the delivery of 750 rads of irradiation to all the major lymph node–bearing areas at a rate of approximately 25 rads per minute. The total nodal irradiation is delivered 24 hours after the last dose of cyclophosphamide. Other centers have used total body irradiation from 300 to 600 rads, and others have employed additional drugs such as Myleran and procarbazine; all of these methods have been successful in reducing the graft rejection rate to less than 10%. The Seattle group employs unirradiated donor buffy coat transfusions after the marrow transplant for four to five days. Recently cyclosporine has been reported by several European centers to be effective in reducing graft rejection.

MARROW PROCUREMENT

Donors should have a complete physical examination, complete blood count, liver and renal function tests, electrocardiogram, and chest film prior to being accepted. In the event of more than one donor, an individual who is younger, of the same sex, and of the same blood group as the patient should be chosen.

The donor is usually admitted to the hospital a day before the procedure. On the morning of donation the patient is taken to the operating room and, under general anesthesia, the marrow is aspirated from the posterior and, if necessary, anterior iliac crests. During the aspirating procedure the marrow is mixed with tissue culture media (TC 199, Difco Labs) that contains 5000 units of preservative-free heparin per 100 ml of tissue culture media. The total volume of the marrow that is taken will depend on the size and weight of the patient and donor, and on the cellularity of the marrow. Manual cell counts need to be performed during the procedure, and the final cell concentration should be greater than 3×10^{-8} nucleated cells per kg of recipient weight. Cell yields below this are correlated with an increased incidence of rejection. Once the marrow has been collected, it is screened through two sizes of metal mesh screens placed on the bottom of cut-off syringes and then placed in a standard blood transfer pack. If there is no major blood group incompatibility between the donor and recipient, the marrow is transfused immediately.

POST-TRANSPLANT SUPPORTIVE CARE

ENVIRONMENT

After the marrow infusion, most patients remain pancytopenic for three to four weeks. During this period of time, patients should be nursed in single rooms and individuals involved with the care of the patient should observe careful handwashing techniques. Conventional reverse isolation techniques are probably of little value. Patients nursed in laminar air flow with gut decontamination and sterile food may have a decreased incidence of graft-versus-host disease (GVHD) and serious infections.

HYPERALIMENTATION

Because of infections and oral mucositis, most patients are unable to meet their caloric needs orally. Hyperalimentation is therefore needed in the majority of patients. We use standard hyperalimentation solutions and attempt to provide 80% to 90% of the patient's caloric needs parenterally.

TRANSFUSIONS

In the majority of patients, adequate blood product support can be provided with packed red blood cell transfusions and random donor platelet transfusions. To avoid the risk of engraftment of lymphocytes in these products, all blood products are irradiated with 2500 rads.

Occasionally patients will become refractory to random donor platelets and require single donor platelets. The marrow donor is usually the best donor in this situation, although other family members may be used.

It is our practice to attempt to keep the hemoglobin in the range of 10 gm/dl and the platelet count above 20,000.

TRANSPLANT-RELATED COMPLICATIONS

GRAFT REJECTION

Failure of engraftment, or graft rejection, is a problem that is seen primarily in marrow transplantation for aplastic anemia. In the early series of patients reported by Seattle the rejection rate was approximately 30%, and other centers reported rates that were even higher. In analyzing their data, two factors were consistently related to graft failure: (1) patients who had been transfused with blood products prior to undergoing preparation for transplantation had a much higher rate of rejection than those who were untransfused; and (2) those patients who received greater than 3×10^{-8} of nucleated cells had a much lower rejection rate. Other factors such as patient/donor sex or age have not proved to be of significant prognostic value. Several methods have been developed to circumvent this problem and they have been alluded to in the section on preparative regimens.

INFECTIONS

Infections are the second major post-transplant complication. Many patients with aplastic anemia may already be infected at the time they come to transplantation, and the majority of patients will become clinically septic within the first few days after receiving their marrow graft. Preventive measures are usually not successful in preventing infections in these profoundly immunosuppressed patients. The use of laminar air flow in conjunction with gut decontamination with nonabsorbable antibiotics and sterile food and linen has been shown to decrease infections but has not improved survival.

Management

The most common organisms that infect patients during the first 30 post-transplant days are staphylococcal species, gram-negative gut flora, and fungi. Therefore, when patients become febrile, empiric broad-spectrum antibiotics should be started. It has been our practice to start patients on a semisynthetic penicillin such as ticarcillin at 3 gm every four hours, an aminoglycoside such as gentamicin or tobramycin at 5 mg/kg/day in three divided doses, and a cephalosporin such as cefazolin at 1 gm every six hours. Peak and trough blood levels of the aminoglycoside should be obtained to prevent renal toxic effects and ototoxicity and to ensure therapeutic blood levels. Prior to the institution of antibiotic therapy, patients should have blood, urine and throat cultures obtained. Frequently, in spite of the clinical appearance of sepsis, no positive cultures will be obtained and the antibiotic choice must remain empiric. If the patient continues to be clinically septic after the institution of triple antibiotic coverage, we add amphotericin B, starting at 0.1 mg/kg/day and increasing the dose by 0.1 mg/kg/day up to 0.5 to 0.7 mg/kg/day; when this dose has been reached, the drug is given on an every-other-day schedule. The drug is administered over three to four hours. In patients who have positive cultures, antibiotic choice can, of course, be guided by the sensitivity reports. Patients who have persistently positive blood cultures in spite of optimal antibiotics should be considered for granulocyte transfusions. To avoid the risk of serious pulmonary reactions, granulocytes should be separated from amphotericin by as much time as possible. When granulocytes are started, they should be continued until the patient is culture negative and the absolute granulocyte count is over 500/dl.

Herpes simplex infections in the oral and genital regions can develop during the early post-transplant period. The antiviral drug acyclovir given intravenously at a dose of 10 mg/kg/dose every eight hours is usually effective in suppressing these infections. Occasionally, repeated 10-day courses may be necessary.

After the granulocyte count has increased to greater than 500/dl, the risk of serious bacterial and fungal infections is reduced except in those patients who have significant GVHD. These patients often require corticosteroids (2 to 4 mg/kg) and other immunosuppressive measures to control the process and, hence, are at continued risk for bacterial and especially fungal infections. In addition, the return of humoral and cellular immunity is delayed in these patients, further aggravating the situation.

INTERSTITIAL PNEUMONIA

Interstitial pneumonia is a major problem after the first 30 post-transplant days. The incidence is lowest in those patients who do not receive radiation as part of the preparative regimen and in those patients who have identical twin (syngeneic) donors. Other risk factors include older age and the presence of GVHD. About 80% of the cases are either idiopathic or related to cytomegalovirus (CMV). Rarely other viruses or *Pneumocystis* can be the cause of interstitial pneumonia. Patients present with steadily increasing hypoxia with a paucity of physical findings. The chest film usually shows a progressively worsening picture of interstitial infiltrates.

Management

Patients with severe GVHD have a very high mortality rate and to date there has been no effective treatment. Antiviral drugs have not proved effective, and the use of high titer immune plasma of globulin has not been successful. There has been some early evidence that the prophylactic use of high titer CMV immune globulin may be effective in preventing the development of interstitial pneumonia.

Herpes zoster infections can occur in up to 50% of patients following transplantation. The peak incidence is at five months. The majority of these patients are still very immunocompromised and at risk of cutaneous and visceral dissemination. It is our practice to start these patients on acyclovir in the same doses used for herpes simplex infections and to treat for 10 days. In most patients this is adequate treatment. Occasionally, patients will reactivate their disease and require second and even third courses of the drug.

GRAFT-VERSUS-HOST DISEASE (GVHD)

Acute GVHD. GVHD is the third major complication of marrow transplantation. It results from the reaction of an immunologically competent donor against an immunologically compromised host. The effector cells are thought to be donor-cytotoxic T lymphocytes. The incidence of severe GVHD is between 40% and 70% in fully HLA identical allogeneic transplants. The severe form is seen in approximately 25% to 30% of patients. The target organs are the skin, the gastrointestinal tract, and the liver. The clinical manifestations of the disorder range from a mild macular skin rash, mild gastrointestinal discomfort and asymptomatic liver functional abnormalities to a fulminant and often fatal form with massive epidermolysis, liver failure, and large quantities of diarrhea. Death in these patients is most often from intercurrent bacterial, fungal, or viral infections. A grading system for the degree of organ involvement has been developed by the Seattle group and is used by most transplant centers. Grades 1 and 2 are considered the mildest forms, and grades 3 and 4 are the most severe forms which are associated with the highest mortality. Advancing age appears to be the greatest risk factor.

Methotrexate given intermittently over the first 100 post-transplant days has been the most commonly used method of attempting to prevent GVHD. It is given at 15 mg/m^2 on the first post-transplant day and at 10 mg/m^2 on day +3, +6, +11, and then weekly thereafter. Most groups have also added prednisolone at 0.5 to 2 mg/kg/day to the methotrexate regimen. Antithymocyte globulin has also been used by some centers but the results have been inconsistent.

Cyclosporine has been employed by many groups, usually starting two to three days prior to marrow infusion and continuing for the first three to six months post transplant. However, its place in the prevention and treatment of acute GVHD remains to be established. Several groups, including our own, have been exploring the use of anti–T cell monoclonal antibodies in an attempt to remove the T cells from the marrow prior to infusion. Preliminary results in fully matched patients look promising. Finally, the Seattle group has reported a decreased incidence of grade 2–4 acute GVHD in patients cared for in a laminar air flow environment.

Chronic GVHD. The chronic form of GVHD can occur in up to 30% of patients any time after the first 100 post-transplant days. It may develop as an extension of the acute form of the disease, after a quiescent period, or de novo. This syndrome may involve multiple organ systems including the skin, liver, gastrointestinal tract, eyes, lungs, hematopoietic system, and musculoskeletal system. The disorder has many of the characteristics of a collagen vascular disease. These patients as well as those with the acute form of the disease have a marked delay in the return of their immune function and, hence, they are at high risk for developing serious overwhelming infections. Most patients suffer from chronic skin rashes, hyperpigmentation and hypopigmentation, loss of subcutaneous tissues, dry mouth and eyes, chronic diarrhea, and liver disease manifested by elevations of the transaminases, alkaline phosphatase, and bilirubin. Many patients are thrombocytopenic and may have low white blood counts, but interestingly, they are not usually anemic. Some suffer from muscle weakness and cramps and occasionally joint effusions.

Treatment has been most successful with the use of oral prednisone, usually in doses of 1 to 2 mg/kg/day. Azathioprine in doses of 1.5 mg/kg/day has been used by the Seattle group in addition to prednisone and initially appeared to improve survival; however, a subsequent randomized trial has failed to confirm their earlier results. The latter patients were treated earlier and were usually placed on prophylactic trimethoprim-sulfamethoxazole, and received more aggressive supportive care. In any event, the survival of these patients has improved in recent years.

FOLLOW-UP

The length of hospitalization will vary for each patient and depend on several factors including the rapidity of engraftment, the severity of infections, the presence of GVHD and its severity, and the nutritional status of the patient. Most patients will spend a total of 40 to 60 days in the hospital. In younger individuals, for those in good general condition prior to undergoing transplantation, and in those with few complications, the period may be shorter. Once individuals are released from the hospital, most require close outpatient follow-up for at least two additional months. The patient's graft status and GVHD must be monitored closely. It is the practice of most transplant centers to keep patients under close observation for the first three months after marrow transplantation and then to return them to their referring physician.

COST

The cost of the procedure can be quite variable, depending primarily on the length of stay in the hospital and the number of transplant-related complications that the patient experiences. In spite of rising medical costs, the cost for most transplants has remained relatively constant and is in the range of $75,000 to $100,000. When one compares this with the cost of repeated hospitalizations to treat complications of severe aplastic anemia, it appears to be cost-effective.

Because of its complexity, and the need for highly trained medical and paramedical support, this is not a procedure that is likely to be easily transported to community hospitals. At present it is limited to those institutions that have the necessary experienced staff and facilities to care for these patients.

CLINICAL RESULTS AND CONCLUSIONS

Over the last decade the clinical results for allogeneic marrow transplantation have improved. Long-term survival ranges from 40% to around 70%. This can be attributed to several factors including earlier transplantation and better supportive care during the period of pancytopenia. The development of methods to prevent graft rejection has clearly been the most important factor in improving the clinical results in aplastic anemia.

While a great deal of progress has been made over this period of time, GVHD and the lack of a histocompatible donor continue to be major problems in the field. If one could obviate GVHD, the limitations of age and histocompatibility could be removed. As discussed previously, few patients over the age of 40 are successfully transplanted; this is primarily due to the increased incidence of GVHD. In fact, the mortality associated with the procedure rises rapidly after the age of 20.

There have been occasional reports of successful transplant between less than fully matched patients and in a few patients using unrelated fully matched donors. However, by and large, these attempts have not been successful. Attempts at removing donor T cells from the marrow have been successful in fully matched patients, but the results in mismatched patients have been disappointing and clearly much more work needs to be done in this area. These problems are currently being worked on in many marrow transplant centers and it is hoped we will see some positive results in the near future. Until these problems are worked out, individuals who are over the age of 40 and those without histocompatible donors should be considered for treatment with alternative forms of therapy such as antithymocyte globulin.

REFERENCES

Champlin R, Ho W, Bayever E, et al: Treatment of aplastic anemia: results with bone marrow transplantation, antithymocyte globulin and a monoclonal anti T-cell antibody. *In* Young N, Levine A, Humphries R: Asplastic Anemia, Stem Cell Biology and Advances in Treatment. Alan R. Liss Inc, New York, 1984, pp 227–238.

Forman S, Hows J: Bone marrow failure. *In* Blume K, Petz L (eds): Clinical Bone Marrow Transplantation. Churchill-Livingstone, New York, 1983, pp 215–214.

Ramsay NKC, Kim T, Nesbit ME, et al: Total lymphoid irradiation and cyclophosphamide as preparation for bone marrow transplantation in severe aplastic anemia. Blood 55:344–346, 1980.

Spruce W, McMillan R, Beutler E: Bone marrow transplantation for the treatment of severe aplastic anemia. Clin Hematol 12:285–310, 1983.

Storb R, Thomas ED, Buckner CD, et al: Marrow transplantation for aplastic anemia. Semin Hematol 21:27–35, 1984.

Sullivan K: Graft versus host disease. *In* Blume K, Petz L (eds): Clinical Bone Marrow Transplantation. Churchill-Livingstone, New York, 1983, pp 91–120.

Thomas ED, Storb R: Technique for human marrow grafting. Blood 36:507–515, 1970.

Young N, Speck B: Antithymocyte and antilymphocyte globulins: clinical trials and mechanisms of action. *In* Young N, Levine A, Humphries R: Aplastic Anemia, Stem Cell Biology and Advances in Treatment. Alan R. Liss Inc, New York, 1984, pp 221–226.

Zaia JA: Infections. *In* Blume K, Petz L (eds): Clinical Bone Marrow Transplantation. Churchill-Livingstone, New York, 1983, pp 131–168.

2 · IRON DEFICIENCY

Virgil F. Fairbanks
MAYO CLINIC AND MAYO FOUNDATION

DEFINITIONS AND DIAGNOSTIC CRITERIA

Iron deficiency is the condition in which total body iron content is less than normal for a person's age and sex. Three stages of iron deficiency are recognized: (1) iron depletion, wherein the normal iron storage pools of ferritin and hemosiderin are markedly reduced or absent but blood hemoglobin and serum iron concentrations are normal and no physiologic effects of iron deficiency are demonstrable; (2) iron deficiency without anemia, wherein the iron storage pools are absent, serum iron concentration may be reduced, and such effects of iron deficiency as decreased work tolerance or epithelial changes may be demonstrated although there is no anemia or morphologic change in erythrocytes; and (3) iron deficiency anemia.

In general, as iron deficiency progresses, it is reflected in the sequence of abnormalities in laboratory test results shown in Table 1.

While Table 1 shows the general pattern in which changes of iron deficiency evolve, exceptions are common. It is not unusual for the serum iron concentration (SI), total iron binding capacity (TIBC), and transferrin saturation to be normal even when anemia and microcytosis are evident. Consequently, these assays are of limited diagnostic value. Serum ferritin assay, now generally available, should supplant assay of SI as a diagnostic test. Normal values for serum ferritin vary between laboratories, depending on the method used. For a commonly used immunoradiometric assay, a value of 10 µg/L or less is usually diagnostic of iron deficiency. A major limitation of the ferritin assay is that the serum ferritin concentration is usually elevated in the presence of chronic disease, such as rheumatoid arthritis, infections, and malignancies including lymphomas and leukemias, and this elevation may obscure concomitant iron deficiency.

Review of a Wright-stained blood film, when interpreted in the context of the clinical history, often suffices for the diagnosis of iron deficiency anemia. However, thalassemias and hemoglobinopathies are so prevalent in our society that one must be careful not to mistake these for iron deficiency. Thalassemic disorders are especially common in those of Italian, Greek, or Asian descent, and in American blacks. Of the nearly one million Indochinese refugees now resettled in the United States, nearly 30% have either a thalassemia or a hemoglobin E disorder, or both, and these are not readily distinguished from iron deficiency anemia by examination of peripheral blood film. Furthermore, erythrocytic hypochromia and microcytosis are also characteristic of chronic disease in the absence of iron deficiency. Since it may be hazardous to administer iron to patients with these disorders, proper diagnosis is important.

PATHOPHYSIOLOGY

Iron deficiency develops when the loss of iron, by bleeding or excretion, exceeds the gain of iron from intestinal absorption of food iron or medicinal iron given orally or parenterally. In very young children, iron deficiency may also develop when the iron demand of body growth exceeds the iron gain. Iron deficiency in children may be due either to inadequate iron intake (as when the diet is mostly milk) or to bleeding, or both. However, *in adults iron deficiency always signifies blood loss* unless, with rare exceptions, proven otherwise. One interesting exception merits note. The iron deficiency that commonly develops many years following subtotal gastric resection with gastrojejunostomy is usually due to markedly reduced absorption of food iron, mostly heme. Such patients absorb medicinal iron readily and thus are easily treated.

Normal adult men lose about 1 mg of iron daily, mostly in exfoliated intestinal epithelial cells. Whereas premenopausal women lose, on average, approximately an additional 1 mg of iron daily from menstrual bleeding, their dietary iron intake is often insufficient to compensate for this aggregate daily iron loss of about 2 mg. Furthermore, the iron cost of the average full-term pregnancy is nearly 1000 mg, and this exacerbates the tenuousness of iron balance.

CLINICAL ASPECTS

TISSUE EFFECTS

Because iron is an important component of numerous enzymes, especially those of the Krebs cycle, and of cytochromes, and because many of these enzymes are very sensitive to iron depletion, histopathologic changes and dysfunction of many organs and tissues accompany iron deficiency even in the early stages of its evolution. Epithelial atrophy or metaplasia occurs in the oral and pharyngeal mucosa, and may be manifested as glossitis or angular cheilitis or the formation of postcricoid pharyngeal webs. Such webs are characteristic of the syndrome of sideropenic dysphagia (Paterson-Kelly or Plummer-Vinson syndrome). Carcinomas also occur in the postcricoid area, with an increased frequency in those who have had chronic iron deficiency. Koilonychia, or "spoon nails," also occurs more frequently in persons with chronic iron deficiency than in the general population. The koilonychia may be due to impairment of an iron enzyme. Not all koilonychia is the result of iron deficiency, as it seems also to occur as a hereditary trait in some families.

PHYSIOLOGIC EFFECTS

Impaired exercise tolerance of iron-deficient rats and humans has been demonstrated by various techniques. This effect has been demonstrated both prior to

Table 1. STAGES OF IRON DEFICIENCY

	Hemoglobin Concentration (gm/dl)	Hypochromia	MCV	Serum Iron Concentration	Serum Ferritin Concentration
Iron depletion (early or latent iron deficiency)	N	N	N	N	L
Iron deficiency without anemia	N	N	N	N to L	L
Early iron deficiency anemia	10–12	N to Sl	N to L	N to L	L
Moderate iron deficiency anemia	8–10	Sl to Mod	L	L	L
Marked iron deficiency anemia	<8	Mod to Mk	L	L	L

Abbreviations: N, normal; L, low; Sl, slight; Mod, moderate; Mk, marked.

and after onset of anemia. While most studies have confirmed the reduction in exercise tolerance, some have not.

Human neonates who are iron deficient exhibit reduction in normal response to stimuli and may have somewhat retarded neurologic maturation.

Phagocytic activity of leukocytes is impaired in iron deficiency, and reduction in activity of some leukocyte enzymes has been reported. An as yet unresolved issue is whether iron deficiency improves or worsens the host response to infections. The impairment in phagocytic activity may be compensated by the depriving of the microorganism of iron, which it also demands for proliferation and full expression of virulence.

SYMPTOMS AND SIGNS

Many of the symptoms of iron deficiency are the same as in any other anemia: fatigue, palpitations, tinnitus, and headaches. Pica or pagophagia (compulsive ice eating) is common, as is compulsive eating of earth, clay, or laundry starch. Pallor may be evident when anemia is severe. The spleen is palpable in perhaps 5% to 10% of cases. Dependent edema may occur if severe anemia has led to cardiac decompensation. Koilonychia may be due to iron deficiency, but is very rare in North America. Besides the changes in erythrocytes described earlier, mild leukopenia is observed in about 10% of cases, but the leukocyte count is rarely less than 3.0×10^9/L. The differential is normal. Thrombocytosis is common in children with iron deficiency anemia. In adults, platelets may be slightly less than normal, or, if bleeding is active, they may be increased.

Surprisingly, patients with iron deficiency anemia, even when marked, often admit to few subjective symptoms of fatigue or functional impairment. This is true of other anemias as well, for example, pernicious anemia, and testifies to the extraordinary physiologic mechanisms that exist to maintain normal or near-normal oxygen delivery even in the face of substantial hemoglobin deficits. Yet often such patients acknowledge, soon after treatment has been initiated, that they "feel much better."

MANAGEMENT

PLAN

Short-Term and Long-Term Goals. The two major management goals are: (1) discovering and, if possible, correcting the cause of iron deficiency; and (2) treating the disease. These two goals should be pursued simultaneously; once iron deficiency is diagnosed, it is not appropriate to delay treatment while other diagnostic studies are undertaken. Table 2 lists well-recognized anatomic sources of blood loss. Besides these, coagulation disorders may precipitate bleeding from any of the organs listed in Table 2; such bleeding may be an important clue to the presence of an otherwise silent anatomic lesion.

Indications for Hospitalization. Iron deficiency anemia per se is treated on an ambulatory basis. Indications for hospitalization depend on the cause of blood loss and the requirements for surgery. Since for most of these conditions surgery is elective, it is usually prudent to treat the anemia until a normal blood hemoglobin concentration has been attained before undertaking sur-

Table 2. SOURCES OF BLOOD LOSS

Respiratory Tract
- epistaxis
- telangiectasia
- infection
- neoplasm
- idiopathic pulmonary hemosiderosis

Alimentary Tract

Esophagus	Biliary tract
varices	trauma
hiatus hernia	cholelithiasis
	neoplasm
Stomach	aberrant pancreas
varices	ruptured aneurysm
ulcer	intrahepatic bleeding
carcinoma	
gastritis	Colon
leiomyoma	ulcerative colitis
angiodysplasia	amebiasis
	carcinoma
Small bowel	telangiectasia
ulcer	angiodysplasia
aberrant pancreas	diverticulum
Meckel's diverticulum	
telangiectasia	Rectum
angiodysplasia	hemorrhoids
polyp	ulceration
carcinoma	
regional enteritis	
helminthiasis	
vascular occlusion	
intussusception	
volvulus	
leiomyoma	
Unspecified	
long-distance running	

Genitourinary Tract

Kidney	Uterus
hematuria	menstruation/menorrhagia
neoplasm	adenomyomas
inflammatory disease	carcinoma
Goodpasture's disease	
hemoglobinuria	
paroxysmal nocturnal hemoglobinuria	
paroxysmal cold hemoglobinuria	
march hemoglobinuria	
other	

Phlebotomy
- blood donation
- therapeutic (e.g., in polycythemia vera)
- self-induced

gery. This requires six to eight weeks or longer, and necessitates patience on the part of physician, surgeon, and patient.

NONPHARMACEUTICAL MEASURES

Transfusion. Transfusion of packed erythrocytes is rarely indicated. However, in severely anemic elderly persons who are likely to have compromised circulation to brain, heart, or other vital organs, transfusion is warranted. In this circumstance, transfusion must be given cautiously to avoid rapid increase in blood volume that may *induce* congestive heart failure. Besides this hazard, transfusion may transmit hepatitis, AIDS, or other diseases. It should not be undertaken casually. No arbitrary rule should be used to define the need for transfusion, since each case must be considered individually. Even for most elderly patients, transfusion usually should not be considered if the blood hemoglobin concentration is above 7 gm/dl. The compensatory physiologic mechanisms for anemia are remarkably effective even for anemias of this degree. When transfusion is indicated, the volume of erythrocytes transfused should be restricted to that which relieves distressing symptoms. No attempt should be made to transfuse to normal hemoglobin concentration; the residual hemoglobin deficit should be corrected by iron therapy.

Diet. It is not practical to attempt to treat iron deficiency by dietary means. Even red meat, liver, and other relatively iron-rich foods are extremely poor sources of iron compared with a single tablet of a ferrous compound. To obtain a therapeutic iron intake from food, one would need to eat several pounds of beef or liver each day, at a substantial price in dollars, in elevation of blood cholesterol, and in weight gain. A well-balanced diet is appropriate to ensure adequate intake of protein and other nutrients.

DRUG THERAPY

Selection of Drugs

Oral Therapy. Hundreds of preparations are available for oral administration in the treatment of iron deficiency, and many of these are of proven efficacy. The most effective and the most economical compounds are simple ferrous salts such as ferrous sulfate, ferrous gluconate, or ferrous fumarate. There is little if any advantage in administering a ferrous salt in combination with any other ingredient such as ascorbic acid, molybdenum, or liver extract, or in combination with many other hematinics. "Shotgun therapy," as exemplified in Trinsicon and many other combination hematinics, is deplorable. An iron-cobalt combination, formerly widely marketed, was clearly a dangerous product in consequence of the significant toxicity of ionic cobalt.

The ideal iron preparation is a simple ferrous salt that disintegrates rapidly in gastric juice, so that a high concentration of iron is presented to the duodenal mucosa, where iron is most efficiently absorbed. Unfortunately, many commercial iron preparations are either in extended-release or enteric-coated form, and thus they make iron available at levels of the intestinal lumen where absorption is not very efficient. Many pharmacists erroneously believe that enteric-coated ferrous compounds cause fewer side effects, such as pyrosis, and therefore dispense enteric-coated preparations when a ferrous salt is prescribed generically. But such medication is often ineffective. In order to avoid this problem, one must prescribe by brand name a ferrous salt one knows is not enteric-coated, or specify "non–enteric-coated" on the prescription. Trivalent iron is not absorbed, but must first be reduced to the ferrous form. Furthermore, insoluble precipitates of ferric hydroxide form from ferric salts within alkaline intestinal contents, so ferric compounds should never be used in therapy of iron deficiency. Table 3 compares several commercial preparations of iron for oral treatment of iron deficiency.

The conventional therapeutic dose of iron is 50 to 70 mg thrice daily between meals. A very satisfactory form is a tablet of ferrous sulfate, exsiccated, 0.2 gm, which contains 65 mg of iron. Table 3 compares several alternative medications. Treatment should be continued at this dose level until the anemia is repaired, and then for six months thereafter to replete iron stores. Thus, a

Table 3. COMPARISON OF ORAL AND PARENTERAL IRON THERAPY

Therapy	Iron Content	Cost to Patient, 1986 ($/gm Fe)	Response Rate	Toxicity
Oral				
Beef	1 mg/oz	125.00	slow	none
Pills	*mg/pill*			
ferrous sulfate	65	0.77	rapid	
ferrous fumarate	66	0.45	rapid	
ferrous gluconate	37	1.35	rapid	mild gastro-
Simron	10	26.00	variable	intestinal
Trinsicon	90	4.18	rapid	symptoms
Geritol	50	2.58	rapid	
Vitron-C	66	1.21	rapid	
Parenteral	*mg/ml*			
Iron dextran (Imferon)	50	106.00	rapid	pain, fever, arthralgia, death
Transfusion (1 unit)	250 (approx.)	533.00	immediate	fever, hepatitis, renal failure, AIDS, death

full course of oral therapy usually is about eight months. While this may seem unduly long, it is necessary because iron absorption is markedly attenuated after anemia has been corrected. If bleeding continues, then iron therapy may need to be continued indefinitely.

For most patients, this treatment is practical, efficient, convenient, and economical. A few patients experience gastrointestinal side effects. These can usually be alleviated by switching to another form of oral iron, such as ferrous fumarate or ferrous gluconate. The latter of these contains less iron. But many patients do respond satisfactorily to lower doses of medicinal iron, and ferrous gluconate, even with its much lower iron content, is a reasonable alternative. Very rarely, adult patients may be encountered who, for psychologic reasons, cannot swallow pills of any kind. For these, ferrous sulfate solution USP (also called ferrous sulfate elixir USP) may be prescribed. This contains 32 mg of iron per 4 ml, so the proper dose for adults is two teaspoonsful thrice daily. The patient must be warned that this preparation is likely to stain the teeth. It may be taken through a straw, and the mouth rinsed afterward.

Parenteral Therapy. Iron dextran, or Imferon, is the only available parenteral form of iron. Many decades of experience with this substance attest to its efficacy and its relative safety, although serious and even lethal consequences may occur. Iron dextran is a dark brown solution that contains 50 mg/ml of iron. It may be administered by either intramuscular or intravenous route. In 1981–1982, as the result of a change in manufacturing technique, a high frequency of adverse effects occurred, especially with one batch of iron dextran, Lot 3511 ML. That lot was recalled, the manufacturer returned to the former method of production, and physicians were advised not to inject more than 2 ml intramuscularly or intravenously. Although a high frequency of adverse effects has not been seen with subsequent lots of iron dextran, the manufacturer had not yet rescinded these advised restrictions by March 1986.

Table 4. APPROXIMATE COST OF IRON DEXTRAN THERAPY*

	Total Cost of Drug ($)	Cost of Each Injection ($)	Number of Office Visits	Total Cost ($)
Intravenous (total dose)	143.00	20.00	1	163.00
Intramuscular				
10 ml/day	143.00	5.00	3†	158.00
2 ml/day	143.00	5.00	15	218.00

*Based on retail charge of $9.53 for each 2 ml ampule and $5.00 for each office visit for intramuscular injection by a nurse, or $20.00 for intravenous infusion, and a total dose of 1500 mg of iron, or 30 ml of iron dextran. Entries are rounded off to nearest dollar.

†Counts 5 ml injected into each buttock as a single injection.

Physicians are thus placed in a quandary as to whether they can justifiably administer intramuscular doses in excess of 2 ml (100 mg Fe). Table 4 illustrates the therapeutic and economic dilemma posed by this restraint. To the approximately $60 additional cost resulting from multiple injections, one must also add the greater inconvenience of numerous office visits, the increased costs of transportation, and the discomfort of numerous injections rather than a few or one. Since there appears to be at present no sound basis for limiting the dose of iron dextran to 2 ml per day, very likely many physicians will elect to use larger doses or intravenous total dose administration, on the principle of "compassionate use."

A simple rule may be used to calculate the total dose of iron dextran to correct anemia:

iron dextran dose required (in mg Fe) = venous blood hemoglobin deficit (gm/dl) × lean body weight in pounds

For example, a woman who weighs 120 pounds and whose venous blood hemoglobin concentration is 8 gm/dl has a hemoglobin deficit of (12 gm/dl − 8 gm/dl =) 4 gm/dl and therefore requires (4 × 120 =) 480 mg of iron just to alleviate the anemia. To this should be added about 1000 mg of iron to replete iron stores, thus making a total dose of 1480 mg of iron, or (1480 ÷ 50 =) 30 ml of iron dextran, or 15 ampules altogether. (This simple and easily remembered calculation does not appear at first sight to make sense. It depends upon some coincidences in conversion of kilograms to pounds and the estimated whole blood volume in ml/kg.) As a precaution against anaphylactic reactions, an initial test dose of 0.5 ml of iron dextran should be given by the route intended. If this does not induce anaphylaxis, then the planned course of therapy may be instituted after a few hours of observation or on the next day.

Adverse Effects

Oral Medications. There are no serious adverse effects from medicinal iron administration orally *to iron-deficient patients.* On the other hand, if the diagnosis is in error, as in a thalassemic patient misdiagnosed as being iron-deficient, continued oral iron therapy may result in chronic iron overloading, with the very serious effects of hemochromatosis. Therefore, when response to oral iron therapy is incomplete after eight weeks, administration of iron must be stopped and the diagnosis reexamined.

Many iron-deficient women have small children in their homes. Ingestion of a child's handful of iron tablets may cause serious iron poisoning in a small child. Patients must be warned to *keep iron pills* in a "child-proof" container and *well out of reach of children.*

Minor side effects of iron therapy are noted by about 10% of patients. These may include "heartburn," nausea, constipation, or mild diarrhea. Patients should be warned that their stools will be black while they are taking iron medication, but it is poor psychology to suggest to them in advance that the iron pills "may cause stomach upset." If these symptoms occur and are troublesome, the strategy should be first to reduce the frequency of administration to twice daily; if this fails, switch to a preparation with a lower iron content such as ferrous gluconate. These measures usually suffice, and often the dose can subsequently be increased to the optimal level. One must avoid the temptation to reduce the iron dose to homeopathic levels, as in some commercial iron preparations, or to administer with meals or antacids, since absorption will then be markedly retarded.

Parenteral Medications. Minor acute side effects of iron dextran therapy include arthralgias, generalized urticarial rash, edema and tenderness at injection site, and fever. These manifestations usually subside after a few days. More troublesome effects are generalized lymphadenopathy and splenomegaly. There may be marked leukocytosis, pleocytosis of the cerebrospinal fluid, or mild hepatic dysfunction. These abnormalities may persist for several days or a few weeks. Brownish staining of the skin over the buttocks in the area of the injection is a minor and very common cosmetic effect that is long-persisting. Thrombophlebitis may occur in veins infused with iron dextran solution. This seems less likely to occur if the iron dextran is administered in isotonic saline rather than in 5% dextrose solution, and if the needle used in the infusion is free of iron dextran on its exterior surface.

The most serious side effect of iron dextran is death from anaphylactic shock. Fortunately, this complication has a low incidence. Yet all physicians and nurses who administer this drug must be aware of this possible outcome and prepared to treat promptly with vasopressors such as epinephrine should a patient's blood pressure drop precipitously following iron dextran administration. There is no evidence of a higher frequency of anaphylactic reactions following intravenous as opposed to intramuscular injections, or large doses rather than small doses. One might anticipate a higher total frequency of anaphylactic reactions in patients given many small doses of iron dextran than in those given a few large doses. However, this is speculation. In a few well-documented instances, sarcomas have developed at sites of intramuscular injection of iron dextran. It seems unlikely that the sarcomas were coincidental, although this is a possibility. The risks of lethal anaphylactic shock and sarcomas, as complications of iron dextran therapy, must compel physicians to use this therapy judiciously and selectively rather than indiscriminately.

PERIODIC EVALUATION

Second Diagnostic Look. A second opinion may be warranted in a small proportion of cases if there is uncertainty of diagnosis or if the patient does not respond to treatment as anticipated, i.e., if the anemia persists despite six to eight weeks of adequate treatment.

Follow-up Visits. Iron deficiency anemia has a high relapse rate because many of the causes of blood loss persist or cannot be corrected surgically. The frequency of follow-up examination must be determined for each patient individually: if bleeding is known to be persisting, follow-up visits may need to be as short as a few weeks; if the bleeding lesion has been corrected, reexamination every few years suffices.

Routine Laboratory Tests. Routine laboratory tests on revisits will ordinarily include at least measurement of venous hemoglobin concentration (or hematocrit), and often serum ferritin assay as well.

PATIENT COMPLIANCE

Patient compliance with oral iron therapy may be inadequate when the patient is of poor socioeconomic status or when there is a language barrier, principally because of ineffective communication between physician and patients. In many communities this is a common cause of therapeutic failure. The patient, not the disease, is refractory. Efforts must be made to amend this problem; if the patient remains refractory, parenteral iron therapy may be indicated.

Other common causes of therapeutic failure are: (1) use of enteric-coated or prolonged-release preparations (often unknown to the physician); (2) inappropriate prescription of an iron preparation that contains very little iron; (3) the rate of blood loss exceeds the rate of iron gain from oral or parenteral therapy; and (4) the diagnosis of iron deficiency is wrong.

Malabsorption of iron is often considered as a cause of therapeutic failure. It is extremely rare, except in patients who have a general malabsorption syndrome such as sprue.

Finally, for unknown reasons, some iron deficiency anemia patients who have been treated with iron dextran are unable to utilize efficiently the iron given in that form. It is sequestered at the injection site or in the phagocytic cells of the reticuloendothelial system. They remain anemic; their erythrocytes are hypochromic and microcytic, and they have low serum iron and ferritin concentrations, although an iron stain of bone marrow shows abundant iron in the phagocytic cells. Most such patients respond readily to simple ferrous salts taken orally.

PREVENTIVE MEASURES

The principal preventive measure is to ensure adequate iron intake in the two groups who are most likely to have negative iron balance: babies and women of the reproductive years. Iron supplementation of infant formulas is generally accepted practice. It is a reasonable precaution to give daily iron supplements to every young woman who menstruates or is pregnant or post partum.

Additional iron fortification of wheat flour and other foodstuffs consumed by the entire population seems unwarranted in view of the probable increased risk of hemochromatosis that this practice would entail.

REFERENCES

Beutler E, Fairbanks VF: The effects of iron deficiency. *In* Jacobs A, Worwood M (eds): Iron in Clinical Medicine II. Academic Press, New York, 1980, pp 393–425.

Cook JD: Iron. Churchill-Livingstone, New York, 1980.

Fairbanks VF, Fahey JL, Beutler E: Clinical Disorders of Iron Metabolism, 2nd ed. Grune & Stratton, New York, 1971.

Pollitt E, Leibel RL: Iron Deficiency: Brain Biochemistry and Behavior. Raven Press, New York, 1982.

3 · MEGALOBLASTIC ANEMIA

David Steinberg
LAHEY CLINIC MEDICAL CENTER

DEFINITION

In one standard textbook of hematology, almost an entire page is devoted to an attempt to define megaloblastic anemia precisely. The more pragmatic clinician views megaloblastic anemia as a group of disorders resulting from impaired synthesis of DNA that share certain characteristic morphologic features. The majority of patients with megaloblastic anemia are deficient in either vitamin B_{12} or folic acid, and this discussion is limited to those deficiencies.

DIAGNOSTIC CRITERIA

A low level of hemoglobin, although typical, is not always found with megaloblastic anemia. Occasionally, large red blood cells will be seen with a normal hemoglobin; a patient may have megaloblastic anemia yet not be "anemic." Neutropenia and thrombocytopenia may occur but are rarely severe.

An increased mean corpuscular volume (MCV) has become such a well-recognized clue to the presence of megaloblastic anemia that it has become important to recognize that the MCV may be normal in patients with vitamin B_{12} and folate deficiency. This typically occurs when a patient also has iron deficiency or thalassemia or an inflammatory disorder. Also, an increased MCV does not necessarily indicate the presence of megaloblastic anemia, since large red cells can be seen with liver disease, with reticulocytosis, after splenectomy, and with a variety of other disorders.

The blood smear is a neglected, inexpensive, but potentially valuable diagnostic tool. Megaloblastic red cells typically are large and oval and show considerable variation in size and shape. The neutrophils in megaloblastic anemia are hypersegmented; a six-lobed granulocyte strongly suggests the diagnosis.

A bone marrow examination is not always necessary; however, when other data leave the diagnosis in doubt, examination of the bone marrow is the most accessible means of viewing the panoply of megaloblastic abnormalities. Erythroid activity is exuberant with nuclear cytoplasmic dissociation. The cytoplasm of the erythrocytes turns pink as it gradually fills with hemoglobin, while the nucleus, defective in its maturation, remains large and immature. Abnormal configurations of the red cell nucleus are also evident. The most striking abnormality of leukocytes, the giant band form, may be an important clue because, in some instances, abnormalities of erythrocytes are minimal.

Most patients with vitamin B_{12} deficiency will have abnormal results on the Schilling test; this test not only documents impaired absorption of vitamin B_{12} but also differentiates the malabsorption syndrome from pernicious anemia, because in pernicious anemia vitamin B_{12} absorption is corrected with intrinsic factor. About 50% of patients with pernicious anemia will have intrinsic factor antibodies, which are usually seen only in pernicious anemia.

It is critical to determine whether megaloblastic anemia is a result of vitamin B_{12} or folic acid deficiency. Serum levels of vitamin B_{12} and folic acid are important in determining the relevant deficiency, but neither can be viewed in isolation or accepted as an absolute standard. Borderline serum levels of vitamin B_{12} can be difficult to interpret, and both false-positive and false-negative results occur. A low level of vitamin B_{12} is less reliable when indications for performing the test are marginal and the patient lacks other classic features of vitamin B_{12} deficiency. Serum folate levels may also be misleading because they are sensitive to recent dietary changes. Folate levels of erythrocytes give a better measure of chronic tissue stores.

PATHOPHYSIOLOGY

Vitamin B_{12} deficiency is almost always a result of malabsorption. Only vegans, strict vegetarians who also avoid such animal products as eggs and milk, become deficient in vitamin B_{12} because of their diet.

Pernicious anemia, an immunologic disorder affecting the stomach, is the best known cause of vitamin B_{12} deficiency. In pernicious anemia, a lack of gastric intrinsic factor results in diminished vitamin B_{12} absorption in the ileum; a lack of gastric intrinsic factor also explains the vitamin B_{12} deficiency seen after total gastrectomy and occasionally after partial gastrectomy. Disorders of the small intestine, such as Crohn's disease, the malabsorption syndrome, and extensive resection of the small bowel, are also associated with vitamin B_{12} deficiency. More exotic causes of vitamin B_{12} deficiency include selective vitamin B_{12} malabsorption (Imerslund's syndrome), anatomic abnormalities of the small intestine with bacterial overgrowth, pancreatic insufficiency, and utilization of vitamin B_{12} by the fish tapeworm, *Diphyllobothrium latum*.

Stores of folic acid are less ample than stores of vitamin B_{12}, and megaloblastic anemia resulting from folic acid deficiency is commonly caused by a poor diet. Persons who are particularly prone to the development of folic acid deficiency include alcoholics and older persons subsisting on substandard diets, such as tea and toast. Folic acid deficiency is found in impoverished parts of the world, especially when folic acid is destroyed by subjecting food to prolonged cooking. It can also be seen in conjunction with diseases of the small bowel, such as the malabsorption syndrome; with certain drugs, such as anticonvulsant agents and birth control pills; and when folic acid requirements are increased, such as in pregnant women, in patients with hemolytic anemia or exfoliative dermatitis, and in patients undergoing dialysis.

CLINICAL ASPECTS

The evaluation of anemia is often erroneously thought of as largely a laboratory exercise. The astute clinician, however, is aware of the setting and clinical features associated with the various anemias and is alert to clues in the patient's history and physical examination that will indicate the most appropriate laboratory tests. The clinical settings likely to be associated with megaloblastic anemia include a history of total or subtotal gastrectomy, the malabsorption syndrome, alcoholism, Crohn's disease, anatomic abnormalities of the small intestine, severe pancreatic disease, and instances when folate requirements are needed in excess.

The clinical features of megaloblastic anemia are a result of the anemia itself and of the underlying disease causing anemia. Anemia develops slowly, allowing the patient to adapt to even extremely low levels of hemoglobin. I have often marveled at how well some patients in their 80s have tolerated hemoglobin levels as low as 5 gm/dl. Abnormalities caused by anemia include pallor, fatigue, lightheadedness, shortness of breath, tachycardia, and a systolic flow murmur. Anemia may also lower a patient's threshold for symptoms from other problems, such as congestive heart failure, angina pectoris, and intermittent claudication.

Pernicious anemia is associated with some well-recognized clinical features, such as glossitis with a sore, smooth tongue, and characteristic neurologic features that may include parasthesias in the hands and feet, loss of position and vibratory sense, an ataxic gait, and disturbances of mentation, which, in the extreme, have been called "megaloblastic madness."

Patients with megaloblastic anemia from the malabsorption syndrome may have loss of weight; diarrhea; fatty, foul-smelling feces; and findings associated with malabsorption of other nutrients, such as bleeding from vitamin K deficiency and osteomalacia due to vitamin D deficiency.

MANAGEMENT

The goal of treatment is to control immediate and threatening complications and then to provide therapy that will replace stores of vitamin B_{12} or folic acid and that will meet the necessary daily requirement of these nutrients. In most instances of vitamin B_{12} deficiency, treatment must continue throughout the patient's life to prevent relapse.

TRANSFUSION

Transfusions of packed red blood cells should be given to patients with megaloblastic anemia only in exceptional circumstances. Anemia usually develops slowly, allowing most patients, even older ones, time to adapt surprisingly well to extremely low levels of hemoglobin. In addition to the usual dangers of blood transfusion, anemic patients are in a high cardiac output state and are at risk for the development of transfusion-induced pulmonary edema, which can be fatal. Transfusions of red cells should, therefore, be reserved for potentially life-threatening cardiac or central nervous system complications. When used, transfusions should be given in small amounts and slowly over several hours. The patient should be monitored for signs of congestive heart failure and should usually be given a diuretic.

VITAMIN B$_{12}$

Because vitamin B$_{12}$ deficiency is almost always due to malabsorption of the vitamin and not to reduced dietary intake, it is said treatment should be parenteral administration of vitamin B$_{12}$. Although I believe it is prudent to use injections of vitamin B$_{12}$, massive doses of vitamin B$_{12}$ taken orally can be effective. Vitamin B$_{12}$, 300 µg a day taken orally, can produce both a good hematologic response and normal serum vitamin B$_{12}$ levels. Lower doses, such as 150 µg a day, can produce a good hematologic response but may result in inadequate serum levels. Doses of vitamin B$_{12}$ higher than 300 µg a day have been effective when taken at less frequent intervals. Low doses of vitamin B$_{12}$ have been prescribed orally with intrinsic factor. This treatment cannot be recommended. Although most patients respond to treatment, some do not, and in some of the patients who respond, treatment ultimately fails.

Oral. Although large oral doses of vitamin B$_{12}$ can be effective, I strongly advise parenteral therapy. Daily oral vitamin B$_{12}$ therapy demands a reliable patient. Many vitamin B$_{12}$–deficient patients are older, and some of them are forgetful. Treatment must continue for life. Less compliance failure and fewer relapses occur with a periodic injection given by a nurse, physician, or relative than when the patient is depended on to take vitamin B$_{12}$ pills every day. Some experts believe vitamin B$_{12}$ injections more reliably replete vitamin B$_{12}$ reserves.

Parenteral. Cyanocobalamin and hydroxocobalamin are two parenteral preparations of vitamin B$_{12}$. The greater the amount of either cobalamin given, the greater the percentage lost in the urine; however, hydroxocobalamin is absorbed more slowly, is bound to tissue more tightly, and is associated with less urinary loss. Hydroxocobalamin is, therefore, retained more efficiently by the body and is theoretically the preparation of choice. However, for practical purposes, both cobalamins are effective and inexpensive. Injections of vitamin B$_{12}$ should be given by the intramuscular or deep subcutaneous route.

The goal of vitamin B$_{12}$ therapy is to replace vitamin B$_{12}$ reserves and to provide the necessary daily requirement of 2 to 5 µg. Specific treatment programs vary. Different authors advise their own favorite regimen, so it is easy to become confused. Fortunately, many effective, nontoxic, and inexpensive ways exist to treat vitamin B$_{12}$ deficiency, and it is hard to go wrong.

Stores of vitamin B$_{12}$ can be replenished with 1000 µg of vitamin B$_{12}$ injected daily or perhaps every other day for two weeks. Alternatively, 1000 µg can be given once a week for six weeks. The physician has some flexibility in adjusting the program to the patient's circumstances, since these regimens probably provide an excessive amount of vitamin B$_{12}$.

It is probably wise to continue to give a large dose of vitamin B$_{12}$ if a patient has appreciable neurologic damage. A reasonable recommendation is 500 to 1000 µg of vitamin B$_{12}$ weekly or every other week for six to 12 months. Although scientific documentation is not ample enough to be dogmatic about how much vitamin B$_{12}$ to give, it is reasonable for the clinician to be generous because vitamin B$_{12}$ is nontoxic, and the neurologic damage from vitamin B$_{12}$ deficiency can be crippling.

Patients should be advised that treatment with vitamin B$_{12}$ is to continue for life and that treatment must continue even when they feel better. Although satisfactory maintenance therapy can be achieved with 100 µg of vitamin B$_{12}$ once a month, I tend to recommend 1000 µg each month. Two successful alternative maintenance programs are 1000 µg of hydroxocobalamin every two or three months and eight injections of 1000 µg of hydroxocobalamin over two to three weeks once a year. I suspect a monthly injection is less likely to be forgotten and may be a more reliable form of treatment. I would, therefore, advise as maintenance treatment 1000 µg of vitamin B$_{12}$ once a month for life.

A widespread problem in vitamin B$_{12}$ therapy is that it is often given to patients who do not need it. It is used as a nonspecific tonic for conditions other than vitamin B$_{12}$ deficiency, such as fatigue, anorexia, and depression. In one epidemiologic study, the amount of vitamin B$_{12}$ sold was three times that estimated as necessary to treat vitamin B$_{12}$ deficiency in that population. It is dishonest to give vitamin B$_{12}$ therapy when it is not needed, and the use of vitamin B$_{12}$ as a placebo diverts attention from the patient's real problem.

FOLIC ACID

Most patients will respond to treatment of folic acid deficiency with 1 mg of folic acid a day taken orally. When folic acid deficiency is due to a poor diet, treatment can be stopped after three or four weeks if the patient resumes a normal diet. It is important to be certain that the patient has folic acid deficiency and not vitamin B$_{12}$ deficiency because treatment of vitamin B$_{12}$ deficiency with folic acid may improve hematologic parameters but can lead to crippling neurologic disease.

4 · HEMOLYTIC ANEMIA

Ernest Beutler
SCRIPPS CLINIC AND RESEARCH FOUNDATION

DEFINITION AND DIAGNOSTIC CRITERIA

Hemolytic anemia exists when there is pathologic shortening of the red cell life span of such a degree that bone marrow response is unable to maintain a normal red cell mass. Compensated hemolysis is said to exist when red cell life span is shortened, but the increased activity of the bone marrow is able to maintain a normal hemoglobin concentration in the blood.

The most direct and definitive means of demonstrating the shortening of red cell life span is to perform a ^{51}Cr red cell survival and excluding, by appropriate means, bleeding as a cause of apparent shortening of the red cell life span. Secondary manifestations of hemolysis include hyperbilirubinemia, decreased serum haptoglobin levels, increased serum lactate dehydrogenase levels, and, most important of all, reticulocytosis. The presence of a persistent reticulocytosis in a nonbleeding patient with a stable hemoglobin is excellent evidence that hemolysis is present.

PATHOPHYSIOLOGY

Red cell life span may be shortened because of an intrinsically defective erythrocyte, a normal erythrocyte circulating in an inclement environment, or a combination of these two factors.

Intrinsic defects of the red cell are, with the exception of paroxysmal nocturnal hemoglobinuria (PNH), all hereditary in nature. Included are hereditary spherocytosis and the closely related defects ovalocytosis and pyropoikilocytosis, red cell enzyme deficiencies such as G6PD deficiency and pyruvate kinase deficiency, and the hemoglobinopathies. An acquired clonal disorder of the hematopoietic stem cell, PNH is an intrinsic red cell defect in which the erythrocyte is uniquely sensitive to hemolysis by complement.

Extracorpuscular factors that lead to increased red cell destruction include the production of autoantibodies in autoimmune hemolytic anemia and abnormalities in the vasculature giving rise to microangiopathic hemolytic anemia. The latter disorder occurs particularly as a consequence of disseminated intravascular coagulation as a result of systemic abnormality, such as severe sepsis or disseminated neoplasia.

CLINICAL ASPECTS

Patients with hemolytic anemia may manifest pallor, weakness, palpitations, and jaundice. Darkening of urine is characteristic of some types of hemolytic disease (e.g., hemoglobinuria in PNH and excretion of dark pigments in patients with unstable hemoglobin); in others urine may be normal (e.g., hereditary spherocytosis). The degree of jaundice varies considerably, and the absence of clinical jaundice does not exclude the diagnosis of hemolytic anemia. Gallstones are common complications of hemolytic anemia. Abdominal pain may occur, particularly during severe hemolytic episodes. In some types of hemolytic anemia (e.g., sickle cell disease, hereditary spherocytosis, pyruvate kinase deficiency), chronic leg ulcers may be present.

MANAGEMENT

The first priority in a patient with hemolytic anemia is establishing the etiologic factor of hemolysis. In this diverse group of disorders, management and prognosis depend entirely upon the cause.

Hereditary Spherocytosis, Ovalocytosis, or Pyropoikilocytosis. Hereditary spherocytosis, the most common of this group of disorders, is characterized by an increased osmotic fragility and by autosomal dominant inheritance. The disorder is relatively benign and cured by splenectomy. Traditionally, this operation has been recommended for all but elderly patients with hereditary spherocytosis, unless a serious contraindication to surgery exists. Severity of the disease varies considerably, and advice regarding splenectomy should be individualized. Family studies should be conducted and other affected individuals counseled about their disorder, thus sparing them much unnecessary treatment with hematinics and providing the benefits of splenectomy when needed.

Patients with hemolytic ovalocytosis also benefit from splenectomy. The situation is less clear in pyropoikilocytosis, which is very rare.

Red Cell Enzyme Defects. Over a dozen different red cell enzyme defects have been described. Their inheritance may be autosomal recessive, as in pyruvate kinase deficiency, glucose phosphate isomerase deficiency, or pyrimidine 5'-nucleotidase deficiency; sex-linked, as in G6PD deficiency and phosphoglycerate kinase deficiency; or autosomal dominant, as in increased adenosine deaminase activity. Results of splenectomy are variable, even within a single type of enzyme deficiency. Response is usually quite favorable in pyruvate kinase deficiency and glucose phosphate isomerase deficiency, but much less so in G6PD deficiency.

Genetic counseling is particularly important in some red cell enzyme deficiencies, such as triose phosphate isomerase deficiency, that are associated with severe neuromuscular disorders. Prenatal diagnosis is usually feasible.

Hemoglobinopathies. The most common clinically significant hemoglobinopathy is sickle cell disease and associated disorders. These are discussed in Section V, Chapter 5. Other abnormal hemoglobins also cause shortening of red cell life span. Particularly prominent are the so-called unstable hemoglobins. Shortening of red cell life span occurs with homozygous hemoglobin C disease and with certain other stable mutant hemoglobins. The mode of inheritance varies but is usually autosomal dominant in the unstable hemoglobins. Splenectomy is not recommended. Management consists of general medical support. Transfusion is rarely necessary.

Paroxysmal Nocturnal Hemoglobinuria (PNH). The severity of paroxysmal nocturnal hemoglobinuria varies from the fulminating course fatal within a month to a chronic, mild hemolytic state, lasting for many years and occasionallly even resolving entirely. No satisfactory treatment exists. Iron administration may be useful when iron deficiency develops because of urinary iron loss. Transfusion with washed red cells is given as needed. Corticosteroids and androgens have been thought to be helpful. In severe cases, bone marrow transplantation provides the potential of cure.

Autoimmune Hemolytic Anemia. Autoimmune hemolytic anemia may arise as an idiopathic disorder and occurs as a frequent complication of lymphomas and of subacute disseminated lupus erythematosus. Initial management consists of administration of steroids. If the response is not adequate or relapse occurs, then use of immunosuppressive agents such as cyclophosphamide, splenectomy, or both are recommended. When the disorder is secondary, treatment of the underlying disease should be the first goal.

Identification of the offending antibody is of critical importance. Patients with this disease sometimes become severely anemic and require transfusion. This can be accomplished most successfully with an understanding of the specificity of the circulating antibodies, which could destroy transfused erythrocytes.

Microangiopathic Hemolytic Anemia. When resulting from sepsis or generalized neoplasia, microangiopathic hemolytic anemia is best managed by directing therapy at the underlying disorder. Microangiopathic hemolysis may also occur as a result of mechanical trauma to red cells occurring secondary to valve prostheses. This frequently milder form of the disease can usually be managed by administering iron when iron deficiency occurs as a result of renal iron loss. If it becomes sufficiently severe, it may require surgical correction of the valvular problem.

5 · SICKLE CELL DISEASE AND THE THALASSEMIAS

Ernest Beutler
SCRIPPS CLINIC AND RESEARCH FOUNDATION

DEFINITION AND DIAGNOSTIC CRITERIA

Sickle cell disease is a collective term applied to the hemolytic disorders that occur when a patient inherits the gene for sickle cell hemoglobin together with a second gene for sickle cell hemoglobin or another gene that enhances sickling. Such a gene may be that for hemoglobin C or beta-thalassemia. It is to be distinguished from sickle cell trait, in which sickle cell hemoglobin is inherited with the normal hemoglobin A, giving rise to the almost entirely benign carrier state.

Thalassemias are hereditary anemias characterized by an absolute or partial defect in synthesis in one of the globin chains. Unlike the sickling disorders and the other hemoglobinopathies, abnormal globin chains are not usually produced, although there are exceptions that are noted below.

PATHOPHYSIOLOGY

The sickling disorders are due to the production of a mutant beta globin chain in which the glutamic acid normally occupying the sixth position from the N terminus of the chain has been replaced by a valine. Hemoglobins containing this mutant chain have a marked propensity to aggregate when they are in the deoxy conformation. This results in marked distortion of the red cells into forms that resemble sickles or holly leaves. Sickled cells are rigid, and their failure to deform results in their sequestration in the spleen and in other organs. The occlusion of small blood vessels by sickle cells is responsible for the painful crises that occur in this disease.

Thalassemias arise from a defect in the synthesis of either alpha chains or beta chains. In the former in-

Table 1. EFFECTS OF LOSS OF ALPHA GENE FUNCTION

No. of Alpha Genes	Designation	Clinical Consequence
4	Normal	None
3	Silent carrier	None or minimal anemia and microcytosis
2	Alpha-thalassemia minor	Mild microcytic anemia
1	Hemoglobin H disease	Severe microcytic hemolytic anemia and splenomegaly
0	Hydrops fetalis	Fetal death with macerated stillborns

stance, they are designated alpha-thalassemias, while in the latter they are designated beta-thalassemias. In the more severe forms of beta-thalassemia, not only are the cells poorly filled with hemoglobin because of the defect in hemoglobin synthesis, but free globin chains of the type produced normally appear in the cytoplasm of the erythroid cell since they can find no partner with which to combine. Such free chains damage the red cell membrane and lead to premature destruction. Free gamma chains (in the newborn) or beta chains (in the adult) also have the capacity to combine with themselves, forming homotetramers designated hemoglobin Barts in the case of gamma chains and hemoglobin H in the case of beta chains.

Normal humans have four alpha chains in their genome. Loss of function of only one of these is a barely perceptible event, while loss of all four alpha genes is lethal before or at the time of birth. The effects of the loss of function of different numbers of alpha genes are summarized in Table 1. The most common cause of loss of alpha gene function is gene deletion, but there are other causes as well. Particularly important is a defect in the stop codon of the alpha chain in which the reading of the gene continues beyond its normal termination point, giving rise to an elongated but unstable globin molecule. This hemoglobin, Constant Spring, is one of the more common causes of alpha-thalassemia.

Each genome has only two beta globin chains; loss of function of these genes is usually due to a defect in splicing of introns from the messenger RNA or in control sequences upstream from the gene. Such defects may result in total loss of beta chain production, or in its diminution. Unequal crossing over between the beta and the delta globin gene may produce a fusion hemoglobin designated hemoglobin Lepore, which is transcribed at a markedly diminished rate. Thus, hemoglobin Lepore gives rise to a thalassemic state.

CLINICAL ASPECTS

Sickle cell disease is characterized by anemia and all of the symptoms that are common to a lowered hemoglobin concentration of the blood. Leg ulcers are a relatively frequent complication. Strokes may occur, particularly in children, and in adults pulmonary hypertension is a sequela of sickle cell disease. Other abnormalities that may occur in various sickling disorders include aseptic necrosis of the femoral head, renal papillary necrosis with attendant hematuria, pulmonary emboli, splenic infarcts, and, most common of all, painful crises.

The milder forms of thalassemia, i.e., loss of the function of only one or two alpha genes or of only one beta gene, are of no clinical consequence. Their diagnosis is important chiefly for the purposes of genetic counseling and to prevent needless and possibly harmful treatment with iron preparations. The more severe forms of thalassemia are characterized by pallor, hepatosplenomegaly, and hyperostosis of the bones giving rise to a mongoloid appearance. Children with thalassemia grow poorly and are subject to frequent infections.

MANAGEMENT

PLAN

Patients with sickle cell disease should be encouraged to live as normal a life as possible. Preparation for nonstrenuous employment is essential during childhood and adolescent years. In many patients with sickle cell disease the manifestations may be relatively mild, and they are able to lead a relatively normal life. Interruptions are caused by periodic painful crises. A few of these, accompanied by prolonged pain and fever, may require hospitalization, but many can be managed on an outpatient basis. In contrast to patients with the sickle cell diseases, it should be emphasized that persons with sickle cell trait are entirely normal and require no special medical attention.

The most severe thalassemic disorders are usually fatal in childhood. These children require frequent transfusion, which often can be given on an outpatient basis. Cardiac failure due to iron overload is often a terminating event. Intercurrent infections may be treated in either the outpatient or the inpatient setting. Splenectomy may ameliorate the disease and should be carried out in most cases. In a few patients, bone marrow transplantation has been successfully performed.

NONPHARMACOLOGIC MEASURES

In both sickle cell disease and thalassemia, blood transfusion may play a major role. In the case of sickle crises, good hydration and maintaining body warmth are important.

DRUG THERAPY

In most patients with sickle cell disease, the most frequent complication is the painful crisis. As in the case of other diseases with chronic pain, the danger of addiction to narcotics is very real. Whenever possible, pain control should be achieved with nonnarcotics, using analgesics such as aspirin. Sedation with phenothiazine derivatives, for example, may also be useful. Although many drugs have been studied for putative antisickling effect, no drug is available that can be used therapeutically in practice to decrease sickling. Instead, the physician must depend upon general measures such as hydration and occasionally blood transfusions. Immunization against pneumonia is commonly given to patients with sickle cell disease because repeated infarction of the spleen and loss of splenic function increase susceptibility to pneumococcal infection.

Drug therapy of severe thalassemia consists chiefly of removing the iron burden by the administration of desferrioxamine. Although this chelating agent may be administered together with blood transfusions, efficient removal of iron requires that it be given daily by prolonged subcutaneous infusion via a portable infusion pump.

PATIENT INFORMATION AND EDUCATION

Sickle cell centers have been set up in many major cities. These provide resources for patient and family education with regard to sickle cell disease. Informational material about thalassemia may be obtained from the Cooley's Disease Foundation.

PERIODIC EVALUATION

It is not necessary to see patients with sickle cell disease or thalassemia frequently when they are doing well. Routine visits may be spaced three to six months apart. At this time a complete blood count should be obtained. It is important that the patient maintain a relationship with his or her physician so that help may be obtained promptly if and when complications occur.

PATIENT COMPLIANCE

Patient compliance is a problem, particularly with iron chelation therapy using desferrioxamine. The importance of the treatment to the patient should be emphasized.

PREVENTIVE MEASURES

Genetic counseling is of major importance both in sickle cell diseases and in thalassemia. This should be carried out by a physician or genetic counselor with a thorough understanding of the intricacies of the genetics of these disorders and laboratory back-up to perform appropriate studies.

SOCIOECONOMIC ASPECTS OF MANAGEMENT

It is necessary to marshal community resources to aid patients with these diseases when they exist in severe form. However, major emphasis should be placed on self-reliance and adaptation to the disease state in such a way that as near-normal a life style as possible may be pursued.

6 · POLYCYTHEMIA: PRIMARY AND SECONDARY ERYTHROCYTOSIS

William Gray Hocking
MARSHFIELD CLINIC

DEFINITION AND DIAGNOSTIC CRITERIA

Erythrocytosis simply refers to an elevated red cell mass (RCM). At sea level the normal RCM for adult females is 23 to 29 ml/kg of body weight and for males 26 to 32 ml/kg of body weight. Erythrocytosis may be primary, that is, resulting from an autonomous proliferation of erythroid progenitors due to an intrinsic cellular abnormality, or it may be secondary to enhanced stimulation of erythropoiesis. Polycythemia indicates an increase in proliferation of all hematopoietic cell lines, but this term is often used interchangeably with erythrocytosis. Relative erythrocytosis is characterized by an elevated hematocrit but a normal RCM and is due to a reduction in plasma volume.

The diagnosis of true erythrocytosis is established when the RCM exceeds the upper limit of normal. Polycythemia rubra vera (PRV) is diagnosed when a patient has manifestations of a myeloproliferative syndrome such as splenomegaly, thrombocytosis, leukocytosis, or an elevated leukocyte alkaline phosphatase and secondary erythrocytosis is excluded by finding a normal arterial oxygen saturation, a normal P_{50}, and no evidence of renal disease or an erythropoietin-producing tumor. A carboxyhemoglobin level should be measured in patients who smoke. On occasion the distinction between primary and secondary erythrocytosis may not be possible at the time of initial evaluation.

PATHOPHYSIOLOGY

Erythrocytosis can be classified according to the pathophysiologic mechanism for elevation of RCM (Table 1). Primary erythrocytosis is related to autonomous proliferation of erythroid progenitors. Rarely this appears as an isolated erythrocytosis without other manifestations of a myeloproliferative syndrome, but the majority of patients with primary erythrocytosis have PRV.

The secondary forms of erythrocytosis can be further classified as physiologically appropriate or inappropriate. The physiologically appropriate causes are those related to decreased tissue oxygenation, which results in an increase in erythropoietin production and red cell mass as a compensatory mechanism. Physiologically inappropriate secondary erythrocytosis is due to the production of erythropoietin or rarely another erythroid-stimulating substance by a neoplasm or by the kidney in certain pathologic states (Table 1).

A rise in RCM produces two important and opposing physiologic effects: an increase in oxygen-carrying capacity and an increase in blood viscosity. In a normovolemic person, systemic oxygen transport is optimal at a hematocrit between 0.40 and 0.45 and any rise in hematocrit above this level results in an overall reduction in systemic oxygen transport despite the increased red cell mass. This reduction is mediated by the increased blood viscosity, which impairs cardiac output and possibly oxygen delivery at the tissue level. In hypervolemic states, however, the optimal hematocrit for oxygen delivery may be as high as 0.55 to 0.60. When RCM rises above the point at which viscosity becomes the limiting factor for oxygen transport, the elevated RCM becomes detrimental.

CLINICAL ASPECTS

POLYCYTHEMIA RUBRA VERA (PRV)

In PRV the clinical manifestations resulting from impaired oxygen delivery may be headache, dizziness, vertigo, tinnitus, visual disturbances, angina pectoris, or intermittent claudication. In addition, symptoms due

Table 1. CLASSIFICATION OF ERYTHROCYTOSIS

Primary autonomous erythropoiesis: polycythemia rubra vera
Secondary
  Physiologically appropriate (decreased tissue oxygenation)
    High altitude
    Chronic lung disease or alveolar hypoventilation
    Cardiovascular right-to-left shunt
    High oxygen affinity hemoglobinopathy
    Congenitally decreased erythrocyte 2,3-diphosphoglycerate
    Carboxyhemoglobinemia
    Histotoxic (e.g., cobalt)
  Physiologically inappropriate (normal tissue oxygenation)
    Tumors producing erythropoietin or other erythropoietic substances
      Renal cell carcinoma
      Cerebellar hemangioblastoma
      Hepatoma
      Uterine leiomyoma
      Ovarian carcinoma
      Pheochromocytoma
    Renal diseases
      Cysts
      Hydronephrosis
      Bartter's syndrome
      Transplantation
    Adrenocortical hypersecretion
Relative polycythemia (Gaisböck's syndrome, spurious or stress erythrocytosis)

to the myeloproliferative process are frequent and include easy bruisability or other manifestations of a bleeding diathesis, abdominal fullness or early satiety from splenomegaly, and pruritus.

A physical examination shows a ruddy face often with congested mucosa and conjunctiva. Approximately 75% of patients will have splenomegaly and 30% hepatomegaly. Hypertension frequently accompanies PRV.

Laboratory Findings. A modest leukocytosis with a left shift and mild basophilia is frequent. Moderate thrombocytosis is seen in 50% of patients. The peripheral blood smear is normal early in the disease, but with the development of myelofibrosis and extramedullary hematopoiesis, striking peripheral blood abnormalities appear. The bone marrow is not diagnostic in PRV but generally reveals trilineal hyperplasia, decreased or absent iron stores, and an increase in reticulin fibers. The leukocyte alkaline phosphatase score is elevated in about 75% of patients.

Complications. A variety of complications may occur in patients with PRV. These include thromboembolic episodes, hemorrhage, gout, and peptic ulcer disease. Two long-term complications are of particular importance. Acute leukemia develops in up to 12% of patients with PRV, and this incidence is partially dependent upon the type of treatment the patient has received. Postpolycythemic myeloid metaplasia ("spent" PRV) occurs frequently in patients with long-standing PRV and is characterized by progressive organ enlargement and ineffective hematopoiesis.

SECONDARY ERYTHROCYTOSIS

The clinical manifestations in these patients are due to the underlying disease state (e.g., chronic obstructive lung disease) or to impaired tissue oxygen delivery.

RELATIVE ERYTHROCYTOSIS

This syndrome, also known as Gaisböck's syndrome or stress erythrocytosis, generally occurs in middle-aged males who are mildly obese and hypertensive. The incidence of thromboembolic complications may approach 30%.

MANAGEMENT

POLYCYTHEMIA RUBRA VERA

The management of this disease requires an individualized approach. Emphasis should be placed on establishing an accurate diagnosis, since this is the only form of erythrocytosis in which myelosuppressive therapy may be indicated. The patient's age, sex, presenting manifestations, and hematologic status are all of importance in determining treatment.

Phlebotomy. All patients should undergo a rapid reduction in hematocrit by phlebotomy until the hematocrit is between 0.42 and 0.46. In patients with normal cardiovascular function, this can be accomplished by phlebotomy of 450 ml every other day until the desired hematocrit is reached. In patients who are elderly (generally over 65) or who have underlying cardiovascular disease, smaller phlebotomies (200 to 300 ml) twice weekly should be done to reduce the hematocrit. The blood removed can be replaced with a normal saline solution. In patients requiring urgent phlebotomy because of ischemic complications or the need for urgent surgery, intensive phlebotomy with appropriate volume replacement should be considered. Elective surgical procedures should be delayed until the hematocrit is normal and any other manifestations of PRV are controlled.

Repeated phlebotomies will lead to iron deficiency. This may have the benefit of producing a microcytic, hypochromic polycythemia with a normal hematocrit. However, a variety of clinical manifestations may result from iron deficiency including glossitis, dysphagia, and generalized weakness. In addition, microcytic red blood cells exhibit increased intrinsic viscosity, which may impair oxygen transport even with a normal hematocrit. While there are no clear guidelines, severe iron deficiency (e.g., MCV < 70) should be avoided. When a decision is made to replace iron, this should be done slowly and with frequent monitoring of the hematocrit, since the requirement for phlebotomy will increase.

Myelosuppressive Therapy. After initial lowering of the patient's red cell mass, a decision regarding the necessity of myelosuppressive therapy must be made. In general, cytotoxic therapy should be avoided in younger patients, particularly women of childbearing age, whenever possible. However, phlebotomy does not control many of the manifestations of the myeloproliferative process such as severe pruritus, splenomegaly, hyperuricemia, or thrombocytosis. In some patients, a requirement for frequent phlebotomies may represent an unacceptable inconvenience. Most important, the risk of both thrombotic and hemorrhagic complications is increased in patients treated by phlebotomy alone. For all of these reasons, consideration must be given to suppressing the panmyelosis. The optimal approach to myelosuppression remains controversial. One of the major concerns in using myelosuppressive therapy is the leukemogenic potential of these treatments. While both chlorambucil (Leukeran) and radioactive phosphorus (^{32}P) are equally effective in controlling PRV, ^{32}P appears to have a lower leukemogenic potential. In addition, ^{32}P has the advantage of requiring only a single injection, which may be effective for six to 24 months and does not require frequent monitoring of the blood counts after control is achieved. Recently hydroxyurea has been introduced as an alternative form of myelosuppression; this appears to have a lower leukemogenic potential but has the disadvantage of requiring more frequent monitoring of the blood counts.

In summary, myelosuppressive therapy should be avoided whenever possible in young patients, particularly those under 40. In elderly patients with PRV, the risk of thromboembolic disease is high and the risk of long-term complications lower, and myelosuppressive therapy should be given in the majority of these patients. Radioactive phosphorus in a dose of 2.3 mCi/m² body surface area is an effective form of therapy with a lower risk of leukemogenesis than alkylating agents. Treatment with ^{32}P is optimal for older patients or where compliance or follow-up visits are difficult. Hydroxyurea requires daily administration and close hematologic monitoring but may be the drug of choice in younger patients with PRV. Alkylating agents such as chlorambucil should be avoided.

Management of Complications. Hyperuricemia in PRV should be treated with allopurinol and not a uricosuric agent. Allopurinol is given in a dose of 300 mg daily in patients with normal renal function.

Pruritus may be severe; although it is usually improved by myelosuppressive therapy, in some cases it will persist. The H_1-antihistamines are generally ineffective. Cyproheptadine (Periactin), which has both antihistamine and antiserotonin effects, may be effective in a dosage of 4 mg q.i.d. In some patients the H_2-blocker cimetidine (Tagamet) has been effective either alone or when given in combination with cyproheptadine.

Follow-up. Once the hematocrit has been normalized, the approach to follow-up will depend upon the decision to employ myelosuppressive therapy. In patients who do not receive myelosuppressive treatment, follow-up at three- to four-week intervals is necessary. In patients treated with ^{32}P, blood counts should be monitored on a monthly basis. For the initial two to three months after treatment, additional phlebotomy may be necessary. However, once the disease is controlled, patients can be followed at two- to three-month intervals. Patients who are treated with either hydroxyurea or an alkylating agent require more frequent monitoring, depending upon the individual circumstances. Usually it will be necessary to check a blood count at least every other week. Once the disease becomes stable on a well-established regimen, follow-up at three- to four-week intervals may be possible. It is important to document regression of organomegaly as well as to monitor the patient for recurrence. A complete blood count with differential and platelet count should be obtained at each visit.

SECONDARY ERYTHROCYTOSIS

Phlebotomy may be necessary in patients with secondary erythrocytosis. In physiologically inappropriate secondary erythrocytosis, it is appropriate to reduce the hematocrit to 0.42 to 0.46 by phlebotomy. The decision to phlebotomize patients with physiologically appropriate secondary erythrocytosis is more difficult, since these patients suffer from decreased tissue oxygenation and may require some increase in red cell mass to compensate for this. The problem in these patients is to determine the optimal hematocrit. Unfortunately there are no easily measurable parameters other than the overall clinical condition of the patient to assist in this determination. Most patients in this category will benefit from a red cell mass that is moderately increased in the range of 0.55 to 0.60, and this should be the initial goal of phlebotomy. It may be possible to determine in an individual patient by empiric trial an optimal hematocrit range, but these patients should not have their hematocrit lowered to the normal range. It is worth emphasizing that patients with secondary erythrocytosis should not receive myelosuppressive treatment.

In some forms of secondary erythrocytosis, elimination of certain causative or aggravating factors may lead to improvement. In carboxyhemoglobinemia ("smoker's erythrocytosis"), cessation of smoking will lead to correction of the erythrocytosis. Patients with alveolar hypoventilation will benefit from weight reduction. In general, diuretic therapy should be avoided, since this may contract plasma volume and exacerbate hyperviscosity. In paraneoplastic erythrocytosis, removal of the tumor will eliminate the erythrocytosis. Likewise, correction of benign renal lesions associated with erythrocytosis will usually reverse the erythrocytosis.

The follow-up of patients with secondary erythrocytosis is dictated principally by the underlying medical condition rather than the erythrocytosis.

RELATIVE ERYTHROCYTOSIS

Both smoking cessation and control of hypertension are beneficial in these patients and may reduce the excess mortality from thromboembolic disease. Diuretics should be avoided, since these patients already have a low normal or reduced plasma volume. Drugs that act as renin antagonists would theoretically be the optimal therapy for hypertension in these patients. The role of phlebotomy is not well defined. However, since these patients have been shown to have reduced cerebral blood flow with hematocrits in excess of 0.46, phlebotomy to this level may be beneficial if other measures are unsuccessful in controlling the hematocrit.

REFERENCES

Balcerzak SP, Bromberg PA: Secondary polycythemia. Semin Hematol 12:353–382, 1975.
Berk PD, Goldberg JD, Silverstein NM, et al: Increased incidence of acute leukemia in polycythemia vera associated with chlorambucil therapy. N Engl J Med 304:441–447, 1981.
Golde DW, Hocking WG, Koeffler HP, Adamson JW: Polycythemia: mechanisms and management. Ann Intern Med 95:71–87, 1981.
Tharling EB: Paraneoplastic erythrocytosis and inappropriate erythropoietin production: a review. Scand J Hematol [Suppl] 17:7–166, 1972.
Wasserman LR: The treatment of polycythemia vera. Semin Hematol 13:57–78, 1976.

7 · BLOOD TRANSFUSION

Mary C. Baldauf
MARSHFIELD CLINIC

Transfusion therapy consists of providing the specific component to treat a patient's condition. A few decades ago, hemotherapy consisted of whole blood transfusion. Advances in preservation and processing have made the components of one unit available to meet the needs of many patients. The basic indications for blood transfusion are the restoration of blood volume in acute hemorrhage, the maintenance of oxygen-carrying capacity, and the correction of deficiencies of platelets or coagulation factors.

COMPATIBILITY TESTING/BLOOD UTILIZATION

Tests are done prior to red cell transfusion to ensure that the patient receives compatible blood. During a crossmatch, the patient's serum is tested against the donor's red cells. The crossmatch includes methods that demonstrate ABO incompatibility and clinically unexpected antibodies. Donor units have been screened for unexpected antibodies. A compatible crossmatch will not prevent immunization to red cell antigens, nor can it predict normal survival of the transfused cells.

For the patient unlikely to receive a transfusion, the doctor may order a type and screen, consisting of an ABO, Rh, and antibody screen. The patient's sample is retained in the laboratory; in the event of transfusion, the specimen is available for testing. Should a dire emergency occur, type-specific blood may be issued. The patient requiring immediate transfusion may receive type O packed red cells. Once the patient's type is determined, the patient may then receive type-specific blood.

Blood utilization review is an area of concern for hospitals and transfusion services. Policies often include a blood ordering schedule that specifies the blood orders for surgical cases. The medical staff may identify transfusions for review by comparing transfusions prescribed by a physician against a list of predetermined criteria.

In order to reduce the cost of hospitalization, transfusions may be performed as an outpatient service. This requires close communication between patient, physician, and laboratory. All aspects of the transfusion require close supervision, and the facility must be able to respond to adverse patient reactions. The patient should receive post-transfusion instructions that mention the signs and symptoms of delayed hemolytic reactions.

RED CELLS

Red cells provide oxygen-carrying capacity to the tissues. Red cells may be dispensed as packed red cells, prepared from whole blood by sedimentation or centrifugation, and having a hematocrit between 70% and 80% and a volume of 250 ml. Newer preservative solutions (Adsol, Fenwal) dilute the packed cells with an additive. The hematocrit of these units is 55% to 60% and the volume is 350 ml.

Biochemical changes occur in stored blood. Blood collected in ACD (acid citrate dextrose) or CPD (citrate phosphate dextrose) can be stored for 21 days. The addition of adenine, CPDA-1, allows a 35-day red cell storage. The anticoagulant/additive solution Adsol increases the shelf-life to 42 days. During storage, both the percentage of viable cells and the plasma pH decrease. Red cell ATP and 2,3-DPG decrease. Plasma hemoglobin and potassium increase. For these reasons, it may be preferable to select a unit with a short shelf-life when transfusing neonates, or patients unable to tolerate these metabolites.

Red cells should be transfused through a 170-micron filter. A microaggregate filter may aid the multiply-transfused patient by reducing the fibrin and debris in stored blood. It may be necessary to dilute a unit of packed red cells with normal saline to establish a flow. Units collected in anticoagulant/nutrient solutions require no predilution. Other intravenous solutions or medications should not be mixed with blood.

When blood is transfused, the patient's blood volume increases by that amount. If hypovolemia is not present, the blood volume returns to normal in about one day. However, patients with congestive failure or renal disease may have difficulty regaining a normal volume. For these patients, the transfusion must be slow, and may be dispensed in several aliquots. An anticoagulant/nutrient solution may be removed prior to transfusion to decrease the volume.

The effect of transfusion is dependent upon many factors. Whole blood produces greater volume expansion, but red cells give a greater increase in hemoglobin. The increment from a transfusion will depend upon the patient's condition, the presence of bleeding, active red cell destruction, and the hematocrit of the donor units. One should expect an increment of approximately 3% in the hematocrit and 1 gm/dl in hemoglobin for each unit the patient receives. A blood transfusion may decrease the person's ability to produce red cells. An increase in hemoglobin will suppress erythropoietin.

The decision to transfuse is based on the patient's clinical condition rather than a given level of hemoglobin. Signs and symptoms may include dizziness, weakness, or shortness of breath.

Autologous transfusion provides a safe alternative for the healthy patient who will have elective surgery. Blood may be stored in the liquid state, or units may be frozen. Patients donating multiple units may benefit from supplemental iron. At least 72 hours should elapse from the time of the last donation until the surgery. Intraoperative blood salvage is another means of autologous transfusion. In cases where contamination is minimal, cells may be recovered, washed, and transfused in surgery.

Leukocyte-poor red cells are red cells with 70% of the original white cells removed and 70% of the red cells remaining. There are many methods of preparation, including inverted centrifugation, nylon wool filtration, and centrifugation and cooling followed by microaggregate filtration. These units may reduce the incidence and severity of febrile nonhemolytic reactions.

Washed red cells are red cells that have been suspended in saline, centrifuged, and concentrated. Once prepared, cells must be transfused within 24 hours. Washing removes a significant portion of plasma and white cells. Many physicians prescribe washed cells to patients with paroxysmal nocturnal hemoglobinuria to prevent hemolysis, but this practice has been challenged.

Frozen red cells are cryopreserved with glycerol and may be stored for three years. After thawing and deglycerolization, the product may be stored for 24 hours at 1 to 6° C. Because the plasma is removed, this product may be used to transfuse IgA-deficient patients with anti-IgA antibodies. Frozen cells enable a facility to preserve rare units. Autologous donations may be cryopreserved for long intervals.

Whole blood (450 ml) may be used to restore volume in the patient with massive hemorrhage. If this is not available, red cells may be supplemented with crystalloid. Fresh frozen plasma may provide needed coagulation factors. Patients whose blood volume is replaced may require platelets.

There is no standard definition of fresh whole blood. This may refer to blood less than 24 hours old or units five days old or less. Although the whole blood may restore blood volume, platelets and coagulation factors in fresh blood may be insufficient to correct problems in these areas.

PLATELETS

Platelet concentrates consist of the platelet-rich plasma separated from blood within six hours of collection. Random platelet concentrates are prepared by the centrifugation of whole blood. Each unit contains 5.5×10^{10} or more platelets and should increase the platelet count by 5000 to 6000/mm^3 in an average adult. Platelets may be made by apheresis. The single donor platelet concentrate contains 3×10^{11} platelets, the equivalent of six or more random units.

Platelets are used in the treatment of hemorrhage with thrombocytopenia. In certain patients with thrombocytopenia, platelet transfusion may prevent hemorrhage. A dilutional thrombocytopenia occurring after massive transfusion may require platelets. The patient with a functional platelet abnormality may benefit from platelets during bleeding episodes or in preparation for surgery. There is little benefit in transfusing platelets to patients with idiopathic thrombocytopenic purpura because of the rapid destruction of the transfused product.

As the platelet count decreases, the chance of hemorrhage increases. If the level of 20,000/mm^3 is used, the frequent transfusion necessary to maintain this level may result in sensitization. In using a lower level, the physician must weigh the risk of hemorrhage against that of sensitization. The thrombocytopenic patient undergoing surgery should have prophylactic platelet transfusion. A platelet count of 100,000/mm³ should be adequate.

Fever, active bleeding, infection, and drugs influence the survival of platelets. Sensitization may result in the rapid removal of platelets from the circulation. A one-hour post-transfusion platelet count may be obtained to evaluate the increment of a platelet transfusion. The sensitized patient may benefit from an HLA-matched product from a blood relative or nonrelated donor. For the unsensitized patient, random platelets may be used as an initial source of platelets, reserving the single donor product for when refractoriness to random platelets occurs.

ABO antigens are expressed on platelets. When available, ABO-compatible platelets should be transfused. ABO-incompatible platelets are hemostatically effective, but may show a decreased recovery. The ABO-incompatible plasma in pooled concentrates may be removed by centrifugation.

Rh antigens are not expressed on platelets; however, red cell contamination may occur in either random or single donor platelets. There is a small risk of immunization to red cell antigens. For this reason it is preferable to give Rh-negative platelets to Rh-negative women in the childbearing years.

FRESH FROZEN PLASMA

Fresh frozen plasma (FFP) is separated from whole blood and frozen within six hours of collection and contains optimal levels of clotting factors. It is stored at −18° C or lower and has a dating period of 12 months. FFP is thawed at 30 to 37° C and should be transfused promptly. After thawing, the shelf-life is 24 hours. The volume is 225 to 250 ml. Isohemagglutinins are present in plasma, and patients should receive type-compatible plasma. FFP is transfused through a blood filter. Because FFP can transmit hepatitis, there is safer alternative therapy for volume expansion.

FFP is a source of coagulation factors for patients with coagulation protein deficiencies. The transfusion of FFP to patients receiving warfarin sodium will restore factors II, VII, IX, and X in situations requiring rapid treatment, such as hemorrhage. FFP may be transfused alone or as the replacement fluid during plasma exchange for patients with thrombotic thrombocytopenic purpura. Other indications include antithrombin III deficiency and massive blood transfusion. Immune globulin is replacing FFP as a source of immunoglobulin in patients with humoral immune deficiency.

CRYOPRECIPITATE

Cryoprecipitate (cryoprecipitated antihemophilic factor) is the cold insoluble portion of plasma remaining after the plasma has been thawed. Each unit contains an average of 80 IU of factor VIII and at least 150 mg of fibrinogen.

The dosage of factor VIII is calculated by determining the patient's blood volume and then plasma volume. Weight (kg) × 70 ml/kg = blood volume; blood volume (ml) × (1.0 − hematocrit) = plasma volume (ml). Plasma volume (ml) × [desired factor VIII level (%) − initial factor VIII level (%)] = number of units of factor VIII. Therapy is given every eight to 12 hours to maintain factor VIII levels.

Cryoprecipitate may be used in the management of von Willebrand's disease and factor VIII deficiency. Cryoprecipitate is a source of fibrinogen for the treatment of hypofibrinogenemia.

VOLUME EXPANDERS

Plasma substitutes prepared from pools of human plasma are a source of volume and colloid. They have been heat-treated to inactivate the hepatitis virus.

Normal serum albumin (NSA) is an aqueous solution containing the normal serum albumin component of blood. NSA (25%) is dispensed in a 50-ml vial, and NSA (5%) in 250- and 500-ml vials. NSA expands the circulating blood volume and is used in the treatment of shock, surgery, burns, and liver failure. The use of albumin as a source of protein for the patient with cirrhosis, malabsorption, or nephrosis is not warranted. Care must be taken when transfusing NSA to patients at risk for circulatory overload.

Plasma protein fraction (PPF) contains 5% plasma proteins that are 88% albumin, 7% alpha globulin, and 5% beta globulin. PPF is dispensed in 250- and 500-ml vials. It is used in the treatment of shock and as a source of protein for osmotic effect. Severe hypotension has been reported with the rapid infusion of PPF. Neither NSA nor PPF contains clotting factors and will not be of help in the correction of coagulopathies.

GRANULOCYTES

Leukocytes are collected by apheresis; a 250-ml concentrate should contain at least 1×10^{10} granulocytes and platelets, lymphocytes, red cells, and plasma. The donor may receive a sedimenting agent, hydroxyethyl starch, or corticosteroids to increase the number of granulocytes in the collection. Red cell contamination is present, and the product should be ABO- and Rh-compatible with the recipient. A crossmatch is performed on these units. Because granulocytes are short-lived, the cells should be transfused soon after collection.

The neutropenic patient with infection who has not improved with antibiotics may receive leukocyte transfusion. Leukocytes are given daily for at least four to six days or until a clinical improvement or severe reaction occurs. Because cells rapidly leave the circulation, a post-transfusion cell count is not a good indication of the effectiveness of therapy. The best indication is an improvement in the patient's condition.

Severe pulmonary reaction may occur during leukocyte transfusion. Signs and symptoms include dyspnea, tachypnea, cough, and fever. Hypotension and shock may result. The leukocytes must be infused slowly. A patient may need to receive premedication with steroids and nonaspirin antipyretics to lessen the symptoms. Because of the large number of lymphocytes present, this product is often irradiated before it is transfused. The physician must weigh the benefit of leukocyte transfusion against the possibility of pulmonary reactions, cytomegalovirus infection, and sensitization when this product is prescribed.

FACTOR CONCENTRATES

Antihemophilic factor is available as a sterile, dried concentrate. It is produced by the fractionation of pooled fresh frozen plasma and is used in the treatment of hemophilia A. The half-life is nine to 15 hours. This concentrate replaces the missing clotting factor necessary to correct or prevent bleeding episodes. Each bottle has the activity printed on the label. This is used in the calculation of the dosage.

A 5% level of factor VIII is needed to prevent spontaneous hemorrhage. Following trauma or surgery, a level 30% or more of normal may be needed for hemostasis. This should be maintained throughout the period of healing. Patients with severe hemorrhage involving the nervous system, the pharynx, or the retroperitoneum may require 80% to 100% of normal levels to stop the bleeding. Factor VIII level assays are important in monitoring therapy.

Factor IX complex contains clotting factors II, VII, IX, X, and other proteins. Factor IX complex is used for the treatment of factor IX deficiency or the treatment of bleeding episodes in patients with factor VIII inhibitors. Large doses of prothrombin complex concentrates may cause myocardial infarction or disseminated intravascular coagulation. The formula for factor VIII dosage may be used for factor IX calculation.

The patient's weight and clinical condition, the presence of inhibitors, and the degree of deficiency all need to be considered when prescribing concentrates. Factor concentrates are produced from large donor pools. Although the product is tested for hepatitis B surface antigen, cases of hepatitis may occur. Acquired immune deficiency (AIDS) may occur in the hemophilic receiving lyophilized concentrates. These risks may be minimized by treating patients with single donor products when possible. Heat-treated factors now available may reduce the risk of viral transmission.

IMMUNE GLOBULIN

Immune globulins are sterile solutions of antibody-specific gamma globulin prepared from pooled plasma. These are given as intramuscular injections.

Rh immune globulin is used to prevent immunization to the D (Rh$_o$) antigen in Rh-negative women. Rh immune globulin is given to an Rh-negative mother within 72 hours of delivery of an Rh-positive infant, or after abortion, or following amniocentesis. In addition to the post-delivery dose, a dose may also be given at 28 weeks' gestation. One vial of Rh immune globulin is sufficient to prevent sensitization from a fetal-maternal hemorrhage, 15 ml packed red cell volume. If a large bleed is suspected, the amount of fetal cells in the mother's circulation may be determined by the acid elution stain. Should the bleed exceed 15 ml packed red cell volume, additional vials of immune globulin must be given.

Varicella zoster immune globulin contains IgG antibodies to varicella zoster. It can reduce the mortality and morbidity from varicella in immunodeficient children and should be given after exposure, prior to signs of disease.

Immunoglobulin is available against other viral diseases including hepatitis and rubella.

ADVERSE REACTIONS

Untoward effects may occur as a result of transfusion. If the patient receiving a transfusion has adverse signs or symptoms, the transfusion should be stopped and the physician notified. A serologic investigation may be of help in determining the cause of the reaction.

HEMOLYTIC REACTIONS

Immediate Reactions. An immediate hemolytic reaction may be caused by red cell hemolysis. The patient may have fever, chills, chest pains, hypotension, or nausea. The only signs in the anesthetized patient may be hypotension or generalized bleeding. The most common cause of acute intravascular hemolysis is ABO incompatibility. Immunologic events will trigger both complement and coagulation systems. Disseminated intravascular coagulation and acute renal failure may develop.

The laboratory investigation should include a clerical check to verify that the patient identification was correct. A visual check for free hemoglobin comparing pre-transfusion and post-transfusion serum and a direct antiglobulin test may confirm red cell hemolysis. Later, ABO and Rh compatibility testing and antibody screen may be done on pre- and post-transfusion specimens. Bacterial contamination, heat or osmotic stress, or donor red cell abnormalities are other causes of hemolysis. If immune hemolysis is not present, these possibilities may be checked.

Therapy consists of maintaining blood pressure and renal urinary output. Although mannitol has been used in the management of hemolytic reactions, furosemide, 80 to 120 mg given intravenously, will improve renal blood flow and result in diuresis.

Delayed Reactions. The delayed hemolytic reaction occurs several days to two weeks after transfusion. The reaction may be the result of a primary immunization. As antibody is produced, red cells are destroyed. Delayed hemolysis may occur as an anamnestic response. The production of high levels of IgG antibodies destroys transfused cells. The patient may have fever, jaundice, or hemoglobinuria. Laboratory results may show a decreased hemoglobin, a positive antiglobulin test, or a red cell alloantibody. Once the alloantibody is identified, the patient should receive blood that is negative for the antigen to which his is sensitized.

IMMUNE REACTIONS WITHOUT HEMOLYSIS

The febrile nonhemolytic reaction occurs when the patient's temperature increases 1° C or more in association with transfusion. The reaction occurs most often in the multiply-transfused patient or in the woman who has had several pregnancies. The mechanism is due to antibodies against leukocytes, granulocytes, or platelet antigens. If the patient has benign reactions, fever and discomfort may be prevented by premedication with antipyretics prior to transfusion. The patient with severe reactions may benefit from a leukocyte-poor blood product.

The anaphylactic reaction occurs after the patient receives a small amount of blood. The patient may have respiratory distress, hypotension, nausea, cramps, or diarrhea. Unconsciousness and shock may follow. The reaction occurs most often in the IgA-deficient patient with anti-IgA antibodies. These patients may receive blood from IgA-deficient donors, frozen deglycerolized red blood cells, or autologous transfusions.

Allergic reactions may result from blood transfusions, and may be due to allergens in the donor's plasma. The patient may itch, or develop erythema or hives. These symptoms respond to treatment with antihistamines. If no other signs or symptoms are present, the transfusion may be continued. A washed red cell product may benefit the patient with severe reactions.

Graft-versus-host disease (GVHD) occurs when immunocompetent lymphocytes from the donor unit engraft in the patient. The patient may have skin rash, diarrhea, liver dysfunction, and marrow suppression. The treatment of GVHD is investigational. A radiation dose of 1500 to 3000 rads to blood products will prevent lymphocytes from dividing, yet not affect platelet, granulocyte, or red cell function.

INFECTIOUS DISEASE

Transfusion-associated hepatitis is a serious complication of blood transfusion. Donor blood has been screened for hepatitis B surface antigen. Non-A, non-B hepatitis accounts for most transfusion-acquired cases. Two to 25 weeks following transfusion, patients may have weakness, nausea, or joint pain. Some may have no symptoms and only elevated liver enzymes. Although most patients do not develop jaundice, certain patients with non-A, non-B hepatitis may develop chronic active hepatitis or cirrhosis. If the physician reports these cases to the laboratory, the donors transmitting non-A, non-B may be identified.

Cytomegalovirus infection may be transfusion-acquired and is a special concern for the neonate and the immunocompromised patient. Although there is no ideal test to determine CMV infectivity of donor blood, some centers may offer CMV antibody-negative units.

Malaria may be transmitted by blood transfusion. The donor history includes questions about travel in malaria-endemic areas. Syphilis may be transmitted by blood products that have been stored at room temperature or those transfused shortly after donation. Federal law requires that donor units be screened for syphilis. Acquired immune deficiency syndrome has been reported as the result of blood transfusion. Units are now routinely screened for HTLV-III antibodies. Bacterial contamination of a unit of blood may result in sepsis or shock.

OTHER PROBLEMS

Blood transfusion may result in hypervolemia. Anticoagulant/additive solutions add 100 ml of volume to a unit of red cells. The patient with congestive heart failure or edema should receive concentrated red cells. Transfusion should be slow and may be dispensed in small aliquots at a rate of 1 ml/kg of body weight per hour.

The chronically transfused patient may develop hemosiderosis. Each unit contains 250 mg of iron, which may deposit in the heart, liver, or glands. Chelating agents may remove iron without decreasing hemoglobin.

REFERENCES

American Association of Blood Banks: Technical Manual, 9th ed. J. B. Lippincott Co, Philadelphia, 1985.
Consensus Conference: Fresh-frozen plasma. JAMA 25:551–553, 1985.
Mollison PL: Blood Transfusion in Clinical Medicine, 7th ed. Blackwell Scientific Publications, Boston, 1983.

8 · IMMUNODEFICIENCY

William R. Friedenberg
MARSHFIELD CLINIC

DEFINITION AND DIAGNOSTIC CRITERIA

Immunodeficiency diseases are rare disorders in which there is a defect in host defense against infection. The primary immunodeficiency disease can be divided into four types (Table 1), although many patients have defects in more than one category.

PATHOGENESIS

Normal immunity requires cooperation among the various populations of lymphocytes, antibodies, complement, and phagocytic cells that participate in the inflammatory process. Patients with defects in cell-mediated immunity (CMI) are most susceptible to viral, fungal, and mycobacterial infections, whereas patients deficient in antibodies, complement, or phagocytic cell function usually present with bacterial infections. Many patients suffer from both kinds of infections.

A patient with an increased incidence of infections, unusual or severe infections, or chronic diarrhea, and an infant with failure to thrive, should have screening tests performed (Table 2). If the clinical suspicion is strong or a screening test is abnormal, additional tests are indicated (Table 2).

CLINICAL ASPECTS AND MANAGEMENT

Patients with CMI defects (and family members) should not receive live attenuated vaccines. They must be protected from exposure to viral infections. Prophylactic and therapeutic maneuvers similar to those with neutropenia (Chapter 9) are indicated in patients with CMI defects as well as antibody, complement, and phagocytic cell deficiencies.

DEFECTS IN CMI

Severe Combined Immunodeficiency Disease (SCID). Patients with SCID develop failure to thrive within a few months of birth. A transient rash, which may be graft-versus-host disease, frequently occurs in the first few days of life followed by persistent oral moniliasis in the neonatal period. Diarrhea and pneumonia due to *Pneumocystis carinii* occur frequently. Patients sometimes

Table 1. PRIMARY IMMUNODEFICIENCY DISEASES

Abnormal Cell-Mediated Immunity	Antibody Deficiency	Complement Deficiency	Phagocytic Cell Dysfunction
Severe combined immunodeficiency disease (SCID)	Bruton's agammaglobulinemia	Classic pathway defects	Chemotactic defects
Nezelof's syndrome	Transient hypogammaglobulinemia	Alternate pathway defects	Phagocytic and killing capacity defects
DiGeorge's syndrome	Common variable hypogammaglobulinemia	Deficient activation of complement components	
Chronic mucocutaneous candidiasis	Miscellaneous		
Wiskott-Aldrich syndrome			
Ataxia telangiectasia			
Duncan disease			

have a positive family history. There is usually severe lymphopenia (<1000 lymphocytes/mm³), with the number of mature T cells low. Some patients have normal B cells, but immunoglobulin levels are usually low. A very rare patient may have agranulocytosis with SCID (reticular dysgenesis). The disease can be inherited in an autosomal or sex-linked recessive way. Half the autosomal recessive cases are associated with a deficiency of the enzyme adenosine deaminase (ADA).

Unless treated with a bone marrow transplantation from an HLA identical sibling or unrelated HLA identical donor, SCID is usually fatal in the first few years of life. In those patients without an HLA identical donor, there have been a few successful transplants of fetal tissue (liver, thymus, thymic epithelium) and non–HLA identical bone marrow transplants. Transfusions of frozen irradiated red cells have been used as a source of ADA in patients with this deficiency with some success.

Combined Immunodeficiency with Predominant T Cell Defect (Nezelof's Syndrome). These patients have severe T cell deficiency with normal B cells and immunoglobulin levels. Some patients have purine–nucleoside phosphorylase deficiency. In vitro T cell responses to mitogens and antigens are absent and immunoglobulin levels are normal. There have been some in vitro improvements in cellular function with infusion of irradiated red cells and plasma from normal donors, but the clinical course in these patients has not been changed.

DiGeorge's Syndrome. Patients with this syndrome fail to develop the third and fourth pharyngeal pouches, causing a congenital malformation in the development of the thymus and parathyroid glands. These infants have neonatal tetany, hypocalcemia, cardiac defects, and abnormalities of the ears, nose, mouth, and great vessels. The T cell defect is variable, with significant depression of CMI and normal B cells. Fetal thymic implants, fetal thymic epithelium, and fetal thymus in a Millepore diffusion chamber have been effective, suggesting a deficiency in thymic hormones.

Chronic Mucocutaneous Candidiasis. These patients have a variety of immune abnormalities: (1) deficiency in lymphocyte responses to a variety of antigens including *Candida;* (2) intact cellular immunity except for a defect in responding to *Candida;* (3) lack of macrophage-inhibiting factor production by lymphocytes after stimulation with *Candida;* and (4) abnormal neutrophil and monocyte chemotaxis.

Many of these patients have associated abnormalities including endocrinopathies, pernicious anemia, and granulomatous disease. Systemic infection occurs infrequently. Treatment with topical agents such as nystatin can suppress infection in mildly affected patients. More severely affected patients can be treated with oral ketoconazole. If there is deep-seated tissue infection or fungemia, IV amphotericin B is indicated. Agents that stimulate T cell function such as transfer factor or thymosin have occasionally been beneficial.

Wiskott-Aldrich Syndrome. Wiskott-Aldrich syndrome (eczema, impaired humoral and cell-mediated immunity, and thrombocytopenia) is inherited as an X-linked recessive trait. Most patients die of infection, a smaller proportion from bleeding or a lymphoma. These boys do not respond well to polysaccharide antigens and lack serum isohemagglutinins. The T cells progressively decrease until profound lymphopenia occurs at approximately 6 years of age. Bone marrow transplantation has been successful in correcting the eczema and lymphocyte dysfunction, but the thrombocytopenia persists. Splenectomy has been useful in improving the platelet count.

Ataxia-Telangiectasia. Ataxia-telangiectasia is an autosomal recessive trait that becomes evident when in-

Table 2. IMMUNE DEFICIENCY EVALUATION

CMI	Antibody Deficiency	Complement Deficiency	Phagocytic Cell Dysfunction
Screening			
CBC	Serum protein electrophoresis	Total hemolytic complement (CH_{50})	Nitroblue tetrazolium (NBT)
Skin tests	Quantitative immunoglobulins		CBC
(Delayed type hypersensitivity)	Immunization with typhoid and tetanus		
*Extensive Evaluation**			
Surface analysis of peripheral blood or tissue lymphocytes' phenotype		C3	Chemotaxis
		C4	Phagocytic index
		Factor B	Bactericidal index
Lymphocyte functional analysis			IgE level

*Many other tests may be indicated based upon abnormalities detected or clinical suspicion. Specific reference labs may be necessary for very specialized tests.

fants begin walking with an ataxic (cerebellar) gait. Telangiectasias appear at approximately the fifth year on the bulbar conjunctivae or on the flexure surfaces of the arms. Patients have repeated sinopulmonary infections and frequently develop lymphoproliferative diseases. Immunoglobulins are low, with a prominent defect in helper T cells and normal suppressor T cell activity. No successful treatment exists.

Duncan Disease. This disease occurs when patients with Epstein-Barr (EB) virus infection develop B cell lymphoproliferative disease, marrow aplasia, fatal progressive mononucleosis, or agammaglobulinemia. Prior to their exposure to EB virus, these patients appear to be immunologically normal, but following the infection, B cells and immunoglobulins decrease and T cells become natural killer cells. Originally this was felt to be an X-linked recessive trait, but subsequently affected female patients have been found. There is no effective treatment.

ANTIBODY DEFICIENCY

Bruton's Agammaglobulinemia. This is an X-linked recessive disorder. Boys present with a pyogenic infection six to nine months following birth when maternally transmitted immunoglobulin disappears. Frequently the pyogenic infections involve the sinopulmonary tree. Chronic diarrhea due to enterovirus may dominate the clinical picture. Usually all three major immunoglobulin classes are below 100 mg/dl. These patients do not respond to standard immunizations. Natural antibodies to blood group substances are absent. B cells are absent or in very low numbers in the peripheral blood, but normal numbers of pre-B cells are found in the bone marrow. Germinal centers are not found in lymphoid tissue, and plasma cells are rare. Cell-mediated immune function is normal.

Treatment with gamma globulin reduces the infection rate, days in the hospital, and chronic debility. Previously, replacement therapy with intravenous plasma required a large volume with an increased risk of hepatitis. Intramuscular injection was painful, limiting the large volumes necessary. Currently, immunoglobulin preparations have been developed for intravenous use (Gamimune, Sandoglobulin) that meet acceptable standards for antibody structure and function, stability, safety, effective half-life, and a minimum of side effects to patients. The usual dose is 100 mg/kg intravenously every month, which provides an increase of approximately 200 mg/dl in serum IgG just before the next injection. Larger or more frequent doses can be given to increase the IgG level to 500 to 1000 mg/dl to try to prevent recurrent sinopulmonary infections or to eliminate already established infections. The intravenous products are superior to the intramuscular form but very expensive.

Transient Hypogammaglobulinemia of Infancy. Normally there is a gradual decrease in the serum IgG level as an infant catabolizes maternally derived IgG, with the nadir occurring between the third and the sixth months. Other tests of the immune system, including IgM and IgA levels, are normal. This syndrome may represent delayed normal maturation of the immune response and, by definition, all infants recover by 1 to 2 years of age.

Common Variable Hypogammaglobulinemia. This disorder may be familial but occurs equally in males and females, with no specific mode of inheritance. Patients usually present with pyogenic infections. Some develop spruelike syndromes, frequently secondary to *Giardia lamblia*. Other patients have nodular lymphoid hyperplasia in the gastrointestinal tract, approximately one third have pernicious anemia, and there is a high incidence of gastrointestinal neoplasms. *Mycoplasma* infections can cause progressive rheumatoid-like illness. Noncaseating granulomas can be found in many organs without any organisms being recovered.

Three pathogenetic mechanisms have been postulated: (1) a defect in the intrinsic nature of the B cell; (2) an excess of T suppressor cells; and (3) autoantibodies to T or B cells.

These patients benefit from prophylactic treatment with intravenous gamma globulin as described for patients with Bruton's agammaglobulinemia.

Miscellaneous. There are patients with: (1) normal immunoglobulin levels who are unable to respond to stimulation with specific antigens; (2) IgG subclass deficiencies; (3) severe hypogammaglobulinemia with thymoma, some of whom respond to thymectomy; (4) X-linked hypogammaglobulinemia who also have growth hormone deficiency; (5) autosomal recessive agammaglobulinemia with an immunoglobulin (IgG or IgA) deficiency with increased IgM; (6) absence of serum IgA, which occurs in one of 700 people in the general population. Although many of these latter patients are apparently healthy, there are some who have frequent infections and autoimmune disease. Low serum IgA may also occur secondary to the administration of phenytoin. Patients without IgA may have angioedema or anaphylaxis with transfusion.

COMPLEMENT DEFICIENCY

Complement deficiencies may be: (1) in the classic pathway; (2) in the alternative pathway; or (3) due to defective activation of the complement components. Patients with apparently normal cellular and humoral immunity who are suspected of immunodeficiency should have their complement system assayed for abnormalities. The entire complement system can be measured by the total hemolytic complement assay and is available in many clinical laboratories. If there is a marked depression of one of the essential complement components, the total hemolytic complement will be low. Complement components can be assayed using commercial kits, and such factors as C3 may be deficient in patients with recurrent infections. In addition to analyzing for deficiencies of C3, C4, and factor B, assays of the generation of chemotactic factors can determine the functional integrity of the classic or alternate pathway. Fresh frozen plasma can replenish complement components during episodes of infection.

PHAGOCYTIC CELL DYSFUNCTION

The most common defect in phagocytic cell activity is quantitative rather than qualitative, i.e., neutropenia (Chapter 9). Since neutrophils and macrophages provide the first line of defense against bacterial invasion, qualitative defects in the ability of these cells to migrate to the site of inflammation (chemotaxis) or to engulf (phagocytosis) and kill microorganisms (bactericidal capacity) are associated with serious infections. Serum inhibitors have also been described that inhibit phagocytic cell function.

Chemotactic Defects. The ability of neutrophils to respond to chemoattractants can be measured in a Boyden chamber. Many drugs have been associated with abnormal chemotaxis, as have patients with diabetes mellitus, renal failure, infections, and burns. Congenital abnormalities with abnormal chemotaxis include the lazy leukocyte syndrome, congenital ichthyosis, hyperimmunoglobulinemia E syndrome (Job's), Schaumann's syndrome, actin dysfunction, the Chédiak-Higashi syndrome, and others.

Phagocytic and Killing Capacity Defects. Defective phagocytosis has been seen in: (1) the actin dysfunction syndrome; (2) severe iron deficiency; (3) infection; (4) malnutrition; and (5) severe hypophosphatemia. Defects in oxygen metabolism, such as occur in chronic granulomatous disease, myeloperoxidase deficiency, Chédiak-Higashi syndrome, Down's syndrome, and others, cause an inability to effectively kill ingested microorganisms. There have been patients reported with isolated defects in killing specific organisms such as *Staphylococcus aureus*.

Fortunately congenital neutrophil dysfunction syndromes are rare, because effective treatment is lacking. Antibiotics, prophylactic and therapeutic, are the mainstay of treatment. Those patients who have serum inhibitors may be candidates for plasmapheresis to try to reduce inhibitory proteins. Granulocyte transfusions may sometimes be useful. If there is concomitant T cell dysfunction, such agents as transfer factor or thymosin may be tried in order to improve cellular immunity and possibly phagocytic cell function as well. Ascorbic acid has been used to try to improve neutrophil function.

CONCLUSION

Treatment of the immunodeficiency diseases requires accurate assessment of the immune system and an understanding that the four limbs of immunity are interdependent and require cooperation in order to keep microorganisms at bay. Since treatment other than bone marrow transplantation is rarely curative, the long-term goal should be palliation with a reduction in the rate and severity of infections.

REFERENCES

Bellanti JA, Dayton DH (eds): The Phagocytic Cell in Host Resistance. Raven Press, New York, 1975.

Good RA (ed): The American Journal of Medicine (Intravenous Immune Globulin and the Compromised Host), Vol 76(3A). Technical Publishing, New York, March 30, 1984.

Hill HR: Immunodeficiency diseases. Prog Clin Pathol 8:205–238, 1981.

Rosen FS, Cooper MD, Wedgwood RJP: The primary immunodeficiencies (two parts). N Engl J Med 311:235–242, 1984; 311:300–310, 1984.

Waldmann TA: The regulation of the human humoral response and functional assays for its assessment. Birth Defects 19:31–36, 1983.

9 · NEUTROPENIA

William R. Friedenberg
MARSHFIELD CLINIC

DEFINITION AND DIAGNOSTIC CRITERIA

Neutropenia is defined as a reduction in the absolute number of circulating neutrophils, calculated by multiplying the percentage of neutrophils (segs and bands) times the total white cell count. The normal absolute neutrophil count is dependent upon age and race, and should be considered abnormal in Caucasian adults if <1600 mm^3. Progressive neutropenia with counts <1000 mm^3 are associated with an increasing incidence of infection (Table 1). Many neutropenic disorders should be treated only when they become symptomatic.

PATHOPHYSIOLOGY

Neutropenia may be secondary to reduced production of neutrophils from the bone marrow, ineffective production, abnormal distribution, an increase in destruction, or combinations of these (Table 1). Many tests

Table 1. DIFFERENTIAL DIAGNOSIS OF NEUTROPENIA

Pathophysiology
Disorders of combined or complex pathophysiology
  Benign chronic neutropenia
  Chronic severe idiopathic neutropenia
  Pseudoneutropenia
  Infection
  Drugs or chemicals
  Cyclical neutropenia
Ineffective or decreased production of neutrophils
  B$_{12}$ or folic acid deficiency
  Malignancy—lymphoma, leukemia, etc.
  Aplastic anemia
  Others
Distribution disorder—hypersplenism
Autoimmune neutropenia (antibody- or lymphocyte-induced)
  Felty's syndrome
  Idiopathic
  Associated with malignancy
  Others
Complement activation neutropenia
  Sepsis
  Dialysis or cardiopulmonary bypass

Degree of Neutropenia

Mild:	1000–1600/mm^3
Moderate:	500–1000/mm^3
Severe:	<500/mm^3

(neutrophil mobilization, bone marrow) have been used to establish a diagnosis, but they should be used selectively.

CLINICAL ASPECTS AND MANAGEMENT

A careful history and physical examination narrows the possible diagnoses considerably. A patient seen for a periodic exam who has mild neutropenia may have a viral infection. In addition to stopping all drugs possible, the patient should return in several weeks for a repeat count prior to an extensive evaluation because many of these patients will return to normal.

Severe neutropenia is a life-threatening condition. Neutropenic patients should be managed at home, if possible, because infections acquired in the hospital are frequently more difficult to eradicate. If additional immune defects are present (hypogammaglobulinemia, lymphocyte dysfunction, splenectomy), the patient will be at higher risk.

Patients should use a soft toothbrush, mouthwashes, and water picks. Bactrim DS, 1 tablet twice a day (in adults), can reduce the incidence of sinopulmonary infections. Preoperative short-term prophylactic antibiotics should be given. Patients should be warned to see a physician at the first hint of infection. Febrile patients should receive broad-spectrum antibiotics after cultures are obtained. In patients who do not respond to antibiotics, granulocyte transfusions may be used. Gamma globulin can be given to patients who also have severe hypogammaglobulinemia. Hospitalized patients do not benefit by having visitors wear masks, gloves, and gowns, but good handwashing prior to entering a private room is good practice. Laminar air flow rooms are expensive and relatively ineffective. Rectal temperatures and examinations should be avoided. Stool softeners and a high-fiber diet may decrease problems with hemorrhoids and perirectal abscess. Long-term indwelling catheters (Hickman) require meticulous attention to sterile technique. The patient's age, underlying illness, and prior treatment will help determine the extent of treatment of an infection.

The treatment of neutropenia requires the specific diagnosis of the cause. Even mild improvements in absolute neutrophil count can be associated with a reduction in infections and the symptoms associated with neutropenia.

DISORDERS OF COMPLEX OR COMBINED PATHOPHYSIOLOGY

Benign Chronic Neutropenia (BCN). Patients with chronic mild to moderate neutropenia in the absence of other diagnoses (Table 1) have BCN. These patients have good bone marrow reserves and do not have frequent infections. No treatment is necessary.

Chronic Severe Idiopathic Neutropenia. These disorders are frequently congenital and associated with other abnormalities. They respond poorly to prednisone and splenectomy, but may improve with lithium, which increases production of neutrophils from bone marrow reserves.

Pseudoneutropenia. These patients have an increased marginal pool, are asymptomatic, and demonstrate a dramatic response to epinephrine. They do not need treatment.

Infections. Sepsis can cause severe neutropenia. Appropriate cultures should be obtained and treatment of the presumed infection initiated.

Drug- or Chemical-induced Neutropenia. Some drugs are notorious for producing agranulocytosis (phenylbutazone, phenothiazines), but all drugs should be suspect. While other etiologic factors are being evaluated, all medications possible should be discontinued. Most patients will rapidly improve after stopping the suspected causative agent.

Cyclical Neutropenia. These patients develop severe neutropenia every 21 days, lasting only three to four days. When neutropenic, they feel tired and may get mouth sores. Splenectomy, androgens, steroids, and lithium have been tried with occasional clinical improvement.

DISORDERS OF INEFFECTIVE OR DECREASED PRODUCTION OF NEUTROPHILS

Disorders such as pernicious anemia may be associated with mild neutropenia but rapidly resolve with vitamin B_{12} replacement therapy. Disorders of production such as aplastic anemia and acute leukemia require treatment of the underlying disease.

DISORDERS OF DISTRIBUTION

Hypersplenism is a common cause of neutropenia that may be isolated or associated with anemia or thrombocytopenia. If the patient is symptomatic, splenectomy should be performed.

AUTOIMMUNE NEUTROPENIA

Antibody-induced neutropenia has been difficult to diagnose because of the lack of a reliable test, such as is available for autoimmune hemolytic anemia (direct Coombs' test). Patients with Felty's syndrome (rheumatoid arthritis, splenomegaly, and neutropenia) improve in 30% to 70% of cases following splenectomy. Lithium has been shown to be effective in some patients with this disorder. Occasional patients may improve with cytotoxic agents or steroids. They should not be treated unless they become symptomatic.

COMPLEMENT ACTIVATION NEUTROPENIA

Complement may be activated with sepsis, hemodialysis, and cardiopulmonary bypass. Activated complement (C5a) causes granulocyte aggregation, neutropenia, and tissue damage. Large doses of steroids may be helpful when this occurs. Patients on hemodialysis who develop neutropenia during dialysis may benefit by changing the dialysis membrane.

REFERENCES

Brown AE: Neutropenia, fever, and infection. Am J Med 76:421–428, 1984.

Dale DC, Fauci AS, Guerry IV D, Wolff SM: Comparison of agents producing a neutrophilic leukocytosis in man. J Clin Invest 56:808–813, 1975.

Kyle RA: Natural history of chronic idiopathic neutropenia. N Engl J Med 302:908–909, 1980.

Rossof AH, Robinson WA: Lithium Effects on Granulopoiesis and Immune Function, Vol 127 (Advances in Experimental Medicine and Biology). Plenum Press, New York, 1980.

Williams WJ, Beutler, E, Erslev AJ, Lichtman MA: Hematology, 3rd ed. McGraw-Hill Book Co, New York, 1983.

10 · INHERITED DISORDERS OF COAGULATION

Karen A. Bringelsen
Gerald S. Gilchrist
MAYO CLINIC AND MAYO FOUNDATION

Table 1. NOMENCLATURE AND FUNCTION OF FACTOR VIII AND VON WILLEBRAND FACTOR

	Factor VIII	von Willebrand Factor
Prior terminology	Antihemophilic factor (VIIIC, VIIIC:Ag)	Factor VIII–related antigen (VIII:Ag) Ristocetin-Willebrand cofactor
Proposed abbreviations (protein, antigen)	VIII,* VIII:Ag†	vWF,* vWF:Ag†
Principal biologic activity	Procoagulant cofactor	Interaction of platelets with the vessel wall Carrier for factor VIII in plasma
Clinical disorder due to deficiency	Hemophilia A	von Willebrand's disease
Inheritance	X-linked recessive	Autosomal
Cellular site of biosynthesis	Not certain	Endothelial cells and megakaryocytes

*Detected by functional assay.
†Detected by immunologic assay.

DEFINITION

The inherited disorders of blood coagulation are characterized by an absence, deficiency, or abnormality in one of the plasma factors necessary for normal hemostasis. Congenital deficiencies of all the factors are recognized, with factors VIII and IX the most common. A better understanding of the coagulation mechanism and plasma components has led to more effective management of hemorrhagic disorders.

PATHOPHYSIOLOGY

The coagulation mechanism is a complex cascade of enzymatic reactions causing sequential activation of clotting factors and resulting in a localized fibrin clot. For purposes of laboratory evaluation, the mechanism is divided into four parts:

1. The intrinsic system, activated by contact of blood with foreign surfaces, requires factors XII, XI, IX, VIII, and platelet phospholipid for activation of factor X.

2. The extrinsic system, activated by exposure of blood to injured tissue, in the presence of factor VII results in activation of factor X.

3. The final common pathway, initiated by activated factor X, results in a localized fibrin clot and requires the presence of factors V, II (prothrombin), and fibrinogen.

4. Consolidation of the fibrin clot occurs through the action of the fibrin-stabilizing factor (factor XIII).

FACTOR VIII DEFICIENCY

Factor VIII, abnormal in hemophilia A and von Willebrand's disease, is a complex molecule. The smaller component, factor VIII, is the coagulant protein or antihemophilic factor. The larger component is a polymeric protein, von Willebrand factor (VWF). Functionally, VWF is necessary for normal platelet/vessel interaction. Its activity is measured by its ability to aggregate normal platelets in the presence of ristocetin.

Table 1 summarizes the proposed new nomenclature for the factor VIII complex and the functions of factor VIII and von Willebrand factor.

HEMOPHILIA A (CLASSIC HEMOPHILIA)

Deficiency of factor VIII is an X-linked trait. The severity of the deficiency and bleeding is variable, but generally consistent within the members of one family.

"Spontaneous" bleeding into joints and soft tissues occurs in patients with severe deficiency (factor VIII of less than 1%). There is potential for serious physical disability with its attendant social and economic problems. Patients with moderate deficiency (2% to 5% of normal) generally bleed only after trauma, but "spontaneous" bleeding does occur. In mild deficiency (6% to 30%), bleeding usually occurs only with significant trauma or surgery. Hemophilia may be suspected from the family history, the bleeding pattern, and an abnormal partial thromboplastin time (PTT) with a normal prothrombin time. The diagnosis is confirmed by specific factor VIII assay. With a mild deficiency of 20%, the PTT may be normal, but the coagulant level is still too low for hemostasis following surgery or trauma.

VON WILLEBRAND'S DISEASE

Deficiency of von Willebrand factor is autosomally inherited, affecting males and females equally. Bleeding is usually mucosal and cutaneous, although joint bleeding does occur with very low factor VIII levels. Epistaxis is especially troublesome in youngsters. Menorrhagia may be severe.

The diagnosis may be difficult because of the variability in clinical severity and laboratory values in the same patient at different times. This variability is in part due to release of stored VWF from endothelial cells in response to physiologic stressors such as exercise or pregnancy. Varying degrees of prolongation of bleeding time, abnormal ristocetin-induced platelet aggregation, and reduced levels of factor VIII, VWF, and VWF:Ag are found.

At least three variants or types of von Willebrand's disease are recognized as detected by differences in the polymer pattern on agarose gel electrophoresis. Type I has a reduced concentration of normal polymers. Type IIA shows absence of large polymers. In type IIB, large polymers are present on platelets but absent in the plasma, and ristocetin-induced platelet aggregation is increased. Type III is a homozygous state in which almost no VWF is synthesized.

CORRECTION OF FACTOR VIII DEFICIENCY

Treatment of bleeding episodes usually requires replacement of factor VIII by products derived from human plasma. Fresh frozen plasma (FFP), cryoprecipitate, and lyophilized factor VIII concentrate are used, each with advantages and disadvantages.

Fresh frozen plasma (FFP), derived from individual donors, contains all the plasma clotting factors and is useful in the treatment of patients with any coagulation factor deficiency. It contains 0.7 to 0.9 units/ml coagulant activity (1 unit is the amount of coagulant activity in 1 ml of plasma with 100% activity). The use of FFP is limited by the large volumes necessary to reach hemostatic factor levels.

Cryoprecipitate is prepared from single donor units of plasma, stored frozen at $-20°$ C, and thawed just prior to administration. Each 20- to 30-ml bag contains approximately 100 units of factor VIII, although the actual amount may vary with the blood bank's extraction and thawing techniques. It has the advantage of exposure to fewer donors and lessens the risk of hepatitis and possibly AIDS.

Lyophilized factor VIII concentrates are extracted from the pooled plasma of thousands of donors. In the United States, concentrates are produced and marketed by a number of pharmaceutical companies. Each lot of concentrate is assayed for factor activity and the activity content is noted on the container. Concentrate can be stored at room temperature and is easily reconstituted. The disadvantage of concentrates is the increased risk of transfusion-related illness.

Dosage Calculations. One unit of factor VIII per kilogram of body weight will raise the circulating factor VIII level by about 2%. The circulating half-life is approximately 12 hours. To raise the factor VIII level to 50% in a 20-kg child with severe hemophilia (VIII <1%) requires:

$$\text{dose} = \frac{\text{weight (kg)} \times \text{rise required}}{2} = 500 \text{ units}$$

Since the increment in factor VIII and the half-life vary, the plasma level can be assayed before, 30 minutes after, and eight to 12 hours after infusion to measure in vivo recovery and decay. This is particularly important in patients undergoing major surgery where satisfactory levels of factor VIII activity must be maintained. Doses calculated to maintain adequate hemostasis are repeated every eight to 12 hours depending on the clinical situation, the peak level, and the estimated half-disappearance time.

Von Willebrand's disease may be treated with fresh frozen plasma or cryoprecipitate. For immediate treatment of major bleeding in patients with low levels of factor VIII, the dose should be calculated as above. However, infusion of plasma or cryoprecipitate stimulates an exaggerated rise of factor VIII in the plasma some hours after transfusion that persists for up to 48 hours. Therefore, to treat minor bleeding or in preparation for surgery, 10 to 15 ml/kg FFP or 1 bag/10 kg cryoprecipitate is used. Smaller doses may be effective, particularly if the baseline factor VIII level is above 3%. We monitor factor VIII levels to assure adequate hemostasis.

DDAVP (desmopressin), a synthetic analogue of vasopressin, is an alternative means of increasing factor VIII levels in mild hemophilia and type I von Willebrand's disease. A dose of 0.3 µg/kg IV in 50 ml saline given over 15 to 30 minutes will release stored factor VIII and increase the baseline level two- to fivefold. Circulating half-life is similar to that achieved with blood products. The dose may be repeated in 48 hours after storage sites have been replenished. DDAVP is useful for patients with mild factor VIII deficiency in whom hemostatic levels can be achieved. It is also useful in type I von Willebrand's disease where the polymers are normal but quantitatively decreased. DDAVP is contraindicated for patients with type IIB disease, in whom it may cause thrombocytopenia due to platelet aggregation by abnormal polymers. It is, therefore, extremely important to determine the type of von Willebrand's disease, before using DDAVP. The individual response is variable, and all patients must have their response to DDAVP measured prior to its use in a treatment situation.

FACTOR IX DEFICIENCY (HEMOPHILIA B, CHRISTMAS DISEASE)

Deficiency of factor IX is an X-linked trait very similar in its clinical manifestations to factor VIII deficiency. The factor IX molecule, smaller than VIII, is distributed beyond the intravascular space. Thus, 1 unit/kg of factor IX raises the level by about 1%. To raise the level to 50% in a 20-kg child with factor IX of less than 1% requires 1000 units of factor IX. Although factor IX has a half-life of about 24 hours, the first phase of disappearance is rapid. Therefore, to maintain hemostatic levels, infusion every 12 hours is necessary.

Fresh frozen plasma and heat-treated lyophilized prothrombin complex concentrates are used for factor IX replacement. Concentrates are also prepared from large donor pools and contain other vitamin K–dependent factors, II, VII, and X.

Although we prefer to treat patients with mild deficiencies and young children with FFP, the volumes necessary can make this impractical, if not impossible. Severely affected individuals and those with major trauma and surgery are treated with concentrates although the risk of hepatitis is increased.

FACTOR XI DEFICIENCY (HEMOPHILIA C)

Fresh frozen plasma is the only product containing factor XI. The dosage calculation is the same as for factor VIII; however, the in vivo half-life is 40 to 80 hours and hemostasis can be maintained with less risk of volume overload. Transfusion of 10 ml/kg will attain a level of about 20% and the dose may be repeated every six to eight hours if tolerated to achieve a stepwise increment in plasma levels. If higher levels are necessary, a partial exchange transfusion or plasmapheresis may be necessary to avoid circulatory overload.

OTHER COAGULATION FACTOR DEFICIENCIES

The remaining clotting factor abnormalities are rare. They are inherited in autosomal recessive fashion. Clinical manifestations vary, but in general are not as severe as in severe hemophilia A or B. Table 2 summarizes the management of these disorders.

Table 2. RARE AUTOSOMAL FACTOR DEFICIENCIES

Deficiency	Bleeding Profile	Replacement Product	Dose
Factor XII, Hageman factor	No bleeding clinically	None necessary	
Factor XIII, fibrin-stabilizing factor	Initial hemostasis with delayed bleeding	Fresh frozen plasma	2–3 ml/kg weekly
Factors II, VII, X	Usually very mild	Fresh frozen plasma Prothrombin complex concentrates (Factor IX conc.)	Similar to Factor IX concentrate
Factor V	Mild	Fresh frozen plasma	Similar to Factor IX

MANAGEMENT OF SPECIFIC PROBLEMS

JOINT BLEEDING

Hemarthroses may occur spontaneously with only the "wear and tear" of normal daily activity. At the onset of bleeding, patients are aware of a tingling, stinging, or stretching sensation before there is pain and are instructed to treat immediately. The factor level is increased to ±40%, although 20% has been found to be effective in some patients. The dose is repeated in 24 hours if signs and symptoms have not begun to resolve. Local measures using Ace wraps and ice may be helpful. Prolonged immobilization is discouraged unless pain has become severe with joint distention. Physical therapy is important to preserve joint function and should begin as soon as bleeding has stopped.

Aspiration of a joint is usually unnecesasry unless there is marked distention with severe pain. There is usually little difficulty distinguishing between hemarthrosis and septic arthritis.

Many patients have a particular "target" joint that bleeds repeatedly with resulting synovitis. The hypervascular synovium is subject to frequent hemorrhage, developing chronic synovitis and debilitating hemophilic arthropathy if untreated. Vigorous replacment therapy is given with a five-day course of prednisone, 40 mg/m²/day. Daily infusions to maintain the factor level between 3% and 5% may be beneficial. Surgical synovectomy may prevent permanent joint damage. Joint replacement in older patients has restored function but is reserved for patients in whom pain is a major problem.

MUSCLE AND SOFT TISSUE HEMORRHAGE

Most soft tissue hematomas are superficial, resolving with local measures of pressure and ice. One replacement infusion to raise factor level to 30% is usually sufficient.

Hemorrhage within a closed compartment may result in nerve compression and permanent loss of neuromuscular function. Iliopsoas hemorrhage presents a typical picture of femoral nerve compression with loss of sensation over the anterior thigh, loss of patellar reflex, decreased quadriceps strength, and pain in the abdomen, in the hip, or over the femoral ring. Pain on extension of the hip, but not with flexion and rotation, distinguishes iliopsoas bleeding from hip hemarthrosis, which is painful with any motion. Iliopsoas hemorrhage may be confirmed by ultrasound. Prompt factor replacement to 40% to 60% is necessary. A series of infusions is usually required. Activity must be resumed cautiously, since rebleeding may occur.

HEAD INJURY

Any significant injury requires immediate factor replacement to a level of 100% prior to evaluation. A prolonged headache or seizure, whether or not accompanied by neurologic signs, should be considered evidence of intracranial bleeding and treated promptly.

ORAL BLEEDING AND EPISTAXIS

Persistent oral bleeding in toddlers is a common problem and may require red cell transfusion. Nosebleeds and bleeding gums are most common in von Willebrand's disease. Factor replacement to 50% will promptly stop bleeding, and Amicar, 100 mg/kg, every six hours for a few days will prevent clot dissolution. Retropharyngeal hematomas potentially compromise the airway and require vigorous treatment and hospitalization for observation.

HEMATURIA

Hematuria is common in adolescents and often persists in spite of adequate factor replacement. Various treatment programs have been used, including bed rest for 24 to 48 hours. Prednisone, 40 to 60 mg/m²/day in divided doses, will usually control hematuria within 48 hours. The dose is then tapered and stopped over the next three days.

GASTROINTESTINAL HEMORRHAGE

Except in von Willebrand's disease, gastrointestinal bleeding is uncommon in any of the inherited bleeding disorders. Appropriate diagnostic procedures should be done to identify the cause. Factor replacement may be necessary prior to endoscopy.

CIRCULATING INHIBITORS

Approximately 10% of severely affected patients with severe hemophilia A develop circulating inhibitors. The presence of such an inhibitor may be suspected and confirmed by an inhibitor assay when the response to treatment is less rapid or less complete than usual.

Low titer inhibitors with no anamnestic response to infusion can usually be treated with larger doses of factor replacement to neutralize the inhibitor and raise the factor level.

Potent inhibitors (>5 Bethesda units) may show a sharp rise with every replacement infusion and no increment in the factor level. In most situations standard prothrombin complexes, Konyne or Proplex, are used in an effort to bypass factor VIII in the clotting cascade. The usual dose is 50 to 70 units/kg of factor IX.

Autoplex and FEIBA are prothrombin complex concentrates developed specifically to bypass the need for factor VIII in patients with a factor VIII inhibitor. A dose of 50 to 100 units/kg is needed to control serious hemorrhage.

Exchange transfusion or exchange plasmapheresis has been helpful in temporarily lowering the titer of circulating inhibitor and allowing massive infusion of factor VIII to be given.

Porcine factor VIII is available as an investigational agent and may be used in an emergency. Sensitivity develops rapidly.

DENTAL MANAGEMENT

Regular professional care must be a part of every hemophiliac's treatment plan. Minor procedures such as prophylaxis and dental restorations usually do not need factor replacement. Whenever possible, local anesthetic infiltration is preferable to a regional block. Extraction of permanent teeth or regional block anesthesia requires factor replacement to 50% within an hour prior to the procedure. With careful packing of a tooth socket and Amicar to stabilize the clot, no further replacement is usually needed.

Amicar (epsilon-aminocaproic acid, EACA), an antifibrinolytic agent, is useful for prevention of clot dissolution in oral bleeding, epistaxis, and menorrhagia. It is available in tablets and liquid and given in a dose of 100 mg/kg every six hours for seven to 10 days. It is contraindicated in the presence of hematuria, since clots may form in the renal collecting system, and if there is evidence of active intravascular coagulation (DIC).

SURGICAL PROCEDURES

Emergency surgical procedures may be undertaken after sufficient factor replacement to achieve a 100% level. If a factor assay cannot be performed, a normal APTT will give some evidence of adequate replacement.

All major surgery should be performed at a center where experienced personnel and adequate laboratory and blood bank facilities are available. Prior to surgery, an inhibitor assay must be done to exclude the possibility of a circulating antibody to the clotting factor. Postoperatively a factor level above 30% must be maintained for at least 10 to 14 days and longer if complications such as infection occur or if physical therapy is required.

PAIN CONTROL

Pain is a problem for most moderately and severely affected patients. In the past, drug abuse and addiction have been major problems. A goal of early control of bleeding is to prevent pain and reduce the need for analgesics.

Acetaminophen is most commonly used for control of pain. When necessary, narcotics should be used in adequate doses to relieve pain, but discontinued as soon as possible.

Nonsteroidal anti-inflammatory agents, such as ibuprofen, are especially helpful in chronic hemophilic arthritis. Although the bleeding time may be slightly prolonged, the platelet effect is transient compared with aspirin. There is no increase in the incidence or severity of bleeding episodes if used for short periods of time.

Aspirin and aspirin-containing products are contraindicated. A single dose of aspirin will alter platelet function by irreversibly inhibiting platelet cyclo-oxygenase. In vitro platelet aggregation may be affected for five to seven days, making laboratory evaluation of platelet function impossible. Patients should be cautioned to read labels on all over-the-counter medications. A list of aspirin-containing products is available from the National Hemophilia Foundation. Nonacetylated salicylates, such as methylcholine salicylate, do not have a platelet inhibitory effect and may be useful in control of arthritic pain.

COMPLICATIONS OF THERAPY

Allergic and febrile reactions may occur with administration of any blood product. These can usually be managed and prevented with antihistamines prior to infusion for patients with previous reactions. Rapid infusion of concentrate can produce a feeling of lightheadedness, which might be confused with a reaction.

Isoagglutinins in cryoprecipitate and concentrate can cause hemolytic anemia with spherocytes and a positive antiglobulin test. Blood group–specific products are available and recommended when patients require large volumes.

Transmission of viral illness is a risk with all blood products, but especially those from pooled plasma. Transfusion-acquired hepatitis occurs despite rigorous screening for the virus. All patients newly diagnosed and those who are HbSAb-negative should be immunized against hepatitis B. There is no donor screening test for non-A, non-B hepatitis.

Acquired immunodeficiency syndrome (AIDS) is a potentially very serious problem for the hemophilic population. Concentrates are now heat-treated during preparation in an effort to reduce transmission of the HTLV III virus thought to be implicated in AIDS. The selection of product for replacement therapy will be influenced by knowledge of the local plasma donor population. If the clinician estimates that there is little risk of AIDS transmission, then cryoprecipitate may be selected because of reduced hepatitis risk. Heat-treated concentrates may be preferred in situations where it is considered that single donor products would provide no particular advantage.

COMPREHENSIVE CARE

The management of a patient with hemophilia must encompass far more than control of hemostasis. Comprehensive hemophilia centers provide interdisciplinary care and utilize the services of hemophilia nurse specialists, hematologists, orthopedists, physical therapists, physical medicine and rehabilitation specialists, oral surgeons, geneticists, and socal workers. Specialized coagulation laboratories, blood banks, and facilities for inpatient services including surgery are available.

Most patients with severe and moderate disease are evaluated annually by appropriate team members. We assess the patient's general health, problems, and progress. Activity, school and work attendance, and social and economic problems are addressed. The team members review and revise the treatment program with the patient and communicate with primary physicians, employers, schools, and community services.

We stress the importance of early treatment of bleeding and provide each patient with a management plan including recommendations for factor replacement and treatment of various types of bleeding episodes. The individual's treatment plan is kept on file in his physician's office and local emergency room. The patient should also carry with him information concerning diagnosis, factor levels, and phone numbers for the clinic where he is registered.

Patients are asked to send monthly records of all bleeding episodes, documenting site of bleeding, factor replacement, and response to treatment for review by the nurse specialists and hematologist. In this way, problems can be identified and families or physicians contacted if changes in management appear indicated.

HOME THERAPY

Home care with self-infusion of factor replacement products has many advantages and can be a major step in normalizing a hemophilic patient's life.

Patients and families must be carefully selected and trained in all aspects of care as well as in specific techniques of self-infusion. The success of home care programs in many centers is due to careful supervision by the center. Many potential hazards exist, such as inadequate or excessive treatment, poor IV techniques, greater risk of hepatitis among household members, and illegal use of intravenous equipment. Few of these problems actually occur. There is usually an initial increase in product usage that diminishes with experience. Most adults are taught to self-infuse, although another family member should be familiar with the procedure. Children are encouraged to help mix concentrates and gradually become self-sufficient by age 9 years or even younger. Parents can be taught to infuse youngsters as soon as the child's veins are adequate in size and the child is cooperative.

Ordinarily patients are given enough product and supplies for four infusions and restock when their supply is down to one infusion. Patients carry a letter that can be used for treatment in an emergency situation or as authorization for carrying intravenous equipment.

EDUCATIONAL RESOURCES

Information about hemophilia and its management is available from the National Hemophilia Foundation, 19 West 34th Street, Suite 1204, New York, NY 10001. The Foundation publishes a wide variety of pamphlets and brochures on all aspects of hemophilia for patients, families, teachers, physicians, nurses, and anyone interested in hemophilia.

The World Federation of Hemophilia, 1170 Peel Street, Room 1126, Montreal, Quebec, Canada H3B 2T4, publishes a "Guide for Traveling Hemophiliacs," listing comprehensive centers located in over 40 countries.

REFERENCES

Bowie EJW: Von Willebrand's disease: state of the art. Scand J Hematol [Suppl] 40:431–440, 1984.

Gill FM: Congenital bleeding disorders: hemophilia and von Willebrand's disease. Med Clin North Am 68:601–615, 1984.

Hilgartner M: Hemophilia in the Child and Adult. Masson Publishing USA, Inc, New York, 1982.

Lusher JM, Shapiro SS, Palascak J, et al: Efficacy of prothrombin complex concentrates in hemophiliacs with antibodies to factor VIII—a multicenter therapeutic trial. N Engl J Med 303:421–425, 1980.

Warrier AI, Lusher J: DDAVP: a useful alternative to blood components in moderate hemophilia A and von Willebrand's disease. J Pediatr 102:228–233, 1983.

11 · PLATELET DISORDERS

Robert McMillan
SCRIPPS CLINIC AND RESEARCH FOUNDATION

Platelets are important in hemostasis; a significant quantitative or qualitative platelet abnormality will result in bleeding. Treatment varies, depending upon the cause of the thrombocytopenia or the nature of the qualitative platelet defect; the therapeutic approach will be discussed according to the etiologic factor. Table 1 lists the disorders commonly associated with thrombocytopenia or abnormal platelet function.

DIAGNOSTIC APPROACH TO THROMBOCYTOPENIA

Thrombocytopenia may be due to (1) decreased platelet production as a result of marrow damage or infiltration; (2) ineffective platelet production due to toxins (e.g., alcohol) or to vitamin deficiencies (e.g., megaloblastic anemia); (3) redistribution of the platelet mass into an enlarged splenic pool; or (4) increased destruction of circulating platelets after their release from the bone marrow.

A complete history must be taken with specific attention to the onset, duration, and severity of bruising, petechiae, or mucosal bleeding. The occurrence of a recent infection or transfusion may be relevant. Drug exposure must be carefully documented. A review of systems may suggest other diseases associated with thrombocytopenia such as infection, collagen disease, lymphoma, or leukemia. A physical examination should document the degree of bruising and bleeding from mucous membranes and the presence or absence of enlarged lymph nodes or hepatosplenomegaly. Initial laboratory studies should include complete blood count, platelet count, blood smear, and bone marrow aspiration and biopsy. Additional laboratory studies such as coagulation tests, antinuclear antibodies, or cultures may also be needed, depending on the clinical presentation.

The type of thrombocytopenia can usually be defined after this initial evaluation (see Table 1).

DECREASED PLATELET PRODUCTION

Illnesses that result in decreased platelet production, such as aplastic anemia, marrow infiltration, and megaloblastic anemia, can easily be diagnosed from the bone marrow examination. The diagnosis of toxic marrow suppression by alcohol or drugs requires a careful history, since the bone marrow is not always helpful in this circumstance. The absence of splenomegaly rules out thrombocytopenia due to splenic pooling. Finally, the combination of thrombocytopenia with an increased percentage of large platelets on the peripheral smear and normal or increased megakaryocytes in the bone

Table 1. PLATELET ABNORMALITIES

Diminished Platelet Production
Aplastic anemia (congenital, acquired)
Marrow infiltration
    Hematologic tumors (leukemia, lymphoma, myeloma)
    Solid tumors (prostate, breast, lung, GI)
    Myelofibrosis
    Infection (TB, fungus)
    Miscellaneous (sarcoid, lipid storage)
Marrow suppression
    Drugs (chemotherapy, thiazides, alcohol)
    Radiation
Ineffective production (megaloblastic anemia)
Paroxysmal nocturnal hemoglobinuria

Platelet Redistribution
Congestive splenomegaly
Other (Gaucher's disease, lymphoma, myelofibrosis)

Platelet Destruction
Infections (bacterial, viral)
Disseminated intravascular coagulation
Thrombotic thrombocytopenic purpura
Giant hemangioma
Platelet loss (massive bleeding, cardiac bypass)
Antibody-mediated
    Chronic ITP
    Drugs (quinidine, quinine, gold, sulfas)
    Isoantibodies (neonatal purpura, post-transfusion purpura)
    Secondary (lymphoma, collagen disease, solid tumors, infection)

Abnormal Platelet Function
Acquired
    Drugs
    Uremia
    Paraproteinemias
Hereditary
    Glanzmann's thrombasthenia
    Bernard-Soulier syndrome
    Storage pool disease
    Others

Thrombocytosis
Benign
    Infection, inflammation
Malignant
    Polycythemia vera
    Chronic granulocytic leukemia
    Myelofibrosis
    Thrombocythemia

marrow suggests either destructive thrombocytopenia or platelet loss.

DESTRUCTIVE THROMBOCYTOPENIA

Nonimmune causes of destructive thrombocytopenia such as infection, disseminated intravascular coagulation (DIC), thrombotic thrombocytopenic purpura (TTP), and a giant hemangioma can be diagnosed on the basis of history, physical examination, and appropriate laboratory testing (e.g, coagulation studies, cultures). Platelet loss due to massive bleeding with replacement by stored blood (usually greater than 10 units) or by surgery requiring extracorporeal perfusion results in a laboratory picture indistinguishable from other forms of destructive thrombocytopenia. Since the bone marrow has essentially no platelet reserve, thrombocytopenia due to these causes may persist from three to five days.

ANTIBODY-MEDIATED THROMBOCYTOPENIA

Antibody-mediated thrombocytopenia may require additional evaluation. Immune thrombocytopenia due to drugs or alloantibodies can be diagnosed after a careful history. Greater than 70% of the cases of drug-induced immune thrombocytopenia are due to the following eight drugs: quinidine, quinine, gold salts, sulfonamides, sulfonamide derivatives, chlorothiazide, chloroquine, and rifampin. Patients with the syndrome of post-transfusion purpura have usually received a transfusion within seven to ten days of the onset of thrombocytopenia. Neonatal purpura is diagnosed from the history of a mother with normal platelet counts having a thrombocytopenic child. Specific tests for alloantibodies and drug-dependent antibodies are available in selected institutions. Antibody-induced thrombocytopenia is also seen in combination with a variety of diseases including collagen vascular disease, solid tumors, lymphoma, and certain infections particularly of viral origin (e.g., mononucleosis).

IDIOPATHIC THROMBOCYTOPENIC PURPURA

The final form of immune thrombocytopenia, and probably the most common, is idiopathic thrombocytopenic purpura (ITP), which is a diagnosis of exclusion. This may present as an acute self-limited syndrome, usually in children and often following a viral illness (acute ITP), or as a more insidious disease occurring most commonly in women between the ages of 20 and 40 years (chronic ITP), which almost always requires specific treatment.

MANAGEMENT

GENERAL TREATMENT

Thrombocytopenic patients may present with bruising and petechiae ("dry purpura") or with bleeding from mucosal surfaces ("wet purpura"). Mucosal bleeding, particularly from the gastrointestinal or genitourinary tracts, suggests very low platelet counts and the risk of central nervous system (CNS) bleeding. Patients with severe mucosal bleeding should be hospitalized and treated with platelet transfusions regardless of the cause of thrombocytopenia. Antiplatelet drugs such as aspirin, dipyridamole, or Anturane as well as antihistamines should never be used in thrombocytopenic patients. If patients are on these agents at the time of diagnosis, they should be discontinued.

PLATELET TRANSFUSION

It is unusual for thrombocytopenic patients to develop significant bleeding until the platelet count drops below 5000 to 10,000/mm³. Bleeding may occur at higher counts if the patient is taking aspirin or other antiplatelet drugs. Platelet transfusions should be given as often as necessary to control life-threatening bleeding but not with the aim of maintaining a predetermined platelet count. In patients with production defects, platelet transfusions are needed about two to three times a week. Platelets may be needed every four to six hours in the face of rapid platelet destruction.

Random donor platelets are used as the preferred platelet source. Usually 6 to 8 platelet packs are given (one pack = 5.5×10^{10} or more platelets). An increase in the platelet count of 5000 to 10,000/mm³/platelet pack one hour after transfusion should be seen unless platelet destruction is occurring (sepsis, DIC, antiplatelet antibody). ABO-matched platelet concentrates give a somewhat higher increment but this is of minor clinical importance. Rh-negative patients may be sensitized to Rh antigen if platelets from Rh-positive donors are given. If evidence of alloimmunization develops (40% to 70% of recipients, usually due to anti-HLA antibodies) as manifested by the lack of an increase in the platelet count after transfusion, either family donors or HLA-matched family or HLA-matched unrelated donors may be required. Platelets can be obtained from these donors by apheresis methods. Usually 5 to 10 units of platelets can be obtained and donors may be used on multiple occasions. Factors such as infection, splenomegaly, mucositis, DIC, and others may also affect platelet increments after transfusion.

SPECIFIC THERAPY

PRODUCTION DEFECTS

In patients with reduced or ineffective platelet production, treatment of the thrombocytopenia requires specific therapy of the primary disorder. Suppression of production by alcohol or myelosuppressive drugs is treated by stopping the drug. Patients with megaloblastic anemia should receive the appropriate vitamin supplementation. Treatment of aplastic anemia or infiltrative diseases is covered in other chapters of this book. Platelet transfusions should be given as needed for treatment of severe bleeding; however, the risk of alloimmunization should always be weighed against the relatively short-term benefits of platelet transfusion.

SPLENIC POOLING

Specific therapy is rarely needed in these patients, since the platelet count is rarely less than 30,000/mm³. However, should platelet counts become dangerously low, splenectomy can be considered. Surgery will commonly result in improvement of the platelet count. Many patients with splenic enlargement have complex causes for their thrombocytopenia (e.g., lymphoma patients may have any combination of marrow infiltration, splenomegaly, and immune thrombocytopenia).

PERIPHERAL DESTRUCTION OF PLATELETS

Treatment of many of the common causes of platelet destruction consists of treating the primary disease (infection, DIC, TTP, giant hemangioma).

In patients with immune thrombocytopenia due to drugs, stopping the agent will in most cases result in normalization of the platelet count within one to three weeks. An exception is gold, which may require several months to be spontaneously eliminated from the body; for this reason, treatment with dimercaprol is required. The usual dose is 2.5 to 5.0 mg/kg IM once or twice daily until the platelet count responds. This may require treatment for several days.

Chronic ITP and Secondary Immune Thrombocytopenia. The types of specific therapy are described in the order we would use them based on either their relative effectiveness or lack of dangerous side effects.

Corticosteroids. Prednisone (1 mg/kg/day or the therapeutic equivalent) is started at the time of diagnosis. Most patients respond within one to two weeks. If the platelet count becomes normal, the dose is maintained for one to two additional weeks and then tapered as follows: 10 mg/week until the dose reaches 0.5 mg/kg and then 5 mg/week thereafter. A complete remission is rare (10% to 15% of patients), and most patients become thrombocytopenic as the steroids are tapered.

In patients on larger doses of steroids, we monitor the serum potassium weekly and observe for signs of gastric irritation and the onset of mental symptoms (steroid psychosis). Antacids one hour after meals and before bed are suggested. Give supplemental potassium if needed.

If a complete remission does not occur with corticosteroids, splenectomy is recommended in adults. Some physicians give a short therapeutic trial of vincristine (1 mg/week for four weeks) prior to surgery to see if a complete remission can be obtained.

Splenectomy. About 70% of patients with chronic ITP will achieve a complete remission and an additional 10% will attain "safe platelet counts" after splenectomy. An increase in the platelet count occurs within hours after surgery and usually peaks within two weeks. A complete remission is more likely in patients who respond to corticosteroids, have recent onset of their disease, attain platelet counts above 500,000/mm³ after surgery, or are less than 60 years of age. If a complete remission does not occur, the presence of an accessory spleen should be ruled out (technetium scan), although this is extremely uncommon. Patients who fail splenectomy should receive a second trial of corticosteroids (see above) to see if "safe counts" (greater than 20,000/mm³) can be achieved with doses of prednisone (5 to 10 mg/day) that are acceptable for long-term administration. In children, splenectomy should be postponed, if possible, until at least the age of 6 years because of the risk of overwhelming septicemia in children without a spleen. Pneumococcal vaccine should be administered to all patients who undergo splenectomy, preferably prior to surgery.

Additional therapy is required in patients who fail to respond to corticosteroids and splenectomy and who are unable to maintan "safe platelet counts" (greater than 20,000/mm³) on acceptable doses of corticosteroids. The agents listed below should be tried in the order in which they are listed. Usually these agents are added to moderate doses of corticosteroids (e.g., 30 to 40 mg prednisone); then, if a response occurs, the corticosteroids are tapered. Initially, patients should be followed at weekly intervals with complete counts.

Vinca Alkaloids. Initially vincristine (1 to 2 mg IV every seven days for four to six weeks) is suggested. A response usually occurs within seven to ten days, but in most patients thrombocytopenia reappears within two to three weeks. Occasionally, long-term complete remissions are obtained, but this is uncommon. In some patients, an acceptable platelet count can be maintained with intermittent infrequent therapy with vincristine, although if frequent doses are required, peripheral neuropathy usually occurs. Vinblastine (5 to 10 mg/week IV) may be equally useful in some patients, and this agent carries a low risk of peripheral neuropathy. Some physicians feel that if vinca alkaloids are infused over a period of six hours, they are more effective.

Colchicine. About 25% of refractory patients respond to this agent. Dosage is limited by gastrointestinal side effects (diarrhea). Suggested dosage is 0.6 to 1.2 mg PO four times daily. A therapeutic trial of one to two months should be given if possible.

Danazol. This modified androgen is given in a

dosage of 200 mg PO two to four times daily. Responses are noted within one to six weeks. Approximately 50% of refractory ITP patients will have a beneficial effect. If no improvement is noted within two months, it is unlikely to occur.

Cyclophosphamide. This chemotherapeutic agent should be given at doses of 50 to 200 mg/day PO or 0.5 to 1.0 gm IV every three to four weeks. A response usually occurs within two to six weeks, and complete unmaintained remissions have been reported in 25% to 40% of patients with refractory chronic ITP. If normal platelet counts are achieved, treatment is continued for four to six additional weeks and then discontinued. While on Cytoxan, patients should drink at least 2 liters of fluid daily to prevent cystitis, and their blood count should be monitored at least once a week. If relapse should occur, the risk of using additional courses of cyclophosphamide (small risk of developing acute leukemia) must be weighed against the benefit achieved with the drug, the severity of the patient's thrombocytopenia, and the availability of alternative therapy.

Azathioprine. This is the safest immunosuppressant agent for long-term maintenance therapy. Daily doses of 1 to 4 mg/kg are given initially and then the dosage is tapered to maintain safe platelet counts. A response occurs slowly over three to 12 months, and complete remissions are unusual. Neutropenia occurs at higher dosages.

Therapy During Pregnancy. Since the IgG antiplatelet antibody in ITP crosses the placenta, the infant is at risk for thrombocytopenia. Corticosteroid therapy is indicated if the mother has marked thrombocytopenia; but unless the situation is life-threatening, additional therapy (splenectomy, immunosuppressants) should be withheld until after delivery.

Therapy may be required to protect the child at the time of delivery. The mother should receive corticosteroids (30 to 40 mg daily) during the last three to four weeks of pregnancy regardless of her platelet count because this may prevent severe thrombocytopenia in the child. At the time of delivery, the major risk to the infant is CNS bleeding during vaginal delivery. Cesarean section theoretically reduces this risk. At the time of delivery, a scalp vein platelet count should be performed on the infant as soon as the maternal membranes have ruptured. Capillary tubes containing EDTA instead of heparin should be used to collect the specimen. We deliver vaginally if the fetal count is greater than 50,000/mm³. Prompt cesarean section is indicated if the fetal count is less than 50,000/mm³. The scalp puncture site should be observed carefully so that excess bleeding does not occur. We monitor the child's platelet count for at least one week, since delayed thrombocytopenia may occur. If the infant becomes thrombocytopenic after delivery, corticosteroids (hydrocortisone, 10 mg IM every 12 hours, followed two to three days later by oral prednisone, 1 to 2 mg/kg/day) should be given until the platelet count becomes normal. If thrombocytopenia is severe, platelet transfusions will maintain the infant until the maternal antibody clears from the child's circulation. Exchange transfusion is never indicated.

Therapy for CNS Bleeding. If CNS bleeding is suspected (usually in children), a CAT scan of the head should be obtained to localize the site of bleeding. If posterior compartment bleeding is noted, emergency splenectomy followed by a craniotomy should be performed. If the bleeding is in the hemispheric regions, the need for surgery depends upon the patient's neurologic status and response to specific therapy for the thrombocytopenia.

Temporizing Therapy. A temporary increase in the platelet count can be obtained in ITP patients using intravenous gamma globulin (0.4 gm/kg/day IV for five days) or by plasmapheresis (3-liter exchange daily for three to five days). These forms of therapy should be reserved for critical circumstances in which a temporary increase in the platelet count will allow time for other therapeutic manipulations. Both treatments are expensive.

Patients with secondary immune thrombocytopenia associated with collagen diseases, lymphoproliferative disorders, and solid tumors are treated in the manner described for chronic ITP except that specific therapy may also be indicated for treatment of the primary illness.

Acute ITP. Acute ITP improves spontaneously in one to two months. Therapy is not needed unless extremely severe thrombocytopenia or life-threatening hemorrhage occurs. Platelet transfusions should be given as described earlier. Corticosteroids do not shorten the duration of the thrombocytopenia or improve survival and most physicians advise against their use. Some physicians use them in doses of 1 mg/kg/day during the first two to four weeks for the possible beneficial effect on "capillary integrity." More recently, successful responses to intravenous gamma globulin (0.4 gm/kg/day for five days) have been reported, and if specific therapy is required, this agent is the treatment of choice.

Alloimmune Purpura. Two forms are seen: post-transfusion purpura and neonatal purpura. Post-transfusion purpura occurs in patients (usually women) who lack a common platelet antigen (usually Pl^A1) and develop antibodies against these antigens when transfused. Thrombocytopenia occurs suddenly about one week after transfusion and may persist for several weeks. Since thrombocytopenia is usually profound with significant bleeding, treatment is required. Intravenous gamma globulin (0.4 gm/kg/day IV for five days) should be given initially; if no response occurs, perform plasma exchange (3 liters daily for up to five days) to clear antibody from the circulation. Corticosteroids (1 to 2 mg/kg/day) may control the process or shorten the duration of thrombocytopenia in less severe cases.

Transfused platelets are usually removed rapidly and should be avoided if possible because they may cause severe reactions. However, at times they may be necessary to prevent death from CNS bleeding.

Neonatal thrombocytopenia is due to the transfer of the mother's antiplatelet antibodies, which develop against antigens on the child's platelets, to the child, with resulting thrombocytopenia. Antibodies are usually against the Pl^A1 antigen. The first child is often affected and the mortality rate is high (30% to 40%). In mothers who have delivered previous thrombocytopenic children, subsequent pregnancies should be monitored by measuring antiplatelet antibodies using the father's platelets as the target. In mothers who develop high antibody levels, consideration should be given to cesarean section. The child should be watched carefully after delivery, since severe thrombocytopenia may develop over the first few days after delivery. Corticosteroids (hydrocortisone, 10 mg IM every 12 hours, and after two to three days oral prednisone, 1 to 2 mg/kg/day) should be given until the platelet count normalizes. We give platelet transfusions for active bleeding; if available, the mother's platelets are the best choice, since they lack the antigen. However, they *must be washed* to remove the antiplatelet antibody, which would be present in the plasma. Exchange transfusion is unnecessary, since thrombocytopenia is self-limited.

THROMBOCYTOSIS

Thrombocytosis is commonly seen in myeloproliferative disorders (see Chapter 18) as well as various infectious, inflammatory, or neoplastic disorders. In these latter conditions, the increased platelets seldom cause symptoms.

PLATELET DYSFUNCTION

Platelet function disorders are of two groups: hereditary and acquired disorders. Acquired disorders may be drug-induced or associated with uremia, paraproteinemia, preleukemia, or acute leukemia. Many drugs inhibit platelet function as well. In normal persons this is usually of no consequence. However, in patients with coagulation disorders, uremia, or thrombocytopenia, or in patients receiving heparin or coumarin anticoagulants, impairment of platelet function by drugs may result in serious bleeding. These drugs include aspirin, indomethacin, phenylbutazone, sulfinpyrazone, and the semisynthetic penicillins (e.g., carbenicillin). There is no specific treatment for acquired platelet function disorders other than treatment of the primary disease if possible and the transfusion of fresh blood or platelet concentrates for treatment of significant hemorrhage. In patients with lifelong hereditary disorders (such as thrombasthenia, storage pool disease), avoid platelet transfusions unless absolutely necessary to prevent the development of alloimmunization.

12 · *HEMOCHROMATOSIS*

Ralph Green
CLEVELAND CLINIC FOUNDATION

DEFINITION AND DIAGNOSTIC CRITERIA

Hemochromatosis is the manifestation of a group of disorders of iron storage in which there is progressive accumulation of iron that leads to organ damage. Hereditary (idiopathic) hemochromatosis (HH) arises from a genetic defect that causes absorption of inappropriate quantities of iron, which ultimately results in damage to the parenchymal cells of the liver, pancreas, heart, gonads, and other organs. Damage to the organs that bear the major burden of iron deposition may result in cirrhosis, diabetes, cardiopathies, and sterility. The major diagnostic criteria of HH include demonstration of increased total body iron stores with a predominantly parenchymal cell deposition and with no apparent cause of secondary iron overload. Evaluation of iron stores is achieved by measurement of serum transferrin saturation and ferritin concentration. Of the two, transferrin saturation is the more reliable, and a value of greater than 60% repeated on at least two occasions is highly suggestive of HH, which should then be confirmed by liver biopsy. Similar iron storage disease also occurs as a result of ineffective erythropoiesis (e.g., thalassemia) and as a complication of repeated blood transfusion in patients with congenital and acquired refractory anemias.

PATHOPHYSIOLOGY

The underlying metabolic defect leading to inappropriate iron absorption is not known and the mechanism of iron-induced tissue injury remains unexplained. There is evidence that when iron accumulates in excess of the cell's capacity to store the metal innocuously, membrane damage occurs either through iron-induced lipid peroxidation or through the release of lysosomal enzymes.

CLINICAL ASPECTS

HH is usually diagnosed between the ages of 40 and 60 years, although it may become manifest at a younger age and juvenile forms of the disease have been described. The disease is more common (5:1 male preponderance) and also presents at a younger age in men than in women. Clinical presentation may vary, but diabetes, weakness, malaise, and weight loss are common. Other presenting features include skin pigmentation ("bronzed diabetes"), abdominal pain, refractory congestive heart failure or arrhythmia, asymptomatic liver enlargement, abnormal liver enzyme tests, arthritis with prominent involvement of the metacarpophalangeal joints, and gonadal hypofunction. An abnormal value may be found on routine transferrin saturation measurement. The inheritance pattern for HH is autosomal recessive and the gene frequency in the United States is estimated to be around 7%. The disease should therefore be suspected in blood relatives of known hemochromatosis patients, particularly in their siblings, and appropriate screening tests should be carried out as described later.

MANAGEMENT

PLAN

The short-term goal of management is to remove accumulated iron stores; the long-term goal is to maintain a low body iron burden, thereby preventing or arresting damage to vital organs and, in some instances, allowing actual reversal of such damage.

There are two approaches that may be used for the management of patients with iron overload: (1) phlebotomy, which is the treatment of choice for HH; and (2) injection of iron-chelating drugs, which is the only available form of treatment for transfusion iron overload. Phlebotomy may be carried out during a clinic visit or by a blood bank. Administration of iron-chelating drugs is best achieved with slow subcutaneous infusion pump devices on a home health care basis, sometimes supplemented with intravenous infusion of the drug at the time of blood transfusion. To initiate a treatment regimen with iron chelators, it is useful to keep the patient in hospital for a day or more to monitor both the therapeutic response to the drug (24-hour urine iron) and the possible occurrence of acute untoward side effects (anaphylaxis). Hospitalization is also useful for instructing the patient in home use of the SC infusion pump.

NONPHARMACOLOGIC MEASURES: PHLEBOTOMY

Phlebotomy is the fastest, safest, and cheapest method to treat HH. Phlebotomy consists of two phases. In the first or intensive phase, frequent phlebotomy is carried out until accumulated stores are removed. During the second or maintenance phase, which is lifelong, phlebotomy is less frequent and designed to prevent iron reaccumulation.

A phlebotomy program should be started as soon as the diagnosis of HH has been established. The program should be as brisk as can be tolerated by the patient until excess iron has been removed in order to arrest or prevent development of the complications of iron overload. Such a program may consist of the removal of 500 ml blood once, twice, or even three times a week. The rationale is to produce a mild to moderate anemia, which stimulates erythropoiesis and thereby mobilizes iron stores, making them available for removal by further phlebotomy. The rate of phlebotomy during the intensive phase should be controlled by both subjective and objective criteria. However, unless post-phlebotomy weakness becomes incapacitating, it is best to be guided by an objective measure, such as measurement of either the hemoglobin concentration or the hematocrit before each phlebotomy. If the hemoglobin concentration is above 11 gm/dl (or the hematocrit greater than 35%), then phlebotomy may be carried out. This is an inexpensive way to monitor the frequency of venesection during the intensive phase of phlebotomy and also provides a safeguard against overtreating. It can be used to indicate when iron stores are depleted and the patient is ready to enter the maintenance phase of less frequent phlebotomy. Iron is usually the rate-limiting factor for erythropoiesis. When the hemoglobin concentration fails to rise above 11 gm/dl for a sustained period, this signals depletion of the body iron store, with the rare exception of a coexistent cause of anemia (e.g., folate deficiency). The time taken to achieve depletion of the body iron store varies with the original size of store and the frequency of phlebotomy. At a rate of 500 ml phlebotomy per week, approximately 10 gm storage iron are removed in a year. A fall in serum iron concentration signals incipient depletion of the iron store, at which point the brakes may be gently applied and the frequency of phlebotomy reduced to once every other week.

During the maintenance phase, a less frequent schedule of phlebotomy every two to four months is established, depending on the rate of iron reaccumulation. The rate of iron absorption in HH is usually between 2 and 4 mg per day.

Phlebotomy is usually well tolerated and often results in disappearance of several symptoms with a general improvement in the patient's sense of well-being. Moreover, there is convincing evidence that phlebotomy prevents the progression of several of the complications of iron overload and that survival is undoubtedly prolonged. The complications most amenable to reversal are diabetes, cardiopathy, and pigmentation. The symptoms of arthropathy and hypogonadism (impotence and sterility), once present, show little or no amelioration in response to iron removal. Although hepatic fibrosis decreases, cirrhosis is probably irreversible. However, there is evidence that the risk of developing hepatoma may be eliminated by iron removal, providing cirrhosis has not yet developed.

DRUG THERAPY

Phlebotomy is the treatment of choice for HH but it may be precluded in some patients who are unable to tolerate venesection because of incapacitating cardiovascular complications such as syncope or angina. Occasionally, coexistence of an unresponsive anemia, by limiting the erythropoietic drive to mobilize iron stores, precludes phlebotomy. Very rarely, unduly fragile or inaccessible veins in an elderly or extremely obese patient may render regular phlebotomy difficult. In such situations, chelation therapy provides an alternative method for iron removal. Iron chelation is the only available method for treating iron storage disease that results from blood transfusion. The iron chelator deferoxamine (DF) may be used effectively to treat the iron overload that results from transfusion of patients with congenital or acquired refractory anemias. For maximum clinical efficacy, it is necessary to administer DF by slow infusion, either IV, SC, or by a combination of both routes. Although somewhat less efficient than the IV route, SC infusion is preferred because it may be carried out at home using a small portable pump. One to 4 gm DF is dissolved in distilled water and the drug is injected via a 25- or 27-gauge butterfly needle inserted under the skin of the anterior abdominal wall. It is usually more convenient for patients to administer the drug over an eight- to 12-hour period during sleep. To achieve negative iron balance in patients receiving 1 unit of blood each week (200 mg iron), it is necessary to remove iron at a rate of almost 30 mg per day. In practice, this requires use of the pump five to seven times per week. Intravenous administration of the drug may be used in addition when the patient receives blood transfusion. In this situation, up to 4 gm DF may be given over two hours.

Administration of vitamin C enhances urinary excretion of iron in response to DF. However, there is evidence to suggest that ascorbic acid may aggravate the cellular damage that occurs in iron overload, and cardiac deterioration has been reported in patients who were treated with vitamin C. The vitamin should therefore be given only if there is clear evidence of deficiency, obtained by measurement of leukocyte ascorbate, or if administration of the vitamin substantially augments otherwise inadequate iron excretion. In any event, megadoses should be shunned and small amounts should be given only *after* DF infusion has begun.

Indications for the Use of Iron Chelators. In patients with HH, the indications for using iron chelation treatment in place of phlebotomy are uncommon and have been described previously. Sometimes iron chelation may be used in conjunction with phlebotomy to augment iron removal in a patient who may be able to tolerate only sporadic phlebotomy. For patients with transfusion overload, where iron chelation offers the only therapeutic approach, the indications for starting treatment vary. For children with severe thalassemia and other congenital anemias requiring regular transfusion, chelation treatment is mandatory for prevention of lethal cardiac complications at an early age (see Section V, Chapter 5). Treatment should begin as soon as the child is able to cooperate and preferably not later than age 5. Chelation therapy is recommended in adults with acquired transfusion-dependent anemias if they have diseases with a reasonably good prognosis, such as stable aplastic anemia or acquired sideroblastic anemia. In the author's experience, the decision to treat iron overload may be postponed until the patient has received 40 to 50 units of blood (equivalent to loading of approximately 10 gm of iron), a level beyond which organ damage is much more likely to occur.

Adverse Effects. Complications of DF are infrequent and usually mild. The most troublesome are local irritation, pain, swelling, and discoloration at subcutaneous injection sites. To alleviate irritation, hydrocortisone (1 mg/ml) may be added to the infusion. Rare but more serious complications include neutropenia, hypotension, and ocular cataracts, and regular slit lamp examination is advisable in recipients of high-dose regimens. Eighth nerve hearing impairment has also been described in such patients.

PATIENT INFORMATION AND EDUCATION

Patients should be informed of the risks and complications of iron overload, the importance of reducing the body iron burden by phlebotomy, and the need to continue phlebotomy throughout life. They should be advised that impotence and arthropathy, once present, are most unlikely to remit; they should also be instructed to report the development of right upper quadrant pain, weight loss, ascites, or any general deterioration of health that could signal the onset of hepatoma. Patients should also receive instruction concerning the preventive measures described later. A Hemochromatosis Foundation has recently been established that provides patient education in the form of literature and newsletters.*

PERIODIC EVALUATION

In HH, the frequency of follow-up visits is determined by the rate of phlebotomy. If this is being carried out by a blood bank, then the patient should be seen by his physician at least once or twice a month during the intensive phase of phlebotomy and once every six months during the maintenance phase.

A hemoglobin or hematocrit is done before each

phlebotomy, and serum iron should be measured once a month. The value of serial serum ferritin measurement is questionable. In the absence of marked liver disease it can provide an index of the rate of iron removal (1 ng/ml serum ferritin represents approximately 10 mg storage iron), but its greatest value may lie in the observation that serum ferritin may rise in patients with hepatoma. Measurement of the serum alpha-fetoprotein level is an insensitive screen for detection of hepatoma.

PATIENT COMPLIANCE

Appropriate education of patients together with their sense of improved well-being usually results in good patient compliance for phlebotomy. Iron chelator treatment, on the other hand, may give rise to compliance problems and considerable attention may need to be directed to patient and family education.

PREVENTIVE MEASURES

Risk Factor Modification. Restricting dietary iron is unnecessary, although it is important to emphasize to patients that they should not take any mineral or vitamin supplements, including "tonics," containing iron. A well-balanced high-protein diet is recommended during the intensive phlebotomy phase. The patient should be advised that alcohol and vitamin C increase iron absorption and that tea taken with meals will inhibit iron absorption.

Family Counseling. Patients should be informed of the genetic nature of HH, and all first-degree blood relatives should be screened by serum measurement of transferrin saturation and ferritin. Siblings are particularly at risk. Because of close linkage between the gene for HH and the HLA antigens, HLA typing is a useful although expensive method to pick out family members who may be at risk. This is particularly useful to identify younger siblings and children who, because of genotype, should be screened every two years to detect early onset of iron loading. Because of the high gene frequency for HH, HLA typing is also useful to identify heterozygotes for purposes of genetic counseling.

SOCIOECONOMIC ASPECTS OF MANAGEMENT

Phlebotomy is relatively cheap but often long drawn out. By comparison, iron chelation treatment is expensive, both because of the price of a pump and because of the high cost of DF. To keep down the costs of laboratory tests, a simple hemoglobin or hematocrit with only monthly serum iron measurement need be carried out during intensive phlebotomy.

REFERENCES

Crosby WH: Hemochromatosis: the unsolved problems. Semin Hematol 14:135–143, 1977.
Edwards CQ, Dadone MM, Skolnick MH, et al: Hereditary haemochromatosis. Clin Haematol 11:411–435, 1982.
Halliday JW, Powell LW: Iron overload. Semin Hematol 19:42–53, 1982.
Ley TJ, Griffith P, Nienhuis AW: Transfusion haemosiderosis and chelation therapy. Clin Haematol 11:437–464, 1982.
McLaren GD, Muir WA, Kellermeyer RW: Iron overload disorders: natural history, pathogenesis, diagnosis, and therapy. CRC Crit Rev Clin Lab Sci 19:205–266, 1983.

---

*Hemochromatosis Research Foundation, Inc., P.O. Box 8569, Albany, NY 12208.

13 · INFECTIOUS MONONUCLEOSIS

Donald G. Norris
CLEVELAND CLINIC FOUNDATION

DEFINITION AND DIAGNOSTIC CRITERIA

Infectious mononucleosis is a viral illness seen primarily in adolescents and young adults caused by the Epstein-Barr virus (EBV). The signs of fever, pharyngitis, and lymphadenopathy added to the symptoms of malaise, lassitude, and anorexia lead the clinician to suspect the diagnosis of infectious mononucleosis.

Supportive laboratory data of lymphocytosis with 10% or more atypical lymphocytes help confirm the diagnosis. The confirmatory diagnostic test is a positive heterophil test to horse red blood cells (Monospot test) or recent antibody production to the Epstein-Barr virus. In most clinical situations the Monospot is confirmatory by six to 10 days, but it may take up to two weeks in some situations.

PATHOPHYSIOLOGY

The causative agent, Epstein-Barr virus, is a DNA virus of the herpes class. The virus has tropism for the B lymphocyte; after invading the cell and its nucleus, it has the ability to replicate as an intracellular parasite or remain latent indefinitely. The viral replication and host responses to the virus cause the striking clinical finding of cervical adenopathy (at times massive) and enlargement of other lymphoid organs, especially the spleen.

Antibody response to the Epstein-Barr virus is clinically detectable as early as six to 10 days, but is most commonly positive in the second week of illness. The full cellular immune response, which finally stops the proliferation of the virus, is seen in most cases to be active by the fifth to sixth week of infection. Clearly, the acute clinical manifestations of the disease are gone by the time of the cellular immune response.

CLINICAL ASPECTS

The clinical manifestations of Epstein-Barr virus infection vary widely with age. There is a subclinical, asymptomatic variety seen in young children that is undetectable fom other viral illnesses.

The disease seen in adolescents and young adults may also be subclinical, but the usual illness is striking. The main symptoms are universal: malaise and fatigue, sweats, and a sore throat and related anorexia. Other symptoms are similar to other viral illnesses, i.e., headache, chills, cough, and myalgia.

The universal clinical sign is adenopathy, which can be so extensive as to cause respiratory difficulty. Also seen is fever and pharyngitis. Splenomegaly is seen in nearly 50% of cases and hepatomegaly and/or liver tenderness in 25% of cases. A skin rash is rare, but becomes quite common when the patient is exposed to ampicillin.

MANAGEMENT

PLAN

The short-term goal of therapy is to make the definitive diagnosis and relieve any anxiety that a malignant process is present. Supportive care and encouragement of rest, along with proper nutrition and fluid therapy for the acute illness, is mandatory.

The long-term goal is the return of the patient to full employment, school, or other activities. Frequently, the adolescent is unwilling to restrict activity, but the nature of the illness soon curbs the return to work because of exhaustion. Patients are frequently so tired that even the most motivated of students are unable to keep up, and temporary withdrawal from school may be necessary. The management of the student-athlete requires special consideration, especially for contact sports. It is recommended that athletic participation be reinstituted in a gradual way under close supervision.

Hospitalization. There is almost no need to hospitalize the patient with infectious mononucleosis. Hospitalization is necessary to manage complications of the disease, listed below.

1. Airway obstruction is due to massive lymphoid hypertrophy. This is the only true indication for the use of corticosteroids in infectious mononucleosis. This occurs in less than 0.5% of cases.

2. Splenic rupture occurs in 0.1% to 0.2% of cases of mononucleosis. Frequently the diagnosis of infectious mononucleosis is made after the splenic rupture.

3. Severe anorexia and dehydration is another rare complication where hospitalization and supportive fluids are mandatory.

4. Hematologic abnormalities such as neutropenia, thrombocytopenia, and true bone marrow aplasia may necessitate hospitalization.

5. Neurologic sequelae, such as meningoencephalitis, Guillain-Barré syndrome, or seizures, are extremely rare. Hospitalization for diagnostic and supportive measures is indicated.

Otherwise, the vast majority of patients may be cared for at home or at college with the provision that adequate supervision is available.

DRUG THERAPY

There is no indication for antibiotic therapy in infectious mononucleosis. No data are available to indicate the use of antiviral agents. Corticosteroids, although used by some practitioners, are indicated only in acute airway obstruction.

PATIENT INFORMATION AND EDUCATION

Efforts to inform the teenager and college student about infectious mononucleosis are important to ensure their understanding of the possible complications of the illness and their role in managing the acute illness and the prolonged malaise that is so common. The early return to study and work can be self-defeating and be associated with a prolongation of symptoms.

PERIODIC EVALUATION

Repeated observation during the acute illness may be necessary to assess the potential for complications and reassure the patient of recovery.

It may be necessary to extend the observations

through the convalescent malaise, again primarily for reassurance.

PREVENTIVE MEASURES

Careful hand, dish, and utensil washing is important to prevent the spread of infectious mononucleosis among family members and school friends. The spread of infectious mononucleosis is facilitated by close or intimate contact. Because of the long incubation period (45 to 60 days), the source of infection is difficult to pinpoint.

SOCIOECONOMIC ASPECTS OF MANAGEMENT

The primary socioeconomic problem of infectious mononucleosis is prolonged loss of school time and work time. School officials and employers must be informed of the illness. It is sometimes necessary to interrupt high school and college for a semester to allow recuperation. This can place unusual financial burdens on the patient and the family.

REFERENCES

Crampacker CS: The Paul-Bunnell test revisited. Rev Infect Dis 4:1069–1070, 1982.
Kieff E, Dambaugh T, Heller M, et al: The biology and chemistry of the Epstein-Barr virus. J Infect Dis 146:506–517, 1982.
Maki DG, Reich RM: Infectious mononucleosis in the athlete. Am J Sports Med 10:162–173, 1982.
Weary PE, Cole JW, Lindsay LH: Eruptions from ampicillin in patients with infectious mononucleosis. Arch Dermatol 101:86–91, 1970.

14 · PRELEUKEMIC OR MYELODYSPLASTIC SYNDROMES (PL/MDS)

Robert V. Pierre
MAYO CLINIC AND MAYO FOUNDATION

DEFINITION AND DIAGNOSTIC CRITERIA

Preleukemic or myelodysplastic syndromes (PL/MDS) are stem cell disorders characterized by cytopenias and dyspoiesis of one or more of the normal bone marrow cell lines, i.e., dyserythropoiesis, dysgranulopoiesis, and dysmegakaryocytopoiesis. The disorders may be primary or secondary to chemotherapy and/or radiation therapy.

Diagnostic criteria have been described by the French-American-British group (FAB). The primary diagnostic features are the numbers of blasts (types I and II myeloblasts) in the peripheral blood and bone marrow; the presence of dyserythropoiesis (dysplasia, megaloblastoid maturation, or pathologic ringed sideroblasts); dysgranulopoiesis (excess blasts, abnormal nuclear characteristics such as the pseudo–Pelger-Hüet anomaly, cytoplasmic abnormalities such as degranulation, or abnormal granules); and dysmegakaryocytopoiesis (micromegakaryocytes, large platelets, defective granulation).

Table 1. FAB CLASSIFICATION OF PL/MDS

	% Blasts in Peripheral Blood	% Blasts in Bone Marrow
Refractory anemia (RA)	<1	<5
Refractory anemia with ringed sideroblasts (RARS)	<1	<5
Refractory anemia with excess blasts (RAEB)	<5	>5 – <20
Chronic myelomonocytic leukemia (CMML)*	<5	>5 – <20
RAEB in transformation (RAEB-T)†	>5	>20 – <30

*Peripheral blood must contain at least 1000 monocytes/µl.
†Auer rods may be present.

The FAB classification consists of five types of PL/MDS (Table 1).

PATHOPHYSIOLOGY

PL/MDS are clonal stem cell disorders in which an abnormal multipotent stem cell line develops in the bone marrow and produces abnormal red cells, white cells, and platelets. Production from the normal bone marrow stem cells is suppressed by inhibitory factors elaborated by the PL/MDS cell lines. The resulting decreased or ineffective production results in anemia, neutropenia, and thrombocytopenia; in addition, many of the neutrophils and platelets are defective in function.

CLINICAL ASPECTS

PL/MDS disorders may occur at any age but are most common in the elderly. They are most frequently discovered in the work-up of a refractory anemia or incidental to examination for other reasons. Patients may also present with infections due to neutropenia or bleeding manifestations secondary to thrombocytopenia or defective platelet function. It is important to distinguish these disorders from potentially reversible disorders with which they may be confused, such as vitamin B_{12} or folic acid deficiency, or drug or chemical marrow toxicity. They must also be distinguished from erythroleukemia or smoldering acute leukemia.

The median survival of patients with PL/MDS is approximately two and a half years; 25% progress to acute nonlymphocytic leukemia (ANLL). The remainder die of complications secondary to their cytopenias, unless other causes supervene.

MANAGEMENT

PLAN

Currently, there is no effective therapy for PL/MDS. Although some consider these disorders to be an early stage of ANLL, traditional aggressive antileukemic chemotherapy has proved to be effective in only a small number of young patients and rarely in older patients. Therefore, the primary plan of care is supportive care and management of complications until the cytopenias become life-threatening or the process evolves to ANLL, at which time more aggressive forms of therapy can be considered. Patients can be managed as outpatients unless a severe bleeding or infectious episode requires hospitalization.

NONPHARMACOLOGIC MEASURES

Transfusion of packed red cells may be required to maintain satisfactory hemoglobin levels to permit reasonable activity. Platelet transfusions may be used to control a specific bleeding episode, but are not a useful long-term therapy.

DRUG THERAPY

There is no uniformly effective drug therapy for this group of disorders at the present time. Vitamin B_{12} and folic acid therapy has no effect unless a concomitant deficiency is present. Patients with RARS should receive a trial of pyridoxine therapy (100 mg/day), since a small number may show improvement in their hemoglobin levels. A trial of androgen therapy may be warranted in transfusion-dependent patients, since a few may increase their erythroid values sufficiently to eliminate the need for transfusions. Corticosteroid therapy (60 mg/day) may transiently elevate erythroid, neutrophil, or platelet levels and is therefore useful in the management of patients with acute complications. However, long-term corticosteroid therapy is not indicated and is usually ineffective. Iron therapy is indicated only when iron deficiency can be documented and should be stopped when the iron deficiency is corrected. Long-term iron therapy in the absence of iron deficiency is ineffective and may contribute to the development of tissue hemosiderosis.

There is a growing trend to label the disorder in patients under the age of 25 years with one of the advanced stages of PL/MDS (e.g., RAEB, CMML, or RAEB-T) as acute nonlymphocytic leukemia (ANNL) and to treat it as such. On the other hand, young patients with RA or RARS should be treated conservatively as are the older patients. Bone marrow transplantation has also proved successful in the management of young patients. When the disease process converts to ANLL, conventional therapy should be given if the patient's age, general status, and personal and family desires support such an approach.

Recent experimental therapy approaches with so-called cell maturation agents, such as low-dose cytosine arabinoside or cis-retinoic acid, have shown promising results with the production of complete or partial responses. Additional studies are required before the role of these agents in the management of PL/MDS is defined.

PATIENT INFORMATION AND EDUCATION

It is important that patients be informed of the nature of the disorder so that they will enter into a follow-up program and avoid continued medical shopping for an answer to their chronic illness, which may lead to trials of expensive and ineffective forms of therapy.

PERIODIC EXAMINATION

The intervals for follow-up visits will depend on the patient's performance status and need for transfusions. Asymptomatic patients may be seen at six-month to one-year intervals. A complete bone count and peripheral blood smear examination should be obtained, and if significant changes are observed, a repeat bone marrow examination should be done.

PATIENT COMPLIANCE

Patient compliance is usually excellent provided the patient has been adequately informed of the progressive nature of the disorder.

PREVENTIVE MEASURES

Since the cause of primary PL/MDS is unknown, preventive measures are not possible. However, secondary PL/MDS may be decreased or avoided if use of alternate therapies to chemotherapy or radiation are used whenever possible. Likewise, minimizing chemotherapy or radiation dosage when feasible may be helpful. Avoidance of exposure to hydrocarbons, solvents, and other possible agents that are toxic to marrow in the work or hobby environment may also minimize the risks.

SOCIOECONOMIC ASPECTS OF MANAGEMENT

PL/MDS are long-term disorders that are invariably fatal owing to progression to ANLL or from complications resulting from the chronic cytopenias. They place a great economic and emotional burden on both the patient and the family.

REFERENCES

Bennet JM, Catovsky D, Daniel MT, et al: Proposals for the classification of the myelodysplastic syndromes. Br J Haematol 51:189–199, 1982.
Juneja SK, Imbert M, Jouault H, et al: Haematological features of primary myelodysplastic syndromes (PMDS) at initial presentation: a study of 118 cases. J Clin Pathol 36:1129–1135, 1983.
Pierre RV: Preleukemic states. Semin Hematol 11:73–92, 1974.
Weber RFA, Geraedts JPM, Kerkhofs H, et al: The preleukemic syndrome. I. Clinical and haematological findings. Acta Med Scand 207:391–395, 1980.
Zittoun R: Subacute and chronic myelomonocytic leukemia: a distinct haematological entity. Br J Haemtol 32:1–7, 1976.

15 · ACUTE LEUKEMIA

Ellis J. Van Slyck
HENRY FORD HOSPITAL

DEFINITION AND DIAGNOSTIC CRITERIA

Acute adult leukemia is classified as either acute nonlymphocytic (ANLL, 85%) or acute lymphocytic (ALL, 15%) and is diagnosed by bone marrow aspiration and biopsy. The typical case has a high total marrow cellularity and a preponderance of immature forms; significant numbers of patients, usually over the age of 50, may have few leukemic blasts in the marrow, a disease process referred to as "smoldering" leukemia.

PATHOPHYSIOLOGY AND CLINICAL ASPECTS

The symptoms of acute leukemia are related to the degree of suppression of normal circulating blood elements. Fatigue, weakness, headache (anemia), abnormal bleeding (thrombocytopenia), and fever with or without signs of local infection (neutropenia) may occur

Table 1. CORRELATION OF MORPHOLOGIC AND CYTOGENETIC ABNORMALITIES IN NONLYMPHOCYTIC LEUKEMIA

FAB Type*	Most Frequent Chromosomal Change
M1 (myeloblastic)	t (9;22)
	+8
M2 (myelobastic with differentiation)	t (8;21)
	+8
	−5 or 5q−
	−7 or 7q−
M3 (promyelocytic)	t (15;17)
M4 (myelomonocytic)	11q abnormalities
	+8
	7q−
M4 Eo†	inv(16) or 16q−
M5 (monocytic)	11q abnormalities
	inv (16) or 16q−
M6 (erythroblastic)	complex abnormalities
	5q− and −7
Megakaryoblastic	−7
2° leukemia (therapy-related)	−5 or 5q−
	−7 or 7q−

*FAB = French-American-British classification.

†M4Eo = subtype of myelomonocytic leukemia with increased eosinophils.

in any combination. Central nervous system (CNS) involvement can occur early in acute lymphocytic leukemia (ALL) and may occasionally be the presenting symptom. Patients who fail to respond to treatment usually die from resistant infection, but some die from uncontrolled bleeding.

When possible, all new cases of acute leukemia should have cytochemical stains and cytogenetic analysis to aid in treatment choices and outcome predictions (Table 1). The recent reclassification scheme (FAB: French-American-British) for both ALL and ANLL has been well accepted as an additional aid in treatment planning. Overall, chemotherapy produces a complete remission in about 60% of ANLL patients.

Acute lymphocytic leukemia (ALL) does not respond to treatment as well in adults as in children. Although about 70% of patients achieve a complete remission, it may last only a few months. Besides age, other high-risk factors that have a poor prognosis for response include an initial white blood cell count >50 × 10⁹/L, the presence of a mediastinal mass, CNS involvement, FAB L3 subtype, immunologic subtypes T cell or B cell, and leukemias that have abnormal chromosomes.

MANAGEMENT

PLAN

The immediate therapeutic goal is to treat infection, if present, and anemia, if severe and symptomatic. Occasionally, abnormal bleeding will require early platelet transfusions. After the particular features of a case have been reviewed, the physician undertakes multidrug chemotherapy with the intent to produce a complete remission. The long-term goal is to produce a durable remission; if attained, this will usually last from 12 to 24 months before relapse. In about 5% of patients, it is permanent. Knowing that the risk of death from induction chemotherapy increases with age and con-

comitant disease (i.e., heart, kidney, or lung disease), the physician may employ supportive measures only, since the use of chemotherapy in nontoxic (non-marrow-suppressive) doses in the fragile elderly patient is of little or no value.

Indications for Hospitalization. Every newly diagnosed patient with acute leukemia must be hospitalized for administration of blood products, chemotherapy, and/or antibiotics, any one or all of which may be indicated. In most new cases, a protracted period in the hospital in excess of a month is needed to accomplish the first induction chemotherapy and to manage related toxic effects. After remission has been attained and so-called consolidation treatment completed, which usually requires additional hospital admissions, the patient can be treated in the physician's office during the maintenance phase. Visiting nurses can render service when the patient is at home by checking the status of an indwelling venous catheter or looking for signs of infection or bleeding, but their services are generally not needed after the first month of consolidation or maintenance treatment.

NONPHARMACOLOGIC MEASURES

Modified isolation while in the hospital, limited contact with relatives and friends while at home, and avoiding crowds are wise measures. When the absolute number of circulating neutrophils (polymorphonuclears and bands) is below 0.5 × 10⁹/L, it is advisable to isolate the patient and require nurses and other attendants to wear face masks and wash hands before each entry into the patient's room.

Other measures that are commonly employed in the neutropenic leukemic patient include daily skin cleansing, use of antiseptic mouthwash, and the placement of indwelling intravenous catheters.

DRUG THERAPY

Acute Nonlymphocytic Leukemia (ANLL)

Remission Induction and Consolidation. The drugs known to be active in destroying myeloid blasts are cytosine arabinoside, daunorubicin (daunomycin), doxorubicin (Adriamycin), 6-thioguanine, and VP16-213 (etoposide). Vincristine and prednisone, of proven use in ALL, may also have some activity in ANLL; other drugs are currently under investigation, including *m*-AMSA, 5-azacytidine, and mitoxantrone.

An established drug combination for remission induction is the "TAD" regimen (6-thioguanine, cytosine arabinoside, and daunorubicin). This treatment is intense and is particularly effective in younger patients. In patients over 60 years of age, I generally reduce the dose of each drug by 25%. An alternate regimen with proven benefit is a combination of vincristine, doxorubicin, cytosine arabinoside, and prednisone ("AdOAP"). This regimen is particularly helpful for cases in which the classification of leukemic cell type is not known. Etoposide, which has shown significant antileukemic activity, particularly in monocytic types, is currently being used effectively in combination with the aforementioned drugs.

The patient's marrow state must be assessed after the induction treatment, and if leukemic cells are still present seven to 10 days after its completion, a second course is given. If, on the other hand, the marrow recovers with no residual evidence of leukemia, consolidation treatment with the same drugs at a 25% reduction in dose is given twice, usually a month apart. Failure to consolidate remission leads to early relapse in many patients.

Maintenance Therapy. Central nervous system (CNS) prophylaxis for ANLL has not been found to be necessary. The value of maintenance therapy in delaying or preventing relapse is controversial. Most hematologists currently give monthly courses of moderate chemotherapy on an outpatient basis for at least 12 to 18 months; this treatment usually consists of cytosine arabinoside subcutaneously for five days and 6-thioguanine orally for five days.

Patients under age 50 who have an available HLA matched donor are candidates for a bone marrow transplant after they have attained remission. Current data indicate that patients in this group, particularly those under age 20, enjoy longer disease-free remissions than patients treated with maintenance chemotherapy. However, 30% of these patients die during or shortly after the transplant process, due to sepsis, interstitial pneumonia, or severe graft-versus-host disease. Furthermore, the evidence is still not clear that overall survival is favorably affected by bone marrow transplants.

Elderly ANLL patients with fewer than 50% blasts and less than normal marrow cellularity have a poor remission rate and high treatment-associated mortality rate when given standard remission induction regimens. To these patients, I usually offer only supportive treatment until the disease becomes fully expressed. Occasionally, a patient may obtain a complete and durable remission from a 14- to 21-day course of low-dose cytosine arabinoside.

Acute Lymphocytic Leukemia (ALL)

Remission Induction. Many drugs are active in reducing the leukemic lymphoblast cell burden. These include corticosteroids, vincristine, anthracycline drugs, L-asparaginase, methotrexate (MTX), cytosine arabinoside, cyclophosphamide, carmustine (BCNU), and the antipurines 6-mercaptopurine and 6-thioguanine. Several newer drugs are also under investigation, such as *m*-AMSA (amsacrine), VP-16-213 (etoposide), VM-26 (teniposide), 2-deoxycoformycin, aclacinomycin, and mitoxantrone. Unfortunately, the available agents, singly or in combination, rarely produce long remissions in adults. For induction treatment, a combination of vincristine, prednisone, and daunomycin (or doxorubicin) is as effective as any combinations currently known.

Early CNS leukemia occurs in perhaps 10% of adult ALL cases and affects many additional patients later, whether in systemic remission or not. The prophylactic use of intracranial radiation to a total dose of 24 Gy, repeated intrathecal (IT) injections of 15 mg methotrexate, or high-dose intravenous methotrexate (100 to 300 mg/kg) with citrovorum factor rescue will all greatly reduce CNS leukemia. In the adult, IT methotrexate alone appears to be sufficient for this purpose. Thus, a lumbar puncture is performed shortly after induction therapy is initiated to establish the presence of leukemic cells, and methotrexate prophylaxis is started intrathecally simultaneously. Ideally, an Ommaya reservoir should be placed for the repeated intraventricular administration of methotrexate, since it provides easy access to the cerebrospinal fluid and attains predictably high levels of methotrexate. In patients with CNS leukemia, Ommaya reservoir placement should be mandatory. Five or six doses of IT methotrexate are given prophylactically over three weeks during the induction period.

Maintenance. Most ALL patients in remission will relapse within one to two years. Many combinations of drugs and schedules have been used as continuation, consolidation, and maintenance therapy, and the consensus is that the more intense the treatment, the longer the remission duration; however, no one particular regimen has proven superiority. All or most of the drugs listed under "Remission Induction" are used cyclically in a complex fashion, with time allowed for marrow recovery after each treatment pulse. This regimen will continue for two or three years. The L10 protocol of Schauer et al. may be referred to as a guide to this phase of treatment, although the schema represents maximum intensity. If relapse occurs, a second remission can often be obtained by using (1) the original induction regimen; (2) sequential, high-dose cytosine arabinoside and asparaginase; or (3) high-dose methotrexate (3 to 6 gm/m^2) with citrovorum factor and vincristine. For patients under age 40 with an HLA-matched donor, a bone marrow transplant during second remission should be offered.

Adverse Effects. Antileukemic drugs produce many side effects in addition to expected, marked marrow aplasia. Most patients experience a few, several, or all of the following: nausea, vomiting, diarrhea, stomatitis (methotrexate), alopecia (Adriamycin), peripheral neuropathy, autonomic dysfunction (vincristine), cardiomyopathy (Adriamycin), pancreatitis (asparaginase), liver dysfunction (6-thioguanine), and anaphylaxis. When chemotherapy is given, antiemetics (Reglan, high-dose bolus methylprednisolone, Compazine, Haldol, or Torecan, etc.) are also usually required. Monilial oral infections, which occur commonly when corticosteroids are combined with marrow depressants, are treated with Mycostatin oral suspension or lozenges. Extravasation of irritating intravenous agents is promptly treated with local hydrocortisone injections, after the irritant has been aspirated via the in situ needle. When vesicants such as the anthracycline drugs are involved, cold compresses are applied for 24 hours, to be followed later by warm compresses.

Management of Complications. Infections are an inevitable consequence of leukemia treatment. Sepsis or pneumonia often without cough or sputum are the most common infections. Although prophylactic antibiotic usage is controversial and not generally recommended, it is imperative to hospitalize the patient and start broad-spectrum antibiotics promptly when a fever of >101° F or when sudden weakness or other deterioration of the neutropenic patient's clinical state suggests bacterial invasion. The antibiotic regimen (usually an aminoglycoside with an antipseudomonal penicillin, such as ticarcillin or mezlocillin) should be started even before blood and urine cultures and a chest film are obtained. Fungal infections with *Candida* and *Aspergillus* continue to emerge as serious problems, as may gram-positive infections.

Severe anemia and thrombocytopenia usually appear during induction chemotherapy and require replacement therapy with red cells and platelet donations. Opinions differ about when platelet transfusions are indicated. Some clinicians favor using them when the patient's platelet count falls below a predetermined value such as 20×10^9/L. I prefer to use 8 to 10 units of random donor platelets when clinical signs of bleeding from the skin or mucous membranes appear. This usually occurs when the platelets are less than 10×10^9/L, although the critical number may vary widely. Following chemotherapy, platelet transfusions may be required every three or four days. However, applying the latter criteria ensures that overall platelet usage will be economical and maximally effective, thus retarding the development of resistance. Single donor platelets (HLA-matched if available) should replace random donor platelets when the latter no longer produce an incremental increase in the recipient platelet count or control bleeding.

PATIENT INFORMATION AND EDUCATION

With few exceptions, patients with newly diagnosed acute leukemia should be told about their diagnosis promptly. After a suitable interval, perhaps 24 hours or longer, a lengthy orientation session between the physician and patient should be arranged.

PERIODIC EVALUATION

Patients in complete remission should be evaluated each month for drug toxicity or early signs of relapse before the next course of maintenance treatment is started. A brief examination and peripheral blood counts with differential usually suffice. Unexpected findings, usually cytopenias in the blood, mandate a progress bone marrow examination to provide clear evidence of excessive toxicity or relapse.

PATIENT COMPLIANCE

To effectively complete induction and consolidation, treatment requires extraordinary compliance from the patient. This is best obtained by always having the patient placed in the same designated area of the hospital where nurses with special knowledge and experience in this field are working. Furthermore, when readmissions become necessary, it helps assuage the patient's anxiety if he or she is familiar with the surroundings and faces. This constructive attitude tends to carry over to outpatient maintenance treatment.

SOCIOECONOMIC ASPECTS OF MANAGEMENT

Unfortunately, the cost of the intensive treatment of acute leukemia is very high. Few patients could pay their expenses without major third party support, and many patients exhaust their own resources during the course of their illness.

REFERENCES

Gale RP: Progress in acute myelogenous leukemia. Ann Intern Med 101:702–705, 1984.

Gale RP, Foon KA, Cline MJ, et al: Intensive chemotherapy for acute myelogenous leukemia. Ann Intern Med 94:753–757, 1981.

Jacobs AD, Gale RP: Recent advances in the biology and treatment of acute lymphoblastic leukemia in adults. N Engl J Med 311:1219–1231, 1984.

Schauer P, Arlin ZA, Mertelsmann R: Treatment of acute lymphoblastic leukemia in adults: results of the L-10 and L20M protocols. J Clin Oncol 1:462–470, 1983.

Van Slyck EJ, Rebuck JW, Waddell CC, et al: Smoldering acute granulocytic leukemia: observations on its natural history and morphologic characteristics. Arch Intern Med 143:37–40, 1983.

16 · CHRONIC LYMPHOCYTIC LEUKEMIA

Joseph J. Mazza
MARSHFIELD CLINIC

DEFINITION AND DIAGNOSTIC CRITERIA

Chronic lymphocytic leukemia (CLL) is probably the most common type of leukemia seen by the practicing internist and the clinical hematologist. The disease is seen most commonly in patients over the age of 50, and the majority of these patients are asymptomatic when the diagnosis is made. The diagnosis of CLL is often made serendipitously when an abnormal peripheral smear or differential is reported from a routine hemogram. The hallmark of the disease is an absolute lymphocytosis (>15,000 per mm³) with or without other hematologic abnormalities, i.e., thrombocytopenia and anemia. Physical examination is quite variable, depending upon the stage of the disease. Generalized lymphadenopathy and splenomegaly are frequently found in patients with more advanced stage disease.

PATHOPHYSIOLOGY

The WBC may be greater than 100,000 per mm³ with 90% or more of the cells being lymphocytes. These lymphocytes appear as small or medium size cells with morphologic characteristics on light microscopy of mature, well-differentiated lymphocytes. Usually there is a scant amount of cytoplasm and the degree of pleomorphism is minimal. The bone marrow aspiration and biopsy show a preponderance of monotonous-appearing mature lymphocytes with relatively few myeloid elements. Usually, however, the myeloid cell lines are morphologically normal and show no maturation abnormalities. Occasionally the marrow contains increased numbers of large plasmacytoid-appearing lymphocytes with more generous amounts of cytoplasm and a decreased nuclear cytoplasmic ration. These cases are sometimes found in association with a monoclonal gammopathy, and serum protein electrophoresis should be obtained in these instances.

Most cases of CLL represent a malignant proliferation of B lymphocytes, and only a small percentage of cases have shown a proliferation of T cells or other less differentiated immature B cells. The type of B cell that proliferates in CLL is not of follicular center origin but rather a noncleaved lymphocyte that is normally found in the medullary portion of the lymph node along the sinusoids. Biopsy of the node shows a diffuse infiltration with effacement of the normal nodal architecture and a histopathologic picture of a diffuse, well-differentiated lymphocytic lymphoma. CLL cells have a very low turnover rate and have only a small amount of surface immunoglobulin, usually IgM and IgG. These B cells are immunologically incompetent and show resistance to blast transformation in vitro with a variety of mitogens or lectins.

CLINICAL ASPECTS

Clinically, CLL is characterized by a protracted course, which usually requires no chemotherapeutic intervention initially. Staging of the disease is of limited value, since the presentation and findings at the time of diagnosis may be remarkably variable. However, staging does aid in predicting duration of survival, with stage III (anemia) and IV (thrombocytopenia) patients having a significantly shorter survival than do patients with stage 0 (lymphocytosis) and I (lymphadenopathy) disease. Staging might also be helpful in determining what treatment modalities are most appropriate. It is not unusual to have patients with CLL present with no peripheral adenopathy or splenomegaly and yet have a white blood cell count in excess of 100,000 per mm^3 with an accompanying anemia and thrombocytopenia. The marrow in this instance will show marked hypercellularity with virtual replacement of the myeloid elements by sheets of mature, well-differentiated lymphocytes. By the same token, patients may present with marked peripheral adenopathy and an enlarged spleen and yet have only a modest lymphocytosis with no anemia or thrombocytopenia. The most important guidelines as to when one should initiate chemotherapy are:

1. The onset of symptoms referable directly to the tumor masses, i.e., large bulky peripheral nodes, marked splenomegaly, or bulky abdominal tumors.

2. Progression of anemia and/or thrombocytopenia.

3. The development of serious complications secondary to the lymphoproliferative process, i.e., systemic infection or hemolytic anemia.

Because the majority of patients with the diagnosis of CLL develop significant hypogammaglobulinemia during the course of their disease, they are at risk of developing serious systemic infections. Usually these infections are bacterial and pyogenic in nature and commonly present as pneumonitis. Viral infections, especially herpes zoster, are not uncommonly seen because of the generalized immunosuppressed state of these patients. Autoimmune hemolytic anemia and immune thrombocytopenia may occur in CLL and be of a magnitude to cause serious clinical problems. Fortunately, both these complications usually respond to prompt intervention with corticosteroids.

MANAGEMENT

The clinical course of CLL is characterized by a protracted indolent phase during which time the patient is entirely asymptomatic and requires no treatment or supportive care. During this time it is sufficient to follow the course of the proliferative process with hemograms every three to six months. There is no specific WBC level that one should use to indicate when chemotherapy should be initiated.

Alkylating agents with or without corticosteroids have been the mainstay of therapy for CLL over the past two decades (see Table 1). Other agents have been tried with limited success when conventional or standard treatment fails to control the proliferative process. Modalities of therapy used in the past have included total body irradiation,^{32}P, and thymic radiation. Radiation therapy to the spleen and bulky tumor sites in conjunction with chemotherapy is a commonly used means of palliation in advanced stage disease. Currently, biological response modifiers and monoclonal antibodies are being tried in the treatment of CLL, and early preliminary data are available on some of these agents. However, further evaluation in multicenter group studies will be necessary to determine their efficacy.

Frequently, low-dose chlorambucil is all that is necessary to control the WBC and improve the hemoglobin and platelet levels in early stage disease patients. Chlorambucil given in low doses (2 to 4 mg/day) appears to be equally as effective as a larger dose intermittently. When the disease does not come under control with such treatment, it is common to begin a more aggressive treatment program using cyclophosphamide and vincristine in conjunction with high-dose corticosteroids on a cyclic basis, repeating the treatment every three to four weeks for an extended period as long as the treatment remains effective and is tolerated by the patient. The addition of an anthracycline (e.g., doxorubicin) to a combination of the above agents (CVP) has not increased the efficacy of this treatment program while it has increased the toxicity significantly.

The immune-mediated hemolysis and/or thrombocytopenia seen with CLL is treated with prednisone (1 to 2 mg/kg/day), continued until the hemoglobin and platelet count return to more normal levels. A tapering dose schedule can be used to avoid the complications of hypercortisolism once improvement in the hematologic parameters has occurred.

Survival data are somewhat difficult to assess in CLL because of the protracted indolent phase and the insidious onset of signs and symptoms. The median survival for all patients following the diagnosis of CLL is five to six years. Early stage (0-I) patients have a median survival of ten years or more, whereas patients

Table 1. CURRENT TREATMENT PROGRAMS FOR ACTIVE CLL

Chlorambucil: 30 mg/m² on day 1 only
Prednisone: 80 mg/day PO × 5 days
 *Repeat q2-wk intervals × 18 cycles
Cyclophosphamide: 300 mg/m² PO daily × 5—days 1–5
Vincristine: 1.2 mg/m² (max 2.0 mg) IV on day 1 only
Prednisone: 100 mg/m² PO daily × 5—days 1–5
 *Repeat q3-wk intervals × 12 cycles

Eastern Cooperative Oncology Group, EST 2480.
*Intervals between cycles can be lengthened and duration of treatment can be extended, depending on patient's response, tolerance, and counts.

with advanced stage disease (III and IV) will have a more progressive course and die within two years.

REFERENCES

Foon KA, Schroff RW, Bunn PA, et al: Effects of monoclonal antibody therapy in patients with chronic lymphocytic leukemia. Blood 64:1085–1093, 1984.

Huang A, Laszlo J, Brenchman W: Lymphoblastoid interferon trial in chronic lymphocytic leukemia. Proceedings of the American Association of Cancer Research, 23:113, March 1982 (Abstract #441).

Phillips EA, Kempin S, Passe S, et al: Prognostic factors in chronic lymphocytic leukaemia and their implications for therapy. Clin Haematol 6:203–222, 1977.

Rai KR, Sawitsky A, Cronkite EP, et al: Clinical staging of chronic lymphocytic leukemia. Blood 46:219–234, 1975.

Spiers ASD: Rarer forms of chronic lymphocytic leukemia. Clin Ca Briefs 6:3–12, 1984.

17 · CHRONIC MYELOGENOUS LEUKEMIA

Joseph J. Mazza
MARSHFIELD CLINIC

DEFINITION AND DIAGNOSTIC CRITERIA

Chronic myelogenous leukemia does not occur with the frequency of chronic lymphocytic leukemia but can be expected to account for 15% of all cases of leukemia in Western countries. The disease occurs with peak incidence in the third to sixth decades and is characterized by leukocytosis and splenomegaly in the majority of cases. Differentiation from agnogenic myeloid metaplasia is required.

PATHOPHYSIOLOGY

Both radiation and chemical exposure are capable of inducing damage to the hematopoietic stem cells, resulting in chromosomal abnormalities and eventual leukemia. Studies from the atom bomb experience leave no doubt about a cause and effect relationship between radiation and eventual leukemia.

CLINICAL ASPECTS

Signs and symptoms of chronic myelogenous leukemia (CML) develop slowly and may be vague and nonspecific. Generalized weakness, malaise, weight loss, and decreased exercise tolerance are frequent, common early symptoms. Left upper quadrant fullness and early satiety are those symptoms associated with an enlarged spleen. Features of hypermetabolism, such as warm skin and fever, may also be seen early in the disease. All of these symptoms will increase in severity if the disease remains untreated.

The most consistent abnormality in CML is the chromosomal hallmark known as Philadelphia chromosome, the deletion of a portion of the long arm of chromosome 22 that has been translocated to chromosome 9. This abnormality can be detected at any stage of the disease and persists throughout the chronic stable phase. As patients enter an accelerated phase of disease, a multitude of additional chromosome abnormalities may develop that are not always predictable or uniform. Although this chromosome abnormality will be seen in 90% of cases, a small percentage of patients will be PH− and exhibit a clinical course different from the PH+ counterparts. The former patients respond less favorably to therapy and are more difficult to control. Evolution into the accelerated phase occurs more rapidly and survival is generally shorter.

A moderately to markedly increased white blood cell count ranging from 50 to 300 × 10^9/L is characteristic of this disease. A significant number of early or blast cells are usually not found in the peripheral smear, and polymorphonuclear leukocytes and bandforms predominate in the differential white blood count. It is not uncommon to see an increased platelet count during the early stages of CML. Mild to moderate anemia is almost always present at the time of diagnosis and is usually normocytic and normochromic. Serum uric acid and vitamin B_{12} are increased owing to the increased proliferation of granulocytes in the marrow. Bone marrow with increases in granulocytes is the rule. In addition, there are usually increased numbers of eosinophils and basophils. A very characteristic finding in CML is the presence of a low leukocyte alkaline phosphatase score.

MANAGEMENT

NONPHARMACOLOGIC MEASURES

Radiation therapy to the spleen has been used as an effective means of achieving rapid regression of an enlarged symptomatic spleen and to control the progression of the disease. Radiation is no more effective than chemotherapy in causing regression of splenomegaly. Bone marrow transplantation has recently been shown to be an effective method of therapy for patients with CML. It has been used for patients in both the chronic as well as the accelerated phase, and has been suggested as the treatment of choice for a young patient with CML in the chronic phase who has an HLA identical donor.

DRUG THERAPY

Once the diagnosis of CML is established and myelosuppressive therapy is instituted, patients should be followed closely with frequent blood counts and examinations to monitor the effects of therapy. The CBC and spleen size are most commonly followed for this purpose.

The two most commonly used myelosuppressive agents to treat CML are busulfan (Myleran) and hydroxyurea (Hydrea). Busulfan used at a dose of 6 to 8 mg/day PO will usually lower the WBC and decrease the size of the spleen in four to six weeks. When the WBC is decreased by 50% of the pretreatment level, it is prudent to cut the dose of busulfan by 50%. Busulfan should be temporarily discontinued when the WBC approximates the upper limit of the normal range. Low-dose busulfan can be used to maintain a normal WBC, and frequently as little as 2 to 4 mg weekly is all that is needed for maintenance therapy. However, maintenance therapy should be adjusted and titrated for each patient. Hydroxyurea used in a similar manner is equally effective in lowering the WBC and platelet count and improving the hemoglobin in CML. An initial dose of 1000 to 1500 mg/day PO is usually sufficient to improve the hematologic parameters. As with busulfan, careful, frequent follow-up counts are required every two weeks until there is a significant fall in the WBC. Appropriate timely adjustments can be made in the dose schedule as the disease comes under control and when the counts return to normal.

Usually, all the manifestations of CML respond promptly to therapy and are easily controlled by appropriate adjustments in medication during the chronic stable phase. However, after a period of one to five years, during which time the patient is asymptomatic and the hemogram is entirely normal, the disease will enter an accelerated phase when control will become increasingly more difficult and the signs and symptoms of the myeloproliferative process will again become apparent. There is a fall in the hemoglobin and platelet count and a significant rise in the WBC. The leukocytosis is almost always accompanied by an increase in the degree of immaturity on the differential count, and sometimes basophilia will be noted. As this phase of the disease progresses (accelerated), the hematologic picture will become more characteristic of a "subacute leukemia" and will eventually evolve into a more acute phase within a matter of weeks. During the accelerated phase, the disease usually becomes more refractory to therapy. Although reversion back to a more stable chronic phase can sometimes be achieved by aggressive chemotherapy, this stable transition is usually short-lived (four to six months), and increased refractoriness to treatment will again occur.

Once the transformation of the chronic disease is complete, numerous complications commonly seen in other acute leukemias ensue; supportive care measures and aggressive multidrug chemotherapy regimens are necessary to induce a remission. The complete remission rate in patients with acute phase CML (blast crisis) is significantly lower than in other acute nonlymphocytic leukemias, and the duration of the complete remission is considerably shorter. Approximately 20% to 30% of patients who develop the acute blast phase of their disease will have morphologic characteristics of acute lymphoblastic leukemia (ALL).

REFERENCES

Armitage JO, Klassen LW, Patil SR, et al: Marrow transplantation for stable phase chronic granulocytic leukemia. Exp Hematol 12:717–719, 1984.

Auclerc G, Jacquillat C, Auclerc MF, et al: Post-therapeutic acute leukemia. Cancer 44:2017, 1979.

Bolin RW, Robinson WA, Sutherland J, et al: Busulfan versus hydroxyurea in long-term therapy of chronic myelogenous leukemia. Cancer 50:1683, 1982.

Rowley JD: Ph¹ Pos. Leukemia, including chronic myelogenous leukemia. Clin Haematol 9:45, 1980.

Speck B, Bortin MM, Champlin R, et al: Allogeneic bone marrow transplantation for chronic myelogenous leukemia. 1:665–668, 1984.

18 · CHRONIC MYELOPROLIFERATIVE DISEASES

Murray N. Silverstein
MAYO CLINIC AND MAYO FOUNDATION

The chronic myeloproliferative diseases (MDS) include polycythemia vera (PRV), agnogenic myeloid metaplasia (AMM), primary thrombocythemia (PT), and chronic myelogenous leukemia (CML). These four diseases have close interrelationships. All of these lesions are clonal hemopathies. This chapter will deal only with agnogenic myeloid metaplasia and primary thrombocythemia, since polycythemia vera and chronic myelogenous leukemia will be dealt with elsewhere in this volume.

Agnogenic Myeloid Metaplasia

DEFINITION AND DIAGNOSTIC CRITERIA

AMM is a chronic myeloproliferative process characterized as follows: (1) splenomegaly; (2) leukoerythroblastic blood reaction (i.e., myeloid immaturity and normoblasts in the peripheral blood); (3) abundant presence of teardrop red cells in the peripheral blood; and (4) bone marrow biopsy demonstrating either reticulin or collagen fibrosis.

PATHOPHYSIOLOGY

AMM is highlighted by an inexorable increase in spleen size and the concomitance of hypersplenism and hypermetabolism.

CLINICAL ASPECTS

Clinically, 20% of patients with AMM are asymptomatic when first seen and 80% of patients manifest symptoms. Of the symptomatic patients, 60% have symptoms of anemia, 22% have symptoms of pressure from the enlarged spleen, and 16% have symptoms of bleeding.

MANAGEMENT

PLAN

There is no cure currently for AMM. In asymptomatic patients, newer experimental methods of management, including the use of antifibrosing agents such as penicillamine and colchicine, are under trial at our institution. Since these agents are entirely experimental, they will not be considered in depth in this treatise. These agents are used in an attempt to delay or inhibit the fibrotic process occurring in the bone marrow.

Long-range goals include the management of complications of this disease, especially the treatment of anemia, the control of bleeding, the control of pressure from splenomegaly, and the treatment of portal hypertension. Any of these problems may lead to hospitalization, and splenectomy may be indicated for all of these complications.

NONPHARMACOLOGIC MEASURES

Nonpharmacologic measures that are employed in the disease include the procedure of splenectomy, the use of radiation therapy, and the use of platelet transfusion. Splenectomy is indicated in patients with the following: (1) painful mechanical splenomegaly; (2) refractory hemolytic anemia; (3) refractory thrombocytopenia; and (4) portal hypertension. Splenectomy should be performed only by a capable senior surgeon with experience in this disease. All patients must be reasonable surgical risks with regard to their cardiac, hepatic, renal, and metabolic findings and should have a full coagulation survey. Patients with qualitative platelet problems or thrombocytopenia may be operated upon with the addition of platelet transfusions and a preoperative cortisone preparation. For patients with disseminated intravascular coagulation, splenectomy or any other surgical procedures are absolutely contraindicated. All patients with mechanical splenomegaly will benefit greatly from splenectomy. Sixty per cent of patients with refractory hemolytic anemia, 50% of patients with refractory thrombocytopenia, and 70% of patients with portal hypertension will have gratifying results from splenectomy.

Radiation therapy may be useful in the following situations: (1) in patients with mechanical splenomegaly who are not splenectomy candidates; (2) in patients with acute splenic infarction for the control of pain; and (3) in patients who develop ascites on the basis of implants of myeloid metaplasia in the peritoneum.

DRUG THERAPY

Drug therapy in AMM currently is utilized to control anemia or the hypermetabolic consequences of the disease. Since drug trials for antifibrosing agents in early AMM are only experimental, these will not be considered here.

When a patient with AMM develops anemia, one must initially obtain a red cell mass and plasma volume. Although many patients with AMM may have hemoglobin levels of 7 to 9 gm, the red cell mass is often found to be normal when blood volume studies are obtained. Plasma volume in such patients will be markedly expanded because of the enlarged spleen. This dilutional form of anemia does not require treatment. In those patients in whom there is defined reduction in red cell mass, our studies have revealed that in 95% of the cases the anemia will be normocytic and normochronic. Ninety-five per cent of the time, the mechanism of this anemia is the result of ineffective erythropoiesis. Androgens are indicated in this situation, and I have felt that oxymetholone in doses of 50 mg three to four times a day is helpful. An androgen trial should continue at least three months, since some late responders have been observed. Liver function studies should be carefully monitored with weekly aspartate aminotransferase and alkaline phosphatase determinations. If these enzyme levels increase three to four times over baseline, the androgen should be discontinued.

Prednisone is indicated in the preoperative preparation of patients for splenectomy who are either thrombocytopenic or have platelet function qualitative abnormalities. Prednisone is also the drug of choice for thrombocytopenia. I have employed it in this situation in doses of up to 60 mg per day. Those patients with hemolytic anemia (i.e., 50% of the normocytic, normochromic anemic patients) may require doses of 20 to 30 mg/day. The usual precautions must be taken with prednisone therapy to allay the onset of latent diabetes, peptic ulcer disease, or osteoporosis.

Recently, hydroxyurea (HU) has been employed in patients with mechanical splenomegaly or hypermetabolic symptoms. HU is given in doses of 0.5 gm twice to three times a day and has been somewhat successful in allaying splenectomy in some patients with a huge, painful spleen. Likewise, hydroxyurea has been helpful in controlling the hypermetabolic aspects of the disease.

PERIODIC EVALUATION

Periodic evaluation of patients is indicated about every four to six months.

PREVENTIVE MEASURES

Since AMM has no genetic consequences, family counseling is not necessary.

SOCIOECONOMIC ASPECTS OF MANAGEMENT

Socioeconomic aspects of management may be a major issue in patients with AMM, especially those who require splenectomy or long-standing drug therapy for this chronic process.

Primary Thrombocythemia (PT)

DEFINITION AND DIAGNOSTIC CRITERIA

PT is characterized by the following: (1) a platelet count in excess of $750 \times 10^9/L$; (2) splenomegaly; (3) profound bone marrow megakaryocytic hyperplasia; (4) absence of the Philadelphia chromosome; and (5) absence of an increased red cell mass.

PATHOPHYSIOLOGY

The disease occurs in two groups: (1) patients older than 60 years of age, and (2) young females in their 20s. In elderly patients, the combination of an increased platelet count and degenerative vascular disease may be lethal and lead to thrombosis, hemorrhage, or death. In younger patients, the high platelet count of itself may produce no serious threat unless the patient is traumatized or requires surgery.

CLINICAL ASPECTS

In older patients, i.e., greater than 50 years of age, 20% are asymptomatic and 80% have symptoms. Of the symptomatic patients, 60% have symptoms of hemorrhage and 40% have thrombotic episodes. Splenomegaly is found in 80% of patients, and 20% of patients autoinfarct their spleens. Microcytic hypochromic anemia occurs in 60% of patients, and the mature neutrophilic leukocytosis is seen in 80% of patients. X-ray evidence suggesting "duodenal ulcer" is seen in up to 40% of patients.

MANAGEMENT

PLAN

In older patients, the short- and long-term goals are to keep the platelet count below 650,000. In younger patients, the goal of treatment is to educate them that they have the disease and that they should wear a Medi-Alert bracelet defining this disease. Additionally, young females are advised not to use oral contraceptive agents because of possible vascular complications.

NONPHARMACOLOGIC MEASURES

In older patients who are experiencing acute hemorrhage or thrombosis, or in younger patients who have had a severe trauma or are being prepared for surgery or obstetric delivery, platelet pheresis is the nonpharmacologic treatment of choice. Pheresis on a cell separator should be continued until the platelet count drops below $650 \times 10^9/L$.

DRUG THERAPY

Drug therapy is indicated in all older patients, i.e., postmenopausal females and males above the age of 50. There is no clear-cut drug of choice in primary thrombocythemia in 1986. Hydroxyurea is a very efficacious agent, however, in high platelet syndromes. I favor doses of 1 to 2 gm/day orally initially, and when the platelet count is below 650,000, I would discontinue the drug. Many patients will require a titrated, low-dose continuing treatment program with hydroxyurea.

In patients older than 65 years of age, ^{32}P is a very effective agent. It is usually given in doses of 2.3 mCi/m² intravenously. Patients should be rechecked six weeks after intravenous ^{32}P to determine if a further smaller dose will be required to bring the platelets to optimal levels.

No significant side effects with ^{32}P therapy have been reported; however, the question of whether such treatment increases the risk of acute leukemia in the future has been fully answered.

We have strongly advised no drug therapy in younger patients to lower the platelet count in this disease, since all available agents may have a leukemogenic potential. Young patients tolerate extremely high levels of thrombocythemia without clinical consequence in our experience.

PATIENT INFORMATION AND EDUCATION

Patients with primary thrombocythemia are well informed of their disease and easily educated as to their problem.

PERIODIC EVALUATION

Periodic follow-up is mandatory; usually I see older patients at four- to six-month intervals, and younger patients at yearly intervals. A hemoglobin count, red blood cell count, white blood cell count, leukocyte differential, and platelet count are obtained.

SOCIOECONOMIC ASPECTS OF MANAGEMENT

Socioeconomic aspects of management of the disease are not difficult in primary thrombocythemic patients. Treatment is usually economically affordable, and survivorship in these patients is quite excellent to date.

REFERENCES

Silverstein MN: Primary or hemorrhagic thrombocythemia. Arch Intern Med 122:18, 1968.

Silverstein MN: Control of hypersplenism and painful splenomegaly in myeloid metaplasia by irradiation (Editorial). Int J Radiat Oncol Biol Phys 2:1221, 1977.

Silverstein MN: Primary thrombocythemia. In Williams WJ, et al (eds): Hematology, 3rd ed. McGraw-Hill Book Co, New York, 1983, p. 218.

Silverstein MN: Agnogenic Myeloid Metaplasia, 1st ed. Publishing Science Corp, Boston, 1985.

Silverstein MN, ReMine WH: Splenectomy in agnogenic myeloid metaplasia. Blood 53:515, 1979.

19 · HODGKIN'S DISEASE

William L. White
MAYO CLINIC AND MAYO FOUNDATION

DEFINITION AND DIAGNOSTIC CRITERIA

Hodgkin's disease, first described over 150 years ago, remains an uncommon disorder of unknown cause. Controversy over the years has focused on an infectious versus a malignant origin of the disease. Today, Hodgkin's disease is viewed as a malignancy affecting lymphoid tissue. Variations in the histologic picture are unified by the presence of the Reed-Sternberg cell, although controversy remains over monocyte-macrophage versus lymphocyte derivation.

PATHOPHYSIOLOGY

Prevalence of Hodgkin's disease has peaks in young adults and in middle age. Pathologic subtypes include lymphocyte predominant, mixed cellularity, and lymphocyte depletion based on cellular composition, and the nodular sclerosis subtype characterized by distinctive collagenous bands partitioning the lymph node into smaller nodules. These subsets are determined by the cells accompanying the Reed-Sternberg cells and can be thought of in terms of numbers of lymphocytes, the degree of cytologic polymorphism, and the presence or absence of collagenous bands.

CLINICAL ASPECTS

Patients usually present with painless enlargement of cervical and/or mediastinal nodes. Clinical presentations above the diaphragm account for about 90% of presenting manifestations. The extent of involvement at presentation is clearly the most important determinant of the treatment plan and prognosis. The Ann Arbor staging classification (Table 1) is widely accepted.

Most investigators recommend bone marrow biopsy, chest film, and either a CT scan or lymphangiogram as necessary pretreatment tests. CT is noninvasive, permits detection of disease in the upper abdomen, and offers the potential for detection of visceral involvement. I regard CT of the abdomen and pelvis as the primary presurgical method for infradiaphragmatic staging. Some radiation oncologists feel that they can tailor their treatment fields better with lymphangiography (LAG), reflecting the multidisciplinary factors that we must keep in mind; if LAG is to be done, it should precede laparotomy.

MANAGEMENT

PLAN

The objective of treatment is cure with the least possible toxic effects using radiation or chemotherapy. Both modalities are usually administered in the Outpatient Department.

NONPHARMACOLOGIC MEASURES

The concept of surgical staging and its application followed the recognition that patients could be cured by radiotherapy but preceded the recognition that combination chemotherapy was also capable of cure. Chemotherapy has gradually attained wider application in this disease, and those patients for whom chemotherapy is indicated do not require surgical staging. Patients with clinical stage IIIB, IVA or IVB disease, those with massive mediastinal adenopathy who are to receive chemotherapy, elderly patients, and those with complicating medical illnesses are examples of patients who do not require exploration. In addition, in my opinion, patients with extensive clinical stage IIIA disease, e.g., those with grossly positive CT scans of the abdomen and pelvis and/or LAGs, do not require exploration (see later).

Table 1. ANN ARBOR STAGING CLASSIFICATION OF HODGKIN'S DISEASE

Stage	Definition
I	Involvement of a single lymph node region
II	Involvement of two or more lymph node regions on the same side of the diaphragm (II), which may be accompanied by localized involvement of an extra-lymphatic organ or site (II_E)
III	Involvement of lymph node regions on both sides of the diaphragm (III), which may also be accompanied by involvement of the spleen (III_S) or by localized involvement of an extralymphatic organ or site (III_E)
IV	Diffuse or disseminated involvement of one or more extralymphatic organs or tissues, with or without associated lymph node involvement

The absence or presence of systemic symptoms of fever, sweats, and weight loss is designated by the suffix letter A or B.

In asymptomatic patients with localized disease (stages I and IIA), radiation is the preferred treatment and is designed to include adjacent lymph node sites that are at risk to harbor occult tumor. For patients presenting with disease above the diaphragm, this means radiation of the mantle field, which includes all node-bearing sites above the diaphragm, as well as treatment to para-aortic nodes with a flag to include the splenic pedicle. If the spleen has not been removed, then it must be treated. For the occasional patients presenting with disease in the groin, radiation therapy will include the pelvis as well as the para-aortic field and the splenic pedicle. The more extensive the process within the abdomen, the more likely it will be that chemotherapy is used.

Exception to the above approach is justified in the patient with bulky mediastinal disease because there is risk of local recurrence within the treated field or marginal recurrence or relapse in the lung. Treatment to the mantle combined with prophylactic radiotherapy to the pulmonary parenchyma or chemotherapy, perhaps followed by radiation therapy directed at pretreatment sites of bulky disease in an effort to consolidate the response, are the alternatives to be considered. I generally favor the radiotherapy approach when possible and consolidation radiotherapy when chemotherapy is the primary modality.

DRUG THERAPY

The role of combination chemotherapy is established in treating patients with stages IIIB, IVA, and IVB disease. The MOPP program consisting of nitrogen mustard, vincristine (Oncovin), procarbazine, and prednisone has been the mainstay of treatment. It has been reported that two thirds of patients who attained complete remission have remained alive without recurrence of disease. BCVPP (BCNU, cyclophosphamide, vinblastine, procarbazine, prednisone) offers the advantage of single monthly injections and less gastrointestinal and neurologic toxicity. Remission induction rates for MOPP and BCVPP are comparable at approximately 75%, with a survival advantage recently reported for BCVPP. ABVD (doxorubicin [Adriamycin], bleomycin, vinblastine, DTIC) is still another active program. Recent studies alternating MOPP and ABVD to test the efficacy of sequential non-cross-resistant drug combinations suggest improved remission induction at about 90% and fewer relapses, and further such studies are in progress to confirm the value of this intensive approach. These are the three main chemotherapy programs that we use in newly diagnosed patients.

Duration of chemotherapy is usually a minimum of six months, although a longer period of therapy may be required. Patients should receive a minimum of two cycles after attainment of complete remission but no less than six cycles even in those who respond quickly.

Patients with symptomatic disease of limited extent (I-IIB) are uncommon. As a general guideline, the greater the bulk of the tumor and the more impressive the systemic symptoms, the more reasonable it is to give chemotherapy.

After mantle radiotherapy, all patients should have periodic assessment of thyroid function to detect and treat preclinical or symptomatic hypothyroidism. Other potential radiation-induced side effects include pneumonitis, pericarditis, and myelopathy. It is hoped that ovarian function can be preserved by oophoropexy during staging laparotomy if it is necessary to treat the pelvis.

Complications. The major delayed complications of therapy include second malignancies, notably acute nonlymphocyte leukemia and non-Hodgkin's lymphoma. Leukemia may be more likely following MOPP than ABVD, perhaps because the latter contains neither an alkylating agent nor procarbazine, and it is more common after combined modality therapy. Almost all men treated with MOPP are sterile; this effect may be less complete in young women. Hormonal therapy to suppress gonadal function while patients are receiving chemotherapy may minimize this toxic effect. Utilization of sperm banks prior to treatment should be considered and has been successful on occasion.

PERIODIC EVALUATION

Patients who have relapsed following initial radiation therapy can be effectively treated with chemotherapy. In other words, prior radiation therapy is not an adverse prognostic factor in dealing with relapse. Unfortunately, prior chemotherapy is an adverse factor. Most relapses will occur within the first several years. The duration of the initial remission is important, relapse in the first year being particularly unfavorable. Available programs for use in relapse, usually identified under the unfortunate and insensitive title of "salvage programs," can be found by referring to the selected references.

SUMMARY

Hodgkin's disease is a potentially curable malignancy affecting lymphoid tissue. The relative predictability of the disease in involving lymph nodes in contiguous fashion combined with knowledge of the tumoricidal dose of radiation allows delivery of radiation therapy with curative intent in properly staged patients with limited disease. Many patients with advanced disease can be effectively and curatively treated by intermittent combination chemotherapy. Given the serious potential consequences of combined modality treatment, this approach can be advised only selectively now.

REFERENCES

DeVita VT, Simon RM, Hubbard SM, et al: Curability of advanced Hodgkin's disease with chemotherapy. Ann Intern Med 92:587–595, 1980.

Hoppe RT: Stage I-II Hodgkin's disease: current therapeutic options and recommendations. Blood 62:32–36, 1983.

Santoro A, Bonadonna G, Bonfante V, et al: Alternating drug combinations in the treatment of advanced Hodgkin's disease. N Engl J Med 306:770–775, 1982.

Symposium on Contemporary Issues in Hodgkin's Disease: Biology, staging and treatment. Cancer Treat Rep 66:601–1071, 1982.

White WL: Hodgkin's disease and the non-Hodgkin's malignant lymphomas. *In* Fairbanks VF (ed): Current Hematology, Vol 1. John Wiley and Son, New York, 1981, pp 398–450.

20 · NON-HODGKIN'S LYMPHOMAS

William L. White
MAYO CLINIC AND MAYO FOUNDATION

The non-Hodgkin's lymphomas are much more diverse and less predictable than is Hodgkin's disease. Radiation therapy can be effective in patients with localized disease, but in general chemotherapy plays a bigger role in management. Patients with low-grade lymphomas are especially challenging; a number of them do well in spite of us. Those with lymphomas of unfavorable prognosis present a challenge in a different way: we simply need to do better. Chemotherapy programs for these patients are very complex and potentially quite dangerous; they should be administered carefully relative to patient characteristics, physician familiarity, and availability of supporting services.

DEFINITION AND DIAGNOSTIC CRITERIA

The term "non-Hodgkin's lymphoma" (NHL) serves to distinguish these lymphoid malignancies from Hodgkin's disease, but that is where the usefulness of this term ends. These disorders range from unfavorable, aggressive tumors, potentially curable, to relatively indolent tumors, likely incurable, characterized by long survival despite minimal or no therapy.

PATHOLOGY

A consensus classification (known as the "working formulation") is now being used by hematopathologists in an effort to allow us all to speak the same language, especially important for investigational purposes, but a modified Rappaport classification based on growth pattern (nodular or follicular versus diffuse) and cell composition (small, large, or mixed populations of lymphocytes) serves us well in day-to-day practice. Nodular lymphomas are generally favorable; diffuse lymphomas are unfavorable with the exception of diffuse, well-differentiated lymphocytic lymphomas. A judgment about the histologic type is the starting point for staging and treatment decisions.

While most non-Hodgkin's lymphomas are B cell tumors, perhaps 10% are of T cell immunotype. These disorders can be broadly grouped into (1) cutaneous T cell lymphomas (mycosis fungoides, Sézary syndrome), (2) peripheral T cell lymphomas, (3) lymphoblastic lymphomas, and (4) HTLV-associated leukemia/lymphoma.

CLINICAL ASPECTS

Painless lymphadenopathy is the most common presenting sign; secondary manifestations related to sites of lymph node enlargement include superior vena caval obstruction, pleural effusions, back pain, obstructive uropathy, neurologic signs secondary to spinal cord compression, and obstructive lymphedema of the lower extremity due to pelvic lymphadenopathy. Furthermore, extralymphatic involvement is seen much more often than in Hodgkin's disease, particularly among the unfavorable lymphomas, and common sites include skin, bone, gastrointestinal tract, thyroid, and testes.

The Ann Arbor staging system (see Chapter 19) is commonly used, but the implications of the stages for non-Hodgkin's lymphomas are not as clearly defined as in Hodgkin's disease. The majority of patients with the non-Hodgkin's lymphomas have advanced disease at presentation.

The bone marrow is often positive in the lymphocytic (non-large-cell) lymphomas.

Lymphangiography (LAG) is an accurate procedure in the assessment of opacified nodes, but a problem in the nodular lymphomas is that mesenteric nodes, which are not opacified by LAG, are commonly involved; a negative LAG in that setting is not very reassuring. I favor computed tomography (CT) as the major infradiaphragmatic staging method. If CT is positive, then this information is helpful in future assessment of progression of disease or response to therapy. If CT is negative, then LAG can be considered, depending on the circumstances and recognizing its limitations.

Because of evidence indicating nonlocalized disease in most patients, the staging laparotomy is uncommonly a consideration in NHLs. Exploratory (as distinguished from "staging") laparotomy is not so uncommon in our experience because we see a number of patients, often elderly, whose primary diagnosis is established in this way; in such circumstances removal of the spleen is of doubtful benefit, and it should not even be considered if in the surgeon's judgment there is concern that postoperative convalescence would be complicated as a result. Open biopsies of the liver, on the other hand, can be obtained easily and are sometimes useful.

The cutaneous T cell lymphomas consist, classically, of mycosis fungoides and Sézary syndrome, and both are uncommon malignancies.The initial cutaneous lesions may be clinically and histologically nonspecific, and a number of years might pass before a firm diagnosis is established. Staging classifications and prognosis relate to the type of skin lesion (limited or generalized plaques, cutaneous tumors, generalized erythroderma), and whether there is involvement of peripheral blood, lymph nodes, and viscera.

MANAGEMENT

PLAN

Treatment options for NHLs consist of radiation and chemotherapy, but the relative predictability of Hodgkin's, which lends itself to effective management by radiation, is not a characteristic of the NHLs.

TREATMENT

Patients with stage I diffuse large-cell lymphomas who have radiosensitive disease can be cured by the radiation oncologist. Patients with high-grade undifferentiated lymphomas should not be included here. An important stumbling block in diffuse large-cell lympho-

mas is the lack of a predictable dose-response curve for radiation therapy. There are also observations in support of multi-agent chemotherapy for such patients with encouraging response rates, and the entire approach to staging and therapy in this situation may have to be reevaluated if additional experience is confirmatory.

Follicular Lymphomas. There is serious doubt that follicular lymphomas are ever localized. Continued application of sophisticated laboratory technology, such as flow cytometry, in association with clinical correlations will ultimately prove that they are not, I believe. In the meantime, it is said that perhaps 10% of these patients do have localized disease and do well following radiotherapy. Observations of long-term response must be tempered by a knowledge of the natural history of this disease in selected patients in whom initial treatment is deferred in spite of the presence of extensive involvement (see below).

Some patients with a favorable NHL histologic type have indolent disease and may show signs of spontaneous regression without therapy. Not only may they regress spontaneously, they may also transform to more aggressive histologic types, usually into the diffuse large-cell lymphomas. Available information suggests that immediate versus deferred therapy has no influence on subsequent transformation, but this has not been tested prospectively. Among patients with low-grade lymphomas given no initial therapy, the median time to treatment has been on the order of one to three years based on limited data. Actuarial survival rates of approximately 80% have been reported at three and five years in different studies. In asymptomatic patients who have no indication of organ compromise, the patient is entitled to a full discussion of the pros and cons of deferred versus immediate therapy; my own choice is to defer and to observe at not more than three-month intervals in the first year, gradually extending the interval thereafter if there is continuing stability.

Patients. Patients with favorable nodular lymphomas who require therapy have been successfully treated with single drugs, combination chemotherapy, aggressive radiation therapy, and combined modality programs. No convincing evidence exists to indicate that aggressive therapy is better. Oral chlorambucil (Leukeran) may be given as a single agent. I have usually used intermittent intravenous cyclophosphamide (Cytoxan) in combination with oral prednisone. Another well-known combination is the CVP regimen consisting of Cytoxan, vincristine (Oncovin), and prednisone. Median survival of responding patients is in excess of five years, but a pattern of continuous late recurrences is typical.

Small Lymphocytic Lymphomas. Patients with diffuse well-differentiated (small lymphocytic) lymphomas have disorders very much like chronic lymphocytic leukemia with a similar prognosis. These patients, too, often do not require immediate therapy. In day-to-day practice I usually treat these patients initially with nonaggressive programs when there is evidence of progressive or symptomatic disease or a likelihood of complications.

Diffuse Large-Cell, Mixed, or Undifferentiated Lymphomas. In contrast to patients with low-grade lymphomas, patients with stages II to IV unfavorable prognosis lymphomas, e.g., diffuse large-cell, mixed, or undifferentiated histologic types, require aggressive chemotherapy. It may seem a paradox that patients with unfavorable disease may in fact experience prolonged disease-free survival, but successful induction of a complete remission, documented by careful restaging, clearly is associated with cure in some patients, perhaps 20% to 30%. Nonetheless, somewhere between 20% and 60% of patients do not achieve complete remission, and their outlook is poor.

Numerous combination chemotherapy programs have been used with complete response rates varying from 40% to as high as 80%. Programs have consisted of nitrogen mustard or Cytoxan in combination with vincristine, procarbazine, and prednisone (MOPP, COPP); CVP drugs in combination with Adriamycin (CHOP, COPA), bleomycin (CPOB, COPB), or both (BACOP, CHOP-bleo) and all five plus procarbazine (CAP-BOP, COP-BLAM); and several high- and low-dose methotrexate programs (M-BACOD, m-BACOD, COMLA, Pro-MACE). Methotrexate-based programs demand attention to such details as renal function, hydration, third-space collections, and urinary alkalinization. Some programs are identically composed but differ in dosage and/or schedule of administration of medications. It is not possible to suggest an optimal regimen to be used in clinical practice. There are too many variables to be taken into account including the characteristics of the patients themselves, such as age and capacity to tolerate aggressive therapy, the familiarity of the physician with these complex and potentially very toxic programs, and the nature and expertise of the supporting services. As a group, these patients are older, bone marrow reserve is diminished relative to younger patients, and other complicating medical illnesses are more frequent.

Cutaneous T-Cell Lymphomas. The cutaneous T cell lymphomas are approached differently. There are four treatment modalities: (1) topical nitrogen mustard; (2) PUVA (photochemotherapy with psoralen and ultraviolet A light); (3) electron beam radiation; and (4) chemotherapy. Topical therapy is most useful in early cutaneous disease. PUVA therapy has been more helpful in patients with plaque disease as opposed to those with tumor stage or generalized erythroderma. The advantage of electron beam therapy is its superficial penetration. The likelihood of attaining complete remission is related to the extent of skin involvement and is about 95% in patients with limited plaque disease. A number of chemotherapy agents are active in the cutaneous T cell lymphomas, including chlorambucil, cyclophosphamide, methotrexate, doxorubicin, and bleomycin. A higher response rate for combination chemotherapy programs has not yet clearly translated into better long-term results. Thus far, the most appropriate therapy relative to stage has not been defined, but once visceral involvement is evident, late in the evolution of the disease, the median survival is approximately one year.

Complications. Complications are similar to those described for Hodgkin's disease.

REFERENCES

Horning SJ, Rosenberg SA: The natural history of initially untreated low-grade non-Hodgkin's lymphomas. N Engl J Med 311:1471–1475, 1984.

Johnson GJ: Hodgkin's disease and non-Hodgkin's lymphoma. *In* Fairbanks VF (ed): Current Hematology, Vol 2. John Wiley and Son, New York, 1982, pp 51–91.

Miller TP, Jones SE: Initial chemotherapy for clinically localized lymphomas of unfavorable histology. Blood 62:413–418, 1983.

White WL: Hodgkin's disease and the non-Hodgkin's malignant lymphomas. *In* Fairbanks VF (ed): Current Hematology, Vol 1. John Wiley and Son, New York, 1981, pp 398–450.

Winkler CF, Bunn PA Jr: Cutaneous T-cell lymphoma: a review. CRC Crit Rev Oncol Hematol 1:49–92, 1983.

21 · MULTIPLE MYELOMA AND RELATED DISORDERS

Robert L. Longmire
SCRIPPS CLINIC AND RESEARCH FOUNDATION

DEFINITION AND DIAGNOSTIC CRITERIA

Plasmacytic myeloma is a malignancy of plasma cells producing a detectable serum or urine abnormality in nearly all cases. Diagnosis depends on combinations of findings, including tissue plasmacytomas, bone marrow plasmacytosis, monoclonal serum proteins greater than 3.5 gm for IgG or 2.0 gm for IgA, light-chain excretion on urine protein electrophoresis, lytic bone lesions, anemia, hypercalcemia, and renal insufficiency.

Other monoclonal gammopathies in addition to plasmacytic myeloma include IgM disorders and benign monoclonal gammopathies (BMG). Malignant lymphomas make up one third of these cases of monoclonal gammopathies with much less frequent occurrence in chronic lymphocytic leukemia, extramedullary plasmacytoma, and indeterminant causes. The disease of Waldenström's macroglobulinemia also makes up one third of the monoclonal gammopathies; this disease is characterized by lymph node and marrow infiltrations and characteristic plasmacytoid lymphocytes. Hyperviscosity syndrome is seen most commonly in this disorder.

Benign monoclonal gammopathies or monoclonal gammopathies of undetermined significance should not be treated but rather followed periodically. Approximately 10% will progress to symptomatic disease. Follow-up at three-month intervals with quantitative immunoglobulins or serum protein electrophoresis for at least one to two years is required before determining that the disease is not progressive.

PATHOPHYSIOLOGY

The disease course varies from indolent to plasma cell leukemia with IgG kappa disease survival being longer than with other heavy- and light-chain types. The major survival determinant is total tumor burden (disease stage); this is directly proportional to the quantity of M-protein in serum or urine. Serial determination of M-protein is the best indicator of tumor burden and treatment efficacy.

Myeloma is quantifiable using a staging system of I (lowest tumor burden), II, or III (highest tumor burden). These stages are based on determinations of hemoglobin, calcium, and protein quantities and are of prognostic importance. Because renal disease may be independent of tumor mass, stages are further classified as A or B depending on the creatinine of less or greater than 2.0 mg/dl.

CLINICAL ASPECTS

Myeloma is usually symptomatic at the time of diagnosis. The disease is suspect in patients over the age of 50 who present with bone pain and with the laboratory findings of anemia, hyperproteinemia, hypercalcemia, proteinuria, azotemia, and lytic bone lesions. Overt disease should be established by a combination of tests including bone marrow examination and serum and urine electrophoresis. Additional evidence may be gained with quantitative immunoglobulins, immunoelectrophoresis, chemistry determinations for calcium, kidney function, and x-ray examination of bone. Because most lesions are purely lytic, a bone scan is of little help and should be normal.

MANAGEMENT

Myeloma is a systemic, bone marrow disorder requiring systemic therapy. Chemotherapy is the treatment of choice; radiation therapy may be useful for palliating painful bone lesions but is not indicated for primary therapy.

PLAN

Myeloma is not a curable disease but a treatable disease with remissions expected in approximately 50% of cases for periods of time varying from one to five years.

NONPHARMACOLOGIC MEASURES

Radiation therapy is useful for palliating painful bone lesions, but caution must be observed that doses not be excessive to cause myelosuppression of the degree that drug therapy cannot be employed.

DRUG THERAPY

Chemotherapy should be withheld in selected patients with stage IA, which encompasses solitary bone plasmacytoma and "indolent" or "smoldering" myeloma. A solitary bone lesion can be treated with radiation to the area. Indolent and smoldering myeloma are asymptomatic, may show depression of normal serum immunoglobulins, and have small amounts of urinary light-chains, but have no anemia, azotemia, hypercalcemia, or recurrent infections. Smoldering myeloma has no lytic bone lesions; indolent myeloma may have up to three. Follow-ups to detect progressive disease are required in all three myeloma variants.

Melphalan and prednisone (MP) have been the standard therapy agents for myeloma. More recently, combination therapies have shown superiority and may improve remission rates and duration of survival. More intensive regimens using vincristine, cyclophosphamide, doxorubicin, and prednisone (VCAP) or substituting BCNU (VBAP) or melphalan (VMCP) have been reported to increase the response rates to greater than 60%, although an overall survival advantage has not been demonstrated. Failure of these programs indicates a need for entrance into investigative protocols with agents such as interferons, infusion chemotherapy, or experimental drugs.

Adverse Effects. Chemotherapy may contribute to anemia, thrombocytopenia, infections, acute leukemia, and adverse prednisone effects such as overt diabetes, osteoporosis, congestive heart failure (CHF), mental changes, muscle weakness, and other catabolic events. Doxorubicin myocardiopathy is a threat requiring monitoring by cardiac ejection studies to prevent intractable CHF.

Outpatient treatment is to be stressed, but hospital care for complications may be necessary. Severe hypercalcemia, infections with leukopenia and pulmonary or meningeal disease, intractable pain, hyperviscosity, acute renal failure, and fractures or incipient fractures of weight-bearing bones may require specific hospital therapy. Continued ambulation and maintenance of an anabolic state, whenever possible, is vital to preserve function and aid in preventing hypercalcemia.

COMPLICATIONS OF MYELOMA

Complications of myeloma are usually reversible by control of total tumor burden; their early recognition and treatment prevents morbidity and mortality. Hypercalcemia, in oriented patients, may be treated at home with oral hydration, salt tablets, and furosemide to increase calciuria. Prednisone or indomethacin decreases bone resorption by blocking osteoclast activating factor. Hyperviscosity may cause bleeding diathesis, retinopathies, hypervolemia, or neurologic signs and symptoms. Prompt plasmapheresis of 4 to 6 units of plasma is most effective with IgM (80% intravascular), but is helpful in IgA polymerization and IgG_3 aggregation. Acute renal failure, usually seen at diagnosis or disease progression, requires dialysis if the myeloma seems amenable to treatment and palliation. Renal failure, with myeloma control, needs chronic dialysis. Orthopedic intervention to preserve weight-bearing is often necessary in advanced lytic cases; early ambulation helps avoid contributing to hyerpcalcemia. Hyperuricemia, present in 50% of diagnosed patients, contributes to acute renal failure. Allopurinol, plus alkalizing urine with bicarbonate, may forestall dialysis.

Immune dysfunction, marrow infiltration, and chemotherapy all contribute to infections being the leading cause of death in myeloma. Patients are particularly vulnerable to the meningococcus and pneumococcus. Another complication of therapy is the recognition of acute leukemia occurring after alkylator therapy with an incidence up to 20% at 48 months.

PERIODIC EVALUATION

Criteria of response to chemotherapy are greater than 50% (Myeloma Task Force) or 75% (Southwest Oncology Group) reduction in serum or urine protein. Improvement is indirectly indicated by a rise in hemoglobin and normalization of normal immunoglobulins and decreasing bone marrow plasma cells. Approximately 45% of patients reach a plateau or stable phase with therapy. At this time, survival may be prolonged without active therapy until the abnormal protein begins to rise. During this time, follow-up should be no longer than six-week intervals with blood counts and determinations of the offending protein. The importance of serially determining the quantitative protein is the single superior guide to tumor burden. Effective therapy and patient status must be stressed. Chemotherapy should not be used in indolent smoldering and plateau myeloma or with solitary plasmacytoma because of the dangers of infections and bleeding.

PATIENT COMPLIANCE

To obtain maximum compliance, patients and their families should be educated to prognosis, treatment, side effects of treatment, complications, and need for adequate nutrition and ambulation.

REFERENCES

Alexanian R: Localized and indont myeloma. Blood 56:521–525, 1980.

Bergsagel DE, Rider WD: Cancer, Principles and Practice. J.B. Lippincott Co, Philadelphia, 1982.

Kyle RA, Greipp PR: Smoldering multiple myeloma. N Engl J Med 302:1347–1349, 1980.

Salmon SE, Wampler SB: Multiple myeloma: quantitative staging and assessment of response with a programmable pocket calculator. Blood 49:378–389, 1977.

Salmon SE, Haut H, Bonnet JD, et al: Alternating combination chemotherapy and levamisole improves survival in multiple myeloma: a Southwest Oncology Group study. J Clin Oncol 1:453–461, 1983.

22 · CANCER OF THE LUNG

James K. Weick
CLEVELAND CLINIC FOUNDATION

DEFINITION AND DIAGNOSTIC CRITERIA

Lung cancer remains the number one cause of cancer deaths in the United States; it is the leading cause of cancer deaths in males and is expected to replace breast cancer as the leading cause of cancer deaths in the female. Unlike many cancers that have remained constant or decreased slightly in recent years, death rates due to lung cancer continue to increase dramatically, especially in females. The new cases of lung cancer in 1986 will be 149,000 with 130,000 deaths in this population. This represents 25% of all cancer deaths and 5% of all deaths in the country regardless of cause.

Unfortunately, lung cancer is usually diagnosed in an advanced stage, creating a low cure rate. Spread to regional lymph nodes or distant metastasis is seen in approximately 70% of all patients so that the five-year survival rate in the aggregate is only 10% to 15%.

There is overwhelming evidence that tobacco smoking is the cause of 30% to 40% of all deaths from cancer. Epidemiologic studies have demonstrated conclusively a consistent association between smoking and lung cancer; analyses of cigarette smoke reveal many mitogens and carcinogens that may be absorbed, be metabolized, and cause genetic change. Recent studies have been designed to examine the possible association of lung cancer with exposure to the cigarette smoking of others (passive or involuntary smoking). This evidence at the present time is very suggestive but not conclusive.

PATHOPHYSIOLOGY

The pathologic classification most widely accepted for lung cancer is that used by the World Health Organization. In order of prevalence, four major pathologic types account for more than 90% of all lung cancer: squamous (epidermoid) carcinoma and adenocarcinoma are the most frequent cell types (30% each) of cases followed by large-cell undifferentiated carcinoma (15%) and small-cell undifferentiated carcinoma (25%).

Epidermoid cancer is more common in males and is almost exclusively a smoker's disease. This tumor is usually found centrally in the chest and this location may contribute to early symptoms, possible earlier detection, and a higher five-year survival rate.

Adenocarcinoma is increasing in frequency especially among women. Unlike the central location of the epidermoid tumor, the adenocarcinoma is more often peripheral and tends to present with either regional or metastatic spread. Such patients may present with brain, bone, or liver metastases.

The least common cell type is a large-cell undifferentiated lung cancer. Like the adenocarcinoma, the large-cell tumor is peripherally diagnosed in 60% of cases and may be indistinguishable from an adenocarcinoma with the exception that the primary tumor is often larger in size than the adenocarcinoma.

The above three types of tumors constitute what is commonly referred to as non-small-cell bronchogenic carcinoma. Other rarer primary lung tumors include carcinoid tumor, sarcomas, and lymphomas.

Small-cell undifferentiated (oat cell) carcinoma behaves quite differently from the aforementioned tumors. Oat cell tumors are usually located in the submucosa and as such may have a lower diagnostic yield on sputum cytologic examination than the epidermoid tumor. The small-cell cancer is usually central in its location with a very rare occurrence in the periphery. Clinical features are usually of short duration because of the rapid growth rate and the frequent metastatic nature of this tumor. It is this early metastatic potential and rapid growth rate that gives small-cell cancer the poorest prognosis of all cell types of bronchogenic tumors. This tumor is also the cell type most often associated with ectopic hormone production (ACTH, ADH) and associated paraneoplastic syndromes.

CLINICAL ASPECTS

Ongoing trials are examining the usefulness of screening methods for detecting early stage lung cancer by the use of periodic chest films and sputum cytologic examination in high-risk individuals, namely middle-aged persons who have been chronic cigarette smokers. To date, it has been established that such measures can detect presymptomatic early tumors, especially the squamous cell variety, and that the resectability is improved over the control subjects who were tested less intensively. There are no conclusions, however, that lung cancer mortality has been reduced as a consequence of these screens, but the trials continue with further observation. Abnormal radiographs are more likely to be seen in early peripheral lesions than in the more central tumors of squamous and small-cell varieties. There are no biochemical markers that have been shown to be effective for early detection.

The signs and symptoms of localized bronchogenic cancer include cough, sputum production, shortness of breath, wheezing, and hemoptysis.

Signs and symptoms of more advanced disease might include hoarseness, chest pain, difficulty swallowing, and pericardial effusion, all indicating invasion of the mediastinum or chest wall. Less commonly, the initial symptoms may be those suggesting metastatic involvement of the brain, bones, or liver.

The most common diagnostic tool for establishing histologic type of lung cancer is the fiberoptic bronchoscope, which will establish diagnosis in a majority of patients either through direct biopsy, brush biopsy, or aspiration cytology. In more peripheral lesions, a percutaneous transthoracic needle aspiration or biopsy done under fluoroscopic or CT guidance has been reported to be effective in between 50% and 80% of cases. In those instances in which neither of these measures yields diagnostic information, a mediastinoscopy and/or exploratory thoracotomy may be required.

A major advance in selecting treatment options was adopted when the American Joint Commission established a staging classification for lung cancer based upon the size of the primary tumor (T), the involvement of the regional lymph nodes (N), and the presence or absence of distant metastases (M). The staging is based on physical examinations, roentgenograms, and biopsies and permits standardized communications about cancer patients as well as being useful in determining prognosis and treatment planning strategies. The evaluation of the primary tumor (T) is usually made by the chest roentgenogram, although tomograms and CT scans may also be useful. The most favorable lesions are thus <3 cm in diameter (T1) contrasted with the T3 tumor, which is defined as a tumor extending into an adjacent structure such as the chest wall, diaphragm, or mediastinum; a T2 tumor is intermediate in severity with a diameter >3 cm. Hilar and mediastinal lymph nodes are best detected either through roentgenograms or more accurately with a CT scan. Mediastinoscopy, performed through a small suprasternal incision, is usually reserved for patients in whom a thoracotomy is being considered or for whom diagnostic tissue may be required.

The determination of metastatic lesions at the time of diagnosis is not recommended for all asymptomatic patients with non-small-cell cancer. The routine application of brain and bone scans, liver scans, and abdominal CT scans may be expected to give positive results in fewer than 10% of cases.

The TNM staging system is of most utility for staging non-small-cell cancer. As earlier stated, small-cell lung cancer is nearly always metastatic at its presentation and systemic therapy is therefore indicated in the majority of these cases. Such metastatic disease is usually seen in the head, the liver, or the bone in percentages varying from 10% to 30% of cases. Because of this high incidence, it is generally recommended that radiographic methods be used for a baseline determination of organ involvement using CT scans of the head and abdomen as well as a radionuclide bone scan and a bone marrow aspiration and biopsy.

In addition to the TNM classification, inoperable lung cancer is classified as either limited or extensive disease. In this classification, limited stage refers to lesions confined to a single hemithorax and regional nodes that may be treated in a single radiation therapy port. All other disease is classified as extensive.

When surgery is contemplated, the assessment of pulmonary function is of critical importance. A predicted postoperative forced expiratory volume (FEV_1) of at least 800 cc is required before a pneumonectomy can be safely performed. Chronic hypercapnea due to intrinsic lung disease is usually a relative contraindication for any lung resection.

MANAGEMENT

PLAN

The goals of all therapy in lung cancer should be to eradicate the tumor through surgery, if possible, or to palliate the tumor through radiation therapy and chemotherapy when indicated. Hospitalization is required if surgical therapy is being contemplated. Unless the performance status of a patient dictates that a hospitalization is necessary, preoperative assessment including bronchoscopy and even mediastinoscopy may be performed in the outpatient department. It may be expected that an uncomplicated surgical procedure should require no more than seven days' hospitalization with any subsequent therapy being performed in the outpatient department, including chemotherapy and radiation therapy. The exception to this statement is the use of medication usually requiring hospitalization such as *cis*-platinum.

NONPHARMACOLOGIC MEASURES

Despite advances in both chemotherapy and radiation therapy, the treatment of choice for non-small-cell lung cancer remains surgical resection unless there is a contraindication to such proposed surgery.

The type of operation to be performed should be determined by the diagnostic measures mentioned in preceding sections. The general goal is to resect all tumor and preserve as much normal lung function as possible. The preferred operation generally is a lobectomy or a segmental resection. A pneumonectomy is generally reserved for extensive disease that is resectable and/or very central lesions.

In tumors that are considered to be stage I cancer (T1N0, T2N0, or T1N1), the five-year survival from surgery alone may be as high as 70%. Surgical treatment is less effective in those cases that are pathologic stage II (T2N1), in which the survival is estimated to be approximately 35%. As expected, stage III disease carries a worse prognosis with five-year survival between 10% and 15%. This stage includes patients with distant metastases, mediastinal lymph node metastases, and any primary tumor that is T3 in size.

As in many solid tumors being investigated at the present time, the role of adjuvant or preventive therapy is not established for lung cancer. In cases in which surgical resection has been accomplished, many patients will relapse and die within two years of the "curative" operation. The rationale for preventive or adjuvant therapy is to kill micrometastases at a time when the tumor might be expected to be more susceptible to such therapy.

Postoperative irradiation is frequently used in those persons who are found to have hilar or mediastinal lymph node involvement at the time of surgery. Randomized trials comparing radiation with no further therapy are lacking; nonrandomized trials do suggest that survival is improved with postoperative radiation in those patients with positive mediastinal lymph nodes.

The treatment of patients with regional unresectable stage III non-small-cell lung cancer is even more controversial, i.e., should patients receive only radiation or should they receive radiation plus chemotherapy or even chemotherapy alone. To date, no combination of chemotherapeutic agents has been found to be clearly effective in this group of persons. We therefore recommend that radiation be used or that the patient be entered on a clinical protocol that may help in the future to establish which of these methods of therapy is to be preferred.

The above considerations have largely been for cases of non-small-cell lung cancer (adenocarcinoma, squamous carcinoma, and large-cell carcinoma) and do not pertain to small-cell or oat cell cancer. Because the majority of these tumors have undergone distant metastases at the time of diagnosis, neither surgery nor primary radiation therapy is the treatment of choice. Rather, initial chemotherapy is indicated and will be discussed later. Despite surgery and radiation efforts for the non-small-cell tumors, recurrence in distant sites is the usual failure in operated patients and it is these recurrences that require systemic treatment.

Most patients with non-small-cell lung cancer present either with "limited" stage III disease (confined to the thorax) or with "extensive" stage III disease (metastatic). The average survival for such patients undergoing radiation therapy is less than one year with an occasional survival to five years. The optimal dose and schedule for the radiation of non-small-cell tumors has not been established. It is generally agreed that doses between 50 Gy and 60 Gy are required for curative treatment. Many physicians are engaged in investigation at the present time to determine whether chemotherapy offers an advantage to established radiation practices in limited unresectable non-small-cell disease.

The primary treatment of small-cell bronchogenic carcinoma differs markedly from the non-small-cell tumor mentioned above. Fewer than 1% of all patients operated on for small-cell cancer can be expected to survive five years. In the unusual instance in which there is a peripheral solitary pulmonary nodule of small-cell histologic type, there may be expected a five-year survival approaching 35% following surgery only.

Radiation therapy has a definite role in the management of small-cell cancer when used in conjunction with chemotherapy. Although very effective chemotherapy is available for limited disease, initial treatment failures frequently occur in the chest whether this area has been irradiated or not. This may be due to inadequate doses of radiation or using an inadequate radiation field to sterilize foci of residual tumors. Conflicting reports exist, but the best long-term survival at present is reported from investigators who use effective chemotherapy together with concomitant radiation therapy.

DRUG THERAPY

Because the important prognostic features in unresectable lung cancer are the stage of disease and performance status, and because the majority of lung cancers are not operable at the time of diagnosis, there is an obvious need for improved systemic therapy. Chemotherapy agents that have shown activity as single agents in non-small-cell cancer include doxorubicin, mitomycin, vinca alkaloids, cyclophosphamide, etoposide, and cisplatin. Used singly, these agents might be expected to be effective in 10% to 30% of cases but only for a very short time. More recently, these agents have been combined in numerous trials throughout the country. Although the survival benefit is lacking to prove the superiority of combination programs over single agents, preliminary reports suggest that the response rates are on the order of 30% to 50%, with average response durations between five and ten months and improved survival as high as two years for advanced metastatic disease. Because of the uncertainty as to which is the better regimen, if in fact any combination regimen is to be favored, we attempt to place patients on comparative protocols. In those instances in which patients prefer not to be treated on protocol, we generally use outpatient chemotherapy with vinblastine and mitomycin, a remarkably well tolerated regimen, and reserve regimens using platinum compounds and anthracyclines for treatment failures with the first regimen. Other common programs nationally include the inpatient treatment monthly using vinblastine or vindesine together with platinum or the CAP regimen, which uses intravenous cyclophosphamide, Adriamycin, and platinum. Comparison trials of these regimens are currently under investigation and will require several more years before definitive statements can be made.

The drug therapy of small-cell lung cancer is more firmly established than it is for non-small-cell tumors. The medications active against small-cell lung cancer are very similar to those of non-small-cell cancer with the addition of methotrexate, nitrogen mustards, and nitrosourea compounds. As single agents, these compounds are effective in 30% to 40% of all cases. Combination chemotherapy is superior to single-agent therapy and shows definite improvement in response rates as well as long-term survivors in both limited and extensive disease. The most common combination of agents employed for the outpatient treatment of small-cell lung cancer is Cytoxan, Adriamycin, and vincristine. Equally beneficial results have been noted using a different combination employing Cytoxan, methotrexate, and CCNU or Cytoxan, Adriamycin, and etoposide.

In addition to the chemotherapeutic approach to small-cell lung cancer, there is a role for radiation therapy, especially to the brain. There are sufficient data to show that the relapse rate in the brain is significantly decreased when 30 Gy is delivered over two weeks. There is no evidence, however, that survival is changed whether the radiation is given in a preventive fashion or when cranial metastases appear. It has recently been reported that local recurrence in the chest cavity is a significant problem in those persons who have responded to chemotherapy, and for this reason investigations are underway to administer chest radiation to those persons who have previously responded to chemotherapy. In either small-cell or non-small-cell tumors, many investigators will continue therapy for at least two years in responding patients. This has been an empiric determination and is not based on sound experimental data.

Other approaches to the treatment of lung cancer involve the use of monoclonal antibodies, reinduction, or intensification chemotherapy; all of these are attempts to kill any cells resistant to the primary therapy.

The complications of chemotherapy agents for the management of lung cancer are few and are generally expected to be the acute toxic effects seen with the use of these powerful agents. Additionally, long-term toxic effects are seen especially with Adriamycin in which there may be dose-limiting cardiotoxicity for this valuable agent. The remainder of the side effects are very predictable and are treated in greater detail by Dr. Kardinal in Chapter 31.

PATIENT INFORMATION AND EDUCATION

It is the obligation of any treating physician for neoplastic disease to obtain informed consent before embarking on therapy protocols, be it chemotherapy, radiation, or surgery. We supply oral summaries of all planned treatments to the patients and their families for consideration as well as presenting options of therapy. As important as the physical treatment of lung cancer is the psychological treatment. Of value to me in the management of these complications are nurse clinicians, social workers, and members of the Department of Psychiatry who are available to counsel and console. Regular weekly meetings are held for both inpatient and outpatient family members and patients for information of educational meetings.

PERIODIC EVALUATION

In patients who are operated on for cure, we recommend follow-up visits with chest films at three-month intervals for the first two years followed by semiannual visits for two years and annual visits thereafter. The follow-up visits for patients on active therapy for either chemotherapy or radiation therapy will vary according to the frequency of treatments but are generally arranged at three- to four-week intervals. All patients undergoing chemotherapy receive blood counts before each treatment. Depending on the expected toxicities of the chemotherapy agents, other chemistry tests may be required.

PATIENT COMPLIANCE

Generally speaking, the patient with advanced malignancy is a very motivated patient trying to get better and will be totally in compliance so long as he or she is fully aware of expected toxicities or side effects and believes that he or she has a reasonable chance for improvement. The patient with advanced disease who is failing available treatment becomes a more difficult problem; this does not imply poor patient compliance but rather a necessary reassessment from time to time as to the expected goals of such treatments.

PREVENTIVE MEASURES

In no other malignancy is prevention more possible. There can be no doubt that the primary prevention of lung cancer is through control of cigarette smoking.

SOCIOECONOMIC ASPECTS OF MANAGEMENT

It is estimated that the cost of cigarette smoking annually is in excess of $80 billion. This represents $27 billion spent on cigarettes and $55 to $60 billion for medical care costs and activity losses directly attributable to smoking-induced disease. A reduction in lung cancer can be achieved through educational programs aimed at restricting the promotion of cigarettes. Until such measures are effective in reducing tobacco abuse, lung cancer will remain the most lethal neoplasm in the United States.

REFERENCES

Bunn PA Jr: Lung cancer: the current approach to diagnosis, staging and treatment. Sieber and McIntyre, Inc, Chicago, 1983.
Eiseman B, Robinson WA, Steele G Jr: Follow-up of the Cancer Patient. Thieme-Stratton Inc, New York, 1982.
Livingston RB: Small cell carcinoma of the lung. Blood 56:575–584, 1980.
Loeb LA, Ernster VL, Warner KE, et al: Smoking and lung cancer: An overview. Cancer Res 44:5940–5958, 1984.
Van Houtte P, Salazar OM, Henry J: Radiotherapy in non-small cell lung cancer: recent progress and future perspectives. Eur J Cancer Clin Oncol 20:997–1006, 1984.

23 · TUMORS OF THE INTESTINAL TRACT— UPPER GI TRACT, CARCINOID SYNDROME, AND LOWER GI TRACT

*Kirk V. Shepard**
*Ronald M. Bukowski**
James W. Manier†
*CLEVELAND CLINIC FOUNDATION
†LOVELACE MEDICAL CENTER

Esophageal Cancer

DEFINITION AND DIAGNOSTIC CRITERIA

Factors that appear to play an etiologic role in the development of esophageal cancer are cigarette smoking and alcohol abuse. Approximately one third of patients with achalasia or lye strictures will subsequently develop esophageal cancer after a latency period sometimes as long as 30 to 35 years. Patients with a Barrett's esophagus or Plummer-Vinson syndrome also have an increased incidence of carcinoma of the esophagus.

PATHOPHYSIOLOGY

Ninety-eight per cent of esophageal cancers are squamous cell carcinomas that occur most commonly in the lower third of the esophagus, whereas 2% of the cancers are adenocarcinomas that usually occur at the gastroesophageal junction. Esophageal cancer most frequently occurs in the sixth decade of life with a strong male preponderance.

CLINICAL ASPECTS

Dysphagia, particularly for meat and bread, is the most common symptom upon presentation. The most frequent sites of distant metastases in an order of declining frequency are the lymph nodes, lungs, liver, pleura, and bone.

Esophagoscopy will obtain a histologic diagnosis in about 95% of the patients. Panendoscopy (esophagoscopy, bronchoscopy, and an ENT exam) is being performed more frequently to rule out second primary tumors in the upper airways and oral cavity that can be seen in up to 10% of the patients.

MANAGEMENT

PLAN

Short-term goals include proper staging of the tumor and an attempt to resect the cancer if localized to the region of the esophagus. If the tumor is unresectable or metastatic, radiation therapy or chemotherapy should be initiated if indicated. Long-term goals include postoperative follow-up with the surgeon to screen for recurrent cancer. The prevention and management of the possible adverse effects of surgery, radiation therapy, and chemotherapy are also important components of care.

NONPHARMACOLOGIC MEASURES

Fewer than half of the patients have resectable cancer of the esophagus. Although surgical resection still remains the most definitive treatment of cancer of the esophagus, studies directly comparing surgery with radiation therapy are lacking. Radiation therapy can be used with either a palliative or curative intent in the treatment of esophageal cancer. Curative radiation produces five-year survival rates below 10%. Whether combined modality treatment with radiation therapy and surgery is better than either modality alone is currently a question that has not been conclusively answered. If relief of dysphagia is not successful with the above-mentioned therapy, endoscopic dilation or insertion of a stent can sometimes relieve the obstruction in the esophagus. A gastrostomy or jejunostomy can also palliate patients who are unable to swallow, and food and fluids can be placed directly in the stomach or small intestine through a tube.

DRUG THERAPY

There are a number of chemotherapy drugs used to treat esophageal cancer with overall response rates above 20%: cisplatin, bleomycin, mitomycin, and 5-fluorouracil. Doxorubicin, methotrexate, and lomustine have generally shown a lesser degree of activity.

Combination chemotherapy with these drugs has appeared to sometimes increase the response rate and response duration of the treatment when compared with single-agent therapy. At the present time, studies are lacking that establish whether chemotherapy and radiation are better than radiation alone, or whether chemotherapy and surgery are better than surgery alone. Preoperative chemotherapy combined with radiation therapy has been studied, and some patients were found without tumor at surgery. Further studies of combined modality treatment in cancer of the esophagus are warranted.

Adverse Effects of Chemotherapy. Common toxic effects seen with most chemotherapy drugs are nausea, vomiting, diarrhea, alopecia, stomatitis, and myelosuppression, especially leukopenia and thombocytopenia. The severity of the nausea and vomiting, most commonly seen with cisplatin, can be decreased with recently developed antiemetic regimens with drugs such as metoclopramide, phenothiazines, steroids, and diphenhydramine. Alopecia occurs in almost all patients receiving doxorubicin despite attempts to lessen this effect with scalp tourniquets and scalp hypothermia. Care also must be taken to avoid injection of doxorubicin or mitomycin outside the vein because serious extravasation injuries can occur. The cardiomyopathy from chronic doxorubicin use is uncommon if the cumulative dose remains below 450 mg/m^2. Pre- and posthydration with saline and monitoring of renal function are necessary to limit the renal toxicity secondary to cisplatin. Bleomycin does not cause significant myelosuppression, but can cause pulmonary edema and fibrosis at any dose, particularly if the cumulative dose exceeds 250 mg/m^2.

PERIODIC EVALUATION

After "curative intent" surgery, periodic follow-up should be approximately every three months with examination and a complete blood count, serum chemistries, and chest film. During chemotherapy or radiotherapy, the patient's symptoms are recorded and measurable or evaluable lesions are followed by physical exam, x-ray films, or scans to evaluate the effectiveness of the treatment program.

PREVENTIVE MEASURES

In China, where the incidence of esophageal cancer is high, preclinical disease has been discovered by screening methods using cytologic brushing. In this early stage of cancer, a 93% three-year survival rate has been achieved by surgical resection. In the United States, where esophageal cancer is rarer, screening methods would not be cost-effective. Studies are needed to examine screening methods in high-risk patients such as excessive drinkers or smokers, or patients with a history of nontropical sprue, tylosis, lye ingestion, or achalasia.

Stomach Cancer

DEFINITION AND DIAGNOSTIC CRITERIA

Ninety-five per cent of all gastric malignancies are adenocarcinomas. One of the most striking differences between countries in the frequency of a tumor is shown by the persistently high rate of stomach cancer in Japan and Chile as compared with the declining rate of stomach cancer in the United States over the past three decades. The reason for this geographic disparity is unknown, but thought perhaps to be related to differences of the environment, especially of the diet.

PATHOPHYSIOLOGY

Although the vast majority of gastric malignancies are adenocarcinomas, other tumors found in the stomach are lymphomas, leiomyosarcomas, squamous cell carcinomas, adeno-adenoacanthomas, and carcinoids.

CLINICAL ASPECTS

The peak incidence of stomach cancer is in the fifth decade of life. It is twice as common in men as in women. At presentation, most stomach cancers involve the pylorus and antrum of the stomach. Of the four morphologic types of stomach cancer, three fourths of the tumors are ulcerating with the remainder being polypoid, scirrhous, or superficial spreading. Unfortunately, few stomach cancers are confined only in the wall of the stomach; approximately three fourths of the patients have evidence of spread to the lymph nodes, one half to the peritoneum, and one third to the liver. As one might guess, only 5% to 10% of the patients are cured of the stomach cancer by surgery. After a "curative intent" operation, the most common sites of recurrence are local and regional lymph node relapses. Other sites of distant metastases are the lungs, ovaries (Krukenberg's tumor), pleura, bone, genitourinary tract, adrenals, and brain.

To establish the diagnosis, gastroscopy is more reliable than are upper gastrointestinal barium studies. In all patients with a gastric ulcer, at least seven endoscopic biopsies should be obtained. Approximately one fifth of gastric ulcers that appear benign visually by gastroscopy will have malignant pathologic changes. Cytologic examination by a gastroscopic brush should increase the chances of diagnosing malignancy.

MANAGEMENT

PLAN

If stomach cancer is diagnosed at an early stage, curative surgery may be attempted. Short-term goals include postoperative healing and dealing with possible problems secondary to the gastrectomy, such as diarrhea and indigestion. Long-term goals after the operation include possible supplementation with vitamin B_{12} and iron sulfate and appropriate screening for recurrent tumor.

If the stomach cancer is metastatic, the chances for long-term survival are markedly diminished. Goals include psychological and social support from the medical team and the patient's friends and family. Other goals include the initiation of palliative chemotherapy or radiation therapy and the control of the side effects of treatment.

NONPHARMACOLOGIC MEASURES

If the cancer appears to be confined to the region of the stomach by clinical staging, then "curative intent"

surgery is the treatment of choice with either a subtotal gastrectomy or a total gastrectomy. Palliative surgery is not indicated in stomach cancer with distant metastases unless the patient presents with a local obstruction or hemorrhage. Local obstruction from stomach cancer is a later and less common complication than from colorectal cancer where palliative surgery is indicated at diagnosis to prevent obstruction.

Of all patients undergoing curative intent surgery for stomach cancer, approximately 5% to 15% will be alive for five years. If the tumor is confined to the stomach wall, approximately one half of the patients will be alive for five years. If the tumor has spread to the lymph nodes, less than 10% will be alive at five years. Patients with unresectable stomach cancer have a median survival of four to six months.

The use of radiation therapy has been largely limited to a palliative role, particularly in the treatment of patients with locally unresectable stomach cancer.

DRUG THERAPY

The question as to whether adjuvant chemotherapy should be given after the resection of the stomach cancer has not been conclusively answered. Conflicting results of studies concerning the use of adjuvant chemotherapy in stomach cancer do not permit a statement about benefit and it cannot be recommended except in investigational studies.

Patients who present or relapse with metastatic stomach cancer are treated with chemotherapy. The antineoplastic drugs that are the most active in treating stomach cancer are 5-fluorouracil, mitomycin, doxorubicin, nitrosoureas, and, more recently, cisplatin. In most studies, combination chemotherapy for stomach cancer with the drugs mentioned has significantly increased the response rate, response duration, and survival times of the patients when compared with treatment of single-drug chemotherapy.

Adverse Effects of Chemotherapy. The common toxic effects seen with the chemotherapy drugs used for stomach cancer are covered in the preceding section on cancer of the esophagus.

MANAGEMENT OF COMPLICATIONS OF GASTRECTOMY

A *vitamin B_{12} deficiency* can occur after gastrectomy because the stomach produces intrinsic factor, which is necessary for the absorption of vitamin B_{12} in the ileum of the small bowel. Patients who have had a large portion of their stomach resected are therefore treated prophylactically with parenteral vitamin B_{12}. Surgical resection of the stomach can result in a lactose intolerance, or malabsorption of fat. The *dumping syndrome* is a rapid emptying of the gastric remnant into the small bowel. This syndrome causes the patient to feel early satiety, nausea, cramping, diarrhea, lightheadedness, and diaphoresis. The dumping syndrome can be relieved by eating frequent small meals that are restricted in fluids and carbohydrates. Because there is some evidence that the syndrome is mediated by serotonin, cyproheptadine, a serotonin antagonist, has improved the symptoms of some patients when taken before meals. The dose of this drug is usually individualized according of the patient's symptoms. The therapeutic range is 4 to 20 mg/day, with most patients requiring 12 to 16 mg/day.

PREVENTIVE MEASURES

A number of possible risk factors for the development of stomach cancer have been identified: lower socioeconomic class, male sex, colder climate, and blood group A. Polypoid lesions of the stomach consist of adenomas that should be excised because of their tendency for malignant change, and hyperplastic polyps that can be left in place because of their low malignant potential.

An increased frequency of stomach cancer has also been reported in patients with pernicious anemia, achlorhydria, and postgastrectomy states. There also appears to be an increased incidence of stomach cancer in relatives of patients with stomach cancer. It is not known whether this familial tendency to develop stomach cancer is hereditary or related to environmental factors. Population screening for stomach cancer by barium studies, gastroscopy, or cytologic sampling has been shown to be of value only in populations with a very high frequency of stomach cancer, such as Japan. Periodic endoscopic examinations and cytologic sampling of the stomach have not yet been shown to be cost-effective or to improve the dismal prognosis of groups of patients with pernicious anemia or postgastrectomy patients who subsequently develop stomach cancer.

Pancreatic Cancer

DEFINITION AND DIAGNOSTIC CRITERIA

During the past three decades, the incidence of adenocarcinoma of the exocrine pancreas has increased.

PATHOPHYSIOLOGY

Over 90% of pancreatic cancers are adenocarcinomas of ductal cell origin. Seventy-five per cent of the tumors originate in the head of the pancreas with the remaining tumors originating in the body or the tail of the pancreas. The cancer may be multifocal within the pancreas in up to one fifth of the cases.

CLINICAL ASPECTS

The peak age of incidence is approximately 60 years. It is two to three times more common in males than in females. Presenting symptoms are weight loss and anorexia, with tumors of the pancreatic head usually presenting with jaundice, and tumors of the body or tail presenting with poorly localized pain. Less than one fourth of the patients will have a palpable abdominal mass on physical examination. Pancreatic cancer usually metastasizes before the diagnosis has been established. The most common sites of metastases are the regional lymph nodes, liver, lungs, peritoneum, and other intra-abdominal organs.

Because of the vague and insidious symptoms of pancreatic cancer, it is often difficult to diagnose. Computerized tomography and ultrasonography of the pancreas are the most reliable radiographic techniques in localizing the tumor. Fine-needle biopsy of a pancreatic lesion is a reliable means of obtaining tissue when used by experienced hands, but laparotomy is often needed to establish a pathologic diagnosis.

MANAGEMENT

PLAN

Short-term goals after the establishment of pancreatic cancer include deciding whether the patient is a candidate for surgery, radiation, or chemotherapy. Long-term goals should concentrate on proper control of pain, possible postoperative effects such as diabetes mellitus, steatorrhea, and the psychosocial problems of the patient and family.

NONPHARMACOLOGIC MEASURES

More than 90% of pancreatic cancers are incurable by surgery. Less than 10% of the patients who undergo an attempted curative resection with a total pancreatectomy or a pancreatoduodenectomy live for five years. Tumors of the pancreas presenting with impending obstruction can be successfully palliated with bypass surgery, although the patient survival time is probably not prolonged beyond the median survival of three to six months in patients not undergoing surgery. Radiation therapy can also be used in a palliative manner, particularly in patients who are inoperable or who have symptomatic distant metastases.

DRUG THERAPY

The role of adjuvant therapy after an attempted curative resection has not been established in pancreatic cancer. Clinical trials have been difficult to complete in this setting, although one large study showed an improved survival for those patients who received 5-fluorouracil and local radiation therapy after surgery when compared with surgery alone. Studies are currently being performed to determine the effectiveness of adjuvant therapy after curative surgery for pancreatic cancer.

Pancreatic cancer is not as responsive to chemotherapy as are gastric or esophageal cancers. The response rates to single agents and combination chemotherapy programs are usually below 20%. The most commonly used drugs are 5-fluorouracil, mitomycin, doxorubicin (Adriamycin), streptozotocin, and perhaps nitrosoureas. There is some preliminary evidence that the combination of radiation therapy and 5-FU may increase the survival of patients with locally metastatic pancreatic cancer, but this needs to be confirmed in future studies.

Adverse Effects of Chemotherapy. The common toxic effects seen with the chemotherapy agents used to treat pancreatic cancer are covered in the preceding section on cancer of the esophagus.

PERIODIC EVALUATION

Follow-up should be similar to what is outlined in the preceding section for cancer of the esophagus.

MANAGEMENT OF COMPLICATIONS OF SURGERY

Postoperatively, the most serious complications of pancreatoduodenectomy are biliary leaks, gastrointestinal tract hemorrhage, infections, and renal failure. Leaks from the biliary tract or the pancreatic stump may also cause problems for months after the surgery. The problems unique to a total pancreatectomy are the development of "brittle" diabetes or exocrine insufficiency, which can usually be managed by insulin and pancreatic preparations that contain pancreatic enzymes, predominantly lipase, amylase, and protease.

PREVENTIVE MEASURES

Unfortunately, because of the lack of information about the etiologic factors or predisposing conditions that cause pancreatic cancer, no screening or preventive measures are currently used for pancreatic cancer.

Carcinoid Tumors

DEFINITION AND DIAGNOSITIC CRITERIA

Carcinoid tumors are uncommon neoplasms that are usually diagnosed incidentally.

Paradoxes encountered in management of these patients include conservative surgical treatment for early disease, whereas in patients with distant metastases aggressive approaches may be indicated. Additionally, the best medical management is frequently no treatment at all, except for attempts to control distressing symptoms.

PATHOPHYSIOLOGY

In view of the widespread distribution of enterochromaffin cells, carcinoid tumors have been identified in sites such as GI and biliary tracts, bronchopulmonary tree, thymus, and ovary, but the majority are found in the appendix and small intestine. Benign and malignant forms of the tumor and the other common GI APUD (amine precursor uptake and decarboxylation) tumors, namely islet cell carcinoma, cannot be distinguished purely by microscopic examination and routine use of hematoxylin and eosin staining.

CLINICAL ASPECTS

The most dramatic manifestation ocurring in 25% of carcinoid tumors is the carcinoid syndrome. This is characterized by the presence of cutaneous flushing, diarrhea, vasomotor instability, bronchoconstriction, endocardial and mesenteric fibrosis, telangiectasias, and arthropathy in variable degrees. The clinical features of the syndrome were originally felt to be secondary to the production of 5-hydroxytryptamine (serotonin) by the neoplasm, but are now known to be secondary to a wide variety of amine and peptide hormones, including histamine, bradykinin, prostaglandins, vasoactive intestinal polypeptide (VIP), calcitonin, and ACTH, allowing the syndrome to occur with other APUD tumors. The occurrence of the syndrome generally requires that the tumor products have access to the systemic circulation with no intervening hepatic detoxification (e.g., presence of hepatic metastases).

MANAGEMENT

PLAN

If localized, carcinoid tumors are managed by surgery and may be curable. Metastatic disease requires pharmacologic or chemotherapeutic intervention.

NONPHARMACOLOGIC MEASURES

Tumors localized to the bowel or to regional lymph nodes are best managed with surgery, either with simple removal for tumors less than 1 cm or with more aggressive cancer operations for tumors over 2 cm, e.g., right hemicolectomy. In instances of lymph node spread, aggressive surgery with resection of involved and adjacent lymph node areas may be beneficial.

Initial therapy of metastases should be surgical resection. Areas producing intestinal obstruction can be removed, and if solitary or localized liver metastases are present, wedge resection or hepatic lobectomy can be performed.

DRUG THERAPY

The carcinoid syndrome can be quite distressing, and pharmacologic therapy can be useful in controlling these symptoms. Since the exact mechanism of production of the syndrome is poorly understood, empiric use of various agents is often employed. Drugs reported to be of value include adrenergic blocking agents (clonidine, propranolol), inhibitors of serotonin synthesis (alpha-methyldopa, parachlorophenylalanine), peripheral serotonin antagonists (cyproheptadine), histamine receptor antagonists (cimetidine), and corticosteroids.

With the presence of systemic symptoms (such as weight loss, impairment of performance status), or with an increasingly severe carcinoid syndrome, hepatic artery occlusion, regional chemotherapy, or systemic chemotherapy may be indicated. In patients with carcinoid heart disease or high urinary 5-HIAA level (>150 mg/24 hr), median survivals are short, and earlier therapy may be warranted. Hepatic artery ligation or occlusion via a percutaneous approach may be quite useful to control symptoms of the carcinoid syndrome. Regional chemotherapy via hepatic artery infusion has been re-

Table 1. CHEMOTHERAPY FOR PATIENTS WITH METASTATIC CARCINOID TUMORS

Drug(s)	Schedule	CR + PR
Doxorubicin	60 mg/m^2 IV (repeat q3 wk)	21%
5-Fluorouracil + Streptozotocin	400 mg/m^2 IV d1–5 500 mg/m^2 IV d1–5 (repeat q6 wks.)	33%
5-Fluorouracil + Cyclophosphamide	400 mg/m^2 IV d1–5 1000 mg/m^2 IV d1,22 (repeat q6 wk)	26%
5-Fluorouracil + Doxorubicin + Cyclophosphamide + Streptozotocin	400 mg/m^2 IV d1&8 30 mg/m^2 IV d1 75 mg/m^2 PO d1–14 400 mg/m^2 IV d1&8 (repeat q4 wk)	35%

ported, but the overall value of this approach is difficult to assess, with most reports being in only small groups of patients. Systemic chemotherapy is now undergoing critical evaluation, with several large cooperative groups (Eastern Cooperative Oncology Group, Southwestern Oncology Group) investigating this approach. Agents that have produced response rates in excess of 20% include doxorubicin, 5-fluorouracil, and cyclophosphamide. Combinations of drugs evaluated include streptozotocin in combination with 5-fluorouracil, and cyclophosphamide plus streptozotocin. Objective responses occur in 20% to 35% of patients and improvement in the carcinoid syndrome can be seen.

Carcinoma of the Colon and Rectum

DEFINITION AND DIAGNOSTIC CRITERIA

Cancer of the colon and rectum affected approximately 138,000 in 1985 and is a leading cause of cancer mortality in the United States. In addition to adenocarcinoma, primary tumors of the lower intestinal tract may rarely be lymphomas, lipomas, hemangiomas, leiomyomas, and their respective malignant counterparts. Adenomatous polyps are neoplastic polyps and have potential to produce an adenocarcinoma. Epidemiologic data have implicated high animal fat, protein, and beef plus a low fiber intake as important etiologic factors in colorectal cancer. It has been suggested that these diets favor the establishment of a bacterial flora in the colon that may convert acid and neutral sterols into carcinogens.

PATHOPHYSIOLOGY

Recent studies support the concept that adenocarcinoma of the colon arises from dysplastic changes in the mucosa, which then develop into adenomatous polyps. There is a direct relationship between the size of the polyp, the dysplasia, and the subsequent development of the adenocarcinoma.

CLINICAL ASPECTS

The position of the tumor will largely determine the symptoms in the patient with primary colon cancer. Because of the smaller circumference of the left colon, symptoms of left colonic carcinoma are those of obstruction (changing bowel habit, pain and bloating, or rectal bleeding); lesions of the right colon, because of a larger luminal circumference, more often present as occult blood in the stool and iron deficiency anemia. Indications for metastatic disease may include fever, malaise, anorexia, and weight loss. Findings on physical examination to be observed include rectal or abdominal masses, ascites, and enlargement of the liver. We normally include the following tests in the evaluation of a patient suspected with carcinoma of the colon: a complete blood count, liver chemistries, urinalysis, and chest film. Proctosigmoidoscopy and colonoscopy are usually required for histologic confirmation of pathologic lesions. The determination of carcinoembryonic antigen (CEA) may be used to follow the patient with known cancer.

MANAGEMENT

PLAN

An initial attempt should be made to evaluate the patient and establish extent of disease by the above methods. Long-term goals include care of the patient through continued postoperative follow-up to identify early recurrence of the tumor.

NONPHARMACOLOGIC MEASURES

The treatment of choice for all colorectal cancer is curative surgery. The extent of surgical resection is determined by the tumor location, the pattern of the lymph drainage, and the blood supply. Left and right colon tumors require a hemicolectomy if anatomically possible. Rectal tumors within 5 cm of the dentate line require an abdominal-perineal resection. In the event curative operations are not possible, palliative surgery including local resection of the tumor and proximal colostomy may be of symptomatic relief. Localized tumors of the colon may be expected to have an 80% five-year survival, whereas this number decreases to 30% with lymph node involvement beyond the colon.

Radiation has been employed as a preoperative measure in both colon and rectal cancer, but there are no data present in any randomized study to show long-term benefits from this procedure.

DRUG THERAPY

The role of chemotherapy either in an adjuvant (preventive) setting or in advanced disease has not been established for colorectal cancer. The objective response rates using 5-fluorouracil have been between 10% and 20%, and these responses have generally been short in duration. National studies are in progress to determine if new agents may be of benefit in this prevalent disease, but to date no beneficial agents have been identified. New approaches to drug delivery being studied include arterial or venous infusion percutaneously or via implanted pump devices.

After curative resection, follow-up should be at intervals of three months for the first two years, then every six months for three years, and yearly for life. If radiation therapy or chemotherapy is the treatment being utilized, then follow-up will be more often, usually at monthly intervals. Follow-up examinations are similar to initial presentations and include blood counts, fecal occult blood studies, liver chemistries, CEA, and, if any of these are abnormal, then either instrumentation of the colon or a CT scan for extracolonic recurrences.

PATIENT INFORMATION AND EDUCATION

Both the American Cancer Society and the National Institutes of Health provide information data for patients and family members about colorectal cancer.

PATIENT COMPLIANCE

As with most malignancies, the patient who has had colorectal carcinoma recently diagnosed will usually take a very active part in rehabilitation and follow-up procedures. High interest in methods to detect the disease was found in all socioeconomic levels surveyed.

Patient compliance with stool occult blood testing has been evaluated in a number of studies. In patients who have been motivated by prior information about the importance and the aims of screening, compliance is about 80%. In groups who have not received such information, compliance has dropped as low as 15%.

PREVENTIVE MEASURES

High-risk groups for development of colorectal cancer include persons over 40 years of age, persons with adenomatous polyps, persons with universal ulcerative colitis over seven years in duration, as well as patients with a family history of colorectal cancer or one of the familial polyposis syndromes. Currently, data from mass population screening programs are not available as to the cost-benefit effectiveness or whether in fact early detection has been beneficial in improving survival rates. Mention was made earlier in this section about the possibility of various environmental and diet factors being responsible for the cause of colon cancer.

SOCIOECONOMIC ASPECTS OF COLORECTAL CANCER

The overall five-year survival for colorectal cancer approximates 50% and has changed very little in the last 25 years. With the high incidence of this tumor nationally, it is obviously a major health problem today for which earlier methods of detection and better treatments of advanced disease are required.

REFERENCES

Bukowski RM, Stephens R, Oishi N, et al: Phase II trial of 5FU, Adriamycin, cyclophosphamide, and streptozotocin (FAC-S) in metastatic carcinoid (for the Southwest Oncology Group). Proc. ASCO 2:130, 1983.

Engstrom P, Lavin P, Folach E, et al: Streptozotocin + fluorouracil vs. Adriamycin for metastatic carcinoid tumors. Proc. AACR, 24:139, 1983.

Johnson LA, Lavin P, Moertel CG, et al: Carcinoids: the association of histologic growth pattern and survival. Cancer 51:882–889, 1983.

Lightdale PJ, Winawer SJ: Malignant tumors of the colon and rectum. *In* Conn RB: Current Diagnosis 7. W.B. Saunders Co, Philadelphia, 1985, pp 682–686.

Moertel CG, Grenville GS: Alimentary tract cancer: large bowel. *In* Holland JE, Frei E III: Cancer Medicine. Lea and Febiger, Philadelphia, 1982, pp 1830–1858.

Moertel CG, Hanley JA: Combination chemotherapy trials in metastatic carcinoid tumor and the malignant carcinoid syndrome. Cancer Clin Trials 2:327–334, 1979.

Moertel CG, Sauer WG, Dockerty MD, et al: Life history of the carcinoid tumor of the small intestine. Cancer 14:901–912, 1961.

Pearse AGE: Th diffuse neuroendocrine system and the APUD concept. Med Biol 55:115–125, 1977.

Schein PS, Smith FR, Woolley PV, et al: Current management of advanced and locally unresectable gastric carcinoma. Cancer 50:2590–2596, 1982.

Shepard KV, Levin B: Gastrointestinal malignancies. *In* Gitnick G (ed): Current Gastroenterology. John Wiley and Sons, New York, 1984, pp 325–354.

Sugarbaker PH, MacDonald JS, Gunderson LL: Colorectal cancer. *In* DeVita VT, Hellman S, Rosenberg SA (eds): Cancer Principles and Practice of Oncology. J.B. Lippincott Co, Philadelphia, 1982, pp 643–710.

Winawer SJ: Neoplasms of the large and small intestine. *In* Wyngaarden JB, Smith LH Jr (eds): Cecil Textbook of Mecicine, 17th ed. W.B. Saunders Co, Philadelphia, 1985, pp 761–770.

Winawer SJ, Sherlock P: Malignant neoplasms of the small and large intestine. *In* Sleisenger MH, Fordtran JS (eds): Gastrointestinal Diseases, 3rd ed, Vol 2. W.B. Saunders Co, Philadelphia, 1983, pp 1220–1246.

24 · GENITOURINARY TUMORS

Stuart J. Tipping
MARSHFIELD CLINIC

Renal Cancer

DEFINITION AND DIAGNOSIS

Renal cancers occur at any age but are most frequent between the ages of 50 and 80 years. Males are affected three times as often as females. Urban living and cigarette smoking are the only suggested risk factors.

CLINICAL ASPECTS

The classic triad of flank pain, hematuria, and palpable mass occurs in only 5% of patients. The majority of patients will have at least one of these symptoms. Thirty per cent of patients will present with systemic symptoms that may include weight loss, fever, anemia, erythrocytosis, thrombocytosis, elevated sedimentation rate, abnormal liver function tests, or hypercalcemia. Excretory urography with nephrotomography is a frequent first step. Careful history and physical, chest film, urinalysis, complete blood count, and chemistry panel should be done. CT scan of the abdomen is the single best means of evaluating a renal mass; not only is it the most accurate means of determining lymph node and liver involvement, but it also provides information about renal vein and inferior vena cava extension. Angiography is used to define the vascularity preoperatively.

MANAGEMENT

NONPHARMACOLOGIC MEASURES

For localized or regional tumors, radical nephrectomy offers five-year survivals of between 35% and 70%. Radiation therapy and adjuvant chemotherapy are of no proven benefit. Over half of the patients with renal cell carcinoma have distant metastases at the time of presentation. Nephrectomy for palliation of pain and hematuria may be considered in these patients. Spontaneous regression of metastases following nephrectomy is so rare that it does not justify the surgical risk. Radiation therapy is effective in palliating symptoms from brain and bone metastases.

DRUG THERAPY

Progestational agents and androgens have a low response rate with relatively little toxicity. Investigational trials hold the best hope of treatment advancement.

PERIODIC EVALUATION

Postoperatively, patients should be followed quarterly for the first year, semiannually until the fifth year, and thereafter annually with examinations, urinalysis, CBC, liver and renal function tests, and chest film.

Bladder Cancer

DEFINITION AND DIAGNOSIS

Bladder cancer is twice as common in males and has its peak incidence in the fifth to seventh decades. There are many risk factors including smoking, pelvic radiation, previous cyclophosphamide therapy, and aromatic amine chemical exposure in the rubber and cable industry.

CLINICAL ASPECTS

Gross hematuria is the presenting symptom in 75% of patients. Nearly all patients have at least microhematuria. Bleeding is characteristically intermittent. Bladder irritability with frequency, urgency, and dysuria occurs in about a third of the patients and is associated with advanced disease. The initial evaluation includes history and physical examination, urine cytology, urinalysis, CBC, chemistry panel, chest film, and intravenous urogram. The diagnosis is established by cystoscopy with biopsy.

MANAGEMENT

NONPHARMACOLOGIC MEASURES

Patients with superficial tumors may be treated with transurethral resection and intravesical chemotherapy. Patients with infiltrating tumors may receive preoperative radiation therapy followed by radical cystectomy. The use of preoperative radiation is being questioned and is used less frequently. Pelvic lymphadenectomy does not improve survival but does provide prognostic information. For poor surgical candidates, radiation therapy alone may be employed but with a lower cure rate.

Carcinoma in situ appears to have a different natural history. It is usually multifocal, persistent, and recurrent with a very high likelihood to evolve into invasive cancer. It frequently involves the urethra and ureter. For patients with a localized area of carcinoma in situ, transurethral resection with close follow-up may be considered. Patients with multifocal carcinoma in situ, particularly high-grade, diffuse, and symptomatic, may come to radical cystectomy, urethrectomy, or ureterectomy.

DRUG THERAPY

The use of adjuvant chemotherapy is investigational. Chemotherapy for advanced disease has had limited success. Cisplatin, cyclophosphamide, doxorubicin, 5-fluorouracil, vinblastine, and methotrexate are active agents. Combination chemotherapy has not yet shown improved survival over single agents.

PERIODIC EVALUATION

Patients with all stages of disease should be followed quarterly for two years, then semiannually for the next three years, and thereafter yearly; follow-up should include a physical exam, cystoscopy, urine cytology, urinalysis, CBC, chemistry panel, and chest film. An IVP should be performed on a periodic basis.

Prostate Cancer

DEFINITION AND DIAGNOSIS

Prostatic carcinoma is rare before the age of 50 and increases steadily in frequency to age 70. The cause is unknown. Subclinical or latent cancer of the prostate is a frequent finding at autopsy of elderly men.

CLINICAL ASPECTS

An asymptomatic prostatic nodule noted on physical exam is a common presentation. Symptoms of bladder neck obstruction or bone pain suggest advanced disease. The patient should be evaluated with history and physical examination, urinalysis, CBC, complete chemistry profile, bone scan, and intravenous pyelogram. Prostatic acid phosphatase is elevated in two thirds of patients with metastatic disease and is rarely elevated in localized tumors. CT scan of the pelvis or lymphangiography may be used to evaluate pelvic nodal disease.

MANAGEMENT

NONPHARMACOLOGIC MEASURES

Those patients with a normal gland by exam who are found to have carcinoma on transurethral resection are classified as stage A. If there are less than 5 mm of tumor on aggregate chips, the patient is considered to have stage A1 disease. Those rare patients with a low stage but a high histologic grade should receive further treatment; the remainder need no further therapy and have a normal survival. The only recommended follow-up is frequent examination of the prostate. If further malignancy is found on needle biopsy or transurethral resection, or if there is diffuse disease on initial resection, they are considered stage A2. Patients with a palpable prostatic nodule are classified as stage B disease. Those with a 1 cm or less nodule are stage B1; involvement of an entire lobe or with multiple nodules in more than one lobe is considered B2. Patients with tumor extending beyond the capsule of the gland are stage C. Patients with B1, B2, and C stage tumors frequently undergo lymphangiography or pelvic lymphadenectomy for pathologic staging prior to definitive therapy.

Treatment of early stage prostate cancer varies from institution to institution. Patients with A2, B2, or C tumors frequently receive radiation therapy but radical prostatectomy is an option. Patients with B1 tumors and possibly younger B2 patients may benefit most from radical prostatectomy, although again radiation is certainly an option. Patients with one or more lymph nodes involved (stage D1) or distant metastases (D2) undergo bilateral orchiectomy as palliative therapy.

DRUG THERAPY

Diethylstilbestrol (DES), 1 to 3 mg/day, may be used as an alternative to orchiectomy in those patients who do not have risk of cardiovascular disease. Low-dose radiation to the breasts should be given prior to DES therapy to prevent painful gynecomastia. Luteinizing hormone releasing factor is currently under clinical trial and may become useful once generally available. Aminoglutethimide plus hydrocortisone or megestrol may produce responses in up to 20% of patients. Primary hormonal failures are less likely to respond to secondary hormonal treatments. Chemotherapy agents of use include 5-fluorouracil, doxorubicin, mitomycin C, dacarbazine, and cyclophosphamide.

PERIODIC EVALUATION

Those patients with localized carcinoma of the prostate should have history and physical examination with special attention to the prostate every three to four months for two years and thereafter semiannually. A CBC and serum acid phosphatase should be obtained with each visit.

Testicular Cancer

DEFINITION AND DIAGNOSIS

Carcinoma of the testicle is a relatively rare tumor. Cryptorchidism is the largest single risk factor. Orchiopexy before the age of 6 years may reduce the risk, but 20% of tumors occur in the contralateral testis, suggesting testicular dysgenesis may be etiologic. A testicular mass is the most frequent presenting symptom.

CLINICAL ASPECTS

Any patient presenting with a solid testicular mass should undergo an inguinal orchiectomy. Transscrotal incision or needle biopsy is contraindicated. Ninety per cent of malignant tumors are of germ cell origin. Initial evaluation should include history, physical, CBC, chemistry panel, chest film, serum alpha-fetoprotein level, beta-hCG level, and LDH. Ultrasound of the testicle may be used to distinguish a solid from a cystic mass. Postoperatively, repeat serum markers, intravenous urogram, CT scan of the abdomen and chest, or whole lung tomograms complete the initial evaluation.

MANAGEMENT

NONPHARMACOLOGIC MEASURES

Forty to 50% of all tumors are seminomas. About 10% of apparently pure seminomas will have detectable levels of beta-hCG. The presence of elevated alpha-fetoprotein or hCG levels suggests nonseminomatous elements and requires treatment as such. Lymphangiography should be performed on all patients with early stage disease. Most patients with seminoma without lymph node involvement (stage I) are treated with radiation therapy to the groin and the ipsilateral pelvic and periaortic nodes. Management of stage II (lymph node–positive) patients is controversial. The standard of therapy for patients felt to have retroperitoneal node involvement with seminoma has been irradiation to the pelvic, abdominal, mediastinal, and supraclavicular nodes. Chemotherapy similar to that used for nonseminomatous tumors has been found effective in seminomatous tumors, but patients who have received extensive radiation are unable to tolerate these regimens. It has therefore been recommended and is under investigation to treat extensive stage II patients with chemotherapy possibly followed by radiation to bulk disease.

Nonseminomatous germ cell tumors consist of embryonal cell carcinoma, mature or immature teratoma, choriocarcinoma, and a small number of yolk sac tumors. The current recommendation for stage I disease is close observation with monthly chest roentgenogram and serum markers with CT scan of the abdomen every three months for a total of two years. Retroperitoneal lymph node dissection is the standard treatment for limited stage II disease; those patients with bulky stage II or visceral disease are best treated with chemotherapy possibly followed by subsequent surgery.

DRUG THERAPY

Testicular cancer ranks as one of the more successful chemotherapy stories. Programs containing cisplatin, vinblastine, and bleomycin for patients with recurrent or metastatic disease are now curing a majority of patients; additionally, VP-16, doxorubin, and high-dose cisplatin are being investigated for efficacy in high-risk patients.

PERIODIC EVALUATION

Following chemotherapy, those patients whose markers have returned to normal but who have evidence of a residual mass should have surgical resection. Negative beta-hCG or alpha-fetoprotein does not rule out the possibility of tumor. Those patients undergoing resection after chemotherapy may have benign mature teratoma, benign fibrous tissue, or residual carcinoma. Patients with residual carcinoma or immature teratoma require further chemotherapy.

Seminoma patients are followed initially on an every two-month basis for two years, then every six months for two years, and then annually. Patients with clinical stage II and III nonseminomatous tumors should be followed on a monthly basis for one year and then every two months for the second year. At two years the risk of recurrence is reduced to 10%. Patients are then followed on an every four- to six-month basis for two years and subsequently on a yearly basis. A physical examination, chest film, and serum markers are done at each visit. The overall survival for patients with germ cell tumors is approximately 90%.

REFERENCES

Elwin EF, Lenze PL, Kennedy BJ: Germ-cell testicular cancer in adults. N Engl J Med 301:1370–1379; 1420–1426, 1979.
Friedell GH, Greenfield RE, Hilgar AG: Urinary bladder cancer. Semin Oncol 6:145–265, 1979.
Harris DT, Maquire HC: Renal-cell cacinoma. Semin Oncol 10:365–431, 1983.
Murphy GP, Gaeta JF, Pickren J, et al: Current status of classification and staging of prostate cancer. Cancer 45:1889–1896, 1980.
Paulsen DF, Perez CA, Anderson T: Genito-urinary malignancies. In DeVita VT, Hellman S, Rosenberg SA (eds): Principles and Practice of Oncology. J.B. Lippincott Co, Philadelphia 1982, pp 732–816.

25 · GYNECOLOGIC TUMORS

Stuart J. Tipping
MARSHFIELD CLINIC

Carcinoma of the Uterine Cervix

DEFINITION AND DIAGNOSTIC CRITERIA

The mortality of cervical cancer has declined by 50% over the past 40 years owing to early detection and treatment. It has been determined that risk factors include intercourse before age 16, frequent intercourse, and intercourse with multiple partners.

PATHOPHYSIOLOGY

The process by which a cervical cancer appears is long, requiring five to ten years. Malignancies begin with cervical intraepithelial neoplasia (CIN), which may be continuum of dysplastic changes from mild to carcinoma in situ. These premalignant changes are asymptomatic, usually not visible, and best detected by a Papanicolaou smear.

CLINICAL ASPECTS

Early stage invasive cancer is often asymptomatic: discharge and postcoital spotting may occur. More advanced stages may result in pelvic pain and bleeding. The diagnosis of microinvasive cancer is usually made by a cone biopsy. The initial evaluation for all patients with suspected invasive cancer should include a careful pelvic examination, laboratory testing with CBC, chemical survey, chest film, and intravenous urogram. Barium enema and sigmoidoscopy should be performed in all advanced stage patients and those with symptoms referable to these regions. Optional studies include lymphangiography and CAT scanning.

MANAGEMENT

PLAN

Advocates exist for both radical surgery and radiation therapy in the treatment of carcinoma of the uterine cervix depending on clinical staging. Cure rates vary from 95% in very limited disease (I) to 5% in disease with spread to distant organs (IVB).

NONPHARMACOLOGIC MEASURES

Microinvasive cancer (stage IA) is best treated with a total abdominal hysterectomy. Radical hysterectomy or radiation for stages IB and IIA therapy are equally effective. Stage IIB, IIIA, and IIIB cervical cancers are usually managed with radiation therapy alone. Stage IVA and IVB patients with disease limited to the pelvis still have some potential for cure treated with aggressive radiation therapy. If distant metastases are present, then patients are generally treated only with palliative radiation therapy.

DRUG THERAPY

Chemotherapy in advanced carcinoma of the cervix can produce responses in 20% to 30% of patients, with little effect on overall survival. Active agents include bleomycin, cisplatin, mitomycin, doxorubicin, and methotrexate.

FOLLOW-UP

Most treatment failures occur within the first two years. We recommend that the patient be seen every two months for the first year, and in gradually increasing intervals over the next two years to semiannually at five years, and yearly thereafter. These follow-up exams should include a Pap smear, blood counts, yearly chest roentgenogram, and a urogram every 12 to 18 months. If any recurrence is detected, this patient should be restaged thoroughly.

PATIENT INFORMATION AND EDUCATION

It is recommended that all women over the age of 20 or those women under age 20 who are sexually active have two Pap smears one year apart. If these are initially negative, Pap smears should be repeated every three years with a pelvic examination. If dyplasia is detected, the woman should be referred to a gynecologist for culposcopic evaluation and biopsy.

Endometrial Cancer

DEFINITION AND DIAGNOSTIC CRITERIA

Endometrial cancer is the most common malignancy of the female genital tract. Eighty per cent of patients are postmenopausal with a peak incidence in the sixth and seventh decades. Risk factors are related to prolonged estrogen stimulation unopposed by progestins. These factors include obesity, diabetes mellitus, hypertension, infertility, and the Stein-Leventhal syndrome. Exogenous estrogen clearly increases the risk of these tumors.

PATHOPHYSIOLOGY

The endometrium proliferates in response to estrogen, producing a continuum of changes ranging from cystic hyperplasia to atypical hyperplasia to carcinoma in situ. The treatment of these hyperplasia in the premenopausal woman is the induction of ovulation or the addition of progestational agents. In the postmenopausal patient, hysterectomy is the treatment of choice unless the source of exogenous estrogen can be removed.

CLINICAL ASPECTS

Abnormal vaginal bleeding is the most frequent symptom, and in fact postmenopausal bleeding should be considered to be endometrial cancer until proven otherwise. The Pap smear may be positive in 10% of cases but an endometrial biopsy or D and C is required in most instances. The initial evaluation should be identical to that of carcinoma of the cervix; initial staging requires fractional D and C, uterine sounding, examination under anesthesia, and IVP.

MANAGEMENT

PLAN AND NONPHARMACOLOGIC MEASURES

Definitive therapy depends upon both stage and grade of the tumor. In general, stage I and well-differentiated tumors (confined to the uterus) are managed with total abdominal hysterectomy. If the tumor is poorly differentiated, radiation therapy is generally added preoperatively. Stage II patients (extension to the uterine cervix) are treated with preoperative external and intracavitary radiation followed by total hysterectomy and bilateral salpingo-oophorectomy. Stage III patients (extension to the vagina or perimetrium) are best treated with radiation therapy. In stage IV, patients have involvement of the bladder, rectum, or structures outside the pelvis, and no generalized statement about therapy is available. Radiation is usually employed to control the pelvic symptoms, and hormonal or chemotherapy may be combined with radiation.

DRUG THERAPY

Progestational agents are frequently employed as systemic therapy either as an adjunct or for metastatic cancer; responses in 40% of patients have been reported. Chemotherapeutic agents used in treatment of this disease include doxorubicin, cyclophosphamide, cisplatin, 5-fluorouracil, and methotrexate.

PERIODIC EVALUATION

The frequency of follow-up exams and tests for endometrial cancer are identical to those of cervical cancer.

Ovarian Cancer

DEFINITION AND DIAGNOSTIC CRITERIA

Carcinoma of the ovary accounts for 20% of all gynecologic tumors but is the most lethal of this group of tumors, accounting for approximately 50% of all cancer deaths in gynecologic malignancies. The risk is increased in those with a prior history of carcinoma of the breast or endometrium. A higher incidence has been noted in industrialized countries.

PATHOPHYSIOLOGY

Most ovarian carcinomas are of epithelial histologic type, with cystoadenocarcinoma and adenocarcinoma predominating; histologic grade is an independent prognostic factor. Stage for stage, patients with well-differentiated tumors have a better response to therapy and survival than do those with poorly differentiated or undifferentiated tumors. Sex cord and germ cell tumors are less common.

CLINICAL ASPECTS

The most frequent first symptoms are increased abdominal girth, pelvic pressure, or nonspecific abdominal pain. The physical exam will usually reveal the presence of ascites or a pelvic mass. In a postmenopausal woman, any adnexal mass should be considered malignant until proven otherwise. In a premenopausal woman, masses up to 6 cm that are not malignant may be found, but any larger mass or one enlarging on a monthly exam should be biopsied. The initial evaluation of a patient with an ovarian mass is similar to that previously mentioned for carcinoma of the cervix and endometrium; CT scan or ultrasound can help assess the extent of disease preoperatively and can assist in follow-up evaluation.

MANAGEMENT

NONPHARMACOLOGIC MEASURES

The tendency of ovarian cancer is to spread throughout the peritoneal cavity, resulting in peritoneal and diaphragmatic implants and ascites. Metastasis outside the abdomen is a late finding. At the time of surgical exploration, all patients should have peritoneal washings done as well as a careful examination of all peritoneal surfaces. Unless further childbearing is desired, the treatment for limited disease is total abdominal hysterectomy and bilateral salpingo-oophorectomy. With advanced disease, maximum debulking of the tumor should be performed, since those with minimal residual disease may be cured with combination chemotherapy.

DRUG THERAPY

The use of adjuvant therapy for those with early stage disease is still controversial. It has been established that intermittent melphalan chemotherapy reduces recurrence but does not appear to affect survival. Patients with advanced or residual disease are usually treated with combination chemotherapy, which often includes cyclophosphamide, doxorubicin, and cisplatin for six to 12 monthly cycles. Patients who are clinically in remission after chemotherapy are advised to have a second laparotomy to evaluate for residual disease. Those patients who have no tumor upon reexploration are followed in a manner similar to that recommended for cervical and uterine cancers. Therapy should be changed in patients with residual disease at second laparotomy. Options include abdominal radiation or the use of other active agents such as methotrexate, 5-fluorouracil, and hexamethylmelamine.

REFERENCES

Disaia PJ, Creasman WT: Clinical Gynecologic Oncology. C.V. Mosby Co, St. Louis, 1981.
Perez CA, Knapp RC, Young RC: Gynecologic tumors. In DeVita VT, Hellman S, Rosenberg SA (eds): Principles and Practice of Oncology. J.B. Lippincott Co, Philadelphia, 1982, pp 823–914.
Richardson GS, Scully RE, Nihrui N, et al: Common epithelial cancer of the ovary. N Engl J Med 312:415–424; 474–483, 1985.
Ulfelder H (ed): Carcinoma of the cervix. Semin Oncol 9:249–387, 1982.
Young RC (ed): Ovarian carcinoma. Semin Oncol 11:209–332, 1984.

26 · TUMORS OF THE SKIN: MALIGNANT MELANOMA

Roger H. Herzig
CLEVELAND CLINIC FOUNDATION

DEFINITION AND DIAGNOSTIC CRITERIA

Melanoma is a malignant neoplasm of melanocytes, cells of neural crest origin that migrate to the skin, uveal tract, and ectodermal mucosa early in gestation. Melanocytes in the epidermis elaborate the melanin that results in skin pigmentation.

A changing skin lesion is the most common sign of melanoma. Rapidly growing lesions are often inflammatory, whereas lesions that grow so slowly as to seem imperceptible are often benign. A skin lesion that doubles in size within six months is highly suspicious. Growth may be associated with a change in color, bleeding, itching, ulceration, or the development of an enlarged lymph node. A definite change in a mole or skin lesion, no matter how trivial, should signal the possibility of melanoma.

PATHOPHYSIOLOGY

Invasive melanoma may progress in a stepwise fashion from a nonmalignant precursor, the dysplastic nevus, the melanoma in situ, to invasive melanoma; or it may begin in situ. Melanoma is classified according to its noninvasive component: superficial spreading (70%), nodular melanoma (15% to 30%), lentigo maligna (4% to 10%), acral lentiginous (2% to 8%), mucosal lentiginous (rare), or unclassifiable.

The histologic characteristics of the melanotic lesion are important prognostically: the *thickness* (Breslow depth) of the tumor is the most important indicator; in general, the greater the depth of the *level of invasion* (Clark's level) into the layers of skin, the worse the prognosis. *Ulceration* portends poorer survival. A number of other characteristics, including growth pattern, mitotic activity, regression, lymphocytic reaction, pigment, cell type, vascular invasion, associated nevi, and solar degeneration, have been studied and shown to have only a modest impact on prognosis.

CLINICAL ASPECTS

Clinical features of malignant melanoma are also important prognostically. The extent of disease affects survival. Patients with disease limited to skin (stage I) have a better prognosis than do patients with lymph node involvement (stage II) or distant metastases (stage III). Within each stage, certain factors are predictive. For patients with stage I disease, increasing age, male sex, and anatomic site (trunk) adversely affect prognosis. Overall, combining the pathologic and clinical variables in a multivariant analysis from eight centers worldwide, the most significant variables (in descending order) for patients with stage I disease were: tumor thickness, tumor ulceration, tumor site, and patient's sex. Thus, thin lesions, without ulceration, occurring on an extremity in a woman have the best prognosis. For patients with stage II disease, similar multifactorial analyses have shown that survival has improved when there is only a single metastatic lymph node. Finally, for patients with stage III disease, the number and site of metastases correlated with survival, a single metastasis and nonvisceral sites having the better prognoses.

MANAGEMENT

GOALS

Management is highly dependent on the stage of the melanoma and the prognostic variables mentioned above. There is sufficient justification to biopsy any suspicious pigmented lesion.

NONPHARMACOLOGIC MEASURES

Any patient who is concerned about the potentially malignant nature of a skin lesion should have a biopsy. The biopsy may be incisional or excisional, but it must be full-thickness. Local control of a primary melanoma consists of a wide excision of the tumor or biopsy site. The risk of local recurrence is related more to tumor thickness than the margins of excision.

Local recurrences are not influenced by the width of the surgical margin, but are influenced by the thickness, ulceration, and site of the primary lesion. The optimal treatment of local recurrences is not known. A single local recurrence can probably be surgically excised without further therapy. Patients with multiple local recurrences, or patients with poor prognostic features, may be considered for isolated limb perfusion, hyperthermia, or high-dose fractionated radiation therapy.

Regional lymph node metastases are the most common presentation of metastatic melanoma. Any lymph node enlargement should be investigated; there is considerable controversy concerning whether a prophylactic (early) lymph node dissection or delayed lymph node dissection may be necessary. In general, patients with multiple poor prognostic variables should have early lymph node dissection. The dissection, if positive, would help identify patients with a poor prognosis who might be eligible for newer adjuvant therapy trials of chemotherapy, radiation therapy, or immunotherapy.

The treatment options for the patient with metastatic (stage III) melanoma are: no treatment, surgery, radiation therapy, chemotherapy, hyperthermia, systemic immunotherapy, and hormonal therapy. No therapy should be considered for patients who are terminally ill, who are of advanced age, or who are asymptomatic with a slow-growing lesion in a favorable site. Supportive care (e.g., pain relief) in symptomatic patients with rapidly progressive disease or with disease unresponsive to other therapy is indicated. Surgery and radiation therapy may be quite effective palliative treatments, especially for patients with skin, subcutaneous, lymph node, bone, or brain metastases.

DRUG THERAPY

Chemotherapy has not been very effective. Imidazole carboxamide (DTIC), alone or in combination with other drugs, has a response rate of about 20%. However, the use of high-dose chemotherapy with intravenous melphalan and autologous bone marrow rescue is a promising experimental approach, with approximately 60% of patients with multiple visceral metastases responding. Hyperthermia is an investigational treatment for solitary hepatic metastases or superficial lesions. Hormonal therapy has not been beneficial, nor has systemic immunotherapy with interferon or nonspecific therapy with BCG or *C. parvum*. Monoclonal antibodies, if cytotoxic, made for a specific individual patient, are an exciting new avenue of research.

PERIODIC EVALUATION

The patient with melanoma must be followed closely for the development of disseminated disease. A complete history and physical examination are most important in evaluating a patient. The history and physical examination are the most sensitive, specific, and cost-effective means of evaluating possible disseminated disease. In the absence of signs or symptoms, a minimum number of laboratory and diagnostic tests should be ordered. Serum tests of liver function and measurement of lactic dehydrogenase are important screening tests. A chest film should routinely be obtained. CT scans are helpful for evaluating patients with *suspected* disseminated disease. Radionuclide scans, although often used, are not indicated for routine screening, since the yield is less than 1%. A novel technique for detecting metastatic disease is the use of radiolabeled monoclonal antibody to melanoma antigens.

The most common clinical sites of distant metastases are skin and subcutaneous tissue, lymph nodes, lung, liver, brain, and bone. At autopsy, involvement of heart, pancreas, adrenals, kidneys, and thyroid is frequently found, but is usually clinically inapparent. The frequency of follow-up is dependent upon risk of recurrence. Patients with stage I thin (< 0.76 mm) lesions are a low-risk group and require yearly follow-up. Stage I patients with lesions > 0.76 mm require more frequent follow-up (every three months for two years, every four months for an additional year, and every six months thereafter). The vast majority of metastases occur within three years. Stage II patients (with lymph node metastases) who progress to distant sites usually do so within one to two years. Therefore, these patients should be followed every three months for the first two years, every six months for an additional three years, and then yearly.

Familial Dysplastic Nevus Syndrome

Dysplastic nevi, with an autosomal dominant inheritance, are the clinical markers and histogenic precursors of melanoma in numbers of many melanoma-prone families. Recent estimates indicate 32,000 people have familial dysplastic nevi, and as many as 4,600,000 people in the United States may have an acquired dysplastic, preneoplastic nevus. Members of families with hereditary melanoma with acquired melanocytic precursors are several hundred times more likely to have melanoma than are persons in the general population. Since dysplastic nevi fall between the common acquired nevi and malignant melanoma, they provide an opportunity to manage melanoma earlier in its natural history when cure is possible. The importance of the dysplastic nevi in facilitating detection and prevention of melanoma is undisputed. The clinical characteristics of the dysplastic nevi also fall between the characteristics of the common acquired nevi and malignant melanoma. Thus, the dysplastic nevi have qualities that fall in a spectrum of findings, of which no single feature is known to be reliably predictive. However, there are some clinical features that should raise the possibility of dysplastic nevi, especially in patients with familial melanoma. Dysplastic nevi range in size from 6 to 15 mm, which usually is larger than common moles. They most often occur after puberty (later than moles), and the distribution, while often similar to common moles, also occurs on the more unusual sites of the scalp, buttocks, and female breast. The color, shape, and texture of the lesion may be a clue. Irregular, variegate-colored macular lesions are often dysplastic. The presence of or development of black in lesions that otherwise appear dysplastic must be biopsied to exclude the diagnosis of melanoma, since one fifth to one third of primary melanomas have remnants of dysplastic precursor.

Dysplastic nevi have been classified into four types, with increasing risk of developing melanoma: A—nonfamilial dysplastic nevi, with no family history; B—familial history of dysplastic nevi; C—personal history of dysplastic nevi and melanoma, but family history of neither; D—family history of one (type D1) or at least two (type D2 or B-K mole syndrome) family members with both dysplastic nevi and melanoma.

Treatment and management of patients from high-risk groups with dysplastic nevi include excisional biopsy of two or three representative lesions to confirm the diagnosis. Any nevi suggestive of melanoma should also be removed. Serial, total body skin examinations with photographs should be performed every six months by a physician and monthly by the patient. Excision of any changing lesions should be performed. Prophylactic excision is not recommended, except for scalp lesions, for lesions occurring in patients with impaired immune function, or in patients with inadequate access for appropriate follow-up. Exposure to sunlight should be minimized. As always, the key to early diagnosis is a *changing lesion*.

REFERENCES

Balch CM, Murad TM, Soong S-J, et al: A multifactorial analysis of melanoma: prognostic histopathological features comparing Clark's and Breslow's staging methods. Ann Surg 188:732–742, 1978.

Balch CM, Soong S-J, Shaw HM: A comparison of worldwide melanoma data. *In* Balch CM, Milton GW, Shaw HM, Soong S-J (eds): Cutaneous Melanoma: Clinical Management and Treatment Results Worldwide. J.B. Lippincott Co, Philadelphia, 1985, pp 507–518.

Greene MH, Clark WH, Tucker MA, et al: Acquired precursors of cutaneous malignant melanoma: the familial dysplastic nevus syndrome. N Engl J Med 312:91–94, 1985.

Lazarus HM, Herzig RH, Graham-Pole J, et al: Intensive melphalan chemotherapy and cryopreserved autologous bone marrow transplantation for the treatment of refractory cancer. J Clin Oncol 1:359–367, 1983.

McGovern VJ, Murad TM: Pathology of melanoma: an overview. *In* Balch CM, Milton GW, Shaw HM, Soong S-J (eds): Cutaneous Melanoma: Clinical Management and Treatment Results Worldwide. J.B. Lippincott Co, Philadelphia, 1985, pp 29–53.

Mihm MC Jr, Fitzpatrick TB, Lane-Brown MM, et al: Early detection of primary cutaneous melanoma: a color atlas. N Engl J Med 289:989–996, 1973.

27 · BRAIN TUMORS

Robert F. Saul
GEISINGER MEDICAL CENTER

DEFINITION AND DIAGNOSTIC CRITERIA

Primary central nervous system tumors caused an estima'ed 12,000 deaths in the United States in 1984. This was less than the anticipated 175,000 patients who died from stroke, but still represents a sizable number. Fewer neurologic illnesses cause greater fear in patients than the diagnosis of malignant brain tumor. Fifteen thousand primary brain tumors are diagnosed in the United States annually, and of these, approximately 45% are found to be malignant glioma. Men slightly outnumber women, and the peak incidence is in the sixth and seventh decades. Genetic and viral causes have been explored, but to date no clear etiologic factor has been found.

PATHOPHYSIOLOGY

Astrocytomas (gliomas) are classified by grades I to IV with grades III and IV being most malignant. Gliomas infiltrate neural tissue, making early diagnosis difficult and total removal impossible. Although they may originate anywhere in the central nervous system, these tumors are confined almost entirely to the supratentorial area in adults. Occasionally, metastases may occur to the spinal cord and the cauda equina.

CLINICAL ASPECTS

The clinical history and examination are still the most important clues to the diagnosis after a lesion is seen neuroradiologically. I most commonly see the middle-aged man or woman brought in by a family member. There may be a history of a progressive loss of use of one side of the body, which is frequently accompanied by a change in mental status. Headache is not a common presenting complaint. The key to the diagnosis is the history of a slowly progressive neurologic dysfunction. However, a small number of gliomas may hemorrhage into a zone of necrosis and produce a clinical picture indistinguishable from an ischemic infarction or a hypertensive hemorrhage. One third of the patients will present with seizures. Obstruction of the ventricular system may cause the patient to present with severe headaches, nausea, vomiting, ataxia, and papilledema. Meningeal gliomatosis may be indistinguishable from pseudotumor cerebri initially. After several months it is apparent that pseudotumor is not the correct diagnosis, as the patient then begins to develop focal neurologic signs and symptoms.

MANAGEMENT

NONPHARMACOLOGIC MEASURES

Management of a suspected malignant glioma depends on the patient's general physical and mental condition to withstand either a stereotaxic biopsy or a craniotomy. The correct diagnosis must be made, since metastatic cancer, cerebral abscess, giant aneurysm, meningioma, and chronic isodense subdural hematomas are in the differential. Less commonly, tuberculomas and syphilitic gummas may have a similar appearance on CT. The CT will show the tumor 98% of the time, but occasionally an early infiltrating mass will be missed. NMR is now being used with success in some of the "CT"-negative lesions, and is recommended when clinical suspicion is high.

Fifty per cent of malignant gliomas are isodense or of low density on an unenhanced CT, but, in almost every case, will enhance with contrast. Usually extending "fingers" of edema produce a shift of the ventricles or the choroid plexus. The forepart of the brain is the most common site, with frontal and temporal lobes equally affected. These tumors are rarely seen in the occipital lobes.

Deep-seated thalamic lesions are best approached by stereotaxic CT-guided biopsy. Frontal and temporal masses, especially nondominant hemisphere tumors, should be reached through a craniotomy with the intent to debulk as much of the tumor as possible. Surgery is still the mainstay to therapy. The goals of the surgical procedure, according to Shapiro, are (1) establishing a diagnosis, (2) debulking the tumor, (3) improving symptoms, (4) buying time for other therapeutic modalities to work, and (5) increasing tumor sensitivity to radiation and chemotherapy by stimulating surviving cells to undergo mitosis.

Following surgery, whole head radiation therapy (RT) up to 60 Gy is recommended. For surgically inaccessible lesions, radiation port can be coned down to deliver 20 Gy. The other 40 Gy rads can be given to the whole brain through the regular ports. We have found that radiation after surgery will provide the patient an extra three to six months of quality life. Recently, however, I have had some patients with particularly aggressive tumors who survived less than four months after the diagnosis was made. A CT scan should be done one to two weeks postoperatively to help the radiotherapist see the resection site and the boundaries of the remaining tumor.

DRUG THERAPY

Chemotherapy is still investigational and is not routinely employed at all institutions. Nitrosoureas are the mainstays of therapy. Our results have generally been poor, failing to prolong the quality of life beyond what radiation has already accomplished. Cooperative groups have shown a median survival of 50 weeks in some patients treated with surgery, radiation, and carmustine (BiCNU). Direct intracarotid injections of BiCNU have shown some promising responses in patients at other institutions. However, the complications of seizures, retinal infarction, and cerebral edema have occurred in almost half of some groups of patients treated. One must consider this approach in relation to the needs of the patient.

Generally, I place all patients on dexamethasone, in doses of 2 to 4 mg every six hours, to control edema. This does seem to sometimes improve a hemiparesis caused by the mass effect, and I have observed reduction in the number of seizures in many patients. All patients are placed on anticonvulsants. Phenytoin is the drug of choice for generalized major motor seizures, and carbamazepine for partial seizures with complex symptoms. The latter drug is used mainly for lesions involving the temporal lobe.

Adult patients taking 300 mg to 400 mg of phenytoin a day in one to three divided doses will generally reach therapeutic levels, but should be monitored regularly. Carbamazepine must be increased gradually because of sedation and diplopia. Begin with 200 mg a day, adding 100 mg (½ tablet) every day as tolerated, until reaching 800 mg to 1200 mg a day, in four divided doses. Elderly patients may require less. The half-life of carbamazepine is about 12 hours and is best given in four doses. Phenytoin may be given once a day, but I recommend twice daily, in case the patient is forgetful, thereby averting the loss of a total daily dose.

COMPLICATIONS

Operative complications, including herniation, postoperative infections with secondary cerebral abscess, or osteomyelitis of a bone flap, occasionally occur. Intracerebral hemorrhage, secondary to necrosis and edema, may also develop. Subdural hematomas can occur after a large debulking procedure. Seizures or toxic reactions to anticonvulsants are not uncommon. Possibly a third of patients living three years or longer will experience white matter degeneration from radiation. Neuropsychological changes may also occur secondary to the radiation. When postoperative meningitis is suspected after the patient has been discharged, a CT scan should be done, before any lumbar puncture, to determine the degree of possible swelling and shift of the ventricles.

PERIODIC EVALUATION

I generally see the patient at monthly intervals if no chemotherapy is given. A repeat CT scan is done several months postradiation. The patient's history and the clinical exam will often determine the need for a CT at an earlier date. It is recommended that patients receiving chemotherapy should have repeat CT scans at two- to six-month intervals until stabilization is reached.

I do not recommend reoperation on any patient even after all the therapeutic choices have been exhausted. Reoperation is not proven to be of benefit and can lead to further neurologic demise.

Finally, above all, the patient's family needs to be told what to expect. The patient should get his or her life in order, and be allowed to participate in the choice of therapy. I inform all my patients of the options and expectations of therapy. The physician should constantly offer support, and let the patient know that he will attend to any complications. When a tumor defies all attempts to thwart its recurrence, the patient needs to be allowed to die with dignity. Heroic measures are not indicated in these patients. The ability to terminate therapy can be learned with experience, and although never easy, it is best handled on an individual basis, governed by the doctor-patient-family relationship.

REFERENCES

Apuzzo MLJ, Chandrasoma PT, Zelman V, et al: Computed tomographic guidance stereotaxis in the management of lesions of the third ventricular region. Neurosurgery 15:502–508, 1984.
Greenburg HS, Ensminger WD, Chandler WF, et al: Intra-arterial BCNU chemotherapy for treatment of malignant gliomas of the central nervous system. J Neurosurg 61:423–429, 1984.
MacCabe JJ: Glioblastoma. *In* Vinken PJ, Bruyn GW (eds): Handbook of Clinical Neurology, Vol 18. Elsevier, New York 1975, pp. 49–71.
Shapiro WR: Treatment of neuroectodermal brain tumors. Ann Neurol 12:231–237, 1982.
Walker MD: Malignant neural tumors. *In* Johnson RT (ed): Current Therapy in Neurologic Disease. C.V. Mosby Co, St. Louis, 1985, pp 210–216.
Walker RW, Posner JB: Central nervous system neoplasms. *In* Appel SH (ed): Current Neurology, Vol 5. John Wiley and Sons, New York, 1984, pp 285–322.

28 · SOFT TISSUE AND BONE SARCOMAS

G. Thomas Budd
CLEVELAND CLINIC FOUNDATION

Soft Tissue Sarcomas

DEFINITION AND DIAGNOSTIC CRITERIA

The term "sarcoma," originally applied to "fleshy tumors," is an imprecise term referring to malignant tumors composed primarily of connective tissue cells, usually derived from the embryonic mesoderm. Sarcomas are best considered as being of either soft tissue or bony origin.

PATHOPHYSIOLOGY

Soft tissue sarcomas may arise from fibrous tissue (fibrosarcoma), muscle (rhabdomyosarcoma, leiomyosarcoma), synovium (synovial cell sarcoma), adipose tissue (liposarcoma), nerve (malignant schwannoma), vascular or lymphatic tissue (angiosarcoma, malignant hemangiopericytoma, lymphangiosarcoma), or other connective tissues (malignant fibrous histiocytoma, giant cell sarcoma, Kaposi's sarcoma, mesothelioma, clear cell sarcoma, epithelioid sarcoma, alveolar soft part sarcoma). Differentiation between these malignancies is often difficult, and while a specific histologic diagnosis should be sought, of more value to the clinician is an estimation of histopathologic grade, an important indicator of biologic aggressiveness. Because of the difficulties involved in making a histogenic diagnosis and because of the importance of tumor grade, soft tissue sarcomas are generally considered as a group when reporting treatment results and making clinical decisions.

In the majority of cases of soft tissue sarcoma, no etiologic factors can be identified. No major role for a hereditary factor in the development of most cases of soft tissue sarcoma is present. The strongest etiologic link with a carcinogen has been that between hepatic angiosarcoma and vinyl chloride; this tumor is also associated with exposure to the radioactive radiologic contrast agent Thorotrast. Soft tissue and osteogenic sarcomas have been seen as a late complication of radiation therapy, appearing in the radiation field 10 years or more after high-dose radiation therapy. Trauma and foreign bodies have played roles in legal proceedings out of proportion to their roles in the pathogenesis of soft tissue sarcoma. Viruses have been shown to cause soft tissue sarcomas in a variety of animal models, but clear evidence of a viral etiology has not been found in humans. Ongoing studies of viral and cellular oncogenes may aid in our understanding of these tumors on the molecular level and represent an exciting avenue for future research.

CLINICAL ASPECTS

Soft tissue sarcoma typically presents as a painless mass. Soft tissue sarcomas may present in virtually any organ, owing to the ubiquitous presence of connective tissue, but the proximal portion of a lower extremity is the most frequent site. Forty per cent of cases will present in the lower extremity, with head and neck, retroperitoneal, other truncal, and upper extremity presentations each representing about 15% of cases. Nodal metastases are unusual except in synovial cell sarcoma, rhabdomyosarcoma, and epithelioid sarcoma. Prophylactic lymph node dissection is not routinely necessary.

The diagnosis of all sarcomas, like that of any malignancy, is a histologic diagnosis. The biopsy procedure is of great importance, because an improperly performed biopsy can compromise or complicate definitive treatment. In general, needle biopsies yield insufficient material to assure the determination of histologic subtype and tumor grade and should be performed only to confirm recurrence or metastasis of an already characterized primary lesion. Cutting needle biopsies are somewhat more definitive, but should not be considered adequate in routine practice.

Soft tissue sarcomas are characterized by a "pseudocapsule" of fibrous tissue compressed by the centripetal growth of the tumor. Malignant cells are contained in this layer of compressed tissue so that enucleation will leave residual tumor cells behind. Because excisional biopsy is inadequate therapeutically and can compromise tissue planes, it is generally contraindicated in all but some small (less than 3 cm) lesions. Incisional biopsy is the biopsy procedure of choice in the majority of cases of soft tissue sarcoma. The biopsy site must be completely resected at the time of the definitive procedure, so the placement of the biopsy site must be chosen with care, keeping in mind such considerations as the future use of skin grafts and the assurance of good hemostasis so as to prevent the development of a large hematoma contaminated with tumor cells. Incisional biopsies of extremity lesions should be done longitudinally along the involved muscle group. Appropriate radiologic studies of the primary lesion include CT scan, xerogram or soft tissue x-ray film, and in some cases angiography. Bone scan, bone x-ray films, and electromyographic studies are indicated in selected cases. Chest roentgenogram and chest CT or tomography should be performed to rule out pulmonary metastasis.

MANAGEMENT

NONPHARMACOLOGIC MEASURES

Surgical resection is the mainstay of local treatment. The surgical procedure must be guided by the knowledge that soft tissue sarcomas tend to spread along structures within an anatomic compartment. Surgical procedures may be classified as (1) excisional biopsy: removal of all gross tumor and pseudocapsule (recurrence rate 80% or more); (2) wide excision: removal of the tumor with a several centimeter margin of uninvolved tissue but not removing the entirety of the involved anatomic compartment (50% local recurrence rate); or (3) radical local excision: removal of the entire anatomic compartment containing the tumor (local recurrence rate 20% or less). The addition of high-dose megavoltage radiation therapy to a wide excision may yield local recurrence rates similar to those obtained by radical local excision. Local control is more difficult to achieve with nonextremity tumors and postoperative radiation therapy is often given to such patients.

With adequate treatment, then, less than 20% of patients should suffer local recurrences; 80% of the local recurrences occur in the first two years postoperatively. Follow-up of patients after therapy is guided by the tendency of these tumors to recur locally or in the lungs during the first two years. Physical examinations and chest films at two- to three-month intervals are recommended during the first two postoperative years, every three to six months for the next three years, and yearly thereafter.

Despite the success of local treatment of soft tissue sarcoma, the five-year survival in most series has been approximately 50%, owing to the development of distant metastases. These metastases nearly always present initially in the lungs, although retroperitoneal sarcomas may spread first to the liver. Approximately 20% of patients presenting with pulmonary metastases may be salvaged by an aggressive combination of surgical resection and chemotherapy.

DRUG THERAPY

Postoperative chemotherapy in high-grade (grades II to III) soft tissue sarcoma is a controversial subject. Most randomized studies have been unable to show an improved survival in patients receiving adjuvant chemotherapy compared with patients who are followed closely and treated aggressively at the time of relapse. A survival advantage for adjuvant chemotherapy in patients with extremity sarcomas has been shown in an NCI study in which patients receiving chemotherapy have a projected actuarial five-year survival of 86% as compared with 51% for those patients randomized to observation. Further investigation of how chemotherapy may be best integrated with local therapy is needed.

Current chemotherapy of soft tissue sarcoma is based on the activity of doxorubicin (Adriamycin), which can produce responses in 25% to 30% of patients when used as a single agent. There is substantial clinical evidence for an increasing response rate with an increasing dose of Adriamycin, and the maximally tolerated dose of this drug should be used. Other agents used include DTIC (dacarbazine), cyclophosphamide, actinomycin D, vincristine, and cisplatin. Combinations of these agents produce response rates of 30% to 50%. Adriamycin-containing combinations have been uniformly superior to the regimens not including this drug. The median survival of patients treated for metastatic soft tissue sarcoma with chemotherapy is just under one year, but a small number will have complete and prolonged responses.

Bone Sarcomas

DEFINITION

Over 85% of bone tumors seen will be benign. Even the most common malignant bone tumor, osteogenic sarcoma, is rare, with only 2500 cases diagnosed yearly in the United States. The next most common malignancy of bone is chondrosarcoma, a tumor that typically presents in the proximal extremity of an adult. The third most common malignant bone tumor is Ewing's sarcoma, an aggressive tumor that most commonly presents in a teenager and may produce systemic symptoms of fever and weight loss.

PATHOPHYSIOLOGY

The diagnosis of osteosarcoma is a pathologic one with incisional biopsy being the procedure of choice in most cases. The histologic hallmarks are osteoid production in the presence of malignant cells. Histologic differentiation from a recent fracture or myositis ossificans may be difficult, and radiologic and physical examinations should be considered when making the diagnosis. Lymph node metastases are unusual, while hematogenous spread tends to produce pulmonary metastases in a typical subpleural distribution.

CLINICAL ASPECTS

Osteogenic sarcoma typically presents as a painful bone lesion in a patient between the ages of 10 and 25 years. A late peak in incidence is seen in adulthood, due largely to osteosarcoma secondary to Paget's disease of bone, radiation, or chronic osteomyelitis. Osteosarcoma most commonly occurs in the metaphysis of a long bone of an extremity, with the majority of cases occurring about the knee and the shoulder.

MANAGEMENT

NONPHARMACOLOGIC MEASURES

Surgery has been the classic approach to the control of the primary tumor, with a 10-cm margin proximal to any physical or radiographic evidence of disease being sought. Limb salvage procedures, often involving bone allografts or endoprostheses, are now being used, often in conjunction with preoperative or postoperative chemotherapy. Surgery may also be useful for resecting pulmonary metastases.

DRUG THERAPY

The role of chemotherapy as a postsurgical adjuvant is an area of controversy. Uncontrolled studies employing adjuvant chemotherapy with high-dose methotrexate or doxorubicin-containing regimens have shown a marked improvement in the five-year survival rate to 40% to 50% as compared with historical series indicating a 20% survival rate with surgery alone. Prospective, randomized trials have proved difficult to perform, but no improvement in overall survival has been shown for adjuvant chemotherapy, although relapse-free survival may be improved. Proponents of chemotherapy have now begun trials employing preoperative drug treatment, tailoring the postoperative adjuvant program according to the results of preoperative chemotherapy. This approach has resulted in a two-year disease-free survival of over 90%.

A variety of chemotherapeutic agents have been used in the treatment of metastatic osteosarcoma, including high-dose methotrexate with leucovorin rescue, doxorubicin, cisplatin, bleomycin, cyclophosphamide, and dactinomycin. Response rates of 20% to 60% have been reported.

In no other tumor system can the use of a multimodal approach to therapy be shown to be of more importance than in the treatment of soft tissue and bone sarcomas. With modern techniques of surgery, radiation, and chemotherapy, the prognosis of these tumors has improved greatly, and every effort should be made to ensure that patients with these tumors are treated in a setting that allows multi-modality therapy to be given by a team of physicians familiar with these tumors.

REFERENCES

Edmonson JH: Role of adjuvant chemotherapy in the management of patients with soft-tissue sarcomas. Cancer Treat Rep 68:1063–1066, 1984.

Lange B, Levine AS: Is it ethical not to conduct a prospectively controlled trial of adjuvant chemotherapy in osteosarcoma? Cancer Treat Rep 66:1699–1703, 1982.

Rosen G, Nirenberg A: Chemotherapy for osteogenic sarcoma: an investigative method, not a recipe. Cancer Treat Rep 66:1687–1697, 1982.

Rosenberg SA: Prospective randomized trials demonstrating the efficacy of adjuvant chemotherapy in adult patients with soft tissue sarcomas. Cancer Treat Rep 68:1067–1078, 1984.

Sears HF (ed): Soft tissue sarcomas. Semin Oncol 8:129–240, 1981.

29 · BREAST CANCER

Joseph D. Purvis
CLEVELAND CLINIC FOUNDATION

DEFINITION AND DIAGNOSTIC CRITERIA

Breast cancer is among the most common malignancies in the United States, accounting for one fourth of all cancers and one fifth of all cancer deaths in women. Its clinical behavior is very heterogeneous. Some patients have indolent disease, and may live for many years with metastatic disease. Other patients, with apparently early disease, rapidly develop visceral metastases and die despite aggressive therapy. This has led to heated controversies about management, evoking emotional arguments even from experienced investigators at times. We now understand some of the prognostic factors that account for divergent clinical behavior, but many questions remain. Our current challenge is to attempt to answer these questions while providing the best of individual care.

Breast cancer should be suspected in any woman with a palpable mass in the breast even though the majority of breast lumps are benign. False-negative mammograms do occur, especially in young women with dense breasts. It is certainly true that breast cancer is uncommon under the age of 30. Unfortunately, young women are likely to have more aggressive, hormone receptor-negative disease. Therefore, any palpable mass should be aspirated or biopsied, even in the presence of a negative mammogram. Needle aspiration cytology can rapidly confirm the presence of benign cyst or malignancy, eliminating the need for more invasive procedures. Likewise, a mammogram suggestive of malignancy should be pursued, even in the absence of a palpable mass.

PATHOPHYSIOLOGY

The causes of breast cancer are largely unknown. Family history, early menarche, the presence of some subtypes of benign breast disease, older age at first pregnancy, and late menopause are all risk factors for the development of breast cancer. While dietary fat intake may play a role, the data suggesting this are inconclusive and should be interpreted with caution.

Although squamous breast cancer does occur, nearly all breast cancers are histologically adenocarcinomas, of which about two thirds are infiltrating duct carcinomas. Most other histologic types seem to carry a somewhat better overall prognosis. These include medullary, lobular invasive, papillary, tubular, and mucinous carcinomas. The diagnosis of inflammatory breast cancer is made clinically by the presence of warmth and skin redness with induration and a demarcated border, and pathologically by the presence of tumor cells in dermal lymphatics. Histologically, inflammatory breast cancer is most often a poorly differentiated adenocarcinoma.

CLINICAL ASPECTS

Both clinical and pathologic staging are used in the assessment of patients with breast cancer. These systems are well described in most textbooks and therefore will not be presented here. Clinical staging systems are most useful in comparing groups of patients who have not had comparable axillary node dissections for staging, whereas pathologic staging tends to predict overall prognosis somewhat better. In patients with apparently localized disease, the most important prognostic factors are (1) extent of axillary nodal involvement, (2) estrogen and progesterone receptor values, and (3) size of the primary tumor. Primary tumor size in excess of 3 cm carries a worse prognosis, as does the presence of four or more involved axillary nodes. In addition, estrogen and progesterone receptor-negative tumors have a predilection for early and visceral-dominant recurrence, and carry a worse general prognosis. Estrogen (ER) or progesterone receptor values of less than 3 femtomoles (fm) are considered negative; values between 3 and 10 are considered borderline; and values over 10 are considered positive. The likelihood of a hormonal response increases with rising receptor values, with values of ER greater than 100 corresponding to a response rate over 50% in advanced disease. Patients with strongly positive estrogen receptors are more likely to have positive progesterone receptors. Generally, about 65% of premenopausal patients have negative receptor values and about the same percentage of postmenopausal patients

have positive receptors. In some series the relapse rate for patients with negative receptors and no axillary involvement was similar to that for patients with positive receptor values and axillary node involvement, indicating that both factors are important indicators of prognosis.

Prior to local therapy, patients should be evaluated for the presence of distant metastatic disease. This should include a careful history and physical examination with particular attention to regional lymph nodes, skin, bone tenderness or pain, and liver size. Laboratory evaluation should include CBC and liver enzymes (AST, LDH, alkaline phosphatase). In the absence of bone pain or tenderness, bone scans usually do not show metastatic disease. However, benign abnormalities are frequent enough that a baseline bone scan is helpful in high-risk patients. Liver or brain scans are rarely positive in the absence of clinical evidence of metastases. Because lung metastases are often asymptomatic, an initial chest film should be done. An elevated LDH in the absence of evaluation of AST should raise the question of marrow involvement, even with normal blood counts. A sector scan of the chest wall can detect internal mammary node enlargement in the patient with an inner quadrant tumor and axillary involvement.

Patients with metastatic disease should have a complete baseline evaluation in order that response to therapy can be assessed. This should include laboratory studies as indicated above along with serum calcium. Although it should not be used as a primary marker, an elevated CEA value may be of assistance in evaluating response to therapy. Bone and liver scans are useful here, as well as x-ray films of spine and femurs (full length) if the bone scan suggests involvement. Lytic disease in the pelvis or skull can sometimes provide a measurable lesion to assess response.

MANAGEMENT

PLAN

The initial goals of management should be staging and treatment planning. In patients with localized disease, assessment of prognostic factors will permit consideration of systemic adjuvant therapy and possible participation in investigational programs. If mastectomy has been performed, reconstruction should be an important part of the overall treatment plan. The long-term goals for such patients include observation for second primary cancers as well as recurrence, since a significant proportion will achieve long-term disease control.

Metastatic breast cancer is not considered to be a curable disease. However, the majority of patients respond to therapy, and some patients (usually hormone responders) can live well with metastatic disease for as long as 10 years or more. The short-term goal here is to obtain a partial or complete remission of systemic disease; the long-term goal is control of disease with minimum morbidity.

NONPHARMACOLOGIC MEASURES

The traditional treatment for local breast cancer has been surgery. The original Halsted radical mastectomy and the extended radical mastectomy of Urban were based on the theory that regional lymph node involvement was an important cause of systemic relapse. It now appears that regional lymph node involvement is an indicator rather than a determinant of biologic behavior. Since there are several local treatment options that provide good local control, the treatment decision should be based on the patient's desires as well as the clinical situation. For the patient with multifocal disease, a large tumor (which would preclude a good cosmetic result from wide excision), or a reluctance to make the time commitment required by radiation therapy, a modified radical mastectomy with subsequent reconstruction may be the best option. Hospitalization can be shortened to as little as two days if the patient is willing to manage a small drain and return for outpatient evaluation. Immediate reconstructive surgery, especially for low-risk patients, is currently being evaluated.

Evidence has now emerged indicating that wide local excision with axillary staging followed by radiation therapy as suggested by Hellman and others provides freedom from local relapse that is equivalent to that seen with modified radical or radical mastectomy. This technique, although it requires five to seven weeks of daily treatments, can provide excellent cosmetic results without the necessity for subsequent reconstruction. Axillary dissection is done here for staging in order that appropriate decisions can be made concerning systemic therapy.

In recent years, the question has been raised as to whether patients would fare as well with wide local excision (partial mastectomy or "lumpectomy") and axillary dissection without radiation therapy. Clinical trials are underway to answer this question, but it will be several years before meaningful results are available. Presently, such treatment should be considered investigational, but may be appropriate for selected patients. Possible candidates for such treatment include the older patient with limited disease and strongly positive hormone receptor values.

For the patient with inflammatory carcinoma or with locally extensive disease, the most effective local therapy is radiation therapy, which is often able to provide local control in these patients for whom control of systemic disease is so crucial. Radiation therapy is often of benefit for local problems due to metastatic disease, such as spine metastasis (with or without spinal cord compression), brain metastasis, or painful bone metastasis.

DRUG THERAPY

The patient with metastatic breast cancer should be evaluated carefully before a choice of therapy is made. With few exceptions, biopsy proof of the presence of metastatic disease should be obtained, since benign diseases (such as hepatic cysts or osteoporosis with vertebral collapse) can occasionally mimic metastasis on scan or x-ray film. Sites of involvement and rate of progression should be assessed, if possible. Reasonable attempts to obtain hormone receptor studies are warranted, since conversion from receptor-positive to receptor-negative is seen. Because tamoxifen binds competitively to the estrogen receptor, patients who have been taking tamoxifen within the previous two to four weeks will show a negative estrogen receptor on biopsy.

Combination Chemotherapy. Combination chemotherapy is essential for the patient with negative hormone receptors, hormone-refractory disease, progressive visceral disease, or inflammatory breast cancer. Useful combinations without doxorubicin include CMF with or without VP (cyclophosphamide, methotrexate, 5-fluorouracil, vincristine, and prednisone). Complete and partial response rate (CR + PR) of 50% to 65% are seen with such combinations, and responses are usually of significant palliative benefit. Adriamycin-based combinations such as FAC (5-fluorouracil, doxorubicin, cyclophosphamide) can produce responses in as many as 70% of patients, and may produce longer responses. However, doxorubicin also adds to the toxicity of such programs the risk of cardiotoxicity and substantial hair loss. A review of the literature by Livingston suggested that anthracyclines such as doxorubicin might be particularly active against receptor-negative breast cancer; however, this is as yet unconfirmed by clinical trial. Unless the patient is participating in a clinical trial, the choice of chemotherapy program is a matter of individual clinical judgment.

Hormonal Therapy. The premenopausal patient with receptor-positive or bone and soft tissue-dominant disease may be a good candidate for hormonal therapy. The initial hormonal therapy of choice is oophorectomy, which is usually done surgically rather than by radiation. Tamoxifen, 10 mg b.i.d., is a possible choice for the patient who declines ovarian ablation, but there is at least a theoretical possibility that rising FSH and LH levels could increase ovarian estrogen and overcome the competitive binding by tamoxifen. Patients who respond to an initial hormonal manipulation should be considered for further hormonal therapy, since the best predictor of a hormonal response is a prior hormonal response. Second-line hormonal options include tamoxifen, "medical adrenalectomy" with aminoglutethimide, 250 mg b.i.d. twice weekly, then 250 mg q.i.d., hydrocortisone, 20 mg AM, 20 mg PM, 40 mg h.s. for two weeks, then 10 mg AM, 10 mg PM, and 20 mg h.s.; and fluoxymesterone, 10 mg b.i.d. Surgical adrenalectomy and hypophysectomy are not commonly used because of their morbidity and the availability of other treatments, especially combination chemotherapy.

The postmenopausal patient with positive hormone receptors or indolent disease is a candidate for additive hormonal therapy. In such patients, tamoxifen is commonly used because of its lack of significant side effects or drawbacks, other than expense. Diethylstilbestrol (DES), 5 mg t.i.d., is as effective at a much lower cost. However, DES is associated with a substantial incidence of vascular and cardiac side effects. Interestingly, about one fourth or more of patients who respond to DES will again respond when the drug is withdrawn once progression occurs. Other additive hormones include fluoxymesterone, megestrol acetate, and aminoglutethimide.

Simultaneous Hormonal Therapy and Chemotherapy. Simultaneous hormonal therapy and chemotherapy can be used in the patient with rapidly progressive disease and positive receptor values, but has not been shown to be better than chemotherapy alone. Although a trial of eight weeks is usually required to assess for hormonal response, progression or lack of response may require the addition of chemotherapy without an adequate hormonal trial. Under these conditions it may be best to continue both treatments until progression occurs.

Palliative radiation therapy, although very effective, should not be substituted for systemic therapy. The patient who requires radiation therapy more than eight weeks after a change of therapy probably has progressive systemic disease and should be evaluated for such.

Special Considerations. Systemic adjuvant chemotherapy for patients with involved axillary nodes continues to be controversial. Several programs such as CMF, CMFVP, and FAC seem to produce improvements in disease-free survival and possibly survival for premenopausal patients with involved nodes. Unfortunately, the best-controlled studies seem to have been done with marginal dose levels. The Southwest Oncology Group has shown CMFVP to be superior to oral melphalan in both pre- and postmenopausal patients for survival as well as median survival, but this study antedates common availability of receptor testing. Adjuvant hormonal therapy is not new, but needs to be reevaluated. We know that oophorectomy was ineffective in unselected patients, but most premenopausal patients are receptor-negative. The Europeans have provided some data, although preliminary, that suggest that tamoxifen alone may benefit postmenopausal receptor-positive patients. Currently, patients who are eligible should be offered participation in adjuvant trials in an attempt to answer the following questions: (1) Does oophorectomy add to chemotherapy for premenopausal ER-positive patients? (2) Does tamoxifen add to chemotherapy, or is tamoxifen alone as effective as chemotherapy for postmenopausal patients with positive receptors? (3) Is Adriamycin-base aggressive chemotherapy more effective for receptor-negative disease? (4) Might systemic therapy be more effective if given immediately after, or even before, surgery? (5) Is there a role for adjuvant therapy for ER-negative stage I patients?

Premenopausal patients with involved nodes who are ineligible for or decline participation in such trials should be offered chemotherapy with or without oophorectomy, depending on receptors and individual judgment. Postmenopausal patients with positive receptors and involved nodes can be offered tamoxifen, combination chemotherapy, both, or observation, depending on the situation. Patients with negative receptors should be considered for chemotherapy, unless precluded by medical condition or the patient's wishes.

PATIENT INFORMATION AND EDUCATION

Patient education should be focused toward several ends. The general public needs to understand the value of self-examination and mammography, especially for high-risk groups. Better knowledge of options for treatments and reconstruction may help patients who would otherwise delay evaluation because of fear and pessimism about treatment. Women with localized breast cancer need to be helped to understand the various treatment options available so that they can be actively involved in decisions about their treatment. Patients with advanced disease need clear explanation of appropriate treatment options, goals of treatment, and possible side effects.

PERIODIC EVALUATION

Patients with localized disease should be seen at two- to three-month intervals during the first year, increasing to four- to six-month intervals after two years, depending on risk status. Follow-up evaluation should include an interim history and physical, CBC, and liver enzymes. Chest roentgenograms should be done every six months for three years and yearly thereafter. Patients with a history of breast cancer should have yearly mammography to screen for a second primary cancer. Bone, liver, and brain scans should be done if metastasis is suggested by history, examination, or laboratory testing. Patients with metastatic disease should be followed at 1- to 3-month intervals, depending on remission status and pace of their disease.

PATIENT COMPLIANCE

Patient compliance is largely a function of the success or failure of patient education. Patients who understand their disease and who are getting adequate support usually comply well with treatment, especially if they have been participants in decision-making.

PREVENTIVE MEASURES

Although a number of risk factors for the development of breast cancer are known, there are currently no effective preventive measures. We can hope, however, that a deeper understanding of the cellular biology of breast cancer will provide us with means to decrease the morbidity and mortality of this common disease.

SOCIOECONOMIC ASPECTS OF TREATMENT

Breast cancer is an exceedingly expensive disease for our society, in terms of lives and productivity lost as well as cost of medical care. Early detection and better treatment offer the promise of significant improvements, but many questions remain unanswered. The challenge is to find answers to these questions in an environment of rapidly diminishing dollars for biomedical research.

REFERENCES

Bonnadonna G, Valagussa P: Adjuvant systemic therapy for resectable breast cancer. J Clin Oncol 3:259–275, 1985.

Croton R, Cooke T, et al: Oestrogen receptor and survival in early breast cancer. Br Med J 283:1289–1291, 1981.

Fisher B, et al.: Five-year results of a randomized clinical trial comparing total mastectomy and segmental mastectomy with or without radiation in the treatment of breast cancer. N Engl J Med 312:665–673, 1985.

Fisher B, et al: Ten-year results of a randomized clinical trial comparing radical mastectomy and total mastectomy with or without radiation. N Engl J Med 312:674–681, 1985.

Harris JR, Hellman S, Silen W: Conservative Management of Breast Cancer. J. B. Lippincott Co, 1983.

Henderson IC, Canellos CP: Cancer of the breast: the past decade. N Engl J Med 302:17–30, 78–90, 1980.

Livingston, RB: Breast cancer and response to chemotherapy: a possible relationship of hormone receptors and doxorubicin. Cancer Treat Rev 9:229–236, 1982.

30 · TUMOR LYSIS SYNDROME

Jane A. Gehlsen
MARSHFIELD CLINIC

DEFINITION

The tumor lysis syndrome is a metabolic derangement that is the direct result of the death of a large number of malignant cells. Generally, the involved tumors have a very rapid growth rate and are exquisitely sensitive to therapy, but rarely, this syndrome may occur from spontaneous tumor necrosis. The reported malignancies resulting in this syndrome include leukemias, lymphomas, adenocarcinoma of unknown primaries, medulloblastomas, and small-cell carcinomas of the lung.

PATHOPHYSIOLOGY

The metabolic derangements seen in tumor lysis syndrome include hyperkalemia, hyperphosphatemia, and hyperuricemia; it is thought that these abnormalities are the direct result of the liberation of intracellular contents into the patient's circulation. Hypocalcemia, which may be quite profound, is due to the effects of hyperphosphatemia; metastatic calcifications may result when the calcium and phosphorus product exceeds 58.

Metabolic studies have shown that abrupt tumor lysis releases such a potassium load that the kidney's normal excretory system is overloaded. If the patient has underlying renal disease, this situation is worsened. Phosphorus balance studies on patients with acute lymphoblastic leukemia revealed a urinary phosphorus excretion four times greater than the daily phosphate intake. The rise in urinary phosphate levels parallels serum levels. Thus, there is an absolute increase in phosphorus and its only source is the dying tumor itself. Similarly, hyperuricemia occurs as a consequence of the release of intracellular nucleic acids.

CLINICAL ASPECTS

Patients with tumor lysis syndrome have different presenting features. Hyperkalemia has been linked to sudden death within 48 hours of chemotherapy and may cause cardiac arrhythmias. Hypocalcemia may be associated with symptoms of tetany. Hyperuricemia is frequently of such degree to exceed the solubility of uric acid in the kidney, producing obstruction in the collecting ducts by urate crystals. These patients present with oliguric or anuric renal failure. The syndrome occurs in the five to seven days after cancer treatments.

MANAGEMENT

The goal of therapy for tumor lysis syndrome is to correct the associated laboratory abnormalities. Any ongoing treatment of the tumor should be discontinued in order to prevent further release of intracellular contents.

Hyperkalemia. Potassium-binding resins, such as Kayexalate in a dose of 20 to 50 gm in 100 to 200 ml of 20% sorbitol solution every four hours, or 50 gm Kayexalate and 50 gm sorbitol as a retention enema held for 30 to 60 minutes, are quite effective in reducing serum potassium levels. Potassium-wasting diuretics (Lasix, 20 to 40 mg orally or intravenously every six hours) are also effective in depleting potassium stores. In hyperacute hyperkalemia, insulin and glucose infusions (10 to 20 units of regular insulin in 25% or 50% glucose solutions) as well as calcium infusions (500 to 1000 mg calcium chloride or calcium gluconate) intravenously will initially decrease the potassium levels by driving the potassium intracellularly.

Acidosis. Any acidosis that is present should be corrected, since it exacerbates the hyperkalemia.

Hypocalcemia. Hypocalcemia can be quite profound and may necessitate the use of intravenous calcium supplementation. This can be supplied as either calcium gluconate or calcium chloride 500 to 1000 mg intravenously as needed. Phosphate-binding antacids (Amphojel or Basaljel, 30 ml orally every four hours) are useful to bring down the serum phosphorus level.

Hyperuricemia. Acute renal failure, if present, is generally due to the complications of hyperuricemia. In such cases, aggressive hydration with normal saline at 200 to 500 ml/hr, allopurinol 300 mg orally acutely followed by dose adjustment based on the patient's kidney function, and alkalinization of the urine are indicated. Alkalinization can be accomplished with the use of bicarbonate, 325 to 650 mg orally or 44 mEq intravenously every two to four hours until the urine pH is 7. Carbonic anhydrase inhibitors (acetazolamide, 125 to 250 mg orally every four hours) can also be used as an aid to urinary alkalinization. Once the urinary pH reaches 7.4, more than 95% of the uric acid is in the soluble form. Urine pH above 7.4 does not improve uric acid clearance and merely produces a more marked degree of systemic alkalosis. In patients who do not respond to medical management, dialysis must be considered.

Complications of Treatment. The administration of alkalinizing agents can decrease the amount of ionized calcium and increase the incidence of tetany. Allopurinol administration has been associated with xanthine nephropathy. Calcium infusions have been associated with metastatic calcification and may contribute to the renal impairment.

PREVENTIVE MEASURES

The most effective way of treating the tumor lysis syndrome is to anticipate which patients are at risk and to monitor them carefully post-treatment. Treating any underlying hyperuricemia and renal impairment before treatment only improves the patient's chances of successfully tolerating the chemotherapy and reduces the morbidity and mortality associated with this syndrome.

REFERENCES

Arseneau JC, Bagley CM, Anderson T, et al: Hyperkalemia, a sequel to chemotherapy of Burkitt's lymphoma. Lancet 1:10–14, 1973.

Cohen LF, Balow JE, Magrath IT, et al: Acute tumor lysis syndrome. A review of 37 patients with Burkitt's lymphoma. Am J Med 68:486–491, 1980.

Garnick MB, Mayer RJ: Acute renal failure associated with neoplastic disease and its treatment. Semin Oncol 5:155–165, 1978.

Vogelzang NJ, Nelimark RA, Nath KA: Tumor lysis syndrome after induction chemotherapy of small cell bronchogenic carcinoma. JAMA 249:513–514, 1983.

Zusman J, Brown DM, Nesbit ME: Hyperphosphatemia, hyperphosphaturia and hypocalcemia in acute lymphoblastic leukemia. N Engl J Med 289:1335–1340, 1973.

31 · PRINCIPLES OF OUTPATIENT CHEMOTHERAPY

Carl G. Kardinal
Marilyn Bateman
OCHSNER CLINIC AND ALTON OCHSNER MEDICAL FOUNDATION

In the 40 years since the introduction of nitrogen mustard, cytotoxic chemotherapy has evolved into one of the major treatment modalities for cancer. Diseases once uniformly fatal, such as acute lymphocytic leukemia, Hodgkin's disease, and advanced testicular cancers, are now regularly cured by aggressive drug treatment. Despite these rather dramatic advances, cancer chemotherapy seems to have a largely negative image with the public as well as with many health professionals. To some extent this is justified in that the toxic effects associated with treatment are real, and the response rates are low in certain tumors, such as melanoma, non-small-cell lung cancer, and gastrointestinal tract cancers. Increasing doses result in increasing responses for most chemotherapeutic agents, but unfortunately toxicity is also strongly dose-related. The safe and effective dose range is often quite narrow.

Over the past few years there has been a changing pattern in cancer care. At the present time, 85% of cancer patients in the United States are diagnosed and treated in the community. The community physician, therefore, must become acquainted with the safe handling and administration of cytotoxic drugs, as well as the anticipation, recognition, and management of chemotherapeutic toxicity.

HANDLING OF CYTOTOXIC DRUGS

As a rule, cancer chemotherapeutic agents act by interfering with DNA or RNA synthesis, intercalating with DNA base pairs, or interrupting cellular protein synthesis. Because of this, it is not surprising that many of these agents have been found to be carcinogenic, mutagenic, or teratogenic. The possible risks to health care personnel of chronic low-dose exposure to antineoplastic drugs has been an issue of increasing concern. To date there are no studies documenting actual risks of handling such materials. However, there have been

Table 1. NIH RECOMMENDATIONS FOR THE SAFE HANDLING OF INJECTABLE ANTINEOPLASTIC DRUG PRODUCTS

All preparations should be performed in a Class II (vertical) laminar flow safety hood.

Safety hood or other work surface should be covered with plastic-backed absorbable paper.

Personnel should wear disposable gloves, closed front gown with cuffed sleeves, and if a safety hood is not available, should also wear a mask.

To avoid aerosolization:

1. An alcohol sponge should be wrapped around the needle and vial top during withdrawal from the vial septum.
2. Alcohol sponge or dry sterile gauze should be placed over needle tip when ejecting air from syringe.
3. Vials with reconstituted drugs should be vented to reduce internal pressure.
4. Wrap neck of glass ampulla with alcohol sponge before breaking.

Needles should be recapped rather than clipped before disposal.

Syringes and IV bottles containing antineoplastic drugs should be labeled: Caution—Cancer Chemotherapy. Dispose of Properly.

During drug administration, protective outer garments should be worn, such as a surgical gown and gloves.

Modified from Zimmerman PF, Larsen RK, Barkley EW, et al: Recommendations for the safe handling of injectable antineoplastic drug products. Am J Hosp Pharm 38:1693–1695, 1981.

uncontrolled reports of the presence of urinary mutagens and an increase in lymphocyte sister chromatid exchange frequency in chemotherapy nurses. In addition, a few agents such as doxorubicin, mitomycin C, and nitrogen mustard are vesicants that can cause varying degrees of local tissue necrosis or irritation of the skin or mucous membranes on direct contact.

Despite the inadequate data to confirm risk, the National Institutes of Health has published recommendations for the safe handling of cytotoxic drugs; these are summarized in Table 1.

DISPOSAL OF ANTINEOPLASTIC WASTES

The National Institutes of Health (NIH) has elected to dispose of all antineoplastic agents as hazardous wastes. In fact, the Environmental Protection Agency (EPA) has officially designated as hazardous wastes seven antineoplastic agents: chlorambucil, cyclophosphamide, daunorubicin, melphalan, mitomycin C, streptozotocin, and uracil mustard. Because of the similarities between these seven agents and other cytotoxic drugs, it seems reasonable to adopt the NIH policy that all such agents are hazardous wastes. *Trace-contaminated* materials, such as needles, syringes, empty drug vials, gloves, gowns, and alcohol swabs, should be incinerated. *Bulk-contaminated* materials, such as unused intravenous solutions and expired or unused antineoplastic drugs, should be incinerated at an off-site hazardous waste incinerator that has an EPA permit, or in an EPA-approved sanitary landfill. Each state has its own solid and hazardous waste agency. These agencies should be consulted for variations in local policy.

MANAGEMENT OF SPILLS

Personnel cleaning spills should wear protective gowns, gloves, and masks. The spill should be contained by absorbent gauze pads or other absorbent disposable material. Decontaminate with clean water at least three times. Consider all absorbable material used as hazardous wastes and dispose of accordingly. In case of direct skin or eye contact with drug, wash the affected area with soap and water or flush eyes with copious amounts of water.

MANAGEMENT OF SHORT-TERM TOXICITY

The management of acute and short-term toxic effects of chemotherapeutic agents, such as bone marrow suppression and gastrointestinal toxicity (nausea and vomiting, stomatitis, and diarrhea), is of immediate concern to the practicing physician and, along with alopecia, is the major concern of patients as well. Perry and Yabro have comprehensively reviewed the toxicity of chemotherapy, including the delayed and long-term effects.

BONE MARROW SUPPRESSION

The most serious and potentially life-threatening toxic effect of cancer chemotherapy is leukopenia (granulocytopenia) with complicating bacterial or fungal sepsis. *Thrombocytopenia* may also occur but is rarely less than 25,000/μl, the range usually associated with overt bleeding complications. However, leukopenia with a total white count of less than 1500/μl and a granulocyte count of less than 500 to 1000/μl is very common. Bacterial or fungal infections occurring during these episodes can be overwhelming and rapidly fatal. All patients receiving chemotherapy must be warned that if fever spikes to 100.5° F (38° C), or if they have a rigor, they must call immediately regardless of the time of day. The CBC must be checked and neutropenic patients must be hospitalized without delay. After appropriate cultures have been taken, patients must be started on intravenous bactericidal antibiotics. A matter of a few hours may make the difference in patient survival. The use of prophylactic antibiotics in afebrile, nonseptic leukopenic patients is not recommended.

To date, there is no simple means of evaluating bone marrow granulocyte reserves, and one is left with the less than perfect CBC as the only practical indicator. There is a steep dose-response curve for most chemotherapeutic agents. Although the most common error of the inexperienced practitioner is undermedicating, one must constantly be aware of the risk of profound granulocytopenia.

GASTROINTESTINAL TOXICITY

Nausea and vomiting have been recognized to be frequent complications of cancer chemotherapy since the introduction of nitrogen mustard in the late 1940s. However, it was not until the late 1970s with the increasing use of cisplatin that the magnitude of the problem became truly apparent. Cisplatin in combination with vinblastine and bleomycin (PVB) is curative treatment in 75% of patients with disseminated testicular cancer, but the regimen is very difficult to tolerate. One report shows as many as half of the patients treated with PVB miss appointments or otherwise delay therapy because of the severe nausea and vomiting, and a few patients even refuse further treatment, which may cost them a chance for cure. When a patient is unwilling to take potentially curative treatment because of severe nausea and vomiting, the problem is truly of major proportions. Approximately 10% of patients who have experienced chemotherapy-induced nausea and vomiting will develop *anticipatory vomiting*, i.e., they will start

Table 2. CLASSIFICATION OF CHEMOTHERAPEUTIC DRUGS BASED UPON THEIR EMETIC POTENTIAL

Severely Emetogenic	Moderately Emetogenic	Minimally Emetogenic
Cisplatin	Doxorubicin	Cytarabine
Nitrogen mustard	Daunorubicin	Methotrexate
Dacarbazine	Cyclophosphamide	Vinca alkaloids
Streptozotocin	Procarbazine	Bleomycin
Combinations* with	Mitomycin C	Melphalan
doxorubicin: CAF,	Actinomycin D	Busulfan
AC, FAM	BCNU, CCNU	Chlorambucil
		Hydroxyurea
		5-Fluorouracil

*CAF = Cytoxan, Adriamycin, 5-FU
AC = Cytoxan, Adriamycin
FAM = 5-FU, Adriamycin, Mitomycin C

vomiting on the way to the clinic or in the waiting room prior to receiving treatment. Clearly, the most critical time to control nausea and vomiting is prior to the first dose of chemotherapy. Once a patient has experienced severe chemotherapy-induced emesis, it will continue to be a problem throughout the course of treatment.

Some cytotoxic drugs are among the most potent emetogenic agents known, whereas others have minimal emetic potential (Table 2). Recognizing the emetic potential of the agents used is of extreme importance in design of appropriate antiemetic regimens. Antiemetic therapy should be started prior to the administration of a chemotherapeutic drug to prevent nausea and vomiting; therapy given after the onset of nausea and vomiting is considerably less effective. Antiemetic regimens that are useful in patients receiving drugs of minimal or moderate emetic potential are listed in Table 3.

The difficult problem is the control of nausea and vomiting associated with the use of the severely emetogenic agents and drug combinations. Useful regimens are listed in Table 4. We have found that administration of cisplatin alone or in combination requires complex management, and patients given cisplatin are usually admitted to the hospital for 24 to 48 hours to assure adequate hydration and emesis control. Cisplatin regimens are the only ones that we consistently give on an

Table 3. ANTIEMETIC REGIMENS FOR USE WITH MINIMALLY OR MODERATELY EMETIC CHEMOTHERAPEUTIC AGENTS*

Phenothiazine	
Prochlorperazine	10 mg IM or PO or 25 mg suppository q 4–6 hr
Chlorpromazine	25–50 mg IM or PO or 100 mg suppository q 4–6 hr
Promethazine	25–50 mg IM or PO or 50 mg suppository q 4–6 hr
Butyrophenones	
Haloperidol	1–2 mg IM or PO q 3 hr × 2 doses
Droperidol	5 mg IM followed by 2.5 mg q 4–6 hr
Cannabinoids	
Tetrahydrocannabinol	5–15 mg/m² PO q 4–6 hr
Nabilone	2 mg PO q 4–6 hr
Benzodiazepine	
Lorazepam	2–8 mg PO q 3–4 hr × 2 doses

*All antiemetic regimens should start 30 minutes prior to the administration of the chemotherapeutic drug, and should be continued on a regularly scheduled basis. Antiemetics should not be given p.r.n.

Table 4. COMBINATION ANTIEMETIC REGIMENS FOR USE WITH SEVERELY EMETIC CHEMOTHERAPEUTIC AGENTS*

Metoclopramide	1–2 mg/kg IV q 2 hr × 2–3 doses
Dexamethasone	20 mg IV × 1 dose
Diphenhydramine	50 mg IV × 1 dose
Secobarbital	100 mg PO or IM
Chlorpromazine	25–50 mg PO or IM q 3–4 hr × 2 doses
Droperidol	2.5–5 mg IV q 3–4 hr × 3 doses
Dexamethasone	20 mg IV × 1 dose
Diphenhydramine	50 mg IV × 1 dose

*All antiemetic regimens should start 30 minutes prior to the administration of the chemotherapeutic drug, and should be continued on a regularly scheduled basis. Antiemetics should not be given p.r.n.

inpatient basis. All other chemotherapeutic regimens can be managed in the outpatient clinic.

Stomatitis may be a troublesome side effect of chemotherapy and is most commonly seen with the use of methotrexate, 5-FU, actinomycin D, doxorubicin, and bleomycin. Stomatitis is occasionally the dose-limiting toxic effect and may be so severe as to interfere with the patient's nutritional intake. As a rule stomatitis is relatively easy to manage, responding rapidly to modest dose reductions or temporary discontinuance of the chemotherapeutic drugs. Topical anesthetics such as viscous lidocaine prior to fluid or food ingestion may be helpful. We have found a suspension of liquid Maalox with equal parts of elixir of Benadryl (5 to 10 ml), swish and swallow, every two to three hours, to be soothing. A complicating infectious stomatitis, especially that caused by *Candida albicans,* should not be overlooked.

Diarrhea is a less frequent gastrointestinal side effect than emesis or stomatitis. Drugs most commonly associated with complicating diarrhea are 5-FU and cisplatin. Diarrhea is also a frequent complication associated with the use of high-dose metoclopramide as an antiemetic. The diarrhea is generally self-limiting, but may be severe and even bloody, particularly with high-dose 5-FU or methotrexate. Fluid and electrolyte loss may be severe enough to require parenteral fluid replacement. As a rule, however, diarrhea responds to simple regimens such as temporary discontinuance of the chemotherapeutic drug and symptomatic treatment with diphenoxylate or loperamide.

NURSING ASPECTS OF CHEMOTHERAPY ADMINISTRATION

PATIENT AND FAMILY EDUCATION

Prior to administration of the first course of chemotherapy, the patient education process should be well underway; it should continue throughout treatment based upon reassessment of need, changes in the treatment regimen, and toxic effects experienced. An explanation of common side effects must be offered so that the patient becomes a participant in his care. The way in which expected side effects are presented may adversely influence response to treatment. A positive yet realistic approach will reassure and increase the patient's hope that chemotherapy will be beneficial.

Just as patient assessment can be accomplished quickly and systematically, patient teaching can be incorporated into each contact with the patient. Obtaining the informed consent to initiate treatment affords an excellent opportunity to present information to the patient and family members. However, this information is often not retained and should never be considered a substitute for continued individualized teaching.

VASCULAR ACCESS

Most patients receiving chemotherapy will require frequent venipunctures for drug administration as well as for laboratory tests. For those patients whose therapy will be short-term (six courses or less), venous access is not generally a problem in skilled hands. Cannulation should be relatively trauma-free if site selection is prudent and rotation of sites is regularly practiced. The smallest scalp vein needle that is practical, usually 23- or 21-gauge, should be used for drug administration. The avoidance of antecubital veins and veins over joints is urged, especially when administering vesicants such as doxorubicin, mitomycin C, and nitrogen mustard to prevent long-term complications from a drug extravasation. Veins in the forearm are generally preferred. Veins in the dorsum of the hand can also be used cautiously if there is no evidence of venous sclerosis above the chosen site that might produce drug pooling. Vigilant observation of the venous site is essential during the administration of chemotherapeutic drugs so that early manifestations of vesicant drug leakage into the tissue can be detected. This will enable the practitioner to immediately institute treatment, avoiding a possibly disabling complication from corrosive tissue damage. With any evidence of possible drug extravasation, further drug administration should be immediately terminated. Treatment should be instituted as outlined below.

1. Aspirate any drug remaining in the needle if possible.

2. With the needle still in place, infiltrate the area with a corticosteroid such as dexamethasone or Solu-Cortef subcutaneously using a 24-gauge needle.

3. Remove the needle and apply a sterile dressing of topical corticosteroid cream.

4. Apply ice packs to the area for 20 minutes four times a day for 48 hours.

VENOUS ACCESS DEVICES

The long-term treatment required by some patients will exhaust available peripheral venous access and render chemotherapy administration impossible. In these patients with impaired venous integrity, an implantable venous access device may be placed and easily managed in the patient within the community setting. Implantable venous access devices are basically of two types:

1. Central venous catheters with external access such as the Hickman or Broviac catheters.

2. Implanted infusion ports such as the Infusaport and PortaCath.

Hickman catheters require daily heparinization and sterile dressing changes, since part of the catheter exits the skin. The infusion ports require less care, since the entire device is implanted under the skin and heparinization is required only every two to four weeks or at the time of each drug administration.

Attention to the management of the acute and

short-term toxic effects of chemotherapy will make it much easier for patients to comply with treatment and, in turn, allow greater ease of drug administration and, ultimately, greater response to treatment. Chemotherapeutic drugs can be safely handled in the private physician's office. However, one must be constantly aware of the need for good technique and of the potential hazards to patients and medical personnel.

REFERENCES

Frei E, Canellos GP: Dose: a critical factor in cancer chemotherapy. Am J Hosp Pharm 38:1686–1693, 1981.

Holland JF: Breaking the cure barrier. J Clin Oncol 1:75–90, 1983.

Jones RB, Frank R, Mass T: Safe handling of chemotherapeutic agents: a report from the Mount Sinai Medical Center. Ca 33:258–263, 1983.

Kardinal CG: Cancer chemotherapy: historical aspects and future considerations. Postgrad Med 77:165–174, 1985.

Laszlo J: Antiemetics and Cancer Chemotherapy. William and Wilkins, Baltimore, 1983.

Perry MC, Yabro JW: Toxicity of Chemotherapy. Grune and Stratton, New York, 1984.

Vaccuri PL, Tonat K, DeChristoforo R, et al: Disposal of antineoplastic wastes at the National Institutes of Health. Am J Hosp Pharm 41:87–93, 1984.

Zimmerman PF, Larsen RK, Barkley EW, et al: Recommendations for the safe handling of injectable antineoplastic drug products. Am J Hosp Pharm 38:1693–1695, 1981.

32 · UNPROVEN METHODS OF CANCER THERAPY

Neil M. Ellison
GEISINGER MEDICAL CENTER

The term "unproven methods of cancer therapy" implies that no reproducible scientific evidence supports the clinical use of the treatment in question. This strict definition could include any drug being tested in a well-designed phase I or II study. For the purposes of this discussion, it will refer to those nostrums that eschew scientific confirmation of objective benefit. Synonyms for these treatments include quackery or the more euphemistic "metabolic," "unorthodox," or "unconventional" therapies.

Cancer is the most feared disease in America. Surgery, radiation therapy, and chemotherapy have respectively been referred to as "cut, burn, and poison" by unconventional therapists. Skepticism for these treatments is present even in some conventional physicians. Cancer patients in complete remission who are treated with curative intent by these modalities often live in continuous fear of recurrence. Up to 55% of conventionally treated patients have reportedly considered or did use an unproven therapy. These treatments are often pressed upon them by well-meaning but poorly informed relatives, friends, or health care providers, as well as those charlatans who will reap financial gain from the treatments. Unproven methods will continue to come and go until all cancer can be prevented or cured by relatively nontoxic therapies. Their primary dangers include a delay of or substitution for possible curative or palliative therapies, toxic effects, and a drain on emotional or financial resources of patients and their families.

WHY PATIENTS SEEK UNPROVEN METHODS

Disillusion with the health care provider is a common reason why patients leave conventional therapists. Often, this is because the patient or family was told, *or perceived they were told*, that the disease was "terminal" or that "nothing else can be done."

Conventional therapists must realize that patients need to be involved in their own health care. Therapeutic options must be discussed with the patient, who will then make the final decision with physician guidance. Good nutrition, exercise programs, and self-help groups should be encouraged. This allows patients and families to be active participants in their own health care and improves their psychological attitudes toward the treatments.

COMMON SIMILARITIES OF UNPROVEN TREATMENTS

Several of the more common nostrums in use today will be described later in this chapter. However, since these will surely submerge as others surface, it is important to identify their similarities.

1. Treatment based on unproven theories.

2. Claim for harmless (painless, nontoxic) treatment. If cure is not claimed, then at least pain relief, increased appetite, increased sense of well-being, and prolongation of life are promised.

3. Claims are published only in the mass media and not in reputable "peer review" scientific journals.

4. Major proponents are not recognized experts in cancer treatments. Famous nonmedical personal testimonials are often used.

5. Claim that only specially trained physicians can produce results with the treatment or that the method of drug preparation is a secret and available only to the unconventional therapist.

6. Claim for a scientific, medical, and governmental conspiracy that prevents the ready availability of the purported cancer cures.

ANECDOTAL CURES OR REMISSIONS WITH UNCONVENTIONAL THERAPIES

One of the most fascinating aspects of cancer quackery is that cases can be found where a cancer regressed or a patient improved while receiving the unproven treatment. Patients often bring reports from lay journals that describe an individual with cancer who was treated with an unproven method and lived for years after the physician "told them they only had weeks." Similarly, National Cancer Institute (NCI) retrospective case reviews of various cancer nostrums demonstrated an occasional "response." Three scientific explanations for these phenomena exist besides the possibility of surreptitious coadministration of conventional therapies.

First is the variable natural history of malignancy. Complete spontaneous remissions may occur as often as 1 in 10,000 patients and more frequently for partial spontaneous remissions.

Second is the placebo effect. Numerous studies

report that about one third of patients with pain will experience a subjective improvement with placebo. More important, when placebo is compared with chemotherapy in double-blind studies, objective tumor shrinkage as well as toxic side effects such as diarrhea, vomiting, stomatitis, leukopenia, and thrombocytopenia are observed in the placebo-treated group. This supports the natural waxing and waning of tumors and indicates that many side effects attributed to conventional therapies are really systemic manifestations of the malignancy.

The third possibility is observer measuring error. When 16 experienced oncologists were asked to accurately measure various-sized spheres under a thin foam layer, both inter- and same-observer error could be assessed. By assuming various measurements as "baseline" and others as "follow-up," a greater than 50% "shrinkage" of the products of the diameters of the same-sized mass was observed about 7% of the time and greater than 50% "growth" was observed about 18% of the time. These measuring errors occurred in the ideal situation, since guarding, anxiety, and discomfort are not traits usually ascribed to foam pads.

SPECIFIC UNCONVENTIONAL THERAPIES

LAETRILE

Laetrile refers to amygdalin, a D-mandelonitrile-β-D-glucosido-6-β-D-glucoside found naturally in a variety of plants. Most commercial Laetrile is extracted from apricot pits. It is falsely claimed to be a vitamin (B_{17}), the deficiency of which results in the development of malignancy. The "scientific rationale" supporting its use states that it is preferentially metabolized by cancer cells to its components, benzaldehyde and hydrogen cyanide. Normal cells supposedly can enzymatically detoxify the lethal hydrogen cyanide more easily than cancer cells. Laetrile will therefore preferentially kill cancer cells. None of these claims were supported by scientific studies specifically addressing these issues.

In 1978, the National Cancer Institute (NCI) published the results of its retrospective Laetrile evaluation. Over 440,000 letters were sent in order to solicit cases showing a beneficial Laetrile response from the estimated 70,000 Laetrile users or their families in the United States. Only six of the submitted cases were assessed to have had a complete or partial response during the Laetrile treatment period. Several factors other than Laetrile could have explained the response, but Laetrile anticancer activity was possible.

The NCI used these six cases as part of the rationale for a prospective Laetrile trial that was initiated in 1980. Laetrile was given in a "metabolic regimen," which included megadose vitamins, minerals, enzymes, and special dietary restrictions—a treatment plan designed in conjunction with the Laetrile advocates. This study evaluated 178 patients and was decidedly negative in terms of antitumor response, extension of life span, or palliation of cancer-related symptoms. Pharmacologic studies indicated that significant plasma cyanide levels occurred after Laetrile administration and symptoms of cyanide poisoning were noted.

VITAMIN C

Vitamin C has attained much notoriety in the lay press as a cancer treatment. In the 1950s it was observed that some groups of cancer patients had subnormal plasma and leukocyte ascorbic acid levels. In the 1970s, Cameron and Pauling first postulated that ascorbic acid acted to maintain the stromal ground substance in order to resist malignant invasion or dissemination and to induce a generalized enhancement of host resistance. They then reported their observations on 100 "terminally ill" cancer patients treated with 10 gm of vitamin C daily. When compared with 1000 historic controls, the ascorbic acid–treated group survived 4.16 times longer and had an "improved quality of life." It is noted that the controls were not shown to be well-matched for known prognostic features. With this beneficial vitamin C effect as a background, Mayo Clinic investigators performed the mandatory double-blind prospectively randomized studies necessary to confirm Cameron and Pauling's initial observation. In the Mayo Clinic studies, vitamin C– and placebo-treated patients were well matched for age, sex, primary tumor site, performance status, tumor grade, and previous antineoplastic therapies. No difference was noted in median survival of either group or in subjective measurements of improved appetite, strength, activity level, or decreased pain.

It should be noted that megadose vitamin C therapy is not innocuous. It can precipitate sickle crises in hemoglobin SS disease, cause hemolysis in patients with G6PD deficiency, cause false-negatives in stool guaiac testing, and interfere with vitamin B_{12} absorption.

ENZYMES

Several products consisting of proteolytic enzymes from animal and plant tissues are being sold in health food stores and pharmacies as cancer therapies. They are sometimes used orally or parenterally, but are primarily administered as enemas. Unsubstantiated claims include direct lysis of cancer cells and decreased metastatic frequency. Perianal irritation can occur after enzyme enema use, and anaphylaxis is possible, especially with parenteral use.

COFFEE ENEMAS

Coffee enemas are claimed to "stimulate the liver to cleanse the blood" as well as being a quick and easy method of "general detoxification." One cup of freshly brewed coffee is mixed with one quart of water. Instant coffee, cream, sugar, and hot coffee are to be avoided. Deaths reported following coffee enemas are most likely due to fluid and electrolyte problems caused by hypotonic enemas.

DIETS

Numerous diets have been recommended as effective cancer treatments. These diets often stress ingestion of fresh fruits, nuts, and vegetables, and decreased intake of animal protein and fats, especially pork and beef. Alcohol and refined sweets are frequently prohibited. Some diets, such as the Grape Diet or the Gerson Diet, place more severe limitations on the patient. Although diets vary, most unfounded cancer therapies rely on them to some degree as an adjunct to the specific treatments.

It may be emphatically stated that no diet has ever been proven of value as a cancer treatment. This does not belittle the value of a well-balanced diet with adequate caloric, protein, vitamin, and mineral intake in the maintenance and support of the cancer patient. Well-nourished individuals are more capable of dealing with infections or other acute body stresses. The key to tumor response is an effective cancer therapy. The use of an ineffective treatment in a well-nourished cancer patient is of no value.

FREEDOM OF CHOICE

All of the proponents of the unproven methods of cancer therapy claim that patients should have the freedom to choose alternative treatments from those offered by conventional therapists. This is an attractive idea for the American public as evidenced by general support of Laetrile legalization. Freedom of choice, however, must be based upon a comprehensive understanding of the proven benefits and toxicities of all of the treatments. Any rational person would choose a "long shot" therapy that was nontoxic if nothing better was offered by orthodox medicine. The "long shot" of unproven therapy is compatible solely with a placebo response or natural variability of malignancy. All of these unproven cancer treatments also have demonstrated toxicities, inconveniences, or expenses. Cancer patients should be protected from the purveyors of these treatments. This is best achieved by an understanding physician who is willing to discuss alternative therapies as well as maintain a supportive role, especially at the time of tumor diagnosis or progression.

REFERENCES

Cameron E, Pauling L: Supplemental ascorbate in the supportive treatment of cancer: prolongation of survival times in terminal human cancer. Proc Natl Acad Sci USA 73:3685–3689, 1976.

Ellison NM, Byar DP, Newell GR: Special report on Laetrile: the NCI Laetrile review. N Engl J Med 299:549–552, 1978.

Moertel CG, Hanley JA: The effect of measuring error on the results of therapeutic trials in advanced cancer. Cancer 38:388–394, 1976.

Moertel CG, Fleming TR, Rubin J, et al: A clinical trial of amygdalin (Laetrile) in the treatment of human cancer. N Engl J Med 306:201–206, 1982.

Moertel CG, Fleming TR, Creagan ET, et al: High dose vitamin C versus placebo in the treatment of patients with advanced cancer who have had no prior treatment. N Engl J Med 312:137–141, 1985.

Subcommittee on Unorthodox Therapies, American Society of Clinical Oncology: Ineffective cancer therapy: a guide for the layperson. J Clin Oncol 1:154–163, 1983.

33 · NONMEDICAL SUPPORT FOR CANCER PATIENTS AND THEIR FAMILIES

A. Dale Gulledge
CLEVELAND CLINIC FOUNDATION

Cancer for many patients, families, and physicians is equated with unrelenting pain, treatment futility, and difficult death. I intend to highlight some of the common concerns and difficulties of supporting the family and patient who are dealing with malignancy.

Living is a process, an experience, and not an object or a thought. It is unique to each person and death represents finitude. Since living is unique to each person, we need to learn what life has meant to the patient in terms of successes, guilt, or failure, what life means now, and what is important in the future. Anxiety about cancer or death often means a person has realized living is finite; therefore, learning one has cancer becomes a period of time when decisions are made—large and small—to finish unfulfilled tasks. It is in the attempt to fulfill these decisions that real purpose and meaning may be first realized.

It has long been recognized that the physician must never allow the cancer or dying patient to be deprived of hope. The Greeks said that the most horrible of all ills was not to die, "but to die alone." Patients should be treated in the warmest possible way, with a touch, a handshake, or the laying on of hands, which often offsets the fear of being untouchable; for the patient, a touch or caress is perhaps the oldest preverbal means we possess in communicating our solace and intent for comfort.

In efforts to preserve life and restore health, the physician sometimes may fail to give enough consideration to his other obligation, namely, to relieve suffering and to allow the patient, if he is to die, to die with some comfort and dignity. It is often overlooked that as physicians our training predisposes us to "save lives" and treat the sick, and that our modern medical training may encourage us to see our role as scientists applying particular skills to solve a problem, rather than dealing with people. This often takes on added significance when we may regard the geriatric or the terminally ill patient with cancer as failure of our skills; often they may be consigned to the younger or more inexperienced physician.

FEARS OF THE PATIENT

What do patients tell us that is important for a physician to know, and what do these patients fear the most? One sample of patients listed their fears as (1) abandonment by others, (2) pain, and (3) shortness of breath. Questions far outnumber answers, whenever the patient is cared for; when dealing with the terminally ill cancer patient, the physician may find that the most difficult situations usually occur at the bedside.

CONCERNS OF THE PATIENT

At the time of diagnosis, areas that have been identified of major concern to the patient with newly diagnosed cancer include the following: truth, competence, compassion, concerns about dependence, grief, anger, self-esteem, guilt, pleasure, and comfort. Despite family concerns to the contrary, nearly all patients prefer the truth concerning the diagnosis of cancer. Telling the truth is merely the beginning of a long process but does establish an open and honest way to provide a firm basis on which to expand this relationship. Likewise, competence is a most reassuring trait of the physician caring for the cancer patient. Still the most highly valued and esteemed attribute in physicians and nurses alike is compassion. This attribute is a quality that can neither be feigned nor contrived. It is quite likely that the physician as well as the patient may go through feelings of shock, denial, outrage, hope, and devastation, the stages of dying described by Kübler-Ross. In the hospital setting, the risk of dehumanization is undoubtedly increased because of the tendency to turn to other testing or other treatments in order to avoid the difficulties that we as physicians have in dealing with our own helpless feelings as we care for the terminal cancer patient. We may rationalize that it is difficult to talk with a patient about private matters because there are too many staff or visitors present in the room during rounds.

PHYSICAL NEEDS

Dependency, grief, depression, and anger are all powerful emotions that are usually present at some time during the course of illness of a patient with cancer. It is extremely important that the physical needs of the terminal cancer patient be met. These needs are likely to include narcotic medications to relieve pain, and many physicians are in error in not knowing what the pharmacology of narcotics may be. The designation of "p.r.n." may demean the patient by almost forcing him or her to beg for pain medication in order to justify its use. Since the goal of adequate analgesic control is pain relief, the ideal administration is therefore to provide a dose in frequency that is adequate to remove pain if possible and prevent its return. The fear of addiction by a patient is almost never justified, by experience. Other necessary details are attention to personal hygiene, including mouth care, and management of infection, odors, secretions, hemorrhage, and nutrition.

Physical and psychological factors go hand-in-hand in pain control; a broad range of therapeutics needs to be constantly explored and improved, ranging from narcotics, neurosurgical procedures, and meditation to biofeedback, if adequate pain palliation is to be accomplished. Nurses often have more skill in relating to physical and often psychological relief of suffering, and more input by them is very necessary in any aspects of the care. Pain teams have been developed throughout the country, but there still remains a dearth of disciplined attention to the needs of the cancer patient.

COMMUNICATION

A skill that may be overly rated is talking with the cancer patient. Most studies emphasize that the ability to listen to the patient is much more valuable than the ability to say something to the patient. The real question is not what you tell your patients, but what your patients tell you. Communication is more than just words. A pat on the arm, a wave, a wink, a grin are often important reassurances, as may be skillful and careful back rubs or a gentle but thorough physical examination. Many patients, although having a malignancy, are still very interested in life and may not want to always talk about cancer, death, and dying.

Similarly, the cancer patient has no more desire to see sour, somber faces than does anyone else. Gentleness and appropriate sense of being often bring considerable relief to both patient and staff.

Unfinished business is that part of living in which the terminally ill patient is concerned with reconciliation, resolution of conflicts, and the pursuit of specific remaining hopes. Dying may perhaps best be identified as "coming together time," where patient, family, and staff all help each other share the burdens and pleasures along with the appropriate good-byes. At no other time is it more important that the treatment be unique and individualized. This can only be accomplished by getting to know the patient and his needs and interests, proceeding at his pace, and allowing him or her to shape the manner in which he or she exists. We are fortunate that there is no "best way to die." Dying has as many pathways and styles as living. Whatever attachments the dying patient has, it must be remembered that these are found among the living, not the dead; thus it is important to focus on life issues rather than inappropriate fears or concerns. Perhaps it could all be summarized by the statement that our role in caring for our patients and teaching our staff is to learn that we cure sometimes, comfort infrequently, and succor always. In the words of Francis Peabody, the secret of the care of the patient is "in the caring for the patient."

NEEDS OF SPOUSES

Commonly unmet needs of the spouses surrounding death are: (1) to be with the dying person at the moment of death; (2) to be helpful to the dying individual; (3) to be assured of the patient's comfort; (4) to be daily informed of the patient's condition; (5) to be privately informed of the impending death; (6) to be comforted and supported by the family; and (7) to feel acceptance and support from the medical staff. Many spouses feel that the hospital or medical staffs do not meet their needs in one or more of these categories, indicating that the hospital system for dying may not always be compatible with survivors' needs. The terminally ill patient and family members often benefit from help from professional teams, which are able to communicate openly with each other and thus facilitate an easeful dying. The family members may need help in letting the patient go. No preparation for death can be made while all energy is devoted to raging. When patients are consciously suffering, especially with pain, preparation for death is most difficult. Relentless pain consumes patient and family and virtually prevents any real communication or planning.

It is not uncommon in the hospital that policies fail to meet the spouse's needs at the time of death, and further do not encourage or assist family members to anticipate autopsy, funeral, or legal needs surrounding the dying process. Autopsy permissions frequently are requested by strange house officers, especially when death occurs at night or on a weekend, resulting in considerable emotional turmoil. Patients may die alone, with relatives at home or out of the room in another area of the hospital, because a physician or nurse or someone else has advised the family members that they need not stay longer or that they will be called if needed. If this occurs it may create unnecessary subsequent guilt feelings in the survivors as well as anger at the hospital and the health care providers for failure to recognize the single need for kinfolk to be with a loved one at the moment of actual death. Legal counseling and funeral counseling are not often available to family members who require them.

PREPARATION FOR DEATH

Too often, no preparations are made for the death of the terminally ill cancer patient. In many instances, the patient, members of the family, the medical staff, and often the primary physician appear to be caught unaware by impending death. Failure to prepare for the obvious can make for a disturbing rather than an easeful death. Easeful does not imply an absence of feelings of sadness, of melancholia, or of loss. Such feelings are appropriate for this phase of living. By easeful is meant the absence of distressingly dysphoric feelings of hostility, guilt, remorse, blandness, excessive depression, or helplessness. A disturbing death creates ill feelings in survivors, causes defensive arrogance or painful guilt in the medical staff, and portends for both physical as well as psychosocial maladaptive problems for the surviving family members in the future. It has been found that less than 30% of the people involved actually discuss any element of dying between themselves. Oftentimes there is no discussion of wills, possessions, remains, or funerals, and no instructions for the future for family members, unless there has been open communication about the possibility of dying between the patient and family members. If this is as common a problem as it seems to be, active preparation for financial, legal, or advisory events, which invariably accompany a death, needs to be something that is entered into by the majority of patients and family members.

Timing is important because terminally ill patients reach a stage where they have less ability and interest to participate actively in final preparations as a result of drug therapy, organic brain disorders, or regressive behaviors. These problems of acknowledgment and communication may be compounded when the medical staff is unprepared for the death (because of its suddenness or unexpectedness) or when the physician or nurse has not accepted that death is near. On some occasions physicians may signal the patient or the family member that a new treatment is available or that a turn for the better is occurring, arousing expectations for improvement and postponing confrontation and preparation. By the same token, the opposite posture is just as injurious. Premature announcements that nothing can be done or signals indicating that the physician is withdrawing efforts to help the patient or family may produce feelings of abandonment. Helplessness in patient and family members can lead to despair or unacceptable behaviors. Thus, either giving up on a patient prematurely or failing to confirm the terminal nature of an illness while continuing to give active support can lead to a rather disturbing death. More frequently the medical staff may be aware that a patient is dying but may not openly communicate to the patient or to the family that death is near so that sufficient time for adequate last-minute preparations can be enacted.

Sexism is another fact of preparation for death. In this regard, physicians frequently feel obliged to inform male cancer patients of their diagnosis and prognosis on the basis that "men need to know" in order to be able to put their affairs in order. This "value concept" clearly relates to a man's position in the family as an economic provider and a property manager. However, the position is frequently reversed for women—male physicians have more of a need to "protect" women from knowing too much and do not feel a need to inform them as frequently of the gravity of the situation. In this value-laden posture, dying women are left to learn on their own, and may receive information or statements from physicians that are contradictory to what they are perceiving in their own bodies and in behavior of others.

Preparation for death is frequently interrelated with a family member's feelings that all has been done that could be done and that no reasonable stone was left unturned. This feeling of exhausting the medical possibilities is certainly related to the concept of Laetrile—"no stone left unturned." A trusted medical or physician advocate who is seen as the patient's personal advocate and not a representative of another allegiance is critical here for appropriate behaviors and decision-making. Home care services and special institutional services, such as hospices, constitute one of the major areas to helpfully prepare family or a patient. Present public policies, which often involve third-party payment systems and economic job-related practices allowing people time off to care for a dying family member, may militate against home dying, especially in a nuclear, small, independent middle-class family. There is little doubt that patients and families may control events in a terminal illness better at home, but it is only if they feel safe with adequate medical and social supports. Fear may well drive many patients (via their own choice, or that of their families) into the hospital; physicians may inadvertently but powerfully aid in this process. Certainly dying is hard enough on all concerned, yet fear of potential medical complications or "felt absence" of needed support can only aggravate the problem.

REFERENCES

Abrams RD: Not alone with Cancer. A Guide to Those Who Care: What to Expect; What to Do. Charles C Thomas, Publisher, Springfield, IL, 1974.

Hackett TP: Psychological assistance for the dying patient and his family. Annu Rev Med 27:371–378, 1976.

Hardy RE, Green DR, Jordan HW, et al: Communication between cancer patients and physicians. South Med J 73:755–757, 1980.

Lack S: The hospice concept—the adult with advanced cancer. *In* Proceedings of the American Cancer Society: Second National Conference on Human Values and Cancer, Chicago, IL, September 7–9, 1977. American Cancer Society, Inc, New York, 1978, pp. 160–166.

Lee R, Spencer PSJ: Antidepressants and pain. J Intern Med Res 5 [Suppl. 1]:146–156, 1977.

McKegney FP, Bailey LR, Yates JW: Prediction and management of pain in patients with advanced cancer. Gen Hosp Psychiatry 3:95–101, 1981.

THE DIGESTIVE SYSTEM

NIRMAL S. MANN
OLIN TEAGUE VA CENTER
AFFILIATED WITH SCOTT AND WHITE CLINIC

1 · ESOPHAGEAL DISORDERS AND DISORDERS OF GASTROINTESTINAL MOTILITY

Theodore W. Burns
OCHSNER CLINIC AND ALTON OCHSNER MEDICAL FOUNDATION

The orderly, timely transport of ingested material through the gastrointestinal tract is dependent on proper function of GI muscle. In recent years, improved diagnostic techniques have allowed better characterization of GI motility, providing a better understanding of the normal and abnormal states and a rational basis for therapy in many diseases.

DISORDERS OF ESOPHAGEAL STRIATED MUSCLE

Hypopharyngeal and upper esophageal abnormalities result in the inability to deliver ingested food from the mouth to the thoracic esophagus. This may be caused by defects in neural control or in skeletal muscle function, or by intrinsic muscular disorders (see Table 1). Symptoms include inability to initiate swallows, difficulty in clearing ingested food from the hypopharynx, nasopharyngeal regurgitation, and tracheal aspiration. True abnormalities of cervical esophageal function should be differentiated from patients with globus hystericus syndrome who perceive a "lump in the throat" but who have no difficulty in swallowing.

In patients with cervical dysphagia, clues to the diagnosis lie in the history, and objective evidence can be gained by physical examination and by videotaped or cineradiographic studies of barium swallows.

Management

The greatest success is achieved when the symptoms are secondary to an underlying treatable illness such as myasthenia gravis or a thyroid disorder. Gradual improvement of dysphagia caused by stroke can occur during the recovery phase and in tumor patients whose malignant disease can be successfully treated.

Patients with cricopharyngeal spasm often go years without diagnosis and adequate treatment. Traditional measures include skeletal muscle relaxants such as diazepam (Valium) or antispasmodics, but these are generally ineffective. Anecdotal evidence supports the use of esophageal bougienage with a large-caliber bougie (size 50 to 54 French). Such treatment is safe in proper hands and often provides prompt, lasting relief. In patients with persistent symptoms in whom an abnormal cricopharyngeus is confirmed by radiographic or manometric studies, cricopharyngeal myotomy is usually helpful. Myotomy has also been used with some success in patients with symptoms of cricopharyngeal dysfunction secondary to myositis or collagen vascular disease. Following cricopharyngeal myotomy, care must be taken to prevent gastroesophageal reflux, which, in the absence of a functional cricopharyngeus, can lead to aspiration.

In patients with progressive degenerative conditions of the nerves or muscles or those with severe dysphagia following head and neck surgery, there is often little treatment to offer, and chronic aspiration or malnutrition frequently occurs. Ultimately, even saliva can become a problem and nutrition is best maintained by nasogastric feeding tube or gastrostomy.

SMOOTH MUSCLE DISORDERS OF THE ESOPHAGUS

For purposes of this discussion, smooth muscle disorders will be classified as primary, secondary, or those associated with gastroesophageal reflux.

Table 1. ETIOLOGY OF CERVICAL DYSPHAGIA

Neurogenic
- CNS malignancy or infection
- Amyotrophic lateral sclerosis
- Multiple sclerosis
- Huntington's chorea
- Parkinson's disease
- Poliomyelitis
- Cerebrovascular accidents

Myogenic
- Cricopharyngeal spasm
- Myasthenia gravis
- Myotonic dystrophy
- Polymyositis, dermatomyositis
- Oculopharyngeal muscular dystrophy
- Thyroid disease
- Amyloidosis

Miscellaneous
- Surgery
- Trauma
- Zenker's diverticulum

ACHALASIA

Achalasia is characterized by absence of peristalsis in the esophageal smooth muscle and a hypertensive lower esophageal sphincter (LES) that fails to relax completely with swallows. Symptoms are progressive dysphagia and regurgitation of previously ingested material when reclining or bending. Early in the disease course, chest pain may accompany dysphagia (vigorous achalasia).

Diagnosis is generally apparent on barium swallow, and manometric studies confirm the diagnosis. Endoscopy is important to rule out "secondary achalasia," due to malignancy at or near the gastroesophageal junction.

Management

The overall objective of treatment for achalasia is to eliminate the resting high pressure at the LES to allow emptying of the esophagus in the upright position even in the absence of effective peristalsis. This can be satisfactorily achieved nonoperatively by pneumatic dilatation or by an open surgical myotomy.

Pneumatic dilatation usually results in prompt resolution of symptoms, although recurrence may require repeat dilatation months or years later. Occasionally patients fail dilatation altogether. Dilatation is complicated by perforation in about 5% of cases, and gastroesophageal reflux is an infrequent sequela.

The open myotomy is an operative approach to incise the hypertensive circular muscle, and provides long-lasting symptomatic relief. Predictably, the incidence of gastroesophageal reflux is higher after myotomy than after pneumatic dilatation and can become a formidable complication.

Recently, smooth muscle relaxation with calcium channel blockers has been found to be effective in some patients with achalasia. Such an approach would require lifelong medical treatment, but may be an alternative to surgery in poor-risk patients.

My colleagues and I favor pneumatic dilatation as a first step. If this treatment fails within days or weeks, we repeat the procedure. Patients who have repeat failures or frequent recurrences should undergo myotomy by an experienced esophageal surgeon. We reserve medical treatment for those who are poor surgical risks in whom dilatation fails or who refuse dilatation. Nifedipine (Procardia), 10 mg sublingually (by puncturing the capsule) before meals, appears to be the most effective medication.

DIFFUSE ESOPHAGEAL SPASM (DES) AND RELATED DISORDERS

Diffuse esophageal spasm is defined as the presence of high-amplitude simultaneous waves in the esophageal body associated with pain or dysphagia. More recently, other peristaltic disorders such as high peristaltic pressure (nutcracker esophagus) have been described in patients with similar symptoms but no evidence of true spasm. Diagnosis of spasm is confirmed when patients exhibit the characteristic spasm on x-ray or manometry coincident with an episode of dysphagia or chest pain.

Management

Treatment of DES is directed toward decreasing the frequency and intensity of spastic waves. Smooth muscle relaxants including nitroglycerin, hydralazine (Apresoline), calcium channel blockers, and anticholinergics have been used with limited success. The response to such agents is highly variable and cannot be predicted for a given patient. In my experience, sublingual nitroglycerin or sublingual nifedipine used as needed has been most successful.

Symptoms of DES and related disorders often wax and wane over years; medical therapy and reassurance are usually adequate treatment. When symptoms are persistent and severe, dilatation of the esophageal body with a bougie (size 50 or 54 French) or even pneumatic balloon can be effective. Surgical myotomy of the smooth muscle segment can be successful but is rarely necessary.

SECONDARY MOTOR DISORDERS

A number of systemic illnesses have been associated with abnormalities of esophageal smooth muscle. The best described is progressive systemic sclerosis (scleroderma), approximately 80% of such patients manifesting the classic low LES pressure and weak peristaltic wave. Patients generally suffer severe, complicated, unrelenting gastroesophageal reflux and must be treated with a compulsive lifelong program of antireflux measures. Blocking gastric acid production with cimetidine (Tagamet) or ranitidine (Zantac) is helpful in symptomatic treatment and may decrease stricture formation. Smooth muscle stimulants such as metoclopramide (Reglan) have little effect on the fibrotic esophageal muscle but may assist in improving gastric emptying. Stricture formation is common, and dilatation should be carried out at the first sign of dysphagia and repeated as necessary to maintain patency of the distal esophagus. Despite a few favorable reports of antireflux surgery in scleroderma patients, such procedures usually result in an achalasia-like syndrome with aperistalsis and a surgically created distal high-pressure zone. Aggressive, continuous medical therapy usually provides acceptable control of reflux complications.

The most serious secondary motor disorder is the achalasia-like illness produced by some tumors at or near the LES. Such patients present with severe, rapidly progressive dysphagia and weight loss. Manometric and fluoroscopic findings are similar to those of primary achalasia. Endoscopic examination with biopsy is usually diagnostic. Such tumors are rarely resectable surgically; chemotherapy or radiation has been shown to reverse motility defects in some cases.

GASTROESOPHAGEAL REFLUX

Often thought of as a peptic disorder, gastroesophageal reflux is more properly considered as a defect in esophageal motility. Reflux of any potentially injurious substance including acid, pepsin, bile, and alkaline small intestine secretions can result in symptoms and mucosal injury. The underlying defect is that of a poor muscular barrier at the LES and poor peristaltic clearance mechanism in the esophageal body. In many patients, concomitant delayed gastric emptying is a contributing factor.

Diagnosis can usually be made on the basis of clinical history. For patients whose presentation is less specific or who have complications or poor response to treatment, a rational approach to evaluation and treatment is shown in Figure 1.

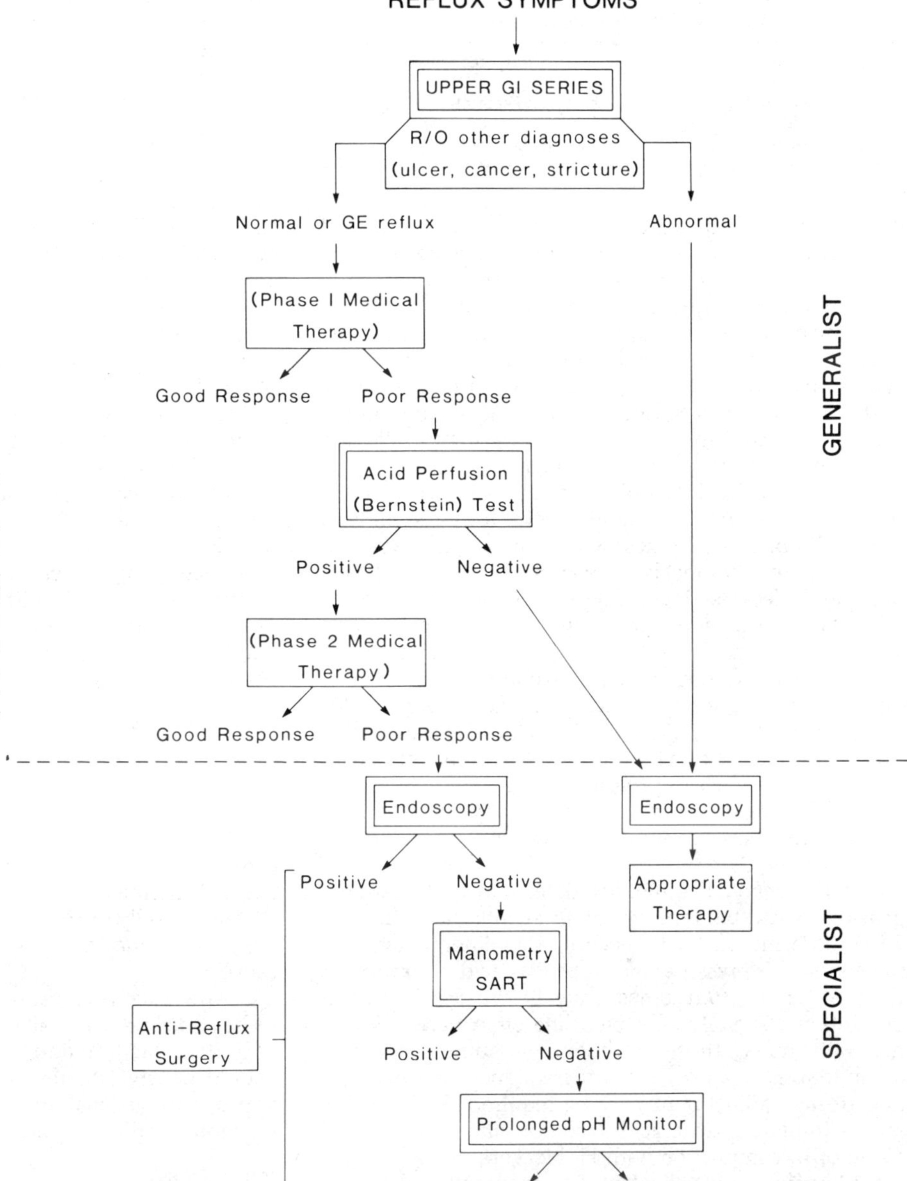

Figure 1. A proposed scheme for the use of diagnostic tests in patients with gastroesophageal disease. Appropriate treatment is recommended at various stages, depending on the complexity of the individual patient. (From Richter JE, Castell DO: Gastroesophageal reflux. Pathogenesis, diagnosis, and therapy. Ann Intern Med 97:93–102, 1982. By permission.)

Management

Gastroesophageal reflux is usually a chronic, recurring illness. A therapeutic plan should be considered with two objectives in mind: first, immediate measures to alleviate symptoms and protect inflamed mucosa; second, a long-term plan to minimize chronic reflux. Thus, the following recommended measures to alter the patient's habits and life style should be encouraged as permanent changes.

In obese patients, weight loss frequently results in rewarding improvements in reflux symptoms. Regulation of the meal schedule and meal size are also important. Multiple small feedings are rarely practical on a long-term basis, but three balanced meals daily are preferable to one or two large meals. It is most important to avoid the popular habit of eating a single large meal in the evening. Activities that require bending or stooping, such as housework and gardening, should be done in the fasting state. Patients should avoid reclining for at least three hours after meals to allow adequate time for gastric emptying. Meals that are high in fat further delay gastric emptying and may provoke symptoms.

Certain substances by their very nature, such as citrus juices, tomato products, and sweets, can produce symptoms of reflux even in the absence of acid. Additionally, foods such as alcohol, peppermint, chocolates, and fats all reduce LES pressure and may precipitate reflux. Cigarette smoking decreases LES pressure and should be eliminated. Many classes of drugs inhibit LES pressure and may aggravate reflux or interfere with effective therapy (Table 2). An effort should be made to eliminate these or to find suitable substitutes.

Bed elevation is important, whether or not nocturnal symptoms are prominent. Creating a 6- to 8-inch

Table 2. DRUGS THAT DECREASE THE PRESSURE OF THE LOWER ESOPHAGEAL SPHINCTER

Progesterone	Alpha-adrenergic antagonists
Theophylline	Dopamine
Prostaglandins E_1, E_2, A_2	Diazepam (Valium)
Anticholinergics	Meperidine, morphine
Beta-adrenergic agonists	Calcium channel blockers

drop from head to foot decreases nocturnal reflux and improves acid clearance, significantly reducing the total time of acid contact with esophageal mucosa.

There is little firm evidence to support the efficacy of antacids in gastroesophageal reflux. Nonetheless, antacids are preferable to drinking milk or snacking for symptomatic relief, as they effectively neutralize gastric acid and may increase LES pressure. An alginic preparation (Gaviscon) is as effective as antacids in relieving symptoms and many patients prefer it.

Histamine H_2 Antagonists. In recent years, medications have become increasingly useful for patients with reflux. Numerous studies with cimetidine (Tagamet) and ranitidine (Zantac) have documented relief of heartburn and decreased antacid requirements. However, relief lasts only while the patient is medicated and symptoms generally recur promptly after cessation of therapy. The dosage schedule recommended for ulcer disease can be recommended for reflux (Tagamet, 300 mg q.i.d. or Zantac, 150 mg b.i.d.), but the duration of therapy should be two to three months. In patients with severe disease such as progressive systemic sclerosis or reflux following myotomy for achalasia, therapy should be maintained on a continuous basis, either in full doses or nocturnally.

Bethanechol. The motility defects in gastroesophageal reflux can be improved with agents that stimulate GI smooth muscle. Bethanechol, a cholinergic agonist, increases LES pressure and improves acid clearance. A dose of 25 mg four times daily before meals and at bedtime is generally effective. Side effects are few and generally reflect those of cholinergic stimulation such as abdominal cramps, urinary frequency, or diarrhea, and dosage adjustment may be required. Bethanechol may stimulate gastric acid secretion and can be used alone or in conjunction with H_2 blockers.

Metoclopramide (Reglan). This agent stimulates GI motility by dopaminergic inhibition and by direct stimulation of acetylcholine release. The standard dose is 10 mg before meals and at bedtime; this may be increased to 20 mg or decreased if side effects are encountered. Metoclopramide can also be used as needed in single doses of 10 to 20 mg. Side effects can be a problem and may limit this agent's usefulness; they include restlessness, anxiety, extrapyramidal reactions, and lethargy and are more frequent in young people.

In patients with reflux symptoms but no signs of complications, I recommend the life style changes described above and regular antacids; cimetidine or ranitidine can be added if needed for symptomatic relief. For those with ulceration or severe symptoms, promotility agents may be needed. Subjects with concomitant suspected or proved gastric stasis often benefit from metoclopramide with or without H_2 blockers.

Patients with very low LES pressures are frequently refractory to medical management and tend to suffer complications of ulceration and stricture. For these, antireflux surgery can be effective in restoring resting LES pressure, resolving symptoms, and healing ulcerated mucosa.

MISCELLANEOUS ESOPHAGEAL DISORDERS

DIVERTICULA

Esophageal diverticula are generally acquired rather than congenital and occur most frequently in the midesophagus. Those proximal to the upper and lower sphincters (called "pulsion diverticula") are generally associated with sphincter dysfunction.

Zenker's diverticulum may be associated with cervical dysphagia and pharyngeal regurgitation. Treatment of a symptomatic Zenker's diverticulum consists of surgical excision or diverticulopexy. Many surgeons include a cricopharyngeal myotomy because of the suspected cricopharyngeal dysfunction that probably gives rise to this diverticulum.

Epiphrenic diverticula are usually associated with LES dysfunction. Treatment should be directed toward the LES rather than the diverticulum per se. Abnormalities such as high pressure or incomplete relaxation are frequently observed. Although myotomy and diverticulectomy may be necessary to achieve relief, careful dilatation under fluoroscopy or over a guidewire may be sufficient.

RINGS AND WEBS

Thin mucosal folds that partially occlude the lumen of the esophagus may be found at any level. The most common of these is Schatzki's ring located at the mucosal junction of the esophagus and stomach. A less common location for mucosal folds is the cervical esophagus. When associated with iron deficiency anemia (Paterson-Kelly or Plummer-Vinson syndrome), there is a high incidence of squamous carcinoma in the cervical esophagus.

After confirmation of the diagnosis by endoscopy, webs and rings are easily treated by passage of a bougie (size 50 French). In addition, patients with cervical webs should be investigated for iron deficiency and treated appropriately. Dilatation results in symptomatic relief for months to years and may be repeated as needed.

INFECTIONS

The two most common infections of the esophagus are candidiasis and herpesvirus infection, usually occurring in immunocompromised hosts. Characteristic symptoms of esophageal infection include odynophagia and severe pyrosis, usually abrupt in onset. Diagnosis is best made by endoscopy with cytologic brushings and biopsies. The treatment of choice for superficial candidal esophagitis is ketoconazole (Nizoral), 400 mg as a single daily dose; nystatin, 250,000 units swallowed every two to four hours, is also effective. Ketoconazole should not be given together with H_2 antagonists because these agents reduce its absorption. If the infection is invasive, therapy must be systemic with amphotericin B.

Management of herpesvirus infection is discussed in Section IV, Chapter 21.

PHYSICAL INJURIES

Mucosal injury may be caused by drugs, radiation, or caustic chemicals. The most common injury is the acute mucosal ulceration produced by intraesophageal dissolution of tetracycline capsules or other medications. Odynophagia is common and substernal burning persists for several days. Treatment consists of the physician's reassurance and frequent antacids. Symptoms generally resolve over several days, and patient education is important to prevent recurrence.

Radiation therapy for thoracic malignancies may result in acute esophagitis, which is generally self-limiting and treated symptomatically with antacids and topical anesthetics. Occasionally, radiation therapy must be temporarily interrupted to allow symptoms to ameliorate. Indomethacin prophylactically reduces radiation esophagitis in animals, but there is no information regarding its use in humans.

Acid or Alkaline Ingestion. A more serious physical injury is that caused by ingestion of strong acid or alkalized solution. While acids produce a superficial burn, alkali rapidly penetrates into mucosa, causing necrosis and vascular thrombosis. If the patient survives the acute injury, alkaline injury frequently results in long, severe esophageal strictures of the esophageal body and a high incidence of squamous carcinoma. Treatment of acid ingestion consists of intake of large quantities of water, early endoscopy to assess the degree of damage, and observation of the patient for perforation of esophagus or stomach.

Because of the potential for heat production, neutralizing agents such as water should not be administered after alkaline ingestion. Soon after admission, careful endoscopy can confirm the injury. Experimental evidence suggest that early corticosteroids are helpful, but control studies are lacking. Antibiotics are indicated when infection is suspected or if corticosteroids are used; antibiotic treatment should be directed toward the oral flora with agents such as penicillin. In the absence of perforation, mediastinitis, or peritonitis, dilatation can be begun early in an attempt to prevent stricture, but most physicians recommend frequent barium swallows to detect strictures early rather than prophylactic dilatation. Long-term care includes dilatation as needed and surveillance for squamous carcinoma in the years following injury.

GASTRIC MOTILITY DISORDERS

Abnormal gastric motor function results in alterations in the rate of gastric emptying. The two most common clinical problems are (1) rapid emptying of liquids (dumping syndrome), usually after vagotomy and partial gastrectomy; and (2) delayed solid emptying (gastric stasis) in the absence of gastric outlet obstruction. The most common causes of gastric stasis are diabetic gastroparesis, postvagotomy states, and idiopathic (see Table 3 for additional causes). Gastric stasis can sometimes be confirmed by x-rays after barium-food mixtures but is best objectively demonstrated in the nuclear-labeled, solid-phase emptying test.

Management

Rapid emptying of liquids can usually be satisfactorily controlled by dietary manipulation. Symptoms occur when a high caloric load is delivered to the small bowel rapidly. Thus, ingestion of high caloric liquids such as soft drinks and fruit juices should be restricted. Fluid should be low in calories and taken with meals.

Reclining immediately after meals may also delay liquid emptying. Although surgical maneuvers such as interposition of reverse jejunal loops between the stomach and duodenum have been used in severe cases, such drastic measures are seldom indicated. Some recent work with pectin suggests that it also may produce symptomatic relief when ingested with meals.

Gastric stasis syndromes may be more difficult to manage. In those occasional patients in whom a reversible cause is found (Table 3), correction of the underlying illness or withdrawal of the offending drug may be all that is necessary. In most cases, however, dietary and life style changes must be made and appropriate medications used.

Long-term measures for gastric stasis include a diet low in fat and low in vegetable fiber, particularly in patients with a history of bezoar formation. The daily meal pattern should include three or four balanced meals daily. The general measures recommended for patients with gastroesophageal reflux may provide improvement even when pyrosis is not a complaint. In patients with symptomatic reflux associated with gastric stasis, cimetidine or ranitidine may help inhibit acid and water secretion.

Metoclopramide. This is a useful agent in many patients with gastric stasis as an antiemetic, a smooth muscle stimulant, or both. However, many people get no benefit at all from this medication and many others are intolerant of side effects. I generally begin patients on a 10-mg dose taken 30 minutes before meals and increase dosage gradually up to 20 mg until improvement occurs or side effects become apparent. If side effects are experienced at the initial dose level, the drug can be gradually reduced until an accepted level is

---

Table 3. ETIOLOGY OF DELAYED GASTRIC EMPTYING

Pharmaceutical Agents and Hormones
  Opiates, including endorphins and narcotics
  Anticholinergics
  Tricyclic antidepressants
  Beta-adrenergic agonists
  L-Dopa
  Aluminum hydroxide antacids
  Gastrin, cholecystokinin, somatostatin
Acute or Transitory Gastric Retention
  Postoperative ileus
  Viral gastroenteritis
  Hyperglycemia and other metabolic abnormalities
  Elemental diets
  Total parenteral nutrition
  Cigarette smoking
Chronic or Prolonged Gastric Retention
  Diabetes mellitus
  Postgastric surgery
    Truncal vagotomy with or without pyloroplasty
    Superselective or gastric vagotomy with or without pyloroplasty
    Antrectomy or subtotal gastrectomy
  Gastroesophageal reflux
  Achlorhydria and atrophic gastritis
  Anorexia nervosa
  Gastric ulcer disease
  Amyloidosis
  Progressive systemic sclerosis
  Idiopathic intestinal pseudo-obstruction
  Systemic lupus erythematosus
  Dermatomyositis
  Myotonic dystrophy
  Progressive muscular dystrophy
  Familial dysautonomia
  Idiopathic gastroparesis–gastric dysrhythmias

found. Metoclopramide liquid (1 mg/cc) is particularly convenient for dosage adjustment. Anticholinergics may not only contribute to gastric stasis but inhibit the effects of metoclopramide, and should be restricted if possible.

While most gastric stasis syndromes are chronic, recurrent acute exacerbations are common in diabetics. These may be associated with poor glucose control and are generally self-limiting. During these episodes, patients should be maintained without oral intake, and nasogastric suction may be necessary to relieve vomiting. Fluid and electrolyte balance must be corrected and blood sugar controlled. Metoclopramide is given IV, beginning at 10 mg and increasing gradually to 20 mg if necessary. In patients intolerant of metoclopramide, bethanechol, 5 mg SQ, may be helpful. As the nausea resolves, refeeding should begin in the form of liquid preparations such as Ensure or Isocal, and metoclopramide is administered PO. Advancement to full diet should be gradual. Although a low fat diet is desirable, fat is a major source of calories in the diabetic and a severe restriction is often not possible.

Refractory patients with idiopathic or postvagotomy gastric stasis may benefit from surgical intervention. Antrectomy and gastroduodenostomy or gastroenterostomy have been employed with some success in patients with gastric dysrhythmias. However, diabetics frequently fail to improve with such procedures, and I prefer jejunal feedings to maintain nutrition in severe cases. This can be accomplished by nasoenteral intubation or surgical jejunostomy.

DISORDERS OF BOWEL MOTILITY: IRRITABLE BOWEL SYNDROME

Irritable bowel syndrome (IBS) is the most common disorder seen by gastroenterologists in the United States. The classic symptoms are cramping abdominal pain with constipation, diarrhea, or both in the absence of organic disease. The underlying abnormality appears to be that of abnormal propulsion in the gut, affecting the colon and probably small bowel as well. Treatment is directed at psychologic factors, bowel irregularity, and abdominal pain.

Management

Although stress or anxiety may clearly provoke symptoms, the disease itself frequently becomes an additional source of stress as the patient becomes increasingly alarmed by the severity of the symptoms and the absence of abnormalities in x-rays and lab tests. To alleviate this source of concern, the physician must convince the patient of the accuracy of the diagnosis and emphasize the good prognosis. Adequate time spent in patient education often alleviates anxiety and allows the patient to gain insights into the environmental and psychologic factors that may provoke and affect bowel habits. Follow-up visits should be encouraged and a warm, trusting relationship between patient and physician established.

Sedation. For patients in whom anxiety or stress is severe, mild sedatives or tranquilizers are often helpful. Combination products such as Librax or Donnatal may be particularly helpful; occasionally, a modest dose of a tricycline antidepressant, equivalent to 50 mg amitriptyline at bedtime, can be dramatically effective in alleviating anxiety and improving bowel habits, especially in patients with diarrhea.

Constipation. Constipation in IBS is treated in a manner similar to that of idiopathic constipation, discussed in Section I, Chapter 5. The increases in dietary fiber and fluids should be encouraged as a lifelong change. Additionally, symptoms of flatulence, bloating, and cramping pain generally improve as constipation is alleviated.

Diarrhea. Diarrhea in IBS patients usually occurs on arising in the morning, in the postprandial periods, or during times of emotional stress. Several alterations in diet and judicious use of anticholinergics are effective. Stimulants such as coffee, tea, and chocolates should be restricted. Raw vegetables, nuts, seeds, and meals high in fat or spices may all provoke diarrhea. Psyllium preparations can be substituted as a fiber source. A lactose-free trial is also recommended initially. After two weeks of a severly restricted diet, patients may gradually add restricted foods to determine their tolerance. Anticholinergic agents given in doses sufficient to dry the mouth before meals often eliminate postprandial diarrhea. IBS patients are also effectively controlled with Lomotil or Imodium, but my colleagues and I reserve the use of these agents for times such as dining out, meetings, and travel, when diarrhea would pose a serious inconvenience or embarrassing social situation. We find that patients appreciate having the option to use antidiarrheals, and the confidence they promote is a psychologic boost.

Abdominal pain usually improves with correction of bowel habits. When necessary, anticholinergics are generally effective for cramping pain. During exacerbation or stressful periods, we encourage patients to use anticholinergics on a regular schedule, rather than as needed, until symptoms subside. Heating pads and warm tub soaks also help relieve abdominal pain and promote relaxation.

The general pattern of symptoms is one of remissions and relapses, and treatment measures must be frequently reinforced. For the occasional patient who receives no improvement from these measures, reevaluation for other possible diagnoses is indicated.

REFERENCES

Burns TW: Colonic motility in the irritable bowel syndrome. Arch Intern Med 140:247–251, 1980.

Dodds WJ, Hogan WJ, Helm HF, et al: Pathogenesis of reflux esophagitis. Gastroenterology 81:376–394, 1981.

Ricci R, McCallum R, Ricci DA, et al.: Effect of metoclopramide in diabetic gastroparesis. J Clin Gastroenterol 7:25–32, 1985.

Richter JE, Castell DO: Gastroesophageal reflux. Ann Intern Med 97:93–102, 1982.

Schuster M (ed): Symposium on gastrointestinal motility disorders. Med Clin North Am 65:1109–1411, 1981.

2 · IDIOPATHIC INFLAMMATORY BOWEL DISEASE

J. Thomas Danzi
GUTHRIE CLINIC

DEFINITION AND CLINICAL PATTERNS

The spectrum of diseases included in the idiopathic inflammatory bowel disease (IBD) classification includes ulcerative colitis, ulcerative proctosigmoiditis, and Crohn's disease of the gastrointestinal tract. The exact etiology of these disorders is unknown.

ULCERATIVE COLITIS

By definition, ulcerative colitis is an idiopathic inflammation involving the mucosa of the colon. Approximately 95% of cases of mucosal ulcerative colitis (MUC) have rectal involvement. In most cases the colonic involvement is uniform. It may extend to the total colon (universal ulcerative colitis) or from the rectum to the transverse or left colon, or may be limited to the rectum and sigmoid colon (ulcerative proctosigmoiditis). The mucosal inflammation is characterized endoscopically by loss of normal submucosal vascular markings. The edema of the mucosa results in it having a granular appearance. In addition, the mucosa can demonstrate varying degrees of erythema and friability. The so-called touch friability of the mucosa involved with ulcerative colitis can be demonstrated by gently applying a biopsy forceps or cotton ball to the involved lining. Typically, the mucosal uclerations are small or fine in appearance. Large, linear, or stellate ulcerations are not characteristic of MUC. A histologic diagnosis of ulcerative colitis is supported by the demonstration of crypt abscesses, goblet cell depletion, and a mucosal inflammatory cellular infiltrate. Most IBD experts favor the endoscopic over the histologic features in establishing a diagnosis of MUC.

CROHN'S DISEASE

A definition of Crohn's disease is more difficult because this disease can involve any part of the digestive system from the mouth to the anus. Additionally, the inflammation of the involved segment may be mucosal only, transmural (TMC), or predominantly submucosal or serosal in location. It is important to note that the extent of histologic involvement with Crohn's disease tends to correlate with clinical features. Predominant mucosal disease is commonly associated with diarrhea, blood loss anemia, and toxicity symptoms; submucosal involvement typically results in strictures, fistulas, and signs of protein calorie malnutrition.

An important distinguishing feature of Crohn's disease is the fact that the involvement can be segmental or nonuniform in character. This is in contrast to the uniform colonic involvement with ulcerative colitis. Another important characteristic of Crohn's disease involving the colon is that the rectum is spared. Indeed, approximately 50% of patients with colonic Crohn's disease have a normal rectal segment. This is an important differential diagnostic criterion for Crohn's disease versus ulcerative colitis.

The histologic features of Crohn's disease include the variable mucosal involvement, preservation of goblet cells within the mucosa, deep and longitudinal mucosal ulcerations, and granulomatous inflammation. However, demonstration of granulomatous inflammation is not required for a diagnosis of Crohn's disease because it is present in only 50% of cases.

Endoscopic features of Crohn's disease include submucosal edema with its resulting mucosal granularity; irregular thickening of the mucosa, producing a "cobblestone" appearance; large linear or stellate ulcerations amid the abnormal mucosa; and areas of normal mucosa, often identified adjacent to areas with abnormal mucosal features.

CLINICAL ASPECTS AND DIAGNOSTIC CRITERIA

Ulcerative colitis and Crohn's disease have important clinical similarities. Both diseases are characterized by a natural history of spontaneous exacerbations and remissions and are associated with well-recognized extraintestinal manifestations. These occur in the skin (pyoderma gangrenosum, erythema nodosum) the eye (uveitis, episcleritis), and the joints (large joint migratory arthritis, synovitis), and usually parallel the activity of the colonic inflammation. Other extraintestinal manifestations are recognized with both types of IBD, but their association does not usually parallel the activity of inflammation within the digestive tract. These include primary sclerosing cholangitis, chronic active hepatitis, ankylosing spondylitis, and nephrolithiasis. The two diseases differ in the rate of surgical cure and in the risk of progressing into colon cancer. A total proctocolectomy with ileostomy is practically curative of ulcerative colitis, but does not cure Crohn's disease of the colon. Clinical recurrence rate of Crohn's disease may approach 100% in a lifetime. Farmer's group at the Cleveland Clinic demonstrated that 40% of all patients with Crohn's disease needed a second operation within 15 years after the initial surgical procedure. Long-standing ulcerative colitis (a history of disease of more than ten years' duration) has been documented to be a premalignant condition. Certain features, including universal colitis (total colonic involvement), more severe manifestations, and onset at an earlier age (adolescent universal colitis), contribute to the likelihood of development of colon cancer. The incidence of colon cancer reaches about 20% per decade beginning after the first ten years of mucosal ulcerative colitis. In contrast, although selected patients with colonic Crohn's disease may have an increased risk of developing colon cancer, this risk is less than the seven to ten times that of patients with long-standing ulcerative colitis.

The clinical aspects of ulcerative colitis and Crohn's disease include symptom groupings that can be helpful from a diagnostic standpoint. Ulcerative colitis and its limited version, ulcerative proctosigmoiditis, most commonly present with a sudden onset of bloody diarrhea, anorexia, and gradual weight loss. The diarrhea may occur mostly at night. Characteristically, the stool is bloody and contains mucus. Crohn's disease of the colon usually presents with the same clinical features. Physical examination may demonstrate tenderness to palpation over the colonic area. Inspection of the perianal and perineal areas for fistula is an important diagnostic step. Confirmation of such a physical finding lends support to a diagnosis of Crohn's colitis.

Crohn's involvement of the small bowel or upper digestive tract has a different symptom complex. Commonly, an individual has diarrhea but usually without bloody stools. A tendency to nocturnal bowel movements may be observed. Abdominal pain, often crampy in nature, is a frequent complaint. In addition, the insidious signs of anemia and varying degrees of protein caloric malnutrition may be observed. The physical examination may be more helpful in establishing this diagnosis than it is for colonic inflammatory bowel disease. Frequently, the abdominal examination reveals a palpable, firm, tender bowel loop, usually in the right lower quadrant. Demonstration of abdominal mass is suggestive of an associated internal fistula. Inspection of the perianal and perineal areas for fistulas is important; these types of fistulas more likely indicate ileocolonic Crohn's disease than small intestinal disease alone.

The diagnosis of IBD is confirmed by the endoscopic features most commonly visualized by proctosigmoidoscopy. The initial examination is best achieved in a "nonprepped" manner, to allow for inspection of mucosal features in an "all-natural" state and enable fresh stool specimens to be obtained in order to exclude an infectious etiology. In addition, the unprepared state eliminates the risk of giving an enema to an individual with severe colitis. This latter point is important because of the potential risk of developing a toxic megacolon from such a preparation. A proctosigmoidoscopic examination can be performed with either the rigid or flexible instrument. I routinely use the rigid sigmoidoscope for the initial inspection because it allows ulcerative colitis to be distinguished from Crohn's disease and ulcerative proctosigmoiditis from ulcerative colitis in most cases. The lack of significant air insufflation with the rigid instrument is an important consideration when the extent and severity of colitis are unknown. The use of a flexible sigmoidoscope for follow-up evaluation, and after there has been improvement of clinical symptoms, is appropriate in my view.

MANAGEMENT

Therapy for inflammatory bowel disease requires a multifaceted approach. The main therapeutic aim for these chronic diseases is to induce and maintain a remission. Successful treatment of Crohn's disease or ulcerative colitis is one of the biggest challenges in the field of medicine.

SHORT-TERM GOALS

The main short-term goal is the induction of remission, i.e., the resolution of acute symptoms and any associated complication. A clinical resolution may precede any histologic improvement by four to six weeks. It is therefore important that therapeutic measures be continued to achieve remission of an acute episode of IBD. Part of short-term therapy includes evaluation and treatment of any associated anemia, state of dehydration, or electrolyte imbalance. Another aspect of management of an acute episode is maintenance of normal nutritional status. This includes preventive measures to maintain a normal protein caloric state or to correct variable protein, caloric, or mineral imbalances.

LONG-TERM GOALS

There are multiple goals in long-term management of both ulcerative colitis and Crohn's disease. The first is the recognition of an intestinal or extraintestinal complication. The presence of either manifestation of IBD is a good indication that a gastroenterologist should be consulted. A second important aspect concerns the surveillance for cancer. With the recognized premalignant potential of long-standing ulcerative colitis and Crohn's disease, how does one develop a screening program to detect early colonic cancer? The histologic evaluation of rectal biopsies for mucosal dysplasia has been shown to be predictive of colonic cancer in a patient with ulcerative colitis (quiescent colitis at the time of biopsy) and the absence of a radiologic or endoscopic diagnosis of cancer. Colonoscopic biopsy technique has now been utilized in an attempt to further increase the yield of premalignant changes. Most IBD experts currently recommend the start of a cancer surveillance program after the seventh year of colitis. A total colonoscopy should be performed during remission, with multiple biopsies. If marked dysplasia is demonstrated histologically, strong consideration should be given to a prophylactic total colectomy. If mild to moderate dysplasia is demonstrated on the biopsies, yearly colonoscopy is recommended. If the histologic evaluation reveals no changes of dysplasia, a colonoscopic reevaluation is advisable every two years.

INDICATIONS FOR HOSPITALIZATION

Some indications for hospitalizing the patient include the presence of a complication (intestinal or extraintestinal), intractability of symptoms, and severity of symptoms with impending toxicity and associated conditions such as anemia, dehydration, or malnutrition. A decision to hospitalize should be based not on a "cookbook" type of list but on sound clinical judgment. Certainly, the medical necessity for intravenous steroid therapy, total parenteral nutrition for either primary or adjuvant therapy, or intensive therapy and observation of acute colitis or toxic megacolon are classic illustrations of the need for hospital admission.

INDICATIONS FOR SURGERY IN IBD

The indications for surgical intervention in either ulcerative colitis or Crohn's disease include (1) failure of medical therapy for severe colitis or toxic megacolon; (2) suspected colonic perforation; (3) intractability of disease, uncontrolled colonic hemorrhage, complications of medical therapy, or associated growth retardation in children; (4) intestinal complications unresponsive to medical therapy, a colonic stricture resulting in obstruction, or failure to exclude a colonic cancer as its cause; (5) progressive extraintestinal complications; and (6) the premalignancy potential of the disease.

It is beyond the scope of this chapter to discuss the specific types of operations recommended. However, it is important to know the surgical thinking in your area regarding a continent ileostomy for ulcerative colitis but not Crohn's disease; an ileorectal anastomosis for

Crohn's disease or ulcerative colitis; and the approach to a toxic megacolon (decompressive for a loop ileostomy with a blow-hole colostomy or resective for a total proctocolectomy with an ileostomy). In this way, in your discussions with patients, your surgical approach will agree with that of your colleagues. This continuity of thinking lends confidence to patients and their families.

HOME HEALTH CARE

IBD patients are using home health care more frequently now. With help from the agencies providing such, it is now possible for both total parenteral and enteral nutrition to be achieved in the home. This capability has enabled many patients with severe forms of either disease to secure nutritional support along with home total parenteral nutrition (nothing by mouth) while continuing their employment or education. I found this extension of the medical therapy for IBD to be especially helpful in adolescent patients. In addition, home health care services enable an ostomy patient to receive the assistance of an enterostomal therapist. This ancillary medical care can be invaluable when dealing with skin problems (infection or allergic reactions), odor control, or high ostomy output states. In addition, the psychologic counseling that comes with these visits can be tremendously helpful to selected individuals.

NONPHARMACOLOGIC THERAPY

The nutritional aspects of management of IBD patients have only recently become better understood. There are both preventive and therapeutic aspects. Studies have demonstrated that 40 to 50 kcal/kg of ideal body weight (IBW) and 1 to 1.5 gm of protein/kg of IBW are required daily to provide adequate nutrition to the average 70-kg patient with IBD. In addition, certain nutritional deficiencies can result from the inflammatory process itself or from the treatment. The best way to supply the many vitamins, minerals, and trace elements that IBD patients require is through high-potency vitamin formulas or prenatal vitamin compounds. It is important that the formulary used contains 1 mg each of iron and folic acid, along with an adequate supply of zinc and calcium.

Many IBD patients require prolonged periods of bowel rest to assist in the healing of their disease. During this time the use of elemental dietary formulas is an accepted way to supply nutritional needs. Many patients are able to ingest these preparations by drinking them slowly and by combining them with various flavoring mixtures to increase palatability. With this approach, I have been able to supply total nutritional requirements while achieving "basic" bowel rest and enabling individuals to continue their educational or vocational needs as outpatients.

Certain patients with IBD require total parenteral nutrition (TPN) because of the severity of their disease or the presence of complications. Individuals with severe colitis, toxic megacolon, or internal fistulas or those requiring surgery can benefit from the clinical application of TPN. In addition, home TPN may be a necessity for patients with short bowel syndrome or as a primary therapy for resistant growth retardation. Driscoll's review of this topic is an excellent reference article for those utilizing this form of therapy in IBD.

DRUG THERAPY

The pharmacologic therapy for IBD seems confusing and complex when first reviewed, but becomes easier to understand in terms of specific indications for each known disease entity.

Medical therapy for ulcerative proctosigmoiditis involves the use of local steroid preparations, either in a foam, enema, or suppository delivery package.

Sulfasalazine. If symptoms are uncontrolled with the above medication, the addition of sulfasalazine in a dosage of 1 to 2 gm daily is recommended. The amount of sulfa medication may be increased to 4 gm daily in unresponsive cases. I usually continue this sulfa therapy for three to four weeks after symptoms have resolved. I then withdraw the local steroid preparations and reduce the sulfasalazine dosage to 1 to 2 gm daily. Since this disease represents a limited variety of ulcerative colitis, I recommend that patients continue on this low-dose sulfa therapy to try to prevent a recurrence. I do not routinely prescribe antidiarrheal medications for ulcerative proctosigmoiditis unless patients have severe tenesmus. It is preferable to observe their responses to the anti-inflammatory medications and render therapeutic decisions appropriately. Certain patients do not respond to this pharmacologic treatment and require oral steroids to induce a remission. The steroid usage is identical to that described below for ulcerative colitis.

Pharmacologic therapy for ulcerative colitis involves two separate aspects: (1) the induction of a remission and (2) its maintenance. Sulfasalazine has been proved in many well-controlled studies to be effective for both aspects, whereas oral corticosteroid therapy has been shown to be effective only in inducing a remission. All patients with active symptoms should receive 4 gm of sulfasalazine unless they have a known allergy to the medication.

Steroid Medications. Oral steroid medications should be added in cases of inability to control active symptoms or when there is progression to a severe colitis with impending toxic megacolon. Since the clinical indication for steroid usage implies severe disease, steroid therapy should be instituted in the 40- to 60-mg daily range for prednisone or its appropriate hydrocortisone IV equivalent.

With the resolution of the acute symptoms, the corticosteroid medications can be withdrawn slowly over a period of four to six weeks while the sulfasalazine is continued in the same dosage. I regularly maintain the patient on 4 gm per day of sulfasalazine for a total of three months after a remission has been induced, and then reduce the dosage to one half for maintenance therapy. There is general agreement that unless there is a specific contraindication to long-term sulfasalazine maintenance therapy, all patients with chronic ulcerative colitis should continue to receive 2 gm daily for a minimum of one year.

Pharmacologic therapy for Crohn's disease varies depending on the site of involvement and the presence of a complication such as an internal or external fistula. Medical therapy for Crohn's disease has been shown to be effective only in inducing a remission and not in preventing a relapse (maintenance treatment). Both the American and European Cooperative Crohn's Disease Studies have demonstrated (1) the effectiveness of sulfasalazine in inducing a remission with Crohn's colitis or ileocolitis, but not ileitis alone; and (2) the effectiveness of oral steroids for Crohn's ileitis and ileocolitis, but not for colitis alone. However, steroids are indicated for use in combination with sulfasalazine in treating severe colitis, toxic megacolon, and the presence of fistulas. The medications are used as described for ulcerative colitis.

6-Mercaptopurine or Metronidazole. There is evidence that these agents may be valuable in treating the fistula complications of this IBD. The main concern with their use has been the high incidence of side effects, their carcinogenic potential, and the length of time required for healing. I have found little clinical applicability for either drug in my practice.

Adverse Effects. An understanding of the adverse effects of each drug used to treat the various types of IBD is imperative. The various local steroid preparations are not associated with any serious side effects and have not been shown to have any adrenal suppression activity. The use of sulfasalazine is associated with a high incidence of troublesome reactions, including anorexia; nausea or vomiting; headache; various skin eruptions; a generalized allergic reaction with fever, skin rash, arthralgias and lymphadenopathy; bone marrow toxicity with neutropenia or a granulocytosis; anemia related to either folate deficiency or red blood cell enzyme deficiencies; hypospermia or abnormal sperm function; hepatic dysfunction and granulomatous hepatitis; and allergic pulmonitis.

Because sulfasalazine has a prominent role in therapy for all types of IBD, allergy to it poses a difficult issue. Recently, some patients have been desensitized to sulfasalazine with small initial amounts of the drug (⅛ to ¼ tablets) for several days, and then slowly increased dosage. The drug is then tolerated by approximately 75% of these individuals.

The adverse effects of long-term steroid therapy are well known. Fortunately, the use of steroids for IBD is usually short term, except for those unfortunate individuals with extensive small bowel disease. Patients on steroid therapy should receive a steroid "prep" preoperatively and continue with the IV form postoperatively.

Use of 6-mercaptopurine is associated with up to a 10% incidence of significant side effects, including variable types of bone marrow suppression, severe acute pancreatitis, and sepsis. There is a known association of cancer development, namely, lymphoma, with this medication.

The long-term use of metronidazole in Crohn's disease is associated with paresthesias and the development of a metallic taste. In addition, there are mutagenic and carcinogenic risks with long-term use of this drug.

Before prescribing any type of therapy for the patient with IBD, it is important to be aware of any other concomitant diseases or medications. This will assist in recognizing such problems as worsening control of a diabetic on steroids, increased blood pressure in a known hypertensive patient on corticosteroid medications, a progressive anemia in a patient with a pyruvate kinase deficiency receiving sulfasalazine, or the development of an exfoliative dermatitis in a patient receiving sulfasalazine.

Antibiotics. A few clinical circumstances require the use of broad-spectrum antibiotics to treat IBD. A patient with Crohn's disease who has a toxic megacolon, severe colitis with possible colonic perforation, and an intraabdominal abscess associated with an inflammatory mass may be a candidate for antibiotic therapy. However, there is no literature to attest to the effectiveness of this type of therapy in IBD. There *is* much literature reflecting concern about indiscriminate use of broad-spectrum antibiotics in IBD patients, because of the risk of an antibiotic-associated colitis or a *Clostridium difficile* infestation causing an exacerbation of the disease.

Complications. Management of the complications of IBD includes therapy for toxic megacolon, uncontrollable hemorrhage, and obstructive symptoms related to a stricture of the involved segment of the GI tract.

Toxic Megacolon. This is the most dramatic complication associated with either ulcerative colitis or Crohn's disease. If the possibility of toxic megacolon is always borne in mind for a patient with severe colitis, the likelihood of missing this important diagnosis should be reduced. The clinical presentation includes a toxic appearance and commonly a lessening of the bloody diarrheal movements. This observation could be misinterpreted as a clinical improvement instead of a sign of clinical deterioration. In the presence of the previously described clinical findings, a plain abdominal x-ray should be ordered. The radiologic diagnosis of toxic megacolon can be established by a single abdominal x-ray demonstrating a segmental or total colonic diameter greater than 7 cm. However, not uncommonly a diagnosis is made by observing the radiographs over a period of a few hours. A progressive increase in colonic diameter, the loss of haustral markings, and a thumb-printing pattern indicative of edema and thinning of the colonic mucosa are features observed with this condition.

The management of toxic megacolon includes (1) intensive monitoring of vital signs; (2) intestinal decompression by either nasogastric or small bowel suction; (3) radiologic observation for colonic diameter increase and the presence of free peritoneal air; (4) prompt surgical consultation; and (5) frequent physical reevaluations. In addition, the patient and family should be notified of the seriousness of this complication and the high likelihood of the need for surgery.

There is no set length of time that an individual with toxic megacolon should be observed and treated medically before surgery is instituted. As a general rule, I observe a patient for 24 hours. If there has been no significant improvement in vital signs, physical examination findings, and radiologic features, I then recommend surgery. However, if within that time there is worsening in any of the clinical features, I favor earlier operation. In my opinion, toxic megacolon is a surgical disease, and the role of the internist is one of diagnosis, preparation for surgery, and prevention.

Colonic Hemorrhage. In my experience, it is the rare patient who has a severe colonic hemorrhage associated with an acute flare-up of IBD. Therapy for this complication is directed at the primary inflammation in the intestinal tract, as previously outlined. If the hemorrhage continues unabated or is so profuse that adequate volume maintenance cannot be maintained, an emergency operation is indicated. It is important in this clinical situation to perform flexible sigmoidoscopy or colonoscopy, if a toxic megacolon is not suspected, to make sure the rectum is not the site of the hemorrhage.

Obstructive Symptoms. Obstructive symptoms in a patient with either ulcerative colitis or Crohn's disease usually indicates a stricture complication. It is important to ensure that the stricture is benign, related to either chronic or acute inflammatory reaction, and not malignant. If the obstructive symptoms do not resolve, surgical resection is necessary.

PERIODIC EVALUATION

The follow-up evaluation is important to detect any adverse effects of either the disease or its treatment. The second diagnostic evaluation of an individual with initially uncomplicated ulcerative colitis or Crohn's disease is usually done within three to four weeks of the first visit. At this time, the clinical response to therapy can be determined and appropriate adjustments made. A proctosigmoidoscopic examination is not necessary at this time if the initial diagnosis is secure and clinical improvement has been noted. However, if there has been no response, a repeat distal colon evaluation is appropriate to reconfirm the diagnosis and to exclude an infectious etiology.

As part of this evaluation, laboratory studies should be performed, including complete blood count and sedimentation rate tests. These tests yield valuable data about the inflammation index and the red and white blood cell levels. Any anemia can be detected, and the follow-up evaluation of the WBC count is important for patients receiving sulfasalazine. The level should always be above 4000 in these individuals. If the WBC count decreases below this amount and is reconfirmed, the sulfa drug should be discontinued to avoid possible bone marrow effects. Patients whose IBD is exacerbated should be reevaluated monthly until a remission has been achieved. Once this is accomplished, I see these individuals every six months as needed to check the CBC and sedimentation rate and to obtain a complete blood chemistry profile. I perform follow-up proctosigmoidoscopy two to three months after a clinical response has been achieved, to evaluate endoscopic healing and response to maintenance therapy for patients with ulcerative colitis.

PATIENT COMPLIANCE

An estimated 95% or more of individuals with either ulcerative colitis or Crohn's disease are very compliant regarding their therapy. Younger patients adapt less well to successful management because of frustration over the effects of the disease on their life style; also, they tend to seek earlier surgical intervention for their chronic disease. This may be appropriate for ulcerative colitis, but with the known recurrence rate of Crohn's disease, it may result in future difficulties and a need for subsequent surgery.

PATIENT EDUCATION

The natural history of the disease, the possibility of multiple complications, the cancer risk, and the potential adverse reactions from the medications make it a prerequisite that the patient be well informed. Many of the answers are supplied in easy-to-read, professional brochures from the National Foundation for Ileitis and Colitis, 44 Park Avenue South, New York, NY. In my experience, a well-informed patient seems to tolerate the complications of IBD better, and the family is more understanding of the potential need for long-term hospitalizations and surgery.

FAMILY COUNSELING

Half of the patients with IBD are female, and will become or want to become pregnant during the course of their illness. This fact poses many difficult questions for the clinician. What is the effect of pregnancy on the course of IBD? Does the varying level of activity of either ulcerative colitis or Crohn's disease influence the outcome of the pregnancy? Can steroids or sulfasalazine be continued throughout the pregnancy without affecting the fetus or delivery date?

Mogadam and colleagues, reviewing retrospectively 324 patients, concluded that the course of IBD was not adversely affected by either pregnancy or the puerperium. In addition, exacerbations of IBD during or after pregnancy were more common in individuals having active symptoms at the time of conception. These authors suggested that therapy for the specific IBD be continued throughout the pregnancy, since the risk of relapse was shown to be lower in pregnant patients with inactive IBD symptoms. With the exception of severe Crohn's disease, the activity of the IBD did not seem to influence the pregnancy or fetal mortality rate. The authors concluded that either form of medical therapy could be used during the pregnancy with the same indications as in a nonpregnant individual. Moreover, Peppercorn has suggested that sulfasalazine therapy can be continued throughout pregnancy and in nursing mothers because the medical literature does not indicate a risk of fetal complications or neonatal jaundice arising from its use.

REFERENCES

Danzi JT: Free Yourself From Digestive Pain: A Guide to Preventing and Curing Your Digestive Illness. Prentice-Hall, Englewood Cliffs, NJ, 1984.

Driscoll RH Jr, Rosenberg IH: Total parenteral nutrition in inflammatory bowel disease. Med Clin North Am 62:185–201, 1978.

Farmer RG, Hawk WA, Turnbull RB Jr: Clinical patterns in Crohn's disease: a statistical study of 615 cases. Gastroenterology 68:627–635, 1975.

Kirsner JB, Shorter RG: Recent developments in nonspecific inflammatory bowel disease (second of two parts). N Engl J Med 306:837–848, 1982.

Lock MR, Farmer RG, Fazio VW, et al: Recurrence and re-operation for Crohn's disease. N Engl J Med 304:1586–1588, 1981.

Mogadam M, Korelitz BI, Ahmed SW, et al: The course of inflammatory bowel disease during pregnancy and postpartum. Am J Gastroenterol 75:265–269, 1981.

Peppercorn MA: Sulfasalazine: pharmacology, clinical use, toxicity and related new drug development. Ann. Intern Med 101:377–386, 1984.

3 · PREMALIGNANT LESIONS OF THE GASTROINTESTINAL TRACT

Robert G. Norfleet
MARSHFIELD CLINIC

The gastrointestinal tract is a major site of cancer. In the United States, about 217,800 patients were expected to have GI cancer in 1986, which corresponds to 23% of all cancer. Surgical resection usually offers the only hope for cure, although radiation and chemotherapy may benefit the patient. The outcome depends on the stage of the cancer at the time of operation. The clinician must recognize premalignant conditions so that cancer can be detected when cure is still possible.

"Premalignant" means that the patient's risk of developing cancer is higher than expected, but not that cancer is inevitable. All patients should have their risk for cancer assessed. Once a high-risk situation is recognized, the clinician must decide if screening and/or surveillance is indicated. Surveillance means the screening test is repeated at appropriate intervals. The following conditions justify screening or surveillance:

1. The disease should be common in the population to be screened.

2. The disease should cause significant morbidity if not treated.

3. Effective treatment must be available for the disease.

4. Treatment applied before symptoms occur should benefit the patient more than if the disease were treated in the stage of early symptoms.

Table 1 outlines the GI conditions generally considered to be premalignant.*

COLORECTAL CANCER

Let us apply the principles of screening, discussed above, to colorectal cancer. First, it is very common in the U.S., with 140,000 new cases and 60,000 deaths predicted in 1986. Since 98% occur after age 40 and 95% after age 50, this group can be screened selectively.

Second, we have effective screening tests. Digital examination of the rectum is simple, safe, and inexpensive and should detect about 12% of colorectal cancers. In men, prostate cancer should also be detected. It is advisable to perform this test yearly in people 40 years of age and older.

The stool blood test is inexpensive and safe. It must be used with care to attain favorable sensitivity and specificity. Our experience shows sensitivity of 35% for colonic adenomas and 75% for carcinomas, and we suggest this test should be repeated yearly after age 50.

*Those meeting the criteria discussed above are considered here; for the reader interested in more details or in the disorders not discussed, see Sherlock et al.

We mail Hemoccult II kits and instructions to our patients before their periodic health examinations. If occult blood is found, the patient is questioned about symptoms and whether the test was done properly. About 25% of our patients do not test properly—usually because of "hemorrhoidal" bleeding. A positive test should be evaluated carefully.

Screening proctosigmoidoscopy is advisable at ages 50 and 51 and then every 3 to five years for Americans without symptoms. We use only the 65-cm fiberoptic sigmoidoscope, which can detect about 75% of all colorectal neoplasms. Patients are more comfortable with this instrument and more likely to allow future examinations. The yearly digital examination is included with sigmoidoscopy.

The third condition for successful screening is that effective treatment must be available. Surgical or endoscopic excision of localized cancer is curative. Since about 95% of colorectal cancers begin as adenomatous polyps, aggressive detection and treatment of these lesions will reduce the incidence of cancer ("secondary prevention").

There are considerable data to support the last condition for successful screening: treatment of the asymptomatic patient is better than waiting until symp-

Table 1. PRECANCEROUS CONDITIONS OF THE GASTROINTESTINAL TRACT

Colon
  Inflammatory bowel disease
    Ulcerative colitis*
    Crohn's disease
  Adenomatous polyps*
  Previous colon cancer*
  Hereditary, nonpolyposis conditions (cancer family syndrome, hereditary gastrocolic cancer, hereditary site-specific colonic cancer, and Muir-Torre syndrome)*
  Familial polyposis coli*
  Gardner's syndrome*

Pancreas
  Chronic calcific pancreatitis
  Hereditary pancreatitis
  Multiple endocrine neoplasia I (pituitary, adrenal cortex, pancreas, and parathyroid)

Stomach
  Severe atrophic fundic gastritis (type A gastritis)
    Pernicious anemia
  Gastric polyps*
  Gastric resection

Liver, Gallbladder, and Biliary System
  Hemochromatosis
  Alpha-1 antitrypsin deficiency
  Wilson's disease
  Cirrhosis
  HB_sAG-positive chronic active hepatitis
  Primary biliary cirrhosis
  Chronic cholelithiasis

Esophagus
  Barrett's esophagus*
  Achalasia
  Plummer-Vinson syndrome*
  Tylosis (keratosis palmaris et plantaris or dyskeratosis congenita)*
  Lye burns of the esophagus*
  Alcohol and tobacco abuse

Small Intestine
  Celiac sprue
  Peutz-Jeghers syndrome
  Crohn's disease
  Alpha-chain disease
  Periampullary villous adenoma and carcinoma in familial polyposis and Gardner's syndrome

*Special screening and/or surveillance recommended.

toms develop. Americans have been educated and warned about the early symptoms of colorectal cancer, yet the five-year cure rate has remained at 42% for the past 30 years. Patients in whom a colon cancer is discovered while asymptomatic have usually a more localized form of cancer and higher survival rates.

HIGH-RISK PATIENTS

There are subgroups of patients at higher risk (see Table 1). We should identify them during their health assessments for special surveillance programs. Inflammatory bowel disease is discussed in Chapter 2. Patients with a history of adenoma or cancer of the large bowel and those with a first-degree relative who has colorectal cancer (and possibly adenoma) deserve additional surveillance. The yearly rectal examinations and stool blood tests should begin at ages 30 and 40, respectively. Every two years fiberoptic sigmoidoscopy should be alternated with either colonoscopy or barium enema examinations, beginning at age 40. During colonoscopy, all polypoid lesions are treated.

If the family history indicates that many relatives have colon cancer or polyps at an early age, the diagnoses of familial polyposis coli, Gardner's syndrome, or one of the hereditary, nonpolyposis syndromes should be considered (see Table 1). Familial polyposis is an uncommon, autosomally dominant condition in which adenomas develop in the second decade of life. By the third decade hundreds stud the mucosa, and progression to cancer is almost inevitable. We advise total colectomy with ileostomy or ileoanal anastomosis. Some choose subtotal colectomy with ileorectal anastomosis, but proctoscopy every three to six months with treatment of all polyps and yearly CEA determinations are then advised.

The family must be counseled and evaluated. I recommend fiberoptic sigmoidoscopy with biopsy of any mucosal abnormality beginning at 15 years of age. If normal, this should be repeated every two years until age 30 to 40 years before it can be concluded that the patient does not have the disease. If adenomas are found, the patient should be referred for surgery and informed that his or her children have a 50% chance of inheriting the disease.

Familial polyposis coli and Gardner's syndrome also impose risk for adenomas elsewhere in the GI tract, especially in the periampullary region. A serum alkaline phosphatase determination each year may prove helpful. Some clinicians recommend upper GI endoscopy with biopsy of the papilla of Vater and/or barium meal roentgenographs, but a satisfactory risk-cost-benefit ratio has not been established.

PANCREAS

Even though 25,500 cases of pancreatic cancer and 24,000 deaths were expected in the U.S. in 1986, neither good screening tests nor effective treatment are available at this time. We do not recommend special testing for the precancerous conditions listed in Table 1.

GASTRIC CANCER

The incidence of stomach cancer is decreasing in the U.S., but 24,700 new cases and 14,300 deaths were expected in 1986. Patients with type A gastritis (severe fundic gastritis, achlorhydria usually progressing to pernicious anemia and parietal cell antibodies) are at extra risk of gastric cancer. A gastric ulcer in these patients should be considered malignant and treated surgically.

Gastric polyps are usually discovered for GI bleeding or nonspecific symptoms. Gastroscopic polypectomy is advised. No further follow-up is needed for nonneoplastic polyps, but neoplastic lesions are followed with periodic gastroscopy.

Patients having gastric resection for benign disease were thought to be at special risk. However, recent studies show no increase in cancer of the gastric stump, so we do not recommend surveillance.

LIVER, GALLBLADDER AND BILIARY SYSTEM

For 1986, 13,600 new cancers and 10,600 deaths were predicted in the U.S. The conditions with increased cancer risk are given in Table 1. Serum alpha-fetoprotein is an inexpensive and nonvasive screening test that will detect about 85% of cases of hepatocellular carcinoma. No benefit from mass screening has yet been reported, so it is not used routinely at our clinic.

Chronic cholelithiasis nearly always precedes gallbladder cancer. Since the risk from cholecystectomy is about equal to that of cancer, cholecystectomy is not recommended for this reason alone.

ESOPHAGEAL CANCER

Mass screening programs using esophageal brushes to obtain cytology specimens are effective in areas where the disease is common (Northern China and Northern Iran), but are not advised in the U.S. where only 9300 new cases with 8800 deaths were expected in 1986. Americans at high risk (see Table 1) can be selectively screened using esophagoscopy with biopsy and/or brushing for cytologic material. In Barrett's esophagus the squamous cell mucosa changes to columnar, probably from chronic gastroesophageal reflux. The risk of adenocarcinoma is estimated to be 10%, and most advise screening these patients although benefit has not yet been shown. Currently we advise yearly esophagoscopy with biopsies for dysplasia.

We evaluate each patient with achalasia before treatment to detect the rare malignancy of the esophagogastric junction that may mimic achalasia. After successful treatment, the risk of esophageal cancer does not warrant surveillance. The Plummer-Vinson syndrome (iron deficiency anemia and esophageal webs) has become rare. Such patients are at increased risk of both esophageal and hypopharyngeal cancer, which may be diminished if iron and vitamin deficiencies are corrected.

Tylosis is a rare genetic disorder (autosomal dominant transmission) with extraordinary calluses of the palms and soles and extraordinary risk of squamous cell carcinoma of the esophagus. These patients deserve yearly esophagoscopy with biopsy of any lesion. Family members should be sought and evaluated. Patients with lye burns are usually followed for stricture. Before strictures are dilated, we advise esophagoscopy with biopsy, and repeat the examination if bougienage becomes difficult.

SMALL INTESTINE

Despite having very rapid cell turnover, the small intestine is seldom affected by cancer: only 2200 cases and 800 deaths were predicted for 1986. The best method of evaluation, barium contrast radiography, lacks sensitivity or specificity and is not recommended for surveillance.

Celiac sprue is characterized by malabsorption of most nutrients, a typical but nonspecific lesion of the small bowel mucosa, and improvement after gluten-containing cereal grains are eliminated from the diet. From 11% to 13% of sprue patients may develop malignancy, usually nine or more years after diagnosis, regardless of the control of the disease. About one half develop histiocytic lymphoma, and most of the rest develop squamous cell carcinoma of the esophagus or adenocarcinoma of the small intestine.

The Peutz-Jeghers syndrome is an inherited (autosomal dominant) association of melanotic spots in or about the mouth and hamartomatous polyps, usually of the small intestine. The extra risk of malignancy is small, so screening is not advised.

REFERENCES

Cancer Statistics, 1986: CA 36:9–25, 1986.

Greenlaw RH, Norfleet RG: Evaluation of the patient with a positive Hemoccult test. Wis Med J 79:17–18, 1980.

Griner PF, Mayewski RJ, Mushlin AI, et al: Selection and interpretation of diagnostic tests and procedures: principles and applications. Ann Intern Med 94:553–600, 1981.

Norfleet RG, Roberts RC: Hemoccult screening for colorectal neoplasms: report of a mail-out project without dietary restriction in a prepaid health plan. Wis Med J 82:23–26, 1983.

Sherlock P, Morson BC, Barbara L, et al: Precancerous Lesions of the Gastrointestinal Tract. Raven Press, New York, 1983.

4 · PEPTIC ULCER DISEASE

Richard R. Babb
PALO ALTO MEDICAL CLINIC

Peptic ulcer disease has been and continues to be a significant health problem in the United States. It has been estimated that 10% of the population will suffer from a peptic ulcer during their lifetime. Approximately 500,000 new cases can be expected to occur annually, and this, coupled with 400,000 hospital admissions and 150,000 operations for ulcers per year, has led to an annual cost of over 2 billion dollars.

For the purposes of this chapter, a peptic ulcer is considered as a hole in the lining of the stomach and proximal duodenum bathed by acid and pepsin. The exact cause of this disorder varies from patient to patient, depending on the interplay among genetic, anatomic, and social factors.

PATHOPHYSIOLOGY

Gastric acid (HCl) is secreted by parietal cells located in glands throughout the stomach. One can measure acid secretion both in the resting state (basal acid output, or BAO) and/or after stimulation (maximal acid output, or MAO). Although acid is required for the development of a duodenal ulcer, the exact cause in any given patient is highly variable and depends on the interplay among numerous aggressive and defensive factors. If there is extreme hyperacidity, an ulcer may result despite adequate mucosal defensive mechanisms. If mucosal reparative processes are inadequate, an ulcer may result despite low-to-normal acid levels.

Physiologic abnormalities in many, but not all, patients with duodenal ulcer include an increased number of parietal cells, increased acid secretory drive, increased sensitivity of parietal cells to gastrin, decreased inhibition of gastrin release, and rapid gastric emptying. Potential defensive defects include abnormalities in mucus and bicarbonate production, mucosal cell turnover rate, and gastric microcirculation.

Combined with the above endogenous defects, peptic ulcers may develop if risk factors such as heredity, cigarette smoking, certain beverages, drugs, and perhaps stress are present.

Evidence derived from family and twin studies, measurement of blood group and ABO secretion status, serum pepsinogen I levels, and analysis of genetic syndromes such as multiple endocrine adenomatosis type I shows that heredity can have an important role in the pathogenesis of peptic ulcer disease. These studies have led to an increasing awareness of the possible subtypes of peptic ulcer disease and the "genetic heterogeneity" involved in their etiology.

Cigarette smoking has numerous gastrointestinal effects including accelerated gastric emptying, potentiation of gastrin-stimulated acid response, decreased gastric mucosal blood flow, decreased gastric prostaglandin synthesis, and decreased pancreatic HCO_3^- secretion—all of which could lead to an increased incidence of peptic ulcer disease in the smoker as compared with the nonsmoker. Indeed, clinical studies have shown this to be the case, smokers having not only a higher incidence of peptic ulcer disease but also a slower healing rate once an ulcer occurs.

The role of diet in causing and perpetuating peptic ulcer disease has become less controversial over the past few decades. There is no evidence that various types of food are significant. Beverages, however, may be important. Coffee (be it regular or decaffeinated), tea, and popular soft drinks such as Tab, Coca-Cola, and 7 Up are gastric acid stimulants and their excessive use may increase the risk of peptic ulcer disease. The role of alcohol is not clear, but in a recent study beer, white wine, and whiskey caused acid secretion.

It is difficult to ascertain whether drugs are an added risk factor. The role of acetylsalicylic acid (aspirin) and nonsteroidal anti-inflammatory drugs such as indomethacin (Indocin) and phenylbutazone (Butazolidin) is more certain for gastric than for duodenal ulcer. Patients taking these drugs for an extended period have a relatively high incidence of gastric and even duodenal erosions. Besides breaking the gastric mucosal barrier, these drugs may induce inhibition of the synthesis of mucosal prostaglandin, and thus loss of its cytoprotective action. The role of corticosteroids in peptic ulcer disease remains elusive and debatable. Experts disagree. One review states that corticosteroids increase the risk of peptic ulcers, and my own opinion is that this is so.

Gastric Ulcer

Although pathophysiologic mechanisms may be the same for duodenal and gastric ulcers, several factors that facilitate the development of a gastric ulcer should be noted. These include abnormalities in pyloric sphincter control leading to duodenogastric reflux, delayed gastric emptying with antral stasis, and changes in mucus and HCO_3^- secretion. Some postulate that against this background the presence of substances such as HCl, bile, alcohol, or drugs leads to damage of the gastric mucosal barrier, back diffusion of H^+ into the gastric mucosa, and anatomic changes resulting in an ulcer.

DIAGNOSIS

Most patients with peptic ulcer disease complain of upper abdominal pain. Usually this has a burning quality, is in the epigastric or right upper quadrant areas, and is relieved by food. I find that many patients have already tried antacids with good results. Pain awakening the patient at night and going into the back may herald a penetrating ulcer, and marked nausea or vomiting often serves as a clue to a pyloric channel ulcer.

At this point, one may treat the patient and go no further in the diagnostic evaluation. This decision obviously depends on the patient and the specific circumstances.

Further evaluation includes laboratory measurement of blood count and kidney, liver, and electrolyte function and fiberoptic endoscopy or upper GI radiography. Because of the expense, relative discomfort, and increased risk from endoscopy, I usually proceed with radiography. If a *duodenal* ulcer is visualized, no further tests are done. If an ulcer is not seen, if signs of gastric outlet obstruction are noted, or if response to medical treatment is poor, endoscopy may be required. Some consider that every patient with a *gastric* ulcer should have endoscopy, whereas others recommend endoscopy only if the ulcer does not appear benign by radiographic criteria, or fails to heal after a trial of medical therapy. Approximately 5% of radiographic benign ulcers are found to be malignant at surgery, and (rarely) a malignant ulcer will initially seem to heal. Patients believed to have a benign gastric ulcer by careful radiographic criteria should be treated and followed closely. Repeat barium studies should be done in four to six weeks, and depending on ulcer size, one expects at least 50% healing. Future radiographic examinations should be made until healing is complete. If there is any suspicion about malignancy or doubt about the healing rate, or if the patient remains symptomatic despite appropriate treatment, endoscopy with numerous biopsies from the ulcer rim and brush cytology is indicated.

MANAGEMENT

Patients with an uncomplicated duodenal ulcer and those with a benign gastric ulcer are initially treated the same way, bearing in mind, however, the possibility of gastric cancer. Over a period of one year, gastric and duodenal ulcers will recur in over 50% of treated patients; however, with more time, patients have fewer and fewer recurrences. Repeated endoscopy has shown that many patients become asymptomatic with treatment, and yet still have an ulcer crater; others continue to have symptoms although the ulcer has healed.

GENERAL PRINCIPLES

Patients should be carefully questioned as to their dietary likes and dislikes, habits, and drug ingestion. Foods or beverages that exacerbate the ulcer pain should be discontinued. I try to allow dietary freedom but ask that they not overindulge or eat a meal at bedtime. I urge patients to avoid smoking and acid stimulants such as caffeine, coffee of any kind, tea, and alcohol. During the initial and subsequent visits, I try to ascertain patients' emotional health and the role of stress in their lives. Psychologic counseling may be needed. I make every effort through words and pictures to educate the patient as to the nature of peptic ulcer disease and the rationale for my advised therapy.

Antacids. When used in appropriate doses and given at an optimal time, antacids are effective in neutralizing gastric acid. The most popular are combinations of magnesium and aluminum hydroxide. These agents react with HCl to form a salt and water:

$$Mg(OH)_2 + 2\ HCl \rightarrow MgCl_2 + 2\ H_2O$$
$$Al(OH)_3 + 3\ HCl \rightarrow AlCl_3 + 3\ H_2O$$

Antacids are most effective in terms of acid neutralization when given one and three hours after meals. Using in vitro techniques, Sleisenger and Fordtran have shown that antacids vary greatly in their neutralizing capacity, and the amount of antacid needed to control gastric acidity varies from one product to another. Moreover, patients may require different amounts of the same antacid to achieve acid neutralization.

There is no "cookbook recipe" for antacid use. Doctors should avail themselves of tables now published in journals or standard textbooks of gastroenterology* (Tables 1, 2, and 3) for the appropriate dose of any given antacid. Cost and sodium content likewise differ for various antacids and are usually mentioned in these tables.

Since clinical trials using endoscopy show that most ulcers heal in six weeks, I treat for that length of time, using approximately 30 cc of an aluminum-magnesium hydroxide combination one and three hours after meals and at bedtime.

---

*See Sleisenger MH, and Fordtran JS: Gastrointestinal Disease: Pathophysiology, Diagnosis, Management, 3rd ed. W. B. Saunders Co, Philadelphia, 1983.

Table 1. NEUTRALIZING CAPACITY, SODIUM CONTENT, AND COST EFFECTIVENESS OF LIQUID ANTACIDS

Antacid	Acid Neutralizing Capacity	Volume Containing 140 mEq	Sodium Content	Monthly Cost of Therapy	Composition	Manufacturer
	mEq/ml	*ml*	*mg/5 ml*	*$*		
Maalox TC	4.2	33	1.2	44	Aluminum hydroxide, magnesium hydroxide	W. H. Rorer, Inc., Fort Washington, PA
Titralac	4.2	33	11.0	35	Calcium carbonate, glycine	Riker Laboratories, Northridge, CA
Delcid	4.1	34	1.5	57	Aluminum hydroxide, magnesium hydroxide	Merrell-National Laboratories, Cincinnati, OH
Mylanta II	3.6	39	1.1	63	Aluminum hydroxide, magnesium hydroxide, simethicone	Stuart Pharmaceuticals, Wilmington, DE
Camalox	3.2	44	2.5	55	Aluminum hydroxide, magnesium hydroxide, calcium carbonate	W. H. Rorer, Inc., Fort Washington, PA
Gelusil II	3.0	47	1.3	74	Aluminum hydroxide, magnesium hydroxide, simethicone	Parke-Davis, Morris Plains, NJ
Basaljel ES	2.9	48	23.0	101	Aluminum carbonate	Wyeth Laboratories, Philadelphia, PA
Maalox Plus	2.3	61	2.5	68	Aluminum hydroxide, magnesium hydroxide, simethicone	W. H. Rorer, Inc., Fort Washington, PA
Gelusil	2.2	64	0.7	80	Aluminum hydroxide, magnesium hydroxide, simethicone	Parke-Davis, Morris Plains, NJ
Riopan Plus	1.8	78	0.7	78	Aluminum hydroxide, magnesium hydroxide, simethicone	Ayerst Laboratories, New York, NY
Amphojel	1.4	100	7.0	114	Aluminum hydroxide	Wyeth Laboratories, Philadelphia, PA
Phosphaljel	0.3	466	12.5	498	Aluminum phosphate	Wyeth Laboratories, Philadelphia, PA

From Drake D, Hollander D: Neutralizing capacity and cost effectiveness of antacids. Ann Intern Med 94:215–217, 1981. By permission.

SIDE EFFECTS

Many patients quickly grow tired of the taste and inconvenience of proper antacid use and prefer the medication discussed below. Sodium bicarbonate may cause edema and alkalosis. Calcium-containing antacids can lead to hypercalcemia, acid rebound, and the milk-alkali syndrome (alkalosis, hypercalcemia, and renal insufficiency). Magnesium products can cause diarrhea, and since a small amount is absorbed, patients with impaired renal function may develop symptoms of hypermagnesemia. In contrast, aluminum hydroxide may lead to constipation. Although some aluminum is likewise absorbed, the long-term medical sequelae are not known. Finally, long-term use of aluminum-containing antacids may lead to a phosphorus-depletion syndrome characterized by decreased phosphorus absorption, hypophosphatemia, hypercalciuria, and symptoms of anorexia, fatigue, bone pain, osteomalacia, and even congestive heart failure.

Anticholinergic Agents. These drugs reduce gastric acidity by inhibiting the action of acetylcholine on the parietal cell. Although some studies have shown them to be effective in the treatment of peptic ulcer disease, side effects of their use are common and have diminished their popularity. They may cause dry mouth, constipation, and urine retention and should not be given to patients suffering from glaucoma, chronic obstructive pulmonary disease, gastric outlet obstruction, or prostatism. I rarely use this type of medication.

A standard low dose of propanthaline (Probanthine) seems to inhibit acid secretion as effectively as a much larger, more toxic dose. Moreover, when combined with cimetidine (Tagamet), acid secretion is inhibited more than with either drug alone. Although not yet available in the U.S., a new anticholinergic agent, pirenzepine, shows promise as an antiulcer drug and thus far has fewer side effects than the older agents.

H_2-Receptor Antagonists. These drugs have become extremely popular in the treatment of peptic ulcer disease because of their efficacy and safety. By selectively blocking one of the two histamine receptor sites in the body, i.e., the H_2-receptor on the parietal cell, these agents markedly inhibit gastric acid secretion, in both the fasting and postprandial states. Pepsin secretion is also inhibited and the volume of gastric secretion is reduced. Numerous clinical trials have shown that cimetidine (Tagamet) and ranitidine (Zantac) are effective agents to peptic ulcer disease and hypersecretory states of gastric acid. Since most patients with ulcers have a recurrence within one year of healing, and some seem to have one attack after another, these H_2-antagonists have also been used for long-term maintenance therapy with good results. The unanswered question is how long such therapy should be continued, since once the drug is stopped the natural history of the ulcer disease reasserts itself, and recurrences are noted yet again.

I prescribe cimetidine, 300 mg PO four times a day, for the initial treatment of patients with active ulcer disease. In those who have a history of numerous recurrences (this is a highly individual decision), one may use a 400-mg dose of cimetidine at bedtime for a prolonged period once the ulcer is healed.

Patients using cimetidine have been remarkably free of serious toxicity. As might be expected, some note a rash, dizziness, or diarrhea. Neutropenia, hepatitis renal dysfunction, and endocrine abnormalities such as gynecomastia and decreased libido and sperm counts may occur, but are rare. A more serious problem is mental confusion, especially in the elderly. This may manifest itself very subtly with only minimal changes in mood, or may be quite overt with delirium.

Table 2. NEUTRALIZING CAPACITY, SODIUM CONTENT, AND COST EFFECTIVENESS OF TABLET ANTACIDS

Antacid	Acid Neutralizing Capacity	Dose Containing 140 mEq	Sodium Content	Monthly Cost of Therapy	Composition	Manufacturer
	mEq/tablet	*tablets*	*mg/tablet*	*$*		
Camalox	16.7	8	1.5	54	Aluminum hydroxide, magnesium hydroxide	W. H. Rorer, Inc., Fort Washington, PA
Basaljel	15.4	9	2.0	68	Aluminum carbonate	Wyeth Laboratories, Philadelphia, PA
Mylanta II	11.0	13	1.3	85	Aluminum hydroxide, magnesium hydroxide, simethicone	Stuart Pharmaceuticals, Wilmington, DE
Tums	10.5	13	2.7	56	Calcium carbonate	Norcliff Thayer, Inc., Tuckahoe, NY
Alka II	10.5	13	2.0	58	Calcium carbonate	Miles Laboratories, Inc., Elkhart, IN
Riopan Plus	10.0	14	0.3	76	Aluminum hydroxide, magnesium hydroxide, simethicone	Ayerst Laboratories, New York, NY
Titralac	9.5	15	0.3	57	Calcium carbonate, glycine	Riker Laboratories, Inc., Northridge, CA
Gelusil II	8.2	17	2.1	107	Aluminum hydroxide, magnesium hydroxide, simethicone	Parke-Davis, Morris Plains, NJ
Rolaids	6.9	20	53.0	86	Aluminum carbonate	Warner Lambert Company, Morris Plains, NJ
Maalox Plus	5.7	25	1.4	106	Aluminum hydroxide, magnesium hydroxide; simethicone	W. H. Rorer, Inc., Fort Washington, PA
Digel	4.7	30	10.6	101	Aluminum hydroxide, magnesium hydroxide, simethicone, magnesium carbonate	Plough, Inc., Memphis, TN
Amphojel	2.0	70	7.0	360	Aluminum hydroxide	Wyeth Laboratories, Philadelphia, PA

From Drake D, Hollander D: Neutralizing capacity and cost effectiveness of antacids. Ann Intern Med 94:215–217, 1981. By permission.

Drug interactions with cimetidine due to changes in liver blood flow and inhibition of hepatic microsomal enzymes occur and should be remembered. Drugs studied include warfarin (Coumadin), diazepam (Valium), chlordiazepoxide (Librium), theophylline, lidocaine, propranolol (Inderal), and phenytoin (Dilantin). These combinations may lead to increased drug blood levels and toxicity.

Ranitidine may be used in a dose of 150 mg twice a day. There have been reports that this agent appeared to heal ulcers not responding to cimetidine. Although one might expect better compliance with this drug as compared with one taken four times a day, this has not been the case in published reports. Initially, ranitidine was thought to have fewer side effects and drug interactions than cimetidine. One might consider its use in preference to cimetidine in elderly patients, individuals with previous CNS symptoms, or those already on multiple drug therapy.

Occasionally, patients with arthritic complaints require the use of ulcerogenic medication despite peptic ulcer disease. There is now evidence that the concomitant use of H_2-antagonists often heals such ulcers and allows drugs such as aspirin to be continued.

Sucralfate. Sucralfate (Carafate) is the aluminum salt of a sulfated disaccharide. It does not reduce acid secretion, as do the H_2-antagonists, nor neutralize gastric acid, as do the antacids. Rather, in the acid environment of the stomach, the aluminum ions dissociate from the disaccharide molecule. The latter forms a thick, pastelike substance that attaches to the ulcer base. This coating presumably prevents the diffusion of acid and allows healing to occur. Sucralfate also has antipepsin activity, absorbs bile acids, and stimulates prostaglandin synthesis. It appears to be effective in the healing of peptic ulcers at a rate comparable with that of antacids and H_2-antagonists. It is poorly absorbed and very safe. Dosage is 1 gm 30 to 60 minutes before meals and at bedtime. Theoretically, this drug should not be used with antacids or H_2-antagonists since its ability to form a paste depends on an acid pH.

Other Drugs. The results of a recent review of pertinent literature show that tricyclic antidepressants such as trimipramine (Surmontil) and doxepin (Sinequan) are effective antiulcer drugs. Mechanisms of action include H_2-receptor antagonism, anticholinergic effects, possible cytoprotective activity, and relief of associated anxiety or depression. Substituted benzimidazoles such as omeprazole inhibit gastric secretion by blocking the proton pump located within the parietal cell. Preliminary studies from Europe show that the drug, when given once a day, causes marked acid suppression and ulcer healing.

Considerable investigation into the antiulcer properties of prostaglandin compounds is being carried out both in the U.S. and abroad. These drugs have been

Table 3. PRACTICAL VOLUMES OF ANTACID NEEDED ACCORDING TO NEUTRALIZING CAPACITY

Antacids	Acid Neutralizing Capacity*	Volume†			
		40 mEq	80 mEq	100 mEq	140 mEq
	mEq/mL		*mL*		
Maalox TC	4.2	10	20	25	35
Titralac	4.2	10	20	25	35
Delcid	4.1	10	20	25	35
Mylanta II	3.6	10	20	30	40
Camalox	3.2	15	25	30	45
Gelusil II	3.0	15	25	35	45
Basaljel ES	2.9	15	30	35	50
Maalox Plus	2.3	15	35	45	60
Gelusil	2.2	20	35	45	65
Riopan Plus	1.8	20	45	55	80
Amphojel	1.4	30	60	70	100
Phosphaljel	0.3	130	270	470	335

*Adapted from *Ann Intern Med.* 94:215–217, 1981.
†Suggested practical volumes to the nearest 5 mL.

used both PO and IV and show an inhibitory effect on acid secretion. They also appear to have a cytoprotective effect, perhaps due to the stimulation of both gastric HCO_3^- and mucus.

INTRACTABILITY

Despite use of the treatment techniques noted above, 10% to 20% of patients with peptic ulcer disease do not heal with therapy. In this event, I ask the following questions: (1) Are the complaints due to peptic ulcer disease? (2) What was the initial evidence for peptic ulcer disease? (3) Was fiberoptic endoscopy done? (4) Has the patient truly been taking the prescribed medications? (5) Are poor health habits such as smoking or abuse of caffeine, coffee, or alcohol playing a role? (6) Is the patient ingesting ulcerogenic medication? and (7) Is there any evidence of the Zollinger-Ellison syndrome (see below)? If the answers to these questions are not helpful and the patient is maintaining an adequate treatment program, one should begin to substitute drugs: e.g., try ranitidine instead of cimetidine, or vice versa; add antacids to H_2-antagonist therapy; try sucralfate; and so on. Occasionally, when medical treatment is unsuccessful and the patient remains symptomatic or has increasing recurrences, surgery is required.

COMPLICATIONS

Acute *bleeding* may occur in 15% to 20% of patients over a 25-year period. They must be carefully evaluated and adequately transfused, depending on the severity of the hemorrhage. Most patients stop bleeding spontaneously and there is no convincing evidence that H_2-antagonists help in this situation, although they are commonly used. Therapeutic endoscopy with the laser is available in some medical centers. If hospitalization is required, a surgeon should be involved with therapeutic decisions from the start.

Over the long term, 6% to 10% of patients may suffer with an acute ulcer *perforation*. Usually the history and physical examination show that an acute and overwhelming event has taken place, the abdomen being rigid and tender. Surgery is almost always required with careful attention to nasogastric suction and fluid and electrolyte balance. Gastric outlet *obstruction* may be difficult to diagnose, but a history of postprandial vomiting in a patient with known ulcer disease, a succussion splash on examination, and an abnormal amount of fluid in the stomach when aspirated are helpful clues. Radiographic studies and fiberoptic endoscopy are usually diagnostic. One should try to ascertain whether the obstruction is due to peptic ulcer disease and not cancer or a perigastric inflammatory process. At times, medical therapy suffices, including IV fluids, nasogastric suction, and acid suppression, but in my experience most of these patients eventually need surgery.

Zollinger-Ellison Syndrome

Since 1955, when Zollinger and Ellison first described two patients with fulminating ulcer disease, gastric hypersecretion, and non-beta islet cell tumors of the pancreas, much has been learned about this uncommon cause of peptic ulcer. It is now clear that this syndrome (ZES) results from the secretion of gastrin by intra-abdominal tumors ("gastrinomas") located in the pancreas or nearby organs.

Most of these patients have persistent pain and diarrhea related to the hypersecretory effects of gastrin, and do not respond well to usual ulcer therapy over a long period. Some 15% to 25% have associated multiple endocrine neoplasia type I. Since most tumors are malignant and many have metastasized by the time of surgery, the cure rate is less than 20%. Diagnosis requires demonstration of an elevated serum gastrin, often the use of provocative tests utilizing secretin or calcium in order to rule out causes of elevated serum gastrin other than ZES, and gastric acid hypersecretion. If these tests are compatible with a diagnosis of ZES, one must next attempt to localize the tumor site and ascertain whether there is metastatic spread.

MANAGEMENT

Management of ZES has become extremely complicated and somewhat controversial. With the advent of antiulcer drugs such as the H_2-antagonists, many patients can be treated medically and perhaps spared unnecessary surgery. What are the best imaging tests for tumor localization? Who should be operated on and when? If the tumor is unresectable at surgery, should a total gastrectomy be done? Should a selective proximal vagotomy be done instead?

In my opinion, patients suspected of having ZES should be sent to a medical center where doctors experienced in diagnosis and treatment of this uncommon entity reside. The important task for most of us is to recognize the possibility of ZES before a catastrophe occurs. This syndrome should come to mind when a patient with peptic ulcer disease shows signs of multiple endocrine disorders, has a positive family history, complains of diarrhea, does not respond to the usual medical treatment, and/or has radiographic evidence of enlarged gastric folds, multiple ulcers, or ulcers beyond the duodenal bulb. Finally, a screening serum gastrin assay should be done in any patient scheduled for ulcer surgery.

SURGERY

Most patients with uncomplicated peptic ulcer disease respond to medical therapy; however, perhaps

10% to 15% eventually require surgery because of either intractability or the complications mentioned above.

The type of operation selected depends on the anatomic location of the ulcer, concurrent complications, the patient's overall health and personal preference, and the surgeon's experience. The goal is to reduce acid and thus heal the ulcer, while at the same time selecting an operation that will minimize postoperative complications. Possible operations (with ulcer recurrence rates in parentheses) include subtotal gastrectomy without vagotomy (1% to 4%), truncal vagotomy and drainage procedure (3% to 10%), truncal vagotomy and antrectomy (1% to 2%), and selective proximal vagotomy (3% to 20%).

There are now three types of vagotomy operations: (1) truncal vagotomy; (2) selective vagotomy, where the hepatic branch of the anterior vagus and the celiac branch of the posterior vagus are preserved; and (3) superselective vagotomy or selective proximal vagotomy, where the hepatic and celiac branches are preserved and only the proximal stomach is denervated, leaving the antrum alone. This latter operation has succeeded in preventing most postvagotomy and drainage complications, but it is technically difficult and in some series has an ulcer recurrence rate of over 20%.

Surgery for a gastric ulcer includes a partial gastrectomy or wedge excision of the ulcer, either with or without one of the above vagotomy procedures.

It is estimated that 80% to 90% of patients are satisfied with the results of ulcer surgery. Long-term complications are numerous, however, and include weight loss, diarrhea, dumping, hypoglycemia, anemia, steatorrhea, osteopenia, bezoar formation, gastritis, and perhaps an increased incidence of gastric cancer.

As noted, some patients suffer an ulcer recurrence, depending on the initial operation. There are several reasons for this including ulcerogenic drugs, hypercalcemia, or a missed ZES, but the most common cause is an incomplete vagotomy or inadequate gastric resection. In some cases H_2-antagonists can be used with success; in others a second operation is necessary.

Dyspepsia

Many patients complain of upper abdominal gas, bloating, and discomfort. The exact cause of these symptoms often defies analysis, and successful treatment can be exceedingly difficult.

My approach is to question the patients carefully. When do the symptoms occur? What is meant by gas? Can they describe the discomfort in terms of burning or cramps? Does it awaken them at night? What are their health habits in terms of diet and beverages? Have they had abdominal surgery? Have they lost weight? I then try to decide whether the dyspeptic symptoms might be related to an anatomic disease of the upper abdomen, to dietary factors, or to stress. If after a careful history and physical examination the cause of these complaints is still uncertain, upper gastrointestinal radiography including a small bowel series and even fiberoptic endoscopy should be done. Occasionally, tests to measure gastric emptying may be required.

I have seen patients in consultation labeled "chronic dyspeptic" who after careful evaluation were diagnosed as having food sensitivity or allergy, peptic ulcer disease, duodenitis, or partial small bowel obstruction, and who responded to appropriate treatment.

Some patients feel dyspeptic because of too much caffeine, lactose, wheat, or carbohydrate in their diet. Poor gastric emptying can be helped with metoclopramide (Reglan). Antiulcer therapy benefits those with peptic ulcer disease or duodenitis. Anticholinergics sometimes give relief to those with gas and bloating related to dysmotility in the small bowel.

A large number of patients with dyspepsia remain, however, for whom no specific precipitating factor or anatomic abnormality can be found. Often they are emotionally disturbed, angry, or under considerable stress. Drug therapy is rarely successful over the long term, but can be tried for symptomatic relief. I try to teach these patients to understand how emotions can cause physical symptoms, and many are content to accept this, returning only when the dyspepsia once again becomes intolerable. If their emotional health improves, their gastrointestinal symptoms often do too.

REFERENCES

Grossman MI, Kurata JH, Rotter JL, et al: Peptic ulcer: new therapies, new diseases. Ann Intern Med 95:609–627, 1981.
Isenberg JI: Peptic ulcer. DM 28:1–55, 1981.
Jensen RT: Zollinger-Ellison syndrome: current concepts and management. Ann Intern Med 98:59–75, 1983.
Stabile BE, Passaro E: Recurrent peptic ulcer. Gastroenterology 70:124–135, 1976.

5 · MALABSORPTION AND MALDIGESTION

Chesley Hines, Jr.
OCHSNER CLINIC AND ALTON OCHSNER MEDICAL FOUNDATION

I hav finally kum tu the konklusion, that a good reliable sett ov bowels, iz wurth more tu a man, than enny quantity ov brains.

JOSH BILLINGS, *His Sayings*, 1866

FAT MALABSORPTION AND MALDIGESTION

The clinical manifestations of fat maldigestion/malabsorption are variable, the classic one being malodorous diarrhea associated with weight loss. However, these may not always be present. In fact, neither weight loss nor diarrhea may be a symptom of maldigestion/malabsorption. The manifestation may be so subtle as to be an unexplained anemia, particularly one due to deficiencies in iron, folic acid, or a combination of the two. Table 1 lists the clinical manifestations of the

Table 1. MALDIGESTION/MALABSORPTION SYNDROME

Clinical Features	Substance Malabsorbed
Weight loss	Calories
Steatorrhea	Fat
Diarrhea	OH fatty acids
Abdominal distention	Sugars
Anemia	Iron, vitamin B_{12}, folic acid
Edema	Protein
Tetany	Ca, Mg
Osteomalacia	Vitamin D, Ca
Bleeding and bruising	Vitamin K

maldigestion/malabsorption syndrome and the associated malabsorbed or maldigested substances.

It is easier to evaluate the patient with suspected fat maldigestion/malabsorption in terms of three major categories: intraluminal defects, mucosal defects, and lymphatic obstruction (Table 2).

INTRALUMINAL DEFECTS

Most patients with intraluminal defects (maldigestion) have one of the problems listed in Table 3.

The evaluation of a patient with suspected fat maldigestion/malabsorption can be facilitated by utilizing the schema shown in Figure 1. Utilizing this workup, one would suspect either hepatic or pancreatic problems if the fecal fat is abnormal and the D-xylose is normal. In a patient with liver trouble as the cause of the fat maldigestion, abnormalities will certainly be evident on routine liver chemical profiles such as the bilirubin, SGOT, SGPT, and alkaline phosphate (Fig. 2).

In a patient with elevated fecal fats but a normal D-xylose and normal liver studies, the most likely cause is pancreatic insufficiency. To evaluate the pancreas, the secretin test and probably endoscopic retrograde cannulation of the pancreatic duct (ERCP) should be performed (Fig. 3). Representative values of the secretin test in patients with pancreatic diseases versus controls are shown in Table 4. Treatment of pancreatic insufficiency is by administration of oral pancreatic enzymes, e.g., pancrease, 2 to 4 capsules per meal.

In patients with bile salt deficiency not due to liver abnormalities, the D-xylose might be abnormal, since bacteria can utilize D-xylose. Evaluation of these patients is outlined in Figure 4 (*see heavy arrows*).

MUCOSAL DEFECTS

The most common causes of maldigestion/malabsorption due to mucosal defects are listed in Table 5. Evaluation of these patients is outlined in Figure 5 (*see heavy arrows*).

Table 2. THREE BROAD CATEGORIES FOR FAT MALDIGESTION/MALABSORPTION

Intraluminal defects (maldigestion)
   Pancreatic lipase deficiency
   Bile salt deficiency
Mucosal defects (malabsorption)
   Small bowel disease
   Small bowel resection
   Small bowel bypass
Lymphatic obstruction (impaired transport)
   Lymphoma
   Lymphangiectasia

Table 3. INTRALUMINAL DEFECTS (MALDIGESTION)

Pancreatic lipase deficiency
   Chronic pancreatitis
   Cystic fibrosis
   Carcinoma of pancreas
Bile salt deficiency
   Severe liver disease
     Primary biliary cirrhosis
     Extrahepatic biliary tract obstruction with secondary biliary cirrhosis
Interruption of enterohepatic circulation of bile salts
   Distal ileectomy
   Ileal bypass
   Diseased terminal ileum
Bacterial overgrowth (bile salt deconjugation)
   Postgastrectomy blind loop syndrome
   Jejunal diverticula
   Strictures
   Fistulas
   Scleroderma and pseudo-obstruction

Celiac disease, tropical sprue, Whipple's disease, and giardiasis require special mention not only because of their importance, but also because of their uniqueness. Although most people with *Giardia lamblia* infestations are asymptomatic, giardiasis can cause diarrhea ranging from acute to chronic to full-blown malabsorption syndrome, particularly in patients with IgA deficiency. Giardiasis is a common cause of traveler's diarrhea not only in tropical and subtropical climates but also in temperate zones. Leningrad, Russia, and Aspen, Colorado, are locations particularly well known for giardiasis. The parasite is particularly common in mountainous streams where beavers reside, since the beaver seems to be the animal host for the parasite. Diagnosis is made by stool examination, duodenal aspiration, or crush biopsy of the duodenal mucosa. Treatment is very effective with either quinacrine hydrochloride (Atabrine), 100 mg three times a day for five to seven days, or metronidazole (Flagyl), 250 mg three times a day for five to seven days.

Celiac disease (nontropical sprue or gluten-sensitive enteropathy) occurs in individuals whose small intestinal mucosa is sensitive to gluten (the protein present in wheat, barley, and rye). Diagnosis is made by small intestinal biopsy. Treatment is very effective when patients avoid the use of any foods containing wheat, barley, or rye. An interesting skin disease, dermatitis herpetiformis, is associated with celiac disease. Tropical sprue is very similar to celiac disease (or nontropical sprue) in some ways, but uniquely different in others. Tropical sprue occurs only in southeastern Asia, the Indian subcontinent, Puerto Rico, Cuba, Haiti, the Dominican Republic, and the Caribbean coastal areas of Mexico, Guatemala, Colombia, and Venezuela. Other Caribbean islands are not affected by this disorder. The disease appears to be infectious and responds to broad-

Table 4. VALUES OF SECRETIN TEST IN PATIENTS WITH PANCREATIC DISEASES VS. CONTROLS

	Volume	HCO_3
Normal	2 cc/kg	85 mEq/L
Pancreatic insufficiency	2 cc/kg	<85 mEq/L
Carcinoma of pancreas	<2 cc/kg	85 mEq/L

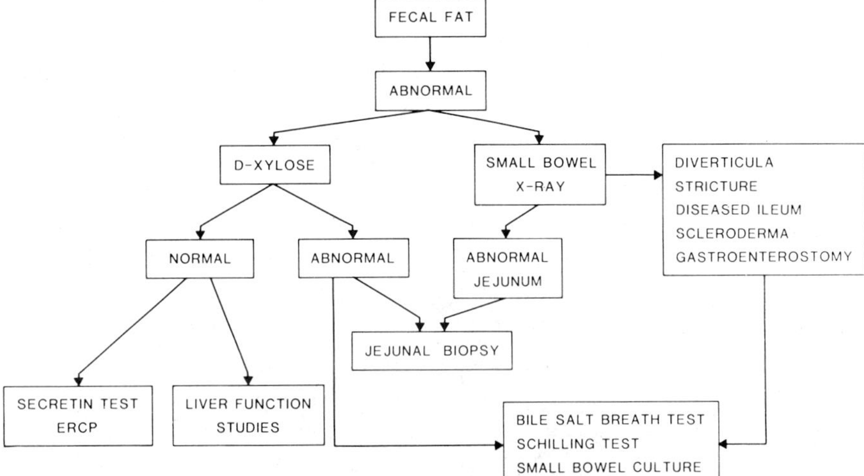

Figure 1. Evaluation of a patient with suspected fat maldigestion/malabsorption.

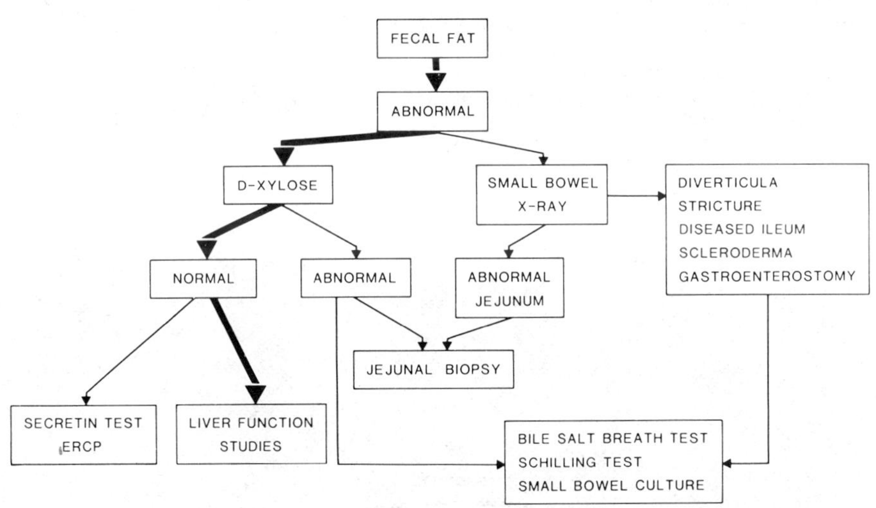

Figure 2. Abnormalities evident on routine liver chemical profiles.

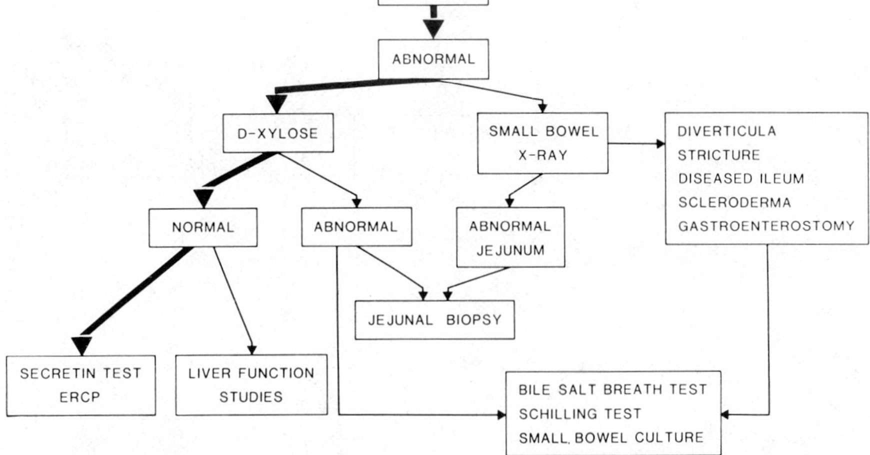

Figure 3. The secretin test and probably the ERCP (endoscopic retrograde cannulation of the pancreatic duct) should be performed.

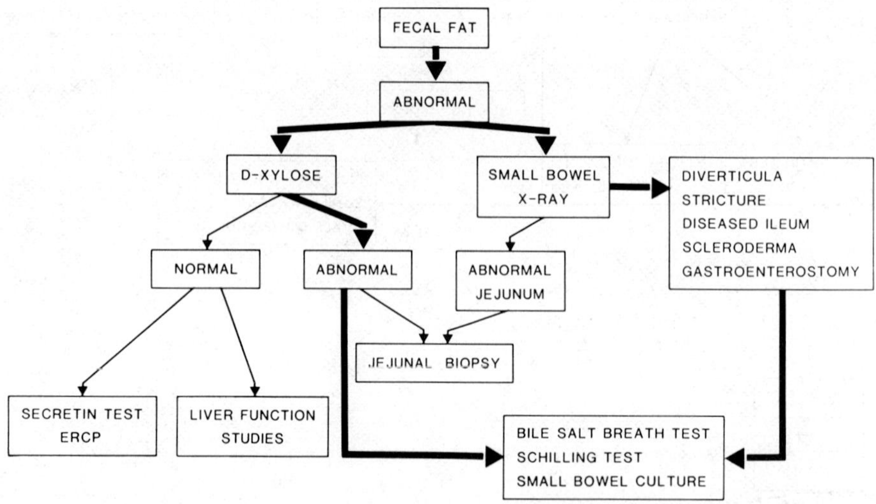

Figure 4. Evaluation of patients with bile salt deficiency not due to liver abnormalities.

Figure 5. Evaluation of patients with mucosal defects.

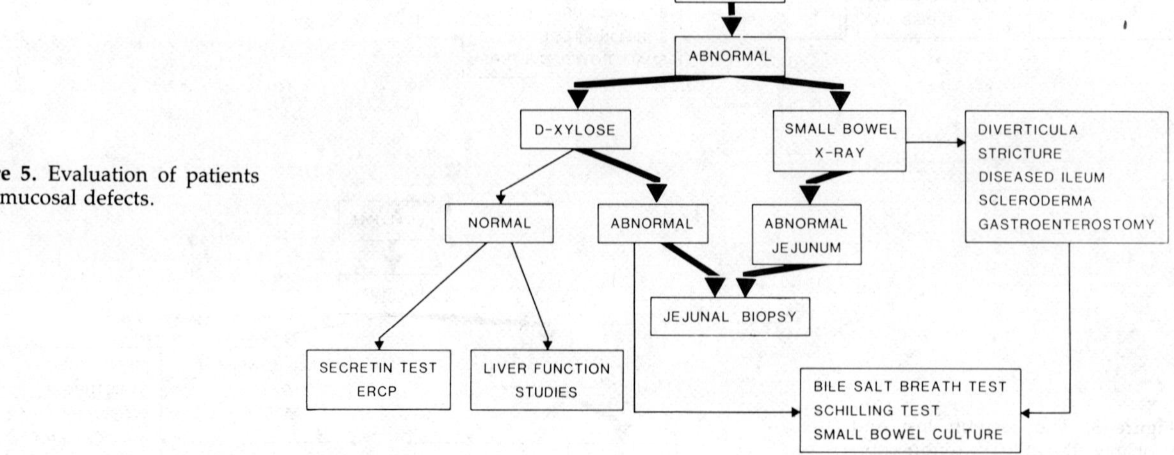

Table 5. MUCOSAL DEFECTS (MALABSORPTION)

Small bowel disease
  Celiac disease (nontropical sprue)
  Tropical sprue
  Whipple's disease
  Eosinophilic gastroenteritis
  Crohn's disease
  Giardiasis (especially with IgA deficiency)
Small bowel resection
Small bowel bypass

spectrum antibiotics. It also involves the ileum, and causes deficiency of B_{12} and at times of folic acid if it involves the jejunum. (Interestingly, it responds to the administration of folic acid as well as to antibiotics.) Celiac disease involves the duodenum and jejunum primarily, causing anemias due to iron deficiency, folic acid, or a combination of the two.

Whipple's disease characteristically involves men over the age of 40 and may be responsible for any of the following symptoms or a combination of them: (1) intestinal malabsorption; (2) fever; (3) increased skin pigmentation; (4) anemia; (5) lymphadenopathy; (6) arthralgia and arthritis; (7) pleuritis; (8) endocarditis; and (9) CNS symptoms. Diagnosis is made by a small bowel biopsy that reveals a characteristic periodic acid–Schiff (PAS)-positive material. Etiology appears to be infectious and responds to long-term administration of antibiotics, either penicillin or tetracycline.

LYMPHATIC OBSTRUCTION

A less common cause of fat malabsorption is lymphatic obstruction. This disorder most commonly results from lymphoma or lymphangiectasia.

CARBOHYDRATE MALABSORPTION

The major carbohydrate malabsorption to consider is lactose malabsorption. Ingested lactose is broken down in the small intestine by the mucosal enzyme lactase into glucose and galactose, which are then absorbed. Lactase deficiency rarely is present at birth but more commonly occurs with the approach of maturity. Lactose malabsorption (lactase deficiency) is so common that it can truly be said that people who can comfortably ingest lactose in adulthood are in the minority compared with the world's population. Nationalities with high incidences of lactose intolerance are as follows:

Chinese	Africans and their
Japanese	descendants
Thais	Southern Italians
Indonesians	Greek Cypriots
Filipinos	Pakistanis
Australian Aborigines	American Indians
New Guineans	Eskimos
Fijians	Jews
Arabs	Indians

Nationalities with low incidences of lactose intolerance are as follows:

Northern Europeans and their descendants

Scandinavians	Swiss
British	Poles
Irish	Czechs
Germans	French
Dutch	Northern Italians

When lactose is not digested, it creates an osmotic diarrhea by its large molecular size. Fermentation of the lactose also creates considerable gas formation, which is associated with abdominal bloating and flatus. Diagnosis can be made quite easily by the lactose tolerance test or by asking the patient to avoid ingestion of lactose in the diet. Treatment consists simply of avoidance of dairy products in the diet or addition of synthetic lactase products to dairy products.

REFERENCES

Drude RB, Hines C: The pathophysiology of intestinal bacterial overgrowth syndromes. Arch Intern Med 140:1349–1452, 1980.

Hines C Jr: Milk intolerance—mimic of the irritable bowel syndrome. J La State Med Soc 129:125–127, 1977.

Hines C Jr: Vitamins: absorption and malabsorption. Arch Intern Med 138:619–621, 1978.

Sleisenger MH (ed): Malabsorption and nutritional support. Clin Gastroenterol 12:12(2), 1983.

6 · PARASITES OF THE GASTROINTESTINAL TRACT

Frederick W. Heiss
John A. Shea
LAHEY CLINIC MEDICAL CENTER

Intestinal parasites are a major cause of disease in many parts of the world. The relatively low incidence of these diseases in North America is largely a result of the favorable climate, advanced methods of sanitation, attention to the problem by public health officials, and good medical care. Nonetheless, intestinal parasites continue to be found in the United States, and failure to consider them in a differential diagnosis can lead to severe complications and even death. Physicians are likely to encounter these parasitic diseases regardless of the location of their practice, because of the large numbers of Americans who travel, work, and live in endemic areas, such as those in the military services, the Peace Corps, and missionary work. In recent years, emigration from southeast Asia, the Caribbean, and Central and South America has brought a large number of persons who have a high prevalance of intestinal parasites into the U.S. In addition, the incidence of intestinal parasitic disease is increased in homosexual men because of their anal-oral sexual practices. Patients with acquired immune deficiency syndrome (AIDS), both naturally acquired and induced by drugs, are at risk of developing severe and disseminated forms of parasitic disease.

Few specific or pathognomonic clinical features permit a ready diagnosis of intestinal parasites. These organisms are well adapted to their human host, and the majority produce minor or no symptoms. Occasionally, however, moderate or severe disease results. The most common symptoms include diarrhea, abdominal distress, and fever. Identification of anemia and eosinophilia by laboratory tests may also be an indicator. The patient may discover the offending organism with the passage of stool. Diagnosis is usually made when the physician considers it and performs the appropriate diagnostic studies. Even though many laboratories lack the experienced personnel with expertise to establish a reliable parasitologic diagnosis, facilities are available for referral of specimens for analysis. Multiple parasitic infections may be present simultaneously. Intestinal parasites should be suspected particularly when the patient has traveled or lived in an endemic area. These diseases are gratifying to treat because cure can usually be expected, and newer drugs provide effective and safe therapy. This chapter briefly reviews the clinical aspects of intestinal parasites and their therapy.

Intestinal parasites are divided into three broad groups or phyla: Protozoa, Nemathelminthes (roundworms), and Platyhelminthes (flatworms).

PROTOZOAL DISEASES

Protozoa are primitive, unicellular organisms of the animal kingdom that frequently are parasites of man and occasionally are important pathogens. Members of this group include a variety of amebas of which only the species *Entamoeba histolytica* is an important pathogen. Other species, such as *Entamoeba hartmanni* (formerly known as "small race" of *E. histolytica*), *Entamoeba coli*, *Endolimax nana*, and *Iodamoeba bütschlii*, are nonpathogenic and do not require treatment. The finding of these organisms in the stool, however, suggests ingestion of fecally contaminated material and should prompt a careful search for pathogenic organisms.

AMEBIASIS

Amebiasis is acquired by ingestion of contaminated food and water containing the cyst stage of *E. histolytica*. Fecal-oral transmission occurs among homosexual men, a group commonly found in recent years to be infected. *E. histolytica* is endemic in most countries and a history of travel is not necessary for the diagnosis to be considered.

Amebiasis is a disease with diverse clinical manifestations. Most individuals who pass cysts are asymptomatic, but overt disease can occur at any time. The mechanism for this change in virulence is poorly understood. Patients receiving treatment with corticosteroid agents and other immunosuppressive drugs are particularly at risk. The clinical course does not have characteristic features, and gastrointestinal symptoms range from alternating diarrhea and constipation associated with crampy abdominal pain, anorexia, loss of weight, and malaise to severe dysenteric colitis. Although amebiasis is a rare cause of inflammatory bowel disease in North America, it should always be considered in the differential diagnosis.

Intestinal amebiasis is diagnosed by finding the organism, either cysts or trophozoites, in the stool or aspirated rectal material. At least three fecal specimens collected over a seven- to ten-day period should be examined by temporary direct smear, stained permanent film, and a concentration method. Techniques for preservation of specimens are available for referral to centers expert in parasitologic diagnosis. Many substances, such as barium, antacids, antidiarrheal agents, and enema preparations, interfere with and invalidate fecal analysis. Antibodies resulting from invasive disease can be detected by a variety of serologic tests. Indirect hemagglutination, complement fixation, and immunofluorescence are the most sensitive.

The most frequent extraintestinal site of infection with *E. histolytica* is the liver, where abscess formation is the result. Other locations in descending order of frequency are the skin, lungs, and brain. Only 50% of patients with amebic abscesses in the liver have demonstrable intestinal infections. Amebiasis should be considered in the diagnosis of an abscess demonstrated by one of the several imaging techniques now available. Amebic abscess is proved only by finding trophozoites in aspirated material, although they are not usually demonstrated. This often is not necessary, and treatment with drugs should proceed in the presence of typical signs and symptoms and a positive finding on serology. Clinical improvement should occur in a few days with appropriate drug therapy in the usual uncomplicated infection. Patients not responding may require administration of broad-spectrum antibiotics for pyogenic organisms, diagnostic or therapeutic aspiration, and open surgical intervention.

Treatment. Treatment of amebiasis depends on the clinical course of the disease and whether invasion of tissue or luminal parasites is the object of therapy. Metronidazole (Flagyl), emetine, and dehydroemetine are tissue-active drugs. Iodoquinol (Yodoxin), diloxanide furoate (Furamide), and paromomycin (Humatin) are poorly absorbed and are active against cysts in the bowel lumen.

Treatment of asymptomatic patients with cysts in the stool is usually recommended, although controversy exists, particularly in highly endemic areas. Drug therapy theoretically removes the risk of potential intestinal disease, abscess in the liver, and contamination of other individuals. Moderately to severely ill patients require hospitalization and supportive measures such as transfusions, fluids, and nutritional replacement. Fulminating disease may require surgical intervention. Most abscesses in the liver encountered in patients in the U.S. are diagnosed early, are relatively small, and are responsive to drug therapy alone. Percutaneous aspiration is usually acceptable, however, for large abscesses that have the potential for rupture, for abscesses that do not respond promptly to drugs alone, or when the diagnosis is uncertain. Serial scanning usually shows gradual resolution over a period of two to four months or longer. Proof that treatment with drugs has been curative should be confirmed by analysis of follow-up stool specimens.

GIARDIASIS

For a discussion of giardiasis, see Section IV, Chapter 15.

DIENTAMOEBA FRAGILIS

Dientamoeba fragilis, recently reclassified as a flagellate, is infrequently the cause of flatulence, diarrhea, and chronic, low-grade discomfort in the lower part of the abdomen. Children in day care centers and persons living under close conditions (communes, for example) or traveling in foreign countries are often among those infected. Only the trophozoite stage has been observed, and *D. fragilis* is thought to inhabit the mucosal crypts of the colon. Unless fresh stools are examined immediately or are preserved for later examination on stained slides, the parasite is frequently overlooked.

BALANTIDIUM COLI

Balantidium coli, a large ciliate protozoan, can rarely be the cause in humans of dysentery similar to that caused by *E. histolytica*. Pigs and other mammals may be the source of infection in man. Cysts, trophozoites, or both are found in the stools.

ISOSPORIASIS

Isospora belli (intestinal coccidiosis) may cause a mild, self-limited diarrheal illness in humans, although a more chronic infection with malabsorption and fever may be seen. Specialized techniques for stool examination and biopsy of small intestine are required for diagnosis. The disease should be considered in the immunocompromised patient, particularly in those with AIDS.

Cryptosporidia are other protozoa related to coccidial parasites. Unlike *Isospora*, this organism does not invade the mucosa and appears only to infect the microvillus membrane of epithelial cells. Infection with this parasite can be seen in AIDS patients, and data are accumulating to suggest that cryptosporidiosis is a relatively common self-limited illness in immunocompetent patients. Diagnosis is by light and electron microscopy of the small intestine, and by special techniques for examination of stools using sugar flotation and phase contrast microscopy. Spiramycin (Rovamycin) appears to be an effective treatment.

HELMINTHS

Worms that infect the intestinal tract are found in two phyla: Nemathelminthes, which includes the class Nematoda or roundworms; and Platyhelminthes, which includes the class Trematoda (flukes) and subclass Cestoda (tapeworms). Those considered here either cause major disease or spend most of their life cycle in the intestinal tract. Others that might be considered intestinal parasites are excluded because of the rarity of their diagnosis in North America. For these reasons, the trematodes (flukes) are not presented.

HELMINTHS: NEMATODA (ROUNDWORMS)

ASCARIASIS

Ascaris lumbricoides, a large (usually 15 to 35 cm in length) worm, is the most common roundworm found in man. Its distribution is worldwide, particularly in tropical and subtropical areas. Adult roundworms usually inhabit the jejunum, where the female lays eggs. Infection is acquired by ingestion of food and water contaminated with eggs from the soil. In the intestine, larvae hatch from eggs, penetrate the intestinal wall, and migrate through mesenteric lymphatics or portohepatic venules to the heart and then to the lungs. Larvae penetrate alveoli, are subsequently swallowed, and settle in the intestines where they develop into the adult form. Migration of larvae produces respiratory symptoms, which are infrequently diagnosed in the United States, although Löffler's syndrome may occur.

Adult worms produce disease when they migrate to aberrant locations. Overcrowding of parasites, fever, certain drugs, and anesthesia are factors associated with this phenomenon. Adult worms may exit by way of the anus, or they may exit through the mouth and enter the respiratory tract, to the alarm of patients or parents. Migration into the biliary tree, pancreatic duct, and appendix produces dysfunction in these areas. Intestinal obstruction is a frequent cause of the acute abdomen seen in children in tropical countries.

The diagnosis of ascariasis is occasionally made by identifying adult worms passed spontaneously. Ova are found on stool examination but are absent when only male worms are present. Adult worms are occasionally identified by typical radiographic features after a barium meal.

Because of the potential seriousness of migration of adult worms, all infections should be treated. Patients known to have ascariasis should be treated before receiving anesthesia.

ENTEROBIASIS (PINWORM INFECTION)

Enterobius vermicularis is the most common helminthic disease diagnosed in the U.S. The infection is more prevalent in children than in adults and in family clusters, schools, and institutions. Infection is acquired by ingesting eggs in contaminated objects or by swallowing them after they have been disseminated in the air. Larvae hatched from eggs in the duodenum migrate to the cecum, where they molt into adults and reside. Gravid females travel to the perianal skin and deposit eggs. The only clinical manifestation is pruritus ani. Reinfection results when a finger touches the mouth after contact with the anus.

The diagnosis is suggested by pruritus ani. Mothers often discover worms on the perianal skin or on the surface of stool. The most reliable diagnostic examination is the Scotch tape test, performed shortly after the patient arises in the morning and before bathing or defecating.

The infection is treated with either pyrantel pamoate (Antiminth) or mebendazole (Vermox). All members of the household should be treated simultaneously, but diagnostic tests are not needed. Although washing hands and cleaning fingernails after defecation and before meals are encouraged, more extensive measures are unnecessary and probably ineffective. Patients should be seen after two weeks for additional treatment to eliminate reinfection.

TRICHURIASIS (WHIPWORM INFECTION)

An estimated 2 million persons in the U.S. are infected with *Trichuris trichiura*. Infection is most common in southern states and in children because of frequent soil ingestion. Concomitant infection with other species of worms is not uncommon, indicating the existence of poor environmental hygiene.

Ingested eggs hatch into larvae, which descend into the cecum and proximal colon, and mature into adults 30 to 50 mm in length. Adults attach to the intestine by burying the anterior portion of their bodies into the mucosal epithelium without producing appreciable injury. Symptoms, as with other helminthic infections, depend on the extent of infection; most people are asymptomatic. Symptomatic infections usually occur in children, diarrhea and dysentery being the most common symptoms. When infections are extremely heavy, rectal prolapse may occur, exposing a mucosa covered with small worms. Eosinophilia and anemia may be seen in chronically ill children.

Diagnosis is made by identification of characteristic eggs on stool examination or by visualization of worms on prolapsed rectal mucosa or proctologic examination. Typical radiographic features have been seen on air contrast barium enema examinations.

Mebendazole is the treatment for trichuriasis. Patients with light, asymptomatic infections do not require treatment, but medication may be indicated to relieve anxiety.

STRONGYLOIDIASIS

Infection with *Strongyloides stercoralis* is usually seen in warm climates and often occurs in the southern U.S. It is acquired when skin comes into direct contact with infective (filariform) larvae in feces, soil, or water, and larvae penetrate into cutaneous blood vessels. After reaching the lung, larvae migrate to the alveoli, where they molt, become immature adults, ascend the airways, and are swallowed. In the duodenum and jejunum, they penetrate and become embedded in the mucosal epithelium. After maturation, the worms produce eggs parthenogenically and release them into the epithelium. Noninfective larvae in the first stage hatch in the epithelium, enter the intestinal lumen, and subsequently are passed in the feces.

Because of the potential for internal autoinfection, strongyloidiasis can become a serious disease. Noninfective larvae in the intestines may metamorphose into infective (filariform) larvae, which reenter the host and thus increase the amount and severity of the disease. Diminished host defenses appear to play an important role in determining the severity of strongyloidiasis. Patients who are debilitated and immunocompromised as a result of malignant disease, malnutrition, or treatment with corticosteroid agents or immunosuppressant drugs may have an overwhelming and even fatal infection.

Most infected persons are asymptomatic carriers. Duodenitis causes abdominal pain similar to that of peptic ulcer disease. Diarrhea and eosinophilia may infrequently occur. Vomiting, acute abdominal pain, severe diarrhea, and malabsorption are seen in severe infections.

Diagnosis is usually established by identification of motile larvae in freshly passed stools. Larvae may also be recovered by duodenal aspiration or with the string test (Enterotest).

All patients with strongyloidiasis require treatment because of the risk of autoinfection. In endemic areas, patients should be screened for infection before receiving immunosuppressive therapy. Thiabendazole (Mintezol) is the drug of choice; this drug kills the adult form but not larvae or eggs. Retreatment is indicated if reexamination reveals parasites two weeks after treatment.

HOOKWORM INFECTION

Hookworm disease is caused by two species of roundworms: (1) *Necator americanus* (American hookworm) and (2) *Ancylostoma duodenale* (Old World hookworm). Virtually all infections originating in the U.S. are due to *N. americanus*. Although these hookworms are an important cause of disease in developing tropical and subtropical countries, their prevalence in the U.S. has decreased and the disease is no longer a serious public health problem. Hookworm is commonly found in warm rural areas with low standards of sanitation and where the inhabitants often go barefoot. Hookworm infection is diagnosed by finding eggs in the feces. Quantification of fecal eggs permits estimates of the intensity of infection.

Infection begins when infective-stage filariform larvae from the soil penetrate the exposed skin of the host. Larvae migrate by way of lymphatics and the venous circulation to the lung and alveoli, ascend the airways, and are swallowed. Most adult worms are found in the jejunum where, as a result of their feeding, minute ulcerations are produced, leading to chronic loss of blood.

Chronic anemia from blood loss is the major consequence of hookworm infection. Anemia develops only when the infection is heavy and dietary intake of iron is inadequate. With massive infection, anemia can be severe and even fatal. Persons with light infections who are asymptomatic do not require treatment with drugs. The heavy migration of larvae through the lungs may cause pneumonitis and coughing. Pruritus, erythema, swelling, and rash ("ground itch") occur at the site of skin penetration.

Treatment is with mebendazole or pyrantel pamoate. Although *N. americanus* and *A. duodenale* differ in their responses to drugs, this is not important in practice. Concomitant anemia and nutritional deficiencies should be corrected at the time of drug therapy. Unless the infection has been severe, follow-up stool examinations and retreatment are not necessary.

HELMINTHS: CESTODA (TAPEWORMS)

DIPHYLLOBOTHRIASIS

The fish tapeworm, *Diphyllobothrium latum* is found most commonly in temperate climates with cold water lakes. Infection is acquired when uncooked or poorly cooked fish containing the infective larvae stage of the worm is ingested. Adult tapeworms are attached to the upper intestinal mucosa by a small scolex and may grow to a length of 10 m. Because of the parasite's ability to absorb vitamin B_{12} and folic acid from the host, megaloblastic anemia may occur. This is infrequent, however, and may be more of a problem in persons in whom there is already a deficiency of these vitamins. The patient usually becomes aware of infection after passing segments or strands of proglottids with the stools. Diagnosis can also be made by identifying eggs in the feces. As with other tapeworm infections, the parasite may occasionally be demonstrated by barium studies.

TAENIASIS (BEEF TAPEWORM AND PORK TAPEWORM INFECTIONS)

These tapeworms occur worldwide, but most infections diagnosed in the U.S. are caused by the beef tapeworm, *Taenia saginata*, while the pork tapeworm, *T. solium*, is usually seen only in travelers and immigrants. Humans are the only definitive hosts and become infected by eating raw or undercooked meat containing cysticerci. The tapeworm attaches itself to the upper small intestine by means of a scolex or head; the body is composed of segments or proglottids. The worm may reach a length of 5 m or more. Probably few or no symptoms result from infection; reports to the contrary are unsubstantiated. Patients become aware of the parasite when proglottids work themselves through the anus, causing an unpleasant crawling sensation. Diagnosis is usually made by identifying retrieved segments on stools, skin, or undergarments.

Cysticercosis occurs when humans become the intermediate host of *T. solium* by being infected with larvae (cysticerci) developing from ingested eggs. This is not caused by *T. saginata* because its eggs are only infective for herbivorous animals. Many tissues may be involved, but cerebral cysticercosis is mainly responsible for serious symptoms. Effective drug therapy with praziquantel (Biltricide) is now available. Theoretically, autoinfection is possible by eggs released from the adult tapeworm during therapy and regurgitation into the stomach. For this reason, some precautions during treatment are advisable (see later).

HYMENOLEPIASIS (DWARF TAPEWORM INFECTION)

Hymenolepis nana is the most frequent tapeworm found in the U.S. It is most commonly seen in children who live in crowded, unsanitary areas, in institutions, or in southern states. It is much smaller than other tapeworms, measuring 25 to 40 mm. Embryos liberated from ingested eggs penetrate intestinal villi and develop into larvae, which are released and mature into adult worms. The worm burden can be increased by internal autoinfection. Clinical symptoms are related to mucosal irritation and include abdominal cramps and diarrhea. Diagnosis is made by identifying characteristic eggs in the feces.

Drug Therapy for Tapeworms. The drug of choice for all adult tapeworms is niclosamide (Niclocide). Since this agent causes the worms to be digested, retrieval of the scolex for identification and proof of cure is usually not possible. All tapeworms except *H. nana* are treated with a single dose of the drug. *H. nana* requires treatment on five consecutive days to ensure that all stages of the tapeworm are killed. Patients with *T. solium* should take an antiemetic before the niclosamide in addition to a saline purge two hours after ingesting these agents, to eliminate dead segments and reduce the likelihood of cysticercosis. When the scolex is not recovered, cure should be confirmed by multiple stool examinations three months after treatment.

DRUG THERAPY

Tables 1 and 2 list first-choice and alternative drugs and recommended doses for the previously discussed intestinal parasites. Since the physician is unlikely to be familiar with many of these agents, package inserts should be reviewed carefully before they are prescribed. Consultation regarding parasitic diseases and certain antiparasitic drugs not routinely obtainable in the U.S. is available from the Centers for Disease Control, Parasitic Disease Drug Service, Atlanta, GA 30333 (telephone 404-329-3311). Patients should be informed of the investigational status and adverse effects of unapproved drugs, or approved drugs used for unapproved indications.

ADVERSE EFFECTS OF ANTIPROTOZOAL DRUGS

Metronidazole. Metronidazole is a nitroimidazole compound that is amebicidal in the intestines and extraintestinal tissue sites, and is available in oral and intravenous forms. The incidence of adverse reactions is low and serious reactions have not been reported. Minor GI disturbances (nausea, diarrhea) are most frequent. Other untoward reactions are unpleasant taste, furry tongue, glossitis, stomatitis, dizziness, ataxia, headaches, urticaria, vaginal and urethral burning or discomfort, and dark urine. When metronidazole is taken with alcohol, a reaction similar to one associated with disulfiram (Antabuse) may occur. Temporary decreases in total leukocyte counts have been reported. Peripheral neuropathy can occur with prolonged use.

Metronidazole is carcinogenic in rodents and mutagenic in bacteria. Long-term studies in humans, however, have not shown evidence of these effects. Nevertheless, this drug usually should not be given to pregnant women, particularly in the first trimester.

Emetine and Dehydroemetine. Adverse reactions occur in 50% to 75% of patients treated with these tissue amebicidal salts of an ipecac alkaloid. Dehydroemetine, which is available from the CDC, may be somewhat less cardiotoxic than emetine. They are administered by subcutaneous or deep intramuscular injection; intravenous injection may cause severe toxic reactions. The most serious adverse reactions are cardiovascular and include arrhythmias, precordial pain, dyspnea, hypotension, gallop rhythm, cardiomegaly, congestive heart failure, and even death. Hospitalization is mandatory; patients require monitoring of blood pressure and baseline and serial electrocardiograms. Changes seen on the EKG are those of conduction delay, and if these are observed, the drug should be discontinued. The changes may be prolonged (average, six weeks). Muscle weakness and cellulitis at the site of injection are frequent accompaniments. Other adverse reactions are nausea, vomiting, diarrhea, headache, skin lesions, and peripheral neuropathy.

Unless other treatment is ineffective, these drugs should not be used during pregnancy, in patients with renal or heart disease, or in children. Since the drugs are eliminated slowly, six to eight weeks should elapse before a second course of therapy is begun.

Chloroquine Phosphate. Chloroquine phosphate (Aralen phosphate) is a tissue amebicide useful for treating amebic abscess in conjunction with emetine or dehydroemetine, because the drug is deposited in considerable amounts in liver tissue. Toxic effects are infrequent during short periods of therapy, are reversible, and are dose related. Mild headache, abdominal distress, diarrhea, pruritus, psychic stimulation, and interference with visual accommodation have been reported. Prolonged use can result in skin eruptions, depigmentation of hair, partial alopecia, localized discoloration of skin, blood dyscrasias, toxic psychoses, neuromyopathy, vertigo, tinnitus, nerve conduction deafness, and damage to the cornea or retina. The drug should be administered with caution in patients with liver disease and deficiency of glucose-6-phosphatase dehydrogenase (G6PD). Chloroquine is contraindicated in patients with psoriasis or porphyria and in patients with changes in the retina or visual fields. Congenital defects may occur and the drug should not be used during pregnancy.

Table 1. DRUG TREATMENT OF INTESTINAL INFECTIONS*

Infection	Drug†	Adult Dose	Pediatric Dose
Amebiasis (*Entamoeba histolytica*)			
Asymptomatic			
Drug of choice	Iodoquinol	650 mg t.i.d. × 20 d	30–40 mg/kg/d in 3 doses × 20 d
Alternatives	Diloxanide furoate	500 mg t.i.d. × 10 d	20 mg/kg/d in 3 doses × 10 d
	Paromomycin	25 to 30 mg/kg/d in 3 doses × 7 d	25–30 mg/kg/d in 3 doses × 7 d
Mild to moderate intestinal disease			
Drug of choice	Metronidazole	750 mg t.i.d. × 5–10 d	35–50 mg/kg/d in 3 doses × 10 d
	plus iodoquinol	650 mg t.i.d. × 20 d	30–40 mg/kg/d in 3 doses × 20 d
Alternative	Paromomycin	25–30 mg/kg/d in 3 doses × 7 d	25–30 mg/kg/d in 3 doses × 7 d
Severe intestinal disease			
Drug of choice	Metronidazole	750 mg t.i.d. × 5–10 d	35–50 mg/kg/d in 3 doses × 10 d
	plus iodoquinol	650 mg t.i.d. × 20 d	30–40 mg/kg/d in 3 doses × 20 d
Alternatives	Dehydroemetine	1–1.5 mg/kg/d IM (max. 90 mg/d) for up to 5 d	1–1.5 mg/kg/d (max. 90 mg/d) IM in 2 doses for up to 5 d
	plus Iodoquinol	650 mg t.i.d. × 20 d	30–40 mg/kg/d in 3 doses × 20 d
OR	Emetine	1 mg/kg/d (max. 60 mg/d) IM for up to 5 d	1 mg/kg/d in 2 doses (max. 60 mg/d) IM for up to 5 d
	plus Iodoquinol	650 mg t.i.d. × 20 d	30–40 mg/kg/d in 3 doses × 20 d
Hepatic abscess			
Drug of choice	Metronidazole	750 mg t.i.d. × 5–10 d	35–50 mg/kg/d in 3 doses × 10 d
	plus iodoquinol	650 mg t.i.d. × 20 d	30–40 mg/kg/d in 3 doses × 20 d
Alternatives	Dehydroemetine	1–1.5 mg/kg/d (max. 90 mg/d) IM for up to 5 d	1–1.5 mg/kg/d (max. 90 mg/d) IM in 2 doses for up to 5 d
	followed by Chloroquine phosphate	600 mg base (1 gm) daily × 2 d, then 300 mg base (500 mg) daily × 2–3 wk	10 mg base/kg (max. 300 mg base)/d × 2–3 wk
	plus Iodoquinol	650 mg t.i.d. × 20 d	30–40 mg/kg/d in 3 doses × 20 d
OR	Emetine	1 mg/kg/d (max. 60 mg/d) IM for up to 5 d	1 mg/kg/d in 2 doses (max. 60 mg/d) IM for up to 5 d
	followed by Chloroquine phosphate	600 mg base (1 gm) daily × 2 d, then 300 mg base (500 mg) daily × 2–3 wk	10 mg base/kg/d (max. 300 mg base/d) × 2–3 wk
	plus Iodoquinol	650 mg t.i.d. × 20 d	30–40 mg/kg/d in 3 doses × 20 d
Giardiasis (*Giardia lamblia*)			
Drug of choice	Quinacrine	100 mg t.i.d. p.c. × 5 d	2 mg/kg/t.i.d. p.c. × 5 d (max. 300 mg/d)
Alternatives	Metronidazole	250 mg t.i.d. × 5 d	5 mg/kg t.i.d. × 5 d
	Furazolidone	100 mg q.i.d. × 7–10 d	1.25 mg/kg q.i.d. × 7–10 d
Dientamoeba fragilis			
Drug of choice	Iodoquinol	650 mg t.i.d. × 20 d	40 mg/kg/d in 3 doses × 20 d
OR	Tetracycline	500 mg q.i.d. × 10 d	10 mg/kg q.i.d. × 10 d (max. 2 gm/d)
Balantidium coli			
Drug of choice	Tetracycline	500 mg q.i.d. × 10 d	10 mg/kg q.i.d. × 10 d (max. 2 gm/d)
Alternative	Iodoquinol	650 mg t.i.d. × 20 d	40 mg/kg/d in 3 doses × 20 d
Isosporiasis (*Isospora belli*)			
Drug of choice	Trimethoprim-sulfamethoxazole	160 mg TMP, 800 mg SMX q.i.d. × 10 d, then b.i.d. × 3 wk	

*Adapted from Drugs for parasitic infections. Med Lett Drugs Ther 26:27–34, 1984.

†Generic and trade names of drugs: iodoquinol (Yodoxin); diloxanide furoate (Furamide); paromomycin (Humatin); metronidazole (Flagyl); chloroquine phosphate (Aralen); quinacrine (Atabrine); furazolidone (Furoxone).

Table 2. DRUG TREATMENT OF INTESTINAL HELMINTHIC INFECTIONS*

Infection	Drug†	Adult Dose	Pediatric Dose
Ascaris lumbricoides (Roundworm)			
Drug of choice	Mebendazole	100 mg b.i.d. × 3 d	100 mg b.i.d. × 3 d for children >2 yr
	OR Pyrantel pamoate	11 mg/kg once (max. 1 gm)	11 mg/kg once (max. 1 gm)
Alternative	Piperazine citrate	75 mg/kg (max. 3.5 gm)/d × 2 d	75 mg/kg (max. 3.5 gm)/d × 2 d
Enterobius vermicularis (Pinworm)			
Drug of choice	Pyrantel pamoate	A single dose of 11 mg/kg (max. 1 gm); repeat after 2 wk	A single dose of 11 mg/kg (max. 1 gm); repeat after 2 wk
	OR Mebendazole	A single dose of 100 mg; repeat after 2 wk	A single dose of 100 mg for children >2 yr; repeat after 2 wk
Trichuris trichiura (Whipworm)			
Drug of choice	Mebendazole	100 mg b.i.d. × 3 d	100 mg b.i.d. × 3 d
Strongyloides stercoralis			
Drug of choice	Thiabendazole	25 mg/kg b.i.d. (max. 3 gm/d) × 2 d	25 mg/kg b.i.d. (max. 3 gm/d) × 2 d
Hookworm			
Ancylostoma duodenale,	Mebendazole	100 mg b.i.d. × 3 d	100 mg b.i.d. × 3 d for children >2 yr
Necator americanus	OR Pyrantel pamoate	11 mg/kg once (max. 1 gm)	11 mg/kg once (max. 1 gm)
Tapeworms (Adult or Intestinal Stage)			
Diphyllobothrium latum (fish),			
Taenia saginata (beef),			
Taenia solium (pork)			
Drug of choice	Niclosamide	A single dose of 4 tablets (2 gm) chewed thoroughly	11–34 kg: a single dose of 2 tablets (1 gm); >34 kg: a single dose of 3 tablets (1.5 gm)
	OR Praziquantel	10–20 mg/kg once	10–20 mg/kg once
Alternative	Paromomycin	1 gm q 15 min × 4 doses	11 mg/kg q 15 min × 4 doses
Hymenolepis nana (Dwarf tapeworm)			
Drug of choice	Niclosamide	A single daily dose of 4 tablets (2 gm) chewed thoroughly × 5 d	11–34 kg: a single dose of 2 tablets (1 gm) × 5 d; >34 kg: a single dose of 3 tablets (1.5 gm) × 5 d
	OR Praziquantel	15–20 mg/kg once	15–20 mg/kg once
Alternative	Paromomycin	45 mg/kg once/d × 5–7 d	45 mg/kg once/d × 5–7 d

*Adapted from Drugs for parasitic infections. Med Lett Drugs Ther 26:27–34, 1984.

†Generic and trade names of drugs: mebendazole (Vermox); pyrantel pamoate (Antiminth); piperazine citrate (Antepar); thiabendazole (Mintezol); niclosamide (Niclocide); praziquantel (Biltricide); paromomycin (Humatin).

Iodoquinol. Iodoquinol (diiodohydroxyquin) is an organic iodine compound that acts against amebas in the intestinal lumen. Occasional adverse reactions include nausea, abdominal cramps, diarrhea, pruritus ani, rash, acne, and slight enlargement of the thyroid. Although rare, optic atrophy and loss of vision can result after prolonged use (months) and in high doses. Liver disease and sensitivity to iodine are contraindications.

Diloxanide Furoate. Diloxanide furoate is a relatively safe luminal amebicide available through the CDC. Excessive flatulence is the most common side effect. Infrequent adverse effects are esophagitis, nausea, vomiting, diarrhea, abdominal cramps, pruritus, urticaria, albuminuria, and vague tingling sensations. Its safety during pregnancy and for young children has not been determined.

Paromomycin Sulfate. Paromomycin sulfate is an aminoglycoside active against amebas in the intestinal lumen. GI disturbances are frequent. Rash, headache, vertigo, and vomiting are occasionally reported. Paromomycin is rarely ototoxic and nephrotoxic.

Quinacrine. Although quinacrine is still often considered the drug of choice for giardiasis, the frequency and potential for adverse reactions from its use have led many to prefer metronidazole for this infection in recent years. Mild and transient headache, dizziness, and GI symptoms may occur. Reversible and infrequent reactions include pleomorphic skin eruptions and neuropsychiatric disturbances (nervousness, vertigo, irritability, emotional change, nightmares, and transient psychoses). Convulsions and transient toxic psychosis are rarely noted. Quinacrine may temporarily cause yellow coloration of the skin and urine. Other adverse reactions described after long-term use are aplastic anemia, hepatitis, exfoliative dermatitis, and reversible corneal edema or deposits. The drug may exacerbate psoriasis, porphyria, and G6PD deficiency. Since it crosses the placenta, it should not be used in pregnancy.

ADVERSE EFFECTS OF ANTHELMINTICS

Mebendazole. Mebendazole has the broadest spectrum of the anthelmintic drugs. Usually less than 10% of the drug is absorbed. Transient abdominal pain and diarrhea are occasional adverse reactions. Except for leukopenia, which occurs rarely, systemic toxicity has not occurred. Because teratogenic effects have been observed in rats, mebendazole is contraindicated during pregnancy. Safety has not been established in children under 2 years of age.

Thiabendazole. Thiabendazole is the drug of choice to treat strongyloidiasis and is well absorbed after oral administration. Common adverse effects are dizziness, giddiness, nausea, and vomiting. Occasional untoward reactions include leukopenia, crystalluria, rash, hallucinations, olfactory disturbances, and the Stevens-Johnson syndrome. Shock, tinnitus, intrahepatic cholestasis, and convulsions are rarely seen. Other reported reactions are lymphadenopathy, anaphylaxis, angioedema, and the appearance of ascarides in the mouth and nose. The drug should be used cautiously in patients with impaired function of the liver or kidneys. Its safety during pregnancy and lactation has not been established.

Pyrantel Pamoate. Pyrantel pamoate is a drug of choice for *Ascaris lumbricoides*. Occasional adverse reactions include anorexia, nausea, vomiting, abdominal pain, diarrhea, headache, dizziness, rash, fever, and increased liver enzymes. Experience with the drug in patients under 2 years of age is limited, and safety during pregnancy has not been determined.

Piperazine. Piperazine (Antepar) is readily absorbed from the intestine and most of it is excreted in the urine. Nausea, vomiting, diarrhea, dizziness, and allergic reactions occasionally occur with therapeutic doses. With larger doses, with inadvertent overdose, or in patients with renal insufficiency, ataxia, hypotonia, visual disturbances, and exacerbation of epilepsy have occurred. Epilepsy and renal and hepatic insufficiency are contraindications.

Niclosamide. Niclosamide is the drug of choice for all the previously discussed tapeworms. It kills the scolex and proximal segments of the worm on contact. The incidence of side effects is low; nausea, vomiting, abdominal discomfort, diarrhea, dizziness, headaches, and rash may occur.

REFERENCES

Cline BL: Current drug regimens for the treatment of intestinal helminth infections. Med Clin North Am 66:721–741, 1982.

Drugs for parasitic infections. Med Lett Drugs Ther 26:27–34, 1984.

Marsden PD (ed): Intestinal parasites. Clin Gastroenterol 7:1–243, 1978.

Wolf MS: The treatment of intestinal protozoan infections. Med Clin North Am 66:707–720, 1982.

7 · *GASTROINTESTINAL BLEEDING*

Surinder K. Mann
Nirmal S. Mann
OLIN TEAGUE VA CENTER
(AFFILIATED WITH SCOTT AND WHITE CLINIC)

Gastrointestinal bleeding is a major medicosurgical emergency. Overt blood in the vomitus or stool is an unnerving sight for patients and relatives, and even for physicians. The amount of blood mixed with vomitus or stool appears to be more than it really is. The goals of treatment of GI bleeding are to stabilize the patient, to try to locate the site and nature of the bleeding lesion so that specific treatment may be started promptly, and to prevent future episodes of bleeding. There are multiple causes of GI bleeding. The natural history of bleeding episodes from different etiologies may be different. It is important to remember that the bleeding may often stop spontaneously, e.g., as in drug-induced gastritis, and in such cases early and unnecessary surgery should be avoided. In other cases, e.g., aortoduodenal fistula, bleeding is not likely to respond to medical therapy, and early surgery is the only hope.

Hematemesis, or bloody vomitus, may be bright red when bleeding is brisk or when the bleeding lesion is at a location where gastric acid does not come in contact with it, or it may resemble coffee grounds when blood has been altered by gastric acid. Melena refers to black, foul-smelling stools that result from degradation of blood. They generally are due to bleeding from the upper GI tract, i.e., from above the ligament of Treitz. However, lesions in the small bowel, cecum, and ascending colon may also cause melena. The term hematochezia is used to denote bright red rectal bleeding or bloody diarrhea. Hematochezia generally is due to distal lower GI bleeding. It may be seen in some cases of upper GI bleeding, if the bleeding is brisk, and particularly when the small bowel transit time is reduced owing to the irritative effect of blood. Sometimes, there is no gross bleeding, and blood is detected by testing the stool with chemical reagents. In such cases, the patient may present with signs and symptoms of chronic anemia.

PATIENT ASSESSMENT AND RESUSCITATION

In a suspected case of GI bleeding, rapid clinical assessment should be carried out. It is very important to evaluate the severity of bleeding by checking the vital signs and determining hemoglobin and hematocrit. No diagnostic work-up can safely be carried out if the patient is in shock. Blood should be sent for typing and cross-matching, and for usual chemistry, blood count, and clotting studies. If the patient is in shock, blood transfusion should be given. In a case of acute blood loss, the hematocrit may not accurately reflect the magnitude of loss during the first few hours, as plasma volume may take a few hours to expand. During this period, the hematocrit will underestimate the severity of bleeding. Clinical tests such as the "tilt test" are important. Tachycardia, hypotension (systolic BP below 100 mm Hg), or a postural drop in blood pressure of 15 mm Hg indicates significant blood loss. Excessive blood transfusion should be avoided, especially in cases of upper GI bleeding from varices, because portal hypertension may become aggravated and cause more bleeding. Depending on the cardiac status and age of the patient, whole blood or packed cells should be given. Transfusion of whole blood also improves both coagulation and oxygenation. We do not give transfusions to stable patients who have a hematocrit of 35 and in whom the bleeding appears to be easing off and rebleeding seems unlikely. When a patient needs a transfusion, we aim for a hematocrit of about 35 to provide reasonable reserve and adequate medical "reaction time" should bleeding recur.

If on initial evaluation the patient is not in overt or impending shock, a quick history is obtained and a rapid physical examination performed. As a presenting feature, hematemesis rather than melena suggests bleeding varices, esophagitis, Mallory-Weiss tear, acute gastritis, or gastric ulcer. Melena rather than hematemesis suggests duodenitis, duodenal ulcer, or hematobilia. Physical examination should look for stigmata of cirrhosis, presence or absence of epigastric tenderness, or cutaneous signs associated with enteric vascular anomalies. At this stage possible sites and lesions can be considered, but no firm opinion should be formed before definitive diagnostic procedures are performed. In 50% of patients with acute upper GI bleeding, the source is from a lesion other than that identified previously.

The next step is to determine whether bleeding is occurring in the upper or lower tract. Upper GI bleeding usually presents as hematemesis or melena; nasogastric (NG) aspirate may show blood (gross or occult), BUN is elevated, and bowel sounds are hyperactive. However, melena can occur in lesions of the small bowel, cecum, or ascending colon. A negative NG aspirate means that active bleeding is not occurring in the esophagus, stomach, or antrum; NG aspirate may be negative for blood in a bleeding duodenal ulcer, which may present with melena. If NG aspirate is negative for blood and has bile in it, a duodenal ulcer is less likely. Lower GI bleeding usually presents with hematochezia, although bright red rectal blood can be seen in cases of massive upper GI bleeding, when small bowel transit time is shortened. In lower GI bleeding, NG aspirate is negative for blood, and BUN and bowel sounds are normal. When the increased BUN is due to blood in the gut, it generally does not exceed 80 mg/dl; a BUN of 100 mg/dl or higher associated with increased serum creatinine indicates intrinsic renal disease.

Acute Upper Gastrointestinal Bleeding

Acute U.G.I. bleeding is a common problem; about 250,000 patients are admitted to hospitals in the United States each year. The causes are listed in Table 1. In one endoscopic study the major sources of upper GI bleeding were duodenal ulcer, acute erosive gastritis, gastric ulcer, varices, and Mallory-Weiss tear. In hospitalized patients with serious underlying illnesses such as uremia, respiratory failure, sepsis, congestive heart failure, and intensive burns, or who have undergone neurosurgical procedures or are on multiple gastrotoxic drugs, the problem of upper GI bleeding due to acute erosive gastritis, acute erosive duodenitis, and acute stress ulcers is becoming increasingly important.

Every effort should be made to find the site and nature of the lesion before therapy is begun. However, if the patient's condition does not allow invasive diagnostic work-up and he or she cannot be rapidly resuscitated, empirical therapy may be tried on the basis of the most likely diagnosis.

Fiberoptic Endoscopy and Barium X-ray. We believe that fiberoptic esophagogastroduodenoscopy (EGD) is the diagnostic procedure of choice in acute upper GI bleeding. In our experience it is likely to give useful information in 95% of cases. If emergency EGD fails to reveal a site of bleeding in the esophagus, stomach, duodenal bulb, or postbulbar area, and if we suspect colonic bleeding, we immediately perform fiberoptic colonoscopy after a rapid cleansing of the colon. Barium x-ray studies are unhelpful in diagnosing acute, superficial, bleeding lesions such as gastritis, esophagitis, or Mallory-Weiss lesions.

Before performing emergency EGD, we insert a large-bore orogastric tube and carry out vigorous ice-saline lavage, because cold fluids reduce gastric blood flow even though they may impair coagulation. In many patients gastric lavage reduces the rate of bleeding, and it becomes easier to perform EGD. However, even if bleeding continues after gastric lavage, we still perform EGD. In our experience, this is a safe procedure with a very low complication rate. It is contraindicated only in patients with acute myocardial infarction, shock, or serious cardiac arrhythmia or who are generally in very poor condition.

Angiography. Angiography is a useful procedure that is currently underutilized in the evaluation of upper GI bleeding. It can be performed even if the patient is in shock or is uncooperative for EGD. If active bleeding is occurring, selective mesenteric angiography may localize the site of bleeding in many patients with vascular malformations, hematobilia, and esophageal varices. Intravenous vasopressin infusion is effective in controlling bleeding, but if diagnostic angiography has been done we do not object to leaving the intra-arterial catheter in place for subsequent intra-arterial vasopressin infusion. Moreover, angiographers may attempt to stop the bleeding by injecting Gelfoam or autologous clot.

MANAGEMENT OF UPPER GASTROINTESTINAL BLEEDING

Varices. Upper GI bleeding from gastric and esophageal varices carries a high mortality. No really satisfactory treatment is available for long-term management of varices. Varices are more likely to bleed when the portal pressure is above 20 mm Hg. Recurrent bleeding from varices is common; the economic implications are obvious, as an inordinate burden is placed on blood banks.

Vasopressin. The treatment and prevention of bleeding from varices is directed toward reducing portal pressure. After initial resuscitation, we use vasopressin, a vasoconstrictor that reduces head pressure on the mesenteric arterial side, thereby reducing portal hypertension. It has no effect on the esophageal veins. We use vasopressin as an infusion, starting at a rate of 0.2 units per minute. If there is no effect within two hours, we gradually increase the amount to 0.8 units per minute. Depending on the rate of bleeding, trial of vasopressin is carried out for six to 12 hours. When this agent has succeeded in controlling the variceal bleeding, it is important not to stop it abruptly but to taper it off gradually. We believe there is no particular advantage to giving vasopressin intra-arterially; however, if mesenteric angiography has been done in the diagnostic work-up we do not object to intra-arterial infusion. Before the infusion is started, an EKG should be taken, and cardiac status should be monitored during vasopressin infusion. This therapy should be stopped if myocardial ischemia appears. The side effects of vasopressin are myocardial infarction, ischemic bowel infarction, and (owing to its antidiuretic effect) worsening of ascites. This agent has a favorable effect on portal vein blood flow, so that liver infarction fortunately is rare. To counteract the adverse effects of vasopressin on coronary circulation, some authors have suggested the concomitant use of nitroglycerin as a 2% ointment (15 to 30 mg) every four hours. More recently a long-

Table 1. CAUSES OF UPPER GASTROINTESTINAL BLEEDING

1. Peptic ulcer disease
   a. Duodenal ulcer
   b. Gastric ulcer
   c. Postpartial gastrectomy marginal ulcer
2. Esophageal and gastric varices
3. Acute erosive gastritis, duodenitis, stress ulcers
4. Acute esophagitis
   a. Reflux esophagitis
   b. Barrett's esophagus
   c. Bile reflux esophagitis
   d. Monilial esophagitis
   e. Radiation esophagitis
   f. Herpes esophagitis
   g. Crohn's disease
5. Mallory-Weiss tear and Boerhaave's syndrome
6. Neoplasms
   a. Polyps
   b. Carcinoma
   c. Leiomyoblastoma
   d. Lymphoma
   e. Hemangioma
   f. Melanoma
   g. Metastatic tumor
7. Hematologic diseases: bleeding disorders, anticoagulant therapy
8. Vascular and elastic tissue disorders
   a. Hereditary hemorrhagic telangiectasia
   b. Arteriovenous malformation
   c. Angiodysplasia
   d. Scleroderma
   e. Blue rubber bleb nevus syndrome
   f. Ehlers-Danlos syndrome
   g. Pseudoxanthoma elasticum
   h. Fabry's disease
   i. Vasculitis of various etiologies
   j. Aneurysm of splenic artery rupturing into stomach
   k. Submucosal microaneurysms of branches of gastric artery
   l. Amyloidosis
9. Arterioenteric fistulas
10. Acute pancreatitis
    a. Associated gastritis
    b. Mallory-Weiss tear (vomiting)
    c. Splenic vein occlusion, left-sided portal hypertension and varices
    d. Hemosuccus pancreaticus
    e. Pseudohematobilia
11. Hematobilia
    a. After penetrating injury to liver
    b. After liver biopsy
    c. After choledochoduodenostomy
    d. Hepatobiliary neoplasms
    e. Hepatic artery aneurysm
    f. Hepatic abscess
    g. Choledocholithiasis
    h. Percutaneous transhepatic biliary drainage
    i. Endoscopic papillotomy
    j. Hepatobiliary parasitic disease
    k. Portal hypertension
    l. Idiopathic
12. Ménétrier's disease
13. Long distance runners
    a. Bowel ischemia due to sympathetic vasoconstriction
    b. Jarring effect on abdominal viscera
    c. Endogenous corticosteroid release due to stress

acting analogue, glypressin (Terlipressin), has been used. It is claimed to have fewer side effects, and is given as a bolus dose of 2 mg IV every six hours. Propranolol and somatostatin have been claimed to lower portal pressure, but we consider these two drugs as experimental and of unproved benefit for variceal bleeding at this time.

If the patient continues to bleed in spite of vasopressin (as is the case in 40% to 50% of those with variceal bleeding), we have to choose from (a) balloon tamponade, (b) injection sclerotherapy, (c) therapeutic shunt, (d) devascularization and transection, (e) transesophageal ligation, and (f) endoscopic laser, or heater probe.

Balloon Tamponade. Some patients who fail to respond to vasopressin benefit from balloon tamponade, and vice versa. If used improperly, balloon tamponade is a dangerous weapon with a high complication rate, but if all the precautions are taken it can be a useful therapeutic modality for temporary control of variceal bleeding. It can successfully control hemorrhage in 80% of cases, but rebleeding rate is high as soon as the balloons are deflated. It can, at best, be considered a stopgap measure. Two types of tubes are available: (1) with gastric and esophageal balloons, i.e., Sengstaken-Blakemore (SB) tube; (2) with gastric balloon alone, i.e., Linton tube. We prefer the former. A modification of the SB tube is available with a fourth lumen to perform suction above the esophageal balloon. Before the tube is passed, the balloons are checked for any leaks. The tube is well lubricated and passed through the nose. About 50 cc of air is injected into the gastric balloon, and the position is checked by x-ray. If the position is confirmed to be in the stomach below the gastroesophageal junction, a total of 250 cc of air is initially injected and traction applied with a traction device. At first only the gastric balloon is inflated and ¾-lb traction is applied. If the bleeding does not stop, the amount of air in the gastric balloon is increased to 350 cc and traction is increased to 1½ lb. If bleeding still continues, the esophageal balloon is inflated to a pressure of 35 mm Hg, and if necessary to 45 mm Hg. Barium, antacids, or nutrition should not be given by SB tube. Continuous suction above the esophageal or gastric balloon should be carried out to prevent aspiration pneumonia. Sometimes, if the gastric balloon is improperly positioned, it may slip up and cause suffocation; a pair of scissors should be at hand to cut the tubes and deflate the balloons. Never inflate the esophageal balloon without inflating the gastric balloon. The traction should be released for 30 to 45 seconds every six hours or so to prevent pressure necrosis of the gastroesophageal junction. If proper precautions are not taken, complications may arise, such as esophageal rupture due to improper positioning, suffocation due to displacement of balloon, aspiration pneumonia, pressure necrosis, or mediastinitis.

Injection Sclerotherapy. In some medical centers, if treatment with vasopressin fails, injection sclerotherapy is carried out in cases of acute variceal bleeding. Percutaneous transhepatic obliteration of varices has been successfully performed, but rebleeding and portal vein thrombosis are serious problems. We predict that this method will not become widely acceptable.

Endoscopic injection sclerotherapy has recently become popular. We recommend the use of a flexible endoscope. The procedure is performed in the usual manner after administering topical pharyngeal anesthesia. In contrast to diagnostic EGD we use slow IV Valium, 5 to 10 mg, when we perform endoscopic injection sclerotherapy. We recommend the use of a retractable needle. Many sclerosing agents have been used: e.g., sodium morrhuate 5%, sodium tetradecyl sulfate 0.1% to 1.0%, ethanolamine oleate 5%, polidocanol 5%, liquid paraffin, and phenolized almond oil. We use 5% sodium morrhuate. The injection can be paravariceal or intravariceal. We prefer the former, but if active bleeding is not controlled this way we inject it into the vein. Sometimes excessive bleeding may occur after intra-variceal injection; in such cases, balloon tamponade is used for immediate control of hemorrhage. We use 2 to 3 ml of 5% sodium morrhuate at each site that is actively bleeding or seems to have recently bled (presence of rent with a clot). Usually four to five separate injections are made as an emergency measure. No attempt is made to obliterate nonbleeding varices. Various investigators have reported a 80% to 90% success rate in controlling acute variceal hemorrhage by sclerotherapy. However, on long-term follow-up, the survival rate was not improved. The complication rate after injection sclerotherapy is 7%, including esophageal ulcer, esophageal stenosis, large pleural effusion, esophageal necrosis, mediastinitis, pyothorax, and lipoid pneumonia.

It has been claimed that elective sclerotherapy and obliteration of esophageal varices is effective in reducing recurrent hemorrhage from esophageal varices. Table 2 lists surgical risk categories as classified by Childs. Elective injection sclerotherapy may be an acceptable approach in class C patients (those with bilirubin greater than 3 mg/dl, albumin less than 3 gm/dl, hepatic encephalopathy, or ascites), where shunt surgery carries a high operative mortality. We accept the efficacy emergency injection sclerotherapy for bleeding varices, but are not convinced that elective injection sclerotherapy of nonbleeding varices (especially in class A or B patients) is an acceptable substitute for definitive elective therapeutic shunt surgery. We believe it is impossible to obliterate all the actual or potential portosystemic esophageal anastomotic sites. Since injection sclerotherapy does nothing to ameliorate portal hypertension, new esophageal varices appear after injection sclerosis; worse still, gastric, duodenal, mesenteric, and colonic varices may appear, which are more difficult to diagnose and treat.

Shunt Surgery. The purpose of the shunt is to decompress part or all of the mesenteric circulation, thereby reducing or eliminating the possibility of variceal bleeding. Many well-designed prospective studies have established that patients with prophylactic shunts (those performed in patients with portal hypertension and varices who have not bled from varices) do not have increased survival, and these shunts are not recommended.

Therapeutic shunts are those performed on patients who have had documented bleeding from esophageal varices. Shunting prevents rebleeding, but patients may die from liver failure and hepatic encephalopathy, especially after a total shunt, and the survival rate is not improved. Therapeutic shunts are emergency or elective. Emergency shunts carry a mortality rate of 50% and even higher in class B and C patients; the average mortality rate of elective shunt surgery is 10%. Temporary control of variceal bleeding can be achieved by vasopressin and balloon tamponade in about 90% of cases. In the remaining 10%, emergency injection sclerotherapy may be attempted.

Central shunts are more effective in portal decompression, but the incidence of post-shunt encephalopathy is higher; in selective shunts, the incidence is lower. The types of shunts performed are (1) portocaval end-to-side, (2) portocaval end-to-side with arterialization of the hepatic end of the portal vein, (3) portocaval side-to-side, (4) portocaval double end-to-side, (5) proximal end-to-side splenorenal, (6) proximal side-to-side splenorenal, (7) central end-to-side splenorenal, (8) distal splenorenal (Warren), (9) portorenal, (10) mesocaval, and (11) coronocaval. Taking into consideration operative mortality, effective control of bleeding, and the incidence of post-shunt encephalopathy, the distal splenorenal (Warren) shunt is the recommended procedure at this time. A few years ago, the umbilical vein–femoral vein shunting procedure performed under local infiltrative skin anesthesia was used as a temporary measure. We believe the availability of emergency injection sclerotherapy has supplanted that procedure.

Devascularization and Transection. A new stapling device allows the surgeon to perform concurrent transection and stapling of the distal esophagus; this procedure can be combined with ligation of the gastric coronary vein. Initial results are encouraging. Extensive devascularization of the esophagus and stomach combined with esophageal transection (Sugiura procedure) is an effective method of controlling variceal bleeding. The mortality rate for elective surgery is about 2%, but rises to above 20% for the emergency procedure.

Transesophageal Ligation. Some surgeons have attempted direct transesophageal ligation of varices to control recurrent bleeding. Operative mortality and rebleeding rates are high, and esophageal leaks are a

---

Table 2. SURGICAL RISK CATEGORIES (Childs' criteria as modified by Pugh et al)

Class A (≤6 points) = good risk
Class B (7–9 points) = moderate risk
Class C (≥10 points) = poor risk

Scored Points*	1	2	3
Bilirubin (mg %)	1–2	2–3	≥3
Albumin (gm %)	3.5	2.8–3.5	<2.8
Prothrombin time (sec. prolonged)	1–4	4–6	≥6
Encephalopathy (grade)	none	1–2	3–4
Ascites	absent	slight	moderate

*Points are totaled for all five parameters.
From Pugh RNA et al: Br J Surg 60:646–649, 1973.

significant cause of postoperative morbidity. We do not recommend this procedure.

Endoscopic Laser. Since laser does not require tissue contact, it has been used for bleeding varices. Immediate hemostasis has been claimed in 90% of cases, with a rebleeding rate of 20%. However, the equipment is not portable and is expensive. We do not recommend laser treatment.

ACUTE EROSIVE GASTRITIS AND STRESS ULCERS

In many cases of acute erosive gastritis, especially drug or alcohol-induced gastritis and duodenitis, massive bleeding is uncommon. Moreover, in a large percentage of such patients bleeding tends to be self-limited. In addition to blood replacement in such patients, medical treatment must be continued and surgery avoided. However, stress ulcers and Curling's ulcers can bleed massively, and Cushing's ulcers can be deep and even perforate. When the bleeding is very active, oral antacids cannot be given, but they can be administered if bleeding has eased after gastric lavage. We recommend Mylanta II, 15 ml every two hours, to keep gastric pH above 5. Some studies have shown that parenteral cimetidine or ranitidine is ineffective in controlling upper GI bleeding. Our opinion is that, in the face of active and brisk hemorrhage from stress ulcers, oral antacids cannot be given. We administer cimetidine, 300 mg IV every six hours; after the bleeding has been controlled, oral antacids can be added. Vasopressin in the same IV dose used for varices has been tried, with variable results. Selective intra-arterial infusion of vasopressin into the left gastric artery is reportedly effective in 90% of patients. Somatostatin and prostaglandin analogues are experimental drugs used in acute, erosive gastritis.

Stress ulcers occur in a setting of sepsis, debility, and multiple organ failure. The mortality rate is high, because of the seriousness of the underlying diseases. In such a setting, stress ulcers should be prevented by antacid and/or cimetidine or ranitidine therapy. In the clinical studies reported, cimetidine is less effective than antacids. This may be because H_2-blockers, while blocking the production of hydrochloric acid, also interfere with intramucosal generation of bicarbonate; oral antacids do not. Antacids and H_2-blockers can be given orally, but not within two hours of each other, as antacids impair their absorption. If, after the above measures, patients continue to bleed, surgery should be performed. Most surgeons recommend vagotomy plus pyloroplasty, and oversewing of bleeding points. Near-total gastrectomy and vagotomy have been recommended for extensive and diffuse lesions. However, the operative mortality is high (above 30%). Some surgeons have performed gastric devascularization, which has controlled the bleeding in 90% of patients, but operative mortality was nearly 40%.

Since most patients with stress hemorrhage have serious underlying disease and are usually poor risks for surgery, nonoperative methods to control the bleeding have been explored. As already mentioned, we do not recommend endoscopic laser photocoagulation because of its expense and the nonportability of the equipment. Equally effective and inexpensive is endoscopic electrocoagulation, which can be monopolar, bipolar, by heater probe, or by electrofulguration (sparking). Because of its low expense, efficacy, and simplicity,

we recommend monopolar electrocoagulation, which should be carried out if discrete bleeding lesions numbering ten or less are seen on endoscopy. Obviously, multiple diffuse bleeding erosions cannot be treated by endoscopic electrocoagulation. In such cases, endoscopic spraying of coagulants or cyanoacrylates has been tried, but this is ineffective in the face of brisk bleeding. We predict that endoscopic topical therapy with clotting factors and tissue adhesives will disappear from medical practice in the near future, as will the use of microiron particles and electromagnets. There is no controlled study of levarterenol applied topically to the gastric mucosa, but uncontrolled studies have reported it to be effective. It can be endoscopically sprayed: Norepinephrine (Levophed), 8 mg in 100 ml of saline. It has been suggested that in alcohol-induced gastritis, bleeding is due to portal hypertension as well as local injury. It is obvious that portal pressure must be reduced (by using vasopressin) to control hemorrhage from alcohol-induced gastritis in cirrhotic patients.

PEPTIC ULCERS

Duodenal, gastric, and marginal ulcers are responsible for upper GI bleeding in 40% to 50% of patients. On endoscopy, if the lesion is not briskly bleeding, we recommend aggressive treatment with antacids (especially for duodenal ulcer). Although some studies have shown H_2-blockers to have no beneficial effect, we combine IV cimetidine, 300 mg every six hours, with antacids. Patients who continue to bleed (i.e., require more than 4 to 5 units of blood per 24 hours) or rebleed on medical treatment are surgical candidates. The presence of visible vessel on endoscopy, hypertension, rare blood type, advanced age, a history of chronic intractable ulcer disease, and previous massive upper GI bleeding are all indications for early surgery. If the bleeding stops and does not recur, there is no indication for emergency surgery and the patient can be maintained on antacids, cimetidine, sucralfate, carbenoxolone sodium, or prostaglandins. Elderly patients, who are poor risks, should undergo oversewing of the bleeding point, truncal vagotomy, and pyloroplasty. Some surgeons have reported good results after ligation of the bleeding site and highly selective vagotomy. In younger, good-risk patients, partial gastrectomy and vagotomy should be performed. In cases of bleeding gastric ulcers, the rate of rebleeding is high after oversewing and vagotomy plus pyloroplasty. For these patients, therefore, it is recommended that gastric resection (including the ulcer) without vagotomy should be performed. In proximally located gastric ulcers, near the gastroesophageal junction, oversewing of the bleeding ulcer, vagotomy, and pyloroplasty are performed.

For elderly, poor-risk patients who continue to bleed, we recommend endoscopic monopolar electrocoagulation. This procedure is performed even if active hemorrhage has stopped, but there is a visible vessel seen on endoscopy in the base of the ulcer. Angiographic embolization of the bleeding artery with autologous blood clot or Gelfoam has been successfully performed, but technically is a difficult procedure.

MALLORY-WEISS SYNDROME

The typical history of vomiting and retching before hematemesis is present in only 50% of patients. Any condition that predisposes to vomiting may cause Mallory-Weiss tear. This lesion is responsible for about 15% of episodes of upper GI bleeding. The linear laceration usually involves the esophagus near the gastroesophageal junction, but may extend into the stomach. Sometimes the only manifestation is submucosal hematoma. If the process extends deeper, perforation of the esophagus and mediastinitis may result (Boerhaave's syndrome). The linear ulcer may be seen on barium meal examination, but endoscopy is preferable. Sometimes the lesion is well seen on selective angiography of the left gastric artery. The hemorrhage is arterial in origin. Many patients stop bleeding on their own and rebleeding is not a problem. However, if active hemorrhage continues, selective infusion of vasopressin (0.4 to 0.8 units per minute) into the left gastric artery or transcatheter embolization of the bleeding lesion may be successful. Technically, it is a difficult procedure, and in patients who are poor surgical risks we recommend endoscopic monopolar electrocoagulation. Rarely, surgical oversewing of the lesion may be necessary.

ACUTE ESOPHAGITIS

Some of the cases of esophagitis are listed in Table 1. It is unusual for esophagitis to cause massive upper GI bleeding; most patients stop bleeding spontaneously. If hemorrhage continues, suture ligation of the bleeding site, vagotomy, and hiatal hernia repair may be necessary. In elderly, poor-risk patients, endoscopic monopolar electrocoagulation may be attempted if few discrete bleeding lesions are seen. We have seen bright red hematemesis in a few cases of monilial esophagitis, which responded well to oral viscous nystatin (Mycostatin), 5 ml (500,00 units) four times daily.

NEOPLASMS

Massive upper GI bleeding from neoplasms is extremely rare; sarcomas, leiomyosarcomas, and leiomyoblastomas may bleed. Appropriate resection is recommended. If the malignancy is unresectable, selective arterial embolization, endoscopic electrocoagulation, or endoscopic laser photocoagulation may be attempted.

VASCULAR ANOMALIES

Hemangiomas, angiodysplasia, or venous ectasia may rarely be responsible for upper GI hemorrhage. The bleeding is painless and massive. Diagnosis can be made by selective angiography (when active bleeding is occurring), radioactive scanning, or endoscopy. Angiographic arterial embolization, surgical ligation of the bleeding artery, surgical resection, and endoscopic electrocoagulation or laser are the therapeutic modalities available. Recurrent hemorrhage is common.

ARTERIOENTERIC FISTULAS

The primary arterioenteric fistulas are due to arterial aneurysms and are better diagnosed by angiography, but can be suspected on endoscopy. All arterioenteric fistulas are due to arterial aneurysms and are better diagnosed by angiography, but can be suspected on endoscopy. All arterioenteric fistulas, whether primary or secondary, produce a premonitory episode of bleeding before massive hemorrhage occurs. Arterioenteric fistulas involving the small vessels may cause recurrent bleeding for many years. Treatment consists of surgical resection.

Upper GI bleeding from secondary arterioenteric (particularly aortoduodenal) fistulas is more common. Any patient who has a prosthetic aortic graft and develops upper GI bleeding (or lower GI if the fistulas are in the small bowel) should be presumed to be bleeding from aortoduodenal fistula until it is proved otherwise. The fistula results from a false aneurysm or localized infection. As in primary cases, there may be an episode of premonitory bleeding, sometimes accompanied by back pain in cases of aortoduodenal fistula. Angiography is of no value in diagnosing secondary arterioenteric fistulas. On endoscopy, the characteristic lesion is a deep defect in the third or fourth portion of the duodenum, with bile-stained base (the bile-stained graft). In some cases, computed tomography with contrast medium shows gas in the retroperitoneal tissues around the prosthesis. After the diagnosis is made or suspected, surgery should be performed promptly; valuable time should not be lost in unnecessary diagnostic procedures. A high operative mortality is seen in such patients.

ACUTE PANCREATITIS

The combination of serious acute pancreatitis and massive upper GI bleeding carries a mortality rate of at least 30%. The various mechanisms of bleeding in acute pancreatitis are listed in Table 1. Splenic vein occlusion in cases of acute or chronic pancreatitis may cause left-sided portal hypertension and esophageal varices, which may bleed. In such cases, bleeding varices can be cured by splenectomy; if active bleeding persists after splenectomy, oversewing of bleeding varices may be performed, and shunt surgery is unnecessary. When we perform emergency EGD in cases of upper GI bleeding with known acute pancreatitis, and when no lesion is seen in the esophagus, stomach, or duodenal bulb, we pay particular attention to the ampulla of Vater. If blood is seen coming out of the ampulla, the diagnosis is either hemosuccus pancreaticus or pseudohematobilia. The former is seen in cases of acute hemorrhagic or acute necrotizing pancreatitis, when a large pancreatic arterial branch communicates with the pancreatic ductal system directly or via a communicating pseudocyst. Pseudohematobilia results when a pseudoaneurysm of the pancreaticoduodenal artery ruptures into the pancreatic ductal system.

Both pseudohematobilia and hemosuccus pancreaticus can be confirmed by angiography. Treatment consists of surgical ligation of the artery. In poor-risk patients, selective angiographic embolization may be attempted. In cases of hemosuccus pancreaticus, when laparotomy is performed to control the bleeding and medical treatment of acute hemorrhagic pancreatitis has failed, concomitant partial or near-total pancreatectomy should be considered if the patient's general condition allows it.

HEMATOBILIA

The various causes of hematobilia are listed in Table 1. Patients present with melena and jaundice in addition to the clinical features of the underlying condition. Hematobilia can be suspected on duodenoscopy, and the diagnosis confirmed by angiography. The treatment of choice is surgical ligation of the hepatic artery branch. In poor-risk patients, angiographic arterial embolization may be done. Rarely, especially if hematobilia is secondary to liver abscess, partial hepatic resection may be necessary. The mortality rate of surgery for hematobilia is about 15%.

Acute Lower Gastrointestinal Bleeding

Lower GI bleeding is defined as bleeding from a site below the ligament of Treitz. Unlike the situation in the upper GI tract, there has been a reduction in mortality in lower GI bleeding, because better diagnostic methods are available to localize the site and nature of the lesion. However, patients presenting with massive lower GI hemorrhage generally are older and may have other complex medical problems. Every effort should be made to locate the site and determine the nature of the lesion before definitive treatment is carried out, whether the bleeding is massive, non-massive, occult, acute, chronic, bright red, or melenic. The causes are listed in Table 3, the most common being diverticula and angiodysplasia.

In patients with massive lower GI bleeding, mesenteric angiography usually localizes the site of hemorrhage. Even if the bleeding has stopped, mesenteric angiography may show angiodysplasia, which can also be diagnosed by colonoscopy. Radioactive scan can be used as a screening procedure before mesenteric an-

giography. If the bleeding has stopped for 48 hours, double-contrast barium enema and/or colonoscopy should be performed. In many cases when barium enema is negative or shows only diverticulosis, colonoscopy can detect additional lesions such as cancer, polyps, colitis, or angiodysplasia. However, it is difficult to perform meaningful colonoscopy in the face of massive torrential lower GI bleeding. In such cases, angiography defines the site and nature of some lesions, such as diverticulum, angiodysplasia, and cancer. Moreover, intra-arterial infusion of vasopressin can be given.

MANAGEMENT OF LOWER GASTROINTESTINAL BLEEDING

DIVERTICULOSIS

Diverticulosis is common in Western countries, especially after the age of 40. Bleeding from diverticula occurs in about 5% of patients with diverticulosis. It is the most frequent cause of lower GI bleeding, because diverticula are so common. Bleeding is often massive and painless. In many patients, hemorrhage may stop spontaneously and not even recur. In patients who continue to bleed, intra-arterial vasopressin (0.2 to 0.6 units per minute) is effective in 90%. Segmental resection is recommended in patients who do not respond to vasopressin or who have recurrent bleeding.

VASCULAR ABNORMALITY; ANGIODYSPLASIA

Vascular abnormalities may occur with or without any skin lesion. Those associated with skin lesions may be found in the upper and lower GI tract, e.g., Osler-

Table 3. CAUSES OF LOWER GASTROINTESTINAL BLEEDING

1. Diverticulosis
   a. Right colon
   b. Left colon
   c. Small bowel
   d. Meckel's diverticulum
2. Hemorrhoids
   a. Without portal hypertension
   b. With portal hypertension
3. Anal fissure
4. Ischemic bowel disease
   a. Occlusive
      i. Mesenteric thrombosis
      ii. Embolism: myocardial infarction, rheumatic heart disease, infectious endocarditis, atrial myxoma
      iii. Vasculitis: SLE, rheumatoid arthritis, periarteritis nodosa, allergic sepsis, radiation, thromboangiitis obliterans, oral contraceptives
      iv. Miscellaneous: fibromuscular hyperplasia, aortic aneurysm, trauma, amyloidosis, celiac axis compression
      v. Venous occlusion:
   b. Nonocclusive
      i. CHF, digitalis, cardiac arrhythmia, aortic insufficiency
      ii. Large AV fistula
      iii. Aortoiliac steal syndrome
5. Inflammatory bowel disease
   a. Ulcerative colitis
   b. Ulcerative proctitis
   c. Crohn's disease
   d. Diversion colitis
6. Infectious bowel disease
   a. *Shigella*
   b. *Salmonella*
   c. *E. coli*
   d. *Campylobacter*
   e. *Yersinia*
   f. Pseudomembranous colitis
   g. *Pseudomonas*
   h. Amebiasis
   i. Tuberculosis
   j. *Vibrio parahaemolyticus*
   k. Viruses
   l. Rectal schistosomiasis
7. Intussusception and volvulus
8. Neoplasms
   a. Primary { carcinoma / lymphoma / sarcoma
   b. Metastatic melanoma
   c. Polyps
9. Vascular and elastic tissue disorders
   a. Hereditary hemorrhagic telangiectasia
   b. AV malformation
   c. Angiodysplasia
   d. Scleroderma
   e. Blue rubber bleb nevus syndrome
   f. Ehlers-Danlos syndrome
   g. Pseudoxanthoma elasticum
   h. Fabry's disease
10. Arterioenteric fistula
11. Miscellaneous
   a. Uremic colitis
   b. Uremic cecal ulcer
   c. Endometriosis
   d. Fecaliths, stercoral ulcer
   e. Pneumatosis cystoides intestinalis
   f. Nongranulomatous ulcerative ileojejunitis and colitis
   g. Ulcerative celiac disease of small bowel and colon
   h. Colonic necrosis and inflammation in pancreatitis
   i. Radiation enteritis and colitis
   j. Drugs, e.g., vincristine-induced cecal ulceration
   k. Anticoagulants and coagulopathy
   l. Small bowel, cecal, and sigmoid varices
   m. Eosinophilic enteropathy

Weber-Rendu. They may be seen endoscopically or angiographically. They may cause massive recurrent bleeding. If they are localized, surgical resection may be carried out; generally, however, they are diffuse, and endoscopic electrocoagulation or laser is recommended. Two types of lesions are not associated with any skin lesion: arteriovenous malformation (AVM) and angiodysplasia. AVM occurs in younger patients predominantly in the small bowel. The recommended treatment is segmental resection, but arterial embolization may be attempted. The more common lesion, angiodysplasia, occurs in older patients and may be associated with aortic stenosis. It is more common in the right colon, but may also occur in the sigmoid and upper GI tract. It is best diagnosed by angiography, especially when active bleeding is occurring. It can be identified endoscopically as a small, bright red, flat area with small vessels radiating from it, giving it a stellate appearance. The bleeding may stop, but may be chronic or recurrent. Intra-arterial vasopressin (0.2 to 0.6 units per minute) may be effective. Before right hemicolectomy is done for a nonbleeding lesion, other causes of recurrent bleeding should be diligently excluded. In poor-risk patients, endoscopic electrocoagulation or laser may be effective.

INFLAMMATORY BOWEL DISEASE

In ulcerative colitis, there may be diffuse oozing of blood, and massive bleeding may require total colectomy. In Crohn's disease massive hemorrhage may occur and sometimes be severe enough to require resectional surgery. Bleeding from ulcerative proctitis may respond to corticosteroid enema.

ISCHEMIC BOWEL DISEASE

The occlusive variety of ischemic bowel disease may produce markedly acute abdomen with radiologic features of mucosal edema and thumb printing. Resectional surgery is often indicated, especially if bowel gangrene is imminent. Venous occlusive disease should be treated by heparinization, but if the bowel becomes nonviable, resection is recommended. Surgery should be avoided in cases of nonocclusive hemorrhagic necrosis, and underlying cardiac disease should be treated. However, a large AV fistula or the aortoiliac steal syndrome may need to be treated surgically.

INFECTIOUS BOWEL DISEASE

Massive lower GI bleeding is uncommon in these disorders. Underlying disease should be treated with chemotherapy. Pseudomembranous colitis may bleed profusely and responds well to vancomycin, given 500 mg PO every six hours for seven to ten days.

INTUSSUSCEPTION AND VOLVULUS

Bright red bleeding may occur with this condition. Usually, surgery is required; volvulus may sometimes be corrected by barium enema or colonoscopy. Recurrent sigmoid volvulus may require resection of the redundant sigmoid.

NEOPLASM

Massive lower GI bleeding is uncommon in cases of carcinoma. Small bowel lymphoma and metastatic melanoma may bleed profusely and require surgical resection. Polyps may cause chronic hemorrhage, which can be managed by colonoscopic polypectomy. However, in a given case polyps may not be the cause of the bleeding, and other lesions should be excluded.

ARTERIOENTERIC FISTULAS

Bleeding is usually massive with arterioenteric fistulas. In a patient with aortic prosthesis, this lesion should be suspected until it is proved otherwise. Immediate surgical resection is indicated after angiography.

HEMORRHOIDS

Hemorrhoids are a common cause of bright red bleeding. Massive bleeding is rare in these cases. Treatment is with stool softeners and sitz baths. In intractable cases, hemorrhoidectomy, banding, or cryosurgery may be indicated.

MISCELLANEOUS

Bleeding from endometriosis should be treated with surgical resection. Pneumatosis cystoides intestinalis is treated by breathing oxygen or with metronidazole (250 mg three times a day for seven days). Bleeding from stercoral ulcers secondary to fecaliths occurs in older people; constipation should be prevented in such patients by usual methods. Massive lower GI bleeding can occur in some cases of nongranulomatous ulcerative ileojejunitis and colitis. Prednisone, 60 mg in four divided doses, may give dramatic results, but the long-term prognosis is poor. Radiation colitis may respond to corticosteroid enema. Bleeding colonic varices may require portal decompression by shunt surgery, but resection of the bleeding segment may be necessary.

GASTROINTESTINAL BLEEDING IN ELDERLY PATIENTS

The same general principles apply to elderly patients as to other age groups. However, significant associated disease makes GI bleeding a specially challenging proposition. Invasive diagnostic procedures carry a higher complication rate in the elderly. Since emergency surgery carries a high mortality rate in elderly patients, every effort should be made to transform an emergency situation to an elective procedure. Nonsurgical procedures such as endoscopic injection sclerotherapy, angiographic arterial embolization, endoscopic electrocoagulation, and endoscopic laser therapy may play an important role in the elderly, poor-risk patient.

REFERENCES

Brandt LJ, Boley SJ: The role of colonoscopy in the diagnosis and management of lower intestinal bleeding. Scand J Gastroenterol 19(Suppl 102):61–70, 1984.
Larson DE, Farnell MB: Upper gastrointestinal hemorrhage. Mayo Clinic Proc 58:371–387, 1983.
Mann NS, Mann SK: Fiberoptic panendoscopy in acute upper GI bleeding. Am J Procto Gastro Colo Rect Surg 29:26–31, 1978.
Swain CP, Salmon PR: Gastrointestinal bleeding—upper gastrointestinal tract. Scand J Gastroenterol 19(Suppl 102):53–60, 1984.
Wilson JL, Powell E, Rodning CB: Upper gastrointestinal bleeding in the elderly. J Fam Pract 17:783–801, 1983.

8 · CHOLECYSTITIS AND CHOLELITHIASIS

William D. Carey
CLEVELAND CLINIC FOUNDATION

DEFINITIONS

The most common manifestation of gallstones (cholelithiasis) is inflammation (cholecystitis), which may be acute or chronic. Cholelithiasis and cholecystitis are often considered synonymous, but are not. The mere presence of gallstones does not imply that the gallbladder harboring the stones will contain any of the pathologic findings of cholecystitis, nor that the patient will develop symptoms. In fact, *most* gallstones are completely asymptomatic and remain that way indefinitely. Moreover, the formation of gallstones is not primarily due to a defect of gallbladder structure or function but to *hepatic* abnormalities of cholesterol and/or bile acid synthesis and secretion. Finally, acute cholecystitis can occur in the absence of gallstones, so that stones are not necessary for the expression of gallbladder disease. The indisputable linkage is that gallstones are by far the most common precursor of cholecystitis. In this chapter we will focus on the dual problem of gallstones and cholecystitis, remembering that these are separable but nevertheless commonly linked events.

What makes gallstones so important is their prevalence. In the United States, gallbladder disease is the fifth leading cause of hospitalization; 800,000 Americans each year are discovered to have gallstones; 400,000 cholecystectomies are performed; and 3000 people die annually after biliary tract surgery.

PATHOPHYSIOLOGY OF CHOLESTEROL GALLSTONES

Cholesterol gallstones form because of the inability of certain biles to maintain cholesterol in solution. They are likely to form if increased amounts of cholesterol are secreted into the bile, or if there is a decrease in the factors that "solubilize" cholesterol. These factors are primarily bile acids and certain proteins. It is clear that most patients who have gallstones do not have symptoms. In one of the few long-term follow-up studies in the U.S., only 18% of individuals with asymptomatic gallstones developed symptoms over a period of 20 years. This attack rate becomes important when therapeutic decisions need to be made. The accepted mechanism by which gallstones are thought to produce symptoms is via obstruction of the cystic duct by the stones. If a gallstone impacts temporarily in the cystic duct, it sets up, in effect, a closed-loop obstruction. Moreover, if the obstruction lasts long enough, bacterial contamination and proliferation can occur, which can lead to infection. When the stone then disimpacts, the episode subsides. Recently it has been shown that patients whose gallstones are buoyant or "floating" are at higher risk of developing acute cholecystitis. This is presumably due to the floating stones' increased susceptibility to becoming impacted in the cystic duct.

Acute cholecystitis can occur in the absence of gallstones, a condition called *acalculous cholecystitis*. It is particularly likely to be seen after major trauma or in the postoperative state. It is thought to occur when biliary flow is diminished, during which time the bile may become more viscous and resistant to flow, setting up a functional obstruction in the cystic duct. Other possible mechanisms include (1) impairment of blood flow and gallbladder hypoxia during or after trauma, (2) increased demand placed on the gallbladder by excretion of blood breakdown products, (3) infection, and (4) fat embolization to the gallbladder. It is reported more often in men. In one series, acalculous cholecystitis accounted for 2% of the cholecystectomies performed.

CLINICAL ASPECTS

Many symptoms have erroneously been attributed to gallstones, and many patients who have had cholecystectomy for gallstones have found to their surprise that the symptoms are not relieved. Perhaps the likeliest gastrointestinal syndrome to be incorrectly attributed to gallstones is irritable bowel syndrome. A knowledge of the symptoms produced by cholecystitis is imperative. *Episodic pain* is the hallmark of acute cholecystitis. Recurrent bouts of pain followed by pain-free intervals is the expected pattern. The location of the pain is variable, but most commonly in the right upper quadrant or epigastrium; other sites are also identified. Occasionally the patient complains of chest pain that may radiate into the neck or arm. When this pattern occurs, it is often mistaken as the pain of myocardial ischemia until appropriate tests exclude this diagnosis. *Radiation* of the pain is frequent, and again the sites of radiation are quite varied, the most characteristic being into the right infrascapular region.

The pain of acute cholecystitis is usually severe and lasts four to eight hours. There may be a feeling of residual soreness for a day or two and then the patient is well until another random attack occurs. The term "biliary colic" is considered by some to be a misnomer since colic implies a cyclic waxing and waning of pain (such as the pain of a bowel obstruction). Careful observations of the nature of the pain of cholecystitis reveals that in only 10% of cases is there any fluctuating feature; in the rest the pain either reaches its peak within an hour and stays at maximal intensity until it wanes, or is of maximal intensity at the outset. It seems useful to take note of these pain patterns, but we will use the term biliary colic in this discussion. Associated features of the pain of acute cholecystitis include restlessness (90%), vomiting (76%), and sweating (70%). Jaundice, dark urine, or light stools may be present if the gallstone has passed through the cystic duct into the common duct and caused extrahepatic large duct obstruction. In addition, once cystic duct obstruction has been present for 24 hours or more, there is increasing likelihood of bacterial infection. Therefore, signs of sepsis may be present in acute cholecystitis. Occasionally a patient with cholecystitis develops attacks of acute pancreatitis. Certain features formerly held to be suggestive of acute or chronic cholecystitis are now

known to be unrelated. Fatty food intolerance is as likely to be reported by those without cholelithiasis as by those with gallstones, and therefore does not seem to predict the presence of either stones or cholecystitis.

MANAGEMENT

PLAN

The major short-term goal of management of acute cholecystitis is the alleviation of pain and the prevention of complications. Many minor and moderate attacks may be handled on an outpatient basis. Major attacks that prompt an emergency visit to office or hospital are most often handled by parenteral use of narcotic analgesics. Hospitalization may be necessary. In such cases it must be decided whether immediate surgery is necessary. In cases where sepsis is present, including emphysematous cholecystitis (due to gas-forming bacteria), surgery should be performed as soon as the patient is medically stable. Early cholecystectomy may be preferred in most patients, since controlled trials have demonstrated that this is not more hazardous than waiting, and early surgery means reduced hospital time and fewer days lost from work. Antibiotics are administered to the seriously ill hospitalized patient with acute cholecystitis, since bile samples from such individuals have at least a 75% chance of being infected. Those with acute pancreatitis secondary to cholelithiasis or cholecystitis should have early surgery if the attack of pancreatitis does not resolve after a few days. Otherwise, surgery in such patients is probably best deferred until resolution of the pancreatitis.

Recurrent Biliary Colic

The patient who has had one or more recent episodes of biliary colic should be considered for definitive treatment even if currently asymptomatic. The best treatment available today is cholecystectomy. The operation is safe and effective wherever good surgical expertise is available. It has a low operative and perioperative mortality, it effects a virtual cure for the underlying disease, and it involves little long-term morbidity. It can be done safely even in quite elderly patients, provided the cardiopulmonary systems are reasonably compensated. For patients ill with acute cholecystitis who are in too precarious a condition to undergo general anesthetic, cholecystotomy with extraction of the gallstones can be accomplished, using light general anesthesia or even local anesthetic. There is little reason to challenge the conventional view that the majority of patients with symptomatic cholelithiasis are best treated by operative means.

Asymptomatic Gallstones

Little evidence is available concerning the natural history of asymptomatic gallstones in various ethnic groups. Moreover, the impact of other diseases on gallstone behavior is poorly documented. The few available studies report the different rates with which asymptomatic gallstones later become symptomatic. These differences may be due both to the populations studied and to methodologic differences. One review of the long-term outcome for untreated Scandinavian patients with cholelithiasis showed that nearly 50% of asymptomatic patients eventually required surgery. In a more recent study from the U.S., only 15% of these individuals developed symptomatic cholelithiasis requiring surgery, leading the authors to conclude that the risk of developing symptoms in an individual with asymptomatic cholelithiasis is greatly overestimated. Clearly, more studies are needed to establish the true risk for different populations of developing symptoms of biliary colic.

MEDICAL DISSOLUTION

Many studies have demonstrated the ability of chenodeoxycholic acid (Chenix) to dissolve certain gallstones. The best known of these is the National Cooperative Gallstone Study, a large multicenter study that compared the therapeutic efficacy of a daily dose of 375 mg of chenodeoxycholic acid (CDCA) with a dose of 750 mg of CDCA. A third group of patients received a placebo medication. After therapy lasting up to two years (shorter if gallstone dissolution occurred), only 14% of the group receiving the higher dose achieved complete gallstone dissolution. It is apparent that at least a twofold increase in the success of therapy can be achieved by administering a total daily dose of 15 mg/kg/day. However, even this is a poor outcome compared with conventional (i.e., surgical) therapy, which is 100% effective. Until better pharmacologic treatment becomes available, medical dissolution of gallstones will be relevant to only a relatively small group of patients. The recent demonstration of very rapid gallstone dissolution (less than eight hours) by infusion into the gallbladder of methyl-tert-butyl ether may revolutionize gallstone therapy if broad experience confirms its efficacy and safety.

Are there any subgroups for whom the results of medical dissolution are better? For patients whose gallstones are buoyant ("floating gallstones"), CDCA has an 80% likelihood of achieving complete dissolution; hence, for these individuals medical therapy appears to be an attractive alternative to surgery. There is preliminary evidence to suggest that patients with buoyant gallstones are more likely to become symptomatic than those with nonbuoyant stones. Only 10% of patients have buoyant gallstones.

Other cautions are necessary before we can embrace medical dissolution therapy. Obese patients are relatively refractory to treatment. Also, gallstones over 2 cm in maximal diameter are unlikely to dissolve. In addition, the administration of CDCA requires attention to dosing schedules and to the minimization of side effects. The latter consist principally of cramps and diarrhea, which are dose related and can be minimized by using a low dose initially (250 mg b.i.d.) and increasing it gradually to the target dose of 15 mg/kg/day (usually between 1000 mg and 1250 mg divided in two doses). Approximately 10% of patients develop mild or moderate liver test abnormalities, so that monitoring of liver tests (particularly SGOT) is mandatory. Liver test abnormalities may be seen in 5% to 10% of cases. The pattern of liver dysfunction suggests mild hepatocellular injury, in that the transaminases (SGOT, SGPT) rise. Interestingly, liver biopsies from patients taking CDCA usually reveal mild changes of cholestasis rather than the anticipated hepatocellular changes. The transaminase elevations are usually mild and respond promptly to a lowering or discontinuation of the dose. Reports of permanent liver injury are rare. We have found that individuals with pretreatment elevations of liver enzymes are particularly likely to develop further rise in these enzymes in response to treatment. If the pretreatment SGOT is more than twice the upper limit of normal, CDCA should not be used. Another bile acid with the same therapeutic efficacy as CDCA, ursodeoxycholic acid, is devoid of the troublesome side effects noted above, but is not yet available for clinical use in the U.S. Finally, recurrence of gallstones after therapy is ended may occur in patients who have achieved gallstone dissolution. Therefore, life-long surveillance by ultrasonography is required, and retreatment with full therapeutic dosages is necessary when gallstones recur.

At present I agree with the American College of Gastroenterology that CDCA therapy "appears especially appropriate only for the small group of patients who have floating radiolucent gallstones, are over the age of 60, and have increased surgical risk factors. . . . Other patients should be evaluated on an individual basis, with consideration given to simple observation for silent gallstones, and to direct intervention if bile duct obstruction occurs."

Medical therapy is, for the most part, well tolerated. About 10% to 20% of patients given CDCA develop diarrhea when given a full therapeutic dose (15 mg/kg/day). This diarrhea is frequently explosive, with associated cramps, and is somewhat unpredictable. This problem can be minimized by starting with a low dose and increasing it gradually over a period of several weeks. Most prescribe 250 mg by mouth twice a day for the first two weeks. After this, increasing the total daily dose by a single pill (250 mg) each week until the full therapeutic dose is reached is often sufficient to avoid most episodes of diarrhea and cramps. If the patient develops these symptoms during therapy, it is useful to omit the pills for a day and then resume. If the episodes are frequent, it is best to cut back the dosage to the highest that can be tolerated, recognizing that a sharp drop-off in efficacy is to be expected if the total daily dose falls much below the ideal. There is some evidence that administration of the entire dose at bedtime increases slightly the rate of gallstone dissolution.

Other side effects are quite uncommon. One major study showed a slight (10%) increase in LDL cholesterol in response to CDCA. However, in this study the placebo group also showed a rise in cholesterol levels (albeit less than with the drug), making the results hard to interpret. We, and most others, have found no rise in serum cholesterol levels after up to two years of treatment. Nonspecific gastroenterologic complaints such as dyspepsia and flatulence may also be reported from time to time, and a few patients have developed leukopenia that cleared upon cessation of the drug.

CDCA is a bile acid, and as such may disrupt the integrity of the gastric mucosa. Thus, the drug theoretically may interfere with ulcer healing. We have treated many patients who have peptic ulcer disease and asymptomatic gallstones with CDCA, but we delay the gallstone treatment until there is definite ulcer healing (demonstrated by endoscopy). It has been my practice to leave patients with recently healed ulcer disease on ulcer prophylaxis therapy (with sucralfate or an H_2-receptor antagonist) while they are receiving CDCA treatment. The accumulated evidence to date does not suggest that CDCA lives up to its theoretic potential for producing ulcer disease, since this is not a reported complication of therapy. CDCA, like all bile acids, is absorbed in the distal ileum. Therefore, it is to be expected that patients with distal ileal disease will malabsorb CDCA. When this happens, increased amounts of bile acids reach the colon and produce diarrhea. For this reason, the use of CDCA in an individual with Crohn's disease of the distal ileum is unwise.

Complications of drug therapy respond promptly to dose reduction or discontinuation. If complications of cholelithiasis emerge during treatment, cholecystitis (or choledocholithiasis) is the result. If there are infrequent mild attacks of cholecystitis and the patient is willing, continued medical treatment may be justified. A single major attack, or many mild attacks, make long-term therapy unreasonable. In these cases, I urge the patient to undergo definitive surgery unless the risks involved are prohibitive.

PATIENT INFORMATION AND EDUCATION

It is very important for all medical therapy, but particularly for long-term therapy that does not greatly alter symptoms, that patients be highly motivated. In view of the known risks of patient noncompliance with a variety of therapies, it is essential that patients actively want to be treated. I almost never initiate a recommendation of medical therapy for gallstones, but present patients with the options and possible outcomes. Only when they indicate a strong preference for this form of therapy do I begin a program. Thus, such patients are highly selected and tend to be highly motivated. I give each patient as much information as possible. I also enlist their help in altering dosages within certain defined limits, to try to reduce to a minimum the troublesome diarrhea that CDCA can produce.

PERIODIC EVALUATION

Follow-up is essential for safety. I do not write refillable prescriptions, to ensure that I see patients at the desired intervals. Since the major safety concern is to recognize liver toxicity that produces no symptoms, it is mandatory that liver tests be checked. Most liver dysfunction occurs within the first few months of therapy. I set up return appointments two, four, and six weeks after starting therapy, and check a complete blood count, bilirubin, SGOT, and alkaline phosphatase. If the patient seems to be getting along well, the visits are then reduced to every three months. Since the drug is very slow-acting, there is no reason to check the gallbladder at frequent intervals. I order an ultrasound or oral cholecystogram nine months after therapy, and an oral cholecystogram at 16 months. The reason for the latter at this time rather than an ultrasound is that I find an oral cholecystogram more accurate for assessment of change in stone size. If there has been no change in the size of the stones by 16 months, I ordinarily abandon pharmacotherapy. If, on the other hand, the stones are still present but definitely smaller, continued treatment is warranted. Although 24 months of therapy is usually sufficient to dissolve most stones capable of dissolution by this drug, some patients demonstrating progressive reduction in stone size may need a few extra months of treatment.

Postdissolution monitoring is necessary. It has been shown that within a short time after discontinuation of therapy, the gallbladder bile reverts to a supersaturated state. It has further been shown that gallstone reformation occurs in at least half (and probably all) patients whose gallstones have been medically dissolved if they are followed for a long enough period. On a yearly basis, therefore, ultrasonography should be done. If gallstones reform, another course of therapy should be given. By regular surveillance of such high-risk patients, recurrent stones should be discovered when quite small and will not require such a protracted course of therapy the second time around. There is little direct evidence of this, however.

REFERENCES

Gracie WA, Ransohoff DF: The natural history of silent gallstones: the innocent gallstone is not a myth. N Engl J Med 307:798–800, 1982.

Pearlman BJ, Schoenfield LF: Gallstones. The present and future of medical dissolution. Med Clin North Am 62:87–105, 1978.

Schoenfield LJ, Lachin JM: Chenodiol (chenodeoxycholic acid) for the dissolution of gallstones. The National Cooperative Gallstone Study: a controlled trial of efficacy and safety. Ann Intern Med 95:257–282, 1981.

Tangedahl T: The present status of agents for dissolving gallstones. Am J Gastroenterol 80:64–66, 1985.

Tangedahl T, Carey WD, Ferguson DR, et al: Drug and treatment efficacy of chenodeoxycholic acid in 97 patients with cholelithiasis and increased surgical risk. Dig Dis Sci 28:545–551, 1983.

9 · DIVERTICULOSIS AND DIVERTICULITIS

Blaine W. Cobb
GUTHRIE CLINIC

Colonic diverticula are extraordinarily common. In some studies, over 50% of aged westernized populations have diverticulosis. Although described in the 1800s and classified in the early 1900s, these intestinal outpouchings are seen with increasing frequency in 20th century autopsy and radiographic studies. Diverticula are unusual in "underdeveloped" countries and correlate with a decreased dietary fiber intake in Western populations. These epidemiologic findings have prompted more recent physiologic investigations suggesting a motility basis for diverticular disease. Reviews dealing with this topic tend to focus on pathology and pathophysiologic concepts. This chapter will minimize these considerations and focus on medical (especially outpatient) management.

DEFINITION

Diverticulosis refers to the presence of outpouchings of colonic mucosa and muscularis mucosae through defects in the colonic wall. As such, these are pseudodiverticula. True diverticula, congenital in nature, may occur in the cecal area. Diverticula may range up to 25 cm in diameter but are usually a few millimeters. The sigmoid region is involved in 95% of cases. The descending, transverse, and ascending colon are involved in order of decreasing frequency. In a radial sense, the diverticula are located between the antimesenteric and the mesenteric taenia coli.

PATHOPHYSIOLOGY

Current notions regarding the etiopathology of diverticular disease center on motility and colonic wall abnormalities. Pathologically, smooth muscle hypertrophy is frequently seen in patients with diverticula. The most popular theory, therefore, is that the high-amplitude contractions of the irritable bowel syndrome (IBS) are accompanied by muscular hypertrophy and eventual herniation of mucosa at a site of relative colonic wall weakness—the area of wall penetration by intramural blood vessels. Many patients with diverticular disease, however, have no history of abdominal pain and show normal results from motility studies. A primary colonic wall abnormality may be dominant in these patients (as in Marfan's syndrome). The alternative explanation, however, is that high-pressure contractions generating the diverticula do not occur continuously and were simply not demonstrated at the time of study.

CLINICAL FEATURES

Most patients with diverticular disease are asymptomatic. When symptoms are present, they are most commonly due to abnormal motility, similar to those seen in IBS. Crampy lower abdominal discomfort related to meals, bowel movements, or flatus is frequent. The pain may be accompanied by constipation or, less commonly, diarrhea. Patients characteristically have had these symptoms for months or years before seeking medical help, and many will have had previous sigmoidoscopic and barium contrast studies.

Complications of diverticular disease include those attributable to perforation, hemorrhage, or obstruction. With free perforation, generalized peritonitis is produced, causing pain, fever, rebound tenderness, guarding, and ileus. Confined perforation may result in the mild, localized pain (frequently left lower quadrant [LLQ]) of diverticulitis or more severe discomfort with palpable mass, high fever, and toxicity of pericolonic abscess. Rarely, right-sided abdominal pain may occur and arouse suspicions of acute appendicitis, cecal diverticulitis, or Crohn's disease. Obstruction of the sigmoid region may accompany an acute episode of diverticulitis or may occur gradually as scarring from diverticulitis produces luminal narrowing. Abdominal distention, increasing constipation, and crampy lower abdominal pain are often present, and sigmoid carcinoma is the most frequent consideration in differential diagnosis. Pneumaturia, recurrent urinary tract infection, passage of gas from the vagina, or a site of cutaneous fecal drainage suggest the possibility of fistulization from colonic diverticula to bladder, vagina, or skin. Hemorrhage from diverticula is characteristically sudden in onset, accompanied by crampy abdominal pain, and often of transfusion-requiring proportion. Spontaneous cessation of bleeding is the rule. Approximately one half of bleeding diverticula appear to be located in the ascending colon, whereas most diverticula are in the sigmoid region. Angiodysplasia may present in a similar fashion; carcinoma and inflammatory bowel disease are other possibilities.

MANAGEMENT

OUTPATIENT

Asymptomatic Diverticulosis. This is usually discovered when gastrointestinal studies reveal the characteristic outpouchings as an incidental finding. For each of these individuals, there are an estimated four to five patients with asymptomatic diverticula in the general population. Furthermore, only 25% of those with radiographically documented diverticula develop symptoms. It is quite clear, therefore, that an asymptomatic course is the "norm" for most people with diverticula. Whether they should be treated or not is controversial. At present there are no prospective controlled studies to indicate benefit, in terms of decreased further production of diverticula or reduction of symptoms, from any particular therapy.

On the basis of epidemiologic studies as well as motility patterns, arguments have been made for putting this group of patients on a high-fiber diet. However, this is frequently accompanied by an increase in stool frequency, decrease in stool consistency, and occasionally increased flatus and abdominal distention—thus producing a symptomatic patient from a previously asymptomatic one. Until properly conducted studies show otherwise, there is no need to treat patients who have asymptomatic diverticula. They should be reassured that their condition is common and in most cases normal for age. The potential complications of diverticular disease should be mentioned but with the emphasis that in most cases these will never materialize. Pamphlets explaining the features of this disorder are quite helpful as quick reference material for patients. The theoretical pros and cons of high-fiber therapy should be discussed, along with the fact that there is no evidence of particular dietary benefit, including avoidance of popcorn, nuts, seeds, and so forth. There is no need for regular follow-up apart from a general medical evaluation. Barium enemas need not be repeated provided patients remain symptom-free. Annual hemoccult tests and periodic sigmoidoscopy for colorectal cancer detection should be carried out as for the general population, and patients should be reassured that their diverticula are not accompanied by an increased risk of colonic cancer.

Abdominal Pain. Abdominal pain, with or without alteration of bowel habit, is the most common symptom associated with colonic diverticulosis. The major issue facing the clinician is whether the pain is (1) referable to the colon and (2) if so, due to a "functional" abnormality, an inflammatory complication of diverticular disease, or an unrelated process (e.g., colonic carcinoma, Crohn's colitis). The abdominal pain occurring in association with diverticulosis appears to be indistinguishable from that found in IBS. "Spastic" colon and "spastic" diverticulosis, therefore, differ only by the finding of diverticula with the latter. The pain associated with spastic diverticulosis is intermittent, usually lower abdominal (frequently LLQ) in location, lasting minutes to a few hours, and often related to meals—occurring 30 to 60 minutes postprandially (perhaps the "gastro-colic reflex"). The pain is usually crampy in nature, not related to body position and usually bears some relationship to bowel movements or flatus (e.g., relief with flatus; worse before, with relief after bowel movement; accompanied by constipation). Abdominal exam (plus pelvic exam in females) may reveal tenderness with deep palpation, and occasionally a palpable, slightly tender but mobile LLQ mass corresponding to the sigmoid colon. A proctosigmoidoscopy (preferably flexible) should be performed to address the issue of a mucosal inflammatory or neoplastic process. A complete blood count should be done to determine the presence or absence of anemia or leukocytosis. A barium enema should be performed on an outpatient basis unless a satisfactory colonic contrast study or colonoscopy has been done within the previous three years, to exclude the possibility of inflammatory or neoplastic disease proximal to (flexible) sigmoidoscopic investigation. (Despite introduction of the full operating length of a sigmoidoscope, colonic mucosa proximal to midsigmoid colon may not be reached.)

Treatment of these patients is similar to that advocated for IBS. Symptoms are thought to be related to high-amplitude colonic contractions and not the diverticula per se. Anticholinergics, sedatives (especially benzodiazepines), and analgesics have their various advocates. None have been shown to be efficacious in terms of significant pain relief over the long term. Heat applied to the abdomen during the most severe episode may be helpful. High-fiber diets have been touted in view of the demonstration of lower intraluminal colonic pressures during administration. Unfortunately, there is no consensus regarding benefit in terms of reduced frequency, duration, or severity of pain when this type of diet is given. Constipation seems to improve, however. Current recommended treatment, therefore, is highly individualized and largely empiric. Patients with *diverticula and abdominal pain but without constipation* are prescribed an inexpensive (usually generic) anticholinergic, e.g., dicyclomine HCl, 10 to 20 mg t.i.d. before meals. It is frequently helpful to administer the drug in terms of the pattern of discomfort (i.e., if pain occurs only in the morning, one dose before breakfast may suffice; if it occurs throughout the day and into the evening, q.i.d. administration may be necessary). Doses are pushed to a satisfactory therapeutic effect or toxicity (usually dry mouth, visual blurring). Patients with *constipation and abdominal pain* are treated with high-fiber diets: bran initially, then supplements such as Metamucil, 1 tbsp b.i.d. If constipation persists, it is frequently helpful to add a stool softener: mineral oil, 1 tbsp b.i.d., is inexpensive and effective, and may be increased to 4 to 6 tbsp daily as needed. There is no "toxicity" but it should be avoided in patients with neurologic defects involving swallowing, in view of the danger of aspiration. Capsules may be substituted, e.g., Colace, Kasof, or Surfac, but are more expensive. Fiber supplements may similarly be increased without "toxicity" until a successful bowel habit is achieved using this individualized fiber-plus–stool softener regimen. If constipation is relieved by this approach but pain persists, anticholinergic therapy is begun at a low dose, e.g., dicyclomine HCl, 10 mg every morning, and increased to either effect or toxicity as previously described. In theory, calcium-channel blocking agents (verapamil, nifedipine) may be effective in disorders accompanied by increased smooth muscle contraction. There have been no reported trials of these agents in symptomatic diverticular disease, however.

Diarrhea. Diarrhea is less likely than constipation or abdominal pain in diverticulosis, but it does occur. Again, treatment is similar to that for patients with IBS who have this symptom. Anticholinergics are administered initially, especially if abdominal pain is present. Dosage, frequency, timing, and increments in treatment are the same as described for management of abdominal pain. Fiber supplementation may be tried, but patients must be advised to ignore the "laxative" label these products carry and recognize that these fibers absorb water. Loperamide may be given, 2 to 4 mg one or two times daily, if anticholinergics are ineffective or produce toxicity.

Follow-up is frequent during the initial phase of treatment, until such time as an effective therapy or combination of therapies is found. Two-week to one-month intervals are appropriate to assess these initial modifications. Thereafter, there should be annual general medical evaluation, including hemoccult testing and proctosigmoidoscopy. Patients should be reassured that some abdominal pain is to be expected and that intensified drug or dietary treatment may have adverse effects (and also be expensive). They should be advised that one formed bowel movement daily is not a sign of health per se.

Diverticulitis. A minority of patients with colonic diverticula develop the probably overdiagnosed syndrome known as diverticulitis. Abdominal pain is the most common initial symptom and is more constant and localized than that seen without colonic microperforation. Constipation, diarrhea, or no change in bowel habit may be noted. Fever may occur, especially with a more extensive suppurative process. Physical exam may demonstrate abdominal distention; absent bowel sounds with adynamic ileus; and a tender, immobile LLQ midline or rarely RLQ mass, or may reveal only slight tenderness with vigorous LLQ palpation. Rectal exam may show tenderness, with or without a rectosigmoid mass, or may be entirely negative. Hematochezia or hemoccult-positive stools are unusual and should raise the possibility of mucosal disease, especially carcinoma. Provided there are no signs of generalized peritonitis suggesting free perforation, abscess (palpable mass with localized peritoneal signs), or obstruction, the disorder may be managed on an outpatient basis. A CBC with differential WBC count often shows leukocytosis and/or a left shift. Microcytic anemia should alert the clinician to the possibility of neoplastic or chronic inflammatory bowel disease, whereas an entirely normal WBC count and differential argue for the absence of true diverticulitis. Erect and supine plain films of the abdomen should be obtained if abdominal distention, vomiting, or a large tympanitic mass is present, to exclude findings of obstruction or volvulus. Proctosigmoidoscopy should be performed, but the timing of this study is highly individualized. For patients with hematochezia or hemoccult-positive stools and signs of diverticulitis but in whom outpatient management is feasible, a cautious exam using no or minimal air insufflation is carried out; the primary concern is to exclude sigmoid carcinoma.

Mucosal findings are minimal on sigmoidoscopic exam in patients with diverticulitis, because the inflammatory process is predominantly extracolonic, related to microperforation. Diffuse or patchy mucosal erythema, submucosal hemorrhage, and mucopus may be noted. Pain and luminal narrowing are frequently present in the area of active disease, the latter more commonly due to smooth muscle hypertrophy or contraction than to extraluminal mass effects. Diverticula are usually seen but the precise site of perforation is practically never apparent, owing to narrowing or obstruction of the ostium by edema or fecalith. The examination should be terminated if severe pain or difficulty in passage are encountered; a repeat exam after resolution of the inflammatory process is preferable to iatrogenic exacerbation of the disease by insistence upon full insertion of the sigmoidoscope. In patients with a hemoccult-negative rectal exam, proctosigmoidoscopy may be deferred until signs of inflammation have abated.

Treatment of the outpatient should include a liquid or low-residue diet, this being an historical and empiric recommendation more than a scientific one. There is no evidence that physical activity need be proscribed. Physical measures (e.g., heat) may be helpful for pain relief, and mild analgesia (e.g., aspirin, acetaminophen [Tylenol], pentazocine, or propoxyphene) should be permitted. Narcotic analgesics have traditionally been avoided beause of their tendency to produce constipation. Antibiotics have not been shown to provide unequivocal benefit to these patients, but agents usually prescribed are ampicillin, 500 mg. q.i.d.; tetracycline HCl, 500 mg q.i.d.; trimethoprim-sulfamethoxazole, 1 tablet b.i.d.; or metronidazole, 250 mg t.i.d. In general, however, the least expensive single-antibiotic regimen should be given, there being no evidence that multiple drug therapies designed to cover the colonic microflora are superior. Most (70% to 90%) of patients may be expected to improve clinically in two to three days with this approach. A regular diet is then allowed. Antibiotics are continued for a total of seven to ten days. Patients should be followed closely during the period of treatment and cautioned to contact the physician promptly should vomiting or signs of toxicity (high fever, confusion) supervene. Reexamination in three to five days should reveal lessening of abdominal tenderness and no signs of an abscess (enlarging, tender abdominal mass on abdominal or rectal exam). Provided this is the case, treatment can be continued on an outpatient basis; otherwise, admission should be arranged. A second follow-up is appropriate two weeks from the time of initial evaluation. Signs of active inflammation should be absent, and sigmoidoscopy, if not previously done or unsatisfactorily performed, should be undertaken. At this time, mucosal erythema, submucosal hemorrhage, narrowing, and spasm may persist, but marked tenderness is generally absent. A barium enema (full-column) should be scheduled to exclude pathology proximal to the sigmoidoscopic end point, for reasons previously mentioned. Frequently, this can be done the same day as the two-week evaluation but after sigmoidoscopy. The fluoroscopist should be alerted to the recently treated diverticulitis so that colonic overdistention is avoided.

One half to three fourths of patients treated for diverticulitis have no further attacks. Treatment and follow-up should revert to that previously described for asymptomatic or symptomatic diverticular disease. Recurrences when remote (i.e., months to years) should be managed in a similar fashion. Early recurrence (i.e., in a few weeks) should prompt careful evaluation for an abscess or obstruction. If results are negative, outpatient management is again followed. A third episode (second early recurrence) prompts hospitalization and surgical consultation.

Obstruction. Obstruction may occasionally present in a gradual manner in patients with recurrent diverticulitis. The slow progression of obstructive symptoms noted in these patients is presumably due to scarring, nearly always in the sigmoid region, with progressive luminal narrowing. Abdominal pain, crampy in nature, with abdominal distention and relief by bowel movement or flatus, is the usual symptom. When seen as outpatients, these individuals may have a palpable, stool-filled sigmoid or transverse colon. The primary concern is sigmoid carcinoma, and flexible sigmoidoscopy as well as barium enema are mandatory. If sigmoid narrowing but normal mucosa and diverticula are found, a resolved inflammatory etiology is likely. If diverticula are absent and pelvic exam, barium enema, or sigmoidoscopy suggest extrinsic sigmoid compression, CT scan or ultrasonography study should be carried out. Individuals may be managed on an outpatient basis if the above studies are negative and incomplete obstruction is found. A low-residue diet supplemented by stool softeners (e.g., mineral oil, 1 tbsp b.i.d.) should be tried. Anticholinergic or other agents tending to cause constipation should be stopped. If symptoms persist despite these measures, surgical resection is indicated.

Fistulas. Fistulas may form between the colon and urinary bladder, vagina, small intestine, or adjacent segment of large intestine, or may communicate to the skin. Pneumaturia and recurrent urinary tract infection strongly suggest a vesicocolic fistula and should prompt sigmoidoscopic and barium enema studies. Sigmoidoscopy does not usually help to visualize the site of communication per se; cystoscopy is more likely to demonstrate the site. Barium enema frequently reveals the site of a tract; IV pylography is usually unrewarding. These patients are not usually particularly symptomatic aside from symptoms of persistent urinary tract or vaginal infection. Symptoms of colonic obstruction may be present, with narrowing at or just distal to the site of fistulization. Crohn's colitis should be considered in these patients, as well as actinomycosis. Outpatient management is restricted to short-term treatment of urinary tract or vaginal infection based on appropriate cultures, and low-residue diet plus stool softeners if a colonic stricture is found. Elective admission for surgical correction should be arranged.

INPATIENT

Diverticulitis. Diverticulitis with signs of toxicity, abscess, obstruction, or free perforation necessitates prompt hospitalization. Those initially treated as outpatients in whom the above signs develop during treatment should also be admitted for more intensive evaluation and treatment. NPO and IV fluids are the rule. Nasogastric suction is begun if vomiting and ileus are present. Because macroperforation and abscess are more likely in these ill patients, two- or even three-drug antibiotic administration is advisable. Ampicillin-clindamycin, cefazolin-gentamicin, ampicillin-clindamycin-gentamicin, and IV metronidazole are some of the regimens currently used at our institution for these cases. Glucagon, 1 mg IV, may be useful for relief of abdominal pain to the extent that spasm plays a role. Anticholinergics should be avoided; parenteral meperidine may be needed for pain relief. Plain-film of the abdomen should be obtained and followed serially if findings suggest obstruction. Surgical consultation should be obtained if any evidence of obstruction or free perforation appears. The timing of proctosigmoidoscopy and barium enema is similar to that for outpatients, and these should generally be performed before discharge. If an abdominal mass suggesting an abscess is present, CT scan or ultrasound should be ordered and surgical consultation obtained if suspicions are confirmed. Most hospitalized patients (70% to 85%) respond to medical treatment; surgery is required in the remainder for abscess, obstruction, perforation, or fistula. Assuming a satisfactory medical course, hospitalization is usually for five to ten days, with follow-up as for outpatients.

Bleeding. Hemorrhage from juxtadiverticular vessels is probably the first or second most common cause of hemodynamically significant (transfusion-requiring) colonic hemorrhage (angiodysplasia of the colon is equally common). The usual case presents with sudden onset of passage of gross blood, accompanied by crampy abdominal discomfort. Physical exam may reveal tachycardia and hypotension (orthostatic or supine), but abdominal findings are usually unremarkable. Rectal exam should be performed, but usually reveals only gross blood. Arrangements for hospitalization should be prompt. A nasogastric tube is placed and aspirated material checked for freedom from gross blood and clots; if blood is found, emergency upper endoscopy should be performed. Large-bore central lines should be placed and isotonic crystalloid solutions administered. Blood needs to be typed, crossed, and transfused if there is orthostatic or supine hypotension or a stat HgB/Hct less than 10 gm/30%. Emergency proctosigmoidoscopy should be carried out, but usually reveals only blood and clots in the lumen. If hemodynamic instability is present, emergency arteriography is done with selective injection of superior and inferior mesenteric vessels. If the patient is hemodynamically stable, a technetium sulfur colloid scan may be done if bright red blood continues from the rectum. An in vitro labeled RBC scan should be done if the sulfur colloid scan is negative or if the bleeding is not thought to be currently active. The patient is kept NPO. If arteriography shows a site of intraluminal extravasation, vasopression infusion, embolization, or surgical resection should be carried out. If scans are positive and the patient becomes unstable hemodynamically, selective arteriography should be done and arteriographic control or surgery planned. If scans are positive but the patient remains stable, colonoscopy should be performed to determine the nature of the bleeding site. It is rare to see active extravasation from diverticula endoscopically, but colonic carcinoma, arteriovenous malformation, or inflammatory bowel disease may be recognized. A positive scan in a site of diverticula without bleeding at the time of endoscopy is strong indirect evidence of spontaneously remitting diverticular bleeding. If arteriography and scans are negative, colonoscopy should be carried out before discharge. If no diverticula and no other abnormalities are found at colonoscopy, a barium enema (air contrast) is advisable to exclude a mucosal lesion missed at endoscopy.

Recurrent bleeding should be approached in an identical fashion. If scans are again positive in an area of demonstrated diverticular formation, a strong case is made for corresponding surgical resection. Segmental resection is advisable when a definite bleeding site is identified; however, patients with recurrent bleeding and diverticula plus angiodysplasia may require total colectomy with ileoproctoscopy for control.

REFERENCES

Almy TP, Howell DA: Diverticular disease of the colon. N Engl J Med 302:324–331, 1980.

Almy TP, Naitove A: Diverticular disease of the colon. *In* Sleisenger MH, Fordtran JS (eds): Gastrointestinal Disease: Pathophysiology, Diagnosis, Management, 3rd ed. W. B. Saunders Co, Philadelphia, 1983, pp 896–912.

Eastwood MA, Smith AN, Brydon WG, et al: Colonic function in patients with diverticular disease. Lancet 1:1181–1182, 1978.

Lehman GA, Buchner DM, Lappas JC: Anatomical extent of fiberoptic sigmoidoscopy. Gastroenterology 84:803–808, 1983.

Painter NS, Truelove SC, Ardran GM, et al: Segmentation and the localization of intraluminal pressures in the human colon, with special reference to the pathogenesis of colonic diverticula. Gastroenterology 49:169–177, 1965.

10 · HEPATITIS

Douglas B. McGill
Jorge Rakela
MAYO CLINIC AND MAYO FOUNDATION

An extraordinary number and variety of agents including viruses, bacteria, drugs, chemicals, and radiation can cause inflammatory disease of the liver. Often the precise factors are not known, as, for example, in the hepatitis observed after jejunoileal bypass surgery. It is convenient to consider acute and chronic hepatitis separately. Inevitably, the distinction is sometimes arbitrary, and what is thought to be acute hepatitis may simply be an acute flare-up of an underlying, long-established chronic condition.

Acute Hepatitis

DEFINITION AND DIAGNOSTIC CRITERIA

The World Health Organization has settled on the definition of acute hepatitis as a condition in which inflammatory disease of the liver has been present for less than six months in an individual not known to have had liver disease before.

PATHOPHYSIOLOGY

Necrosis of liver cells and varying degrees of inflammation are the central histopathologic features of the disease. There is associated mesenchymal response, with Kupffer cell and fibroblastic proliferation, resulting in new collagen, more or less plasma membrane injury with "leakage" of intracellular enzymes, and reparative efforts by parenchymal cells characterized as "regeneration." The nature of the attack may be cytolytic by direct action of the offending agent, or immunologic. It may be (1) vascular, in which case ischemia produces more necrosis than inflammation; or (2) biochemical, related to metal overload, as in the copper and iron storage disorders, Wilson's disease and hemochromatosis, respectively.

ETIOLOGIC AGENTS

A number of exotic viruses are known to affect the liver, such as Marburg, Ebola, and Lassa fever viruses. The more ordinary agents (A; B; non-A, non-B; Epstein-Barr; cytomegalic; herpes simplex; coxsackie; toxoplasmosis; and yellow fever) do exhibit somewhat different patterns of injury and response. There is much overlap, however. Toxins well known to damage the liver include phosphorus, carbon tetrachloride, methylenedianiline, *Amanita phalloides*, toluene, and trichlorobenzene. Perhaps the most common cause of hepatotoxicity in our overmedicated society is that owing to drugs. Isoniazid is the prototype for hepatitis, while chlorpromazine and erythromycin estolate are classic cholestatic agents. Other well-known hepatitis-producing drugs are halothane, methotrexate, and phenytoin. Usually the picture is mixed, with both hepatitic and cholestatic features. Ethanol, the most abused drug, is a special case by virtue of its potential for harm and widespread use.

CLINICAL ASPECTS

Clinical features of hepatitis range all the way from mild, clinically inapparent disease to fatal, or so-called fulminant, hepatitis. The disease is usually anicteric. There may be no symptoms, the evidence of liver cell injury being reflected in abnormal aminotransferases on routine screening. Symptoms, when present, are usually nonspecific and "flu-like": malaise, anorexia, nausea, vomiting, fatigue, arthralgias, weakness, and headache in various proportions. The differential diagnosis of acute hepatitis should include acute cholecystitis, malignant disease whether primary or secondary, right heart failure, right lower lobe pneumonia, and Wilson's disease. The course may be protracted or brief, depending on the agent, the dose, and discontinuance of the offending agent.

MANAGEMENT

PLAN

The goal of management should be to identify and neutralize or remove the etiologic agent, and to support the patient and the liver until regeneration has occurred.

A more subtle and difficult goal is that of preventing chronic disease and cirrhosis. In most instances hospitalization is unnecessary even when viral disease, presumptive or proved, is established. The indication for hospitalization should be that the patient requires the type of nursing care that cannot be provided at home. Often during the early course of the hepatitis it is impossible to predict whether a patient will deteriorate significantly before recovery. He or she can be monitored at home and hospitalized if complications develop. The most dreaded of the earliest complications is encephalopathy, manifested initially by transient confusion, unusual sleepiness, and slurred speech. This is an unfavorable prognostic sign and should prompt immediate hospitalization for the kind of supportive care that will likely be necessary.

NONPHARMACOLOGIC MEASURES

Nonpharmacologic measures, in the absence of specific therapy, are the only course. Bed rest was so strongly endorsed to another generation that absolute recumbency, to favor liver blood flow, was mandatory. There were never experimental data to support such an approach, and ample clinical evidence has accumulated to indicate that bed rest has no special virtues. Many patients feel so ill that anything else is unthinkable. When patients feel well enough, they should be encouraged to be up and about. Reassurance as to the transient nature of debilitating symptoms is important, bearing in mind that depression is often a feature of prolonged hepatitis. The dietary prescription is simple. Patients should be encouraged to eat, since they generally do better with nutrients. There is no rationale for a low-fat diet, with its attendant requirement for a high carbohydrate intake, and physicians should stop torturing patients by making them drink large volumes of unpleasant-tasting sweet liquids. Patients should be encouraged to eat whatever they feel like, and no more. Failure to eat or drink is an indication for hospital admission so that intravenous fluids and glucose may be given. Obviously, complications such as infection and hemorrhage should be promptly treated.

DRUG THERAPY

Unfortunately, there is no specific treatment for any form of hepatitis. Corticosteroids are to be avoided in patients with acute viral hepatitis since controlled studies have demonstrated that they do not help. In principle, steroids may do harm by encouraging viral replication. (+)-Cyanidanol-3, a putative free radical scavenger, offered modest promise for acute viral hepatitis, but trials have been disappointing. A number of antiviral agents are undergoing tests in the United States and abroad, including ribavirin, interferon, adenine arabinoside, and acyclovir. Some have been shown to have modest success in reducing viral markers but little clinical benefit, and their use at present is still highly experimental. Antiemetics and sedatives may help, bearing in mind that the sick liver metabolizes drugs slowly and inefficiently, so that undermedication is generally preferred. Alcohol should be proscribed in the course of acute hepatitis, although there are no hard data to support this recommendation; it simply makes sense when faced with a known hepatotoxin to avoid

administration of a second. If the cause of the hepatitis is a jejunoileal bypass, it should be taken down.

PERIODIC EVALUATION

While at home early in the course of acute viral hepatitis, patients should keep in frequent touch with the physician. When feeling better, as often happens with the appearance of jaundice, they should be encouraged to stay away from work until visible icterus has largely cleared. After clinical improvement, there is little reason for blood testing more often than every two weeks or so. Return of serum bilirubin and liver enzymes to normal or near-normal should be documented. Aminotransferases (ALT or GPT and AST or GOT) are exceedingly high during the first few days of acute hepatitis, owing to viral infection; they may be equally high after toxic exposure. The AST is usually less than 300 IU in patients with acute alcoholic hepatitis, and the ALT is usually less than 50% of the AST. After viral hepatitis, aminotransferases may remain modestly elevated in the ½ to two times' normal range for up to a year, so-called benign transaminitis. Fluctuations are most common after non-A, non-B disease. It is reasonable to document this, but return to work or school should not be delayed while waiting for complete normalization of enzyme profiles. Cirrhosis, i.e., fibrosis with architectural distortion, may develop under cover of normal or near-normal biochemistries, but there is no known way to prevent this. In most instances of acute hepatitis, liver biopsy is not necessary for diagnosis, determination of prognosis, or documentation of return to normal.

PREVENTIVE MEASURES

It is important to know how the patient contracted hepatitis. Obviously, alcoholism should be treated, and other drug use examined, and job changed if chemical toxins were responsible. If viral infection is proved or suspected, later infection with another virus is possible, so hygienic circumstances should be improved.

Family counseling is vital in respect to prophylaxis against viral infection. The recommendations of the Public Health Department are reasonable and should be followed.

Type A Hepatitis. When type A hepatitis has been diagnosed, immune serum globulin (ISG) is recommended for contacts in private households (both permanent and temporary household members) and in large institutions such as prisons or institutions for the mentally retarded. ISG is not necessary for casual contacts of a single case in schools, offices, factories, or hospitals, and is no longer recommended in outbreaks of hepatitis spread by a common vehicle (water, food, sewage, etc.). Experience has demonstrated that a dose of 0.02 ml/kg (1 to 2 ml) given as soon as possible provides effective protection in most circumstances. It should not be given more than two weeks after exposure. There is considerably more emotion than reason regarding gamma-globulin prophylaxis. As long as supplies are adequate, there is no compelling reason to restrict its use among very concerned and worried contacts who cannot be otherwise reassured.

Non-A, Non-B Hepatitis. There are no data available to govern the use of commercially available ISG in patients having contact with persons suspected of having non-A, non-B hepatitis. Several authors consider that immunoprophylaxis should be provided for sexual contacts of those with acute disease, accidental needle-stick exposures, and neonates of mothers with acute or chronic non-A, non-B hepatitis. The exposed person may receive gamma-globulin, 0.06 ml/kg IM in one dose.

Type B Hepatitis. Treatment to prevent hepatitis B infection after exposure to hepatitis B virus should be considered in the same three situations mentioned in the case of non-A, non-B disease. The primary goal of postexposure prophylaxis for exposed infants is prevention of the B virus carrier state. The baby should receive 0.5 ml of hepatitis B immune globulin (HBIG) IM within 12 hours of birth, and 0.5 ml (10 μg) of hepatitis B vaccine IM at the same time in a different site. The vaccine should be repeated at one month and six months, 10 μg each time. Because the efficacy of this regimen depends on administering HBIG as soon as possible on the day of birth, hepatitis B surface antigen–positive mothers must be identified before delivery. Testing for HBsAg and anti-HBs is recommended at 12 to 15 months to monitor the final success or failure of therapy. A child who is HBsAg-positive is likely to be a chronic carrier. On the other hand, if anti-HBs is demonstrated, protection has been achieved. After exposure to blood containing HBsAg, via needle or bite, a single dose of HBIG should be given as soon as possible, 0.06 ml/kg, or 5 ml for adults. If the individual chooses not to receive Heptavax-B, the dose should be repeated at one month. Ideally, Heptavax-B, 1 ml or 20 μg IM, should be given as soon as possible, with a second and third dose at one and six months, respectively. The same general approach should be offered to patients who have had sexual contact within the previous week or two with HBsAg-positive persons.

SOCIOECONOMIC ASPECTS OF MANAGEMENT

A major problem in our society is the manner in which we respond individually and collectively to the modern leper, i.e., the HBsAg carrier. People who are obviously suffering from hepatitis, but not identified as virus shedders, experience the same societal disapproval, albeit relatively transiently. Extensive discussions, reassurance, support, and sometimes legal guidance are necessary for the chronic HBsAg carrier. This is particularly true if the carrier is HBeAg-positive, implying a greater degree of infectivity or "infectiousness." A carrier state is recognized for non-A, non-B disease, which may turn out to be as prevalent, or indeed more prevalent, than B carriage. The social problems engendered will be very great.

Chronic Hepatitis

DEFINITION AND DIAGNOSTIC CRITERIA

Patients with chronic hepatitis have signs, symptoms, or histologic evidence of liver disease for more than six months. Despite the variety of names that suggest precise identification as disease entities, there is often meager scientific foundation for classification. This is a particularly severe problem when the etiology is not known, as is often the case with chronic liver disease. In the final analysis, chronic hepatitis is a biopsy diagnosis, and histology may only hint at the cause. Some diseases are relatively discrete, such as the syndrome of primary biliary cirrhosis (PBC) with its hepatitic component, or alpha₁-antitrypsin deficiency with its hepatitis. Most chronic hepatitis evolves toward cirrhosis, a stage that may be masked by biopsy sampling error. In the last decade it has become conventional to divide chronic hepatitis not otherwise categorized into two broad groups: chronic active and chronic persistent hepatitis. These may simply be at opposite ends of a severity spectrum, and no etiologic implications are intended by these terms. Either histologic disorder may be due to virus, drug, or "autoimmune" factors.

PATHOPHYSIOLOGY

The necroinflammatory change implied by the term chronic hepatitis may lead ultimately to liver failure. The associated collagen synthesis, which with zones of collapse produces distortion of hepatic architecture, results in portal hypertension with its untoward physiologic consequences, particularly ascites and bleeding esophageal varices. Cirrhosis implies that the lesion for practical purposes is irreversible, and further suggests the potential for malignant degeneration, an event that may be very common if the cause is hepatitis B, or unusual in PBC. Alternatively, the process may be mild and static for years.

CLINICAL ASPECTS

Patients with chronic hepatitis may have no symptoms even in later stages, or may present with acute fulminant disease as the final episode in a long history of a variably symptomatic chronic illness. Physical findings and laboratory tests generally mirror the severity of the necroinflammatory change.

MANAGEMENT

PLAN

The short-term goals are first to identify, if possible, an etiologic factor such as is present in Wilson's disease or hemochromatosis. The second goal should be to reverse the process if it has not already progressed to cirrhosis, bearing in mind that evidence is accumulating to indicate that one may suppress inflammation without halting the steady progress toward cirrhosis. The longer-term goal in patients with well-established disease is to correct and modify all factors that may contribute to worsening liver health, such as infection, bleeding, anemia, malnutrition, and electrolyte depletion.

NONPHARMACOLOGIC MEASURES

The required diet will be indicated by the presence or absence of complications such as ascites, edema, or encephalopathy. Adequate nutrition must be maintained with a diet that is calorically sufficient and provides protein of high biologic value, to about 1 gm/kg/day. Protein restriction may be necessary to treat encephalopathy, and sodium restriction may be important. Other dietary manipulations are not necessary. Patients should be encouraged to rest periodically throughout the day to the extent necessary to treat or avoid fatigue; if they feel well, there is no need for rest. Obviously, patients with hemochromatosis require phlebotomy, and other rare conditions need treatment as appropriate.

DRUG THERAPY

All patients with chronic hepatitis should be considered candidates for prednisone therapy, but the decision whether to treat is often difficult. Patients whose disease is due to the hepatitis B virus should not receive prednisone unless they are very ill, since possible harm exceeds possible benefit. They can respond to corticosteroids, but in higher doses than usually required, and they relapse sooner when treatment is discontinued. This is true, also, for patients with non-B disease who have established cirrhosis at the time they are first treated. There is no doubt that individuals with severe chronic active hepatitis, as manifested by aminotransferase levels of tenfold or greater, who have signs and symptoms of progressive and severe liver disease, respond to corticosteroid therapy and have a high mortality rate if not treated. It is less clear that patients with modest disease should be treated, since they do not face the same mortality risk and do experience complications of corticosteroids. The decision should be based on clinical symptoms, laboratory tests (chiefly serum bilirubin, aminotransferase, and protein levels), and assessment of liver histology by an experienced liver pathologist. Any one indicator is probably insufficient justification to begin treatment. With treatment, remission can be expected in approximately 80% of patients, and the drug should be continued for at least 12 months. At a maintenance dose of 20 mg of prednisone daily for one year, serious complications are relatively few. Equal results can be achieved with a lower dose of prednisone (e.g., 10 mg a day) and 50 mg of azathioprine daily. Careful monitoring for bone marrow toxicity is essential. Patients who do not respond may develop all the complications of severe liver disease, including edema, ascites, jaundice, encephalopathy, GI bleeding, and sepsis. Such patients are usually cared for in the hospital, but often recover sufficiently to allow outpatient follow-up and management.

PATIENT INFORMATION AND EDUCATION

As with all serious chronic diseases, patients do best if they are fully aware of the reasons for various therapies and know what to expect from them.

PERIODIC EVALUATION

It often happens that patients are subjected to frequent laboratory follow-up, less because there is important therapy depending on the results than because neither physician nor patient knows exactly what else to do. Once the pattern of illness is understood and treatment begun, biochemical monitoring at more than three- to six-month intervals is unnecessary, as long as the patient feels well. One may wonder about the presence of esophageal varices, but in the absence of bleeding, endoscopy for documentation is not required. It is difficult to steer an intermediate course between reasonable solicitousness and the appearance of abandonment.

PATIENT COMPLIANCE

This is not usually a problem in patients with severe chronic hepatitis. If the disease is mild, no therapy is available or necessary; if it is severe, patients are likely to follow whatever program is prescribed.

PREVENTIVE MEASURES

Close contacts of patients found to be ill with chronic hepatitis type B should be treated as for acute hepatitis. Counseling about alcoholism is essential, if that is the problem. Family members should be screened for Wilson's disease or hemochromatosis as appropriate.

REFERENCES

Alter HJ: Hepatitis B. Semin Liver Dis 1:1–87, 1981.
Czaja AJ: Diagnosis and treatment of chronic hepatitis. Comp Ther 10:58–63, 1984.
Schiff L: Diseases of the Liver, 5th ed. J. B. Lippincott Co, Philadelphia, 1982.
Seeff LB, Koff RS: Passive and active immunoprophylaxis of hepatitis B. Gastroenterology 86:958–981, 1984.
Zakim D, Boyer TD: A Textbook of Liver Disease. W. B. Saunders Co, Philadelphia, 1982.
Zuckerman AJ: Infectious agents as causes of liver disease. Semin Liver Dis 4:277–374, 1984.

11 · CIRRHOSIS OF THE LIVER

Luis A. Balart
OCHSNER CLINIC AND ALTON OCHSNER MEDICAL FOUNDATION

DEFINITION AND DIAGNOSTIC CRITERIA

Hardening and shrinkage of the liver were recognized by the Greeks and Romans long before more detailed descriptions of cirrhosis began to appear. Laennec's role in the evolution of our present knowledge was cemented by his brilliant suggestion that scarring in the cirrhotic liver developed because of the deposition of new connective tissue. This observation led to our currently accepted criteria for the definition of cirrhosis, which includes three main principles: (1) hepatic parenchymal necrosis leading to (2) deposition of connective tissue and (3) regeneration of liver cells in a nodular manner. Cirrhosis, then, can be simply defined as an alteration of the original architecture of the liver by regenerating nodules surrounded by fibrous septae, which disturbs both the gross and histologic appearances of the organ. The diagnosis of cirrhosis is a histologic one based on accepted morphologic criteria. One must guard against the common temptation of making the diagnosis on purely clinical grounds in other

Table 1. ETIOLOGIC CLASSIFICATION OF CIRRHOSIS

Alcoholic cirrhosis
Cirrhosis due to infectious processes
  Chronic viral hepatitis: type B; non-A, non-B
  Congenital syphilis
  Parasitic infections: schistosomiasis
Cirrhosis due to autoimmune processes
  Autoimmune or "lupoid" chronic active hepatitis
  Primary biliary cirrhosis
Cirrhosis due to nutritional disorders
  Jejunoileal bypass for obesity
Cirrhosis due to metabolic or genetic disorders
  Galactosemia
  Tyrosinosis
  Glycogen storage diseases
  $Alpha_1$-antitrypsin deficiency
  Wilson's disease
  Hemochromatosis
  Rendu-Osler-Weber syndrome
  Abetalipoproteinemia
Secondary biliary cirrhosis
Congestive cirrhosis
  Cardiac
  Venous outflow obstruction
Chemically induced cirrhosis
  Following predictable or unpredictable toxic injury

than the most advanced and obvious stages of the disease (see "Clinical Aspects").

Despite the commonly accepted belief that a morphologic classification, i.e., macronodular versus micronodular cirrhosis, can be used to shed light on the etiology, reality dictates the contrary and to the clinician this approach is usually of little help. I favor a classification based on etiology (Table 1). This serves two very important functions. First, it forces one to think about the multiplicity of entities causing cirrhosis, thus making likely a more accurate diagnosis. Second, it allows for more rational and intelligent management decisions once the correct diagnosis has been made.

PATHOPHYSIOLOGY

Because the liver has a large amount of blood flowing through it (25% of cardiac output) and has a central role in endogenous metabolism and metabolism of drugs, cirrhosis can cause alterations in almost every organ system in the body. Only the most important of these will be reviewed here.

CARDIOVASCULAR FUNCTION

Cardiovascular function in cirrhosis is characterized by increased cardiac output, increased blood volume, and decreased peripheral resistance. As the heart rate increases to match oxygen demand, a hyperdynamic state similar to that seen in sepsis results. The renal circulation is characterized by decreased cortical flow leading to reduced glomerular filtration rate and plasma flow, which in turn impairs tubular function. In most patients with cirrhosis, renal blood flow is not generally affected until ascites develops. In these patients, renal plasma flow decreases and can lead to renal failure. Hepatic hemodynamic changes reflect impaired portal venous perfusion, resulting in portal hypertension and reduced hepatic blood flow. Changes in the pulmonary vasculature are characterized by shrinking around the pulmonary capillaries or perfusion of poorly ventilated areas, leading to arterial hypoxemia.

HEMATOLOGIC ABNORMALITIES

Many hematologic abnormalities both in formed elements and in coagulation factors can be seen in cirrhosis. Megaloblastic anemia is common in alcoholics but bears no direct relationship to the presence or absence of cirrhosis. Hemolytic activity of one degree or another is almost always present in cirrhotics and is proportional to the size of the spleen. Other factors, including folate deficiency, protein malnutrition, and availability of iron, combine to make the anemia of cirrhosis truly a multifactorial problem. Leukopenia and thrombocytopenia can result from a direct toxic effect in alcoholics or as part of hypersplenism.

The most common coagulation defects include reduction of factor VII, factor V, prothrombin, and factor X. In contrast, the activity of factor VIII in plasma is usually normal or slightly increased. Even in the absence of disseminated intravascular coagulation (DIC), fibrinogen is usually decreased. Although rare in patients with cirrhosis, clinically severe DIC does, of course, lead to accelerated fibrinogen consumption. In most cases, some evidence of DIC is present without an increase in fibrin split products. In advanced cirrhosis, increases in plasminogen activator inhibitor lead to fibrinolysis and bleeding diathesis.

ALBUMIN SYNTHESIS

Albumin synthesis is reduced in approximately one third of cirrhotic patients; however, the albumin concentration itself is not proportional to the capacity of the liver to synthesize it. Although the relationship between synthesis of albumin and cirrhosis, particularly in patients with ascites, has not been well defined, it is known that removal of agents causing parenchymal damage (e.g., alcohol), as well as resumption of adequate nutrition, leads to an increase in the rate of albumin synthesis.

ENDOCRINE ABNORMALITIES

Endocrine abnormalities in cirrhosis are more marked in alcoholic cirrhosis. In men, both hypogonadism and feminization occur in a high proportion of patients. In women, severe gonadal failure with oligomenorrhea, loss of secondary sexual characteristics, and infertility can result from failure of the ovaries.

CLINICAL ASPECTS

Cirrhosis may remain asymptomatic for long periods; indeed, in some patients it may be first noted at autopsy. In the United States, unsuspected cirrhosis is found in approximately 20% of autopsies. The rate of asymptomatic cirrhosis is, of course, dependent on the skills, experience, and diligence of the clinician in searching for its presence. In general, clinical manifestations can be grouped into two categories: those associated with hepatic parenchymal failure, and those associated with portal hypertension, such as ascites and portosystemic shunting. However, since it is important to recognize subclinical liver disease, conditions that are suspicious for occult liver disease should be kept in mind. These include incidental physical findings such as spider angiomata, splenomegaly, gynecomastia, or pigmentation; nonhepatic manifestations of the disease in alcoholics; incidental abnormal liver tests, positive autoimmune markers, or positive hepatitis B serology; autoimmune diseases, inflammatory bowel disease, neurologic diseases, systemic infections, and endocrinopathies; and hereditary liver diseases such as hemochromatosis, Wilson's disease, and alpha$_1$-antitrypsin deficiency in relatives of patients.

Particular attention should be given to the signs and symptoms of the treatable forms of cirrhosis, which can often be subtle and therefore missed. In hemochromatosis, endocrinologic manifestations, such as testicular atrophy and gynecomastia are more common than in other forms of cirrhosis. Abdominal pain, pigmentation (slate gray or bronze), and the invariable presence of a large liver are other common findings. In Wilson's disease, clinical manifestations can often be primarily neuropsychiatric or hematologic (choreoathetosis, hemolysis). In autoimmune forms of chronic active hepatitis seen in young women, the initial presentation may include oligomenorrhea.

The final diagnosis of cirrhosis should be based on a thorough history and physical examination, tests of liver function and of necroinflammatory activity, and appropriate tests directed by the etiologic considerations and confirmed by biopsy material.

MANAGEMENT

Management of the cirrhotic patient necessarily takes a very different route in each individual according to the underlying disease entity. Thus, in a patient with hemochromatosis or Wilson's disease, where the underlying disorder is treatable early, appropriate management in most instances results in improvement or remission of disease, thus avoiding serious and tragic complications. In other instances, such as in cirrhosis due to chronic viral hepatitis or in primary biliary cirrhosis, management consists largely of prompt recognition of complications and their proper therapy. Unfortunately, most patients in this latter group die. A simple outline for a plan of management for any patient with suspected cirrhosis should include the following elements:

1. Accurate diagnosis, preferably with histologic confirmation.

2. Identification and removal of the offending agent or appropriate treatment of the underlying disorder.

3. Prompt recognition and treatment of complications.

In general, people with stable cirrhosis can be followed adequately in the outpatient clinic.

TREATABLE DISORDERS

Measures aimed at eliminating progression to cirrhosis are of paramount importance in idiopathic hemochromatosis, Wilson's disease (hepatolentricular degeneration), chronic active hepatitis of the autoimmune type, and alcoholic hepatitis.

WILSON'S DISEASE

Wilson's disease, the inherited disorder in which degeneration of the basal ganglia, corneal pigmentation (Kayser-Fleischer rings), and hematologic disorders are variably accompanied by cirrhosis, is due to a specific defect in copper mobilization and transport. This leads to accumulation of excess amounts of copper in the liver

and other organs. Treatment is directed at the removal of excess copper in patients as well as in affected asymptomatic relatives. Penicillamine is the treatment of choice, 250 mg three to four times a day, resulting in the excretion of large amounts of copper in the urine. Once copper stores become depleted, a maintenance dose should be continued. Side effects of penicillamine unfortunately are worrisome and include the nephrotic syndrome, leukopenia, and the lupus-like syndrome. Because this disease is hereditary, genetic counseling is of paramount importance.

ALCOHOLIC HEPATITIS

Because of the potentially reversible nature of alcoholic liver disease, it is important to make as accurate a diagnosis as possible. This may require histologic confirmation in some cases. Complete abstention from alcohol, by whatever means are most suitable for the individual patient, is imperative. In most instances, treatment in a special unit combining medical and psychologic aspects of therapy is necessary. Outpatient follow-up should take place often enough to ensure continued abstention.

MANAGEMENT OF COMPLICATIONS OF CIRRHOSIS

For the most part, complications in cirrhosis patients are life-threatening, demanding prompt recognition and, usually, hospitalization. The practitioner must be always aware of the dangerous consequences of even minor illnesses in cirrhotic patients.

Upper Gastrointestinal Hemorrhage

Upper gastrointestinal hemorrhage requires prompt localization of the source of bleeding via flexible endoscopy, as many cirrhotic patients may be bleeding from sites other than esophageal varices, making management drastically different. In an outpatient setting, it is not unusual to be confronted by an otherwise stable patient with melena, positive stools, or a falling hemoglobin. In this situation, one cannot simply assume that varices are responsible and neglect to look for alternative treatable bleeding sites, such as duodenal or gastric ulcers. If found, these lesions should be treated as in any patient, with H$_2$-blockers, until healed. We recommend that long-term prophylaxis be continued in an attempt to decrease the incidence of recurrence, especially in the case of duodenal ulcerations. This can be achieved by administering a nighttime dose of either cimetidine or ranitidine. Treatment of variceal hemorrhage is slightly more problematic since traditionally some type of portosystemic shunting procedure has been recommended for patients who are good surgical risks. This decision can often be difficult if patients are marginal candidates (Childs B category*) or if the site of bleeding cannot be unequivocally ascertained. In these patients, a waiting period can often improve surgical risks or result in a more accurate diagnosis if rebleeding should occur. The introduction of injection sclerotherapy has provided a safe, inexpensive, and effective treatment alternative for patients who are not suitable surgical candidates (Childs C category*). Scler-

---

*See Table 2, Section VI, Chapter 7.

otherapy can be carried out using available fiberoptic instruments and readily available sclerosing agents, usually with a minimal hospital stay or in an outpatient treatment unit. The goal of sclerotherapy is to cause sclerosis and fibrosis of esophageal varices and thus reduce the risk of rebleeding. Several randomized trials have shown the efficacy of this form of treatment in decreasing the risk of bleeding and reducing the need for transfusions.

Ascites

Central to the problem of ascites formation is the inability of the kidneys to excrete sodium, and its accumulation in the peritoneal cavity as a result of elevated portal pressures. Ascites forms in the cirrhotic patient in direct proportion to the amount of sodium retained. Investigation of ascites should be pursued vigorously until its etiology is ascertained, since it often has nonhepatic causes. Classification into transudative and exudative processes is very useful clinically, as this generally facilitates further evaluation. This can be accomplished with ease and confidence by measuring serum albumin and ascites albumin concentration and subtracting these two values. A difference of greater than 1 mg% implies a transudative process. Since transudates are most common and form when there is portal hypertension, this simplifies the diagnostic approach to the patient with ascites by avoiding exhaustive and time-consuming evaluations.

Therapeutic measures useful in the management of ascites are generally aimed at decreasing the oral intake of sodium and increasing its renal excretion. Bed rest and dietary sodium restriction (less than 2 gm per day) are effective in mobilizing ascites fluid and may be all that is required in some patients. Compliance can easily be checked by monitoring urinary sodium concentration and weight. Diuretic use becomes necessary in many patients but must always be closely monitored to avoid electrolyte imbalances and volume contraction.

Because mobilization of ascites fluid is limited to approximately 900 ml per day, losses of more than 1 kg of weight per day can be assumed to be occurring at the expense of circulating volume. Contraction of circulating volume may cause symptoms and clearly should be avoided. An exception to this rule is the patient with peripheral edema, in whom rapid and large losses can occur without compromising intravascular volume. Spironolactone is the diuretic of choice, 50 to 100 mg daily, a maximum of 300 to 400 mg at times being necessary. Diuresis usually occurs with a delay of 24 to 48 hours after commencing spironolactone. If there is no response, furosemide can be added with caution (20 mg once or twice a day).

Hyponatremia in the cirrhotic is a common finding that is usually well tolerated. Markedly low serum sodium or rapidly falling levels can be generally managed with fluid restriction; it is rarely necessary to administer hypertonic saline. Finally, in truly refractory ascites, a peritoneojugular (LeVeen) shunt may be the only viable therapeutic alternative. However, it must be stressed that only when all other avenues have been exhausted should this form of treatment be considered, as there are complications associated with its use.

Peritonitis

Spontaneous bacterial peritonitis (SBP) can at times complicate ascites and should be suspected clinically in a cirrhotic patient with unexplained fever or abdominal pain or tenderness, or in any patient who suddenly worsens. Its presence is suspected by the finding of ascites polymorphonuclear leukocyte counts greater than 300 per cu nm. Gram stain of the ascites fluid can be helpful if positive. The ultimate diagnosis rests on bacteriologic confirmation, *E. coli* being the most frequent organism found. Broad-spectrum coverage in suspected cases is indicated until the diagnosis can be confirmed. I prefer a combination of aminoglycoside and a synthetic penicillin, continued for ten days.

Encephalopathy

Hepatic encephalopathy is a clinical syndrome in which cerebral dysfunction occurs in a setting of advanced liver disease and, presumably, systemic shunting of portal blood. The suspected pathophysiologic basis of the cerebral dysfunction is the accumulation of toxic substances or false neurotransmitters (ammonia, octopamine). Of late, imbalances between branched-chain and aromatic amino acids have been described as an alternative explanation for the encephalopathy. Clinically, the syndrome can range from mild confusional states, reversal of the normal day/night sleep ratio, and postprandial somnolence to asterixis, flaccid paralysis, and coma. Precipitating factors should be diligently sought, including GI bleeding (at times occult), sedative or hypnotic use or abuse, infection, constipation, and electrolyte imbalances. The last-named are usually precipitated by diuretic use, where alkalosis and hypokalemia can frequently trigger encephalopathy. Elevated blood ammonia or abnormally high CSF glutamine levels are helpful in diagnosis. Of course, other causes of encephalopathy such as hypoglycemia, CNS trauma, or infection must always be ruled out by appropriate tests. This is especially important in the alcoholic patient in whom CNS trauma can be often missed.

Treatment of hepatic encephalopathy should first aim to identify and eliminate the precipitating problem. Oral administration of neomycin, 1 gm four times a day, or lactulose, 15 ml three times a day, has proved effective. Lactulose can be increased up to 150 ml daily if needed and can also be given as an enema. Side effects to look out for are diarrhea, hypovolemia, and electrolyte disturbances. Dietary protein restriction should be the mainstay of any treatment regimen for prevention of recurrent encephalopathy. Generally, 40 to 60 gm of protein per day is sufficient to maintain positive nitrogen balance and help prevent encephalopathy. Intravenous and orally administered amino acid mixtures, enriched with branched-chain amino acids, have not been widely used because of their general lack of improvement over established methods and their great expense. Use of these mixtures, however, becomes of value in providing adequate nutritional support to cirrhotic patients without precipitating encephalopathy.

12 · PANCREATITIS

Surinder K. Batra
HENRY FORD HOSPITAL

DEFINITION

Pancreatitis, the inflammatory disease of the pancreas, is classified for clinical purposes as (1) acute, (2) chronic, or (3) chronic with acute exacerbations. Acute pancreatitis may further be classified as (a) mild, (b) moderate, or (c) severe; mortality is less than 5% in the mild and may reach 75% in the severe variety. The diagnosis of chronic pancreatitis implies that there is some permanent impairment of the endocrine and/or exocrine function of the pancreas. The etiologic factors associated with acute pancreatitis are listed in Table 1.

PATHOPHYSIOLOGY

Regardless of the trigger mechanism by which pancreatic enzymes are activated within the substance of the pancreas, it results in a process of autodigestion and further tissue destruction.

Elastase, activated by the trypsin, breaks down collagen and is believed to be responsible for vascular damage, which implies high risk of hemorrhagic pancreatitis. Phospholipase A is also activated by trypsin or bile acids and causes marked pancreatic necrosis. Lipase activated by bile is responsible for fat necrosis in pancreatic and surrounding tissue during acute pancreatitis.

Acutely inflamed pancreas releases kallikrein-kinins (bradykinin and kallidin), which are responsible for vasodilatation, edema, and pain, thus promoting shock. Transient hyperglycemia results from insult to the islets of Langerhans and is associated with an increased level of glucagon and not a reduction of insulin. Calcium sequestration in areas of fat necrosis is responsible for the transient hypocalcemia observed in acute pancreatitis. Arterial hypoxia and adult respiratory distress syndromes may occur in severe pancreatitis owing to intrapulmonary right-to-left shunting and microthrombi, secondary to subclinical disseminated intravascular coagulation. Renal function impairment may result from hypovolemia, shock, or increased renal vascular resistance.

The association between alcohol abuse and pancreatitis is well established. Alcoholic pancreatitis is a disease of younger males aged 30 to 50 years. The mortality rate of alcoholic pancreatitis is 7%, and that of acute pancreatitis secondary to gallstones is 20%.

CLINICAL ASPECTS

There are no specific clinical features that readily distinguish pancreatitis from a variety of other diseases. However, epigastric or left upper quadrant pain of progressively increasing intensity is the most common feature. Other clinical manifestations of acute pancreatitis in decreasing order of frequency are epigastric pain,

Table 1. ETIOLOGIC FACTORS ASSOCIATED WITH ACUTE PANCREATITIS

Most Common*
Alcohol abuse
Cholelithiasis
Idiopathic

Less Common
Abdominal trauma
Penetrating peptic ulcer disease
Postoperative factors
Injection into pancreatic duct
Hyperlipidemia, types I, IV, or V
Hereditary factors
Hypercalcemia
Drugs: thiazides, sulfa drugs, rifampin, isoniazid, oral contraceptive agents, and steroids
Postrenal transplantation
Ductus divisum
Viral infections: mumps, HB_sAg, infectious mononucleosis
Scorpion bite: Tityus Trinitatis
Parasites: roundworm
Connective tissue diseases

*Responsible for about 90% of cases.

tachycardia, nausea and vomiting, fever, abdominal ileus, tenderness and guarding, hypotension and shock, jaundice, abdominal mass, pleural effusion, ascites, tetany, and skin lesions such as Grey Turner's or Cullen's sign.

The most prominent and common clinical manifestation of chronic pancreatitis is abdominal pain. Occasionally, there may be no symptoms until steatorrhea or diabetes mellitus appears.

LABORATORY DIAGNOSIS OF ACUTE PANCREATITIS

Serum Amylase. Almost all patients with acute pancreatitis have an elevated serum amylase level, but this may be missed if they are seen after 48 hours of onset. Hyperamylasemia in an appropriate clinical setting clinches the diagnosis. An elevated level of serum amylase may also be observed in other acute abdominal conditions, but levels usually do not exceed 500 IU.

Serum Lipase. Serum lipase levels usually rise early in the course of the pancreatitis and remain elevated for five to seven days after onset.

Amylase/Creatinine Clearance Ratio. Amylase and creatinine in serum and spot urine samples obtained at the same time are used to calculate the amylase/creatinine clearance ratio, expressed as a percentage and used to establish the diagnosis of acute pancreatitis. A level of up to 4 is normal, whereas a level above 6 is another indication of acute pancreatitis. Because of its low specificity, this test is of very limited value.

Isoamylase Fractionation of Amylase. Fractionation into pancreatic and salivary types is more sensitive and specific for the diagnosis of acute pancreatitis, but is time-consuming and expensive.

Serum Trypsin–Like Immunoreactivity. This is one of the newer tests for the diagnosis of pancreatitis. Immunoreactivity is elevated in both acute and chronic pancreatitis.

The prognosis in acute pancreatitis is related to the initial severity and cause of the disease. The ultimate outcome has been predicted accurately in 96% of cases by Ranson and Pasternack (Table 2). The mortality in

Table 2. DIAGNOSTIC CRITERIA SERVING TO ASSESS PROGNOSIS

At Admission
  Age over 55 years
  WBC over 16000/mm^3
  Blood glucose greater than 200/dl
  Serum lactic dehydrogenase over 350 IU/liter
  Serum glutamic oxaloacetic transaminase over 250 Sigma Frankel
    units/liter

During Initial 48 Hours
  Hematocrit drop of more than 10 percentage points
  BUN rise of more than 5 mg/dl
  Arterial oxygen tension less than 60 mm Hg
  Base deficit greater than 4 mEq/liter
  Serum calcium level less than 8 mg/dl
  Estimated fluid sequestration more than 6 liters

patients with less than three *positive* factors was 0.9%, with three to four 16%, with five to six 40%, and with seven or more factors 100%.

LABORATORY DIAGNOSIS OF CHRONIC PANCREATITIS

Patients presenting with steatorrhea and diabetes mellitus who have pancreatic calcifications on a plain film of the abdomen require no further investigations.

The secretin-pancreozymin test is a very sensitive one for patients with suspected chronic pancreatitis, but its associated technical difficulties limit its use to very few laboratories.

Endoscopic retrograde cholangiopancreatography findings may vary from blunting and dilatation of the secondary pancreatic ductules to narrowing of the main duct in late stages of chronic pancreatitis.

MANAGEMENT

ACUTE PANCREATITIS

The short-term goals of treatment are (1) to prevent or stop further autodigestion of the pancreas and (2) to prevent development of local or general complications. The long-term goal is to prevent recurrence.

All patients with acute pancreatitis require hospitalization and an assessment of the severity of the episode. If the attack is mild, they may be treated safely with analgesics and nothing by mouth (NPO). For patients with moderate and severe pancreatitis, treatment consists of general supportive measures such as adequate analgesics to relieve pain, careful and frequent monitoring of vital signs, and correction and maintenance of fluid and electrolyte balance. To prevent further autodigestion, the concept of "placing the pancreas at rest" has evolved over the years. Many modalities such as NPO, nasogastric suction, anticholinergics and H$_2$-blockers, aprotinin (Trasylol), and glucagon have been used to achieve the objective. Multiple prospective randomized trials have shown that anticholinergics, H$_2$-blockers, aprotinin, and glucagon are of little value in the management of acute pancreatitis. Prophylactic antibiotics are of no value.

Surgical treatment of severe pancreatitis consists of open or closed peritoneal lavage or pancreatic resection. Peritoneal lavage does not improve survival but may delay the onset of complications in patients with severe pancreatitis. Pancreatic resection carries a high mortality and morbidity rate associated with secondary infection and hemorrhage. Life-threatening complications of acute pancreatitis such as shock, sepsis, respiratory insufficiency, renal insufficiency, and intra-abdominal hemorrhage should be recognized early and treated appropriately. Surgical intervention may be required for pancreatic pseudocyst or obstruction of the GI tract or biliary tree after the diagnosis has been established by ultrasonography, barium contrast study, or endoscopic retrograde cholangiopancreatography.

Follow-up and Prevention of Recurrence. At an appropriate time during hospitalization, usually while the attack is subsiding, patients should be told the cause of and prognosis for the pancreatitis. If the cause is suspected to be alcohol, patients should be cautioned against imbibing and may even need a referral to the substance abuse counselor. If deemed appropriate and not done earlier, ultrasonography to detect gallstones is indicated. Elective cholecystectomy is preferred during the same hospitalization. Shortly after discharge from the hospital, serum cholesterol, triglyceride, and calcium levels should be measured.

CHRONIC PANCREATITIS

Goals of management are (1) abstinence from alcohol, (2) pain control, (3) maintenance of adequate nutrition, and (4) control of diabetes mellitus.

Complete abstinence from alcohol is not only the goal but the rule of management of chronic pancreatitis. Considerable time may have to be spent with the patient reemphasizing this necessity; if necessary, the substance abuse counselor should work with the patient. Life expectancy is decreased by continuous use of alcohol.

Pain Control. The control of pain of chronic pancreatitis may be the most difficult and frustrating management problem. These patients appear to have very low pain thresholds. Every effort should be made to control pain with nonopiate drugs. Propoxyphene (Darvon) and its compounds may be habit-forming and dangerous if combined with alcohol. Acetaminophen without codeine can be used. Occasionally, narcotics (meperidine, morphine, or even codeine) may be required for adequate pain relief. Celiac ganglion block by alcohol or procaine may provide pain relief up to six months. Intractable pain requires surgical procedures such as distal pancreatectomy, longitudinal pancreaticojejunostomy, or subtotal pancreatomy. Total pancreatectomy is reserved for patients who obtain inadequate relief from other less extensive procedures. Insulin-dependent diabetes is a dreaded complication of resective procedures, and many centers are evaluating islet cell autotransplantation in the hope of preserving endocrine function.

Maintenance of Adequate Nutrition. Diet depends on the degree of pancreatitis. Adequate nutrition must be ensured with a diet containing at least 80 to 100 gm of protein and 80 to 100 gm of fats. Total parenteral nutrition or enteral feedings may be needed in patients with severe malnutrition. A medium-chain triglyceride (MCT oil) is needed for patients with severe steatorrhea, as it is absorbed intact. If steatorrhea and malnutrition persist, supplementation of pancreatic enzymes should be considered. Adequate pancreatic supplement therapy with the most potent available preparations, pancrelipase (Ilozyme, Viokase, or Cotazyme), one or two tablets before eating, three to six tablets with meals and two to four with snacks, is necessary to control steatorrhea. These enzyme supplements occasionally help with pain relief also. There is some evidence that the effect of pancreatic enzyme supplements is enhanced when used with H_2-receptor antagonists or antacids. Sometimes antidiarrheal agents such as Lomotil or Imodium may be tried. Impaired absorption of vitamin B_{12} requires parenteral supplementation.

Control of Diabetes. Mild diabetes may be managed with oral hypoglycemic agents. Most patients end up requiring 15 to 40 units of insulin. Caution is advised in the use of insulin, as hyperglycemia may be brittle. Because of low glucagon reserves, patients with pancreatic diabetes mellitus are extremely insulin sensitive and prone to develop marked hypoglycemia.

Once stable, patients are seen every four to six weeks by their personal physician and two to three times a year by the specialist. A better prognosis is seen in patients who refrain from drinking alcohol, eat good nourishing food, and have a clear understanding of steatorrhea and diabetes mellitus.

REFERENCES

DiMagno EP: What is appropriate nonoperative treatment of acute pancreatitis? Dig Dis Sci 24:337–338, 1979.

Grendell JH, Cello JP: Chronic pancreatitis. *In* Sleisenger MH, Fordtran JS (eds): Gastrointestinal Disease: Pathophysiology, Diagnosis, Management, 3rd ed. W. B. Saunders Co, Philadelphia, 1983, pp 1485–1515.

Moosa AR: Diagnostic tests and procedures in acute pancreatitis. N Engl J Med 311:639–642, 1984.

Ranson JH, Pasternack BS: Statistical methods for quantifying the severity of clinical acute pancreatitis. J Surg Res 22:79–91, 1977.

Soergel KH: Acute pancreatitis. *In* Sleisenger MH, Fordtran JS (eds): Gastrointestinal Disease: Pathophysiology, Diagnosis, Management, 3rd ed. W. B. Saunders Co, Philadelphia, 1983, pp 1462–1485.

13 · COMMON ANORECTAL PROBLEMS IN INTERNAL MEDICINE

Terry C. Hicks
J. Byron Gathright, Jr.
John E. Ray
Bernard T. Ferrari
OCHSNER CLINIC AND ALTON OCHSNER MEDICAL FOUNDATION

The internist frequently is confronted with a patient suffering from anorectal complaints. Making the correct diagnosis and instituting the appropriate therapy can often challenge the physician, since anorectal symptomatology may have a myriad of pathologic etiologies. The cornerstone to success is a systematic approach to the problem and the maintenance of appropriate follow-up care. This ensures that nonresponders are reevaluated and that their therapy is adjusted appropriately, and

also this provides a safeguard against missing a potentially life-threatening diagnosis.

Pruritus Ani

Pruritus ani is the unpleasant cutaneous sensation that leaves the patient with a nearly uncontrollable desire to scratch. The classic complaint is itching but, as the process progresses, increasing skin damage may lead to symptoms of burning and soreness. The causes of pruritus ani are extremely diverse and the physician's familiarity with them is crucial if treatment is to be successful. Some of the major etiologies are listed in Table 1.

A careful history can often identify the etiology. Attention should be paid to oral and perianal medications, diet, and systemic diseases. The physical examination should reveal the degree of skin involvement and help identify possible anatomic causes (fissures, fistulas, anal papillae, and skin tags). For completeness, sigmoidoscopy and anoscopy should be performed. Occasionally, microscopic evaluation of perianal skin scrapings may be of value. Pinworms may be identified by the standard scotch tape test, and Wood's lamp may help identify fungi or specific bacteria as the offending agents.

If history, physical exam, and laboratory studies can identify the etiology, a specific therapy can be instituted. However, the cause is usually not determined and the condition is diagnosed as idiopathic pruritus ani. Treatment must be individualized to meet the specific degree of perianal disease encountered.

CLINICAL MANAGEMENT

The following can serve as a therapeutic guideline.

1. Physician/patient rapport: the physician should fully explain the cause (if known) and reassure the patient that in idiopathic pruritus the therapeutic measures employed will probably relieve symptoms. This often helps to achieve patient compliance.

Table 1. MAJOR CAUSES OF PRURITUS ANI

Personal hygiene: poor cleansing habits with exposure to residual irritating feces, or (conversely) overmeticulous cleaning with excessive rubbing and soap utilization; obesity
Dietary: coffee, alcohol, citrus, milk, spices, tea, chocolate, colas
Systemic disease: diabetes, leukemia, aplastic anemia, liver disease
Diarrheal states: irritable bowel, Crohn's disease, chronic ulcerative colitis
Dermatologic: contact dermatitis (especially "-caine" preparations), psoriasis, lichen planus, reaction to oral antibiotics (especially tetracycline)
Infectious: fungal (dermatophytosis, candidiasis), viral, bacterial (erythrasma), parasites (scabies, pinworms, pediculosis)
Anatomic disorders: fissures, cryptitis, skin tags, ectropion, fistulas, hypertrophied anal papillae, hemorrhoids
Neoplasms: extramammary Paget's disease, intraepidermal carcinoma (Bowen's), other anal tumors
Clothing: tight clothing (underwear and girdles) or clothing materials that fail to allow proper ventilation
Radiation: postirradiation changes
Idiopathic

Table 2. PATIENT CARE HANDOUT FOR TREATMENT OF PRURITUS ANI

1. Hygiene is extremely important. Our goal is to keep the perineal skin clean, dry, and slightly acidic.
2. During bath or shower, wash outside the anal area, applying Balneol with fingertips or wet cotton. Do not use soap in the anal area (it is alkaline and may increase discomfort). Pat dry, or use a hair dryer. Avoid abrasive trauma from vigorous rubbing.
3. Following each bowel movement, wipe with Tucks or moist pads. Be sure not to leave the pads in contact with the skin for a prolonged period. Always avoid the use of toilet paper on irritated skin.
4. During the day, apply a thin cotton pledget directly in the anal crease. It should be small enough so that you are not conscious of its presence. You may dust the cotton with baby powder or cornstarch if needed. It is important to change the pledget often during the day.
5. Soaking in a warm sitz bath for 20 minutes can provide relief. A capful of liquid bleach added to the bathwater may be helpful, especially in the evening. Be sure to dry the anal area thoroughly afterwards.
6. After cleaning and drying the anal area, apply a small amount of hydrocortisone cream as per your prescription.
7. It is important to keep the stool soft, large, and nonirritating so that it can pass through the anal canal without causing mechanical or chemical trauma. This can be accomplished by the following:
   a. Metamucil, Hydrocil, or Konsyl. Take _____ tablespoons in _____ glasses of water or juice _____ times a day.
   b. Eat a high-fiber diet that includes:
      - 8 to 10 glasses of water or juice a day
      - plenty of fruits and vegetables
      - bran cereal every day
   c. Avoid foods that cause bowel irritation, are mucus-producing, or aggravate drainage, including: dark colas, pepper, citrus fruits and juices, coffee (regular or decaffeinated), beer and alcoholic beverages, nuts, popcorn, milk, and foods known to produce gas or indigestion. You may have 7 Up, ginger ale, or other light-colored soft drinks.
8. Wearing cotton gloves to bed can be of some benefit if you scratch yourself while sleeping.
9. Intermittent recurrences of this disease are common. Don't become despondent over this; just be sure to reconsult your doctor so that appropriate corrections in therapy can be made.

2. Instructions: A printed treatment guide for the patient can be most effective (Table 2).

Techniques of cleansing, drying, and medication application should be carefully explained. Dietary changes should include a systematic elimination of potential offending agents and an increase in bulk. An increase in fluid intake is a useful adjunct. If symptoms continue despite aggressive therapy, reevaluation is required. If a formal course of therapy has been unsuccessful over a period of three to four weeks, the physician should be prepared to obtain a biopsy.

Fissures

An anal fissure is a linear ulcer in the anal canal. Fissures are most frequently present in the posterior midline and occasionally in the anterior midline. These lesions reportedly are extremely painful; patients describe them as a cutting, tearing, or burning sensation, especially during or immediately after defecation. In our experience, the lesions are not always painful. Bright red blood often may be present in small amounts. A classic fissure triad has been described as (1) the anal ulcer, (2) a hypertrophic papilla, and (3) the sentinel pile. The sentinel pile represents fibrosed external hemorrhoidal tissue present at the distal fissure margin; the hypertrophic papilla is located at the proximal margin.

The etiology of these lesions appears to be multifactorial. Trauma to the canal from dry, hard, large-caliber stools appears to be the primary factor. Abnormal anal manometric studies have been noted in fissure patients, but these abnormalities may be a reaction to the injured epithelium rather than a primary cause.

A classic history usually leads to the proper diagnosis, but it is always necessary to separate the buttocks and adequately inspect the lower anal canal to confirm the diagnosis clinically. Often the application of a topical anesthetic to the area gives the patient enough comfort to allow a gentle digital examination; however, excessive spasm may make this examination impossible. If the examiner finds lesions in the lateral positions or a broad-based ulcer, other medical conditions must be considered as the source of the lesion, including Crohn's disease, ulcerative colitis, syphilis, leukemia, and tuberculosis.

CLINICAL MANAGEMENT

To obtain the maximal response from therapy for fissure disease, one must understand its cyclic nature. Often the patient who initially follows the treatment plan and becomes asymptomatic will at some future point fail to maintain stools of appropriate caliber and softness, and experience an acute recurrence.

Initial supportive measures include stool softeners containing psyllium, a high-fiber diet, and frequent sitz baths (especially after bowel movements). For most patients the application of topical steroidal creams is beneficial; remember that, to be useful, these agents must come into contact with the lesion. A supply of finger cots and careful instructions as to the location of the fissure will aid in correct application. Suppositories are of no use in the treatment of anal fissure disease, because after insertion they lie above the levators and have no contact with the diseased area below.

Most fissures respond to this conservative approach and no further therapy is needed. Patients who fail to respond to therapy or whose pain cannot be controlled are surgical candidates. The lateral internal sphincterotomy is the preferred surgical procedure. Performed under local or regional anesthesia, the procedure consists of partial division of the internal (nonvoluntary) sphincter muscle. Lateral anal internal sphincterotomy cures nearly all patients with chronic fissure disease (not associated with inflammatory bowel disease) and yields less than a 3% complication rate.

Fissures found to be laterally situated or wide-based require biopsy to rule out a systemic disease as their source. Whether patients are treated medically or surgically, a sigmoidoscopy should be included as part of the evaluation process, either at the time of surgery or after improvement has occurred.

Hemorrhoids

Hemorrhoids are thought to represent discrete vascular cushions. They are consistently found in the left lateral, right anterior, and right posterior positions, but smaller groups often are noted between these positions. The exact cause of hemorrhoids is highly speculative but the primary culprit appears to be excessive straining. Other factors such as lack of venous valves, erect posture, chronic constipation, pregnancy, and lack of bulk in the diet also play important roles. The function of hemorrhoids appears to be twofold: (1) to aid in maintaining continence and (2) to prevent excessive trauma to the anal canal at the time of defecation.

Hemorrhoids are either internal or external. The internal cushions arise above the dentate line and are covered by nonsensitive mucosa; external hemorrhoids arise below the dentate line and are covered by well-innervated epithelium. The external group are of clinical significance when a thrombosis occurs in this plexus. Internal hemorrhoids may bleed or prolapse, which can lead to subsequent strangulation, ulceration, and perianal discomfort. A clinical staging system exists for internal hemorrhoids. First-degree hemorrhoids represent enlarged cushions that do not prolapse. Second-degree hemorrhoids prolapse through the anal canal during defecation but spontaneously reduce themselves. Third-degree hemorrhoids protrude with straining and require manual reduction. Fourth-degree hemorrhoids represent permanent tissue prolapse.

CLINICAL MANAGEMENT

Hemorrhoids are part of the normal anatomy and, if not symptomatic, require no surgical treatment. Often hemorrhoidal complaints may actually represent another problem (e.g., fistula, abscess, fissure, pruritus, or rectal prolapse), and these alternative diagnoses must be carefully evaluated. Even if hemorrhoids are truly symptomatic, other colorectal pathology must be ruled out (e.g., colon, cancer, anal cancer, or inflammatory bowel disease); thus, a complete work-up should include proctosigmoidoscopy and anoscopy. For patients who are candidates for surgery and are over 40 years of age, a preoperative barium enema is in order.

INTERNAL HEMORRHOIDS

Asymptomatic internal hemorrhoids require no treatment. Symptomatic internal hemorrhoids should be treated on the basis of the severity of symptoms and degree of enlargement. Five major modalities are available and should be individualized to the patient's needs: (1) bowel habit education plus dietary changes; (2) banding; (3) cryosurgery; (4) sclerotherapy; and (5) hemorrhoidectomy.

Table 3 contains our present recommendations for treatment of internal hemorrhoids.

Diet and Education. Patients should avoid straining with bowel movements or spending excessive time on the toilet. They should also be advised of the relationship between excessive exercise and increasing hemorrhoid symptoms. Increased fluid intake and increased

Table 3. TREATMENT OF INTERNAL HEMORRHOIDS

Primary hemorrhoids	Conservative treatment with bowel habit education and dietary changes.
Secondary hemorrhoids	Banding; bowel habit education and dietary changes
Third-degree hemorrhoids	Banding, or surgery if severe; bowel habit education and dietary changes
Fourth-degree hemorrhoids	Hemorrhoidectomy; bowel habit education and dietary changes
Acute strangulated hemorrhoids	Urgent treatment (surgery may be necessary)

fiber intake along with psyllium seed products for stool softening may decrease straining. Avoidance of constipating foods, such as dairy products, may also be of some value.

Banding. This technique is appropriate for all secondary and uncomplicated third-degree hemorrhoids, and for some patients whose medical condition prevents them from undergoing formal hemorrhoidectomy. Utilizing adequate exposure with the anoscope, redundant hemorrhoidal tissue is grasped with forceps that have been passed through a special channel in the banding ligator. The ligator is then fired, placing a strong rubber band around the hemorrhoidal tissue. Necrosis and sloughing follow in approximately five days. Fixation of the remaining hemorrhoidal tissue occurs by scarring, thus preventing future prolapse of the residual cushion. It is imperative that the tissue be grasped above the dentate line as this area is insensitive to superficial pain. If the patient encounters severe pain after the rubber band placement, it indicates that the band has been placed too far distally and should be immediately removed.

It is our practice to do one group of hemorrhoids at a visit, spacing the visits approximately three to four weeks apart. After banding, patients may sense a mild discomfort for two or three days. This can be relieved by mild analgesics that are nonconstipating. Patients should avoid aspirin-containing compounds and alcohol, and use a stool-softening agent. Complications are rare, but on occasion significant bleeding has been reported after banding.

Cryosurgery. Despite dismal results, commercially available kits are still produced for cryosurgery. Bleeding, pain, increased drainage, and sphincter damage have all been reported with cryosurgery. Most centers have therefore abandoned this treatment for internal hemorrhoids.

Sclerotherapy. Sclerotherapy, the injection of a sclerosing solution into the proximal area of an internal hemorrhoidal group, is a long-recognized treatment for prolapsing hemorrhoids. Complications such as excessive sloughing of tissue, abscess formation, and (more rarely) prostatic or urethral injury make sclerotherapy an unwise choice for physicians who are not well schooled in the technique.

Hemorrhoidectomy. Patients with severe third-degree, fourth-degree, or strangulated hemorrhoids are candidates for hemorrhoidectomy. This procedure is much dreaded by many patients, but if performed by a qualified surgeon it can be accomplished with minor pain, and it offers the most complete and lasting relief of symptoms.

THROMBOSED EXTERNAL HEMORRHOIDS

External hemorrhoids are rarely symptomatic unless a thrombosis occurs. A thrombosis presents as a bluish subcutaneous nodule that is initially painful. The natural course of the thrombosis is a gradual decrease in discomfort over a three- to four-day period, with resolution in one to three weeks. Treatment is adjusted to the degree of patient discomfort. For lesions seen in the first 48 hours that are still painful, surgical unroofing is in order. The clot evacuation must be accompanied by excision of an adequate ellipse of skin; incision and forcible extrusion of the clot allow the skin edges to reseal and the clot to reform. The use of incision rather than excision can also lead to incomplete clot evacuation.

Excision can be performed under local anesthesia in the office or emergency room. Postoperative therapy includes a psyllium seed product to soften the stool, sitz baths, and a nonconstipating pain medication.

Thrombosed external hemorrhoids that are not painful may be treated conservatively. Measures include increased bulk in the diet (psyllium seed products), increased fluid intake, and sitz baths (especially after bowel movements).

Anal Suppurative Disease (Abscess-Fistulas)

Reddened, painful swelling around the anus most often heralds a perianal abscess or fistula. Antibiotic therapy may be appropriate in patients with certain systemic disease (e.g., diabetes, impaired immunity, cardiac or vascular prostheses), but prompt and adequate surgical drainage is mandatory in all cases.

Examinations under anesthesia may permit primary fistulotomy, eliminating the need for a second operation and ensuring adequate drainage. If surgical intervention is to be delayed, partial relief of symptoms may be attained by incision of the most fluctuant point of the mass after infiltration of the skin with a local anesthetic. Ethyl chloride "freezing" is painful, provides poor anesthesia, and should be avoided.

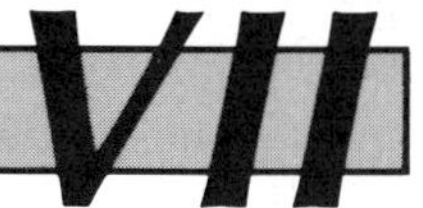

ENDOCRINE DISORDERS

RANDY LINDE

1 · HYPOTHALAMIC DISORDERS

Ronald P. Monsaert
GEISINGER MEDICAL CENTER

Hypothalamic Hypopituitarism

DIAGNOSTIC CRITERIA AND CLINICAL PRESENTATION

The isolation and synthesis of hypothalamic releasing hormones and the use of pharmacologic agents as probes of the neuroendocrine system reveal a far more complex organization than had been anticipated at a time when the pituitary was thought to be "the master gland." Some patients with isolated or multiple pituitary hormone deficiencies are now recognized to have releasing factor impairment, either due to disease localized to the hypothalamus or stalk, or due to inadequate or inappropriate input from other areas in the central nervous system. Hypothalamic hypopituitarism is any loss of pituitary trophic hormone secretion due to loss of releasing factor(s).

Etiologies include primary or metastatic neoplasms, infiltrative lesions, trauma or functional defects arising from significant changes in weight (gain or loss), psychologic trauma, and intensive athletic training. These functional defects are commonly manifest as primary or secondary amenorrhea, delay of puberty, or growth retardation.

True precocious puberty may also be a consequence of hypothalamic disease and should be differentiated from precocious thelarche (breast development), precocious adrenarche (sexual hair growth), and puberty initiated by autonomous secretion of sex steroids from ovarian or adrenal lesions.

Localization of trophic hormone deficiency to the hypothalamus may be suggested by results of testing with releasing factors, by coexistence with other hypothalamic disorders such as diabetes insipidus, or by findings on CT scan or other neuroradiologic studies.

MANAGEMENT

Evaluation and management is usually done in an outpatient setting, but patients with symptoms of an intracranial mass lesion may require hospitalization. Surgery may be considered for some lesions near the hypothalamus, such as craniopharyngioma. However, most hypothalamic tumors are best managed by radiation therapy, since surgery in this area is associated with considerable morbidity and mortality.

DRUG THERAPY

The goal of therapy is to replace absent hormone secretion if possible in a manner consistent with normal physiology. Thyroid deficiency is treated with L-thyroxine (0.1 to 0.15 mg daily), which should be instituted gradually in the elderly or in patients with ischemic heart disease. Hydrocortisone (20 mg q AM, 10 mg q PM) should be administered to those with ACTH deficiency, and as much as 300 mg per day should be given during stress.

Replacement of gonadal steroids in men can be accomplished with testosterone enanthate or cypionate (100 to 300 mg IM q two to four weeks). With these agents the incidence of hepatic toxicity is significantly less than with synthetic oral anabolic agents. Gynecomastia, however, may limit patient compliance. Testosterone therapy must be interrupted and gonadotropins administered if spermatogenesis is desired, although puberty and spermatogenesis have also been initiated with chronic intermittent gonadotropin-releasing hormone (GnRH). More traditionally, puberty can be initiated with testosterone (50 to 100 mg IM q three to four weeks) in boys with psychologic difficulties as a result of constitutional delay of puberty.

In females, treatment is accomplished with ethinyl estradiol (10 to 20 μg) or conjugated estrogens (0.6 to 1.2 mg) daily for 25 days, and a progestational agent (medroxyprogesterone, 5 to 10 mg) on days 16–25 or 21–25 to avoid endometrial hyperplasia. The substantial risk of osteoporosis in untreated patients usually outweighs any contraindications for its use in younger patients. Preliminary data on exercising amenorrheic women suggest that bone density often remains normal, but gonadal steroids should be considered in those with functional amenorrhea who are sedentary. Ensuring a calcium intake of 1.5 gm per day or 1500 mg per day in amenorrheic women is also important to prevent negative calcium balance. Gonadotropin therapy should not be undertaken by physicians unfamiliar with its use. As in males, GnRH therapy has been successful in initiating puberty and ovulation, but requires referral to a center

435

and is administered by a sophisticated drug delivery system.

Children with true precocious puberty should probably be referred to centers for GnRH analogue therapy. This appears to be far superior to any other agent, desensitizing the pituitary to native GnRH and thus halting puberty until a suitable age. GnRH and GnRH analogue therapy appear safe, but long-term side effects are as yet unknown.

Growth hormone should be replaced in patients with a capacity for growth and growth hormone deficiency. Growth hormone is given intramuscularly (0.08 to 0.1 mg/kg) three times a week and should be discontinued when growth is no longer recorded, when the epiphyses close, or when a desirable height is reached.

Diabetes Insipidus

DEFINITION

Diabetes insipidus (DI) is a disorder of reduced urinary concentrating capacity due to absent or deficient secretion of vasopressin (complete or partial hypothalamic DI) or impaired renal responsiveness to vasopressin (nephrogenic DI).

PATHOPHYSIOLOGY

Secretion of arginine vasopressin (AVP) results in augmented water absorption from the collecting tubules of the kidneys. AVP is secreted in response to increasing plasma osmolality, decreased plasma volume, decreased blood pressure, and various neural and pharmacologic stimuli. Reduced secretion results in polyuria, increasing plasma osmolality, and subsequent dehydration, hypotension, and death. If thirst mechanisms are intact, the patient can compensate by augmenting water intake and maintain a relatively normal state of hydration.

The etiologies of DI are similar to those of hypothalamic hypopituitarism although frequently the pathogenesis remains obscure. Recently a group of patients with idiopathic DI was found to have serum antibodies against neurons in the supraoptic and paraventricular nuclei, suggesting an autoimmune etiology.

CLINICAL ASPECTS

Patients with intact thirst mechanisms notice excessive thirst (usually for cold liquids) and polyuria of 3 to 30 liters per day. Typically, patients are able to date the onset, which is usually abrupt. Occasionally there are hypopituitarism or neurologic problems such as headache or diplopia. Differentiation of hypothalamic from nephrogenic DI and other polyuric states such as primary polydipsia requires an assessment of changes in urine osmolality or urine flow in response to water deprivation and vasopressin administration (dehydration tests) or to infusion of hypertonic saline (Hickey-Hare test). Further precision of diagnosis can be obtained by performing plasma AVP levels during these indirect tests. A therapeutic trial with vasopressin is occasionally helpful.

MANAGEMENT

NONPHARMACOLOGIC MEASURES

In patients with intact thirst mechanisms and free access to water, liquids form a mainstay of therapy. A low-sodium diet reduces symptoms to a small degree.

DRUG THERAPY

Vasopressin is indispensable to therapy for complete hypothalamic DI. Available in three forms, the best is dDAVP, a solution (0.1 to 0.2 ml) delivered to the posterior nasal mucosa by a rhinyl catheter. Satisfactory antidiuresis may last 24 hours, but most patients require two doses a day and are advised to occasionally wait for a return of diuresis before readministering this agent, to avoid overtreatment. dDAVP can be used parenterally (2 to 4 μg) in unconscious or postoperative patients, during a water deprivation test, or when an upper respiratory infection precludes adequate nasal absorption. dDAVP has virtually no pressor effects but unfortunately is expensive.

The least expensive preparation, pitressin tannate in oil (2.5 to 5 units), has the advantage of a long duration of activity (24 to 72 hours). Its disadvantage is that it must be given IM and the adverse effects include abdominal pain, headache, increased blood pressure, uterine cramps, and exacerbation of coronary artery disease. Care must be taken to mix the small pellet of vasopressin thoroughly before injection. Lysine vasopressin (Diapid) is an intranasal preparation effective for about three hours; it is moderately expensive.

Patients with partial DI may have a significant antidiuresis with chlorpropamide (250 to 500 mg per day) as a single agent or given to reduce the dosage of dDAVP. Hypoglycemia necessitating an altered eating schedule or even precluding the use of this agent is more likely to occur with concomitant use of sulfonamides, salicylates, nonsteroidal anti-inflammatory agents, and other drugs. Hydrochlorothiazide (50 mg once or twice per day) is also a useful adjunctive agent (as are other thiazides), and a potassium supplement should be coadministered when necessary. Clofibrate and carbamazepine may also be helpful, but should be reserved for special circumstances because of the more serious potential toxicity.

PATIENT INFORMATION AND EVALUATION

Patients should be instructed to wear a health-alert bracelet. Management of patients with impaired thirst usually requires a strict schedule for vasopressin administration and a predetermined amount of fluid intake, which should be modified according to changes in insensible fluid losses.

PERIODIC EVALUATION

Adequacy of therapy can be monitored by checking serum osmolality, and in most cases this is adequately reflected by serum sodium. These levels should be normalized, and sleep and work schedules should not be disturbed by polyuria. Patients with impaired thirst should initially be seen at least weekly in the outpatient setting, with appropriate laboratory studies and body weights. Well-controlled patients can be seen every three to four months, and a general assessment of neuroendocrine systems should be performed yearly to make sure that the cause of DI has not involved other hormonal or neurologic functions.

Inappropriate ADH Secretion

DEFINITION

The syndrome of inappropriate secretion of antidiuretic hormone (SIADH) was described by Schwartz and Bartter in 1957 as hyponatremia with plasma hypo-osmolality and inappropriately elevated urinary osmolality. Urinary sodium excretion is greater than 20 mEq/L; renal, adrenal, and thyroid function are normal; there should be no evidence of volume depletion, edema, or overt cardiac or hepatic decompensation.

PATHOPHYSIOLOGY

Plasma vasopressin levels are normally suppressed (<1 pg/ml) when ambient plasma osmolality is less than 280 mOsm/kg and rise briskly as plasma osmolality increases. In patients with SIADH, however, four different patterns of AVP responses have been found. Most patients display erratic fluctuation of AVP levels that appear independent of osmotic control. One third of patients regulate AVP levels in response to osmotic stimuli, but the set point for release is lower than normal plasma osmolality. Unfortunately no pattern of secretion seems related to any specific cause of SIADH.

CLINICAL ASPECTS

Patients may present with anorexia, weakness, lethargy, confusion, seizures, or coma. Both the degree and rate of development of plasma hypo-osmolality determine the development of symptoms, which are largely due to cerebral edema from water intoxication.

Laboratory findings include low levels of serum sodium, osmolality, chloride, BUN, creatinine, and uric acid. Urine should be hypertonic to plasma with urinary sodium in excess of 20 mEq/L. Plasma or urine AVP levels are usually detectable, although not necessarily elevated, but are not needed to establish the diagnosis.

The most important causes of SIADH are listed in Table 1.

MANAGEMENT

NONPHARMACOLOGIC MEASURES

Patients with seizure or coma from hyponatremia should be admitted to a constant observation area and treated with an infusion of 200 to 300 ml of hypertonic saline (3% to 5%) over two to three hours. Furosemide (40 mg IV) can be given concurrently, especially when there is a risk of congestive heart failure. Less acute situations should be managed with fluid restriction (500 to 1000 ml per 24 hours). Once the patient is stabilized and the serum sodium reaches 128 to 132 mEq/L, fluid restriction can be modified to maintain these values, and evaluation and treatment of the underlying disorder can begin.

Table 1. SOME CAUSES OF SIADH

Malignant Disease	**Thoracic Disease**
Carcinoma of lung, pancreas, duodenum, bladder, ureter, prostate	Pneumonia, pulmonary abscess
	Tuberculosis
Mesothelioma	Empyema
Thymoma	Cystic fibrosis
Lymphoma, leukemia	Pneumothorax
Ewing's sarcoma	Asthma
Carcinoid	Positive-pressure breathing
Central Nervous System Disorders	**Drugs**
Meningitis, encephalitis, brain abscess, Rocky Mountain spotted fever	Vasopressin, oxytocin
	Thiazide diuretics
	Chlorpropamide
Guillain-Barré syndrome	Vincristine, vinblastine, cisplatin
Head trauma, post-transphenoidal surgery	Phenothiazines, MAO inhibitors
Cerebral hemorrhage	Carbamazepine
Cavernous sinus thrombosis	Clofibrate
Cerebellar and cerebral atrophy	Nicotine
Shy-Drager syndrome	**Miscellaneous**
Acute intermittent porphyria	Idiopathic
Delirium tremens	Hypothyroidism
	Acute psychosis

DRUG THERAPY

Occasionally SIADH does not remit or therapy aimed at its etiology is unsuccessful, so that long-term outpatient management is necessary. Some cooperative patients can be readily treated with continued fluid restriction. Others, however, do not tolerate this and may be given the tetracycline derivative demeclocycline (900 to 1200 mg per day) in divided doses. Demeclocycline produces reversible nephrogenic DI within a few days and fluid restriction can be withdrawn. Potential adverse effects include photosensitivity, nausea, bacterial superinfection, and azotemia, which is usually reversible. Significant polyuria may develop, and dehydration and volume depletion is a possibility. Similarly, lithium carbonate, 600 to 900 mg per day, may be effective by inhibiting the AVP effect on the kidney. Neurologic toxicity is a frequently reported side effect, and lithium probably should not be used except in unusual situations.

Furosemide (40 mg PO per day) together with a high sodium diet may be effective in the outpatient setting. Unlike thiazide diuretics that do not interfere with free water reabsorption, furosemide promotes free water clearance. As with IV furosemide use in the acute setting, care must be taken to avoid hypokalemia and volume depletion.

Urea produces an osmotic diuresis and has been shown to alleviate SIADH acutely and chronically by IV or PO administration. Oral doses of crystalline urea (30 gm) dissolved in 100 to 200 ml of water can correct SIADH and allow the patient free access to water during therapy. Urea is generally innocuous; however, it may be irritating to gastric mucosa and can be given with an antacid.

PERIODIC EVALUATION

Progress can be monitored by serum sodium or osmolality. Body weight is also useful to follow, a weight gain usually indicating excessive water retention. It is appropriate to discontinue therapy at intervals to see whether SIADH has been self-remitting or whether therapy aimed at its etiology has been effective.

REFERENCES

Givens JR (ed): The Hypothalamus. Year Book Medical Publishers, Chicago, 1984.

Streeten DHP, Moses AM, Miller M: Disorders of the neurohypophysis. *In* Isselbacher KJ, Adams RD, Braunwald E, et al (eds): Harrison's Principles of Internal Medicine, 9th ed. McGraw-Hill Book Co., New York, 1980, pp 1684–1694.

Yen SSC: Clinical applications of gonadotropin-releasing hormone and gonadotropin-releasing hormone analogs. Fertil Steril 39:257–266, 1983.

Zerbe RL, Robertson GL: A comparison of plasma vasopressin measurements with a standard indirect test in the differential diagnosis of polyuria. N Engl J Med 305:1539–1546, 1981.

Zerbe RL, Stropes L, Robertson GL: Vasopressin function in the syndrome of inappropriate antidiuresis. Annu Rev Med 31:315–327, 1980.

2 · HYPOPITUITARISM

Charles Abboud
MAYO CLINIC AND MAYO FOUNDATION

GENERAL PRINCIPLES

The anterior pituitary gland is composed of a number of different types of cells, each of which has distinctive endocrine functions (Table 1). In hypopituitarism, failure can affect one (monotropic), more than one (multitropic), or all of the anterior pituitary hormones (pantropic). For each hormone affected, the failure can be partial or complete. In the evolution of pituitary disease, hypopituitarism can progress from monotropic to multitropic or pantropic failure, and for each hormone the failure can progress from a partial to a complete one. In the diagnostic assessment, the physician should elucidate the type and degree of hormone deficiency.

The hypothalamus regulates the endocrine functions of the anterior pituitary gland through its regulatory hormones (Table 1). Anterior pituitary failure can be *primary* (due to inherent disease of the pituitary gland) or *secondary* (due to hypothalamic disease). The

Table 1. HYPOTHALAMIC PITUITARY HORMONES

Pituitary Cell	Pituitary Hormone	Hypothalamic Regulatory Hormone
Somatotroph	Growth hormone (GH)	Growth hormone inhibitory hormone (somatostatin)
		Growth hormone–releasing hormone (GHRH)
Lactotroph	Prolactin (PRL)	Prolactin inhibitory hormone (Dopamine)
Gonadotroph	Follicle-stimulating hormone (FSH)	Gonadotropin-releasing hormone (GnRH)
	Luteinizing hormone (LH)	
Corticotroph	Corticotropin (ACTH) β-lipotropin (β-LPH) β-endorphin (β-END)	Corticotropin-releasing hormone (CRH)
Thyrotroph	Thyrotropin (TSH)	Thyrotropin-releasing hormone (TRH)

Table 2. CAUSES OF HYPOPITUITARISM

Primary: Pituitary Disease
Neoplasms
　Pituitary tumors
　Craniopharyngioma
Vascular
　Postpartum necrosis
　Pituitary apoplexy
Inflammatory
　Autoimmune hypophysitis
Iatrogenic
　Surgery
　Radiotherapy
Idiopathic
Secondary: Hypothalamic Disease
Functional
　Nutritional (starvation, obesity)
　Anorexia nervosa
　Psychosocial dwarfism
　Hormones, e.g., glucocorticoids
　Drugs, e.g., vincristine
　Systemic disease
　Thyroid disease
　Adrenal disease
Organic
　Tumors (primary or metastatic)
　Trauma (stalk section)
　Inflammatory, e.g., sarcoidosis
　Infiltrative, e.g., histiocytosis X
　Vascular
　Idiopathic
　Congenital, e.g., Kallmann's syndrome
Extrasellar disease
Meningioma
Optic glioma
Carotid aneurysm
Chordoma

causes of hypopituitarism are listed in Table 2. Primary disease of the pituitary gland is always organic. Hypothalamic disease, however, can be organic or functional. In evaluating hypopituitarism, the physician should be particularly aware of its functional causes since they are common, easily identified, and potentially reversible.

Treatment of hypopituitarism is based on (1) removal of the cause and (2) substitution of the deficient hormone. There are three potential ways to substitute for a given pituitary hormone deficiency: (a) Administer the hypothalamic regulatory hormone. At present, this is feasible only for gonadotropin-releasing hormone (GnRH) in the management of hypothalamic hypogonadism. The future holds exciting possibilities for the use of other regulatory hormones as therapeutic options in patients with secondary hypopituitarism. (b) Administer the anterior pituitary hormone. This has been limited to the use of growth hormone to promote linear growth in growth hormone–deficient children or adolescents, and to the use of gonadotropins in hypogonadism to promote fertility. (c) Administer the hormone of the affected target gland or one of its synthetic analogues. This is the most practical and effective means of hormone replacement in target gland failure because of its cost advantage, ease of administration, and prolonged action.

ACTH DEFICIENCY

This is a potentially life-threatening deficiency and its treatment takes precedence over that of all other anterior pituitary hormones. ACTH deficiency results in decreased secretion of cortisol and adrenal androgens by the adrenal cortex. Aldosterone secretion by the zona glomerulosa is, however, primarily under the control of the renin-angiotensin system. Aldosterone secretion is usually unaffected in hypopituitary patients unless they are subjected to severe salt depletion.

The goal of treatment in ACTH deficiency is to restore a eucortisol state. This is achieved by administration of cortisol, or one of its glucocorticoid analogues, in a dose equivalent to day-to-day normal cortisol production and in a way that mimics normal circadian rhythm. In addition, the dose is increased during periods of stress to mimic the normal increased production of cortisol in such situations.

Glucocorticoid therapy can be given as hydrocortisone, 20 to 30 mg/day, cortisone acetate, 25 to 37.5 mg/day, or prednisone, 5 to 7.5 mg/day. Two thirds of the dose is given in the morning and the other third in early or midafternoon. Each dose is given with a meal or snack to prevent gastric irritation. High-potency, long-acting glucocorticoids such as dexamethasone are not recommended for glucocorticoid replacement. In the child with ACTH deficiency, hydrocortisone (7.5 to 15 mg/day in two divided doses), or its equivalent is given. It is critical to avoid excess glucocorticoid in children since it leads to decreased responsiveness to growth hormone and to a decrease in linear growth.

Complications are rare with the doses described above. Some patients may have insomnia or irritability after therapy is begun and for these the dosage should be reduced. Follow-up of the adequacy of the daily dose consists of assessing the patient's feeling of well-being and examining for evidence of glucocorticoid deficiency or excess. Measurement of serum cortisol or ACTH is not helpful in this regard.

SPECIAL CONSIDERATIONS

Stress. Each patient is taught the standard steroid stress precautions. Under conditions of stress (e.g., acute illness, fever, moderate to severe trauma), the dose should be increased to two to three times the usual daily replacement dose and given in divided doses daily until the stress subsides, when the patient can be returned to the usual daily replacement dose. The patient is told that if it is difficult to decide about the need for increased glucocorticoid administration during a given period of stress, it is better to err on the side of overreplacement.

Vomiting. Each patient is told that in the event of vomiting, injectable steroids should be used and medical attention sought promptly. Hydrocortisone hemisuccinate (Solu-Cortef), 100 mg IM, or dexamethasone, 4 mg IM, may be taken. Parenteral cortisone acetate should not be used in situations necessitating rapid replacement because absorption, and therefore the onset of action, is not dependable. Patients should always carry with them an injectable steroid for emergency treatment, especially if they plan to travel in areas where good medical care may not be available promptly. They should be instructed in self-injection technique.

Medical Identification. All patients on maintenance glucocorticoid therapy should wear an appropriate medical identification bracelet or necklace explaining glucocorticoid replacement and the need for increased steroid dosage during periods of stress.

Acute ACTH Deficiency. In acute ACTH deficiency, such as occurs in pituitary apoplexy, therapy is instituted promptly after the diagnosis is suspected. A blood sample is drawn for serum cortisol and serum ACTH. Parenteral soluble glucocorticoids and supportive care are given simultaneously with the assessment and the correction of precipitating factors. Hydrocortisone, 100 mg, is given IV, followed by 50 to 100 mg every six hours on the first day, 50 mg every six hours on the second day, and 25 mg every six hours on the third day, tapering to maintenance dose by the fourth to fifth days.

Perioperative Glucocorticoid Therapy. Hydrocortisone phosphate or hemisuccinate, 100 mg IM, is given on call in the operating room; 50 mg IM or IV in the recovery room; and then 50 mg every six hours for the first 24 hours. If progress is satisfactory, the dose can be reduced to 25 mg every six hours for 24 hours and then gradually tapered to maintenance dose by the third to fifth days. However, if fever, hypotension, or other complications occur, the dose of hydrocortisone is increased to 200 to 400 mg/day in divided doses every six hours, followed by gradual tapering to maintenance dose.

Partial ACTH Deficiency. If ACTH deficiency is partial, the patient may be able to secrete enough cortisol to take care of day-to-day needs and thus may not need daily replacement therapy. The patient with partial ACTH deficiency must be educated to use glucocorticoids during periods of stress and to undergo periodic assessment, because of the potential for progression to complete ACTH deficiency.

Psychotic Behavior. Some patients with hypopituitarism of long duration may exhibit euphoria or psychotic behavior with full replacement doses of glucocorticoids. For these, the minimal replacement dose necessary should be used.

Diabetes Insipidus. In patients with diabetes insipidus, concomitant lack of cortisol may prevent polyuria and polydipsia because cortisol is needed for free water clearance. In these, glucocorticoid therapy permits the clinical emergence of diabetes insipidus.

TSH DEFICIENCY

The goal of treatment is to replace normal thyroid function by administration of thyroid hormone. Two general types of thyroid hormone preparations are available: (1) thyroproteins derived from animal thyroids (thyroid extract, USP); and (2) synthetic hormones, which include L-thyroxine (T_4), L-triiodothyronine (T_3), or a combination of the two. Synthetic preparations are preferred because of their uniform potency. T_4 is the agent of choice because it does not lead to abrupt increases in serum T_3 concentration, which could be dangerous in older patients or those with coexisting heart disease. T_4 therapy is associated with a stable T_3 concentration because of the constant generation by peripheral tissues of T_3 from administered T_4.

The usual replacement dose of L-thyroxine is between 0.1 and 0.2 mg/day. To establish the appropriate dose, the physician uses the clinical assessment accompanied by serum free T_4 levels. Since we are dealing with secondary or tertiary hypothyroidism, measurement of TSH is of no value in this regard.

Endogenous T_4 production is decreased in the elderly. Therefore, a reduction of 20% to 40% in replacement dose is often required in elderly patients to avoid subtle manifestations of hyperthyroidism.

In an otherwise healthy young patient with hypopituitarism, or in hypopituitarism of recent onset, thyroid hormone replacement therapy can be initiated at the replacement dose. If, however, the hypopituitarism is severe or of long standing, or if there is coexistent ischemic heart disease, a sudden increase in metabolic rate may tax cardiac reserve. In these patients, therapy is initiated with 0.025 mg of T_4/day, and the daily dose is increased slowly by 0.025 mg of T_4 every two to three weeks until the maintenance dose is achieved. In selected patients it is wise to evaluate the electrocardiogram before proceeding to the next level of replacement. If anginal symptoms develop before the full replacement dose is achieved, the final replacement dose must be balanced between that which does the most to relieve symptoms of hypothyroidism and that which does not produce angina.

SPECIAL CONSIDERATIONS

Unrecognized ACTH Deficiency. Administration of thyroid hormone to treat TSH deficiency in a patient with unrecognized ACTH deficiency may precipitate addisonian crisis, because thyroid hormone accelerates cortisol metabolism and increases the need for cortisol. It is therefore critical that the ACTH-cortisol axis be evaluated in any patient with TSH deficiency; if ACTH deficiency is found to be present, glucocorticoid replacement should be instituted before T_4 therapy.

Partial TSH Deficiency. In patients with partial TSH deficiency, the physician has two therapeutic options. The first is to use small doses of T_4 to achieve the euthyroid state, to monitor the patient periodically, and to adjust the replacement dose as needed. This option requires frequent reevaluation since the progression of partial to complete TSH deficiency may be unpredictable. The second option is to give full replacement doses of L-thyroxine, which obviates the need for frequent monitoring after the euthyroid state is achieved.

Juvenile Hypothyroidism. In childhood and juvenile hypothyroidism, full replacement therapy is started promptly after the diagnosis of hypothyroidism is made, to optimize normal intellectual development and physical growth. It is important to avoid supraphysiologic levels of thyroid hormone replacement because this accelerates bone age and ultimately reduces growth hormone responsiveness.

Hypopituitary Coma. If hypopituitary coma or precoma is present, the urgency of thyroid hormone replacement is more acute and is to be approached in a fashion similar to that for myxedema coma. A dose of 400 μg of L-thyroxine is given parenterally followed by a daily dose of 50 μg. This is optimally done in an intensive care unit with continuous EKG monitoring. The hazard from this abrupt increase in circulating thyroid hormone levels is the precipitation of myocardial ischemia and ventricular arrhythmia. This disadvantage is outweighed by the very poor survival rate in these patients if replacement is accomplished by small, gradual increases in thyroid hormone dosage.

GONADOTROPIN DEFICIENCY

The aim of treatment is to restore gonadal function. This is accomplished by (1) reversing the cause of the hypopituitarism; (2) if this is not feasible, by replacing gonadal steroids; (3) and, when indicated, by restoring fertility potential by administration of gonadotropins or GnRH.

In all patients with gonadotropin deficiency, the physician should consider the possibility of functional hypothalamic hypogonadism. If present, this is generally reversible by simple direct means such as psychiatric and supportive care in anorexia nervosa, correction of nutritional abnormalities in starvation and obesity, thyroid hormone replacement therapy in primary hypothyroidism, or dopaminergic agents in hyperprolactinemic states. Otherwise, the treatment of gonadotropin deficiency is as described below.

Females. In premenopausal women, estrogen therapy is indicated for maintenance of secondary sexual characteristics, prevention of osteoporosis and possibly of coronary artery disease, and preservation of a general sense of well-being. A variety of estrogen preparations can be used, including ethinyl estradiol, 0.02 to 0.05 mg/day, or conjugated estrogens (Premarin), 0.625 to 1.25 mg/day.

It is prudent to use the lowest possible dose that produces the desired clinical effects. Because of the increased risk of endometrial cancer and occasional development of cystic changes in the breasts in women on long-term estrogen therapy, estrogen should be given cyclically for 25 days of each month (day 1 to day 25), accompanied in the last ten days by a progestational agent such as medroxyprogesterone acetate, five to ten mg/day (day 16 to day 25). This regimen induces menstrual bleeding and prevents endometrial hyperplasia. Alternatively, one of the oral contraceptive preparations can be used in cyclic fashion.

It is not known whether the increased risk of thromboembolism, hyperlipidemia, and carbohydrate intolerance and the other known risks associated with the use of estrogen in normal women also arise in hypopituitary patients. However, the benefits of restoring normal physiologic function in these women warrant the use of replacement therapy, after careful consideration of the appropriate contraindications for and precautions needed for such therapy.

It is still controversial whether the advantages of estrogen replacement therapy outweigh the disadvantages after the time of expected menopause. The potential benefits and risks should be discussed frankly and fully with the postmenopausal patient to help her decide for or against this therapy.

It is important to ask about the patient's libido. Decreased libido often results from absence of adrenal androgens and may not be corrected by estrogen replacement. Restoration of libido can be accomplished by IM administration of a long-acting androgen such as testosterone enanthate, 50 mg every one to two months. The lowest effective dose should be used to avoid development of hirsutism, acne, and other evidences of hyperandrogenicity.

In prepubertal girls, estrogen should be started only after consideration of psychosocial development, height, and the need for growth hormone therapy. Since estrogen can cause premature epiphyseal closure, therapy should be withheld as long as practical to allow for optimal linear growth. Conjugated estrogen is given in a dose of 5 to 10 mg PO/day as long as is necessary to induce maximal breast development. The patient is then placed and maintained on one of the oral contraceptives in standard cyclic fashion.

Infertility. With gonadotropin deficiency, infertility can be due to an inadequate luteal phase or to anovulation. Euprolactinemic luteal insufficiency can be reversed successfully with vaginal administration of progesterone (25 mg b.i.d. after ovulation). Hyperprolactinemic luteal insufficiency or anovulation can be reversed by suppression of hyperprolactinemia by bromocriptine. If euprolactinemic anovulation is present and the patient has withdrawal bleeding in response to progesterone, stimulation of gonadotropin secretion by clomiphene will result in ovulation. Clomiphene is an antiestrogen compound believed to act by binding to estrogen receptors in the hypothalamus. In response to clomiphene, the secretion of FSH and LH is increased, leading to stimulation of follicular development and ovulation. Clomiphene is usually started with a dose of 50 mg PO daily for five days, commencing on the fifth day of spontaneous or progestin-induced menstrual bleeding. If ovulation does not occur with this dose, it can be increased in a stepwise fashion to a maximal dose of 200 mg per day for a five-day cycle. Three to four cycles are required before this therapy can be regarded as a failure.

In persons with primary pituitary disease, gonadotropin therapy consisting of human menopausal gonadotropin (hMG, Pergonal), an FSH-rich preparation obtained from the urine of postmenopausal women, and human chorionic gonadotropin (hCG), can be used to induce ovulation. hMG is first given to initiate follicular growth and maturation in a dose of 150 units IM daily for 10 to 14 days. This is monitored by daily measurement of plasma estradiol and, when feasible, by ultrasound of the ovaries. When plasma estradiol levels reach 500 to 1000 pg/ml and the ultrasound of the ovaries shows a maturing follicle, 10,000 units of hCG is injected IM to induce ovulation. This form of therapy is expensive and hazardous, and may lead to the hyperstimulation syndrome (ovarian enlargement, abdominal distention, ascites, pleural effusion, and shock) and to multiple births. Therefore, it should be undertaken only under the direction of physicians who have experience in this therapeutic regimen.

Alternatively, in hypothalamic hypogonadism, pulsatile GnRH therapy, when it becomes available and approved for use by the FDA, can be used. This stimulates gonadotropin secretion, follicular maturation, and ovulation and can be monitored by plasma estradiol levels and ultrasound of the ovaries with less morbidity.

Males. In the adult male, testosterone therapy is required to restore and maintain libido, potency, secondary sexual characteristics, muscle strength and other androgen-dependent anabolic processes. Testosterone can be given orally or parenterally. Oral preparations, such as methyltestosterone or fluoxymesterone, are not recommended because of their greater cost, variability in absorption, and known association in a small percentage of patients with the development of cholangiolitic hepatitis, peliosis hepatis, or hepatoma. Parenteral testosterone preparations do not have these drawbacks and are the preferred agents for replacement therapy. They can be given as testosterone enanthate or cypionate, 100 to 300 mg IM every two to four weeks, or as testosterone propionate, 25 to 50 mg IM two to three times a week. Patients are taught self-injection to reduce cost. Effectiveness of therapy can be monitored by patients' clinical state and by assay of plasma levels of testosterone. Overdosage leads to salt and fluid retention, edema, excessive sexual stimulation, priapism, gynecomastia, aggressive behavior, polycythemia, and worsening of benign prostatic hypertrophy. If these symptoms develop, the dose can be adjusted downward. Androgen therapy is contraindicated in patients who have carcinoma of the prostate or breast.

Longstanding Hypogonadism. In longstanding hypogonadism, psychosocial defenses in patients' relationships occur that may affect their life style, including marital status, choice of marital partner, occupation, and so forth. Testosterone therapy may lead to major problems of adjustment. These must be carefully considered and discussed with patients before therapy is begun.

Androgen-Dependent Tumors. With testosterone therapy, there is increased risk of growth of androgen-dependent tumors in middle-aged and elderly patients. Those in this age group should have a prostate check every six months while on testosterone therapy.

Hypopituitary Adolescents. In hypopituitary adolescents who have hypogonadism and a lack of growth hormone, therapy is initiated with growth hormone until reasonable height is achieved before testosterone therapy is started. Testosterone is then given as 100 to 150 mg/meter^2 surface area every one to three weeks. This should result in normal pubertal growth and sexual development.

Infertility. Fertile men who are about to undergo surgical or radiotherapeutic ablative treatment that is potentially destructive to the hypothalamic-pituitary unit may wish to consider placing sperm in a sperm bank where it might be kept viable for several years.

Exogenous gonadotropins have been used successfully to induce spermatogenesis and fertility. hMG is available in ampules containing 75 units of FSH and 75 units of luteinizing hormone (LH) per ampule; hCG is supplied as 5000 to 20,000 USP units per vial. The most satisfactory program is to stop testosterone exogenous therapy and initiate gonadotropin therapy: hMG, 75 units and hCG, 2000 units IM three times a week. Restoration of full spermatogenesis may take 12 to 18 months, at which time spermatogenesis can be maintained by hCG alone. Impregnation often occurs with total sperm counts below 20×10^6/ml. After successful conception, the male is switched back to testosterone parenteral therapy. Gonadotropin therapy should be initiated and followed by experienced endocrinologists.

In hypothalamic hypogonadism, pulsatile GnRH therapy, when it becomes available in the future, can be used successfully to initiate and maintain spermatogenesis and fertility potential.

GROWTH HORMONE DEFICIENCY

In hypopituitary adults, the lack of growth hormone is a common finding but there is no evidence of associated clinical or biochemical disturbances. There is therefore no indication for growth hormone replacement.

In children, the lack of growth hormone leads to decreased linear growth, insulin sensitivity and hypoglycemia, or alternatively to insulin resistance and glucose intolerance. Growth hormone replacement can reverse these abnormalities. Traditionally, growth hormone replacement has been limited to use in the hypopituitary child or adolescent with significant growth retardation prior to epiphyseal closure, and has been available either from the National Pituitary Agency or from commercial sources. Because of possible contamination by the agent that causes Jakob-Creutzfeldt disease, this source of growth hormone is no longer available. Genetically engineered growth hormone has been released and is given intramuscularly or subcutaneously with the usual dose of 0.1 to 0.2 international units/kg three times per week until a height of at least 5 feet, 4 inches is achieved. In general, the younger the patient when the therapy is initiated, the better is the response.

Careful attention to concomitant hormone deficiencies is in order. Physiologic thyroid and glucocorticoid replacement are essential for maximizing growth hormone responsiveness. The physician, however, should avoid supraphysiologic replacement with glucocorticoid or with thyroid hormone because of interference with the growth-promoting effect of growth hormone therapy. Sex steroid therapy should be delayed until an acceptable height is achieved.

PROLACTIN DEFICIENCY

Prolactin is not available for substitution therapy. Prolactin is needed only in the management of a lack of postpartum lactation. No satisfactory form of therapy is available for this problem.

REFERENCES

Abboud CF: Laboratory diagnosis of hypopituitarism. Mayo Clin Proc 61:35–48, 1986.

Kaltenborn KC, Jubiz W: Quadruple injection of hypothalamic peptides to evaluate pituitary function in normal subjects (clinical investigation). West J Med 142:37–41, 1985.

Report of the Committee on Growth Hormone Use of the Lawson Wilkins Pediatric Endocrine Society, May, 1985. Degenerative neurologic disease in patients formerly treated with human growth hormone. J Pediatr 107:10–12, 1985.

Van Vliet G, Bosson D, Robyn C: Effect of growth hormone–releasing factor on plasma growth hormone, prolactin and somatomedin C in hypopituitary and short normal children. Horm Res 22(1–2):32–45, 1985.

3 · ACROMEGALY

Lawrence V. Basso
Maurice Fox
PALO ALTO MEDICAL CLINIC

DEFINITION

Excess production of growth hormone leads to overgrowth of bones and soft tissues. When the growth hormone excess occurs after puberty, acromegaly results. If the growth hormone hypersecretion begins prior to epiphyseal fusion, excessive linear growth causes gigantism. Acromegaly accounts for about 15% of all pituitary tumors.

PATHOPHYSIOLOGY

A hypothalamic etiology is supported by the following evidence: (1) In a subset of patients with acromegaly, somatostatin can inhibit growth hormone release. (2) Dopamine agonist drugs such as bromocriptine (Parlodel) also suppress growth hormone production in some patients with acromegaly. (3) Growth hormone–releasing factor secreted ectopically induces the development of growth hormone–secreting pituitary tumors.

CLINICAL ASPECTS AND DIAGNOSTIC CRITERIA

Clinical evaluation has to define the abnormalities caused by the consequences of excess growth hormone, a space-occupying mass in the sella turcica, and possible deficits of other pituitary hormones and their target glands. At diagnosis the pituitary tumor is greater than 1 cm in diameter in 85% of cases. In adults the diagnosis is infrequently made before ten years of the disease state have elapsed. The typical patient is middle-aged. Early findings are quite subtle and feature soft tissue swelling, coarseness of facial features, and acral enlargement. Patients are often unaware of the facial changes until old photographs are used for comparison.

Headache may at times be unrelenting. Arthralgias may progress to severe osteoarthritis involving the hips and shoulders. Cardiomegaly may be associated with congestive heart failure. Some degree of glucose intolerance occurs in 45% of acromegalic patients, but retinopathy and other complications of diabetes are unusual. Hypercalciuria is common, and kidney stones occur. Long-standing acromegaly can eventually result in osteoporosis, as trabecular bone is diminished despite increased cortical bone thickness. Mild hyperphosphatemia, commonly observed, has no known pathophysiologic effects and decreases with treatment.

Amenorrhea and impotence occur because of decreased gonadotropin production. Prolactin levels are elevated in approximately one third of patients, but galactorrhea is relatively uncommon. Hypermetabolism with tests showing normal thyroid function is commonly seen. Hypothyroidism results secondary to loss of thyroid-stimulating hormone (TSH). Very rarely, hypersecretion of TSH by the pituitary gland results in hyperthyroidism. The cell most resistant to loss of function by adjacent pituitary tumor is the corticotroph. Sudden loss of all pituitary function, including growth hormone secretion, happens rarely with infarction of the tumor, causing a serious condition known as pituitary apoplexy. Acromegaly can be seen in association with the familial multiple endocrine neoplasia type 1 syndrome. Tumors producing growth hormone–releasing factor (GRF) with secondary development of either a pituitary adenoma or hyperplasia are very rare and have been described with bronchial carcinoids, pancreatic islet cell tumors, and hypothalamic tumors.

With the advent of high-resolution (1 mm) multiplanar computed tomographic scanning with contrast enhancement and coronal views, intrasellar and suprasellar tumor extension can be measured accurately. This is of particular importance in the patient with visual abnormalities. CT scanning of the pituitary is necessary for appropriate planning of therapy and follow-up after a specific treatment modality has been initiated.

MANAGEMENT

PLAN AND NONPHARMACOLOGIC MANAGEMENT

The goal is reduction of growth hormone levels to the normal range, but safe elimination of the tumor without causing hypopituitarism cannot always be accomplished. Surgical removal via transsphenoidal adenomectomy is the optimum therapy, but transsphenoidal hypophysectomy is often necessary. This procedure is widely available in most community hospitals. Seventy-five per cent of patients achieve normal growth hormone levels immediately after surgery, but larger tumors, especially those with suprasellar extension, frequently recur. Surgical mortality is lower than 1%. Morbidity is also infrequent and includes CSF rhinorrhea, meningitis, sinusitis, nasal-oral fistula, and dental problems. Diabetes insipidus is the most common complication (15% to 20% incidence) and can last from three days to several weeks. Following surgery the long-acting arginine vasopressin derivative desmopressin acetate (dDAVP), given sublingually or intramuscularly, can control polyuria and hypernatremia. The complications of transsphenoidal surgery are directly proportional to the size and erosive properties of the tumor and inversely proportional to the experience of the surgeon. The greatest advantage of surgery is the rapidity with which growth hormone levels can become normal. Transfrontal hypophysectomy is required only in rare cases when there are gross visual field cuts, extensive suprasellar extension, cranial nerve palsies, increased CSF pressure, or erosion of the tumor into the cavernous sinus.

Results of radiation therapy for the patient with acromegaly depend largely upon regional expertise and enthusiasm. Most radiotherapy departments use a supervoltage of 5000 rads delivered uniformly to the pituitary gland over six weeks, taking special care to avoid the eyes and optic nerves. Normal growth hormone levels are reached in 70% of patients in five years and in 80% in five to ten years after completion of therapy. The incidence of hypopituitarism approaches 30%. Experience with heavy-particle or proton-beam irradiation is limited to two centers in the United States. In general the results are similar to supervoltage irradiation, but the entire course of treatment can be completed in just one week. Complications of radiation therapy are rare, fortunately, and they include damage to the optic nerve or innervation of the extraocular muscles and temporal lobe epilepsy due to focal radiation necrosis. The complication rate may be slightly higher with heavy-particle or proton-beam irradiation than with conventional radiation.

Speed in achieving normal growth hormone levels is an important factor in patients with diabetes, congestive heart failure, or severe arthritis. In general, we suggest that transsphenoidal hypophysectomy be the initial treatment of choice. Radiation therapy can always be elected secondarily if the surgeon leaves tumor remnants or if there is a recurrence after the initial surgical procedure. Surgery, on the other hand, becomes extremely difficult after radiation has been given because of tissue changes brought about by radiation therapy. In the authors' experience, about 50% of patients require secondary supervoltage radiation therapy in order to normalize growth hormone levels completely. This is probably because many patients with acromegaly have rather large macroadenomas, making transsphenoidal hypophysectomy only partially effective. Moreover, recurrence of these tumors can be explained by the fact that surgery is aimed only at resection of the pituitary tumor, although the etiology may be hypothalamic.

DRUG THERAPY

Drug therapy has been a major therapeutic disappointment. Levodopa (L-dopa) was the first dopamine agonist shown paradoxically to lower growth hormone levels in patients with acromegaly, but the large doses required made it impractical. Subsequently bromocriptine has been used with variable and controversial success. Those patients who respond with lower growth hormone levels require 20 to 40 mg per day, doses that often produce intolerable side effects including nausea, nasal stuffiness, and postural hypotension. Bromocriptine therapy in the acromegalic patient should be considered as third-line treatment only after transsphenoidal hypophysectomy and radiation therapy have been unsuccessful or only partially successful.

High-dose estrogens have been used in one study to antagonize somatomedin-C levels. In this group of five patients there was no change in growth hormone levels, but somatomedin-C levels were reduced, and there was improvement in metabolic status, with documentation of decreased bone resorption, lower serum phosphate, and a 20% decrease in the fasting blood glucose. This form of therapy is still being investigated. Long-acting derivatives of somatostatin or of GRF may also hold some hope in the future for reducing growth hormone levels in the acromegalic patient.

PERIODIC EVALUATION

Hypopituitarism following surgery generally occurs within several months and tends to be associated with larger pituitary tumors. In contrast, it may take several years to see hypopituitarism following radiation therapy. The incidence of hypopituitarism is about 10% to 15% following surgery and about 30% following radiation therapy. Corticotrophic evaluation using insulin-provoked hypoglycemia and metyrapone is recommended at least yearly following therapeutic intervention. Thyroid evaluation is performed using a free T_4 radioimmunoassay because total T_4 may be spuriously low, related to an effect of growth hormone on T_4 binding to thyroid-binding globulin. Gonadotropin-releasing hormone (GnRH) may be used to evaluate gonadotroph function. Prolactin levels should be checked every six months following therapy in those patients who initially presented with hyperprolactinemia. Following treatment, growth hormone levels should be checked before and after an oral glucose load every six months until they have been normalized. The patient has achieved remission when the growth hormone level is 10 ng per ml or lower and suppresses with glucose to under 5 ng per ml. Failure of thyrotropin-releasing factor (TRF) to elevate growth hormone level in a patient who previously responded to TRF is another signal of remission.

Glucose intolerance may require oral sulfonylurea agents or insulin and improves as the growth hormone level comes into the normal range. Ongoing evaluation of the patient for signs and symptoms of heart failure and hypertension with institution of appropriate therapy is essential. Patients with acromegaly have a 15% to 25% incidence of malignancy, especially colonic cancers, and periodic evaluation for precancerous colonic polyps is indicated. Following stabilization of the patient and documentation that the tumor is in remission, plastic surgical reconstruction of the face, nose, and lower jaw can be carried out safely.

If the etiology of acromegaly is hypothalamic and only the pituitary gland is treated with either irradiation or hypophysectomy, a high recurrence rate would be expected. In actual fact this is not the case. This suggests that either (1) there is not always a hypothalamic factor involved or (2) hypopituitarism is more common following a specific therapeutic intervention than previously recognized and indeed hypopituitarism may be part of the natural history of the disease.

REFERENCES

Eastman RC, Gorden P, Roth J: Conventional supervoltage irradiation is an effective treatment for acromegaly. J Clin Endocrinol Metab 48:931–940, 1979.

Jadresic A, Banks LM, Child DF, et al: The acromegaly syndrome. Q J Med 51:189–204, 1982.

Nelson DH: Growth hormone secreting tumors. In O'Dell WD, Nelson DH (eds): Pituitary Tumors. Futura Publishing Co, Mount Kisco, New York, 1984, pp 209–231.

Wass JAH: Growth hormone neuroregulation and the clinical relevance of somatostatin. Clin Endocrino Metab 12:695–724, 1983.

Williams RA, Jacobs HS, Kurtz AB, et al: The treatment of acromegaly with special reference to trans-sphenoidal hypophysectomy. Q J Med 44:79–98, 1975.

4 · PROLACTINOMA

M. Saeed-uz-Zafar
Raymond C. Mellinger
HENRY FORD HOSPITAL

DEFINITION AND DIAGNOSTIC CRITERIA

Current concepts of the management of prolactinoma, a benign lactotroph cell pituitary tumor, have evolved only over the past 15 years. Diagnosis rests on the demonstration of a persistently increased serum prolactin concentration along with evidence by computer tomography (CT) of a pituitary tumor. Since patients with primary thyroid failure and pregnant women may have hyperprolactinemia and pituitary enlargement, these conditions must be excluded. Diagnosis of prolactinoma is particularly difficult in patients with moderate hyperprolactinemia (100 ng per ml or less) and large pituitary tumors, for hyperprolactinemia in such cases may be a consequence of pressure on the pituitary stalk (pseudoprolactinoma). Ultimately, the diagnosis of prolactinoma requires histochemical evidence.

PATHOPHYSIOLOGY

The hypothalamus exercises control over prolactin synthesis and secretion through the inhibiting influence of dopamine. Pharmacologic agents that are dopamine agonists rapidly reduce prolactin secretion and the size of most prolactinomas. In some patients, hyperprolactinemia may be the result of failure of normal control by dopamine. The frequent recurrence of prolactinomas after successful surgery suggests that hypothalamic dysfunction may also underlie adenoma development by the lactotrophs (proloctin-secreting cells). However, the fact that bromocriptine fails to control either prolactin secretion or tumor growth in some patients suggests the existence of intrinsic abnormalities of the lactotrophs.

CLINICAL PRESENTATION

In addition to galactorrhea in women, increased prolactin secretion commonly causes hypogonadism in either sex. A large prolactinoma may crowd out other pituitary cells, but prolactin excess also alters the secretion of gonadotropins and modifies their effect on sex hormone secretion. Prolactinomas may cause headache and impaired visual fields, but some patients are asymptomatic. In women, tumors are often detected because of amenorrhea, infertility, or galactorrhea. Impairment

of other pituitary function occurs infrequently. In men, pubertal failure, impotence, or infertility are common, but galactorrhea is rare. In fact, males may not recognize symptoms of a prolactinoma until it causes headache, visual impairment, or other disturbances of the endocrine system. Bone demineralization can occur in affected men and women.

EVALUATION

CT can demonstrate pituitary tumors as small as 3 mm, disclose any suprasellar extension, or reveal features of the "empty sella syndrome." Those tumors smaller than 1 cm are termed microadenomas, and larger tumors are macroadenomas. In men, prolactinomas are usually large by the time of diagnosis, and a plain lateral radiograph, although not adequate to demonstrate a suprasellar tumor, may suffice for their demonstration. Although frequently recommended, comprehensive anterior pituitary evaluation is unnecessary unless the tumor is very large or there is evidence of hypothalamic encroachment. Hyposecretion of anterior pituitary hormones other than gonadotropins is very rare in these patients. Similarly, evaluation of visual fields is necessary only with suspected suprasellar extension. Tests to stimulate or suppress the elevated prolactin levels provide no additional information, but a serum prolactin level above 200 ng per dl strongly supports the diagnosis of prolactinoma rather than idiopathic hyperprolactinemia or pseudoprolactinoma.

MANAGEMENT

The natural history of these tumors is not known with certainty; some may enlarge very slowly. Even without treatment, prolactin levels may return to normal after a number of years, but we are not aware of any patient in whom residual prolactinoma after surgery resolved spontaneously.

Treatment goals are (1) elimination or reduction of tumor mass, (2) correction of hyperprolactinemia, (3) restoration of secondary hormone deficiencies, and (4) prevention of recurrence.

Methods of treatment include bromocriptine (Parlodel), transsphenoidal adenomectomy (TSA), and pituitary irradiation.

NONPHARMACOLOGIC MEASURES

Surgery. Experience with TSA for prolactinoma is extensive. With this procedure, microadenomas can be removed totally, serum prolactin levels returned to normal, and impaired pituitary function restored. Initial cure rates of 80% for microadenomas are reported from some centers, and the rate seems to vary inversely with the serum prolactin level. Only about 20% of patients with macroadenomas and a serum prolactin level exceeding 500 ng per dl have normal serum prolactin concentration after TSA. Moreover, 50% of microadenomas and 80% of macroadenomas are reported to recur within four years. Despite misgivings about long-term benefits, surgical adenomectomy may be indicated in (1) patients with severe headaches or visual impairment (particularly during pregnancy), (2) those who fail to respond to or cannot tolerate pharmacologic therapy, (3) those who prefer surgical treatment, and (4) those

with microadenomas who have a high probability of surgical remission.

The major preoperative decisions are the optimal timing and extent of surgery. Assessment of the response to bromocriptine is an essential part of this evaluation, since the response may be so satisfactory that surgery can be avoided. Very rarely, while the serum prolactin level normalizes with bromocriptine, the prolactinoma enlarges. Patients who fail to respond to pharmacologic agents may require near-total hypophysectomy. In women who anticipate pregnancy, planned surgical adenomectomy may be postponed until a few months before conception. After surgery, persistent hyperprolactinemia should be controlled with bromocriptine. Even patients in biochemical and clinical remission need to have their serum prolactin level determined annually. Additional CT scanning is not indicated in the absence of symptoms if the prolactin concentration remains normal.

Adrenal steroids, which are often administered postoperatively by the surgeon, can usually be tapered after five to seven days without encountering adrenal insufficiency. Transient diabetes insipidus and abnormalities of thirst are frequent after TSA. Antidiuretic hormone (ADH) deficiency, with characteristic polyuria and polydipsia, commonly occurs 12 to 24 hours after surgery. In some patients a disturbance of thirst sensation independent of ADH secretion causes polydipsia or hypodipsia, and in others the syndrome of inappropriate ADH secretion (SIADH) may develop one to two weeks postoperatively. Postoperative ADH deficiency may require desmopressin (dDAVP), 2 to 4 μg subcutaneously every 12 to 24 hours.

Anterior pituitary function is changed little by TSA. Serum cortisol should nonetheless be measured after withdrawal of adrenal steroids since some patients encounter adrenal insufficiency. The need for adrenal steroids should be proved and never assumed. Patients with prolonged ADH deficiency must be taught the interpretation of thirst and polyuria and the indications for intranasal administration of dDAVP. Persistent hypogonadism must be treated with sex steroids. Postoperative cerebrospinal fluid rhinorrhea, an uncommon sequela of transsphenoidal adenomectomy, should be corrected surgically to avoid potentially fatal meningitis.

Radiation. If the serum prolactin level remains elevated, treatment with bromocriptine or radiation or both is indicated. Pituitary irradiation does not achieve prompt reduction of prolactin secretion but may have delayed effects. Significantly lowered prolactin levels have been observed some years after high-voltage radiation. At present, such therapy is adjunctive to bromocriptine treatment or is administered after surgery because remission is incomplete. Infrequently, radiation is administered to a patient who is unresponsive to bromocriptine and refuses TSA. Older patients with large tumors may benefit from radiation, especially if there are no local symptoms. Although radiation therapy may impair pituitary function, this complication has not been reported after radiotherapy for prolactinoma.

DRUG THERAPY

Bromocriptine, a semisynthetic ergot alkaloid, inhibits prolactin secretion by normal lactotrophs as well

as by prolactinomas. The most commonly used therapy for almost all patients with hyperprolactinemia, bromocriptine, usually reduces prolactin secretion and causes a rapid decrease in tumor size, which is the result of decreased cell volume.

Treatment is initiated at a dose of 1.25 mg given with food at bedtime. If well tolerated, the dose is increased in a stepwise fashion every two to three days to a total of 5 or 7.5 mg in divided doses daily. Further increases are made until a normal prolactin concentration is achieved. Maximum dose rarely exceeds 20 mg, but higher amounts have been used. Ninety per cent of patients respond with a normal serum prolactin level, restoration of menses, or sexual potency. Fertility is achieved in 90% of women able to tolerate the drug, and only a rare patient is unresponsive. If hyperprolactinemia is readily brought under control, CT need not be repeated for a year unless headaches or visual impairment are encountered. Men with secondary hypogonadism may require supplemental testosterone indefinitely despite control of hyperprolactinemia.

Although the manufacturer admits to a 68% incidence of adverse symptoms, these side effects generally do not prevent effective therapy. Some patients experience intolerable nausea from the drug, but no other effective medication is available in the United States. Headache, dizziness and fatigue, abdominal cramps, nasal congestion, constipation or diarrhea, and palpitations have all been reported. Severe postural hypotension occurs very rarely, and Raynaud's phenomenon has been observed. Alcohol ingestion is said to increase the incidence of side effects.

Since many patients with a prolactinoma seek treatment for infertility, the possible teratogenic effects of bromocriptine is a concern. However, a review of nearly 2000 pregnant women taking bromocriptine at the time of conception showed that the incidence of fetal abnormalities was not increased. Infertile patients are instructed to have three regular menstrual periods before attempting to conceive, and bromocriptine is discontinued as soon as pregnancy is diagnosed.

The most important risk of pregnancy for a woman with prolactinoma is enlargement of the tumor, which can occur when prolactin secretion is physiologically stimulated by estrogen. Serious enlargement of microadenomas during pregnancy occurs in less than 1% of patients but has been reported in 20% of those with macroadenomas and suprasellar extension. In the latter cases, TSA is recommended before pregnancy is undertaken, although attempts to reduce the adenoma with medical therapy seem reasonable. When an enlarging prolactinoma causes headaches or visual impairment, bromocriptine treatment is reinstituted. A number of patients have received the drug throughout pregnancy and delivered normal infants. If tumor enlargement cannot be controlled, TSA, abortion, or induced delivery are therapeutic options.

Bromocriptine cannot be resumed post partum if breast feeding is planned for the newborn. Should lactation, persistent amenorrhea, and elevated prolactin levels continue after weaning, bromocriptine therapy is resumed.

PATIENT INFORMATION AND EDUCATION

Patients must be reassured that a prolactinoma is a benign tumor. The mechanism of the symptoms must be explained to provide the necessary background for choosing among treatment options. The patient should be informed that although a microadenoma per se may require no treatment, secondary hypogonadism is associated with significant sequelae. The patient should know that despite the possibility of an early cure through surgery, the chance of recurrence is strong. Complications of surgery, radiation, or pharmacologic therapy must be described in detail, and the patient must be informed that effective medical treatment probably will be required indefinitely. In every case, the need for periodic evaluation of pituitary function is lifelong.

Patient compliance is excellent if therapy is successful and side effects are not severe. Women who are inclined to neglect treatment, considering hyperprolactinemia a natural means of birth control, must be advised against this course.

SOCIOECONOMIC ASPECTS

The management of prolactinoma is never inexpensive. Bromocriptine is costly, and prolonged treatment is usually needed. Neither pituitary irradiation nor TSA is inexpensive. Furthermore, none of these treatments is reliably curative, and none obviates the need for long-term periodic evaluation.

REFERENCES

Grossman A, Cohen BL, Charlesworth M, et al: Treatment of prolactinomas with megavoltage radiotherapy. Br Med J 288:1105–1109, 1984.

Hardy J, Beauregard H: Prolactin-secreting adenomas: transsphenoidal microsurgical treatment. *In* Robyn C, Harter M (eds): Progress in Prolactin Physiology and Pathology. Elsevier-North Holland Biomedical Press, Amsterdam, 1978, pp 361–370.

Serri O, Rasio E, Beauregard H, et al: Recurrence of hyperprolactinemia after selective transsphenoidal adenomectomy in women with prolactinoma. N Engl J Med 309:280–283, 1983.

Vance ML, Evans WS, Thorner MO: Bromocriptine. Ann Intern Med 100:78–91, 1984.

Zafar MS, Rogers S, Boulos R, et al: Enlargement of prolactinoma despite normal prolactin levels during bromocriptine therapy. Proceedings, IV International Congress on Prolactin, Charlottesville, NC 1984, p 153.

5 · HYPOTHYROIDISM

Paul F. Gilliland
SCOTT AND WHITE CLINIC

DEFINITION AND DIAGNOSTIC CRITERIA

Hypothyroidism is the clinical state that occurs as a consequence of an inadequate amount of thyroid hormone at the cellular level. The diagnosis is established by demonstrating a subnormal level of "free" thyroxine (T_4), measured directly or derived mathematically from serum T_4 and resin triiodothyronine (T_3) uptake.

PATHOPHYSIOLOGY

Inadequate production of thyroid hormone may arise from defects within the thyroid (primary), pituitary (secondary), or hypothalamus (tertiary). When caused by Hashimoto's thyroiditis, primary hypothyroidism may be infrequently associated with other autoimmune endocrine deficiency states, including adrenal insufficiency. By contrast, secondary hypothyroidism frequently occurs in conjunction with impaired secretion of other pituitary hormones.

CLINICAL ASPECTS

Most patients seek medical attention early in the course of the disease, when the clinical findings are minimal and nonspecific. A high index of suspicion should be directed at individuals with a personal or family history of thyroid disease or surgery, radioactive iodine therapy, radiation therapy to the head or neck, or pituitary disease. Because the likelihood of coexisting adrenal insufficiency is much higher in secondary and tertiary hypothyroidism, it is very important to distinguish these types from primary hypothyroidism.

MANAGEMENT

PLAN

The goal is to replace thyroid hormone safely in a dose that approximates normal endogenous production. Most people can be treated on an outpatient basis, but hospitalization is mandatory if the patient has myxedema coma.

DRUG THERAPY

Synthetic levothyroxine sodium (L-T_4) (Synthroid, Levothroid) is considered the drug of choice by most endocrinologists. Because of a plasma half-life of seven days, the occasional omission of a dose does not significantly alter plasma levels. Synthetic L-T_4, like endogenous T_4, is converted to T_3 at extrathyroidal sites. A free T_4 level or index correlates well with the metabolic status of treated patients and varies little with the time of sampling in relation to the dose. Because bioavailability varies, the use of generic L-T_4 is not recommended; in fact, the two name-brand products also are probably not interchangeable.

The usual daily replacement dosage of synthetic L-T_4 is 0.1 to 0.15 mg for adults. Rare patients may require as little as 0.05 mg or 0.075 mg; equally rare are those who require 0.2 to 0.4 mg. As a general rule, elderly patients need a smaller dosage. In young adults or juveniles free of other disease, treatment can be started with the full replacement dosage in contrast to patients with known heart disease or diabetes mellitus or those who are older than 40 years. In these patients, I start with 0.025 mg per day and increase by increments of 0.025 mg per day every two weeks until the full replacement dosage is reached.

Synthetic liothyronine sodium (L-T_3) (Cytomel) has a comparatively rapid onset of clinical effects of one to three days. Serum T_3 varies markedly according to the time of sampling in relation to hormone ingestion because of rapid absorption and fast degradation. These features make it very difficult to monitor the dosage, and patients may have transient symptoms of thyrotoxicosis several hours after ingestion of the medication. If several doses are forgotten, the patient may develop symptoms of hypothyroidism. For these reasons, L-T_3 is not recommended for long-term management of hypothyroidism.

Preparations containing both L-T_4 and L-T_3 (Thyrolar, Euthroid) were marketed when it was not known that T_4 is converted to T_3 at extrathyroidal sites. Some patients have symptoms of transient thyrotoxicosis several hours after ingestion of this medication because of rapid absorption of the T_3 component. When the patient is taking these combination preparations, routine thyroid tests do not correlate well with metabolic status. There is no longer a rationale for using these agents.

Thyroid USP is derived from thyroid glands of domestic animals slaughtered for human consumption. Since the former United States Pharmacopeia (USP) standards required only an assay for organic iodide but not for biologic potency, previous preparations contained varying amounts of T_4 and T_3. There were well-documented instances of thyroid USP preparations that were essentially devoid of biologic activity. New USP standards, effective January 1985, require chromatographic assay of the T_4 and T_3 content, and although this should result in a more consistent preparation, its use is not recommended for the same reasons pertinent to synthetic T_4 and T_3 combinations. This also applies to purified thyroglobulin (Proloid), which is derived from hog thyroid glands.

Excessive dosage may produce thyrotoxicosis. Inadequate dosage due to use of a poor preparation or incorrect judgment results in an incomplete remission of hypothyroidism.

The coexistence of angina pectoris and hypothyroidism is an especially difficult problem because treatment for hypothyroidism can increase myocardial oxygen demand and result in myocardial infarction or fatal arrhythmia, even if the thyroid dosage is subnormal. Coronary artery bypass surgery has been advocated in these patients before the institution of L-T_4 therapy.

In a patient with suspected adrenal insufficiency, therapy should be withheld pending evaluation, since treatment can precipitate addisonian crisis.

The catabolism of vitamin K–dependent clotting factors increases with L-T_4 therapy, resulting in an enhanced anticoagulant effect from warfarin and its derivatives. Unless studies have been done to determine the effect of hypothyroidism on the pharmacokinetics of specific drugs, one should assume that the metabolism of the drug might be increased by the institution of thyroid therapy, so that increased dosage of the drug, such as digoxin, may be required.

Complications. Coma is a life-threatening complication that may occur when a patient with myxedema is subjected to trauma, opiates, or infection. Treatment with intravenous thyroid hormone is mandatory because the mortality rate with oral administration is approximately 90%. The use of L-T_4 is recommended because a parenteral preparation is commercially available. A single dose of 0.5 mg L-T_4 is given to replete the peripheral thyroid pool. Intramuscular injection is not recommended because absorption in the face of hypotension is unpredictable. Approximately half of the predicted daily oral replacement dose is given IV on a daily basis until the patient is alert and well enough to take the medications PO, usually three to six days. The severe physiologic and metabolic defects that may accompany myxedema coma, such as hypoventilation, hypotension, hypothermia, dilutional hyponatremia, hypoglycemia, and hypoadrenocorticism due to coexisting primary or secondary adrenal insufficiency, require supportive therapy.

PERIODIC EVALUATION

If pretreatment laboratory data are unavailable, the only way to determine whether a treated patient is incapable of producing adequate amounts of thyroid hormone is to discontinue the thyroid preparation and obtain a serum T_4 six weeks later. Sometimes a patient may provide historical information that is sufficiently convincing to avoid cessation of therapy, such as an improvement in symptoms starting several weeks after institution of therapy and a return of hypothyroid symptoms several weeks after previous cessation of therapy. On the other hand, continuation of therapy is rarely harmful, even if the patient never had hypothyroidism, providing the dosage is not excessive.

When the patient is treated with T_4, an assay of free T_4 is routinely used to monitor therapy. The value should be in the upper one fourth of normal range or just above normal. If the patient has primary hypothyroidism, the proper dosage of T_4 should reduce thyroid-stimulating hormone (TSH) to the normal range. Traditional TSH assays are not sufficiently sensitive to detect excessive dosage of thyroxine, but new, highly sensitive TSH assays can be used to detect an excessive or insufficient replacement dosage in patients with primary hypothyroidism.

PATIENT EDUCATION AND COST

The patient should be advised that lifelong therapy is expected. Forgetting several doses produces few if any symptoms, so that the patient has no feedback to serve as a reminder that medication has been forgotten. It is advisable for the patient to take a dose at the same time each day so that taking L-T_4 becomes a habit, but it makes no difference what time of day the tablet is ingested. Fortunately, Synthroid 0.1-mg tablets are sold for 12¢ each, which amounts to only $3.60 for a one-month supply.

REFERENCES

Blum M: Myxedema coma. Am J Med Sci 264:432, 1972.
DeGroot LJ, Larsen PR, Refetoff S, et al: Adult hypothyroidism. *In* DeGroot LJ (ed): The Thyroid and Its Diseases, 5th ed. New York, John Wiley & Sons, 1984, pp 585–595.
Hennesey JV, Burman KD, Wartofsky L: The equivalency of two L-thyroxine preparations. Ann Intern Med 102:770–773, 1985.
Holvoet G, Gillebert TC, Piessens J, et al: Coronary artery surgery in patients with myxoedema. Acta Cardiol (Brux) 9:139–145, 1984.
Mangini RJ (ed): Drug Interaction Facts. Applied Therapeutics, San Francisco, 1983, pp 43, 95, 363.
Sawin DT, Herman T, Molitch M, et al: Aging and the thyroid. Am J Med 75:206–209, 1983.

6 · HYPERTHYROIDISM

Thomas F. Nikolai
MARSHFIELD CLINIC

Hyperthyroidism is the excess production of thyroid hormones by the thyroid gland. Thyrotoxicosis is the condition in which there is an excess of thyroid hormone action, either of exogenous or endogenous source. Treatment of thyrotoxicosis or hyperthyroidism is related to the correct diagnosis and classification as outlined in Table 1.

DIFFUSE TOXIC GOITER (GRAVES' DISEASE)

Graves' disease is a syndrome that includes hyperthyroidism, exophthalmus, pretibial myxedema, and acropachy in different combinations. Pretibial myxedema and acropachy almost never occur unless significant exophthalmus is present. Exophthalmus occurs in only about half the patients with hyperthyroidism but may occur alone.

The clinician and the patient have a choice of three commonly used forms of treatment, each being effective but all having drawbacks. These include thionamides, radioactive iodine, and near-total thyroidectomy. These treatments may be supplemented in some cases by adrenergic blocking agents, iodine, and other drugs.

NONPHARMOCOLOGIC MEASURES

Radioactive Iodine Therapy. Radioactive iodine (^{131}I) has become the treatment of choice for many clinicians because it is very effective, easily administered, and almost devoid of side effects except for a high incidence of hypothyroidism. The fear that ^{131}I-induced tumors, leukemia, and genetic damage will occur has been dispelled. ^{131}I therapy in children has not induced cancers, and no reproductive difficulties, other health problems, or congenital abnormalities in their offspring have occurred later in life.

A 20% to 50% incidence of hypothyroidism occurs within the first year after therapy, increasing another 2% to 3% annually thereafter. This complication is easily recognized and treated, so that this rarely leads to problems later in life except in those who do not take replacement therapy. Thyroid storm has been reported rarely after ^{131}I therapy.

Radioactive iodine therapy is contraindicated in pregnancy. Therefore, all women of childbearing age should have a highly sensitive pregnancy test done before being given such therapy. A total dose of 6 to 15 mCi ^{131}I is usually given. Total dose is calculated by the following equation: the size of the thyroid in grams ×

Table 1. CLASSIFICATION OF THYROTOXICOSIS ACCORDING TO RADIOACTIVE IODINE UPTAKE

Elevated iodine uptake
  Diffuse toxic goiter (Graves' disease)
  Toxic multinodular goiter (Plummer's disease)
  TSH induced
    TSH-producing pituitary adenoma
    Partial pituitary resistance to thyroid hormone
    Acromegaly
Malignancy
  Trophoblastic tumor
  Embryonal testicular tumor
Neonatal hyperthyroidism—maternal transplacental transfer of
  thyroid-stimulating immunoglobulin
Supressed iodine uptake
  Thyroiditis
    Silent (lymphocytic thyroiditis with spontaneously resolving
      hyperthyroidism)
    Subacute thyroiditis (deQuervain's)
  Excessive ingestion of thyroid hormone
    Iatrogenic
    Factitious
  Iodine induced (jodbasedow)
  Metastatic follicular carcinoma of thyroid
  Struma ovarii

0.1 mCi ^{131}I per gram × 100 over the percentage of the ^{131}I uptake. Patients with severe heart disease, severe hyperthyroidism, and other serious illness are best treated with larger doses of ^{131}I to ensure that the first dose controls the hyperthyroidism. About 5% to 10% of patients require more than one dose, a few patients being extremely resistant and needing up to five doses for control.

As it usually takes two to four months to gain control of hyperthyroidism after ^{131}I therapy, patients with severe hyperthyroidism and other illness also need beta-adrenergic blockers, thionamides, or both. Patients should be followed with serum thyroid tests at one- to three-month intervals, depending on the severity of the illness. Once hypothyroidism has developed, it is almost always permanent, and lifelong thyroid replacement is needed.

Surgery. Subtotal thyroidectomy is also an effective and relatively safe therapy for hyperthyroidism. Patients should be rendered euthyroid with thionamides or pretreated with beta-adrenergic blockers to prevent postoperative thyroid storm, although the latter used alone has resulted in a few cases of thyroid storm. After control of the hyperthyroidism is achieved preoperatively, iodine in the form of a saturated solution of potassium iodide is given as two to three drops t.i.d. for seven to ten days to reduce the vascularity of the gland before surgery while continuing the thionamides.

The major problems of subtotal thyroidectomy include hypothyroidism, recurrent laryngeal nerve injury with vocal cord paralysis, hypoparathyroidism, and recurrent hyperthyroidism. Hypothyroidism is very common, varying from 20% to 30% within the first two years after surgery. Thereafter, a slow rate continues, generally related to the size of the thyroid remnant and the frequent occurrence of autoimmune lymphocytic thyroiditis. With an experienced surgeon, there is no more than a 1% incidence of permanent postoperative hypoparathyroidism. Transient postoperative hypocalcemia is much more common and may require oral calcium, 2 to 4 gm daily for several weeks, to prevent

tetanic symptoms. Vocal cord paralysis occurs at a rate of one in 500 to 1000. This is almost always unilateral and is due to inadvertent damage to the recurrent laryngeal nerve or its blood supply. There is moderate hoarseness and weakness of the voice, which often improves with time. No treatment is generally required unless the paralysis is bilateral.

DRUG THERAPY

Antithyroid Drugs. Multiple thionamides are available throughout the world, but only propylthiouracil (PTU) and methimazole (Tapazole) are used in the United States. These drugs work by blocking organification of iodide and are not influenced by the degree of iodine uptake. PTU (but not methimazole) also blocks peripheral T_4 to T_3 conversion, an additive effect in decreasing serum T_3 levels in hyperthyroidism. An additional effect of these drugs in Graves' disease is a decrease in circulating thyroid-stimulating immunoglobulin (TSI) levels.

A dose of 300 to 400 mg daily of PTU, or 30 to 40 mg per day of methimazole in two to four divided doses, is effective, but doses twice as large should be started when severe hyperthyroidism or large goiters are present. If initial treatment is effective, there is usually a dramatic reduction in serum T_4 and T_3 levels within two to four weeks, and levels may normalize within one to two months. Some physicians combine PTU and L-thyroxine in doses of 75 to 150 μg daily at this point, especially in patients with large goiters, to prevent TSH production and further increase in thyroid size. Failure to respond within two to four weeks is an indication to increase the dose by 50% to 100%. With an effective response, these drugs are continued for 12 to 18 months. The dose can be decreased by 50% at one- to three-month intervals as long as a stable and normal level of T_4 is maintained.

Adverse reactions to thionamides occur in up to 10% of treated patients. The most severe reaction, agranulocytosis, occurs in about five of 1000 treated cases and may be heralded by fever, sore throat, skin rash, or malaise.

Thionamides are most often used in children, in pregnant women, and to prepare hyperthyroid patients for thyroidectomy. There appears to be a subset of patients identified by positive TSI titers and HLA-DR3 antigen who predictably relapse within one year after PTU therapy. Those with small goiters and mild hyperthyroidism have less chance of relapse after PTU.

Beta-Adrenergic Blockers. Although some of the symptoms and signs of hyperthyroidism are decreased and the patient feels improved after taking beta-adrenergic blockers, the basic abnormality in hyperthyroidism is not changed. Atenolol is given in a once-daily dose of 50 to 200 mg or propranolol in divided daily doses of 40 to 200 mg, the former being advantageous because it can be taken once daily and has fewer side effects.

Corticosteroids. Corticosteroid therapy causes a rapid alleviation of thyrotoxicosis by an unknown mechanism different from that of PTU and iodides and also by inhibiting peripheral T_4 to T_3 conversion. Corticosteroids need only be used in severe thyrotoxicosis with impending or actual thyroid storm.

Other Therapy. Other drugs such as reserpine and

guanethidine have long been used as supplemental therapy for hyperthyroidism and in thyroid storm, but now are usually replaced by beta-adrenoreceptor blockers.

Iodine is best used as adjunctive therapy in thyroid storm (see below) and to prepare patients for thyroid surgery, since the thyroid escapes from its effects within a few weeks. Usually much more is given than necessary, which only increases the chance of side effects.

Lithium carbonate is quite effective in thyrotoxicosis, inhibiting secretion from the thyroid. A dose of 600 to 1200 mg daily is used, achieving serum levels of 0.5 to 1 mEq/L.

OPHTHALMOPATHY

The ophthalmopathy of Graves' disease varies from just barely discernible to severe changes that result in optic neuritis and blindness. Protective glasses with colored lenses and side shields are often needed. Elevation of the head of the bed may reduce orbital edema. Artificial tears should be used liberally and regularly if corneal exposure appears excessive. Corticosteroid therapy provides dramatic relief in severe exophthalmus, using doses of prednisone in the 20- to 40-mg range initially with gradual tapering for a three- to six-month course. More severe ocular involvement requires larger daily doses of prednisone, 80 to 120 mg, tapering rapidly during the first two to four weeks to 40 to 60 mg and then gradually for a four- to eight-month course.

Orbital radiation up to 2000 rads focused on the retro-orbital contents to avoid the eye and the putuitary is also effective in the more severe forms. Surgical decompression by the transantral route is used for severe residual exophthalmus and as an emergency procedure when papilledema and rapid visual loss occur. A common complication of this procedure is diplopia, which may require later correction by eye muscle surgery.

PRETIBIAL MYXEDEMA (DERMOPATHY)

Spontaneous resolution may occur in pretibial myxedema. In most instances no therapy is indicated except for cosmetic reasons. The most effective treatment is intralesional corticosteroid injection or topical corticosteroid creams with occlusive dressing and follow-up at two- to four-week intervals.

THYROID ACROPACHY

No treatment is indicated for thyroid acropachy, nor has any been shown to be effective.

TOXIC MULTINODULAR GOITER (PLUMMER'S DISEASE)

The hyperthyroidism resulting from toxic multinodular goiter is due to multiple autonomous functioning nodules. Autonomy of function appears to be the end result of long-standing nontoxic, multinodular goiter in about 10% of patients. The symptoms and signs of thyrotoxicosis develop insidiously over years.

Thyroid levels generally are less elevated than in Graves' disease. The thyroidal uptake of iodine is quite variable, often being in the high-normal range and rarely in the high ranges seen in Graves' disease.

Radioactive iodine appears to be the ideal therapy for toxic multinodular goiter; larger doses, 10 to 30 mCi, are required. PTU is effective but does not result in permanent remission. Surgery is also effective but often contraindicated because many of the affected patients are elderly with many other medical problems. Surgery is probably best used to debulk extremely large goiters, to relieve obstructive neck and thoracic inlet conditions, and to resolve the question of malignancy in rapidly growing nodules.

TOXIC UNINODULAR GOITER

Only about 2% to 3% or less of all cases of hyperthyroidism are due to a single "hot" nodule. The "hot" nodule rarely causes hyperthyroidism unless it is larger than 2.5 to 3 cm. Only about 5% to 10% of euthyroid "hot" nodules progress to hyperthyroidism in five to ten years.

Treatment of toxic uninodular goiter consists of either ^{131}I therapy or surgical excision. The former is effective in ablating the hyperfunctioning nodule, although a small residual nodule is often left; the dose required is 15 to 30 mCi. Surgery removes the hyperfunctioning nodule and one need not worry about a residual nodule.

OTHER CAUSES OF HIGH RADIOACTIVE IODINE UPTAKE (RAIU) THYROTOXICOSIS

A thyroid stimulator other than TSH, human chorionic gonadotropin (hCG), has been shown to cause mild hyperthyroidism in some patients with molar pregnancy, choriocarcinoma, and testicular embryonal carcinoma. Treatment consists of ablation of the primary tumor or of the thyroid.

Excess TSH secretion from a pituitary adenoma or in a syndrome called "partial pituitary resistance to thyroid hormone" also causes hyperthyroidism. Treatment consists of removal of the pituitary tumor in the former and ablation of the thyroid by ^{131}I or surgery in the latter.

Maternal transplacental transfer of TSI results in transient hyperthyroidism in newborn infants of mothers with active or inactive Graves' disease who have appreciable serum titers of TSI.

LOW RADIOACTIVE IODINE UPTAKE THYROTOXICOSIS

Iatrogenic thyrotoxicosis is easily corrected by reducing the dose of thyroid hormone by about 15% to 25%, rechecking thyroid function in two to four weeks, and continuing to readjust the dosage until correction has been achieved. Some physicians prefer to stop thyroid hormone for three to five days before starting the patient on reduced doses.

Factitious thyrotoxicosis, the surreptitious ingestion of thyroid hormone, is uncommon and extremely hard to uncover. Patients usually have psychiatric illness and are often related to the medical profession, e.g., physicians, physicians' wives, nurses, and other paramedical personnel.

Silent thyroiditis is also known as lymphocytic thyroiditis with spontaneously resolving hyperthyroidism and painless thyroiditis. These patients have typical symptoms and signs of thyrotoxicosis, a suppressed RAIU, little or no thyroid pain or tenderness, and a normal or only slightly enlarged thyroid gland. The incidence varies from rare to 20% of all cases of thyrotoxicosis in different areas of the U.S. A similar syndrome called postpartum thyroiditis occurs within one to six months of delivery. Sedatives, tranquilizers, and beta-adrenergic blockers relieve symptoms in those with mild to moderate thyrotoxicosis. Prednisone for one month reduces the thyrotoxic phase to one to two weeks. Relapse does not occur, but 10% to 15% of patients have recurrent episodes of silent thyroiditis one to three years apart.

Subacute thyroiditis is easily recognized, since all patients with thyrotoxicosis have a moderately or markedly tender thyroid gland and an elevation of the sedimentation rate above 50 mm per hour. Aspirin or other nonsteroidal anti-inflammatory drugs control mild cases, but prednisone should be used in those not responding to this therapy or in severe disease. Beta-blocking drugs often control symptoms of transient hyperthyroidism.

IODINE-INDUCED THYROTOXICOSIS (JODBASEDOW)

In some patients, small doses of iodine induce thyrotoxicosis, which usually disappears after the iodine source is discontinued. This form of thyrotoxicosis was first found in people with multinodular goiters in iodine-deficient areas, but is now recognized to occur even in iodine-sufficient areas and in people without thyroid disease. To prevent it, iodine treatment should not be given for nontoxic goiters, since there is no actual iodine deficiency in our society now.

SPECIAL CONDITIONS

THYROTOXICOSIS IN PREGNANCY

Hyperthyroidism in pregnancy is uncommon. It occurs in only about one of 2000 pregnancies and is almost always due to Graves' disease. There is a slight increase in neonatal mortality, low-birth-weight infants, and possibly increased fetal wastage.

Treatment for thyrotoxicosis during pregnancy consists of either subtotal thyroidectomy during the first and second trimesters or thionamide therapy throughout pregnancy. Thionamides or propranolol can be used to prepare a pregnant patient for thyroid surgery. They should be titrated carefully during pregnancy, keeping the free thyroxine index in the upper range of normal or slightly elevated, since these agents cross the placenta and may affect the fetal thyroid.

THYROID STORM

Thyroid storm is a life-threatening condition, usually with markedly increased levels of thyroid hormone, that appears to be precipitated in hyperthyroid patients by acute stress, surgery, or infection. Patients develop manic behavior, marked tachycardia, high fever, extreme restlessness, heart failure, confusion, and marked weight loss. When thyroid storm is recognized, patients must be hospitalized immediately and aggressive therapy instituted. Treatment consists of iodine, propranolol, corticosteroids, thyroid blockers, oxygen, and IV fluids. PTU should be started at least one hour before iodine to prevent use of the iodine to produce more thyroid hormone. If heart failure is present, diuretics and digitalis are also needed. Aspirin should not be used, as it displaces T_4 from albumin and may actually worsen the condition. PTU is given initially in massive doses, 900 to 1200 mg daily, PO or by stomach tube, if necessary, followed by 600 to 1000 mg daily in divided doses. We give iodine in the form of SSKI, ten drops PO three times a day, or as sodium or potassium iodine, 1 g IV every six to eight hours. Propranolol should be given PO, 40 to 80 mg q.i.d., or IV, 1 mg per min for a total dose of 2 to 10 mg and repeated every three to four hours. Routine measures should be used to control the high fever. Most patients show a dramatic response within 24 to 48 hours.

REFERENCES

Dunn JT: Choice of therapy in young adults with hyperthyroidism of Graves' disease. Ann Intern Med 100:891–893, 1984.

Hamilton CR Jr, Maloof F: Unusual types of hyperthyroidism. Medicine 52:195–215, 1973.

Nikolai TF, Coombs GJ, McKenzie AK, et al: Treatment of lymphocytic thyroiditis with spontaneously resolving hyperthyroidism (silent throiditis). Arch Intern Med 142:2281–2283, 1982.

Utiger RD: Treatment of Graves' disease. N Engl J Med 298:681–682, 1978.

Volpé R: The pathogenesis of Graves' disease: an overview. Clin Endocrinol Metab 7:3–29, 1978.

7 · GOITER AND THE SINGLE THYROID NODULE

Neal M. Friedman
LOVELACE MEDICAL CENTER

Evaluation of a thyroid nodule or other goitrous enlargement poses a diagnostic challenge. Approximately 4 % of the general population in the United States will have at least one palpable thyroid nodule. The key question is whether a patient could have thyroid cancer, which fortunately is usually of low virulence and curable if treated early. Many other thyroid abnormalities cause nodules that may not require treatment.

PATHOPHYSIOLOGY

The most common goiter is a nontoxic multinodular gland. Iodine deficiency was once the most common etiology, but iodination of salt has made this a rare problem in most developed areas of the world. The most common etiology today is chronic thyroiditis. Multinodular goiters arise from the multiplication of heterogeneously functioning epithelial cells that then form new follicles of rapidly dividing cells. A degree of autonomy of growth or function occurs in each thyroid follicle, which may eventually form a nodule as it enlarges. Thyroid-stimulating hormone or growth-stimulating immunoglobulins may be the trophic factors.

CLINICAL ASPECTS

As with any clinical problem, the most important facts come directly from the patient. Important historical points include family history, radiation exposure, length of time that the thyroid has been enlarged or enlarging, pain, change in voice, or difficulty breathing or swallowing. Ingestion of goitrogens should be asked about, including foods in the cabbage family, lithium, and high-dose iodides, such as those found in water purification tablets. Symptoms of hypo- or hyperthyroidism should be sought.

The thyroid and neck should be carefully inspected and palpated. When examining the thyroid gland, the physician should stand directly behind the patient, who should be seated in a comfortable position. The patient should then swallow a sip of water, and, as the thyroid moves, the isthmus and both lobes should be carefully palpated with both hands. Single and prominent nodules should be carefully measured and documented. A search should be made for signs of thyroid dysfunction.

Nodules less than 1 cm in diameter are rarely malignant and need only periodic observation. All nodules greater than 1 cm in diameter in a functional patient of any age should be evaluated as described subsequently to exclude carcinoma. High-risk individuals can be directly considered for surgical biopsy. This is especially true in patients with a solitary nodule and previous thyroid irradiation exposure or otherwise unexplained cervical lymphadenopathy. Young males should also be considered at high risk.

Patients with a family history of multiple endocrine neoplasia type II should be evaluated for medullary carcinoma, which may present as a nodule or a diffuse goiter. Dynamic testing of calcitonin should be performed with either calcium or pentagastrin, and total thyroidectomy should be performed if any abnormal elevation occurs.

The following discussion applies to patients who have a normally functioning thyroid gland with a single nodule, a multinodular goiter in which there is one prominent nodule, or a goiter with a high suspicion of cancer.

MANAGEMENT

THYROID SCAN AND ULTRASONOGRAPHY

Thyroid scanning with either technetium or ^{123}I has been the most frequently used test in recent decades despite growing evidence that radionuclide scanning is a poor predictor of carcinoma. Nodules are categorized on scan as being hot, warm, or cold. Hot nodules are rarely malignant, although nodules that are hot by technetium scan but cold by ^{123}-I scanning have been reported. Several reviewers have pointed out that cold and warm nodules have the same rate of malignancy. Thus, a cold nodule is not presently recognized as being a higher-risk lesion than a warm nodule. The important differentiation is between a hot and a nonhot nodule.

Thyroid ultrasonography is widely utilized and is the most sensitive technique. Unfortunately, an ultrasonographic picture is in most situations nonspecific. Approximately 20% of cold nodules are simple cysts and have a greater than 95% chance of being benign if they measure less than 3 cm in diameter. A mixed lesion or complex cyst is of greater concern. Most of these represent hemorrhagic cysts; however, the risk of carcinoma is approximately 25%.

It is my opinion that obtaining a scan or an ultrasonogram or both is not helpful or cost-effective before performing a fine-needle biopsy. Locally, the total cost of a biopsy and an interpretation is equal to that of a scan or an ultrasonogram. I have found it more cost-effective to perform an ^{123}-I scan if a microfollicular adenoma is found on biopsy or to obtain an ultrasonogram if a cystic lesion is determined to be present and complete resolution of the nodule does not occur after drainage.

FINE-NEEDLE BIOPSY

The most cost-effective and accurate method of evaluting nodules is the fine-needle biopsy. This is an office procedure that is non-traumatic and carries minimal risk of local hematoma and mild discomfort. We perform fine-needle biopsies using a 21- to 23-gauge needle, a disposable 20-cc syringe, and a Cameco syringe pistol. For large-needle biopsies we use an 18-gauge needle. The patient is first placed in a supine position with the neck hyperextended. The skin over the nodule is carefully sterilized with povidone-iodine (Betadine) and alcohol and anesthetized locally with lidocaine (Xylocaine). The needle is then inserted into the thyroid nodule as deeply as possible, and at least three to five passes are made at three different angles from the medial and lateral sides, to ensure adequate sampling from all areas.

Cytologic specimens are aspirated into the needle and syringe. One or two drops from the syringe are placed on a clean slide and smeared with a cover slip. The slide is immediately fixed in 95% ethyl alcohol and stained by the Papanicolaou method. The syringe and needle are then carefully washed out with normal saline, and the specimen is taken to the cytology laboratory and passed through a millipore filter. Large pieces of tissue on the filter are processed into a cell block. The remaining material is then processed onto a slide and stained as described previously. We have found that material obtained by this technique is frequently superior to that seen in direct smears.

Slides are interpreted by a pathologist and the attending endocrinologist. Nodules are classified into one of several categories: "not suspicious for malignancy," "suspicious for malignancy," or "malignant." Specimens that are indeterminate are an indication for rebiopsy, usually with a large needle.

Benign Nodules. Most benign nodules ("not suspicious for malignancy") fall into the classification of *colloid goiter*. The greater the amount of colloid, the more likely it is that the nodule is benign. We have come to call these nodules *macrofollicular adenomas*. Subacute thyroiditis and chronic lymphocytic thyroiditis can also be identified. However, differentiation of these from lymphoma or anaplastic carcinoma may be difficult. The size and staining patterns of nuclei must be examined carefully.

Microfollicular or Hürthle Cell Adenomas. This particularly perplexing subgroup must be considered "suspicious for malignancy." These adenomas account for approximately 20% of all biopsy specimens. Frequently the differentiation between a benign and malignant process is difficult, even on histologic grounds, and may rest solely on evidence of capsular invasion or distant spread. A thyroid scan may be helpful in that about 10% of follicular nodules are hot and may be considered benign. If the adenoma is warm or cold, surgical biopsy is indicated for definitive diagnosis.

Papillary Adenocarcinomas. These tumors are accurately diagnosed through biopsy. They have little or no colloid and are highly cellular, with papillary formations. The presence of psammoma bodies is pathognomonic. Other types of cancers such as medullary, anaplastic, or metastatic carcinoma can be diagnosed by fine-needle biopsy as well.

SUMMARY

When a patient presents with a single or prominent nodule, the first step should be to perform a fine-needle biopsy. If the cytologic specimen appears malignant, an immediate surgical procedure should be performed for definitive diagnosis and treatment. Biopsies that appear "suspicious for malignancy" should also be excised unless they are classified as a microfollicular or Hürthle cell neoplasm. In this situation, an [123]-I scan is helpful. If the lesion appears cold or warm, the nodule should be surgically removed. If the nodule appears hot, it should be followed at six-month intervals by palpation. Hot lesions that are enlarging also need to be evaluated every six months for excessive hormone secretion. The best single laboratory value to follow is the T_3 radioimmunoassay. Surgical removal or ablation with ^{123}I should be performed when the value is clearly elevated.

Although a biopsy is the most accurate and economic method of evaluating single or prominent nodules, the technique is not 100% accurate. As many as 5% to 10% of all carcinomas may be missed with a single biopsy. Our practice is to place all patients with a benign biopsy result on a suppressive dose of L-thyroxine for 6 to 12 months. The nodule is then followed and carefully palpated and measured. Nodules that are difficult to palpate can be most carefully observed through ultrasonography.

If at the end of 12 months the nodule has not decreased in size by at least 50 % or to less than 1 cm in diameter, a second thyroid biopsy should be performed. If this appears "malignant" or "suspicious for malignancy," the nodule needs to be excised. Otherwise, the patient should stay on thyroid hormone suppression and be followed indefinitely at 12-month intervals. If at any time the nodule measurably enlarges as shown by palpation or ultrasonography, it should be surgically removed, repeat biopsy not being necessary. All patients on chronic suppression should have a yearly measurement of thyroxine and protein binding to avoid iatrogenic hyperthyroidism. If this occurs, the nodule should be evaluated for autonomy and, if present, thyroid hormone should be withdrawn.

REFERENCES

Gharib H, Goellner JR, Zinsmeister AR, et al: Fine-needle aspiration of the thyroid: the problem of suspicious cytologic findings. Ann Intern Med 101:25–28, 1984.

Hamberger B, Gharib H, Melton LJ, et al: Fine-needle aspiration biopsy of thyroid nodules: impact on thyroid practice and cost of care. Am J Med 73:381–384, 1982.

Miller JM: Needle biopsy of the thyroid: methods and recommendations. Thyroid Today 5:1–5, 1982.

Studer H: Pathogenesis of goiter: a unifying hypothesis. Thyroid Today 4:1–7, 1984.

Van Herle AJ, Rich P, Ljung BM, et al: The thyroid nodule. Ann Intern Med 96:221–232, 1982.

8 · THYROIDITIS

Bruce R. MacKay
Ferrol J. Lee
GUTHRIE CLINIC

DEFINITION

The term thyroiditis encompasses bacterial, viral, and immune inflammatory reactions with attendant pain, swelling, and thyroid dysfunction (Table 1).

HASHIMOTO'S THYROIDITIS

Hashimoto's thyroiditis (HT), also known as struma lymphomatosa, is the most common type of thyroiditis and is an autoimmune disorder. Cell-mediated immunity may be more important in the pathophysiology and ultimate destruction of thyroid tissue, but the antithyroglobulin (ATA) and antimicrosomal (AMA) antibodies are extremely useful as diagnostic markers. HT clusters in families and is seen in association with other autoimmune disease. It has four principal variants, the features of which are listed in Table 1. In the oxyphil variant, RAIU values are often in the upper-normal range, presumably because of an associated organification defect in thyroid hormone synthesis, and scans characteristically show a somewhat mottled pattern within a normal outline of the gland.

Atypical presentations of HT include subacute onset with rapid growth of a goiter, which may be painful and clinically mimic de Quervain's thyroiditis. HT that has been clinically stable may rarely give way to classic Graves' disease, or more often may coexist with typical Graves' disease, a condition known as "hashitoxicosis." At times the glandular configuration may mimic a multinodular goiter or rarely a solitary nodule, and fine-needle aspiration cytology may be necessary to confirm the diagnosis.

Although HT is usually well tolerated and a benign condition, it can be found in conjunction with papillary carcinoma and is associated with an increased incidence of lymphoma of the thyroid gland. The physician must also be alert to associated autoimmune endocrine disorders.

Drug Therapy

Untreated, the natural history of HT is progressive enlargement of the gland with ultimate hypothyroidism and eventual atrophy. Therapy consists of a suppressive/replacement dose of L-thyroxine (T_4), 0.1 to 0.2 mg daily, but is best determined by remeasurement of T_4 and thyroid-stimulating hormone (TSH) after eight weeks of treatment and every three to six months thereafter until values are stable within the normal

Table 1. CLINICAL AND LABORATORY FEATURES OF THYROIDITIS

	Juvenile*	Oxyphil*	Fibrous*	Silent*	de Quervain's	Acute	Riedel's
% of all thyroiditis	5	60	10	15	10	<1	<1
F/M	15:1	20:1	10:1	15:1	2:1	1:1	2:1
Age/yrs.	<20	20–50	40–60	<20	<20	–	30–60
Goiter	+	+ + +	+ +	±	+ +	+	+ +
	N	firm	hard	nontender	tender	tender	hard
	sym.	sym.	sym.	sym.	asym.	asym.	fixed
Thyrotoxicosis	–	–	–	+ +	+	–	–
Hypothyroidism	+	+ +	+ + +	–	±	–	+
RAIU	N	N or incr.	decr.	decr.	<2%	N	N or decr.
Antibodies							
ATA	±	+ +	+ + + +	+	±	–	–
AMA	+ +	+ + + +	+ + +	+	±	–	–
Aspiration cytology	lymphs	lymphs, oxyphils	plasma cells	lymphs	PMN, giant cells	PMN, bacteria	nondiagnostic
Therapy	T_4	T_4	T_4	beta-blockers	aspirin, beta-blockers	drainage, antibiotics	surgery

*Hashimoto's variants.

F/M = female:male ratio; + = degree of presence; − = absent; sym. = symmetric; asym. = asymmetric; RAIU = radioactive iodine uptake; N = normal; incr. = increased; decr. = decreased; T_4 = L-thyroxine; PMN = polymorphonuclear leukocytes.

range. Most goiters decrease by 30% to 50% after three to six months of suppressive therapy. Almost all patients should be treated and therapy is usually lifelong. A euthyroid individual with a small goiter and low antibody titers can be followed safely without therapy, but should be made aware of symptoms of hypothyroidism.

SILENT THYROIDITIS

Silent thyroiditis with spontaneously resolving hyperthyroidism is an important variant of HT. These patients present with signs, symptoms, and laboratory findings of thyrotoxicosis, but a very low RAIU. If a goiter can be identified, it is painless, small, and nontender. The thyrotoxicosis, while limited to several weeks, often recurs within one to two years and is particularly prone to reappear in the postpartum period. Symptoms usually are readily alleviated by beta-blocking drugs. Long-term follow-up has shown an increase in goiter size and more characteristic findings of HT in 50% of cases.

SUBACUTE THYROIDITIS

Subacute thyroiditis, also known as de Quervain's or granulomatous thyroiditis, is a viral-mediated, relatively acute inflammation of the thyroid. There may be a prodrome, but most often there is rather abrupt pain in the anterior neck in conjunction with an asymmetric, firm, tender goiter. Pain on swallowing is minimal, while referred pain into the retroauricular area, vertex, and back of the neck is common. Systemic features are usually mild, but occasionally there may be high fever and prostration. Because the inflammatory process results in leakage of preformed T_4 and T_3 from damaged acinar cells and colloid, mild thyrotoxicosis may occur. Laboratory diagnosis hinges on an elevated sedimentation rate and the inability of the damaged cells to concentrate radioiodine. Fine-needle aspiration biopsy, though infrequently needed, is diagnostic.

Drug Therapy

Aspirin or nonsteroidal anti-inflammatory drugs such as ibuprofen (Motrin), 600 mg b.i.d., relieve pain and systemic symptoms. Hyperthyroidism is readily controlled by atenolol (Tenormin), 50 mg daily. Rarely the thyrotoxicosis and systemic symptoms may be severe, in which case prednisone in a tapering dosage from 40 mg daily is indicated. The overall course of the illness lasts several weeks, 95% of patients ultimately regaining normal thyroid histology and function.

ACUTE THYROIDITIS

Acute thyroiditis is rare and usually due to contiguous infection or a bacteremia-induced staphylococcal abscess. Diagnosis is made by aspiration. Therapy consists of parenteral culture-specific antibiotics and resection or aggressive drainage.

RIEDEL'S STRUMA

Riedel's struma is an equally rare, unexplained, chronic inflammatory process characterized by a dense fibrosis replacing thyroid tissue and extending to involve adjacent structures. The process is most easily confused with an infiltrating anaplastic carcinoma. Management consists of surgical release of the trachea and great vessels.

REFERENCES

Doniach D, Bottazzo GF, Russel RCG: Goitrous autoimmune thyroiditis (Hashimoto's disease). Clin Endocrinol Metab 8:63–80, 1979.
Nikolai TF, Brosseau J, Kettrick MA, et al: Lymphocytic thyroiditis with hyperthyroidism (silent thyroiditis). Arch Intern Med 141:1455–1458, 1981.
Volpé R: Subacute (de Quervain's) thyroiditis. Clin Endocrinol Metab 8:81–95, 1979.
Woolf P: Transient painless thyroiditis with hyperthyroidism: a variant of lymphocytic thyroiditis? Endocr Rev 1:411–420, 1980.

9 · THYROID CANCER

Ferrol J. Lee
Bruce R. MacKay
GUTHRIE CLINIC

DEFINITION AND DIAGNOSTIC CRITERIA

There are four types of thyroid cancer. The well-differentiated forms are the papillary and follicular malignancies, and the remaining types are medullary and anaplastic thyroid carcinoma. Infrequently the thyroid gland may be the site of metastatic carcinoma or a primary lymphoma.

PATHOPHYSIOLOGY

External irradiation to the thyroid is an important cause of thyroid cancer and exhibits latent periods of 10 to 30 years. The younger the patient at the time of irradiation, the greater is the likelihood of developing cancer.

Chronic stimulation of the thyroid with thyroid-stimulating hormone (TSH), as seen in chronic iodide deficiency, or long-term administration of goitrogenic drugs can produce thyroid malignancy. The only well-documented hereditary thyroid malignancy is medullary carcinoma of the thyroid (MCT). Of these malignancies, 10% to 20% are associated with multiple endocrine neoplasia type II (MEN II).

CLINICAL PRESENTATION

Patients usually present with a single thyroid nodule. A rapidly expanding, painful, and immobile goiter, dysphagia, shortness of breath, and hoarseness are rarely seen except in undifferentiated malignancies.

Papillary carcinoma, accounting for over 60% of all thyroid malignancies, has a peak incidence in the third to fourth decade and is the most common thyroid malignancy in childhood. Women are more commonly affected than men in a ratio of 3:1. This tumor is slow-growing, and metastases are usually limited to regional lymph nodes.

Follicular carcinoma, which represents 15% of thyroid malignancies, has its peak incidence in the fourth to fifth decade. Because of the angioinvasive nature of these tumors, metastases occur distantly to the lungs and bones, as well as locally. The bone lesions are usually osteolytic and not associated with elevations of alkaline phosphatase.

MCT accounts for 2% to 8% of thyroid cancers. When sporadic the tumor is usually confined to one lobe, whereas in familial MCT it is usually bilateral. The diarrhea and flushing associated with MCT may respond to prostaglandin inhibitors or antihistamines. These tumors metastasize to nodes in the neck, lungs, soft tissue of the mediastinum, and liver. Many patients have elevated basal calcitonin levels and nearly all have elevations with provocative testing, using either pentagastrin or calcium infusion. These tests must be used to screen first-degree relatives of patients with the MEN II syndrome for C-cell hyperplasia, the premalignant harbinger of MCT, which can then be treated by complete thyroidectomy.

Anaplastic tumors generally occur in persons in the seventh to eight decade. They are very locally aggressive and pulmonary metastases are usually present.

PROGNOSIS

Well-differentiated thyroid cancer can be indolent for decades without causing symptoms. In papillary carcinoma confined to the thyroid and cervical nodes, there is a 90% 10-year survival and a 70% 20-year survival. If the cancer is extrathyroidal, survival rates are 50% at 10 years and 40% at 20 years. In follicular carcinoma without capsule invasion, survival rates are similar to those for papillary carcinoma. If there is capsular or vascular invasion, the survival rate is 35% at 10 years and 15% at 20 years.

MANAGEMENT

SURGICAL THERAPY

Surgery is the mainstay of therapy for thyroid carcinoma. We favor a subtotal thyroidectomy, with resection of the involved lobe, isthmus, and most of the remaining lobe, but with particular care to preserve parathyroid function. Remaining thyroid tissue is then ablated with radioactive iodine (^{131}I). This approach eliminates the 7% recurrence rate in the unresected lobe. There is a 2% incidence of unilateral recurrent nerve injury and a 5% to 15% incidence of permanent hypoparathyroidism in patients who have a near-total thyroidectomy, although these risks can be substantially minimized by an experienced thyroid surgeon.

In patients with extrathyroidal, well-differentiated thyroid cancer, a modified neck dissection is added in an effort to remove all nodes and soft tissue that contain malignancy.

Patients with MCT should have a total thyroidectomy and probably a radical neck dissection if cervical lymph node metastases are present. In the absence of distant metastases, this approach improves the 10-year survival rate from 43% to 67%.

The treatment of choice in poorly differentiated carcinoma is total thyroidectomy. Unfortunately, excision is possible in only one third of patients.

RADIOACTIVE IODINE

Radioactive iodine is used both to ablate normal thyroid tissue (which must be accomplished before metastasis can be detected by scanning) and to destroy metastatic thyroid cancer. On the day after surgery, L-triiodothyronine (Cytomel) is started, 25 µg t.i.d. Eight weeks after surgery, Cytomel is stopped. Two weeks later, a 24-hour RAIU is performed. If the uptake in the neck at 24 hours exceeds 1%, the patient is treated with 30 mCi of ^{131}I, which over a period of three to four months ablates remaining normal thyroid tissue in 80% of patients; the remainder need a second 30-mCi dose. Cytomel is resumed five days post ^{131}I.

When the uptake in the neck is less than 1%, the patient should have a total body scan using 1 to 2 mCi of ^{131}I. If there is no clinical or scan evidence of metastases, the patient should be rescanned in one year. If this scan is negative, repeat scans are performed only if there is clinical suspicion of recurrent disease. If metastases are seen on scan, the patient is hospitalized and treated with 150 mCi of [131]I. This dose does not usually cause side effects. When pulmonary metastases are present, the total dose of ^{131}I is adjusted so as to avoid radiation pneumonitis. [131]I therapy for metastases should be repeated at four- to six-month intervals as long as the metastases continue to concentrate ^{131}I and there is no evidence of bone marrow suppression or pulmonary fibrosis. Approximately 80% of metastatic thyroid cancers accumulate [131]I. In the remaining cases, efforts to induce ^{131}I uptake should be attempted with a low-iodide diet and bovine TSH injections. If there is still no uptake, ^{131}I therapy will probably be of no benefit. This therapy is ineffective in the treatment of patients with MCT or anaplastic thyroid carcinoma.

When the total body scan is negative, a baseline serum thyroglobulin level is obtained. Elevation of these levels in patients who have had thyroid ablation strongly suggests a recurrence of thyroid cancer, and can be seen in the presence of a normal total body ^{131}I scan.

CONVENTIONAL RADIOTHERAPY AND CHEMOTHERAPY

External radiation can be palliative in patients with stage III or IV thyroid cancer and should be considered when a tumor does not accumulate [131]I. Chemotherapy is recommended in thyroid malignancies only if other therapeutic modalities have failed and there is rapid progression of the tumor.

THYROID HORMONE THERAPY

All patients with thyroid cancer should be given lifetime treatment with exogenous thyroid hormone. L-Thyroxine (Synthroid), 0.15 to 0.2 mg a day, prevents hypothyroidism and suppresses TSH, thus eliminating its growth-stimulating effect on malignant thyroid cells. After the patient has taken exogenous thyroid hormone for four to six weeks, serum T_4 should be in the upper range of normal or slightly above. The adequacy of suppression can be confirmed by a TRH stimulation test or supersensitive TSH assay.

REFERENCES

DeGroot LJ: Thyroid neoplasia. *In* DeGroot LJ (ed): Endocrinology. Grune & Stratton, New York, 1979, pp 509–518.

DeGroot LJ, Larsen PR, Refetoff S, et al: Thyroid neoplasia. *In* The Thyroid and Its Diseases, 5th ed. John Wiley & Sons, New York, 1984, pp 773–818.

Friedman EW, Schwartz AE: Well-differentiated thyroid cancer. *In* Krieger DT, Bardin CW (eds): Current Therapy in Endocrinology 1983–1984. B.L. Decker, Philadelphia, 1983, pp 92–98.

Mazzaferri EL: The thyroid. *In* Mazzaferri EL (ed): Endocrinology. Medical Examination Publishing Co, New Hyde Park, NY, 1980, pp 219–245.

Refetoff S, Lever EG: The value of serum thyroglobulin measurement in clinical practice. JAMA 250:2352–2357, 1983.

10 · PARATHYROID DISORDERS

Melvin A. Block
SCRIPPS CLINIC AND RESEARCH FOUNDATION

Primary Hyperparathyroidism

DEFINITION AND DIAGNOSTIC CRITERIA

Diagnosis is based on persistent hypercalcemia, elevation of serum parathyroid hormone (PTH) levels in most cases, and no other cause for these findings. The carboxy-terminal (biologically inactive segment of PTH) assays usually reflect the presence or absence of parathyroid hyperfunction, but midmolecule (toward the biologically active end) assays are more accurate and are becoming increasingly available. Most laboratories now provide a normogram, which categorizes serum PTH levels in hypercalcemia relative to the likelihood of primary or secondary hyperparathyroidism or other cause, including malignancy.

CLINICAL PRESENTATION

Clinical clues include a family history of the disease, previous radiation therapy to the head and neck, calcium oxalate nephrolithiasis or nephrocalcinosis, metabolic bone disease (osteoporosis, spontaneous fractures, cystic bone disease of the von Recklinghausen variety, "brown" tumors of bone or soft tissues), and complications of hypercalcemia. The last-named include muscle weakness and myalgias, reduced mental acuity, polyuria, hypertension, constipation, peptic ulcer disease, and acute pancreatitis. Anemia is an infrequent finding. A clinical classification is listed in Table 1.

Malignancies must be excluded as a cause of hypercalcemia, including carcinoma of the lung, breast, kidney, or pancreas; lymphoma, leukemia, multiple myeloma; and certain soft tissue malignancies. Hypoalbuminemia should register a suspicion of malignancy as the cause of hypercalcemia, whereas an elevated level of 1,25-vitamin D favors a diagnosis of hyperparathyroidism. Other conditions that can produce hypercalcemia include sarcoidosis, immobilization, or ingestion of excess amounts of vitamin D or A or calcium.

Benign familial hypocalciuric hypercalcemia, an autosomal dominant condition, occurs often enough to

**Table 1. PRIMARY HYPERPARATHYROIDISM:
A CLASSIFICATION**

1. Sporadic (95%)—single (90%) or multiple (10%) parathyroid gland
   involvement
2. Hereditary (5%)
   Multiple endocrine neoplasia I and IIA syndromes—multiple
   gland involvement nearly always present
   Autosomal dominant—multiple gland involvement usually
   Autosomal recessive—single gland involvement usually

require exclusion, especially for patients with uncomplicated hypercalcemia. This is done by showing urine calcium levels over 100 mg per 24 hours and a urine calcium-creatinine clearance ratio over 0.01. Serum magnesium levels in benign familial hypercalcemia are elevated or at the upper limit of normal, contrasting with depressed levels in primary hyperparathyroidism. This life-long entity causes no evident health problems, and no treatment is necessary. However, neonates born of affected parents may have severe hyperparathyroidism, requiring total parathyroidectomy.

MANAGEMENT

NONPHARMACOLOGIC MEASURES

Surgery is the definitive treatment for primary hyperparathyroidism and consists of identification and removal of a single enlarged parathyroid gland for approximately 85% of patients. For the remaining patients with multiple gland involvement, treatment involves removal of all enlarged parathyroid glands when two or three are enlarged, or either subtotal parathyroidectomy or total parathyroidectomy with autotransplantation when all glands are enlarged. Exploration by an experienced surgeon results in correction of primary hyperparathyroidism in more than 95% of cases.

Decision-making depends on whether there are complications of hypercalcemia and on the overall medical status of the patient. For patients with complications of hypercalcemia, exploration is advisable unless more serious medical problems take priority on a temporary or long-term basis. The advisability of surgery in uncomplicated hyperparathyroidism is not clear-cut. However, there has been an increasing tendency to recommend surgical correction, especially if the serum calcium level exceeds 11 mg/dl on occasion, because (1) in most patients, accentuated bone demineralization is halted by control of the disease; (2) in at least 20% of patients, hypercalcemia progresses and this can be abrupt; (3) many patients do not comply with advice for periodic evaluations; (4) nonspecific but significant manifestations of hypercalcemia, especially weakness and reduced mental acuity, may not be appreciated until after the problem is corrected; and (5) the risks involved are extremely low and, with hospitalization usually requiring only two days, costs have been reduced.

Severe hypercalcemia with associated toxicity requires urgent exploration of the parathyroid glands to avoid a fatality. Manifestations include severe weakness, stupor, seizures, gastrointestinal disturbances, and polyuria. Malignancy and other causes of hypercalcemia should be excluded rapidly by a complete physical examination and basic laboratory tests (chest x-ray, hematologic survey, intravenous pyelogram). There may not be time to wait for the results of a serum PTH level test. Preparation for surgery includes IV hydration and reduction of serum calcium levels by IV administration of mithramycin, 25 μg per kg in 1000 cc of fluid IV over one hour, which can be repeated on a daily basis, or calcitonin, 10 to 20 MRC or by intravenous administration over one hour or as 4 to 8 MRC or IV every six to 12 hours. After adequate hydration is achieved, IV furosemide (40 mg once or twice daily) is given to increase calcium excretion and reduce serum calcium levels. An indwelling catheter in the urinary bladder permits close monitoring of urinary output and hydration. Surgery usually can be undertaken within several days of recognition of the hypercalcemic crisis.

The place of preoperative localization studies has not been precisely defined. Currently, no test is dependable in localizing slightly enlarged parathyroid glands (those less than 200 mg). Improving resolution will probably make ultrasonography most cost-effective. Thallium-201 scans are more expensive than ultrasonography and have a significant but unspecified false-negative rate. The thallium-technetium subtraction scan can be of particular value in identifying ectopic parathyroid tumors. Although rare, mediastinal parathyroid tumors are a serious problem for patients who are elderly or have severe hypercalcemia; if a prolonged neck exploration fails, they have to endure the risks of the disease and another operation. Knowledge of a probable ectopic tumor can permit immediate exploration of the mediastinum if the initial neck exploration is unsuccessful. Intraoperative use of ultrasonography can be of value in locating enlarged parathyroid glands.

My preference is to evaluate all parathyroid glands at surgery and remove those that are grossly abnormal. Although the finding and removal of a single enlarged gland and the recognition of a normal gland on the same side of the neck usually resolves the problem, an additional parathyroid tumor is present in the contralateral neck or mediastinum in at least 3% of patients. In all cases, an enlarged supernumerary parathyroid gland, often ectopic and in the superior mediastinum accessible through the neck incision, should be sought and removed if found. There is a spectrum of enlargement of multiple parathyroid glands. With gross involvement of one, two, or three glands, only the obvious parathyroid tumors should be removed. Consideration may be given to biopsy of remaining glands, but tissue devitalization and consequent permanent hypoparathyroidism must be avoided. Therefore, biopsy of normal appearing glands is performed only in problem cases.

For patients in whom all glands are involved by hyperplasia (usually those with multiple endocrine neoplasia, MEN), it is preferable to preserve 50 to 150 mg of viable parathyroid tissue. This is successful in over 90% of cases and avoids a three-month period of hypocalcemia if total parathyroidectomy with autotransplantation is performed. If all glands are greatly enlarged, making preservation of a part of one gland technically difficult, all glands should be removed and 50 to 150 mg autotransplanted. Numerous locations can be used for parathyroid autotransplantation. The forearm facilitates subsequent monitoring of activity by determining levels of PTH in venous blood from the site. Ten to 15% of the latter procedures are unsuccessful. Some surgeons prefer to freeze parathyroid tissue rather than perform immediate autotransplantation because of the fear of persistent hypercalcemia from an overlooked hyperplastic supernumerary ectopic parathyroid gland.

A challenging problem for the surgeon is the slightly enlarged gland causing primary hyperparathyroidism, especially difficult to assess if surrounded by fat. Fortunately, the darker than normal color often permits recognition of one or more hyperplastic glands.

Less than 1% of patients who have single parathyroid gland enlargement develop hyperfunction of a parathyroid gland considered to be grossly normal at the initial operation. Subtotal parathyroidectomy for patients with multiple gland involvement results in control of the disease in approximately 92% of cases.

The morbidity of parathyroid surgery is low, permanent hypoparathyroidism or recurrent laryngeal nerve damage occurring in less than 1% of cases. Persistent or recurrent hyperparathyroidism results from failure to identify and remove a single hyperfunctioning parathyroid gland or an adequate amount of hyperfunctioning parathyroid tissue in multiple gland involvement. In such cases, it is necessary to try to localize the residual hyperfunctioning tissue, guided by information gained at previous surgery. Noninvasive studies, in addition to those previously described, include computerized tomography and magnetic resonance imaging of the mediastinum and neck. Invasive studies include selective venous sampling for PTH levels, arteriography, and digital subtraction angiography. In general, further surgery is justified in the presence of significant disease. Second operations are technically difficult and demand an experienced surgeon.

DRUG THERAPY

The nonoperative treatment of primary hyperparathyroidism is, in general, unsatisfactory but may be helpful in mild cases of hypercalcemia and in patients who are not surgical candidates. Dietary measures, which include phosphate feeding (1 gm of inorganic phosphorus divided into four doses daily), restriction of dairy products to once daily, and a large fluid intake, are of some value. Salt intake should be increased to avoid intravascular volume depletion from polyuria. Long-term therapy with calcitonin and steroids has not been satisfactory. Conjugated estrogens have been reported to be useful in controlling serum and urine calcium levels with a reduction in bone turnover.

Secondary Hyperparathyroidism

DEFINITION AND DIAGNOSTIC CRITERIA

Renal insufficiency as well as any cause of chronic hypocalcemia is a stimulus for parathyroid hyperplasia. Unpredictably, this can result in secondary hyperparathyroidism with intense pruritus, renal osteodystrophy with severe bone pain, muscle weakness, and soft tissue calcifications with ulceration. Tertiary hyperparathyroidism occurs if the parathyroid hyperplasia becomes autonomous and continues even after renal-transplantation, with the potential for injury to the new kidney.

MANAGEMENT

NONPHARMACOLOGIC MEASURES

If an operation is necessary for secondary or tertiary hyperparathyroidism, total parathyroidectomy with autotransplantation of 20 to 25 thin slices of parathyroid tissue is commonly performed. Every effort is made to remove all parathyroid tissue, including thymic tissue, through the neck incision. Alternatively, excised parathyroid tissue can be frozen for later use, because in a few cases residual hyperplastic parathyroid tissue makes autotransplantation unnecessary, at least at the time. Recurrent hyperparathyroidism occurs in 8% of cases following total parathyroidectomy and autotransplantation. For this reason, some surgeons prefer subtotal parathyroidectomy when it is technically possible (there has to be at least one parathyroid gland small enough to permit partial removal and preservation of the desired 50 to 150 mg of viable tissue). Another problem following total parathyroidectomy with autotransplantation has been invasive growth of the autotransplant, suggesting malignancy. Subtotal parathyroidectomy obviates the period of temporary hypoparathyroidism after total parathyroidectomy with autotransplantation. I have selected the extent of removal of the parathyroid gland primarily on the basis of gross enlargement and color at the time of operation, removing those glands that show gross evidence of hyperplasia, up to subtotal parathyroidectomy.

DRUG THERAPY

Medical therapy now minimizes the occurrence of secondary hyperparathyroidism in patients with advanced renal failure. The same measures are used to treat manifestations of established secondary hyperparathyroidism, especially renal osteodystrophy. Treatment includes dietary restriction of phosphorus and the use of phosphate-binding antacids to control hyperphosphatemia, calcium supplementation, and administration of vitamin D.

Hypoparathyroidism

DIAGNOSTIC CRITERIA

Hypoparathyroidism is due to a heterogeneous group of disorders and can be classified broadly into two major groups: (1) deficient PTH production and (2) end-organ unresponsiveness to PTH (pseudohypoparathyroidism), which results in an excess of PTH production. All hypoparathyroid patients are subject to the deleterious effects of hypocalcemia.

CLINICAL PRESENTATION

Acute hypocalcemia is more evident in young patients and is manifested by paresthesias and neuromuscular irritability (with Chvostek and Trousseau signs present) that can lead to tetany and laryngeal stridor. Chronic hypocalcemia may result in cataracts and reduced mental acuity.

The clinical states in which hypoparathyroidism is due to a deficiency of PTH production are listed in Table 2. Pseudohypoparathyroidism is also a heterogeneous group of disorders characterized by target organ resistance to a variety of hormones whose actions are mediated by cyclic AMP. In most cases the clinical presentation is dominated by PTH insensitivity, with resistance to other hormones remaining subclinical. In the largest subgroup of patients with this disorder, skeletal or somatic abnormalities constitute characteristic features of Albright's osteodystrophy. A separate group of patients with skeletal or somatic manifestations of pseudohypoparathyroidism but with normal serum calcium and PTH levels have been designated as having pseudopseudohypoparathyroidism. In some cases of the latter, blood calcium and PTH levels vary from low to normal. Thus, features of pseudohypoparathyroidism and pseudopseudohypoparathyroidism can coexist in the same patient or different members of the same family. Genetic counseling is sometimes appropriate.

MANAGEMENT

DRUG THERAPY

Treatment of hypoparathyroidism relates to control of hypocalcemia. In acute symptomatic hypocalcemia, in which serum calcium levels are usually less than 7 mg/dl, 10 to 20 cc of 10% calcium gluconate given IV slowly over 10 to 15 minutes usually provides correction. This is repeated either intermittently or as 20 to 40 cc in 1000 cc of IV fluids given over eight hours as a continuous infusion. Serum calcium levels are monitored periodically. For mild temporary hypocalcemia, or to provide long-term management after acute symptomatic hypocalcemia has been controlled, oral calcium is given. Calcium carbonate powder, 2 or more teaspoons in water q.i.d. or Os-Cal 500, two to four tablets taken t.i.d. or q.i.d. has been preferred for this purpose. The dose is adjusted to serum calcium levels. For patients with hypocalcemia following thyroid or parathyroid surgery, calcium alone is given. Oral vitamin D therapy is initiated in such cases only when it is evident that calcium administration is inadequate or that hypoparathyroidism is permanent.

Table 2. HYPOPARATHYROIDISM SECONDARY TO PARATHYROID HORMONE DEFICIENCY

Post-treatment
  Temporary ("hungry bone syndrome," suppressed parathyroid glands)
  Following thyroid or parathyroid surgery
  Following radioactive iodine therapy (rare)
Neonatal
  Associated with maternal hyperparathyroidism (transient)
  Hypomagnesemia
  DiGeorge's syndrome (congenital aplasia)
Idiopathic
  Autosomal recessive
  Autosomal dominant
  Autoimmune (including autoimmune pluriglandular syndrome)
  Associated with chemotherapy for malignancy (2 reports)

Vitamin D is needed to treat permanent hypoparathyroidism. Preparations include vitamin D_2 (calciferol), 50,000 to 100,000 or more units daily with a biologic effect that lasts up to six weeks, or dihydrotachysterol (Hytakerol), 0.2 to 0.4 mg three times daily, with an effect lasting up to two weeks. For a more predictable and rapid effect without prolonged action, 1,25-dihydroxycholecalciferol or calcitriol (Rocaltrol) is given, a daily dose of 0.5 to 1.5 µg PO, but this is expensive. It is necessary to adjust the dose on the basis of periodic serum calcium determinations, and the frequency of testing is decreased as stability is achieved. Supplementary oral calcium also is needed in some cases. To ensure normal serum phosphate concentrations, aluminum-containing antacids are used to bind phosphate. Urine calcium levels are determined occasionally, and dietary salt restriction and a thiazide diuretic are prescribed to avoid hypercalciuria.

In pseudohypoparathyroidism, treatment is directed toward increasing intestinal calcium absorption by administering vitamin D, as discussed above. In addition to monitoring serum calcium levels, it is advisable to evaluate patients regularly for hypothyroidism.

PERIODIC EVALUATION

Serum calcium and phosphate levels should be determined two to three times each year. Parathyroid function can return up to one year after surgery. Hypercalcemia, either as parathyroid function returns or from overdosage of medications, is manifested by nausea, vomiting, weakness, polyuria, and stupor.

Carcinoma of the Parathyroid Gland

DIAGNOSTIC CRITERIA AND CLINICAL PRESENTATION

The diagnosis of parathyroid carcinoma requires anatomic evidence of direct invasion of adjacent tissues and/or metastasis. The presence of increased mitoses in parathyroid cells alone is insufficient evidence for the diagnosis. Parathyroid carcinoma is usually hormonally active, and very high levels of serum calcium and a palpable neck mass make the diagnosis likely. Parathyroid carcinoma has been reported in two members of families with hereditary hyperparathyroidism. Death usually results from the effects of uncontrolled hypercalcemia rather than local effects of the malignancy. Acute pancreatitis with hypercalcemic crisis may be the terminal event.

MANAGEMENT

NONPHARMACOLOGIC MEASURES

Cure requires operative excision including at least a partial thyroidectomy and removal of adjacent tissue. A regional lymph node dissection is justified; metastases occur in one third of the patients. Removal of as much carcinoma as possible is justified even in the presence of metastases because of the difficulty of controlling hypercalcemia.

DRUG THERAPY

Streptozotocin, mithramycin, calcitonin, phosphate therapy, and reduced oral calcium intake effected by limiting dairy products are all used in the effort to control hypercalcemia. Diphosphonates inhibit bone resorption and have been used to reduce serum calcium levels, although only etidronate disodium (Didronel) is currently available, and this agent has not generally produced good results.

Unusual Parathyroid Problems

PRIMARY HYPERPARATHYROIDISM IN PREGNANCY

Women with more than marginal hypercalcemia should undergo surgical correction of primary hyperparathyroidism, preferably after the first trimester of pregnancy. Maternal and neonatal morbidity and the risk of fetal loss are sufficient to justify this policy. Patients with minimal hypercalcemia, especially if this is recognized late in pregnancy, can be managed medically until after delivery.

PARATHYROID CYST

This unusual lesion may stimulate a thyroid nodule and is most frequently evident as a palpable nodule in young women. Aspiration usually provides clear fluid containing elevated PTH levels and low thyroxine levels, confirming the diagnosis. In most cases there is no evidence of hyperparathyroidism, and aspiration of fluid resolves the problem. The lesion should be distinguished from cystic degeneration of a parathyroid adenoma producing hyperparathyroidism. Rarely, benign cysts are associated with an adenoma producing primary hyperparathyroidism.

REFERENCES

Block MA, Cerny JC: Endocrine system. *In* Beahrs OH, Beart RW Jr (eds): Therapy Update Service, General Surgery. Harwal Publ, Media, PA, revised 1984, pp 1–47.

Block MA, Frame B, Kleerekoper M, et al: Surgical management of persistence after subtotal parathyroidectomy for primary hyperparathyroidism. Am J Surg 138:561–566, 1979.

Editorial: Medical management of primary hyperparathyroidism. Lancet 2:727–728, 1984.

Gaz RD, Wang C: Management of asymptomatic hyperparathyroidism. Am J Surg 147:498–502, 1984.

Van Dop C, Bourne HR: Pseudohypoparathyroidism. Annu Rev Med 34:259–266, 1983.

11 · ADRENOCORTICAL INSUFFICIENCY

Frederick S. Sunderlin
GEISINGER MEDICAL CENTER

DEFINITION

Adrenocortical insufficiency is present when the adrenal cortex is unable to elaborate either glucocorticoids, aldosterone, or both in response to the body's requirements. Primary adrenal failure (Addison's disease) occurs when 90% or more of the adrenal gland mass is destroyed. Idiopathic atrophy on an "autoimmune" basis is the most common etiology and is associated with an increased incidence of other autoimmune endocrinopathies, including Hashimoto's thyroiditis and, in children, hypoparathyroidism and mucocutaneous candidiasis. Granulomatous diseases (tuberculous and fungal infections), adrenal hemorrhage due to anticoagulant therapy or overwhelming sepsis (Waterhouse-Friderichsen syndrome), metastatic carcinoma, and infiltrating processes such as amyloidosis are uncommon causes. Secondary adrenal insufficiency results from inadequate production of adrenocorticotropic hormone (ACTH). This can occur with hypopituitarism of any cause including selective ACTH deficiency, but it is seen most commonly when the hypothalamic-pituitary-adrenal axis is suppressed by pharmacologic doses of glucocorticoids. Isolated aldosterone deficiency is rarely caused by an enzymatic defect in aldosterone biosynthesis and more often is secondary to defective renin secretion (hyporeninemic hypoaldosteronism).

DIAGNOSTIC CRITERIA

The short ACTH (cosyntropin [Cortrosyn]) test is an excellent screening tool. The diagnosis of glucocorticoid deficiency is established when the plasma cortisol fails to increase by $\geq$ 7 µg/dl to an absolute value of $\geq$ 20 µg/dl one hour after intravenous injection of 0.25 mg of cosyntropin. In the absence of previous exogenous steroid use, subnormal responses should be followed by repetitive ACTH infusions, an insulin tolerance test, or metyrapone testing to determine whether the defect is primary or secondary to ACTH deficiency.

Isolated aldosterone deficiency is demonstrated by the failure of aldosterone to rise in response to volume depletion with normal cortisol secretion, which is shown by ACTH testing. Simultaneous plasma renin activity is measured to determine whether this condition is adrenal or renal in etiology.

CLINICAL ASPECTS

Chronic adrenal insufficiency usually presents insidiously. The most common features are fatigue, anorexia with weight loss, orthostatic hypotension, and fasting hypoglycemia. Hyperpigmentation in the flexor creases, pressure points, and mucous membranes is characteristic of primary adrenal destruction. Salt craving and muscle cramps reflect electrolyte imbalance from mineralocorticoid deficiency. Laboratory studies may be normal with mild disease. Hyperkalemia, hyponatremia, and metabolic acidosis are characteristic of advanced disease. Similar findings accompany secondary adrenal insufficiency, but electrolyte disturbances are less common since aldosterone secretion is preserved. Hyperpigmentation is lacking, and typically there are deficiencies of other pituitary hormones.

Isolated aldosterone deficiency presents with hyperkalemia resulting in weakness and occasionally cardiac arrhythmias. Chronic renal insufficiency and diabetes are frequent predisposing factors.

MANAGEMENT

The management objective in adrenal insufficiency is adequate replacement of steroids both during stress and during periods of well-being.

Daily maintenance therapy usually consists of hydrocortisone (30 to 40 mg) or cortisone acetate (37.5 mg) in divided doses, two thirds in the morning and one third in the late afternoon. With primary adrenal insufficiency, mineralocorticoid is provided as 9 α-fluorocortisol (fludrocortisone [Florinef]), 0.05 to 0.1 mg daily. If a parenteral mineralocorticoid is needed, deoxycorticosterone acetate, 2 to 5 mg intramuscularly may be used. Children should receive hydrocortisone 20 mg/m² in a similar divided schedule. Mineralocorticoid replacement for children is typically 0.1 to 0.2 mg of fludrocortisone, with the addition of salt to the baby's formula if treating an infant with mineralocorticoid. Patients with secondary adrenal insufficiency do not need mineralocorticoid replacement, as aldosterone secretion is preserved.

Isolated aldosterone deficiency is treated solely with fludrocortisone, 0.1 to 0.2 mg daily. Beta blockers, prostaglandin synthetase inhibitors, converting enzyme inhibitors, potassium-sparing diuretics, and potassium supplements should be avoided.

Acute adrenal insufficiency is a medical emergency in which a few minutes may mean the difference between life and death. Hydrocortisone sodium succinate (Solu-Cortef), 100 mg IV push followed by 100 mg every eight hours in an IV infusion of dextrose and saline for volume replacement, is life saving. In stressful situations, 300 to 400 mg of hydrocortisone or its equivalent per day is sufficient; as the patient improves, the dose may be reduced by half each day until the maintenance dose is achieved. When the patient is receiving more than 100 mg of hydrocortisone per day, there is no need to give a mineralocorticoid.

Surgery requires stress doses of steroids, including 100 mg of soluble hydrocortisone by IV infusion during surgery and in the immediate postoperative period. This should be decreased by 50% each postoperative day until maintenance levels are reached, assuming an uneventful course.

Pregnancy usually requires no alteration of maintenance dosages. If significant vomiting develops, injectable steroids may be necessary. Labor and delivery should be treated as a stress; guidelines cited previously should be followed.

PATIENT INFORMATION AND EDUCATION

Patient education is critical, and it should be stressed at every visit that medication is essential for survival and must be taken daily. Patients should carry identification that includes the diagnosis, medication, physician's name, and telephone number. Injectable hydrocortisone hemisuccinate (50 to 100 mg) or dexamethasone phosphate (4 mg) should be available for emergency use if oral intake is not tolerated. Criteria for dosage adjustments during stress should be clearly spelled out. Daily dosage should be doubled for mild illness with temperatures 38 to 39°C and tripled for temperatures greater than 39°C, with gradual tapering to maintenance daily dosage as the infection resolves. If fluids are not tolerated IV administration of dextrose and saline may be necessary. Supplemental salt ingesting may be necessary when exercising, particularly in hot weather.

PERIODIC EVALUATION

Periodic evaluation should include serum electrolytes, patient education, and two-position blood pressure determinations to assess intravascular volume status. Underreplacement results in weight loss, fatigue, headache, postural hypotension, and hyperkalemia. Overzealous replacement appears clinically as insomnia, hypertension, edema, hypokalemia, and cushingoid features.

PREVENTION

Suppression of the hypothalamic-pituitary-adrenal axis by pharmacologic doses of steroids may occur after only a few weeks of therapy. There is great variability in the dose and duration of therapy necessary to cause suppression. For those self-limited disorders in which steroids are given for less than two weeks, they may be abruptly stopped. If withdrawal of chronic high-dose steroid therapy is attempted, a gradual tapering is preferred. No one formula works for all patients, but slow tapering over two to eight weeks to a maintenance physiologic replacement dose can usually be accomplished with patient monitoring. Once the patient is stable on a physiologic dose, he or she may be switched to hydrocortisone (20 mg daily each morning), which allows ACTH production to occur. By following 8 AM plasma cortisol levels over the next few months, endogenous steroid production can be assessed and the maintenance dose of hydrocortisone stopped when cortisol secretion returns to normal (> 10 μg/dl). As recovery of the entire axis may take up to 12 months, a safe approach would be to regard patients previously treated with steroids for longer than a few weeks as having the potential for adrenal insufficiency during periods of *stress* and to take appropriate precautions for at least one year following discontinuation of high-dose steroid therapy.

REFERENCES

Dixon RB, Christy NP: On the various forms of corticosteroid withdrawal syndrome. Am J Med 68:224–230, 1980.

Lindbolm J, Kehlet H, Blickert-Toft M, et al: Reliability of the 30-minute ACTH test in assessing hypothalamus-pituitary-adrenal function. J Clin Endocrinol Metab 47:272–274, 1978.

Schambelan M, Sebastian A, Biglieri EG: Prevalence, pathogenesis and functional significance of aldosterone deficiency in hyperkalemic patients with chronic renal insufficiency. Kidney Int 17:89–101, 1980.

Streeten DHP, Anderson GH, Dalakos TG, et al: Normal and abnormal function of the hypothalamic-pituitary-adrenal system in man. Endocr Rev 5:371–394, 1984.

12 · CUSHING'S SYNDROME

Alan L. Burshell
Lawrence Blonde
OCHSNER CLINIC AND
ALTON OCHSNER MEDICAL FOUNDATION

DEFINITION AND DIAGNOSTIC CRITERIA

Cushing's syndrome is a constellation of clinical manifestations caused by glucocorticoid excess. Exogenous glucocorticoids are the most common cause of this syndrome.

The diagnosis of Cushing's syndrome requires the demonstration of cortisol excess. Since levels of adrenocorticotropic hormone (ACTH) and cortisol fluctuate throughout the day, single cortisol levels are not sufficient for the diagnosis. Generally, Cushing's syndrome can be excluded if the level of 24-hour urine-free cortisol is less than 100 μg or if the level of 8:00 AM plasma cortisol (following 1 mg of dexamethasone at 11:00 PM) is less than 5 μg/dl.

PATHOPHYSIOLOGY

Seventy per cent of adults with endogenous Cushing's syndrome have Cushing's disease. Surgical resection of a pituitary microadenoma can cure these patients, and recently it has been demonstrated that corticotropin-releasing factor (CRF) testing returns to normal after removal of a pituitary microadenoma. However, there are well-documented cases of pituitary hyperplasia, recurrences, and beneficial responses to cyproheptadine, which suggest that in some patients the primary defect may be hypothalamic. Furthermore, there appear to be two patterns of cortisol secretion that may correlate with hypothalamic and pituitary disease, respectively.

In general, ACTH can be suppressed in patients with Cushing's disease, but this requires a higher dose of glucocorticoid than that required in normal patients. This has been termed a set-point abnormality.

Patients with the ectopic ACTH syndrome have higher levels of ACTH that do not respond to CRF or glucocorticoids. The elevated ACTH results in enlargement of the adrenals, with more secretion of cortisol, androgens, and potent mineralocorticoids. Frequently, manifestations of mineralocorticoid excess predominate in these patients.

Glucocorticoid-secreting adrenal adenomas cause ACTH suppression, which results in atrophy of the androgen-secreting normal adrenal tissue. Adrenal carcinomas tend to be large and secrete all of the adrenal steroids, particularly the androgens and their precursors.

Nodular adrenal hyperplasia has features common to both Cushing's disease and adrenal adenomas. The fact that nodular adrenal hyperplasia is bilateral suggests that ACTH may have stimulated the adrenal growth. However, the low ACTH levels are more compatible with the presence of adrenal adenomas.

CLINICAL ASPECTS

Patients with Cushing's disease cannot be distinguished from those with an adrenal adenoma on clinical grounds alone. In Cushing's disease, the pituitary lesions are small and thus seldom cause visual-field defects or destroy other pituitary cell types. Patients with adrenal carcinoma usually present with a palpable abdominal mass, and affected women have hirsutism and virilization. Patients with the ectopic ACTH syndrome caused by bronchogenic carcinoma frequently present with weight loss, hypokalemic alkalosis, and hyperpigmentation. Other causes of the ectopic ACTH syndrome, such as a bronchial carcinoid, may be more difficult to differentiate from Cushing's disease. Patients with Cushing's syndrome of any etiology may have centripetal obesity, thin skin with bruises and purple striae, excessive lanugo hair growth, menstrual irregularities, hypertension, edema, hypokalemia, glucose intolerance, muscle weakness, osteoporosis, and psychologic problems.

Because of the reliance on laboratory tests in the evaluation of Cushing's syndrome, certain pitfalls must be avoided. Depressed patients do not have normal dexamethasone suppression test results. If Cushing's syndrome is suspected in a depressed patient who has abnormal suppression test results, an insulin-induced hypoglycemia test should be performed. In patients with Cushing's syndrome, there is no increase in the cortisol level after hypoglycemia, whereas depressed patients have a normal response. Phenytoin (Dilantin) and other agents that induce hepatic microsomal enzymes increase the metabolism of dexamethasone and therefore may give false-positive results on dexamethasone testing. If the drug cannot be discontinued, a test measuring the level of 24-hour urine-free cortisol or a suppression test using hydrocortisone and measuring plasma corticosterone is appropriate. Alcoholics with liver disease occasionally have clinical features and laboratory results compatible with Cushing's syndrome. Results of the laboratory studies, however, become reliable after a period of abstinence. An injection with long-acting glucocorticoid can cause clinical features of Cushing's syndrome but with suppressed cortisol levels and a low 24-hour urine-free cortisol level. A similar pattern can be seen with periodic Cushing's syndrome. If there is an abnormal elevation of corticosteroid-binding globulin, the plasma cortisol levels may be elevated after dexamethasone suppression, but all urine studies measuring glucocorticoid production will be normal.

MANAGEMENT

The first priority is to identify the specific etiology so that appropriate therapy can be selected. This is usually accomplished in an outpatient setting. If the patient's serum cortisol fails to suppress adequately after an overnight dexamethasone test, a two-day, "low-dose" dexamethasone suppression test may confirm the diagnosis, and an ACTH level and "high-dose" suppression test often identify the specific etiology. Computed tomographic scanning of the pituitary is performed for suspected Cushing's disease, as is CT imaging of the adrenals for suspected adrenal neoplasm. Occasionally, the results of these tests are equivocal, and additional studies, such as a metapyrone test, ACTH stimulation test, or CRF stimulation test, may help clarify the diagnosis.

THERAPY

Cushing's Disease. Transsphenoidal adenomectomy is the treatment of choice. Failure to demonstrate a pituitary or sellar abnormality on CT scanning is not a contraindication to surgery, although the small size of most ACTH-secreting pituitary adenomas poses technical problems for the neurosurgeon. If a tumor is found at the time of exploration, it is resected. If no tumor is discovered, near total hypophysectomy may be appropriate for older patients. Preoperative petrosal sinus ACTH sampling has been used to localize an adenoma such that, if no tumor is identified at the time of surgery, hemihypophysectomy is performed on the side of the higher ACTH levels. This approach may successfully resolve Cushing's disease without resulting in the loss of other pituitary functions, and it is therefore particularly advantageous for younger patients.

Nearly 80% of patients with microadenomas (<1 cm in diameter) are cured by transsphenoidal surgery. Unfortunately, less than 50% of patients with larger lesions (macroadenomas) can expect this procedure to be curative. Tumors with marked suprasellar extension may require a transfrontal approach, and postoperative radiation therapy is almost always required. At our institution, we do not recommend repeat surgery for patients with persistent or recurrent Cushing's disease; we prefer radiation therapy, bilateral adrenalectomy, or chemotherapy (see below).

All patients require glucocorticoid coverage during surgery and perioperatively. We administer 2 mg of dexamethasone one hour prior to surgery and provide 300 mg of hydrocortisone during the 24-hour period, commencing with the induction of anesthesia. Glucocorticoid coverage is gradually tapered to replacement levels over five to seven days. After successful surgery, replacement therapy is frequently needed for a year or longer. During this interval, the suppressed pituitary recovers the capacity to secrete ACTH, in turn stimulating the adrenal cortex to recover its ability to secrete cortisol.

Diabetes insipidus, usually transient, is the most common surgical complication. Additional complications, which are encountered only rarely, include meningitis, hemorrhage, cerebrospinal fluid leak, blindness, and death.

Bilateral adrenalectomy is infrequently required. Although this procedure almost always cures Cushing's disease, it produces permanent adrenal insufficiency requiring lifelong corticosteroid replacement therapy. Adrenalectomy is also associated with the risk of subsequent development of Nelson's syndrome, an ACTH-secreting pituitary macroadenoma with invasive local growth and severe hyperpigmentation.

External radiation (4000 to 5000 rad) to the pituitary has been most successful in therapy for children with Cushing's disease. Only about 50% of adult patients have had a successful response when evaluated one year after therapy. Thus, the success rate for radiation therapy is lower than that for transsphenoidal surgery. Additionally, there is a variable post-treatment delay prior to the amelioration of symptoms, and therapy may result in pituitary hormone deficiencies. A combination of irradiation with pharmacologic therapy has allowed earlier clinical improvement.

Adrenal Adenoma. Since wound healing may be a significant problem in patients with Cushing's syndrome, a flank incision is often preferred. Patients usually require the same preoperative and postoperative glucocorticoid management as those with Cushing's disease. However, if bilateral adrenalectomy is performed, mineralocorticoid replacement is necessary. High doses of hydrocortisone have significant mineralocorticoid action, but fludrocortisone (Florinef), 0.1 mg/day, should be administered as the hydrocortisone dose is tapered below 100 mg/day.

Adrenal Carcinoma. Although surgical resection should be attempted, in 75% of cases complete resection is precluded by local invasion of the inferior vena cava and other structures. Postoperative therapy usually involves a trial of mitotane (o,p'-DDD, Lysodren). Radiation may be considered for a symptomatic localized tumor. The enzyme inhibitors (aminoglutethimide and metyrapone) are not adrenolytic and are utilized when gluco- or mineralocorticoid levels remain elevated in spite of therapy with mitotane.

Ectopic ACTH Syndrome. Ideally, this disorder is treated by removing the tumor that is secreting ACTH. However, this frequently is not possible, and the patient may require therapy to reduce the elevated glucocorticoid levels. This can be accomplished with aminoglutethimide or metyrapone or both (or even, on occasion, adrenalectomy).

PHARMACOLOGIC AGENTS

The serotonin antagonist cyproheptadine can decrease ACTH levels and lower the production of cortisol in some patients with Cushing's disease; however, many patients do not respond to this agent. In addition, cyproheptadine is not curative; therefore, Cushing's disease will recur if the medication is discontinued. The same is true for the dopamine agonist bromocriptine. Therefore, these drugs are rarely used in the initial management of patients with Cushing's disease.

Metyrapone and aminoglutethimide are expensive and, since they block the synthesis of cortisol, ACTH levels rise and ever-increasing dosages are required when they are used to treat Cushing's disease. However, in patients with the ectopic ACTH syndrome or an adrenal tumor, these agents may be useful clinically, and in selected patients they may accomplish a temporary decrease in cortisol levels and thus help prepare a patient with severe cushingoid signs for surgery. Metyrapone, 250 to 500 mg every six hours with food or milk, may allow normalization of cortisol levels for several weeks prior to surgery. Aminoglutethimide, which blocks early steroidogenesis, is the more effective of the two agents. Therapy is initiated at a dose of 250 mg b.i.d. and gradually increased to 1 to 2 gm/day. Hydrocortisone, 20 mg b.i.d., should be provided to treat resultant adrenal insufficiency. The other major toxicity is dermatologic eruption.

Mitotane has been used most often in patients with adrenal carcinoma. Mitotane destroys adrenal cells and alters steroid metabolism so that serum cortisol or urine-free cortisol determinations, rather than measurements of urine 17-hydroxycorticosteroids, must be utilized to assess therapy. Treatment of adrenal carcinoma requires a daily dose of ≈ 10 gm or more, which must be attained gradually. Evidence of therapeutic benefit may be delayed for a significant interval beyond the initiation of treatment. Lower doses (2 to 4 gm/day) have been used (often in combination with radiation) in therapy for patients with Cushing's disease.

Mitotane therapy causes anorexia, nausea, vomiting, depression, malaise, and diarrhea. However, since it is the only agent that is adrenolytic, patients with adrenal cancer should be encouraged to persist with therapy. Finally, in some patients, treatment results in adrenal insufficiency and necessitates glucocorticoid replacement.

PERIODIC EVALUATION

Follow-up visits after surgical therapy for Cushing's syndrome are required in order to (1) determine whether the treatment was successful, (2) follow and educate the patient about adrenal insufficiency, (3) evaluate the patient's pituitary hormone status, (4) help with psychologic problems that may be associated with alterations in glucocorticoid levels, and (5) reassess the need for antihypertensive or hypoglycemic medications, or both, that may have been required for the manifestations of Cushing's syndrome.

Patients are generally seen one week after hospital discharge and then at monthly intervals. At each visit an 8 AM serum cortisol level is obtained after the patient has not taken any glucocorticoid for the previous 24 hours. Once the 8 AM cortisol level is ≥ 12 μg/dl, an ACTH (cosyntropin [Cortrosyn]) stimulation test can be performed. When there is a normal response to this test, the glucocorticoid therapy can be discontinued. It frequently takes a year or more before these patients recover normal function of the hypothalamic-pituitary-adrenal axis. During this time, they should receive the same treatment and follow the same precautions as other patients with adrenal insufficiency.

REFERENCES

Aron DC, Findling JW, Fitzgerald PA, et al: Cushing's syndrome: problems in management. Endocr Rev 3:229–244, 1982.
Boggan JE, Tyrrell JB, Wilson CB: Transsphenoidal microsurgical management: report of 100 cases of Cushing's disease. J Neurosurg 59:195–200, 1983.
Chrousos GP, Schulte HM, Oldfield EH, et al: The corticotropin-releasing factor stimulation test: an aid in the evaluation of patients with Cushing's syndrome. N Engl J Med 310:622–626, 1984.
Crapo L: Cushing's syndrome: a review of diagnostic tests. Metabolism 28:955–977, 1979.
Fitzgerald PA, Aron DC, Findling JW: Cushing's disease: transient secondary adrenal insufficiency after selective removal of pituitary microadenomas; evidence for a pituitary origin. J Clin Endocrinol Metab 54:413–422, 1982.

13 · HIRSUTISM

Lawrence V. Basso
Randy Linde
PALO ALTO MEDICAL CLINIC

DEFINITION AND DIAGNOSTIC CRITERIA

In our appearance-conscious society, excessive hair is a common complaint among women. An objective diagnosis of hirsutism rests on finding increased amounts of coarse hair on the face or body, usually in the second or third decade of life. An important study, in which 400 women who did not report hirsutism were examined, found the normal hair distribution shown in Table 1.

Mild androgen excess causes hirsutism and complexion changes. Moderate to severe androgen excess leads to virilization, which includes temporal balding, thinning of scalp hair, deep voice, male body habitus, and clitoromegaly. Male pattern balding without increased facial or body hair or anovulation is a most unusual manifestation of androgen excess. The development of hirsutism during pregnancy or menopause occurs often enough for it not to be considered pathologic in most cases.

PATHOPHYSIOLOGY

The differential diagnosis of hirsutism is summarized in Table 2. The principal androgens in women are dehydroepiandrosterone (DHEA) and dehydroepiandrosterone sulfate (DHEAS) (mainly adrenal) and testosterone (50% by direct ovarian secretion, 50% by adrenal secretion of testosterone and of androstenedione, which is peripherally converted to testosterone). Free androgens constitute the active hormonal pool, with only 1% to 2% of testosterone normally in the unbound state. Sex hormone–binding globulin (SHBG) is lowered by a high level of testosterone, thereby increasing the proportion that is free in hyperandrogenic states.

Table 1. NORMAL FEMALE HAIR DISTRIBUTION

Location	% of Patients
Arms and legs	84
Linea alba	35
Face (upper lip)	26
Chest (excluding sternum)	17
Chin	10
Sternum	<3

Table 2. DIFFERENTIAL DIAGNOSIS OF HIRSUTISM

Ovarian causes
   polcystic ovary syndrome (PCO); hyperthecosis; androgen-secreting
     tumor
Adrenal causes
   congenital adrenal hyperplasia; Cushing's syndrome;
    androgen-secreting tumor
Increased sensitivity of the pilosebaceous unit to androgen
   e.g., increased 5α-reductase activity
Drug effects
    e.g., androgens, corticosteroids, phenytoin, minoxidil, diazoxide
Idiopathic

Androgen receptors are found on the skin in the hair follicles and the sebaceous and sweat glands. These sites metabolize androgens, and in particular convert free testosterone by 5α-reductase to the most potent androgen, dihydrotestosterone. Cutaneous pubic fibroblasts of many hirsute women contain far more 5α-reductase activity than is present in normal women. Intracellular metabolism of dihydrotestosterone to androstanediol glucuronide may also play a role in the development of hirsutism, and concentrations of this metabolite are frequently elevated in women with idiopathic hirsutism.

Thus, hirsutism occurs as a consequence of increased production of, or sensitivity to, androgen.

CLINICAL ASPECTS

To determine the etiology of hirsutism in a specific patient, the following questions must be asked:

1. What is the ethnic background and family history?
2. Did hirsutism begin at puberty or later in life?
3. Is hair growth progressive?
4. Is the patient virilized?
5. Is there associated failure of ovulation?

Laboratory evaluation should be done to rule out tumor and to establish the most likely cause. Although testing of total serum testosterone and DHEAS levels is sufficient for many patients, the following are also occasionally indicated: urinary cortisol and ketosteroid determinations, serum SHBG and free testosterone, androstenedione and gonadotropin levels, and ACTH stimulation testing to prove an adrenal enzyme deficiency. When tumor is suspected, ultrasound of the ovaries and CT scan of the adrenals are indicated.

MANAGEMENT

NONPHARMACOLOGIC MEASURES

Long-term medical treatment may ultimately prevent new hair growth but will have no effect on hair already present. Bleaching, plucking, waxing, chemical depilatories, or shaving can bring about short-term improvement. Electrolysis may provide long-term benefit but is painful, costly, and time-consuming and may leave scars. Nonetheless, this is widely used and often helpful for mild hirsutism never brought to a physician's attention. Techniques using radiofrequency energy for depilation usually leave less if any residual scarring, but produce a burning sensation and are relatively untested. As yet there is no proven permanent method of non-pharmacologically preventing excessive hair growth, other than removing a pituitary, ovarian, or adrenal neoplasm. Ovarian wedge resection for polycystic ovary syndrome is rarely indicated and often of only temporary benefit.

DRUG THERAPY

Idiopathic Hyperandrogenism. The ideal medication would block a final common pathway of hair growth. The failure of any one available agent to reduce hair growth in all patients is indirect proof of the variety of pathogenic mechanisms in hirsutism. The antiandrogen cyproterone acetate has been widely used in Europe, but it produces a number of side effects, including suppression of the pituitary-adrenal axis, and is not FDA-approved. Cimetidine (Tagamet) is also an antiandrogen, but its use is limited by a paucity of clinical studies and often precluded by expense. The most promising agent is spironolactone (Aldactone), which competes for the androgen receptor on the hair follicle but also inhibits ovarian steroidogenesis and increases peripheral conversion of testosterone to estradiol. The dose ranges from 50 to 200 mg daily; larger doses produce a greater antiandrogenic effect. Although some patients report a response within two months, a therapeutic trial should be continued for at least six months. Some oligomenorrheic women develop ovulatory cycles while taking spironolactone. We have observed one virilized woman with congenital adrenal hyperplasia who reported a diminution of hair growth in only two weeks on just 25 mg BID, and all features of masculinization regressed within two months.

Ovarian Hyperandrogenism. The time-honored treatment for ovarian hyperandrogenism is a combination oral contraceptive. An agent containing as little as 30 or 35 μg of estradiol usually produces good results (Loestrin 1.5/30 or Demulen 1/35). The progestin suppresses luteinizing hormone (LH) levels, which in turn lowers the serum testosterone. The estrogen increases SHBG, lowering free testosterone levels. Clomiphene citrate is indicated for ovulation induction in women with the polycystic ovary syndrome but is not used as therapy for hirsutism. Although we do not prescribe medroxyprogesterone acetate (Provera), this drug has been given to individuals who cannot take estrogen, 10 mg TID, gradually tapered after the first month of treatment. The mechanism of action is a suppression of LH and an increase in testosterone clearance. Long-acting Depo-Provera given IM is controversial and not FDA-approved for this use. The effects of the lower dose "progesterone-only" oral contraceptives (Micronor-QD or Ovrette) on hair growth have not been sufficiently studied.

Adrenal Hyperandrogenism. In adrenal hyperandrogenism, a bedtime dose of dexamethasone can be used to lower the nocturnal ACTH surge. The dosage, usually 0.25 to 0.5 mg, should be the lowest effective dose that does not obliterate the pituitary-adrenal response to stress or cause cushingoid changes. Suppression of urinary 17-ketosteroids or serum DHEAS to the normal range is necessary for a therapeutic response.

Combination Therapy. A combination of these drugs is often the most effective means of treatment. We have had particularly good results using both a low-dose oral contraceptive and spironolactone.

Adverse Effects

Spironolactone infrequently causes breast enlargement or tenderness or mild hypotension; these problems resolve with lower doses or discontinuation. Women are warned of the necessity for birth control since this drug may be teratogenic. Oral contraceptives can exacerbate hypertension, morbid obesity, hyperlipidemia, or vascular headache and thus are relatively contraindicated in patients with these disorders. Infrequently, nonmorbid obesity or diabetes mellitus is worsened by oral contraceptives. Hyperprolactinemia, active liver disease, or previous deep vein phlebitis are absolute contraindications, as is cigarette smoking in women over 35 years of age. We rarely prescribe oral contraceptives for women over 35 and never for those over 40, because of potentially increased cardiovascular morbidity. Medroxyprogesterone can cause weight gain, amenorrhea, and headaches. Dexamethasone is a potent glucocorticoid and excessive doses result in striae, bruising, moon facies, glucose intolerance, and hypertension.

Periodic Evaluation and Compliance

We suggest follow-up every three to six months to ensure continuity. If a patient is willing, some form of objective reassessment is used, e.g., photography or weighing hair shaven from a designated area after one week's growth. Most patients report improvement rather accurately, however, and the patient's perceived improvement is the goal of treatment, as hirsutism by itself does not threaten health. Compliance is rarely a problem, although loss of therapeutic efficacy occurs and may demand a change in treatment.

REFERENCES

Biffignandi P, Massucchetti C, Molinatti GM: Female hirsutism: pathophysiological considerations and therapeutic implications. Endocr Rev 5:498–509, 1984.

Ferriman D, Gallwey JD: Clinical assessment of body hair growth in women. J Clin Endocrinol Metab 21:1440–1447, 1961.

Futterweit W: Polycystic Ovarian Disease. Springer-Verlag, New York, 1984.

New MI, Levine LS: Congenital Adrenal Hyperplasia. Springer-Verlag, Heidelberg, 1984.

14 · MALE HYPOGONADISM AND IMPOTENCE

Peter C. Walther
SCRIPPS CLINIC AND RESEARCH FOUNDATION

DEFINITION AND DIAGNOSTIC CRITERIA

Hypogonadism refers to a state of inadequate testosterone production or utilization in peripheral tissues. It is a leading cause of organic (nonpsychogenic) impotence. Impotence is the inability to obtain or maintain an erection satisfactory for sexual intercourse. Virtually all men occasionally experience inability to maintain an erection during intercourse. Most sexual dysfunction therapists believe true impotence is not present until there is failure in at least 50% of attempts. Today we are seeing increasing public awareness of impotence as a treatable problem, even as a common and popular topic for TV and radio talk shows.

PATHOPHYSIOLOGY AND CLINICAL ASPECTS

The clinical presentation of hypogonadism may vary from isolated loss of libido to overt eunuchoidism. The etiology may be hypothalamic, pituitary, or testicular. Decreased testosterone production with a low serum luteinizing hormone (LH) implies a disorder of the pituitary or hypothalamus that can be either congenital or acquired in origin. Gonadotropin-releasing hormone (GnRH) is available clinically and can be used to determine pituitary responsiveness to exogenous stimulation. When serum LH is normal or elevated, hypogonadism is secondary to a primary testicular disorder.

Hypogonadism is the most common identifiable cause of pathologic gynecomastia, a painless enlargement of the male breasts. Other leading causes include drugs (e.g., digitalis, cimetidine, spironolactone, and a wide variety of CNS agents), marijuana, and testicular and human chorionic gonadotropin (hCG)-producing nontesticular tumors. At puberty, 60% to 70% of boys experience physiologic gynecomastia and most are unaware of it. Systemic diseases such as renal failure, hepatic disorders, and hyperthyroidism also produce gynecomastia.

Primary testicular failure peaks in incidence in the fifth decade of life and has multiple causes including viral orchitis, trauma, epididymitis, granulomatous disease, radiation exposure, alcoholism, or drugs (especially those used in chemotherapy). Recent studies have shown a qualitative defect in testicular response to LH in aging and severe systemic illness.

Pertinent history in a man with impotence includes a general medical review with emphasis on erectile characteristics, libido, partner participation, alcohol, smoking, and other recreational drug use. One needs to ask specifically about the presence and quality of nocturnal or early-morning "full bladder" erections. Hypogonadism invariably includes some degree of decreased libido. Primary loss of interest is due to reduced production or utilization of testosterone. Job-related, marital, and family stress all contribute to secondary loss of interest in sex and potential impotence without abnormalities of testosterone production.

The physical examination should exclude abnormalities of the neurologic and vascular systems. Sacral reflex arcs such as the bulbocavernosus reflex and anal tone should be tested. Peripheral pulses in the lower extremities should be recorded. Signs of alcohol abuse, loss of secondary male characteristics, gynecomastia, and reduced testicular size should be noted. While normal testicular size is highly variable, a longitudinal diameter less than 3.5 cm should alert one to the possibility of testicular failure.

The laboratory evaluation begins with measurement of serum testosterone. Normal values vary depending on local laboratory methods, but 500 to 600 ng/dl is the mid-range, decreasing to 350 to 400 ng/dl by age 70. The lower limit of normal is poorly established, but generally a value below 300 ng/dl is considered abnormal. The clinical history is important in relating serum testosterone levels to abnormal sexual function. In the absence of diminished libido, reduced serum testosterone rarely implicates hypogonadism as a cause of impotence. In patients with abnormal serum proteins (e.g., thyroid disease, severe liver disease, or nutritional deficiencies), a measurement of total and free testosterone is of more value. Normal values also vary among laboratories, but free testosterone should be 80 to 210 pg/ml. This test is of limited value.

Serum LH is of practical value only when there is a question of a low testosterone level. It is rare to see hypogonadotropic hypogonadism in an adult if there has been no previous pituitary surgery or radiation. As a general rule, a borderline low serum testosterone level in conjunction with normal serum LH in an adult male with impotence means that testicular function is normal. GnRH can be used to measure pituitary reponsiveness, a normal response to a 100-μg dose given IM or IV being a several-fold increase in LH levels. Failure to respond suggests pituitary dysfunction. Similarly, hCG can be used to measure Leydig cell function, with 5000 U given daily IM for four days and serum testosterone measured immediately before and after treatment. A normal response is at least a doubling of testosterone levels.

Hyperprolactinemia is a rare cause of male impotence; when this is present the patient may have a pituitary tumor that can be quite large. In my experience with over 400 new patients with sexual dysfunction, only four elevated serum prolactins were found, and this low incidence has been corroborated in other larger series. It is not cost effective to obtain a serum prolactin without evidence of diminished libido, gynecomastia, or signs of pituitary disease.

Routine use of specialized testing to evaluate impotence is now commonplace. There is a simple test to measure the presence of erections during sleep. Just before the patient retires for the night, a ring of stamps is placed around the base of the penis, overlapping by one stamp, which is then moistened to secure the ring. If the ring is not broken at a perforation, it can be assumed the patient did not have an erection during the night. It often takes five to ten nights to ensure adequate reproducibility of this test. Nocturnal penile tumescence monitoring in a sleep center is a more accurate measurement of erections during rapid eye movement sleep, presumably a time free of psychogenic impotence.

Sophisticated electromyographic equipment is utilized to measure sacral nerve function objectively and minutely. This procedure, sacral evoked potentials, measures the time interval between a stimulus applied to the penis, with transit through the sacral spinal reflex centers, and a response recorded in the perineal musculature and/or cerebral cortex. Noninvasive vascular evaluations can be performed using a Doppler stethoscope to measure arterial wave forms and absolute pressures of penile arteries. Intracorporeal (penile) injections of papaverine (30 mg) and phentolamine (0.5 mg) are being used increasingly as both a diagnostic and therapeutic maneuver. They cause intense local vasodilation, producing an erection usually 50% to 70% of normal. This injection may become a standard functional test of penile arterial sufficiency. Specialized angiographic visualization of the arterial and venous penile vasculature, first developed in Europe, is slowly becoming available in the United States. All these tests are difficult to perform and usually require the patient to be referred to a sexual dysfunction center specializing in sophisticated diagnostic testing.

MANAGEMENT

NONPHARMACOLOGIC THERAPY

Sexual therapy is indicated for any patient with psychogenic impotence. Performance anxiety is the most common nonorganic cause of impotence, and marital disharmony is much more common than generally appreciated. Often the primary physician, by taking the time to listen and reassure, can treat these anxious men. It is often effective to focus the man's efforts on participating with his partner, and proscribing intercourse for a fixed period, usually four to twelve weeks. These sensate focus exercises allow the couple to concentrate on each other without fear of performance failure.

Surgical treatment of erectile failure is reserved for patients who fail to respond to more conservative treatments, but is highly effective at reestablishing normal erections in the appropriate patient. Diabetes is the leading cause of impotence in men undergoing surgical treatment of impotence. Vascular disease is the second most common cause, and a variety of other conditions including radical pelvic surgery make up the remaining groups. Great advances have been made in the materials used in penile prostheses. Complications such as infection and mechanical failure, previously as high as 30%, now range from 3% (semirigid) to 12% (inflatable). In the near future microvascular techniques will be widely available for reconstruction of penile arteries and obliteration of abnormal venous outflow as alternatives to penile implants.

DRUG THERAPY

Hypogonadism, whether due to pituitary or testicular failure, is best treated with an injectable testosterone ester in an oil preparation. The two most useful preparations are testosterone enanthate and testosterone cypionate. I favor the enanthate since it is longer acting and more evenly absorbed. A therapeutic trial can be given with 300 mg IM every three weeks for three doses. Response should be prompt, with increased libido noted first. The absorption and decay curves of injected testosterone suggest that a maximal response should occur by days five to seven, but the biologic effect may not be seen for two to three weeks. A small but significant number of patients think they need only "a shot to get them going" and are unwilling to face up to the complex personal and social problems that are often the root of the sexual dysfunction. These patients report a good response to the first injection but none to subsequent injections. Most then become receptive to other forms of therapy. I have varied the dose between 200 and 400 mg and the timing from two- to four-week intervals, titrating to the individual patient's needs.

Higher or more frequent doses are unnecessary. Usually the first three doses are given in the office; if treatment is continued, the patient or his partner is taught self-injection. The anterior thigh is a convenient and safe site.

Oral androgen replacement is also therapeutic but should not be used in the long term. The 17-alpha-alkyl-substituted androgens (such as methyltestosterone) are the most frequently used agents in doses ranging from 10 to 20 mg per day.

It is rare to see isolated hypogonadism as the sole cause of sexual dysfunction. One must look for additional factors, as outlined earlier, and treat them in addition to simply replacing testosterone. Strict blood sugar control in diabetic patients, including the use of insulin, may restore erectile potency. A multifactorial rationale includes reversal of peripheral neuropathy and an improved sense of well-being. Antihypertensive medications commonly produce impotence. Prazosin HCl (Minipress), as single therapy, seems to produce the lowest incidence of impotence, but overall I have been unimpressd by attempts to recover potency with changing medications. Greatest success might come by controlling hypertension with nonpharmacologic means such as weight loss, stress reduction, and biofeedback.

Bromocriptine is the drug of choice for hyperprolactinemia. Treatment is begun at 2.5 mg b.i.d., occasional patients requiring as much as 10 to 15 mg per day.

Impotence secondary to alcohol excess requires total cessation of alcohol use for at least six months. At best, only 50% of these patients recover normal sexual function. More commonly seen, however, is the patient with episodic erectile failure produced by acute intoxication. Education and counseling is helpful for this group of individuals.

Treatment of gynecomastia is best directed at the cause. Physiologic breast enlargement of puberty can be ignored. A careful drug history is usually sufficient to identify and remove the offending agent. Patients should be encouraged to stop taking alcohol and marijuana. Hyperthyroidism and neoplasia can be treated by medical and/or surgical means.

As mentioned previously, intracorporeal (penile) injections of papaverine and phentolamine can produce a partial erection (50% to 70%) in men with neurologic and psychologic impotence. It is being used at an increasing number of centers, but is still considered experimental at this time.

ADVERSE EFFECTS OF THERAPY

Surgical treatment of impotence carries well-defined risks. Infection occurs in 1% of nondiabetic patients and in 2% to 3% of diabetics. Once diagnosed, an infected prosthesis requires complete removal and it is often three to six months before it can be replaced. The inflatable prosthesis, since it is a hydraulic system, has several points where leaks can occur. A leak requires surgical correction since the prosthesis will not function without fluid. There is the additional risk and cost of anesthesia for every operative procedure.

Injectable testosterone carries few risks. Occasional patients complain of slight gynecomastia, but in my experience this has not necessitated discontinuance of therapy. Testosterone ester preparations do not produce hepatic dysfunction as do the oral androgens. Patients with prostatic enlargement and voiding difficulties must be warned of the risk of exacerbating the underlying disease and even necessitating a prostatectomy. This has only occasionally been a problem in my practice. Cancer of the prostate at any stage is an absolute contraindication to any androgen replacement. Testosterone therapy does not, however, cause prostate cancer. Patients on such therapy long term should be examined at six- to 12-month intervals.

Testosterone replacement therapy, whether given IM or PO, often produces infertility. In younger patients, usually with abnormalities of the hypothalamic-pituitary axis, sophisticated treatment with GnRH or with hCG and human menopausal gonadotropins (hMG) is required to treat hypogonadism while promoting fertility.

Oral androgens sometimes help to reverse impotence, but are not suitable for long-term therapy since they cause hepatic dysfunction. Frequent (three-month) liver enzyme determinations are necessary to monitor this type of drug therapy. I have not used synthetic androgens, commonly favored by body builders, for replacement therapy.

Bromocryptine has several troubling side effects, nausea being the most common, with orthostatic hypotension next. In most patients these effects disappear with continued use of the medication at a low dose (2.5 mg b.i.d.).

REFERENCES

Griffin JE, Wilson JD: The testis. *In* Bondy PK, Rosenberg LE (eds): Metabolic Control and Disease, 8th ed. W. B. Saunders Co, Philadelphia, 1980, pp 1535–1578.

Mallory TR, Wein AJ: The etiology, diagnosis and surgical treatment of erectile impotence. J Reprod Med 20:183–194, 1978.

Rabin D, McKenna TJ: Clinical Endocrinology and Metabolism. Grune & Stratton, New York, 1982, pp 49–54.

Shrom SH, Lief HI, Wein AJ: Clinical profile of experience with 130 consecutive cases of impotent men. Urology 13:511–515, 1979.

Streem SB: The endocrinology of impotence. *In* Bennett AH (ed): Management of Male Impotence. Williams & Wilkins Co, Baltimore, 1982, pp 26–45.

15 · MULTIPLE ENDOCRINE NEOPLASIA (MEN)

A. Mary McCarroll
SCRIPPS CLINIC AND RESEARCH FOUNDATION

DEFINITION

Multiple endocrine neoplasia encompasses three distinct multiglandular syndromes: MEN I, MEN IIa, and MEN IIb, observed in families and sporadically in individuals (Table 1). Inheritance is by autosomal dominant mode with equal number of males and females affected.

Table 1. MULTIPLE ENDOCRINE NEOPLASIA: GLANDULAR INVOLVEMENT FREQUENCY (%)

Men I		Men II	IIa	IIb
Parathyroid	80	Thyroid	90	100
Pancreas	75	Parathyroid	40	1
Pituitary	56	Adrenal medulla	20	50

PATHOPHYSIOLOGY

Various models have been proposed, including Wermer's original gene mutation theory, Knudson's mutation model for tumor formation, Pearse's APUD (*a*mine *p*recursor *u*ptake *d*ecarboxylation) cell concept, and a theory that the tumor might release substances trophic for other glands.

CLINICAL FEATURES

The most common combination of three-gland involvement in MEN I is hyperparathyroidism, gastrinoma, and nonfunctioning pituitary adenoma. Multiglandular involvement of the parathyroid glands is common but carcinoma is rare. Pancreatic lesions typically involve the gastrin- or insulin-secreting cells with peptic ulceration or fasting hypoglycemia. Many pancreatic tumors are malignant. Most pituitary tumors are (1) nonfunctioning, (2) benign, and (3) recognizable on radiographic screening or because of headache, visual disturbance, or excessive secretion of growth hormone, ACTH, or prolactin.

MEN IIa consists of multifocal hyperplasia or neoplasia of the C cells of the thyroid, parathyroids, and adrenal medulla. MEN IIb (mucosal neuroma syndrome) consists of hyperplasia or neoplasia of the C cells of the thyroid and adrenal medulla, a marfanoid habitus, and multiple mucosal neuromas on the eyelids, lips, and gastrointestinal tract. There is no clinically relevant parathyroid disease. Most cases of MEN I are silent until 15 years of age and most are diagnosed after the age of 25 years, but screening studies for hereditary medullary carcinoma of the thyroid (MCT) should begin as early as 2 years of age in family members at risk and be continued annually until the patient is approximately 40 years of age. The C-cell and adrenomedullary dysfunctions follow less aggressive courses in MEN IIa, while it is unusual for a person with MEN IIb to survive beyond 40 years.

MANAGEMENT

EVALUATION

MEN I. An appropriate screening for MEN I includes fasting serum calcium and phosphate (parathyroid); fasting plasma gastrin, insulin, and glucose with calculation of the insulin: glucose ratio (pancreas); and basal serum prolactin, early morning cortisol, and free thyroxine (pituitary).

MEN II. Annual screening should start at 2 years of age. The combined calcium gluconate–pentagastrin test or a ten-minute calcium infusion are equally satisfactory provocative tests for calcitonin release. A normal basal value is considered to be less than 100 pg/ml, with a normal stimulated value as high as 250 pg/ml. Prospec-

tive studies have not shown conversion of a negative to a positive test after the age of 35, so that the frequency of screening can then be decreased. Adrenomedullary disease must be evaluated and treated before thyroid disease. Two techniques appear to be most sensitive for diagnosing early adrenomedullary abnormalities. The first is the measurement of 24-hour excretion of urinary epinephrine and norepinephrine with calculation of the epinephrine:norepinephrine ratio. The second is the [131]metaiodobenzylguanidine (MIBG) scan. The risks of other provocative tests make their use unjustifiable.

TREATMENT

MEN I. Treatment is surgical for the most part and should be done only by a person well trained and experienced in endocrine surgery.

Parathyroid. It is essential for the surgeon to expose all four glands and to resect three and one half glands (subtotal parathyroidectomy), as the likelihood of persistent or recurrent hyperparathyroidism is great. An alternative procedure preferred by some is total parathyroidectomy with immediate autotransplantation.

Pancreas. Cimetidine or ranitidine can be used to control hyperacidity, but gastrinomas are generally best treated by total gastrectomy with or without resection of the tumor. An effective preoperative localization procedure is percutaneous transhepatic portal system venography and venous sampling for immunoreactive gastrin. Approximately 75% of patients have multiple lesions, of which nearly half are malignant. Thus, only about one patient in four with the Zollinger-Ellison syndrome has a chance of being cured by the removal of a single excisable pancreatic tumor. Since hypercalcemia can increase gastrin and gastric acid secretion in hyperparathyroidism, parathyroidectomy and remeasurement of serum gastrin and gastric acid production should precede surgery for gastrinoma. If possible a solitary lesion of the pancreas should be removed after a meticulous search has been made for other lesions and about 10% of the distal pancreas has been examined microscopically to rule out microadenomatosis. Some patients may be cured by removal of a solitary lesion. In the younger asymptomatic family member in whom the condition is diagnosed as the result of screening, exploration of the pancreas is indicated.

The definitive treatment for insulinoma is pancreatic exploration and excision of abnormal beta-cell tissue, preceded by percutaneous transhepatic portal system venography and venous sampling for immunoreactive insulin. Family screening may disclose asymptomatic patients with mild hyperinsulinemia. The finding of supernormal levels of a second islet hormone, e.g., glucagon, increases the probability that malignancy exists and is a relative indication for exploration of the pancreas in such patients. The incidence of malignancy in MEN I is about 20%.

Pituitary. Treatment for the most part is surgical, by the transphenoidal approach. Bromocriptine therapy for prolactinoma has improved management considerably when surgery has been unsuccessful or not feasible, and is used by an increasing number of endocrinologists as first-line therapy.

MEN II

Pheochromocytoma. There are two equally acceptable surgical approaches: (1) routine bilateral adrenalectomy; (2) unilateral adrenalectomy with preservation of the remaining adrenal gland if it appears normal radiologically and by palpation. Alpha- and beta-blockade is employed before surgery. Intraoperative blood pressure elevations can be managed with either phentolamine or nitroprusside infusion; tachyarrhythmias can be treated with propranolol. Aggressive blood and fluid replacement is generally advocated and appears to be beneficial.

Medullary Thyroid Cancer. Total thyroidectomy with central node dissection is the only effective treatment because this is always a bilateral disease. The same surgery is performed in those who convert from a negative provocative test to a positive one. Care must be taken to preserve some parathyroid tissue. Chemotherapy is ineffective in eradicating this disease, although some patients have had a reduction in tumor mass after treatment with doxorubicin (Adriamycin), cisplatinum, or radiotherapy. Adjunctive radioactive iodine therapy at the time of surgery prevents recurrence in those with localized disease but does not influence the outcome in those with metastases.

PERIODIC EVALUATION

If MEN is diagnosed, first-degree family members should be screened as soon as possible. Subsequently both they and the propositus should have repeated reevaluations. There are no rules for the frequency of these nor for the precise screening protocol to be followed. Frequency is determined, at least partly, by ease and cost of testing, family pattern of involvement, and individual age and willingness. In MEN I and II lifelong follow-up is essential to detect recurrent disease and to monitor hormone replacement therapy.

REFERENCES

Graze K, Spiler IJ, Tashjian AH, et al: Natural history of familial medullary thyroid carcinoma: effect of a program for early diagnosis. N Engl J Med 299:980–985, 1978.

Knudson AG: Genetics and etiology of human cancer. In Harris H, Hirschhorn K (eds): Advances in Human Genetics, Vol 8. Plenum Publishing Corp, New York, 1977, pp 1–66.

Pearse AGE: Common cytochemical properties of cells producing polypeptide hormones, with particular reference to CT and the thyroid C-cells. Vet Rec 79:587–590, 1966.

Wells SA, Baylin SB, Linehan WM, et al: Provocative agents and the diagnosis of medullary carcinoma of the thyroid gland. Ann Surg 188:139–141, 1978.

Wermer P: Genetic aspects of adenomatosis of endocrine glands. Am J Med 16:363–371, 1954.

16 · PLURIGLANDULAR AUTOIMMUNE SYNDROME

A. Mary McCarroll
SCRIPPS CLINIC AND RESEARCH FOUNDATION

DEFINITION

Dysfunction of two or more endocrine glands on the basis of an autoimmune mechanism constitutes the pluriglandular autoimmune (PGA) syndrome (Table 1). In making the diagnosis, causes of multiple glandular insufficiencies other than autoimmunity must be considered. These include hypopituitarism, infiltrative disorders such as hemochromatosis and sarcoidosis, and a syndrome described in middle-aged males that has been given the acronym POEMS to indicate its principal features: polyneuropathy, organomegaly, endocrinopathy, M protein, and skin changes.

PATHOPHYSIOLOGY

Autoimmunity is strongly suggested by lymphocytic infiltration in the involved endocrine glands and by circulating organ-specific and non–organ-specific autoantibodies in affected persons and their first-degree relatives. PGA type I is not associated with an increased incidence of any specific human leukocyte antigen (HLA), but B8 and DR3 are often present in Caucasian patients with PGA type II, suggesting a separate pathogenesis for these syndromes. As might be expected if chromosome 6 influences pathogenesis, there is a higher prevalence of disease in relatives whose HLA genotype is identical to that of the proband. A possible etiology is that the autoimmune phenomenon follows a primary insult to the target gland, such as from viruses or chemicals, with overt disease occurring in genetically predisposed individuals.

CLINICAL ASPECTS

PGA syndrome type I usually begins in childhood as mucous membrane, ungual, or cutaneous candidi-

Table 1. PRINCIPAL MANIFESTATIONS OF THE PLURIGLANDULAR AUTOIMMUNE SYNDROMES

PGA Type	Manifestations
I	Chronic mucocutaneous candidiasis, hypoparathyroidism, adrenal insufficiency
II	Adrenal insufficiency, autoimmune thyroid disease, insulin-dependent diabetes mellitus
III	Autoimmune thyroid disease, pernicious anemia, insulin-dependent diabetes mellitus

asis. There is a female predominance. Although siblings are often affected, members of successive generations are not. Family studies suggest an autosomal recessive trait, but sporadic cases also occur. Hypoparathyroidism almost always precedes the onset of adrenal insufficiency. Endocrine failure usually occurs within a few years of the onset of mucocutaneous candidiasis. Other commonly reported autoimmune disorders in affected persons include ovarian failure, juvenile-onset pernicious anemia, chronic active hepatitis, and malabsorption syndromes.

PGA type II starts most frequently in the third or fourth decades with adrenal insufficiency associated with autoimmune thyroid disease or insulin-dependent diabetes mellitus or both. As in PGA type I there is a female predominance, and both familial and sporadic cases occur. Although other endocrine diseases occur much less often than with PGA type I, an increased prevalence of Sjögren's syndrome, autoimmune thrombocytopenic purpura, and rheumatoid arthritis has been reported.

PGA type III affects adults and consists of autoimmune thyroid disease occurring without adrenal insufficiency but with insulin-dependent diabetes mellitus (type III-A), pernicious anemia (type III-B), or vitiligo, alopecia, or other organ-specific autoimmunity (Type III-C). Autoimmune hypopituitarism has been described as part of this syndrome.

MANAGEMENT

The criteria for diagnosis and management of the PGA syndrome are those of the individual endocrinopathies. There is a striking uniformity in the sequence of appearance of the various disease components of PGA I. When a child presents with mucocutaneous candidiasis or hypoparathyroidism or both, she or he should be screened regularly for (1) adrenocortical insufficiency with AM plasma cortisol estimations, (2) chronic active hepatitis with liver function studies and antibodies to smooth muscle, and (3) malabsorption syndromes. Although this situation is unusual, the endocrinopathies may not present until the third or fourth decades, so long-term follow-up is critical.

Treatment of chronic active hepatitis and mucocutaneous candidiasis is difficult. The former may respond to immunosuppressive agents. Mild candidiasis fre-

quently responds to nystatin. However, most dermatologists now use ketoconazole as first-line treatment for severe cases instead of combined amphotericin B with transfer factor.

The prevalence of autoimmune adrenal insufficiency among patients with autoimmune thyroid disease is very low. Only if other factors are present and recognized as being associated with an increased risk of developing adrenal insufficiency, for example, insulin-dependent diabetes mellitus or a positive family history of PGA type II, should a patient with primary hypothyroidism be evaluated more thoroughly for latent adrenal insufficiency.

On the other hand, the risks of developing thyroid disease and insulin-dependent diabetes mellitus are significantly increased in a patient with autoimmune adrenal insufficiency. The most efficient and cost-effective approach to the management of these patients is to evaluate them for specific disorders at periodic intervals. This principle can also be applied to PGA type III.

PATIENT INFORMATION AND EDUCATION

Twenty-five per cent of patients with hypofunction of one gland have another end organ–specific or nonspecific autoimmune disease. Continued suspicion of other glandular hypofunction must be maintained in following such patients, who should be fully informed of this significant risk and impressed with the need to wear a Medic-Alert bracelet and to return for regular and long-term follow-up. Family members must be made aware of the high prevalence of endocrinopathies among first-degree relatives. They should be evaluated by means of a subjective questionnaire and informed of the early symptoms of the major disorders for which they are at risk. Clinical and biochemical screening should be initiated if suggestive symptoms appear.

PREVENTIVE MEASURES

The value of elevated circulating antiorgan antibodies as predictors of eventual endocrine gland failure has not been established in either patients or their first-degree relatives. Routine HLA typing and assessment of humoral and cellular immune profiles of relatives are not recommended since inheritance is complex and sporadic cases occur.

REFERENCES

Bardwick PA, Zvaifler NJ, Gill GN, et al: Plasma cell dyscrasia with polyneuropathy, organomegaly, endocrinopathy, M-protein, and skin changes. The POEMS syndrome. Medicine 59:311–322, 1980.

Eisenbarth GS, Lebovitz HE: Mini review: immunogenetics of the polyglandular failure syndrome. Life Sci 22:1675–1684, 1978.

Eisenbarth GS, Wilson PW, Ward F, et al: The polyglandular failure syndrome: disease inheritance, HLA type, and immune function. Studies in patients and families. Ann Intern Med 91:528–533, 1979.

Trence DL, Morley JE, Handwerger BS: Polyglandular autoimmune syndromes. Am J Med 77:107–116, 1984.

Wilson PW, Buckley CE III, Eisenbarth GS: Disordered immune function in patients with polyglandular failure. J Clin Endocrinol Metab 52:284–288, 1981.

17 · HORMONES AND CANCER

George E. Dailey III
SCRIPPS CLINIC AND RESEARCH FOUNDATION

DEFINITION

The possible interactions of hormones and cancer are legion. Two important questions facing clinicians are: (1) do exogenous hormones cause cancer? and (2) what are the clinical presentations and potential utility of tumorous hormone production?

MANAGEMENT

HORMONAL TREATMENT

Endometrial and Breast Carcinoma. The first question is most relevant for carcinoma of the endometrium and breast in women and carcinoma of the prostate in men. Unopposed estrogen therapy increases the risk of endometrial carcinoma four- to ninefold. Extensive data in several thousand women suggest that adding cyclic progestin therapy nullifies the risk, perhaps below that of women not supplemented at all (e.g., conjugated estrogen, 0.625 mg PO qd days 1–25 and medroxyprogesterone acetate [Provera], 10 mg PO qd days 16–25). Despite the fact that most breast carcinomas possess estrogen (and often progesterone) receptors, there are few data to suggest that estrogen administration increases the de novo risk of breast carcinoma. Concomitant progesterone cycling may be additionally protective for the breast. Evidence suggests that oral contraceptives decrease the risk of benign breast disease. I am particularly careful to order a baseline mammogram before beginning estrogen supplementation. Absolute oncologic contraindications to estrogen therapy include a personal history of breast, endometrial, or possibly ovarian cancer or melanoma, since estrogen receptors have been found in all of these tumors. A remote history of breast cancer or positive family history must be weighed against the risk of not treating.

The use of tumor estrogen and progesterone receptor status is useful in guiding therapy and determining prognosis. Estrogen receptor–negative breast tumors respond better to combination chemotherapy. Patients with estrogen receptor–positive tumors have a longer disease-free survival from initial surgery. Ameliorating hormonal therapy involving castration, hypophysectomy, adrenalectomy, antiestrogens, and adrenal steroid blocking agents have all proved useful. Tamoxifen (10 mg PO b.i.d.), the prototypic antiestrogen, has been especially successful and well tolerated in postmenopausal metastatic breast cancer.

Prostatic Carcinoma. Microscopic foci of prostatic carcinoma are seen in 20% to 40% of males aged 70 to 79, but clinical disease is limited to 0.8%, indicating that many tumors never reach biologic significance. Testosterone is probably a necessary factor for the development of prostatic carcinoma since the disease does not occur in castrated animals. Nonetheless, as with breast cancer, there are no substantive data implicating physiologic doses of testosterone replacement therapy (e.g., testosterone enanthante in oil, 300 to 400 mg IM q three to four weeks) with an increased risk of prostatic carcinoma. Orchiectomy and estrogen therapy provide significant though sometimes limited remissions in men with metastatic carcinoma of the prostate. New hormonal therapies include antiandrogens (e.g., flutamide, not yet available) and gonadotropin–releasing hormone analogue (leuprolide [Lupron], 1 mg subcutaneously daily), the latter producing profound and long-lasting suppression of pituitary gonadotropin secretion.

Other genitourinary carcinomas with hormonal relationships include ovarian and vaginal carcinoma. Maternal exposure to diethylstibestrol (DES), formerly used in pregnancy, results in a small but definite risk of vaginal adenocarcinoma in female offspring. Particularly careful surveillance is needed in these young women.

PRODUCTION OF HORMONES BY TUMORS

Hormone production by a tumor can serve as a reliable marker for (1) screening disease, (2) monitoring therapy, and (3) detecting recurrence. The prototype of such a tumor is choriocarcinoma of pregnancy with production of human chorionic gonadotropin (hCG). It is estimated that each tumor cell secretes 1 pg per 24 hours. Radioimmunoassay techniques can detect as few as 1×10^6 cells (1 mm^3), signaling the need to initiate treatment.

Testicular carcinomas may secrete β-hCG or α-fetoprotein and these may prove useful for monitoring therapy. Medullary carcinoma of the thyroid reliably produces calcitonin, permitting detection of very early disease. This is particularly important in families with a history of this condition as well as those with pheochromocytoma or hyperparathyroidism (multiple endocrine neoplasia). Screening should begin in the first decade of life for families at risk.

ECTOPIC HORMONE PRODUCTION

Production of hormones by tissues not normally thought to produce them is defined as ectopic hormone production. Tumor localization is sometimes possible by selective venous sampling. Such procedures have been useful in patients with ectopic production of ACTH that result in Cushing's syndrome. In this instance, the excess ACTH production may arise in the head, chest, abdomen, or pelvis. Ultimately, development of monoclonal antibody labeling should permit more accurate localization and selective tumor treatment.

Sensitive immunostaining techniques have shown that tumors may produce hormones in the absence of measurable plasma levels. For example, islet cell tumors of the pancreas may contain insulin, glucagon, somatostatin, growth hormone–releasing hormone, vasoactive intestinal peptide (VIP), pancreatic polypeptide, and many other peptide hormones.

When sufficient quantities of bioactive hormone are released, a resulting clinical syndrome may be difficult to distinguish from overproduction by the eutopic or normal source. Examples include ectopic ACTH syndrome, tumoral hypoglycemia, and feminization or precocious puberty from ectopic β-hCG production.

Hypercalcemia ultimately develops in 10% of all malignancies, and most are associated with demonstrable osseous metastases. Others may be connected with a humoral substance causing hypercalcemia, including prostaglandins or osteoclast-activating factor (OAF) associated with lymphoid malignancies, or a substance with parathyroid hormone–like properties. Although low levels of PTH immunoreactivity may be measurable in patients with hypercalcemia, the distinction between primary hyperparathyroidism and malignancy is rarely difficult.

REFERENCES

Dailey GE: Hypercalcemia and malignancy. Practical Reviews in Internal Medicine (Audio tape series) 8:9–12, 1979.

Gambrell RD Jr: Clinical use of progestins in the menopausal patient: dosage and duration. J Reprod Med 27:531–538, 1982 (Suppl 8).

Gambrell RD Jr, Maier RC, Sanders BI: Decreased incidence of breast cancer in postmenopausal estrogen-progestogen users. Gynecol 62:435–443, 1983.

Guidelines for the cancer related health checkup in California. CA 30:224–229, 1980.

Lippman ME: Endocrine responsive cancers of man. *In* Wilson JD, Foster DW (eds): Williams Textbook of Endocrinology, 7th ed. W. B. Saunders Co, Philadelphia, 1985, pp 1309–1326.

18 · INFERTILITY

Randy Linde
PALO ALTO MEDICAL CLINIC

DEFINITION AND DIAGNOSTIC CRITERIA

Infertility, defined as the inability to conceive after one year of unprotected intercourse, occurs in 15% to 20% of the population. Failure to conceive can be due to nonmedical factors, such as incorrect mechanics of intercourse or use of a sperm-damaging lubricant. Sperm counts fall temporarily after coitus, reducing the number of sperm presented to the cervix if conception is attempted too often. Although counseling and reassurance may suffice in these unusual situations, an evaluation should be considered in most cases of infertility.

PATHOPHYSIOLOGY AND CLINICAL ASPECTS

Male. In approximately 40% of infertile couples there is a demonstrable male component. Usually idiopathic, identifiable causes include Klinefelter's syndrome, in utero exposure to diethylstilbestrol (DES), primary or secondary hypogonadism, orchiopexy for cryptorchidism, herniorrhaphy, exposure to chemicals or radiation or heat, trauma, mumps orchitis, epididymitis, chronic prostatitis, or medication such as sulfasalazine or anabolic steroids. The most frequent physical finding is the varicocele, a dilated venous plexus generally palpable only on the left, although occasionally bilateral as shown by venography.

Female. Hypothalamic amenorrhea is usually secondary to anorexia, endurance exercise, or stress, although infrequently it is congenital. The polycystic ovary (PCO) syndrome, congenital adrenal hyperplasia (CAH), and virilizing ovarian and adrenal tumors often result in infertility. Ovarian dysgenesis and premature ovarian failure result in primary and secondary amenorrhea. Anovulation may also arise as a consequence of the resistant ovary syndrome, thyroid disease, hyperprolactinemia, or serious systemic disease. Deficient corpus luteum progesterone production leads to an inadequate luteal phase. Damage to the mucinous glands from a cone biopsy or cryosurgery can lead to inadequate production of mucus, as can cervicitis. Antisperm antibodies are found in the cervical mucus of 5% to 10% of infertile women. Uterine abnormalities include congenital absence, a small body from DES exposure, Asherman's syndrome, and leiomyomata. Fallopian tube dysfunction accounts for 25% to 35% of all cases of infertility and is caused by pelvic inflammatory disease, endometriosis, or adhesions from previous surgery. Risk factors include use of an intrauterine device or multiple partners. Infrequently the tubes may be congenitally absent or anomalous.

MANAGEMENT

SCREENING EVALUATION

A semen analysis is done first since other testing is unnecessary if azoospermia is found. The evaluation proceeds with basal body temperature recording, postcoital testing at midcycle, hysterosalpingography (HSG) between cycle days 10 and 12, and an endometrial biopsy done during the late luteal phase. Although other tests such as hysteroscopy, laparoscopy, cervical mucus-sperm migration assay, and a hamster egg-sperm penetration assay may be required, this initial battery establishes a prognosis at minimal inconvenience and expense. I advise a screening evaluation in a younger couple and a complete evaluation with advanced maternal age. Laparoscopy can then be performed as an outpatient procedure with general anesthesia. Morbidity is minimal, and this is the only reliable test for diagnosing endometriosis, as an HSG can produce false-negative or false-positive results.

NONPHARMACOLOGIC MEASURES

Male. Varicocelectomy is done with ligation of varicosed testicular veins while the patient is under general anesthesia. This often results in improvement in sperm motility and morphology, yet it increases conception rates by only 10% to 20%. Vasovasostomy requires a microsurgical reconstruction of the ligated vas deferens and is often requested by a man who has remarried. Local experience suggests that reappearance of sperm in the ejaculate occurs often, but fertility occurs in only a minority of these cases. In vitro fertilization is occasionally successful in male infertility despite quantitative or qualitative sperm defects.

Female. Surgical management of endometriosis and pelvic adhesions has become a specialty of its own. A variety of techniques have been developed, including laser fimbrioplasty and methods to avoid postoperative intra-abdominal scar formation. The ideal candidate for in vitro fertilization is a woman with either absent oviducts or previously unsuccessful tubal surgery in whom the ovaries and uterus are normal. Skilled centers average a 10% to 20% completed pregnancy rate with no discernible increase in congenital malformations.

DRUG THERAPY

Male. In oligospermia, normal gonadotropins portend a better than even chance of improving the semen analysis with a three- to six-month course of clomiphene citrate taken as either 25 or 50 mg daily or for 25 days each month. Pregnancy rates are significantly lower, suggesting that sperm function is abnormal and not corrected. Slightly less favorable odds apply to the use of tamoxifen citrate, which has fewer side effects but has not been effective in clomiphene-resistant patients. Human chorionic gonadotropin (hCG, 1500 to 2000 IU every two to five days) with or without human menopausal gonadotropin (hMG, or Pergonal, 75 IU three times weekly) is best reserved for hypogonadotropic hypogonadism. This treatment is unpredictable and less successful in idiopathic oligospermia than clomiphene. Testosterone-rebound therapy is reserved for oligospermic men with elevated gonadotropins. An intramuscular injection of testosterone enanthate, 200 mg daily, is administered weekly for 20 weeks; semen is analyzed after four weeks of treatment since rarely an improvement will be noted that should prompt discontinuation of therapy. If azoospermia occurs after ten injections, the dose is dropped to 100 mg weekly for another ten weeks, with the median duration of rebound to improved seminal parameters taking three to four more months. Treatment is time-consuming and inconvenient, but a man who demonstrates an improvement with the first course of injections is likely to respond to subsequent courses.

Ovulatory Factors. Patients with hypothalamic amenorrhea have traditionally been treated with injections of hMG and hCG to stimulate ovarian function. Luteinizing hormone–releasing hormone (LHRH) can now be administered with a portable infusion pump that releases pulses at 90-minute intervals, reproducing the hormonal sequences that occur in spontaneous menstrual cycles with concomitant ovulation and conception. An IV dose of 2.5 or 5 µg mimics physiologic gonadotropin release, but phlebitis or bacteremia may occur, and an indwelling IV catheter can be troublesome. A dose of 10 to 15 µg delivered subcutaneously every 90 minutes prevents these complications but produces a conception rate of about 65% as opposed to nearly 100% with the IV route. Both Ferring and Autosyringe make pumps for this purpose, although the latter are somewhat bulky. The pump should be continued for two weeks after ovulation to provide added luteal support, but reduced luteal phase progesterone production has nonetheless been reported at low rates of LHRH infusion.

Anovulation in women with PCO generally responds to clomiphene, 50 mg on cycle days five to nine. The dose can be increased by 50-mg increments or by giving seven to ten days of treatment each cycle until ovulation is achieved.

Uterine Factors. For luteal phase inadequacy our center employs progesterone delivered as 25-mg vaginal suppositories twice daily, beginning three days after ovulation has occurred by thermic or urine LH (First Response, Ovusticks) monitoring. Clomiphene treatment is successful less often, although indicated if an endometrial biopsy shows glandular stromal asynchrony. Treatment with hCG requires an injection every three days and interferes with the pregnancy test.

Cervical Factors. Insufficient secretion of cervical mucus is managed with a low dose of estrogen during the follicular phase, with the aim of enhancing production of mucus without preventing ovulation. Conjugated estrogen (Premarin, 0.3 mg) or ethinyl estradiol (Estinyl, 20µg) on days 3 to 12 of the cycle can be used, but these are more likely to suppress ovulation than DES (0.1 mg). The use of DES is frowned on by many physicians because of its deleterious effects when given during pregnancy, but no untoward effects are known to occur when DES is given before conception. Viscous mucus might be thinned with daily use of a mucolytic agent such as glyceryl guaiacolate. *Mycoplasma* infection is treated by giving both partners doxycycline, 100 mg twice daily, for the first ten days of the cycle. Antisperm antibody suppression can be attempted with 96 mg prednisolone, administered daily for five days, given to the affected partner three weeks before ovulation, when the immunosuppressive effect will be greatest. Conception rates are poor, however, and treatment often is outweighed by potential side effects. Intrauterine insemination may cause intense abdominal cramping or anaphylaxis, but this procedure or in vitro fertilization bypasses cervical mucus and is thus the ultimate treatment for an abnormality refractory to other therapy.

Peritoneal Factors. Danazol (Danocrine), 400 mg twice daily for six months, is standard therapy for endometriosis. When the LHRH agonists become FDA-approved, these agents will likely replace danazol as suppressants of pituitary gonadotropin secretion.

Adverse Effects

Male. Clomiphene infrequently causes side effects, with men reporting aggressiveness, nipple sensitivity, and scotomata. In large doses this agent has an antifertility effect, reducing sperm counts. Human chorionic gonadotropin may cause gynecomastia; combined hCG–hMG treatment is uncomfortable, costly, and inconvenient. Testosterone for rebound spermatogenesis rarely produces adverse effects, although salt and water retention, prostatic growth, or testicular atrophy could occur. Oral methyltestosterone is not used because of its potential to cause obstructive jaundice.

Ovulatory Factors. Treatment with hMG and hCG to induce ovulation is painful and costly, and it requires daily observation, frequent pelvic examinations, serial estradiol assays, and ultrasound evaluation. Even in experienced centers the ovarian hyperstimulation syndrome occurs in mild form in 3% to 6% of treated women and is severe in almost 1% of patients. Multiple gestations occur in 20% of conceived cycles with gonadotropin therapy. Clomiphene increases the multiple gestation rate only slightly, but doses of 150 mg or more can exert an antiestrogenic effect on cervical mucus, and clomiphene can also induce an inadequate luteal phase or cause ovarian cyst formation.

Complications of the LHRH pump include spontaneous abortion and multiple gestations, the latter probably induced by using 60-minute pulses or excessive doses of LHRH in early studies. The spontaneous abortion rate has been reported to be as high as 40%, but the rate appears exaggerated because these cycles were observed with β-hCG levels to confirm early pregnancies that would likely be unnoticed in the general population. There are no reported congenital anomalies with the pump, although cytogenetic studies of abortus material are pending. The pump should be avoided in women who are substantially underweight or have PCO. In the former group, there is an increased risk of prematurity and underweight offspring, and in the latter group, ovulation and conception rates have been disappointingly low.

Peritoneal Factors. Danazol invariably produces weight gain and fluid retention and may also induce hirsutism and acne.

PATIENT INFORMATION AND EDUCATION

At a preliminary interview attended by both partners, it should be explained that about 25% of infertile couples conceive without medical evaluation, while a greater number fail to conceive despite therapeutic intervention. All alternatives should be aired before embarking on a course that can be painful or hampered by complications and may produce only frustration. Medical insurance companies generally lend little support toward diagnosis and treatment, and some procedures such as in vitro fertilization can be prohibitively expensive.

On occasion infertility can serve as a source of immense frustration or even as the catalyst for divorce. Both partners should have joint and private access to the physician to discuss personal feelings and problems. If stress seems excessive, referral to a marriage counselor, social worker, psychologist, or psychiatrist is indicated.

PERIODIC EVALUATION

One couple in 20 have a normal evaluation. Under this circumstance, repeat testing should be considered. A variety of qualitative sperm defects not assessed by the hamster egg assay probably account for many of these cases. If a problem has been identified and treated, periodic checks are necessary until pregnancy is achieved. Intuitively obvious for abnormalities of sperm or cervical mucus, this also applies to endometriosis and a "second look" laparoscopy after a course of danazol or surgical intervention. Once treatment has started, conception may take six to 12 months, and a couple should return at least every six months to retain continuity.

ALTERNATIVE OPTIONS

In past years, infertile couples have turned to adoption when patience or prognosis for conception reached a low level. With lengthy waiting lists for adoption, artificial insemination by donor for couples with male infertilty and, to a far lesser extent, the use of surrogate mothers for couples with female infertility have become alternatives. A genetic background of the semen donor or surrogate mother should be available to the prospective parents and kept as part of the future child's medical record. The identity of the surrogate mother or semen donor should, however, remain absolutely confidential. The long-term emotional and legal complications of these procedures remain controversial.

REFERENCES

Bain J, Schill W-B, Schwarzstein L: Treatment of Male Infertility. Springer-Verlag, Berlin, 1982.
DeCherney AH, Polan ML: Reproductive surgery. *In* Speroff L (ed): Seminars in Reproductive Endocrinology. Thieme-Stratton, New York, 1984, pp 101–221.
Keller DW, Strickler RC, Warren JC: Clinical Infertility. Appleton-Century-Crofts,, Norwalk, CT 1984.
Speroff L, Glass RH, Kase NG: Clinical Gynecologic Endocrinology and Infertility, 3rd ed. Williams & Wilkins Co, Baltimore, 1983.
Wentz AC, Givens JR, Anderson RH, et al: Manual of Gynecologic Endocrinology and Infertility. Williams & Wilkins Co, Baltimore, 1979.

19 · ORAL CONTRACEPTION

George T. Schneider
OCHSNER CLINIC AND ALTON OCHSNER MEDICAL FOUNDATION

A need for contraception has been recognized from earliest recorded history. Today contraception is particularly important because of the unprecedented growth in the world's population following World War II as a result of a steady birth rate and a decline in death rates. About 80 million people (equivalent to the population of Mexico) are added to this planet every year. Unfortunately 90% of this growth is in the less developed countries and results in political and economic turmoil that has a direct influence on the interests of the United States, involving also increased immigration.

Oral contraception began two decades ago and has become the most popular method of fertility control in most countries where multiple techniques are available. An estimated 50 million women in developed and developing countries now use the "pill," and numerous prospective studies have shown a significant reduction of various complications following a decrease in the amount of steroid components in the pill, especially estrogen.

PATHOPHYSIOLOGY

The combination pill, consisting of estrogen and progesterone, prevents ovulation by inhibiting gonadotropin secretion. The estrogen component exerts negative feedback, suppressing secretion of follicle-stimulating hormone (FSH). The progesterone component suppresses secretion of luteinizing hormone (LH). Ovarian function is thus diminished. The endometrium is also altered, undergoing a certain degree of atrophy, and cervical mucus is thickened, thus inhibiting sperm transport. Estrogen also provides stability to the endometrium, preventing unwanted irregular sheddings (breakthrough bleeding).

CLINICAL ASPECTS

PROBLEMS

We routinely advise gynecologic followup including Pap smear every nine to 12 months in patients taking oral contraceptives, but for people who fall into various high-risk categories we advise visits every three to six months. Some conditions completely contraindicate pill use, with rare exceptions (Table 1).

The increased risk of thromboembolic disease such as pulmonary embolism or cerebellar thrombosis has been established, but this is associated with higher pill estrogen content than is generally prescribed today. This complication is more likely to occur in women who have predisposing conditions such as hypertension, diabetes, obesity, advancing age, prolonged immobilization, or varicose veins or who indulge in excessive smoking.

A significant reduction in thromboembolic phenomena has been effected by a decrease of estrogen content to 50 μg and below. If the administering physician has any suspicions regarding thromboembolism, the antithrombin III blood level should be measured before prescribing the pill, since this can detect an unsuspected abnormal clotting tendency if the level is below normal. Ideally, pills should be terminated at least three weeks before any contemplated elective surgery, to lessen the risk of postoperative thrombosis.

The increased risk of development of coronary artery disease in pill users who smoke should be strongly emphasized. The synergism between smoking and birth control pills can be partly explained by the latter's effects on lipoproteins used for cholesterol transport. The risk of coronary heart disease increases with a decrease in high-density lipoprotein (HDL) levels and also with an increase in low-density lipoprotein (LDL). Combination estrogen and progesterone pills increase LDL, whereas only high-dose pills improve HDL levels. An increase in triglycerides is also common among pill users. All these factors become clinically significant after the age 30 to 35.

The presence of an estrogen-dependent neoplasm or suspected carcinoma of the breast is also a definite contraindication, as is a known or suspected pregnancy.

Steroids are contraindicated in patients with acute hepatitis or markedly impaired liver function until that function returns to normal.

The minor contraindications to pill use (Table 2) should be discussed with patients before oral contraceptives are administered.

The use of pills in patients over the age of 35 carries an increased risk because of the greater number of complications in this group. However, in my experience patients who are in good health, do not smoke, and do not have any of the above-named problems can continue

Table 1. MAJOR CONTRAINDICATIONS TO USE OF ORAL CONTRACEPTIVES

1. Thrombophlebitis, thromboembolic disorders, coronary occlusion, cerebral vascular disease, or a past history of these conditions
2. Markedly impaired liver function
3. Known or suspected carcinoma of breast or endometrium or any estrogen-dependent neoplasm
4. Undiagnosed abnormal genital bleeding
5. Known or suspected pregnancy

Table 2. MINOR OR ARBITRARY CONTRAINDICATIONS TO USE OF ORAL CONTRACEPTIVES

1. Age over 35	5. Hyperlipidemia
2. Migraine headaches	6. Cigarette smoking
3. Hypertension	7. Elective surgery
4. Gestational diabetes	

to take birth control pills over age 35. In general, however, other forms of contraception are advised for this age group.

Migraine headaches increase in some patients, remain unchanged in an equal number, and improve in a smaller number.

An elevation in blood pressure occurs in some women taking oral contraceptives in direct proportion to the amount of estrogen content. This is probably due to salt and water retention and an alteration in renin-angiotensin aldosterone mechanisms. Predisposing factors include familial tendency, age, obesity, and previous toxemic pregnancy. Hypertension may develop at any time while the patient is taking the pill and is usually reversible when the pill is discontinued.

A decrease in glucose tolerance has been observed in a significant percentage of patients on oral contraception; thus, prediabetic and diabetic patients should be carefully monitored while taking the pill.

BENEFITS

Before a practitioner prescribes a pill, all the above potential complications must be evaluated against the known benefits of the pill for each individual patient. No contraceptive pill has been associated with a higher mortality rate than that of pregnancy itself. Moreover, there are other distinct but less tangible benefits, such as the patient's complete freedom from pregnancy-related concern. Other benefits include reduction in the overall incidence of ovarian cancer, fibrocystic breast disease, endometrial cancer, pelvic inflammatory disease, and ectopic pregnancy. Additional advantages include relief from dysmenorrhea, improvement in menstrual regularity, reduction in menstrual blood loss, temporary control of endometriosis, and the reduction of side effects that accompany polycystic ovary syndrome.

PATIENT COUNSELING

When a woman chooses to use an oral contraceptive rather than alternative means of birth control, selection of an appropriate type is an important factor. Our therapeutic principle is to use the pill that gives effective contraception and the greatest margin of safety for the individual patient. Current evidence supports the view that there is greater safety with combination pills containing 50 μg of estrogen, or preferably less. Pills with less than 25 μg of estrogen combined with progesterone are associated with excessive breakthrough bleeding and a slightly higher rate of failure. Breakthrough bleeding problems should be minimal with a new oral contraceptive formulation, the so-called "triphasic product." Those most commonly used are Tri-Phasil, Ortho-Novum 7-7-7, and Tri-Norinyl, all of which have been found to have no significant effect on the glucose tolerance curve. At present these drugs seem to be the best overall solution to the hazards of oral contraceptive use.

REFERENCES

American College of Obstetricians and Gynecologists: Technical Bulletin No. 41, Oral Contraception, pp 441–445, July 1976.

Böttinger LE, Boman G, Eklund G, et al: Oral contraception and thromboembolic disease and the effects of lowering estrogen content. Lancet 1:1097–1101, 1980.

Gambrell RD Jr: Hormones in the etiology and prevention of breast and endometrial cancer. South Med J 77:1509–1515, 1984.

Speroff L, Glass RH, Kase NG: Clinical Gynecologic Endocrinology and Fertility. 3rd edition. Williams & Wilkins Co, Baltimore, 1983, pp 409–449.

World Population and Fertility Planning Technologies: The Next 20 Years Summary. Congress of the United States, Office of Technology Assessment Bulletin. Washington, D.C., 1982 (Superintendent of Documents, U.S. Government Printing Office, Washington, DC).

20 · MENOPAUSE

V. K. Piziak
SCOTT AND WHITE CLINIC

DEFINITION AND DIAGNOSTIC CRITERIA

During the menopause, declining ovarian function results in a lower level of estrogen production, with subsequent chronic stimulation of follicle-stimulating hormone (FSH) and luteinizing hormone (LH) release from the pituitary and gonadotropin-releasing hormone (GnRH) from the hypothalamus. Marked serum FSH elevation (> 50 μu/ml) is diagnostic of the menopausal state.

CLINICAL ASPECTS

The hormonal changes of menopause result in a number of signs and symptoms that can be divided into the following categories: vasomotor, genitourinary, emotional, skeletal, and dermatologic. The most common symptoms are vasomotor, occurring in an estimated 75% of patients with menopause. Atrophy of the genitourinary epithelium also occurs. The epithelium becomes progressively thinner and more easily traumatized. Because lubrication and local defense mechanisms are compromised, the postmenopausal woman is more susceptible to vaginal infections and urethritis. Symptomatic osteoporosis affects 25% to 30% of women in the United States. An accelerated bone-mass loss results, particularly during the first three to five years after menopause. The emotional aspects of menopause are in part due to estrogen loss and in part related to the patient's coping with aging and its various changes. In addition, there is a documented decrease in the total amount of sleep and in the REM phase of sleep experienced by postmenopausal women.

MANAGEMENT

Hormone replacement therapy should be used to relieve specific symptoms as well as to help preserve bone mass and the urogenital tissue. Some symptoms, such as vasomotor events or emotional lability, may be treated for a definite period of time, with gradual reduction and elimination of estrogen therapy. Some patients may wish only this limited amount of therapy. Vaginal atrophy may require an indefinite interval of therapy in order to provide long-lasting success, and preservation of bone mass requires early institution of hormone and long-term therapy. Therapeutic goals should be discussed with the patient and should incorporate her preference.

DRUG THERAPY

In the majority of women, estrogen therapy diminishes or eliminates vasomotor symptoms. When estrogens are contraindicated, alkaloids of belladonna (Bellergal 1 to 4 tablets daily), clonidine (Catapres, 0.1 mg twice daily), or propranolol hydrochloride (Inderal, 40 mg twice daily) are sometimes effective. These may be increased until vasomotor symptoms diminish, as long as hypotension is not a problem. Estrogen therapy either taken orally or applied topically as a vaginal cream (1 gm two to three times weekly) is generally effective in alleviating most symptoms of urogenital atrophy. Estrogen diminishes the trabecular bone loss associated with menopause, and it retards the loss of skin collagen, thus preserving the resiliency of the skin. Estrogen administration also increases total sleep and the proportion of REM sleep.

The minimal effective dose of oral estrogen should be given for 21 to 25 days per month and then stopped for five to seven days to allow for withdrawal bleeding in patients who have a uterus. A dose of 0.625 mg of conjugated estrogen is sufficient to preserve bone mass. In women with a uterus, a progestational agent such as medroxyprogesterone acetate (Provera, 10 mg) should be added daily for the last 10 to 12 days of estrogen therapy.

COMPLICATIONS OF MANAGEMENT

A minority of women may develop hypertension or glucose intolerance on hormone replacement. There have been no increases in venous thrombotic events in women receiving postmenopausal estrogen-progestogen replacement therapy, and recent studies have shown no increase in the incidence of myocardial infarction.

The greatest concern for patient and physician is the induction of neoplastic changes in the breast and uterus that may occur with prolonged estrogen therapy. Increased incidence of endometrial carcinoma in patients taking unopposed estrogen has been documented. Progestational agents antagonize the uterine proliferative effect of estrogen, and when given for 10 to 12 days of the cycle, they reduce the incidence of endometrial carcinoma to the level observed in untreated patients. A prospective study indicates that there is no significant increase in breast cancer in women using combination estrogen-progestogen therapy.

Estrogens are absolutely contraindicated in patients with cancers of the breast or endometrium, undiagnosed vaginal bleeding, acute liver disease, or acute vascular thrombosis. Patients with a history of thromboembolic disease or a family history of breast cancer should be treated on an individual basis, depending on their risk of significant complications of menopause.

PERIODIC EVALUATION

Pretreatment evaluation should include a history, with emphasis of estrogen deficiency symptoms, risk factors for osteoporosis, previous estrogen-responsive cancer, thrombophlebitis, migraine headaches, benign breast disease, and family history of cancer of the breast or uterus. Physical examination should include blood pressure measurement, breast and pelvic examinations, and a Pap smear. A pretreatment endometrial biopsy is indicated if there is abnormal uterine bleeding or a family history of endometrial carcinoma. Baseline mammography should be performed. At a follow-up visit, four to six months after the pretreatment evaluation, the patient should have weight and blood pressure recorded, and relief of symptoms should be documented. Subsequent visits may be made at yearly intervals and should include additional breast and pelvic examinations and mammography. An endometrial biopsy should be performed if other than expected bleeding occurs.

PATIENT INFORMATION AND EDUCATION

The increasing life span of women has made the postmenopausal period equivalent in length to the reproductive years in many women. It has become imperative to consider the risks and benefits of hormonal replacement during this period and to educate our patients about them so that an informed decision can be made. Emphasis should be placed on proper nutrition and adequate calcium intake—at least 1 gm of elemental calcium per day for the premenopausal woman and the woman on estrogen replacement, and 1.5 gm of elemental calcium per day for the postmenopausal patient not on estrogen replacement. It should be emphasized that regular exercise and the avoidance of cigarette smoking and excessive alcohol intake are also important in the preservation of bone mass.

REFERENCES

Gambrell RD Jr: The menopause: benefits and risks of estrogen-progestogen replacement therapy. Fertil Steril 37:457–474, 1982.

Hammond CB, Maxson WS: Current status of estrogen therapy for the menopause. Fertil Steril 37:5–25, 1982.

Hammond CB, Ory SJ: Endocrine problems in the menopause. Clin Obstet Gynecol 25:19–38, 1982.

Piziak VK, Shull BL: Menopausal hormone replacement. Hosp Pract Feb. 15, 1985; 82GG–82RR.

Ryan KJ: Postmenopausal estrogen use. Annu Rev Med 33:171–181, 1982.

21 · COMMON GYNECOLOGIC PROBLEMS IN INTERNAL MEDICINE

George T. Schneider
OCHSNER CLINIC AND ALTON OCHSNER MEDICAL FOUNDATION

Often the obstetrician-gynecologist becomes the "family doctor" for the young female patient who is first seen as an obstetric patient. It is equally true that the family physician or internist is often called on to treat common gynecologic problems throughout a patient's lifetime, especially if she remains single, has no children, or does not develop a rapport with a gynecologist. The most common management problems include infection, contraception, the premenstrual syndrome, dysmenorrhea, and gynecologic cancer.

CLINICAL ASPECTS

VAGINITIS

Vaginitis is an inflammation of the vaginal mucous membrane, usually involving the cervix and vulva, which occurs in most women at some stage of life. The overwhelming majority of vaginal infections, particularly in women of childbearing age, are caused by *Candida albicans*, *Trichomonas vaginalis*, and *Gardnerella* (*Haemophilus vaginalis*). Other causes include herpesvirus type II, papillomavirus, *Chlamydia trachomatis*, *Mycoplasma* T strains, and toxic shock syndrome. Precise identification of the causative organism is essential for effective treatment, because many symptoms, such as vaginal discharge, itching, and irritation, are common to all three, and more than one organism is often found simultaneously in the same patient. Moreover, because these organisms are transmitted sexually, it is often important to include in the examination a culture for gonorrhea when this is suspected in a particular patient.

We utilize a Thayer-Martin culture medium, especially when multiple sex partners are suspected.

Infections occur, albeit less commonly, in postmenopausal women, but atrophic vaginitis is a major cause of vaginal irritation in this age group. Supervised use of supplementary cycling estrogen with progesterone in patients who still have a uterus or application of local vaginal estrogenic cream can ameliorate atrophic vaginitis.

Candidiasis. Candidal organisms can be identified on a saline wet mount, with potassium hydroxide, or frequently from a Pap smear. Confirmation can be obtained with a culture on Sabouraud's or Nickerson's medium. The introduction of the imidazole group of antifungal agents—clotrimazole (Gyne-Lotrimin), and miconazole (Mycelex-G, Monistat 7)—has been a great boon in the treatment of *C. albicans* vaginal infections. Improvement in the potency of these agents has shortened the necessary course of treatment. Vaginal creams, tablets, and suppositories are all effective. Vaginal acidification also helps combat yeast infections, especially in preventing recurrence, and we often prescribe the use of boric acid vaginal capsules, 10 grains (0.6 gm) inserted vaginally every night for two to three weeks. A pharmacist can easily make these capsules. In acute, painful cases, gentian violet applied to the inflamed tissues also alleviates discomfort rapidly.

In patients with chronic recurrences, it is important to rule out diabetes mellitus and to identify individuals with a low renal glucose threshold. These patients, although not diabetics, spill urinary sugar at their peak level of glucose absorption. A reduction of dietary free sugar in these individuals may help reduce recurrences. The patient with candidiasis should be advised to wear cotton underwear and if possible to discontinue any prolonged antibiotic therapy, such as for chronic acne. Birth control pills may have to be discontinued for a time.

Trichomoniasis. This motile, pear-shaped, flagellated protozoan can be identified from saline smear or Pap smear. Culture is not usually necessary. Metronidazole (Flagyl) is the drug of choice for *Trichomonas* infection. Different clinicians prescribe various dosages ranging from 250 mg three times a day for seven to ten days to a single 2-gm dose that has been found reliable. During this therapy and for 24 hours afterward patients should be advised not to drink alcohol, to avoid an Antabuse-like effect. Since infection is transmitted by sexual contact, the sexual partner should always receive treatment. A medicated cleansing douche such as povidone-iodine (Betadine) also helps reduce inflammation.

Gardnerella (Haemophilus vaginalis) *Vaginitis.* There is still some controversy regarding the role of bacteria in vaginitis. *H. vaginalis* is the most frequently implicated organism but it may act synergistically with anaerobic bacteria. *H. vaginalis* can normally be identified under saline smear by the presence of "clue cells," large, desquamated epithelial cells that appear stippled because they are covered with small gram-negative bacilli that can also be cultured in Casman broth medium. Therapy with a sulfa vaginal cream such as Sultrin or AVC cream for ten days or two weeks is usually satisfactory, and we usually prescribe a Betadine douche before application. However, resistant organisms, especially in the presence of concomitant infections, require additional therapy such as metronidazole, ampicillin, or tetracycline.

Herpesvirus Type II. One of the most distressing and painful causes of vaginitis is herpesvirus type II. Its incidence has increased rapidly in the last decade and the virus may have oncogenic potential, having been linked to the development of dysplasia and carcinoma of the cervix. The disease is spread primarily by sexual contact, and symptoms usually appear three to seven days after exposure to the virus. Fortunately, the condom has proved a fairly effective prevention against direct exposure. Primary lesions may be extensive and appear as indurated papules with vesiculation and ulceration. The initial attack may persist for seven to ten days, depending on the patient's immune response. Recurrences are not uncommon since the virus migrates to central nerve ganglia. The frequency of recurrence depends on the patient's susceptibility. Diagnosis is usually made by recognition of the ulcers and confirmation of the organism on a Pap smear of exfoliated epithelial cells from the vagina, cervix, or vulva. Cultures can also be obtained by unroofing the blister and culturing the fluid.

The presence of herpesvirus in the vagina during labor and delivery poses a significant threat to the fetus. Herpes cultures are begun at weekly intervals as of 36 weeks, and if positive within one week of expected delivery, cesarean section is advised to prevent contamination in the birth canal. Most laboratories can give a fairly reliable preliminary report within 48 hours.

Many remedies for herpesvirus have been recommended but as yet none has been completely satisfactory. Symptomatic relief can be obtained with aluminum acetate (Domeboro Powder) solution and Betadine washings. Acyclovir (Zovirax Ointment 5%) is available for direct application and seems to be helpful when applied frequently, up to six times daily. Oral acyclovir has been approved recently for chronic recurrences.

For severe cases and for patients at risk of disseminated herpes, intravenous acyclovir, 5 mg/kg, can be infused over one hour every eight hours for a total dose of 15 mg/kg/day for five to seven days. We have used laser therapy on the superficial ulcerations of primary infections, and when performed early this has shortened the period of acute pain.

Toxic Shock Syndrome. This syndrome occurs most frequently in menstruating women and is characterized by a desquamating rash, fever, hypotension, and multisystem involvement. Toxin-producing strains of *Staphylococcus aureus* have been cultured from vaginal or other specimens in almost all cases. The possible association between this syndrome and the use of vaginal tampons in menstruating women is still controversial. However, in suspected cases it is wise to culture specimens from the cervix and vagina for the presence of *S. aureus* and to advise patients to discontinue tampons.

NONORAL CONTRACEPTION

1. The intrauterine device (IUD) is the second most frequently used form of medical contraception in the Third World, but in the United States it has proved less than ideal. Extensive media coverage of various adverse side effects has made a considerable impact on its acceptance and use. No member of our department recommends an IUD for nulliparous women because of

the possibility of infection. Whether the new medicated devices (e.g., those containing progesterone) are a significant improvement remains to be seen.

2. Barrier methods, especially the condom and diaphragm, are still used successfully by many individuals. The vaginal sponge is considered to be in a period of trial.

3. Vaginal foams and suppositories are an alternative form of vaginal contraception and are relatively successful if used properly.

4. Tubal sterilization is an increasingly prevalent method of fertility control that is intended to be permanent and was popularized by the development of the laparoscope. Various occluding devices can be applied through the scope, or ligation can be performed fairly easily through a mini-laparotomy. This procedure has sometimes been performed indiscriminately during the last decade, especially in younger women. The need for surgical reversal has increased as patients change their minds following altered marital status or the death of a child.

5. Various types of periodic abstinence are also utilized in the U.S., but success rates vary owing to the unpredictability of ovulation in many women.

PREMENSTRUAL SYNDROME

The premenstrual syndrome (PMS) may be defined as a cyclical recurrence of symptoms in the premenstrual period that disappear completely at or soon after the onset of bleeding, and are absent during other phases of the menstrual cycle. Manifestations of PMS are varied and range in severity from mild to incapacitating. Because there are strong psychologic components in this syndrome, it is important that physicians spend a considerable amount of time in discussion with patients. Therapy should be individualized according to a relatively simple classification—the somatic group and the psychologic group. For the somatic or "bloated" group, diet and exercise are important together with avoidance of caffeine and reduced intake of salt. Diuretics should be used minimally and only under supervision. For the psychologic group, reassurance is most important, and mild sedation can occasionally be added. Prostaglandin inhibitors are helpful in the dysmenorrheic portion of the syndrome, and sometimes progesterone vaginal suppositories are successful. This may alleviate the volatile changes in endorphin levels that have been implicated as a cause of this syndrome. Vaginal progesterone suppositories are not commercially available in the U.S. and must be prepared by a pharmacist. The use of progesterone is still controversial and dosage also varies: ideally, that which produces the best results with the minimal dosage. The severity of PMS naturally varies from cycle to cycle, and thus the dosage of progesterone can vary from cycle to cycle, from 25 to as much as 600 mg daily. Therapy should be initiated approximately three days before the usual onset of symptoms but not before ovulation has occurred. Side effects consist of local vaginal irritation and perhaps a slight increase in the incidence of yeast vaginitis, but there are no reports of any serious side effects.

DYSMENORRHEA

Two forms of medical therapy have been considerably successful: (1) hormonal treatment in the form of birth control pills and (2) prostaglandin synthetase inhibition.

Presumably, a thinner endometrium resulting from use of the pill produces less prostaglandin precursor and ultimately less prostaglandin at the time of progesterone withdrawal. In our patients whose symptoms are not controlled with the usual analgesics or antiprostaglandins, a short two- to three-month course of low-dose estrogen birth control pills frequently provides reassurance that menstruation can be pain free.

The prostaglandin synthetase inhibitors have also proved effective for this disorder. The three products most commonly used in our department are ibuprofen (Motrin), 600 mg every four to six hours; mefenamic acid (Ponstel), 250 mg three to four times daily; and naproxen sodium (Anaprox), 275 mg three to four times daily. Patients are advised to take these medications on a full stomach.

CANCER PREVENTION

One of the most valuable benefits for the internist who conscientiously practices primary gynecologic care is the ability to detect cancer early.

A careful breast examination should always be included in the annual physical or gynecologic examination, and monthly self-examination of the breasts should be encouraged. Any suspicious lesions can be evaluated further with mammography or biopsy and occasionally by using newer techniques such as xerography, ultrasonography, and light transillumination.

The development of cervical cytology has markedly improved the early detection of carcinoma of the cervix. Pap smears can be obtained easily through a small speculum and are frequently done by public health nurses when physicians are not available. Abnormal reports, of course, should be followed by colposcopic examination. For the internist who is adept at pelvic examination, ovarian cancer can be detected on annual examination. Finally, endometrial cancer, which is increasing in incidence over cervical cancer, can be screened by small endometrial biopsy instruments, such as a Novak curette.

REFERENCES

Driscoll CE: Genital herpes. The Female Patient. 9:41, 1984.

Faratian B, Gaspar A, O'Brien PM, et al: Premenstrual syndrome: weight, abdominal swelling, and perceived body image. Am J Obstet Gynecol 150:200–204, 1984.

Helgerson SD, Mallery BL, Foster LR: Toxic shock in Oregon. JAMA 252:3402–3404, 1984.

Reid RL, Yen SSC: The premenstrual syndrome. Clin Obstet Gynecol 26:710–717, 1983.

Schneider GT: Vaginal infections. Postgrad Med 73:255–260, 1983.

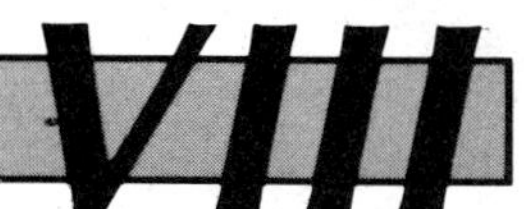

DISORDERS OF THE KIDNEY AND UROGENITAL TRACT

K.K. VENKAT
NATHAN LEVIN

1 · CLINICAL APPROACH TO THE PATIENT WITH RENAL DISEASE

Julio E. Figueroa
OCHSNER CLINIC AND ALTON OCHSNER MEDICAL FOUNDATION

The clinical evaluation of patients with renal disease includes an informative history and an adequate physical examination, obtaining the least number of laboratory studies needed to develop a working diagnosis, developing a plan of therapy and follow-up, and monitoring changes in the patient's condition.

After the initial clinical evaluation, usually the problem can be categorized into one of ten symptom complexes or renal syndromes characteristic of the most common renal diseases (Table 1). These syndromes can be developed further to include specific renal conditions that would cause the particular syndrome. Further studies are done to either rule out or corroborate the more specific diagnosis.

NEPHROTIC SYNDROME

A variety of glomerulonephritides cause the nephrotic syndrome (Chapter 4). The patient with the nephrotic syndrome usually presents with a history of swelling with anasarca, ascites, or other symptoms of volume overload. Occasionally, an observant patient will notice excessive foaming of the urine in the bowl. Lassitude, weight gain, and shiny skin may also be noticed.

Physical examination reveals varying degrees of edema, ascites, evidence of pleural effusion, and rarely, when severe, the presence of horizontal white lines across the nail beds.

The sine qua non of the nephrotic syndrome is *heavy* proteinuria (>3.5 gm/24 hr). This may diminish as serum albumin concentration decreases to very low levels. The other laboratory abnormalities of the nephrotic syndrome (hypoalbuminemia and hypercholesterolemia) may not be present in the early stages. Once the diagnosis of the nephrotic syndrome is made, I try to determine if the causative glomerulopathy is primary or secondary to systemic disease. In adults, renal biopsy is usually necessary to make a definitive diagnosis in order to institute therapy. Between 10% and 30% of patients with the nephrotic syndrome have renal vein thrombosis with or without pulmonary emboli. This condition, therefore, must be kept in mind, and when suspected, renal vein angiography may be necessary. It should also be remembered that the nephrotic syndrome may be a paraneoplastic manifestation of carcinomas and lymphomas.

NEPHRITIC SYNDROME

Puffiness of the face or a change in color or appearance of urine usually brings the patient with this syndrome to the office. General malaise, swelling, and headaches suggest anemia, significant proteinuria, or hypertension, respectively. The nephritic syndrome is usually caused by various forms of proliferative glomerulonephritis (Chapter 4). The term "rapidly progressive glomerulonephritis" is used when renal function deteriorates rapidly in patients with the nephritic syndrome. Such a course is usually associated with crescentic glomerulonephritis (Chapter 4).

The most helpful laboratory study is the routine urinalysis, which reveals hematuria and the presence of

Table 1. COMMON RENAL SYNDROMES

Nephrotic syndrome	Hypertensive renal disease
Nephritic syndrome	Obstructive renal disease
Recurrent hematuria	Nephrolithiasis
Asymptomatic proteinuria/hematuria	Cystic renal disease
Tubulointerstitial disease	Renal failure

granular and cellular (red cell or mixed cell) casts. Proteinuria may be moderate or severe; a nephrotic picture can accompany the nephritic urinary sediment. A fresh specimen of urine is necessary for an accurate evaluation of the urinary sediment. Old specimens, especially if the pH is alkaline, may give misleading results since the formed elements may disappear.

The next most important laboratory study in this syndrome is the determination of blood urea nitrogen (BUN) and serum creatinine. The presence of azotemia signifies severe nephritis and requires prompt evaluation. Once again, the nephritic syndrome must be further categorized as either primary or a manifestation of systemic disease. Early renal biopsy followed by appropriate treatment may make the difference between recovery of renal function and end-stage renal failure, particularly when the picture is one of rapidly progressive renal failure associated with crescentic glomerulonephritis.

In the nephritic as well as the nephrotic syndrome, measurement of the so-called immune markers may give a clue to the cause of the renal disease. These studies include measurement of serum complement (C'3, C'4, and CH50), antinuclear antibodies, anti-DNA antibodies, antistreptolysin titer or some other indication of a recent streptococcal infection, and protein electrophoresis to identify abnormal proteins in the serum.

RECURRENT HEMATURIA

Recurrent gross hematuria may occur in patients with IgA nephropathy (Berger's disease), Alport's syndrome, benign familial hematuria, and polycystic kidney disease. Hematuria from these conditions should be differentiated from that due to urologic causes such as malignancies and calculi. If the cause of hematuria is not obvious after urologic evaluation (Chapter 10), kidney biopsy should be considered.

ASYMPTOMATIC PROTEINURIA/HEMATURIA

Discovery of proteinuria and/or microscopic hematuria on routine urinalysis is not an uncommon presentation of renal disease. By definition these patients have less than nephrotic range proteinuria and normal renal function as measured by creatinine clearance. Isolated proteinuria may be postural: urinary protein excretion is abnormal in the upright position, but not in recumbency. Postural or orthostatic proteinuria is benign and does not progress to renal failure, but pathologic proteinuria may also have a postural component. IgA nephropathy and nonspecific mesangial proliferative glomerulonephritis may cause asymptomatic proteinuria and/or microscopic hematuria. Progressive renal failure is uncommon in these disorders. However, other glomerular, tubulointerstitial, vascular, and cystic disorders of the kidney that may later cause renal deterioration may present initially with asymptomatic urinary abnormalities. Patients with this syndrome should be followed carefully. Progressive increase in proteinuria or deterioration of renal function should prompt consideration of kidney biopsy. Determination of insurability or employability are other indications for kidney biopsy in patients with asymptomatic urinary abnormalities.

TUBULOINTERSTITIAL DISEASE

Patients with tubulointerstitial diseases may come to the physician's office with a history of acute or gradual deterioration of renal function, recurrent urinary tract infections, a picture of nephrogenic diabetes insipidus, salt-losing nephritis, or other clinical manifestations of tubular dysfunction. Acute renal colic due to the passage of necrotic papillary tissue is occasionally seen in analgesic nephropathy. I emphasize the need for the clinician to inquire vigorously about drug use, particularly analgesics, nonsteroidal anti-inflammatory agents, and antibiotics. Chronic back pain, chronic headache, or peptic ulcer disease with gastrointestinal bleeding may give a clue to the diagnosis of analgesic nephropathy.

Laboratory evaluation usually reveals a bland urinary sediment and mild to moderate proteinuria. Eosinophils in the urine sediment may be seen when the disease is caused by an acute hypersensitivity reaction to drugs such as methicillin. Fever, malaise, azotemia, and at times nephrotic range proteinuria may occur in acute tubulointerstitial nephritis.

The investigation of chronic tubulointerstitial nephritis must include visualization of the entire genitourinary system to rule out structural abnormalities that may be reversible. Partial or complete obstruction of urinary drainage, vesicoureteral reflux, staghorn calculi, or necrotic papillae are examples of abnormalities commonly seen. Specific tubular defects can be diagnosed by appropriate laboratory studies (see later).

HYPERTENSIVE RENAL DISEASE

Primary hypertension is an important cause of significant renal disease particularly in black patients. The history is usually one of sustained hypertension for years, poor control of blood pressure, and noncompliance with either medications or follow-up. The presenting symptoms may be those of uncontrolled or malignant hypertension or uremia. The physical findings are those of sustained long-standing hypertension including funduscopic vascular abnormalities that range from sclerosis to exudates, hemorrhages, and papilledema. Cardiomegaly, hyperkinetic precordium, and very elevated diastolic blood pressure are also seen.

Important laboratory abnormalities include moderate proteinuria, hematuria, and occasionally casts, elevation of the BUN and serum creatinine, electrocardiographic evidence of left ventricular hypertrophy, and prominence of the left ventricle on a chest x-ray film. Hyperreninemia is usually indicative of malignant hypertension or significant renal arterial stenosis.

When a patient with hypertensive renal disease presents with sudden or recent worsening of the hypertension, unilateral or bilateral renal artery stenosis must be ruled out. A renal scan may be of help if the disease is unilateral. Visualization of the renal arteries becomes mandatory and can be done by either digital subtraction angiography or conventional renal arteriography.

Patients with malignant nephrosclerosis secondary to hypertension may present with a syndrome of diffuse intravascular coagulation, which can be diagnosed on the basis of laboratory studies.

OBSTRUCTIVE RENAL DISEASE

Obstruction of the urinary tract is either complete or partial and can occur at any level of the genitourinary system. If the obstruction is partial, the presenting complaint is frequency of urination and polyuria. Measurement of specific gravity demonstrates the presence of isosthenuria, which assumes significance in the absence of renal failure. In contrast, complete bilateral urinary tract obstruction is associated with severe oliguria or anuria. A history of sudden anuria preceded by polyuria, particularly in the elderly male, suggests obstructive uropathy secondary to prostatic disease.

Laboratory studies reveal a bland urinary sediment unless the obstruction is associated with infection. If the obstruction is relatively sudden, and the patient is seen soon after its development (less than 48 hours), visualization of the urinary tract may be possible using infusion intravenous pyelography or a renal scan. However, the diagnosis of long-standing obstruction resulting in renal failure requires either ultrasonography or retrograde pyelography. Hydroureteronephrosis is usually demonstrated unless the obstruction is due to retroperitoneal fibrosis or tumor infiltration of the retroperineum. Under these circumstances, caliectasis may not be very prominent, but a mass effect can usually be demonstrated on ultrasonography or computed tomography of the retroperineal space.

NEPHROLITHIASIS

The patient with nephrolithiasis usually gives a history of renal colic. Occasionally, the presenting complaints are symptoms of urinary tract infection without renal colic, and a diagnosis of renal calculi or nephrocalcinosis is made with a plain x-ray film of the abdomen. Rarely, patients with renal tubular acidosis develop severe hypokalemia, and may present with severe muscle weakness before the nephrocalcinosis is detected. Physical examination may vary in these patients depending on the presenting symptoms. Laboratory studies of importance include a urinalysis, which may reveal hematuria, pyuria, bacteriuria, and specific crystals. A scout film of the abdomen may demonstrate nephrocalcinosis or radiopaque stones (calcium or cystine stones). Radiolucent (uric acid) stones will not be seen unless contrast material is injected. Measuring the daily excretion of calcium, oxalate, phosphate, uric acid, and cystine in the urine will help make a specific diagnosis. First morning urine pH and capillary blood gases are helpful as screening tests for renal tubular acidosis. At times these studies may be normal, and a challenge with ammonium chloride is necessary in order to demonstrate inability to produce maximally acidic urine. The effect of dietary calcium and sodium intake on urinary excretion of calcium may be important in determining the type of hypercalciuria responsible for the stone disease. When hypercalcemia is present, studies for hyperparathyroidism and malignant disease are necessary. Serial renal tomograms can help in the follow-up of patients with radiopaque renal calculi by allowing measurement of stone growth or detecting formation of new stones.

CYSTIC RENAL DISEASE

Isolated cysts of the kidneys are usually discovered as an incidental finding on a scout film of the abdomen or on an intravenous pyelogram (IVP). These cysts are of no consequence but must be differentiated from solid tumors utilizing ultrasonography.

Multicystic disease, however, is clinically significant and may present in several ways. Gross hematuria or urinary tract infection is the most common initial presenting symptom of polycystic kidney disease. Abdominal pain secondary to bleeding into a cyst, enlargement of the abdominal girth, and hypertension of mild degree are also common manifestations. Plain x-ray film of the abdomen may show renal calculi, and an intravenous pyelogram may show splaying of the calyceal system and enlargement of the kidneys. However, the definitive diagnosis of adult polycystic kidney disease is made by renal ultrasound. Polycystic kidney disease may occur early in life, but usually presents itself in the fourth to eighth decade of life. Because it is an autosomal dominant genetic trait, this condition rarely skips a generation, and family history is usually positive. Multiple cysts in other organs, such as the liver, the ovaries, and the lungs, are common. The association of polycystic kidney disease and berry aneurysms of the brain is also well documented.

Medullary cystic disease of the kidneys (familial nephronophthisis) must be distinguished from medullary sponge kidney, which is a benign condition. Medullary sponge kidneys are usually asymptomatic, but may present with renal calculi or urinary tract infection. Medullary cystic disease presents with polyuric isosthenuria, terminal hypertension, insidious development of anemia, azotemia, and bland urinary sediment with little proteinuria. Definitive diagnosis of sponge kidney is usually made by IVP with visualization of ectasia of the collecting ducts in the pyramids. Uremic medullary cystic disease is more difficult to diagnose clinically, but can be associated with medullary calcinosis, as well as tubular abnormalities.

RENAL FAILURE

ACUTE RENAL FAILURE

Renal failure is either acute or chronic. Although oliguria was felt to be necessary for the diagnosis of acute renal failure (ARF) we now know that in many instances patients are not oliguric. Nonoliguric ARF is usually due to nephrotoxins such as aminoglycosides. When ARF occurs, one must determine whether the azotemia is caused by prerenal factors, such as volume depletion or hypotension, or by acute tubular necrosis (ATN). The measurement of urinary sodium, creatinine, and osmolality may distinguish between prerenal azotemia and ATN (Chapter 2). The urinary sediment may show pigment casts, which are characteristic of ATN, or may give other clues as to the cause of the renal

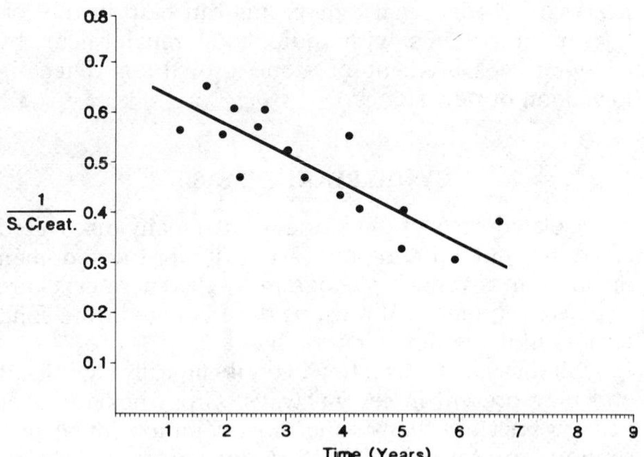

Figure 1. Graph showing the slope of the inverse of serum creatinine (1/s. creat.) over a period of time in a patient with chronic renal failure.

failure. When the presenting picture is one of severe oliguria or anuria, one must consider obstructive uropathy, occlusion of the renal vessels, or cortical necrosis. Renal ultrasound for detection of hydronephrosis is indicated when obstruction is suspected. A renal scan will help determine the presence or absence of blood flow and therefore prognosis for recovery of function.

CHRONIC RENAL FAILURE

Patients with chronic renal failure may come to the office complaining of malaise, lassitude, anorexia, nausea, vomiting, metallic taste, or diarrhea. A family physician may refer the patient because of newly discovered anemia. Physical examination usually reveals hypertension, pallor, and uremic fetor. The uremic frost is rarely seen nowadays because of earlier diagnosis. Small kidneys by ultrasonography or tomography will help differentiate between acute and chronic renal failure. Normal size or enlarged kidneys in patients with chronic renal failure may be due to renal vein thrombosis, diabetes, or infiltrative diseases of the kidney. Decline of renal function in chronic renal failure is best followed by plotting the slope of the inverse of serum creatinine (1/s. creat.) versus time (Fig. 1). As shown, 1/s. creat. usually declines linearly over time in progressive renal failure irrespective of etiology. Thus the time at which a certain value of serum creatinine will occur in the future can be predicted. Decline of renal function more rapidly than predicted should prompt consideration of potentially reversible factors that might be accelerating the renal failure (e.g., volume depletion, uncontrolled hypertension, obstruction, nephrotoxins).

Renal Function Tests

TESTS OF GLOMERULAR FUNCTION

The 24-hour creatinine clearance is the most useful simple test although much potential for inaccuracy ex-

ists. Accurate, complete collection is necessary. Use of the serum creatinine alone may be misleading; due to the influence of muscle mass on the serum creatinine concentration, both the initial diagnosis and the progression of renal failure may be misjudged in small-framed elderly individuals.

The BUN:serum creatinine ratio is a useful tool in the differentiation of renal failure caused by intrinsic renal disorders from prerenal azotemia. The normal value for this ratio is approximately 10:1. Increase in the ratio suggests decreased renal perfusion, which might result from a variety of causes, e.g., hypovolemia, cardiac failure. Alternatively, gastrointestinal bleeding or other causes of protein catabolism could account for an increase in this ratio. In intrinsic renal disorders, such as ATN, the ratio is usually normal because both BUN and serum creatinine increase proportionately. Poor protein intake may result in a low value for this ratio in patients with acute or chronic renal failure.

TUBULAR FUNCTION

Concentrating ability is measured without relying on patient compliance by the use of injected vasopressin in oil (10 IU IM the night before) combined with prescribed fluid restriction. The specific gravity or preferably osmolality is measured in the first voided urine the next morning. Urinary acidification can be evaluated by measuring baseline blood gases, serum electrolytes, and urinary pH, and then administering calcium chloride or ammonium chloride. Remeasurement of blood values will confirm absorption of the hydrogen ion load. Urinary pH decrease should occur in the next two to six hours. In some instances measurement of excretion of urinary ammonium and titratable acid may be necessary in addition.

Imaging Studies in the Evaluation of Renal Function and Renal Disease

The IVP is still the most commonly used imaging study in the diagnosis of renal diseases. It is important to recognize that this study is not a renal function test, but rather a test to visualize the structure of the kidney and the genitourinary system. The contrast material used is potentially nephrotoxic, particularly in patients with preexisting azotemia, diabetes mellitus, or paraproteinemias. Therefore, it is important to use this test sparingly under those circumstances. Hydration prior to and after IVP, and the use of osmotic diuretics at the time of the test, may be useful to minimize nephrotoxicity.

Radioisotope renal studies are helpful to demonstrate normal or altered renal blood flow. Radioiodine hippurate scintiscanning can help in the diagnosis of renal artery stenosis when the lesion is unilateral. Bilateral stenosis may be missed by this study. Early or incomplete obstruction can be seen using technetium glucoheptonate. This compound is also useful in determining glomerular blood flow as well as in showing the structural details of the kidneys.

Renal ultrasound is a safe, noninvasive procedure. It is valuable in showing the presence of two kidneys, the size of each kidney, abnormal masses (solid or cystic), as well as caliectasis secondary to obstruction. Ultrasound has simplified renal biopsies. It is now possible to consistently biopsy the lower pole of the kidney with little danger of puncturing the large blood vessels or the renal pelvis.

Computerized tomography (CT) is a highly sophisticated but expensive technique, which for the most part is not necessary in the diagnosis of renal diseases. It is helpful when the question of a renal mass arises and the ultrasound is not conclusive. In some situations injection of contrast material is required at the time of CT, and this limits the value of this test in patients with renal failure. The role of magnetic resonance imaging of the kidneys in the diagnosis of renal diseases is currently being evaluated.

Renal arteriography and venography have specific uses in the clinical evaluation of patients with renal disease, and for the most part are procedures that need to be done in the hospital. In contrast, digital subtraction angiography can be done in outpatients, and has been used to visualize the renal arteries when vascular stenosis is suspected. The risks of toxic effects to the kidneys from the contrast material is the same in digital angiography and conventional arteriography. However, the risk of intra-arterial catheter insertion and possible dislodging of plaques or clots in the arteries can be avoided by venous digital angiography.

The Use of Renal Biopsy

Since the introduction of percutaneous renal biopsy in the United States by Robert Kark and his associates in Chicago in the late 1950s, this procedure has been most helpful in the clinical evaluation of patients with renal disease. At first performed as a blind procedure, later guided by image intensifiers and more recently by ultrasonography, renal biopsy is now a very safe procedure. However, the procedure still has to be performed in the hospital because of the necessary observation for significant bleeding after biopsy.

The indications for renal biopsy have changed since the original studies by Kark and associates. Initially, biopsies were done primarily to learn about the natural history and histopathologic abnormalities in renal disease. The present state of the art does not make it necessary to biopsy patients indiscriminately. In the pediatric population, for instance, renal biopsies are seldom needed in the diagnosis of nephrotic syndrome or acute glomerulonephritis. In the adult population, however, the nephrotic syndrome still requires renal biopsy in order to make a specific diagnosis so that prognosis and potential therapy can be evaluated. The importance of a renal biopsy in these conditions is unquestionable. Rapidly progressive renal failure of

uncertain etiology is another absolute indication of renal biopsy.

Recent studies in patients with systemic lupus erythematosus with renal involvement suggest that renal biopsy may not be helpful in the clinical evaluation. There are, however, patients with this condition in whom the specific renal abnormality is not clear on the basis of the clinical picture. In these cases a biopsy is needed to determine the degree of activity of the disease and to decide on treatment. Whatever the controversies concerning the indications for renal biopsy, it is imperative when biopsy is performed that the tissue is handled properly, and that studies for light microscopy, immunofluorescence, and electromicroscopy are performed. Otherwise, a definite diagnosis may not be possible and the procedure, which carries some risk, would not be of the greatest benefit to the patient. As with any other delicate procedure, a renal biopsy should be performed by an expert, preferably a nephrologist.

REFERENCES

Coe FL: Clinical and laboratory assessment of the patient with renal disease. *In* Brenner BM, Rector FJ (eds): The Kidney, 3rd ed. W.B. Saunders Co, Philadelphia, 1986, pp 703–734.

Danovitch GM, Nesserison AR: The role of renal biopsy in determining therapy and prognosis in renal disease. Am J Nephrol 2:179–184, 1982.

Harrington JT, Kassirer JP: Renal vein thrombosis. Ann Rev Med 33:255–262, 1982.

McCluskey RT: The value of renal biopsy in lupus nephritis. Arthritis Rheum 25:867–875, 1982.

2 · ACUTE RENAL FAILURE

Richard M. Finkel
LAHEY CLINIC MEDICAL CENTER

DEFINITION

Acute renal failure represents impairment of renal function of sudden onset, occurring under a wide variety of circumstances. Acute renal failure in adults is usually due to the clinical syndrome of acute tubular necrosis (ATN), which occurs either after hypoperfusion of the kidneys (ischemic ATN) or after exposure to nephrotoxins (nephrotoxic ATN). It should be noted that although the term ATN is used commonly, in many patients with this disorder histologic examination of the kidneys does not reveal necrosis of the tubular epithelium. ATN should be differentiated from prerenal acute renal failure–transient renal failure caused by decreased blood volume, hypotension or congestive heart failure, and postrenal acute renal failure caused by obstruction of the urinary tract. Besides ATN, other intrinsic renal disorders such as rapidly progressive glomerulonephritis and acute interstitial nephritis may cause acute renal failure. The principal causes of acute renal failure are shown in Table 1. This chapter is limited to the discus-

Table 1. PRINCIPAL CAUSES OF ACUTE RENAL FAILURE

Prerenal Causes
Hypotension from any cause
Hypovolemia due to hemorrhage or loss of fluid and electrolytes
Congestive heart failure, cardiac tamponade

Impairment of Renal Autoregulation
Nonsteroidal anti-inflammatory agents (NSAIA), captopril (Chapter 8)

Renal Causes
Ischemic acute tubular necrosis (ATN): Same prerenal factors as above
  when not corrected quickly
Nephrotoxic ATN: Aminoglycosides, radiocontrast agents, hemoglobi-
  nuria and myoglobinuria, heavy metals and organic solvents
Rapidly progressive glomerulonephritis
Acute interstitial nephritis
Vascular disorders: Renal arterial or venous occlusion, atheroembolic
  disease, malignant hypertension, systemic sclerosis, thrombotic
  thrombocytopenic purpura, hemolytic uremic syndrome
Hepatorenal syndrome
Miscellaneous: Hypercalcemia, multiple myeloma, acute uric acid ne-
  phropathy

Postrenal Causes
Infravesical obstruction: Urethral stricture, prostatic hypertrophy,
  prostatic malignancy
Ureteric obstruction: Calculi, retroperitoneal fibrosis, retroperitoneal or
  pelvic malignancy

sion of the clinical features, differential diagnosis, and management of ATN.

DIAGNOSIS

The diagnosis of acute renal failure is made by recognition of a rapid rise in the level of blood urea nitrogen (BUN) or serum creatinine. Acute increase in the serum level of creatinine is a more reliable indicator of renal failure because it is not influenced by gastrointestinal bleeding or by protein intake, as is the level of BUN. Acute renal failure may develop in virtually any acutely ill patient. Thus, it is wise to monitor the serum level of creatinine and urine output closely in such patients, particularly if other complications are developing. One of the pitfalls in the diagnosis of renal failure is that large deficits in renal function may produce only small changes in the serum level of creatinine. This is especially true for the patient with small muscle mass whose daily production of creatinine is low and whose normal serum level of creatinine is at the low end of the normal range. For example, a 50% increase in the serum level of creatinine from 0.8 mg/dl to 1.2 mg/dl might not attract much attention because both values are within normal limits. However, this increase in serum level of creatinine indicates that a 33% loss in renal function has occurred if it is not caused in part by laboratory variation. Urine outputs may also be deceptive because approximately one third of the patients with ATN have high or normal urine output rather than the more classic oliguria.

In oliguric ATN, renal tubular concentrating ability and conservation of sodium are profoundly disturbed. Thus, the ratio of urine creatinine to plasma creatinine is low, the urine osmolality is close to that of plasma, and the sodium concentration of urine is high. In patients with prerenal acute renal failure, the kidney is underperfused, but concentrating ability and conservation of sodium are well preserved. Thus, the ratio of urine creatinine to plasma creatinine is high, the urine osmolality is high, and sodium concentration of urine is low. Typical values for these parameters are shown

in Table 2. It is important to determine the composition of urine in oliguric patients before administration of mannitol or loop diuretics because these agents will modify the findings. When the results are equivocal, it is often helpful to calculate the renal failure index (RFI) or the fractional excretion of sodium (FENa) as shown in Table 2. RFI and FENa are usually greater than 2 in oliguric ATN and less than 1 in oliguria of prerenal origin, but exceptions do occur. Microscopic examination of the urine is helpful in the differential diagnosis of acute renal failure. In ATN the urinary sediment typically contains large numbers of tubular cells, tubular cell casts, and coarsely granular casts. Hematuria and RBC casts are unusual in ATN and are suggestive of other renal disorders such as glomerulonephritis.

PATHOPHYSIOLOGY

ATN is most often a result of surgical stress, sepsis, hypotension, hemorrhage, major trauma, and exposure to nephrotoxins. A variety of theories have been developed based on data from experimental models to explain the pathogenesis of ATN. Major factors that have been proposed are a back leak of glomerular filtrate across injured tubular epithelium, obstruction of tubular lumen by casts or debris, and disruption in intrarenal hemodynamics with consequent cortical ischemia. However, for most patients with acute renal failure, the respective roles of these factors remain uncertain.

CLINICAL ASPECTS

A commonly overlooked prerenal factor in patients with renal failure is sodium depletion. The most important findings associated with sodium depletion are diminished skin turgor, absence of edema, low venous pressure, and loss of weight. Usually, records of intake and output will show that negative fluid balance has occurred in the recent past. If oliguria is present, the urine will have a prerenal composition (Table 2). Other prerenal factors, such as volume contraction caused by loss of blood, hypotension, and congestive heart failure, are easily recognized. Nonsteroidal anti-inflammatory agents (NSAIA) may precipitate acute renal failure in patients with any of the prerenal factors mentioned, probably by inhibiting the renal synthesis of vasodilatory prostaglandins (Chapter 8).

Exclusion of obstructive uropathy is of great importance in any patient with rapidly failing renal function. The presence of anuria or wide fluctuations in hourly urine output should suggest this possibility. As with ATN, normal urine outputs do not exclude the diagnosis. In fact, many patients with partial bilateral urinary tract obstruction have polyuria. Percussion and palpation of the suprapubic area may reveal evidence of enlargement of the bladder in patients with obstruction of the lower urinary tract. Catheterization of the bladder will readily confirm or rule out this possibility. Physical examination is not as helpful in the diagnosis of obstruction of the upper urinary tract, although occasionally palpation of the flanks will reveal renal enlargement due to hydronephrosis. The presence of hydronephrosis is easily confirmed by renal echography. A plain radiograph of the abdomen may provide useful information in patients with obstruction from calculi.

Table 2. COMPOSITION OF URINE IN OLIGURIC PATIENTS

	Prerenal Azotemia	Acute Tubular Necrosis
Urine osmolality*	>400 mOsm/kg	<300 mOsm/kg
Urine sodium*	<20 mEq/L	>40 mEq/L
$\dfrac{\text{Urine creatinine (mg/dl)}}{\text{Serum creatinine (mg/dl)}}$	>40	<20
Renal failure index (RFI)† $$\dfrac{\text{urine sodium (mEq/L)}}{\text{urine creatinine (mg/dl)/serum creatinine (mg/dl)}}$$	<1	>2
Fractional excretion of Na (FENa)† $$\dfrac{\text{urine sodium (mEq/L)/serum sodium (mEq/L)}}{\text{urine creatinine (mg/dl)/serum creatinine (mg/dl)}} \times 100$$	<1%	>2%

*Performed on spot urine samples.
†Performed on simultaneously obtained spot serum and urine samples.

MANAGEMENT

PREVENTIVE MEASURES

Attempts have been made to prevent ATN or to shorten its course by giving a variety of agents, including mannitol, loop diuretics, and dopamine. Unfortunately, most of the data about these agents come from inadequately controlled studies. Thus, it is still unclear which patients, if any, may exhibit improved renal function from these drugs. However, increase in urine output sometimes seen with these agents can be beneficial even if renal function does not improve because nutritional supplements and parenterally administered medications can be given with less chance of fluid overload.

In the acutely ill patient, even a transient drop in blood pressure or urine output may indicate the presence of a serious complication that can result in ATN. Hypertensive patients may suffer severe loss of renal perfusion when the blood pressure drops to levels considered normal in other patients. Prompt recognition and correction of sodium depletion, loss of blood, congestive heart failure, and sepsis in the hypotensive or oliguric patient may prevent prerenal failure from developing into ATN.

Aminoglycoside antibiotics are the commonest cause of nephrotoxic ATN. Greater care must be exercised in giving these drugs to the elderly, to patients with contracted blood volume, and to patients with preexisting renal disease. The use of tobramycin in place of gentamicin may questionably provide the patient at risk with an extra margin of safety. Although monitoring serum levels of aminoglycosides and using doses modified for reduced renal function are helpful, these measures do not rule out the occurrence of aminoglycoside nephrotoxicity. One factor that likely affects this is the accumulation of aminoglycosides in the renal cortex. It is important to review the result of the morning serum creatinine before giving aminoglycosides to patients at risk. If standing orders for aminoglycosides are left, one or two doses may be given before it is realized that the serum level of creatinine has increased. As already discussed, even a slight increase in the serum level of creatinine may indicate that a major change in renal function has occurred.

DRUG THERAPY

If a patient is oliguric and either has no obvious prerenal factors or does not respond promptly to correction of prerenal factors, it is reasonable to administer mannitol, 12.5 gm to 37.5 gm, intravenously. If the patient is volume expanded, the dose should be limited to 12.5 gm to avoid congestive heart failure. Patients who are volume expanded or euvolemic may be given a loop diuretic such as furosemide intravenously. Single doses of greater than 200 mg or multiple large doses administered over a short period of time offer no particular advantage and may cause ototoxicity. Dopamine, an inotropic catecholamine, may be given to oliguric patients with inadequate cardiac output or unstable blood pressure at rates up to 30 µg/kg/min provided that any preexisting volume contraction has been corrected. Improvement in cardiac output may result in improved renal blood flow and urine output. A further increase in urine output may occur if furosemide is given with dopamine.

HYPERKALEMIA

Hyperkalemia should be anticipated in patients with ATN because the capacity to excrete potassium is negligible. In addition, release of potassium from cells may occur as the result of metabolic acidosis or cellular breakdown from abscesses, necrosis, hemolysis, or rhabdomyolysis. It is important to review orders for medications, intravenous fluids, and nutritional support and to discontinue any agents that may be contributing to hyperkalemia, such as potassium-sparing diuretics and potassium salts.

Patients with a rising serum level of potassium or a potassium of 6 mEq/L or greater should be watched closely for cardiac toxicity. Cardiac monitoring allows prompt recognition of cardiotoxic effects of hyperkalemia such as peaking of the T wave or widening of the QRS complex. Although 10% calcium gluconate, 10 to 50 ml, given intravenously can reverse cardiac toxicity, it does not lower the serum level of potassium. Intravenous calcium should be given cautiously in patients receiving digitalis. Sodium bicarbonate, 44 to 88 mEq/L, administered intravenously is effective in shifting potassium from extracellular fluid into the cells, as is glucose, 25 to 50 gm, with 5 to 10 units of regular insulin given intravenously. Sodium polystyrene sulfonate (Kayexalate), a cation exchange resin, is effective in removing potassium. Fifty grams of this drug may be given as an enema in 150 ml of 70% sorbitol or 10% glucose, or 15 to 20 gm may be given orally with 20 ml of 70% sorbitol solution up to four times a day. Patients who require repeated doses should be monitored for congestive heart failure, since 1 mEq of sodium is returned to the patient for every mEq of potassium that is removed. When conservative measures fail to control hyperkalemia, hemodialysis can be used to promptly lower the serum level of potassium.

METABOLIC ACIDOSIS

The serum level of bicarbonate should be maintained between 18 and 20 mEq/L. Losses of sodium should be replaced with sodium bicarbonate rather than sodium chloride when the level of bicarbonate is below 18 mEq/L. If sodium chloride is given before treatment of metabolic acidosis, an expansion of intravascular volume occurs, which makes it more risky to administer sodium bicarbonate. The use of lactate or lactated Ringer's solution is inappropriate since the conversion of lactate to bicarbonate may be impaired, and the potassium present in Ringer's solution is contraindicated. Correction of bicarbonate to above 22 mEq/L is undesirable since most patients with acute renal failure are hypocalcemic, and the hypocalcemia may become symptomatic if acidosis is completely corrected. In patients with impaired ventilation, however, it may be necessary to maintain the bicarbonate at a higher level to prevent severe acidosis. Normally, alveolar hyperventilation compensates for metabolic acidosis. However, patients with ATN often have a variety of respiratory complications that may prevent compensation. Under these circumstances the blood pH may fall precipitously. If the pH drops below 7.30 despite optimal respiratory support, it is necessary to maintain the bicarbonate at 25 mEq/L or above.

VOLUME OVERLOAD

Patients with ATN are frequently volume expanded because of fluids given before recognition of renal failure and because of fluids required for nutritional support and parenterally administered medications. Stability of body weight usually implies that lean body mass lost because of catabolism is being replaced by fluid. Early recognition and treatment of fluid overload will prevent congestive heart failure or hypertension. Overload is less likely in patients with nonoliguric renal failure or in the oliguric patient whose urine output increases in response to loop diuretics. Daily observation of weight, presence or absence of edema, records of intake and output, blood pressure, neck veins or central venous pressure, and the cardiorespiratory status are helpful in identifying overload. In patients with compromised left ventricular function, monitoring of pulmonary capillary wedge pressure is helpful in establishing optimal volume status.

Hyponatremia. Hyponatremia is a frequent finding in patients with ATN and most often is due to fluid overload with an excess of water. The appropriate treatment is rigid restriction of fluids, not administration of salt. Medications must be given in the minimum possible volume. Fluids used to keep intravenous lines patent should be avoided by use of heparinized peripheral venous catheters. Sometimes fluid is given to patients with ATN because the patient "looks dry" or out of concern that the patient may become dehydrated. It is important to realize that dry skin does not mean dehydration. Dryness of the surface of the tongue may result from breathing through the mouth rather than from dehydration. Careful observation of these patients will usually reveal that they are not "dry" but instead are overloaded with fluid. When conservative management fails to control volume overload or hyponatremia, dialysis should be instituted.

UREMIA

Uremia may develop in patients with ATN if not properly managed. The most frequent manifestations are anorexia, nausea and vomiting, platelet dysfunction, pericarditis, and toxicity to the central nervous system. Although urea by itself is not toxic, it is a useful marker. The higher the level of BUN, the greater the likelihood of uremia. To prevent uremia, the BUN should be kept below 100 mg/dl. Patients with high output renal failure who are not catabolic may never become this azotemic and thus can be managed by conservative measures. However, patients with oliguria commonly attain this level of BUN unless dialysis is instituted. High levels of BUN may develop in patients who are catabolic within four or five days, requiring early intervention with dialysis.

A stepwise increase in urine output is a good prognostic sign. It indicates that the patient is entering the diuretic phase of ATN and that eventual return of renal function may occur. Improved urine output is helpful in managing metabolic acidosis and volume overload. However, glomerular filtration rate often remains low for several days. Levels of BUN and serum creatinine continue to rise, and uremia may develop. Resolution of oliguria, therefore, is not a reason to withhold dialysis. A decline in the daily increment of BUN and serum creatinine indicates, however, that the glomerular filtration rate is improving and levels of BUN and serum creatinine may soon fall. In these patients a greater degree of azotemia can be tolerated for brief periods in anticipation of improved renal function.

Hemodialysis. Hemodialysis is preferable to peritoneal dialysis in patients who are catabolic because clearance of metabolic end products is so much greater. It is also much more effective than peritoneal dialysis in the treatment of hyperkalemia. Hemodialysis is the procedure of choice if rapid removal of a dialyzable nephrotoxin is desired or when recent abdominal surgery or abdominal adhesions make peritoneal dialysis more hazardous. Hemodialysis is also preferable in patients with borderline respiratory status who might not tolerate distention of the abdomen with dialysate.

Peritoneal Dialysis. Peritoneal dialysis is tolerated better by patients with cardiovascular instability. It is also useful in the treatment of patients with active bleeding, since anticoagulation is not required. In addition, the disequilibrium syndrome seen with the rapid corrections achievable with hemodialysis does not occur with peritoneal dialysis.

NUTRITION

Patients with ATN should be given sufficient calories and essential amino acids to minimize negative nitrogen balance and consequent loss of lean body mass. If the patient can eat, is not oliguric, and is minimally catabolic, adequate nutrition can be maintained easily. Patients with aminoglycoside nephrotoxicity often fall into this category. These patients should receive at least 25 kcal/kg/day. If caloric intake is inadequate, a preparation of glucose polymers (Polycose) can be given as a supplement. An intake of protein of 0.5 gm/kg/day will meet essential amino acid needs providing it is a high-quality protein. Eggs and milk are the best sources, but meat, poultry, and fish are also satisfactory. Intake of protein should be raised to 1 gm/kg/day to replace losses of amino acids in patients undergoing hemodialysis and 1.5 gm/kg/day in patients undergoing peritoneal dialysis to replace losses of protein.

If the patient has oliguria, a nonfunctioning gastrointestinal tract, and a brisk catabolic rate, it is much more difficult to maintain adequate nutrition. Patients with postoperative or post-traumatic renal failure usually fall into this category. These patients require 50 kcal/kg/day. Parenteral nutrition is provided by a catheter placed in the superior vena cava, which is used only for nutrition and is carefully maintained by a nutrition team to avoid infection. This catheter allows administration of hyperosmolar solutions of glucose and amino acids. A typical infusion would contain 35% glucose, 3.5% amino acids, and multivitamins and would be administered at a rate of approximately 80 ml/hour. Additional calories can be given as a 10% or 20% fat emulsion. These preparations provide 1.1 and 2 calories/ml, respectively. Because they are isotonic, they can be given by way of a peripheral vein. In patients who show a brisk anabolic response to this program, hypokalemia, hypomagnesemia, and hypophosphatemia may develop. This is the opposite of what is usually seen in ATN. Therefore, these serum levels must be watched closely and electrolyte supplements should be added as necessary. The positive fluid balance caused by nutritional support and fluids required for parenterally administered medications must be dealt with by appropriate degrees of ultrafiltration during hemodialysis. Recently, slow continuous ultrafiltration (SCUF) with highly permeable hemofilters has been used in the treatment of acute renal failure. SCUF can remove large volumes of plasma ultrafiltrate containing urea and other uremic toxins. This technique permits the administration of adequate amounts of parenteral hyperalimentation without the risk of fluid overload and may reduce dialysis requirements.

DIURETIC PHASE

If recovery from ATN is to occur, it often does so within two weeks. However, recovery depends on resolution of the underlying disease and may take as long as several weeks. Large urine outputs may occur, which can cause appreciable losses of sodium, potassium, and water. The levels of urine sodium and potassium provide a useful guide for replacement, but until these results are available, urine output can be replaced with 0.45% saline solution. Some of the sodium is given as sodium bicarbonate if the patient is acidotic. If the serum level of potassium is below 4 mEq/L, potassium is given in concentrations of 10 to 20 mEq/L.

COMPLICATIONS

Infection is a common cause of death in patients with acute renal failure. Central venous catheters require meticulous care and indwelling urinary catheters should be avoided. Any sputum or discharge from wounds should be gram-stained and cultured promptly. Blood cultures should be obtained if fever, unexplained hypotension, or any other unexplained deterioration in the patient's status occurs. Nephrotoxic antibiotics should be avoided unless no alternative is available. As with any renally excreted drug, doses of antibiotics should be modified for reduced renal function.

Another important cause of morbidity is gastrointestinal bleeding, either caused by duodenal ulcer or multiple gastric ulcers. Stools should be monitored periodically for occult blood. Prophylactic use of cimetidine or antacids may be helpful. For most patients with acute renal failure, aluminum hydroxide is preferable to magnesium-containing antacids, since these may aggravate hypermagnesemia commonly present in these patients. Since aluminum hydroxide binds phosphate, it may have an additional advantage in controlling hyperphosphatemia. To prevent calcification of tissue, it is best to keep the level of phosphate low enough so that the calcium-phosphate product is below 70.

Mortality rate varies fom 30% to 70%, depending on the setting in which ATN develops. Higher figures are seen in postoperative patients, in patients who have experienced trauma, and in patients with multiple organ dysfunction. The mortality in nonoliguric ATN is much lower than in oliguric ATN. Many patients with less complicated disease, however, will recover clinically adequate renal function if given careful fluid and electrolyte management and nutritional and dialytic support.

REFERENCES

Kirschenbaum MA, Nissenson AR: Acute renal failure. *In* Gonick HC (ed): Current Nephrology, Vol 5. Wiley Medical Publication, New York, 1982, pp 241–270.

Levinsky NG, Bernard DB, Johnston PA: Mannitol and loop diuretics in acute renal failure. *In* Brenner BM, Lazarus JM (eds): Acute Renal Failure. W.B. Saunders Co, Philadelphia, 1983, pp 712–722.

Miller TR, Anderson RJ, Linas SL, et al: Urinary diagnostic indices in acute renal failure: a prospective study. Ann Intern Med 89:47–50, 1978.

Schrier RW, Conger JD: Acute renal failure: pathogenesis, diagnosis, and management. *In* Schrier RW (ed): Renal and Electrolyte Disorders, 2nd ed. Little, Brown & Co, Boston, 1980, pp 375–408.

Wesson DE, Mitch WE, Wilmore DW: Nutritional considerations in the treatment of acute renal failure. *In* Brenner BM, Lazarus JM (eds): Acute Renal Failure. W.B. Saunders Co, Philadelphia, 1983, pp 618–642.

3 · CHRONIC RENAL FAILURE

K.K. Venkat*
Nathan W. Levin*
Antoine Kaldany†
John A. D'Elia†
*HENRY FORD HOSPITAL
†JOSLIN CLINIC

DEFINITION AND DIAGNOSTIC CRITERIA

Chronic renal failure (CRF) is defined as slowly progressive decline in the glomerular filtration rate (GFR) over many months or years. This is in contrast to acute renal failure (ARF) in which the GFR declines suddenly over a short time and is reduced for days to weeks. The term "chronic renal insufficiency" is sometimes used to refer to the earlier stages of CRF (serum creatinine < 5 mg/dl). Acute renal failure in the presence of CRF may occur when chronically diseased kidneys are subjected to acute insults such as dehydration, hypotension, uncontrolled hypertension, nephrotoxins, obstructive uropathy, and infection. Whereas ARF is usually reversible if the patient survives the underlying illness, CRF is generally progressive.

The clinical diagnosis of renal failure (acute or chronic) is usually based on the detection of elevated blood urea nitrogen (BUN) and serum creatinine values. However, it should be remembered that these values rise above the normal range only after the GFR has decreased to less than 50% of normal. Measurement of the GFR (usually by determination of the endogenous creatinine clearance) is thus required for the diagnosis of the initial stages of renal failure. Serum creatinine is more reliable than BUN measurement in the estimation of GFR because the latter is influenced by dietary protein intake. The serum creatinine value at any level of renal function is determined by the muscle mass of the individual. Since the muscle mass can change, especially in the later stages of renal failure because of poor nutritional intake, periodic measurement of the creatinine clearance is recommended in the follow-up of patients with CRF. The use of the plot of the reciprocal of the serum creatinine (1/s. creat.) versus time in monitoring the progression of renal failure is discussed later in this chapter.

In the azotemic patient the differentiation of CRF from ARF can be difficult. Past records showing elevated serum creatinine, presence of broad urinary casts, radiologic evidence of renal osteodystrophy, and small echogenic kidneys on ultrasonography are pointers to the diagnosis of CRF. Anemia and altered serum calcium and inorganic phosphate concentrations are not reliable because these abnormalities may be seen in both ARF and CRF. Also, anemia may be lacking in some patients with CRF (especially in patients with polycystic kidney disease). Renal ultrasonography should be part of the evaluation of all patients with renal failure because in addition to giving information on the size and echogen-icity of the kidneys, it also helps to exclude remediable obstructive uropathy (shown by the presence of hydronephrosis).

ETIOLOGY OF CRF

A wide variety of renal diseases can cause CRF (Table 1). On a worldwide basis, the commonest cause of CRF, especially in younger patients, is glomerulonephritis of different types. Hypertension is an important cause of CRF in the black population in the United States. The greater prevalence and severity of hypertension in blacks is a major reason why the percentage of blacks in the dialysis population is much higher than in the general population. Diabetic nephropathy is an increasingly important cause of CRF. Approximately 40% of type I and 6% to 20% of type II diabetics develop renal failure, and about 25% of patients currently entering dialysis/transplantation programs in this country are diabetics.

PATHOGENESIS OF UREMIC SYMPTOMS

The symptoms of uremia are for the most part due to the accumulation of toxic nitrogenous end products of metabolism normally excreted by the kidney. Although urea (or urea nitrogen) and creatinine are commonly measured to assess the degree of renal failure, there is evidence that these substances themselves are not toxic and are only markers for other unidentified nitrogenous toxins of similar molecular weight (less than 200 daltons). The "middle molecule" hypothesis incriminates toxins of larger molecular weight (1000 to 5000 daltons) in the pathogenesis of uremic symptoms. Studies until now, however, have not established a clear relationship between uremic symptoms and accumulation of specific middle molecule fractions. Alterations in sodium, potassium, and water balance due to defective renal excretion, acidosis resulting from impaired hydro-

---

Table 1. CAUSES OF CHRONIC RENAL FAILURE

Glomerulopathies
Primary—focal segmental glomerulosclerosis; membranoproliferative glomerulonephritis; membranous nephropathy; crescentic glomerulonephritis (types I, II, and III); nonspecific proliferative glomerulonephritis; IgA nephropathy (uncommon)
Secondary—systemic lupus erythematosus; vasculitides including polyarteritis, Wegener's granulomatosis, Henoch-Schönlein purpura; Goodpasture's syndrome; diabetes mellitus; amyloidosis; heroin abuse; poststreptococcal glomerulonephritis (uncommon); acquired immunodeficiency syndrome; sickle cell anemia

Chronic Tubulointerstitial Diseases
Chronic bacterial pyelonephritis acquired in early childhood especially in association with vesicoureteric reflux; analgesic abuse; chronic hypercalcemia; chronic hyperuricemia; oxaluria; heavy metals (lead, cadmium, beryllium, platinum); idiopathic

Vascular Disease
Hypertensive nephrosclerosis; atherosclerotic renal artery stenosis; progressive systemic sclerosis; hemolytic uremic syndrome

Hereditary and Developmental Disorders
Polycystic kidney disease; medullary cystic disease (nephronophthisis); Alport's syndrome and other hereditary nephritides; renal hypoplasia-dysplasia; Fabry's disease; oxaluria type I and II; cystinosis

Urologic Causes
Urinary tract obstruction; vesicoureteric reflux; recurrent stone formation (especially infection-associated "staghorn" calculi)

Miscellaneous
Multiple myeloma and other paraproteinemias; radiation nephritis; irreversible acute renal failure (ischemic or nephrotoxic)

---

gen ion excretion, anemia caused by a number of factors, alterations in calcium/phosphate homeostasis, and endocrine and immunologic abnormalities all contribute to the uremic syndrome. Some of the adaptive changes developing with progressive renal failure have also been implicated in the pathogenesis of uremia: parathormone (PTH) and natriuretic hormone, whose production is increased in CRF in an "attempt" to correct abnormalities in calcium/phosphate/vitamin D balance and sodium balance, respectively, have been incriminated as uremic toxins by some authors. Failure of the normal endocrine function of the kidney (decreased erythropoietin and 1,25-dihydroxyvitamin D_3 production) also causes some of the manifestations of the uremic state. Increased renin secretion from diseased kidneys contributes to hypertension in 15% to 20% of patients with CRF.

THE PROGRESSIVE NATURE OF CHRONIC RENAL DISEASE

While the progression of chronic renal disease to end-stage renal failure (ESRF) may be due to the persistence of the original cause, there is now evidence suggesting that once renal injury is initiated, it can progress owing to other factors. Adaptive increase in glomerular filtration (glomerular hyperfiltration) in nephrons initially undamaged has been shown to cause progressive sclerosis of these glomeruli. The higher the protein intake, the greater is the degree of glomerular hyperfiltration in the remnant nephrons. This postulated mechanism is probably of greater importance in renal failure caused by glomerular diseases. The altered calcium/phosphate balance in CRF favors soft tissue calcification, which in the kidney may cause progression of renal damage. Hypertension, which almost invariably accompanies chronic parenchymal renal disease, can itself cause further renal injury. These mechanisms form the basis for the recommendation of dietary protein and phosphate restriction and meticulous blood pressure control to slow the progression of CRF.

PATHOPHYSIOLOGY OF CRF

SALT AND WATER BALANCE

Until the creatinine clearance reaches less than 10 ml/min, adaptive changes in the undamaged nephrons enable patients with CRF to remain in salt and water balance despite decreased renal function and unlimited salt/water intake. However, such patients cannot adjust quickly to acute increases or decreases in salt and water intake and may become overhydrated or dehydrated repetitively under these circumstances with resultant acute worsening of renal function. Patients with chronic tubulointerstitial nephropathies, obstructive uropathy, polycystic kidney disease, and medullary cystic disease tend to be renal "salt wasters" and may require increased sodium intake to maintain sodium balance. In advanced CRF with urine volumes of less than 1000 ml/24 hours, sodium and water retention will develop leading to peripheral and pulmonary edema, dilutional hyponatremia, and hypertension unless salt and water intake are restricted.

POTASSIUM BALANCE

Until the advanced oliguric stage of renal failure is reached, most patients with CRF remain in potassium balance despite normal dietary potassium intake. Increased aldosterone production leading to increased potassium excretion through remaining undamaged nephrons and the colon is the major adaptive mechanism in this regard. Patients with diabetic nephropathy and chronic tubulointerstitial diseases may exhibit type IV renal tubular acidosis (RTA) in which aldosterone secretion is defective as a result of renin deficiency (hyporeninemic hypoaldosteronism) or an adrenal cortical abnormality, or the renal tubules may be resistant to aldosterone action. Such patients may manifest hyperkalemia even with mild to moderate renal insufficiency. Acidosis, excessive potassium intake, the use of potassium-sparing diuretics (triamterene, amiloride, spironolactone), drastic dietary salt reduction (by limiting sodium availability in the distal nephron for exchange with potassium), and insulin deficiency in diabetics may also contribute to hyperkalemia in early renal failure. Patients with advanced renal failure are very vulnerable to exogenous or endogenous potassium loading, which may result in life-threatening hyperkalemia.

ACID-BASE BALANCE

In patients with glomerular diseases, metabolic acidosis due to impaired renal hydrogen ion excretion usually becomes manifest when the creatinine clearance is reduced to less than 30 ml/min. The metabolic acidosis tends to be of the high anion gap type in these patients. In patients with chronic tubulointerstitial diseases, normal anion gap RTA develops earlier in the course of CRF and with advanced renal failure changes to high anion gap metabolic acidosis. Metabolic acidosis contributes to bone disease in uremic patients and also tends to aggravate hyperkalemia.

CALCIUM, PHOSPHATE, VITAMIN D, AND MAGNESIUM METABOLISM

Phosphate retention due to decreased renal excretion occurs in the earliest stages of renal failure. Elevation of serum phosphate causes the serum ionized calcium level to fall. Defective hydroxylation of 25-hydroxyvitamin D_3 to 1,25-dihydroxyvitamin D_3 (1,25-D_3) by the diseased kidney leads to a reduction in the serum level of the latter form of vitamin D. Since 1,25-D_3 regulates intestinal calcium absorption, its decreased synthesis also contributes to hypocalcemia. The fall in serum calcium due to these factors causes parathyroid hyperplasia and increased PTH secretion (secondary hyperparathyroidism). Since the parathyroid glands have receptors for 1,25-D_3, fall in the serum level of this metabolite may also be a stimulus for secondary hyperparathyroidism. In the earlier stages of CRF (until the creatinine clearance has fallen below 30 ml/min), increased PTH secretion is able to normalize serum phosphate levels by increasing phosphate excretion through undamaged nephrons. The correction of hyperphosphatemia, increased renal production of 1,25-D_3, and mobilization of skeletal calcium resulting from increased PTH secretion maintain the serum calcium also in the normal range in early renal failure. When the creatinine clearance has fallen to less than 30 ml/min, hypocalcemia and hyperphosphatemia become manifest despite these adaptive mechanisms. Elevation in the serum calcium/phosphate product favors the development of metastatic (soft tissue) calcification. Secondary hyperparathyroidism, which develops as a compensatory mechanism in the early stages of CRF, is detrimental to the skeleton: hyperparathyroid bone disease (osteitis fibrosa) is a major cause of morbidity in the later stages of CRF and in dialysis patients. Sometimes secondary hyperparathyroidism is so marked that hypercalcemia may develop.

Mild hypermagnesemia (serum magnesium 2.0 to 3.0 mEq/L) due to defective renal magnesium excretion becomes manifest when the creatinine clearance falls below 30 ml/min. Severe hypermagnesemia may develop if magnesium-containing antacids and laxatives are used.

HEMATOLOGIC CHANGES

Normochromic, normocytic anemia develops in CRF from a combination of factors: reduced erythropoietin production by the diseased kidneys, inhibition of bone marrow response to erythropoietin by uremic toxins, shortened red cell life span, and the bleeding tendency of uremia.

Qualitative platelet dysfunction is common in the later stages of CRF, leading to prolongation of the bleeding time. Uremic toxins such as guanidinosuccinic acid interfere with platelet aggregation. Abnormal platelet factor 3 release and platelet adhesiveness have also been reported in uremia. Thrombocytopenia occurs occasionally in advanced renal failure.

Defective granulocyte phagocytic function and abnormalities in cellular and humoral immunity have been described in CRF. These changes may be responsible for increased susceptibility to infections and for the increased incidence of malignancies in patients with CRF.

ENDOCRINE ABNORMALITIES

Abnormalities in thyroid function tests (decreased thyroxine and triiodothyronine levels with normal TSH level) without clinical or physiologic evidence of hypothyroidism are common in patients with advanced CRF and in dialysis patients. The prevalence of goiter is also increased in these patients. Growth retardation in children, impotence, amenorrhea, galactorrhea, and sterility are other endocrine problems in the uremic population.

HYPERURICEMIA

Serum uric acid is elevated in CRF owing to decreased urinary excretion of uric acid. Although the serum uric acid level commonly exceeds 10 mg/dl in advanced renal failure, secondary gout is rare in these patients. Crystalline arthropathy is more commonly due to pseudogout in this population.

CARBOHYDRATE METABOLISM

Mild glucose intolerance due to insulin resistance (pseudodiabetes) is common in nondiabetic CRF patients. When diabetics develop CRF, insulin requirements decrease owing to decreased catabolism and excretion of insulin by the diseased kidneys. A syndrome of spontaneous hypoglycemia probably due to defective gluconeogenesis has been described in cachectic patients with ESRF.

HYPERLIPIDEMIA

Type IV hyperlipoproteinemia with hypertriglyceridemia is a common abnormality in patients with advanced CRF and in those on dialysis. Hypercholesterolemia is much less common. Decreased high-density lipoprotein cholesterol and apoprotein C-II (less commonly apoprotein A-I and A-II) has also been reported. These abnormalities may contribute to arteriosclerotic cardiac, cerebral, and peripheral vascular disease, which is a major problem in these patients.

CLINICAL ASPECTS

The "uremic syndrome" affects all organ systems. As already described, many of the biochemical and hematologic abnormalities of CRF do not develop until the creatinine clearance is below 30 ml/min. Symptoms of uremia usually do not appear until the creatinine clearance is below 5 to 10 ml/min. The clinical features of CRF are shown in Table 2. Many uremic symptoms are rarely seen nowadays because of the institution of dialysis before these symptoms appear.

MANAGEMENT OF CRF

There are three aspects to the management of the patient with CRF. The first is therapy of the cause whenever possible. Examples are corticosteroid and cytotoxic therapy of primary and secondary forms of glomerulopathies; interdiction of analgesics, other drugs, and toxins causing CRF; and the correction of obstructive uropathy. Such measures might stabilize or improve renal function. Second, one should always seek to identify and treat potentially reversible factors that might be aggravating renal failure irrespective of the primary cause. Volume depletion due to poor salt and water intake, vomiting/diarrhea and overzealous diuretic therapy, uncontrolled hypertension, use of nephrotoxic drugs (aminoglycosides, nonsteroidal anti-inflammatory agents, radiocontrast agents), urinary tract infection, and urinary tract obstruction are examples of reversible causes of acute on CRF. Disproportionate elevation of BUN compared with the serum creatinine should suggest the possibility of prerenal azotemia due to volume depletion superimposed on CRF. Deterioration of renal function at a rate faster than predicted by the slope of 1/s. creat. versus time plot (see later) should also dictate a search for the above-mentioned causes of acute on CRF. The remainder of this chapter will deal with the third aspect of the management of CRF—"nonspecific" dietary and drug therapy irrespective of the etiology.

NONPHARMACOLOGIC MEASURES: DIETARY MANAGEMENT OF CRF

Dietary Protein Restriction. Until a few years ago this restriction was imposed only after uremic gastrointestinal or neurologic symptoms had developed, or after the BUN exceeded 70 to 80 mg/dl. Considerable experimental evidence has now accumulated suggesting that a high dietary protein intake causes glomerular hyperfiltration and progressive glomerulosclerosis in nephrons initially partially or completely undamaged by the primary renal disease. The beneficial effect of dietary protein restriction in slowing the course of CRF is well

Table 2. CLINICAL FEATURES OF CHRONIC RENAL FAILURE

	Clinical Problem	Mechanism
Cardiovascular	Hypertension	Increased extracellular fluid volume in 80% to 85% of patients. Increased renin production in 15% to 20%. Decreased production of vasodilatory prostaglandins and kinins by kidney may play a role.
	Congestive heart failure	Hypertension, anemia, salt and water excess, greater prevalence of arteriosclerotic heart disease, (?) primary cardiomyopathy due to uremic toxins.
	Pericarditis with or without effusion (often hemorrhagic)	Pericardial inflammation due to deposition of uremic toxins.
Pulmonary	Pulmonary edema	Salt and water excess, increased pulmonary capillary permeability due to uremic toxins.
	Pleurisy with or without effusion (often hemorrhagic)	Same as in pericarditis.
Renal	Polyuria, nocturia, and increased thirst in the initial stages of CRF	Defective renal tubular concentrating ability.
	Oliguria/anuria in the later stages	Marked reduction in GFR.
Gastrointestinal	Stomatitis, parotitis, hiccups, anorexia, nausea, vomiting, erosive gastritis and colitis, pancreatitis (rare)	Accumulation of nitrogenous uremic toxins.
Neuromuscular	CNS-emotional lability, difficulty in concentrating, insomnia, myoclonus, asterixis, psychosis, seizures, stupor, coma, tetany (rare); peripheral neuropathy	Accumulation of uremic toxins. Hypocalcemia causes tetany and may cause seizures.
Osteodystrophy	Bone pain, fractures, bone deformity, proximal muscle weakness	Metabolic acidosis worsens bone disease.
	Secondary hyperparathyroidism (osteitis fibrosa)	Effect of PTH on skeleton.
	Rickets in children	Deficiency of active form of vitamin D.
	Osteomalacia (rarely seen before institution of dialysis)	Aluminum accumulation in bone from ingested aluminum-containing phosphate binders or from aluminum-contaminated dialysate.
Metastatic Calcification	Vascular (may contribute to cardiac, cerebral, and peripheral vascular disease)	Increased calcium/phosphate product.
	Articular—pseudogout	Increased calcium/phosphate product.
	Visceral—renal, pulmonary, myocardium. May contribute to dysfunction of these organs	Increased calcium/phosphate product.
	Cutaneous—may be partly responsible for itching	Increased calcium/phosphate product.
General	Fatigue	Anemia, uremic toxins.
	Itching	Uremic toxins, calcium/phosphate deposition in skin, dry skin.
	Weight loss	Anorexia.
	Growth retardation in children	Uremic toxins, endocrine changes, deficiency of active vitamin D.
	Loss of libido, impotence, amenorrhea, sterility	Endocrine dysfunction. Zinc deficiency has been incriminated in impotence in dialysis patients.
	Galactorrhea (rare)	Prolactin excess.

documented in experimental animals and in a small number of human clinical studies. "Early" dietary protein restriction (when serum creatinine exceeds 2.5 to 3.0 mg/dl) is now becoming common practice. A daily intake of 0.5 to 0.6 gm/kg of high biological value protein is recommended for this purpose. However, it is difficult to obtain compliance with such a diet in asymptomatic patients with early renal failure. Some authors have suggested that protein restriction of this magnitude can be imposed even on patients with heavy proteinuria and renal failure; reduction in proteinuria and improvement in serum albumin has been reported subsequently. Dietary supplementation with essential amino acids or ketoanalogues of such amino acids has been shown to have a favorable effect on the course of CRF, and this form of therapy is now being evaluated in controlled clinical studies. When dialytic therapy is instituted for ESRF, dietary protein intake is increased to 1 to 1.5 gm/kg/day to avoid protein malnutrition, which is common in the dialysis population.

Phosphate Intake. Hyperphosphatemia contributes to secondary hyperparathyroidism, bone disease, and possibly the progression of CRF by the deposition of calcium and phosphate in the kidneys. Since protein foods have a high content of phosphate, early dietary protein restriction helps also in control of phosphate intake. Limiting the intake of phosphate-rich milk and dairy products should be emphasized. Patients with advanced renal failure (serum creatinine >5 mg/dl) should restrict their daily phosphate intake to about 750 mg.

Salt and Water Intake. Since, in general, salt and water balance is maintained until the end oliguric phase of CRF develops, restriction of salt and water intake is usually not required earlier in the course of CRF. As already discussed, decreased dietary salt and water intake may in fact predispose to dehydration with consequent worsening of renal function and hyperkalemia in patients with CRF. Patients with "salt-wasting" renal diseases may require dietary salt and water supplementation to avoid volume depletion and aggravation of renal failure.

Hypertensive patients require restriction of salt intake to 5 gm/day or 85 mEq of sodium/day (no added salt diet). Stricter dietary sodium restriction is impractical and this level of sodium intake is permitted even in patients on dialysis. Once urine output has fallen to less than a liter/day, daily water intake should be restricted to equal the sum of the urine volume and estimated insensible losses (approximately 600 ml/day).

Potassium Intake. Since potassium balance is maintained till advanced oliguric renal failure develops, dietary potassium restriction is usually not required earlier. Patients with type IV RTA may require potassium restriction even in early CRF. Mild hyperkalemia requires restriction of potassium intake to 2 gm or 26 mEq/day. In terminal oliguric renal failure and in patients on dialysis, potassium intake is limited to 1.5 gm or 20 mEq/day to avoid hyperkalemia. Some patients with chronic tubulointerstitial diseases may have renal potassium wasting and may require dietary potassium supplementation.

Carbohydrate and Saturated Fat Intake. Hypertriglyceridemia is a common problem in the later stages of CRF and in dialysis patients. Restriction of carbohydrate calories to 35% of the total caloric intake is helpful in decreasing triglyceride levels. Limitation of saturated fat intake is also recommended in CRF patients because atherosclerotic cardiovascular disease is a major problem.

ANTIHYPERTENSIVE DRUG THERAPY

Hypertension is common in patients with CRF and contributes to progressive renal damage and cardiovascular disease. Blood pressure control is thus a critical aspect of the management of these patients. Since salt and water excess is the major factor causing hypertension in this population, dietary salt restriction and diuretics should be the initial therapeutic measures. Thiazides and chlorthalidone are generally ineffective when the creatinine clearance is less than 30 ml/min. Potassium-sparing diuretics are best avoided in patients with renal insufficiency because of the risk of hyperkalemia. The loop diuretics (furosemide, ethacrynic acid, or bumetanide) and metolazone are the only effective diuretics in patients with significant renal failure, but the dose of these drugs needs to be increased in such patients. Guidelines for their use in renal impairment are described in Chapter 8. If the addition of antihypertensive drugs is required, agents such as guanethidine, which lower renal blood flow, should be avoided. Prazosin, hydralazine, methyldopa, clonidine, beta-blockers, and calcium channel antagonists (nifedipine, diltiazem) can be used alone or in appropriate combinations. Minoxidil and captopril should be considered for refractory hypertension. Captopril should be used with caution in patients with renal failure because of the risks of hyperkalemia, neutropenia, proteinuria, and further impairment of renal function. The use of antihypertensives in renal failure is discussed in Chapter 8.

One should aim to maintain the blood pressure as close to normal as possible without producing symptomatic postural hypotension and drug side effects. In younger patients the target should be 110 to 120/70 to 80 mm Hg and in older patients 140 to 150/80 to 90 mm Hg.

DRUG THERAPY FOR CALCIUM, PHOSPHATE, AND VITAMIN D ABNORMALITIES

Serum calcium and phosphate values should be maintained in the normal range throughout the course of renal failure and in patients on dialysis to minimize the risks of secondary hyperparathyroidism, bone disease, and soft tissue calcification. The dietary measures described are by themselves insufficient to correct calcium/phosphate/vitamin D abnormalities in patients with advanced renal failure. Calcium supplementation (calcium carbonate 1000 to 2000 mg/day) is required when the serum calcium falls to the lower range of normal. Some authors recommend calcium supplementation earlier in the course of renal failure even if the serum calcium is normal in an attempt to suppress hyperparathyroidism. Hyperphosphatemia, if present, should be corrected with aluminum hydroxide (see below) before calcium supplementation is begun to avoid the risk of soft tissue calcification.

Phosphate binder therapy is instituted when the serum phosphate approaches the upper limit of normal. Aluminum hydroxide (300 to 1200 mg) after each meal and snack binds dietary phosphate and prevents its absorption. Various aluminum hydroxide preparations in tablet, capsule, and liquid form are available (Amphojel, Alu-Cap, Alu-Tab, AlternaGEL, Basaljel, Dialume, Nephrox). Patient compliance with phosphate binder therapy is generally poor because of the taste and the constipation that it invariably causes. If a patient dislikes one preparation of phosphate binder, he should be encouraged to try an alternative formulation and laxatives should be prescribed. Magnesium-containing antacids and laxatives are generally avoided in CRF because of the risk of hypermagnesemia.

Calcium carbonate itself is phosphate-binding. Since high-dose aluminum hydroxide therapy leading to aluminum accumulation in the skeleton and brain has been associated with osteomalacia and dementia, the use of high-dose calcium carbonate therapy alone or in combination with low-dose aluminum hydroxide therapy has been recommended for phosphate control. A few studies have reported success with this approach but further experience is needed.

Vitamin D supplementation is needed when hypocalcemia persists despite calcium carbonate therapy. Clinical, biochemical, or radiologic evidence of progression of parathyroid bone disease is another indication for vitamin D therapy. Some authors have recommended "prophylactic " vitamin D supplementation beginning in early renal failure to minimize secondary hyperparathyroidism, and this approach is currently being evaluated in controlled clinical studies. Calcitriol (1,25-dihydroxyvitamin D_3, Rocaltrol—0.25 to 2 μg daily), calcifediol (25-hydroxyvitamin D_3, Calderol—20 to 100 μg daily), and dihydrotachysterol (1α-hydroxyvitamin D_3, Hytakerol—0.5 to 1.25 mg daily) are all effective in correcting hypocalcemia in CRF patients, with calcitriol being the most effective. In order to avoid metastatic calcification, vitamin D therapy should be instituted only after hyperphosphatemia is corrected. The serum calcium and alkaline phosphatase levels should be monitored closely in patients on any of these vitamin D metabolites. Hypercalcemia may be preceded by a rapid fall in alkaline phosphatase level. Hypercalcemia should be avoided because it can aggravate renal failure and favor metatastic calcification. Progression of parathyroid bone disease despite vitamin D therapy and the development of hypercalcemia limiting the use of vitamin D are indications for subtotal parathyroidectomy.

MISCELLANEOUS MEDICAL THERAPY

Metabolic Acidosis. Serum bicarbonate levels should be maintained above 20 mEq/L with sodium bicarbonate (650 to 1300 mg t.i.d. or q.i.d.) to avoid the adverse effect of acidosis on bone disease and hyperkalemia.

Type IV RTA. Dietary potassium restriction, the use of loop diuretics to increase renal potassium excretion, and correction of acidosis with sodium bicarbonate are usually sufficient. Some patients require cation exchange resin therapy (Kayexalate). Mineralocorticoid supplementation (Florinef, 0.1 to 1 mg daily) may be used, but salt retention and fluid overload are potential problems.

Symptomatic Therapy. Uremic pruritus may respond to hydroxyzine, cyproheptadine, or diphenhydramine. Correction of hyperphosphatemia and the use of skin lotions and creams to avoid dry skin are also important. Institution of dialysis may relieve pruritus but some patients have aggravation of this symptom during hemodialysis. Ultraviolet light therapy to the skin is sometimes helpful in patients with severe pruritus. Although dramatic relief of pruritus has been reported following parathyroidectomy, the results are not consistent.

The use of phenothiazines or metoclopramide may be required for the relief of uremic nausea and vomiting.

Adjustment of Drug Dosage. A very important aspect of the management of CRF is to adjust the dose of any drug prescribed to the level of the patient's renal function. This subject is discussed in detail in Chapter 8.

PLANNING FOR ESRF THERAPY

Plans for dialysis and/or renal transplantation should begin well before ESRF and uremic symptoms develop. This subject is dealt with in Chapter 9.

MEDICAL FOLLOW-UP OF THE PATIENT WITH CRF

Patients with early renal failure (serum creatinine 2 to 5 mg/dl) should be seen every three to six months, and those with more advanced renal failure require monthly or bimonthly visits. Blood pressure, urinalysis, 24-hour urine protein and creatinine clearance, hematocrit, BUN, serum creatinine, electrolytes, calcium/ inorganic phosphate, alkaline phosphatase, total protein and albumin, triglycerides, and cholesterol should be checked during these visits. Skeletal x-ray films, bone densitometry, and PTH measurements are recommended annually in patients with advanced renal failure and in those on dialysis to assess the status of renal osteodystrophy and secondary hyperparathyroidism.

When a number of serum creatinine measurements are available over a period of time, the 1/s. creat. versus time plot can be created (see Fig. 1, Chap. 1). The 1/s. creat. usually declines linearly in the course of CRF, and by extending the plot, the time at which a certain value of serum creatinine will be reached can be predicted. Following the 1/s. creat. versus time plot is thus helpful in planning for eventual ESRF therapy. In addition, decline of renal function more rapidly than predicted by the 1/s. creat. plot may be a clue to the presence of reversible factors aggravating renal failure. This plot also allows the managing physician to measure the impact of interventions aimed at slowing the course of CRF (e.g., control of hypertension and hyperphosphatemia; dietary protein restriction).

PATIENT AND FAMILY EDUCATION

As in any chronic disease, this is a very important part of the management of CRF. The progressive nature of CRF and the eventual development of ESRF should be explained. The favorable effect of dietary protein and phosphate restriction and blood pressure control in slowing the progression of CRF should be stressed. The fact that disabling bone disease may be preventable by control of calcium/phosphate/vitamin D balance by diet and drugs should be emphasized. Patients should be encouraged to comply with dietary restrictions and medical therapy even though they are asymptomatic. Home blood pressure monitoring should be taught. The dietitian should meet periodically with the patient and the person responsible for preparing the patient's meals. Dietary restrictions become critical when the advanced oliguric stage of CRF is reached and in patients on dialysis. Patient and family education in regard to treatment alternatives for ESRF is discussed in Chapter 9.

REFERENCES

Barsotti G, Giannoni A, Morelli E, et al: The decline in renal function slowed by very low phosphorus intake in chronic renal failure patients following a low nitrogen diet. Clin Nephrol 21:54–59, 1984.

Brenner BM, Rector FC (eds): The Kidney, 3rd ed. W.B. Saunders Co., Philadelphia, 1986, pp 1553–1790.

Brenner BM, Stein JH (eds): Chronic Renal Failure. Churchill-Livingstone, New York, 1981.

Hostetter TH: Progressive glomerular injury: roles of dietary protein and compensatory hypertrophy. Pharmacol Rev 36:101S–108S, 1984.

Psychological Aspects

A. Dale Gulledge
Lilian Gonsalves-Ebrahim
Jeffery C. Hutzler
CLEVELAND CLINIC FOUNDATION

THE NONCOMPLIANT PATIENT IN CHRONIC RENAL FAILURE

Inability to adhere to the prescribed medical regimen can be a major problem in patients with chronic medical problems, particularly end-stage renal disease. Whether the patient goes on to chronic hemodialysis, chronic ambulatory peritoneal dialysis (CAPD), or renal transplantation, compliance will be a major factor in the success of the treatment selected.

Patients can undermine treatment in a variety of ways. They may follow diets poorly, take medications only sporadically, refuse to be physically active, or refuse suggestions for increased bed rest. They may not show up for appointments, use alcohol or drugs inappropriately, and in various ways cause a disruption of their treatment program. These patients may use poor judgment in their diabetic treatment or other medical treatment programs. All of these behaviors may result in an unstable medical picture, ranging from excess fluid intake between dialysis procedures to life-threatening states of coma, seizures, and eventually death.

The patient who is noncompliant for these and other reasons may have one of several psychiatric disorders. The following are some conditions frequently encountered in the chronic renal patient.

DEPRESSION

Depression results from both a biochemical and a psychological cause. In part, it is due to a depletion of central nervous system biogenic amines (serotonin, norepinephrine, and dopamine). It is also a result of declining psychological ability, disturbed interpersonal relations, and intrapsychic conflicts.

The diagnosis of depression is straightforward (Table 3). A brief mental status examination will, in a majority of cases, point to depression. Patients who are depressed have disturbed sleep; often they have difficulty falling asleep and then wake within one or two hours off and on throughout the night. Therefore they frequently show initial insomnia, middle insomnia, and terminal insomnia (wakening at four or five o'clock in the morning and being unable to fall back to sleep). These patients often complain bitterly over relatively minor medical and physical problems, seem uninterested in their usual activities, and may withdraw from family and friends. They become irritable.

Management of Depression

Depression is commonly and successfully treated with *psychotherapy* and *antidepressant medication*. Psychotherapy defines problems in the patient's life. These often involve the changing roles experienced by a person with chronic illness, such as becoming an ineffective spouse, and other concerns, such as changes in sexual interest and ability, fears of increased dependency upon others, and losing an occupation. Once these problems are identified, problem-solving can begin. The patient can learn that these problems are common and are open to solutions through change in behavior and attitudes. The patient then becomes involved in learning new behaviors, which result in changes that alleviate the underlying conflict. Psychotherapy is the most effective tool in solving problems of noncompliance and is always used in conjunction with any form of chemotherapy.

Antidepressant medication is extremely effective (85% of major depression responds to this treatment). The heterocyclics are the most frequently used antidepressants in patients with chronic renal failure. Table 4 includes three commonly used heterocyclics and the initial dose used in medically ill patients.

One of these heterocyclics can be chosen, begun at low levels (25 mg q.h.s.), and increased by 25-mg increments every five to seven days, hoping to achieve

Table 3. CRITERIA FOR MAJOR DEPRESSION

Sad or depressed mood
Four of the following symptoms that have continued for two weeks or
   more:
  Poor appetite
  Insomnia or hypersomnia
  Slowing of motor activity (or agitation)
  Decreased interest in activities
  Fatigue
  Feelings of worthlessness
  Decreased concentration (can't read or watch TV for 30–45 minutes)
  Wishing to be dead or suicidal thinking

Table 4. EXAMPLES OF ANTIDEPRESSANTS AND INITIAL DOSES IN MEDICALLY ILL PATIENTS

Drug	Initial Dose	Notable Side Effects
Doxepin	50 mg at bedtime PO	Sedation
Desipramine	50 mg at bedtime PO	Few except dry mouth
Trazodone	100 mg at bedtime PO	May lower seizure threshold

a total dose of about 100 to 200 mg/day. This medication is usually given at bedtime to facilitate sleep. Monitoring serum levels is helpful with only a few of these medications (i.e., desipramine, nortriptyline).

It usually takes from two to four weeks to see clinical improvement. These drugs are effective but require patience. They should be increased carefully to achieve therapeutic effects.

DEPRESSION PRESENTING AS DEMENTIA

An important constellation of symptoms in considering depression in an end-stage renal disease patient is the disorder of "pseudodementia." This presents very much like an organic dementia: the patient suffers severe difficulty with his or her memory, is unable to remember to take medication, forgets relatives' names, appears confused and disoriented, and feels unsure as to where he or she is or what the date is. He may not be able to do simple calculations. He may look disheveled.

A high degree of suspicion should occur for pseudodementia when the patient answers questions with statements like "I don't know" or "It doesn't matter." Frequently this patient has suffered a recent loss in life, such as the death of a spouse, relative, or pet. The patient may be feeling abandoned by his family. He may also look depressed, with sighing respirations and a defeated appearance with bowed head and little psychomotor activity.

Patients with pseudodementia respond very well to psychotherapy and chemotherapy. It is important to make this diagnosis (or even overdiagnose it), since this condition is highly treatable and dramatic results can be achieved with a return to a normal state of intellectual function.

DELIRIUM

Delirium is a major cause of noncompliance. Patients who develop this disorder are suffering from disturbed brain function caused by drug intoxication, metabolic derangement, structural CNS lesions, or other physical causes. They have a generalized clouding of consciousness and are often uncooperative because cerebral function is impaired. They may have difficulty orienting themselves or be unable to interpret new environments, and so may become belligerent and angry, particularly in the hospital.

The causes of delirium are as numerous as there are derangements in metabolic state, or medications. The diagnosis is made by brief mental status examination testing the brain functioning. Table 5 lists questions that will elicit deficits in acute brain dysfunction (delirium).

Management of Delirium

Delirium is treated by correcting the underlying medical cause. While this is being done, medication can

**Table 5. MINI–MENTAL STATUS QUESTIONS FOR
SUSPECTED DELIRIUM**

Place: Where are you?
Time: What is the month, day, year?
Circumstance: Why are you in the hospital?
Person: What is your middle name? What is your address?
Serial Sevens: Subtract 7 from 100 and keep subtracting from the
  remainder.

be given to decrease the anxiety of these patients, ease their disturbed behavior, manage their hallucinations (usually visual), and calm their hyperaroused state. Haloperidol is the drug of choice in most cases, and the patient can be given 1 or 2 mg IM or PO. If the patient becomes sedated or clears in approximately two hours, no repeat medication need be given. However, if the patient remains confused and disoriented and combative, the medication can be increased to 5 mg IM or PO, again waiting for approximately two hours to see whether there is a response. A total of about 10 mg over six hours can be given, but if the patient continues to require increasing doses of haloperidol, a psychiatric consultation should be requested. Furthermore, if haloperidol is required beyond three days, a psychiatric consultation should also be requested.

MAJOR PSYCHIATRIC DISORDERS (PSYCHOSES)

Psychosis is defined as a loss of contact with reality or distortion of reality in a major way. One of the most common psychoses occuring in the end-stage renal disease patient is caused by medications or drugs. Steroids often induce tremendous changes in mood, mimicking manic (elevated mood) or severe depressed states. Patients often are dependent on analgesics, particularly narcotics, and can become addicted and then toxic from these medications, developing a drug-induced psychosis. Patients also may abuse minor tranquilizers such as Valium, Librium, Ativan, and others in an attempt to deal with chronic anxiety and boredom. They may become physically addicted to these medications and have a withdrawal psychosis up to a week to ten days after being in the hospital without them. Any drug can cause toxic effects or drug-induced psychosis. Therefore, any time a patient demonstrates bizarre behavior, the first rule of thumb is to go to the family to get a clear history of the patient's drug intake and then review his or her chart.

In a minority of cases, a patient may demonstrate a schizophrenic disorder with bizarre delusions ("My body is rotting" or "I have worms in my belly that are eating me"). These patients often have auditory hallucinations with the voices accusing them of something or making derogatory or "dirty" remarks.

If a schizophrenic disorder is suspected, a psychiatric consultation should be requested. This will allow the joint management of the end-stage renal disease patient with a schizophrenic disorder by the psychiatric arm of the renal team. The schizophrenic disorders are also treated with major tranquilizers such as haloperidol, thioridazine, thiothixene, or chlorpromazine.

Another major psychiatric disorder is the bipolar affective disorder (manic-depressive disorder). This manifests itself by grandiose or elevated mood, resulting in inappropriate behavior. The patient may spend money he does not have, act inappropriately sexually, or behave in a grandiose way inappropriate to his background. These patients speak very rapidly, are easily irritable, and often do not pay attention to their medical regimen.

This condition is best treated with the use of lithium carbonate, which must be monitored closely for blood levels, particularly in end-stage renal disease patients. It is even more difficult to manage patients who are on dialysis with this medication, but it can be done with careful liaison between the psychiatrist and the nephrologist.

PSYCHIATRIC COMPLICATIONS ASSOCIATED WITH DIALYSIS

It is well known that severe stresses confront the chronically ill dialysis patient. Issues of intimacy, autonomy, personal responsibility, and quality of life need to be resolved and dealt with on an almost daily basis. It is not surprising, then, that the rate of psychiatric symptoms in this population is three to five times greater than in the general population. Common psychiatric problems include anxiety responses to treatment, depression, passive noncompliance with medical demands, and psychotic states secondary to metabolic or "functional" causes. Marital discord, spouse or patient fatigue, and wish to terminate dialysis are other psychological issues facing dialysis patients. It is also important to remember that the patient on dialysis has a profound effect on family and dialysis staff.

THE DEPRESSED DIALYSIS PATIENT

Depression is a response to loss—real, threatened, or fantasized. The physician facing the depressed dialysis patient must explore several issues, i.e., attitude toward dialysis, changes in life style, loss of biological drives, medical problems, current medications, premorbid personality and coping styles, and history of affective disorders in the patient and family. Reserpine, alpha-methyldopa, clonidine, beta-blockers, alcohol, and chronic opiate and tranquilizer use are well known to cause depression. Dialysis patients are commonly treated with these medications, and a careful review of drug use and onset of depression is in order. Presence of a dysphoric mood and vegetative signs and symptoms—namely, loss of appetite and weight, fragmented sleep, psychomotor retardation, anhedonia, fatigue, lack of concentration, and suicidal ideation—indicate a major depression and usually necessitate a drug trial of antidepressants. Second generation antidepressants such as maprotiline and trazodone may offer an advantage for the depressed dialysis patient, since their cardiovascular and anticholinergic side effects and toxicity are less than those of imipramine and amitriptyline. The dialysis patient is on an average of ten medications compared with an average of six for a nondialyzed hospital patient. Thus, the physician must be aware of drug-drug interactions and use clinical judgment when prescribing antidepressants. This is probably best done by using daily small and divided doses and gradually increasing the dose until a therapeutic and maintenance level is achieved. An antidepressant trial should be continued for at least two to six weeks at the maximum tolerated dose before deciding to change medications.

THE CONFUSED DIALYSIS PATIENT

Psychoses associated with dialysis infrequently occur and are usually delirium-confusional states. Electrolyte imbalances and drugs such as barbiturates, anticholinergic agents, antihistamines, sedatives, and steroids are common causative factors. Careful assessment for other metabolic problems should also be made. Sedatives such as benzodiazepines and barbiturates should be discontinued and fluid and electrolyte balances corrected. Frequent reassurance and reorienting to assist with reality testing can be done by the patient's physician, nurse, and family. A clock, a calendar, familiar photographs, and an unobtrusive light during the night are some helpful environmental measures. Nursing intervention at night is kept to a minimum in order to reduce sleep disruption. If the patient is frankly psychotic with visual hallucinations, we prefer to begin to titrate and use haloperidol 1 mg PO, q.i.d. If the patient is extremely agitated, parenteral haloperidol 5 mg IM every hour until sedation occurs often is indicated; the latter drug regimen is commonly used in stress-induced, acute psychotic states.

COMPLIANCE ISSUES

The renal patient is suspended in a state of limbo between the world of the sick and the world of the well, belonging to neither, yet a part of both. The dialysis patient's recurrent health problems not only interfere with the normal pattern of life but also throw the patient back into the sick role. This conflict led Abram to refer to the "independence-dependence conflict" of the renal patient. Abram maintained that we need to meet "the patient where he is—allowing him to live his life as he sees fit." The majority of patients are torn between the fear of jeopardizing their lives and the need to comply with medical restrictions. They often "test limits" and learn to operate with some latitude of freedom in determining compliance with diet, fluid intake, and other medical demands. Pathologic food and fluid binges are behaviors often seen in dialysis patients. This noncompliance allows a means, although somewhat self-defeating, of displacing some of the anger, frustration, and hostility generated by the stress of dialysis and also serves as an expression of the lack of control over one's life. The tragic irony appears to be that the patient's attempts at autonomy through noncompliance are precisely the behaviors that are most likely to require more care while alienating staff and generating more hostility. It is important to remember that this independence-dependence conflict is a common human situation. Helpful interventions include helping the patient and his significant others work toward a compromise of the competing demands.

EFFECTS OF DIALYSIS ON THE FAMILY

Spouses share many stresses with their spouse patients, i.e., the possibility of death of the ill spouse, enormous medical expenses, lost personal opportunities for work, recreation and travel, and changes in the marital relationship. These stresses appear to be intensified with diabetic patients, where progressive loss of body parts and function forces the healthy spouse to take a more active role in the patient's dialysis routine.

ETHICAL ISSUES

Most patients receiving chronic dialysis consider terminating treatment if "the quality of life" available to them is not sufficient. This raises several questions and often renders the dialysis staff guilty, angry, or helpless. Although there are no clear guidelines to the patient's rights in accepting or refusing medical care, it is important to ascertain that the patient making such a request is *competent*. Competency includes answering the following questions: (1) Does the patient understand the nature of the act and its consequences, i.e., without dialysis he/she will die? (2) Is the patient psychotic? (3) Is the patient suffering from a suicidal depression? (4) Is the patient in severe pain that could interfere with his/her rational thinking? A psychiatrist is best suited for determining the patient's competency with regard to withdrawal of dialysis. He or she can openly and honestly discuss the implications of such a decision with the patient, family, and dialysis staff and help alleviate some of the guilt and helplessness.

TRANSPLANTATION

Confrontation with maintenance hemodialysis can produce an almost psychological stalemate in living. Dietary restrictions, multiple medications, fluid restrictions, and time on "the machine" may contribute to a situation where the patient and family see dialysis as a stress rather than a relief from illness. Looking for an alternative existence, the patient often sees successful kidney transplantation as a means to escape these restrictions in living, viewing the transplant as an opportunity for a "new life." However, cessation of dialysis does not necessarily mean no more medications, doctors, or even hospitalization. For many successful patients, transplantation does not automatically mean return to vigor, work, and independence, or absence of anxiety, depression, or resentment.

During the first week or so, the newly transplanted patient can usually benefit from expressing his guilt at having received a kidney at someone else's expense, while verbalizing his fears about dysfunction of the allograft. Assuring the patient that these are common feelings is helpful at this stage; as kidney function improves, optimism begins and thoughts turn to home and escape from the confinements of the hospital. With continuation of successful renal function, life becomes better and begins to expand, while interactions with family and staff improve. Buchanan has noted several important themes in patients following successful kidney transplantation. These include hesitancy to leave the dependent sick role, the need for social skills to reenter society, concerns about reentering the work force, continued opportunity to vent feelings about prior and current health care providers, the importance of being needed rather than needing, maintenance of hope during periods of rejection, continued need for detailed information about their condition, and the need to escape feelings of uniqueness in terms of both physical and psychological symptoms.

Diabetic patients generally experience more problems with psychosocial adaptation following transplantation. Although diabetic patients show improvement in self-esteem, independence, control, depression, and anxiety after a successful transplant, they frequently do not return to work, school, or recreation when follow-up evaluations are made five to nine years later. As Peterson notes, consultation for the diabetic patient following transplantation is often for the primary problem of "difficulty in coping" because of progressive debilitation, manifested as acute depression or behavioral problems. This emphasizes that psychiatric morbidity in the diabetic patient often parallels the course of physical disability, with compliance often being a major problem.

The patient may view his future as a vicious cycle, that is, one of dialysis, hope, transplantation, rejection, frustration, failure, and return to dialysis. Common fears of the patient may include the following: (1) fear of the unknown; (2) fear that he may not have a donor; (3) pain of surgery; (4) transplantation rejection; (5) lack of confidence in rehabilitation; and (6) long-term health problems.

FAMILY DONOR DECISION-MAKING

Simmons et al. indicate that the vast majority of family members who donate report little or no ambivalence regarding the basic question of donation, although concerns about surgery are frequent. The family's communication style and efforts tend to be *the major initial influence* on donor recruitment, although the decision to donate in most situations is "instantaneous and immediate."

Some well-matched potential donors will decide not to donate. Certainly all donors have misgivings about giving up part of their body in exchange for something less than a cure for their relative, and some potential donors undergo the medical evaluation while secretly hoping for a medical reason to justify not donating. Others indicate their reluctance by not returning for appointments for evaluation. If the decision is made not to donate, special guidance by the transplant team can help that family member avoid the tendency toward feelings of guilt, impaired self-esteem, and self-recrimination.

Effective confidential process to protect the feelings of the non-donor is necessary, and the physician in charge must be careful that undue pressure is not exerted on the potential donor because of the needs of the patient. Perhaps one of the best ways to minimize pressure by the physician on the potential donor is to limit contact between the physician and family members during the decision-making period. Even when a family member is unable to donate for medical reasons, subsequent counseling and support may be needed because of feelings of bitterness or guilt, which may produce a decline in comfort or effectiveness in intrafamilial relationships.

REFERENCES

Abram H: The "uncooperative" hemodialysis patient. *In* Levy GB (ed): Living or Dying. John Wiley and Sons, New York, 1984.

Blogget C: A selected review of the literature of adjustment to hemodialysis. Int J Psychiatry Med 11:97–124, 1981–1982.

Buchanan D: Group therapy for kidney transplant patients. Int J Psychiatry Med 6:523–531, 1975.

Gulledge AD, Buszta C, Montague DK: Psychosocial aspects of renal transplantation. Urol Clin North Am 10:327–335, 1983.

Peterson L, Perl M: Diabetic patients and the impact of renal transplantation. Psychosomatics 23:173–185, 1982.

Simmons RG, Hickory D, Kjellstrand CM, et al: Donors and nondonors: the role of the family and the physician in kidney transplantation. *In* Castenuovo-Tedesco P (ed): Psychiatric Aspects of Organ Transplantation. Grune & Stratton, New York, 1971.

Simmons RG, Kamstra-Hennen L, Thompson CR: Psychosocial adjustment five to nine years posttransplant. Transplant Proc 13:40–43, 1981.

Simmons RG, Klein S, Simmons RL: Gift of Life: The Social and Psychological Impact of Organ Transplantation. John Wiley and Sons, New York, 1977.

4 · PRIMARY GLOMERULAR DISEASES

Jorge A. Velosa
MAYO CLINIC AND MAYO FOUNDATION

The primary glomerular diseases constitute a heterogeneous group of disorders in which pathologic lesions in the glomeruli are either the sole or the predominant feature. As the disease progresses, there are concomitant tubular, interstitial, and vascular changes that together are referred to as "parenchymal renal disease."

Grouping patients by the common patterns of clinical presentation is a useful working approach to glomerular diseases. During the initial evaluation of a patient with possible glomerular disease, the physician thinks in terms of these broad categories of clinical syndromes and simultaneously explores the possibilities of systemic disorders that may underlie the renal clinical syndrome. Six major clinical syndromes can result from glomerular disease: the nephritic syndrome, rapidly progressive glomerulonephritis, the nephrotic syndrome, recurrent hematuria, asymptomatic proteinuria/hematuria, and chronic renal failure. The characteristics of these syndromes are described in Chapter 1. The term "chronic glomerulonephritis," is used when any type of glomerular disease leads to progressive renal damage resulting in end-stage renal failure. The major primary glomerular diseases are discussed in this chapter. Glomerulopathies secondary to systemic diseases are dealt with in Chapter 6.

Acute Poststreptococcal Glomerulonephritis

DEFINITION AND DIAGNOSTIC CRITERIA

Poststreptococcal glomerulonephritis (PSGN) may be defined as an acute nephritic syndrome that occurs after group A (beta-hemolytic) streptococcal pharyngeal or skin infection and is associated with elevated antibody titers against streptococcal exoenzymes and with reduced serum complement levels. This disease is self-limited and has an excellent prognosis. The latent period between the development of glomerulonephritis and the preceding streptococcal infection is usually one to three weeks. Urinalysis reveals proteinuria, erythrocytes, leukocytes, and casts, including red blood cell casts. The antistreptolysin O (ASO) titer becomes elevated (more than 200 Todd units) within one to three weeks after the onset of infection and may remain elevated for several months. With cutaneous infections, elevation of antibodies to streptococcal deoxyribonuclease B (ADNase-B) occurs more frequently than elevation of ASO antibodies. More than 90% of patients with PSGN have a reduced level of total hemolytic complement or of C3 during their first weeks of illness, after which, almost invariably, this returns to normal in less than eight weeks.

PATHOPHYSIOLOGY

The presence in the glomeruli of immune complexes presumably composed of streptococcal antigens and antibodies to these antigens induces the histologic changes and the clinical manifestations. These complexes initiate an inflammatory response mediated by complement, neutrophils, and macrophages.

MANAGEMENT

Patients with PSGN should be seen frequently until the acute nephritic syndrome resolves. Urinalysis, blood urea nitrogen (BUN) and serum creatinine, serum total complement and C3, blood pressure, and weight are monitored during this period. Patients are asked to maintain a daily record of their weight. They should be reassured about the likelihood of spontaneous recovery and the excellent prognosis of PSGN. Hospitalization is indicated for the treatment of severe renal failure, severe hypertension with volume overload, or acute heart failure. Generally, most patients without complications are ambulatory.

The management of acute PSGN is essentially non-pharmacologic, unless complications develop. Sodium intake is restricted even if the patient has no complications. If acute renal failure develops, sodium intake is restricted to 40 to 60 mEq a day, protein is restricted to 30 to 40 gm of high biological value protein a day, and fluids are restricted to replacement of urine output plus insensible losses. There are no specific drugs for the treatment of acute PSGN. If there is evidence of throat or skin streptococcal infection, penicillin treatment is indicated.

Severe hypertension and edema can occur owing to sodium and water retention secondary to decreased glomerular filtration. Severe hypertension may cause congestive heart failure and hypertensive encephalopathy. Diuretics and antihypertensive drugs are used if these complications develop. Acute renal failure due to rapidly progressive PSGN is fortunately rare; hemodialysis or peritoneal dialysis is indicated in these patients.

Renal biopsy is indicated if the nephritic or the nephrotic syndrome persists, if the serum complement does not normalize, or if the renal function continues to be impaired, eight to 12 weeks after the development of the disease. If urinalysis, 24-hour urine protein excretion, creatinine clearance, serum complement, and blood pressure are normal after two to three months of observation, no further follow-up is indicated. If there are residual renal changes, the patient is seen one year later to establish whether the condition is entering a chronic phase.

Crescentic–Rapidly Progressive Glomerulonephritis

DEFINITION AND DIAGNOSTIC CRITERIA

The term "crescentic–rapidly progressive glomerulonephritis" (CRPGN) is used here to describe a clinicopathologic syndrome characterized by rapid decrease in renal function during a short period, usually weeks or a few months, and by the presence of crescents in 30% or more of the glomeruli in the renal biopsy specimen.

Patients with primary CRPGN may be divided into four groups: (1) those with antibodies to glomerular basement membrane (GBM) with or without pulmonary hemorrhage; (2) those with idiopathic immune complex–mediated RPGN; (3) those with idiopathic CRPGN of unknown pathogenesis; and (4) those with CRPGN superimposed on other well-recognized primary glomerular diseases, e.g., membranoproliferative glomerulonephritis, PSGN, membranous glomerulopathy, and IgA nephropathy. Crescentic glomerulonephritis can also occur as a complication of systemic diseases such as systemic lupus erythematosus (SLE), Wegener's granulomatosis, and other types of vasculitis.

Antiglomerular Basement Membrane Antibody-Mediated CRPGN

Two groups of patients have this type of glomerulonephritis. In one, the glomerulonephritis is associated with pulmonary hemorrhage, widely recognized as Goodpasture's syndrome, whereas in the other, glomerulonephritis is the only clinical manifestation.

DEFINITION AND DIAGNOSTIC CRITERIA

Anti-GBM antibody-mediated glomerulonephritis is characterized by abrupt onset, presence of crescents, and demonstration of the linear deposition of IgG along the GBM by immunofluorescent study of the kidney biopsy. The diagnosis of anti-GBM disease is supported by demonstration of antibody to GBM in the serum. Renal biopsy is, however, necessary because there are false-positive and false-negative results in the detection of circulating anti-GBM antibodies.

PATHOPHYSIOLOGY

Anti-GBM antibodies bind with the endogenous antigens they are directed against and lead to glomerulonephritis. The glomerular injury is mediated by complement activation and participation of both neutrophils and macrophages. Fibrin deposition in the Bowman's space seems to initiate glomerular crescent formation.

CLINICAL ASPECTS

Goodpasture's syndrome occurs most often in young adult males. An association between exposure to hydrocarbons and the development of anti-GBM antibodies has been described. In Goodpasture's syndrome, pulmonary hemorrhage occurs owing to antibody-mediated injury of the pulmonary basement membrane. Hemoptysis occurs in most but not all patients. With severe pulmonary hemorrhage, the mortality rate is as high as 30%. Pulmonary involvement may precede, follow, or occur simultaneously with renal disease. Renal involvement usually leads rapidly to end-stage renal failure.

MANAGEMENT

Early treatment is of critical importance for success. Thus, the short-term goal is to establish the diagnosis as soon as possible and to initiate therapy as soon as the diagnosis is made. When the serum creatinine level has increased to 6 mg/dl or more, the chances of recovery of renal function are slim with any type of therapy. For patients with Goodpasture's syndrome who have active hemoptysis or severe respiratory failure, the overriding consideration is the control of these complications because they are the main limiting factors for survival of the patient.

Hospitalization is necessary for all patients. Intensive care management is mandatory if the patients have serious respiratory complications. Open renal biopsy may be necessary if the patient cannot cooperate for percutaneous needle biopsy. Artificial ventilation and tracheostomy may be necessary for treatment of respiratory failure.

Intensive plasma exchange to remove anti-GBM antibody appears to be beneficial for arresting pulmonary hemorrhage and for recovery of renal function. The patient is given daily plasma exchanges of 3 to 4 liters for the first few days, followed by every-other-day exchanges for one to three weeks. If there is no response by two weeks, discontinuation of therapy is justified.

Plasma exchange therapy is combined with prednisone (1 mg/kg/day) and cyclophosphamide (2 to 3 mg/kg/day). Most nephrologists administer intravenous "pulse" methylprednisolone therapy (see below) before commencing high-dose oral prednisone. Prednisone and cyclophosphamide should be gradually tapered off over several months.

In the past, bilateral nephrectomy was performed in patients with severe pulmonary hemorrhage and renal failure in an attempt to remove the source of the antigen against which anti-GBM antibodies are directed. Another indication for this procedure was to hasten the disappearance of the circulating antibody in patients awaiting renal transplantation. Since plasma exchange and immunosuppressive therapy are effective, bilateral nephrectomy is no longer indicated in the treatment of this disease.

Plasma exchange has significant hazards: infection (local and systemic), procoagulant deficiencies with bleeding, thrombocytopenia, hepatitis, and hypocalcemia. Adverse effects of pulse methylprednisolone include acute arrhythmias, hypertensive crisis, manic-depressive psychosis, aggravation of diabetes, infection, and possibly cataracts. Adverse effects secondary to cyclophosphamide are predisposition to opportunistic infections, marrow toxicity, gonadal toxicity, and hemorrhagic cystitis.

Patient follow-up is determined largely by the residual renal function. Unfortunately, many patients do not recover renal function because when they are hospitalized their serum creatinine levels are already above 6 mg/dl. Such patients require maintenance dialysis. Renal transplantation can be considered after tests for anti-GBM antibodies in the blood have been consistently negative. In the presence of circulating antibody, fulminant glomerulonephritis usually recurs in the transplanted kidney. Patients who have recovered renal function need close follow-up initially. If their condition remains stable for two to three months, visits every three months for the first year and every six to 12 months thereafter are appropriate.

The following tests are done during the periodic evaluations: urinalysis, measurements of serum creatinine, hemoglobin, hematocrit, and chest roentgenogram. Serum anti-GBM antibody determination is obtained during the first year of follow-up, and the glomerular filtration rate is measured three to six months after hospital dismissal and every year thereafter.

Immune Complex–Mediated and Unknown Pathogenesis CRPGN

DEFINITION AND DIAGNOSTIC CRITERIA

Patients with idiopathic immune complex–mediated CRPGN have, by definition, evidence for deposition of immune complexes in the glomeruli in the form of granular deposits of immunoglobulin and complement on immunofluorescence, or electron dense deposits on electron microscopy. The other important part of the definition is the exclusion of other primary glomerulopathies (e.g., membranoproliferative glomerulonephritis, IgA nephropathy, PSGN) or systemic disorders (e.g., SLE) that may have similar immunopathologic findings.

In idiopathic CRPGN of unknown pathogenesis, evidence for immune complex–mediated or anti-GBM antibody-mediated glomerular injury is lacking. In addition, there is no evidence of systemic vasculitides such as Wegener's granulomatosis, which can cause similar glomerular changes. ·

CLINICAL ASPECTS

Patients present with the acute nephritic syndrome, with rapid decrease in renal function but often without edema or hypertension. Patients are usually older than those with anti-GBM antibody glomerulonephritis, and may have constitutional symptoms such as fever, malaise, and arthralgias. Hemoptysis and pulmonary infiltrates may occur, and their presence suggests the clinical impression of Goodpasture's syndrome, but the immunopathologic and serologic findings are usually decisive in the differential diagnosis.

MANAGEMENT

Urgent diagnosis and immediate initiation of treatment are critical. Patients require immediate hospitalization for diagnosis and treatment as well as for management of the renal failure. A diet restricted in sodium, protein, and potassium should be adjusted to the degree of renal insufficiency; fluid should be restricted to the maintenance of adequate fluid balance.

Although controlled studies have not been published, there is anecdotal evidence that methylprednisolone "pulse" therapy may be effective. In patients with serum creatinine levels higher than 5 to 6 mg/dl, I give pulse therapy with methylprednisolone (approximately 20 to 30 mg/kg) intravenously over 20 minutes daily for three days, followed by oral prednisone, 1 to 1.5 mg/kg/day for four to six weeks, and then decrease the dose gradually over several months. A response usually occurs within five to 10 days and may continue for a few weeks. In patients with functioning kidneys and serum creatinine levels less than 5 to 6 mg/dl, satisfactory results have been obtained with conventional oral prednisone therapy; "pulse" therapy is optional. These patients are treated initially with 1 to 1.5 mg/kg/day of prednisone for four to six weeks, after which the dose is reduced gradually over several months. In my experience, patients with CRPGN and associated symptoms suggestive of a systemic disease respond well to glucocorticoid therapy. It is unclear if plasma exchange and cyclophosphamide are effective in these forms of CRPGN, but these measures have been used empirically in severely ill patients.

I discuss the serious nature of this type of renal disease, as well as the indications, limitations, and adverse effects of the therapeutic modalities with the patients and their families. Dietitians instruct patients and close relatives on the appropriate dietary restrictions, when indicated.

Close follow-up is necessary because there is a tendency for reactivation of the disease. Depending on the degree of renal function loss, I schedule visits every one to two months for the first six months and then every two to three months thereafter. If the patient's condition remains stable for a year, I recommend periodic visits every six months. Patients with irreversible end-stage renal failure are maintained on dialysis and evaluated for renal transplantation.

IgA Nephropathy

DEFINITION AND DIAGNOSTIC CRITERIA

In IgA nephropathy, mesangial deposition of IgA is consistently demonstrated in glomeruli. Some authors regard IgA nephropathy as a form of Henoch-Schönlein purpura with pathologic changes limited to the kidney.

PATHOPHYSIOLOGY

Mesangial deposition of immune complexes is probably responsible for the glomerular changes and triggers the periodic episodes of hematuria, but the nature of the antigens and antibodies involved in the formation of the immune complexes is poorly understood.

CLINICAL ASPECTS

The most frequent clinical presentation is recurrent episodes of gross hematuria (about 70% to 80% of the patients) closely related in time to a viral upper respiratory infection or a gastrointestinal syndrome. The diagnosis in the remainder of the cases is made during the work-up of asymptomatic, persistent hematuria and/or proteinuria. The serum IgA level is elevated in about 50% of the patients. Characteristically, the serum complement levels are normal, and this feature is of importance in differentiating IgA nephropathy from PSGN. Renal survival, determined from the time of presentation to the time of end-stage renal failure, has been calculated at about 90% at 10 years and 75% at 20 years.

MANAGEMENT

I recommend a low-salt diet for the rare patient with severe nephrotic syndrome and for the patient with hypertension. Patients with decreased renal function are advised to follow a restricted protein diet based on the degree of deterioration of renal function. No specific drug therapy has been beneficial in IgA nephropathy.

Patients with recurrent episodes of gross hematuria need reassurance about the benign nature of these episodes and the underlying disease. The emphasis on the benign characteristics of this disease are balanced by the emphasis on follow-up. If renal biopsy is not performed at the initial presentation of the disease, it should be considered in patients who have more than a 25% reduction in renal function, or who excrete more than 3 gm of urine protein in 24 hours at some time during their follow-up.

The Nephrotic Syndrome

The nephrotic syndrome is the result of abnormal permeability of the glomerular capillary wall, which allows large amounts of plasma proteins to pass into the urine. Proteinuria of sufficient magnitude induces hypoproteinemia. Hypoalbuminemia triggers the pathophysiologic processes responsible for the clinical and laboratory findings in the nephrotic syndrome, including edema and hyperlipidemia. Several primary glomerular diseases produce the nephrotic syndrome: minimal-lesion glomerulopathy, focal segmental glomerulosclerosis, membranous glomerulopathy, and, less frequently, membranoproliferative glomerulonephritis and crescentic glomerulonephritis. Glomerulopathies secondary to systemic diseases such as SLE, metabolic disorders such as diabetes mellitus and amyloidosis, drugs such as gold, penicillamine, captopril and heroin, and malignancies such as carcinomas and lymphomas may also cause the nephrotic syndrome.

MANAGEMENT

The short-term goal is to keep the patient ambulatory and working while a remission of the nephrotic syndrome either is induced by treatment or occurs spontaneously. The long-term goal is to induce a long-lasting remission. Realistically, this is possible only in patients with the minimal-lesion glomerulopathy, in a few patients with focal segmental glomerulosclerosis, and perhaps in a few patients with membranous glomerulopathy. In practice, many patients with the nephrotic syndrome do not respond to treatment and require symptomatic management, regardless of the type of glomerulopathy.

The vast majority of patients with the nephrotic syndrome can be managed as outpatients. The most frequent indication for hospitalization is treatment of anasarca associated with severe hypoalbuminemia that has rendered the patient bedridden. Other reasons for hospitalization are venous thrombosis associated with pulmonary emboli, acute thrombosis of the renal veins, and acute renal failure resulting from profound volume depletion due to severe hypoalbuminemia.

Dietary management is very important in the treatment of all nephrotic patients. In fact, patients with a mild to moderate nephrotic syndrome may be managed with just dietary salt restriction of about 2 gm of sodium chloride per day. In addition, the dietary intake of cholesterol and saturated fats is restricted. Calories are usually not restricted, unless the patient is obese. Recent studies have challenged the old practice of prescribing a high-protein diet. Furthermore, in patients with the nephrotic syndrome and impaired renal function, restriction of protein intake has been advocated, hoping to decrease the rate of renal function loss. I recommend a daily intake of 1.0 gm of high biological value protein per kilogram of body weight for patients with normal renal function and without severe hypoalbuminemia, and 0.7 gm of high biological value protein per kilogram per day for patients with impaired renal function.

Elastic stockings are useful for control of edema by applying mild hydrostatic pressure to the lower extremities, thus helping to mobilize fluid. Most patients with the nephrotic syndrome require diuretics for control of edema at one time or another. For patients with mild nephrotic syndrome and normal renal function, hydrochlorothiazide (50 to 100 mg/day) is often sufficient to control the edema. For patients with severe nephrotic syndrome or for those with decreased renal function, the more potent loop-acting diuretics, such as furosemide, bumetanide, or ethacrynic acid, are indicated. Some patients with severe hypoalbuminemia are unresponsive even to large doses of these potent diuretics. Under these circumstances, the addition of small amounts of metolazone (5 to 10 mg/day) usually restores diuresis. Patients with severe hypoalbuminemia and edema have difficulty in mobilizing fluid from the interstitial compartment into the vascular compartment. An effective maneuver to mobilize fluid from the interstitial compartment is to infuse hyperoncotic albumin intravenously (25 gm once or twice a day) while simultaneously administering a potent diuretic (e.g., furosemide, 40 to 80 mg intravenously). The effect of the infused albumin is very transient because it is rapidly excreted in the urine.

It is important to consider the adverse effects of diuretics. Vigorous diuresis may lead to intravascular volume depletion, orthostatic hypotension, and, in some situations, impairment of glomerular filtration rate and acute renal failure. Hypokalemia and hyponatremia are common in patients taking diuretics and may be severe in patients taking loop-acting diuretics in combination with metolazone. Rarely, patients may develop an acute allergic interstitial nephritis secondary to thiazides or furosemide.

Nephrotic patients have an increased tendency for developing deep venous thrombosis in the legs and thrombosis of one or both renal veins. Unilateral or bilateral renal vein thrombosis has been found most frequently in patients with membranous nephropathy, but it can occur in any patient with the nephrotic syndrome. Pulmonary emboli may be a complication of either deep vein thrombosis or renal vein thrombosis. I administer anticoagulants in two situations: (1) when patients develop definite pulmonary emboli and (2) when patients with acute renal vein thrombosis have associated impaired renal function. I limit long-term anticoagulation to patients with demonstrated pulmonary emboli, and I do not give anticoagulants to patients who have chronic renal vein thrombosis.

Infections may complicate the nephrotic syndrome. Patients with the nephrotic syndrome seem to be more susceptible to gram-positive and gram-negative encapsulated organisms. Thus, pneumococcal vaccine may be indicated in patients with severe, long-standing nephrotic syndrome, particularly children.

The following laboratory tests are performed periodically during the long-term follow-up of nephrotic patients: urinalysis, 24-hour urine protein excretion and creatinine clearance, total serum proteins, serum albumin, cholesterol and triglycerides, and hemoglobin and hematocrit. If diuretics are being used, the serum electrolytes should also be monitored. If patients have significant renal function loss, additional tests such as the determination of serum alkaline phosphatase, calcium, and phosphorus are performed.

There are definite socioeconomic implications for patients with severe nephrotic syndrome unresponsive to treatment. They cannot continue working and their social activities are limited owing to dietary restrictions and edema.

Minimal-Lesion Glomerulopathy

DEFINITION AND DIAGNOSTIC CRITERIA

In minimal-lesion glomerulopathy, the glomeruli are usually normal on light microscopy and immunofluorescence studies and electron microscopy reveals fusion of the podocytes, the characteristic lesion of this syndrome.

PATHOPHYSIOLOGY

In the nephrotic syndrome caused by this glomerulopathy in both humans and experimental animals, the predominant type of protein excreted in the urine is albumin, which is a negatively charged molecule. Alterations of the structural and functional integrity of the glomerular capillary wall, especially the loss of its normal negative electric charge, appear to be critical for the development of albuminuria.

CLINICAL ASPECTS

Minimal-lesion glomerulopathy is the most common cause of the nephrotic syndrome in children. It occurs much less frequently in adults. Characteristically, minimal-lesion glomerulopathy manifests clinically as a full-blown nephrotic syndrome with heavy proteinuria, hypoalbuminemia, and hyperlipidemia, with normal renal function and blood pressure and an "inactive" urinary sediment.

MANAGEMENT

The vast majority of patients with this glomerular disease respond to corticosteroid therapy. The regimen that I use is the administration of prednisone, 1 mg to 1.5 mg/kg daily in a single dose for four weeks; if proteinuria has subsided at four weeks, the dosage of prednisone is decreased on a daily or alternate-day schedule, and after four additional weeks, the treatment is discontinued. Alternatively, 2 mg/kg of prednisone may be administered every other day as initial therapy. If proteinuria does not subside with four weeks of prednisone therapy, a response can be obtained in some patients by continuing the initial dose for another two to four weeks.

Steroid-dependent patients have relapses as glucocorticoid therapy is reduced, or within two weeks after the therapy has been discontinued. For patients with frequent relapses of the nephrotic syndrome (more than three relapses a year), treatment with cytotoxic agents is a reasonable option. Cyclophosphamide (1 to 2 mg/kg daily) or chlorambucil (0.1 to 0.2 mg/kg daily), in combination with glucocorticoids for eight to 12 weeks, reduces the frequency of and sometimes eliminates relapses in about 80% of patients.

Glucocorticoids can produce significant side effects. Growth retardation is a major problem in children. Cushingoid changes are to be expected in almost all patients. Other side effects include hypertension, skin striae, infections, and gastrointestinal bleeding. Cyclophosphamide toxicity includes bone marrow suppression, cystitis, gastrointestinal irritation, alopecia, and infections. Most of the immediate complications are reversible or avoidable. Long-term side effects secondary to cyclophosphamide include sterility, amenorrhea, menopausal symptoms, leukemia, neoplasms, lung fibrosis, ovarian fibrosis, and chromosomal damage. Azoospermia appears to occur when the cumulative dose exceeds 150 and 250 mg/kg. Gonadal toxicity may be reversible. Acute toxicity with chlorambucil is dose-related and includes leukopenia, gastrointestinal irritation, seizures, and infections. Long-term effects include azoospermia, ovarian fibrosis, amenorrhea, and leukemia. Cumulative doses of chlorambucil higher than 11 to 14 mg/kg provide no additional beneficial effects to the patient and increase both the acute and long-term toxicity.

The patient is reassured that this type of glomerulopathy almost never causes renal failure, but is warned about the recurrence of the nephrotic syndrome. The side effects associated with the medications are discussed, and the patient is alerted to potential serious complications.

Patients who received prednisone or cytotoxic agents for a short period usually comply with the treatment program. Most patients comply with the diuretic program because of the problems with edema or anasarca. Patients tend to use more diuretics than necessary and may have to be reminded of this problem. As for many other medical problems, dietary compliance is the most difficult to obtain. In this regard, short visits with the dietitian and follow-up by the dietitian usually help to obtain the patient's cooperation.

In children with the nephrotic syndrome, corticosteroid therapy is usually begun without performing a kidney biopsy because minimal-lesion glomerulopathy is the commonest cause; response to corticosteroids is used as a valid test for the diagnosis of this disease. In adults with the nephrotic syndrome, minimal-lesion glomerulopathy is uncommon, and kidney biopsy is usually performed before commencing therapy. Diagnostic reevaluation, including kidney biopsy, is indicated in children if the nephrotic syndrome does not respond to eight weeks of prednisone therapy, if renal function worsens, or if cytotoxic drug therapy is considered.

Focal Segmental Glomerulosclerosis

Focal segmental glomerular sclerosis (FSGS) is an important primary glomerular disorder causing the nephrotic syndrome. It is more frequent in adults than in children.

DEFINITION AND DIAGNOSTIC CRITERIA

FSGS is a pathologic diagnosis made in the setting of the nephrotic syndrome resistant to corticosteroids. Light microscopy shows that segmental sclerosis, with or without hyalinosis, is present in some glomeruli, while other glomeruli are normal.

CLINICAL ASPECTS

Overall, FSGS is found in 10% to 20% of patients with the nephrotic syndrome. A few patients have asymptomatic proteinuria; their clinical course is relatively benign. Patients with massive proteinuria usually have a clinical course characterized by relatively rapid deterioration of renal function, so-called malignant FSGS.

MANAGEMENT

The short-term and long-term goals in patients with asymptomatic proteinuria involve observation only. The short-term goal in patients with the nephrotic syndrome is to determine whether they are responsive to corticosteroids. The long-term goal for patients who are corticosteroid-resistant is to establish a dietary and diuretic program that would maintain the patient ambulatory and working. Most patients with FSGS and the nephrotic syndrome remain ambulatory. Patients with massive proteinuria, however, often require hospitalization for treatment of severe edema.

The results of drug therapy in FSGS have generally been disappointing. For patients with symptomatic nephrotic syndrome and serum creatinine levels less than 3 mg/dl, I recommend a six- to eight-week course of prednisone, 1 to 1.5 mg/kg/day. About 20% of patients respond by either normalization or a significant reduction of urine protein. In most of the responders, the nephrotic syndrome is either steroid-dependent or frequently relapsing.

Preliminary studies at the Mayo Clinic have shown that some patients with FSGS respond to meclofenamate, one of the nonsteroidal anti-inflammatory agents, with a significant reduction in the proteinuria and stabilization of renal function. Controlled studies, however, are required to confirm the efficacy of this drug in FSGS. Cyclosporine A, widely used in transplantation, is currently under investigation in nephrotic syndrome, including FSGS.

I discuss with the patients the progressive nature of the disease and the options available for treatment of eventual end-stage renal failure. Patients with asymptomatic proteinuria are informed about the benign nature of their disease.

Patients should be reevaluated after completion of six to eight weeks of corticosteroid treatment to assess whether there has been a response to therapy. For the patient with asymptomatic proteinuria, a follow-up visit every year is adequate. For the patient with moderate to severe nephrotic syndrome on corticosteroid therapy or diuretic therapy, reevaluation every six months is appropriate. The patient with massive proteinuria needs frequent visits and hospitalizations for control of edema.

Idiopathic Membranous Glomerulopathy

DEFINITION

Idiopathic membranous glomerulopathy is defined by the immunopathologic findings on renal biopsy. Typically, light microscopy shows diffuse and uniform thickening of the capillary wall of the glomeruli without appreciable cell proliferation. Immunofluorescence reveals diffuse granular deposition of IgG and C3 in the glomeruli. Under the electron microscope, widespread electron dense deposits are seen in the subepithelial location in the glomerular capillary wall.

The glomerular damage results probably from the in situ formation of immune complexes in the glomerular capillary wall. While most of the cases in the United States are idiopathic, membranous glomerulopathy can be caused by drugs such as gold, penicillamine and captopril, and by SLE. Also, when the nephrotic syndrome occurs in patients with carcinomas, membranous glomerulopathy is the usual pathologic finding. Older patients with this glomerulopathy should be investigated for malignancies.

CLINICAL ASPECTS

Membranous glomerulopathy is the most frequent lesion underlying the nephrotic syndrome in adults. Clinically, membranous nephropathy is most often associated with heavy proteinuria and the biochemical manifestation of the nephrotic syndrome, but about 20% of the patients may have asymptomatic proteinuria only. The association of renal vein thrombosis and the nephrotic syndrome occurs more commonly with membranous glomerulopathy than with other glomerular diseases.

MANAGEMENT

The short-term and long-term goals for patients with asymptomatic proteinuria involve observation. For patients with the nephrotic syndrome, the short-term and the long-term goal is to establish a dietary and diuretic program to keep the patient ambulatory and fully employed. Long-term observation is necessary because some patients have recurrence of the nephrotic syndrome, others will have persistent nephrotic syndrome, and still others will suffer renal insufficiency leading to end-stage renal failure.

The United States Collaborative Study of Adult Nephrotic Syndrome compared oral prednisone therapy with placebo in idiopathic membranous glomerulopathy in a prospective, randomized, double-blind trial; patients receiving prednisone had a slower progression of renal insufficiency. Based on these results, most nephrologists recommend prednisone, 2 mg/kg, on alternate days for two months, for nephrotic patients with membranous glomerulopathy and serum creatinine levels less than 3 mg/dl. After this, prednisone is tapered off over four to six weeks.

I discuss the natural history of membranous glomerulopathy and the possible benefits and limitations of treatment with corticosteroids with the patients. I emphasize the benign nature of asymptomatic proteinuria and convey a hopeful attitude regarding spontaneous remissions. To patients with severe persistent nephrotic syndrome, I convey a more guarded prognosis.

For patients with asymptomatic proteinuria, a follow-up visit every one or two years is adequate. In patients treated with prednisone, a determination of the response, or lack of it, should be made at the end of the treatment period. If the patient continues to be nephrotic, dietary and diuretic management is emphasized. Subsequently, visits every six months to a year may be adequate, depending on the severity of the nephrotic syndrome.

Membranoproliferative Glomerulonephritis (Mesangio-capillary Glomerulonephritis)

DEFINITION AND DIAGNOSTIC CRITERIA

The term "hypocomplementemic glomerulonephritis" was applied in the past to membranoproliferative glomerulonephritis (MPGN) because persistent decrease in C3 complement was thought to be an invariable feature of this disease. However, many patients have normal serum complement levels throughout the illness; thus, the diagnosis, as in other primary glomerular diseases, is based on pathologic findings. Light microscopy shows increased glomerular cellularity, double-contour of the glomerular capillary wall, and accentuation of the lobular architecture of the glomerulus. Based on immunofluorescence and electron microscopy, some nephropathologists recognize three types of MPGN, but the most widely accepted types of MPGN are type I and type II. In type I MPGN, immunofluorescence reveals granular deposition of C3 and IgG in the glomeruli, and electron microscopy shows electron dense deposits and interposition of the mesangial cells in the subendothelial space in the glomerular capillary wall. Type II MPGN is characterized by the isolated deposition of C3 complement in the glomeruli on immunofluorescence and a very dense lamina densa of the GBM on electron microscopy. For this reason type II MPGN is also known as dense deposit disease. The cause and pathogenesis of MPGN are poorly understood.

CLINICAL ASPECTS

Both types of MPGN are more common in children than in adults. Type I MPGN is usually slowly progressive, although it may remain stable for years in some patients. Some studies indicate that the median renal survival to end-stage renal disease ranges from nine to 12 years in both children and adults. Type II MPGN appears to be more aggressive, and the median survival to end-stage renal disease varies from five to ten years. Type II is also more frequent in young patients and may be associated with partial lipodystrophy. In both forms of MPGN, proteinuria and microhematuria are almost always present. C3 levels are decreased in more than 80% of the patients with MPGN; levels of C3 are decreased more persistently in type II than in type I MPGN.

MANAGEMENT

Asymptomatic patients need only observation until chronic renal failure develops. For patients with hypertension or the nephrotic syndrome, the short-term goal is to control these two clinical problems. The long-term goal involves keeping the patients normotensive to avoid target-organ damage and controlling the edema to keep the patients functional. The vast majority of patients with MPGN can be maintained ambulatory. In rare cases, severe hypertension may necessitate admission to the hospital for appropriate control. Other patients need hospitalization for control of edema.

As in other chronic progressive renal diseases, dietary measures are very important. Hypertensive patients benefit from salt restriction, usually to less than 90 mEq/24 hours. Adjustment of protein intake in nephrotic patients is discussed under the general approach to the nephrotic syndrome.

No clearly established form of treatment is available for MPGN. High-dose, long-term alternate-day steroid therapy, long-term anticoagulation, and/or the use of antiplatelet drugs have been reported to decrease the rate of progression of renal failure in some studies.

Patients are informed of the variable but usually progressive course to end-stage renal failure. As in any other progressive renal disease, I inform patients of the recent experimental and clinical studies suggesting that the rate of progression of chronic renal disease may be slowed by dietary protein restriction. I also emphasize that control of hypertension is very important in order to avoid additional renal function loss secondary to hypertension.

Diagnostic reevaluation is necessary only when the patient is losing renal function at a faster rate than would be predicted according to the natural history of the disease. This problem is a rare occurrence, and under these circumstances I usually perform a renal biopsy again. Follow-up visits are usually scheduled every six months for patients with progressive renal impairment and every year for patients who have a relatively stable course. Evaluation for dialysis and renal transplantation begins when the patient approaches end-stage renal failure. MPGN, especially type II, can recur in the transplanted kidney, but this is not an absolute contraindication for transplantation.

REFERENCES

Donadio JV: Treatment of glomerular-disease with anticoagulant, antiplatelet, and nonsteroidal anti-inflammatory agents. *In* Robinson RR (ed): Nephrology—Proceedings of the IXth International Congress of Nephrology. Springer-Verlag, New York, 1984, pp 1486–1497.

Garovoy MR: Immunogenetic associations in nephrotic states. Contemp Issues Nephrol 9:259–282, 1982.

Glassock RJ, Cohen AH, Adler S, et al: Primary glomerular diseases. *In* Brenner BM, Rector FC Jr (eds): The Kidney, 3rd ed. W. B. Saunders Co, Philadelphia, 1986, pp 929–1013.

Kim Y, Michael AF, Fish AJ: Idiopathic membranoproliferative glomerulonephritis. Contemp Issues Nephrol 9:237–257, 1982.

Quadracci LJ, Striker GEB: Glomerulonephritis due to other infections. *In* Massry SG, Glassock RJ (eds): Textbook of Nephrology, Vol I. Williams & Wilkins Co, Baltimore, 1983, pp 6.19–6.26.

5 · TUBULOINTERSTITIAL NEPHROPATHY AND URINARY TRACT INFECTIONS

John P. Parker
Richard A. Dart
Douglas P. Duffy
MARSHFIELD CLINIC

Tubulointerstitial Nephropathy

A wide array of diseases of diverse causation can result in tubulointerstitial nephropathy (TIN). Glomeruli are spared until the advancing lesion results in secondary glomerulosclerosis. In the United States, glomerular diseases remain among the major causes of end-stage renal disease. However, about 25% of end-stage renal disease is due to analgesic abuse nephropathy (AAN), vesicoureteral reflux (VUR), complicated pyelonephritis, and polycystic kidney disease. Tubulointerstitial diseases are divided into acute and chronic disorders on the basis of both clinical and pathologic findings (Table 1). Acute pyelonephritis most commonly presents with fever, flank pain, pyuria, and bacteriuria. Acute TIN may present with deteriorating renal function and features of a hypersensitivity reaction. The presentation of chronic TIN is frequently subtle with the patient having progressive azotemia of undetermined cause. In chronic TIN, the major clinical and physiologic abnormalities are polyuria due to loss of normal urine concentration, urinary salt loss, early hyperkalemia due to defective potassium excretion, and normal anion gap metabolic acidosis due to defective hydrogen ion excretion. Urine sediment in chronic TIN is frequently sparse, although in papillary necrosis sloughed papillae may be observed. Hypertension is generally a late feature.

CHRONIC TUBULOINTERSTITIAL NEPHROPATHIES

The causes of chronic TIN are shown in Table 1. Only the more common forms of chronic TIN are discussed below.

Vesicoureteral Reflux

DEFINITION

Vesicoureteral reflux (VUR) is defined as the retrograde flow of urine from the bladder into the ureter, the renal pelvis, and potentially the renal parenchyma.

Table 1. PRINCIPAL CAUSES OF TUBULOINTERSTITIAL NEPHROPATHIES

Acute	Chronic
Acute bacterial pyelonephritis	Chronic bacterial pyelonephritis
Drug hypersensitivity (Table 2)	Obstructive uropathy—with or without urinary infection
Infection-associated, but without actual renal infection: streptococcal and staphylococcal infections, viral infections, diphtheria, Legionnaire's disease	Vesicoureteral reflux (VUR) with or without urinary infection
Idiopathic	Drugs—analgesic nephropathy; lithium
	Metabolic—hypercalcemia; hyperuricemia; hypokalemia; oxalate; oxalosis and oxaluria
	Heavy metals—lead, cadmium
	Hereditary—polycystic disease, Alport's syndrome
	Miscellaneous—Sjögren's syndrome; Balkan nephropathy; sarcoidosis; lymphomatous, leukemic, or myelomatous infiltration of kidney; radiation nephritis; idiopathic

PATHOPHYSIOLOGY

The balance of evidence to date suggests that renal damage from VUR usually occurs in infancy and early childhood, and is usually associated with reflux of infected urine into the renal parenchyma.

CLINICAL ASPECTS

Urinary tract infection (UTI) in early childhood (before 5 years of age) is the most common marker for VUR. Whether reflux of sterile urine can cause progressive renal damage remains in question. Overall, the evidence for this is not convincing. Mild reflux does not cause progressive renal damage and generally disappears after treatment of UTI. Moderate and severe reflux does cause renal scarring, which generally begins before the age of 5 and leads to chronic renal failure one to three decades later.

MANAGEMENT

The first UTI in a child should be treated with appropriate antibiotics, depending on sensitivities, and requires a work-up that includes excretory urography and voiding cystourethrogram (VCU). If severe reflux is documented, corrective surgery is advised in children before the age of 5 years. After age 5, the indications for surgery are unclear. This is particularly true in the adult when azotemia is associated with proteinuria greater than 1 gm/day. These patients frequently have focal glomerulosclerosis, and correction of the reflux does not stop progression of glomerular disease. The presence of nephrotic range proteinuria in these patients indicates a poor prognosis. Some authors claim that long-term suppressive antibiotic therapy to prevent recurrent UTI is sufficient to prevent renal damage.

Suggested management of the adult with a history of VUR includes yearly serum creatinine or creatinine clearance, urinalysis, and urine culture. In the presence of proteinuria, the 24-hour urinary protein excretion is measured. UTI should be treated promptly. Recurrent UTI may require long-term suppressive therapy with antimicrobial agents. Blood pressure should be monitored yearly and maintained in the normal accepted range with antihypertensive therapy.

Analgesic Abuse Nephropathy

DEFINITION

Since the first description in 1950 by Zollinger, it has been recognized that chronic and sufficient ingestion of the mixed analgesics phenacetin, aspirin, and acetaminophen can cause papillary necrosis and chronic tubulointerstitial disease. The development of analgesic abuse nephropathy (AAN) usually requires ingestion of greater than 1 gm of phenacetin in combination with other analgesics per day for a few years, with the average affected patient having taken a total of 2 to 4 kg. Aspirin alone can cause the disease but this is distinctly unusual and it is the combination of analgesics that is more likely to be responsible.

PATHOPHYSIOLOGY

Phenacetin is metabolized to acetaminophen, which concentrates along the medullary gradient, a process accentuated by dehydration. Aspirin uncouples oxidative phosphorylation and inhibits synthesis of prostaglandin E from arachidonic acid. Ischemia of the renal papillae results from the combined adverse effects on oxidative metabolism and the decreased medullary blood flow from decreased prostaglandin E. This leads to ischemic papillary necrosis and chronic interstitial fibrosis and inflammation.

CLINICAL ASPECTS

The patient frequently presents with azotemia of undetermined cause. Typically urinalysis shows low specific gravity with minimal or no proteinuria and a fairly unremarkable sediment. Pyuria with or without infection is fairly common and nocturia may have been present for years. There may be a history of one or more bouts of ureteral colic attributed to a stone but actually caused by sloughed papillae. The detection of papillary necrosis by intravenous pyelography supports the diagnosis of AAN. These patients have multiple functional complaints, particularly headaches. Frequently the use of analgesics is denied, in which case an interview with family members may be helpful.

MANAGEMENT

Critical to management is diagnosis! AAN should be considered in any patient with chronic headache who has any of the following: long-standing nocturia, sterile pyuria, a history of renal colic, or azotemia. These patients should be questioned about intake of analgesics. The mainstay of treatment is complete abstinence from all mixed analgesics. Nonsteroidal anti-inflammatory drugs should also be avoided. It should be remembered that drugs such as Darvocet-N and Parafon Forte contain acetaminophen. The complete avoidance of these drugs cannot be overemphasized and usually leads to stabilization or improvement of renal function. If analgesic abuse continues, progressive renal damage may occur, leading to end-stage renal failure. Patients with AAN have had a marked increase in the incidence of transitional cell carcinoma of the uroepithelium. It is therefore recommended that urine be submitted for yearly cytologic examination.

Lithium

DEFINITION

Lithium produces vasopressin-resistant nephrogenic diabetes insipidus by inhibiting the vasopressin-mediated increase of cyclic AMP in the collecting duct. Lithium toxicity has also been associated with progressive renal damage caused by chronic TIN.

MANAGEMENT

The benefit of lithium must be weighed against its risk. Use of lithium has allowed many patients with bipolar affective disorders to return to society as productive individuals. Clearly in these patients the benefit outweighs the small risk of taking the drug. However, internists and psychiatrists caring for these patients must clearly understand the potential risks and monitor serum lithium levels, which should be kept between 1 and 1.5 mEq/L until therapeutic response occurs and between 0.6 and 1 mEq/L for maintenance therapy. Since the renal tubular handling of lithium is similar to that of sodium, volume depletion and the use of thiazide diuretics may lead to increased tubular reabsorption of lithium leading to toxic blood levels. Patients should be advised to maintain good salt intake and hydration, and diuretics should be avoided. If azotemia develops, lithium should be discontinued.

Urate Nephropathy

DEFINITION

Urate nephropathy is a form of chronic TIN resulting from deposition of sodium urate in the tubules and interstitium of the kidney. This chronic disorder should be distinguished from acute renal failure resulting from sudden elevation of serum uric acid as seen in patients receiving chemotherapy for malignancies. Uric acid calculi and calcium oxalate stones with a nidus of uric acid are other renal disorders associated with hyperuricemia and hyperuricosuria.

CLINICAL ASPECTS

Urate nephropathy is a manifestation of prolonged and sustained hyperuricemia with or without gout. However, the relative roles of uric acid deposition per se and coexisting hypertension and arteriolar nephrosclerosis in the causation of TIN are controversial. Secondary hyperuricemia as seen in saturnine gout from ingestion of "moonshine" whiskey may also cause chronic TIN, although in this disorder, renal damage from the lead content of the illicit liquor may be of greater importance (see later).

MANAGEMENT

Whether asymptomatic hyperuricemia should be treated to prevent gout, uric acid calculi, and renal damage is an unresolved issue. In the absence of these complications, hyperuricemia of less than 12 mg/dl in men and women probably does not require therapy. If uric acid values are higher than these limits, or if any of the above-mentioned complications are present, allopurinol therapy is indicated. A dose of 300 to 400 mg/day is used if renal function is normal, while 100 to 200 mg/day is sufficient in patients with azotemia.

Lead Nephropathy

Chronic TIN with progressive renal impairment has been described in association with lead intoxication from chronic occupational or accidental exposure to lead or ingestion of lead-containing "moonshine" whiskey. Hyperuricemia or gout frequently coexists in these patients. Although elevated serum lead levels may be helpful, the diagnosis is best made by demonstrating 24-hour urinary lead excretion of more than 1000 μg following administration of disodium calcium edetate. Long-term administration of edetate may improve renal function if instituted early in the course of renal disease.

Acute Tubulointerstitial Nephritis

The causes of acute TIN are shown in Table 2. This discussion will be limited to acute TIN resulting from antibiotics and nonsteroidal anti-inflammatory agents (NSAIA). These drugs are the most common causes of this disorder in an outpatient setting. Neither the incidence nor the exact mechanisms involved in the pathogenesis of acute TIN secondary to antibiotics or NSAIA are completely known. Prostaglandin E_2 synthesis in the interstitial cells of the medulla may be inhibited by aspirin and other NSAIA, leading to medullary ischemia and necrosis. Additional postulated mechanisms include antibody and cell-mediated immune phenomena, where the drug acts as an antigen or hapten. With the proliferation and widespread use of a variety of antibiotics and NSAIA, it could be expected that the occurrence of acute allergic and/or toxic TIN secondary to these drugs would rise.

Table 2. PRINCIPAL CAUSES OF DRUG-INDUCED ACUTE TUBULOINTERSTITIAL NEPHRITIS

Penicillin and semisynthetic analogues	*Nonsteroidal anti-inflammatory agents (NSAIA)*
Penicillin G	Fenoprofen
Penicillin V	Ibuprofen
Methicillin	Naproxen
Ampicillin	Phenylbutazone
Nafcillin	
Oxacillin	*Miscellaneous drugs*
Carbenicillin	Phenytoin
	Thiazides
Other antimicrobial agents	Furosemide
Rifampin	Allopurinol
Sulfonamides	Cimetidine
Cephalosporins	
Sulfamethoxazole-trimethoprim	

With short courses of either of these types of drugs, the occurrence of acute TIN may be underestimated because the symptoms may be subclinical and the condition can resolve without overt manifestation. On the other hand, a full-blown presentation of fever, arthralgias, rash, eosinophilia, eosinophiluria, and azotemia with or without proteinuria, within one to 30 days of use of antibiotics or NSAIA, is highly suggestive of drug-induced acute TIN. With NSAIA, the nephrotic syndrome may occur together with acute TIN. Pretreatment information of allergy to the drug in question may be helpful. However, prior uncomplicated use of a drug does not preclude the occurrence of acute TIN on subsequent use. Since these drugs may be associated with adverse renal effects, urinalysis and the serum creatinine should be checked periodically during their use, especially in patients with preexisting renal disease. If fatigue, minor arthralgias, fever, skin rash, proteinuria, or azotemia occurs during the use of these drugs, an acute allergic and/or toxic reaction to the drug should be considered. Urinalysis might show microhematuria and a Wright stain of the sediment may reveal eosinophiluria. Eosinophilia occurs in some patients. Conversely, eosinophiluria, elevated blood eosinophils, or an elevation of the creatinine may not be present despite the clinical manifestations described, in which instance one should still be suspicious of drug reaction and consider termination of the use of the potentially offending agent(s).

MANAGEMENT

If significant abnormalities such as proteinuria, azotemia, or eosinophiluria persist three to five days after the cessation of the presumed offending agent(s), a short course of corticosteroids should be considered. There is controversy as to the effectiveness of prednisone. If used, a dose of 20 mg t.i.d. or an equivalent dose of other steroids is recommended daily for seven to ten days with rapid tapering and discontinuation over another seven to ten days. In most instances, discontinuing the drug and/or addition of the steroids will satifactorily resolve the problem. Persistence of abnormalities, especially after steroid therapy, should prompt consideration of referral to a nephrologist, since permanent damage or previously unrecognized renal disease may warrant more intensive investigation such as renal biopsy.

Urinary Tract Infections

DEFINITION AND DIAGNOSTIC CRITERIA

Significant bacteriuria is identified by quantitative urine culture from an early morning clean catch, midstream-voided specimen showing 100,000 or more bacterial colony-forming units (cfu) per milliliter of urine. In a catheterized specimen, 10,000 or more cfu/ml is significant. Acute pyelonephritis is bacterial invasion of the kidney and may present with bacteriuria, flank pain, fever, or more toxic constitutional symptoms including septicemia. Cystitis is infection confined to the bladder and may be an acute problem or recurrent owing either to relapse with the same bacteria or reinfection with a different organism. Asymptomatic bacteriuria is defined as the presence of a significant number of bacteria in the urine without accompanying symptoms. Bacteria seen in unspun urine at low power usually indicate UTI and this finding correlates with a significant culture. Pyuria is defined as 5 or more WBC/hpf in a centrifuged specimen of urine, and is present in about 75% of UTI. Hematuria (more than 2 to 3 RBC/hpf) may occur in uncomplicated cystitis, but may be indicative of complicated UTI, e.g., UTI associated with obstruction, calculi, or tumor.

PATHOPHYSIOLOGY AND EPIDEMIOLOGY

The majority of UTI follow ascending bacterial colonization of the urinary tract by enteric bacteria. Structural genitourinary abnormalities such as obstruction and VUR, the shorter urethra in females, pregnancy, the postpartum period, diabetes mellitus, preexisting nonbacterial TIN, and sickle cell anemia predispose to UTI. In sexually active females, coitus may contribute to transient bacteriuria. Other factors that have been implicated in the pathogenesis of UTI include periurethral bacterial colonization, decreased IgA levels in cervicovaginal secretions, and certain surface-fimbriated *E. coli* and *Proteus* strains, which are more adherent to the epithelial cells of the vagina and urethra.

The spectrum of pathogenic bacteria in acute UTI is as follows: *E. coli* in approximately 90%, *Proteus* 3%, multiple organisms 3%, and *Pseudomonas, Enterococcus, Enterobacter, Klebsiella* and others in the remainder. *Proteus* has a predilection for upper tract involvement and stone formation. Staphylococcal bacteremia may lead to hematogenous spread of infection to the kidney. Recurrent UTI has a slightly different spectrum, with *E. coli* in about 80%, *Proteus, Klebsiella*, and gram-positive bacteria being slightly more common than listed above. A past history of childhood UTI with recurrent UTI in adult life may suggest structural abnormality of the urinary tract such as VUR. Sterile pyuria can be seen with chlamydial urethritis, genitourinary tuberculosis, and nonbacterial TIN.

After respiratory infection, UTI is the most common infectious illness in the general population. Among schoolgirls, the prevalence of bacteriuria is 2%, and this rises about 1% per decade. In pregnancy, the prevalence is about 6%, depending upon age, parity and socioeconomic group, and about 25% of pregnant women with asymptomatic bacteriuria develop pyelonephritis. In schoolboys UTI has a prevalence of 0.05%, and this rises little until prostatic hypertrophy becomes evident in middle age. In the elderly, the prevalence in males is around 10%, and in females 15%, depending on health, sanitation, and whether the individual lives alone or in an institution. The prevalence rises even further with hospitalization and instrumentation of the urinary tract.

CLINICAL ASPECTS

The clinical features of lower UTI such as cystitis, urethritis, and prostatitis are discussed in Chapter 10. The typical presentation of acute upper UTI is with fever, chills and flank pain, usually associated with frequency, urgency, and dysuria from involvement of the lower urinary tract. The occurrence of ureteric colic should suggest the presence of urinary calculi or papillary necrosis. However, symptoms may be limited to the lower urinary tract even in patients with acute pyelonephritis. Chronic pyelonephritis may present as recurrent episodes of acute pyelonephritis, but symptoms can be nonspecific: intermittent low grade fever and weight loss may occur without urinary tract symptoms. While there is good evidence that UTI occurring before the age of 5 years (especially when associated with VUR) can lead to progressive renal scarring and renal failure, it is doubtful if recurrent UTI in adults causes progressive renal damage unless associated with other structural abnormalities of the urinary tract.

Diagnosis of UTI is based on urinalysis and urine culture (Chapter 10). The differentiation of UTI limited to the bladder from pyelonephritis can be difficult. Flank pain and high fever and chills usually indicate upper tract involvement, but these symptoms may occur in cystitis. Urinary sediment showing white cell casts is indicative of pyelonephritis. The antibody-coated bacteria test involves the examination of the urinary sediment by immunofluorescence microscopy after staining with fluorescein-labeled antihuman globulin. The demonstration of bacteria coated by gamma globulin antibody by this test correlates strongly with the presence of renal infection. However, a significant number of false-positive (usually in patients with prostatitis) and false-negative results occur, and the use of this test is currently limited to epidemiologic investigation only. Bacterial growth in urine specimens obtained by direct ureteric catheterization, or after washing out the bladder with sterile normal saline to which gentamicin and streptokinase-streptodornase have been added, confirms upper tract infection, but these techniques are too cumbersome for routine clinical use. Failure to respond to single-dose therapy for cystitis (Chapter 10) or relapse of infection after a seven-day course of antibiotics is suggestive of involvement of the kidney.

MANAGEMENT

The treatment of lower UTI is discussed in Chapter 10. Otherwise healthy patients with acute nontoxic pyelonephritis can be treated with oral agents as outpatients. Those with persistent nausea and vomiting, high fever and rigors, renal failure and systemic disease such as diabetes, and the elderly, who may present with septicemia with limited systemic signs, require hospitalization for initial parenteral antibiotic therapy followed by conversion to oral agents. In addition to urine culture, blood cultures should be obtained before starting therapy in severely ill patients.

ANTIMICROBIAL AGENTS

A 10- to 14-day course of antimicrobial agents is recommended for pyelonephritis. The choice of the initial therapy should be based on the results of the Gram stain of the urinary sediment. If gram-negative bacilli are present, *E. coli* is the most likely pathogen. Sulfamethoxazole-trimethoprim (one double-strength tablet b.i.d.), cephalexin (500 mg q.i.d.), ampicillin (500 mg q.i.d.), amoxicillin (500 mg t.i.d.), or tetracycline (500 mg q.i.d.) are equally effective alternative oral regimens for *E. coli* pyelonephritis. If gram-positive cocci are seen in the urinary sediment, enterococcal infection should be suspected, and ampicillin or amoxicillin is the preferred agent. Sulfamethoxazole-trimethoprim and tetracyclines should not be used in pregnant women. In severely ill patients, initial intravenous therapy should be with an aminoglycoside (gentamicin or tobramycin 1 to 1.7 mg/kg q 8 hrs) in combination with a cephalosporin such as cefazolin (1 to 2 gm q 6 hrs) or ampicillin (1 to 3 gm q 6 hrs). The results of urine culture should be available within 24 hours and can guide further therapy. It should be noted that the doses given are for adults with normal renal function. In children and in patients with renal impairment, appropriate dose reductions must be made. The use of an aminoglycoside requires measurement of blood levels of the drug to avoid toxic or subtherapeutic levels.

URINE CULTURE

Urine culture should be obtained 48 to 72 hours after starting therapy for pyelonephritis. If bacteriuria persists, the antimicrobial agent should be changed based on the sensitivity report. On the other hand, if clinical and bacteriologic response has occurred, the drug chosen initially can be continued even if the organism is reported to be resistant to it. High fever or positive blood cultures persisting beyond 48 to 72 hours after starting therapy should prompt consideration of urinary tract obstruction or perinephric abscess. Ultrasound or computed tomography evaluation of the urinary tract followed by appropriate urologic intervention is mandatory. Urine should be cultured again two weeks after completion of therapy to confirm bacteriologic cure.

UROLOGIC EVALUATION

Urologic evaluation is indicated in all males and prepubertal females after their first UTI and in postpubertal females after their second or third documented UTI. Relapse of infection after two weeks of antibiotic therapy, UTI associated with diabetes or stone disease, hematuria persisting after eradication of the infection, and UTI due to organisms other than *E. coli* are also indications for urologic evaluation. Intravenous pyelography (IVP) including a post-voiding film of the bladder should be the initial procedure. Voiding cystourethrography (VCU) is indicated in all preschool children with UTI. In patients at increased risk for acute renal failure

following contrast administration (e.g., diabetics with impaired renal function), ultrasound examination combined with VCU is the recommended alternative. If structural abnormalities are documented, urologic consultation should be requested to consider correction of the abnormality.

RELAPSE

If symptomatic UTI relapses after two weeks of therapy, a six-week course of the antimicrobial agent may be effective. In males with relapse, the possibility of chronic prostatitis should be considered. In patients with frequent symptomatic UTI (more than two infections in a six-month period) in the absence of correctable urologic abnormalities, a six-month course of suppressive therapy with sulfamethoxazole-trimethoprim, trimethoprim alone, or nitrofurantoin may reduce the frequency of infection. Smaller doses of these drugs are used for suppressive therapy (half a single-strength tablet of sulfamethoxazole-trimethoprim, 50 mg of trimethoprim, or 50 mg of nitrofurantoin daily at bedtime). Methenamine mandelate, sulfisoxazole, and nalidixic acid have also been used for suppressive therapy. Some patients may require suppressive therapy indefinitely to prevent recurrent symptomatic infections. Long-term suppressive therapy is also indicated in those at risk for progressive renal damage from recurrent symptomatic or asymptomatic UTI (e.g., patients with uncorrectable obstructive uropathy or children with VUR). Suppressive therapy should commence only after eradication of infection with a full course of antimicrobial treatment.

UTI WITH RENAL FAILURE

Treatment of UTI in patients with renal failure is difficult because of decreased excretion of the drugs by the kidney leading to inadequate urinary concentrations. The penicillins, cephalosporins, and aminoglycosides are useful despite renal failure, although their doses should be decreased based on the level of renal function. Sulfamethoxazole-trimethoprim can be used in standard doses when GFR is greater than 30 ml/min and at half the usual dose when GFR is 15 to 30 ml/min. This drug is not recommended in more advanced renal failure. Tetracyclines should be avoided in the presence of renal impairment because of their antianabolic action and low urinary concentration. Nitrofurantoin should be avoided in patients with renal impairment, since toxic metabolites accumulate leading to severe peripheral neuropathy.

ASYMPTOMATIC BACTERIURIA

Treatment of asymptomatic bacteriuria depends on the associated circumstances and should be undertaken only after two cultures have confirmed the presence of infection. Children with asymptomatic bacteriuria should receive treatment similar to that for symptomatic infection followed by IVP and VCU. Asymptomatic bacteriuria in pregnancy should be treated because it is frequently followed by acute pyelonephritis. After eradication of the infection, urine culture should be obtained monthly throughout pregnancy and until three months post partum to detect recurrence of bacteriuria. Patients with recurrent UTI during pregnancy should be investigated by urography three months post partum. A single two-week course of antimicrobial therapy with a nontoxic agent is justified for the treatment of asymptomatic bacteriuria in adult males, nonpregnant females, and the elderly of either sex, but if infection is not eradicated, no further therapy is indicated. Structural abnormalities of the urinary tract should be ruled out in all patients with persistent asymptomatic bacteriuria.

CHRONIC CATHETERIZATION

Chronic catheterization of the bladder is commonly associated with bacteriuria. If asymptomatic, treatment recommendations are as above plus removing the catheter whenever possible. If chronic catheterization is required, the treatment of asymptomatic infection without removing the catheter will only lead to reinfection with more resistant organisms. The use of diapers, condom catheters, or intermittent catheterization instead of indwelling catheters will reduce the occurrence of bacteriuria and symptomatic UTI. Periodic review of catheter care procedures with nursing staff is helpful. In patients with recurrent symptomatic infections due to indwelling catheters, methenamine mandelate (1 gm q.i.d.) coupled with ammonium chloride (1 to 4 gm q.h.s.) and an acid-ash diet to maintain a urinary pH around 5 to 5.5 will significantly reduce the number of symptomatic infections. The urinary pH must be in this range for the methenamine to be converted to formaldehyde, which is the active agent. Methenamine is ineffective in patients with renal impairment.

REFERENCES

Clive DM, Stoff JS: Renal syndromes associated with nonsteroidal anti-inflammatory drugs. N Engl J Med 310:563–572, 1984.

Cotran RS: Tubulointerstitial nephropathies. Hosp Pract 17:79–92, 1982.

Hodson CJ, Cotran RS: Reflux nephropathy. Hosp Pract 17:133–156, 1982.

Pusey CD, Saltissi D, Bloodworth L, et al: Drug associated acute interstitial nephritis: clinical and pathological features and the response to high dose steroid therapy. Q J Med 52:194–211, 1983.

Sobel JD, Kaye D: Urinary tract infections. In Mandell GL, Douglas RG, Bennett JE (eds): Principles and Practice of Infectious Diseases, 2nd ed. John Wiley and Sons, New York, 1985, pp 426–452.

6 · THE KIDNEY IN SYSTEMIC DISEASE

Antoine Kaldany
John A. D'Elia
JOSLIN CLINIC

The variety of systemic diseases that can affect the kidney usually cause glomerular injury. Tubulointerstitial disease secondary to systemic diseases is less common. The clinical manifestations resulting from renal involvement in systemic diseases are similar to those found in primary forms of glomerular and tubulointerstitial diseases. Thus, a search for underlying systemic disease should be part of the evaluation of patients with renal disease. We shall focus in this chapter on the more common forms of renal diseases secondary to systemic disorders.

The Kidney in "Connective Tissue Diseases"

SYSTEMIC LUPUS ERYTHEMATOSUS (SLE)

DEFINITION AND DIAGNOSTIC CRITERIA

Systemic lupus erythematosus (SLE) is a disease of unknown cause that manifests clinically by involvement of many systems and organs. Its salient manifestations include arthritis, dermatitis, cerebritis, myocarditis, serositis, pneumonitis, hepatitis, hemolytic anemia, thrombocytopenia, leukopenia, and nephritis. SLE is characterized by the formation of antibodies directed against nucleoproteins including DNA, and a variety of other endogenous antigens. Tissue injury in SLE is caused by the deposition of antigen-antibody immune complexes in various organs, including the kidney. Complement activation is one of the mechanisms of immune complex–mediated tissue injury and decrease in serum complement levels (CH50, C3, C4) is a common finding in active SLE, especially when there is renal involvement; return of complement values to normal is an indication of subsidence of active SLE. Although most patients with SLE have some morphologic evidence of glomerular involvement, the incidence of clinical renal abnormalities (proteinuria, hematuria, decreased glomerular filtration rate) has been reported to vary from 50% to 75%.

CLINICAL ASPECTS

In most series female:male ratio is approximately 9:1. Lupus nephritis can cause a variety of renal syndromes: asymptomatic proteinuria/hematuria, the acute nephritic syndrome, acute renal failure due to rapidly progressive glomerulonephritis (RPGN), the nephrotic syndrome, and chronic renal failure. Hypertension is commonly associated with the more severe forms of lupus nephritis.

MANAGEMENT OF LUPUS NEPHRITIS

As a first step in the management of SLE nephritis, the physician should establish a comprehensive clinical profile of the patient's disease. This should include an inventory of all the manifestations of SLE and other health data that may alter treatment choices and strategies. The following studies are performed to assess the immunologic activity of SLE: serum complement concentrations (C3, C4, CH50), antinuclear antibody pattern and titer, and anti-DNA antibody titer. The renal status is evaluated by urinalysis and by the measurement of the 24-hour urinary protein excretion and creatinine clearance. We usually perform kidney biopsy to establish the type of lupus nephritis prior to therapy (see later). The value of routine kidney biopsy in the management of lupus nephritis has, however, been questioned recently.

Selection of Treatment Plan

The selection of therapy will, to a large extent, depend on the nature and extent of the kidney lesions in the renal biopsy. All the major pathologic classifications of SLE nephritis are controversial. One classification, advanced by Baldwin et al. in 1977, recognizes four forms of SLE nephritis: (1) minimal or mesangial glomerulonephritis, (2) focal proliferative glomerulonephritis, (3) diffuse proliferative glomerulonephritis, and (4) membranous glomerulonephritis. This classification is clinically useful because clinical presentation, natural history, and response to therapy of lupus nephritis show some correlation with the type of SLE nephritis found on biopsy. However, transition from one type of lupus nephritis to another can occur in the course of the disease. Additional lesions such as glomerulosclerosis, interstitial nephritis and fibrosis, and necrotizing vasculitis may be found superimposed on the primary forms of lupus glomerulonephritis.

Expected Outcomes

Minimal or mesangial glomerulonephritis is probably a pathologic hallmark of SLE and will be found in almost all patients if the kidney biopsy is examined by electron microscopy and immunofluorescence in addition to light microscopy. Clinical renal abnormalities are either absent or minimal in patients with this type of lupus nephritis.

Focal proliferative glomerulonephritis is usually associated with mild to moderate proteinuria and hematuria. Progression to renal insufficiency is uncommon, but may occur after transition to diffuse proliferative lupus nephritis.

Diffuse proliferative glomerulonephritis is usually accompanied by the nephrotic syndrome, hematuria, renal insufficiency, and hypertension. Twenty-five to 30% of patients develop end-stage renal failure (ESRF) within five years of diagnosis. Aggressive therapy to prevent progressive renal failure seems justified in patients with this type of renal involvement.

Membranous lupus nephritis is almost always accompanied by the nephrotic syndrome. If the nephrotic syndrome persists, slowly progressive renal insufficiency is frequently observed.

Departures from the clinical outcome predicted on the basis of renal histologic features are not uncommon in lupus nephritis, and only some of the variations in the expected clinical course result from transition from one type of lupus nephritis to another. The degree of chronic renal injury (glomerulosclerosis, tubular atrophy, and interstitial fibrosis) on the biopsy appears to predict the outcome of the renal disease better than the type of lupus nephritis.

Nonpharmacologic Measures

Patient and family education are key to long-term patient compliance and successful patient management. The unpredictable course of lupus nephritis, the possibility of developing ESRF requiring renal replacement therapy with dialysis/transplantation, and the adverse effects of the drugs used in the therapy of the disease should be clearly explained to the patient and family. The need for regular long-term follow-up should be stressed.

Dietary restrictions should be explicitly communicated: salt restriction in patients with hypertension and protein restriction in patients with renal insufficiency. The importance of blood pressure control in slowing the progression of renal disease should be emphasized. Patients should be instructed to measure blood pressure at home regularly. They should be taught the use of dipsticks to monitor proteinuria and hematuria at home periodically.

Drug Therapy

Selection of Drugs

Mesangial Nephritis. No specific treatment is required for this renal lesion. Extrarenal manifestations of SLE should be treated appropriately.

Focal Proliferative Nephritis. Patients with this type of SLE nephritis and minimal proteinuria and normal renal function are treated similarly to mesangial lupus nephritis. If proteinuria increases progressively or is more than 1 gm/24 hours, or if renal function is impaired, therapy as outlined below for diffuse proliferative lupus nephritis is indicated.

Diffuse Proliferative Nephritis. Early treatment is key to success; remission can generally be induced in patients with serum creatinine <2 mg/dl, whereas treatment failure is likely with advanced renal insufficiency. High-dose corticosteroid therapy (prednisone 60 mg/day) for six to 12 weeks induces remission of the nephrotic syndrome in about 30% to 35% of the patients. Steroids should then be tapered slowly to the lowest possible maintenance dose that will control the renal and extrarenal manifestations of SLE and an attempt should be made to convert the patient to alternate-day steroid therapy. Intravenous "pulse" methylprednisolone therapy (5 to 30 mg/kg/day for three to five days) followed by high-dose oral steroids has been used in patients with RPGN secondary to SLE and there are anecdotal reports of success. If a remission does not occur after two to three months of daily high-dose glucocorticoid therapy, or if the renal function and/or proteinuria deteriorates rapidly during such therapy, a cytotoxic agent (cyclophosphamide, chlorambucil, nitrogen mustard, or azathioprine) should be added to the treatment. Regimens in use include the daily administration of the cytotoxic agents (cyclophosphamide or azathioprine 1.5 to 2.5 mg/kg/day; chlorambucil 0.1 to 0.2 mg/kg/day), administration of cyclophosphamide (500 to 1000 mg/m² intravenously) every three months, and the one-time administration of nitrogen mustard (two doses of 0.2 mg/kg intravenously 48 hours apart). The combined use of cyclophosphamide and azathioprine (1 mg/kg of each drug daily) has also been reported. The recommended duration of cytotoxic drug therapy in patients who respond to it has varied from six to 12 months to the indefinite maintenance of small doses. Cytotoxic therapy usually allows a reduction of the dose of steroids and conversion to an alternate-day program. There is evidence that the alkylating agents (cyclophosphamide, nitrogen mustard, chlorambucil) are superior to the purine analogue azathioprine. Plasma exchange has been used empirically in patients with severe diffuse poliferative lupus nephritis. The efficacy of plasma exchange in this condition is currently being evaluated in controlled clinical studies.

Membranous Nephritis. Early treatment with high-dose oral steroid therapy may induce remissions in some patients. If a response is obtained, steroids should be slowly tapered while monitoring the 24-hour urinary protein excretion. In the absence of remission of the nephrotic syndrome within two months of steroid therapy, steroids should be tapered to the smallest dose sufficient to control extrarenal manifestations of SLE.

The efficacy of cytotoxic agents in membranous lupus nephritis is unclear. Renal vein thrombosis may complicate membranous lupus nephritis and this diagnosis should be considered when proteinuria or renal function deteriorates suddenly. Progression of renal failure is seen mostly in patients with persistently heavy proteinuria and the nephrotic syndrome. This progression is, however, very slow (five-year renal mortality is 10%).

Superimposed Lesions. Progressive glomerular sclerosis leading to renal failure may happen in patients with clinically inactive SLE. There is no known therapy for these slowly progressive, unremitting lesions. Interstitial nephritis (interstitial cellular infiltration, tubular damage, and interstitial fibrosis) is commonly associated with SLE glomerulonephritis. In occasional patients, lupus nephritis may take the course of severe interstitial nephritis (azotemia, renal tubular acidosis, excessive salt and potassium losses) without glomerular disease. Isolated lupus interstitial nephritis may also respond to steroid therapy. Necrotizing vasculitis superimposed on SLE glomerulonephritis usually presents with severe hypertension and rapidly progressive renal failure.

Adverse Effects of Drug Therapy. The adverse effects of prolonged, high-dose steroid therapy are well known. These side effects can be minimized with the following steps: conversion to alternate-day regimen whenever possible; tapering dosage whenever clinically possible; taking the tablets after meals with antacids; and restriction of calorie and carbohydrate intake. The patient should be educated to monitor the stool for occult blood at home. During the use of cytotoxic agents, two main side effects are of concern: bone marrow suppression (which can aggravate preexisting anemia, leukopenia, or thrombocytopenia) and gonadal toxicity leading to sterility. Both high-dose corticosteroid and cytotoxic drug therapy increase the risk of serious opportunistic infection. These adverse effects of immunosuppressive therapy are major causes of morbidity and mortality in patients with SLE. If renal disease progresses despite such therapy, the doses of these drugs should be tapered to avoid their adverse effects and preparations should be made for the treatment of ESRF with dialysis and/or renal transplantation. SLE appears to become inactive once dialysis therapy is initiated. Recurrence of lupus nephritis in the transplanted kidney is very rare.

PERIODIC EVALUATION

The patient should be followed closely initially every four to six weeks to monitor SLE activity, renal status, and response to and tolerance of treatment. The frequency of follow-up visits can be decreased to every three to six months in patients in whom renal and extrarenal manifestations remit following therapy. Meticulous control of blood pressure is important to delay progression of renal failure. The following laboratory tests should be obtained in order to evaluate disease activity and response to treatment during follow-up: WBC, RBC and platelet counts, sedimentation rate, blood urea nitrogen (BUN), serum creatinine, electrolytes, serum calcium and phosphate levels, urinalysis (the treating physician should himself examine the urinary sediment regularly to monitor signs of active nephritis: microscopic hematuria, RBC casts, and other casts), complement profile (C3, C4, CH50), anti-DNA antibody titer, 24-hour urinary protein excretion, and creatinine clearance. Patients should be asked to report promptly any change in proteinuria and hematuria found by dipstick at home.

SYSTEMIC VASCULITIS

The term "systemic vasculitis" encompasses many clinical syndromes characterized by focal necrotizing arteritis in multiple organs. Renal involvement is most commonly observed in polyarteritis nodosa (both the "classic" and the so-called microscopic types), Wegener's granulomatosis, and anaphylactoid purpura (Henoch-Schönlein syndrome).

CLINICAL ASPECTS

The illness is often vague or mild initially. In many patients vasculitis presents with low grade fever, fatigue, weight loss, arthralgias, and myalgias. Some patients have purpuric (or nonpurpuric) skin lesions. Abdominal pain and mononeuritis multiplex may occur. Upper and lower respiratory tract involvement is most commonly seen in Wegener's granulomatosis resulting in nasal discharge, epistaxis, sinusitis, hemoptysis, and pulmonary infiltrates. Renal involvement may result in the acute nephritic syndrome or crescentic RPGN. Hypertension commonly accompanies the renal disease, especially in polyarteritis nodosa.

Laboratory findings include normochromic, normocytic anemia, leukocytosis, elevated erythrocyte sedimentation rate, proteinuria, microscopic hematuria, and red cell casts. Rheumatoid factor and cryolobulins may be present. Hepatitis B surface antigenemia may be associated with systemic vasculitis.

The diagnosis is usually confirmed by renal and visceral angiography, which might show aneurysms in the affected arteries ("macroscopic" polyarteritis), or by biopsy of affected organs (kidney, skin, upper or lower respiratory tract).

MANAGEMENT

Whereas polyarteritis nodosa and Wegener's granulomatosis respond to therapy with corticosteroids and cyclophosphamide, evidence for the efficacy of such therapy in Henoch-Schönlein purpura is lacking.

In patients with fulminant, life-threatening disease, high doses of methylprednisolone given intravenously ("pulse" therapy: 5 to 30 mg/kg/day for three to five consecutive days) may provide the required short-term control of the disease. Oral glucocorticoids (prednisone 1 mg/kg/day) are given either as initial therapy in patients with less severe disease or following "pulse" methylprednisolone therapy. This dose of prednisone is maintained for six to eight weeks, followed by slow reduction in dose and eventual discontinuation of the drug in six to 12 months' time.

Impressive results have been achieved with the use of cyclophosphamide (initial oral dose 2 to 3 mg/kg/day) in combination with corticosteroids. The efficacy of cyclophosphamide is best documented in patients with Wegener's granulomatosis: one-year patient survival rate has improved from 20% to more than 80%. In patients who respond, the dose of cyclophosphamide should be tapered and maintenance doses (0.5 to 1 mg/kg/day) should be continued for two to five years to avoid relapses of vasculitis. Although plasma exchange has been used in vasculitic disorders, its efficacy is uncertain. Urinalysis, blood pressure, creatinine clearance, 24-hour urinary protein excretion, and the sedimentation rate should be monitored regularly during the follow-up of patients with systemic vasculitis. ESRF secondary to systemic vasculitis has been treated successfully with dialysis and renal transplantation in patients without severe extrarenal organ involvement.

PROGRESSIVE SYSTEMIC SCLEROSIS (SCLERODERMA)

DEFINITION AND CLINICAL ASPECTS

Progressive systemic sclerosis (PSS) is a multi-system disorder, predominantly affecting the skin, gastrointestinal tract, heart, lungs, and kidneys. The cutaneous manifestations include marked thickening of the skin, which is tightly bound to the underlying structures, telangiectasia and subcutaneous calcification especially in the digits, and Raynaud's phenomenon. Excessive fibrosis in the esophagus, small and large bowel, lungs, and myocardium is the cause of dysfunction of these organs.

Renal involvement occurs in 45% to 50% of patients with PSS, usually several years after the initial diagnosis of the disease. Occasionally renal disease is the presenting feature of PSS in the absence of cutaneous and other organ involvement. Sudden development of severe hypertension and the rapid development of ESRF within a few weeks thereafter is the typical presentation of "scleroderma kidney." Pathologically, there is involvement of the interlobular arteries by intimal fibrinoid change and thickening that is indistinguishable from the lesions seen in malignant hypertension. Glomerular afferent arteriolar necrosis and ischemic changes in the glomerular capillary tuft are associated features. Renal disease is second only to cardiorespiratory involvement as a cause of death in PSS. Asymptomatic proteinuria, mild hypertension, and slowly progressive renal failure unassociated with hypertension are much less commonly recognized presentations of renal disease in PSS.

MANAGEMENT

In patients with PSS who present with severe hypertension and rapidly progressive renal failure, it has been shown that strict control of hypertension will stabilize or improve renal function if irreversible ischemic glomerular injury has not already developed. Hypertension in PSS is largely renin-angiotensin–mediated; the angiotensin-converting enzyme inhibitors (e.g., captopril) are ideal agents for treating hypertension in PSS. This group of drugs is usually used in combination with beta-blockers and diuretics. Incidental improvement in Raynaud's phenomena and in the skin changes of PSS has been reported with the use of captopril. Minoxidil is another potent agent for the treatment of severe hypertension and some patients require the combined use of captopril and minoxidil. Once an effective antihypertensive regimen has been established, it should be maintained indefinitely. ESRF secondary to PSS has been managed by dialytic therapy, but difficulty in creating hemodialysis accesses is a major problem. Renal transplantation has been performed in a few patients with PSS with good long-term results.

The limiting factor in the management of ESRF by dialysis or renal transplantation in PSS patients is the extent of extrarenal disease in the cardiac, respiratory, and gastrointestinal systems.

The Kidney in Hematologic Diseases

MULTIPLE MYELOMA

DEFINITION AND DIAGNOSTIC CRITERIA

Multiple myeloma represents a neoplastic transformation of plasma cells with the production and secretion of abnormal and unique monoclonal paraproteins.

CLINICAL ASPECTS

Symptoms secondary to anemia and bone disease tend to predominate: fatigue, skeletal pain, pathologic fractures. Radiologically, areas of osteolysis without osteoblastic reaction are characteristic. Bone involvement may lead to hypercalcemia. Normocytic, normochromic anemia is a characteristic feature and bone marrow examination reveals an increased number of abnormal plasma cells. In addition, leukopenia, thrombocytopenia, and hemolysis are not rare. Overproduction of myeloma paraprotein is usually complicated by hypogammaglobulinemia leading to increased susceptibility to infections. Increased blood viscosity due to the paraproteins may cause the "hyperviscosity syndrome."

The scope of renal abnormalities runs a wide gamut: Bence-Jones proteinuria, acute or chronic renal failure due to the precipitation of paraproteins in the renal tubules ("myeloma kidney"), the nephrotic syndrome and progressive renal failure due to amyloidosis or light-chain glomerulopathy, hypercalcemic nephropathy, uric acid nephropathy, increased susceptibility to acute renal failure induced by radiocontrast agents, obstructive uropathy secondary to retroperitoneal plasma cell tumors, and renal infiltration by malignant plasma cells. Reversal of the albumin-globulin ratio, high normal or elevated serum calcium despite renal failure, and proteinuria being more marked with the sulfosalicylic acid test than with the dipstick test (because the dipstick detects only albumin and not the abnormal globulins and light-chains in the urine) are important clues to the diagnosis of multiple myeloma. Serum and urine protein electrophoresis and immunoelectrophoresis to detect paraproteins should be included in the work-up of unexplained renal failure or proteinuria in the older patient.

MANAGEMENT

There are anecdotal reports of improvement in renal function with the use of plasma exchange to remove circulating paraproteins in patients with acute renal failure due to myeloma kidney. Maintenance of adequate hydration and good diuresis minimizes the changes of hypercalcemic or hyperuricemia nephropathy. X-ray contrast agents should be avoided unless absolutely necessary and patients should be well hydrated before and after the use of these agents. Dialytic therapy has been employed in the management of ESRF secondary to multiple myeloma, but the life expectancy depends on the control of the underlying disease with chemotherapy. Some patients have survived three to five years on dialysis.

SICKLE CELL ANEMIA

DEFINITION AND DIAGNOSTIC CRITERIA

The properties of hemoglobin S (HbS) account for the findings in sickle cell disease: under certain conditions, HbS produces a semisolid gel with the formation of tactoids. These conditions include low oxygen tension, increased hydrogen ion concentration, and increased osmolality. Normal conditions in the renal medulla tend to favor sickling: relative hypoxia, low pH, and the maintenance of a hyperosmolar environment for urinary concentration.

CLINICAL ASPECTS

Ischemic damage to the renal tubules due to repeated sickling in the medullary vessels results in inability to concentrate the urine. Hyperkalemic renal tubular acidosis (type IV RTA) due to defective distal tubular hydrogen ion and potassium secretion can also result from tubular damage. Ischemic medullary or papillary necrosis can cause hematuria, which can be recurrent and severe. Hematuria tends to occur much more commonly from the left than the right kidney; the reasons for this are unclear. The concentrating defect and hematuria can occur in both sickle cell trait and sickle cell disease. The nephrotic syndrome and progressive renal failure due to gomerular disease have been reported in sickle cell disease. Membranoproliferative glomerulonephritis and focal segmental glomerulosclerosis are the common lesions. It has been suggested that ischemic tubular injury releases tubular antigens, which in turn cause immune complex–mediated glomerulonephritis.

MANAGEMENT

Prevention of dehydration is the key to avoiding sickling in the medulla with consequent tubular damage. Patients should be encouraged to take adequate amounts of fluids. Persistent severe hematuria has been succesfully treated with aggressive hydration and the use of epsilon-aminocaproic acid (EACA) given either orally or intravenously (5 to 10 gm given over 8 hours). Blood may clot in the ureters leading to obstructive uropathy. Intractable, life-threatening bleeding may necessitate nephrectomy. Both dialysis and renal transplantation have been used successfully in the management of ESRF secondary to sickle cell nephropathy, although an increase in the frequency of sickle cell crises has been reported in some patients after transplantation.

The Kidney in Diabetes Mellitus

DEFINITION

The term "diabetic nephropathy" refers to the specific glomerulopathy that occurs in diabetes mellitus. A number of other urinary tract disorders also occur with increased frequency in diabetics: renal atherosclerosis, urinary tract infections, papillary necrosis, neurogenic bladder secondary to autonomic neuropathy, type IV RTA with hyperkalemia, and radiocontrast agent–induced acute renal failure. We shall deal exclusively with diabetic glomerulopathy in this chapter.

In the early stages of diabetic nephropathy, glomerular enlargement and mesangial expansion occur. Diffuse and uniform thickening of the glomerular basement membrane is the characteristic feature of diabetic nephropathy. Glomerulosclerosis is seen in the more advanced stages. Diabetic glomerulosclerosis can be diffuse or nodular. Diffuse glomerulosclerosis is the more common lesion, but the nodular lesion (Kimmelstiel-Wilson disease) is specific for diabetes mellitus.

PATHOPHYSIOLOGY

The respective roles of hyperglycemia, insulin deficiency, and other endocrine and metabolic abnormalities on the one hand and diabetic microangiopathy per se on the other in the causation of diabetic glomerulopathy have been debated for a long time. There is now evidence to suggest that the metabolic and endocrine abnormalities are probably the more important factors: pathologic changes of diabetic nephropathy have been demonstrated in kidneys from normal donors transplanted into diabetic recipients within a few years after transplantation. Simultaneous kidney and pancreas transplantation in diabetic recipients has prevented the development of diabetic glomerular changes in the renal allograft. These observations suggest that strict control of hyperglycemia in the early years of clinical diabetes mellitus may prevent the later development of diabetic nephropathy.

Considerable attention is now being focused on the role of altered glomerular hemodynamics in the pathogenesis of diabetic nephropathy. Glomerular filtration rate (GFR) is increased in early diabetes and it has been suggested that the increased glomerular capillary hydrostatic pressure associated with the increased GFR may initiate diabetic glomerular injury. Once the glomerular filtration surface has been reduced by mesangial expansion and glomerulosclerosis, adaptive hyperfiltration in the remaining nephrons may injure them progressively.

CLINICAL ASPECTS

Diabetic nephropathy develops in nearly 40% to 50% of patients with type I and 10% to 20% of patients with type II diabetes mellitus. Black patients with type II diabetes mellitus appear to be more prone to develop diabetic renal disease. Diabetic nephropathy is the cause of ESRF in approximately 25% of patients entering dialysis and renal transplantation programs in the United States at present. The clinical course of diabetic nephropathy can be divided into the preazotemic and the azotemic phases.

The Preazotemic Phase. In type I diabetics, the duration of this phase is 10 to 20 years. During this period there is no evidence of renal disease as judged by routine urinalysis and the measurement of BUN, serum creatinine, and creatinine clearance. In the first few years after the diagnosis of type I diabetes, the kidneys are increased in size and the GFR is higher than normal and both these abnormalities can be corrected by control of hyperglycemia with insulin therapy. Recent work has shown that even in the preazotemic phase, small increases in urinary albumin excretion ("microalbuminuria") can be demonstrated either at rest or after exercise in patients who will eventually develop clinical nephropathy. Highly sensitive radioimmunoassay techniques are required to detect "microalbuminuria."

In type II diabetics the apparent preazotemic phase is usually much shorter (a few years). This may be because asymptomatic diabetes mellitus might have been present for many years prior to the diagnosis of the disease. It is not known if renal enlargement, increased GFR, and "microalbuminuria" occur during the preazotemic phase of type II diabetes.

The Azotemic Phase. The first sign of clinical diabetic nephropathy is usually the detection of proteinuria on routine urinalysis. On an average, elevation of serum creatinine occurs within one to two years and ESRF within five years after the development of proteinuria. Once manifest, proteinuria usually increases steadily and soon evolves into the nephrotic syndrome. Hypertension almost invariably accompanies diabetic nephropathy. Uremic symptoms appear to develop earlier in diabetics: they may occur when the GFR has decreased to 10 to 15 ml/min (serum creatinine 5 to 7 mg/dl). Renal failure is usually more advanced than this in nondiabetics before uremic symptoms develop. Blindness from diabetic retinopathy, diabetic gastroparesis, arteriosclerotic heart and peripheral vascular disease, and diabetic neuropathy are common coexisting problems in the azotemic diabetic. Progressive decrease in insulin requirements is a characteristic feature during the course of chronic renal failure in diabetic nephropathy. This results from decreased insulin catabolism and excretion by the diseased kidneys. In type II diabetes, insulin may no longer be required once advanced renal failure has developed.

When proteinuria and azotemia are detected in a long-standing diabetic, diabetic nephropathy is the most likely cause, and kidney biopsy is not indicated. However, the possibility of nondiabetic renal disease should be considered if persistent microhematuria and RBC casts are present, and if renal function declines rapidly over several weeks rather than over many months. The absence of diabetic retinopathy should also lead to consideration of nondiabetic renal disease because diabetic retinopathy and nephropathy almost invariably coexist.

MANAGEMENT

Once proteinuria or azotemia has developed in a diabetic, the internist or diabetologist caring for the patient should enlist the help of a nephrologist. Periodic evaluation of the progression of diabetic retinopathy by an ophthalmologist is also an important part of the management of these patients.

Nonpharmacologic Measures

Sodium restriction (2 gm/day) is an important feature of the diabetic diet when the nephrotic syndrome or hypertension develops. Dietary protein (0.6 to 0.9 gm/kg/day) and phosphate restriction (750 mg/day) are necessary once azotemia supervenes. Potassium and fluid restriction are usually not required until the patient is near ESRF. In patients with type IV RTA, dietary potassium restriction (1.5 to 2 gm/day) may be needed earlier.

Drug Therapy

Antihypertensives. There is now good evidence that strict control of blood pressure retards the progression of diabetic nephropathy. Drug therapy should be adjusted to obtain sitting blood pressure readings as close to 120/80 mm Hg as possible while maintaining standing systolic pressures at a level compatible with daily activities (around 100 mm Hg). Drugs that reduce renal blood flow (e.g., guanethidine) should be avoided. Beta-blockers should be used with caution, since they may mask the symptoms of hypoglycemia. If captopril is chosen, serum potassium should be monitored carefully, since hyperkalemia may develop in patients with type IV RTA and in patients with renal failure. Prazosin, clonidine, methyldopa, nifedipine, and minoxidil (when the hypertension is severe) are safe drugs to use.

Diuretics. The nephrotic syndrome and hypertension are indications for diuretic therapy. In patients with minimally impaired renal function (serum creatinine < 2.5 mg/dl), thiazides may be effective. With more advanced renal failure, loop diuretics (furosemide, ethacrynic acid, or bumetanide) in increasing doses are indicated. Addition of metolazone (5 to 10 mg/day) to loop diuretics may be effective in refractory cases. Potassium-sparing diuretics (spironolactone, triamterene, or amiloride) are best avoided in the azotemic diabetic because severe hyperkalemia can develop.

Hypoglycemic Agents. Insulin requirements decrease progressively with advancing renal failure and insulin dosage will have to be reviewed and adjusted as required. Type II diabetics may not require any insulin once renal failure is advanced. Long-acting oral hypoglycemic agents such as chlorpropamide should be avoided in the diabetic with renal failure because their excretion is delayed and prolonged hypoglycemia may result.

Calcium Supplements/Phosphate Binders. As in any patient with progressive renal failure, these drugs should be added to maintain normal serum calcium and inorganic phosphate levels.

ESRF Therapy in the Diabetic

Since uremic symptoms appear earlier and arteriovenous fistulas for hemodialysis take a long time to develop in diabetics, therapeutic options for ESRF should be discussed early in the course of renal failure (when serum creatinine reaches 4 to 5 mg/dl). Type I diabetics do much better after renal transplantation (especially living donor transplantation) than on dialysis. Every attempt should be made to recruit a living related kidney donor from within the family so that transplantation can be performed electively before dialysis is required. Since diabetic retinopathy appears to stabilize or improve after transplantation, it has been recommended that transplantation should be performed earlier in the course of renal failure in diabetics than in nondiabetics (when creatinine clearance approaches 10 ml/min as compared with less than 5 ml/min in nondiabetics). In practice, however, most diabetics receive transplants only after being on dialysis for a while. Intraocular bleeding secondary to heparinization during hemodialysis may worsen vision already compromised by diabetic retinopathy; careful heparinization during hemodialysis can avoid this complication. It has been suggested that continuous ambulatory peritoneal dialysis (CAPD) is superior to hemodialysis in the management of ESRF in diabetics because heparinization and wide fluctuations in blood pressure are avoided. However, poor vision from diabetic retinopathy and the effects of diabetic neuropathy on the fingers often make it impossible for the patient to do CAPD exchanges.

Type II diabetics above the age of 50 to 55 years have a very high mortality rate from cardiovascular complications after renal transplantation. Therefore, we prefer to manage ESRF in older type II diabetics with hemodialysis or CAPD, and generally advise against transplantation.

Diabetics on dialysis have a higher incidence of access (thrombosis, infection), cardiovascular (arrhythmias, angina, myocardial infarction, congestive heart failure), and peripheral vascular (gangrene) problems than do nondiabetics. Depression tends to be more severe in diabetics also. The services of psychiatrists, vascular surgeons, ophthalmologists, and occupational therapists are frequently required in the care of these patients.

PATIENT AND FAMILY EDUCATION

The progressive nature of diabetic nephropathy and the invariable development of ESRF should be explained to the patient and family. The importance of strict control of blood pressure and dietary protein and phosphate restriction in slowing the progression of renal failure should be stressed. Patients should be instructed on home blood pressure and blood sugar monitoring. They should be told that insulin requirements decrease with advancing renal failure and should be alerted to the possibility of hypoglycemic episodes if insulin doses are not adjusted. Regular follow-up visits with the nephrologist, diabetologist, and ophthalmologist should be emphasized. Therapeutic options for ESRF should be discussed early in the course of renal failure. The fact that type I diabetics do better after renal transplantation than on dialysis should be explained. The superiority of living related donor transplantation should be discussed in an attempt to obtain a donor from within the family.

REFERENCES

D'Elia JA, Kaldany A, Miller DG: Diabetic kidney disease. In Kozak GP (ed): Clinical Diabetes Mellitus. W.B. Saunders Co, Philadelphia, 1982, pp 268–287.

Lee HS, Mujais SK, Kasinath BS, et al: Course of renal pathology in patients with systemic lupus erythematosus. Am J Med 77:612–620, 1984.

Suki WN, Eknoyan G: The Kidney in Systemic Disease. John Wiley and Sons, New York, 1981.

7 · NEPHROLITHIASIS

Stephen B. Erickson
MAYO CLINIC AND MAYO FOUNDATION

DEFINITION AND DIAGNOSTIC CRITERIA

Nephrolithiasis is a relatively common condition, defined as concretions in the renal papillary tips or urinary collecting system. Nephrolithiasis is to be differentiated from nephrocalcinosis, which is calcification of the renal parenchyma. Demographic studies show that the incidence of stones is increasing in white males and is stable in white females. Stone formation in blacks is less common. The stone types are calcium salts (75%), uric acid (15%), calcium, magnesium, ammonium phosphate, or struvite (10%), and cystine (1%). Mixed stone compositions also occur.

PATHOPHYSIOLOGY

Although there are many different clinical causes of nephrolithiasis, the basic pathophysiologic mechanism is the same. In order to form a highly ordered crystal out of randomly moving molecules in urine, energy is required. This energy comes from supersaturation of the urine by the mineral that forms the stone. If the urine is undersaturated with this mineral, there is no driving force for crystallization. However, if the urine becomes saturated with the mineral, a driving force toward crystallization begins. As the urine becomes progressively more saturated, the energy available for crystallization builds until it reaches a level sufficient for heterogeneous nucleation to occur. In heterogeneous nucleation, small crystals form around particles already present in the urine. Once nuclei form, crystal growth and aggregation can occur at lower energy levels. Normal human urine is usually supersaturated with calcium oxalate but undersaturated with uric acid, struvite, and cystine. Inhibitors of crystallization, at least for calcium salts, also are present in normal human urine and may be the reason that most persons do not form calcium-containing stones.

CLINICAL ASPECTS

There are many clinical causes of calcium stones (Table 1). When nephrolithiasis is associated with hypercalcemia, the most frequent cause is primary hyperparathyroidism. The combination of hypercalcemia and

Table 1. CLINICAL CAUSES OF CALCIUM STONES

Cause	Conditions
Hypercalcemias	Primary hyperparathyroidism, sarcoidosis, multiple myeloma, bone metastases, milk-alkali syndrome, vitamin A or D toxicity, immobilization, Cushing's syndrome, hyperthyroidism, Paget's disease of bone
Hypercalciurias	Idiopathic absorptive hypercalciuria—types I and II, idiopathic renal leak hypercalciuria, distal renal tubular acidosis, response to acetazolamide, exogenously administered steroids
Hyperoxalurias	Primary (hereditary) hyperoxaluria—types I and II, pyridoxine deficiency, enteric hyperoxaluria, vitamin C abuse, oxalate gluttony

stones should be considered to be due to hyperparathyroidism until proved otherwise by a vigorous investigation, including a parathyroid hormone assay and consultation with a physician or surgeon with expertise in parathyroid disease. About 5% of calcium stone formers have primary hyperparathyroidism. Treatment is by subtotal parathyroidectomy.

Hypercalciuria is common and, depending on the definition, may occur in as many as 60% of calcium stone formers. Although most hypercalciurias are idiopathic, two causes are hypothesized: hyperabsorption of calcium by the intestine and renal leakage of calcium, with or without bone resorption.

Hyperoxaluria is usually mild and is presumably dietary in origin. Severe hyperoxaluria is uncommon: the usual setting is loss of distal ileum through either inflammatory bowel disease or bowel bypass for the treatment of morbid obesity.

Uric acid stones are most commonly seen in patients who have small volumes of unusually acidic urine, such as occurs after ileostomy. Interestingly, hyperexcretion of uric acid, as seen in gouty patients, is a less common cause.

Struvite stones are formed only in the presence of urinary infections by bacteria that can split urea to ammonia through the action of a bacterial enzyme, urease. The most frequent urinary pathogen, *Escherichia coli*, seldom if ever produces urease. *Proteus mirabilis* is the usual culprit, and recurrent urinary infections due to *Proteus* require urography in search of struvite stones and anatomic abnormalities of the urinary tract.

Cystinuria is an uncommon autosomal recessive inborn error of metabolism. High urinary concentrations of poorly soluble cystine result and usually cause nephrolithiasis. The possibility of cystinuria must be considered particularly in children and adolescents with nephrolithiasis. Studies must also be done in siblings; carriers (parents) do not excrete enough cystine to form stones.

MANAGEMENT

PLAN

In formulating a patient care plan, stone disease should be considered from two different perspectives: surgical activity and metabolic activity. Surgical stone activity refers to episodes of colic, obstruction, or infection. Metabolic stone activity refers to new stone formation, growth of existing stones, or passage of documented gravel within the past year. The common situation wherein adequate roentgenograms do not exist

to allow the determination of metabolic activity is referred to as indeterminate metabolic activity. Thus, stones may be surgically active but metabolically inactive, or vice versa.

The short-term goal of stone treatment is to abolish surgical and metabolic activity. Long-term goals are similar: to maintain metabolic inactivity and treat surgical activity as it occurs.

The pain of ureteral colic is often severe and requires hospitalization so that studies can be done to exclude other causes of pain and to administer narcotics parenterally for the control of pain. Mildly to moderately painful ureteral colic in the absence of infection or high-grade obstruction may be managed by oral analgesics and fluids on an outpatient basis. Most stones that are 5 mm or less in diameter will pass spontaneously. Stones that do not appear likely to pass should be removed, if they are obstructive. The more obstructive the stone, the more urgent its removal, lest permanent renal damage result. Struvite stones associated with infection should also be removed if possible, as it is otherwise difficult to prevent their continued growth. Urinary infection and an obstructive stone together represent an urgent surgical condition. Sepsis during these conditions is common and requires early surgical intervention in conjunction with appropriate antibiotic treatment to control the infection.

NONPHARMACOLOGIC MEASURES

Nonpharmacologic control of metabolic stone activity is both feasible and in the patient's best interest. The mainstay of this program is liquid, preferably water. If properly motivated, many patients will comply with such a program. The admonition "go home and drink a lot of water" is not adequate. The clinician should explain the therapeutic advantages of dilute urine in the avoidance of supersaturation and help the patient set a specific fluid goal compatible with his or her life style. One recommendation is to drink 8 ounces of fluid hourly while awake and just before going to bed. A daily intake of at least 2½ liters of fluid, half of which should be water, is necessary. Data do not exist to state whether hard, soft, or distilled water is preferable. Unless extraordinarily hard, any water is vastly superior to none at all.

Calcium stone formers should prudently restrict their consumption of dairy products. However, to diminish the risk of osteoporosis, a single daily serving of milk, cheese, yogurt, or ice cream is allowed. Other foods need not be restricted on the basis of their calcium content. Concurrent restriction of foods with high oxalate content is important (Table 2). Normally, calcium and oxalate bind to a large degree in the gut, forming an insoluble compound that is subsequently excreted in the feces. Restriction of calcium alone allows excessive absorption of oxalate and an increase in urinary supersaturation with calcium oxalate. Uric acid stone formers should reduce their purine intake by reducing their dietary protein.

DRUG THERAPY

Drug treatment both to prevent metabolic stone activity and to dissolve existing stones has undergone rapid proliferation recently. Before discussing drugs that are helpful to the stone former, one should be aware of

Table 2. FOODS HIGH IN OXALATE CONTENT

Vegetables	Fruits	Miscellaneous
Beets	Cranberry juice	Beer
Carrots	Currants	Chocolate and cocoa
Celery	Figs	Chocolate-flavored
Chives	Gooseberries	beverages
Green beans	Grapefruit	Cola drinks
Greens:	Grapefruit juice	Marmalade
Beet	Grape juice	Nuts
Collard	Orange and	Ovaltine
Dandelion	lemon peel	Peanut butter
Kale	Orange juice	Peanuts
Mustard	Oranges	Tea
Spinach	Plums	Wheat germ
Swiss chard	Prunes	
Turnip	Raspberries	
Okra	Rhubarb	
Parsley	Tangerines	
Parsnips		
Pumpkin		
Sweet potatoes		
Tomatoes		
Tomato juice		
Tomato sauce and paste		

drugs that may accelerate stone formation. A careful drug history is important, since some of the main offenders may not be considered "drugs" by the patient. If used in excess, vitamins A and D may cause hypercalcemia and hypercalciuria. Vitamin C is partly metabolized to oxalate and may cause hyperoxaluria; thus, megadose vitamin C is to be strongly discouraged. Large quantities of absorbable antacids containing sodium bicarbonate or calcium carbonate may produce a variant of the milk-alkali syndrome, resulting in calcareous renal deposits. Baking soda, Tums, and Rolaids are common examples. Corticosteroids cause hypercalciuria and occasionally stones. Acetazolamide produces distal renal tubular acidosis, which may also result in stones.

Drug treatment for calcium oxalate stone formers should be attempted only after the patient has had demonstrable metabolic activity while on an adequate dietary and fluid program. At this point, drug treatment is best considered in relation to the cause of the stone formation.

Thiazides are considered the mainstay of treatment of hypercalciuria. Hydrochlorothiazide, 25 to 50 mg twice daily, will reduce urinary calcium excretion by nearly 50%. Trichlormethiazide (Naqua), 2 to 4 mg twice daily, may be even more effective, although this has not been proved. Chlorthalidone (Hygroton), 25 to 50 mg once daily, is more convenient and essentially as effective as the others. In addition to the common side effects of hypokalemia, hyperglycemia, and hyperuricemia, there is the possibility of thiazide-induced impotence in this predominantly male population.

Recently, cellulose sodium phosphate (Calcibind) has become available for the treatment of hypercalciuria caused by excessive gastrointestinal absorption of calcium. It binds dietary calcium in the gut, making it nonabsorbable. However, it also binds dietary magnesium, causing hypomagnesuria, which may be detrimental. This drug also allows excess oxalate absorption and hyperoxaluria, which is also detrimental. Because of these negative features, although they are correctable, and the nuisance of every-meal-dosage and high cost, I cannot recommend this therapy. The long-term effects of this therapy on bone mineralization are unknown.

Hyperoxalurias are difficult to treat. In primary hyperoxaluria, oxalate excretion can be decreased by pyridoxine, 50 mg three times daily, and neutral phosphate (Neutra-Phos or K-Phos Neutral) containing 500 mg of elemental phosphorus four times daily. (Children's doses must be adjusted by body weight or surface area.) Treatment of enteric hyperoxaluria depends on the urinary composition. In addition to severe restriction of dietary oxalate, alkali therapy such as Polycitra-K, in doses adequate to normalize urinary citrate, may be helpful. Allopurinol (Zyloprim), as much as 300 mg daily, is also helpful in reducing hyperuricosuria. Oral calcium supplements may be used to bind intestinal oxalate, but there is a definite risk of offsetting the gain of lowered urinary oxalate by increasing the urinary calcium. Cholestyramine resin (Questran), 9 gm three or four times daily, may indirectly reduce oxalate absorption in the gut by lessening bile acid–induced bowel inflammation and subsequent oxalate hyperabsorption. Conceivably, cholestyramine may also directly bind oxalate. Gastrointestinal side effects are common.

Hyperuricosuria is common and may facilitate calcium stone formation through the formation of a nidus of sodium urate, around which calcium salts can crystallize. Allopurinol (Zyloprim), as much as 300 mg daily, may be used in this situation, although the other metabolic abnormalities should be treated first. Recently, interest has developed in hypocitraturia as a causal factor in calcium stone formation. Citrate is known to inhibit calcium phosphate and calcium oxalate crystallization. Hypocitraturia may allow crystallization to occur at lower urinary supersaturations. Polycitra-K, 15 ml three times daily or as needed to normalize urinary citrate, appears promising.

If no metabolic abnormality is found, metabolic activity can often be prevented by using neutral phosphate in 500-mg doses four times daily. This therapy is preferred to an alternative treatment of 100 mg of magnesium oxide or hydroxide given twice daily. Either treatment may result in diarrhea, which can be lessened by slowly increasing the dose to achieve therapeutic levels.

Uric acid stones are not only preventable but also dissolvable if they are not too obstructive. The best prevention is to "alkalinize" the urine with sodium bicarbonate or Polycitra to a pH of 6.5, as guided by nitrazine paper testing. At this pH, about 90% of uric acid will be in the soluble urate form. Higher urine pH gains little therapeutically and risks complicating the stone disease by precipitating an insoluble shell of calcium phosphate. To dissolve a urate stone, allopurinol, 300 mg daily, is usually a necessary addition to the program.

The treatment of struvite stones is complete surgical removal and correction of underlying structural problems. When surgery is not feasible or when prophylaxis is indicated, medical therapy should be given. Since all struvite stones result from the production of ammonia through the action of bacterial urease, the bacteria and hence stone formation may be suppressed by an appropriate antimicrobial agent. However, the infection will not be eradicated as long as infected stone material exists. A newer therapy works through the inhibition of urease by acetohydroxamic acid (Lithostat), 250 mg four times daily (if renal function is normal). This treatment may have serious side effects, including hemolytic anemia and venous thromboembolism, and should be used only in complicated and carefully selected cases.

Prevention and dissolution of cystine stones is also possible. For prevention, copious fluid intake (minimum of 4 liters daily) and urinary alkalinization to at least a pH of 7.5, as guided by nitrazine paper testing, are necessary. The same systemic alkalinizing agents used in the therapy of uric acid calculi are employed. Dissolution of cystine stones requires the addition of a chelating agent to the above program. Therapy with D-penicillamine (Cuprimine), four times daily, in doses adequate to lower unbound urinary cystine excretion to 250 mg or less daily is necessary. D-penicillamine has a particular propensity toward toxic reactions and must be used with caution. Among the more feared complications are bone marrow suppression or aplasia, Goodpasture's syndrome, myasthenia gravis, nephrotic syndrome, and pemphigoid-type skin lesions. Consequently, bimonthly follow-up visits, including a complete blood count and urinalysis, are in order, especially early in the course of treatment. Usually, treatment begins with a subtherapeutic dose that can be increased as tolerated.

SURGICAL THERAPY

Important advances are being made in the treatment of surgically active stones and open surgical removal of stones should soon become unusual. This radical change has been brought about by two innovative techniques.

Percutaneous lithotripsy has been available in this country for several years. The kidney is punctured percutaneously, and the opening is dilated. Through this tract various instruments may be introduced, including a stone basket, forceps, flexible nephroscope, ultrasonic lithotrite, or electrohydraulic lithotrite. Stones in the mid to upper ureter, renal pelvis, and lower pole calyces are all removable by this technique. Complications include bleeding and puncture of the renal pelvis. Hospitalization time is only about five days.

Extracorporeal shock wave lithotripsy is now available in the United States. Stones are chipped into tiny fragments by repeated focused hydraulic waves generated by underwater explosions while the patient is precisely positioned in a bathtub-like apparatus. No incision is necessary, but spinal or epidural anesthesia is required. With experience, ureteral stones also may prove susceptible to this technique. Debris usually passes without colic, minimizing hospitalization. Although more experience is necessary to learn the optimal way to proceed, the two techniques are probably complementary rather than competitive. The lower morbidity and more rapid patient recovery characteristic of these procedures justify patient referrals if equipment is not available locally.

PATIENT INFORMATION AND EDUCATION

Without treatment, most stone formers have recurrence of stone formation within 10 years. Thus, prevention is very important and is dependent on patient compliance with treatment. To this end, patient education is invaluable. The patient needs to understand that prevention is a lifelong process. The clinician must realize that daily adherence to diet and fluid programs is difficult, especially since metabolic stone activity is asymptomatic. The patient's motivation may wane between bouts of colic, and periodic follow-up visits are highly desirable not only to check for recurrence but also to reinforce the need for compliance. The patient also needs to understand that passage of old stones, no matter how painful, does not necessarily signify treatment failure (metabolic activity), and compliance must continue.

PERIODIC EVALUATION

Successful treatment programs can be ensured only by periodic follow-up. The first visit should take place within one or two months after colic has resolved. At this first visit, metabolic evaluation should be done to determine the cause of stone formation and to formulate a treatment program. The patient is usually highly motivated and attentive at this time because the memory of stone pain is fresh in his mind. Metabolic investigations should be done on outpatients who are following their usual dietary and activity patterns because these are the conditions under which the stones were made. The period of hospitalization for colic or surgery is an extremely poor time to perform metabolic evaluation because normal fluid, diet, and activity are greatly altered, as is urinary composition.

Timing of the second follow-up visit varies with the suspected metabolic activity of the patient. Usually six months is about the right time. The second visit should include repeated metabolic studies and, most important, a kidney-ureter-bladder film (usually with tomograms) to determine whether new stone material is present. Comparison with previous films is mandatory. Intravenous pyelography is unnecessary unless obstruction or radiolucent stones are suspected. Opaque contrast only obscures opaque stones. If no metabolic activity is present, yearly follow-up is planned. Patients who are metabolically or surgically active stone formers must be seen more frequently.

PATIENT COMPLIANCE

As noted, no amount of treatment will prevent stones if the patient does not follow it. Careful patient education initially, coupled with periodic reinforcement, will help compliance greatly. Especially after stone passage, the patient needs to be reminded that treatment has not necessarily failed. Follow-up studies at such times often are needed to classify the metabolic stone status and reassure the patient that new stones have not formed, lest he lose faith in the program.

PREVENTIVE MEASURES

Prevention of stones should be aimed not only at the patient as outlined earlier, but also, in selected instances, at his family. Idiopathic calcium nephrolithiasis, especially of the hypercalciuric variety, tends to run in families. Males are more usually affected. Although the penetrance is low enough that screening family members is not recommended, the children should be encouraged to drink a lot of fluid and to use moderate amounts of dairy products after bone growth has been completed.

Cystinuria and primary hyperoxaluria are autosomal recessive in transmission. Fortunately, genetic counseling is not necessary because heterozygotes (children) do not make stones, and the chance of finding a heterozygous mate is low, barring consanguinity. However, there is a one in four chance that each sibling is affected, and screening with 24-hour urine cystine or oxalate determination is strongly advised.

SOCIOECONOMIC ASPECTS OF MANAGEMENT

Because of the relatively high prevalence of stone disease in our society, effective prevention has the potential for saving large amounts of money. An active stone former can miss a great deal of work and even jeopardize his employment. Additionally, repeated colicky episodes often require frequent narcotics, and concurrent drug addiction can occur in the most active stone formers. Conversely, dietary restrictions are inexpensive, as is water. Thiazides and sodium bicarbonate are also inexpensive. Even with more expensive medications and office visits, prevention makes fiscal sense, not to mention the alleviation of human misery.

REFERENCES

Coe FL: Nephrolithiasis: causes, classification, and management. Hosp Pract 16:33–45, 1981.

Erickson SB: When should the stone patient be evaluated? Limited evaluation of single stone formers. Med Clin North Am 68:461–468, 1984.

Lemann J Jr: Nephrolithiasis. *In* Massry SG, Glassock RJ (eds): Textbook of Nephrology, Vol 2. Williams & Wilkins Co, Baltimore, 1983, pp 6.266–6.282.

Pak CYC, Peters P, Hurt G, et al: Is selective therapy of recurrent nephrolithiasis possible? Am J Med 71:615–622, 1981.

Smith LH: Urolithiasis. *In* Earley LE, Gottschalk CW (eds): Strauss and Welt's Diseases of the Kidney, Vol 2, 3rd ed. Little, Brown & Co, Boston, 1979, pp 893–931.

8 · TOXIC NEPHROPATHIES AND DRUG USE IN PATIENTS WITH RENAL IMPAIRMENT

Fred E. Husserl
OCHSNER CLINIC AND ALTON OCHSNER MEDICAL FOUNDATION

Toxic Nephropathies

Toxic nephropathy is a significant alteration of renal function caused by drugs or environmental toxins and characterized by acute or chronic excretory and regulatory failure and/or variable proteinuria. A comprehensive list of agents responsible for these nephropathies is presented in Table 1, but the discussion in this chapter is limited to the drugs used commonly in an outpatient setting.

Table 1. TOXIC NEPHROPATHIES

Excretory Function
Acute renal failure
  Tubular necrosis: aminoglycosides, amphotericin B, colistimethate, organic solvents, heavy metals, acetaminophen, iodinated contrast agents
  Glomerulonephritis: organic solvents, sulfas, penicillin
  Interstitial nephritis: nonsteroidal anti-inflammatory agents (NSAIA), methicillin and other penicillins, cimetidine, thiazines, furosemide, allopurinol, sulfas
  Obstructive uropathy:cholecystographic agents, cancer chemotherapy (urate), methotrexate, ethylene glycol (oxalate)
  Autoregulatory imbalance: NSAIA, captopril
Chronic renal failure
  Glomerulonephritis: heroin
  Interstitial nephritis: analgesics, radiation, lead, lithium
  Obstructive uropathy: retroperitoneal fibrosis—methysergide; calculi—calcium/vitamin D, acetazolamide

Regulatory Function
Water retention
  ADH release: narcotics, clofibrate, vincristine, carbamazepine
  ADH action: NSAIA, chlorpropamide, cyclophosphamide
  Diluting abnormalities: diuretics
Water loss
  ADH related: alcohol, lithium, diphenylhydantoin, demeclocycline
  ADH unrelated: lithium, glyburide
Metabolic acidosis
  Increased anion gap: salicylate intoxication, methanol, ethylene glycol, phenformin
  Normal anion gap: acetazolamide, amphotericin B, outdated tetracycline
Metabolic alkalosis
  Mineralocorticoid-like: licorice, carbenoxolone sodium
  Non-reabsorbable anion: carbenicillin
Respiratory alkalosis
  Central stimulation: salicylates

Nephrotic Syndrome
NSAIA, captopril, heavy metals (gold), anticonvulsants, heroin, penicillamine
*Miscellaneous**
Worsening of azotemia: glucocorticoids, tetracycline, diuretics, androgenic steroids
Edema: estrogens, minoxidil, carbenicillin, calcium channel blockers
Hyperkalemia: spironolactone, triamterene, amiloride, potassium penicillin G, captopril, beta-blockers, indomethacin, salt substitutes
Hypermagnesemia: magnesium-containing antacids and laxatives

*Most often seen in patients with impaired renal function.

NONSTEROIDAL ANTI-INFLAMMATORY AGENTS (NSAIA)

As a group these drugs are among the most widely prescribed agents (ibuprofen is now available as a nonprescription analgesic). Renal dysfunction caused by these drugs is well recognized. In subjects with normal sodium/volume balance and unimpaired circulation, prostaglandins do not have a significant effect on renal function. Under those conditions, NSAIA transiently reduce sodium and water excretion, slightly decrease glomerular filtration rate (GFR), and increase plasma renin levels. During volume depletion or decreased renal perfusion, the kidneys depend on increased secretion of vasodilatory prostaglandins to regulate function. In these circumstances the use of NSAIA, which inhibit the cyclo-oxygenase system leading to decreased prostaglandin production, causes significant functional changes. *Indomethacin* is the most frequently reported NSAIA to cause acute renal failure (ARF). However, the use of almost all NSAIA has been associated with ARF. Sulindac has been reported to cause less renal dysfunction than other NSAIA. ARF occurs within one to seven days after starting NSAIA with symptoms of oliguria and weight gain, increasing blood urea nitrogen (BUN) and serum creatinine, and hyperkalemia. Predisposing factors include older age, underlying intrinsic renal disease (especially lupus nephritis), gout, and decreased effective renal plasma flow (nephrosis, congestive heart failure, liver disease with ascites). In such patients at increased risk, all NSAIA should be used cautiously, and urine output, BUN, serum creatinine, and serum potassium should be monitored. The concurrent use of NSAIA and trimaterene has been reported to cause ARF and should be avoided. Renal failure is rapidly reversible in most cases when the drug is stopped, but if acute tubular necrosis (ATN) occurs, dialysis may be necessary. Hospitalization is advised when ATN develops; simultaneously all predisposing factors should be corrected.

Another renal syndrome associated with NSAIA is characterized by heavy proteinuria and progressive renal failure of varying severity. Microhematuria and casts are seen in 50% of these cases and a skin rash occurs in some. Renal biopsy reveals interstitial nephritis and minimal change glomerulopathy. Typically this syndrome occurs several months after NSAIA therapy is begun. Most patients improve after discontinuing the drug, but the resolution of renal failure and proteinuria may take up to one year. This syndrome is believed to be a hypersensitivity reaction to the drug. Corticosteroids are recommended when renal functional loss and proteinuria are severe and do not resolve spontaneously. The occurrence of this syndrome seems to be specific to the class of NSAIA being used; therefore, a carefully monitored trial with a NSAIA belonging to another class can be undertaken if needed. Papillary necrosis has also been associated with NSAIA. Renal function and urinalysis should be checked periodically in patients on long-term NSAIA therapy.

NSAIA should be used with great caution in patients with sodium retention or established hypertension. The need for a diuretic because of edema or increased blood pressure should dictate discontinuation of NSAIA. Potassium levels should be monitored, especially if renal impairment exists; if hyperkalemia is documented, NSAIA should be discontinued. In general, NSAIA should not be used concomitantly with potassium-sparing diuretics, potassium supplements, salt substitutes, or angiotensin-coverting enzyme inhibitors.

RADIOGRAPHIC CONTRAST AGENTS

The administration of radiographic contrast agents may produce ARF ranging from asymptomatic nonoliguric and transient renal dysfunction to an oliguric and rapidly progressive course requiring dialysis. Urinary sodium and fractional excretion of sodium are unexpectedly low in many instances. The pathogenesis is not well defined but includes proximal tubular dysfunction with sloughing, inflammation and vacuolation, and the potential obstruction of tubules by proteinaceous material, uric acid crystals (especially with cholecystographic agents), or oxalate. Vasodilation followed by renin-angiotensin–mediated vasoconstriction and morphologic changes in eythrocytes may also play a role.

In a general patient population, the incidence of radiocontrast-induced ARF is 1%.

Two groups are at great risk of ARF: (1) those patients with preexisting renal disease (45% to 70% incidence) in whom the severity of ARF seems to be directly related to the degree of preexisting renal dysfunction, and (2) diabetics with renal failure. The incidence varies from 50% to 75% if moderately severe renal failure coexists but approaches 100% with severe renal failure (creatinine > 4.5 mg/dl). Other risk factors include multiple myeloma (incidence of 5%) and volume depletion. Proteinuria per se, hyperuricemia, and advanced age do not appear to be independent risk factors.

In patients with these risk factors, alternative diagnostic methods not involving the use of radiocontrast agents should always be considered. However, it should be noted that the incidence rates quoted above are based on retrospective studies. Careful hydration before contrast administration and the injection of mannitol (12.5 to 25 gm IV) during the study, followed by continued hydration to match urine output, decreases the risk of ARF significantly. A screening serum creatinine should be obtained 48 hours after the dye test. Hospitalization is indicated if severe renal failure develops, and dialysis therapy may be required. Although irreversible renal failure may occur, renal function usually improves within seven to 14 days.

LITHIUM

The use of lithium in the treatment of bipolar affective disorders has been associated with the development of nephrogenic diabetes insipidus and chronic tubulointerstitial nephropathy. This subject is discussed in Chapter 5.

GOLD

Nephrotoxicity is characterized by occasional microhematuria and by the nephrotic syndrome, which occurs in 1% to 3%. Tubular damage with subsequent immune response to tubular antigens leading to glomerular injury and membranous nephropathy has been postulated. Withdrawal of gold therapy is indicated if microhematuria or increased proteinuria is documented on two occasions. In general, these findings are reversed by stopping the drug, but if the nephrotic syndrome worsens or persists more than six months, a renal biopsy to establish the diagnosis (and to exclude amyloidosis) is useful. A therapeutic trial with moderate-dose corticosteroids (1 mg/kg) daily for six weeks may be useful in these cases. Reinstitution of gold should be avoided, since the nephropathy tends to recur.

PENICILLAMINE

Penicillamine can cause proteinuria or nephrotic syndrome with normal renal function in 5% to 7% of patients treated for one year, and in 20% of those treated for more than five years. Membranous nephropathy is the common histologic finding. Once the drug is withdrawn, the proteinuria decreases in four to six months and generally will recur if rechallenged.

CAPTOPRIL

Captopril can cause proteinuria in up to 1.2% of patients and 25% of these patients may develop the nephrotic syndrome; the incidence is higher if underlying renal disease exists. The cause is unclear, but again membranous nephropathy is frequently found. Most cases occur before the eighth month of therapy; therefore, first-voided urinary protein dipstick determination should be followed roughly at monthly intervals during this period. If abnormal, 24-hour urine protein quantitation should follow. Generally, mild proteinuria will subside after six months in spite of ongoing therapy. If renal function deteriorates or massive proteinuria ensues, captopril should be discontinued. Captopril has also been reported to cause ARF. Functional autoregulatory impairment leading to ARF is seen in patients with significant renal artery stenosis of either both renal arteries or the renal artery of a solitary kidney. Captopril should be used with extreme caution and under very close supervision in these cases. If ARF occurs, the drug should be discontinued. ARF due to idiosyncratic interstitial nephritis is rare. Hyperkalemia may occur when captopril is used in patients with impaired renal function; NSAIA and potassium-sparing diuretics should not be used concomitantly with this drug. Newer angiotensin-converting enzyme inhibitors (e.g., enalapril) may be free of these side effects.

Use of Drugs in Patients with Renal Impairment

Drug therapy in patients with renal impairment (RI) is difficult and potentially dangerous, since many drugs are excreted, at least in part, by the kidneys. The situation is further complicated by altered volume of distribution, decreased protein binding, and uremia-induced changes in hepatic metabolism. Adjustment of drug dosage and a solid knowledge of drug interactions are essential for safe and effective pharmacotherapy in RI. Medication lists should be reviewed frequently and updated prior to issuing a new prescription.

Dosage modification should be proportionate to the renal handling of a given drug and to the renal function as measured by creatinine clearance and not the serum creatinine. Serum drug levels are useful in guiding therapy of drugs with a narrow therapeutic range; proper timing of samples and adequate knowledge of protein binding and of the activity of metabolites are important in blood level interpretation. Loading doses are required by some drugs to achieve prompt effect. The maintenance dosage can be altered by giving the usual dose at longer intervals or using a smaller dose at standard intervals; both methods are useful, but I emphasize the need to retain the same method for each specific drug and to frequently use the reference tables and available normograms.

ANALGESICS

Since patients with RI are at increased risk for gastrointesinal bleeding, aspirin should be used only in small doses, and for platelet inhibition rather than analgesia. Acetaminophen is used in the usual manner. The doses of propoxyphene should be reduced because of accumulation of toxic metabolites.

ANTICONVULSANTS

Phenytoin can be given with no modification of dose or interval of administration in patients with RI. However, phenytoin is less protein bound in RI, resulting in lower total plasma levels with standard doses. Thus it is essential to monitor both free (unbound) and total plasma phenytoin levels. Carbamazepine requires no alteration, whereas the dose of ethosuximide should be reduced by 15% if glomerular filtration rate (GFR) is <10 ml/min. Trimethadione should be avoided because of its long half-life. Valproic acid should be used very cautiously, since little information is available about its use in RI; decreased plasma protein binding and accumulation of active metabolites dictate careful titration using low dosage if GFR is < 30 ml/min.

ANTIHYPERTENSIVES

Antihypertensives are very frequently prescribed in patients with renal impairment. The initial decrease in GFR associated with antihypertensive therapy is followed by readjustment and long-term stabilization or improvement of renal function. Antihypertensive drugs known to cause significant decrease in renal blood flow and GFR should not be used (e.g., guanethidine, guanadrel). Lipid-soluble beta-adrenergic antagonists are safe and can be given in usual dosage and intervals. Timolol and pindolol are partially excreted by the kidneys but require no change in dose. The lipid-insoluble compounds are excreted by the kidneys. Atenolol dose should be reduced by 50% if GFR ranges from 15 to 30 ml/min and further reductions are required as renal function deteriorates. Nadolol can be given every 36 hours if GFR is 30 to 50 ml/min, every 48 hours if GFR is 10 to 30 ml/min, and at reduced dosage below this limit. Labetalol, a combined alpha- and beta-blocker, causes no change in GFR and requires no change in dose. It can be used in doses of 300 to 400 mg orally for the acute treatment of severe hypertension; response is seen in two to three hours. Rauwolfia derivatives and guanethidine are rarely used owing to their multiple side effects. Alpha$_1$-adrenoreceptor antagonists preserve renal function; both prazosin and indoramin are used in the usual dosage and intervals.

Central alpha-adrenergic agonists do not alter GFR. Clonidine can be used without dose modification in severe RI, and in the treatment of hypertensive urgencies by using a low-dose loading regimen (0.1 mg initially and then every one to two hours until control of pressure is achieved). The new transdermal therapeutic system (TTS) of clonidine administration reduces plasma levels and side effects, and improves compliance by requiring once-a-week application only. Methyldopa requires slight decrease in dose in severe RI owing to the accumulations of active metabolites. Vasodilators such as hydralazine do not change renal perfusion or function and can be used in a twice-a-day regimen without altering the dosage. Minoxidil is very effective in severe refractory hypertension and requires no change in dose; it produces significant sodium retention and tachycardia requiring concomitant diuretic and beta-blocker therapy. Converting enzyme inhibitors like captopril may increase GFR but should be used with caution, since drug-induced granulocytopenia is more frequent when serum creatinine is >3 mg/dl. Captopril may cause hyperkalemia in patients with GFR of <40 ml/min. The risk of ARF in patients with bilateral renal artery stenosis has been mentioned earlier. The starting dose should be reduced, especially in patients on diuretics.

ANTI-INFLAMMATORY AGENTS AND GOUT

The renal complications associated with the use of NSAIA were described earlier. Allopurinol is the drug of choice in gout, since uricosuric drugs are ineffective when GFR is <30 ml/min; the daily dose should generally be decreased to 200 mg if GFR is <50 ml/min and to 100 mg if GFR is <20 ml/min if control by hyperuricemia is effective. Allopurinol may cause ARF secondary to interstitial nephritis. Colchicine is partially eliminated by the kidneys and should be given in a dose of 0.6 mg every 24 hours as maintenance in moderately severe and severe RI. It is the safest drug for acute gout.

ANTIMICROBIALS

The penicillins and cephalosporins are generally excreted by the kidneys. The dose of penicillin G should be reduced if GFR is <20 ml/min for a maximum dose of 10^7 units per day. Ampicillin and amoxicillin are used in the usual dose for urosepsis at any level of GFR, but otherwise should be used in reduced doses every 12 to 18 hours if GFR is <30 ml/min. Caution should be taken in using the combination of amoxicillin/potassium clavulanate in severe RI, since each tablet contains 47 mg of potassium. Cloxacillin, dicloxacillin, nafcillin, and oxacillin require no change in dosage. Cephalothin only requires an increase in dosage interval if the GFR is <10 ml/min. Cephalexin's interval of administration should be increased to every six to 12 hours if GFR ranges from 10 to 50 ml/min and to every 12 to 24 hours if GFR is <10 ml/min. Cephradine should be used in reduced doses if the GFR is <20 ml/min. Cefazolin and cefadroxil should be reduced by 50% if GFR is <50 ml/min and to 25% of the normal dose if the GFR is <10 ml/min, or intervals should be increased to every 24 hours. The tetracyclines with the exception of doxycycline and minocycline should be avoided in moderate or severe RI owing to their antianabolic effects; although the latter two agents can be used in their usual doses in most patients with RI, they may also aggravate azotemia in some.

Sulfisoxazole and sulfamethoxazole should be administered every eight to 12 hours if the GFR is <50 ml/min and every 24 hours in severe RI. Trimethoprim requires a proportional reduction to every 18 and 24 hours, respectively; its use may cause an increase in the serum creatinine by competing with creatinine for the same tubular secretory sites or due to interstitial nephritis. Erythromycin requires no change in dosage due to extensive hepatic metabolism. Lincomycin should be used in normal doses but at 12- to 24-hour intervals if the GFR is <10 ml/min. Clindamycin requires no modification. Chloramphenicol dose need not be decreased even in severe RI unless liver dysfunction coexists. The dose of metronidazole should be given every eight hours if the GFR is <30 ml/min and every 12 hours in severe RI in order to avoid the accumulation of toxic metabolites. Oral vancomycin is not absorbed and requires no change in dose. The excretion of intravenously administered vancomycin is markedly prolonged in patients with RI.

The aminoglycosides (gentamicin, tobramycin, amikacin, streptomycin, kanamycin) should be used with great caution in patients with RI because their excretion is mainly through the kidneys. Ototoxicity and further impairment of renal function due to the nephrotoxicity of these drugs are major concerns. Normograms are available to guide the dosage of aminoglycosides in RI, but the importance of monitoring blood levels and renal function cannot be overemphasized.

Of the antifungal agents, flucytosine should be given every 12 to 24 hours as GFR decreases from 50 to 20 ml/min and every 24 to 48 hours if GFR is <20 ml/min; blood levels are available and should be used to guide therapy and to avoid toxic effects to bone marrow and liver. Griseofulvin and ketoconazole require no dose modification.

Of the antituberculous drugs, rifampin requires no dosage modification, whereas isoniazid requires a 30% reduction of normal dose if GFR is <10 ml/min and the patient is a slow acetylator. Ethambutol can be given daily using 50% of the normal dose if the GFR is <50 ml/min, and approximately 25% of the normal dose can be given in severe renal failure.

CARDIOVASCULAR AGENTS

Careful and closely monitored prescription of digoxin and digitoxin using blood levels makes their use safe in RI. If GFR is <50 ml/min, the usual digoxin maintenance dose should be decreased to 50%, and subsequently to 25% if GFR is <10 ml/min. The loading dose of digoxin should be reduced by 30% to 60% in patients wih RI. Digitoxin has complex pharmacokinetics but in general can be used without modification if GFR is >20 ml/min and with a 25% reduction in dose if GFR is <20 ml/min. Quinidine should be used with caution in patients on digitalis but requires no change in dose. Blood levels should be monitored. Procainamide is difficult to use because of the variable acetylation rate and the accumulation of the parent drug and N-acetylprocainamide (NAPA). When GFR is <50 ml/min, procainamide requires a change of the dose interval to every six to 12 hours, and with GFR of less than 10 ml/min to every 12 to 24 hours. Plasma concentration of procainamide and NAPA should be checked frequently. The dose of disopyramide should be lowered to 150 mg every 12 hours if the GFR is between 10 and 30 ml/min, and to 150 mg every 24 hours if GFR is <10 ml/min; it produces dry mouth and urinary retention complicating the management in patients with RI. Tocainide clearances decrease in patients with RI. If GFR is 10 to 50 ml/min, initial dose of 400 mg b.i.d. may be adequate; with GFR <10 ml/min, 400 to 600 mg/day may suffice. Concomitant cimetidine and allopurinol therapy can increase blood levels significantly. Calcium channel blockers should be used with caution but require no major dosage modification.

DIURETICS

Diuretics are very useful adjuncts in the treatment of patients with RI. Their dose needs to be increased as GFR decreases. The thiazides, with the exception of metolazone, are ineffective if GFR is <25 ml/min. Furosemide, bumetanide, and ethacrynic acid are effective in advanced RI. Upward titration of furosemide to doses ten times the usual is common, whereas ethacrynic acid dose should only be doubled. Bumetanide is sometimes effective in cases refractory to furosemide. A potent diuretic regimen in patients with RI is the addition of metolazone to one of the above loop diuretics. Patients receiving this combination require close monitoring of fluid and electrolyte status. The potassium-sparing diuretics should not be used when the GFR is < 40 ml/min because of the danger of hyperkalemia. Diabetics with associated hyporeninemic hypoaldosteronism are especially prone to the development of hyperkalemia with the use of potassium-sparing diuretics, even if the renal function is only minimally impaired.

IMMUNOSUPPRESSANTS

Only those immunosuppressants used very frequently will be mentioned here. Cyclophosphamide is metabolized to an active metabolite that accumulates when GFR is <10 ml/min, requiring an increase in the interval of administration to every 18 to 24 hours. Azathioprine requires minor adjustments of the dose with severe RI. Allopurinol interferes with the hepatic metabolism of azathioprine. If these two drugs are used concomitantly, the dose of azathioprine should be reduced by 50% to 70%, irrespective of renal function. Prednisone requires no dose modification.

SEDATIVES, TRANQUILIZERS, AND NARCOTICS

Long-acting barbiturates should be avoided because of their accumulation in RI. The benzodiazepines are safe when prescribed carefully and require no change in dosage. The pharmacokinetics of such agents as methaqualone, glutethimide, and methyprylon are not well elucidated and therefore their use should be avoided. The phenothiazines and tricyclic antidepressants are metabolized by the liver and require no major adjustment in dose. Haloperidol is a very useful antipsychotic agent that does not require any adjustment either. Due to the serious side effects associated with lithium therapy, the extensive renal handling, and the lack of extensive clinical experience with its use in RI, this drug should in general be avoided in patients with RI.

Patients with renal failure are very sensitive to the usual dosages of morphine and meperidine, which require careful titration to avoid oversedation. Standard doses of naloxone will reverse this side effect. Codeine will worsen constipation in those taking phosphate binders and also causes excessive sedation. Pentazocine requires no change in dose. Methadone may accumulate in severe RI, requiring an increase in interval of administration. All these agents should be very carefully titrated to obtain the desired narcotic effect without excessive sedation.

MISCELLANEOUS AGENTS

The hypoglycemic drugs, with the exception of tolbutamide, should be avoided if the GFR is <50 ml/min. Cimetidine should be given every eight hours if GFR is <50 ml/min and every 12 hours in severe RI. The dosage interval for ranitidine should be increased to every 18 to 24 hours in patients with significant RI.

Chlorpheniramine requires no modification, whereas diphenhydramine should be given at 12-hour intervals if GFR is <10 ml/min; both agents produce significant sedation.

Active metabolites of clofibriate accumulate in patients with RI. This is associated with the development of toxic myopathy. This drug should be avoided in the presence of RI.

Heparin and warfarin require close monitoring owing to altered hemostatic mechanisms present in RI, but essentially require no modification in the doses.

The three most frequently used anthelmintic agents, mebendazole, thiabendazole, and pyrvinium pamoate, require no change in dose. Propylthiouracil is also used in usual dose and intervals. Theophylline may aggravate nausea but is used without modification.

REFERENCES

Anderson RJ, Bennett WM, Gambertoglio JG, et al: Fate of drugs in renal failure. *In* Brenner BM, Rector FC Jr (eds): The Kidney, 2nd ed. W.B. Saunders Co, Philadelphia, 1981, pp 2659–2708.
Anderson RJ, Schrier RW: Clinical Use of Drugs in Patients with Kidney and Liver Disease. W.B. Saunders Co, Philadelphia, 1981.
Bennett WM, Porter GA, Bagby SP, et al: Drugs and renal disease. Monograph in Clinical Pharmacology. Churchill-Livingstone, London, 1978.
Garella S, Matarese RA: Renal effect of prostaglandins and clinical adverse effects of nonsteroidal anti-inflammatory agents. Medicine 63:165–181, 1984.

9 · DIALYSIS AND TRANSPLANTATION

K. K. Venkat
Nathan W. Levin
HENRY FORD HOSPITAL

Dialysis

Hemodialysis and peritoneal dialysis are standard modes of therapy for patients with end-stage renal failure (ESRF). These procedures are also used for the treatment of acute renal failure and occasionally for the treatment of poisoning. The discussion in this chapter is limited to the consideration of dialytic therapy in the treatment of chronic renal failure. Approximately 80,000 individuals are being treated with dialysis techniques in the United States, 70,000 being on hemodialysis and 10,000 on peritoneal dialysis. Approximately 80% are being treated in hemodialysis centers and 20% at home. Both by federal mandate (for patients falling under the Medicare program) and because of the nature of the field, a dialysis unit is inherently multidisciplinary in nature and its work represents the combined efforts of nephrologists, surgeons, nurses, social workers, dietitians, technicians, and in some cases occupational therapists and psychiatrists. In many cases, bioethical opinion and information are essential in dealing with problems of access to treatment, discharge from treatment, and right-to-die issues. The majority of patients being dialyzed are covered by the federally constituted Medicare program under which there is control of reimbursement for dialysis. A system of end-stage renal disease networks provides information to the federal government through regional offices on the quality of care in individual dialysis units within each network. The federal government strongly supports the concept of home dialysis, in the form of home hemodialysis or peritoneal dialysis.

INDICATIONS AND REFERRAL FOR DIALYSIS

Patients are considered to be suitable for dialysis once they have reached the point of irreversible ESRF. This occurs approximately when the creatinine clearance has reached the level of 5 ml/min or less, although under circumstances of special sensitvity to the symptoms of uremia, dialysis may have to begin earlier than this. At the time dialysis is initiated, the patient is on the verge of uremia, i.e., there are already symptoms as a result of the accumulation of nitrogenous products, acidosis, hyperkalemia, anemia, and possibly bone disease. Clearly it is preferable for the nephrologist who will eventually care for the patient to have the opportunity of examining the patient well before dialysis is begun. There are two good reasons for this: first is the opportunity for favorably influencing the rate of progression of some of the later complications of chronic renal failure, particularly bone disease. The second is the opportunity for the necessary access surgery to be performed early (see below). Consideration for renal transplantation should occur at the same time as the patient is being evaluated for dialysis. This may require referral to a specific transplantation unit.

HEMODIALYSIS

ACCESS

Hemodialysis requires access to the circulation. The ideal access would allow dialysis without the pain of needle puncture, would not be associated with infection, bleeding or thrombosis of the access, and would be easy to use. No such access is available at present and all current approaches have disadvantages. Accesses in use include the internal arteriovenous (AV) fistula; prosthetic bridges between artery and vein consisting of expanded polytetrafluoroethylene, bovine carotid artery, or umbilical vein; and a variety of devices consisting of prosthetic AV grafts from which a "button" projects through the skin allowing direct access to the circulation without repeated needle puncture. The internal AV fistula is considered to be the best method of access because no foreign material is used; but in many patients, especially diabetics, the small size of blood vessels makes it impossible for such fistulas to be created. Even the AV fistulas, which may last for many years, are not free from complications such as infection, aneurysm formation, thrombosis, or stenosis. These problems are more frequent and often occur earlier when prosthetic AV grafts are used. Button devices, which are very popular with patients, appear to be especially prone to occult infection. Because internal AV fistulas may require weeks or months to develop maximal flows, they must be created well before dialysis is planned. Prosthetic AV grafts can be used one to two weeks after they are placed; thus their placement can occur later in the course of renal failure than that of AV fistulas. When a chronic access has not been created in a patient who requires hemodialysis immediately, subclavian or femoral vein catheters may be used as temporary access to the circulation. In patients in whom all access sites have been utilized or have been thrombosed as a result of intravenous drug use, these and right atrial catheters may be the only means of providing access to the circulation.

PHYSICS OF HEMODIALYSIS

Hemodialysis is based on two physical phenomena: dialytic transfer of uremic toxins from the blood into the dialysis fluid based on their relative concentrations on either side of a semipermeable dialyzer membrane; and the removal by convective ultrafiltration of electrolytes, other substances, and water from the blood into the dialysis fluid across the dialyzer membrane. The latter is accomplished by the application of positive pressure on the blood side or negative pressure on the dialysis fluid side of the membrane. Dialysis machines in use now provide a safe means for the preparation of the dialysis fluid by diluting a concentrate containing electrolytes (and usually glucose) to physiologic concentrations, while exerting control over the rate of blood and dialysis fluid flow through the dialyzer, the temperature of the dialysis fluid, and the rate of fluid removal by ultrafiltration. Water used for preparation of dialysis fluid is treated by deionization and/or reverse osmosis to reduce bacterial contamination and to eliminate unwanted minerals and chemicals that may cause adverse effects in dialysis patients. The American Association for Medical Instrumentation (AAMI) guidelines for water quality are widely followed. Other safety features in dialysis machines include detectors for air in the blood returning to the patient (to prevent air embolism) and for blood in the dialysis fluid (indicating rupture of dialyzer membrane). Newer "smart" dialysis machines incorporating microprocessor technology can be programmed to perform automatically a number of manipulations usually performed by nursing and technical personnel.

DIALYZERS

Dialyzers themselves are of various types most commonly composed of coils, hollow fibers, and flat plates. A variety of membranes are used in dialyzers, until now usually cellulose-based, and more recently consisting of other synthetic materials such as polysulfones, polyacrylonitrile (PAN), and polymethylmethacrylate (PMMA). Dialyzers are available in different sizes depending on the clearance and ultrafiltration needs of the patient. Dialyzer reprocessing for reuse based on carefully defined protocols is now a practice in the majority of dialysis units in the United States. AAMI guidelines for this procedure will be available shortly.

DURATION AND FREQUENCY

Decisions as to how long and how often to hemodialyze a patient may be taken empirically based on an impression of patient well-being and an inspection of blood chemistry. Alternatively, these decisions may be derived from a study of the urea kinetics of the patient. In one widely followed scheme, as defined by Gotch and Sargent, a target midweek predialysis blood urea nitrogen (BUN) concentration (approximately 80 mg/dl in our dialysis program) is chosen while prescribing the appropriate dialyzer clearance, the duration and frequency of dialysis, and protein intake. Information required to make these prescriptions is obtained by knowledge of BUN concentrations in the serum before and after a dialysis and before the next dialysis and rate of dialyzer blood flow, and by making assumptions based on previous data on the relationship of protein catabolic rate to protein intake in the stable individual.

With the high-efficiency hollow fiber dialyzers currently in use in many dialysis units, the duration of a dialysis session is usually between two and a half and four hours and the frequency of these sessions is two to three times a week. There is a recent trend toward even shorter dialysis times using higher blood flows than have previously been used, and using dialyzers or combinations of dialyzers with greater clearances.

Heparin anticoagulation to prevent blood clotting in the dialysis lines and the dialyzer is almost always the rule, although citrate and prostacyclins have been used experimentally. A "dry" (edema-free) weight is estimated for each patient; the rate of ultrafiltration of fluid during hemodialysis is adjusted to reduce the patient's weight from its predialysis value to the estimated dry weight. Chronic carriers of hepatitis B surface antigen are dialyzed in isolation to prevent the spread of the infection to other patients and dialysis staff. Hepatitis B vaccination is now recommended for both dialysis patients and personnel.

INTRADIALYTIC PROBLEMS

Intradialytic problems are frequent and to some extent are inherent in the nature of the procedure, its timing, and the materials used to make the dialyzer membranes. Some patients may manifest allergic reactions to certain membranes or to substances used to sterilize the dialyzer; these reactions can range from minor symptoms to anaphylactic shock and respiratory failure. The term "first use syndrome" is often used to describe a series of symptoms that include chest and back pain, pruritus, and general feeling of discomfort occurring during the first use of cellulosic membranes. These symptoms are associated with leukopenia and complement activation, although the cause and effect relationship between the symptoms and the biochemical phenomena has not been conclusively proved. These symptoms are markedly ameliorated by using reprocessed dialyzers. Hypotension to varying degrees is a common intradialytic problem and is associated with

a more rapid removal of solutes and fluid than can be accommodated by the patient's compensatory responses. Cramps, nausea, and vomiting are not infrequent problems during hemodialysis. Hypoxemia occurs during dialysis as a result of reduction in ventilation following carbon dioxide loss from the patient into the dialysate, and to a dialyzer membrane-plasma interaction. Hemodialysis-induced hypoxemia may have adverse effects in the elderly or the cardiopulmonary compromised patient. New approaches to dialysis including sodium modeling, the use of bicarbonate buffer in the dialysate instead of acetate, accurate contol of fluid removal, and automated saline administration in response to hypotension may reduce the frequency of intradialytic symptoms. Major life-threatening problems such as hemolysis, air embolism, and serious electrolyte disorders such as hypo- and hypernatremia have become very rare with the use of dialysis machines with appropriate controls and alarms.

PERITONEAL DIALYSIS

There are three types of peritoneal dialysis in common use. The most widely used type is CAPD (continuous ambulatory peritoneal dialysis), in which a catheter is inserted in the peritoneal cavity and the patient, out of the hospital, infuses sterile peritoneal dialysate through this catheter three or four times a day. The dialysate remains in the peritoneal cavity for four to six hours during the day, and during sleep. After this "dwell" time during which dialysis takes place, the fluid is allowed to drain followed by the infusion of fresh dialysate. CAPD is easy to learn even by pediatric patients and has the merit of not requiring machines. For many patients this is an ideal therapy permitting independence and greater ease of travel, and allowing much less dietary limitation. The major problem with CAPD is peritonitis, usually due to cutaneous organisms (staphylococci), and less commonly due to enteric gram-negative organisms. Recurrent attacks of peritonitis frequently necessitate the removal of the peritoneal catheter and changeover to hemodialysis. The second type of peritoneal dialysis is called CCPD (continuous cycling peritoneal dialysis), in which a machine (a cycler) automatically infuses fluid into and drains fluid from the peritoneal cavity through an indwelling catheter three to four times, usually at night while the patient is sleeping. This may be combined with some exchanges as in CAPD during the day. The third type is called intermittent peritoneal dialysis, in which a patient, usually in a hospital or in a dialysis center, dialyzes for 10 to 12 hours three times a week with multiple dialysis exchanges. Intermittent peritoneal dialysis appears to be associated with poorer survival than CAPD or CCPD, and this, to some extent, may be a reflection of the type of patient for whom this type of treatment is chosen. CAPD may have a special role in the treatment of patients with diabetes and renal failure since it does not require the use of heparin, which some have associated with aggravation of diabetic retinopathy, and because the gradual nature of the treatment does not produce the rapid shifts in intravascular volume for which some diabetic patients have little compensatory response. In order to reduce the rate of infection of the peritoneal cavity in the CAPD patient, a variety of technical solutions is being attempted to reduce the contamination that may occur at the time of changing over from one dialysate bag to another. These techniques may reduce the rate of peritonitis but have not yet solved the problem of infection of the subcutaneous tunnel in which the peritoneal dialysis catheter lies. Patients may go fom CAPD to renal transplantation just as they might from hemodialysis.

MEDICAL PROBLEMS IN DIALYSIS PATIENTS

The mere fact that a patient is being adequately dialyzed may not prevent some of the problems that occur as a direct or indirect result of the uremic state. Dialysis patients are prone to ateriosclerotic heart disease. Arrhythmias are frequent as compared with the general population of the same age, and sometimes result in sudden death. Bone disease is a common problem in the uremic patient. While dialysis itself does not accelerate bone loss, renal osteodystrophy developing in the predialytic period may continue to progress after the initiation of dialytic therapy. Subtotal parathyroidectomy may be required for secondary hyperparathyroidism in dialysis patients, especially in those who are noncompliant with phosphate binder therapy. Where aluminum is not removed from the water used for manufacturing dialysate for hemodialysis, aluminum bone disease (dialysis osteomalacia) is common. When the dialysate is appropriately aluminum-free, this form of bone disease may still occur in some patients who use large doses of aluminum-containing phosphate binders. In this condition, calcification of osteoid is markedly impaired and aluminum deposition in bones can be demonstrated. In general, the anemia characteristic of chronic renal failure is not helped by dialysis, although occasionally the hematocrit may rise slightly, particularly when the anemia has been in part due to blood loss and hemolysis. Anabolic steroids may improve anemia in dialysis patients and are commonly used for this purpose. Access-related complications such as thrombosis, infection, and aneurysm formation continue to be major problems in hemodialysis patients. Hospitalization for declotting or revision of accesses, and for the treatment of access infection in hemodialysis patients and for peritonitis in CAPD patients, is common.

MEDICAL CARE OF THE DIALYSIS PATIENT

Patients on in-center hemodialysis are usually seen by a physician or a nurse clinician on every visit, although this practice may vary widely. A detailed monthly assessment of in-center patients is usually performed with a full physical examination and review of laboratory data. Patients on home hemodialysis or peritoneal dialysis are seen monthly. Blood counts, hepatitis B surface antigen, BUN, serum creatinine, calcium, inorganic phosphate, alkaline phosphatase, electrolytes, ferritin, and liver function tests are checked monthly. Radiolgic examination for renal osteodystrophy is done annually. Dietitians and social workers also meet with the patient on a regular basis. The federal government has mandated the end-stage renal disease networks to ensure that quality of care is appropriate and that all patients have long-term care plans providing evaluation by transplant surgeons and physicians interested in home dialysis. All care plans are reviewed on a regular basis.

As with all chronic illnesses, there is a high incidence of psychiatric and behavioral problems in patients undergoing dialysis. Activities that alleavite these problems include the support of all the members of the dialysis team (physician, nurses, dietitians, social workers) and specifically, when available, the use of occupational therapists, psychiatrists, and psychologists. The aim of such support is to ensure as much rehabilitation as possible. However, the mean age of the dialysis population is over 55 years, and rehabilitation aimed at return to gainful employment is often impractical. However, improvement in the ability to perform the activities of daily life and enhancement of self-expression are the objectives.

RESULTS OF DIALYSIS

It is difficult to compare the survival of patients on the various modalities of dialysis, since random allocation does not occur. Studies correcting for differences in age, race, and the presence of other medical problems besides ESRF (e.g., diabetes mellitus and heart disease) suggest that there is little difference in patient survival with various modalities of dialysis, with the exception that intermittent peritoneal dialysis has inferior results. Although patients on home hemodialysis have the highest survival rates, this may be largely due to selection of highly compliant patients with good family support and without other major medical problems for this modality of dialysis. In the dialysis population as a whole, after the first year the annual mortality rate is aproximately 10%. This rate is much lower in younger ESRF patients without other medical problems and much higher in the elderly, and in those with diabetes mellitus and arteriosclerotic heart disease. Longevity of the dialysis patient is hardly dependent on the procedure. The major cause of morbidity and mortality in dialysis patients is cardiovascular disease. The prevalence of arteriosclerotic heart disease is much greater in dialysis patients than in the general population. It has been suggested that the progression of this type of heart disease may be accelerated in dialysis patients, but this is probably due to the presence of multiple risk factors for coronary atherosclerosis in these patients rather than due to dialysis itself.

COST

The average annual cost (excluding hospitalization) for CAPD, home hemodialysis, and in-center hemodialysis is approximately $18,000, $20,000 and $30,000, respectively. Hospitalization for access problems and peritonitis adds considerably to these costs.

Renal Transplantation

In the three decades since the initiation of renal transplantation in Boston in 1954, this procedure has become an established therapeutic option for ESRF.

Experience and advances in immunosuppression have greatly increased graft survival and reduced morbidity and mortality in renal transplantation. Ideally all patients with ESRF should be looked at as potential candidates for transplantation unless they are clearly unsuitable. If a living donor is available, renal transplantation can be performed before dialysis is initiated. Some have suggested that this may be of particular value in the diabetic patient.

EVALUATION OF THE POTENTIAL TRANSPLANT RECIPIENT

To be a candidate for transplantation, the patient should be preferably between the ages of 5 and 60 years, free of life-threatening problems in organ systems other than the kidneys, and have no evidence of active infection or malignancy. However, older patients may be considered if in good general health, and transplantation has been successfully performed even in infants.

A detailed urologic evaluation including cystoscopy, cystometrogram, and voiding cystourethrogram is performed in all recipients to ensure that there will be no vesical problems following the anastomosis of the allograft ureter to the patient's bladder. Removal of the patient's own kidneys prior to transplantation is required only with a history of recurrent urinary tract infections (especially when associated with vesicoureteral reflux), with severe hypertension uncontrolled by control of extravascular volume by dialysis and optimal antihypertensive drug therapy, and when very large polycystic kidneys are present. Most transplant centers no longer perform routine pretransplant splenectomy as an immunosuppressive measure. Peptic ulcer and cholelithiasis in potential recipients should be treated surgically before transplantation to avoid the risk of severe gastrointestinal hemorrhage and cholecystitis after transplantation. Excision of the affected segment of the colon prior to transplantation should be considered in patients with a definitive history of diverticulitis.

HISTOCOMPATIBILITY MATCHING AND SELECTION OF THE DONOR

Since the major blood group antigens are expressed on the surface of the endothelial cells of the renal vasculature, the donor and recipient must be ABO-compatible. Rh and minor blood group incompatibilities, however, are not important in renal transplantation. Since rejection depends largely on the differences in the HLA antigens of the donor and recipient, the more closely these antigens are matched, the better are the results of transplantation. The favorable effect of matching for the HLA-A and HLA-B locus antigens was documented over a decade ago. More recently the importance of the antigens of the HLA-DR locus has come to be recognized, and matching for these antigens may be more important than matching for the HLA-A and B antigens. Differences in the HLA-D locus antigens other than the DR antigens also affect the outcome of transplantation. However, unlike the HLA-A, B, and DR antigens, which can be identified quickly with serologic techniques, disparity in the other antigens of

the D locus can be recognized only by the mixed lymphocyte culture (MLC) test in which lymphocytes from the donor and recipient are incubated together. The degree of stimulation of the recipient's lymphocytes by the donor's lymphocytes is determined by the amount of radioactive thymidine uptake by the former. The MLC test requires about a week to perform and, as discussed later, is used at present only in living donor transplantation.

In our view, a living related donor should always be sought because the probability of matching for HLA antigens is much higher among close relatives. Siblings completely matched for HLA-A, B, and DR antigens (two-haplotype match) and showing low reactivity in the MLC test with the recipient make the best donors. Transplantation from siblings, parents, and offspring sharing only one half of the HLA antigens with the recipient (one-haplotype match) is less successful. In one-haplotype–matched pairs, the higher the MLC reactivity between the donor and recipient, the lower is the success rate of transplantation. When the living donor is completely mismatched (two-haplotype mismatch) with the recipient, the results are no better than in cadaveric transplantation. Therefore, until a few years ago the use of one-haplotype–matched, highly MLC reactive donors and two-haplotype–mismatched donors was thought to be unjustified, but as described later, following pretransplant donor-specific blood transfusions such donors can be used successfully.

HLA matching improves results in cadaveric transplantation also, but because of the limited availability of cadaver organs, such matching is not insisted upon except in the case of recipients who have rejected previous transplants. Also, since the cadaver kidney can be preserved for only 48 to 72 hours, the selection of a recipient based on low MLC reactivity to the donor is also not possible because this test takes a week to complete. A nationwide computerized organ procurement program to match cadaver donors with potential recipients on the basis of HLA antigens is now being formed in the United States. An absolute requirement for both living donor and cadaveric transplantation is that a crossmatch between the donor's lymphocytes and the recipient's serum should be negative. A positive crossmatch as shown by the lysis of the donor lymphocytes indicates the presence of cytotoxic antibodies against the donor's antigens in the recipient's serum, which can cause hyperacute rejection of the allograft within a few hours after transplantation.

Living related donors should be above the age of legal consent (18 years), and it should be ascertained that the donation is completely voluntary. Donation by minors requires court approval. Declaration of brain death and consent from the next of kin are required prior to removal of organs for transplantation from cadaver donors. Any evidence of renal disease, hypertension, diabetes mellitus or other major systemic diseases, hepatitis B antigenemia, sepsis, and malignancy (except primary intracranial neoplasms) are contraindications for kidney donation. The remaining kidney in the living donor shows compensatory hypertrophy and hyperfiltration. The concern that these phenomenona might eventually lead to significant renal disease in the donor has not been borne out by long-term follow-up.

BLOOD TRANSFUSION AND RENAL TRANSPLANTATION

The recognition of the beneficial effects of pretransplant blood transfusions on graft survival is one of the major factors that have contributed to improved results of renal transplantation in the past decade. Since the patient who has never been transfused has very poor graft survival (30% to 40% at one year), the deliberate transfusion of 5 to 10 units of whole blood or packed red cells within the year preceding transplantation is now a common practice. The effect of blood transfusions might be through the identification of the "strong responder" recipients who form antibodies against the transfused HLA antigens and therefore will be able to receive kidneys only from donors having HLA antigens to which they are nonreactive. Alternatively, and more likely, transfusions might induce suppressor lymphocytes or "protective" anti-idiotypic antibodies. With donor-specific transfusions (DST) in which the recipient is transfused with blood from the potential donor prior to transplantation, the survival of kidneys donated by one-haplotype–matched, highly MLC reactive living related donors has improved to levels achieved with HLA identical donors. Following DST the recipient is screened for the development of cytotoxic antibodies to donor lymphocytes and the transplant is performed only if such antibodies do not develop. Approximately one third of recipients given DST develop such antibodies and therefore cannot receive a kidney from that donor. The administration of azathioprine along with DST has been shown to decrease the formation of these antibodies without impairing the beneficial effect of DST on graft survival. A small number of transplants have been performed from two-haplotype–mismatched related donors and living unrelated donors following DST, with success rates comparable to that obtained with HLA identical donors.

SURGICAL TECHNIQUE OF RENAL TRANSPLANTATION

The allograft is placed extraperitoneally in the right or left lower quadrant of the abdomen. The renal artery and vein are anastomosed to the internal (hypogastric) or external iliac artery and vein of the recipient The ureter is connected to the bladder through a submucosal tunnel to prevent vesicoureteral reflux.

IMMUNOSUPPRESSIVE THERAPY

All recipients of renal allografts except those with an identical twin kidney donor require immunosuppression after transplantation to prevent rejection. Four drugs are currently in use for this purpose: azathioprine (Imuran), corticosteroids (prednisone, prednisolone, or methylprednisolone), antilymphocyte antibodies (antilymphoblast globulin [ALG] or antithymocyte globulin [ATG]) and cyclosporine (Sandimmune). "Conventional immunosuppression" consists of a combination of azathioprine and corticosteriods with or without antilymphocyte antibodies. Since the advent of cyclosporine, this drug, usually in combination with corticosteroids, has replaced conventional immunosuppression in cadaveric renal transplantation in most centers. However, conventional therapy is still widely used in living donor transplantation because excellent results are obtained in this group of recipients even without the use of cyclosporine. A newer regimen called "triple therapy," in which cyclosporine, azathioprine, and corticosteroids are combined in lower than usual doses in an attempt to minimize the side effects of these drugs while retaining their immunosuppressive effect, is currently being evaluated in a number of transplant centers including ours.

A series of cellular and humoral immune phenomena are involved in the rejection of transplanted solid organs. The initial step is the activation of helper T lymphocytes after they bind to the foreign class II HLA antigens expressed on the cells of the allograft. Activated helper T cells produce a macrophage-stimulating factor and also develop receptors for the lymphokine interleukin-1 (IL-1). Stimulated macrophages release IL-1, which acts on helper T cells and causes them in turn to release another lymphokine, interleukin-2 (IL-2). After binding to the class I HLA antigens of the allograft, cytotoxic T lymphocytes develop IL-2 receptors. IL-2 released from helper T cells acts on cytotoxic T cells to cause their proliferation. Helper T cells are themselves acted upon by IL-2 , leading to the release of B lymphocyte growth factors that stimulate antibody production by these cells. The rejection of the transplanted organ is the combined result of the cytodestructive effects of proliferating cytotoxic T cells and activated macrophages, and the action of antibodies directed against the allograft.

The drugs used for immunosuppression interrupt the sequence of events in the rejection response at different points. The major effect of corticosteroids is the blocking of IL-1 production by macrophages. Azathioprine acts nonspecifically to block the proliferation of lymphocytes, and antilymphocyte antibodies cause lysis of lymphocytes. Cyclosporine prevents the release of IL-2 by helper T cells, thus blocking the continued proliferation of cytotoxic T cells and the release of B cell growth factors from helper T cells. In contrast to other immunosuppressive drugs, cyclosporine spares suppressor T cells, which promote tolerance of the allograft.

AZATHIOPRINE

Azathioprine is given initially in a dose of 2 to 2.5 mg/kg/day. This dose is adjusted further based on the blood counts. After the first year following transplantation we gradually decrease the dose to 1.5 mg/kg/day in patients with good graft function. The major side effect of this drug is bone marrow suppression. It has also been implicated in liver dysfunction in transplant recipients.

CORTICOSTEROIDS

Over the last few years much lower doses of corticosteroids are being used in renal transplantation. In our program we now begin with 0.5 mg/kg/day of methylprednisolone as compared with 1.2 mg/kg/day until a few years ago. This dose is gradually decreased to 20 mg/day by four to six weeks and to the indefinitite maintenance level of 10 mg daily or 20 mg every other day by six to nine months after transplantation. Patients experiencing repeated rejections are not converted to alternate-day steroid therapy and require a higher maintenance dose than mentioned above. The side effects of corticosteroids are well known. Weight gain, steroid-induced diabetes mellitus, cataracts, and avascular necrosis of bone, especially in the hip, are particularly troublesome problems in renal transplant recipients.

ANTILYMPHOCYTE ANTIBODIES

Antilymphocyte antibodies have to be administered intravenously (15 to 30 mg/kg/day). They are either given prophylactically during the first three to four weeks after transplantation to prevent rejection or administered to treat established rejection, and are effective used either way. These preparations contain animal proteins and allergic reactions are common during their use: fever, chills, and rarely anaphylaxis. Antilymphocyte antibodies are not completely free of antibodies against other formed elements in the blood, and this can cause leukopenia, thrombocytopenia, and hemolytic anemia. Monoclonal antilymphocyte antibodies directed against specific T cell subpopulations such as the helper T cells and without effect on suppressor T cells are currently being evaluated in clinical studies.

CYCLOSPORINE

Cyclosporine was approved for clinical use in organ transplantation in 1983 and its use has resulted in markedly improved graft survival in kidney, heart, and liver transplantation. The initial oral dose of cyclosporine in our program is 15 mg/kg/day. An intravenous preparation is also available and is used until the patient is able to take cyclosporine orally. We adjust cyclosporine doses based on the serum trough level of the drug measured by radioimmunoassay. Trough level targets in our protocol are: first month, 150 to 200 ng/ml; second month, 100 to 150 ng/ml; and third month, 75 to 100 ng/ml. We have found that after three months, trough levels around 50 ng/ml are sufficient to prevent rejection in most patients. Since the absorption of cyclosporine improves progressively after transplantation and since the trough level targets are decreased with time, the dose of cyclosporine can be decreased steadily in most patients to eventual maintenance doses of 2.5 to 7.5 mg/kg/day. We maintain these doses indefinitely unless cyclosporine nephrotoxicity or the patient's inability to afford the cost of the drug forces the change to conventional immunosuppression. Other programs have successfully replaced cyclosporine with azathioprine three to six months after transplantation, but in a few patients this has resulted in irreversible rejection.

Cyclosporine has a number of side effects. Many of these are not serious: nausea, vomiting, hirsutism, gingival hyperplasia, paresthesias, and tremors. Hepatotoxicity has not been common in our experience, and has consisted of minor abnormalities in liver function tests, which are easily reversed by dose reduction. Hypertension and nephrotoxicity are the major problems during the use of cyclosporine. This drug appears to increase both the incidence and severity of hypertension in renal transplant recipients; the mechanisms underlying this effect are unclear. Nephrotoxicity is encountered at some time during the post-transplant course in the majority of renal allograft recipients. When cyclosporine is used in the immediate postoperative period, the combination of cyclosporine nephrotoxicity and preservation injury of the allograft may result in increased incidence and duration of acute tubular necrosis (ATN), and some grafts may never function. In recipients of nondiuresing kidneys, we use conventional immunosuppression (with ALG) initially and defer the administration of cyclosporine until one week after transplantation This policy has not resulted in any decrease in long-term graft survival. Nephrotoxicity may also take the form of acute or slowly progressive elevations in serum creatinine after good graft function has occurred. It is difficult to differentiate these forms of renal dysfunction from acute and chronic rejection respectively; even kidney biopsy may not be helpful and often one has to rely on the response to reductions in cyclosporine dose to make the diagnosis. The lowest serum creatinine level achieved after renal transplantation is generally higher in cyclosporine-treated recipients when compared with their conventionally treated counterparts. Thus a certain degree of stable renal dysfunction appears to be inherent in cyclosporine therapy. Cyclosporine analogues that may be free of nephrotoxicity are currently being sought. Cyclosporine is very expensive and this is a limiting factor in the use of this drug in patients whose medical insurance does not cover the cost of drugs.

MEDICAL PROBLEMS FOLLOWING RENAL TRANSPLANTATION

ACUTE TUBULAR NECROSIS

Immediate graft function is the rule in living donor transplantation, but initial oliguric ATN is not uncommon in cadaveric transplantation (30% to 50% incidence). The patient is dialyzed regularly during the period of ATN, which usually lasts less than two weeks but can last several weeks, and some grafts never function.

REJECTION

Improved techniques of crossmatching the recipient's serum and donor lymphocytes before transplantation have made hyperacute rejection uncommon. Acute rejection can occur as early as three to five days after transplantation and is uncommon after the first six months. While fever, graft enlargement, graft tenderness, oliguria, weight gain, hypertension, proteinuria, and lymphocyturia may occur, the only consistent abnormality during acute rejection is an unexplained elevation of serum creatinine. The difficulty in differentiating acute rejection from cyclosporine nephrotoxicity was mentioned earlier. Acute rejection is treated with either intravenous boluses of methylprednisolone (250 to 1000 mg/day) for three to five days or increased oral doses of corticosteriods. Steroid-resistant rejection episodes are treated with ALG. Plasma and lymphocytopheresis and local irradiation of the graft have been used in the treatment of steroid- and ALG-resistant rejection, but the efficacy of these measures is questionable. Chronic rejection is characterized by slowly progressive loss of renal function unresponsive to increased immunosuppression, and eventually leads to graft loss. We, like others, have found that a higher percentage of cyclosporine-treated recipients have a totally rejection-free postoperative course than their conventionally treated counterparts (40% vs. 20%).

INFECTIONS

The immunosuppressed transplant recipient is forever at an increased risk of opportunistic infections, but this threat is most marked in the first year after transplantation. Urinary tract infection related to the indwelling bladder catheters is not uncommon in the immediate postoperative period. Infection due to the herpes group of viruses (cytomegalovirus [CMV], herpes simplex, herpes zoster) is most commonly seen during the first three months. ALG-treated patients are especially prone to CMV infection. Since ALG is generally not used in cyclosporine-treated recipients, CMV infection is uncommon in this group of patients. Pulmonary or disseminated infections due to gram-negative bacteria, *Legionella* species, *Pneumocystis carinii*, mycobacteria, *Cryptococcus*, *Aspergillus*, and *Nocardia* may occur in immunosuppressed patients. In addition to infection, rejection, ALG administration, and lymphomas may cause fever in the transplant recipient. Infection in the setting of immunosuppression can be fulminant and an aggressive diagnostic approach including biopsy of affected organs is mandatory. Proper choice of antimicrobial therapy and reduction or withdrawal of immunosuppression are critical for the infection to be overcome. The importance of avoiding repeated courses of antirejection therapy with high-dose corticosteroids and/or ALG, which greatly increase the risk of life-threatening infections, is now well recognized.

HYPERTENSION

Systemic hypertension is a common problem following renal transplantation. In the majority of recipients who are hypertensive at the time of transplantation, the blood pressure remains elevated postoperatively. Less commonly hypertension develops de novo following transplantation. Hypertension may contribute to the increased risk of cardiovascular disease after transplantation. Persistence of renin secretion from the patient's own kidneys, transplant renal artery stenosis, corticosteroids, cyclosporine, and allograft rejection have been implicated in the causation of hypertension after renal transplantation. Difficulty in controlling the blood pressure with drugs, especially when associated with allograft dysfunction, is an indication for transplant renal arteriogram and renin measurements from the native and transplant renal veins. Bilateral native nephrectomy or correction of transplant renal artery stenosis by angioplasty or sugery may be required based on the results of these tests. Captopril therapy in the presence of transplant renal artery stenosis may cause acute renal failure.

CARDIOVASCULAR DISEASE/HYPERLIPIDEMIA

Arteriosclerotic heart disease is the most important cause of morbidity and mortality after the first year following transplantation. Diabetics (especially type II) appear to be at an even greater risk for this complication. For this reason we generally avoid transplantation in type II diabetics older than 50 to 55 years. Hyperlipidemia persists following transplantation with hypercholesterolemia as the principal abnormality.

LIVER DISEASE

Asymptomatic elevation of liver enzymes is common in transplant recipients. Drugs (azathioprine, cyclosporine) and viral infections (CMV, hepatitis B, non-A/non-B hepatitis, herpes simplex, Epstein-Barr virus) may lead to liver disease in these patients, although the cause remains unidentified in the majority of instances. Chronic active hepatitis develops in 2% to 5% of recipients and almost invariably leads to death from liver failure.

NEOPLASIA

Transplant recipients have been estimated to have a 100-fold increase in the risk of developing malignant tumors when compared with the general population. Five to 6% of renal transplant recipients develop malignancies. Skin cancer, carcinoma of the cervix, and malignant lymphomas are the most common tumors in these patients. Early experience with cyclosporine indicated a high incidence of lymphomas, but it now appears that the risk of this complication is no greater than with conventional immunosuppression. Epstein-Barr virus markers have been demonstrated in the B-cell lymphomas that develop during cyclosporine therapy. This suggests that reactivation of Epstein-Barr viral infection in B cells during cyclosporine immunosuppression may cause their malignant transformation. Withdrawal of cyclosporine and treatment with the antiviral drug acyclovir have caused the remission of some of these tumors, but others require the addition of radiotherapy and chemotherapy.

HYPERPARATHYROIDISM

The parathyroid hyperplasia of chronic renal failure does not regress fully after transplantation. Hypercalcemia may develop in the post-transplant period, and subtotal parathyroidectomy may be required. Hypophosphatemia due to hyperparathyroidism and defective renal tubular reabsorption of phosphate is a common post-transplant abnormality, but is usually not severe enough to warrant phosphate supplements.

UROLOGIC COMPLICATIONS

Disruption of the ureteral anastomosis to the bladder may cause leak of urine into the pelvis. Obstructive uropathy leading to graft dysfunction may develop owing to intrinsic narrowing or extrinsic compression of the transplant ureter. The latter is usually due to collection of lymph in the pelvis. These lymphoceles usually disappear with repeated percutaneous aspiration, but occasionally require surgical drainage.

RECURRENT RENAL DISEASE

Most types of primary gomerulopathies affecting the patient's own kidneys have been reported to recur in the allograft causing proteinuria of varying severity and renal insufficiency. The risk of recurrent disease is, however, negligible except in focal segmental glomerulosclerosis, dense deposit type of membranoproliferative glomerulonephritis, and anti-GBM antibody disease (if the antibody is present in the circulation at the time of transplantation). Glomerulopathies can also develop de novo in the allograft and chronic rejection may cause glomerular pathologic changes (transplant glomerulopathy). Recurrence of lupus nephritis in the allograft is rare. Histologic changes of diabetic nephropathy have been demonstrated in the allograft in diabetic recipients within a few years after transplantation.

RESULTS OF RENAL TRANSPLANTATION

In primary cadaveric transplantation with pretransplant blood transfusions and conventional immunosuppression, graft survival at one year is 60% to 70% and 50% to 55% at five years. Cyclosporine immunosuppression has improved graft survival in primary cadaveric transplantation to 75% to 85% at one year. Blood transfusion appears to have an added beneficial effect on graft survival even in cyclosporine-treated patients. Cadaveric retransplantation with conventional immunosuppression in patients who have rejected an earlier transplant is far less successful (one-year graft survival 30% to 40%). Contrary to initial reports, cyclosporine has not significantly improved results in this group of patients. With an HLA identical living related donor and conventional immunosuppression, one-year graft survival is over 90%. Comparable success has been reported with DST and conventional immunosuppression in recipients of less well matched and totally mismatched living donor kidneys. The place of cyclosporine in living donor transplantation is unlcear because conventional immunosuppression and DST result in excellent graft survival, which is difficult to improve upon. It has been claimed that cyclosporine therapy can achieve equally good results even without DST, but more experience is needed before this approach can be accepted. The policy of avoiding excessive immunosuppression has resulted in patient survivals of over 90% at one year in both cadavaric and living donor transplantation. Transplantation in general results in a better quality of life and rehabilitation than does dialysis. The limited availability of cadaver organs is now the main obstacle to the more widespread use of transplantation in the treatment of ESRF. Nationwide enactment of "required request" legislation, which mandates a request for organ donation prior to termination of respiratory and cardiovascular support in brain-dead patients, may help to improve the supply of cadaver organs for transplantation. At present, only a few states have enacted such legislation.

REFERENCES

Cogan MG, Garovoy MR: Introduction to Dialysis. Churchill-Livingstone, New York, 1985.

Hakim RM, Lazarus JM: Medical aspects of hemodialysis. *In* Brenner BM, Rector FC (eds): The Kidney, 3rd ed. W.B. Saunders Co, Philadelphia, 1986, pp 1791–1845.

Hollenberg NK, Tilney NL: Renal transplantation: donor selection and surgical aspects. *In* Brenner BM, Rector FC (eds): The Kidney. W.B. Saunders Co, Philadelphia, 1981, pp 2599–2617.

Strom TB: Immunosuppressive agents in renal transplantation. Kidney Int 26:353–365, 1984.

Strom TB, Tilney NL: Renal transplantation: clinical aspects. *In* Brenner BM, Rector FC (eds): The Kidney, 3rd ed. W.B. Saunders Co, Philadelphia 1986, pp 1941–1976.

10 · COMMON UROLOGIC PROBLEMS IN INTERNAL MEDICINE

Harold A. Fuselier, Jr.
OCHSNER CLINIC AND ALTON OCHSNER MEDICAL FOUNDATION

The most common urologic problem seen in clinical practice is urinary tract infection (UTI). The pathogenesis and risk factors of UTI and the management of upper UTI (pyelonephritis), asymptomatic bacteriuria, and catheter-related UTI are discussed in Chapter 5 of this section. This chapter will deal with lower UTI and other urologic problems commonly encountered by internists.

CYSTITIS

Bacterial cystitis is the most common cause of bladder symptoms and is easy to diagnose and treat. The typical presentation is the occurrence of frequency, dysuria, urgency, frequent voiding of small amounts of urine, and suprapubic pain in young females. Fever, chills, and flank pain are unusual in cystitis and usually indicate renal infection. While hematuria may occur in uncomplicated cystitis, its persistence after treatment of the infection should suggest the possibility of tumor or calculi.

The diagnosis of UTI (upper or lower) requires microscopic examination and culture of urine obtained by proper technique. The midstream, clean catch technique, in which the external genitalia are cleansed well before voiding urine and the initially voided urine is discarded, is sufficient in most patients. Bladder catheterization is indicated only in patients who are unable to cooperate. Suprapubic aspiration of urine from the bladder avoids contamination of urine by urethral and perineal organisms but is seldom required except in very young children. A presumptive diagnosis of UTI can be made by the demonstration of WBC and bacteria by microscopic examination of urine. More than 5 WBC per high power field in the centrifuged sediment of urine is suggestive of UTI. To look for bacteriuria, a drop of uncentrifuged urine is examined after Gram or methylene blue staining. The presence of one or more bacteria per oil immersion field correlates with significant bacteriuria (see below). Reagent strips for quick and indirect detection of bacteriuria (based on the formation of nitrite from urinary nitrate by gram-negative bacteria) and pyuria (based on the action of leukocyte esterases on a substrate) are available, but are not completely reliable.

Urine should be cultured promptly or within 24 hours of refrigeration. Since bacterial contamination is not completely avoided by the midstream, clean catch technique or bladder catheterization, quantitative methods of urine culture are employed to distinguish contamination from actual UTI. The growth of more than 10^5 organisms/ml of urine correlates well with the presence of infection. Less than 10^4 organisms/ml suggests contamination. Bacterial count between 10^4 and 10^5/ml is referred to as low count bacteriuria, and this may be significant under certain circumstances. For example, about one third of female patients with symptomatic cystourethritis may have low count bacteriuria. Prior antimicrobial therapy, diuresis, and infection by fastidious organisms may also result in low count bacteriuria in the presence of infection. Any bacterial growth in urine obtained by suprapubic aspiration should be considered significant. Low count bacteriuria in males and in urine specimens obtained by bladder catheterization may be associated with actual infection because contamination is less likely under these circumstances. It is doubtful if urine culture is cost-effective in uncomplicated cystitis. However, urine culture and sensitivities must be obtained in patients with suspected pyelonephritis, recurrent UTI, or asymptomatic bacteriuria, and if structural abnormalities of the urinary tract are present.

Initial treatment of cystitis is based on the results of the methylene blue or Gram stain of the urinary sediment. If the bacteria are large rods, the most likely bacteria causing infection are the Enterobacteriaceae. *Escherichia coli* alone accounts for two thirds to three fourths of infections. Treatment with sulfisoxazole (0.5 gm q.i.d.), nitrofurantoin (50 mg q.i.d.), ampicillin (250 mg q.i.d.), amoxicillin (250 mg t.i.d.), or sulfamethoxazole-trimethoprim (one double-strength tablet b.i.d.) for seven days will result in a cure in the vast majority of patients. If cocci in pairs or in chains are seen on the stain, enterococcus (group D streptococcus) is the most likely agent and should respond to amoxicillin or ampicillin. Single-dose therapy with 3.5 gm of ampicillin, 3 gm of amoxicillin, 2 double-strength tablets of sulfamethoxazole-trimethoprim, or 2 gm of sulfisoxazole has been shown to be effective in women with uncomplicated cystitis. Single-dose therapy should not be used if symptoms have been present for more than ten days and in men with cystitis. Symptoms suggestive of upper UTI and the presence of obstruction or stone disease are also contraindications for single-dose therapy. Patients are advised to take warm sitz baths, increase oral fluids, and use urinary analgesics such as phenazopyridine (Pyridium) 200 mg two to three times a day for the first day or two as needed. A follow-up urinalysis and urine culture should be done two weeks after starting therapy to confirm eradication of infection.

Sexually active young women frequently contract "honeymoon cystitis." Cases of cystitis occurring shortly after intercourse can be prevented by having the patient void after coitus and drink a large tumbler of water. If this regimen fails, the administration of one double-strength tablet of sulfamethoxazole-trimethoprim after coitus and one the following morning may be effective. Long-term suppressive therapy for recurrent UTI is discussed in Chapter 5.

FEMALE URETHRAL SYNDROME

About 50% of women with frequency, urgency, dysuria, suprapubic pressure, and low backache have significant bacteriuria and these symptoms are due to urethritis coexisting with bacterial cystitis. Twenty to 30% of women with cystourethritis have low count bacteriuria, and these patients also respond well to antimicrobial therapy as recommended for cystitis. In patients with symptoms of urethritis if urinalysis shows pyuria in the face of negative urine culture, chlamydial or gonococcal urethritis should be considered. Gonococcal urethritis is diagnosed by demonstrating gram-negative intracellular diplococci in the urethral smear. If the smear is negative, a urethral specimen is sent for gonococcal culture. Although techniques for rapid detection of chlamydia by immunofluoresence using antichlamydial monoclonal antibodies and for culture of chlamydia from urethral samples are available, these tests are not used routinely. A diagnosis of chlamydial urethritis is usually made by excluding gonococcal urethritis in patients with urethral symptoms and sterile pyuria. Appropriate treatment directed against gonococcal or chlamydial infection will eradicate the symptoms. Genital herpes and vaginitis may also be associated with urethral symptoms. In middle-aged patients with lower tract symptoms, nonbacterial pyuria, and microscopic hematuria, carcinoma in situ of the bladder is a possibility, and urine cytology and cystoscopy should be performed.

About 15% of women with urethral symptoms have none of the above causes and the term "female urethral syndrome" has been applied to them. Urinalysis does not show pyuria in these patients who usually do not respond to antimicrobial therapy. The urologic examination is usually normal or minimal changes in the urethra and trigone are noted during cystoscopy. The diagnosis is usually made after excluding other causes of the lower tract symptoms. This condition can last for years and is frustrating to both patient and physician. Therapy is usually based on supportive measures such as sitz baths, antispasmodics, and urinary analgesics. Urethral dilation is occasionally effective. These patients must be informed that they do not have a serious illness and that symptomatic relief is all that we can offer. A frequent cause of this syndrome that can be easily remedied is atrophic vaginitis due to postmenopausal lack of estrogen production. Local vaginal treatment with topical estrogens (DV Cream, one full applicator at bedtime one to two times per week) provides prompt relief of symptoms.

INTERSTITIAL CYSTITIS

Interstitial cystitis is a frequently overlooked disease in my experience and is often confused with the female urethral syndrome. These patients have marked diurnal frequency and lower abdominal pain that may be relieved by voiding. Urinalysis is usually negative. Many patients report having had a negative cystoscopy, a result of endoscopy with inadequate filling of the bladder. Patients with this history required redistention of the bladder at cystoscopy, which will allow visualization of the characteristic ulcers and mucosal bleeding seen in this disease. Once the preliminary diagnosis of interstitial cystitis is made, the patient must be admitted to the hospital for bladder biopsy to rule out carcinoma in situ. Hydrodistention of the bladder under anesthesia will result in a marked improvement of the symptoms. Antispasmodics (Ditropan, 2.5 to 5 mg four times a day) combined with instillation of DMSO (dimethyl sulfoxide, Rimso-50, 50 ml intravesically) or periodic office dilation of the bladder at four- to eight-week intervals alleviates most of the symptoms. Patients who respond poorly will require repeat hydrodistention of the bladder under anesthesia. The refractory patient with a persisting small bladder capacity and urge incontinence may require augmentation of bladder capacity with small or large intestinal segments.

PROSTATITIS

Infection of the prostate can be acute or chronic. These entities are distinct: chronic prostatitis is not preceded by episodes of acute prostatitis. The causative organisms in acute prostatitis are similar to those causing UTI. Gonococcal prostatitis has become rare since the advent of antibiotics. In chronic prostatitis, in addition to these organisms, *Staphylococcus aureus* and *epidermidis* have been implicated. It has been suggested that chlamydia, mycoplasma, and viruses may play a role in causing chronic prostatitis. Pathogens may reach the prostate by hematogenous spread, by ascending the urethra, or via lymphatics from the rectum. Urethral instrumentation, prostatic surgery, and sexual intercourse with a partner who has vaginal colonization by enteric bacteria are possible risk factors predisposing to prostatitis.

ACUTE PROSTATITIS

High fever, chills, perineal and back pain, and symptoms of cystourethritis are the presenting symptoms of acute prostatitis. Urinary retention may occur. This condition is diagnosed easily: a warm, swollen, and extremely tender prostate is found on rectal examination. The causative organism can almost always be grown on urine culture. Prostatic massage to obtain specimens from the gland for culture is contraindicated in acute prostatitis, since bacteremia may result. It should be remembered that urethral discharge is unusual in acute prostatitis. However, in urethritis due to gonococcal or chlamydial infection, the prostate may be secondarily infected. The presence of prostatic tenderness is the clue to the diagnosis in these patients.

Antimicrobial therapy as recommended for acute UTI is very effective in acute prostatitis because the causative organisms are similar and drugs readily penetrate into acutely inflamed prostatic tissue. However, in acute prostatitis, duration of therapy should be longer—four to six weeks. Severely ill patients require hospitalization. Sitz baths, antispasmodics (Ditropan, 2.5 to 5 mg q.i.d.), urinary analgesics (Pyridium, 200 mg t.i.d.), and laxatives provide symptomatic relief. If urinary retention develops, suprapubic bladder aspiration or temporary suprapubic cystotomy should be used. Urethral catheterization is to be avoided, since it is extremely painful in patients with acute prostatitis. If symptoms do not subside quickly with these measures, the possibility of a prostatic abscess should be considered and surgical drainage may be required.

CHRONIC PROSTATITIS

Unlike acute prostatitis, patients with chronic bacterial prostatitis may be asymptomatic or may have mild but annoying symptoms such as perineal discomfort, low back pain, and intermittent low grade fever. Recurrent UTI may occur in patients with chronic prostatitis in the absence of symptoms referable to the prostate. Rectal examination is usually unremarkable. X-ray examination of the prostate may reveal prostatic calculi. The diagnosis of chronic prostatitis is difficult and requires simultaneous quantitative culture of initially voided urine (urethral specimen), midstream urine (bladder specimen), prostatic secretion expressed by massage, and urine voided after prostatic massage. Chronic prostatitis is diagnosed if either of the last two specimens yields bacterial growth at least tenfold greater than the first two specimens. Fluid expressed by prostatic massage in patients with chronic prostatitis has more than 10 WBC/hpf and numerous lipid-laden macrophages. The normal prostatic secretion has antibacterial property but this is lacking in chronic prostatitis.

Most of the drugs used to treat UTI are ineffective in chronic prostatitis since they do not penetrate well into the gland. Erythromycin, clindamycin, trimethoprim, and rifampin are the exceptions. The first two drugs are useful only in infection by gram-positive organisms. Sulfamethoxazole-trimethoprim (Bactrim or Septra, one double-strength tablet twice a day) for six to 12 weeks is the recommended regimen for chronic prostatitis. It is unclear if the sulfonamide adds to the effect of trimethoprim and rifampin. Even prolonged treatment may not eradicate the prostatic infection and relapses are common. In patients with recurrent UTI secondary to chronic prostatitis, long-term suppressive therapy with smaller doses of trimethoprim-sulfamethoxazole (one half of a single-strength tablet q.h.s.) may be effective. Transurethral resection of the prostate does not usually eradicate all foci of infection within the gland. Total prostatectomy is curative but is associated with considerable morbidity. These surgical procedures are not recommended for the treatment of chronic prostatitis.

PROSTATODYNIA

This condition is characterized by painful lower urinary tract symptoms and low back or perineal ache. The symptoms are similar to chronic prostatitis but urinalysis, urine culture, and culture of prostatic secretion are negative. There is no history of UTI. I go to great lengths to reassure these patients that antimicrobial therapy is not necessary. A post–prostatic massage urine culture, excretory urogram (IVP), and occasionally cystourethroscopy are necessary to convince these patients that they have a neuromuscular disorder of the pelvic floor. Antispasmodics and sitz baths are prescribed for symptomatic relief. Diazepam (Valium), 5 mg two or three times a day, has helped many of my patients. Periodic prostatic massage and nonsteroidal anti-inflammatory drugs are sometimes effective. In refractory cases, the patient is referred for psychiatric evaluation for possible behavior modification.

IMPOTENCE

Patients presenting with impotence should be questioned carefully to determine the exact nature of their problem. Decreased libido, inability to obtain or maintain erection, premature or absent ejaculation, and failure to achieve orgasm may all be referred to as impotence, but each of these symptoms has different causes. Impotence is most often due to psychological factors such as anxiety about sexual performance, depression, and marital discord. If penile erection is normal, loss of libido and failure to achieve orgasm are almost always psychogenic in origin. The organic causes of defective erection include testosterone deficiency, hyperprolactinemia, drugs (beta-blockers, reserpine, clonidine, methyldopa, spironolactone, thiazides, antidepressants, psychotropic drugs, tranquilizers), alcohol or heroin abuse, neurologic disorders that affect penile innervation (temporal lobe lesions, diabetes mellitus, tabes dorsalis, spinal cord disease), damage to nervi erigentes by total prostatectomy or rectosigmoid surgery, and penile vascular insufficiency due to aortoiliac occlusive disease. Absence of ejaculation is usually due to retrograde ejaculation into the bladder and can be caused by sympathectomy or drugs such as guanethidine, phenoxybenzamine, or phentolamine.

The first step in the management of impotence is to identify whether it is psychogenic or organic. In a patient complaining of defective erection, the continued occurrence of penile erection upon waking up or the documentation of normal nocturnal penile tumescence (NPT) during rapid eye movement (REM) sleep points strongly to functional impotence. Sexual dysfunction occurring only with some partners or only under certain cirumstances is evidence against organic impotence. Determination of testosterone, prolactin and gonadotropin levels, measurement of penile blood flow by the Doppler technique or arteriography, and testing the innervation of the penis with conduction studies of the bulbocavernosus reflex may be required in the evaluation of patients with suspected organic impotence.

Reassurance, sexual counseling, and occasionally a placebo or aphrodisiac (Yohimex, 5 mg t.i.d.) are indicated in patients with psychogenic impotence. Some causes of organic impotence can be easily remedied (e.g., testosterone deficiency or drug-induced impotence). Surgical revascularization of the penis in patients with decreased penile blood flow is occasionally feasible. If the organic cause cannot be corrected, referral to a urologist for consideration of a penile prosthesis is indicated.

REFERENCES

Drach GW: Prostatitis and prostatodynia. Urol Clin North Am 7:79–80, 1980.

Meares EM Jr: Prostatitis and related disorders. *In* Walsh PC, Gittes RF, Perlmutter AD, et al (eds): Campbell's Urology, 5th ed. W. B. Saunders Co, Philadelphia, 1986, pp 868–887.

Shortliffe LMD, Stamey TA: Urinary infections in adult women. *In* Walsh PC, Gittes RF, Perlmutter AD, et al (eds): Campbell's Urology, 5th ed. W. B. Saunders Co, Philadelphia, 1986, pp 797–830.

Sobel JD, Kaye D: Urinary tract infections. *In* Mandell GL, Douglas RG, Bennett JE (eds): Principles and Practice of Infectious Diseases, 2nd ed. John Wiley and Sons, New York, 1985, pp 426–452.

METABOLIC DISORDERS

A. CADER ASMAL

1 · TREATMENT OF THE PATIENT WITH TYPE I DIABETES

Richard S. Beaser
John W. Hare
JOSLIN CLINIC

DEFINITION

Diabetes mellitus is a metabolic disorder characterized by an absolute or relative deficiency of insulin. Type I or insulin-dependent diabetes mellitus (IDDM) results from an absolute lack of insulin, in contrast to type II or non–insulin-dependent diabetes mellitus (NIDDM), where the defect is a reduction in insulin action and a relative insufficiency of insulin. The diagnosis of type I diabetes can usually be made clinically based on the symptoms of polyuria, polydipsia, polyphagia and weight loss, and confirmed by the findings of glycosuria, ketonuria, and hyperglycemia. Rarely, an oral glucose tolerance test may be required for confirmation.

PATHOPHYSIOLOGY

There is strong evidence to suggest that IDDM is an autoimmune disease that develops with increased propensity in persons with the HLA genotype DR3 or DR4. At the outset of the disease, up to 70% of people with IDDM have the presence of islet cell antibodies (ICA) and up to 40% or 50% have IA-positive T lymphocytes, suggesting an immune disturbance.

Insulin lack is the hallmark of IDDM. Since insulin is critical to normal anabolic events in muscle, liver, and adipocytes, its deficiency results in major metabolic derangements. Acute insulin deficiency results in increased free fatty acid oxidation, ketone production, and diabetic ketoacidosis (DKA). The chronic hyperglycemia of poorly controlled diabetes contributes to the development of the complications that often accompany this disease.

CLINICAL PRESENTATION

The *classic* type I diabetic patient is a school-aged child of normal body weight, presenting with rapid weight loss, polyuria, polydipsia, polyphagia, and blurred vision. The findings of hyperglycemia, glycosuria, and ketonuria confirm the diagnosis. If untreated, dehydration and ketoacidotic coma ensue.

Type I diabetes may occasionally develop in either obese or nonobese older individuals. In these people the disease onset is often less precipitous, resembling type II diabetes. However, failure to respond to oral hypoglycemic agents may be the initial clue to the true nature of the diabetes.

MANAGEMENT

PLAN

Since there is substantial evidence that improved control reduces the likelihood of diabetic complications, the ideal goal of therapy is the attainment of normoglycemia. However, achieving this ideal can present many practical problems. Therefore, individual ability and interest levels should play a key role in designing a treatment program and setting therapeutic goals.

In the absence of ketoacidosis, hospitalization is not always necessary. Even for the newly diagnosed patient, injection techniques can be taught in an outpatient setting, and control can usually be established easily. Elderly, visually impaired, or otherwise infirm patients may need hospitalization for this purpose. Ultimately, the treatment program for all patients must be "fine-tuned" to their outpatient life style.

NONPHARMACOLOGIC MEASURES
Diet

The three interdependent principles of therapy of type I diabetes are diet, exercise, and insulin. "Diet" often implies a restriction of calories to reduce weight, yet for many persons with type I diabetes, the objective is weight maintenance or even gain. For any prescribed eating plan to be accepted by the patient, it must be carefully tailored to the individual's preferences while meeting the goals of diabetic therapy. It must also, of course, be properly taught to the patient (and his/her family or others interested). Appropriate follow-up is essential both to answer questions and to reinforce compliance. Restructuring the plan may be necessary to increase patient acceptance.

Professional nutritional counseling is the most effective means of providing effective dietary instruction. However, the physician must assess the patient's medical needs and set the goals of therapy. Food quantity should be determined based on desired changes in patient weight. If a person is of average activity, prescribe about 25 kcal/kg of *ideal* body weight to maintain present actual weight, 30 kcal/kg (or more) to promote weight gain, and 20 kcal/kg for weight loss. Adjustments upward or downward by 10% should be made for large or small frames, and unusually active people will require extra calories. After taking a diet history, a dietitian can use standard food exchange lists to design a meal plan with a balance of substances similar to that of type II diabetic diet (carbohydrate 45% to 55%, protein 20%, fat 30% [10% each unsaturated, monounsaturated, saturated]), but with the appropriate quantities for the type I individual. The daily caloric allotment is distributed into meals and snacks, avoiding intake of large caloric loads at once.

Recent trends in dietary management have included eating foods higher in dietary fiber, which blunt postprandial hyperglycemia. In addition, the advent of nonnutritive sweeteners has resulted in greater food variety.

Exercise. Exercise is effective in lowering blood glucose levels in persons with well-controlled diabetes by potentiating the action of insulin. In those with poorly controlled diabetes, however, exercise may paradoxically produce a rise in blood glucose and ketone levels by stimulating glucose production from the liver via a rise in the counterregulatory hormones glucagon and epinephrine. Regular, structured exercise as well as an overall increase in the level of activity in keeping with an individual's physical abilities should be encouraged, since compensatory adjustments in food consumption and insulin dose can easily be made. Conversely, irregular activity and failure to adjust the eating or insulin can accentuate the instability of diabetes control and promote unpleasant hypoglycemic reactions.

PHARMACOLOGIC TREATMENT MODALITIES

Drug Selection

Once it is determined that a person has type I diabetes, therapy with one of the various types of insulin is required. Table 1 outlines the characteristics of the various types of insulin now available. Commercially available insulins have traditionally been pork, beef, or beef-pork mixtures. Recently, human insulins have reached the market (Table 1). All commercially available insulins have impurities, consisting of substances such as proinsulin, glucagon, and somatostatin for the products made by extraction of animal insulins, and bacterial peptides in the synthetic human products.

The quantities of impurities in standard insulin (50 parts per million [ppm]) or purer insulins (5 ppm) are much reduced from levels standard prior to 1972 (10,000 ppm), but still may cause difficulties on occasion (see later). The indications for use of a purer (5 ppm) or same (human) species insulin would be patients with (1) a local allergy to beef-pork, beef, or pork insulin, (2) lipodystrophy, (3) true immunologic resistance to beef and/or pork insulin (not to be confused with overinsulinization and/or poor dietary compliance), and (4) temporary insulin therapy (during surgery or illness). Most newly diagnosed type I patients are now started on human insulin.

Insulin Administration Regimens

The newly diagnosed type I diabetic patient can usually be treated adequately with one daily morning injection of an intermediate insulin (NPH or Lente). Some patients may experience an early reduction in insulin requirements, known as a remission or "honeymoon" period. However, these people will inevitably require a larger dose of insulin again within a year. After five to eight years of diabetes, endogenous pancreatic insulin production may drop to insignificant levels, and the single morning dose will likely need supplementation by additional daily injections. The regimen of insulin administration, the number of daily injections, and the insulin types required are related to the inherent stability of the diabetes. The stability or "brittleness" of blood glucose levels is probably determined by the degree of residual insulin secretory capacity, although the precise cause is often not really known.

Single Dose. The single morning dose of intermediate insulin can be adjusted to correct hyperglycemia at various times of the day. If high prelunch glucose levels occur, they may be treated by substituting regular insulin for some of the morning intermediate insulin. The morning intermediate insulin may also be increased to provide full 24-hour coverage.

Split Dose. Eventually, the single dose may result in hypoglycemia in the afternoon and evening, while failing to control glucose levels throughout the full 24 hours, and a split insulin dose would be indicated. The second injection may consist of regular plus intermediate insulin before supper, especially if the patient has a marked rise in glucose level between supper and bedtime. Alternatively, intermediate insulin given at bedtime would be preferable if fasting or prelunch glucose levels were still high in spite of a presupper dose. When a second injection is added, the morning insulin dose can often be reduced. The total daily insulin quantity, when split, is often divided so that two thirds is prebreakfast and one third is presupper. If a bedtime dose

Table 1. CHARACTERISTICS AND ACTIONS OF COMMONLY USED INSULIN

Action Category	Type	Products Available	Action (hours)	
			Peak	Duration
Rapid	Regular (crystalline)	p, bp, P, P*, B, Hr, Hs	2–4	5–7
	Semilente	b, bp, P	2–8	12–16
Intermediate	NPH (Isophane)	b, bp, B, P, P*, Hr, Hs	6–12	18–24
	Lente	b, bp, B, P, Hr, Hs	6–12	18–24
Slow	Ultralente	b, bp, B	16–18	24–36
	Protamine Zinc	bp, B, P	14–20	24–36

Key: Standard insulins (approximately 50 parts per million [ppm] impurities); b = beef; p = pork, bp = beef/pork mixture. Purified insulins (< 5 ppm impurities): B = beef; P = pork, P* = pork mixture of 30% regular and 70% NPH; Hr = human–recombinant DNA origin; Hs = human–semisynthetic (from porcine) origin.

is used, a slightly higher morning fraction may be used. Within each dose, regular insulin usually consists of one fourth to one third of the total, with the remainder as intermediate insulin.

The total daily insulin dose is about 0.5 units per kilogram of body weight for an adult with type I diabetes of five to eight years' duration. Youngsters and adolescents often need more. In general, when making a change in the program, it is best to underdose initially, then use some home blood glucose monitoring to increase the dose as needed.

Ultralente. The optimal insulin administration plan would mimic the function of a normal pancreas, which secretes a basal level of insulin with supplementary output in response to ingested food. One program that approaches this pattern utilizes Ultralente and regular insulin. Ultralente itself peaks unpredictably, but when used twice daily in moderate doses it may simulate the pancreatic basal output. Approximately 50% of the daily total insulin dose is divided between two doses of Ultralente, given prebreakfast and presupper. The remaining insulin (50%) is given as premeal regular insulin boluses, approximately 20% prebreakfast and 15% prelunch and presupper. (A variation of this program is to give regular insulin premeals, plus intermediate insulin at supper or bedtime.) With daily premeal blood testing, the doses of regular insulin can be titrated to the actual blood glucose levels at the time of injection. This program is especially useful for people with quite unstable diabetes, or with inconsistent life styles.

Mechanical Pumps. When a patient cannot achieve acceptable control using these various injection regimens, the battery-driven mechanical pumps may be used. They simulate the pancreatic basal output with a constant subcutaneous flow of regular insulin, plus give boluses of regular insulin premeals and presnacks. The doses of insulin are similar to those used with Ultralente and regular, with the equivalent of the Ultralente dose being delivered over 24 hours as the basal. As these devices provide a constant insulin infusion day and night, constant home blood monitoring is essential. Obviously, patients must be sufficiently intelligent and motivated to undertake the effort of pump self-management.

Adverse Effects of Insulin

Insulin Allergy. Insulin allergy is usually local, is mild, and disappears spontaneously. It may present as slight, localized erythema, swelling, stinging or itching, or marked swelling, pain, or induration. These reactions usually appear within 15 to 20 minutes of injection, although rarely the response can be delayed. They often subside with continued injections or on switching insulin. Local symptomatic treatment or systemic antihistamines can provide temporary relief. Rarely, the allergy may manifest itself systematically with generalized urticaria or angioedema. Desensitization kits and instructions are available from insulin manufacturers to treat this complication.

Patients newly started on insulin with rapidly improving diabetes control may also develop "insulin" edema of the hands or lower extremities, which usually disappears spontaneously within a few weeks.

Insulin Resistance. True insulin resistance—the requirement of over 200 units of insulin daily for over two or three days—may be due to immunologic or nonimmunologic mechanisms. However, most persons receiving insulin injections develop insulin antibodies (usually IgG) without clinical consequence.

The treatment of immunologic insulin resistance in type I patients includes: (1) switching species; often human insulin may help; (2) a course of prednisone, starting with large doses of about 60 mg daily and tapering over three to four weeks; (3) a trial of sulfated insulin; and (4) passage of time. U-500 insulin is available for those patients requiring extremely large insulin doses.

Hypoglycemia. Insulin may induce hypoglycemia if administered in too great a quantity for the amount of food intake or activity. Although the body will release glucose from the liver's glycogen stores, oral supplementation is often advisable. Should the patient be unable to take oral glucose, subcutaneous or intramuscular injection of glucagon, 1 mg, will cause a blood sugar rise. Patients and their families can be taught to administer glucagon. In a hospital setting, especially if there is stupor or coma, an intravenous bolus of 50% dextrose in water is indicated.

Interference by Concomitant Disease

Almost any illness in a type I diabetic can increase insulin needs and precipitate ketoacidosis. It is, therefore, essential that patients are thoroughly educated in "sick-day" management procedures. Blood glucose and urine ketone levels should be tested every three to four hours, day and night. If the blood glucose is over 240 mg/dl, and the ketones are moderate or high, an incremental dose of regular insulin, up to 20% of the total daily dose, should be given immediately. If the timing is concurrent with a scheduled dose, the increment may be added to the usual dose. Testing, with supplementary insulin administration if necessary, should be continued every three to four hours *around the clock* until the illness subsides. If, after 24 hours of supplementation, the glucose level is not controlled or if the patient cannot hold down food, professional help should be sought.

Interference by Other Medications

Many medications raise blood glucose levels (e.g., glucocorticoids, thiazides) and appropriate insulin dose adjustments can be used to compensate. Beta-adrenergic blockers may mask some of the early signs and symptoms of hypoglycemic reactions and must be used with care, although they are not contraindicated in a well-controlled diabetic patient. The cardioselective beta-blockers may be somewhat safer in this situation. Alcohol, especially if consumed without other sources of calories, suppresses gluconeogenesis and can produce severe hypoglycemia in a person with type I diabetes.

PATIENT EDUCATION

From the previous discussions, it is obvious that the diabetic individual is confronted with learning skills—proper diet, insulin usage, home monitoring, and proper self-care—that are necessary for maintaining his or her good health. An essential part of diabetes therapy is ongoing patient education to equip the individual with these skills, and update them as needed.

PERIODIC EVALUATION OF THE TYPE I DIABETIC PATIENT BEYOND DIAGNOSIS

Office visits play an important role in the lifelong treatment of the type I diabetic patient, both to monitor for complications and to provide guidance on balancing the insulin, eating, and activity levels. Thus, after the initial period of instruction for a new diabetic, physician visits three to four times per year are advised.

At each visit, recent diabetic control should be assessed, including a review of records of home monitoring. Evaluation should also include examination of the eyes for evidence of retinopathy, the carotid and peripheral arteries for evidence of ischemia, and the peripheral reflexes and sensation for evidence of neuropathy. The blood pressure and urinalysis provide a clue as to the existence of nephropathy.

It is often prudent to recommend routine evaluations by an ophthalmologist and a podiatrist as well. Specific findings from the diabetes evaluation might also indicate that additional consultations by a nephrologist or vascular surgeon are needed.

Assessment of Control. Patients should clearly understand that they cannot determine their level of control by the symptoms they feel. Regular assessment of control, based on home blood or urine glucose monitoring plus glycohemoglobin levels, is critical. The glycohemoglobin can greatly assist efforts to maintain good blood glucose levels. This test reflects the average blood glucose level over the previous one to two months. It should be remembered that the glycohemoglobin level is an average, and reveals nothing about daily excursions of glucose levels. Thus, a patient having frequent hypo- and hyperglycemia might show a fairly good average, but home monitoring logs would tell the true story.

Home Monitoring. Home blood glucose monitoring (HBGM) may be used to determine when or why control may be suboptimal. The use of test strips (Chemstrip bG, Visidex) is usually sufficient, but meters provide more accurate results, especially for those with visual impairment or color blindness, or those wanting or requiring this additional accuracy.

For most type I patients, "block blood testing" is useful. Patients should test their blood four times daily (premeals and bedtime) for four days in a row. Additional tests during this block can be performed concurrently with exercise or at night to look for nocturnal hypoglycemic reactions with early morning rebounds. These results should be written down so that the patterns can be examined and the trends remembered later. These blocks can be repeated routinely one to three times per month, but more frequently after a major dosage change or an alteration of life style. Consistent upward or downward trends over a few days can help pinpoint the need for dose adjustments. A realistic goal of therapy is premeal glucose levels between 80 and 130 mg/dl, and under 180 mg/dl one to two hours postprandially, although these levels cannot always be achieved for all patients. In between blocks, less frequent blood testing (once or twice a day) or even urine tests can be performed to be sure that marked hyperglycemia has not occurred.

For patients unwilling or unable to perform HBGM, regular urine testing still provides some useful information. Moreover, some patients may require daily insulin adjustments. Blood testing four times daily every day may be required, with resultant insulin dose adjustments based on algorithms. HBGM can also add flexibility to a patient's schedule of eating and activity.

PATIENT COMPLIANCE

The requirements of patient involvement in the care of his or her diabetes are great, but some people are more willing than others to undertake such a long-term effort. Initial assessment of the patient's abilities determines therapeutic goals at the outset. However, the patient more actively involved in his own care is more likely to maintain appropriate compliance. Fear tactics are rarely helpful.

PREVENTIVE MEASURES

The main goal of therapy of diabetes is the prevention of complications. In addition, it is important to eliminate risk factors of associated diseases by treating conditions, such as hyperlipidemia, hypertension, and avoiding smoking.

FAMILY COUNSELING

The offspring of one type I diabetic parent have a 1% to 5% chance of developing diabetes, which is somewhat greater if both parents are affected. The sibling of a diabetic child has a 5% to 10% chance of developing the disease.

SOCIOECONOMIC ASPECTS OF MANAGEMENT

Diabetes is an expensive disease, and the burden for those with limited means may not be supported by many insurance programs. Thus, financial constraints might manifest themselves as lack of compliance, refusal of educational opportunities, poorer dietary compliance, or decreased frequency of office visits or hospitalizations for regulation. In addition, complications can have an astronomical cost in lost wages and medical expenses. Health care professionals should be sensitive to these economic issues that may confront their patients, and assist the patient in obtaining the proper counseling or social support when financial difficulties provide further complications.

REFERENCES

Arky RA: Clinical correlates of metabolic derangements of diabetes mellitus. *In* Kozak GP (ed): Clinical Diabetes Mellitus. W.B. Saunders Co, Philadelphia, 1982, pp 16–20.

Bolli GB, Gottesman IS, Campbell PJ, et al: Glucose counter regulation and waning of insulin in the Somogyi phenomenon (posthypoglycemic hyperglycemia). N Engl J Med 311:1214–1219, 1984.

Flood, TM, Halford BN, Cooppan R, et al: Dietary management of diabetes. *In* Marble A (ed): Joslin's Diabetes Mellitus. Lea & Febiger, Philadelphia, 1985, pp 357–379.

Galloway JA, deShazo RD: The clinical use of insulin and the complications of insulin therapy. *In* Ellenberg M, Rifkin H (eds): Diabetes Mellitus. Medical Examination Publishing, Inc., New Hyde Park, NY, 1983, pp 519–538.

Marble A: Insulin in the treatment of diabetes. *In* Marble A (ed): Joslin's Diabetes Mellitus. Lea & Febiger, Philadelphia, 1985, pp 380–405.

2 · NON–INSULIN-DEPENDENT DIABETES MELLITUS

Fred W. Whitehouse
Dorothy M. Kahkonen
HENRY FORD HOSPITAL

DEFINITION AND DIAGNOSTIC CRITERIA

Type II or non–insulin-dependent diabetes mellitus (NIDDM) occurs at any age but with increasing frequency after the age of 40 years. It is commonly associated with obesity and a family history of diabetes. However, there is no characteristic genetic pattern and no relation to specific HLA haplotypes as exists in type I diabetes. A subtype occurs in younger people called maturity-onset diabetes in the young (MODY) and is inherited as an autosomal dominant trait.

Diagnosis is confirmed by fasting hyperglycemia (140 mg/dl plasma or greater on more than one occasion) or by plasma glucose levels over 200 mg/dl at one and two hours after oral glucose. Often one fasting plasma glucose over 140 mg/dl and one postprandial level above 200 mg/dl confirm the diagnosis.

PATHOPHYSIOLOGY

NIDDM, although associated with ineffective insulin action, is not characterized by absence of insulin effect. Thus, insufficient insulin secreted by the pancreatic beta cell and ineffectively working at the liver, muscle, or fat cell creates a milieu in which too much glucose is made by the liver (enhanced glucogenesis) concomitant with an increase in peripheral resistance to insulin (diminished glucose utilization). The degree to which inadequate insulin release or enhanced insulin resistance occurs is reflected by the clinical intensity of the diabetic state. On the one hand, there may be minimal peripheral insulin resistance and limited secretory defect in early type II diabetes; on the other, there may be significant peripheral resistance and a major insulin secretory defect mimicking type I diabetes. At times, one may be hard-pressed to differentiate type I and type II diabetes in a specific patient. Measuring fasting and post-stimulatory C-peptide levels in serum may help in definition, but rarely is indicated for proper clinical management. It is important to remember that *non–insulin-dependent* is not synonymous with *non–insulin-requiring*. In our clinical practice only 25% of NIDDM patients are controlled by diet alone or diet and an oral hypoglycemic agent.

CLINICAL ASPECTS

Most often, the patient with NIDDM is asymptomatic or presents problems related to metabolic or vascular complications (namely, neuropathy [burning feet], premature vascular disease such as myocardial infarction or gangrenous toe, furunculosis [recurring boils], or early cataracts). Infrequently, the diagnosis is suspected when patients present with the classic symptoms of diabetes (thirst, increased urination, pruritic genitalia, weight loss, and fatigue). Thirty to 50% of women with NIDDM have had babies with a birth weight over 4000 grams. Obesity is present in 80% of the patients. Peculiar to the person with NIDDM will be the presence of significant hyperglycemia without ketonuria. Hyperosmolar coma rarely occurs and acidosis even less often presents as a complication of an underlying stress.

Diet is the cornerstone of therapy as in all diabetic patients and may alone achieve metabolic control in many patients with NIDDM. Oral hypoglycemic drugs will effectively substitute for insulin in others, but often insulin will be required to relieve symptoms and achieve acceptable biochemical control.

MANAGEMENT

PLAN

Treatment Goals. Although therapy should be individualized, we try to restore the biochemical state as close to normal as possible after correcting the symptoms due to uncontrolled diabetes. Correction of symptoms alleviates discomfort; restoring biochemical normalcy lowers risk for future diabetic complications.

Goals include normal blood glucose, glycosylated hemoglobin (HgbA1c) and serum lipid levels, weight within 120% of ideal body weight, and a tranquil state of mind regarding the presence of an incurable disease. To paraphrase Robert Louis Stevenson, "It is not important to decide whether the hand of cards is a good one or a poor one; rather it is more important to play a poor hand well."

Fasting blood glucose levels should range from 70 to 120 mg/dl while postcibal levels should average below 200 mg/dl. Normal HgbA1c will depend on the method used. Generally, we aim for less than four standard deviations (SD) above the mean of the nondiabetic level. Although hard data are lacking, we prefer that our diabetic patients achieve HgbA1c levels below 9.0% (normal = 4.0%–7.0%). Serum cholesterol and triglycerides should measure less than 220 mg/dl and 160 mg/dl respectively. We encourage a life style with minimal hypoglycemia while accomplishing these goals. The immediate benefit of a normal metabolic state means a state of well-being and no acute complications; the hoped-for long-term benefits include few or no vascular complications.

Ambulatory Treatment. Excepting extraordinary medical circumstances (ketoacidosis, hyperosmolar states, severe complicating medical illnesses) or difficult social situations with the lack of family support, we treat our patients in the *office*, promptly starting diet counseling, instituting insulin or oral hypoglycemic agents as indicated, and establishing methods of self-monitoring of diabetes at home and stepwise education in self-care. For many patients, we will recommend attendance at one of our three-day outpatient diabetes regulation and management programs structured to achieve a small group atmosphere. Assisting patients with NIDDM in a more natural environment together with other diabetic patients offers immediate encour-

Table 1. EDUCATION OF THE PATIENT WITH DIABETES

What every diabetic patient should know:
1. General information about diabetes (including why good control is essential, the risks if uncontrolled).
2. Importance of diet plan and how to incorporate it into the patient's life style.
3. Testing the urine and/or the blood glucose.
4. Proper foot care.
5. Sick-day care.
6. Why one might need an oral agent or insulin.

What the insulin-taking diabetic patient also needs to know:
1. How to take insulin.
2. Type of insulin taken—onset, peak, and duration.
3. Care of syringes, needles, and insulin.
4. Self-monitoring blood glucose.
5. Testing the urine for acetone.
6. Recognizing and treating low blood sugar.
7. How to use glucagon.
8. Sick-day care when using insulin.

agement, giving them the opportunity to "take charge of their own health." In this regard, the patient must be a member of the health care team.

PATIENT INFORMATION AND EDUCATION

The educational process begins with the first encounter between the patient and the health care provider and must be ongoing. We find that a multidisciplinary approach with help from the physician, clinical nurse specialist, diabetes educator, dietitian, social worker, and psychologist offers the patient much support. These contacts should increase the patient's knowledge and understanding of the diabetes management and permit development of independence in self-care. The time to achieve independence varies from patient to patient, but it will occur sooner in the milieu where a structured educational plan exists.

Patients and family members are encouraged to become involved in the educational process early in their care. Contracting is a method of negotiating patients' boundaries of responsibility for health care. Our experience with written contracts is limited, although we have found that patients respond positively to clinical research programs requiring informed consent. Patients and families may be assisted to set realistically achievable goals through contracting, which will also help the health care providers be realistic in their expectations of the patient.

Education of the patient with diabetes should include general information about the disease and specific self-care regimens as outlined in Table 1. Comprehensive hospital programs should include both inpatient and outpatient education programs. Physicians in the community who do not have the support of health care teams available to them need to be aware of these resources and utilize them. Often a patient hospitalized with an acute illness will return shortly after discharge to our outpatient education program for further help with self-care. People do not learn self-care well during an acute illness; however, we want patients with diabetes to be motivated to learn.

NUTRITIONAL MODIFICATION (THE DIET)

In general, patients with type II diabetes eat too many calories, eat too much fat and cholesterol, and often use too much salt. When these patients age, and particularly when they live alone on restricted finances, the physician must stress the importance of a balanced diet. Are fruits, vegetables, and proteins included daily? Is there hidden malnutrition? Many patients with NIDDM are obese. For them, a diet has several purposes: (1) to eliminate extra fat tissue and approach normal body weight, thus lessening peripheral insulin resistance; (2) to ensure an adequate intake of protein and other needed nutrients, yet to supply an adequate intake of carbohydrate for energy; and (3) to restrict calories derived from animal fat, which will lower cholesterol intake.

For weight reduction, we prescribe 20 kcal/kg ideal body weight (IBW) distributed over three meals and a bedtime snack. Patients who use insulin may require a midafternoon snack. For patients who should maintain their weight, we start with 25 to 30 kcal/kg IBW with adjustments in caloric intake depending upon body frame, the degree of physical activity, and previous weight change. When a patient requires weight gain because of a previous illness or a severe loss of weight related to uncontrolled diabetes, we prescribe 40 kcal/kg IBW. As a "rule of thumb" for adequate weight, we suggest:

For women: 100 lb for 5 feet of height plus 5 lb per inch above 5 feet.

For men: 106 lb for 5 feet plus 6 lb per inch above 5 feet

Patients should be less than 120% IBW.

Alcohol yields 7 kcal/gm and is void of nutritional value. Distilled whiskeys average one calorie per ounce per proof. Most wines and beers contain somewhere between 50 and 150 calories per serving. Clearly, patients who need to lose weight should avoid alcohol.

In the United States, the average intake of carbohydrate ranges from 40% to 50% of total calories, which is lower than the world average. This has led to higher intake of fat calories and cholesterol than is safe, which has accentuated the risk of atherosclerosis. We suggest that:

1. Carbohydrates should total 50% to 60% of the daily caloric intake.

2. More carbohydrates should be complex (starches), while fewer simple sugars (oligosaccharides) should be eaten.

3. Higher fiber foods, which slow the absorption of glucose from the gut and blunt the rise of the blood glucose after a meal, should be preferred, since they will satiate the individual and decrease appetite.

4. Highly concentrated oligosaccharides (sweets) should be avoided.

Recent studies have suggested that the rate of carbohydrate absorption may vary greatly from patient to patient and from foodstuff to foodstuff. The glycemic index (Jenkins) gives the areas of the blood glucose response curve for various foodstuffs as a percentage of the area after the same amount of carbohydrate ingested as glucose. These data will guide the patient to those carbohydrates more slowly absorbed.

Adequate protein intake ensures good tissue repair and adequate muscle mass. Ten to 15% of total calories should be protein. We advise from 0.5 to 1.0 gm/kg

IBW of protein daily. Protein should be high quality but not necessarily of animal source. Many high quality proteins come from vegetable sources and are included in the higher fiber diets, especially when legumes and soybean products are used.

The American diet still contains much animal fat and cholesterol. Diabetic patients should lower the dietary fat to less than 30% of total calories and include a greater intake of vegetable than animal fat and limit the cholesterol intake to 300 mg/day. Some vegetable fat sources are preferred because of a greater concentration of polyunsaturated fats. Unexpected sources of fat in the diet can be identified by the amount of meat and cheese eaten. Restricting high-fat meat will restrict saturated fats. "Fast foods," sausage, bacon, and lunchmeats contain much animal fat. Animal and vegetable fat are equal in calories and both should be restricted in weight-reducing diets.

An appropriate dietary prescription, properly understood and followed, is the touchstone of the treatment of the patient with type II diabetes. Since a "tear out" diet is inadequate for the patient, the demands on the average physician together with a lack of familiarity with the details of nutrition make a visit between the patient and a competent nutritionist mandatory. Here the prescribed diet can be reviewed and the major points of dietary modification emphasized. Continuing support by both the physician and the nutritionist will be required to ensure adherence. Both must be patient but persistent in helping the diabetic person with the diet. Socioeconomic issues, such as money available to buy food, an understanding of simple dietary principles, and ingrained cultural habits will affect the success of the diet prescription.

While most diabetic patients may not achieve ideal weight, some weight reduction will decrease peripheral resistance to insulin and improve metabolic control. A weight loss of one pound per week is reasonable. Give the patient a short-term achievable goal rather than one that is perceived by the patient as impossible. While many factors contribute to insulin resistance, and although some patients with type II diabetes have significant degrees of insulin deficiency, some residual endogenous insulin is secreted from the beta cells. Minimizing excess weight takes advantage of endogenous insulin secretion and allows the patient to control the diabetic state either with diet alone or with a minimum amount of medication.

DRUG THERAPY

Insulin. Some NIDDM patients will require insulin for control of hyperglycemia or to prevent symptoms. Some of these insulin-requiring patients have been unsuccessful with diet; others have too great an insulin deficiency to get along without exogenous insulin. Often, the former have been unable to achieve or maintain ideal body weight, which is the most appropriate and effective treatment for type II diabetes.

Insulin preparations commonly used by us are regular (short-acting) and NPH or Lente (intermediate-acting). We rarely use Semilente, Ultralente, or protamine zinc insulins. Most of our patients take beef or mixed beef-pork insulin without incident (see Chapter 1). However, we tend to use human insulin more often for new patients who require insulin. Certainly those few patients with local or systemic immunogenic side effects should use human insulin. Starting insulin can easily be done in an office setting. We prefer one of our three-day regulation and education programs where the insulin prescription can be adjusted daily; then the patient can visit members of the team every few days for appropriate follow-up advice. For type II patients, we rarely use more than two injections of insulin daily. We have no type II patients on continuous subcutaneous insulin infusion systems (CSII) and only a few on multiple daily doses of insulin (MDI). A split mixture of regular and intermediate insulin taken before breakfast and supper is sometimes advised in our NIDDM patients. Often their dose of regular insulin is adjusted by an algorithm related to the capillary blood glucose measured at the time of the insulin injection. However, most NIDDM patients require only one insulin injection daily, usually a dose of intermediate insulin of less than 40 units given before breakfast. At normal or near-normal weight, these patients will require from 0.25 to 0.75 units of insulin/kg/day.

Oral Hypoglycemic Agents. The controversy aroused by the University Group Diabetes Program (UGDP) has abated. Although the findings and recommendations of this study have been questioned, the study did highlight the importance of diet in the management of type II diabetes and placed the use of oral hypoglycemic agents in proper perspective. These drugs increase the sensitivity of the pancreatic beta cell to the usual stimulus for the release of insulin, and they lower peripheral resistance to insulin either by enhancing the number of receptors or their affinity for insulin or possibly by modifying some unidentified postreceptor abnormality to favor an insulin effect.

Oral hypoglycemic agents substitute for insulin in those patients who have moderately diminished beta cell function. In the person with type II diabetes, we first establish a quality diet. If adequate symptomatic and biochemical control is not achieved by diet alone, then insulin should be considered. At this point, the physician and the patient can decide whether the use of one of the oral hypoglycemic agents as a substitute for insulin is appropriate. If used, an oral agent then substitutes for insulin, not for diet.

Six oral hypoglycemic agents are now available (Table 2). The agent of choice should be the drug with which the physician is most familiar. We use chlorpropamide (Diabinese) most often. The patient is started on a dose predicted to be appropriate to need, usually somewhere near the minimum dose. The response to this dosage is judged by monitoring the urine and blood glucose. Usually the patient is seen two weeks after beginning treatment to make an appropriate dosage adjustment. One to two months after the start of oral hypoglycemic therapy, one should judge the effectiveness of the therapy. Failure to control blood sugar values means insulin should be advised.

Side effects of these drugs are uncommon. Hypoglycemia can complicate their use in elderly patients who eat erratically and in patients who overuse alcohol. Because of its long-acting effect, chlorpropamide most commonly causes hypoglycemia. It may also enhance the effect of the antidiuretic hormone, causing water retention and hyponatremia. Hepatic toxicity and bone marrow failure are extremely rare; skin rash and gastric upset occur in less than 1% of the patients.

NIDDM in whom oral agents may be used safely

Table 2. ORAL HYPOGLYCEMIC AGENTS

	Generic Name	Trade Name	Dosage (mg) Minimum	Maximum	Daily Frequency
1st Generation:	Acetohexamide	Dymelor	250	1500	2
	Chlorpropamide	Diabinese	50	500	1
	Tolazamide	Tolinase	100	1000	2
	Tolbutamide	Orinase	500	3000	2
2nd Generation:	Glyburide	Micronase DiaBeta	2.5	20	1–2
	Glipizide	Glucotrol	5.0	40	2

are: (1) over the age of 50; (2) otherwise healthy; (3) free of allergies to sulfonamide preparations; and (4) interested in using an oral agent instead of insulin. Patients in whom the oral agents should not be used generally include: (1) those suspected of having "closet" type I diabetes; (2) a patient with an acute illness; (3) any patient under stress from surgery or infection, or using glucocorticoids; (4) any pregnant patient; and (5) a patient with symptomatic diabetes and fasting hyperglycemia over 250 mg/dl. Caution in the use of oral hypoglycemic agents should include: (1) younger patients with type II diabetes; (2) patients who have complicating parenchymal disease involving liver or kidneys; (3) individuals on a variety of other drugs; and (4) patients who are very old, alcoholic, or not seen regularly by their physician. Whenever the diabetic state is improperly controlled with a maximum dose of an oral agent, insulin should be given. We do not use an oral agent in combination with insulin; data available do not suggest an advantage to combined therapy.

Second generation oral antidiabetic drugs include glyburide (Micronase, DiaBeta) and glipizide (Glucotrol) (Table 2). These drugs have been used for several years in Europe and have some differing characteristics when compared with the "first generation" oral drugs: (1) these drugs are more potent, on a milligram for milligram basis; (2) they do not retain water, which has been noted in some of the first generation drugs; and (3) they have fewer pharmacologic interactions with other drugs such as warfarin (Coumadin) and clofibrate (Atromid-S). It is unclear whether any wider application of these drugs in patients with type II diabetes will be possible, but it is appropriate to test them in patients who fail to achieve biochemical control with one of the older drugs or to use them in patients with new-onset diabetes.

PERIODIC EVALUATION

Monitoring Metabolic Control. Current technology allows more sophisticated monitoring of metabolic control by measuring HgbA1c and by studying accumulated data of capillary blood glucose tests done by the patient. Self-monitoring of blood glucose allows the patient a feeling of personal control over his diabetes. This important advance assists the patient in regulating insulin and improving metabolic control.

The newer self-monitoring strips offer a dry wipe or blot technique. These methods simplify the procedure and avoid skewed results due to over- or underwashing of the strip. Reflectance meters are also available for use. However, a finger or earlobe puncture must still be done and an adequate drop of blood placed properly on the sensitive paper strip. These maneuvers often are difficult for patients to do. The patients must be helped until one is confident of their skill, for inaccurate data are worse than no data. A variety of automatic devices to obtain blood are available, are simple to use, enhance the patient's ability to obtain the proper-sized drop of blood needed, and provide an almost painless method of obtaining a blood specimen. Despite these advantages, 15% of our patients who have been advised to use blood glucose monitoring prefer not to measure their own blood glucose; rather, they test the urine for glucose as a means of self-monitoring. A larger percentage of patients who initially monitor their own blood glucose lose this enthusiasm with time. HgbA1c levels offer another means of evaluation of metabolic control. These levels compare favorably with the mean blood glucose levels, and in NIDDM patients more closely correlate with the fasting blood glucose level than is true in patients with IDDM. While we measure HgbA1c levels every three to six months in IDDM, in our NIDDM patients every six to 12 months seems reasonable. In those patients who require only diet therapy, we often depend on blood glucose alone.

Follow-up Visits. Monitoring your diabetic patients also means checking certain physical and chemical findings regularly. Most of our patients return every three to six months. At these visits, we evaluate weight, blood pressure, pulse, peripheral circulation, and the ocular fundi. Sites of insulin injection are checked for lipodystrophy. We measure the serum cholesterol and creatinine annually. Every one to four years, a complete physical examination is done. One should recall that people with diabetes may fall heir to any illness seen in a person without diabetes.

The detection of any diabetic complications accentuates the need for closer supervision and improved control. The presence of significant retinopathy necessitates regular ophthalmologic evaluations. Foot problems from ischemia and neuropathy will demand close collaboration with a skilled podiatrist. Painful neuropathy should be treated by improved metabolic control, analgesics, and vitamins. Amitriptyline (Elavil) (25 to 100 mg daily) or fluphenazine (Prolixin) (1 to 3 mg daily) may relieve the pain or dysesthesias. Hypertension requires vigorous control to delay deterioration of renal function, as do prompt treatment of urinary tract infections and early correction of obstructive uropathy. End-stage renal disease requires chronic dialysis or transplantation.

REFERENCES

Jenkins DJA: Lente carbohydrate: a newer approach to the dietary management of diabetes. Diabetes Care 5:634–641, 1982.
Lebovitz HE, Feinglos MN: The oral hypoglycemic agents. *In* Ellenberg M, Rifkin H (eds): Diabetes Mellitus: Theory and Practice, 3rd ed.

Medical Examination Publishing Co, Inc, New Hyde Park, NY, 1983, Chapter 28.

National Diabetes Data Group: Classification and diagnosis of diabetes mellitus and other categories of glucose intolerance. Diabetes 28:1039–1057, 1957.

The Physician's Guide to Type II Diabetes (NIDDM): Diagnosis and Treatment. American Diabetes Association, New York, 1984.

Whitehouse FW, Whitehouse IJ, Cox MS, et al: Outpatient regulation of the insulin-requiring person with diabetes (an alternative to hospitalization). J Chronic Dis 36:433–438, 1983.

3 · HYPOGLYCEMIA

Ronald P. Monsaert
GEISINGER MEDICAL CENTER

DEFINITION AND DIAGNOSTIC CRITERIA

Hypoglycemia is a metabolic disorder of many different causes wherein symptoms are engendered by a low blood glucose and reversed by restoration of the euglycemic state. Blood glucose has been observed in otherwise healthy individuals to fall below 40 mg/dl during the course of a fast, during a five-hour glucose tolerance test, and during prolonged exercise without symptoms. Therefore, hypoglycemia cannot be defined on the basis of an arbitrary glucose value. For clinical purposes, a low blood glucose may be defined as less than 40 mg/dl.

Hypoglycemia has been classified into two types: postprandial (reactive) and fasting, depending on whether symptoms occur predominantly a few hours following a meal or in the fasting state.

PATHOPHYSIOLOGY

Blood glucose is supported by a variety of hormonal systems, and the number of these mechanisms underscores the importance of maintaining euglycemia. Since glucose is the primary source of energy for certain tissues, especially the central nervous system, cell dysfunction or death may result from hypoglycemia.

Hypoglycemia may be the result of either inadequate production of glucose or excessive glucose utilization. In the fasting state, glucose levels are supported by conversion of liver glycogen (glycogenolysis) and muscle protein (gluconeogenesis) to glucose. These processes are stimulated by glucagon, catecholamines, cortisol, and growth hormone; thus, deficiencies of these hormones can compromise glucose homeostasis. Similarly, deficiency of a specific enzyme in these metabolic pathways or toxic suppression by ethanol, aspirin, or akee fruit would have similar results. Malnutrition, by causing substrate deficiency, may be associated with hypoglycemia, particularly when accompanied by muscle wasting, hepatic insufficiency, uremia, and so on.

Hypoglycemia may also be caused by excessive utilization of glucose. Surreptitious or immoderate insulin administration of excessive endogenous insulin secretion as from an islet cell tumor will lower blood sugar by facilitating glucose transport across cell membranes. In similar fashion, polypeptide and glycoprotein compounds, known collectively as nonsuppressible insulin-like activity (NSILA and NSILP), augment glucose transport into cells. These proteins have growth-promoting activity and have been noted to be elevated in as many as 37% of non–islet cell tumors associated with hypoglycemia. Some large tumors weighing more than 1 kg consume glucose at a rate that can exceed hepatic output. The hypoglycemia of pregnancy is also due to an obligate glucose drain.

CLINICAL ASPECTS

Symptoms of hypoglycemia may take two forms. Often an acute fall in blood sugar will simulate an adrenergic discharge, and the patient will experience palpitation, sweating, nervousness, and tremulousness. A more gradual or protracted fall will produce neurologic symptoms (neuroglycopenia) such as confusion, headache, coma, cranial nerve deficits, and focal or generalized seizures. Symptoms may be precipitated by exercise.

Administration of glucose should readily relieve all of these symptoms if hypoglycemia is corrected before permanent injury has occurred.

Postprandial Hypoglycemia. Patients with postprandial hypoglycemia usually present with typical adrenergic symptoms. In patients who have had surgery for peptic ulcer disease, this often occurs one and a half to three hours following a meal and may be preceded by the "dumping syndrome." These symptoms are produced by rapid gastric emptying, which alters the usual synchrony between glucose absorption and insulin release.

Postprandial hypoglycemia may also be seen in patients with impaired glucose tolerance, in some children with inborn errors of metabolism, and in an idiopathic form. It is important to demonstrate that patients with symptoms suggestive of reactive hypoglycemia actually have low blood glucose during symptoms because most patients will not satisfy diagnostic criteria. Many patients seem to have typical symptoms following a meal or during a glucose tolerance test, but actually have normal blood glucose at this time. These patients are classified as having nonhypoglycemia or the idiopathic postprandial syndrome.

Fasting Hypoglycemia. Patients with fasting hypoglycemia usually present with symptoms of neuroglycopenia and are more likely to have symptoms during exercise or if they miss a meal. Many patients have been mistakenly sent for neurologic or psychiatric consultation before the true nature of their disorder has been discovered. Some causes of fasting hypoglycemia are classified according to their insulin level (Table 1). Thus, the insulin assay forms a pivotal point in the differential diagnosis.

The clinical presentation may be significant for cachexia in the patient with malnutrition, chronic alcoholism, or certain neoplasms such as hepatoma and adrenal carcinoma. The latter may also be occasioned by frank signs of Cushing's syndrome. Signs of a large intra-abdominal or intrathoracic mass may be apparent in the case of some NSILA-secreting mesenchymal tumors.

Table 1. CAUSES OF FASTING HYPOGLYCEMIA

Insulin Low or Normal
Artifactual (polycythemia vera or chronic myelongeous leukemia)
Inborn and acquired errors of metabolism
Malnutrition, uremia, and substrate deficiency
Pregnancy
Tumors
NSILA-secreting tumors
Drugs, toxins, alcohol
Liver disease
Hormonal deficiencies
Insulin receptor antibody syndrome

Insulin Elevated
Insulinoma
Surreptitious insulin use
Oral Hypoglycemic agents
Autoimmune hypoglycemia syndrome

MANAGEMENT

PLAN

Evaluation of Hypoglycemia. The immediate concerns in the management of the hypoglycemic patient are to temporarily reverse the hypoglycemia and to establish an etiologic factor for this condition. Definitive treatment of hypoglycemia is unique to its causation.

Patients with reactive symptoms can be evaluated in the outpatient setting with a five-hour glucose tolerance test. Patients should be prepared with a 200 gm carbohydrate diet for at least three days prior to testing. Some authorities recommend replacing the 75 gm glucose load with a small breakfast, arguing that this is a more physiologic assessment; but neither the meal composition nor the diagnostic criteria have been firmly established. It is important to document that typical symptoms occur at a time when blood glucose is low so that patients with nonhypoglycemia are thus excluded.

The evaluation of patients with fasting hypoglycemia is more complex and may require a hospital admission, particularly if the patient is having frequent or potentially life-threatening symptoms. Those with mild symptoms may be seen in an outpatient setting following a 12-hour fast, and blood should be obtained for insulin and glucose. A plasma insulin greater than 10 μU/ml in a nonobese insulin-naive patient or an insulin/glucose ratio greater than 0.4 suggests an insulin-mediated cause of hypoglycemia. Liver and kidney function studies, pituitary testing, and a chest x-ray film can be obtained at that time. The patient's history, physical findings, or family history may suggest consideration of additional studies. Patients in health-related occupations or with other access to antidiabetic medication may be suspected of having factitious hypoglycemia. A C-peptide level, insulin antibodies, and urine sulfonyluria assay should be obtained in that setting. If insulinoma is suspected, a proinsulin level, HCG level, and localizing procedures may be warranted. Patients who do not demonstrate hypoglycemia may be admitted for a 72-hour fast and evaluated as above. Most patients with fasting hypoglycemia will fulfill diagnostic criteria in 36 hours of fasting and rarely will other studies such as a tolbutamide tolerance test be necessary.

Surgery. Surgery is definitive therapy for insulinoma and possibly other tumors. Surgery, however, may be of no benefit or be only palliative in the case of malignant insulinoma or in patients with benign beta cell hyperplasia or multiple adenomas. The latter is more common in patients with the MEN I syndrome. It is, therefore, useful to try localizing the lesion preoperatively with an abdominal CT scan and/or pancreatic angiography. Some success has been reported with pancreatic venous sampling, which may be indicated in some patients suspected of having hyperplasia or multiple adenomas, or following a previously unsuccessful operation. This procedure should be left to those with demonstrated expertise; however, the otherwise benign, single, nonlocalizing adenoma may well be found by an experienced surgeon despite the fact that these lesions are usually less than 3 cm in diameter. In the event no tumor is found, an incremental distal pancreatectomy should be performed with frozen sections following each resected segment. The proximal 15% to 20% of the pancreas should be left in situ.

Patients with malignant insulinoma or other cancers may benefit from a debulking procedure if their hypoglycemia is not manageable by diet or drug therapy.

NONPHARMACOLOGIC MEASURES

A diet low in simple sugar with frequent-feeding strategy is appropriate for the usual patient with hypoglycemia. Fructose, however, can usually be added to the diet without causing symptoms. Patients with nonhypoglycemia usually do not respond to this regimen and may be difficult to manage, since they usually have their "hypoglycemia" reinforced by misleading literature in the lay press, may have had an asymptomatic low blood glucose on a prior, carbohydrate-restricted glucose tolerance test, and usually have an abnormal personality profile characterized by hypersomatization and hypochondriacal complaints as determined by MMPI. Demonstration of normal blood sugar during their symptoms is usually reassuring to these patients and helps make them amenable to therapy directed at relieving anxiety and stress.

Patients with mild fasting hypoglycemia may be managed by frequent oral feedings unless and until more definitive treatment can be found. Treatment should be empiric, starting with meals of known caloric content every six hours or more frequently as necessary. Increasing the caloric content may be helpful, but excessive weight gain should be avoided if possible. Since exercise may provoke hypoglycemia, the timing of meals may need to be adjusted to allow recreational activity.

DRUG THERAPY

Glucose. The management of hypoglycemia in the unconscious or seizing patient should be with intravenous glucose infusion, D_5 to D_{50} as necessary. Patients with frequent episodes or those resistant to a frequent oral feeding strategy might also need similar therapy. Note should be made that continuous infusion of more concentrated dextrose solutions are irritating to peripheral veins and should be given by a central catheter. Again, weight gain may be a complication of therapy. Glucose support should not be withdrawn prematurely, especially in the case of sulfonylurea-related hypoglycemia where hypoglycemia may persist for four days or more depending on quantity of ingestion and drug half-life.

Diazoxide. Diazoxide is the most effective hyperglycemic agent available in the management of fasting hypoglycemia. Diazoxide suppresses insulin secretion and augments glycemia by increasing hepatic gluconeogenesis and decreasing peripheral utilization of glucose. Doses (300 to 900 mg/day) orally or by slow intravenous infusion frequently will reverse the hypoglycemia associated with nearly all causes of this syndrome. Often patients can be weaned from frequent feedings or IV glucose support with this single agent. Anecdotal reports suggest that concomitant use of propranolol may be adjunctive. Diuretics must usually be administered with diazoxide because of fluid retention. Patient compliance is further compromised because of hirsutism and weight gain.

Other Agents. Hypoglycemia refractory to diazoxide may present a very real clinical challenge. The following are second-line agents that empirically may be tried alone or in combination. Parenteral glucagon and pharmacologic doses of prednisone (20 to 100 mg/day) may be beneficial because of their glycogenolytic and gluconeogenic properties. Dilantin (300 to 600 mg) appears to act by suppressing insulin secretion. Insulin synthesis appears also to be inhibited by the cytotoxic antibiotic mithramycin (1 mg IV). Mithramycin is toxic to bone marrow, liver, and kidneys. In the case of insulinoma, intravenous infusion of somatostatin may be attempted by groups having access to this not-yet-released octapeptide. Success has also been reported with a longer-acting somatostatin analogue given subcutaneously.

Adjuvant Chemotherapy. Adjuvant chemotherapy for malignant insulinoma is disappointing because it does not prolong life and the agents are very toxic. We reserve chemotherapy for patients whose hypoglycemia is unmanageable by other means or for those who have progressive hepatic metastases or other symptoms from their tumor. Streptozotocin and 5-fluorouracil will be tried initially, followed by Adriamycin if there is no response. Chemotherapy may be useful for other hypoglycemia-associated tumors and radiation therapy should also be considered in selected cases.

Unconscious patients suspected of having hypopituitarism or Addison's disease should be treated with hydrocortisone (300 mg/day IV) after studies have been obtained. In less acute situations, the patient should be maintained on oral hydrocortisone (20 mg in the morning, 10 mg in the afternoon) or equivalent. Pharmacologic doses of adrenal steroids may be helpful in the autoimmune hypoglycemia syndrome should dietary treatment or therapy of its related disease be unsuccessful. One should expect the usual side effects seen with high-dose glucocorticoid therapy.

Patients with reactive hypoglycemia who do not have satisfactory response to diet therapy may benefit from anticholinergic agents such as propantheline (15 to 30 mg) in two or three divided doses. Dry mouth, urinary retention, and blurred vision are commonly recorded side effects. Selected patients may respond to propranolol.

PATIENT EDUCATION

Patients can facilitate at-home management by recording blood glucose obtained by fingerstick and metered estimation. Patients might be advised to check blood glucose at particularly vulnerable times of the day such as before a meal, during the sleeping period, and during or after exercise. They should be advised against using agents that may exacerbate hypoglycemia, such as ethanol. The patient and family should be made to understand that serious morbidity and death may result from untreated hypoglycemia, and patients should be instructed to eat at the first sign of low blood glucose. Driving privileges should be curtailed until a satisfactory period has elapsed without symptoms. Also, a health-alert bracelet may be recommended for the hypoglycemic patient who is managed at home.

REFERENCES

Bauman WA, Yalow RS: Hyperinsulinemic hypoglycemia. Differential diagnosis by determination of the species of circulating insulin. JAMA 252:2730–2734, 1984.

Fajans SS, Floyd JC: Fasting hypoglycemia in adults. N Engl J Med 294:766–772, 1976.

Howell RR: The glycogen storage diseases. *In* Stanbury JB, Wyngaarden JB, Fredrickson DS (eds): The Metabolic Basis of Inherited Disease, 4th ed. McGraw-Hill, New York, 1978, pp 137–159.

Merimee TJ, Tyson JE: Hypoglycemia in man. Pathologic and physiologic variants. Diabetes 26:161–165, 1977.

Service FJ (ed): Hypoglycemic Disorders. G.K. Hall, Boston, 1983.

Service FJ, Dale AJD, Elveback LR, et al: Insulinoma. Clinical and diagnostic features of 60 consecutive cases. Mayo Clin Proc 51:417–429, 1976.

4 · OBESITY

Abdul Cader Asmal
JOSLIN CLINIC

DEFINITION AND DIAGNOSTIC CRITERIA

Obesity may be viewed as a syndrome of disordered energy homeostasis due to an imbalance between caloric intake and expenditure and characterized by excessive body weight and fat.

The degree of obesity is gauged by several indices relating weight to height, of which the most widely used are: (1) relative weight: the ratio of actual to desirable weight; and (2) body mass index (BMI): wt (kg)/ht (m²). The BMI is most closely correlated with total body fat. An estimate of body fat may be obtained clinically by measuring of skinfold thickness (SFT), and in the research setting by using specialized techniques, e.g., densitometry.

Obesity is diagnosed when either the relative body weight is greater than 1.2 (i.e., more than 20% above the desirable weight), the BMI exceeds 30, or the triceps SFT is in excess of 25 mm in females and 18 mm in males. Its severity is quantified as follows: mild 20% to 59%, moderate 60% to 99%, and morbid >100% above desirable weight.

PATHOPHYSIOLOGY

The cause of obesity is multifactorial with a complex interplay between genetic and environmental factors that modulate their effects through regulating either food intake or energy expenditure, or both.

In the pathogenesis of obesity, caloric intake ex-

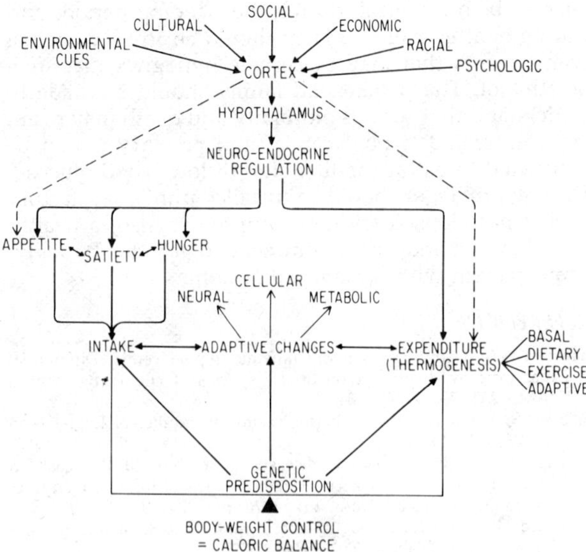

Figure 1. The multiple mechanisms that operate to maintain a fine balance between caloric intake and expenditure to ensure normal weight.

ceeds expenditure. This is not synonymous with an absolute increase in food intake. Increased caloric intake may result from either increased availability (conditioned by economic, social, cultural, and behavioral factors) or increased "need" (induced by genetic or environmentally acquired derangements of appetite-satiety-hunger control) (Fig. 1). While increased intake with constant expenditure promotes weight gain, the slope of this correlation differs among individuals. Thus, two individuals with the same caloric intake and expenditure may gain significantly different amounts of weight. Furthermore, once obesity is established, caloric intake may no longer be excessive either in relative or absolute amounts, but is equaled by expenditure at a new steady state.

The importance of caloric expenditure in the evolution of obesity has not been sufficiently emphasized in the past. Energy expenditure, which may be equated with thermogenesis, falls into four categories: basal, diet-induced, exercise-induced, and adaptive thermogenesis.

It is postulated that differences in thermogenesis might explain the differential weight gain on equivalent dietary intakes. Orderly and efficient thermogenesis is considered to promote caloric conservation, whereas ineffectual thermogenesis, as through operation of futile metabolic cycles, is considered to encourage dissipation of excess calories. Although demonstrated to be important in certain laboratory animals, there is still no conclusive proof that thermogenesis acts as an energy buffer in man.

In the majority of obese patients, the etiologic factor and pathogenesis remain unclear. In a very small proportion, a specific causal mechanism may be identified, e.g., in association with the Laurence-Moon-Biedl syndrome, Cushing's syndrome, insulinoma, hypothyroidism, and hypothalamic lesions.

Pathologically, obesity is divided into two subsets: hypercellular and hypertrophic. Hypercellular obesity classically develops in childhood at a time when adipocytes still retain their capacity to proliferate. It is characterized both by an increase in the number of fat cells as well as by the quantity of lipid per cell. With weight reduction the fat content of individual cells diminishes but the number remains unchanged. This predisposes to weight regain, making the treatment of hypercellular obesity an intractable problem so that about 80% of obese children become obese adults. Hypertrophic obesity usually develops in adult life, often precipitated by events such as marriage, pregnancy, bereavement, or menopause. The lipid content of existing adipocytes markedly increases, but generally there is no increase in fat cell number. Consequently, weight reduction and maintenance are relatively easier in this group.

CLINICAL ASPECTS

The prevalence of obesity depends upon the criteria employed. If obesity is defined in terms of a relative weight (measured divided by ideal weight) >1.2, 14% of American men aged 20 to 74 and 24% of American women in the same age group are obese. The frequency of overweight in both sexes increases with age.

The distribution of excessive body fat may be primarily truncal (android) or peripheral (gynecoid). The association between obesity and disorders such as diabetes, hypertension, hyperuricemia, and hypertriglyceridemia may be greater in females with android rather than those with gynecoid obesity.

The presence of obesity significantly influences the physiology of several systems, including an increase in cardiac output, blood volume, renal blood flow and filtration, a reduction in total peripheral resistance, and an impairment of respiratory function. Obesity induces insulin resistance through both receptor and postreceptor mechanisms with impairment of carbohydrate tolerance or diabetes despite increased insulin secretion. Other hormonal abnormalities include a blunted growth hormone response to secretagogues, a modest elevation in serum T_3 levels, augmented adrenocortical steroid secretion rate, lowered testosterone concentrations in men, and irregular menses. These abnormalities invariably return to normal with weight reduction.

Life insurance statistics have established a relationship between obesity and increased mortality in patients with associated disease such as hypertension, coronary artery disease, diabetes, gallbladder disease, renal calculi, and certain forms of cancer. Prospective studies have confirmed that obesity increases mortality but only if hypertension and hypercholesterolemia are also present. Whether obesity per se is an independent risk factor is unresolved. A relative body weight exceeding 1.2 is accompanied by a 20% increase in relative risk of death, and relative body weight more than 1.6 by a threefold increase in risk compared with age-matched normal weight individuals.

MANAGEMENT OF OBESITY

PLAN

Short-term and Long-term Goals. Because obesity is the outcome of a relative excess of caloric intake over expenditure, treatment has to employ strategies that reverse this trend, and ensure that it remains reversed. Several therapeutic modalities are available to attain these goals: nutrition counseling; behavior modification and psychologic support; exercise instruction; anorectic drugs; surgical procedures, including intestinal bypass and gastric reduction; and miscellaneous approaches of unproven value including hypnosis, acupuncture, and a wide range of drugs (thyroid hormones, human chorionic gonadotropin, cholecystokinin, starch-blockers). The sequence and combination in which they are used depend on the severity of the obesity and the rapidity with which the weight loss is required. A comprehensive program of management provides the best hope of achieving and sustaining the weight reduction.

Indication for Hospitalization. All grades of obesity should be managed in an outpatient setting except under the following circumstances:

1. Morbid obesity, either for definitive gastrointestinal surgery, or as a prelude to surgery for a finite period of intensive weight reduction based on a very-low-calorie diet or total starvation.

2. Moderate or morbid obesity in patients with a severe medical problem: pickwickian syndrome, unstable cardiac rhythms, uncontrollable diabetes.

NONPHARMACOLOGIC MEASURES

Based on the severity of the obesity, a stepwise approach to its management is followed. A hypocaloric diet with pertinent nutritional education forms the basis of all weight reduction programs. The degree of caloric restriction and nutritional balance may vary greatly from diet to diet.

Balanced Hypocaloric Diet. This is the safest and most appropriate diet for the majority of patients who are mildly obese. It is based on a 250 to 500 kcal/day reduction in the estimated calorie requirement. The daily caloric requirement is derived as the product of the ideal body weight (IBW) (kg) and activity level. The IBW is derived from appropriate tables, and caloric expenditure is estimated as follows: 20 kcal/kg IBW/day for sedentary, 25 for moderate, 30 for vigorous activity. Thus, the estimated caloric intake for an individual weighing 70 kg (IBW) who is moderately active is 70 kg × 25 = 1750 kcal/kg/day. This is a weight-maintaining diet. For a moderately active obese patient whose IBW is 70 kg, the diet may be reduced to between 1250 and 1500 kcal/day and would result in a theoretical weekly weight loss of 1/2 to 1 lb (1 lb of fat = 3500 kcal). The diet itself is nutritionally balanced, consisting of 50% carbohydrate, mainly unrefined, 30% fat, balanced between saturated and polyunsaturated, and 20% protein.

The goal of this approach is to establish a subtle and gradual change in the patient's eating behavior and life style, and it is designed to promote a slow but sustained weight reduction. The acronym ACT may help the patient adhere to his dietary plan:

A = *Amount* of food prescribed/24 hours
C = *Consistency* in timing and proportions of food eaten
T = *Types* of food permitted and prohibited

Patients are advised to meet regularly with the dietitian for instruction on food groups and exchanges, avoidance of calorie-dense products, and the judicious use of sugar substitutes. They are encouraged to increase their overall level of activity—such as walking instead of riding, climbing stairs instead of using elevators, avoiding cat naps immediately after meals, and so on. The judicious use of anorectic agents (see later) over a limited period may facilitate the adjustment in life style.

Balanced Low-Calorie Diet. For patients in whom the first approach is ineffectual, a balanced low-calorie diet of not less than 800 kcal/day together with a multivitamin is prescribed. A nutrition educator sees the patients at least weekly and reviews their diaries of daily food intake (amount, type, caloric content, preparation) and eating behavior. Nutritional counseling is reinforced, concepts of behavior modification are introduced, and exercise programs are discussed. Anorectic agents (see later) may also be helpful adjuncts for a limited period. *Low-calorie unbalanced* (low-carbohydrate, low-fat, or fad—emphasizing a single food) *diets are not recommended*.

Very-Low-Calorie Diets (VLCD): 200 to 800 kcal/day. Because of their unacceptable risk-benefit ratio, these diets are used only in moderate to morbidly obese patients under medical supervision. Patients are prescreened by history, examination, EKG, chest film, CBC, SMA, and urinalysis. Those with a recent cardiac infarction, stroke, cancer or insulin-dependent diabetes mellitus (IDDM), significant hepatic or renal disease, on lithium treatment, or suffering from overt psychosis are excluded.

The VLCD are based solely on protein (natural food or milk- or egg-based formula) or a combination of protein (1 to 1.5 gm/kg IBW) and carbohydrate (0.5 gm glucose/kg IBW). Mineral and vitamin supplementation is mandatory (1 multivitamin tablet, 3 to 5 gm NaCL, 3 gm potassium, 400 to 800 mg calcium per day may be adequate). Fluid intake of 1.5 to 2.1 liters daily is necessary. Some commercial preparations are fortified with minerals and vitamins.

Note: (1) The relative efficacy of the exclusively protein versus the protein-carbohydrate combination diet in promoting weight loss remains unresolved. (2) The current VLCD have to be contrasted with the liquid protein diet based on low quality protein hydrolysates of collagen, which caused more than 58 deaths in the late 1970's.

Patients on VLCD are evaluated weekly for weight loss, for management of side effects such as mild postural hypotension, constipation, cold intolerance, dizziness and dry skin, and for reinforcement of nutritional education, behavior modification, and exercise programs. In the short term, patients may lose 2 to 5 kg in the first week and 1 to 2 kg/wk subsequently, with improvement in blood pressure, carbohydrate tolerance, and plasma lipids.

The long-term efficacy has not been as encouraging, with up to 56% of the patients regaining more than half of their weight loss. The diets have been used (under close supervision) from four weeks to a year.

Starvation. Starvation (200 kcal/day) as an approach to the management of obesity has been generally abandoned because of the morbidity and mortality associated with its use and its long-term ineffectiveness.

DRUGS

Of the various classes of pharmacologic agents investigated, the anorexiant drugs are the most effective when used as adjuncts in an overall strategy of weight reduction in patients with a BMI of >30. The anorexiants are structural analogues of amphetamine (excepting mazindol), and are thus pharmacologic stimulants (excepting fenfluramine). Their precise mechanisms of action in appetite suppression are unclear, and it is possible that fenfluramine may exert effects on metabolism independently of its anorectic action.

Drug Selection. A selection of some of the available drugs and their federal scheduling is outlined below.

Schedule II: Amphetamine, dextroamphetamine, methamphetamine.

Schedule III: Benzphetamine, chlortermine, phendimetrazine.

Schedule IV: Diethylpropion (Tenuate, 25 mg t.i.d.), phentermine (Ionamin, 15 to 30 mg daily) fenfluramine (Pondimin, 20 to 40 mg t.i.d.), mazindol (Sanorex, Mazanor, 1 mg t.i.d.).

All anorectic agents have comparable efficacy, but since the Schedule IV compounds have a lower abuse potential, they are the drugs of choice. The nonprescription agent phenylpropanolamine may be as effective with fewer side effects.

Because of its metabolic effects, fenfluramine is preferred in the obese diabetic but contraindicated when there is a history of depression. Mazindol, phentermine, and diethylpropion are contraindicated in patients with a history of agitation. Anorectic drugs should be avoided in patients with significant hypertension or symptomatic coronary disease (including arrhythmias). In appropriately selected patients, the correct drug should be used for finite periods either to facilitate the adaptation to a new meal plan during the initial phase of hypocaloric diet, or to promote continued compliance with the diet at a later stage when the rate of weight loss has reached a discouraging plateau. Therapy should begin with a minimum dose with stepwise increases. In general it should continue for no more than one to two months, and then be tapered off.

Adverse Effects. Most of the compounds may produce excessive pharmacologic stimulation causing insomnia, excitement, agitation, dizziness, tremor, headache, dry mouth, palpitations, hallucinations, confusion, and panic states. Impotence may occur. Fenfluramine produces sedation, drowsiness, and depression, which may be marked on discontinuing the medication. Diarrhea may also occur. These compounds may affect the ability to operate machinery or drive a car.

Contraindications. Obesity often coexists with medical illnesses such as symptomatic coronary disease, severe hypertension, glaucoma, hyperthyroidism, agitation, or depression that contraindicate the use of anorectic drugs. A history of drug abuse, hypersensitivity to sympathomimetics, the use of monoamine oxidase inhibitors (MAOI) within 14 days, and pregnancy are additional contraindictions.

Drug Interactions.

1. Use with MAOI within 14 days may precipitate hypertensive crises.

2. Fenfluramine potentiates the effect of antihypertensives such as methyldopa, and CNS sedatives and alcohol.

3. Mazindol and phentermine antagonize the antihypertensive effect of guanethidine and similar agents, and potentiate pressor response to catecholamines.

Patients on appetite suppressants should not take any medications without consulting their physician or pharmacist regarding possible drug interactions.

SURGICAL MANAGEMENT

Morbid obesity unresponsive to intensive conservative therapy is an indication for either gastric or intestinal bypass surgery. The risk of surgery is high because of associated hypertension, diabetes, coronary disease, or pulmonary hypoventilation. Preoperative evaluation should exclude patients with renal failure and those with significant myocardial, inflammatory bowel, pulmonary, or progressive hepatic disease. Surgery should be performed only in specialized centers.

Although weight loss is inevitable after intestinal bypass surgery, the complications are legion. The overall mortality averages about 2.8% with an acute morbidity characterized by pulmonary embolism, wound infection, intestinal bleeding, renal failure, and pancreatitis. Chronic medical problems include diarrhea, malabsorption of electrolytes (especially potassium, calcium, and magnesium), deranged liver function, syndromes of bacterial overgrowth, renal calculi, and polyarthritis. The use of this approach has progressively declined.

Several types of gastric reduction operations are currently in vogue: they all reduce the effective gastric volume. Although the operative mortality is lower and the chronic complications are fewer than with intestinal bypass, weight loss may not be sustained because of remodeling of the stomach and the patients' consumption of frequent small meals. Vomiting, afferent and efferent loop obstruction, and dumping are some of its later complications.

PATIENT INFORMATION AND EDUCATION

Nutritional counseling with frequent feedback, review, and reinforcement as well as behavior modification and exercise programming should be ongoing processes. Anorectic drugs and surgery are both efficacious but their limitations, adverse effects, and contraindications must be understood by patients. An informed, cooperative, and motivated patient holds the key to the success of any weight reduction program.

PERIODIC EVALUATION

Periodic evaluation is necessary to reinforce knowledge and to monitor weight, blood pressure, and other parameters such as plasma cholesterol, triglycerides, glucose, and electrolytes as necessary. The frequency of evaluation is determined by the severity of the obesity, the strictness of the diet, and the use of adjunctive anorectic drug therapy.

PREVENTIVE MEASURES

While treatment of obesity is focused on the individual, its prevention should be directed to society at large. Society conditions our attitudes to food intake and energy expenditure. Therefore, all of us should rethink our views on nutrition, food advertising and feeding practices, and reappraise our needs for regular physical activity whether in the form of walking for pleasure, aerobics classes, or formal exercise programs. Only a broad-based approach can make a significant impact in reducing the prevalence of obesity at an individual level.

SOCIOECONOMIC ASPECTS OF MANAGEMENT

Because obesity is a social disease, its prevention and treatment should be the concern of society. In 1977 the Fogarty International Conference on Obesity made important recommendations to both the public and private sectors in terms of education, regulation, food services, and financial incentives. Implementation of some of the recommendations would be the first decisive step in the prevention of this common, frequently relapsing, and not uncommonly refractory problem.

REFERENCES

Bray GA: Diet and exercise as treatment for obesity. In Corn HL, DeFelice GA, Kuo P (eds): Health and Obesity. Revere Press, New York, 1983, pp 79–103.

Moss AJ: Caution: very-low calorie diets can be deadly. Ann Intern Med 102:121–122, 1985.

Stunkard AJ: Obesity. W.B. Saunders Co, Philadelphia, 1980.

Vasselli JR, Cleary MP, Van Itallie TB: Modern concepts of obesity. Nutr Rev 41:361–373, 1983.

Wadden TA, Stunkard AJ, Brownell KD: Very low calorie diets: their efficacy, safety and future. Ann Intern Med. 99:675–684, 1983.

5 · ANOREXIA

Meir Gross
CLEVELAND CLINIC FOUNDATION

Anorexia nervosa is a rather baffling disease with a difficult course of treatment that could at times be prolonged. This is a condition that occurs predominantly in adolescent girls at a ratio of 9:1. These teenage girls slowly starve themselves to death. A mortality rate of up to 20% has been cited in the literature. Anorexia can affect one of every 250 girls between the ages of 12 and 18 years.

The typical anorexic girl sees herself as fat even if she is severely emaciated, which is a distortion in the body image. She is constantly preoccupied with her size and appearance. Sometimes this preoccupation is limited to only part of the body, such as hips, breasts, or thighs, with the patient claiming they look too big. The typical anorexic also is preoccupied with foods, counting calories of each food item constantly. They tend not only to limit the amount of calories consumed at each meal but also to make sure they get only the minimal amount; they would prefer to eat only one or two food items regularly and constantly every day. They will choose only foods with low carbohydrates or fat. If they feel they have eaten too much, they might then over-exercise in an obsessive-compulsive manner for prolonged times. They might also try to get rid of the food by abusing excessive amounts of laxatives, diuretics, or enemas. If they feel desperate about giving in to their appetite, they might even induce vomiting voluntarily in order to get rid of the food immediately after meals.

DIAGNOSIS

The diagnostic criteria are best classified in the *Diagnostic and Statistical Manual of Mental Disorders* of the American Psychiatric Association. Of course, any organic reason for severe weight loss in the patient should be considered, but the diagnosis can be made in the practitioner's office even without any complicated tests, just by observing the classic signs and symptoms of the typical anorexic patient. In other words, the diagnosis could easily be made in the first visit at the office, based on the positive signs when observing the patient while taking a medical history.

The *Diagnostic and Statistical Manual* emphasizes that the first and most important sign to watch for is intense fear of becoming obese, which is not reduced in the patient even if the weight loss progresses to a dangerous level. The patients almost always claim to be or feel fat and will refuse to cooperate in bringing up the body weight to a minimal normal weight for age and height. In order to diagnose the patient as suffering from anorexia, one usually observes a weight loss of at least 25% of the original body weight. If the patient is under 18 years of age, the weight loss considered should be calculated from the projected profile of weight gain expected from the growth chart.

PATHOPHYSIOLOGIC CHANGES

As the weight loss progresses, there are typical physiologic changes seen in the anorexic patient. Many of the patients start to complain about feeling too cold even in the summer, the pulse tends to slow down, (bradycardia), and there is reduction in the blood pressure (hypotension) with possible episodes of fainting due to orthostatic hypotension. Newborn-like hair called lanugo may appear on the body, more so on the face and shoulders. Some patients might develop loss of hair (alopecia) of the scalp, which might be quite frightening to the teenager who is concerned about her hair. If the anorexia started beyond adolescence, at older age, severe emaciation could cause a wrinkled skin, making some adult anorexics look older than their chronologic age. If the illness is associated with abuse of laxatives, diuretics, or induced vomiting, hypokalemia may occur causing cardiac arrhythmias, lethargy, or at times cardiac arrest and death. As the weight loss progresses, the fat tissue composition falls below 17% of body fat, at which point the menstrual periods will stop. Amenorrhea may occur even before severe weight loss due to the patient's emotional stress. There is often reduction in luteinizing hormone (LH) and follicle-stimulating hormone (FSH), which consequently results in reduction of the estrogen levels.

The weight loss initially consists of the adipose tissue, then the muscle, and at the third stage there is depletion of the visceral proteins seen by lowering of transferrin in the blood. At this stage, the immunologic system is being compromised with the danger of severe lethal infection that can lead the patient into toxic irreversible shock and death.

MANAGEMENT

It is important first to evaluate the patient in order to assess the level of medical risk involved with the weight loss. The evaluation should be twofold, medical and psychiatric.

RECOMMENDED MEDICAL TESTS

The medical assessment in the office should include first a thorough general physical examination. In addition, a few simple laboratory tests should be done in order to rule out other pathologic changes or physical complications due to the process of anorexia itself so that the patient can be treated properly. Hematologic values including hemoglobin will help to find if the patient is anemic owing to long starvation or unbalanced diet habits. White blood cell count including differential count can give an estimate about the immunoresistance of the anorexic patient. An SMA-18 might show abnormal value of enzymes or abnormal liver functions that are seen in severely anorexic patients. Sedimentation rate and urinalysis are simple screening tests to rule out other pathologic conditions causing the weight loss, such as Crohn's disease, diabetes, or possible malignancy. A purified protein derivative (PPD) test will help to rule out the possibility of tuberculosis of the gastrointestinal tract. Checking the functional thyroid index (FTI) or level of thyroid hormones will help to determine if the loss of weight is due to hyperthyroidism rather than anorexia. Determining cortisol levels in the morning and evening will help to rule out Edison's disease, Sheehan's syndrome, or Simmonds' disease. A stool test will help to rule out a malabsorption syndrome in case the history of the symptoms is suggestive of such a disorder, and the possibility of gastrointestinal parasites could be ruled out as well. If suspicion of a brain tumor exists (such as pituitary, parasellar, or hypothalamic), specific x-ray examinations such as head computerized tomography with contrast medium not only will help in finding such a tumor but also could show evidence for brain atrophy, which can be seen in severely anorexic patients. In a series of 27 anorexic patients at the Cleveland Clinic who had CT scans, six showed mild atrophy of the brain.

If the history is suggestive of any gastrointestinal irregularity, then roentgenographic examination of the whole gastrointestinal tract is recommended, including upper gastrointestinal series, small bowel series, and barium enema examination in order to rule out any defect in the swallowing mechanism, ulcers, tumor, malabsorption, or Crohn's disease. These tests are indicated more for patients who abuse laxatives excessively or who tend to induce vomiting after meals (the bulimic type). In such cases, monitoring of the blood electrolytes and routine electrocardiogram are necessary in order to evaluate the potassium blood level.

NUTRITIONAL EVALUATION

In addition to the above tests, nutritional assessment is very important in evaluating the nutritional status of the patient and realizing how severe the patient's condition is. If the fat tissue composition is less than 17%, it is calculated at what weight the patient will be above 17% fat tissue. Consequently, this weight is recommended to the patient as the goal weight to achieve in order to get back the menstrual periods. Blood transferrin level is checked also as part of the nutritional assessment, since transferrin level gives an estimate of the status of the visceral proteins. If the transferrin level is below normal, the nutritional state of the patient is considered to be poor with the immunologic system being adversely compromised. If the level of the fat tissue composition is below 10% and the transferrin level is below normal, it would be advisable to admit the patient into the hospital for more intensive and urgent care.

INTENSIVE MEDICAL TREATMENT

Admitting the patient into the hospital enables the practitioner to correct various physiologic abnormalities, such as imbalance of the electrolytes, and to provide nutrition by intragastric tubing (nasogastric tube) or, in case of severe malnutrition, by hyperalimentation as total parenteral nutrition (TPN).

If the patient's condition is not acute, dietetic counseling on an outpatient basis will supplement the nutritional evaluation. The dietitian can help the patient plan a specific diet in which the amount of calories is increased gradually. The first goal should be stabilization of the patient's weight with strong emphasis that no further loss of weight is allowed. The next step will be helping the patient build up the weight gradually at the rate of a quarter pound per day. The final step of the dietetic counseling is helping the patient maintain the goal weight once it has been achieved. Basically, anorexic patients do not need any specific medical diet. They can eat whatever they like, providing that their daily consumption is balanced with the necessary nutrients and vitamins.

THE PSYCHOLOGICAL EVALUATION

The other side of the coin in providing proper management to the anorexic is evaluating the patient's emotional needs, finding any evidence for a possible psychopathologic disorder, and treating it accordingly.

During the evaluation, the practitioner can pay attention to changes in the patient's personality that occurred as the weight loss progressed so that the patient can be confronted directly and a referral to a psychiatrist can be made. In severe cases, the following is seen: In order to suppress hunger, the patients involve themselves in many activities. Many fear growing up and facing adult responsibilities and use anorexia to stop the growth process. Many patients have delayed psychosexual development in order to avoid coping with the transition of adolescence. Their interest in sex is decreased and very rarely are they interested in dating or getting married during the illness. Many patients show difficulties in achieving normal adolescence tasks, such as being able to separate from parents and family and become more independent.

The typical obsessive-compulsive behavior should be recognized by the physician, and the patient has to be confronted with it for better sense of reality. Other confrontations should be done in regard to the elaborate ritualistic behavior and the daily rigid routine typical of these patients. Their tendency to be perfectionistic should be dealt with directly as part of the total symptom complex in anorexia nervosa.

PSYCHIATRIC OUTPATIENT THERAPY

Once the patient has been referred to a psychiatrist who treats eating disorders, treatment is on an outpatient basis, mainly individual weekly therapy, family therapy and counseling as recommended by Minuchin (especially in cases where the origin of the emotional distress has to do with faulty family relations), and group therapy. If self-help organizations for patients and parents exist in the nearby locality, referral to such organizations might help, since they are organized after the principles of Alcoholics Anonymous groups.

IN-HOSPITAL PSYCHIATRIC THERAPY

If the nutritional assessment indicates a physical risk, in-hospital therapy should be suggested to the patient. Such a program can provide more intensive psychotherapy including such additional therapies as behavior modification, which is easier to implement in a hospital setting. Also, the effect of the in-hospital milieu is very beneficial to many patients.

In the hospital, a variety of therapies are provided by professionals such as psychiatrists, psychologists, social workers, and nurses. These therapies include biofeedback, assertiveness training, psychoanalytic psychotherapy, and hypnotherapy. Psychopharmacology or use of medication could be used if necessary, as in the case of depression with anorexia nervosa. The author's preference is the use of Triavil, starting with 2-25 size tablets twice a day, increasing gradually to three to four times a day if needed. Triavil includes amitriptyline, which is an antidepressant, and perphenazine, which is a major tranquilizer. This combination was found to be especially beneficial for anorexic patients, since it tends to stimulate the appetite and induce some weight gain in addition to its psychotropic action. The tranquilizing effect of the medication helps patients to accept the fact that they must gain weight and undergo intensive therapy. In low doses it is rare to see the side effects of the tricyclic antidepressants or of the neuroleptic drugs. The most common complaint of patients on Triavil is somnolence. That could be avoided if the medication is started on a low dose and increased gradually.

THE TEAM APPROACH

It is important to coordinate the medical treatment with the psychiatric therapy. In most centers, the pediatrician or the internist is evaluating and treating the medical aspects of the illness, while the psychiatrist is in charge of the psychotherapy. If the program for anorexia nervosa is in a psychiatric unit, the internist is caring for the medical problems on a consultative basis. If the patient is being seen first by the family physician or the internist, it is important to ask for a psychiatric consultation as soon as possible, since the sooner the psychotherapy starts, the better the prognosis.

PSYCHOTHERAPY

Psychotherapy is usually done by a psychiatrist or by a psychologist under the supervision of an expert psychiatrist. The specific technique or modality of psychotherapy should be appropriately chosen according to the age of the patient, and his or her level of sophistication, and readiness for therapy. In the severe stage of malnutrition, patients cannot respond to insight-oriented therapy. They need more support, education and encouragement. The therapist has to differentiate between symptoms of starvation and the central conflict of the patient. Many symptoms of prominent compulsions and obsessions may improve without therapy once the weight is restored to normal.

Once some weight is gained, the therapy can be directed toward analysis of unconscious conflicts. Patients who suffer from anorexia nervosa tend to intellectualize their feelings and often tend to draw the therapist into talking about food, weight, and calories. This should be avoided and limited to the time of the dietary consultation. Common dynamic issues usually shared by many anorexic patients are fear of maturation and facing responsibilities of adult life, avoidance of inner sexual impulses and fear of dating, inability to handle stressful situations, difficulties separating from parents who are too overprotective and involved, and possibly any repressed unconscious memory of a severe traumatic event in childhood. It is important to have patients understand that nobody is perfect, and that they are allowed to make mistakes in the future. These dynamics of the therapy could be dealt with in individual therapy, group therapy, family therapy, or any other parallel therapy that is done at the same time. All these therapies should be coordinated between the various therapists so information about the conflicts of the patient can be shared, and consequently therapeutic goals can be formulated. This kind of team approach was found very successful in many medical centers that treat patients who suffer from eating disorders.

REFERENCES

American Psychiatric Association: Diagnostic and Statistical Manual of Mental Disorders, 3rd ed. Washington, DC, 1980.
Gross M: Anorexia Nervosa: A Comprehensive Approach. The Collamore Press, Lexington, MA, 1982.
Gross M: Anorexia nervosa: an overview. Cleve Clin Q 50:371–376, 1983.
Hsu LKG: Outcome of anorexia nervosa: a review of the literature (1954–1978). Arch Gen Psychiatry 37:1041–1046, 1980.
Minuchin S: Families and Family Therapy. Harvard University Press, Cambridge, MA, 1974.

6 · HYPERLIPIDEMIA

Bruce R. Zimmerman
MAYO CLINIC AND MAYO FOUNDATION

DIAGNOSTIC SCREENING

Interest in hyperlipidemia has been primarily stimulated by epidemiologic studies demonstrating a correlation between increasing atherosclerosis risks and increasing lipid concentrations. The American public has been trained to inquire about their serum cholesterol level no matter what their age or health problem. Bending to this pressure, most physicians obtain cholesterol determinations more frequently than necessary. In my opinion, both serum cholesterol and triglycerides should be measured for screening purposes. Without simultaneously measured triglyceride concentrations, serum cholesterol values are often misinterpreted and several important lipoprotein abnormalities are missed. Screening should be done on healthy young adults once and then not repeated for at least five years unless there

Table 1. TOTAL CHOLESTEROL, PERCENTILES (mg/dl)

	90th Percentile		95th Percentile	
Age (years)	Men	Women	Men	Women
0–19	185	190	200	200
20–24	205	215	220	230
25–29	225	220	245	235
30–34	240	220	255	235
35–39	250	230	270	245
40–44	250	235	270	255
45–49	260	250	275	270
50–64	260	265	275	285
65+	250	275	270	295

Modified from Rifkind BM, Segal P: Lipid research clinics program reference values for hyperlipidemia and hypolipidemia. JAMA 250:1869–1872, 1983.

is a change in health leading to a specific indication for the tests. Screening should not be done on healthy elderly patients previously known to have normal values. Specific indications for screening studies at any age include xanthoma or xanthelasma, a family history of premature atherosclerosis or hyperlipidemia, diabetes, pancreatitis or unexplained abdominal pain, renal failure, and neuropathy. For appropriate screening, the patient should avoid alcohol for 24 hours and be fasting overnight. Interpretation of the results should be based on age- and sex-adjusted values for the laboratory used. Patients found to have values between the 90th and 95th percentile (Tables 1 and 2) should be instructed in a low-fat, low-cholesterol diet with calories adjusted to achieve ideal body weight and have follow-up studies in about three months. Patients with values greater than 95th percentile require a specific diagnosis.

Once elevated lipid values are confirmed, several simple clinical steps should be taken. The medical history and examination should be reviewed with particular emphasis on the dietary and alcohol intake, family history, medications, and a search for xanthoma. Next the hyperlipidemia should be categorized and secondary causes excluded before a specific genetic diagnosis is made. This process is facilitated by dividing the screening tests into these broad groups: (1) chylomicronemia, (2) moderate hypertriglyceridemia, (3) mixed hyperlipidemia, and (4) hypercholesterolemia. Frederickson's types are a parallel method of grouping by phenotype, which contributes no additional information about cause.

Table 2. TOTAL TRIGLYCERIDES, PERCENTILES (mg/dl)

	90th percentile		95th Percentile	
Age (years)	Men	Women	Men	Women
0–9	85	95	100	110
10–14	100	115	125	130
15–19	120	115	150	130
20–24	165	145	200	170
25–29	200	145	250	170
30–34	215	145	265	170
35–39	250	160	320	195
40–44	250	170	320	210
45–49	250	185	320	230
50–54	250	190	320	240
55–64	235	200	290	250
65+	210	205	260	240

Modified from Rifkind BM, Segal P: Lipid research clinics program reference values for hyperlipidemia and hypolipidemia. JAMA 250:1869–1872, 1983.

PATHOPHYSIOLOGY AND CLINICAL ASPECTS

CHYLOMICRONEMIA (TYPES I AND V)

Chylomicrons can be confirmed by finding a creamy layer on top of a serum or plasma specimen stored at about 4° C for 12 hours. They are almost always absent when triglycerides are less than 1000 mg/dl and present when greater than 1500 mg/dl. When triglyceride concentrations are greater than 500 mg/dl, serum cholesterol is usually elevated also.

With persistent chylomicronemia many nonspecific symptoms may occur, including abdominal pain, pancreatitis, mild mental dysfunction, dyspnea, vague arthralgias, and neuralgias. Physical examination findings associated with chylomicronemia are eruptive xanthoma, lipemia retinalis, hepatomegaly, and splenomegaly. Chylomicrons displace water volume and plasma components are artifactually lowered if the chylomicrons are included in the volume used to calculate the concentration. Chylomicrons interfere with the blood O_2 electrode, causing apparent hypoxemia. Hemoglobin, amylase, bilirubin, and chloride measurements may be inaccurate.

Most patients with chylomicronemia have an inherited cause of moderate hypertriglyceridemia aggravated by a secondary factor, of which the most common is poorly controlled diabetes. Excessive alcohol intake, estrogens, contraceptives, thiazide diuretics, and betablockers are also common aggravating factors. An occasional patient with abnormal immunoglobulins from multiple myeloma, other hematologic tumors, or lupus has developed chylomicronemia without an apparent underlying hypertriglyceridemia.

Genetic Chylomicronemia. Less common are the genetic chylomicronemias. Familial lipoprotein lipase deficiency is an autosomal recessive disorder first manifest in early childhood by intolerance of dietary fat and chylomicronemia. Deficiency of apo CII, the lipoprotein lipase activator, is another autosomal recessive disorder with features similar to lipoprotein lipase deficiency. So-called primary type V hyperlipoproteinemia is not well defined. It may be the inheritance of two familial forms of hypertriglyceridemia. Other evidence suggests an abnormal apo E or sialylation of apo CIII. All of these disorders are rare enough to require referral to a lipid research center for definitive classification.

MODERATE HYPERTRIGLYCERIDEMIA (TYPE IV)

Both primary and secondary hypertriglyceridemia are common, particularly triglyceride overproduction secondary to non–insulin-dependent diabetes mellitus (NIDDM, type II), obesity, alcohol, excessive "simple" dietary carbohydrates, nephrotic syndrome, and hypothyroidism. Renal failure, insulinopenic diabetes, and hypothyroidism may reduce triglyceride clearance. Moderate hypertriglyceridemia is associated with no specific symptoms or signs.

Familial hypertriglyceridemia appears to follow an autosomal dominant inheritance pattern and to be due to either overproduction or decreased removal of VLDL-triglycerides, depending on the particular family. Whether atherosclerosis risk is increased in this disorder is controversial.

MIXED HYPERLIPIDEMIA (TYPES IIb and III)

Moderate elevations of both cholesterol and triglyceride concentrations are associated with three genetic abnormalities.

Familial Combined Hyperlipidemia. Familial combined hyperlipidemia is best explained by an overproduction of apo B. Family screening is important to confirm this diagnosis because in affected members about one third have increased LDL alone, one third mixed hyperlipidemia, and the remainder increased VLDL alone. The exact manifestation is modified by factors such as diet, obesity, alcohol, medications, and other diseases. This disorder definitely increases the risk of coronary artery disease but has no specific signs or symptoms. It is a common disorder said to be present in 10% to 20% of myocardial infarction survivors under age 60.

Familial Dysbetalipoproteinemia. Familial dysbetalipoproteinemia is caused by abnormal apo E. The structure of apo E is determined by at least three gene alleles resulting in six phenotypes that can be identified by isoelectric focusing gel electrophoretograms of VLDL. Dysbetalipoproteinemia is specified by the phenotype E-2:E-2, which has about a 1% prevalence in the American population. The apo E present in this disorder is not recognized well by hepatic receptors, resulting in the accumulation of chylomicron and VLDL remnants in some patients. Clinical manifestations of the disorder are rare even though the genotype is common. Exact determinants of the clinical expression are still being defined. The sex of the patients is important, since hyperlipidemia in women inheriting the genotype is rare prior to menopause and estrogen treatment decreases remnant accumulation. Some patients with the phenotype and hyperlipidemia seem to have inherited another form of hyperlipidemia with the interaction between them aggravating both. Hypothyroidism, obesity, and excess alcohol intake also may cause the hyperlipidemia. Patients with dysbetalipoproteinemia may have characteristic tuberous and palmar xanthomas. The development of atherosclerosis is definitely accelerated and occurs more in peripheral arteries. It is not known if people with the genotype but no hyperlipidemia or those heterozygous for E-2 have accelerated atherosclerosis, but in some reports the heterozygotes have an increased prevalence of xanthelasma. Confirmation of the diagnosis of dysbetalipoproteinemia may be difficult because isoelectric focusing is not widely available. Paper electrophoresis is not reliable for this diagnosis. A VLDL-cholesterol:triglyceride ratio ≥ 0.35 has proved reliable. Similar hyperlipidemia and palmar xanthoma are found with primary biliary cirrhosis and occasionally with dysproteinemia.

Familial Lecithin: Cholesterol Acyltransferase Deficiency. Much more rare is familial lecithin:cholesterol acyltransferase deficiency (LCAT deficiency), which may present as a mixed hyperlipidemia. This is an autosomal recessive disorder in which young adults develop minute, grayish corneal dots, normochromic anemia, proteinuria, renal failure, hypertension, and premature atherosclerosis.

HYPERCHOLESTEROLEMIA (TYPE IIa)

Hypercholesterolemia is found with hypothyroidism, the nephrotic syndrome, acute intermittent porphyria, and high dietary fat and cholesterol. When these are excluded and the cholesterol elevation is mild, HDL-cholesterol should be measured to exclude familial hyperalphalipoproteinemia. Patients with high HDL and normal LDL do not have an increased risk of atherosclerosis and require no treatment.

About one person in 500 in the United States will be heterozygous for familial hypercholesterolemia. In the heterozygote, this disorder results in diminished number or function of the LDL receptors. In the homozygote, receptors are almost absent or nonfunctional. Either circumstance results in elevated LDL and a major increase in atherosclerosis risk. About 50% of the men and 30% of the women heterozygotes will have symptomatic coronary artery disease by age 60. Homozygotes usually have coronary artery disease in childhood or adolescence. Other manifestations of this disorder include tendon xanthoma, xanthelasma, and corneal arcus. Homozygous patients have more extensive xanthomatosis with plantar cutaneous xanthoma at points of trauma and digital web xanthoma. Tendon xanthoma are almost specific for familial hypercholesterolemia but can occur in the patient with beta-sitosterolemia or cerebrotendinous xanthomatosis, two very rare disorders.

MANAGEMENT

DIETARY TREATMENT

Except for patients with chylomicronemia and familial hypercholesterolemia, the initial treatment of patients with hyperlipidemia should be diet alone. Several aspects of the diet apply to all patients. Calories should be restricted to achieve ideal weight. Daily dietary cholesterol should be less than 300 mg. Fat should be restricted to 30% or less of total calories with an emphasis on reducing saturated fats to about 10% of calories. In the patient with chylomicronemia and abdominal pain, severe fat restriction is justified because following it the chylomicrons usually clear rapidly. The dietary fats must remain restricted to less than 10 to 20 gm/day in patients with familial lipoprotein lipase deficiency or apo CII deficiency. Addition of medium-chain triglycerides is often helpful in these patients. On the other hand, in patients with secondary chylomicronemia, dietary fat restriction can usually be eased as symptoms clear and the diabetes is controlled or the secondary factor such as alcohol or drugs is removed. Some patients with hypertriglyceridemia are sensitive to simple sugars and restriction of sucrose may be helpful. Patients with hypertriglyceridemia should completely avoid alcoholic drinks.

If followed, dietary therapy is effective in 80% to 90% of patients with hypertriglyceridemia but usually results in only a 10% to 20% reduction in cholesterol in patients with familial hypercholesterolemia. Patients with dysbetalipoproteinemia and familial combined hyperlipidemia usually have a good response to diet but may have residual hypercholesterolemia. If the cholesterol or triglycerides remain above the 90th percentile following diet therapy, then drug treament should be considered.

DRUG CHOICE

Choice of the best drug treatment program depends on the specific diagnosis. Drugs are not effective for familial lipoprotein lipase deficiency or apo CII deficiency. Other forms of chylomicronemia often require immediate initiation of drug treatment in addition to diet because of the risk of pancreatitis. Either gemfibrozil or nicotinic acid is a reasonable choice. Often the drug can be withdrawn after several months when the secondary factors have been treated. Patients with diabetes usually require sulfonylurea or insulin treatment. Moderate hypertriglyceridemia persisting despite dietary therapy raises difficult therapeutic questions. With a family history of premature atherosclerosis and triglycerides greater than 500 mg/dl, drug treatment is warranted. If the triglycerides are between the 90th percentile and 500 mg/dl and studies suggest familial combined hyperlipidemia, drug treatment is probably worthwhile, but may not be if familial hypertriglyceridemia is diagnosed. The drug of choice is gemfibrozil, with nicotinic acid also an effective agent. Dysbetalipoproteinemia responds very well to gemfibrozil or clofibrate. Nicotinic acid is a second choice. Hypercholesterolemia from either familial combined hyperlipidemia or familial hypercholesterolemia responds to the resins cholestyramine or colestipol. Dietary therapy alone is never adequate for familial hypercholesterolemia so I usually initiate drug therapy early, but wait to judge the response to diet for familial combined hyperlipidemia. Often combination therapy using a resin and either nicotinic acid or gemfibrozil is necessary for treatment of hypercholesterolemia. When these drugs are not tolerated, probucol can be used. Mevinolin and compactin are two investigational drugs that show great promise in combination with the resins. D-Thyroxine, neomycin, and beta-sitosterol have been used with limited success. Drugs should not be used in children under the age of 6 years or in pregnant women. Only resin treatment of hypercholesterolemia has been proved to reduce the development of coronary artery disease, so the potential risks and benefits of drug treatment must be carefully balanced. This can only be done with drug metabolism and side effects in mind.

SPECIFIC DRUG INFORMATION

Cholestyramine and Colestipol. The resins cholestyramine (Questran) and colestipol (Colestid) both have similar mechanisms of action and side effects. They bind bile acids in the intestine, increasing their excretion. Increased bile acid synthesis occurs utilizing cholesterol and stimulating development of more LDL receptors and cholesterol reduction. Neither drug is absorbed from the intestine, so there are no serious systemic side effects except fat-soluble vitamin, iron, and calcium deficiencies with large doses. Unfortunately both drugs cause severe constipation in about 20% of patients. This usually subsides if the drug is continued and may be eased by bulk laxatives. Nausea and bloating are common when the drugs are started and can be lessened by a gradual increase to the full dosage. Absorption of other drugs such as thyroxine, digoxin, and thiazides is interfered with, and they should be taken one hour before the resins. The resins are powders that must be mixed with water or juice. Cholestyramine comes in 4-gm packages or with a 4-gm scoop, and colestipol comes in 5-gm units. Usual dosage is 8 or 10 gm twice a day but may be increased to three times a day.

Clofibrate and Gemfibrozil. Clofibrate (Atromid-S) and gemfibrozil (Lopid) are analogues with similar characteristics. Gemfibrozil is the newer drug and is probably more effective in most patients. Both appear to act by increasing lipoprotein lipase and decreasing VLDL synthesis. Gemfibrozil may stimulate AI and AII synthesis. Both cause mild nausea and bloating in some patients, but this usually subsides. Both may cause hepatocellular liver function abnormalities in a small proportion of patients. Cholelithiasis risk is doubled by these drugs and decreased libido occurs in about 12% of men. Both potentiate anticoagulant action. Creatine kinase elevations and myositis occur rarely. The World Health Organization study suggested clofibrate might increase the frequency of some malignancies. Several design problems in this study make it hard to apply the findings to the usual use of the drug. Clofibrate comes in 0.5-gm capsules and is usually given as 1 gm twice a day. Gemfibrozil comes in 300-mg capsules and is usually given as 600 mg twice a day. These drugs should be used in reduced dosage, if at all, in patients with impaired renal function.

Nicotinic Acid. Nicotinic acid increases lipoprotein lipase, decreases lipolysis, and decreases VLDL synthesis, thus lowering both VLDL and LDL. Unfortunately it is not well tolerated by many patients. Almost all patients develop cutaneous flushing at the onset of treatment and when the dose is increased. This usually subsides in a few days and may be attenuated by aspirin taken about one half hour before the nicotinic acid. Gastric irritation is common and may be less if the drug is taken with meals. Hepatotoxicity occurs and may be either hepatocellular or cholestatic. Glucose tolerance may worsen and uric acid may increase. Dry skin, pruritus, and occasionally acanthosis nigricans can be bothersome. The side effects may be lessened by gradually increasing the dose from 100 mg three times a day to a maximum of about 7.5 gm/day. Usually hypertriglyceridemia responds to 1.5 gm/day but hypercholesterolemia requires larger doses.

Probucol. Probucol (Lorelco) is used only infrequently in the United States. Its mechanism of action is not clear, but it is highly lipophilic. In addition to lowering LDL it lowers HDL and apo AI and increases triglycerides, which are undesirable effects. It usually is well tolerated but may cause diarrhea and a mild normochromic anemia. Both dogs and monkeys have died from ventricular arrhythmias induced by this agent. Q-T prolongation preceded the arrhythmias. Absorption of the drug is poor but is increased if taken with meals. It comes in 250-mg capsules and is usually given as 500 mg twice a day.

Other Drugs. Several other drugs have very limited usefulness and will be only briefly discussed. D-Thyroxine (Choloxin) in doses up to 8 mg daily will lower cholesterol, but it has been associated with increased angina pectoris and arrhythmias. It should be used only in patients free of heart disease and intolerant of other cholesterol-lowering drugs. Neomycin lowers cholesterol but can be absorbed in large enough amounts to cause ototoxicity with chronic use. Beta-sitosterol impairs intestinal absorption of cholesterol but has not been very effective in lowering serum cholesterol. Oxandrolone lowers triglycerides and is occasionally helpful in patients with chylomicronemia. Estrogens lower lipids in women with dysbetalipoproteinemia.

OTHER TREATMENT

Patients who are homozygous for familial hypercholesterolemia respond poorly to drug treament. Portacaval shunting, plasmapheresis, and liver transplantation have been tried on an investigational basis. Because these patients have severe atherosclerosis at an early age, they should be referred to a specialty center. Intestinal bypass has been used to treat hypercholesterolemia but accomplishes little more than the resins at the price of operative morbidity and mortality.

PERIODIC EVALUATION

Effective treatment requires close follow-up. Patients with secondary hyperlipidemia often have an underlying primary disorder and must be followed. Patients treated by diet require careful instructions about the details of the diet and regular follow-up to judge the response to diet and continued compliance with the diet. Patients begun on drugs should have lipid studies and additional tests to judge drug effectiveness and side effects in one month. Studies should be repeated again in three months. If gemfibrozil or clofibrate has shown no benefit, it should be stopped. If the resins have not resulted in a serum cholesterol less than the 75th percentile, combination therapy should be considered, adding either nicotinic acid or gemfibrozil. Patients should continue to be seen at least every three months until the lipid response is adequate and the treatment program stable. Thereafter the follow-up program can be individualized. Long-term treatment for hyperlipidemia is expensive for the patient, sometimes costing in excess of $100 per month. Supporting letters to insurance companies may be as important as any other aspect of treatment for the patient.

PREVENTIVE MEASURES

Because the goal in treatment of hyperlipidemia in most cases is reduction of atherosclerosis risk, concentration on the matters already mentioned is not enough. All other atherosclerosis risk factors must be considered. The adverse effects of smoking should be discussed. Hypertension should be treated vigorously, avoiding thiazides and beta-blockers if they are aggravating hypertriglyceridemia. A regular exercise program, designed in light of the patient's cardiovascular status, should be instituted.

When a genetic cause of hyperlipidemia is diagnosed, family screening should be done. Familial hypercholesterolemia can be diagnosed in childhood. Familial combined hyperlipidemia, dysbetalipoproteinemia, and familial hypertriglyceridemia may not be manifest until after age 30.

POPULATION AND SOCIOECONOMIC FACTORS

Epidemiologic studies have clearly demonstrated that even within the normal range, higher cholesterol values are associated with an increased risk of atherosclerosis independent of the primary lipid disorders. Although highly statistically significant, what is not generally appreciated is that the predictability of atherosclerosis based on these values is low. The large numbers of patients studied lead to the highly significant P-values despite low predictability. This has resulted in the calculation of risk ratios based on minor changes in lipid values, which are less than the reproducibility of the tests. This is clearly a ridiculous exercise when applied to the individual patient whose risk would fluctuate greatly from week to week if the studies were repeated. Unfortunately, these studies have tended to focus on isolated lipid values such as total cholesterol, triglycerides, and HDL-cholesterol, ignoring the complex interactions among them. Their interdependence has not always been taken into account in the statistical analysis in the epidemiologic studies leading to the controversy about triglycerides. The atherogenicity of triglycerides is dependent on the lipoprotein particle. Triglycerides in IDL are atherogenic but not those in chylomicrons. Detailed studies of lipoproteins and apoproteins are providing a much better insight into atherosclerosis and lipids. For example, apo AI is a more accurate predictor of atherosclerosis than cholesterol or triglycerides. The patient with high normal lipids might prudently decide to reduce dietary fats and cholesterol. The patient with low or mid-normal range lipids should hope that additional research will be completed before major changes are recommended in the diet of the entire population.

REFERENCES

Goldstein J, Kita T, Brown M: Defective lipoprotein receptors and atherosclerosis. N Engl J Med 309:288–296, 1983.
Havel RJ, Kane JP: Therapy of hyperlipidemic states. Ann Rev Med 33:417–433, 1982.
Kressberg, A: Editorial: Lipids, lipoproteins, apolipoproteins and atherosclerosis. Ann Intern Med 99:713–715, 1983.
Schaefer EJ, Levy RI: Pathogenesis and management of lipoprotein disorders. N Engl J Med 312:1300–1310, 1985.

7 · INBORN ERRORS OF CARBOHYDRATE METABOLISM

Joseph I. Wolfsdorf
JOSLIN CLINIC

The diseases described in this chapter are rare and usually encountered by pediatricians, either during the newborn period or in early infancy. It is recommended that the primary care physician obtain confirmation of the diagnosis and guidance on the management of these disorders by referral to a specialized center.

Glycogen Storage Diseases (Glycogenoses or GSD)

DEFINITION AND DIAGNOSTIC CRITERIA

The glycogen storage diseases or glycogenoses comprise several inherited diseases that have in common some abnormality involving either the structure or metabolism of glycogen or the transformation of glycogen-

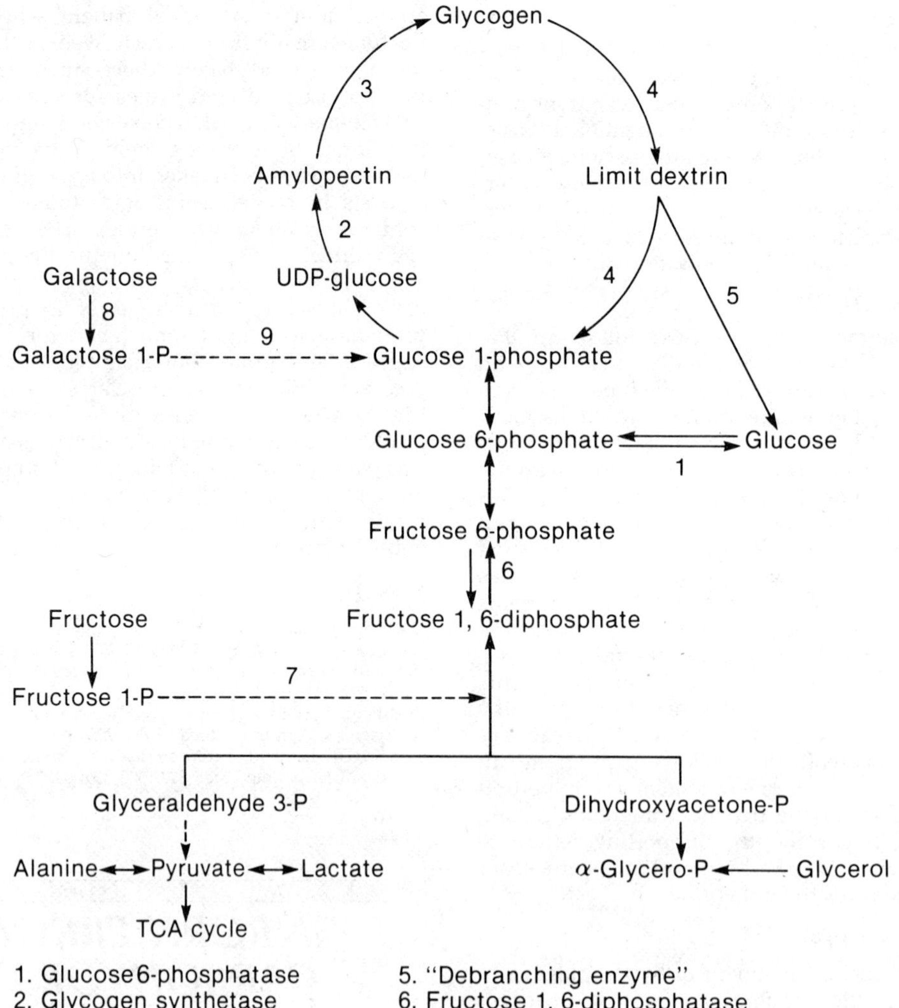

Figure 1. Simplified scheme of the metabolic pathways involved in glycogen synthesis, degradation, and gluconeogenesis.

olytic products, or gluconeogenic substrates, to glucose (Fig. 1). As a result, increased storage of glycogen occurs in several tissues, especially liver and muscle.

The diagnostic criteria and salient clinical and laboratory features of these disorders are summarized in Table 1.

MANAGEMENT

TYPE I

The metabolic and hormonal abnormalities in type I GSD are the consequence of glucose deprivation, which becomes evident a few hours after feeding and is markedly accentuated by fasting. Treatment consists of providing glucose to prevent blood glucose levels from falling below about 70 to 80 mg/dl so the liver is not called upon to produce glucose. When exogenous glucose is provided in adequate amounts, the liver size decreases, the abnormal serum biochemistry reverses to normal or near-normal, the bleeding tendency disappears, and growth and development progress normally.

Treatment should attempt to provide sufficient glucose to maintain the blood glucose concentration above the critical level necessary to suppress the secretion of counterregulatory hormones. This can be accomplished by giving glucose-containing polymers (e.g., Polycose or Hycal) intermittently during the day, and either a 25% or 50% solution of glucose during the night as a continuous infusion via a nasogastric tube or gastrostomy. The rate is kept constant by using an infusion pump. This is begun when the infant no longer readily takes three-hourly feedings at night and becomes susceptible to hypoglycemia when fasted for three to four hours or more. The amount of glucose prescribed is initially calculated to approximate the rate of hepatic glucose production, from the equation

$$Y = 0.0014x^3 - 0.214x^2 + 10.411x - 9.084$$

where Y = mg glucose per minute and x = body weight in kilograms. Subsequently, the quantity of glucose needed is determined by monitoring the clinical and biochemical response to treatment, and adjusting the amount and frequency of glucose administration until clinical and biochemical parameters are both as near to normal as possible. When adequate exogenous glucose is provided in this manner, significant hyperuricemia is usually prevented. In the unusual event that it persists, uric acid levels can be lowered with allopurinol, a xanthine oxidase inhibitor, 5 to 10 mg/kg/day.

The total daily intake of calories is determined largely by the child's appetite (as long as the rate of growth and weight gain are normal) taking into account that the diet prescribed must ensure an adequate intake of protein, fat, minerals, and vitamins to support optimum growth. When adequate glucose is prescribed, limited amounts of milk products and fruit, despite their content of galactose and fructose, respectively, may be used to supply essential nutrients, minerals, and vitamins. Carbohydrate provides about 60% of the daily calories, and the bulk of the carbohydrate is in the form of glucose and glucose polymers.

Recent studies have shown that orally administered uncooked cornstarch appears to act as an intestinal reservoir of glucose that is slowly absorbed into the circulation. This property of uncooked cornstarch has been used to develop a feeding regimen for older children that promises to replace the current method of frequent daytime feedings combined with continuous intragastric glucose overnight. The uncooked cornstarch is given as a slurry in flavored water or in milk, at three- to five-hour intervals during the day and four- to six-hour intervals overnight. The amount given is initially based on the calculated hepatic glucose production rate (see above equation). More experience is needed, however, to determine the optimum schedule and amounts of intermittent uncooked cornstarch feedings for chil-

dren with type I glycogenosis of different ages, and to establish its long-term effectiveness.

The regimen described above should be followed at least until growth and development are complete. The biochemical abnormalities ameliorate by early adulthood; however, some patients develop hepatic adenomas and hepatocellular carcinomas. It is not yet known whether optimal biochemical control of patients with type I GSD can influence the development of hepatic neoplasms or influence their natural history.

TYPE II

There is no specific treatment; at present, only supportive therapy for the cardiac or pulmonary symptoms is available.

TYPE III

Because only a limited amount of glucose can be mobilized from glycogen, a state of glucose deprivation with hypoglycemia develops in infants or young children fasted overnight or longer. This occurs despite increased gluconeogenesis and enhanced hepatic uptake of gluconeogenic amino acids, which results in low levels of several plasma amino acids. Thus, as in type I glycogenosis, continuous replacement of glucose overnight (see earlier), combined with a normal intake of total calories, protein and other nutrients, results in marked amelioration of the clinical and biochemical picture. Because patients with type III GSD have an intact gluconeogenic pathway, frequent ingestion of large quantities of protein to provide a constant source of glucose via hepatic transformation, together with complex carbohydrates in the form of starch, is believed to be more effective than carbohydrate alone in correct-

Table 1. MAJOR CLINICAL AND BIOCHEMICAL ABNORMALITIES OF THE GLYCOGENOSES

Type	Defective Enzyme	Major Clinical Features	Major Biochemical Features	Response to Glucagon*
I	Glucose 6-phosphatase Glucose 6-phosphate translocase	Acidosis and hyperventilation, hepatomegaly, kidneys enlarged, growth failure, bleeding tendency, xanthomatosis, delayed puberty, gout, hepatic adenomas; neutropenia in type Ib	Marked fasting hypoglycemia especially in infants, lactacidemia, hypertriglyceridemia, moderate hypercholesterolemia, liver transaminases often abnormal, abnormal platelet function	Small or no increase in glucose, basal hyperlactatemia increases further
II	Lysosomal α-1; 4-glucosidase (acid maltase)	Muscle weakness, enlarged tongue, cardiomyopathy	Blood glucose, lipids, and uric acid are normal	
III	Amylo-1, 6-glucosidase and/or oligo-1, 4→1, 4-glucan transferase (debrancher enzyme)	Hyperventilation with ketosis, hepatomegaly at times with splenomegaly, growth failure, delayed puberty, myopathy, normal kidney size	Moderate to severe hypoglycemia with ketosis after long fast, normal fasting lactate and uric acid, mild to moderate hyperlipidemia, liver transaminases increased	Normal glycemic response 2 hrs after carbohydrate meal; with more prolonged fast, small or no increase in glucose and no increase in lactate
IV	Brancher enzyme	Cirrhosis of liver, portal hypertension	Increased serum transaminases and 5'-nucleotidase; hypoglycemia does not occur	
V	Muscle phosphorylase	Strenuous muscular exertion causes muscle cramps and myoglobinuria; muscle-wasting in later life	CPK, aldolase, LDH increased after exercise; ischemic exercise does not elevate blood lactate	
VI	Liver phosphorylase	Hepatomegaly	Fasting hypoglycemia either absent or mild; lactate and uric acid normal, may have mild hyperlipidemia	Usually normal glucose and lactate responses
IX	Phoshorylase kinase	Heptomegaly		
X	Protein Kinase	Hepatomegaly		

*Used as a diagnostic test in the glycogenoses associated with hypoglycemia.

ing the disorder. It has been suggested that a specific feeding regimen may result in clinical improvement in those type III patients with significant growth retardation and myopathy. This involves continuous nocturnal feeding of a nutrient mixture consisting of glucose, glucose oligosaccharides, and amino acids (Vivonex), and intermittent daytime feedings high in protein. Continuous nocturnal feeding is accomplished in the same manner as that described for patients with type I GSD.

TYPE IV

There is no treatment other than supportive measures for liver failure. Death usually occurs before the age of 5 years from the complications of cirrhosis.

TYPE V

No specific treatment is known; nevertheless, most patients are able to live a reasonably normal life by modifying their activities. Because muscle pain and stiffness occur during intense or prolonged exercise, patients should be advised not to engage in strenuous exercise. When muscular pain develops, the patient should immediately rest until the pain subsides. Continuing to exercise despite the presence of pain or cramps may result in myoglobinuria due to muscle necrosis, soreness, and swelling lasting several days.

Attempts to provide fatty acids as an alternative metabolic fuel for exercising muscle have not been uniformly efficacious. Recently it has been found that a high-protein diet (25% to 30% of total calories) improved muscle function and increased endurance in a patient with McArdle's syndrome.

TYPES VI, IX, AND X

There is no proven specific treatment for these disorders. A recent report claimed that D-thyroxine, 4 mg daily, caused the liver to shrink, decreased serum triglycerides, and improved growth in a few children with phosphorylase deficiency.

When it does occur, hypoglycemia is only mild; hence, specific dietary measures are not routinely necessary. The enlarged liver regresses when patients reach puberty.

Galactosemia

DEFINITION AND DIAGNOSTIC CRITERIA

Classic galactosemia is an autosomal recessive disorder that results from lack of activity of the enzyme galactose 1-phosphate uridyl transferase (transferase), which converts galactose 1-phosphate to uridyl diphosphate-galactose, an essential step in the pathway of galactose metabolism (Fig. 1).

Galactosemia should ideally be diagnosed before clinical signs appear. Techniques to screen newborns for galactosemia are reliable but not specific; hence, confirmatory testing is necessary. The definitive diagnosis is made by demonstrating very low or absent activity of transferase in erythrocytes. Genetic variants of transferase, such as Duarte and Los Angeles, are not associated with clinical manifestations and can be differentiated by enzyme electrophoresis.

PATHOPHYSIOLOGY

Galactose and galactose 1-phosphate accumulate throughout the body. Galactose itself probably does not damage tissues other than the lens of the eye; galactose 1-phosphate is the toxic substance in tissues such as the brain, liver, and kidney.

CLINICAL ASPECTS

Infants with galactosemia usually appear normal at birth. Symptoms appear a few days after the infant has received milk or a formula that contains lactose; vomiting, jaundice, lethargy, and occasionally diarrhea occur. The child fails to thrive and hepatomegaly is the most common physical finding. Hypoglycemia is common and results from decreased release of glucose from the liver. Fulminant *E. coli* sepsis may develop within the first few days of life. The child may die from liver failure if galactosemia is not promptly recognized and treated. Cataracts form within a few days to weeks but are usually not recognized until later. The child who survives untreated does not thrive, develops cirrhosis and cataracts, and is usually mentally retarded. Despite treatment, hypergonadotropic hypogonadism develops in a high percentage of females with classic galactosemia and it is thought that exposure to galactose in utero or during the neonatal period may damage the ovary. Gonadal function in males appears not to be affected.

MANAGEMENT

Treatment is aimed at controlling the tissue accumulation of galactose metabolites. Urgent attention must also be given to the treatment of the secondary manifestations of the disorder: infections, the bleeding tendency, hyperbilirubinemia, and so on. Both the immediate and long-term treatment involve elimination of galactose from the diet, which is accomplished by avoiding lactose, present in milk and milk products, and substituting a lactose-free formula. Lists of lactose-free foods are available to physicians and parents. Institution of a galactose-free diet rapidly brightens the clinical picture; cataracts, if not already far advanced, may regress. A galactose-free formula may be the sole source of calories until the usual baby foods are added. Many baby foods contain some form of milk and must be avoided. Cereals, vegetables, fruits, and meat are safe.

As the child grows older and the diet becomes more varied, caution must be exercised in selecting new foods. Milk is commonly found in bread, cake, some canned puddings, and various chocolate candies; accordingly, the labels on all food packages must be scrutinized. Parents need to periodically consult a nutritionist to ensure that the child's diet is well-balanced and contains all the nutrients necessary for growth and development. By the time children with galactosemia reach school age, they tend to reduce their intake of the milk substitute, which can then be replaced by water, fruit, or vegetable juices, and a calcium supplement added. Meat, poultry, fish, and eggs are excellent sources of protein, but liver, pancreas, and brain should be avoided because they contain galactose. Labels on cold cuts and other meats that commonly contain fillers should be carefully examined to ensure that no milk or milk products are included. Dietary therapy is lifelong.

MONITORING THERAPY

Biochemical control is monitored by measuring the concentration of galactose 1-phosphate in red cells. In untreated galactosemia this level is about 20 to 100 mg/dl, whereas in treated patients the level should be 0 to 3 mg/dl.

GENETIC COUNSELING

There is a 25% chance of recurrence in any subsequent pregnancy; therefore, genetic counseling should be provided. Transferase is present in cultured amniotic cells from the normal fetus, so it is now possible to detect transferase deficiency before birth. The carrier state can be identified by quantitative assays of enzyme activity in erythrocytes. This service should be offered to members of a family in which galactosemia has been diagnosed.

Galactokinase Deficiency

DEFINITION AND DIAGNOSTIC CRITERIA

Patients with galactokinase deficiency are unable to convert galactose to galactose 1-phosphate (Fig. 1). They have increased blood levels of galactose, galactosuria, and increased excretion of urinary galactitol. These compounds should be sought after milk feedings and not in the fasting state. The diagnosis is confirmed by the absence of galactokinase in erythrocytes. Heterozygotes excrete excessive amounts of galactitol in their urine.

PATHOPHYSIOLOGY AND CLINICAL ASPECTS

The formation of galactitol in the lens causes cataracts; its accumulation in the brain may cause pseudotumor cerebri. Early recognition of the disorder is difficult because there are no systemic symptoms. The cataracts may appear at any age and can also occur in heterozygotes; thus, even partial galactokinase deficiency may be clinically significant.

MANAGEMENT

As in classic galactosemia, dietary galactose must be assiduously avoided. The lenticular cataracts may or may not regress. A lactose-free diet during subsequent pregnancies is recommended to protect the lenses of the fetus.

Hereditary Fructose Intolerance (HFI)

DEFINITION AND DIAGNOSTIC CRITERIA

HFI results from a deficiency of hepatic fructose 1-phosphate aldolase, which catalyzes the conversion of fructose 1-phosphate to glyceraldehyde and dihydroxyacetone phosphate as well as the conversion of fructose 1,6-diphosphate to glyceraldehyde 3-phosphate and dihydroxyacetone phosphate (Fig. 1). Exposure of affected individuals to even small amounts of dietary fructose induces the state of fructose intoxication.

The diagnosis is often suggested by the history, but should be confirmed by performing a fructose tolerance test with the patient fasting. After fructose has been withdrawn from the diet for several weeks, the definitive diagnosis is made by demonstrating very low or unmeasurable levels of fructose 1-phosphate aldolase activity in a biopsy sample of liver.

PATHOPHYSIOLOGY

When patients with HFI are exposed to fructose, severe depletion of cellular inorganic phosphate occurs as fructose 1-phosphate accumulates in tissues lacking the aldolase activity. This induces a severe disturbance of adenine nucleotide metabolism with secondary inhibition of fructokinase and phosphorylase. Glycogenolysis is impaired and leads to hypoglycemia.

CLINICAL ASPECTS

Individuals with HFI do not have symptoms as long as they avoid fructose. The appearance of symptoms virtually coincides with the first ingestion of fructose, usually at the time of weaning when fructose and sucrose are introduced into the diet in the form of fruit, vegetables, and sweetened cereals. Fructose intoxication is expressed as either of two strikingly symptomatic syndromes.

Acute Syndrome. In the acute syndrome, transient abdominal pain and vomiting occur within minutes of exposure to fructose and symptomatic hypoglycemia occurs within an hour. Hepatomegaly is invariably present and is usually associated with jaundice and other evidence of liver dysfunction such as ascites, edema, and a bleeding tendency. In infancy, three dominant symptoms occur: poor feeding, vomiting, and failure to gain weight. If the disorder is not recognized and treated promptly, the severely affected infant with HFI may die of acute liver failure or shock. Withdrawal of fructose always results in dramatic improvement; vomiting ceases, appetite improves within a few days, and the disturbances of liver and renal tubular function disappear within 48 to 72 hours. The acute symptoms tend to be more severe in infants and milder in older individuals.

Chronic Syndromes. If the infant survives and remains untreated, a chronic syndrome develops characterized by severe metabolic derangement, failure to thrive, recurrent vomiting, hepatomegaly, and pronounced liver and renal tubular dysfunction. By 2 years of age, most of these children have acquired a pronounced aversion to foods containing fructose and sucrose so that they tend to avoid foods containing these sugars sufficiently to prevent the symptoms of acute fructose intoxication.

Moderate fructose ingestion by older patients causes persistent hepatomegaly and growth retardation but no acute symptoms. Stringent restriction of fructose (less than 40 mg/kg/day) is necessary to reverse the growth retardation.

LABORATORY FINDINGS

Increased levels of transaminases, abnormal prothrombin time, and serum proteins indicate liver dysfunction. Fructosuria, moderate proteinuria (less than 1 gm/day), aminoaciduria, and acidosis indicate disturbed renal tubular function. The urine contains fructose and gives a positive reaction to tests for reducing substances. The levels of phosphate and potassium in the serum are reduced; magnesium and uric acid levels are increased.

MANAGEMENT

The diagnosis should be suspected in any infant with recurrent intractable vomiting and a history of feeding difficulties. Whenever the diagnosis is suspected, fructose must be immediately withdrawn from the diet. Unless the infant's condition has already deteriorated irretrievably, symptoms and signs typically abate within a few days; hepatomegaly may persist for many months although the liver does gradually become smaller.

Because ingestion of small amounts of fructose is associated with a syndrome of chronic fructose intoxication, it is imperative to rigorously impose a diet that excludes fructose in any form. This is easily accomplished during infancy by nursing or using a formula that contains neither fructose nor sucrose. When weaning occurs, nutritional restrictions must be stringently enforced.

EDUCATION

The parents and ultimately the patient must receive appropriate nutrition education. In addition to sucrose-containing sweets, drinks and cookies, the following should be avoided completely: ham, bacon, lunch meats, sweet potatoes, all fruits and fruit juices (including tomato), bread, sugar-containing cereals, salad dressings, most desserts, catsup, pickles, jam, preserves, and honey. Some potatoes, especially if fresh, certain vegetables such as broccoli, cucumber and gourds, and some varieties of peas and rhubarb may contain small amounts of sucrose or fructose and should

be avoided. Invert sugar, sorbitol, and levulose must never be administered intravenously. These dietary restrictions have to be lifelong. All processed and packaged foods should be viewed with suspicion and the list of contents carefully examined.

Friends and teachers should be given a list of allowable foods and warned of the dangers of sucrose-containing food or drinks.

Treatment of the acute symptoms involves the correction of hypoglycemia by intravenous administration of glucose-containing solutions.

MONITORING

The patient's progress is monitored by careful evaluation of growth parameters, liver size, and biochemical indices of hepatic and renal function. A reduction in linear growth velocity appears to be a sensitive indicator of inadequate dietary compliance.

GENETIC COUNSELING

Because the disorder is inherited in an autosomal recessive fashion, there is a 25% risk of any subsequent children being affected. A dominant pattern of inheritance has also been described and raises the possibility of at least two genetic forms of the disorder. At the present time it is not possible to detect persons who are heterozygous for the abnormality.

Fructose 1,6-Diphosphatase Deficiency

DEFINITION AND DIAGNOSTIC CRITERIA

This rare autosomal recessive disease is due to lack of activity of a key gluconeogenic enzyme (Fig. 1). It shares certain clinical features in common with type I glycogen storage disease. In contrast to the latter, accumulation of glycogen in the liver does not occur; the enlarged liver is due to storage of fat. When these patients fast, blood glucose levels remain normal for about 12 hours, then fall to hypoglycemic levels; lactic acidosis, ketoacidosis, hyperuricemia, and hypertriglyceridemia develop. Glucagon does not elicit a glycemic response. The diagnosis is confirmed by demonstrating lack of fructose 1,6-diphosphatase activity in a liver biopsy specimen.

PATHOPHYSIOLOGY

Because the glycogenolytic pathway is intact, the liver can produce glucose from glycogen as long as it is still available. Once the liver's store of glycogen has been depleted, hypoglycemia occurs because gluconeogenic substrates (lactate, glycerol, amino acids) that enter the pathway below the level of fructose 1,6-diphosphatase cannot be converted to glucose.

When substrates are supplied that are phosphorylated and enter the glycolytic pathway below the level of fructose 1,6-diphosphatase, lactic acid accumulates. Dietary or intravenous fructose causes lactic acidosis;

and, under conditions of catabolic stress, endogenous substrates such as glycerol and amino acids induce lactic acidosis.

CLINICAL ASPECTS

Symptoms usually appear before 6 months of age. Hepatomegaly, hypoglycemia, and lactic acidosis are the major features. Inadequate treatment is associated with failure to thrive.

MANAGEMENT

Meals must be eaten at regular intervals and fasting avoided. During intercurrent illness, a high-carbohydrate diet should be given. A diet containing 50% to 60% utilizable carbohydrate (glucose, maltose, lactose), 10% to 12% protein, and 30% fat is effective in controlling chronic lactic acidosis and hypoglycemia. Sucrose and fructose should be avoided. Circumstances associated with catabolic stress (infection, surgery) can lead to life-threatening hypoglycemia and lactic acidosis, and warrant treatment with parenteral glucose to restore normoglycemia and bicarbonate to correct lactic acidosis.

REFERENCES

Gitzelmann R, Steinmann B, Van Den Berghe G: Essential fructosuria, hereditary fructose intolerance, and hereditary fructose-1,6-diphosphatase deficiency. *In* Stanbury JB, et al (eds): The Metabolic Basis of Inherited Disease, 5th ed. McGraw-Hill, New York, 1983, pp 118–140.

Howell RR, Williams JC: The glycogen storage diseases. *In* Stanbury JB, et al (eds): The Metabolic Basis of Inherited Disease, 5th ed. McGraw-Hill, New York, 1983, pp 141–167.

Segal S: Disorders of galactose metabolism. *In* Stanbury JB, et al (eds): The Metabolic Basis of Inherited Disease, McGraw-Hill, New York, 1983, pp 167–191.

Stanley CA: Intragastric feeding in glycogen storage disease and other disorders of fasting. *In* Walker WA, Watkins JB (eds): Nutrition in Pediatrics: Basic Science and Clinical Application. Little, Brown & Co, Boston, 1985, pp 781–794.

8 · HYPERURICEMIA AND GOUT

Leonard H. Serebro
Thomas E. Weiss
OCHSNER CLINIC AND ALTON OCHSNER MEDICAL FOUNDATION

DEFINITION AND DIAGNOSTIC CRITERIA

Many factors affect serum urate levels, including age, sex, race, diet, drugs, and a variety of diseases. Hyperuricemia is present when plasma urate levels exceed a value of two standard deviations above the mean in a sex- and age-matched healthy population. In general, this implies an upper limit of normal for men of 7 mg/dl and for women 6 mg/dl. By these criteria, between 3% and 20% of Americans have hyperuricemia. Only a minority of patients with hyperuricemia

Table 1. CLASSIFICATION OF ACUTE ARTHRITIS OF PRIMARY GOUT*

Major Criteria
1. Monosodium urate monohydrate microcrystals in joint fluid during attack
2. Tophus (proved)

Minor Criteria
1. Maximum inflammation developed within 1 day
2. More than one attack of acute arthritis
3. Monoarthritis attack
4. Redness observed over joints
5. First metatarsophalangeal joint painful or swollen
6. Unilateral first metatarsophalangeal joint attack
7. Unilateral tarsal joint attack
8. Tophus (suspected)
9. Hyperuricemia
10. Asymmetric swelling without a joint on x-ray examination
11. Subcortical cysts without erosions on x-ray examination
12. Joint fluid culture negative for organisms during attack

*Classification as the acute arthritis of primary gout requires one major criterion or any six of the 12 minor criteria. From the American Rheumatism Association, 1977.

develop gout, which is a disorder characterized by a variable combination of acute and chronic arthritis, soft tissue tophaceous deposits of urate, and urate nephropathy and nephrolithiasis. The diagnostic criteria are shown in Table 1. A definite diagnosis of articular gout can be made by finding urate crystals in joint fluid using a polarizing microscope. Long needle-shaped crystals, which are strongly negatively birefringent, may be seen inside or outside polymorphonuclear leukocytes from joint fluid or in tophi. Even without urate crystals, the presence of six out of 12 minor criteria enable a diagnosis of gout to be made.

PATHOPHYSIOLOGY

Uric acid is the end product of purine metabolism, and plasma uric acid levels may be elevated because of either excessive production or defective removal. Although genetically determined enzymatic defects may rarely cause hyperuricemia, the cause of increased production in the majority of patients is unknown. Renal uric acid excretion occurs by a series of complex processes involving complete glomerular filtration followed by more or less total reabsorption in the proximal tubule. There is subsequently further resecretion and reabsorption. Again, the reasons underlying a defect in excretion in most patients with hyperuricemia are not known. Of the two pathogenetic mechanisms, the majority of patients with hyperuricemia fall into the category of underexcreters, defined as patients who excrete less than 700 mg of uric acid per 24 hours. Overproducers are defined as excreting more than 800 mg of uric acid per day while on a regular diet. The majority of patients are underexcreters, and in some a combination of both mechanisms may coexist.

Both hyperuricemia and gout may be primary, where the precise pathogenetic mechanism is unclear, or secondary to a large number of drugs and diseases that either interfere with removal or increase uric acid production (see Table 2).

CLINICAL FEATURES OF ACUTE GOUTY ATTACK

The acute attack of gout is typically a monoarthritis with sudden onset, often occurring at night, becoming symptomatic early in the morning, and involving the first metatarsophalangeal joint of the big toe (podagra). Podagra occurs at some stage in 90% of patients with gout and is the site of the first attack in 70%. The attack increases rapidly in intensity, often reaching a maximum within four to six hours accompanied by swelling, redness, severe pain, and exquisite tenderness. The patient may not even tolerate a bedsheet touching the affected joint. *After several days to a week or two, the pain may subside even if untreated.* The acute attack may be precipitated by minor trauma, alcohol or purine excess, surgery, dehydration, acidosis, or even initiation of drugs to lower the uric acid. Often no precipitating event is found. The first attacks are painful events of short duration, separated by long symptom-free periods. If no therapy is started, the disease usually worsens. The intervals between attacks decrease and a phase of chronic polyarticular gout may occur. Other joints commonly affected by gout include tarsal joints, ankles, knees, wrists, elbows, and fingers. Olecranon bursitis occurs commonly. Rarely are shoulders, hips, sacroiliac, or other intervertebral joints involved. Deposits of urate (tophi) may form in and around joints and tendons. Urate may be deposited in the glomeruli, tubules, interstitial tissues, or blood vessels of the kidneys. Uric acid kidney stones may form.

Premenopausal women rarely develop gout, and if gout occurs in this setting, glucose 6-phosphatase deficiency (von Gierke's disease) should be excluded. The incidence of gout in postmenopsausal females rises to equal that of men in later years.

Obesity is the common factor associated with diabetes, hyperlipidemia, hypertension, atherosclerosis, and hyperuricemia. If these other risk factors for coronary artery disease are removed, then elevated serum urate level alone is probably not associated with coronary heart disease.

MANAGEMENT

PLAN

Short-term Goal. The immediate goal in detecting a patient with hyperuricemia is to identify the primary or secondary nature of the condition.

Long-term Goal. The long-term goal is the prevention of recurrent attacks of acute gout, nephrolithiasis, and urate nephropathy. The treatment of gout is an outpatient procedure except when the patient also has acute or chronic renal failure or sudden nephrolithiasis.

DRUG TREATMENT

The drugs used in the management of hyperuricemia and gout fall into two categories. First are those used to lower raised plasma uric acid concentrations. These compounds either inhibit uric acid synthesis or promote its excretion. The second category of drugs are those that are used to treat the acute attacks of arthritis and prevent further recurrences.

Hyperuricemia is about 50 times more common than gout. Many patients with hyperuricemia are inappropriately treated with long-term medications, whereas many patients with gout are not adequately treated. After confirming the diagnosis of hyperuricemia by serial urate determinations, we need to define whether the hyperuricemia is primary (no associated disease) or secondary (to another disease or medication, e.g., low-dose salicylates or thiazide diuretic). Our approach to history, physical examination, and laboratory tests is summarized in Table 2.

MANAGEMENT OF THE ASYMPTOMATIC PATIENT WITH HYPERURICEMIA

After patients with secondary hyperuricemia are identified, the primary hyperuricemia patients can be separated into two groups.

The Patient with Hyperuricemia and Normal Renal Function

The risks are gout and tophi, renal disease, and renal stones. If treated, there is risk of side effects and the cost and inconvenience of lifelong drug therapy (especially if not medically indicated) and the likelihood of poor patient compliance.

The patient should be warned of the risk of an acute attack of gout. There are no permanent sequelae from a single attack and long-term therapy is started after the attack resolves. Prudent goals for this patient are moderate decreased dietary purine intake, loss of weight, and control of hypertension and hyperlipidemia.

We believe that elevated urate levels alone do not adversely affect renal function. The renal disease that accompanies hyperuricemia is secondary to poorly controlled hypertension as well as aging, renal vascular disease, and calculi. Prevention of these problems rather than reduction of hyperuricemia should be our aim. Urate nephropathy is probably a late event and very rarely occurs without preceding attacks of acute gout. We prefer to treat our patients after the first attack of acute gout and so prevent urate nephropathy.

The risk of stones increases with the rise in serum urate, reaching 50% at values of 13 mg/dl or higher. In 40% of these patients, stones *preceded* the development of gouty arthritis, sometimes by more than ten years. Both urate and calcium stones may occur, and normalizing the urinary uric acid excretion may prevent both types of stones.

We treat patients with hyperuricemia who have a history of renal stones with allopurinol. Those patients with *primary* hyperuricemia and no history of stones with a serum urate of 10 mg/dl have a 30% risk of developing renal stones. This risk increases as the hyperuricemia increases. Thus, a 24-hour urine uric acid excretion is measured in these patients on a regular diet, as well as in patients with lower than 10 mg/dl who have a family history of gout, kidney stones, or tophi. *If the 24-hour excretion exceeds 1000 mg/day, allopurinol therapy is started* because of the risk of stones developing in these patients if they are not treated.

The risk of tophus formation without a preceding attack of gout is remote, but if one occurs, treatment can be started. A rare indication to treat hyperuricemia is unilateral or early bilateral aseptic necrosis of a major joint in a hyperuricemic patient.

The Patient with Hyperuricemia and Abnormal Renal Function

Patients with both hyperuricemia and renal insufficiency are difficult management problems. Urate can precipitate slowly in the interstitium of the kidney leading to urate nephropathy, or rapidly in the collecting tubules (uric acid nephropathy) leading to acute renal failure. Uric acid can form stones that result in renal obstruction. In contrast, renal failure (acute or chronic) unrelated to urate will result in secondary elevation of serum uric acid. *It is difficult but critical to distinguish these two clinical situations.* Treatment with allopurinol must be given if urate or uric acid nephropathy is the cause of renal dysfunction. Stones must be removed if obstruction is causing renal dysfunction.

Look for history of gout or appropriate clinical conditions for urate nephropathy, e.g., due to increased nucleic acid breakdown such as following chemotherapy or myeloblastic crisis, after marked exercise in poorly conditioned soldiers, or after multiple epileptic seizures. Without evidence to implicate gout and when *no other readily demonstrable cause* exists to explain the renal disease, we start allopurinol to decrease uric acid production because of the *possible* existence of urate nephropathy. Ultrasound evaluation of the renal tract is needed to exclude obstruction secondary to stones.

In acute renal failure, measure the uric acid/creatinine ratio in a spot urine sample. Ratios greater than one suggest increased uric acid production and possible uric acid nephropathy as the cause of the renal failure.

MANAGEMENT OF GOUT

The therapy of gout can be divided into three completely different treatments, each with different goals: (1) treatment aimed at aborting an acute attack; (2) long-term treatment aimed at sustained reduction of the serum urate level below 6.5 mg/dl; and (3) prophylactic treatment aimed at decreasing the frequency of acute attacks until the serum urate level has been stabilized below 6.5 mg/dl for one year.

Treatment of Acute Attack

The aim of therapy is to abort the acute attack of gout in as short a time as possible with a minimum of side effects and risk to the patient. The nonsteroidal anti-inflammatory drugs (NSAID) are our first choice. Indomethacin (Indocin) 50 mg every six hours for four doses followed by 50 mg every eight hours for a week is very effective. It is usually well tolerated, but some patients develop abdominal pain, headache, or other side effects and require substitution of another NSAID or use of Indocin by rectal suppository.

Table 2. EVALUATION OF PATIENT WITH HYPERURICEMIA

History	Physical Examination	Laboratory Tests
Gout or acute attacks of monoarthritis, especially podagra	Look for: Tophi	Guided by findings on history and exam: CBC, BUN, creatinine, electrolytes, calcium, thyroid
Renal stones (urate or calcium)	Synovial effusions	function, FBS and 2-hour postpradial blood sugar
History of renal colic	Anemia	Liver profile (if drug therapy needed)
Kidney disease	Lymphadenopathy	Lipid profile (if obese or other cardiac risk)
Family history	Hepatosplenomegaly	Aspirate synovial fluid or suspected tophi for crystal examination
Gout	Bleeding and bruising	
Hyperuricemia	Hypertension and its sequelae	If history of kidney stones or renal colic, get tomogram of kidney (may need IVP, as urate stones are radiolucent)
Renal Stones	Calculate ideal body weight	
Kidney disease		
Medications causing hyperuricemia		If lead suspected, do calcium EDTA infusion or RBC delta-amino-levulinic acid dehydrase level
Diuretics (especially thiazide)		X-ray suspected periarticular tophi looking for punched out erosions
Salicylates (ask about "over-the-counter" preparations, e.g., Alka-Seltzer—patients are often unaware of salicylate content in these preparations)		24-hour urine uric acid collection if: Serum urate greater than 10 mg/dl and secondary causes of hyperuricemia excluded
Anticancer drugs		In primary hyperuricemia if serum urate is less than 10 mg/dl and family history of gout, hyperuricemia, tophi, or kidney stones
Vitamin—nicotinic acid; ascorbic acid (vitamin C)		
Methotrexate—used in therapy for severe psoriasis		
Alcohol consumption (ask about home-brewed alcohol—may be contaminated by lead, "saturnine gout")		
Obesity (associated with uric acid—may get gout when start to diet)		
Dietary fads—fasting may cause ketosis		
Hematologic disease		
Hemolytic anemia		
Hematologic cancer—leukemia, lymphoma		
Carcinoma		
Radiation therapy for malignant disease		
Endocrinopathies		
Diabetes mellitus, especially ketosis		
Hypothyroid		
Hyperparathyroid		
Diabetes insipidus		
Extensive psoriasis (even untreated)		
Occupational exposure		
Lead		
Beryllium		
Copper		
Mercury		
Platinum		
Post surgery		

Naproxen (Naprosyn) 500 mg every 12 hours and sulindac (Clinoril) 200 mg every 12 hours would be our next choice followed by piroxicam (Feldene), tolmetin sodium (Tolectin), or ibuprofen (Motrin). These NSAIDs are effective in treatment of acute gout and should be swallowed with food (in the middle of a meal). Phenylbutazone is highly effective but its increased toxicity leads us to reserve it for resistant cases.

In elderly patients, lower dosages should be used. Patients with a history of peptic ulceration may need to be given prophylactic ranitidene (Zantac) 150 mg b.i.d. or cimetidine (Tagamet) 300 mg q.i.d. while the NSAID is administered. NSAIDs should be used with care in patients with congestive heart failure, renal insufficiency, and diabetes because sodium retention and decreased renal function may result. Clinoril may be less likely to affect renal prostaglandins and thus is safer in these situations, but renal function still should be monitored.

Alternative therapy for an acute attack is colchicine 0.6 mg given every one to two hours until relief of pain or onset of diarrhea. No more than 12 tablets should be given in any 24-hour period. Patient tolerance is improved by giving colchicine every two hours. Colchicine may be given intravenously, 1 to 2 mg colchicine diluted with normal saline to a volume of 20 ml and injected slowly over five minutes. Care must be taken to avoid extravasation or severe local tissue necrosis can result. No more than 4 mg of intravenous colchicine should be given in one 24-hour period. Colchicine given intravenously produces more rapid relief with less gastrointestinal side effects. Colchicine doses need to be reduced if renal insufficiency is present. Response to colchicine is diagnostically important because only gout and sometimes pseudogout respond dramatically to this form of treatment. The rare patient who cannot tolerate a NSAID or colchicine may need an injection of intramuscular ACTH or cortisone.

Postoperative patients who develop acute gout may be treated with IV colchicine or indomethacin suppositories (given in dosage similar to oral indomethacin).

Long-term Treatment of Gout

The aim of long-term therapy is to slowly achieve and then maintain a *consistent* serum urate level of 6.5 mg or less and requires lifelong therapy for most patients. By achieving this level of serum urate, we will gradually mobilize urate from the joints and other tissues where it has been deposited over the years prior to the first acute attack, thus reversing and preventing the complications of gout. In addition, patients should be encouraged to gradually achieve ideal body weight, stop smoking, reduce hyperlipidemia, and have their blood pressure controlled to prevent renal disease.

Patient Education. The patient must fully understand the goals of long-term therapy for successful compliance. This usually requires *several* education sessions initially, together with reinforcement whenever the patient is seen for follow-up visits. Those few minutes spent reemphasizing the importance of compliance can be very cost-effective therapy.

The pamphlet entitled "Gout" available from the Arthritis Foundation is a useful educational aid.

Dietary Modification. Gouty patients should conform to moderate dietary modification to avoid foods of very high purine content such as sardines, anchovies, liver, kidney, sweetbreads, herring, sheep's heart, mussels, and yeast. There is no need to aim for purine-free diets since patients will usually not comply and good drug therapy is available. Each patient should try to identify any foods that have been implicated in past attacks of gout and eliminate or reduce these foods.

Overeating should be avoided. Alcohol intake should be reduced and "alcoholic binges" avoided. Fasting and *severe* dieting should be avoided. Medications known to precipitate gout should be restricted and salicylates should be avoided. Liberal fluid intake is encouraged.

Long-term Therapy. After the acute attack of gout has completely resolved, the patient is started on moderate dietary purine reduction and educated about gout and its treatment. Drug therapy is started if the serum urate remains above 6.5 mg.

Two types of drugs lower urate levels: *allopurinol* lowers serum urate by diminishing urate production due to the inhibition of xanthine oxidase (the enzyme that converts xanthine to uric acid), and the *"uricosuric" drugs* (probenecid and sulfinpyrazone) decrease serum urate by increasing renal uric acid excretion.

There is widespread agreement that the following gouty patients require treatment with allopurinol: (1) patients with a history of any type of renal stones; (2) patients with decreased renal function; (3) patients with tophi; (4) patients who excrete more than 700 mg uric acid in 24 hours on regular diet; (5) patients whose serum urate remains above 6.5 mg despite use of uricosuric drugs or who develop side effects to them; and (6) patients with myeloproliferative disease prior to chemotherapy.

In other patients either allopurinol or a uricosuric drug can be selected. If a uricosuric drug is used, a 24-hour uric acid collection measurement is needed to assure levels below 700 mg. Otherwise there is a risk of renal stones or urate nephropathy resulting from therapies that increase uric acid excretion.

Our approach is to choose allopurinol first for all patients with gout. Allopurinol can be given in a single daily dose due to the long half-life of its active metabolite oxypurinol. This helps to ensure good compliance in contrast to the two or three times daily doses of uricosuric drugs. There is no cost difference between allopurinol therapy and uricosuric drugs.

The theoretical fears that allopurinol might be carcinogenic because of its derivation from 6-mercaptopurine have not been proved after more than 20 years of usage. Both allopurinol and uricosuric drugs have low toxicity. Although allopurinol toxicity is highest in renal dysfunction patients, it is the only drug of choice for such patients. Allopurinol also obviates the need for a 24-hour urine uric acid excretion prior to therapy.

We start patients on 100 mg allopurinol a day and then increase the dose by 100 mg every two weeks until a dose of 300 mg is reached. This dose suffices for most patients, but we will adjust the dosage to the lowest dose that maintains serum urate below 6.5 mg.

If they are underexcreters, we give patients who develop side effects while receiving allopurinol uricosuric drugs, either probenecid or sulfinpyrazone. Toxicity with allopurinol is rare but includes gastrointestinal intolerance, skin rashes, alopecia, bone marrow suppression, hepatitis, jaundice, and vasculitis. Toxicity is greater in patients with renal insufficiency who should be treated with smaller doses. Skin rashes are more frequent in patients on ampicillin, which should not be given with allopurinol. Rarely oxalate stones occur. CBC and liver function tests are repeated every four to six months. Both allopurinol and uricosuric drugs can precipitate an acute attack of gout especially just after therapy is started, which is why we begin with small doses and gradually increase the dose.

Prophylactic Therapy

Colchicine 0.6 mg b.i.d. is given as prophylactic therapy. We start this when gout is diagnosed and dietary modification is instituted and before starting allopurinol or uricosuric drugs. We continue this dosage after initiation of allopurinol or uricosuric drugs until urate levels are stable below 6.5 mg for about one year. It helps prevent acute attacks after long-term drug therapy has been started and has minimal toxicity at this dosage.

By using this information, we can select the appropriate therapy for patients with hyperuricemia and gout.

REFERENCES

Kelley WN, Harris EDJ, Ruddy S, et al: Textbook of Rheumatology. W.B. Saunders Co, Philadelphia, 1985, pp 489–497; pp 1359–1398.
Weiss TB, Lange, RK: Gout. *In* Conn RB (ed): Current Diagnosis, 7th. ed. W. B. Saunders Co, Philadelphia, 1985, pp 796–799.
Wyngaarden J, Kelley W: Gout and Hyperuricemia. Grune & Stratton, New York, 1976.

9 · *DISTURBANCES IN ELECTROLYTE METABOLISM, DIABETIC KETOACIDOSIS, AND HYPEROSMOLAR COMA*

William L. Black
Abdul Cader Asmal
JOSLIN CLINIC

Disturbances in plasma electrolytes may arise from a variety of causes and different mechanisms. Whereas some may demand immediate correction regardless of cause, e.g., hyper- or hypokalemia, others require appropriate diagnosis for specific treatment, e.g., hyponatremia.

Hyponatremia

A serum sodium above 125 mEq/L rarely requires treament. Below 110 mEq/L, neurologic symptoms usually indicate emergent treatment. Within this range clinical judgment prevails.

PATHOPHYSIOLOGY

Hyponatremia may accompany severe hyperlipidemia (triglyceride levels > 1000 mg/dl) or paraproteinemia (protein concentration > 10 gm/dl) owing to a dilutional effect, or profound hyperglycemia owing to a fluid shift from the intracellular space. In patients with severe cardiac failure, cirrhosis, or nephrotic syndrome, hyponatremia may represent the end stage of the disease. Hypovolemia from osmotic diuresis or diuretic overuse or from extrarenal causes such as emesis, diarrhea, or intestinal fluid sequestration may be associated with hyponatremia if fluid replacement is not matched by salt intake. These entities can readily be recognized. On the other hand, clinical states characterized by excess renal sodium loss, e.g., proximal renal tubular acidosis, Bartter's syndrome, salt-losing nephritis and Addison's disease, or those in which free water clearance is impaired, e.g., oliguric renal failure, hypothyroidism, isolated cortisol deficiency, and the syndrome associated with inappropriate ADH secretion (SIADH), cause the greatest diagnostic and therapeutic dilemmas. SIADH may be due to diseases of the CNS (infection, stroke, porphyria, psychosis) or lungs, malignancies, and many drugs (amitriptyline, antipsychotics, morphine, carbamazepine, chlorpropamide, clofibrate, cyclophosphamide, vincristine, and others. Surgical stress is an equally frequent cause of SIADH.

CLINICAL FEATURES

With salt depletion, the features are those of extracellular fluid dehydration; with impaired water clearance, those of water intoxication. This usually manifests with symptoms such as mental changes, lethargy, confusion, stupor, and convulsions occurring when the serum osmolality falls below 240 mosm/kg.

MANAGEMENT

The hyponatremia due to abnormally raised lipids, proteins, or glucose requires no therapy per se. The hyponatremia of end-stage disease responds to fluid restriction if patients comply; that of extrarenal sodium deficit improves on IV 0.9% saline infusion. The major problem is in distinguishing those patients whose primary defect is one of severe salt loss from those whose defect is one of water clearance. The presence of hypovolemia may aid in the differential. However, as the distinction is rarely clear-cut, one searches for evidence of specific disease entities by checking electrolytes, BUN, creatinine, uric acid, and thyroid and adrenal function (one-hour Cortrosyn stimulation test). In the absence of evidence to the contrary, and in an appropriate clinical setting (see below), one often treats presumptively for SIADH. The diagnosis should be reconsidered if urine sodium, which may be high initially, fails to fall with water restriction of < 500 ml/day. If water restriction is ineffective, demeclocycline in a dosage of between 600 and 1200 mg/day may be used.

When SIADH causes a dangerously low serum sodium, 3% NaC1 should be infused intravenously (with furosemide if heart failure is a concern); 500 ml of 3% saline will raise the serum sodium about 6 mEq/L in a 70-kg man. Given over six hours this usually rescues the patient from immediate danger.

Note: (1) Patients with renal salt loss will need NaCl supplements. (2) Patients with suspected Addison's disease should not be fluid-restricted.

Hypernatremia

Chronic hypernatremia (up to 160 mEq/L) may be well tolerated. Acute hypernatremia, on the other hand, may cause brain shrinkage, rupture of blood vessels, and death.

PATHOPHYSIOLOGY

Hypernatremia most frequently develops in a setting of excessive water loss with or without reduced intake. Fluid loss may be extrarenal (vomiting, nasogastric suction, diarrhea, sweating) or renal in origin. Renal loss may be due to diuretic use, uncontrolled diabetes, high-protein alimentation, hypokalemia, hypercalcemia, lithium and demeclocycline use, and diabetes insipidus (DI). DI itself may be central (idiopathic or secondary to trauma, tumors, granulomas, and infarct involving the pituitary and hypothalamus) or nephrogenic (congenital or secondary to systemic disease, e.g., myeloma, or renal disease, e.g., polycystic or medullary sponge kidney). Dehydration is a feature of these latter states. On the other hand, when hypernatremia is iatrogenic, fluid overload may be manifest. The hypernatremia of hyperadrenocorticism is itself asymptomatic.

CLINICAL FEATURES

When hypernatremia is due to fluid loss, the features may be primarily those of dehydration. With increasing severity, confusion, neuromuscular excitability, seizures, and coma may develop.

MANAGEMENT

The therapy depends on the cause, and in the absence of fluid overload IV 5% dextrose in water may be needed. Any offending drug should be stopped and electrolyte abnormality corrected. The diagnosis of DI is readily made in a hypernatremic polyuric patient with a hypotonic urine. The treatment of cranial DI depends on its severity. Mild DI may be controlled by increasing fluid intake. For moderately troublesome DI, with partial ADH deficiency, oral therapy with chlorpropamide or clofibrate may be effective. These drugs are cheap, are convenient, and carry minimum risk of water intoxication. For chronic disabling DI, the drug of choice is desmopressin. It is best given b.i.d. in amounts just sufficient to control polyuria. Every few days a dose should be held until polyuria and thirst are reestablished to protect against water intoxication. The use of the nasal tube requires manual dexterity. For the acute and usually temporary DI that develops after pituitary adenectomy, treatment with subcutaneous aqueous vasopressin (2 to 10 units every four to six hours) is employed. Mild polyuria should be allowed to develop between doses to prevent water intoxication due to the

occasional release of ADH from damaged neurons. In patients with impaired mental status, frequent determinations of serum Na, daily weights, and fluid balance should be done. For the acute DI that occasionally follows prostatectomy, large volumes of 5% dextrose in water may be required IV over the first six to 12 hours to restore plasma osmolality.

The treatment of nephrogenic DI is less satisfactory. Polyuria can be reduced by salt restriction and the use of hydrochlorothiazide 50 to 100 mg/day.

Hypokalemia

Hypokalemia is unlikely to be a significant problem unless the potassium level falls below 3 mEq/L.

CLINICAL FEATURES

The life-threatening effects of hypokalemia include paralysis, rhabdomyolysis, and arrhythmias. It also causes weakness, ileus, polyuria, and glucose intolerance.

PATHOPHYSIOLOGY

Diuretics (thiazides, loop diuretics, acetazolamide) are the most common cause of hypokalemia. A good history will reveal most of the others, including uncontrolled diabetes, malnutrition, diarrhea (pancreatic cholera, villous adenoma), emesis (or nasogastric drainage), drugs (amphotericin, carbenicillin, gentamicin), the acute effect of insulin, barium poisoning, periodic paralysis, and initiation of therapy for pernicious anemia. Once these causes have been excluded, the problem will lie in one of three categories. If the patient is hypertensive, hyperaldosteronism or some variant is likely, e.g., primary hyperaldosteronism, renin-secreting tumors, both renovascular and malignant hypertension, certain forms of adrenogenital syndrome, Cushing's syndrome (including ectopic ACTH), licorice ingestion, and Liddle's syndrome. Renin, cortisol, and aldosterone levels obtained under standardized conditions may help to further refine the diagnosis. If the patient is normotensive, the problem is to distinguish between organic disease such as Bartter's syndrome or renal tubular acidosis and self-abuse due to surreptitious emesis, diuretics, or laxatives. In patients with abuse, deranged behavior is common and denials must be suspected. Urinary thiazide levels are obtained and patients are hospitalized in a supervised setting. Findings that exclude organic disease include (1) easily corrected hypokalemia that does not recur; (2) low urinary potassium during repletion (assuming the patient is receiving at least 120 mEq/day of sodium; and (3) low urinary chloride (in the alkalotic patient).

Oral potassium repletion is safest. When this is inadequate or impossible (or in emergencies), one can administer 10 mEq/hour IV without special precautions. If needed, up to 40 mEq/hour can be given, watching for EKG evidence of hyperkalemia. Limiting the potassium in any one bottle to 40 mEq/L minimizes the chance of accidental overdose. Total body potassium deficit may amount to several hundred mEq and many days may be required to restore a normal electrolyte balance. The magnesium deficiency that often accompanies hypokalemia should also be corrected.

Hyperkalemia

Hyperkalemia is unlikely to produce clinical problems unless the potassium level is greater than 6.5 mEq/L.

PATHOPHYSIOLOGY

An artificial elevation of potassium levels in serum but not plasma may accompany hemolysis and breakdown of very high levels of leukocytes and thrombocytes during phlebotomy. Release of intracellular potassium occurs in acidosis, in hyperkalemic periodic paralysis, in digitalis poisoning, and after succinylcholine. Large amounts of intravenous glucose can cause fatal hyperkalemia in insulin-deficient diabetics. Drugs such as nonsteroidal anti-inflammatory agents, converting enzyme inhibitors, beta-blockers, as well as heparin may induce hyperkalemia by different mechanisms. Excessive potassium intake can cause hyperkalemia, particularly if excretion is impaired. The route may be oral (salt substitutes, geophagia) or intravenous (banked blood, potassium penicillin, KCl). Damaged cells (hemolysis, crush injuries, tumor lysis) may release large amounts of potassium into the serum. Impaired excretion occurs in oliguric states as a result of potassium-"sparing" diuretics, and in hypoaldosteronism (Addison's disease, congenital adrenal hyperplasia, renin deficiency). Every patient with unexplained hyperkalemia should be evaluated by a one-hour Cortrosyn stimulation test.

CLINICAL FEATURES

Although hyperkalemia can cause confusion, weakness, and paralysis, the major dangers are arrhythmias and cardiac arrest.

MANAGEMENT

Potassium levels above 8 mEq/L should be treated emergently. At lower levels the urgency of treatment is best determined by the presence of EKG changes. Emergency treatment includes:

1. 10 ml of 10% calcium gluconate (unless the patient receives digoxin) IV over two minutes, repeated after five minutes if needed.

2. One ampule (44 mEq) of sodium bicarbonate IV over five minutes, repeated after 15 minutes if necessary.

3. One ampule of 50% dextrose (25 gm) IV over five minutes, along with 10 units of regular insulin IV.

4. 50 gm of Kayexalate and 50 gm of sorbitol in 200 ml of water as a retention enema, repeated hourly as needed.

Only the last measure (or dialysis) actually removes potassium from the body. For a nonurgent situation, potassium restriction and encouraging of salt intake are useful general measures. Fludrocortisone, or if the patient is hypertensive, thiazide diuretics, may be necessary. Potassium-sparing diuretics, nonsteroidal anti-inflammatory agents, and beta-blockers should be avoided.

Diabetic Ketoacidosis (DKA)

DEFINITION

DKA is a medical emergency characterized by dehydration, hyperglycemia, and acidosis. It is diagnosed at the bedside with reagent strips that measure blood and urine glucose and ketone concentrations. It is confirmed later by results that generally show a blood glucose exceeding 300 mg/dl, pH below 7.3, and bicarbonate below 15 mEq/L.

PATHOGENESIS

The insulin lack in DKA promotes muscle protein breakdown and adipocyte lipolysis, thereby increasing the supply of gluconeogenic and ketogenic precursors to the liver. The contrainsulin hormone excess (growth hormone, cortisol, glucagon, and catecholamines) that accompanies the insulin lack amplifies the signal for enhanced ketogenesis and gluconeogenesis, resulting in marked elevation of blood glucose and ketone and lipid levels.

CLINICAL FEATURES

DKA may be the presenting feature of diabetes or supervene in a known diabetic because of omission of or inadequate supplementation with insulin (through ignorance or design) in the face of apparently trivial ailments (cold, gastric upset) or major stress (trauma, sepsis, silent myocardial infarction), which increase insulin need. The symptoms may be those of the precipitating illness or a progression of the polyuria to weakness, vomiting, abdominal pain, and somnolence. Examination may reveal evidence of dehydration, Kussmaul breathing, acetone breath, clouding of the sensorium, and signs of the underlying disease.

MANAGEMENT

The management of DKA should only be undertaken electively in a hospital setting where special medical and nursing staff and adequate laboratory facilities are available. Although there are differences of opinion regarding details, the following guidelines are generally applicable:

1. Document diagnosis at bedside; send off confirmatory tests, including blood glucose, ketone, electrolyte, acid-base, and blood count determinations; and set up an IV line.

2. If coma is present, establish a clear airway,

administer oxygen, consider intubation and possibly gavage.

3. If shock is present, administer a plasma volume expander.

4. Infuse 0.9% saline, the first liter over 15 to 60 minutes.

5. Administer insulin by either continuous IV infusion (0.2 unit/kg stat, 0.1 unit/kg/hour) or by intermittent IM injections (10 units/hour).

6. Identify and treat the precipitating cause, e.g., sepsis.

7. Assess the need for special procedures: CVP line or Swan-Ganz, bladder catheterization, gavage, EKG monitor, etc.

8. Start a flow sheet: vital signs, mental status changes, fluid and electrolyte balance, etc.

9. Replace potassium to maintain serum levels between 3.5 and 5.5 mEq/L.

10. Use bicarbonate only if pH < 7.1, or plasma bicarbonate < 5 mEq/L.

11. Repeat blood glucose and electrolytes hourly initially.

12. Anticipate a 10% fall in blood glucose/hour.

13. When the blood glucose level is 250 mg/dl, switch infusion fluid to 5% dextrose in water (D5W) with 10 mEq KCl, and infuse at the rate of 100 to 300 ml/hour.

14. Restabilize on conventional insulin dose once hydration is complete and oral feeding initiated.

NONPHARMACOLOGIC MEASURES

Saline (0.9%), being isotonic, is the ideal initial replacement fluid for correction of the extracellular dehydration. Its rate of infusion is determined by the severity of dehydration. In severe cases the first liter may be infused over 15 to 30 minutes. Thereafter 2 liters may be infused over the next four hours, and additional liters over four hours each. Precipitation of congestive heart failure, hypernatremia, and hyperchloremic acidosis are some of its disadvantages. For this reason, 0.45% saline may be used after infusing the first liter of 0.9% saline.

With the blood glucose at 250 mg/dl, 5% dextrose in water is infused in place of saline. This solution helps to replete the water deficit, to prevent acute precipitation of hypoglycemia, and to suppress lipolysis and ketogenesis.

Although there may be a potassium deficit up to 500 mEq, this is not reflected in the serum potassium level. Its replacement should be guided by serial plasma potassium determinations and EKG monitoring. Potassium can be replaced at the rate of 0, 10, 20, or 30 mEq/hour when the serum potassium levels are above 5, between 4 and 5, between 3 and 4, and below 3 mEq/L, respectively. The need for potassium increases when 5% dextrose in water or bicarbonate is administered. Oral supplements may be needed for a week after the acute episode.

Bicarbonate usage should be restricted to arterial pH < 7.1 or bicarbonate < 5.0. Under such circumstances 200 mEq may be infused over two to four hours. Excessive bicarbonate infusion can induce an acute metabolic alkalosis with hypokalemia, an intensification of cerebrospinal acidosis, and a worsening of mental status.

The hypophosphatemia of DKA requires no treatment because clinically it produces no manifestations and the biochemical effect of the reduction in 2,3-diphosphoglycerate levels that it induces is balanced by the effect of the acidosis on this substrate.

DRUG THERAPY

Insulin can be administered by either one of two routes, both of which are equally effective:

1. Continuous IV infusion at a dosage of 0.1 unit/kg/hour preceded by a bolus of 0.2 unit/kg establishes a steady-state insulin concentration of between 100 and 140 μU/ml within 30 minutes. This dose suppresses lipolysis, gluconeogenesis, and ketogenesis and achieves a 10% per hour fall in blood glucose level. In patients failing to show the expected response, the infusion rate may be doubled. The IV infusion must be continued for at least 30 minutes after the reintroduction of subcutaneous insulin. A point of technical importance is that since insulin adsorbs to glass and plastic, the infusion line should be preflushed with the insulin solution.

2. Intermittent intramuscular injection of insulin 10 units/hour also achieves a satisfactory steady-state insulin concentration allowing a predictable fall in glucose level. Its ease and safety make the IM approach especially useful to hospitals that lack facilities to monitor the effects of continuous IV infusion. The presence of shock or severe dehydration precludes intramuscular application.

The following caveats need to be noted:

1. Correction of the acute dehydration, hyperglycemia, and acidosis with fluid, electrolytes, and insulin is an urgent problem.

2. Restoration of the metabolic and electrolyte homeostasis to normal can be done more gradually over 12 to 24 hours.

3. An overzealous and imprudent management approach can precipitate iatrogenic problems, e.g., alkalosis or hypo- or hyperkalemia. There is no routine in DKA management, nor is there a substitute for constant vigilance of an everchanging scene.

Hyperosmolar Coma

DEFINITION

The cardinal features of this syndrome are marked hyperglycemia, increased osmolality, and profound dehydration.

PATHOGENESIS

The pathogenesis of hyperosmolar coma, especially in the absence of ketoacidosis, remains unclear and may best be explained by postulating a differential tissue sensitivity to insulin with regard to suppression of lipolysis and promotion of glucose utilization.

CLINICAL FEATURES

The typical patient is elderly and may have no previous history of diabetes. Evidence of an associated or precipitating illness such as myocardial infarction, cerebrovascular accident, or sepsis may be present. Medication such as glucocorticoids, diuretics, phenytoin, propranolol, and others may trigger the onset. Patients with burns or undergoing dialysis or hyperalimentation or hypertonic glucose are at increased risk. Limited fluid access in the setting of dementia and inanition may be a predisposing factor. Physical examination usually reveals profound dehydration and hypotension with varying obtundation and signs of the underlying illness.

MANAGEMENT

The management of hyperosmolar coma is an acute emergency that should only be undertaken in the hospital. As in the case of DKA, the presence of coma or shock will demand immediate appropriate resuscitative measures. Once an intravenous line is set up and appropriate blood samples are taken for glucose, electrolytes, BUN, acid-base and blood count determination, fluid replacement should be instituted. The blood glucose in general exceeds 600 mg/dl and the calculated osmolality 350 mosm/kg. The serum sodium may be high-normal or low, the latter signifying profound dehydration. The serum potassium may be low or normal, and the BUN is invariably high. The bicarbonate level is generally normal or slightly reduced and there is no significant ketonemia.

Although during the evolution of the hyperosmolar state the water deficit may have been significantly greater than the accompanying salt loss, replacement should be initiated with 0.9% saline because of the pressing extracellular fluid depletion. The first liter may be administered over 30 to 60 minutes. If hypotension persists, 0.9% saline should be continued; if not, a switch to 0.45% saline is made. The rate of fluid administration is determined by close surveillance of vital signs. However, following the initial liter of fluid, 2 more liters may be given over the succeeding two hours and 3 over the next six hours in severely dehydrated patients. Thereafter, we give 1 liter every four hours until repletion is complete.

Because of the severe dehydration, intramuscular insulin administration is not favored in hyperosmolar coma. Intravenous insulin is given according to the same protocol as used in DKA, 0.2 unit/kg as initial bolus, followed by 0.1 unit/kg/hour as continuous infusion after preflushing.

Adequate rehydration per se may produce a significant fall in the blood glucose level. When the blood glucose level falls to a level of 200 mg/dl, the infusion may be stopped and sequential glucose determination done to assess further insulin need. Rarely, the insulin infusion rate may need to be doubled when patients fail to respond to the initial dosage regimen.

Serum potassium levels may be variable and should be monitored as closely as in DKA with attention to urine output. The infusion rate of KCl should be varied to keep the potassium levels between 3 and 5 mEq/L (see DKA). Hyperosmolar coma rarely requires the use of bicarbonate replacement unless there is concomitant lactic acidosis and shock. Phosphate replacement is unnecessary.

Hyperosmolar coma carries a mortality of between 15% and 50%, usually because of serious underlying illnesses. Complications such as convulsions, infection, shock, renal failure, thrombophlebitis, and pulmonary embolism should be assiduously sought out and treated.

PREVENTION

Education of the patient and the family is the key to the prevention of acute complication of diabetes. (See Chapters 1 and 2.)

REFERENCES

Brown RS: Potassium homeostasis and clinical implications. Am J Med 77:3–11, 1984.
Fraser R: Disorders of the adrenal cortex: their effects on electrolyte metabolism. Clin Endocrinol Metabolism 13:413–427, 1984.
Moses AM, Notman DD: Diabetes insipidus and syndrome of inappropriate antidiuretic hormone secretion. *In* Stollerman GH (ed): Advances in Internal Medicine, Vol 24. Year Book Medical Publishers, Chicago, 1982, pp 73–99.
Vignati L, Asmal AC, Black WL, et al: Coma in diabetes. *In* Marble A, Krall LP, Bradley RF, et al (eds.) Joslin's Diabetes Mellitus, 12th ed. Lea & Febiger, Philadelphia, 1985, pp 526–553.

10 · DIAGNOSIS AND MANAGEMENT OF ACID-BASE DISTURBANCES

James H. Diaz*
Edward J. Busick†
OCHSNER CLINIC AND ALTON OCHSNER MEDICAL FOUNDATION*
JOSLIN CLINIC†

As life is an acidogenic process, the human body must constantly balance acid output against acid input to remain in acid-base balance at neutral pH. Acidity is determined by the hydrogen ion concentration (H^+) and is best reflected by pH or the negative logarithm of the hydrogen ion concentration. Despite the daily addition of tremendous dietary and metabolic acid loads to body fluids, an efficient system of body buffers helps to maintain body fluid pH within a narrow normal range of 7.35 to 7.45. As cellular metabolism imposes an even greater acid load to cell buffers, intracellular pH is maintained between 6.80 and 7.10.

When food is oxidized, carbon dioxide (CO_2) from carbohydrates and fats and hydrogen ions (H^+) from proteins are added to extracellular fluids in vascular and interstitial spaces. Immediate buffering of acid loads occurs within these spaces to minimize pH changes. Large quantities of acid are then carried to the lungs for rapid excretion as CO_2 gas and to the kidneys for slow elimination as nonvolatile acids. Only the lungs can excrete CO_2 to provide for rapid control of sudden fluxes in H^+ concentration imposed by drugs, diet, or disease.

Unlike the respiratory response, the renal excretion of H^+ ions as nonvolatile acids is slow to develop and may require several days to reach maximum capacity.

Thus, three systems must operate together to maintain acid-base balance at near-neutral pH in body fluids: (1) the body buffers for initial response to acid-base derangements, (2) the lungs to quickly eliminate buffered acids as CO_2, and (3) the kidneys to provide slow elimination of nonvolatile acids and bases.

BUFFERING SYSTEMS

A buffer is really a combination of two related compounds in solution that acts to prevent major fluxes in H^+ concentration when either acid or base is added to the solution. The average H^+ intake is 50 to 80 mEq/day, and the normal adult buffering capacity is 500 to 700 mEq/day, or 10 times the daily intake. If dietary H^+ intake ceases in anuric patients, metabolically produced H^+ ions can be easily buffered for seven to ten days before dialysis becomes necessary.

Most body buffers are combinations of weak acids and strong bases and are called buffer pairs. Common buffer pairs include carbonic acid/bicarbonate and sodium dihydrogen phosphate/disodium hydrogen phosphate. The principal buffer pair in body fluids is carbonic acid/bicarbonate. Buffers in blood, in order of importance, are hemoglobin, bicarbonate, plasma proteins, and phosphate. Intracellular buffers are mainly proteins and phosphate. Renal buffers include bicarbonate, ammonia, and phosphate.

Neutral pH is 7.4 in vitro and 6.8 in vivo at normal body temperature of 37°C. In the carbonic acid/bicarbonate buffer system, the relationship of acidity, as reflected by pH, to neutrality is determined by the Henderson-Hasselbalch equation:

$$pH = pK_a + \log (salt)/(acid)$$

Where:

pK_a = the dissociation constant of carbonic acid of 6.1
salt = bicarbonate (HCO_3^-)
acid = carbonic acid = dissolved CO_2

Thus:

$$ph = 6.1 + \log (HCO_3^-)/CO_2$$

Since:

Normal (HCO_3^-) = 24 mEq/L
Normal Pa_{CO_2} = 40 mm Hg
Dissolved CO_2 = 0.03 × 40 (by Henry's law)

Therefore:

$$pH = 6.1 + \log 24/0.03 \times 40$$
$$= 6.1 + 1.3$$
$$= 7.4$$

Bicarbonate Buffer System. The bicarbonate buffer system maintains the neutrality described by the Henderson-Hasselbalch equation in a unique physiologic way. The concentration of each buffer pair is under separate physiologic control. The carbonic acid (H_2CO_3) concentration is under rapid respiratory regulation via CO_2 elimination. The bicarbonate (HCO_3^-) concentration is under slow renal regulation via HCO_3^- production, retention, or elimination. The bicarbonate buffer system operates best at a pH of 7.4 where the ratio of $HCO_3^-:H_2CO_3$ is 20:1. Although well outside of the buffer system's best working range, a 20:1 ratio of $HCO_3^-:H_2CO_3$ provides a powerful natural safeguard to any acidotic challenge to neutral homeostasis. The greatest strength of the bicarbonate buffer system is its ability to quickly eliminate CO_2 by the lungs and to carefully regulate HCO_3^- through the kidneys. Carbonic anhydrase is the rate-limiting enzyme that catalyzes the bicarbonate reaction in either direction in response to acid-base fluctuations.

Hemoglobin. Hemoglobin is responsible for half of the buffering power of blood, while bicarbonate, proteins, and phosphates provide the rest. Hemoglobin is a good buffer for two reasons. First, it is a protein buffer; second and even more important, it accepts H^+ ions when reduced. Thus, the buffer pair in the hemoglobin system includes the weak acid, oxyhemoglobin, and the base, reduced hemoglobin, which accepts CO_2 to form carbaminohemoglobin.

Proteins. Quantitatively, proteins are the most important buffers in the body because they are found in both extracellular (blood, interstitial fluid) and intracellular compartments. A protein is a good buffer because its molecule often contains a large number of both acidic and basic groups. Basic groups may include amino $(-NH_2)$, ammonia $(-NH_3)$, guanidino, or imidazole groups. Carboxyl groups $(-COOH)$ are the main acidic groups. Regardless of location, most protein buffer systems work best near pH 7.4.

Phosphate Buffer System. The phosphate buffer system with an acid dissociation constant (pK_a) of 6.8 works better in the acid environment of the renal tubule than in blood. In the phosphate system, the buffer pair is composed of sodium dihydrogen phosphate (NaH_2PO_4) as the weak acid and disodium hydrogen phosphate (Na_2HPO_4) as the weak base. In blood and, especially, in tubular fluid, excess H^+ ions combine with phosphate buffers (HPO_4^-) to form dihydrogen phosphate $(H_2PO_4^-)$ releasing HCO_3^- in the process.

Ammonia Buffering. Besides the phosphate buffer system, the kidneys also rely on ammonia buffering to fine-tune acid-base balance. Ammonia (NH_3) produced by tubular epithelium diffuses into tubular fluid and accepts H^+ ions to form ammonium ions (NH_4^+), which are easily excreted as urinary ammonium chloride (NH_4Cl). At the same time, the renal arm of the carbonic acid/bicarbonate system conserves HCO_3^- and expels H^+ ions into the tubular fluid for ammonia titration.

CLINICAL DERANGEMENTS OF ACID-BASE BALANCE

Once body buffers are overpowered by acid or base excess, a variety of acid-base derangements can occur and trigger compensatory phenomena (Table 1). All organ systems are affected. The primary acid-base changes include respiratory acidosis, respiratory alka-

Table 1. PRIMARY ACID-BASE DISTURBANCES

Primary Acid-Base Disturbance	Compensatory Disturbance	Compensating Organ System
Respiratory acidosis	Metabolic alkalosis	Kidneys
Respiratory alkalosis	Metabolic acidosis	Kidneys
Metabolic acidosis	Respiratory alkalosis	Lungs
Metabolic alkalosis	Respiratory acidosis	Lungs

Table 2. CAUSES OF RESPIRATORY ACIDOSIS

Alveolar hypoventilation
   Central nervous system disorder
   Neuromuscular paralysis or disorder
   Thoracic deformity
   Primary pulmonary disease

Ventilation-perfusion mismatching
   Pulmonary embolism
   Cardiorespiratory arrest

losis, metabolic acidosis, and metabolic alkalosis (Table 1).

RESPIRATORY ACIDOSIS

Simple respiratory acidosis results from any condition that produces alveolar hypoventilation, like diaphragmatic paralysis, or promotes mismatching of ventilation and perfusion, like pulmonary embolism (Table 2). In respiratory acidosis, the concentration of dissolved CO_2 in extracellular fluids increases dramatically, the bicarbonate buffer system fails, and the arterial pH drops acutely 0.008 units for each 1 mm Hg rise in Pa_{CO_2}. In persistent respiratory acidosis, the kidneys begin to slowly compensate for the acidosis by secreting more H^+ into the tubular fluid for excretion as $H_2PO_4^-$ and NH_4^+. The kidneys will also reabsorb HCO_3^- to restore the bicarbonate buffer system. With fully compensated respiratory acidosis, the arterial pH will only drop 0.003 units for each 1 mm Hg rise in Pa_{CO_2}.

The systemic effects of respiratory acidosis include tachypnea, peripheral vasodilation, cardiac arrhythmias, and cardiovascular depression, partially offset by increased sympathetic tone. Central nervous system (CNS) responses to respiratory acidosis result from rapid increases in cerebral blood flow causing intracranial hypertension with headache, papilledema, and seizure activity progressing to lethargy, stupor, coma, and death by asphyxiation.

Management. Management of respiratory acidosis is by reestablishment of effective alveolar ventilation and O_2 supplementation. Airway obstruction must be corrected rapidly by endotracheal intubation or tracheostomy. If spontaneous ventilation is not resumed, mechanical ventilation must be instituted. Once the patient is stabilized, diagnostic work-up can continue with CNS evaluation, toxicity screening for analgesic or sedative overdose, and careful exclusion of primary pulmonary disorders (Table 2).

RESPIRATORY ALKALOSIS

Simple respiratory alkalosis is usually the result of alveolar hyperventilation from anxiety, cerebral edema, sepsis, hepatic encephalopathy, salicylate toxicity, or mountain sickness (Table 3). In respiratory alkalosis, the concentration of dissolved CO_2 in extracellular fluid decreases dramatically, the carbonic acid/bicarbonate buffer fails, the arterial pH increases, and the plasma bicarbonate falls 0.5 mEq for each 1 mm Hg fall in Pa_{CO_2}. Bicarbonate levels rarely drop below 15 mEq/L in simple respiratory alkalosis. Bicarbonate levels below 15 mEq/L suggest a mixed acid-base disturbance, like metabolic acidosis with respiratory acidosis. In persistent respiratory alkalosis, the carbonic acid/bicarbonate buffer system will respond by allowing the kidneys to

Table 3. CAUSES OF RESPIRATORY ALKALOSIS

Central hyperventilation
Drug-induced hyperventilation: salicylates, xanthines, progesterone
Mechanical hyperventilation
Miscellaneous: cirrhosis, sepsis

secrete fewer H^+ ions and to filter more HCO_3^- into the tubular fluid.

The systemic effects of respiratory alkalosis are mostly mediated by cerebral vasoconstriction with reduction in cerebral blood flow and may include dizziness, confusion, paresthesias, syncope, and seizures. Potassium (K^+) and calcium (Ca^{++}) ions are also driven intracellularly, resulting in extracellular fluid hypokalemia and hypocalcemia with neuromuscular excitability, tonoclonic convulsions, or tetany. The oxyhemoglobin dissociation curve is shifted leftward, promoting tissue hypoxia. Cardiac arrhythmias may result from profound hypokalemia.

Management. Management of respiratory alkalosis need not be as prompt as for respiratory acidosis. The etiologic factor of respiratory alkalosis should be suspected and determined, since correction of the underlying cause will reverse the acid-base derangements. In mountain sickness and high-altitude pulmonary edema, O_2 supplementation and return to a lower altitude will correct hypoxia and alkalosis. The compensatory respiratory alkalosis of salicylate intoxication may be so severe as to promote dysrhythmias, fatigue, and respiratory arrest. Controlled ventilation may be indicated in such circumstances to permit correction of metabolic derangements and provide normal alveolar ventilation.

METABOLIC ACIDOSIS

Simple metabolic derangements in acid-base balance are more insidious and have slower onsets than respiratory and mixed derangements. Simple metabolic acidosis is caused by the slow accumulation of nonvolatile acids that may complicate severe diarrhea, uremia, or diabetes. In metabolic acidosis, blood and renal buffers are overwhelmed, arterial pH drops, and plasma HCO_3^- is reduced. Respiratory compensation occurs but is incomplete, restoring only 50% to 75% of the acid imbalance through CO_2 elimination.

Metabolic acidosis may be the result of large acid loads (diabetic ketoacidosis, alcoholic ketoacidosis, lactic acidosis, poisoning), loss of alkali by diarrhea or gastrointestinal fistula, or renal dysfunction (Table 4). Differential diagnosis is aided by determination of the

Table 4. CAUSES OF METABOLIC ACIDOSIS

Large acid loads
   Ketoacidosis: diabetes, alcohol
   Lactic acidosis
   Renal dysfunction
   Drug-induced: acetazolamide, amiloride, cholestyramine,
      salicylates
   Iatrogenic: hyperalimentation; acid therapy with HCl,
      ammonium chloride, or arginine hydrochloride

Loss of alkali
   Severe diarrhea
   Gastrointestinal fistulas
   Pancreatic fistula
   Ureterosigmoidostomy

anion gap, which divides the causes of metabolic acidosis into two main categories: anion gap and non–anion gap acidosis. The anion gap represents the negative charges contributed to plasma by anions other than Cl^- and HCO_3^-. The normal anion gap of 8 to 14 mEq/L is determined by the formula:

$$\text{Anion gap} = (HCO_3^- + Cl^-) - (Na^+)$$

In non–anion gap acidosis, metabolic acidosis is usually the result of loss of alkali or accumulation of HCl. In increased anion gap acidosis, metabolic acidosis is due to the accumulation of acid anions other than Cl^-, as in renal dysfunction (PO_4^-, SO_4^-), diabetic ketoacidosis, alcoholic ketoacidosis, lactic acidosis, and salicylate poisoning. In nonketotic acidosis, an elevated serum osmolality with increased anion gap suggests ethylene glycol or methanol poisoning. In nonketotic acidosis, a normal serum lactate with increased anion gap suggests poisoning or overdose with formaldehyde, toluene vapor, iron, dimethyl sulfate, isoniazid, nalidixic acid, or amphotericin B.

The systemic effects of metabolic acidosis may include hyperventilation and CNS depression with fatigability, lethargy, somnolence, and coma. Initial cardiovascular stimulation may give way to cardiovascular depression with bradycardia, hypotension, and shock.

Management. Management of metabolic acidosis should be aimed first at identifying and reversing the cause of the acidosis. When the acidosis is moderately severe (pH > 7.1) and the cause of the acidosis can be treated specifically, alkali replacement with sodium bicarbonate ($NaHCO_3$) is usually not necessary. In acute, severe acidosis (pH < 7.1), intravenous $NaHCO_3$ may be necessary even if the underlying cause of the acidosis can be treated. As total correction of the acidosis is unnecessary and may even be harmful, bicarbonate therapy should be directed at restoring the plasma bicarbonate level to 12 to 15 mEq/L. Bicarbonate therapy should also be directed by its volume of distribution in extracellular fluids and administered according to the formula:

$$\text{mEq } NaHCO_3 = (0.3 \times \text{body weight in kg}) \times (\text{base deficit})$$

Treatment with one half of the calculated amount of $NaHCO_3$ is recommended. Reevaluation of acid-base status by anion gap and arterial blood gas determinations should be undertaken before further alkali therapy.

Total and rapid correction of acute metabolic acidosis may prove harmful for several reasons. First, cerebrospinal fluid (CSF) pH may not equilibrate with a rapidly corrected plasma pH, and CSF acidosis may continue to direct central hyperventilation with alkalemia. Second, CSF acidosis may be further aggravated by HCO_3^- association with H^+ to form H_2CO_3, which then dissociates into CO_2 and H_2O. Large alkali boluses will promote rapid HCO_3^- diffusion across the blood-brain barrier, which is ordinarily resistant to rapid inward diffusion of HCO_3^-. Third, rapid alkalinization may precipitate hypocalcemia with tetany and hypokalemia with dysrhythmias. Lastly, the additional sodium load accompanying $NaHCO_3$ administration may promote fluid overload, causing hyperosmolality and pulmonary congestion. Under most circumstances, alkali

therapy should be slowly titrated and monitored by frequent laboratory determinations of arterial pH and HCO_3^-. A persisting mild acidosis (pH 7.30) is preferable to overcorrection of the metabolic deficit with its additional risks.

METABOLIC ALKALOSIS

Simple metabolic alkalosis may result from abnormal acid losses with gastric outlet obstruction, overzealous administration of alkali, adrenal disorders, steroid therapy, or excessive metabolism of organic acid salts, like ketones and lactate (Table 5). In metabolic alkalosis, plasma HCO_3^- and pH increase, provoking a compensatory respiratory response to hypoventilate and conserve CO_2. The anticipated respiratory compensation is a 0.5 to 1.0 mm Hg increase in $Paco_2$ for each 1 mEq elevation of plasma bicarbonate above normal (23 to 25 mEq/L). In response to the alkalinization of the extracellular fluid, H^+ ions will move from the intracellular to the extracellular compartment in exchange for K^+ and Na^+ to lessen the severity of alkalemia. Renal excretion of excess bicarbonate is, however, ultimately responsible for correction of metabolic alkalosis.

The systemic effects of metabolic alkalosis are largely determined by the underlying cause, like gastric outlet obstruction or Cushing's syndrome, and may include mental confusion, lethargy, weakness, muscle cramping, and cardiac dysrhythmias. Gastric outlet obstruction may result in severe fluid and electrolyte losses in addition to alkalemia. Hyponatremia, hypochloremia, and hypokalemia are common and need correction before surgical management of gastric outlet obstruction from a variety of causes, most commonly peptic ulcer disease and gastric carcinoma.

Management. Management of metabolic alkalosis depends on the proper identification of underlying cause. In gastric outlet obstruction, treatment would consist of correction of fluid losses and ionic deficits, particularly potassium and chloride. Metabolic alkalosis is rarely severe enough to require acid therapy. Fluid and electrolyte replacement is preferred to acid therapy in most cases.

In persistent severe alkalosis, acid may be administered as dilute hydrochloric acid (HCl), ammonium chloride, or arginine hydrochloride. Hepatic biotransformation yields HCl from both ammonium chloride and argenine hydrochloride. Acid therapy with dilute HCl is preferred to ammonium chloride or arginine hydrochloride therapy. Ammonium chloride administration may be contraindicated in hepatic insufficiency, as urea is a byproduct of its metabolism to HCl. Arginine hydrochloride administration may produce severe hyperkalemia with cardiac dysrhythmias as arginine cation displaces intracellular K^+. Should acid therapy be required for alkalosis, the H^+ ion yield of the acid solution

---

Table 5. CAUSES OF METABOLIC ALKALOSIS

Loss of gastric acid	Drug-induced: steroid therapy,
Severe vomiting	licorice ingestion
Gastric drainage	
Gastric outlet obstruction	Miscellaneous
	Bartter's syndrome
Adrenal disorder	Liddle's syndrome
Cushing's syndrome	
Primary hyperaldosteronism	

selected should be determined, and the solution administered according to the formula:

$$\text{Acid required (mEq/L)} = (0.3 \times \text{body weight in kg}) \times \text{desired drop in HCO}_3^- \text{ (mEq/L)}$$

Isotonic HCl solution supplies 150 mEq/L of H^+ ions. The serum HCO_3^- should not be reduced more than 8 to 12 mEq/L during the first 24 hours of acid therapy.

CONCLUSIONS

The diagnosis and management of acid-base disturbances should rest on a sound understanding of body pH and buffer systems, proper identification of the underlying cause of the acid-base derangement, and therapy aimed at helping body buffers gradually restore neutral homeostasis. Treatments that offer a quick fix to acid-base problems may do more harm than good to our patients.

Acknowledgement: The authors gratefully acknowledge and appreciate the advice and recommendations of Alan W. Grogono, M.D., who reviewed this chapter and its formulas.

REFERENCES

Davenport HW: The ABC of Acid-Base Chemistry, 6th ed. University of Chicago Press, Chicago, 1974.
Grogono AW: Acid-base balance. *In* Attia RR, Grogono AW (eds): Practical Anesthetic Pharmacology. Appleton-Century-Crofts, New York, 1978, pp 262–274.
Narins RG, Emmett M: Simple and mixed acid-base disorders: a practical approach. Medicine 59:161–187, 1980.
Siggaard-Anderson O: The Acid-Base Status of the Blood, 4th ed. Williams & Wilkins, Baltimore, 1974.

11 · HYPERCALCEMIA AND HYPOCALCEMIA

Carlos A. Verdonk
SCOTT AND WHITE CLINIC

Hypercalcemia

DEFINITION

Although ionized calcium is the biologically active fraction, elevation of total serum calcium is commonly used to define hypercalcemia. Normal fasting values vary according to laboratory techniques and need to be correlated with the albumin level (0.8 mg/dl change in serum calcium per gm/dl change in albumin). With atomic absorption spectrophotometry, the upper limit of normal (mean ± 2 SD) is 10.1 mg/dl. With the less accurate autoanalyzer methods, the range of normal serum calcium is wider.

PATHOPHYSIOLOGY

Hypercalcemia results from a variety of diseases (Table 1). Malignancy and primary hyperparathyroidism

Table 1. HYPERCALCEMIA: DIFFERENTIAL DIAGNOSIS

Common:	Malignancy
	Primary hyperparathyroidism
Less common:	Thiazides
	Myeloma
	Sarcoidosis
	Vitamin D or A intoxication
	Thyrotoxicosis
Rare:	Lymphomas, lithium, immobilization (children, young adults, Paget's disease), familial hypocalciuric hypercalcemia, granulomatous infections, and milk alkali syndrome

account for 90% of hypercalcemia problems. The most common malignancies are squamous cell carcinoma of the lung, breast cancer, myeloma, and hypernephroma. Sarcoidosis is associated with $1,25(OH)_2$ vitamin D production, and thyrotoxicosis with increased bone turnover. Thiazide-induced hypercalcemia is mild (less than 11 mg/dl) and its mechanism has not been definitely worked out.

CLINICAL ASPECTS

Because of the widespread use of automated chemistry, hypercalcemia has become a problem of serendipity. Hypercalcemia may be associated with a wide spectrum of clinical presentations ranging from asymptomatic to the following syndromes: gastrointestinal (constipation, vomiting), urologic (polyuria, nephrolithiasis), and neurologic (fatigue, confusion, coma).

MANAGEMENT

PLAN

The key to the treatment of hypercalcemia is in making the etiologic diagnosis. The diagnostic work-up needs to be individualized and may include all or some of the following: questioning the patient about family history and vitamin and thiazide use; obtaining thyroid function tests, protein electrophoresis, sedimentation rate, and parathyroid hormone levels (in moderate or severe renal insufficiency, parathyroid hormone assay results require special interpretation because of retention of parathyroid fragments in the circulation); x-ray films of the chest, kidneys, and hands. Bone scan, bone marrow, and vitamin D metabolite levels may be needed in certain cases.

NONPHARMACOLOGIC MEASURES

Dietary measures need to ensure the avoidance of excessive dairy products or calcium supplements. Surgery is the only effective treatment for primary hyperparathyroidism.

DRUG THERAPY

For mild hypercalcemia, treatment of the underlying cause is sufficient. There is no satisfactory long-term drug treatment for primary hyperparathyroidism. In case of thiazide use, up to six weeks may be required for the hypercalcemic effect to wear off.

With severe, symptomatic hypercalcemia, the patient is hospitalized. Intravenous normal saline is given at a rate of 200 to 300 ml/hour to rehydrate the patient and to induce an effective calcium diuresis. Hemodynamic monitoring may be necessary in critically ill patients. Digitalis preparations should be avoided because of adverse interaction with hypercalcemia. Once the patient is rehydrated, furosemide is added (40 to 80 mg every four to 12 hours as needed). An accurate fluid balance record is critical. These measures will result in a decrease of serum calcium of about 2 to 3 mg/dl in 24 hours. Additional measures will often be necessary to buy time while the diagnostic evaluation is being completed. These include: (1) Calcitonin (Calcimar): usual starting dose is 100 units subcutaneously every eight hours and may be increased to 8 units/kg/12 hours. Calcitonin is expensive but safe and well-tolerated and results in a decrease of 1 to 3 mg/dl in serum calcium. Unfortunately, it loses its efficacy after two to three days. (2) Mithramycin is very effective as a temporizing measure in hypercalcemia of any cause, as a single intravenous dose of 25 µgm/kg, which may be repeated every three to seven days for short-term treatment. Monitoring for thrombocytopenia, hepatotoxicity, and nephrotoxicity is essential. (3) Prednisone 40 to 60 mg/day is the treatment of choice for severe vitamin D intoxication and sarcoidosis. However, hypercalcemia may persist for months and prednisone dosage needs to be tapered accordingly. Prednisone is also effective in myeloma and some breast and hematologic malignancies. (4) Oral phosphates (500 mg four times a day) are occasionally used, if renal function is not impaired.

Hypocalcemia

DEFINITION

Although symptoms of hypocalcemia are related to the fraction of ionized serum concentration, its presence is suspected because of a reduction in the total calcium level. Correction for hypoalbuminemia must be made.

PATHOPHYSIOLOGY

Hypocalcemia is due to hypoparathyroidism or to vitamin D deficiency. Hypoparathyroidism results either from surgical intervention in the parathyroid gland area or from hypomagnesemia (malnutrition, cisplatin therapy), autoimmunity, resistance to parathyroid hormone action (pseudohypoparathyroidism), or iron overload. Transient hypocalcemia usually occurs following parathyroid adenoma resection and resolves spontaneously in a few days, except if parathyroid bone disease was present or if permanent hypoparathyroidism was induced. Hypocalcemia from vitamin D deficiency is usually milder and results from chronic renal failure and less commonly from intestinal malabsorption and rarely from dietary insufficiency or vitamin D resistance. Other causes of hypocalcemia include acute pancreatitis, osteoblastic metastases, or massive blood transfusions. Serum phosphorus levels are helpful in the differential diagnosis, since they are increased in hypoparathyroidism and decreased in vitamin D–related problems.

CLINICAL ASPECTS

Patients with hypocalcemia may remain asymptomatic for years or present with paresthesias, tetany, laryngeal stridor, seizures, psychosis, dementia, cataracts, or, rarely, congestive heart failure. Patients with pseudohypoparathyroidism have a peculiar phenotype. In adults with vitamin D deficiency, bone pain and muscle weakness are prominent features.

MANAGEMENT

PLAN

Treatment of hypoparathyroidism consists of vitamin D and calcium supplements, aiming for a serum calcium level that relieves the symptoms while avoiding the problems of chronic overdosing. Vitamin D deficiency is treated by physiologic vitamin D supplementation or by correcting the underlying cause.

NONPHARMACOLOGIC MEASURES

In hypoparathyroidism, dietary manipulations are not very helpful, since dairy products contain as much calcium as phosphorus, which is already elevated.

DRUG THERAPY

Selection of Drugs. *Acute symptomatic hypocalcemia* is readily corrected with 10 to 20 ml calcium gluconate 10% (90 to 180 mg elementary calcium) given IV over five to ten minutes. Similar amounts can then be infused over eight hours and repeated until oral calcium and vitamin D is begun. In magnesium deficiency, magnesium sulfate should be given, 2 ml (8.1 mEq) of a 50% solution IV or IM, and repeated every six hours for a five-day period, with individual adjustment in dosage taking renal function into account.

In *mild chronic hypoparathyroidism*, oral calcium supplements are sufficient. For more severe cases, vitamin D and calcium supplements are necessary. Calcium supplements are given to ensure a total daily calcium ingestion of about 1500 mg. An average American diet contains about 750 mg calcium. The easiest preparation to comply with is calcium carbonate, containing 500 mg elementary calcium per tablet (as Os-Cal or cheaper generic and over-the-counter preparations such as Tums or Titralac containing 200 mg elementary calcium per tablet or Titralac liquid, 400 mg elementary calcium per 5 ml). If hypochlorhydria is present, calcium carbonate is not adequately absorbed and other preparations are used: calcium gluconate (90 mg elementary calcium per 1000-mg tablets, which need to be chewed instead of swallowed), calcium lactate (85 mg elementary calcium per 625-mg tablet), or liquid Neo-Calglucon (115 mg elementary calcium per 5 ml). Compliance with these preparations is more difficult because of the larger number of tablets required. Calcium citrate (Citracal, 200 mg elementary calcium per tablet) has been shown to be effectively absorbed in hypochlorhydria.

Vitamin D preparations are listed in Table 2. Treatment is begun with vitamin D_2 (in my experience, Drisdol, among others, is preferred to unknown generic preparations), 50,000 units daily, or $1,25(OH)_2$ vitamin D (Rocaltrol) 0.25 µg b.i.d., and calcium carbonate 500 mg t.i.d. The time action characteristics of the vitamin D preparations are important: vitamin D_2 reaches maximum effect in four to six weeks (lag time needed for conversion to active metabolites) and adjustments in dosage should not be made more frequently than this lag time. In contrast, $1,25(OH)_2$ vitamin D (Rocaltrol)

Table 2. ORAL VITAMIN D PREPARATIONS FOR CORRECTION OF HYPOCALCEMIA[1,2]

Generic	Brand Name	Strength[3,4]	Approx. Relative Cost	Time to Reach Effect	Usual Daily Dose
Vitamin D_2 (ergocaliferol)	Drisdol Deltalin Calciferol Generic	50,000 U	1	2–6 wks	50,000–100,000 U
1,25$(OH)_2$ vitamin D	Rocaltrol	0.25 and 0.5 µg	3–6	2–4 days	0.25–2.0 µg
Dihydrotachysterol	Dihydrotachysterol USP	0.125, 0.2, 0.4 mg	3–4	1–2 wks	0.2–1.0 mg

[1]A preparation for IM use is available (500,000 U vitamin D_2 per ml (Calciferol)).
[2]25(OH) vitamin D (Calderol) is approved for hypocalcemia of chronic renal failure.
[3]The strength of vitamin D_2 50,000 U capsules varies somewhat according to the manufacturer.
[4]A liquid oral preparation (8000 U/ml) is also available.

reaches maximum effect in two to four days. It has the advantage of easier (every three to six days) titration and rapid reversal of toxicity but is much more expensive. Vitamin D dosage is adjusted to achieve a major change in serum calcium while manipulation of calcium tablets allows finer adjustment of the calcium level and correction of acute hypocalcemic symptoms, should these occur. Some patients achieve satisfactory calcium levels without need for calcium supplements.

Initially, serum calcium levels are obtained twice a week for 1,25$(OH)_2$ vitamin D (Rocaltrol) and every one to two weeks for vitamin D_2, aiming for a serum calcium level close to the lower limit of normal. Because hypercalciuria occurs at lower serum calcium levels than normal in the absence of parathyroid hormone, a 24-hour urine collection for calcium is important. If hypercalciuria (more than 4 mg/kg/24 hours) occurs, one should aim either for a lower serum calcium or, if needed, hydrochlorothiazide 25 mg/day may be added, along with a modest dietary salt restriction. This results in a 1 mg/dl rise in serum calcium and usually satisfactory reduction of the urinary calcium. Phosphate binders are rarely needed.

Drug Interactions. Patient and physician should anticipate the need for possible changes in the drug regimen. With estrogens, thiazides, pregnancy, and lactation, the dosage needs to be reduced. With glucocorticoids, physical stress, or fever, the dosage needs to be increased.

In *vitamin D deficiency*, the effect of vitamin D_2 (ergocalciferol) on rickets or osteomalacia is much stronger than its effect in hypoparathyroidism. Very small doses (400 to 1000 units/day) are effective in the rarely encountered, strictly dietary vitamin D deficiency. In chronic renal failure, 1,25$(OH)_2$ vitamin D (Rocaltrol) is the treatment of choice. For other causes of hypocalcemia from vitamin D deficiency, correction of the underlying cause (such as celiac sprue) or vitamin D supplementation (as in chronic malabsorption) is effective.

Adverse Effects. Hypercalcemia and renal insufficiency result from excessive vitamin D therapy and may occur unpredictably. Intoxication with 1,25$(OH)_2$ vitamin D (Rocaltrol) is rapidly reversed by interruption of the treatment. For severe vitamin D_2 intoxication, saline and a brief course of prednisone are the treatment of choice, but mild hypercalcemia from vitamin D_2 intoxication may persist for months.

PATIENT INFORMATION AND FOLLOW-UP

The patient should know the symptoms of hypercalcemia and the need for lifelong follow-up, with visits every four to six months for serum calcium, phosphorus, creatinine, and if possible 24-hour urine calcium.

PATIENT COMPLIANCE

Patient compliance is maximized with simple drug regimens such as a single dose of vitamin D_2 and b.i.d. or t.i.d. calcium supplements. 1,25$(OH)_2$ vitamin D (Rocaltrol) is preferably given b.i.d. but in the lower dosage range is also effective as a single daily dose.

PREVENTIVE MEASURES

Parathyroid autotransplantation into the forearm may obviate hypoparathyroidism in patients undergoing reexploration for persistent or recurrent hyperparathyroidism with previous inadvertent removal of normal glands.

REFERENCES

Broadus AE: Mineral metabolism. *In* Felip P, Baxter JD, Broadus AE, et al (eds): Endocrinology and Metabolism. McGraw-Hill, New York, 1981, pp 963–1079.
Frame B, Parfitt AM: Osteomalacia: current concepts. Ann Intern Med 89:966–982, 1978.
Mundy GR, Ibbotson KJ, D'Souza SM, et al: The hypercalcemia of cancer: clinical implications and pathogenic mechanisms. N Engl J Med 310:1718–1727, 1984.
Sharp CF, Singer FR: Hypoparathyroidism. *In* Krieger DT, Bardin CW (eds): Current Therapy in Endocrinology. C.V. Mosby, St. Louis, 1983, pp 266–269.

12 · OSTEOMALACIA AND OSTEOPOROSIS

Douglas B. Muchmore
SCRIPPS CLINIC AND RESEARCH FOUNDATION

DEFINITION AND DIAGNOSTIC CRITERIA

The generic term for deficient bone mass is osteopenia, which does not imply a specific cause, structural defect, or clinical presentation. Osteomalacia is defined as failure of normal mineralization of bone matrix and may lead to osteopenia. Osteoporosis simply means that histologically and structurally normal bone is present in a pathologically inadequate amount. A diagnosis of osteoporosis is based on the pathologic fracture, although newer techniques for assessing bone mass are now allowing the clinician earlier confirmation of a suspicion. In contrast, a final diagnosis of osteomalacia depends not on clinical data but rather on histologic evidence of impaired osteoid mineralization.

PATHOPHYSIOLOGY

OSTEOMALACIA

Osteomalacia has many causes, most of which are the result of a disordered vitamin D metabolism (Table 1). Thus, sunlight deficiency, malabsorptive syndromes, hepatic cirrhosis, and chronic renal failure may result in inadequate production, absorption, or metabolic activation of the vitamin. Vitamin D is normally produced in sun-exposed skin or ingested as the inactive prohormone cholecalciferol. It then undergoes sequential hydroxylation at the 1 and 25 carbon atoms in the liver and kidney, respectively. Activated vitamin D acts primarily to stimulate calcium absorption, and vitamin D deficiency results in an inadequate supply of calcium for mineralization of bone matrix. This calcium deficiency also increases parathyroid hormone, which stimulates bone resorption.

OSTEOPOROSIS

The pathogenesis of osteoporosis is less clearly defined. The basic cellular unit of bone is composed of the bone-resorbing osteoclast and the bone-forming osteoblast. These cells work in a closely coordinated sequence of resorption followed by formation. This allows remodeling and repair to occur, and about 5% of the skeleton is renewed annually. The basic defect(s) of osteoporosis result in a mismatch in resorption/formation rates, leading to net bone loss. Bone loss is a normal aspect of aging, occurring in both males and females progressively after the third decade. Dietary calcium deficiency and estrogen deficiency in the female are the two most important causes of osteoporosis. Estrogen deficiency results in calcium malabsorption; this is poorly tolerated by American females whose dietary calcium of 500 mg/day is already insufficient. Additional factors in osteoporosis include race (whites affected, blacks protected), body configuration (obese and large-boned individuals protected), tobacco and alcohol use, family history, exercise patterns, medications (especially corticosteroids), presence of other

chronic disease, high-protein intake, and male hypogonadism.

CLINICAL ASPECTS

Established disease may present with or without symptoms. Height loss of two or more inches, development of kyphosis ("dowager's hump"), or presence of mid-dorsal spinal pain that is worse with bending and better with rest often go unmentioned. On the other hand, vertebral crush fracture is readily appreciated by physician and patient alike, and Colles' fracture of the distal radius presents directly to the orthopedic clinic. The major cause of expense, disability, and death is the hip fracture, affecting over 30% of women who reach the age of 90. Clinical differentiation of osteomalacia from osteoporosis is imprecise, but generalized bone pain is a feature of osteomalacia not often seen in osteoporosis.

When bone disease is suspected, its presence should be confirmed. X-ray films may show demineralization, fracture, or osteomalacia (pseudofractures). Thinning of cortex and accentuation of trabecular pattern are clues to osteoporosis, indicating that more than 30% of bone mineral has been lost. Anterior vertebral wedging or end-plate deformity ("cod-fishing") confirm the diagnosis. Quantitative assessment of bone mineral density is an important adjunct to x-ray examination in management of the disease. Since medullary trabecular bone is far more metabolically active than cortical lamellar bone, it is preferable to choose a technique that will measure trabecular bone density. Thus, single beam photon absorptiometry of the wrist, which is composed primarily of cortical bone, does not accurately reflect vertebral body or femoral neck disease. Two newer techniques are of great value in following response to treatment: dual beam photon absorptiometry and quantitative CT. Neither technique is accurate as a diagnostic screening tool because of overlap between normals and osteoporotics.

Osteomalacia is diagnosed when evidence of bone demineralization is accompanied by a history of known etiopathogenetic mechanisms along with characteristic depression of serum calcium and phosphate, elevation of alkaline phosphatase, and lowering of urinary calcium excretion. However, some patients may not show these findings and the diagnosis is definitively confirmed only with bone biopsy, and then only using undecalcified processing and tetracycline prelabeling of bone matrix so that deposition rates can be measured. In practice, I find that biopsy is rarely needed to assign diagnosis or choose therapy, but the physician's suspicion based on clinical clues is important in this decision.

MANAGEMENT

Once significant osteopenia is demonstrated, its cause should be identified. A breakdown of bone disorders along with recommended initial studies is shown in Table 2. Naturally, treatment is directed to any secondary conditions. Assessment of family history, menstrual status, dairy product intake, tobacco and alcohol use, exercise patterns, and medication records should be routine in the general evaluation of all adult females, especially small-boned Caucasians. A history of malabsorptive symptoms, anticonvulsant use, kidney

Table 1. ETIOLOGY OF OSTEOPENIA

Primary Osteopenia	Osteomalacia
Senile osteoporosis	Vitamin D deficiency
Postmenopausal osteoporosis	Malabsorption
Juvenile osteoporosis	Gastric surgery
Idiopathic osteoporosis	Anticonvulsant drugs
	Chronic liver disease
Secondary osteopenia	Chronic renal failure
Osteoporosis	Aluminum intoxication
Corticosteroid excess	Renal tubular acidosis
Thyrotoxicosis	Hypophosphatemic rickets
Chronic renal failure	Osteitis fibrosa cystica
Chronic liver disease	Hyperparathyroidism
Alcoholism	Malignancy
Tobacco use	Multiple myeloma
Immobilization	Metastatic disease
Weightlessness	
Heparin therapy	
Hypogonadism	
Other chronic disease	

Table 2. RECOMMENDED DIAGNOSTIC EVALUATION OF OSTEOPENIA

Blood
Complete blood count, erythrocyte sedimentation rate, calcium, phosphate, alkaline phosphatase, electrolytes, serum protein electrophoresis, and thyroxine
Parathyroid hormone if calcium is over 10 and 1,25-dihydroxycholecalciferol if osteomalacia is suspected

Urine
Urinalysis with pH
24-hour urinary calcium

Structural studies
Lumbar and thoracic spine films
Quantitative bone mineral assessment (CT scan, dual beam)
Bone biopsy if diagnosis uncertain

disease, gastrointestinal surgery, or inadequate sun exposure alert one to the possibility of osteomalacia.

PLAN

Short-term goals for the acutely symptomatic patient are to reduce pain, promote healing, and preserve functional status. Long-term goals in the patient with established disease include prevention of bone loss and, if possible, rebuilding of lost bone.

The outpatient clinic is the focus for ongoing care. Hospitalization is required for surgical treatment of hip fracture and for a few patients with acute vertebral compression. Ideally, the physician coordinates care with a team that may include a nurse, physical therapist, exercise physiologist, dietitian, social worker, and/or psychologist. Assessment of the individual's present disability and home resources is essential in the older patient with advanced disease. Fear of falling often leads to withdrawal and isolation; in these cases, social and group support may be instrumental in rehabilitation. Approximately 50% of elderly hip fracture patients lose independent care status, underscoring the magnitude of these problems. Home health care may include supportive services, physical therapy, and "fall-proofing" the home environment.

NONPHARMACOLOGIC MEASURES

Dietary Calcium. Prevention and treatment of bone disease hinge on adequate calcium intake. Sources of calcium are summarized in Table 3. A diet history to estimate calcium intake will then direct treatment with calcium-containing foods or supplements. Although the U.S. Recommended Daily Allowance (RDA) for calcium is only 800 mg/day, the premenopausal female requires 1000 mg/day to maintain calcium balance and the estrogen-deficient woman needs 1500 mg/day to meet this goal.

Exercise. Exercise is important in prevention, treatment, and rehabilitation. Intermittent loading exercise, such as walking, stimulates bone formation, whereas bed rest results in rapid bone resorption. Additionally, flexibility and strengthening exercises improve functional status. A cautionary note, however: bending, lifting, and other flexion maneuvers increase vertebral fracture rates and are to be avoided. A combination of extension, strengthening, and walking exercises is ideal. In the acutely symptomatic patient, bed rest is helpful for the first few days; some patients find that custom-fitted soft support corsets subsequently allow greater mobility, but rigid braces are not recommended.

DRUG THERAPY

Calcium Supplements. The younger, premenopausal, active individual who is at risk for bone disease should maintain 1000 mg/day calcium intake. Low-fat dairy products are adequate in those willing, but personal preference or lactose intolerance may dictate use of supplements. Supplements are usually needed in the menopausal individual to reach the 1500 mg/day goal. Calcium carbonate is preferred for reasons of cost, convenience, and high calcium content.

Estrogen. Estrogen replacement treatment should be entertained in every menopausal woman, especially those under age 50. Cyclical estrogen administered with progesterone does not promote endometrial carcinoma. Risk of this therapy to the breast is disputed but likely negligible; a history of breast cancer, however, is an absolute contraindication to this treatment. Endometrial sampling prior to institution of hormonal treatment is preferred by many physicians, and it is indicated in cases of excessive withdrawal bleeding. Dose-response studies show that 0.625 mg/day of conjugated estrogen (e.g., Premarin) administered for the first 25 days of each month is adequate to provide maximum benefit; medroxyprogesterone (Provera) 5 mg is given concurrently on days 16 to 25. Be sure your patient expects to resume menstruation, and counsel her that the bleeding tends to diminish over the first few months.

Sodium Fluoride. Sodium fluoride is the most potent promoter of bone formation, and although not yet approved by the FDA for this purpose, is used as the third-line treatment in severe cases. Dosage is 40 to 80 mg/day. There is no convenient formulation available by prescription (Fluoritabs contain only 2.2 mg), but a combination mineral supplement called Florical (8.3 mg sodium fluoride and 145 mg elemental calcium as carbonate) is available over-the-counter. Side effects of fluoride include gastrointestinal upset and periosteitis. The former limits dosage in about one third of patients, but sprinkling the powder in applesauce and taking it with meals is often helpful. The latter complication occurs rarely, and only after six or more months of high-dose treatment. It presents as an acutely painful heel or large bone metaphysis and responds to drug withdrawal followed by reinstitution of a smaller dose a few weeks later.

Vitamin D. Vitamin D supplementation to a level of 400 to 1200 IU/day (100 to 300% of the RDA) is suggested. Large doses (50,000 IU per week or more) are

Table 3. SOURCES OF CALCIUM

Dietary
Whole milk or nonfat milk (290 mg/8 oz)
Buttermilk (300 mg/ 8 oz)
Cottage cheese (160 mg/ 6 oz)
Yogurt (280 mg/8 oz)
Broccoli (150 mg/spear)
Spinach or rhubarb (200 mg/cup)
Other vegetables (25–50 mg/cup)
Eggs (25 mg each)
Beef or chicken (20 mg/5 oz)
Grains (30 mg/cup)
Fruits (30–50 mg/cup)

Supplemental (percentage elemental calcium)
Calcium carbonate (40%)
Calcium gluconate (9%)
Calcium lactate (13%)
Others (generally about 10%)

not recommended except in deficiency of or antagonism to vitamin D. Of special note, corticosteroids impair production of 1, 25-dihydroxycholecalciferol, and determination of the blood level of this active metabolite followed by supplementation with cholecalciferol or 1, 25-dihydroxycholecalciferol (Rocaltrol) is sensible, although not as yet of proven efficacy.

A problem in medication compliance is the large number of tablets and capsules needed in treatment. However, drug interaction problems are minimal. Other drugs that may be entertained in treatment include anabolic steroids and calcitonin. Finally, judicious use of muscle relaxants and analgesics is appropriate in the acute vertebral compression syndrome.

PATIENT INFORMATION AND EDUCATION

Diet concerns are central, and the services of a registered dietitian are very helpful. The physical therapist and exercise physiologist can work together to tailor a program of strengthening, flexibility, and aerobic conditioning. The nurse or social worker can aid in home needs assessment with particular attention to fracture prevention: removal of throw rugs, avoidance of polished floors, use of nonskid products in the bathroom, training in the use of a cane or walker, use of proper rubber-soled footwear, and so on. A number of patient education materials are available through pharmaceutical houses, and, for the highly motivated individual, Notelovitz and Ware's book is highly recommended.

PERIODIC EVALUATION

Follow-up of the acute fracture patient is tailored to his or her progress. In initiating a multiple-agent regimen for the patient with established disease, the clinician should introduce drugs one at a time, waiting a month or so to observe patient tolerance before adding another agent. Once a regimen is established, review every three to six months is suggested. Spinal x-ray films and bone densitometry are recommended annually, as is follow-up of urinary calcium excretion, routine chemistry, and, if indicated, vitamin D level. Sodium fluoride raises alkaline phosphatase, and response to the drug is monitored by checking the enzyme every three to six months. I would emphasize that patience by physician and patient alike is helpful, since both progression of disease and response to therapy occur over months to years. However, failure to stabilize the disease does warrant diagnostic reevaluation.

PATIENT COMPLIANCE

Most individuals with acutely symptomatic osteoporosis are well motivated to comply with the burdens of a management program. Effective prevention is a greater challenge but may be achievable through increased patient and public education and physician awareness. The traditional view that osteoporosis is inevitable and untreatable is less prevalent now, but it must be eradicated. Targeting information to high-risk groups is bound to be useful.

PREVENTIVE MEASURES

The clinician's interest is focused on prevention, diagnosis, and treatment. To achieve the first goal, early identification of at-risk populations is needed. The threshold value of vertebral bone density below which spontaneous fracture is likely is approximately 1.0 gm/cm^2 (dual beam) or 100 gm/cm^3 (quantitative CT). Measures that augment mature skeletal mass will delay the time when the aging adult's bone density crosses below this critical value. Adequate dietary calcium and good exercise habits are thought to promote mature skeletal mass and thus constitute the basis for a general preventive strategy. In the clinic, identification of individuals at risk, followed by risk factor counseling and modification, are the means to prevent or retard appearance of the disease. Thus an intensive program of exercise, calcium supplements, avoidance of alcohol and tobacco, and early hormonal replacement may be suggested for the females of a small-boned Caucasian family whose matriarchs have withered bones, while no intervention may be appropriate for the husky black male former football star.

SOCIOECONOMIC ASPECTS OF MANAGEMENT

The annual direct costs of osteoporotic fracture care in this country are estimated to exceed three billion dollars; the indirect dollar expenses and psychosocial impact add considerably to this expense. Public, patient, and professional education programs can reduce these costs. The continuing care of the fracture-free patient is not labor-intensive, with two to four annual visits adequate in most cases. Initial bloodwork is mostly part of the routine general evaluation. Inclusion of vitamin D, parathyroid hormone, and urinary calcium will add about $100 to the costs. Spinal density measurement by the newer techniques runs $100 to $200, an amount that is justified by the value of the information to the management program.

REFERENCES

Aloia JF: Exercise and skeletal health. J Am Geriatrics Soc 29:104–107, 1981.

Heaney RP: Prevention of age-related osteoporosis in women. *In* Avioli LV (ed): The Osteoporotic Syndrome. Grune & Stratton, New York, 1983, pp 123–144.

Mundy G: Differential diagnosis of osteopenia. Hosp Pract 13:65–72, 1978.

Notelovitz M, Ware M: Stand Tall! Triad Publishing Co, Gainesville, FL, 1982.

Peck WA, Barrett-Connor E, Buckwalter JA, et al: Osteoporosis (NIH Consensus Panel Statement). National Institutes of Health, Office of Applications Research, Bethesda, MD, 1984.

13 · TRACE ELEMENTS

Ramachandiran Cooppan
JOSLIN CLINIC

Trace elements are substances that are required by the body in minute quantities. Their main role is in enzyme systems in cells. By combining with protein molecules, they confer longevity and increased reactivity to the cells. Because they are required in small amounts, the usual daily requirements are met in a good balanced diet. However, because of this small requirement, deficiency can occur fairly rapidly.

The trace elements considered essential for man are zinc, copper, manganese, iron, iodine, cobalt, molybdenum, chromium, selenium, fluorine, and vanadium. Their exact mechanisms of absorption are not fully understood, although many bind to proteins called thioneines. These are low molecular proteins that bind the trace element and function also in regulation of metal toxicity and intracellular metabolism. Their synthesis occurs in the liver, kidney, and spleen and is inducible. Most of the elements are found in normal dietary foods such as meats, seafood, various legumes, and grains. Excretion pathways vary. Zinc is excreted mainly via pancreatic secretions. Copper is excreted via the bile, and chromium mainly by the kidney.

The whole area of trace element metabolism is still new and changing. Until more definitive evidence of deficiency states is documented, one should be careful about oversupplementation and the claims for therapeutic benefits in various disease states.

IRON

The total body iron in adult males is about 3.45 gm and in females about 2.45 gm. Most of this is in hemoglobin (60% to 70%). The rest occurs as myoglobin and enzymes, and is also stored in the bone marrow, liver, and spleen. Nonheme Fe (iron) occurs in organic and inorganic food and must be reduced to the ferrous state for absorption. Phytate reduces absorption as do calcium and phosphorus together. Tea can form insoluble Fe tannate complexes. Ascorbic acid, however, enhances absorption by maintaining Fe in the reduced form. Daily requirement is 10 mg for men and 18 mg for women. Iron deficiency results in a hypochromic microcytic anemia. (See Iron Deficiency, Chapter 2, Section V.) This is the most common form of anemia worldwide.

Iron Overload. Iron overload can occur as a primary disease with increased absorption (hemochromatosis) or with increased ingestion (iron therapy, alcoholic cirrhosis, Bantu hemosiderosis) or repeated blood transfusion. Primary hemochromatosis results in cirrhosis of the liver together with iron deposition in the skin, heart, pancreas, pituitary, and joints. Over 50% of patients have diabetes mellitus. Hepatomas occur with increased frequency. The diagnosis should be considered especially in patients with diabetes, cardiac disease, and liver enlargement. If the diagnosis is proved, family members should be screened. The plasma iron is elevated >200 μgm/100 ml, with a saturation >70%. Treatment is phlebotomy or by chelating with desferrioxamine. (See Hemochromatosis, Chapter 12, Section V.)

IODINE

About 80% of iodine is found in the thyroid as thyroglobulin, and it is the basis for thyroxine and triiodothyronine. Deficiency still exists worldwide mostly in mountain areas and results in a goiter. In the United States most salt is iodized and so deficiency is uncommon. In fact, the average intake is several times more than the RDA of 150 μgm/day. Chronic toxicity occurs when intake is >2000 μgm/day.

COPPER

This element is involved in many biochemical processes that range from electron transport to formation of collagen and elastin, immune system integrity, amino acid metabolism, hematopoiesis, and central nervous system myelinization. Current estimates suggest that most typical meals in the United States contain only half of the 2 to 3 mg copper required daily. The major dietary sources are whole grain cereals, shellfish, and nuts.

Deficiency is uncommon but can occur when other factors interfere with absorption. High zinc and ascorbic acid intakes or excessive antacid use can reduce the copper available for metabolism. The characteristic signs of deficiency in animals are growth retardation, anemia, hyperlipidemia, hypertrophy of the heart, osteoporosis, and pathologic fractures. The mechanism of the hyperlipidemia is not fully understood but has been noted in humans as well as experimental animals. Menkes' syndrome is a congenital copper deficiency in humans with hypotonia, mental retardation, and cortical blindness.

Hypercupremia is rare alone. Nausea, vomiting, headache, dizziness, hypertension, rapid pulse, and hemolysis can occur. Treatment is cessation of intake and hospitalization for hydration and supportive care.

Wilson's Disease. Wilson's disease is an autosomal recessive copper storage state affecting especially the liver, brain, cornea, and kidney. It is accompanied by reduced serum ceruloplasmin and copper levels and excessive copper sequestration into the liver parenchymal cells. When hepatic saturation occurs, the cornea, kidney, and brain are affected. Manifestations are protean and involve hepatic, neurologic, and psychiatric systems. Onset is in the first decade. In later childhood hepatic disease presents as cirrhosis with hepatosplenomegaly, jaundice, anorexia, and fatigue. Kidney involvement results in renal tubular acidosis and Fanconi syndrome. Kayser-Fleischer rings may be present in the limbus of the cornea as greenish brown discoloration. The serum copper is low (normal 108 μgm/dl) and ceruloplasmin is reduced. However, low levels can also be seen in malnutrition, nephrosis, and newborns. Urinary copper levels are increased (normal <40 μgm/24 hours). A liver biopsy may show increased copper but heterozygotes may have intermediate values (100 to 250 μgm/gm dry weight). Untreated, the disease is fatal. Reduction of copper absorption by avoiding organ meats, shellfish, dried legumes, nuts, and whole grains is important. D-Penicillamine, 250 mg/day, is the drug of choice. Dosage is gradually increased to 2 to 4 gm. Pyridoxine, 25 to 50 mg/day, is added to avoid a deficiency. Toxic reactions include fever, skin rash, leukopenia, and thrombocytopenia. Wilson's disease should always be considered in the differential diagnosis of childhood cirrhosis.

ZINC

Like copper, zinc is involved in many biochemical reactions in the body. Its importance in human nutrition has only recently been recognized. It is a component of many enzyme systems, is essential for synthesis of nucleic acids and proteins, and is an important factor in carbonic anhydrase in red cells.

Clinically, a role is suggested in immunity, taste

acuity, bone calcification and growth, gonadal function, and wound healing. Deficiency in humans is associated with germinal cell injury with oligospermia and infertility.

The total body contains 1 to 2.5 gm, found mainly in bone, teeth, hair, liver, and muscle. The RDA is 15 mg/day for adults and 20 mg for pregnant women. Several surveys show that many diets are below the RDA in the United States. Foods high in zinc include red meats, oysters, eggs, and fish. Diets high in phytate (cereals), fiber, and phosphate (dairy products) impair intestinal absorption. Deficiency can also occur in cystic fibrosis, malabsorption states, alcohol abuse, liver disease, diuretic treatment, and inadequate replacement in total parenteral nutrition.

A syndrome of growth retardation, anorexia, and hypogenesis has been described in children less than 4 years old. Acrodermatitis enteropathica is a recessively inherited disease of zinc absorption. Patients present with alopecia, psoriasiform rash, and growth retardation. Deficiency in adults can present with skin lesions, irritability, and alopecia.

The diagnosis is usually made on the basis of low plasma zinc concentrations. Normal plasma levels are 90 to 100 μgm/dl. Acute stress, trauma, burns, sepsis, and surgery can lower the levels by redistribution from plasma to tissues. Once diagnosed, treatment is zinc sulfate, 220 mg one to three times daily. This is best given on an empty stomach; it is well tolerated and relatively nontoxic. Industrial exposure can result in fever, cough, leukocytosis, and pulmonary infiltration. Toxicity can occur with excessive intake and presents with vomiting, dehydration, abdominal pain, electrolyte imbalance, and renal failure. Hospitalization is needed and treatment is to discontinue the intake and support the patient. Excess intake can also result in a copper deficiency anemia from competitive inhibition of copper absorption. Until more is known about the long-term effects, it is recommended that supplements be used only in patients with convincing evidence of a deficiency.

MANGANESE

Manganese is widely distributed in human tissues (bone, pituitary, liver, pineal) but exact functon is not entirely clear. It activates a number of metal enzyme complexes. It is found mainly in wheat germs, seeds, leafy vegetables, and meat. Deficiency has not been fully identified in humans. Chronic poisoning can occur in miners inhaling dust and presents as an encephalitis with extrapyramidal signs.

COBALT

The major role of cobalt is an essential part of vitamin B_{12}. Humans cannot synthesize this vitamin and obtain it from the diet. The average intake of cobalt is about 300 mg/day and the richest sources are liver, kidney, oysters, and clams. Legumes and cereals are very poor sources. A high intake can result in polycythemia and cardiomyopathy with congestive cardiac failure. Cobalt chloride can lead to a goiter that disappears when intake is discontinued.

SELENIUM

Selenium closely resembles sulfur and is involved in reoxidation of reduced glutathione. It is the least abundant of the essential elements in food and the most toxic. Fish, seafood, and protein-rich plant foods are the major sources. As glutathione peroxidase, it protects cells and membranes against oxidative damage. It also provides protection against mercury and cadmium toxicity. The requirement may increase as the unsaturated fatty acid content of the diet increases. Dietary deficiency may result in a childhood cardiomyopathy and long-term parenteral feeding may also cause a deficiency. Toxic effect can occur from industrial dusts. To date no convincing evidence exists to link this element with the incidence of cancer.

CHROMIUM

Although the biochemical role of chromium has not yet been defined, it is part of the glucose tolerance factor needed for optimal utilization of glucose. It may facilitate the binding of insulin to the cell and thus promote glucose transport. Chromium is poorly absorbed and is excreted in the urine and feces. Total body levels are lower in the United States ($\pm$ 1 to 7 mg) than in the Far East (9 mg). The amount in the hair indicates the chromium status. The major source is foods of plant origin, especially vegetables and whole grain cereals. Low intakes have been associated with reduced glucose tolerance and an increasing incidence of diabetes with age. Other symptoms observed are decreased glycogen stores, retarded growth, and disturbed amino acid metabolism. At present there is inadequate evidence to suggest that supplementation has a beneficial effect in diabetes mellitus.

FLUORINE

Normal formation of bone and teeth is dependent on the presence of fluorine, most of which is concentrated in these tissues. It is widely distributed in sea fish and present in tea and coffee. Fluoridation of water (1 to 2 ppm) provides a readily available source. Fluorine deficiency predisposes to dental caries and possibily to osteoporosis. Excessive fluorine intake (fluoridation >10 ppm) results in fluorosis, which is characterized by mottling and pitting of the permanent teeth and osteosclerosis and exostoses of the spine. Its role in the prevention and treatment of osteoporosis requires further study.

OTHER TRACE ELEMENTS

There are many other trace elements that appear to be necessary for human nutrition in minute amounts. Deficiency states have not been fully documented in humans. Cadmium toxicity can occur in industrial settings or from food intake, as in Japan. Pulmonary emphysema, proteinuria, and anemia can occur. In Japan a syndrome of osteomalacia and nephropathy has been described with food grown with contaminated water. A possible relationship to high blood pressure may exist. Increased vanadium levels may play a role in manic-depressive psychosis. So far, strontium has not been found to be an essential nutrient.

Given the recent trend to use more organic foods and for vitamin and trace element supplementation, patients must be cautioned about excessive therapeutic claims and potential side effects. With a proper balanced diet, there appears to be no good evidence for oversupplementation. In the elderly, the use of One-A-Day vitamins with trace elements may be beneficial provided excess intake is avoided.

REFERENCES

Goodhart RS, Shils ME: Modern Nutrition in Health and Disease, 6th ed. Lea & Febiger, Philadelphia, 1980, Chapter 9.
Mertz W: The essential trace elements. Science 213:1332–1338, 1981.

14 · VITAMINS

Ramachandiran Cooppan
JOSLIN CLINIC

Vitamins are organic compounds that cannot be synthesized in the body and are required in small amounts for the promotion of normal metabolism and maintenance of health. They exert their effects via diverse biochemical mechanisms, including altering the permeability of cell membranes, acting as oxidation-reduction agents, and behaving as coenzymes or enzyme inhibitors.

Food is the best source, and with an adequate diet, supplement should not be needed. The Recommended Daily Allowances (RDA) have been established by the Food and Nutrition Board of the National Research Council. These allowances are higher than the minimum requirements to prevent deficiency. The U.S. RDA is a simplified table of food values for labeling.

Deficiencies should not arise with a balanced diet. However, on a global level, malnutrition resulting in reduced intake remains the major cause. In more affluent societies, fad diets, very strict vegetarianism, and alcoholism are more likely causes. Reduced absorption from malabsorption syndromes and inadequate supplementation with hyperalimentation are also potential causes. Clinical features vary considerably. With the increasing number of elderly people in our society, especially those living alone and with other diseases, reduced intake may become more of a problem. It is estimated that 10% to 12% of the 70- to 80-year group are deficient to some extent in vitamin B, folic acid, vitamins C and D, and iron. Furthermore, other medications complicate the picture. Anticonvulsants interfere with vitamin D hydroxylation and also reduce the absorption of B_6, B_{12}, and folate. Isoniazid can interfere with B_6 absorption. Until we know more about the needs of the elderly, oversupplementation should be avoided and reliance placed on good nutrition.

In general, mild deficiency cannot be diagnosed accurately. Office treatment is satisfactory in patients who are not acutely ill. Severe cases of deficiency require hospitalization.

In the last ten years megavitamin therapy has increased and therapeutic claims far exceed verifiable results. More than 30% of American adults take vitamins and/or mineral supplements at an annual cost of nearly two billion dollars. Diseases in which they are used range from mental illness to cancer and the common cold. It is especially important to avoid excessive fat-soluble vitamins, which tend to accumulate in the body. On the other hand, the use of many medications (e.g., aspirin or antacids) may affect vitamin absorption or activity and accentuate their need.

The role of components such as pangamic acid, laetrile (B_{17}), lecithin, and inositol as vitamins and/or nutrients remains to be established.

FAT-SOLUBLE VITAMINS

Vitamins D, A, K, and E are absorbed like fat in the small intestine. Any condition causing fat malabsorption can result in a deficiency of one or more vitamins. Storage is mainly in the liver and excretion via the feces. Because of their slow metabolism, overdosage can result in toxic effects.

VITAMIN A

Vitamin A is necessary for growth and bone development in children, for dim light vision, and for maintaining the integrity of epithelial and mucous membranes. Retinol is the natural form and beta-carotene the major precursor, being found in yellow and green vegetables. About one third of the beta-carotene is converted to vitamin A. Preformed vitamin A is found in eggs, dairy products, and meat. Protein and zinc are probably needed to mobilize the reserves in the liver. RDA is 800 to 1000 (Retinol equivalent) or 5000 IU/day.

Vitamin A Deficiency. Vitamin A deficiency is a major health problem in many developing countries where inadequate intake is the chief cause. Liver disease and malabsorption are others. Mild deficiency results in night blindness, conjunctival xerosis, and Bitot's spots. Treatment with 5000 to 10,000 IU/daily for ten days is sufficient. A single massive dose of 200,000 IU can also be used. Severe deficiency involves the cornea and progresses to keratomalacia with blindness. Water-soluble vitamin A (100,000 units) is used initially followed by oral dose of 100 to 200,000 units. Concomitant illnesses must be treated.

Hypervitaminosis. Hypervitaminosis occurs with excessive intake, but wide variations exist. Acutely, malaise, headache, irritability, and vomiting occur; with chronic toxicity, carotenemia, weight loss, alopecia, skin, joint, and psychiatric changes result. X-ray films show periosteal bone changes, and treatment is to stop the vitamin.

VITAMIN D

Ergocalciferol (D_2) is derived from yeast and fungal sources. Irradiation of the provitamin, 7-dehydrocholesterol, in the skin produces cholecalciferol (D_3). Storage is in the liver as 25-hydroxyvitamin D [25(OH) D_3], a hydroxylated form. In the kidney, further hydroxylation results in 1,25-dihydroxyvitamin D, the most potent form. Together with parathyroid hormone and calcitonin, it controls calcium absorption, bone mineralization, and regulation of phosphorus metabolism.

Normal requirements are small and usually met with exposure to sunlight. Rickets and osteomalacia result from deficiency. Primary deficiency is rare and may occur in the elderly, alcoholics, food faddists, and institutionalized patients. The usual causes are malabsorption syndromes and inherited or acquired metabolic diseases (vitamin D–dependent rickets, D-resistant rickets, renal osteodystrophy).

Osteomalacia. Osteomalacia may present with very few symptoms and signs. Diagnosis must be pursued aggressively, since the response to treatment is excellent. Apart from an increased serum alkaline phosphatase and a normal or reduced calcium, a bone biopsy remains the best diagnostic tool. With treatment, bone pain improves in two to three months and bone healing occurs in six to 12 months. As far as possible, underlying problems should be treated. Gluten-free diets, pancreatic enzyme replacement, correction of acidosis, and cessation of excessive aluminum hydroxide are potential issues. Ergocalciferol (Calciferol, Drisdol) is an effective replacement therapy. These products can lose potency with long storage, and combinations with folic acid, ascorbic acid, thiamine, and pyridoxine enhance degradation and should be avoided. Injectable ergocalciferol has variable potency and should not be used. Maximum effect is reached in four to ten weeks and the effect lasts six to 30 weeks after cessation. Average dose is 5 to 75 µg in deficiency states. Drisdol capsules contain 50,000 IU of the vitamin. Resistant cases and some of the inherited problems require much larger doses. Osteomalacia responds to 50,000 units on average. Dihydrotachysterol is derived from irradiation of ergosterol, a plant sterol. Because of the A ring rotation when 25-hydroxylated, it acts as a 1,25 form. Use in rickets and osteomalacia is limited. Calcifediol, 25-hydroxyvitamin D, is used in hepatic or renal disease. Calcitriol, $1,25(OH)_2D$, is the most potent form available; absorption is rapid, and half-life is short (three to eight hours). Its general use has been in renal osteodystrophy or vitamin D resistance. Because of the risk of toxicity, increments in dose must be made very slowly and the calcium kept in the lower normal range and the calcium/phosphorus product < 55. Calcium supplements are also needed, and 1 gm elemental calcium is supplied by four (650-mg) tablets of calcium carbonate or 12 (650-mg) calcium lactate tablets. Therapy should be monitored closely with plasma calcium levels and urinary calcium excretion.

Vitamin D Intoxication. Vitamin D intoxication results in hypercalcemia and may present with anorexia, nausea, vomiting, pancreatitis, and cardiac (tachycardia, hypertension, digitalis sensitivity), renal (proteinuria, azotemia, nephrolithiasis), and neurologic (weakness, confusion, headaches) manifestations. Treatment is immediate cessation of the drug and hospitalization in severe cases for hydration and the use of prednisone (30 to 40 mg/daily) if needed for four to six weeks. Calcitonin, 50 to 100 MRC units, can be used subcutaneously daily for five to seven days.

To avoid the problems with toxicity, patients should be advised on drug interactions, strongly urged not to make dose changes, and instructed to return for regular follow-up.

VITAMIN E (TOCOPHEROL)

Of the several forms available, alpha-tocopherol is the most abundant. Although an essential nutrient, exact biochemical functions are not fully understood. Nutritional deficiency occurs in certain genetic and acquired diseases. Vegetable oils (soybean, corn, cottonseed) are richest sources. RDA is 8 to 10 mg daily (12 to 16 units). Fat-dependent absorption occurs and it acts mainly as an antioxidant in stabilizing unsaturated lipids against autooxidation. Use in cardiovascular disease has received a lot of attention but no randomized double-blind studies are available. Some subjective benefit in peripheral vascular disease has been reported. Most diets contain enough, and replacement should be restricted to deficiency states with low blood levels or increased red cell fragility to peroxidase. Situations of prolonged fat malabsorption (celiac disease, tropical sprue, cystic fibrosis, hepatic and biliary disease) can lead to deficiency. Treatment with 5 to 7 mg RDA is sufficient.

VITAMIN K

This fat-soluble vitamin is essential for prothrombin formation. Deficiency occurs with malabsorption of fats or inhibition of bacterial biosynthesis. The symptoms and signs are those of the underlying disease as well as hypoprothrombinemia. Oozing from the gums and frank hemorrhage can occur. Besides the reduction in prothrombin level, the vitamin K–dependent factors VII, IX, and X are also reduced. Treatment is with phytonadione (vitamin K_1) 10 mg IM in severe cases, and in emergencies 10 to 50 mg can be dissolved in 5% dextrose in water and infused at no greater than 1 mg/minute. With oral anticoagulant overdosage, 5 to 20 mg can be given orally. Excessive vitamin K can cause hemolysis, especially with G6PD deficiency.

WATER-SOLUBLE VITAMINS

These include ascorbic acid (vitamin C) and the B group complex: thiamine (B_1), riboflavin (B_2), pyridoxine (B_6), niacin (nicotinic acid), pantothenic acid, biotin, B_{12}, and folic acid. Structurally diverse, these vitamins act as coenzymes or oxidation-inhibiting agents. Metabolism is rapid with excretion in the urine. With normal renal function, toxic effects rarely occur.

ASCORBIC ACID

Ascorbic acid acts mainly as a reducing agent and antioxidant and is involved in the synthesis of collagen. Early deficiency results in malaise, irritability, fatigue, arthralgia, and after five to six months, clinical scurvy. Treatment with 2 to 4 oz fresh or concentrate orange juice is sufficient for mild disease. Scurvy requires 100 mg t.i.d. for a week and then daily for several weeks. The efficacy of large doses in preventing the common cold or cancer is still not established.

FOLIC ACID

Folic acid is found in many plant and animal tissues. It acts as a coenzyme in methylation and other reactions needed for nucleotide synthesis. Minimal adult daily requirement is 50 µg/day, and the liver stores 7.5 mg. A balanced diet provides adequate amounts. Deficiency can result in megaloblastic anemia as well as infertility and glossitis, stomatitis, and malabsorption. It is important to rule out pernicious anemia before using more than 0.4 mg of folic acid, since the neurologic changes due to B_{12} deficiency progress.

THIAMINE (B_1)

Thiamine (B_1) functions as a coenzyme in oxidative decarboxylations. Deficiency results in beriberi with peripheral neuropathy and cerebral (Warnicke-Korsakoff syndrome) and cardiovascular (biventricular failure) manifestations. Primary deficiency occurs with inadequate intake (highly polished rice) and secondarily with increased need (hyperthyroidism, pregnancy, lactation) or impaired utilization (liver disease). In alcoholics, all three factors operate. Elevated blood pyruvate levels and reduced urine thiamine occur late. Treatment with 10 to 20 mg/day for mild neuropathy is sufficient; in advanced cardiac and cerebral forms, 50 to 100 mg SC or IV is given b.i.d. until there is a response. Rare anaphylactic reactions have been reported with intravenous use.

RIBOFLAVIN (B_2)

Riboflavin (B_2) functions as a coenzyme in oxidation-reduction reactions (FAD) and is needed for proper growth and tissue function. Primary deficiency occurs with poor intake of milk and animal protein. Chronic deficiency occurs with liver disease, chronic pancreatitis, chronic diarrhea, and chronic alcoholism. Angular stomatitis, glossitis, and rubeolation of the cornea occur. A urinary excretion of <30 μ/gm creatinine is associated with clinical deficiency. Treatment is with 10 to 30 mg daily in divided doses until a response is noted and then with 2 to 4 mg until recovery.

NIACIN (NICOTINIC ACID)

Niacin (nicotinic acid) also functions as a coenzyme in oxidation-reduction reactions (NAD) and its deficiency results in pellagra. This occurs when corn forms the major part of the diet. Secondary deficiency is seen with liver disease, alcoholism, and chronic diarrheas. Isoniazid therapy and malignant carcinoid tumors are other causes. Clinically, cutaneous (acute, intertriginous, chronic hypertrophy, and atrophic lesions), mucous membrane (mouth, vagina, and urethra), neurologic (organic psychosis and an encephalopathic syndrome), and gastrointestinal (nausea, vomiting, and diarrhea) symptoms and signs occur. Diagnosis is easy in the setting of malnutrition with dermatitis, diarrhea, and dementia. A balanced diet with supplemental niacinamide 300 to 1000 mg/day is given. If necessary, 100 to 250 mg IM or SC can be given two to three times a day.

Nicotinic acid is now used therapeutically to treat hypercholesterolemia in doses up to 7 gm daily. Flushing and pruritus can occur in over 90% of patients with this dose. Use of aspirin 15 to 30 minutes before helps reduce this. Large doses of niacin can cause gastric acidity, cholestatic jaundice, increased uric acid levels, and elevated fasting plasma glucose, and even result in acanthosis nigricans.

VITAMIN B_6

Vitamin B_6 consists of pyridoxine, pyridoxal, and pyridoxamine, which are phosphorylated and function as coenzymes in transamination and deamination. Primary deficiency is rare and secondary deficiency occurs with malabsorption, excessive loss, or inactivation by drugs (isoniazid, hydralazine, corticosteroids, DL-penicillamine). Stomatitis, glossitis, cheilosis, peripheral neuropathy, and lymphopenia result. Several X-linked recessive states with B_6 dependency (adequate pool but defective ability of a protein apoenzyme to bind the coenzyme) exist and present with mental retardation and convulsions. Measurements of plasma pyridoxine (<25 ng/ml) or urinary creatinine (<20 μ/gm) help in diagnosis. Treatment with 50 to 100 mg/day is sufficient. Recently a syndrome of progressive sensory ataxia has been described with doses of 500 mg/day, so care is needed with use of supplements.

VITAMIN B_{12} (CYANOCOBALAMIN)

Vitamin B_{12} (cyanocobalamin) consists of several cobalt-containing compounds. They are part of coenzymes essential for synthesis of nucleic acids. Thus, they affect integrity of neural tissue and cell maturation. Animal tissues are the primary source, and deficiency is rare except in very strict vegetarians. Absorption requires intrinsic factor and calcium ions. Lack of intrinsic factor causes pernicious anemia and subacute degeneration of the cord. The RDA for adults is 6 μg/day. Oral therapy may be needed during pregnancy or in some vegetarians. Pernicious anemia is treated with B_{12} injections for life.

REFERENCES

Goodhart RS, Shils ME: Modern Nutrition in Health and Disease, 6th ed. Lea & Febiger, Philadelphia, 1980, Chapter 6.

15 · PARENTERAL NUTRITION

Donald G. Miller
JOSLIN CLINIC

The successful introduction of parenteral nutrition by Dudrick and his coworkers in 1968 stimulated interest in the field. Further impetus was provided by the pioneering studies of Blackburn and others that showed an alarming incidence of malnutrition in the hospitalized population. These studies suggested the deleterious effects of malnutriton added to those of the acute illness would lead to increased morbidity and mortality. Subsequent studies confirmed that malnutrition impaired patients' immunologic defenses and weakened their resistance to infection. Preoperative nutritional support was then shown to decrease postoperative morbidity and improve wound healing in certain malnourished patients.

In recent years the concept of the nutritional support team has arisen in order to optimize the selection of patients and the provision of nutritional therapy in the hospitalized population. This team is composed of physicians, nurses, dietitians, and pharmacists. In essence, its goal is to provide balanced nutrition with appropriate amounts of calories, protein, fluid, electrolytes, vitamins, and trace elements for variable time periods to patients who are malnourished or incapable of sustaining their nutrition over these periods.

NUTRITIONAL ASSESSMENT

In general, every patient, whether seen in the office or in the hospital, should undergo some form of nutritional assessment. A number of assessment tools, such as weight to height ratios, triceps skinfold thickness, midarm muscle circumference, urinary creatinine and 3-methyl histidine excretion, and serum albumin, transferrin, prealbumin and retinal binding protein, have been developed in order to assess nutritional status. In addition, skin tests for anergy and lymphocyte count have been used. Research techniques include measurement of total body potassium, or nitrogen, and estimates of fat stores using whole body immersion techniques. As a practical approach, however, assessing weight for height, estimating muscle mass by visual inspection, and obtaining serum albumin are probably the most useful screening tests for malnutrition. If the patient is deficient in one or more of these tests (weight/height <85% of normal, or midarm muscle circumference <5th percentile, or albumin <3.5 gm/dl) or has a history of greater than 10% weight loss, one should do further nutritional assessment and decide whether nutritional support is necessary.

ALTERNATIVES TO TPN

Once nutritional support has been recommended, it is necessary to decide on the method. In general, the use of the gastrointestinal tract is easier, more physiologic, safer, and less expensive, and has fewer complications than any type of parenteral nutrition. Therefore, attention should first be given to dietary supplements, tube feedings via nasogastric or nasoduodenal tubes, or via gastrostomy or jejunostomy before the use of parenteral nutrition is considered. If parenteral nutrition is necessary, one must then decide whether to do it via peripheral vein or via a central vein.

INDICATIONS FOR TPN

The indications for the use of parenteral nutrition include the diagnosis of malnutrition or the likelihood of malnutrition because of the inability to feed the patients enterally for a five- to seven-day period *and* the inability to use the gastrointestinal tract for enteral nutrition. Some situations in which this occurs include abdominal surgery or trauma, inflammatory bowel disease, paralytic ileus, intestinal obstruction, fistulas, pancreatitis, and burns.

TYPES OF TPN

Once a decision is made for parenteral nutrition, one can choose between peripheral and central venous access for parenteral nutrition. Central venous access was first developed by Dudrick and is still the favorite approach. Using a high-flow central vein, one can administer very hypertonic solutions of 20% to 45% dextrose and 2.5% to 5% amino acids in a quantity sufficient to meet all nutritional needs. If one uses a peripheral vein for parenteral nutrition, one is generally restricted to isotonic or only slightly hyperosmotic solutions in order to avoid phlebitis. For practical purposes this means one must use mixtures of 5% to 10% dextrose and 10% to 20% fat emulsions as the caloric source. Thus, a peripheral vein limits the amount of nutrients that can be provided unless the patient can tolerate large volumes of fluid.

VASCULAR ACCESS FOR TPN

Access for parenteral nutrition is traditionally gained via percutaneous insertion of a central venous catheter through the subclavian or the internal jugular vein. The catheter must be shown by x-ray film to be in the superior vena cava just above the right atrium. If the catheter is too proximal or loops upward, there is a much higher likelihood of thrombosis. Complications of insertion include hemothorax and pneumothorax but are uncommon for the trained physician. Introduction of Silastic as opposed to polyethylene central venous catheters and the addition of heparin to the TPN solution may lessen thrombogenic complications. Double-lumen or even triple-lumen catheters can be inserted in order to permit simultaneous administration of antibiotics, blood products, and other fluids. The use of catheters with Dacron cuffs and subcutaneous tunnels as well as implantable central venous access devices is probably best reserved for patients requiring long-term parenteral nutrition, such as patients on home parenteral nutrition. It is probably not necessary to routinely change catheters over a wire, but catheter changes are indicated if infection or thrombosis is suspected.

COMPOSITION OF TPN FLUIDS

Once the vascular access is established, one must assess the patient's nutritional needs. Assessment of energy expenditures using indirect calorimetry has suggested that nonstressed patients need probably 25 to 35 kcal/kg/day with an increase of up to 100% for highly stressed patients such as those with burns and extensive trauma. Postoperative patients probably only need a 10% to 25% increase in caloric requirements over and above that of the nonstressed patient. The calories can be provided either as dextrose or as lipid emulsions. In general, lipid emulsions should not constitute more than 60% of the total calories supplied. Some experts favor the use of mixed fuel systems in order to optimize utilization of the energy substrate. In particular, in trauma and burn patients where there appears to be a limit on the patient's ability to utilize carbohydrate, the use of lipid emulsions for energy may be beneficial. There appears to be no contraindication to the use of lipid emulsion in patients with pancreatitis or with pulmonary insufficiency.

Protein hydrolysates have been replaced by defined amino acid solutions as the source of protein. In general, one wants to provide 1 to 1.5 gm/kg/day of amino acids to the patient with the amount being increased for the patients under severe stress. In stress situations, it has recently been shown that amino acid formulas enriched with branch chain amino acids may increase protein synthesis. The use of specially defined branch chain-enriched amino acid solutions with decreased amounts of aromatic amino acids may be useful in patients with chronic liver disease and cirrhosis. It has not been convincingly shown that essential amino acid solutions are better for patients with renal failure than standard amino acid preparations.

In addition to a source of calories and protein, the patients must be provided with adequate amounts of fluid, sodium, potassium, magnesium, phosphorus, and vitamins. A sample TPN formula is shown in Table 1. Patients on long-term parenteral nutrition may also need trace minerals such as copper, zinc, chromium, selenium, and iron, as well as a source of essential fatty acids.

MONITORING TPN

It is important to realize that patients need time to adapt to a parenteral nutrition infusion. In general, for hypertonic dextrose solutions, one increases the rate of infusion by 1 liter/day until one achieves the desired rate of administration. The patient must be watched, using urine or blood tests for glucose in order to avoid hyperglycemia. Hyperglycemia can be corrected by reducing the infusion rate, adding insulin, or substituting fat emulsions for some of the dextrose. In addition, the patient must be monitored for electrolyte abnormalities, particularly hypokalemia and hypophosphatemia, which can develop rapidly within several days owing to the intracellular movement of potassium and phosphorus. Some patients will develop acute elevation of liver function tests, which will respond to a temporary decrease in the rate of infusion of the parenteral nutrition solution. Table 2 shows the laboratory tests used to follow the average patient. In addition, the patient should be followed clinically and with proper laboratory monitoring in order to assess the efficacy of parenteral nutrition. This can be done by assessment of weight, albumin, transferrin, midarm muscle circumference, and triceps skinfold at two- to three-week intervals. In addition, skin tests for cutaneously delayed hypersensitivity can be repeated to see if anergy, if initially present, is corrected. If parenteral nutrition is done via peripheral veins with fat emulsions, the plasma should be checked for lipemia.

Table 1. SAMPLE TPN SOLUTION

500 ml	50% dextrose
500 ml	8.5% amino acids
40 mEq	sodium chloride
20 mEq	potassium chloride
15 mEq	potassium phosphate
4.5 mEq	calcium gluconate
8 mEq	magnesium sulfate
5 mg	zinc chloride
2000 units	heparin
1 ampule	multivitamins (e.g., MVI-12)
1 mg	iron (e.g., Imferon)
1 ampule	trace metals (selenium 100 µgm/day, chromium 15–20 µgm/day, copper 1 mg/day)

Vitamin K 10 mg SQ
Fat emulsion 50–100 gm weekly

Table 2. LABORATORY MONITORING FOR TPN

Initially	
Daily:	Urine or blood glucoses 3–4 times
Daily:	Glucose, electrolytes, phosphorus
M-W-F:	Bilirubin, aspartate aminotransferase, alkaline phosphatase
M-Th:	Calcium, magnesium
After stabilization:	
M-Th:	Electrolytes, glucose, phosphorus
Weekly:	Bilirubin, aspartate aminotransferase, alkaline phosphatase, calcium magnesium, albumin, CBC, prothrombin time
Monthly:	Iron, selenium, zinc

COMPLICATIONS

Complications of parenteral nutrition can be divided into technical, infectious, and metabolic categories. Technical complications are related to the use of peripheral or central venous catheters and include hemothorax, pneumothorax, and laceration of the vein due to catheter insertion. These can be detected by chest film and appropriate measures taken.

Infectious complications include infection at the exit site and catheter-associated bacteremia or fungemia. These complications are minimized with careful aseptic technique and periodic dressing changes. Catheter-associated septicemia is suspected when the patient develops fever with or without leukocytosis. In that situation, blood cultures should be drawn peripherally and through the catheter. At that time, if the clinical suspicion of catheter-associated infection is great enough, the catheter should be replaced over a wire and the original catheter tip also sent for culture. Removal of the catheter is usually sufficient to eradicate the infection and antibiotic therapy is not usually warranted unless the bacteremia has been prolonged. If a catheter change over a wire is not successful or if there is an infection at the exit site of the catheter, the catheter site should be changed. The addition of small amounts of heparin to the parenteral nutrition solution may decrease the thromboembolic complications of parenteral nutrition. If the catheter becomes occluded, one can infuse a small amount of streptokinase or urokinase in order to clear the catheter. If thrombosis develops around the catheter as evidenced by swelling of the face or hands or by development of subcutaneous venous collaterals, the catheter should be removed, a venogram obtained, and if necessary heparin or antithrombolytic therapy given to the patient.

Metabolic complications of parenteral nutrition include electrolyte disturbances, in particular hypokalemia, hypophosphatemia, hypomagenesemia, hypocalcemia, abnormal liver function tests, and various vitamin and trace element deficiencies. These deficiencies can be prevented and corrected with proper monitoring.

CONCLUSION

In recent years the adverse effect of malnutrition upon the patient's response to acute illness has been demonstrated. Prevention and correction of malnutrition, which appears to be highly prevalent in the hospitalized population, can reduce morbidity and mortality. Moreover, in those patients unable to sustain their own nutritional balance, TPN represents a major advance in tiding them over their long- or short-term disability.

REFERENCES

Graham LH (ed): Nutrition and the Surgical Patient. Churchill Livingstone, New York, 1981.

Grant P: Handbook of Total Parenteral Nutrition. W.B Saunders Co., Philadelphia, 1980.

Jeejeebhoy KN: Total Parenteral Nutrition in the Hospital and at Home. CRC Press, Inc, Boca Raton, FL, 1985.

Silk DBA: Nutritional Support in Hospital Practice. Blackwell Scientific Publications, Boston, MA, 1983.

Wright RA, Heyinsfield E: Nutritional Assessment. Butterworths, Stoneham, MA, 1984.

ALLERGIC DISORDERS

JOHN ANDERSON

1 · ANAPHYLAXIS

Alice Marosi
Michael H. Keslin
Stanley Z. Berman
LOVELACE MEDICAL CENTER

DEFINITION

The term "anaphylaxis" was introduced by Portier and Richet in 1902 to describe a fatal systemic reaction to a second injection of a previously tolerated foreign protein. Anaphylaxis may be considered a *clinical syndrome* with a multiplicity of inciting etiologic agents and a variety of pathogenetic mechanisms. If so defined, the distinction between "anaphylactic reactions" (IgE mediated, antigen induced) and "anaphylactoid reactions" (not IgE mediated, not antigen induced) may be eliminated.

PATHOPHYSIOLOGY

The degranulation of tissue mast cells and circulating basophils results in the release of a variety of potent, biologically active mediators. Histamine and the leukotrienes (formerly slow-reacting substance of anaphylaxis, SRS-A) appear to be most important. Mediator release is an active, energy-requiring process influenced by the intracellular concentration of cyclic nucleotides (cyclic adenosine monophosphate, cAMP and cyclic guanosine monophosphate, cGMP). In IgE-mediated reactions, mast cell and basophil degranulation is a result of specific antigen reexposure and previous sensitization (formation of IgE antibodies and their attachment to basophils or mast cells). In non–IgE-mediated anaphylaxis ("anaphylactoid"), previous sensitization is not required and one of several pathogenetic mechanisms may be involved: (1) immune complex– or complement-mediated reactions, (2) alterations in arachidonic acid metabolism, and (3) direct mast cell degranulation. The final common pathway of all these processes is the pharmacologic effect of mediators on various target cells/tissues/organs, inducing increased capillary permeability, smooth muscle constriction, mucous gland secretion, and attraction of inflammatory cells. *These pathophysiologic changes account for the clinical manifestations of anaphylaxis.*

CLINICAL ASPECTS

The most characteristic feature of anaphylaxis is rapid, often unexpected onset and progression to severe, sometimes fatal outcome. In general, the sooner after antigen contact that symptoms occur, the more severe is the reaction. Even initially *mild symptoms may progress to severe* and possibly irreversible stages; prompt treatment should be considered even when symptoms appear to be mild. The potential causes of anaphylaxis are numerous (Table 1).

Prodromal symptoms may or may not be present: feelings of uneasiness, "impending doom," apprehension, generalized weakness, diaphoresis. Subsequently, four organ systems may be involved singly or in combination:

1. *Skin*: flushing, pruritus, urticaria, angioedema.
2. *Respiratory*: hoarseness, stridor, "lump in the throat" (caused by laryngeal edema that may progress to complete upper airway obstruction). Bronchial obstruction is manifested by cough, chest tightness, wheezing, dyspnea. Upper or lower airway obstruction may lead to severe hypoxemia and respiratory failure.
3. *Cardiovascular*: hypotension, shock, arrhythmias (may progress to loss of consciousness and death). Cardiac manifestations may be:
   a. secondary to critical reduction in plasma volume and hypoxia;
   b. caused by the primary cardiac effect of mediators; or
   c. secondary to therapy initiated for anaphylaxis.
4. *Gastrointestinal*: nausea, vomiting, intestinal cramps, diarrhea, fecal incontinence.

Other less common manifestations include uterine cramps, urinary incontinence, seizures. Cardiovascular collapse and upper airway obstruction are the most common causes of death.

History of a previous antigen exposure and clinical suspicion are important diagnostic tools. Diagnosis may be difficult when the cause-and-effect relationship is not obvious (e.g., a patient presenting to the emergency room in shock; hypotension or respiratory arrest during general anesthesia; or sudden vascular collapse in a child or young adult). Cutaneous manifestations, when present, greatly aid diagnosis, but serious reactions may occur without any cutaneous findings.

MANAGEMENT

Short-term goals in dealing with systemic anaphylaxis are: (1) obtain a relevant medical history (Table 1);

591

Table 1. CAUSES OF ANAPHYLAXIS OR ANAPHYLACTOID REACTONS

Antibiotics/Antimycotics
Penicillins*‡
Cephalosporins
Tetracyclines
Nitrofurantoin
Streptomycin
Vancomycin
Chloramphenicol
Bacitracin‡
Neomycin‡
Polymyxin B
Amphotericin B
Kanamycin
Ketoconazole
Spectinomycin

Foreign Protein Agents/Hormones/Enzymes
Antiserum*
ACTH*
Insulin*
Parathyroid hormone
Chymopapain
Chymotrypsin/trypsin
Penicillinase
Relaxin
Seminal plasma*
Vasopressin
Antilymphocyte globulin
Acacia
Protamine
Thyroid-stimulating hormone*

Cancer Chemotherapy
Asparaginase
Cisplatin, including intra-vesical
Cyclophosphamide
Cytosine arabinoside†
Mitomycin
Methotrexate
Melphalan
Mechlorethamine‡
Chlorambucil
Hydroxyurea
Procarbazine
5-Fluorouracil

Venom/Saliva
Hymenoptera venom*
(i.e., bee, wasp, yellow jacket, hornet)
Triatoma (i.e., kissing bug saliva)
Deerfly venom
Rattlesnake venom
Rodent bite*
Tick (*Argas reflexus*)*

Therapeutic Agents
Allergen extracts*
Muscle relaxants (some reactions)
Estradiol
Benzylopenicilloyl polylysine (Pre-Pen)
Tripelennamine
Thiopental
Local anesthetics (some reactions)
Dextran*†
BCG vaccine
Streptokinase*
Modified fluid gelatins
Egg-containing vaccines*
Equine serum antitoxin
Muscle relaxants (e.g., suxamethonium)
Protamine
Chymopapain, papain*

"Health Foods"
Bee pollen
Chamomile tea
Sunflower seeds*
Millet seed*

Blood Products
Whole blood, plasma (including associated anti-IgA antibody)
Cryoprecipitate
Immunoglobulin, including intravenous
Pooled platelet concentrate
Plasma exchange

Dialysis
Ethylene oxide gas
New Cuprophane dialyzers

Diagnostic Agents
Iodinated contrast media
Iophendylate
Sodium dehydrocholate
Sulfobromophthalein

Nonsteroidal Anti-Inflammatory Agents
Acetylsalicylic acid
Indomethacin
Ibuprofen
Fenoprofen
Naproxen
Tolmetin
Benzoates (presumed)
Tartrazine (possibly)

Direct Histamine-Releasing Agents
Opiates (including codeine)
Curare, D-tubocurarine
Iron dextran (?)
Thiamine (?)
Hydralazine
Stilbamidine
Pentamidine
Polymyxin
Deferoxamine
Doxorubicin
Daunorubicin
Hymenoptera venom (some)
"Others" (including some listed elsewhere)

Idiopathic
Hyper-IgE–associated
Gonadotropin suppression responsive
(Inhalation allergen challenge)

Complement Activation
Lidocaine
Protamine
New Cuprophane dialyzers
Gammaglobulin, intravenous
Leukocyte-depleted blood

Occupational Exposure
Inhaled sodium chromate

Recreational
"Alpine slide" (Water slide) (? grass pollen)
Soft drink (? penicillin-like contaminant)
Yew (*Taxus*) needle ingestion
"Running shoe"
Exercise

Table 1. CAUSES OF ANAPHYLAXIS OR ANAPHYLACTOID REACTONS *Continued*

Foods
Milk
Egg white
Shellfish
Legumes (i.e., soybeans, pinto beans, chick-peas)
Buckwheat/grains
Nuts
Citrus fruits
Bananas
Chocolate
Fish
Beets
Potato
Rice
Mango
Cottonseed
Corn
Safflower oil
Sesame seed*

"Unusual"
Albuterol
"Hidden" source penicillin
Metabisulfite, bisulfite
Delayed hypersensitivity skin tests (i.e., *Trichophyton**)
Tetanus toxoid
Ethanol (i.e., acetic acid)
Psyllium*
Mannitol
Insect repellent‡
Cimetidine
Cromolyn
Hydrocortisone
Methylprednisolone

*Apparently IgE mediated.
†Including intraperitoneal.
‡Including topical.

(2) monitor vital signs; (3) make a relevant physical examination; and (4) repeatedly question the patient about specific symptoms. *Long-term goals* consist of a systematic treatment plan (Table 2), adequate nursing support, medical equipment, and drugs.

Indications for hospitalization are few. Most patients can be optimally managed in an emergency-type setting. Severe and rapidly progressing reactions are best managed in an intensive care unit. Home health care revolves primarily around patient information and education (see below).

NONPHARMACOLOGIC MEASURES

A tourniquet may be used, when appropriate, to occlude venous and lymphatic flow from the site of

Table 2. THERAPY FOR SYSTEMIC ANAPHYLAXIS

1. Tourniquet when applicable
2. Place patient in recumbent position and elevate legs
3. Epinephrine, 0.3–0.5 ml* of 1:1,000 solution SQ or IM may repeat every 15 min; if hypotension is present, administer 10 ml of 1:100,000 solution (0.1 ml of 1:1,000 epinephrine in 10 ml of normal saline) IV over 5–10 min‡
4. Diphenhydramine hydrochloride, 50 mg† IM or IV
5. Establish and maintain an adequate airway
6. Oxygen at 4–6 L/min if hypoxia is present
7. IV fluids with normal saline; fluid requirements of up to 10 L within a 12-hr period have been reported
8. Pressor agents for severe hypotension, such as norephinephrine by IV infusion at initial rate of 2–8 µg/min, or dopamine hydrochloride, 2–5 µg/kg/min; titrate dose on basis of response
9. If bronchospasm, aminophylline, 5.6 mg/kg IV loading dose over 10 min followed by maintenance dose of 0.9 mg/kg/hr
10. Corticosteroids such as hydrocortisone, 100 mg IV every 6 hr to prevent protracted anaphylactic reaction
11. Specific antiarrhythmic drugs or cardiopulmonary resuscitation as indicated

*Pediatric dose is 0.01 ml/kg, maximum 0.3 ml.
†Pediatric dose is 1 mg/kg, maximum 50 mg.
‡Continued slow infusion of 1:200,000 solution may be necessary for control.

parenteral antigen exposure. Patients should be placed in a recumbent position and the lower extremities elevated; if patients are hypoxic, administer oxygen.

Maintenance of an adequate airway is essential. Direct visualization of the larynx may be required to assess the presence or severity of laryngeal edema. Advanced techniques of airway management are required for acute, life-threatening pharyngeal or laryngeal edema: endotracheal intubation, cricothyroidotomy, and tracheostomy. Emergency endotracheal intubation should be performed by the oral route unless the oropharynx is obliterated, in which case nasotracheal intubation may be required. A temporary airway can be obtained by percutaneous cricothyroid membrane puncture with an 11-gauge needle or a polyethylene catheter; this provides an adequate airway for a few minutes if high-flow oxygen is attached to the catheter. Complications of this procedure include vocal cord injury, bleeding, and subcutaneous emphysema. Cricothyroidotomy is easier to perform than tracheostomy, which should be attempted only by a skilled surgeon in an operating room setting. Reported complications of cricothyroidotomy include vocal cord damage, mediastinal or subcutaneous emphysema, hemorrhage, cellulitis of the neck, tracheal or laryngeal perforation or laceration, apnea, cardiac arrhythmias, hypotension, subsequent subglottic stenosis, and tracheoesophageal fistula. Cardiopulmonary resuscitation is required in situations of cardiac arrest.

DRUG THERAPY

Epinephrine. Epinephrine, 1:1000 given subcutaneously or intramuscularly in a dose of 0.3 to 0.5 ml, remains the cornerstone of therapy. If anaphylaxis has resulted from parenteral administration of an antigen, 0.1 to 0.2 ml of the above dose may be injected directly into the source of the antigen to retard systemic absorption. Doses of epinephrine may be repeated every 15 minutes if necessary. If vascular collapse occurs, administer slowly a dilute solution of IV epinephrine; optimal doses have not been clearly established. One literature review suggests 10 ml of a 1:100,000 solution (0.1 ml of 1:1,000 in 10 ml of normal saline) IV over five to ten minutes; this represents a 100-μg bolus given at the rate of 10 μg/min. Control of shock may require slow infusion of dilute IV epinephrine (1:200,000 solution).

Patients with hypotension may require large volumes of isotonic saline or plasma expander given IV to help restore adequate circulation. Under these circumstances, optimal management requires an intensive care unit. Pressor agents such as norepinephrine by continuous IV infusion, 2 to 8 μg/min, may be used in patients unresponsive to volume replacement. Cardiac monitoring is advised. If there is cardiac failure, an inotropic agent such as dopamine hydrochloride may be helpful. If lower airway obstruction secondary to bronchospasm occurs, IV aminophylline may be indicated.

Adverse effects of epinephrine include hypertension; increased myocardial oxygen consumption secondary to tachycardia, and increased myocardial contractility resulting in myocardial ischemia; premature atrial contractions; premature ventricular contractions; and other arrhythmias. Intravascular potassium fluctuations may occur. There may be complications with a concomitant

disease or disorder (e.g., elderly patients with preexisting coronary artery disease or hypertension). Interference with a concomitant drug therapy is a possibility. Drug interactions may occur with digitalis, mercurial diuretics, tricyclic antidepressants, certain antihistamines, sodium L-thyroxine, and beta-adrenergic receptor blocking drugs (see below).

Corticosteroids. Agents such as hydrocortisone, 100 to 200 mg IV every six hours, may help prevent protracted anaphylaxis, but are not helpful in the immediate management of a reaction. Cardiac arrhythmias may require treatment with specific antiarrhythmic agents.

Some authors have suggested using antihistamines of the H_2-receptor blocking type (i.e., cimetidine) in conjunction with more classical H_1 drugs. H_2-blocking drugs may be of value in treating vasodilation, decreased peripheral vascular resistance, and increased bronchial secretions.

PATIENT INFORMATION AND EDUCATION

Prompt and immediate treatment can influence the outcome of an anaphylactic/anaphylactoid reaction and may be lifesaving. Patients with previous systemic life-threatening reaction should have drugs available for "self-treatment first aid."

Although alternative drugs (e.g., isoproterenol) and means of administration (e.g., inhalation) have been suggested, injectable epinephrine remains the first drug of choice. Prefilled syringes are commercially available for patient convenience; ANA-KIT* has a prefilled syringe that can deliver two doses of 0.30 ml of 1:1,000 aqueous epinephrine. Patients should be instructed in the use of injectable epinephrine; this may best be performed by knowledgeable personnel in a "one on one" context. Supervised self-administration of SQ saline as a test run may be both informative and reassuring; many find it less objectionable than anticipated. A suitable substitute for ANA-KIT is an auto-self injector— Epi-Pen and Epi-Pen Jr.† These units deliver 0.3 ml and 0.15 ml of 1:1000 epinephrine, respectively, as each device is jammed against the upper thigh. The kit should be available at appropriate times (e.g., in a restaurant, if ingestible food is a factor; in the summer or early fall if stinging insects are the problem; during exercise, if this is a concern). Oral antihistamines and a tourniquet with appropriate instructions should be available.

Timing of epinephrine dosage may vary. Given a history of an immediate severe reaction, many advise immediate administration (e.g., following a bee sting in a previously sensitive patient). Depending on history, current medications, and clinical status before the event, the physician may advise delaying administration until a systemic reaction actually occurs. Patients should be instructed to go immediately to the nearest medical facility for appropriate, definitive evaluation and treatment; ideally, the driver of a vehicle should be someone other than the patient. Epinephrine may be administered if a systemic reaction is noted. Oral antihistamine should be taken immediately following an insect sting in a sensitive patient. An identifying necklace or bracelet

---

*Hollister-Stier Laboratories.
†Center Laboratories.

is advisable (e.g., Medic-Alert), with a notation of the allergic problem.

PERIODIC EVALUATION

A second diagnostic look is of value in ascertaining the status of the patient and may permit confirmation or clarification of the situation (e.g., the location and cause of the airway obstruction). Follow-up visits allow an opportunity to ensure that medical records are current; medications or other factors associated with these reactions should be recorded prominently in the chart. The remote possibility of subsequent serum sickness might be excluded. Routine laboratory tests may not be necessary, but follow-up may be advisable (electrocardiogram or pulmonary function test) if an abnormality is noted during the acute episode. Normal blood pressure may be more readily assessed if not previously recorded. More specific diagnostic tests for etiology (e.g., *Hymenoptera* venom, drug allergy) may best be evaluated by a trained allergist: tests frequently have to be evaluated within the context of the clinical situation. The allergist may also review with the patient any options for specific prophylaxis (i.e., *Hymenoptera* venom immunotherapy).

PATIENT COMPLIANCE

Patient compliance may be evaluated during the follow-up visit. Alterations in life style (exercise, current medications, dietary habits) may be reviewed. Make sure the patient understands what to avoid and how to avoid it.

PREVENTIVE MEASURES

Some necessary precautions are outlined above. Risk factor modification includes avoiding the incriminating agent, taking drugs orally instead of parenterally and choosing chemically and antigenically unrelated drugs. Ensure that the patient knows when and how to self-administer the correct dose of the drug. Premedication regimens may be of value (as with iodinated contrast media reaction history), as may consultation with an allergist in specific situations (i.e., *Hymenoptera* venom immunotherapy, family counseling, desensitization). Previous immunizations should be reviewed as necessary.

Beta-adrenergic blockade has potential theoretical and clinical implications: anaphylaxis may be associated with less than ideal response to treatment in a beta-blocked patient. Some studies indicate that beta-blockade may have been a contributing factor in severe or refractory anaphylaxis associated with food, venom, nonsteroidal anti-inflammatory agents, and immunotherapy for allergic rhinitis. A severe adverse reaction has been associated with haloperidol or hemodialysis concomitant with propranolol.

REFERENCES

Austen KF: Systemic anaphylaxis in man. JAMA 192:108–110, 1965.

Easton JG: Anaphylaxis. *In* Bierman CW, Pearlman DS (eds): Allergic Diseases of Infancy, Childhood and Adolescence. W. B. Saunders Co, Philadelphia, 1980, pp 681–685.

Patterson R, Valentine M: Anaphylaxis and related allergic emergencies including reactions due to insect stings. JAMA 248:2632–2636, 1982.

Sheffer AL, Pennoyer DS: Management of adverse drug reactions. J Allergy Clin Immunol 74:580–588, 1984.

Wasserman S: Anaphylaxis. *In* Middleton E, Reed CE, Ellis EF (eds): Allergy—Principles and Practice, 2nd ed. C. V. Mosby Co, St. Louis, 1983, pp 689–699.

Weiszer I: Allergic emergencies. *In* Patterson R (ed): Allergic Diseases—Diagnosis and Management, 2nd ed. J. B. Lippincott Co, Philadelphia, 1980, pp 374–394.

2 · ALLERGIC AND NONALLERGIC RHINITIS

Hugh L. N. MacKechnie
HENRY FORD HOSPITAL

Allergic Rhinitis

The most common cause of rhinitis symptoms of short duration is the common cold. Patients with allergic symptoms frequently blame them on a "cold" or virus infection. The presence of systemic symptoms such as fever, myalgia, and malaise should help to differentiate viral infections from allergy, although these two often coexist.

Allergic rhinitis may be noted in as many as 10% of the general population. Allergic rhinitis may be seasonal or perennial; often there is a seasonal worsening in patients with perennial symptoms. Also, in view of a priming effect in a season, other allergens that are normally not troublesome, such as dog or cat dander, may produce symptoms. A family history for atopic disease is often found and may be as high as 80% of cases.

PATHOPHYSIOLOGY

Pollen grains and mold spores are trapped in the nose. Studies also suggest that fragments of pollen grains exist and can likely penetrate further and prolong classic allergy seasons. These allergens bind to IgE, which is attached via Fc receptors to the surface of mast cells in the submucosa of the nose. Bridging by allergen of two surface IgE molecules induces membrane changes and increases enzymatic activity, raising cyclic Gmp levels. This action facilitates mediator release. These mediators include histamine, which produces most of the clinical symptoms related to allergic rhinitis. Other mediators include leukotrienes, eosinophil chemotactic factors, and prostaglandins. Histamine exerts a negative feedback on mediator release via H_2-receptors. Raising cyclic AMP levels blocks mediator release. As mediator release is also calcium dependent, a role for calcium channel blocking agents may be forthcoming.

CLINICAL FEATURES

The key to diagnosis (see Table 1) in allergic rhinitis is the history. Symptoms include itching of the nose and often the palate, paroxysmal sneezing, clear rhinorrhea, and congestion. There are often ocular symptoms of tearing, intense itching, and erythema on examination. The nasal mucosa appears boggy and pale, almost as if you could wring the fluid out. Symptoms and signs of asthma may also be present.

Perennial allergic symptoms are most often due to house dust, dust mites, family pets (e.g., dogs, cats, hamsters), and molds. The cockroach has recently been recognized as a potent cause of allergy. Pollen antigens are the cause of most seasonal problems, although molds such as *Alternaria* can peak in August in the Northeast and Midwest, giving the appearance of a seasonal problem. Ragweed season is mid-August to the end of September, but there is no ragweed problem west of the Rocky mountains. Grass season is generally mid-May to mid-July but in the South and Southwest may appear to be perennial. Grasses often share antigens but differ in various regions of the country (e.g., Bermuda grass and Johnson grass are not found in the Midwest or northern parts of the country). Trees generally pollinate in the Midwest from late March or early April to mid-May. Each type of deciduous tree may only pollinate for two to three weeks, but different species tend to pollinate in sequence (e.g., maples after elms). Controversy still exists over whether tobacco smoke is an allergen, but current evidence is against an allergic basis for induced symptoms and favors an irritant role. Occupationally related causes are suggested if symptoms clear when the patient is away from the work site, especially on weekends or on vacation. Foods are an uncommon cause of isolated allergic nasal symptoms in adults.

ALLERGY TESTS AND DIAGNOSIS

A nasal smear can be performed; if it shows more than 4% eosinophils, it is suggestive of allergy. Allergy skin tests may then be performed to confirm a suspected history. Scratch or prick tests are applied first. If these inhalant allergens are negative, intradermal tests may be performed; these are more sensitive than scratch or prick testing and should not be done first since anaphylaxis is a risk, especially for the pollens in a highly sensitive patient. When skin testing cannot be performed (such as in diffuse skin disease or dermographism, or when a skin–histamine positive control test is nonreactive), a radioallergosorbent test (RAST) may be performed. This is an in vitro assessment of specific IgE antibody to allergens coupled to discs; however, it is less sensitive than intradermal testing.

MANAGEMENT

Management of allergic rhinitis should aim to relieve symptoms in the short term and to block recurrence in the long term. Chronic allergic rhinitis may predispose to sinusitis, requiring aggressive medical/or surgical therapy. With a good suggestive history and confirmation by allergy skin testing, avoidance of the suspected allergen (such as feather pillows) is the simplest and most effective treatment. Other likely sources that can easily be avoided include animals, although in the case of occupational exposure this may not be easy. Environmental measures to reduce dust, dust mites, and mold offer additional relief. The mattress should be stripped and vacuumed to reduce the mite content (dust mites tend to feed off human dander, which gathers in mattresses). Plastic covers may be used for old mattresses, or they may be replaced. Damp, musty areas in basements or bathrooms should be dried out; Lysol may help reduce mold growth. Air conditioners are effective in removing pollen grains (10 to 25 μ). Electronic air cleaners can remove dust and mold particles down to 0.1 μ.

When specific avoidance is not possible, the next step is medication. Antihistamines are most effective for controlling the symptoms of rhinorrhea, sneezing, and itching. They are best used on a regular basis

Table 1. DIFFERENTIAL DIAGNOSIS OF ALLERGIC RHINITIS

Condition	Symptoms	Sign	Nasal Smear and Other Tests	Management
Allergic rhinitis	Itching Sneezing Profuse rhinorrhea	Pale, boggy mucosa	Eosinophils (+) skin tests	Antihistamines Beclomethasone spray (Vancenase or Beconase) Flunisolide (Nasalide) Cromolyn sodium (Nasalcrom) Immunotherapy
NARES syndrome	Obstruction Rhinorrhea	Nasal polyps	Eosinophil (−) skin tests	Topical corticosteroid spray
Vasomotor rhinitis	Obstruction Rhinorrhea	Turbinate edema		Antihistamine decongestants (often poor response)
Rhinitis medicamentosa	Severe nasal obstruction			Stop vasoconstrictor spray and apply topical steroids
Rhinitis of pregnancy	Congestion Rhinorrhea	Boggy turbinate of edema		Watch
CSF rhinorrhea		Clear fluid "teapot" sign	Glucose positive	Surgery
Nasal polyps	Congestion Purulent drainage Cough Anosmia	Pale glistening sacs	R/O cystic fibrosis	Corticosteroid sprays Antibiotics Surgery
Sinusitis	Congestion Nocturnal cough	Purulent drainage	polymorphs Sinus x-rays	Antibiotics Drainage Surgery

through a season, but with steady use tachyphylaxis may develop. Cycling two or three different agents often offsets this effect.

The primary side effect of the antihistamines is sedation but this often decreases with continuous use. Perennial symptoms may require treatment only as needed. Serious reactions such as agranulocytosis and neurologic sequelae are uncommon. Many newer agents have not been shown to be safe in pregnancy; this should be discussed with appropriate patients if long-term use is planned. The availability of new, nonsedating antihistamines such as astemizole and terfenadine should help. Clemastine fumarate (Tavist), 1.34 mg, one to two every 12 hours, or chlorpheniramine (Chlor-Trimeton), 8 or 12 mg every eight to 12 hours, is helpful.

When congestion is a complaint, decongestants are helpful. This is best accomplished by the use of combination tablets or capsules such as Tavist-D (clemastine fumarate and phenylpropanolamine HCl) every 12 hours; Dimetapp Extentabs (brompheniramine maleate, phenylephrine HCl, phenylpropanolamine HCl), one every eight to 12 hours; Deconamine (chlorpheniramine and D-pseudoephedrine), one every 12 hours; or Trinaline (azatadine maleate and pseudoephedrine sulfate), one every 12 hours. Extendryl, which also contains scopalamine, is a more effective drying agent and can be tried when the other agents do not control the symptoms. Dimetapp Elixir, for which dosage adjustment is much easier, may be used in those patients unable to tolerate the tablet or capsule form.

Topical corticosteroid-derived sprays are also highly effective. Beclomethasone dipropionate (Beconase or Vancenase), used initially in a dose of two sprays in each nostril three to four times a day, with reductions in dosing every two weeks, is effective for allergic rhinitis. Once the symptoms are under control, one spray in each nostril once daily or on alternate days can often control the problem. Flunisolide (Nasalide spray), used in an initial dose of two sprays in each nostril twice daily, is an alternative. Unlike Vancenase, which is a metered-dose aerosol, Nasalide is a pump aerosol. The propylene glycol preservative in Nasalide often produces severe but transient burning in the nose, lasting several seconds. As it is a liquid, it often penetrates better in the nose and may be preferred where there is obstruction. Patients should be warned that both these types of sprays may produce irritation, dryness, and minor bleeding in the nose. If this occurs, they should discontinue the spray for four to five days and restart at a reduced dosage. These sprays should be discontinued during upper respiratory infections. Long-term studies suggest that there is little risk for atrophic changes in the nose, and the safety of beclamethasone for asthma supports this. Nonetheless, patients should discontinue these sprays for two to three weeks every six months or so. Case reports of nasal septal perforations possibly related to Nasalide are cause for concern. These sprays are useful with supplemental antihistamines for perennial and seasonal allergic rhinitis.

Nasalcrom spray (cromolyn sodium) is of greatest help in seasonal allergic rhinitis or as a preventive for specific allergen exposure, e.g., a cat-sensitive patient visiting a house where there is a cat. It is used as two sprays in each nostril four times a day. The pump aerosol produces a fine mist that is well tolerated.

For severe allergic rhinitis symptoms when none of the above measures have helped, the use of corticosteroids orally or parenterally may be considered. This is generally for a patient with severe seasonal allergic rhinitis that is disabling. Prednisone 25 to 30 mg per day with tapering over two weeks, may allow control of symptoms and restore the effectiveness of the other medications; side effects when this drug is used in this fashion are minimal. Depot injections such as Kenalog, although longer lasting, should be used only rarely, as these are more adrenal suppressive and (especially in younger females) there is an increased risk of fat atrophy at the injection site.

Immunotherapy for inhalent-induced allergic rhinitis constitutes effective long-term management if patients are carefully selected. Initiation of immunotherapy is not recommended until at least a second season of allergic symptoms. Studies have shown that a small number of patients are not troubled in a second year. In a short pollen season such as that of ragweed (mid-August to September), a simple and effective medical program (such as antihistamines, Vancenase) may preclude immunotherapy. For a longer seasonal problem or perennial symptoms, immunotherapy may be initiated. Pollens are the most effective treatment antigens. Dust, molds, mites, roaches, and animal danders are given, but with slightly less effectiveness. Dosage is begun at 1:100,000 w/v or even 1:1,000,000 w/v in extremely sensitive patients, advanced weekly to tolerance or recommended levels. No long-term adverse effects have been shown in the more than 70 years that immunotherapy has been used. Acute reactions, however, are not uncommon and range from mild local swelling to systemic symptoms of anaphylaxis. Patients should be questioned about the presence of any reaction other than mild local swelling lasting a few hours, so that dosage may be modified. Because of the risk of these reactions, immunotherapy is not started in pregnancy but can be continued with a lower dosage, e.g., a 50% reduction in maintenance dosage. If the patient experiences good relief, treatment can be discontinued after two to four years. About half of these patients continue to do well. In those whose symptoms recur, the injections can be restarted.

NARES Syndrome

Presentation of the NARES syndrome (nonallergic rhinitis with eosinophilia) is similar to that of perennial allergic rhinitis, although obstruction and rhinorrhea are the major clinical problems. IgE levels are normal but nasal secretions show a significant number of eosinophils. Allergy skin tests are negative in these patients. Nasal polyps and sinusitis are more common, and x-rays show mucosal thickening. Asthma is a frequently associated problem.

Management is similar to that of allergic rhinitis,

with a good response to topical corticosteroid sprays. Antihistamines and decongestants may be effective.

Vasomotor Rhinitis

Vasomotor rhinitis is a perennial condition with a hyperreactivity to such stimuli as temperature and humidity changes. Stress situations can induce nasal congestion, as does exposure to smoke and other irritants. These patients may have other evidence of vascular instability, such as Raynaud's phenomenon. Nasal obstruction and rhinorrhea are the common symptoms, with turbinate swelling on examination. Nasal polyps and sinus infections are uncommon in this condition, although nasal smears show neutrophils.

This condition may result from an autonomic imbalance where a blockage of alpha-adrenergic stimulation produces nasal congestion. Stimulation of the parasympathetic nerves causes hypersecretion of mucus. With profuse hypersecretion as the major problem, a vidian neurectomy blocking parasympathetic innervation has proved effective, but this should be reserved for severe cases in view of the risk of atrophic changes.

Management is often difficult. Response to antihistamines, decongestants, and even topical or oral corticosteroids is poor.

Drug- and Hormone-Induced Rhinitis

Rhinitis medicamentosa is associated with the abuse of topical vasoconstrictor nasal sprays. There is severe nasal obstruction, continuous use gives less and less relief, requiring patients to use the sprays more and more. Other than a vascular rebound, the underlying pathophysiology is not clear. Management consists of discontinuing the sprays, but often a course of prednisone, 20 to 25 mg per day tapering over four to seven days, is required to prevent patients from restarting the spray. Nasal vasoconstrictor sprays should be restricted to three to five days' maximal use, but with these restrictions may be helpful in the treatment of sinusitis.

Other drugs may result in nasal symptoms, predominantly nasal congestion. Antihypertensive agents such as reserpine, a peripheral alpha-adrenergic blocker, and clonidine, a centrally acting alpha-blocker, can produce nasal symptoms. These alpha-blockers can potentiate the congestive actions of beta-receptors and cholinergic receptors.

During the second or third trimester of pregnancy, many women note increased nasal congestion and rhinorrhea. These symptoms persist through the remainder of the pregnancy and usually abate shortly after birth and delivery. Oral contraceptives may occasionally produce the same problems, but these medications rarely need to be discontinued. Management is symptomatic, but (within the guidelines of safe drug usage during pregnancy, and generally trying to avoid medication) small amounts of chlorpheniramine and/or pseudoephedrine are acceptable. Most pregnant women prefer not to take any medication when the cause of the symptoms is explained.

Hypothyroidism also may have nasal congestion as a major presenting complaint. Patients have been referred for suspected allergic rhinitis whose only other complaint was that of increased fatigue. If the hypothyroidism is of slow onset, even the patient or his family may not notice changes that are obvious to the physician. This form of rhinitis is treated by thyroid hormone replacement.

ANATOMIC CAUSES OF RHINITIS

Injuries to the nose occur commonly and the history may not be dramatic or may have been forgotten. Deviated septa are a common finding, as alterations in nasal air flow or function result in rhinitis symptoms. Surgery is seldom indicated unless the obstruction is severe or facilitates sinus infection. Treatment is symptomatic, with the medications described for the NARES syndrome.

It is important to recognize CSF rhinorrhea in view of the substantial risk of infection. There may be a history of trauma or congenitally weakened membrane, which may rupture following a violent sneeze with an upper respiratory infection. The fluid is clear and often drips from the nose, especially with the patient sitting up and leaning forward ("teapot sign"). The fluid will contain glucose and this can be easily confirmed. Management should be symptomatic and the patient promptly referred to a neurosurgeon for repair of the leak.

Unilateral rhinitis should lead to a search for a tumor or foreign body. Suspicion of a nasopharyngeal carcinoma or other tumor should be high in older patients with unilateral symptoms, and referral to an otolaryngologist should be made. Definitive treatment for a foreign body requires removal, and the availability of rhinoscopy enables this to be done more easily.

Choanal stenosis and adenoidal hypertrophy are not generally problems in the adult population.

Nasal Polyps

Nasal polyps are pale, glistening sacs filled with a mucoid material. Studies have shown that they contain eosinophils, plasma cells, IgA, IgE, and all the mediators of an allergic reaction (histamine, leukotrienes C and D, eosinophilic chemotactic factor of anaphylaxis). In spite of these suggestive features, most polyp patients are not atopic. The incidence of polyps is unknown, but they are estimated to occur in 4% to 7% of patients with rhinitis and asthma. The incidence increases with age.

There is a high incidence in children with cystic fibrosis and immotile cilia syndrome. In adults, there is a high correlation with either a present or future development of asthma induced by aspirin or other nonsteroidal anti-inflammatory agents, although it is uncertain why this occurs. Polyps may result from recurrent episodes of mucosal edema with uneven resolution.

Polyps produce nasal obstruction, especially at night when the patient is lying flat, as they can fall back up into the nose. There is increased postnasal drainage and loss of smell and taste. Rhinorrhea is frequent and may be watery to mucoid. Almost all patients with nasal polyps have radiologic evidence of sinusitis, which relates to the polyps blocking the sinus ostia.

In view of the high rate of recurrence following surgery, polypectomy should be reserved for severe nasal obstruction with sinusitis. Polyps have recurred in only a few months, and in one case a patient had 15 polypectomies over a period of 20 years. In patients in whom surgery is indicated, an ethmoidectomy (the area where most polyps tend to arise) should be considered. In view of the proximity of the ethmoid sinuses to the eye, blindness is a risk from this surgery.

Medical management includes systemic decongestants and combination antihistamine decongestant preparations; with associated sinus infection, antibiotics are required. The polyps often respond dramatically to corticosteroids. In view of the risks of chronic sinusitis and aggravation of asthma control, systemic corticosteroids are justified. Kenalog, 40 mg IM, has proved the most effective, but before use its indications and side effects should be reviewed with the patient. In view of the risks of lipoatrophy in young females, a preparation other than Kenalog should be chosen. Prednisone 40 mg per day with a slow taper over seven to ten days, is often effective. Once the polyps are shrunken, topical cortisone-derived sprays such as Vancenase, Beconase, and Nasalide may often facilitate control and retard recurrence.

Sinusitis

Significant radiographic changes of chronic sinusitis may be found in a significant number of patients with symptoms of chronic rhinitis. These changes include at least 5- to 8-mm mucosal thickening, complete radiologic opacification of a sinus and/or air fluid levels. The presence of associated sinus disease in an asthmatic patient may make the asthma extremely labile and difficult to manage. One study suggests that as many as 60% of children with chronic nocturnal cough and congestion may have sinus infection.

Sinusitis, or inflammation of the mucous membranes lining the sinuses, is a closed-space infection. Thus, any process producing blockage of the ostial openings will predispose to its occurrence once infection is introduced. Predisposing local factors include viral, bacterial, or fungal rhinitis; nasal polyps; foreign bodies; tumors; allergic diathesis; dental infections; barotrauma; diving or swimming in infected waters; and nasal septal pathology. Systemic predisposing factors include im-

motile cilia syndrome, antibody deficiency, chemotherapy, and any generally debilitating condition. Some types of vasculitis, such as Wegener's, can also predispose to sinusitis.

CLINICAL FEATURES

Clinical presentation may be acute (one day to three weeks), subacute (three weeks to three months), and chronic (more than three months). By the chronic stage, epithelial changes are generally irreversible and surgery for drainage, aeration, and removal of infected material is usually required. Acute sinusitis is associated with fever, pain, malaise, and purulent nasal discharge. The pain can be aggravated by bending or stooping. The associated sinus is often tender to palpation. At the other end, chronic sinusitis may be asymptomatic but patients often complain of intermittent cough (especially at night), altered taste, bad breath, and malaise. Confirmation of the diagnosis is best obtained by sinus x-rays. Ultrasound may prove helpful for maxillary sinus involvement, but the sphenoid sinus cannot be visualized by this technique. In view of the sphenoid sinus's strategic location adjacent to the brain stem, cavernous sinus, and sella turcica, disease here should be treated aggressively.

Nasopharyngeal cultures are not helpful in defining the causative bacterial agent. Acute sinusitis is most often due to *Streptococcus pneumoniae*, *Haemophilus influenzae*, or *Bramhamella catarrhalis*. *Staphylococcus aureus* occurs less often, except in Wegener's granulomatosis. Chronic sinusitis has a mixed flora and *S. aureus*, and anaerobes may be up to 40% or more of the organisms found.

MANAGEMENT

Management includes not only antibiotics, but some measure to produce drainage and, in acute sinusitis, pain relief. Topical vasoconstrictor nosedrops may be used several times daily for the first four to five days. Steam also helps to promote drainage by liquefying secretions. An efficient method of obtaining steam is the hot shower. The patient should remain in the room with the hot water turned on for 10 to 15 minutes three to four times a day. "Facial saunas" may also achieve this goal.

Amoxicillin, 500 mg every eight hours for 14 days, is effective against most causes of sinusitis. Alternate antibiotics include trimethoprim-sulfa double-strength tablets, one every 12 hours for two weeks, or doxycycline, 100 mg b.i.d. for the first day then one each morning for two weeks. In view of the increasing resistance of *H. influenzae* to several antibiotics, cefaclor (Ceclor), 500 mg every eight hours, may be an alternate choice. Erythromycin does not penetrate the sinuses well and is less effective against *H. influenzae*.

Follow-up x-rays after the initial two-week course should be ordered routinely. If there has been no change, antibiotics should be changed and treatment continued for another three weeks. If there is still no improvement, otolaryngologic referral should be made for consideration of antral puncture, culture, and lavage. Adenovirus, rhinovirus, and influenza can produce sinus infections, and unusual organisms such as *Pseu-*

domonas should raise the possibility of cystic fibrosis or immotile cilia syndrome. Fungal sinusitis, although uncommon, may suggest an underlying immune deficiency.

Surgical procedures primarily involve improving drainage, such as with nasal antral windows, if simple lavage is not effective. Removal of chronically infected mucosa may also help.

Specific treatment of allergic factors can be effective for long-term management, as can topical corticosteroid sprays to retard regrowth of polyps. In some patients the use of a single Bactrim DS (trimethoprim and sulfamethoxazole) tablet prophylactically at bedtime may control symptoms for a prolonged period.

REFERENCES

Mullarkey MF: A clinical approach to rhinitis. Med Clin North Am 65:977–986, 1981.

Mygind N: Clinical investigation of allergic rhinitis and allied conditions. Allergy 36:195–208, 1979.

Norman PS: Review of nasal therapy: update. J Allergy Clin Immunol 72:421–432, 1983.

3 · URTICARIA AND ANGIOEDEMA

Joseph F. Kelley
CLEVELAND CLINIC FOUNDATION

DEFINITION AND DIAGNOSTIC CRITERIA

Urticaria (hives, wheals) and angioedema are swellings of the skin that occur in an estimated 20% of the population.

Urticariae are raised, sharply demarcated wheals varying in size from a few millimeters to several centimeters, distributed over any part of the body, from just local area involvement to total body rash. These wheals are most often pruritic and red. They may be discrete circles, larger irregular swellings, or confluent areas covering large portions of the body.

The lesions appear within one to thirty minutes of the patient's exposure to an allergen and by definition are evanescent, lasting from a few minutes to a few hours. They characteristically leave no trace unless dilated blood vessels are broken by rubbing or scratching.

Angioedema involves swelling in deeper layers of the skin and usually is not sharply demarcated. It may occur in any part of the body, including the respiratory and gastrointestinal tracts. It generally does not itch but may give a sensation of mild pain or stinging caused by stretching of the outer skin layers. Angioedema may be life-threatening when the pharynx or larynx is involved, causing respiratory distress.

PATHOPHYSIOLOGY

Because avoidance of causative substances is of first importance in management, it is important to be aware of precipitating factors (Table 1). Occurrence of urticaria and angioedema may be mediated by immunoglobulin E (IgE) reactions (allergic), causing local release of histamine and other cellular mediators. This type I immune reaction is most often caused by allergy to drugs, such as penicillin and sulfonamides. It may also be caused by reaction to foods. The most frequent offenders are nuts, seeds, eggs, milk, fish, and shellfish, but any given food may be involved. Rarely the type I immune reaction may be caused by contact, as with pollen, dust, or plant oils. Hives commonly appear with viral infections such as infectious mononucleosis and enteric viruses.

Cholinergic urticaria is common and can be described as small, mildy pruritic hives that appear after exercise or during times of stress. They last briefly and usually require no medication.

In patients who are allergic to stinging insects, a sting may precipitate urticaria and angioedema.

Dermographism and pressure urticaria involve histamine release initiated by physical factors such as pressure on the skin. Warming after exposure to cold may bring on hives (cold urticaria).

Cold urticaria is clinically important because sudden exposures, such as diving into a cold swimming pool or the ocean, may cause massive histamine release resulting in vascular collapse.

Exposure to varying wavelengths of light may cause the appearance of hives (solar urticaria). Mechanical vibrations and contact with water may give rise to vibratory urticaria and aquagenic urticaria respectively.

Within the past few years, there has been interest in food colorings, especially tartrazine (FD & C Yellow No. 5) and related compounds. Foods such as berries often contain direct histamine-releasing substances. Some drugs, such as opiates, barbiturates, and iodinated contrast materials, may nonspecifically cause direct histamine release resulting in hives.

Exercise may produce exercise-induced anaphylaxis. It may also increase body heat, causing the appearance of cholinergic urticaria.

In hereditary angioneurotic edema (HANE), there is an absence of or defect in the C1 esterase inhibitor enzyme.

Hives may also occur with other systemic diseases, such as systemic lupus erythematosus, or other connective tissue disorders. Rarely they may be associated with malignancies, chronic infection such as sinusitis, or intestinal infestations such as giardiasis.

Table 1. URTICARIA AND ANGIOEDEMA: ETIOLOGY

Allergic Reaction	Underlying Disease
Drugs	Viral
Foods	Chronic bacterial infection
Contactants	Infestation
Stinging insect sensitivity	Malignancy
	Connective tissue disease
Physical Factors	
Pressure	**Hereditary Angioneurotic Edema (HANE)**
Cold	Absence of C1 esterase inhibitor
Vibration	Inactive C1 esterase inhibitor
	Lack of specific complement elements
Exercise	
Solar	
Heat	
Cholinergic	

MANAGEMENT

ACUTE DISTURBANCES

Epinephrine. If the urticaria is severe or respiration is impaired, aqueous epinephrine (1:1000 [Adrenalin] 0.3 cc subcutaneously) should be given and repeated in 30 minutes if significant clearing has not occurred. For children, 0.01 mg per kg can be given SQ. An airway and oxygen should be available in case respiratory distress continues.

Diphenhydramine Hydrochloride. Acute urticaria or angioedema requires initial symptomatic treatment. Because by definition both disorders are of short duration, antihistamines are the first line of drugs used. Diphenhydramine hydrochloride (Benadryl) can be used at 50 to 100 mg every four hours in adults and 5 mg per kg orally or IM over 24 hours in children. Other antihistamines such as chlorpheniramine maleate (Chlor-Trimeton) can be used (4 mg every four hours in adults, 1 to 2 mg four times a day in children).

Hydroxyzine. Also known as Atarax or Vistaril, hydroxyzine, preferably in syrup form for speed and predictability of absorption, can be given in a dosage of 10 (1 teaspoonful) to 50 mg four times a day for adults. In children under 6 years, a divided dose of up to 50 mg per day can be used. In children over 6, a divided dose of 50 to 100 mg can be given. Antihistamines should be continued until the episode is controlled and symptoms are gone.

In hereditary angioneurotic edema, epinephrine and antihistamines do not relieve the swelling. Supportive therapy and maintenance of adequate airway must be continued until the swelling subsides.

For patients with sudden violent flares of hives and angioedema, the precaution of carrying epinephrine (Epi-Pen or ANA-KIT) should be strongly encouraged.

Cyproheptadine Hydrochloride. For cold urticaria cyproheptadine hydrochloride (Periactin) is the drug of choice for both acute treatment and preventive management (4 mg three to four times a day for adults, 0.25 mg per kg per day for children, not to exceed the adult dosage of 16 mg per day).

CHRONIC DISTURBANCES

Chronic Urticaria. Chronic urticaria is defined as continuing or recurring urticaria over a six- to eight-week period. Antihistamines are the first line of control. Hydroxyzine can be effective in low doses (10 to 20 mg) often as infrequently as once every one or two days. I advise regular dosage at bedtime whether lesions are present or not, because transient drowsiness usually wears off after seven or eight hours but the antihistamine effect may last for up to three days. Terfenadine (Seldane), a long-acting, relatively nonsedating drug, may also be used for chronic urticaria.

If this does not work, I try other antihistamines (h_1-blocker type, see Table 2). If symptoms continue, addition of an H_2-block drug such as cimetidine (Tagamet, 200 or 300 mg three or four times a day) may be effective. In adults drugs such as doxepin hydrochloride (Sinequan, 10 to 75 mg taken at bedtime) may help. In some cases concomitant theophylline, albuterol, or similar drugs may give added relief.

Corticosteroids. I believe corticosteroids should be used only when the other drugs fail to control symptoms

Table 2. SYMPTOMATIC MANAGEMENT: URTICARIA AND ANGIOEDEMA

Acute
- Aqueous epinephrine
- Antihistamines H_1
  - Diphenhydramine hydrochloride, chlorpheniramine maleate, brompheniramine
  - Hydroxyzine
  - Cyproheptadine

Chronic
- Antihistamines H_1
  - Diphenhydramine hydrochloride, chlorpheniramine maleate, brompheniramine
  - Hydroxyzine
  - Cyproheptadine
- Antihistamines H_2
  - Cimetidine
  - Ranitidine hydrochloride
- Corticosteroids

and then only in conjunction with the other drugs. The dosage should be kept at the lowest possible amount needed to maintain control. I start with an equivalent of prednisone at 20 mg per day. When control is maintained, a steroid dosage every other day should be tried, the aim always being to reduce and discontinue it as soon as possible.

It should be made clear to patients that most chronic urticaria and recurrent angioedema occur in a cyclic nature and that if an underlying cause cannot be found, as is the case in over 80% of patients, the likelihood of the process subsiding on its own is great. The physician should explain that, in the meantime, control of symptoms to allow a normal existence is the goal.

REFERENCES

Buckley RH, Mathews KP: Common "allergic" skin diseases; primer on allergic and immunologic diseases. JAMA 248(20):2611–2622, 1982.

Kaplan AP: Urticaria and angioedema. *In* Middleton E, Reed CE, Ellis EF (eds): Allergy Principles and Practice, vol. II, 2nd ed. C. V. Mosby Co, St. Louis, 1983, pp 1341–1360.

Levinson AI: Urticaria and angioedema. Current approach to common problems. Postgrad Med 76:183–192, 1984.

Schneider SB, Atkinson JP: Urticaria and angioedema. *In* Fitzpatrick ED, et al. (eds): Update–Dermatology in Medicine. McGraw-Hill Book Co, New York, 1983, pp 61–79.

Twarog FJ: Urticaria in childhood: pathogenesis and management. Pediatr Clin North Am 30:887–898, 1983.

4 · ADVERSE REACTIONS TO DRUGS

David A. Mathison
SCRIPPS CLINIC AND RESEARCH FOUNDATION

Patients receive an average of ten drugs during hospitalization and ambulatory patients take an average of two drugs on a regular basis. Adverse reactions occur about once in every 20 courses of drug treatments. Most reactions to drugs are clinically minor, readily recognized by patient and physician, and are reversible when the drug is suspended. However, for the 10% of adverse reactions that are life-threatening and for those reactions in which the relationship to a drug may be somewhat obscure, additional expertise in management is required. This chapter reviews reactions to drugs and the management of patients with a history of reactions to drugs to which they need to be reexposed.

DEFINITIONS AND DIAGNOSTIC CRITERIA

The term "adverse reaction" to drugs encompasses all varieties of unwanted responses.

Toxicity or poisoning is the excess of direct intended drug action resulting from overdosage, be it involuntary or voluntary. Diagnosis depends on measurement of the drug in body fluids or tissues at levels above therapeutic or those usually tolerated.

Side effects are undesirable symptoms or signs resulting from direct but unintended actions, drug-drug interactions, microaggregate embolization, or alteration of bacterial growth resulting in superinfection or malnutrition. Diagnosis is by association of symptoms and signs with known effects of the drugs used, supplemented, when available or needed, by measurement of the drugs in tissue or body fluid at levels in the therapeutic or usually tolerated range.

Immunologic hypersensitivity reactions are those triggered by antibody or sensitized lymphocytes specific to epitopes, the antigen binding sites of the drug, either as a complete antigen or hapten linked to a carrier molecule. Mediator systems and various other cells may contribute beyond the specific antibodies or sensitized lymphocytes and determine the manifestations of the reaction. Diagnosis depends on identification of immune reactants (specific antibodies or immune complexes in fluids; immunoglobulins in tissues; cutaneous immediate, late, or delayed hypersensitivity) and the presence of a putative drug known to be capable of evoking the immunologic reaction.

Anaphylactic or immediate hypersensitivity type I (Coombs and Gell) reaction results from specific antigen combining with IgE antibodies fixed to mast cells or basophils leading to release or synthesis and action of autacoids (histamine, arachidonate metabolites including leukotrienes, prostaglandins, and cellular chemotactic factors). Diagnosis depends on demonstration of specific IgE antibody to the putative drug by a direct cutaneous test for wheal-flare immediate reaction or a test of body fluid by a radioallergosorbent or similar method.

Anaphylactoid reactions have clinical features of anaphylactic reactions but result from nonimmunologic activation of mast cells or autacoids; the term "pseudoallergic" is frequently applied to these reactions. Presumptive diagnosis is based on the appearance of symptoms or signs of anaphylaxis coincident to administration of a drug known to activate mast cells in the absence of specific IgE antibodies.

Mental reactions include (1) the overly dramatic expression of perception of drug actions or side effects as experienced by individuals with histrionic personality organization; (2) somatoform or psychotic reaction with involuntary misattribution of symptoms or signs to drugs rather than to the mental disorder per se; (3) factitious voluntary misuse of a drug to achieve a toxic or side effect; and (4) psychophysiologic reactions, when psychologic factors affect the action of or reaction to a drug. Diagnosis of the mental disorder, according to psychiatric criteria, allows characterization of the reaction.

The term "allergy" was initially coined to apply to immunologic reactions harmful to, rather than protective of, the host, and is restricted in use by some physicians to IgE-mediated reactions. However, over the past 75 years of lay usage the term has come to mean any exaggerated reaction to a substance, situation, or physical or emotional stimulus. As a warning flag, affixing "allergic to" or (better) "adverse reaction to" to a patient or his medical record has merit so long as the drug can reasonably be avoided. When the drug cannot be avoided, for example, when a penicillin drug becomes the agent of choice for a life-threatening infection, the expert clinical allergist-immunologist may be able to help overcome or circumvent the "allergy."

A summary of adverse reactions and the levels of meaning of the word "allergic" can be found in Tables 1 and 2.

CLINICAL ASPECTS

Toxicity may result from overdose or decreased drug inactivation and clearance, as in the elderly or severely ill patient with impaired hepatic or renal function. Alteration in mental status, sleep disturbance, fever, erythema, rash, bleeding diathesis, electrolyte disorders, or deteriorating hepatic or renal function may be clues to drug toxicity. Digitalis, diuretics, antimicrobials, tranquilizers, antihypertensives, anticoagulants, and steroids are the drugs that most frequently account for dose-related toxicity. The margin of safety between optimal therapeutic and toxic levels can be sufficiently narrow for digoxin, theophylline, gentamicin, phenytoin, carbamazepine, and lithium to warrant measurement of serum levels during the initial stages of therapy with these drugs, and again when illness or additional drug therapy supervenes during their long-term use. Management of overdose and organ injury by specific drugs is beyond the scope of this chapter; the reader is referred to the prescribing information for individual drugs.

Table 1. TYPES OF ADVERSE REACTIONS TO DRUGS ACCORDING TO MECHANISM

Toxic—overdose—poisoning
Side effects—drug interactions—superinfections
Sensitivity—"allergic"
    Idiosyncratic—paradoxical
    Immunologic hypersensitivity—"allergic"
        Anaphylactic/IgE mediated—type I*—"allergic"
        Membranolytic/cytolytic—type II
        Serum sickness/immune complex type III
        Delayed hypersensitivity—"allergic" contact type IV
    Anaphylactoid—"pseudoallergic"
Mental
    Overdramatic—histrionic
    Involuntary misattribution—somatoform/psychotic
    Factitious
    Psychophysiologic—psychologic factors affect

*Types of immunologic reactions according to Coombs and Gell.

Table 2. TYPES OF ADVERSE REACTIONS TO DRUGS ACCORDING TO CLINICAL MANIFESTATION

Immediate generalized anaphylactic/anaphylactoid
Febrile
Mucocutaneous
    Pruritus—urticaria—angioedema
    Erythematous macular
    Erythema multiforme
    Erythema nodosum—vasculitis
    Photosensitive
    Eczematous contact dermatitis
Lupus erythematosus–like
Organ specific

Immediate generalized *anaphylactic* or *anaphylactoid* reactions have precipitous onset during or within minutes of administration of the drug, and may include itching, erythema, urticaria, angioedema, asthma, or hypotension.

Fever may develop immediately after a drug is first taken or may increase in a stepwise fashion over the first week of administration. It may be low-grade or hectic and accompanied by constitutional symptoms. The patient may appear less ill than would be anticipated from the height of the fever, though occasionally a septic picture can be mimicked. Phenytoin, barbiturates, and antimicrobials are frequent causes of drug fever. The fever may be expected to subside within a day or two of discontinuing the suspected offending drug. Associated *serum sickness–like* reactions of the skin, lymph nodes, or joints may take longer to subside and, if severe, may warrant corticosteroid therapy.

Rash as a manifestation of reaction to drugs may take several forms. Pruritus or urticaria, with or without angioedema are the common manifestations of mild anaphylactic reaction to penicillin or anaphylactoid reaction to a narcotic or injected radiocontrast media. Chronic urticaria or angioedema may be perpetuated in part by anaphylactoid reaction to ingested vitamin C, citric acid, laxative, aspirin, or nonsteroidal anti-inflammatory drugs, or anaphylactic reaction to trace amounts of penicillin contaminating dairy products or fowl. Fine, erythematous, macular, measles-like eruption reflective of circulating aggregates or immune complexes occurs commonly in patients who have mononucleosis treated with ampicillin, sulfonamides, thiazides, allopurinol, and other agents. Persistent administration of the offending drug may lead to confluent erythroderma and exfoliative dermatitis. Erythema multiforme is characterized by the formation of sharply circumscribed mucocutaneous lesions with annular spread and a clear central "iris" or "target." Antimicrobials, especially sulfonamides, and barbiturates are the drugs most commonly implicated. Erythema nodosum may be caused by sulfonamides, iodides, and oral contraceptives. Small vessel vasculitis, as in Henoch-Schönlein purpura, may follow treatment with penicillin, sulfonamide, tetracycline, or aspirin. Photosensitivity reactions characterized by erythema, edema, and scaling limited to areas exposed to light are most commonly provoked by doxycycline, thiazides, or sulfonamides. Eczematous contact dermatitis is not infrequently traced to lanolin or neomycin contained in ointments or other topical medicaments.

A *lupus erythematosus–like* syndrome has been described following procainamide (most patients develop autoantibodies with prolonged treatment, but only a small proportion develop disease); hydralazine; phenytoin; and others.

Hematopoietic disorders related to drugs include (1) thrombocytopenic purpura associated with quinine, quinidine, thiouracil, and anticonvulsants; (2) agranulocytosis with phenylbutazone and aplastic anemia with chloramphenacol, gold salts, and sulfonamides; (3) Coombs positivity without or with anemia during methyldopa (Aldomet) treatment; and (4) the genetically determined hemoglobinopathies that allow idiosyncratic hemolysis to multiple drugs.

Acute *hepatic injury* may follow halothane or erythromycin estolate (Ilosone) as a hypersensitivity reaction in adults. Liver damage has also been associated with chlorpromazine and sulfonamide administration.

MANAGEMENT

Generalized anaphylactic or anaphylactoid reaction constitutes a medical emergency. Immediate treatment should include epinephrine 1:1000 (1 μg/ml), 0.1 ml/25 kg up to 0.5 ml subcutaneously, and parenteral diphenhydramine (Benadryl), 25 to 50 mg. In cases involving hypotension, dilute IV epinephrine (1:100,000), with close monitoring, is usually necessary. Cimetidine (Tagamet), 300 mg IV, has been advised by some authors as an additional medication. IV saline/colloid "wide open" oxygen by mask or nasal clips is recommended. (See "Anaphylaxis", Sect. 10, Chap. 1.)

Treatment for other adverse reactions in progress includes withholding of the known or putative offending drugs and further pharmacotherapy according to the nature of the reaction (see Sec. X, Chaps. 1 and 3 and Sec. XI, Chap. 11).

The great majority of patients who have had adverse reaction to a drug or chemical can continue throughout their lifetime to avoid subsequent exposure and risk of reaction by substituting alternative drugs. Occasionally, there is critical need for use of a drug or chemical to which a patient has previously reacted. In this circumstance, a carefully taken history can enable the reaction to be categorized as life-threatening or not. Table 3 lists common reactions and the drugs most frequently implicated.

When there is a history of immediate generalized anaphylactic reaction, cutaneous tests for a wheal-flare response indicative of IgE antibodies can be performed. If there is no reaction, the drug can be administered, first by an oral test dose and then, if there is no reaction in 30 minutes, parenterally. If there is a wheal-flare reaction, antihistamine is given, an IV line is placed, and cautious desensitization (controlled anaphylaxis) is undertaken. This should start with the skin test dose, and the dose should be doubled every 20 minutes thereafter (while monitoring for blood pressure drop, respiratory distress, or cutaneous reaction) until a full therapeutic dose is achieved. Once the desensitized state is achieved, the drug should continue to be administered every few hours throughout treatment, since interruption of therapy may allow the anaphylactic state to return.

When there is a history of anaphylactoid reaction, as for parenteral radiocontrast media, pretreatment with prednisone (50-mg doses at six-hour intervals beginning

Table 3. ADVERSE REACTIONS TO DRUGS THAT MUST BE READMINISTERED

Immediate generalized life-threatening
  Anaphylactic
    Penicillin—cephalosporin
    Insulin
    Chymopapain
    L-Asparaginase
    Horse serum
      Antitoxin
      Antithymocyte globulin
    Avian origin vaccines (influenza, measles, mumps rubella, typhus)
    Ethylene oxide–treated hemodialysis membranes
    Protamine (reversal of heparin anticoagulation)

  Anaphylactoid
    Iodinated radiocontrast media—parenteral narcotics
    Succinylcholine
    High-molecular-weight dextran
    Aspirin/nonsteroidal anti-inflammatory agents

Late-delayed life-threatening
  Exfoliative dermatitis
    Thiazides
    Sulfonamides
    Allopurinol
    Gold salts
  Asthmatic
    Aspirin nonsteroidal anti-inflammatory agents
  Organ specific—multiple agents and mechanisms

Non–life-threatening
  Pruritus
  Erythematous macular rash
  Mental

18 hours before the procedure) and diphenhydramine (50 mg parenterally one hour before the procedure) will reduce the risk of life-threatening reaction from about 40% to less than 5%.

For life-threatening cutaneous or other organ-specific reactions, further use of the implicated drug is best avoided.

For non–life-threatening reactions, the implicated drug can be reintroduced at ¹⁄₁₆th of the ordinary dose and doubled, with one, two, or three doses given daily, until the full dose is attained. To allow treatment with a drug to which a patient previously reacted, we give antihistamines, if the previous reaction was pruritus or rash only, or corticosteroids in full therapeutic dose (e.g., prednisone, 40 mg daily) if there were other reactions.

REFERENCES

Goldstein RA, Patterson R: Drug allergy: prevention, diagnosis, treatment. J Allergy Clin Immunol 74:549–644, 1984.

Patterson R, Anderson J: Allergic reactions to drugs and biologic agents. JAMA 248:2637–2645, 1982.

Taffet SL, Das KM: Desensitization of patients with inflammatory bowel disease to sulfasalazine. Am J Med 73:520–524, 1982.

Van Arsdel PP Jr: Adverse drug reactions. *In* Middleton E Jr, Reed CE, Ellis EF (eds): Allergy: Principles and Practice. C.V. Mosby Co, St. Louis, 1983, pp 1389–1414.

5 · ADVERSE REACTIONS TO FOODS

John A. Anderson
HENRY FORD HOSPITAL

DEFINITION AND PATHOPHYSIOLOGY

The term "allergy" has become a lay term commonly used to express a person's feeling that unpleasant effects come from that person's exposure to a chemical agent, although most people are not harmed. It is also a term commonly used in the medical literature to describe all sorts of adverse reactions, regardless of mechanism. "Adverse reaction to food" or "food sensitivity" are better general terms representing clinically abnormal responses attributed to an exposure to food or food additives.

Adverse reactions to foods, therefore, can be broadly classified on the basis of mechanisms. Reactions related to an immunologic event are designated as "food allergy." Reactions that are caused by other mechanisms or represent reactions of unknown cause can be designated "food intolerance."

Food hypersensitivity describes those immunologic food reactions mediated by the presence of IgE antibodies. The most classic of such reactions is anaphylaxis. In this condition, IgE food-reactive antibodies are formed, fixed to tissue mast cells and circulating basophils; later, upon rechallenge with a food allergen, this results in the release of chemical mediators from the mast cells and basophils. These mediators produce the signs and symptoms commonly associated with anaphylaxis. Foods most prone to be associated with anaphylaxis in adults include seafood (particularly shrimp and crab), eggs, fish, peanuts, and nuts.

Anaphylactoid reactions to foods appear to be clinically indistinguishable from the immunologic anaphylaxis reaction. These reactions result from the direct nonimmunologic release of chemical mediators. Examples include reactions to strawberries, Swiss cheese, and wine, as well as "anaphylaxis-like" reactions to food additives (e.g., exacerbation of asthma or shock after sulfite preservative exposure).

Other terms used to classify types of food intolerance reactions include food idiosyncrasy, food toxicity or poisoning, and both pharmacologic and metabolic food reactions.

CLINICAL ASPECTS AND DIAGNOSTIC CRITERIA

PRESENTING SIGNS AND SYMPTOMS

The signs and symptoms with which the physician is confronted, which have a *proved* relationship to diet, and which are based on immune mechanisms, generally resemble other known allergic reactions. These signs and symptoms include those seen with urticaria and angioedema, anaphylaxis, allergic conjunctivitis and rhinitis, bronchial asthma, atopic dermatitis, and a variety of gastrointestinal complaints such as vomiting, abdominal cramps, and diarrhea. Other presenting signs and symptoms, such as headache, muscle ache, joint pain or swelling, fatigue, hyperactivity, "mental disorientation," urinary complaints, and nonspecific GI abnormalities, are most likely to be either unrelated to diet or (if related to diet) to be based on nonimmune mechanisms (food intolerance).

If an adverse reaction to food is seriously considered, the physician should inquire about the timing, frequency, duration, and severity of reaction.

The timing of an adverse food reaction involves establishing the relationship of the adverse reaction to the process of eating as well as the ingestion of or exposure to a specific food. Most food reactions occur within minutes to hours of exposure to the food. If this is the case, the cause-and-effect relationship often can be easily established, particularly if the pattern is repeated several times.

Delayed-onset food reactions (longer than two hours) are most often caused by nonimmunologic mechanisms. However, immunologic reactions may also be manifested late, hours after the allergic exposure. Such reactions may fall into the Gell and Coombs class III (Arthus or antigen-antibody complex) or class IV (cell-mediated or delayed hypersensitivity) category. In addition, it has become clear that significant delayed-onset reactions may occur that are the result of class I (IgE antibody) reactions. In almost all cases in which this occurs, there is an initial immediate response followed hours later by a delayed response. Some of the food-related flares in atopic dermatitis may be due to this mechanism.

The frequency and duration of the food reaction is also important. Urticaria and angioedema that occur intermittently are more likely to be associated with a specific food than is chronic urticartia or angioedema. In chronic urticaria, the cause is more likely to be idiopathic (about 80% of cases).

As a rule, GI signs and symptoms, such as abdominal pain and diarrhea, which occur intermittently with long (months) periods of normalcy without change of diet are not likely to be directly related to food ingestion. When the signs and symptoms are continuous, the relationship to a specific food ingestion may be difficult to predict. In well-controlled studies utilizing double-blind food challenge (DBFC), it has been shown that there may be a poor correlation of symptoms with the history of a specific food sensitivity.

Signs and symptoms that are mild or moderate in nature, but not those that are debilitating, can usually be investigated and managed on an outpatient basis. Severe reactions, especially those that are potentially life-threatening, require special attention.

Often the physician is faced with differentiating from the patient's story those conditions that may fall under adverse reactions to foods (either allergic or intolerance) from conditions that have nothing to do with the content of the diet or have only a secondary relationship to the process of eating. If the initial impression favors an alternative diagnosis (Table 1), the appropriate work-up or specialty referral may be necessary. If adverse reactions to foods are suspected, further work-up is probably needed.

SUPPORTING LABORATORY TESTS IN ADVERSE REACTIONS TO FOODS

Most allergic adverse reactions to food involve IgE mechanisms. Total serum IgE may be helpful as a measure of the overall allergic state or the presence of atopy. If the value is elevated (see Sect. X, Chap. 7), the patient is likely to be atopic, with a greater potential to be allergic to any allergen.

Food allergen–specific immediate-reacting (15 to 20 minutes) IgE prick/scratch/puncture skin testing can be used as a screen for suspected allergic reaction to food. Investigations utlizing DBFC, placebo-specific techniques have shown that patients with a positive blind challenge to a specific food almost always have a corresponding positive immediate-reacting food prick skin test reaction. On the other hand, the same patients may have several positive immediate skin test reactions to foods and still not react *clinically* to that food. A positive prick skin test will correlate with clinical sensitivity 50% to 70% of the time. Patients who have negative food IgE prick skin test reactions, however, almost never have clinical sensitivity to the food (reliability 94% to 100%). Thus, skin testing can be used as a reliable *negative* indicator of the presence of allergic reactions to foods.

The IgE radioallergosorbent test (RAST) and the IgE enzyme-linked immunosorbent assay (ELISA) are in vitro assays of allergen-specific antibody. They give the same information as the immediate-reacting skin test but are less sensitive.

Food allergen–specific IgE RAST or ELISA assays can provide valuable supplementary information. These are the tests of choice when we attempt to validate the

---

Table 1. PRACTICAL APPROACH TO DIAGNOSIS OF SUSPECTED ADVERSE REACTION TO FOOD

Initial Evaluation:
History and physical examination; character of signs and symptoms

Initial Impression:
Timing, duration, and severity of reaction
   Adverse reaction to food: additional studies needed
   Alternate diagnosis, suspected: appropriate work-up, specialty referral or therapy

Suspected Allergic Food Reactions:
Supportive studies
   Total serum IgE
   Direct immediate-reactive IgE allergen-specific prick/scratch/ puncture skin testing
   IgE allergen-specific RAST or ELISA
   Other immunologic tests (types III, IV, II)*

Suspected Food Intolerance:
   Specific studies appropriate to suspected diagnosis (e.g., studies for lactose intolerance)
   Specialty consultation

Diary Confirmation:
   Food diary
   Basic allergen-free diet followed by open challenge
   Specific food elimination followed by double-blind food challenge (DBFC)

---

*Gell and Coombs' classification of immune reactions: Type I—IgE mediated. Type II—antitissue antibodies. Type III—antigen-antibody complex. Type IV—cell mediated.

Table 2. ALLERGEN-FREE DIAGNOSTIC DIET

Only Foods Allowed (avoid coffee, tea, cola, and chewing gum)		
Rice	White potatoes	Water
Barley		Ginger ale (dry)
Rye*	Sweet potatoes, yams	
Corn*	Squash	Sugar (cane or beet)
	Carrots	Salt
Lamb	Spinach	Maple or maple flavor
Bacon (ham)*	Chard	White vinegar
Chicken-turkey	Beets	Olive oil
Beef*	Asparagus	Crisco
	Artichokes	Vanilla extract
Apples	Cabbage	Safflower oil margarine
Pears	Broccoli	
Peaches	Brussels sprouts	Tapioca pearl
Apricots	Lettuce	Arrowroot
Pineapples		Poi
Cranberries	Soy*	
Cherries	Peas*	
Plums, prunes	Beans*	

Possible milk substitutes: I-Soyalac (corn-free), ProSoyBee, Isomil (for infants); Coffee Rich nondairy creamer

Suggested Menu

Breakfast	Dinner	Supper
Rice cereal	Lamb or beef pattie	Chicken or turkey
Milk substitute	Baked potato	Mashed potatoes
Bacon	Lettuce and carrot salad	Peas
Tapioca and peaches	Baked pears	Lettuce and pineapple salad
Apple juice	Ginger ale	Frozen peaches
Water	Water	Water

Format for Physician's Instructions

Stay on basic diet for ______days.   *Result*

Then, on ______, add ______, alone, first thing in AM   __________________________

Next, on ______, add ______, alone, first thing in AM   __________________________

Next, on ______, add ______, alone, first thing in AM   __________________________

Next, on ______, add ______, alone, first thing in AM   __________________________

Adapted from: Methods for Diagnosis of Adverse Reactions to Foods. *In* Anderson JA, Sogn DD, AAAI, and NIAID: Adverse Reactions to Foods. NIH Publication 84-2242, July 1984, pp 123–160.
*Foods safe in *most* (but not all) allergic individuals.

history of a life-threatening anaphylaxis situation. Food IgE RAST and ELISA assays usually correlate with DBFC results in a similar fashion as do the IgE prick skin tests in anaphylactic-sensitive individuals.

Also of practical importance in the evaluation of suspected food intolerance with GI signs and symptoms are tests for lactose intolerance. The need for additional tests (x-rays, blood determinations, cultures, biopsies, and neurologic and psychologic examinations) is probably best determined by the initial evaluation (see Table 1). Food "allergy" tests of no proved value include the cytotoxic food test and the Rinkle type of titration—provocation challenge testing.

FOOD DIARY, ELIMINATION DIETS, AND OPEN DOUBLE-BLIND FOOD CHALLENGE (DBFC)

Following the initial evaluation, the physician must obtain confirmaton of the relationship between a given set of signs and symptoms and a specific food exposure. If the situation involves a self-limited event that may have recurred intermittently, the use of a *diet diary* is appropriate: e.g., for patients who have intermittent attacks of acute urticaria. Patients are directed to record all foods ingested in the 12 hours before the event, concentrating on the last foods eaten. In most situations, however, confirmation requires more intervention. A basic allergen-free diagnostic diet followed by an open

challenge at home can be utilized under these circumstances (Table 2). This diet should include foods that have proved least likely to be associated with allergic symptomatology. Cow's milk, egg, peanut, wheat, and soy are of particular concern. Other foods that may be of importance include fish, seafood (particularly shrimp and crab), nuts, orange, tomato, pork, and celery. Most other foods are tolerated by allergic individuals.

The diagnostic allergen-free diet is used as follows:

1. The suspected allergic patient is placed on the allergen-free diet for two-plus weeks.

2. Foods are then added to the diet, usually at three- to seven-day intervals. The foods most difficult to keep out of a normal diet are tried first (milk, eggs, wheat). Usually a small-to-moderate amount on an empty stomach is given in the first meal. If this first meal is tolerated over a two-hour period, subsequent administration of that food can be given at least twice daily at regular mealtime.

3. After three to seven days, if no change in the clinical status of the patient occurs, the test food can be accepted as a permanent additive to the basic diet, and a second test food challenge is begun. If suspicious signs or symptoms do occur with the challenge of the test food, that food is withdrawn from the diet and the patient is treated until the adverse signs and symptoms are controlled before proceeding.

Usually the patient can be challenged with relatively few foods, depending on the prick skin test reactivity. It is best to define limits to the test period and to restrict the challenge to a few important foods, otherwise the patient is likely to tire of the procedure and compliance will be poor. The nutritional consequence of any long-term dietary manipulation must always be considered. If foods are discovered that cause suspicious signs or symptoms, the open challenge is best repeated. One or two sets of positive food challenges can be given only the *presumptive diagnosis* of food sensitivity.

In some cases the allergen-free diet followed by the open challenge procedure does not suffice. In these special circumstances, the DBFC procedure with placebo should be carried out under controlled conditions. In most cases these difficult situations should be referred to an allergist skilled in such evaluation. The DBFC procedure involves the following:

1. Establishing a baseline period on a basic allergen-free diet or with a nonallergenic protein base food such as Vivonex.

2. Placing patients in a controlled situation so that they can be monitored during the test period by non-biased, trained observers. Any serious signs or symptoms that arise can be promptly managed (e.g., inadvertent onset of anaphylaxis).

3. Patients are challenged with either a specific food or placebo in a double-blind, randomized fashion. The choice of food for challenge is best based on the results of allergy prick skin tests or in vitro RAST/ELISA assays.

4. The challenge is usually graded, beginning with a small dose (20 to 200 mg) and progressing at two-hour intervals (2-10× increases) to a maximum of 8 to 10 gm of food safely tolerated. The food is given either in dehydrated form* using opaque colorless #1-sized gelatin capsules, or hidden in a variety of bland food-stuffs such as Pregestimil and Nutramigen Formula, unflavored or vanilla-flavored regular Vivonex, or solid foods such as hamburger or mashed potatoes.

5. Most adverse reactions (e.g., skin or respiratory tree) occur within a two-hour period. GI adverse reactions may manifest later.

6. All negative DBFC results should be followed with an open challenge using the amount of food normally eaten in the patient's regular diet.

Serial pulmonary function evaluation may be used as an objective end point for evaluating possible sensitivity to food and food additives. Examples include "baker's asthma," in which the baker is given an inhalation of wheat flour, as well as asthmatics suspected of sensitivity to tartrazine, sodium benzoate, gutylated hydroxyanisole/gutylated hydroxytoluene (BHA/BHT), monosodium glutamate, or sulfites.

MANAGEMENT OF PATIENTS WITH PRESUMPTIVE OR DEFINITIVE DIAGNOSIS OF ADVERSE REACTION TO FOOD

PLAN AND GOALS

Once the diagnosis of food sensitivity has been either presumed or definitely confirmed, the best treatment is to advise the patient to *avoid that food or food*

---

*The relative value of challenges with fresh, frozen, or cooked foods is unknown at this time.

additive. In the case of IgE-mediated food allergy, a dose-response relationship does not exist in a strict sense. A very small exposure to food allergen may produce a massive response.

Some evidence exists, particularly concerning food allergy reactions in children, that these children may "lose" their clinical reactions to foods such as milk or egg over a few years, especially if these foods are strictly avoided. However, anaphylactic sensitivity to foods such as fish, seafood, and tree nuts, which begin later in life, may persist for many years in spite of strict avoidance.

Avoidance of food and food additives is not an easy task. It is more easily done in one's own home. Labels on processed foods can be helpful, but "hidden" sources of food allergens are always a problem. Careful investigation and prudent buying, however, may identify safe food products by brand name. The problem of strict allergy avoidance becomes impossible, however, when the susceptible patient must eat away from home, such as in a restaurant. An example of the risks of this situation is the possible shock and severe asthma following exposure to sulfite preservatives sprayed on lettuce in restaurant salad bars.

In the case of food intolerances, a dose-response relationship is more likely to exist: e.g., patients who have primary lactose intolerance. These patients may not be able to tolerate a glass of homogenized milk but may tolerate some processed cheese and yogurt (because of a relatively low level of lactose in these latter dairy products).

DRUG THERAPY

Drugs important for management of the signs and symptoms of food sensitivity include injectable epinephrine for anaphylaxis and asthma, and injectable and oral antihistamines for urticaria/angioedema and nasal rhinitis and conjunctivitis. Other bronchodilators may also be used to treat asthma. Corticosteroids may be helpful for severe anaphylaxis and for immune complex and type IV immune reactions, such as in Heiner's syndrome, as well as for food-induced eosinophilic gastroenteritis and food-induced protein-losing enteropathy.

Orally administered cromolyn sodium *may* be of some help in the management of GI signs and symptoms from adverse food reactions. However, the only commercial form of powdered cromolyn sodium comes in a nondissolvable, 20-mg plastic capsule mixed with 20 mg lactose. Unfortunately, patients with GI symptoms may also have concurrent lactose intolerance.

In patients with a history of food-induced anaphylaxis or food additive anaphylactoid reactions, the use of either a pre-loaded Adrenalin syringe or epinephrine auto-injection for use in emergencies (e.g., for those allergic to stinging insects) is advised. The pre-loaded syringe delivers 0.3 cc and may be repeated for a total of 0.6 cc (Ana-Kit). The auto-injectors (Epi-Pen and Epi-Pen Jr.) are designed to deliver either 0.3 or 0.15 cc of epinephrine through clothing and into the thigh as the device is jammed against the leg.

PREVENTIVE MEASURES

Pregnant women who are atopic or who come from strongly allergic families should be advised of the risk of allergy in their offspring. Allergic manifestations may be modified or prevented if the mother modifies her diet in the last trimester of pregnancy and continues to modify it following the delivery of the child while she is breast-feeding. She should also be advised to avoid introducing certain solid foods into the infant until after the child is either 6 or 9 months of age, and to watch the infant's general environment and exposure to cat, dog, house dust, and mold respiratory allergens. Foods to be avoided in the diet of both mother and infant include those most likely to produce allergen sensitization (cow's milk, egg, peanut, wheat and nuts). Soy probably should be avoided in the mother's diet but still may be used to supplement breast milk or as a substitute for breast milk in the infant, since another suitable and inexpensive substitute for cow's milk formula is not commercially available at present.

REFERENCES

American Academy of Allergy and Immunology Committee on Adverse Reactions to Foods and National Institute of Allergy and Infectious Diseases: Adverse Reactions to Foods. Anderson JA, Sogn DD (eds). U.S. Department of Health and Human Services, NIH Publication 84–2442, July 1984.

Anderson JA: Anaphylaxis and serum sickness. In Rakel RE (ed): Conn's Current Therapy. W. B. Saunders Co, Philadelphia, 1985, pp 583–589.

Bock SA, May CD: Adverse reaction to food caused by sensitivity. In Middleton E, Reed CE, Ellis EF (eds): Allergy—Principles and Practice. C. V. Mosby Co, St. Louis, 1983, pp 1415–1427.

Sampson HA, Albergo R: Comparison of results of skin tests, RAST and double-blind, placebo-controlled food challenges in children with atopic dermatitis. Allergy Clin Immunol 74:26–33, 1984.

Tenth Annual Marabou Symposium: Food sensitivity. Nutr Rev 42: 65–140, 1984.

6 · ALLERGIC REACTION TO INSECT STING

Edward W. Hein
CLEVELAND CLINIC FOUNDATION

DEFINITION AND DIAGNOSTIC CRITERIA

An allergic reaction to an insect sting is an immunologic response (either local or systemic) to one or more of the components of the insect venom. Local reactions are the most common response to insect sting and consist of mild redness, pain, and swelling at the sting site. This type of reaction lasts several hours and then disappears. Occasionally, moderate to severe local reactions extend to larger areas and last for days. Most local reactions are not immunologic in nature but are caused by toxins in the venom. Other toxic symptoms include nausea, vomiting, diarrhea, headache, dizziness, and convulsions.

Severe allergic or systemic reactions begin with similar symptoms but then rapidly progress to hives, swelling, difficulty in breathing, asthma, laryngospasm, or fainting due to a sudden severe drop in blood pressure. These symptoms are typical of those seen in anaphylaxis from any cause.

PATHOPHYSIOLOGY

Members of the Hymenoptera order are responsible for most severe allergic reactions to stinging insects. The Apidae, which include honeybees and bumblebees, are docile and sting in self-defense. Their stingers are barbed and are left behind after stinging, which results in death of the insect. The Vespidae, which include yellow jackets, hornets, and wasps, have smooth stingers and sting multiple times. Fire ants are responsible for severe allergic reactions in areas of the Gulf Coast and southeastern United States.

Other biting insects including mosquito, flea, black fly, chigger, bedbug, kissing bug, sand fly, and deer fly can also cause hypersensitivity reactions. Most of these reactions are local, occur immediately, and are due to toxins. The other reactions are delayed and use non-IgE–immune mechanisms in causing tissue damage. It has been difficult to demonstrate specific IgE antibody against these insects.

The Hymenoptera venom contains many nonallergenic amines and peptides (i.e., histamines and kinins), which have inflammatory and vasoactive properties contributing to the local sting reaction. In allergic sting reactions, allergens in the venom interact with specific IgE antibody to cause problems. The most common venom allergens are phospholipase A, hyaluronidase, acid phosphatase, antigen 5, and melitin. There are differences among insect venom proteins; however, immunologic cross-reactivity has been noted among the vespid venoms.

Patients who are allergic to stinging insects have large amounts of insect-specific allergic antibody (IgE) on the surface of their basophils and tissue-bound mast cells. Upon exposure, the venom allergen interacts with specific IgE antibody to signal the mast cell or basophil to release mediators (histamine, leukotrienes, prostaglandins, kinins, and so forth). This stimulates smooth muscle contraction, vasodilation, and mucus production. Edema, bronchospasm, hypotension, urticaria, anaphylaxis, and ultimately death from cardiovascular failure can occur if there is no medical intervention.

CLINICAL ASPECTS

Reactions to stinging insects may occur in any person whether or not he or she has an allergic background. About 0.4% of the general population has significant allergic reactions to insect stings, but only 25% of these people have atopic histories. Each year 40 to 50 people die because of severe reactions from anaphylactic shock after a sting. This number may be higher in that a significant number of people who die of myocardial infarction or other unexplained deaths have RAST (radioallergosorbent test) evidence of sensitization to Hymenoptera venom. Twenty per cent of the general population have RAST or skin test evidence of sensitization to Hymenoptera venom. This suggests that venom sensitization is common but transient in many of these people and that it often disappears after a few years. Nobody knows the actual risk of severe reaction and positive skin tests. Patients with both a previous history of large local sting reactions and positive skin tests have a 5% to 10% risk of having future systemic sting reactions. Most significantly, patients who have both a history of systemic sting reaction and positive skin tests have a 50% risk of having future systemic sting reactions. Therefore, it is important to recognize the serious potential of even mild generalized symptoms and to make certain that patients with systemic insect sensitivity receive appropriate medical management.

MANAGEMENT

PLAN

When a patient suffers an adverse reaction to an insect sting, the short-term goals are to minimize the size of the reaction and the degree of suffering. The long-term goals are to prevent generalized systemic reactions either by avoiding stings or by interfering with the immune response pharmacologically or immunologically.

NONPHARMACOLOGIC MEASURES

Acute local sting reactions are treated symptomatically. If the stinger is still present, the first step is to remove it by "flicking" it out with a knife blade or similar instrument, taking great care not to squeeze the venom sac and thereby inject more venom into the site. Ice should be applied immediately to the sting site. Folk remedies such as rubbing mud, baking soda, or Adolph's Meat Tenderizer on the sting site have been recommended. No controlled studies have been done to evaluate their effectiveness. If the patient develops hives or other systemic symptoms (breathing difficulties, lightheadedness, palpitations), he or she should go immediately to the nearest emergency room for treatment.

DRUG THERAPY

Patients who are stung find that oral antihistamines such as diphenhydramine hydrochloride (Benadryl), 2 mg/kg (up to 25 mg) or hydroxyzine (Atarax), 0.1 mg/kg (up to 20 mg) help reduce itching and swelling. Antihistamines should be continued for two to three days after the sting to prevent recurrence of swelling. When reactions are extremely large and painful, oral steroids may help reduce swelling. Prednisone, 20 to 40 mg taken each morning, may be useful for several days. Patients who suffer systemic sting reactions or anaphylaxis require prompt medical attention. Antihistamines are adequate to treat generalized cutaneous reactions but alone are ineffective against the threat of progressive anaphylaxis. Epinephrine, intravenous fluids, oxygen, steroids, and bronchodilators may also be needed to relieve symptoms. See Sect. X, Chap. 1 for more specific information on treatment of systemic allergic reactions and anaphylaxis.

These medications should be used cautiously in patients who suffer from cardiovascular diseases, hypertension, diabetes, thyroid problems, and seizure disorders, since the side effects may aggravate these conditions.

EVALUATION

Patients who suffer generalized sting reactions should undergo an evaluation by a well-trained, qualified allergist to see whether they are allergic to stinging insects and whether immunotherapy would be helpful in minimizing or preventing these reactions.

The diagnosis of stinging-insect allergy is generally self-evident. Unless the stinger is found, most people cannot identify the specific insect. Therefore, allergy testing is done with venom concentrations from honeybee, wasp, white-faced hornet, yellow jacket, and yellow-faced hornet. In earlier years testing was done with whole insect bodies; however, controlled studies have shown that these extracts are unreliable and do not distinguish allergic from nonallergic individuals. Now, insect skin-testing extracts contain venom concentrations because they yield a more reliable diagnosis. Allergy skin testing is done first by the scratch or prick method, with a venom concentration of 1.0 μg/ml. If results are negative, a series of intradermal tests is done, starting with venom concentrations of 0.001 μg/ml. The testing is repeated with increasing concentrations until 1 mg/ml is reached or a positive skin test is noted. A negative control with diluent and a positive control with histamine are used. When skin testing is conducted with concentrations greater than 1 μg/ml, nonspecific reactions can occur because the venom concentrations cause nonimmunologic mast-cell mediator release.

In vitro tests are also available for the diagnosis of stinging-insect allergy. IgE-specific antibodies have been measured by RAST and by histamine release from leukocytes. RAST testing may miss 15% to 20% of patients who may be allergic by provocation testing and have positive venom skin tests. Histamine release from leukocytes is generally a costly and time-consuming laboratory procedure too cumbersome for routine diagnostic work. These methods of allergy testing are used in the research setting or when skin testing cannot be done.

PREVENTIVE MEASURES

For patients sensitive to stings, simple precautions decrease the risk of being stung. Food and odors attract insects; therefore, garbage should be well wrapped. Insect-sensitive patients should be wary of outdoor cooking and eating. They should wear leather shoes and slacks when walking in grass or fields, and gloves when gardening. Perfumes, cosmetics, and hair sprays should be avoided. Brightly colored clothing, especially flowery designs, should be avoided. Insect hives in the home or the work environment should be removed. When in the presence of a stinging insect, patients must remain calm.

Some of our patients have found that using large amounts of vitamin B_{12} makes them less attractive to insects. Others have found that Skin-So-Soft (Avon) bath oil repels insects. Controlled studies have not been done to validate these observations.

Patients with serious allergic reactions to stinging insects should always carry medical kits containing epinephrine and an antihistamine. ANA-KIT, marketed by Holister-Steir, contains a syringe loaded with 0.5 cc of epinephrine 1:1000 and several tablets of chlorpheniramine maleate. Also a spring-loaded syringe of epinephrine called Epi-Pen is available in 0.3-cc loads for adolescent and adult patients and 0.15 cc for children. The Epi-Pen is especially helpful for patients who may fear using a standard syringe and needle. If these medications are used, the patient should go immediately to the emergency room for further care, since epinephrine has a short duration of action.

Venom immunotherapy has been shown to provide protection for over 95% of patients with histories of sting anaphylaxis who are subsequently restung while on maintenance therapy. All adults who have histories of systemic reactions and positive allergy tests (skin testing or RAST) are candidates for venom immunotherapy. Therapy is initiated in small doses, beginning with a concentration tenfold more dilute than the one for which the patient had a positive skin-test response or at 0.001 μg/ml. The incremental doses are increased at each injection until a maximum dose of 100 mg is reached. Since the lower concentrations of venom extract are unstable after a few days, our patients receive the entire series of injections at a single visit until the more stable concentrations are reached. When 1.0 cc of the maximum concentration (100 μg/ml) is reached, patients continue on a monthly maintenance program. At this time there is no criterion to determine when to discontinue immunotherapy. Therefore, patients who start venom immunotherapy use it for the rest of their lives.

In children, the indications for immunotherapy are slightly modified. The risk of systemic reaction in children with a history of generalized cutaneous reaction to stings is only 10% as compared with 40% to 60% in the adult population. The incidence of severe systemic reactions in children with milder reactions is less than 1%. Therefore, only children who have respiratory distress or syncope associated with allergic sting reactions are considered for immunotherapy.

Controlled studies showing the effectiveness of immunotherapy with extracts of the biting insects are lacking; therefore, this is not recommended.

Reactions to venom immunotherapy occur no more frequently than those seen with other allergens. Systemic reactions occur in 5% to 15% of patients during the induction phase regardless of the regimen used. They are less common with the higher doses. Large local reactions occur in 50% of these patients, especially in the mid-dose range. These reactions do not indicate an increased risk of systemic reactions with large doses, and the best way to overcome them, unless they are extreme or involve a joint, is to proceed with the prescribed regimen so as to achieve higher doses and better immunity without undue delay. Serious side effects and toxicity from long-term therapy are unknown, although experience with beekeepers who are repeatedly stung and with patients who have received venom immunotherapy for several years suggests that there are none.

SOCIOECONOMIC ASPECTS OF MANAGEMENT

For patients who suffer systemic or generalized allergic reactions to insects stings, the suffering, medical costs, lost school- or workdays, and impact on their families can be very significant and costly. Fortunately, most people who are stung experience local burning, pain, redness, itching, and swelling only. For the smaller number who have more serious allergic reactions, medical treatment is available and its cost is justified, so that this problem is less life-threatening and better tolerated than it used to be.

REFERENCES

Golden DBK, Valentine MD: Insect sting allergy. Ann Allergy 53:444–449, 1984.

Lichtenstein LM, Valentine MD, Sobotka AK: Insect allergy: the state of the art. J Allergy Clin Immunol 64:5–12, 1979.

Patterson R, Valentine MD: Anaphylaxis and related allergic emergencies including reactions due to insect stings. JAMA 248:2632–2636, 1982.

Reisman RE: Insect allergy. *In* Middleton E, Reed CE, Ellis EF (eds): Allergy: Principles and Practice, 2nd ed. C.V. Mosby Co, St. Louis, 1983, pp 1361–1377.

7 · LABORATORY TESTING IN EVALUATION AND MANAGEMENT OF ALLERGIC DISEASES

Henry A. Homburger
MAYO CLINIC AND MAYO FOUNDATION

Relatively few laboratory tests are used routinely by clinicians in the evaluation and management of allergic diseases. Immunoassays for IgE and for allergen-specific IgE antibodies (IgE antibodies) are the mainstays. The usefulness of each test is determined by the clinical context in which it is applied. Tests for IgE and IgE antibodies are ordered principally for diagnosis. The results do not guide therapy or prognosis. The usefulness of test results is determined empirically by whether or not it is difficult to establish an accurate diagnosis of allergic disease or to decide on a particular therapeutic regimen on clinical grounds alone. In children and adults, IgE-mediated immediate hypersensitivity may be the primary mechanism of disease or a contributory factor. Although it is often possible to establish the presumptive diagnosis of an allergic disease on clinical grounds, definitive diagnosis and management by allergen immunotherapy require that the offending allergen(s) be identified. This is particularly important in instances of severe allergic disease that occur in individuals without an atopic background or family history of allergic disease: e.g., occupational asthma, food-induced anaphylaxis, and insect venom hypersensitivity.

CLINICAL APPLICATIONS

IGE TEST AND MULTI-ALLERGEN IGE ANTIBODY TEST

The primary care physician may have difficulty supporting the impression of allergic disease in infants and children. In this situation, measurement of IgE and detection of IgE antibodies to groups of allergens by the multi-allergen IgE antibody test are particularly useful as screening tests.

Table 1. SERUM IgE CONCENTRATIONS IN HEALTHY SUBJECTS

	IgE Concentrations, U/ml*		
	Mean	+1SD	+2SD
Newborn	<12	<12	<12
1–11 mo	<12	12	56
1 year	<12	15	83
2–4 yr	<12	33	130
5–80 yr	20	85	367

*Concentrations based on log transformed data.

The most sensitive laboratory indicator of allergy is an above-normal concentration of IgE in serum. The concentration increases progressively with age, reaching adult levels at approximately 7 years of age (Table 1). Since there is considerable overlap in the frequency distributions of serum concentrations in healthy children and adults compared with those in children and adults with clinically documented allergic disease, it is necessary to use a low cut-off concentration: e.g. the mean +1 standard deviation as a presumptive indicator of allergy to maximize the diagnostic sensitivity of the IgE test in the screening mode (Table 2). The magnitude of elevation of serum IgE concentration is directly proportional to the extent and severity of allergic disease. Individuals with limited end-organ involvement, e.g. those with rhinitis, typically have lesser elevations than those with multi-system disease, such as atopic dermatitis and rhinitis.

Before the multi-allergen IgE antibody test became available, the cost of performing several discrete tests for IgE antibodies in the screening mode was prohibitive. This is no longer true. As a screening test for respiratory allergy to inhalant allergens, the multi-allergen IgE antibody test is highly effective. Positive test results have a high predictive value for allergic disease and agree better with the clinician's impression of allergy than the results of other screening tests (Table 2).

At this time, allergen-immunosorbents of many different classes, such as pollens and foods, are commercially available for use in the multi-allergen IgE antibody test, but few published clinical investigations have documented the usefulness of this test except in the diagnosis of respiratory allergy to seasonal and perennial inhalants. The multi-allergen IgE antibody test should be used cautiously in other clinical situations such as suspected food allergy.

ESTABLISHING ALLERGEN SPECIFICITY BY IGE ANTIBODY TEST

The IgE antibody test is roughly equivalent to the skin test as a means to identify the allergen specificity of an allergic reaction. Each test has certain advantages. The IgE antibody test is convenient, it poses no risk to the patient, and its results are not affected by antihistamine or sympathomimetic drugs. The test is particularly useful in infants and children and in patients with widespread dermatitis or dermographism. It is clear, however, that the diagnostic sensitivity of the IgE antibody test diminishes with the time elapsed following exposure to an allergen. Also, some classes of allergens, e.g., dusts and molds, elicit synthesis of lower titers of IgE antibodies than others, e.g., pollen allergens and insect venoms.

The decision to identify the allergen(s) responsible for clinical signs of allergic disease may be tempered by knowledge that the treatment will not be influenced. For example, asthma is usually treated symptomatically and in many cases it is not possible to identify the allergens that provoke signs and symptoms. In most patients with allergic disease, however, knowledge of the offending allergens is useful clinically in order to decide which allergens should be included in an immunotherapy regimen (as in allergic rhinitis or insect venom sensitivity) or to facilitate avoidance of an allergen (as in cases of anaphylactic sensitivity to foods or drugs).

In respect to hypersensitivity to insect venom, many patients are not able to identify the insect(s) responsible for their allergic reactions. Tests for IgE antibodies are very useful to define the venom allergens to be included in an immunotherapy program, but in some cases the tests reveal antibodies not suspected from the medical history and the clinician must decide whether to include these additional venoms in the regimen. It is known that certain allergenic proteins in Hymenoptera venoms share cross-reactive antigens.

The diagnostic sensitivity of the single-allergen IgE antibody test varies directly with the magnitude of clinical sensitivity. In children and adults with respiratory allergy, positive test results are found in more than 90% of patients in whom allergen provocation tests are unequivocally positive. The same is true for anaphylactic sensitivity to foods, drugs, and insect venom allergens. The presence of detectable levels of IgE antibodies in serum in patients with anaphylactic sensitivity is strong evidence that these antibodies are implicated in causing disease. This is not always the case, however, in patients with lesser degrees of clinical sensitivity. For example, serum IgE antibodies to cow's milk proteins are common in children under 3 years of age, and the presence of IgE antibodies is not per se an indication of allergy to cow's milk.

Measurement of IgE antibodies by the single-allergen IgE antibody test is useful in many clinical situa-

Table 2. PREDICTIVE VALUES OF SCREENING LABORATORY TESTS

	Sensitivity (%)	Specificity (%)	Predictive Value of		
			Positive Test (%)	Negative Test (%)	Efficiency %
Multi-allergen IgE antibody test*	63	96	98	46	71
Combination of single-allergen IgE antibody tests†	64	92	96	50	71
Serum IgE >1SD for age	83	64	87	55	78
Serum IgE >2SD for age	49	76	86	33	56

*Allergens used were short ragweed pollen, timothy grass pollen, and *Dermatophagoides farinae*.
†Single allergens used were same as for multi-allergen test.

tions, including (1) evaluation of children and adults suspected of having allergic respiratory disease, to establish the diagnosis and to define the specificity of allergen sensitivity to pollens, dusts, fungal antigens, and foods; (2) evaluation of insect venom sensitivity; (3) evaluation of food allergy, to confirm the clinical impression of sensitivity to specific foods in patients with anaphylactic sensitivity; and (4) evaluation of suspected drug allergy, to confirm the diagnosis in patients with anaphylactic sensitivity.

There are clinical situations in which measurement of IgE antibodies by the single-allergen or multi-allergen test is not useful, including (1) evaluation of patients following immunotherapy, to assess whether there is residual clinical sensitivity to an allergen; (2) evaluation of insect venom–sensitive patients, to assess the risk of future anaphylactic reactions; and (3) screening for allergic disease before obtaining a thorough allergic disease history.

Typically, in patients treated with parenteral allergen immunotherapy, IgG antibodies are synthesized in high-titer, μg/ml concentrations. These antibodies are known to interfere with measurement of IgE antibodies, but the titers of IgG antibodies do not correlate well with the clinical response to treatment, nor do they indicate when treatment may be discontinued. As noted earlier, tests for IgE or IgE antibodies are not indicated to assess the response to allergen immunotherapy.

REFERENCES

Homburger HA, Yuninger JW: Laboratory testing in the diagnosis and management of allergic diseases. *In* Homburger HA, Batsakis JG (eds): Clinical Laboratory Annual. Appleton-Century-Crofts, E. Norwalk, CT, 1983, pp 351–388.

Liebman WM, Frick OL: Serum IgE levels and RAST for cow's milk protein—use in children with recurrent abdominal pain. Am J Dis Child 135:741–742, 1981.

Ownby DR, Anderson JA, Jacob GL, et al: Development and comparative evaluation of a multiple-antigen RAST as a screening test for inhalant allergy. J Allergy Clin Immunol 73:466–472, 1984.

8 · ALLERGEN IMMUNOTHERAPY

Joseph E. Kelleher, Jr.
John M. O'Loughlin
John A. Saryan
LAHEY CLINIC MEDICAL CENTER

DEFINITION

Allergen immunotherapy, also known as hyposensitization or desensitization, is a treatment used in patients with IgE-mediated respiratory disorders. It consists of injections of antigenic material to which the patient is sensitive. The first successful use of immunotherapy, reported by Noon and Freeman in 1911, was in grass-sensitive hay fever sufferers who were injected with extracts of grass pollen.

A number of immunologic changes have been shown to take place in patients undergoing immunotherapy. In 1935 Robert A. Cooke, the first American proponent of immunotherapy, discovered a blocking antibody in the sera of patients treated with immunotherapy that could inhibit the allergic reaction. This blocking antibody has since been identified as IgG. Blocking antibody titers do not always correlate with improvement in symptoms, and other mechanisms have now been identified, including a decrease in allergen-induced histamine release from basophils in vitro and generation of suppressor T lymphocytes, which decrease allergen-specific IgE synthesis. No one mechanism, however, can explain the clinical benefit seen in all patients.

INDICATIONS AND EFFICACY

Allergen immunotherapy is indicated in the treatment of IgE-mediated rhinitis and asthma. The primary goal is safe and effective relief of signs and symptoms caused by exposure to allergens. Achievement of this goal often involves several steps and considerations.

Foremost is the need to establish that the patient has an IgE-mediated disorder. A thorough history and physical examination are essential. Special attention is given to timing of symptoms, exacerbation of symptoms on exposure to potential allergens, and the patient's environment. Sensitivity to inhaled allergens is confirmed by skin testing. Prick testing is used initially and is followed by the more sensitive intradermal technique if results of the prick test to a suspected major allergen are negative. The radioallergosorbent test (RAST), which measures allergen-specific IgE in the blood, is used infrequently in very young children and in patients with diffuse skin diseases, such as eczema or dermographism.

The basic treatment of allergic rhinitis or allergic asthma involves avoidance of the offending allergens and in most instances use of medications to relieve symptoms. When results of these steps are unsatisfactory, immunotherapy should be considered an adjunct to the treatment program after reviewing the pros and cons with the patient. The potential benefit to be derived from immunotherapy needs to be weighed against such factors as the inconvenience of receiving frequent injections for several years, the expense involved, and the possibility of adverse reactions. Frequently, an intolerance to the side effects of antihistamines, decongestants, or intranasal corticosteroid agents necessitates the use of immunotherapy in allergic rhinitis. Secondary complications of allergic rhinitis, such as sinusitis, middle ear effusions, or nasal polyposis, may be improved with immunotherapy. Patients who have bronchial asthma with a major allergic component are candidates for immunotherapy, especially those who require corticosteroids either in frequent tapering doses or in daily maintenance doses. Immunotherapy should also be considered for allergic patients with frequent upper respiratory tract symptoms that may aggravate their asthma.

Many of the large number of allergens used for immunotherapy have been evaluated in controlled trials. Numerous studies have demonstrated the effectiveness of ragweed and grass pollens in placebo-controlled studies of patients with seasonal allergic rhinitis; improvement was noted in 80% to 90% of patients. Most studies emphasize the importance of using high doses of extract in treatment protocols. The results of treatment of patients with perennial allergic rhinitis are less impressive, but immunotherapy can still be an important part of the overall regimen. Several double-blind controlled studies have reported improvement in both symptoms and bronchial challenge with extracts of house dust, house dust mite, cat pelt, and (to a lesser extent) pollen in the treatment of patients with allergic asthma. Although mold antigens are included in immunotherapy by most allergists, controlled studies are lacking.

METHOD OF IMMUNOTHERAPY

Allergen immunotherapy consists of subcutaneous administration of gradually increasing doses of allergenic extracts of inhaled substances to which the patient has shown sensitivity. Patients given aqueous extracts of ragweed or grass pollens occasionally are unable to receive increasing doses of extract because of large local or possibly mild systemic reactions. In these instances, use of aqueous extracted alum-precipitated extracts (Center-Al), which are absorbed more slowly, often permit patients to receive more antigen while avoiding unwanted side effects. We use aqueous extracts primarily and treat patients with antigens that are impossible or difficult to avoid. Only those inhalant allergens that are implicated by history and confirmed by skin testing are included in treatment. If a patient has symptoms restricted to the spring but shows skin reactions to both ragweed and grass pollens, only the extract of grass pollen is used. Perennial allergens such as feathers and kapok usually are avoidable and are not included in immunotherapy. Animal dander allergen extract immunotherapy may be advocated by some and avoided by other allergists. Extracts of house dust and dust mite are used to treat perennial symptoms. The choice of pollen antigens used depends on the geographic locale. In New England, pollens from ragweed, grass, English plantain, and trees as well as mold spores are the major seasonal allergens.

Currently most extracts of allergens are measured either in protein nitrogen units (1 PNU = 1 μg protein nitrogen) or in weight:volume ratio, neither of which reflects antigenic potency; 1 cc of 10,000 PNU/ml roughly equals 1 cc of 1:50 wgt/vol strength allergenic extract. Extracts of ragweed are required to be labeled as to antigen E content. Efforts are under way to develop similar standardization for other allergens. We employ the PNU system in our own practice. The weakest solution is 10 PNU/ml, with tenfold increases to the strongest solution (10,000 PNU/ml). Most patients are initially given 0.05 ml of the 100 PNU/ml extract. If they show a marked skin test reaction by the prick method or with a dilute intradermal concentration of allergen, the starting dose is 0.05 ml of the 10 PNU/ml solution.

We usually give separate injections of each extract, such as mixed grasses, mixed trees, English plantain, ragweed, mixed molds, house dust, and mites. Administration of single extracts enables us to give the highest tolerable dose for each allergen. Patients whose extracts are sent to and administered at another physician's office follow the same schedule, but we may combine two pollen extracts, such as mixed grasses and mixed trees, in one vial to limit the number of vials.

The dosage schedule for all extracts is shown in Table 1. The dose of ragweed is usually held or reduced during the season between August 15 and the first frost because the combination of exposure to airborne pollen and dose of allergen may result in increased symptoms in some patients. In the spring, we occasionally reduce the dose of allergen in symptomatic patients with sensitivity to tree or grass pollen. Although most extracts of allergen are stable if kept refrigerated, potency is gradually lost with time. Therefore, when new extracts are mailed out, the maintenance dose is reduced by 50% and gradually built back up to prevent reactions.

Immunotherapy is given on a year-round basis. Perennial immunotherapy has consistently been shown to be more effective than preseasonal or coseasonal therapy. Injections are given weekly until the highest tolerated or maintenance dose is reached, and then given every two weeks. The usual maintenance dose is between 0.50 and 1.0 ml of the 10,000 PNU/ml strength, but in some patients this dose is unattainable because of adverse reactions. After one successful season with appreciably diminished symptoms, injections are given every three weeks, and later every four to six weeks. Some patients do not tolerate these increases and may need to be maintained at less than four-week intervals. Immunotherapy is usually given for three to five years. Currently there are no criteria to determine how long the patient will do well after stopping immunotherapy. If the patient is not improved after one to two years of therapy, the injection program is reassessed and often is discontinued.

Allergy injections should be given only when a physician is present. Before each injection, patients are asked whether any appreciable local or systemic reactions occurred with the previous injection (see "Adverse Reactions" below). A separate, disposable tuberculin syringe with a 26- or 27-gauge, 5/8-inch needle is used for each separate antigen or mixture. The vials of extract are color coded according to strength. The patient's schedule is checked and matched carefully with the correct vial of extract before administration. After the outer middle part of the upper arm is cleansed with alcohol, the patient is injected subcutaneously. Make certain that a blood vessel is not entered by first withdrawing the plunger of the syringe.

Table 1. SAMPLE SCHEDULE FOR ADMINISTRATION OF ALLERGEN EXTRACT

100 PNU/ml	1000 PNU/ml	10,000 PNU/ml
0.05 ml*	0.05 ml	0.05 ml
0.10 ml	0.10 ml	0.10 ml
0.20 ml	0.20 ml	0.15 ml
0.30 ml	0.30 ml	0.20 ml
0.40 ml	0.40 ml	0.25 ml
0.50 ml	0.50 ml	0.30 ml
0.60 ml	0.60 ml	0.35 ml
0.70 ml	0.70 ml	0.40 ml
		0.45 ml
		0.50 ml†

*Starting dose.
†Maintenance dose.

ADVERSE REACTIONS AND CONTRAINDICATIONS

The two basic types of adverse reactions to immunotherapy are localized and systemic. These reactions can occur immediately or several hours later, but most occur during the initial build-up period before attaining the maintenance dose. The most common of these reactions is the immediate wheal-and-flare reaction, which occurs within minutes at the site of the injection and subsides within a few hours. In our judgment, swelling greater than 2 cm warrants either holding or reducing the next dose because of the risk of a subsequent anaphylactic reaction. Further increases in the dose of extract are given cautiously and are often reduced from 0.10 to 0.05 ml during the build-up period. Delayed local reactions appear as itchy, erythematous swellings within a few hours after injection. Although these reactions may become painful, they do not lead to systemic reactions. Patients are treated symptomatically with application of ice and administration of antihistamines and aspirin. The degree of discomfort caused by these reactions may require a reduction in dose.

Sometimes patients experience an exacerbation of allergic symptoms several hours after injection of an allergen. If these occur with any consistency they should be considered delayed systemic reactions requiring a reduction in dosage. These reactions must be acknowledged because they result in considerable morbidity and some treatment failures. The most serious of the adverse reactions induced by immunotherapy is the immediate systemic or anaphylactic reaction. The possibility of such a reaction is the main reason why patients are told to remain in the office for at least 20 minutes after receiving their allergy injection(s). The description and treatment of anaphylaxis are well outlined in Section X, Chapter 1. Any physician administering injections of allergens must be prepared to treat anaphylaxis. When a patient receiving immunotherapy experiences such a reaction, subsequent injection of allergens is delayed two to three weeks and all doses of allergen are reduced 50%. Caution is exercised when approaching the dose previously associated with induction of anaphylaxis.

We do not give injections to patients with a fever or to asthmatic patients during an exacerbation. No evidence is available to establish any long-term side effects from administration of aqueous extracts, including harm to the fetus in a pregnant woman receiving immunotherapy. We usually do not initiate immunotherapy during pregnancy because of the increased risk of anaphylaxis during the build-up period, but continue maintenance immunotherapy throughout gestation.

REASONS FOR FAILURE

The reasons why immunotherapy may not be successful are numerous. Not instituting or adequately maintaining environmental controls may result in the apparent failure of immunotherapy or in relapse of symptoms. The continued presence or new acquisition of furry pets in the home is the most common source of this problem. Occasionally patients experience a new sensitivity to an allergen that is not in their treatment regimen. Addition of the new allergen to the immunotherapy program should alleviate this problem. Overreliance on the results of skin tests or RAST without consideration of the patient's history can result in an incorrect choice of antigens and a lack of symptomatic improvement. Inadequate doses of extracts of allergen often lead to treatment failures, as does use of extracts lacking biologic potency. An incorrect diagnosis may also lead to an apparent failure of immunotherapy. Patients with vasomotor rhinitis or intrinsic asthma do not benefit from immunotherapy. Occasionally patients may have unrealistic expectations as to the amount of improvement they will receive from immunotherapy. Complete cures are seldom realized, and months of treatment may be required before improvement is apparent.

OUTLOOK

In the future, we are likely to see safer and more effective forms of immunotherapy. Several newer extracts, including glutaraldehyde-treated allergens (polymerized) and formaldehyde-treated allergens (allergoids), have been effective in controlled trials but are not yet available for clinical use. Both retain their immunogenicity but are far less allergenic than conventional aqueous extracts and less likely to cause local or systemic reactions. Improved standardization of currently used extracts of aqueous allergens should ensure their potency and increase the success rates of immunotherapy.

REFERENCES

Davies RJ: Immunotherapy in respiratory allergy. Thorax 38:401–407, 1983.
Lichtenstein LM, Valentine MD, Norman PS: A reevaluation of immunotherapy. Am Rev Respir Dis 129:657–659, 1984.
Norman PS: An overview of immunotherapy: implications for the future. J Allergy Clin Immunol 65:87–96, 1980.
Patterson R: Clinical efficacy of allergen immunotherapy. J Allergy Clin Immunol 64:155–158, 1979.

9 · THE HYPER-IgE RECURRENT INFECTION SYNDROME

Dennis R. Ownby
HENRY FORD HOSPITAL

DEFINITION

The syndrome of hyperimmunoglobulin E and recurrent infections is a rare form of primary immunodeficiency. The diagnostic features are recurrent and chronic staphylococcal abcesses of the skin, lungs, and other sites associated with serum IgE levels greater than ten times the upper limits of normal (greater than 2000 IU/ml in most laboratories). The recurrent infections typically start during the first year of life and continue.

It should be stressed that the hyper-IgE syndrome

is distinct from the more common clinical problem of patients with secondarily infected atopic dermatitis. The major difference is the frequency, severity, and chronicity of the staphylococcal abscesses at sites beyond the skin. Virtually all patients with the hyper-IgE syndrome will have had multiple episodes of staphylococcal pneumonia and other severe infections. They often also have a history of a pruritic eczematoid rash in infancy, but the distribution is not typical of that found in atopic dermatitis.

Job's syndrome was originally described as occurring in fair-skinned, red-haired girls with "cold" staphylococcal abscesses. Since patients with Job's syndrome also have recurrent deep infections, eczematoid dermatitis, and elevated IgE levels, there is little reason to consider Job's syndrome and the hyper-IgE syndrome as distinct clinical entities. The term Job's syndrome may be more poetic, but the term hyper-IgE recurrent infection syndrome is preferable because of its descriptive nature.

PATHOPHYSIOLOGY

The precise pathogenesis of the hyper-IgE syndrome is unknown. Affected individuals have variable degrees of increased IgE antibody formation, decreased IgG and IgM antibody formation, decreased cell-mediated immunity, and decreased monocyte and neutrophil chemotaxis. None of these immune abnormalities are pathognomonic of the syndrome.

The validity of all hypotheses for the pathogenesis of the hyper-IgE syndrome must await further studies.

CLINICAL ASPECTS

The major clinical features of the hyper-IgE syndrome are summarized in Table 1. The syndrome is rare, fewer than 100 cases having been reported. Patients are usually affected with recurring staphylococcal infections in infancy and continue to have recurring and chronic infections throughout life. While survival well into adulthood is possible, patients may succumb early in life, usually because of recurrent pulmonary infections. Approximately equal numbers of males and females are affected and no racial predominance has been noted.

Table 1. MAJOR CLINICAL FEATURES OF HYPER-IgE AND RECURRENT INFECTION SYNDROME

Present in Virtually all Patients (90 + %)
Recurrent bacterial infections, usually staphyloccocal, involving skin and lungs; other sites may be involved
Elevated serum IgE, 2000 IU/ml
Infections start during first year of life

Commonly Present (50 + %)
Coarse facial features
Cold abscesses
Mucocutaneous candidiasis
Eosinophilia
Current (or history of) eczematoid rash
Elevated erythrocyte sedimentation rate
Abnormal neutrophil chemotaxis
IgE antistaphylococcal antibody

Other
No propensity for either sex or any race
Rarely, common allergic disease such as allergic rhinitis or asthma

The most common major clinical problem is the recurring sinopulmonary infections. Most patients with hyper-IgE have recurrent bronchitis and frequently develop pneumonias from *Staphylococcus aureus* or *Haemophilus influenzae*. Other organisms may be involved less commonly, such as *Streptoccocus* or *Pneumococcus*. The episodes of pneumonia are often complicated by pneumatoceles and empyema. The pneumatoceles resolve slowly and may become chronic. Secondary infections with less common pathogens such as *Aspergillus* may occur in previously damaged areas of the lungs, further complicating the clinical course. Surgical intervention for drainage of empyemas and resection of areas of chronic pneumatoceles are often necessary.

Cutaneous staphylococcal abscesses are the most common finding in the hyper-IgE syndrome. Chronic mucocutaneous candidiasis with onychomycosis and oral and vaginal infections also occur commonly. In addition to these skin infections, younger patients may have an eczematoid dermatitis, usually on the scalp, behind the ears, and in other flexural areas such as the axillae. The rash frequently becomes secondarily infected. Almost two thirds of patients with the hyper-IgE syndrome are said to have coarse facial features: a broad nasal bridge, a prominent nose, and irregular cheeks and jaws.

A variety of other problems have been reported in association with the hyper-IgE syndrome, including osteogenesis imperfecta tarda, cranial synostosis, membranoproliferative glomerulonephritis, and systemic lupus erythematosus. The relationship of these to the syndrome is unclear.

LABORATORY FINDINGS

Total white blood cell counts range from normal to markedly elevated, often with eosinophilia. The latter is usually modest but may become marked at the time of infections. Anemia is sometimes present, presumably related to the chronic infections. Also related to the chronic infections is the typical finding of an elevated erythrocyte sedimentation rate (30 to 60 mm/hr, Westergren).

Evaluation of the humoral portion of the immune system usually shows normal or mildly elevated levels of IgG, IgA, and IgM and a marked elevation of serum IgE. Serum IgE levels are typically several thousand IV/ml, although this feature may not be fully developed in infants and young chidren. Total serum IgD levels are also elevated in patients with hyper-IgE, but the significance of this is not known.

The elevated IgE is polyclonal, with both kappa and lambda chains. Consistent with this, patients often have strongly positive immediate wheal-and-flare responses to common allergens. Somewhat surprising considering this immediate sensitivity to common allergens is the lack of symptoms typical of allergic disease. As previously noted, a large proportion of the IgE may be specific for *Candida* and staphylococcal and other bacterial and fungal antigens. It has not been possible to correlate directly the presence or absence of anti-*Candida* IgE and clinical mucocutaneous candidiasis.

The normal serum concentrations of IgG, IgA, and IgM do not indicate totally normal function of these antibody classes. Levels of antibodies to common immunogens such as diphtheria and tetanus are often low and reimmunization produces a poor anamnestic response. Serum complement studies are usually normal.

MANAGEMENT

Since the precise pathogenesis remains unknown, no specific form of therapy has been developed. A number of experimental attempts at immunologic augmentation have been tried in patients with hyper-IgE, but none has proved of value. Until a specific form of therapy becomes available, the mainstays of treatment are local care, appropriate antibiotics, and prompt surgical drainage. As with all chronic and potentially fatal diseases, a good relationship between the patient and physician is desirable.

Bronchitis and Pneumonia. The most significant clinical problems requiring treatment are the recurring episodes of bronchitis and pneumonia. These episodes almost always require intravenous antibiotics for two or more weeks. Initial therapy should be directed against staphylococci and *Haemophilus* sp. Current appropriate antibiotics include nafcillin, oxacillin, cefazolin, cefamandole, ampicillin, and gentamicin, alone or in combination. The choice of antibiotic should be reviewed as soon as culture results are known. The length of therapy should be individualized, but physicians must remember that these patients do not respond to treatment as rapidly as normal individuals.

The pulmonary infections and the areas of lung damage by infections may become infected with unusual pathogens such as *Aspergillus* and other fungal species. These unusual pathogens may require lung biopsy or surgical excision for proper diagnosis and treatment.

Abscesses. Other serious infections that may occur include abscesses within the abdomen or at other sites. Paradoxically, patients with relatively large abscesses may not appear seriously ill, because of their generally poor local inflammatory responses. The physician must carefully consider any change in the patient's condition.

Patients with the hyper-IgE syndrome frequently require surgical drainage of abscesses. Because of the reduced evidence of inflammation, the threshold for surgical intervention must be lowered for these patients. Relatively benign-appearing masses may be found to be large collections of pus or matts of infected lymph nodes when surgically explored. Early identification and rapid therapy with antibiotics, plus adequate surgical drainage, are the best methods for reducing morbidity.

Skin Infections. Minor skin infections frequently result in the formation of small abscesses. Local care and appropriate oral antibiotics are usually adequate for these minor infections. Chronic oral antistaphylococcal antibiotics may help reduce the frequency and severity of these cutaneous abscesses, but the effectiveness of chronic antibiotics in preventing or reducing more severe infections has not been systematically investigated. The risk of chronic antibiotic treatment seems small, however, compared with the potential benefit.

The chronic eczematoid dermatitis found in patients with hyper-IgE responds poorly to most common treatments such as topical corticosteroids. Treatment of suprainfections of staphylococci or *Candida* may temporarily ameliorate these skin eruptions. The dermatitis usually improves spontaneously with age.

An additional site of infectious problems is the mouth. Patients with hyper-IgE should receive good dental care to reduce gingivitis, caries, and occasional periodontal abscesses.

Another common infectious problem for patients with hyper-IgE is candidiasis. Onychomycosis and oral and vaginal candidiasis typically respond to antifungal drugs such as ketoconazole.

EXPERIMENTAL DRUGS

A number of experimental approaches have been tried to improve the immune function of patients with hyper-IgE, including treatment with levamisole, ascorbic acid, transfer factor, thymopoietin, and both H_1 and H_2 antihistamines. The only one of these evaluated in a prospective double-blind trial was levamisole, and it was ineffective. None of the other experimental therapies can be recommended on the basis of current limited knowledge.

HEREDITY AND FAMILY COUNSELING

Another difficult problem is counseling the family. Parents may be concerned about the risk of hyper-IgE in subsequent offspring. Similarly, as patients become adults, they may be concerned about the risk for their own children. There is little genetic information about the risk of hyper-IgE. Cases in which two siblings were affected and transmission took place from parent to child have been reported. In one series of 20 patients, seven instances of familial occurrence were found. The best genetic hypothesis would be of an autosomal dominant form of inheritance with incomplete penetrance. Considering the seriousness of this condition, the genetic risks, and the lack of any method of prenatal diagnosis, individuals should be cautious in deciding to have children or additional children.

REFERENCES

Buckley RH, Becker WG: Abnormalities in the regulation of human IgE synthesis. Immunol Rev 41:288–314, 1978.
Donabedian H, Gallin JI: The hyperimmunoglobulin E recurrent-infection (Job's) syndrome. A review of the NIH experience and the literature. Medicine 62:195–208, 1983.
Merten DF, Buckley RH, Pratt PC, et al: Hyperimmunoglobulinemia E syndrome: radiographic observations. Radiology 132:71–78, 1979.

DISEASES OF THE SKIN

HERBERT B. CHRISTIANSON
MARILYN RAY

1 · MANAGEMENT OF DECUBITUS AND LEG ULCERS

Donald J. Miech
MARSHFIELD CLINIC

Leg and decubitus ulcers are the most common ulcers of the skin. They may be traumatic, vascular, infectious, neoplastic, drug induced, metabolic, hematologic, or neurologic.

The decubitus ulcer is a traumatic ulcer produced by prolonged pressure. Seventy-five per cent of leg ulcers result from venous stasis; most of the remainder are from arterial insufficiency. However, many have components of both venous stasis and arterial insufficiency. Ulcerating infections can be caused by bacteria or deep fungi such as blastomycosis, coccidioidomycosis, sporotrichosis, cryptococcosis, and maduromycosis. Ulcerating neoplasms include metastases, Kaposi's sarcoma, and squamous cell carcinoma. A rare form of squamous cell carcinoma (epithelioma cuniculatum) on the plantar surface of the foot can be confused with a nonhealing diabetic or infectious ulcer. By their vegetative appearance, drug-induced ulcers from halogens (iodides and bromides) can often resemble a deep fungal infection.

Internal causes of skin ulcers include vasculitis and metabolic, hematologic, and neurologic diseases. Pyoderma gangrenosum, a relentless ulcerative dermatosis, is often diagnosed only after excluding other causes and observing the clinical behavior of the ulcers.

DIAGNOSIS

The clinical history and findings are most important in making a diagnosis. Varicosities and stasis pigmentation suggest venous stasis. Arthritis may suggest rheumatoid vasculitis, systemic lupus erythematosus, or pyoderma gangrenosum.

A biopsy of the edge of the ulcer with intact epithelium may be very helpful in establishing a diagnosis. However, if ischemia is present, a biopsy may extend the ulcer and delay healing. A biopsy is necessary if deep infection, such as mycobacteria or deep fungi, is suspected. A biopsy submitted for culture of the tissue produces a much greater yield than a swab. Also, histologic studies with special stains may serve to identify the organism even before the result of the bacterial culture has returned.

Occasionally blood concentrations for bromides or iodides may uncover a suspected halogen-induced ulcer. A complete medical work-up is indicated for patients with possible hematologic, metabolic, or neurologic diseases. Vascular studies, including vascular flow studies and even arteriograms and venograms, may be important in assessing the extent of venous or arterial impairment.

All ulcers are colonized by bacteria that may thrive under creams and ointments. A culture for aerobic bacterial pathogens rarely adds significant information. Many leg ulcers and decubitus ulcers contain gram-negative pathogens, but antibacterial treatment may merely result in resistant organisms. Many ulcers, especially the vascular or pressure type, need very little antibiotic care unless there is an associated cellulitis.

TREATMENT

The basic principle of treatment is to provide a favorable environment for wound healing—no more, no less!

General Measures. The general measures to be taken involve prevention of any further trauma to the ulcer and keeping the ulcer clean and free of infection. In preventing further trauma one must consider pressure, such as external pressure seen in decubitus ulcers or pressure from localized tissue swelling in the venous ulcer. Many new types of mattresses and beds have been invented to relieve pressure, but nothing replaces good nursing care with frequent turning of the patient. Having the patient lie on a sheet-covered sheepskin may provide sufficient pressure reduction to benefit the decubitus ulcer.

The venous stasis ulcer does not heal if the affected limb continues to swell with stasis edema. Leg elevation and, in many cases, elastic support are the most helpful measures one can prescribe for the healing. One of the most difficult tasks in treating stasis ulcers is to convince the patient that the affected leg *must* be elevated most of the time.

Elastic support of stasis ulcers may be difficult if the ulcer is over a bony prominence. Pulling elastic hose over an ulcer may further traumatize it, but use of elastic or Coban wrap may be helpful during such times.

Specific Measures. A compress to the ulcer can help clean away the fibrin and debris that build up in the ulcer and also can eliminate a substantial amount of the bacterial load. If the ulcer is superficial, cleansing with hydrogen peroxide may be all that is necessary. Compresses of povidone-iodine or dilutions thereof are widely used and are generally quite effective. Occasionally an allergic contact dermatitis develops around the ulcer. The redness and itching that develop can be distinguished from cellulitus. Despite their lack of antibacterial activity, compresses of saline are also widely used to help keep the ulcer base moist and to cleanse the debris. It is important to reduce the bacterial count in an ulcer. Studies have shown a correlation between reduction of bacterial count and healing of leg ulcers. I prefer to use acetic acid compresses (0.5% to 1.0%) in treating patients with the chronic stasis ulcer. These can be left on the ulcer for one to two hours twice daily. Petrolatum should be used to protect the surrounding epithelium, and the compress should be applied to the ulcer *only*. If the patient complains of pain from the acetic acid, a few drops of 1% lidocaine solution without epinephrine can be applied to the ulcer before applying the compress. The acidic environment is hostile to many bacterial pathogens, and cutaneous sensitization has not been observed with acetic acid.

After the compress, a variety of agents have been used. If the ulcer contains extensive fibrotic debris, enzymatic debridement with sutilains ointment (Travase) or the combination of fibrinolysin and desoxyribonuclease (Elase) may be effective. If the ulcer is exudative, dextranomer (Debrisan) granules can be useful. Because of their abrasive nature, the polyethylene granules must not be used in an area of friction or rubbing. When changing a dressing, the granules can be flushed easily from the ulcer, with minimal manipulation of the tissues. One must also consider the size of the ulcer, for dextranomer's main disadvantage is its cost.

For the uncomplicated ulcer, application of 0.25% aqueous gentian violet will suffice after the compress. Its antiseptic effect and rare sensitization make it a reasonable choice, although it may leave the ulcer dry and crusted.

Antibiotic ointments or creams applied to the ulcer produce relatively little antibiotic effect. One study actually showed little difference in healing time between application of silver sulfadiazine (Silvadene) cream and of its vehicle without Silvadene. There is also the increased risk of sensitization in the chronically inflamed area that often surrounds leg ulcers. A topical steroid cream of intermediate potency, such as 0.1% triamcinolone cream, may be used for the common surrounding dermatitis. Care must be taken not to apply the cream to the ulcer, since this can retard the natural healing process.

Semipermeable (oxygen-permeable) polyurethane membranes (such as OpSite) developed for surgical use have been shown to be helpful in some pressure sores and leg ulcers. The occlusive effect can provide significant pain relief. Some animal studies support the benefits of occlusive dressings in wound healing. However, the adhesive material in the dressing can sometimes pull off surrounding intact epithelium when the dressing is removed. Self-treatment with OpSite is almost impossible.

An encouraging recent treatment for ulcers is the hydrocolloid dressing (Stomahesive and Varihesive originally designed for stomal care). DuoDerm (oxygen impermeable) has been developed more recently specifically for leg and decubitus ulcers. It is thinner and more pliable than the stomal dressings and can adhere to the ulcer for as long as seven days. Initial studies show that regeneration of epithelium occurs at about the same rate with wet dressings as with DuoDerm. Most patients reported convenience in management and substantial relief of pain with the hydrocolloid dressings. If adhesive effects are not wanted, Vigilon dressing may be substituted. In our clinic, the hydrocolloid dressing has replaced both the gelcast bandage (Unna boot) and daily compresses in many patients because of increased ease of management and relief of pain.

Skin grafting may be beneficial to reduce the duration of hospital stay. If the ulcer is greater than 3 cm in diameter and has a good granulating base, grafting may be the most appropriate treatment.

Therapy for both pressure and leg ulcers must be tailored to the individual and should be directed at the underlying disease process. The goal of local therapy is to provide an optimal environment for the body's normal healing process.

REFERENCES

Alper JC, Welch EA, Ginsberg M, et al: Moist wound healing under a vapor permeable membrane. J Am Acad Dermatol 8:347–353, 1983.

Friedman SJ, Su WPD: Management of leg ulcers. Am Fam Physician 27:219–226, 1983.

Friedman SJ, Su WPD: Management of leg ulcers with hydrocolloid occlusive dressing. Arch Dermatol 120:1329–1336, 1984.

Geronemus RG, Mertz PM, Eaglstein WH: Wound healing: the effects of topical antimicrobial agents. Arch Dermatol 115:1311–1314, 1979.

Lookingbill DP, Miller SH, Knowles RC: Bacteriology of chronic leg ulcers. Arch Dermatol 114:1765–1768, 1978.

Reddy MP: Decubitus ulcers: principles of prevention and management. Geriatrics 38:55–61, 1983.

2 · ATOPIC DERMATITIS AND NEURODERMATITIS

Tomasz F. Mroczkowski
Patricia K. Farris
Lynn A. Anderson
TULANE UNIVERSITY
SCHOOL OF MEDICINE
in affiliation with
OCHSNER CLINIC AND ALTON OCHSNER MEDICAL
FOUNDATION

Atopic Dermatitis

DEFINITION

Atopic dermatitis is a common skin disorder often associated with a family history of asthma and hay fever. It is believed to result from a lowered cutaneous threshold to pruritus.

PATHOPHYSIOLOGY

Theories attempting to explain the mechanism of the disease can be categorized into three major groups: the inborn error of metabolism, the psychosomatic theory, and the immunologic theory. The last-named is gaining increasing recognition since the vast majority of patients with atopic dermatitis display some immunologic dysfunction. Noted abnormalities include elevated serum IgE levels and functional impairment of T lymphocytes. How these immunologic abnormalities relate to the clinical presentation and pathogenesis of atopic dermatitis remains uncertain.

CLINICAL ASPECTS

Atopic dermatitis is divided into four phases: infantile, childhood, adolescent, and adult. The infantile form has its onset between 2 and 4 months of age and may disappear or become less severe by age 2 to 3 years. It begins with eczematous lesions characterized by erythema, papules, vesicles, oozing, and crusting. Initially, the cheeks and forehead are involved with central facial sparing. Subsequently, the eruption extends to the scalp, trunks, buttocks, and extremities. Associated clinical findings include Dennie-Morgan line, which is an accentuation of the infraorbital skin fold, and the "allergic shiner," which is hyperpigmentation of the periorbital skin. An additional finding in some patients is the "headlight sign" that results from pallor in the central facial region.

In the childhood form, which lasts from 2 years of age to puberty, the lesions tend to be less eczematous and drier. The eruption is characterized by papules that merge and coalesce into plaques. The eruption is located predominantly in the flexural areas, including the posterior auricular fold, neck, antecubital and popliteal fossae, wrists, and ankles. As a result of frequent scratching and rubbing, excoriations, crusting, and lichenification occur. In severe cases there may be associated lymphadenopathy secondary to chronic inflammation and bacterial colonization of the skin.

In the adolescent and adult form, the skin lesions are characterized by areas of hyperpigmentation and lichenification surrounded by dry, crusted papules. Distribution is similar to that occurring in the childhood form: antecubital and popliteal fossae, neck, face, and wrists. It is not uncommon to see a patient in whom only the feet or hands are involved with vesicles or papules on the dorsal and distal phalanges as well as lateral aspects of fingers.

MANAGEMENT

Relief of pruritus is important and aggressive therapy is warranted. Control of the eczematous eruption and treatment of secondary infection are necessary in the acute stage, and exacerbating causes need to be avoided.

NONPHARMACOLOGIC MEASURES

Detection and avoidance of exacerbating factors are crucial to the effective management of atopic dermatitis.

Irritants. The most common source of irritation is frequent bathing and excessive use of hot water and soap. Most atopic patients are very intolerant of woolens and other stiff or rough fabrics. Clothing must be well rinsed and in some instances a change in detergent may be necessary. Cosmetics or other topical preparations containing lanolins, perfumes, preservatives (e.g., parabens and ethylenediamine), analgesics, and antibiotics should be avoided. Mattress and pillow covers should be used, and Dacron or foam rubber filler used in bedding. Dust-catching objects (curtains, shag rugs, toys) should be minimized in the environment. Atopic children should not have pets.

Temperature/Humidity. Patients must learn to prevent increased body temperature. Overabundant bedclothes can induce nighttime itching. Occlusive plastic or nylon garments should be avoided, cotton materials being preferable.

For some individuals, exertional activities or participation in sports must be avoided because the increased sweating caused by strenuous activity may provoke itching. Dry skin due to low humidity may also cause itching, but this can be improved by installing cool mist vaporizers in low-humidity areas.

Chilling or sudden changes in room temperature can also cause pruritus. Both cold and hot weather can be irritants to atopic patients, and measures such as wearing of appropriate clothing, air conditioning, mist vaporizers, and dehumidifiers should be taken to avoid these.

Food/Diet. Controversy surrounds the role of food allergy in the pathogenesis of atopic dermatitis. Certain foods may be best avoided in infancy if their ingestion can be correlated (by history) with clinical flares. Of particular concern are cow's milk products, eggs, broths, wheat, corn, citrus fruits, shellfish, chocolate, and nuts.

Emotional Stress. Psychologic factors may play a role in the course of the disease in certain patients. Stress in the home environment is of particular concern and may require changes.

DRUG THERAPY

The objectives of drug therapy include reduction of inflammation, control of pruritus, prevention or treatment of infections, and dry skin care.

Inflammation. The most effective method of reducing inflammation is through the use of topical steroids. Systemic steroids are rarely used in atopy and may even be contraindicated, in that a severe flare of dermatitis may occur after systemic therapy is discontinued. The newer, more potent topical steroids are nearly as effective as systemic steroids in reducing skin inflammation. The practitioner today is faced with a wide variety of preparations. As with systemic steroids, all topical preparations must be prescribed with caution. Table 1 presents a partial list categorized according to potency, based on the Stoughton vasoconstrictive assay. In the clinical setting, the strength chosen depends, of course, on the location and severity of the dermatitis.

High-potency Steroids. These are recommended for acute flares in limited areas of the body. Patients are instructed to apply the preparation sparingly for short periods (four to six days), to reduce side effects such as striae, telangectasia, and epidermal atrophy. The ointment forms of steroid are usually more potent than their cream analogues, since ointments hydrate the epidermis more effectively than other vehicles, thus allowing greater drug penetration. Steroid gels or lotions contain an alcoholic vehicle and should be avoided because of their potentially irritating properties.

High-potency steroids should be avoided in children and must not be applied on the face, intertriginous areas, or genitalia.

Medium-Potency Steroids. These are recommended for less severe flares and for maintenance therapy in adults.

Low-Potency Steroids. These are the drugs of choice for maintenance therapy in children and for mild dermatitis of the face and intertriginous areas. An important consideration is the base of the preparation. In the winter, preparations containing a moisturizing base are

Table 1. CATEGORIES OF TOPICAL CORTICOSTEROIDS

High Potency for Flares
Amcinonide
Betamethasone benzoate
Betamethasone dipropionate
Desoximetasone
Diflorasone diacetate
Fluocinonide
Halcinonide

Medium Potency for Less Severe Flares
Betamethasone valerate
Clocortolone pivalate
Fluocinolone acetonide
Flurandrenolone
Hydrocortisone valerate
Triamcinolone acetonide

Low Potency for Maintenance Therapy
Desonide
Hydrocortisone

Table 2. ADJUNCTIVE TREATMENT

Anti-infection	Anti-inflammatory	Antipruritic
Vioform HC	Tar	Sarna
	Estargel	Topic Gel
	Psorigel	Eurax Cream
	T/Gel	

recommended to atopic patients in order to overcome the problem of asteatosis. During summer, when the problems of hydration are less important and heat becomes a concern, creams and sprays may be used.

Tar Preparations. An alternative to topical steroids for maintenance therapy is the application of tar preparations (Table 2). Tar is an effective anti-inflammatory agent, but has disadvantages: it has a foul odor, it stains clothing, and it can provoke irritation.

Ultraviolet Light. Ultraviolet light with tar (Goeckerman regimen) or ultraviolet plus psoralens (PUVA) can reduce inflammation and pruritus and may be very helpful in some patients. Phototherapy is available in only some dermatologic settings, which limits its usefulness in outpatient therapy.

Pruritus. Since atopic dermatitis is believed to result from an altered cutaneous threshold to pruritus, it is important to reduce the severity of itching. This helps to minimize chronic skin changes such as lichenification and hyperpigmentation, which result from scratching and rubbing. Approaches to the control of pruritus include topical and systemic therapy, and combinations thereof.

Topical Antipruritics. These include topical high- and medium-potency steroids; 0.5% to 1% phenol, menthol, and camphor in cream or lotion (Sarna lotion); cool soaks; and pramoxine (Prax).

Systemic Antipruritics. These include diphenhydramine, hydroxyzine, cyproheptadine, azatadine, brompheniramine, clemastine, and doxepin. Patients should be informed about the side effects of systemic antipruritics. Sedation is the most frequently reported problem, although this may be beneficial in patients with intense pruritus at night.

Dry Skin. A recently published study demonstrates that there are at least three different types of dry skin among atopic patients: dry skin (1) due to the mild eczematous changes; (2) as a manifestation of ichthyosis vulgaris; and (3) as a result of both eczema and ichthyosis. It is important to differentiate among these three varieties, since patients with ichthyosiform skin do not benefit from topical steroids. Ichthyosis responds to treatment with emollients and desquamatives, as listed in Table 3.

Infection. Patients with atopic dermatitis have a significant colonization of *Staphylococcus aureus* on both involved and uninvolved skin. During an atopic flare, pruritus and subsequent scratching introduce the organism into the skin, with resulting pyoderma. This acute weeping dermatitis should be managed by both drying agents and systemic antibiotics. Wet dressings with cool water or preferably Burow's solution, 1:40 (1 tablet or packet of Domeboro powder in 1 quart of cool water) will provide antimicrobial and astringent effects. Wet dressings should be applied to the involved areas of the skin for about 20 minutes every four to six hours. Caution should be taken not to overdry the skin; we

Table 3. DRY SKIN MANAGEMENT SCHEDULE IN ATOPIC DERMATITIS

Dry skin due to ichthyosis without eczematous changes	**Lubricants** Keri lotion LactiCare lotion	Moisturel lotion Complex 15 lotion/cream Purpose cream Neutrogena hand cream Eucerin cream or lotion
	Desquamatives Carmol 10 lotion Carmol 20 cream Ultra Mide 25 moisturizer	
	Skin Cleansing Cetaphil lotion Alpha Keri soap Aveeno soap Dove soap Neutrogena soap Emulave soap Oilatum	
Mild eczematous changes with or without ichthyosis	**Low-Potency Steroids**: e.g., Hytone 1% or 2.5% creams, Synacort 1% and 2.5% creams, MetiDerm 0.5% cream	
Moderate eczematous changes with or without ichthyosis	**Medium-Potency Steroids**: e.g., Westcort 0.2% cream, Kenalog 0.025% ointment or cream, Aristocort 0.1% ointment or cream	
Severe eczematous changes with or without ichthyosis	**High-Potency Steroids**: e.g., Cyclocort 0.1% ointment or cream, Halog 0.1% ointment or cream, Topicort 0.25% ointment or cream	

therefore restrict the use of wet dressings to two to three days. Systemic antibiotics should be administered at the first sign of pyoderma. Culture should always be taken before starting antibiotic therapy. Initially, we recommend erythromycin, 1.5 to 2 gm per day or cloxacillin, 250 mg four times daily, since most isolates of *S. aureus* are penicillin resistant. The duration of therapy is usually five to ten days; in patients who develop repeated infections, it can be extended for several weeks.

Failure to respond to systemic antibiotic therapy within a few days may suggest antibiotic resistance or perhaps herpes simplex infection. The latter is usually self-limited but sometimes may require the use of oral or intravenous acyclovir (Zovirax).

PATIENT INFORMATION

Patients and their families should be informed that atopic dermatitis is a chronic disease. Most patients improve with time, and long-lasting remissions may occur even in those most severely affected. They should be made aware of factors that exacerbate the disease and of the importance of using prescribed medications regularly.

Neurodermatitis

Neurodermatitis circumscripta (lichen simplex chronicus) is a part of the eczema group closely related to atopy. The etiology is not entirely understood but it is believed that a scratch-itch cycle results in lichenification and thickening of the skin. Emotional instability, tension, and frustration are important factors in the production and continuation of this dermatosis.

In most patients a single area is affected. The individual lesion is usually a well-circumscribed, dry, hypertrophic, lichenified plaque, most often on the neck, wrist, thighs, or perineum. It usually is hyperpigmented, but it can be violaceous, especially in individuals with dark skin. The skin lines are exaggerated and may divide the lesion into rectangular patches.

Other clinical variants are (1) lichenification gigantea, in which large, verrucous patches are localized to legs, groin, and axillae; and (2) polymorphic neurodermatitis, which involves different types of lesions, including nodules, in different parts of the body.

MANAGEMENT

Since the clinically apparent lesion is the result of scratching and rubbing, it is necessary for patients to refrain from such activity. They should be told that if they stop scratching, the skin lesion will disappear. Very light, minimal rubbing (done unconsciously during sleep) may be of great importance.

PHARMACOTHERAPY

Topical corticosteroids are the treatment of choice. High-potency topical steroids reduce pruritus most effectively. They can be applied openly or in occlusive dressings (Saran Wrap or other plastic wraps) to increase penetration. Cordran tape is another effective therapy for neurodermatitis.

Tar preparations may be useful: (1) 5% to 20% liquor carbonis detergens in cream base; (2) 5% crude coal tar in zinc oxide ointment; or (3) Estar gel.

Antihistamines also control pruritus effectively.

REFERENCES

Abramson JS, Dahl MV, Walsh G, et al: Antistaphylococcal IgE in patients with atopic dermatitis. J Am Acad Dermatol 7:105–110, 1982.

Hanifin JM: Clinical and basic aspects of atopic dermatitis. Semin Dermatol 2:5–19, 1983.

Herndon JH Jr: Itching: the pathophysiology of pruritus. Int J Dermatol 14:465–484, 1975.

Kang K, Cooper KD, Vanderbark A, et al: Immuno-regulation in atopic dermatitis. T-lymphocyte subset defined by monoclonal antibodies. Semin Dermatol 2:20–25, 1983.

Uehara M, Miyauchi H: The morphologic characteristics of dry skin in atopic dermatitis. Arch Dermatol 20:1186–1190, 1984.

3 · PSORIASIS

Leonard E. Gately III
TULANE UNIVERSITY SCHOOL OF MEDICINE AND
OCHSNER CLINIC AND ALTON OCHSNER
MEDICAL FOUNDATION

DEFINITION

Psoriasis is a genetically determined, hyperproliferative disease of the skin characterized by erythematous scaling plaques. It is fairly common, with a conservatively estimated incidence of 1% to 2% in the general population.

Although much is known of the histopathology and inflammatory processes involved in psoriasis, the exact mechanism of the pathogenesis of the disease is not completely known. The histologic findings in psoriatic skin consist of parakeratosis in the stratum corneum, an absence of the granular layer, acanthosis (a thickening of the epidermis caused by an increased number of layers of cells), and increased mitotic figures. There is an elongation and clubbing of the rete of the epidermis. Collections of polymorphonuclear leukocytes are found in the epidermis and these are the Munro microabscesses considered diagnostic of psoriasis. There is proliferation and dilatation of the capillaries in the papillary dermis and an associated infiltrate of mononuclear cells.

Currently it is speculated that the changes seen in the epidermis of psoriasis are at least partly due to the actions of leukotrienes and other arachidonic acid derivatives.

The clinical features of psoriasis may vary. Although this condition is generally considered to be nonpruritic, it is not unusual to find patients who complain of itching, occasionally severe. Because there is a genetically determined basis for the occurrence of psoriasis, patients sometimes, but not always, have a family member who also has the disease.

The typical appearance of the psoriatic lesion is of an erythematous plaque with a silvery micaceous scale. Lesions are sharply defined, with an abrupt change from normal skin to the psoriatic plaque at the lesion's edge. In general there is little variation in the appearance of psoriasis except when it is on the palms and soles.

Individual lesions of psoriasis appear similar, but there can be differences in the distribution and size of the lesions. Guttate psoriasis is characterized by small lesions with a diminished scale uniformly distributed over the body. This type is usually seen in children and young adults and following streptococcal infections. The psoriasis if persistent rarely remains guttate and becomes the typical larger scaling plaques.

The typical patient with psoriasis has round or oval plaques 1 to 3 inches in size. Lesions occur over the elbows, knees, legs, sacrum, and scalp and may have a polycyclic edge due to coalescence of several smaller round lesions. On the scalp there can be typical plaques of psoriasis or generalized scaling. Thick hyperkeratotic plaques may occur on the palms and soles in addition to the usual scaling plaques. Painful fissured plaques

may lead to inability to use the hands or to stand for prolonged periods.

An associated arthritis occurs in about 2% of patients with psoriasis and is seronegative. The arthritis can vary from an involvement of the distal interphalangeal joint of the fingers and toes predominantly, to a rheumatoid arthritis–like or severe crippling and deforming arthritis.

MANAGEMENT

Psoriasis is usually a chronic disease with an unpredictable course and is very difficult to treat at times. It can be influenced by outside environmental factors. Psychologic stress can lead to worsening of disease or resistance to treatment. Chronic minor trauma (köbnerization) may give rise to occupationally related psoriasis. Several drugs such as lithium carbonate, beta-blockers, and chloroquine may exacerbate psoriasis, as may rapid withdrawal of corticosteroids. If these external factors can be corrected, the psoriasis may clear or at least become less resistant to therapy.

TOPICAL MEDICATIONS

Steroids. Topical corticosteroid creams and ointments are often the first treatment utilized in typical psoriasis. In general, potent topicals such as Lidex, Halog, or Diprolene are used several times a day, except as noted below. On thick plaques the corticosteroid may be used under occlusion with plastic wrap to enhance penetration of the topical agent. Diprolene is not recommended for use under occlusion.

Potent topical steroids should not be used in the axillae, inguinal folds or on the face, because in these areas the development of cutaneous atrophy, telangiectasia, or striae is more likely. Occasionally, owing to the chronic nature of the eruption, only hydrocortisone 1% to 2½% can be used for prolonged periods in these areas. After chronic use of topical corticosteroids, the patient may no longer respond to these agents.

Tar. The use of other nonsteroidal topical agents in conjunction with corticosteroids can give increased success. This is particularly true for the scalp. At the minimum a daily tar shampoo (T/Gel, Pentrax, Vanseb-T, Ionil T-Plus, Sebutone) is required and usually a topical corticosteroid solution (Halog 0.1%, Valisone 0.1%) twice a day, including occlusion under shower cap at night. For severe, thick scaling of the scalp, warm mineral oil under occlusion at night or P & S Liquid under occlusion followed by morning shampoo is needed.

Topical crude coal tar or more refined varients are effective alone or with topical steroids. Crude coal tar 3% to 5% in Aquaphor or petrolatum applied to remain overnight is very useful but somewhat messy; the odor and staining of sheets and clothes are unacceptable to some patients. The tar gels (Estar, Psorigel) are more acceptable but probably not as effective. The gel base is occasionally irritating and causes burning, particularly on fissured palms and soles. All tars can cause irritation in intertriginous areas and body folds.

Tar Combinations. Tar derivatives can be mixed in some useful combinations. Lidex gel (60 gm) and Estar gel (90 gm) are useful on psoriatic plaques in the scalp and on the body. Three per cent crude coal tar and 5%

salicylic acid in petrolatum are effective in treating hyperkeratotic lesions of the palms and soles. The concentration of the salicylic acid can be increased as needed and tolerated.

Anthralin is a coal tar derivative that can be used in much the same manner as coal tar, except in lower concentrations (¼% to usually no more than 1%) and with more care because of its much greater capacity for burning and irritation, particularly in the genital region.

ULTRAVIOLET LIGHT

Exposure to ultraviolet light is one of the oldest modalities for treating psoriasis. The beneficial effects of sunlight exposure are well known. Ultraviolet-B (UVB) can be used alone with only an emollient or in combination with crude coal tar or anthralin. Small areas can be treated with a movable ultraviolet lamp. Patients with more extensive psoriasis are treated more conveniently in walk-in light boxes lined with fluorescent sunlamp bulbs.

UVB with the use of an emollient to decrease reflection and increase absorption of the light will clear a substantial number of patients with psoriasis. This is very useful for outpatient treatment in people who fail to respond or cease to respond to topical treatment alone. Patients are treated at least three times a week or more frequently. The amount of light used in the initial treatment depends on the skin type of the patient. Patients who always burn on sunlight exposure or those who tan poorly are begun on less light than those who tan well. The initial amount of light is between ½ and 1 minimal erythema dose (MED). A MED is the amount of radiant light energy that causes a detectable erythema 10 to 24 hours after exposure. The exposure time needed for this depends on the power output of the ultraviolet light. In absolute terms the amount of light for 1 MED is 50 to 200 milliwatts per cm², depending on skin type. The amount of light is gradually increased with each treatment unless the previous treatment has resulted in excessive erythema and burning. Clearing occurs at six to eight weeks but this is variable, some patients requiring less and some more time. If the psoriasis is limited in the area of involvement, it may be more economical for patients to purchase a sunlamp for home use. They are instructed to place the lamp 18 to 24 inches from the skin and maintain the same light-to-skin distance throughout treatment. Initial treatment is for 15 to 30 seconds, depending on skin type, and the light is administered daily with an increase of 15 seconds per day. As with clinic treatment, patients should use protective goggles for the eyes and never look into the sunlamp.

Crude coal tar 2% to 3%, tar gels, and anthralin can be used in conjunction with UVB sunlamps. The ultraviolet light greatly enhances the efficacy of crude coal tar in the treatment of psoriasis. Earlier schedules called for prolonged application times of the crude coal tar, but application times of two hours before light exposure give the same effect.

Individuals with extensive psoriasis that does not clear when treated at home may be admitted to the hospital for intensive therapy. While hospitalized, 2% to 3% crude coal tar in Aquaphor is applied daily overnight. In the morning, a Balnetar bath is taken to remove the crude coal tar and the patient receives UVB light exposure daily as above. Following light treatment, topical corticosteroids (Lidex, triamcinolone) in Aquaphor are applied. The addition of UVA light to the tar and UVB does not appear to improve the effectiveness of this treatment.

PUVA

For patients who do not clear with tar and UVB light, oral 8-methoxypsoralen and UVA (PUVA) can be used. The psoralen, 0.6 mg/kg, is given one to two hours before UVA light exposure. More careful measurement of light energy with a lightmeter is required for PUVA treatments. Initial treatment is with ¼ to 1 joule per cm², depending on skin type. Patients are treated two to three days per week, with the UVA light increased ½ joule/cm² every or every other treatment as tolerated. Some patients have a maximal UVA exposure. Severe burns can result from PUVA treatment and great care must be taken. There should be improvement in the psoriasis after two to three weeks, and clearing in one to three months. The combined use of PUVA and UVB light results in faster clearing and smaller cumulative doses of both UVA and UVB.

There are side effects from PUVA. Burning can easily occur, particularly if too large an initial dose is used. This can also cause the psoriasis to flare. Before beginning PUVA the patient should be evaluated for photosensitive diseases such as lupus erythematosus, which can flare with PUVA therapy. Protective glasses must be worn for 24 hours after treatment to prevent additional UVA exposure to the lens of the eye in which the psoralen persists for 12 to 24 hours. Minor complaints of nausea, headache, and dizziness can occur.

The most significant side effect of PUVA therapy is the striking increased risk of skin cancer, particularly in fair individuals. Even more troubling is the increased number of potentially more serious squamous cell carcinomas over the basal cell carcinomas usually seen in actinically damaged skin. In view of these side effects, PUVA should be used only for disabling psoriasis that is unresponsive to other conventional therapies.

METHOTREXATE

Methotrexate is an alternative form of therapy for patients with severe widespread psoriasis or erythrodermic or pustular psoriasis unresponsive to the usual therapies. Careful and close evaluation of the patient is required before and during treatment with methotrexate. Before treatment bone marrow and liver and kidney function should be evaluated and shown to be normal, and white blood cell count, platelet count, and SGOT and SGPT transaminase should be normal. Initially and at three-month intervals the hemoglobin, serum creatinine and creatinine clearance, serum albumin, alkaline phosphatase, and prothrombin time should all be normal on testing.

Methotrexate can cause leukopenia, thrombocytopenia, and anemia, but liver toxicity is the major concern with its use. The hepatotoxicity appears to be related to the total accumulated dose of methotrexate. Liver biopsies are recommended before therapy, after a 1.5-gm cumulative dose of methotrexate, and after 1:0 to 1.5-gm increments in cumulative dose, although not all physicians perform liver biopsies on all patients. Unless needed as a life-saving measure, methotrexate should not be given to patients (1) who have preexisting liver disease, ulcerative colitis, or peptic ulcer disease; (2) whose alcohol intake is heavy; or (3) who are under 50 years of age. Women should be on contraceptives while receiving methotrexate and for three months after cessation of this agent.

Methotrexate may be administered parenterally or orally, 0.2 to 0.4 mg/kg. The drug is given in a single injection or single oral dose at seven- to ten-day intervals initially. Alternatively, 2.5 to 7.5 mg can be given at 12-hour intervals for three doses. This schedule is only marginally superior to the single oral or parenteral dosage and may be more hepatotoxic than single dosage.

Despite the dangers of long-term methotrexate use, it does have a place in the treatment of severe disabling psoriasis, psoriatic erythroderma, and generalized pustular psoriasis. Hydroxyurea is used in severe psoriasis but is less effective. Patients must be carefully and closely followed.

As stated previously, psoriatic arthritis is a rare finding in patients with psoriasis. It is severe and mutilating in some individuals. In brief, therapy is determined by the severity of the arthritis. In mild cases, aspirin or other nonsteroidal anti-inflammatory drugs may suffice. Bed rest initially and physical therapy later are helpful. Methotrexate helps severe psoriatic arthritis, and occasionally prednisone may be required to arrest the progression of a fulminant psoriatic arthritis. Corticosteroids should be avoided if at all possible. Severe psoriatic arthritis is best managed by a rheumatologist.

RETINOIDS

Oral retinoids are the newest drugs in the therapy of psoriasis. Accutane is currently the only retinoid widely available in the United States. Some patients respond to 1 mg/kg of Accutane per day or a combination of PUVA and Accutane.

The aromatic retinoid etretinate, currently available only in Europe, is superior to Accutane in the treatment of psoriasis, particularly pustular psoriasis. It is less effective in erythrodermic psoriasis and less still in plaque psoriasis. Pustular psoriasis requires 1 mg/kg for four to six weeks before this dose is decreased. Etretinate has been used in combination with UVB and with PUVA therapy, and yielded better results than single therapy.

There are many side effects associated with retinoid therapy. Dryness of mucous membranes and peeling of the palms, soles, and face are most common. Alopecia and musculoskeletal symptoms are not unusual. Hepatotoxicity is somewhat greater with etretinate but is not common. Both Accutane and etretinate are teratogenic. Female patients of childbearing potential must use effective contraceptive methods while taking retinoids and for several months after cessation of Accutane. Etretinate has a long half-life of 140 days and is present in significant amounts long after cessation; contraceptive measures may therefore be needed long afterwards.

Psoriasis is a common disorder that varies from localized asymptomatic disease to life-threatening erythrodermic and generalized pustular forms. Patients are best served by careful evaluation and selection of therapy appropriate for the severity of their disease.

REFERENCES

Baker H, Wilkinson DS: Psoriasis. *In* Rook A, Wilkinson DS, Ebling FJG (eds): Textbook of Dermatology. Blackwell Scientific Publ, Oxford, 1979, pp. 1315–1362.

Farber EM, Abel EA, Charuworn A: Recent advances in the treatment of psoriasis. J Am Acad Dermatol 8:311–321, 1983.

Goldyne ME: Leukotrienes: clinical significance. J Am Acad Dermatol 10:659–668, 1984.

Momtaz TK, Parrish JA: Combination of psoralens and ultraviolet A and ultraviolet B in the treatment of psoriasis vulgaris: a bilateral comparison study. J Am Acad Dermatol 10:481–486, 1984.

4 · PEMPHIGUS AND PEMPHIGOID

Marilyn C. Ray
OCHSNER CLINIC AND
ALTON OCHSNER MEDICAL FOUNDATION

DEFINITION

Pemphigus and pemphigoid are blistering diseases. In general, pemphigoid describes a group of relatively benign subepidermal blistering disorders, whereas pemphigus encompasses a more aggressive group of disorders with intraepidermal bullae.

PATHOPHYSIOLOGY

Patients with pemphigus produce IgG antibodies against an antigen contained in the intercellular cement substance in the epidermis. Loss of this substance destroys the cell-to-cell adhesion of the epidermis, and the blisters result from the subsequent cell separation (acantholysis). Pemphigus has been found to be increased in frequency in patients with other immune diseases, such as thymoma and myasthenia gravis. The IgG antibody has been demonstrated in the epidermal cells and sera of patients with pemphigus, and many (but not all) studies demonstrate a positive correlation with titers of antibody and activity of the clinical disease.

Approximately 70% of patients with pemphigoid have IgG antibody (usually IgG, though other classes have been identified) in the serum specific for the basement membrane zone. In contrast to pemphigus, pemphigoid shows no relation between the extent of the clinical disease and the titer of antibodies in the serum. Direct immunofluorescence demonstrates immunoglobulin and complement along the basement membrane, and electron microscopy reveals that the immune deposits have been localized to the lamina lucida.

CLINICAL DIAGNOSIS

The term pemphigus (Greek for bubble) was first used by Hippocrates around 425 BC to describe a group of febrile blistering diseases. From 1860 to 1960, bullous diseases were separated into several smaller groups, and pemphigus is now used to describe two major types of disease, pemphigus vulgaris and pemphigus foliaceus.

PEMPHIGUS VULGARIS

Pemphigus vulgaris (PV) occurs in middle-aged patients and has a predominance in Jewish people. The flaccid bullae of PV usually begin as localized oral or scalp lesions or both. These bullae rupture and leave weeping and often secondarily infected areas. Such a picture can last from days to months. The eruption then spreads and tends to occur on the back, groin, flexures, midsternum, and feet. The mucosal lesions do not heal well and can cause significant pain with resultant weight loss. This disease usually continues to evolve over one to two years and can lead to death if not treated. Mortality rates prior to treatment were over 90% and now are about 30%. Death usually is the result of infection, poor nutrition, or complications of therapy.

A variant of pemphigus vulgaris is pemphigus vegetans, which occurs as heaped-up vegetating lesions in the intertriginous areas, often exuding serum or pus and studded with small pustules. Its course generally is prolonged and, like that of PV, may be fatal if untreated.

PEMPHIGUS FOLIACEUS

The other major type of pemphigus is pemphigus foliaceus (PF), which tends to be a more chronic and benign condition requiring less aggressive therapy than that needed for PV. The age of onset varies more widely than that in PV, and PF can occur in children. Onset is slow, with appearance of a few lesions on the face or scalp, upper chest, and back. The lesions usually appear as crusted plaques in areas where seborrheic dermatitis occurs, though other presentations may occur, including flaccid bullae and, on the face, erythematous scaling lesions. The erythematous lesions may assume a butterfly distribution and simulate lupus erythematosus. Eventually, the lesions spread to involve most of the body surface, so the patient can present with exfoliative erythroderma. In addition to its more benign course, PF differs from PV in the level of blister formation in the epidermis. In PF one finds separation of cells in the superficial (stratum granulosum) layers, whereas in PV the separation and characteristic acantholysis occur first above the basal cell layer of the epidermis. The two major variants of PF are pemphigus erythematosus, which is now considered to be coexistence of lupus erythematosus and PF, and fogo selvagem, an endemic form of PF found in Brazil.

BULLOUS PEMPHIGOID

Bullous pemphigoid (BP) differs from pemphigus in that it tends to be a chronic disease of the elderly, and the level of blister separation is subepidermal with no acantholysis. The disease may last from months to years and is characterized by exacerbations and remissions. The eruption usually starts as a nonspecific urticarial or eczematous eruption, which may continue for several months before generalization occurs with typical large, tense, irregular bullae. The areas of predilection for this eruption are the lower abdomen, groin, thighs, and flexor areas of the forearms. Approximately 75% of patients experience itching and burning. The early lesions of BP may resemble those of erythema multiforme. Mucous membrane lesions occur in about one third of patients, but, in contrast to pemphigus, in BP they do not usually precede the skin lesions.

The subtypes that have variably been described as belonging to the pemphigoid group are localized chronic pemphigoid (Brunsting-Perry pemphigoid), desquamative gingivitis, cicatricial pemphigoid (benign mucosal pemphigoid), vesicular pemphigoid, linear IgA subepidermal bullous dermatoses, and herpes gestationis. A discussion of these pemphigoid variants is beyond the scope of this section, and the reader is advised to consult a good general textbook of dermatology such as Fitzpatrick, *Dermatology in General Medicine*. Whether all of these represent different forms of BP remains controversial, and many regard them as separate diseases with pathogenic mechanisms that happen to involve the same or a closely related anatomic site.

MANAGEMENT

Predictably, the treatment regimens for pemphigus are more aggressive than those for pemphigoid, since pemphigus tends to be a much more serious disease.

The most successful treatments of pemphigus vulgaris and pemphigus foliaceus involve the use of corticosteroids or immunosuppressants or both. Treatment of both major types of pemphigus are discussed together in this chapter, but keep in mind that pemphigus foliaceus is a milder disease than pemphigus vulgaris, requiring smaller doses of these drugs over shorter periods of time. Early, stable pemphigus (i.e., a few localized lesions present) is much more easily controlled with therapy than is more generalized disease. Thus, early diagnosis is important to avoid the well-known side effects observed with long-term use of these agents. The three most commonly used immunosuppressants for pemphigus are azathioprine (Imuran), cyclophosphamide (Cytoxan), and methotrexate (MTX, A-methopterin). In addition, some reports have shown that gold compounds are beneficial.

CORTICOSTEROIDS

The most widely accepted treatment regimen for pemphigus is corticosteroids (i.e., prednisone) followed by an immunosuppressant, which is taken as the steroid is gradually tapered. The initial dose of prednisone varies in the literature from 60 to 360 mg/day, depending on the severity of the disease. High doses of steroid should be avoided if possible. One retrospective study of over 100 patients treated for pemphigus demonstrated that the majority of deaths were due to complications of steroid therapy. Some of these complications include infection, gastrointestinal bleeding, perforation of the duodenum or stomach, and thromboembolic phenomena. Increases in morbidity and mortality rates have been found with doses of prednisone higher than 120 mg/day, but it is not clear whether this is a true association with prednisone or related to more severe pemphigus with a poor prognosis.

Management of the dose of steroid used must be decided on an individual basis, according to the needs of the patient. One study recommends continuing high-dose prednisone until all lesions have healed for a duration of at least six weeks to prevent relapses. After completion of the high-dose treatment, the dose of prednisone is reduced to 40 mg daily for one week, 30 mg daily for one week, 25 mg daily for one week, and then 40 mg on alternate days, at which time an immunosuppressant is added. Another group recommends treatment with prednisone (60 to 100 mg/day), either alone or in combination with immunosuppressants, until the blisters have healed and both the indirect and direct immunofluorescent tests for anti-intercellular cement substance antibodies are negative. If a six- to eight-week course of 60 to 100 mg of prednisone is not effective, the dose may be increased to 150 mg/day. After the disease is controlled, first prednisone is tapered off at a rate of 2.5 mg per week. Second, the immunosuppressant is then tapered off over one to two months. The patient is observed at three- to four-month intervals both clinically and serologically for disease activity. Using this method, one third of this group's patients stayed in a prolonged remission, and in patients who relapsed, the pemphigus antibody could again be found. From this study and others, there is a close correlation between the presence of the pemphigus antibody and clinical disease, demonstrating the importance of following the antibody during treatment of the disease.

IMMUNOSUPPRESSANTS

The pemphigus autoantibodies provide the rationale for use of immunosuppressants. Azathioprine (Imuran), an analogue of beta-mercaptopurine, is a commonly used agent for pemphigus. It has been used successfully alone for localized pemphigus and with steroids for more widespread disease. A dose of 1 mg/kg/day (50 to 100 mg) is used and may be slowly increased at one-month intervals to a maximum of 2.5 mg/kg/day. Hemoglobin, platelet, and leukocyte counts should be followed closely, as patients can develop severe leukopenia or thrombocytopenia or both. Of all immunosuppressants, azothioprine enjoys the most widespread use. Methotrexate is an antagonist of folic acid and has been found to have a limited use in pemphigus vulgaris. It can be used in combination with corticosteroids in an intramuscular dose of 25 to 50 mg/week, but it has a greater effect on the cutaneous lesions than on the mucosal lesions, and some patients even relate that their mucous membrane lesions become more painful. Because methotrexate has long-term side effects, including bone marrow depression, hepatotoxicity, impaired renal function, pulmonary fibrosis, and diarrhea, it should be used only by those with experience. Cyclophosphamide is a synthetic immunosuppressant drug chemically related to nitrogen mustard. It can be used in a dose of 50 to 150 mg/day in combination with steroids. However, it is known to cause numerous adverse reactions, such as alopecia, hemorrhagic cystitis, dysuria, leukopenia, nausea and vomiting, and diarrhea. Weekly evaluations of complete blood count, platelet count, fasting blood glucose, blood urea nitrogen, liver function studies, total protein, and urinalysis should be done. In one study of ten patients

with PV, cyclophosphamide was used with small doses of steroid (10 to 20 mg/day) after initial treatment with high-dose prednisone. The patients' disease was well controlled, and the only complications encountered were alopecia and reversible leukopenia.

Gold sodium thiomalate (Myochrysine) is an antiarthritic drug that can be used with steroids for pemphigus. It has been shown to decrease the titer of pemphigus antibodies. There is a lag of about six weeks between initiation of cryotherapy and evidence of a response, so it is started along with high-dose prednisone, which is tapered while administration of gold sodium thiomalate continues. This can allow some cases to be controlled with gold therapy alone. The initial test dose is 10 mg IM, which is followed by 25 mg the next week and 50 mg IM weekly thereafter. The most common dermatologic side effects of gold therapy are lichenoid eruptions and oral ulcerations. A generalized exfoliative erythroderma may occur. The more toxic effects of gold include nephritis, bone marrow suppression, and pneumonitis. During gold therapy, WBC counts and urinalysis for protein should be performed biweekly, with periodic platelet counts. Gold toxicity is directly related to the total dose administered, and reports of toxicity occur after a total dose of at least 250 mg. The necessary maintenance dose varies among patients. After control is obtained, the dose can be decreased to 25 mg IM bimonthly and then to monthly injections.

PLASMAPHERESIS

An alternative form of therapy using plasmapheresis has been reported, but further evaluation is necessary.

LOCAL CARE

Local care is also important for patients with pemphigus. Bullae heal somewhat more rapidly if the edge of the bulla is incised to make a small opening and the contents are drained. Modified Burow's solution diluted 1:40 (aluminum sulfate, Domeboro) may be used as compresses for oozing or infected lesions for 15 minutes three times a day. Bacterial superinfections should be treated with appropriate systemic antibiotics. For oral lesions, anesthetics such as viscous lidocaine or diphenhydramine hydrochloride (Benadryl) elixir diluted 1:1 with water can be swished in the mouth before eating. For persistent lesions, a topical steroid (fluocinonide, Lidex gel) may be applied locally.

BULLOUS PEMPHIGOID

Systemic Therapy. The treatment of bullous pemphigoid is similar to that of pemphigus; however, since it is not as serious an illness as pemphigus, smaller doses are used for shorter periods. The first drug of choice for bullous pemphigoid is prednisone. Starting doses of 60 to 80 mg/day as a single dose are usually effective and can be tapered when there is no formation of new blisters (about three weeks). The steroid is tapered slowly at 10 mg/week with careful observation for development of new lesions. As with pemphigus, disappearance of the antibody may be used as a sign to start tapering the dose of steroid. Over 90% of patients go into remission, with resolution of both clinical disease and antibodies to pemphigoid (negative direct and indirect immunofluorescent tests). Unlike patients with pemphigus, those with pemphigoid, once in remission, usually do not relapse. To avoid the potential side effects of steroids as previously discussed, immunosuppressants may be employed. Azothioprine (1.0 to 2.5 mg/kg/day), cyclophosphamide (1.5 to 2.0 mg/kg/day), and methotrexate (25 mg IM weekly) have each been used with prednisone in about half its usual starting dose in several studies with good results. Again, azothioprine is the most commonly used of these agents. The same precautions apply to the use of immunosuppressants in pemphigoid as in pemphigus. They should be used only as "steroid-sparing" agents when necessary to avoid the toxicity of high-dose steroids. In addition, both diaminodiphenylsulfone (DDS, Dapsone) and sulfapyridine have been used in some studies as steroid-sparing agents, though their success is not uniformly accepted. Dapsone is usually started in a dose of 50 mg/day after checking for a normal glucose-6-phosphate dehydrogenase level and normal liver functions and performing a complete blood count (CBC). Its most common side effect is hemolysis. The CBC should be checked weekly for the first month of treatment.

Topical Therapy. As in pemphigus, topical therapy for the lesions of BP includes draining the individual blisters and using drying soaks. In addition, a steroid cream such as triamcinolone 0.1% may be added to a shake lotion such as milk of bismuth (MOB) (e.g., 60 gm of triamcinolone cream 0.1% in 240 cc of MOB) as long as bullae are present.

BENIGN MUCOSAL (CICATRICIAL) PEMPHIGOID

Benign mucosal (cicatricial) pemphigoid often is difficult to control. A combination of prednisone with azathioprine or cyclophosphamide, as for BP, or cyclophosphamide alone has been reported to slow the clinical progression. Conjunctival involvement is a particularly troublesome feature of this disease, occurring in 75% of cases, and it eventually leads to blindness in some patients. Rarely, the larynx and esophagus may be involved, requiring surgery for stricture formation. Dapsone has also been used both alone and with steroids to control the disease. Local treatment is identical to that of oral pemphigus, with the use of viscous lidocaine if necessary for pain and topical steroids for decreasing inflammation.

REFERENCES

Diaz LA, Provost TT: Pemphigus and pemphigoid. *In* Provost TT, Farmer ER (eds): Current Therapy in Dermatology. C. V. Mosby Co, St. Louis, 1985, pp 57–63.

Krain LS, Landau JW, Newcomer VD: Cyclophosphamide in the treatment of pemphigus vulgaris and bullous pemphigoid. Arch Dermatol 106:657–661, 1972.

Lever WF: Methotrexate and prednisone in pemphigus vulgaris. Arch Dermatol 106:491–497, 1972.

Lever WF, Schaumberg-Lever G: Immunosuppressants and prednisone in pemphigus vulgaris. Arch Dermatol 113:1236–1241, 1977.

Rosenberg FR, Sanders S, Nelson CT: Pemphigus, a 20-year review of 107 patients treated with corticosteroids. Arch Dermatol 112:962–970, 1976.

Sams WM, Jordan RE: Correlation of pemphigoid and pemphigus antibody titers with activity of disease. Br J Dermatol 84:7–13, 1971.

Williams GH, Dluhy RG, Thorn GW: Diseases of the adrenal cortex. *In* Isselbacher KJ, Adams RD, Braunwald E (eds): Principles of Internal Medicine. McGraw-Hill Book Co, New York, 1980, pp 1711–1736.

5 · *ERYTHEMA MULTIFORME*

Henry W. Randle
SCOTT AND WHITE CLINIC

DEFINITION AND DIAGNOSTIC CRITERIA

Erythema multiforme (EM) is an acute, self-limited, inflammatory disorder of the skin and mucous membranes. It is considered to be an immunologically mediated hypersensitivity reaction to one of a variety of antigens such as drugs or infections. Severe cases may result in major complications and death.

Since there are no specific identifying markers, diagnosis is made on the basis of distinctive skin lesions and a clinical syndrome, supported by histopathologic examination and direct immunofluorescent skin biopsies compatible with a diagnosis of EM.

PATHOPHYSIOLOGY

Erythema multiforme is the final common pathway in response to one of a number of inciting agents. Suspected causes include drugs, infections, chemicals, tumors, and inflammatory disorders. The factors most frequently identified are sulfonamides, penicillin, hydantoins, phenobarbital, herpes simplex, and *Mycoplasma*. Lists in textbooks usually include over 100 potential causes. I find these lists useful in attempting to determine the etiology of EM for individual patients and in counseling them on what substances to avoid in the future to prevent recurrent attacks.

What follows an antigenic stimulus is probably the result of immune complex formation and deposition in the vessels of the skin and mucous membranes. Immunoglobulin M (IgM) and complement (C3) have been found in the microvasculature of the upper dermis (papillary) and granular C3 along the basement membrane. Circulating immune complexes have been demonstrated in serum samples from EM patients in several studies with both monoclonal rheumatoid factor inhibition assay and a C1q-binding radioimmunoassay.

Histologically, this is reflected by involvement of both the epidermis and dermis. Initially there is a sparse lymphohistiocytic infiltrate around dilated blood vessels in the papillary dermis, with necrotic keratinocytes and vacuolar degeneration at the dermoepidermal junction. As serum and red blood cells exude into the dermis and epidermis, this histologic pattern is intensified, producing subepidermal and intraepidermal blisters. In the most severe cases, this degeneration may produce confluent epidermal necrosis and sloughing of large sheets of epidermis. The gray color of the blisters results from the epidermal necrosis, the indurated rings from vascular dilatation and dermal edema, and the purpura from extravasated erythrocytes in the superficial dermis.

CLINICAL ASPECTS

The most striking character of this affection is its appearing on certain special parts of the body. In every instance it is present on the dorsal surfaces of the hands or feet. In the more severe cases . . . on the forearms and legs, and even on the trunk and face . . . The efflorescence . . . consists of flattened papules or tubercles of dark-blue or a brownish-red color between lentils and beans in size . . . giving rise to very trifling subjective symptoms . . . a slight burning sensation or a slight itching . . . concomitant and febrile symptoms are to be observed only in exceptional cases . . . no important complications or sequelae occur in the train of this eruption.

FERDINAND VON HEBRA, 1866

. . . the boy was acutely ill with a temperature of 103° F . . . the eyes are swollen shut, exuding pus; the lips are black with crusted blood . . . the tongue was swollen, bright red and fissured, and the mucous membrane of the mouth was inflamed with small bullous lesions which rapidly broke down leaving a raw and angry surface . . . the trunk, arms, and thighs were thickly set with discrete, oval, brownish purple papular lesions . . . Eleven weeks after the onset of his disease, the sunken, sightless eyes bear witness to the destructive effect of the ophthalmia . . .

STEVENS AND JOHNSON, 1922

In 1866 Ferdinand von Hebra considered a number of previously described acute cutaneous eruptions (erythemas papulatum, tuberculatum, annulare, iris, and gyratum) to be forms of the same disease in different stages. He proposed to combine these erythemas under the single term of erythema multiforme, a malady with distinctive characteristics. Von Hebra did not describe mucous membrane involvement as a part of this disorder. In 1922 two American physicians, Stevens and Johnson, described two children with an acute fever and skin lesions that resembled EM, but who in addition had severe stomatitis and a purulent conjunctivitis that led to permanent visual impairment. These children were very sick with systemic symptoms. Subsequently, this condition became known as Stevens-Johnson syndrome, a severe form of EM. In 1950 Thomas proposed that EM was a disorder with a spectrum of presentations. The mild "typical" EM described by von Hebra should be designated "erythema multiforme minor" (EM minor) and the severe mucocutaneous variety described by Stevens and Johnson should be "erythema multiforme major" (EM major). This classification is useful when we recognize that these two conditions represent limits in a spectrum of the same pathologic process. Some patients with recurrent EM may initially present with EM minor and develop EM major with subsequent episodes.

Most EM patients are young, healthy adults 20 to 40 years of age (range: 1 to 89) with an approximately equal sex distribution. The eruption is recurrent in one third of patients, especially those with mucous membrane involvement and those whose eruption is precipitated by herpes simplex infections.

A prodrome of an upper respiratory illness accompanied by fever, malaise, and headache occurs in one third of cases and may be present for a week or more before the onset of EM. The skin eruption occurs seven to 14 days after the inciting agent. Not only do cutaneous manifestations vary from patient to patient, but they may evolve and change in appearance during the course of the illness in any one patient, thus earning the term "multiforme."

Mild forms (EM minor) are characterized by flat-topped, sharply marginated, dusky red papules 1 to 2 cm in diameter. A few of the larger papules have concentric rings with variable alterations in morphology and color. There may be a central papule, blister, or area of epidermal necrosis with outer rings varying in color—white, gray, blue, red, and pink—giving rise to the terms "iris" or "target" lesions. Typically, though not invariably, a few of the papules will be the target type, and when present are virtually pathognomonic of this disorder. Lesions may coalesce, forming a polycyclic configuration. Individual skin lesions persist for a few weeks and then resolve, leaving scaling and postinflammatory hyperpigmentation, but no atrophy or scarring. Distribution of the lesions of EM minor are characteristically symmetric and acral over the dorsum of the hands, palms, and soles. Later, the eruption moves onto the flexural surfaces and truncal skin, and less frequently onto the neck, ears, and face. Lesions are rarely found on the scalp. When truncal lesions occur, they are far less dense than extremity involvement.

Mucosal involvement is reported in 20% to 60% of patients with EM, but in my experience most patients have some involvement. If an EM diagnosis is suspected, the ocular, oral, and genital surfaces should be carefully examined. The finding of mucosal inflammation can be very helpful in determining a diagnosis of EM. There may be mild conjunctivitis; the lips may have fine superficial scaling with faint erythema or may have confluent erosions with crusting. There may be diffuse erythema in the mouth with irregular ulcerations covered by pseudomembranes. The mouth may be the only site involved in EM. Similar ulcers may be present on the genitalia; the external urethral meatus should be examined for ulcerations, as it is easy to overlook this area.

Patients may be asymptomatic or may complain of mild malaise, itching or burning of the skin, and pain of the mucosal erosions. Fever, myalgia, arthralgias, and headache are rare. Duration is usually less than four weeks.

The above features are grossly exaggerated in EM major. The typical patient has a week of profound constitutional symptoms consisting of fever (103° to 104°F), malaise, and upper respiratory symptoms, followed by the explosive onset of generalized erythematous plaques a few centimeters in diameter with superimposed flaccid bullae. By definition, all EM major patients have mucous membrane involvement, which can include painful hemorrhagic crusted lips, erosion of the entire oral mucosa, and purulent conjunctivitis. In addition, there may be periorbital edema and erythema, corneal erosions, and perforations. In approximately 5% of patients, blindness has been reported. Erosions may extend to any part of the gastrointestinal tract and may lead to esophageal lesions, intestinal bleeding, perforations, and anal ulcers resulting in strictures. The respiratory tract erosions may cause epistaxis, pneumothorax, and pneumonia (also a leading cause of death from EM). Genitourinary erosions may make urination extremely painful to the point of urinary retention, and may subsequently cause strictures of the urethra and vaginal orifice. Occasionally, there is nephritis, myocarditis, pericarditis, and hepatitis. Less serious complications include postinflammatory hyperpigmentation of the skin and shedding of the finger- and toenails. Healing usually occurs in four to six weeks; mortality rates range from 5% to 15%.

To confirm the proper diagnosis, skin biopsies can be performed for both routine histology and direct immunofluorescent examination. Cultures of the throat and sputum may be indicated. Additional tests are suggested by an abnormal clinical examination (primarily to avoid the rare but serious complications), to include chest x-ray for upper respiratory infections, urinalysis for potential nephritis, complete blood count for depressed white blood cell counts, liver function tests for hepatitis, electrolytes for an imbalance, blood cultures if there is evidence of sepsis, and electrocardiogram for myocarditis.

Toxic epidermal necrolysis (TEN) is most likely a variant of severe EM in which there is widespread blister formation so extensive that sheets of skin are lost, much like an extensive burn. Owing to fluid and electrolyte imbalance and secondary sepsis, mortality rates are as high as 25% to 50%.

MANAGEMENT

PLAN

EM minor is considered a benign, self-limiting disorder whereby individuals are treated easily in an outpatient setting. Stevens-Johnson syndrome or EM major is usually a medical emergency, requiring hospitalization and meticulous nursing care for most patients.

NONPHARMACOLOGIC MEASURES

Sometimes EM minor does not require treatment unless there is mucous membrane involvement. If these membranes are involved, patients should avoid hard, hot, acidic, sharp, irritating foods, and consume instead a liquid or soft diet. Adequate hydration must be maintained with frequent mouthwashes (see ''Drug Therapy'' below), ice chips, and perhaps a bedside humidifier. Treatment of EM major varies from the good oral hygiene for EM minor to possible intragastric feeding via nasogastric tube, intravenous fluids, and urinary catheterization. Daily intake and output of fluids and body weight should be monitored. As for a burn victim, meticulous skin care is necessary and burn-wound isolation should be instituted.

DRUG THERAPY

Drug therapy for EM must be a logical approach that considers the potential seriousness of the disorders, the initial inciting agent, the pathophysiology of the problem, and our own personal experience, since controlled, systematic studies of EM treatment do not exist.

For EM minor systemic steroids may be withheld. Treatment is given for symptomatic relief of minor skin and mucous membrane inflammation. If itching is present, an antihistamine (e.g., hydroxyzine, 25 mg four times a day); a medium-strength topical steroid (e.g.,

triamcinolone cream, 0.1% three times daily); and tub soaks with an unscented bath oil are given. For mild cheilitis, I prefer fluocinonide gel 0.05%, applied three to four times daily. Alternatives are white petrolatum or bacitracin ointment. For those with painful mucosal erosions, frequent mouthwashes with Cepacol diluted 1:4 with water several times daily are recommended. A soothing mixture of 1:1 Kaopectate plus diphenhydramine elixir or viscous lidocaine diluted 1:4 with water may alleviate pain. If there is evidence of secondary infection in the oral mucosa, erythromycin, 1 gm/day, can be given for seven days. Ponaris emollient is useful for softening hemorrhagic nasal crusting. For the occasional patient who has edema of the hands and feet with malaise or fever, 10 grains of aspirin is given every four hours.

Since the death rate varies from 5% to 15% and serious ocular sequelae may occur including blindness, I consider EM major a medical emergency. I therefore use prednisone or a prednisone equivalent of 1 to 2 mg/kg of body weight per day, tapered over one to three weeks and withdrawn as healing occurs. For patients with extensive mouth lesions who are unable to take oral medication, parenteral steroids are given. Once this treatment is started, lesions cease spreading. If there is any indication that *Mycoplasma* is the cause, I give erythromycin. Although more extensive than EM minor, the oral lesions are treated the same. For extensive bullous eruptions, tap-water wet compresses may be applied every three hours as tolerated. Some patients cannot tolerate any type of pressure on their skin. For those with extensive erosions and bullae, potassium permanganate baths (or sponge baths) diluted 1:16000 are antiseptic and drying, and help prevent secondary infections of the skin or generalized sepsis. Silver sulfadiazine cream is often applied to ruptured bullae when the patient is removed from the bath if he or she is not allergic to sulfa. Some physicians prefer to treat severe cases in hospital burn units.

The principal morbidity that occurs with EM major is related to the eyes. An ophthalmologic consultation is mandatory to avoid secondary infections, conjunctival scarring, uveitis, perforations of the globe, and subsequent visual impairment. These are managed carefully with wet compresses, frequent irrigations, artificial tears, lysis of adhesions, topical steroids, and topical antibiotics.

For persistent cases in which lesions recur when steroids are discontinued, azathioprine has been used successfully. Levamisole is being studied in clinical trials and appears to offer clinical benefit.

Adverse Effects. Potential problems involved in the use of systemic steroids include masking infections, precipitating secondary infections, masking bowel perforations, and GI bleeding. Some authors report decreased healing and prolonged hospitalization with steroids. Therefore, when steroids are used, patients must be monitored carefully for potential complications. If there is an underlying disease such as diabetes and the patient is receiving insulin, that dosage may have to be modified during steroid therapy.

Management of Complications. EM minor is virtually free of complications other than postinflammatory hyperpigmentation, which requires no therapy. With EM major, however, many deaths have been caused by upper airway complications. These include pneumonia and pneumothorax; thus, the lungs should be monitored closely and subsequent complications treated appropriately. Complications such as esophageal strictures and vaginal and anal stenosis should be treated by the appropriate specialists. In cases in which there are large areas of epidermal necrosis, fluid and electrolyte problems and subsequent dehydration and electrolyte imbalances constitute major problems and should be monitored and treated with appropriate IV fluids. Patients should be evaluated for secondary infections of the skin and for systemic infections.

PATIENT INFORMATION AND EDUCATION

I tell patients that EM is similar to an allergy. Identification and avoidance of precipitating factors are of great importance. Patients should be aware of potential complications so that they can attempt to avoid these. Patients with EM minor do not require follow-up unless there are recurrences. Periodically, those with EM major should be evaluated for potential complications, especially by ophthalmologists for such problems as ocular scarring and inadequate tear production and by urologists for urethral strictures.

Patient compliance depends on appropriate patient education concerning the avoidance of precipitating factors. Patients should avoid drugs that are thought to precipitate their specific EM and should use measures to prevent herpes simplex. These measures should include sunscreens with sun-protective lip preparations, protective clothing, sun avoidance, and salicylates whenever there is fever. Acyclovir ointment (5%) should be used for recurrent herpes simplex infections as soon as noted. Although hospitalization is expensive, it is indicated for most cases of EM major.

REFERENCES

Ackermann AB, Niven J, Grant-Kels JM: Differential Diagnosis in Dermatopathology. Lea & Febiger, Philadelphia, 1982.
Duvic M: Erythema multiforme. Dermatol Clin 1:217–230, 1982.
Huff JC, Weston WL, Tonnesen MG: Erythema multiforme: a critical review of characteristics, diagnostic criteria, and causes. J Am Acad Dermatol 8:763–778, 1983.
Lozada F, Silverman S: Erythema multiforme. Clinical characteristics and natural history in fifty patients. Oral Surg 46:628–636, 1978.
Rasmussen J: Toxic epidermal necrolysis. Med Clin North Am 64:901–920, 1980.

6 · ACNE VULGARIS

John W. Melski
MARSHFIELD CLINIC

PATHOGENESIS

Acne is a disease of the pilosebaceous follicle. A compact plug forms in the infrainfundibulum. The process is called retension hyperkeratosis, and the resulting plug is called the comedo. If the follicular orifice dilates, the "closed" comedo becomes an "open" comedo.

When sebaceous glands are stimulated by androgens, the secretions mix with the products of keratinization to produce sebum. In the anaerobic depths of the plugged follicle, sebum provides nutrients for microbes such as *Propionibacterium acnes*. A variety of potentially harmful products result. Bacterial lipases liberate free fatty acids. Proteases, esterases, neuraminidase, hyaluronidase, and lecithinase are made. Soluble chemotactic factors invite immunologic assault. Finally, the follicular wall ruptures. The microbes are quickly killed, but the inflammatory debris reeks havoc. If the rupture is superficial, a small papule or pustule results. If the rupture is deep, an inflammatory nodule is formed. Nodules may mutilate by progressing to scars, cysts, or sinuses.

EVALUATION

A common error in the management of acne is failure to draw conclusions from the inventory of lesions. Crusts and post-inflammatory macules in the absence of primary lesions suggest habitual picking. Patients need to recognize their role in aggravating and creating blemishes. Clustering may be a clue to the presence of friction or occlusion. Acne flourishes under chin straps, shoulder pads, head bands, sweaty palms, or greasy pomades. The absence of lesions may indicate a quest for perfection that cannot be achieved. Conversely, extensive disease, nodules, and scars are evidence for systemic treatment.

PATIENT EDUCATION

Patients need to know the natural history of their lesions. Unmolested papules and pustules resolve in five to ten days. Nodular lesions may take up to eight weeks. Post-inflammatory redness and pigment may last for months. Scars and cysts are permanent unless surgically corrected. The main purpose of most treatments is to prevent new blemishes, not to accelerate healing of old ones. Patients who apply their medicine only to existing lesions, or who see no improvement when only sequelae are left, have not learned this lesson.

Patients also need to know the time course of treatment response. Some see improvement within a few weeks, but many have to wait longer. Maximal benefit from tetracycline may take three months. Lesions may still appear after 20 weeks of isotretinoin. The virtues of patience and persistence need to be stressed, especially in the treatment of comedones. Papular closed comedones and open "black-heads" do resolve, but slowly.

MANAGEMENT

TOPICAL TREATMENT

Many patients can be successfully managed with topicals alone, and these may be adjunctive even when systemic treatment is required. However, proper application of topicals is not instinctive: it must be taught. It is wise to start slowly. Irritation is common, whereas allergy is uncommon. Small amounts should be applied to small areas until tolerance is demonstrated. Sample quantities provided by most manufacturers are excellent for this purpose. Eventually, all the acne-bearing skin is treated once or twice a day. It is reasonable to restrict treatment to the face when other areas are not of concern. Some patients do well with less frequent application, especially during maintenance. Few patients comply if applications have to be made more than twice daily.

Six factors must be considered when adjusting the potency of topicals: the amount applied, frequency of use, location, concentration, vehicle, and hydration of the skin. Topicals should vanish into the skin. Pea-sized amounts are adequate for each region of the face. The skin near the eyes and corners of the mouth is particularly sensitive. Treatment begins with lower concentrations, and samples can be used for experimentation with higher concentrations. Gels are generally more potent than creams. Dry skin (one-half hour after washing) is less sensitive than wet skin.

Benzoyl Peroxide. Benzoyl peroxide is the single most useful topical for acne. It works as an antimicrobial. Resistant organisms have not been described. Theories that benzoyl peroxide works as a sebostatic or comedolytic have been refuted. Its main indication is inflammatory acne. Suppression of *P. acnes* suppresses harmful bacterial products and thereby follicular rupture also. Benzoyl peroxide is available without prescription and may be the only agent necessary for mild papulopustular acne. It bleaches some fabrics, which restricts its use on the trunk. It also inactivates retinoic acid and must be applied at a different time when used in combination, usually once a day. Irritant reactions are sometimes difficult to distinguish from true allergic reactions. A 5% preparation is a useful starting point for most patients.

Retinoic Acid. Retinoic acid is the only practical comedolytic available. It is useful in all forms of acne because microcomedones are the precursors of inflammatory lesions. However, it may promote follicular rupture and should be combined with an antimicrobial when treating inflammatory acne. Retinoic acid is synergistic with other agents, in part by increasing follicular permeability. Morning use of benzoyl peroxide plus evening use of retinoic acid constitutes an effective program for many patients.

Retinoic acid can be irritating. Patient education is essential for effective use. The increasing order of irritancy is 0.05-cream, 0.1-cream, 0.01-gel, 0.025-gel, and 0.05-solution. The 0.01-gel is a useful starting point for most patients. Maximal benefit may take months, especially when treating predominantly comedonal disease. Peeling doses are not necessary, but doses near tolerance may accelerate response. Retinoic acid may also be used to treat comedones induced by sunlight, tars, and chlorinated hydrocarbons, as well as steroid acne.

Skin treated with retinoic acid has complex interactions with the sun. Tumor formation can be promoted or suppressed, depending on the animal model and experimental conditions. Patients may note a lightening of pigment or interference with tanning. Significant sun sensitivity is distinctly uncommon. Sunscreens have been advised, but this complicates treatment and may be comedogenic. I do not emphasize sun sensitivity.

Topical Antibiotics. Antibiotics are effective, but bacterial resistance following topical use is a concern. Combination with benzoyl peroxide may suppress resistance and increase effectiveness. A topical antibiotic alone may be necessary for those who do not tolerate benzoyl peroxide, such as atopic patients. As with benzoyl peroxide, the main indication is inflammatory acne. Suppression of bacteria may decrease comedo formation, but this is probably a second-order effect. Antibiotics may have direct anti-inflammatory effects.

Topical clindamycin gained early and widespread use. However, topical erythromycin appears to be as effective and does not have the cloud of pseudomembranous colitis associated with clindamycin. Topical tetracycline is also available, but discoloration and fluorescence of the skin are disadvantages and it may not be as effective. All these preparations are available in premixed containers with applicators, and generally are used twice a day.

Other Topicals. A vast number of preparations have been tried but many are ineffective. Antimicrobials such as hexachlorophene, benzalkonium chloride, and povidone-iodine do not penetrate well enough to affect acne flora. Salicylic acid is comedolytic in concentrations that are too irritating for most patients (5% to 10%). Irritants such as sulfur and resorcinol may promote desquamation and resolution of superficial lesions, but this is a nonspecific effect. Claims have been made for anhydrous aluminum chloride, miconazole, azelaic acid, and a variety of other antibiotics.

No topical decreases sebum production. Surface oils can be removed for comfort by soap and water. Astringents may compromise the use of more effective preparations. Abrasives and washing more than twice a day should be avoided.

SYSTEMIC MEDICATIONS

Tetracyclines. Tetracycline can be used alone, but many patients benefit from combination with benzoyl peroxide or retinoic acid. It is relatively inexpensive and remarkably safe. Dose-dependent nausea and vaginal moniliasis are the most common side effects. It is incorporated into growing bones and teeth and should not be used in young children or during pregnancy. To be absorbed, it must be taken on an empty stomach (one hour before or two hours after eating). To avoid esophagitis, it should not be taken less than one-half hour before lying down (e.g., before bedtime). Photosensitivity is rare with the doses used for acne. Demeclocycline has its own peculiar photosensitization and may also cause diabetes insipidus. All but doxycycline may be toxic to kidneys during renal failure. Allergic reactions are distinctly uncommon, but fixed drug eruptions and other cutaneous expressions of allergy have been reported. Other rare sequelae include hematologic abnormalities, pseudotumor cerebri, and hepatic dysfunction in pregnant women with renal failure.

A common error with tetracycline is to use too little for too short a time. Many patients need 1 gm or more of tetracycline a day for many weeks or months to achieve maximal benefit. Tetracycline resistance should be carefully evaluated before other treatments are considered. Patients usually comply with twice-a-day administration. Proper use should be reviewed. Aggravating factors should be sought, including manipulation, psychologic stress, other medications, and comedogenic exposures. Many sequelae of acne are long-lived.

Other Antibiotics. Minocycline has been touted for tetracycline-resistant acne. Its toxicity is similar to that of other tetracyclines. It also induces vestibular dysfunction above doses of 150 mg a day. It can be taken with meals but is much more expensive than plain tetracycline. Studies comparing minocycline with tetracycline are flawed by failure to choose comparable doses or by making comparisons at six weeks rather than 12.

Erythromycin is also effective. Unfortunately, it often has the same side effects in the same patients as tetracycline: nausea and vaginal moniliasis. An occasional patient who does not respond to tetracycline will respond to erythromycin.

Many antibiotics might work but are either too expensive or unsafe for serious consideration. Enthusiasm for clindamycin has come and gone. Ampicillin has testimonial support but has not been carefully studied. Trimethoprim-sulfa combinations have an alarming rate of allergic reactions with regular use. Trimethoprim alone may be effective.

Isotretinoin. Isotretinoin (Accutane) is a remarkable drug that provides salvation for patients with severe acne that other therapies cannot control. Patients who were once hospitalized or treated with dapsone or prednisone are now candidates for cure with isotretinoin, and are best managed by a dermatologist.

Catastrophic birth defects are the most feared complication of isotretinoin, and pregnancy is an absolute contraindication to its use. I repeatedly warn female patients of this and offer to arrange birth control counseling. Treatment should begin only when the patient has a negative pregnancy test after well-established and effective birth control.

Long-term follow-ups on large numbers of patients are not yet available. Side effects during the typical 20-week course are mostly tolerable and manageable. Triglycerides must be monitored: levels above 600 are an indication for stopping isotretinoin at least temporarily, and levels above 400 are an indication for close monitoring, reduced dosage, and dietary restrictions (especially alcohol). I look for, but have not yet seen, other significant laboratory abnormalities, including abnormal liver function tests. Xerosis and cheilitis are concomitants of effective treatment. Atopic patients may get into trouble with staphylococal impetigenization. Decreases in visual acuity require evaluation by an ophthalmologist. Insulin-dependent diabetics may be more difficult to control, and the drug should be used with caution in patients with inflammatory bowel disease.

As the time after initial treatment lengthens, the number of relapses increases. These can be kept to a minimum by using at least 1 mg/kg during initial treatment. When necessary, I alternate the number of 40-mg pills on odd and even days rather than use smaller doses.

Hormone Therapy. In the pre-isotretinoin era, high-estrogen birth control pills (50 µg) with a non-androgenic progestin (norethynodrel, ethynodrel diacetate, or norethisterone) were often used for women with severe acne. This is still an option if the risks are understood by and acceptable to the patient. For patients with less severe disease, the role of hormone therapy is unclear. The definition of normal is too elusive to justify screening all women. Endocrine evaluation should be considered for those with irregular menses two years after the menarche, for older women with infertility, or for women with masculinization. Low-dose evening prednisone (2.5 mg) may be useful for some patients, theoretically those with increased adrenal androgens and elevated DHEAS. I have little enthusiasm for long-term antiandrogen therapy such as spironolactone, cimetidine, or ketoconazole.

Anti-inflammatory Agents. Blanching inflammatory nodules with small amounts of intralesional triamcinolone acetonide (2.5 mg/cc or less) is often appreciated by patients who need a quick fix of an unsightly and painful blemish. It should not replace preventive treatment.

Ibuprofen in doses up to 600 mg four times a day has been shown to augment the benefits of systemic tetracycline. This may be the tip of the iceberg of anti-inflammatory treatments in the future.

SURGERY

Comedo extraction in a patient using topical retinoic acid may accelerate an otherwise slow process. Without retinoic acid, comedones reform.

Some nodules are fluctuant and drain copious amounts of liquefied debris. Most nodules do not benefit from incision and drainage, and scarring may be increased by such efforts. True cysts and sinuses should be suspected when lesions do not resolve after several months. Revision of the acne-scarred face is a topic unto itself.

OTHER TREATMENTS

The improvement that occurs in the summer is not due to ultraviolet light. It may be related to decreased stress. A tan hides blemishes, but the aging and carcinogenic effects of ultraviolet light make it an unattractive cosmetic.

The best cosmetic is none. "Oil-free" is undefined. "Non-comedogenic" refers to laboratory investigations using rabbit ears. In the absence of better data and a deeply ingrained desire for cosmetics on the part of the patient, the practitioner is wise to have a list of non-comedogenic cosmetics available.

Oral zinc has not had reproducable benefits and causes nausea in most patients. Dietary manipulations, other than starvation, do not alter sebaceous secretions. Fried foods should not be smeared on the face but can be safely eaten. Vitamin A is a dangerous substitute for isotretinoin. Cold slushes and sprays and superficial peels may hasten the resolution of some lesions but are an expensive adjunct to natural healing. Steam treatments and "pore minimizers" are a waste of time and money. Radiation cannot be justified.

CONCLUSIONS

Most patients benefit from topical treatment, usually some combination with benzoyl peroxide. Extensive disease, nodules, and scar formation are indications for systemic treatment, usually tetracycline. Isotretinoin should be reserved for patients with objective evidence of severe disease. Patience is a virtue for all treatments. There should be enough time between visits to allow for two menstrual cycles, or two months. More frequent visits can be justified early in treatment to reinforce basic priciples or in order to monitor patients on isotretinoin. Less frequent visits are needed when treatments are stablilized. Practitioners should be willing to spend time with their patients to evaluate and teach them about their disease.

REFERENCES

Chalker DK, Shalita A, Smith JG, et al: A double-blind study of the effectiveness of a 3% erythromycin and 5% benzoyl peroxide combination in the treatment of acne vulgaris. J Am Acad Dermatol 9:933–936, 1983.

Dicken CH: Retinoids: a review. J Am Acad Dermatol 11:541–552, 1984.

Hubbell CG, Hobbs ER, Rist T, et al: Efficacy of minocycline compared with tetracycline in treatment of acne vulgaris. Arch Dermatol 118:989–992, 1982.

Leyden JJ, McGinley KJ, Cavalieri S, et al: *Propionibacterium acnes* resistance to antibiotics in acne patients. J Am Acad Dermatol: 8:41–45, 1983.

Lucky AW: Endocrine aspects of acne. Pediatr Clin North Am 30:495–499, 1983.

Padilla RS, McCabe JM, Becker LE: Topical tetracycline hydrochloride vs topical clindamycin phosphate in the treatment of acne. Int J Dermatol 20:445–448, 1981.

Plewig G, Kligman AM: Acne: Morphogenesis and Treatment. Springer-Verlag, New York, 1975.

Shalita AR, Smith EB, Bauer E: Topical erythromycin vs clindamycin therapy for acne. Arch Dermatol 120:351–355, 1984.

Wong RC, Kang S, Heezen JL, et al: Oral ibuprofen and tetracycline for the treatment of acne vulgaris. J Am Acad Dermatol 11:1076–1081, 1984.

7 · SUNBURN

Joseph F. Seber
MARSHFIELD CLINIC

Sunburn is an acute skin injury caused by ultraviolet (UV) light. The spectrum of ultraviolet light is from 200 to 400 nanometers (nm), just below that of visible light (from 400 to 790 nm). The peak of the sunburn spectrum, from 290 to 320 nm, is known as ultraviolet-B (UVB). The tanning spectrum occurs in ultraviolet-A (UVA), (320 to 400 nm). These two wavelengths act additively to produce their effects.

PATHOGENESIS

Ultraviolet radiation sufficient for sunburn does not produce erythema for at least three hours. Because of this delay, many sunburn victims are unaware that their exposure has been excessive. Redness and edema peak at 24 hours and begin to subside at 72 hours. Dyskeratotic and vacuolated "sunburn" cells are evident in the epidermis. The erythema represents inflammation around the blood vessels in the superficial and deep venous plexus. Mast cells degranulate, histamine levels rise fourfold, and prostaglandin E_2 reaches one and one half times the control values. These changes probably result from direct injury to cellular protein and nucleic acids. Chronic UVB exposure interferes with immune surveillance and promotes squamous- and basal-cell skin cancers. Repeated sunburns are themselves a risk for malignant melanoma.

PREVENTION

Ultraviolet flux varies according to altitude, latitude, time of day, and atmospheric conditions. People susceptible to sunburn are at greatest risk on a clear, sunny day at high noon. Proximity to the equator, elevation above sea level, and wind are also risk factors. Summertime activities before 9:00 AM or after 3:00 PM, when the sun is less intense, are the safest. Those skiing at high altitude should take extra precautions even in winter. Fifty per cent of ultraviolet light reaching the skin is from scattered sunlight, so that sunscreens are important even on cloudy days or when in the shade.

Sunscreens containing para-aminobenzoic acid (PABA), PABA esters, and benzophenones offer substantial protection even for fair-skinned persons. These products are assigned a sun protective factor (SPF) that represents the amount of time required to produce erythema (minimal erythema dose, MED) relative to the time required to produce MED if the sunscreen is not used. Therefore, a sunscreen lotion with an SPF of 15 means that a person can remain in the sun 15 times longer than when not covered with the lotion. If sunlight exposure is anticipated, fair-skinned individuals should apply an SPF-15 sunscreen 15 minutes before exposure. The routine use of sunscreens should be encouraged.

TREATMENT

Many acute sunburns can be controlled adequately with cool wet soaks alone. Terry cloth towels soaked in cool water are placed over the sunburned area. These can be changed every one to two hours. Some advocate the use of topical corticosteroids (0.1% triamcinolone cream) under the soaks to facilitate relief. Although precise investigations show that neither topical nor systemic corticosteroids benefit lab-induced sunburn, many clinicians advise 60 to 80 mg of prednisone each morning for three consecutive days to decrease pain and erythema. It is important to stress that relief for the patient is the primary goal, since it has been shown experimentally that sunburn-induced erythema subsides by 72 hours with no treatment. Finally, aspirin, indomethacin, or other nonsteroidal anti-inflammatory agents are helpful to individuals who know they have a low MED, as these can be taken within the first few hours of sun exposure to prevent much of the erythema.

REFERENCE

Gilchrest BA, Soter NA, Stoff JS, et al: The human sunburn reaction: histologic and biochemical studies. J Am Acad Dermatol 5:411–422, 1981.

8 · HERPES ZOSTER

Elizabeth I. McBurney
OCHSNER CLINIC AND ALTON OCHSNER MEDICAL
FOUNDATION

DEFINITION

Herpes zoster is a cutaneous viral infection caused by the varicella-zoster virus. It is commonly known as shingles, which derives from the Latin word meaning girdle, and refers to the characteristic clinical picture of unilateral, linear vesicles in a dermatomal distribution. There is no seasonal variation in the incidence of the disease. Although a person can contract zoster at any age, the attack rate increases dramatically after the age of 60. Knowledge of this disease and of its complications and therapy is important in the care of the elderly and immunosuppressed patients, as both groups are at greatest risk for herpes zoster and are rapidly increasing in number.

PATHOPHYSIOLOGY

The varicella-zoster virus is a DNA virus and is included in the same group as herpes simplex, cytomegalovirus, and Epstein-Barr. The primary human infection of the varicella-zoster virus causes varicella, or chickenpox. During this infection the virus spreads to the dorsal root or cranial nerve ganglia, where it remains latent, usually for many years. Reactivation of the varicella-zoster virus leads to the clinical illness of herpes zoster. There have been occasional conflicting reports in the literature, suggesting that herpes zoster may in some cases represent exogenous exposure to the varicella-zoster virus rather than the reactivation of endogenous latent virus. Exactly how this virus is triggered or reactivated is not known, but age, trauma, surgery, radiotherapy, use of immunosuppressive drugs, debilitating diseases, and malignancy, such as Hodgkin's lymphoma, are known to be risk factors. The current opinion is that reactivation of the latent virus reflects a generally lowered cellular immunity. Zoster cannot be acquired from other patients with zoster or varicella. A patient with herpes zoster may transfer the virus to a nonimmunized person, resulting in varicella or chickenpox. Four per cent of patients have second attacks, and some have third attacks, usually involving the same dermatome.

CLINICAL CHARACTERISTICS

Diagnosis is usually made on clinical grounds. The cutaneous eruption is preceded by one to five days of pain or paresthesias in the involved dermatome, headache, fever, and lymphadenopathy. Prior to development of the characteristic rash, the pain may be confused with abdominal crisis, pleuritis, renal colic, cardiac disease, sciatica, or Bell's palsy. Occasionally a patient is admitted to the coronary care unit for severe left-sided chest pain, only to be found on rounds 24 hours later to have developed the classic herpes zoster dermatomal vesicular lesions. It is not unusual to have five or six isolated lesions outside the dermatome. Zoster may involve any part of the body, but it appears most frequently in the thoracic dermatomes. However, zoster is not uncommon in the cervical and lumbar dermatomes and in the cranial nerve distribution, especially the ophthalmic branch of the trigeminal nerve. The developing erythematous-based vesicles ultimately develop a crust, although some may rapidly become pustular earlier, and some leave significant pitted scarring. New lesions may continue to appear for up to seven days, and complete resolution generally occurs within two to three weeks.

Dissemination of herpes zoster is generally a mild disorder associated with little morbidity or mortality. Approximately 2% to 4% of all zoster cases in normal hosts disseminate. In 20% to 30% of patients with malignancy, particularly lymphoproliferative disorders, and those with severe immunosuppression, localized herpes zoster disseminates.

There are two clinical syndromes that uniquely involve the cranial nerves. First is herpes zoster ophthalmicus, which involves the trigeminal nerve. Fifty per cent of patients with this syndrome develop ocular complications, the most frequent of which are keratitis, iritis, secondary glaucoma, and extraocular muscle involvement (ptosis). The second cutaneous clinical syndrome is herpes zoster oticus (Ramsay Hunt syndrome), which involves the geniculate ganglion and is characterized by facial nerve paralysis, hearing impairment, dizziness, and the characteristic eruption on the pinna or external auditory canal.

The most dreaded complication of herpes zoster is the development of postherpetic neuralgia, which is generally defined as persistent pain in the affected dermatome two months after resolution of the cutaneous lesions. This is seen with increasing frequency in patients over 60 years of age and is rare in children and young adults. In a few patients, the pain may be so severe as to lead to narcotic addiction, severe depression, or even suicide.

Occasionally a clinical case may be atypical or may mimic herpes simplex. Additional diagnostic studies are required to confirm herpes zoster. A Tzanck smear of the scraping of a vesicle base confirms a viral infection by the presence of multinucleated giant cells but does not differentiate between herpes simplex and herpes zoster. Other laboratory diagnostic tests include direct immunofluorescence staining of cellular material from a fresh vesicle, viral cultures, counterimmunoelectrophoresis, and serologic antibodies.

MANAGEMENT

PLAN

Short-term and Long-term Goals. The primary goals in the management of herpes zoster are fourfold: (1) to isolate the patient to prevent spread of the varicella-zoster virus to susceptible younger patients, pregnant women, and immunosuppressed persons; (2) to minimize the acute pain and discomfort from the cutaneous lesions; (3) to be aware of the possibility of dissemination of a localized disease, particularly in an immunosuppressed patient; and (4) to prevent the development of postherpetic neuralgia.

Indications for Ambulatory Treatment and Hospitalization. Most people with herpes zoster may be treated on an outpatient basis. The exceptions to these are elderly patients with gangrenous necrotic lesions associated with excruciating pain, immunosuppressed patients, those with disseminated zoster, and patients with severe facial zoster and eye involvement.

DRUG THERAPY

Topical. For the patient with uncomplicated herpes zoster, I usually recommend that the lesions be soaked with 1:40 modified Burow's solution (aluminum acetate solution, Domeboro) compresses for 15 minutes three times a day, using a clean washcloth saturated with the solution. After being compressed for 15 minutes, the involved area is dried well, and a lotion composed of 60 gm of triamcinolone cream 0.1% in 120 cc of milk of bismuth is applied. If there is any evidence of secondary infection, the patient is also started on a broad-spectrum antibiotic, such as erythromycin, 250 mg q.i.d.

Systemic Steroids. In multiple studies the need for systemic steroids to prevent postherpetic neuralgia has been well documented. Systemic steroids do not increase the possibility of dissemination, and their use is not contraindicated with eye involvement. Unless contraindicated, systemic steroids should be used in all zoster patients over 40 because of the high occurrence of postherpetic neuralgia in this group. Treatment should be started immediately; it does not influence the healing time of the cutaneous eruption. There are various regimens in the literature. Most recommend tapering doses of oral corticosteroids over a three- to four-week period. Oral prednisone or its equivalent is given: 60 mg daily in a single dose for one week, 30 mg every day for the second week, and 15 mg every day for the third week. Another regimen is prednisone, 40 mg daily with gradual reduction over four weeks. I personally have found it very useful to give 1 cc of triamcinolone acetonide (Kenalog 40) IM weekly, for a total of three weeks. The advantages of IM steroids are two: they permit a measured control over the amount given, and there is no need to instruct elderly persons how to taper oral steroids, which can be confusing to them.

Analgesics. It has been my experience that because the systemic steroids have no effect on the acute pain, the patient requires adequate doses of analgesics. My preferences are acetaminophen with 0.5-grain codeine (Tylenol #3) and oxycodone hydrochloride (Percodan), given once every four hours as needed for pain. Elderly patients should be cautioned about side effects of the analgesics. These can be a problem, particularly during the night if patients get up to go to the bathroom, when they may be disoriented and more likely to fall. I recommend the use of a night light. Patients are advised not to drive or operate equipment such as a snowblower or lawnmower while taking analgesics.

Antiviral Agents. Intravenous acyclovir (Zovirax) has been shown to improve the rate of healing and shorten the duration of pain in acute herpes zoster. It is given in doses of 5 to 10 mg/kg infused at a constant rate over one hour, every eight hours for seven days. Acyclovir has a low toxicity and high efficacy. Unfortunately, since the drug is given IV, patients require hospitalization. Thus the expense of this therapy is reserved for immunosuppressed patients or those with severe localized disease. This drug has not been licensed by the Food and Drug Administration for treating zoster, but many controlled studies in the literature support its use.

The role of oral acyclovir in treating herpes zoster is currently being investigated. Some preliminary British reports suggest that early initiation of oral acyclovir after 96 hours of the eruption can reduce significantly the duration of vesicles, development of new lesions, and acute pain. The dosage evaluated is 400 to 800 mg five times daily for five days. Neither the oral nor IV acyclovir has any influence on the development of postherpetic neuralgia.

Treatment of immunocompromised hosts has shown the efficacy of vidarabine, acyclovir, and alpha-interferon in the therapy for herpes zoster. Each of these drugs has individual toxicity, and all must be given parenterally. Investigations to compare the three agents in a controlled manner are under way, but at present it seems most appropriate to treat severely immunocompromised patients in the earliest states of herpes zoster with IV acyclovir.

Other. Some initial reports have suggested that cimetidine (Tagamet) may be helpful in the treatment of acute herpes zoster. The dose administered is 300 mg q.i.d. for five to seven days. In the few reported cases, cimetidine induced prompt resolution of cutaneous lesions and diminished acute severe pain.

MANAGEMENT OF COMPLICATIONS

A patient presenting with herpes zoster ophthalmicus should be referred immediately to an ophthalmologist. Topical ophthalmic antiviral agents are of unproven efficacy, and topical and systemic steroids are the mainstay of therapy.

The most difficult patient to treat is the one with residual postherpetic neuralgia pain, which may be constant or episodic. The affected dermatome may have a hyperesthetic area, and light touch to the area may trigger severe, stabbing pain. Treatment of established postherpetic neuralgia is less than satisfactory, and prevention of the complication by use of systemic steroids is of great importance. To avoid chronic dependence on narcotic drugs, other modes of therapy for postherpetic neuralgia should be vigorously pursued.

The use of a combination tricyclic antidepressant and a substituted phenothiazine medication may give resolution of pain after a couple of weeks of therapy and it may be necessary to continue for several months. Amitriptyline hydrochloride (Elavil), 75 to 100 mg daily, can be used in combination with perphenazine (Trilifon), 4 mg t.i.d. or q.i.d.; fluphenazine hydrochloride (Permitil), 1 mg t.i.d. or q.i.d., or thioridazine (Mellaril), 25 mg q.i.d. Use of these drugs in elderly patients may be associated with memory lapse, sedation, and hallucination.

It has been reported that relief of pain in patients with acute herpes zoster and postherpetic neuralgia has occurred through intralesional or subcutaneous injection of corticosteroids into the affected dermatome. Triamcinolone acetonide, 200 mg, is added to 100 ml of normal saline to produce a suspension of 2 mg/ml. The mixture is injected subcutaneously via a 25-gauge, 5/8-inch long needle into involved areas. Up to 60 mg of triamcinolone (30 cc of suspension) can be given at each session. Repeated daily injections are administered until desired results are achieved, but little additional benefit can be expected after the first 12 to 14 treatments. If an extensive area is involved, it may require two or three daily injections. Reported complications are few, but they include pain at time of injection, hemorrhages, local atrophy, abscess formation, thrombophlebitis, and vertigo.

Additional therapeutic options for postherpetic neuralgia include local cryosurgery of the involved dermatome, transcutaneous electrical stimulation, surgical excision of the scarred dermatome, and neurosurgical intervention in those patients with intractable pain.

PERIODIC EVALUATION

No follow-up therapy is necessary after resolution of herpes zoster. Because of the increased risk of herpes zoster in patients with cancer, a complete evaluation for underlying malignancy has been advocated in the past for herpes zoster patients. A 1982 Mayo clinic study showed that the incidence of cancer was no greater in that population than in the general population. Subjecting patients who present with herpes zoster to aggressive work-ups for occult cancer does not seem justified on this evidence.

PREVENTIVE MEASURES

Patients with herpes zoster should be advised that they may transfer the virus to nonimmunized persons, resulting in varicella or chickenpox. Transfer of herpes zoster to another patient is not likely. Patients should be isolated from pregnant females and immunocompromised patients.

The role of zoster immunoglobulin has shown no therapeutic advantage in the treatment of cutaneous disseminated zoster. It should be reserved for the prevention and modification of varicella in exposed, susceptible immunocompromised patients.

REFERENCES

Arndt KA: Manual of Dermatologic Therapeutics. Little, Brown & Co, Boston, 1983, pp 101–106.
Koch-Weser J, Hirsch MS, Schooley RT: Treatment of herpes virus infections (first of two parts). N Engl J Med 309:963–970, 1983.
Liesegang TJ: The varicella-zoster viruses: systemic and ocular features. J Am Acad Dermatol 11:165–191, 1984.
Ragozzino MW, Melton LJ, Kurland LT, et al: Risk of cancer after herpes zoster: a population-based study. N Engl J Med 307:393–397, 1982.
Reuler JB, Chang MK: Herpes zoster: epidemiology, clinical features and management. South Med J 77:1149–1156, 1984.

9 · CUTANEOUS MANIFESTATIONS OF RHEUMATOID ARTHRITIS

F. J. Viozzi
O. F. Miller III
GEISINGER MEDICAL CENTER

Rheumatoid arthritis presents classically with acute recurrent attacks of joint inflammation and progressive and chronic joint deformity. The disease attacks other organ systems, including the skin, with a wide spectrum of cutaneous disease. Several of the cutaneous changes demand therapeutic intervention to prevent incapacitation, further disability, or sepsis. Toxicity or allergy to antiarthritic medications accounts for additional cutaneous involvement.

PATHOPHYSIOLOGY

Rheumatoid arthritis and its major serious cutaneous manifestations remain of uncertain pathogenesis, although alterations of the immune response appear to be inseparably related. Patients with immune complex deposition demonstrated in involved vessels often have more significant arthritis and cutaneous disease, higher titers of rheumatoid factor, lower levels of complement, and circulating immune complexes.

CLINICAL ASPECTS

Rheumatoid nodules, the most commonly recognized extra-articular cutaneous manifestation, present as firm, subcutaneous, mobile, usually asymptomatic nodules on the extensor surfaces. Rarely, ulceration follows trauma or pressure.

Vasculitis has protean manifestations varying from nail fold telangiectasia to palpable purpura to severe ulcerations. Nail fold infarcts appear as pustules, crusts, or barely perceptible pigmented streaks on finger pads or nail folds, often in association with Raynaud's phenomenon. Infarcts can remain small and limited or may progress to digital gangrene.

Ulcers pose a diagnostic and therapeutic challenge. In addition to vasculitic ulcers, increased skin fragility predisposes rheumatoids to the development of traumatic and stasis ulcers with unpredictable pain. Vasculitis presents as painful, punched-out, sometimes deep ulcers with overhanging margins. Marginal erythema signals active disease, with possible enlargement of the ulcer and resistance to therapy. A most ominous presentation of vasculitis is the painful supramalleolar ulcer with footdrop and loss of sensory perception in the involved extremity. Pyoderma gangrenosum, a vasculitic variant, presents initially as erythematous hemorrhagic nodules that rapidly ulcerate. Dusky, boggy, necrotic, and undermined borders characterize fully developed classic pyoderma gangrenosum, usually located on the lower extremities or abdomen.

Antirheumatic medications have been implicated in many different cutaneous manifestations varying from hives to life-threatening mucocutaneous exfoliation. A single medication may be associated with a wide range of cutaneous manifestations. Approximately 10% of patients on gold therapy present with nonspecific dermatologic reactions, as well as a more characteristic lichen planus–like eruption. D-Penicillamine has been implicated in pemphigus foliaceus, which may persist despite discontinuation of the drug.

MANAGEMENT

The goals of management in the outpatient setting are long-term reduction of primary disease activity and short-term preservation of tissue and function. Despite the emphasis on outpatient therapy, individuals with vasculitic ulcers, mononeuritis multiplex, pyoderma gangrenosum, or significant secondary infection should be initially hospitalized for treatment and stabilization of disease through the multidisciplinary approach of rheumatology, dermatology, orthopedics, and rehabilitation medicine.

The approach to the nonspecific cutaneous changes involves general skin care, including proper use of soap and emollients. To avoid excessive drying and irritation of the skin, soap and water use should be limited during the less humid, colder months. Nonmedicated emollients contribute to maintenance of soft, pliable skin. Fluorinated topical steroids for irritation should not be employed for intervals longer than two weeks, and if topical steroids are necessary, nonfluorinated hydrocortisone preparations should be substituted wherever possible.

Rheumatoid nodules can be excised if painful or ulcerated from trauma, or on occasion for cosmetic purposes.

Patients with Raynaud's phenomenon should stop smoking and avoid caffeine. Head and extremities should be compulsively protected from cold. Nail fold infarcts can acquire significant size and require surgical or whirlpool debridement, with or without proteolytic agents. If the infarct progresses to digital gangrene,

surgical amputation remains the only option. An area of limited gangrene free of infection and disease activity will often self-amputate. Calcium channel blockers such as nifedipine (Procardia), 10 mg t.i.d., may avert further tissue destruction and afford some pain relief.

In the treatment of ulcers, several aspects of care remain paramount (Fig. 1). All patients with rheumatoid arthritis require proper rest. We stress a daily minimum of one hour, preferably reclining, with the affected extremity elevated. For all ulcers, regardless of cause, the sine qua non of therapy includes elimination or prevention of edema, appropriate debridement, and antibiotics for secondary infection. Eliminate edema with elevation and the application of support stockings or Ace wraps before the patient gets out of bed. Although they are effective, fitted stockings (e.g., Jobst), can be difficult to manage even for the least debilitated. The need for debridement varies with the amount and degree of adherence of debris. Our initial approach includes proteolytic agents or a 40% urea preparation occluded with polyethylene (Saran Wrap) for one to four days before gentle mechanical or whirlpool debridement.

Reepithelialization of the debrided ulcer bed may be enhanced with 1% silver sulfadiazine creme or the Pace technique (10% benzoyl peroxide occluded with polyethylene b.i.d.). Recently we have noted more rapid reepithelialization as well as dramatic pain relief through occlusion with artifical skin dressings (vapor-permeable membranes) applied for periods of up to one week.

Pyoderma gangrenosum poses a unique therapeutic problem. Rest and elevation are indicated. Despite significant necrosis, vigorous surgical debridement often appears to increase disease activity and contribute to ulcer enlargement (the phenomenon of pathergy). Intralesional steroids (triamcinolone acetonide, not exceeding a total dose of 40 to 80 mg at four-week intervals) infiltrated into the advancing borders and base of the ulcer can reduce or halt disease activity.

Systemic steroids remain the therapeutic mainstay of vasculitis and pyoderma gangrenosum, with an initial dose of 80 mg reduced by 25% decrements every two to four weeks once the disease process has been controlled and healing has begun. For severe vasculitic ulceration and pyoderma gangrenosum, closely monitored pulse therapy with large doses of corticosteroids has been effective, but should be carried out only by physicians experienced in this method. Adjunctive therapy is frequently required with one of several options: a minimal trial of eight weeks of dapsone, 200 to 300 mg q.d.; minocycline hydrochloride, 200 mg q.d.; cyclophosphamide, 1 to 2 mg/kg/day; clofazimine, 100 mg t.i.d.; or hyperbaric oxygen. Plasmapheresis with 2-liter exchanges and albumin-electrolyte replacement daily for ten days is indicated for demonstrable cryoglobulins or immune complexes. Further adjunctive measures include calciferol and a calcium supplement to reduce the risk of osteopenia in postmenopausal women (Table 1).

The usual approach to cutaneous reactions from medications is to discontinue them. However, in the presence of cutaneous changes without mucosal involvement, "treating through the reaction" is reasonable. We have repeatedly seen cutaneous reactions resolve without interruption of drug therapy. The

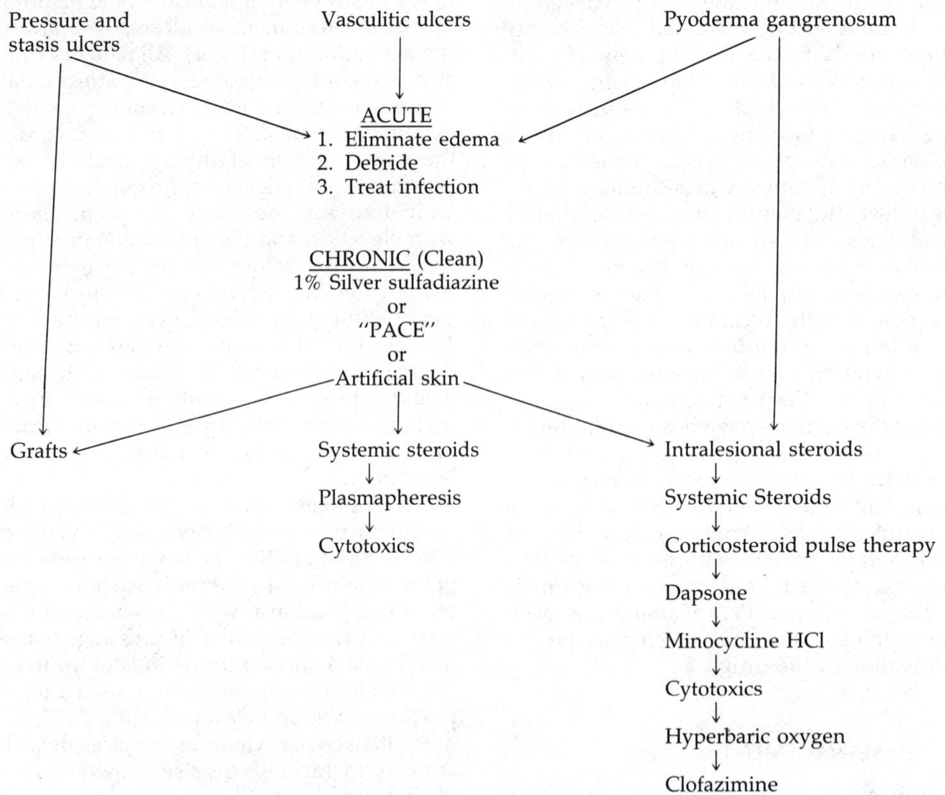

Figure 1. Ulcers associated with rheumatoid disease.

Table 1. USE AND MONITORING OF PHARMACOLOGIC AGENTS

Name	Initial Dose	Increments	Pretreatment	Monitor	Length of Therapy	Reduction
Dapsone	100 mg/day	100 mg q.2 wk to 300 mg/day	Hemoglobin, G6PD	Weekly hemoglobin until stable	2 mo +	25–50 mg q. mo
Minocycline	100 mg b.i.d.	–	–	–	2 mo +	100 mg q. mo
Corticosteroids (Prednisone)	80 mg/day	–	PPD, chest x-ray, blood sugar	Blood sugar, blood pressure	2 mo +	Maintain until response, then 25% every 2 wk
Pulse Methylprednisolone	1 gm daily IV	–	–	Cardiac arrhythmias, infections, CNS side effects	3–5 days	–
Vitamin D (calciferol)	50,000 units 3 days weekly	–	Serum and urine calcium	Serum and urine calcium q.3 mo	Coincident with steroids	–
Calcium (Os-Cal)	500 mg b.i.d.	–	Serum and urine calcium	Serum and urine calcium q.3 mo	Coincident wih steroids	–
Clofazimine	100 mg t.i.d.		Renal function		2–20 wk	–
Cyclophosphamide	1–2 mg/kg/day PO	–	CBC, platelets, urinalysis	CBC, platelets, urinalysis q.3 wk	As needed	–

dermatitis involved can be approached symptomatically or with a short course of prednisone tapered from 60 mg over a 12-day period.

REFERENCES

Jorizzo J, Daniels JC: Dermatologic conditions reported in patients with rheumatoid arthritis. J Am Acad Dermatol 8:439–457, 1983.
Kivden JK, Naevdal A, Milde EJ: Pemphigus and rheumatoid arthritis treated with penicillamine. Scand J Rheumatol 10:95–96, 1981.
Sibbitt WL Jr, Williams RC Jr: Cutaneous manifestations of rheumatoid arthritis. Int J Dermatol 21:563–572, 1982.
Thurtle OA, Cawley MI: The frequency of leg ulceration in rheumatoid arthritis: a survey. J Rheumatol 10:507–509, 1983.

10 · CONTACT DERMATITIS

Carey A. Bligard*
Marilyn C. Ray†
*TULANE UNIVERSITY SCHOOL OF MEDICINE
†OCHSNER CLINIC AND ALTON OCHSNER MEDICAL FOUNDATION

DEFINITION

Contact dermatitis is inflammation of the skin resulting from physical contact with an offending substance. It accounts for considerable morbidity in the general population and a great deal of occupational disease. It may be divided into two major etiologic groups: allergic contact dermatitis and irritant contact dermatitis.

PATHOPHYSIOLOGY

Allergic contact dermatitis (ACD) is classically defined as a delayed reaction from a type IV (cell-mediated) immune response to the sensitizing antigen. A five- to 21-day sensitization period is required. A clinical reaction occurs 24 to 72 hours after reexposure to the contactants. Sensitivity to common contactants may persist for years and is reinforced with each exposure.

Irritant contact dermatitis is caused by direct toxicity of an agent on the skin in a nonsensitized individual. Its intensity varies in proportion to the strength of the inducing agent. In contradistinction to ACD, it does not require previous exposure to the agent; i.e. an agent responsible for an irritant dermatitis has the ability to cause dermatitis in a majority of individuals exposed to it. Strong irritants include acids and alkalies, which may cause severe inflammation in low concentrations. Mild irritants such as detergents may require high concentrations, frequent exposure, or exposure to skin that is already compromised by other underlying conditions. Repeated exposure may induce irritant dermatitis, not because of specifically sensitized T lymphocytes, but because of direct damage to normal barrier function of the skin. The irritant potential of a substance is affected by factors such as thickness of the skin and the degree of maceration (humidity, friction, or pressure affecting the skin). Common causes of contact dermatitis are listed in Table 1. An excellent reference for a complete description of common contactants is *Contact Dermatitis* by Fisher.

CLINICAL ASPECTS

The clinical presentation of ACD is that of an inflammatory process with pruritus, erythema, and edema, which progresses to papules and vesicles with oozing. In the case of irritant contact dermatitis the eruption is limited to the area of contact and lasts only a few days, whereas ACD may occur in different areas over a period of about two weeks. With continued exposure, chronic changes occur with thickening, fissuring, and hyper- or hypopigmentation.

The differential diagnosis of contact dermatitis includes other eczematous processes. Psoriasis, nummular eczema, dyshidrosis, atopic dermatitis, and "id" reactions to dermatophyte infections are the most common diagnoses to be considered. Contact dermatitis to topical medications can complicate the treatment of skin disorders and must be considered when a dermatitis worsens with appropriate treatment.

The most critical part of the diagnostic work-up of contact dermatitis is a thorough history. This must include the date of onset and its relationship to any new activities. The initial location of the eruption may provide a clue to the identity of the contactant. Contact dermatitis commonly begins in exposed areas but may later spread and even become generalized, obscuring the clinical picture. The patient's work (such as chromate sensitivity, seen in cement workers) and hobbies and the effect of vacations on the eruption may all give clues to the etiology.

Physical examination can be suggestive and in some cases even conclusive of the cause of contact dermatitis. One example is eyelid dermatitis, usually a reflection of contactants on the hands that are conveyed to the more easily sensitized eyelid skin. Plant dermatitis tends to occur in linear streaks where the leaves or their resin have brushed the skin. Eczema of the areas frequently in contact with jewelry such as earlobes, neck, and wrists often implicate nickel as the offending sensitizer. Metallic objects may be tested for the presence of nickel by dimethylglyoxime testing solution (obtainable through Westwood Pharmaceuticals, Inc., Buffalo, NY),

Table 1. CONTACT DERMATITIS

Primary Irritant	Allergic
Acids: HCl, H_2SO_4, salicylic acid	Metal: nickel, chromium
Bases: NaOH, NH_5OH	Rubber: paraphenylenediamine
Organic solvents: gasoline, benezene	Plants: *Rhus* (poison ivy)
Detergents: sodium lauryl sulfate	Plastic: Formaldehyde and epoxy resins
Desiccant: CaO_2	Topical preparations
Oxidizers: bleaches, chlorine	Antihistamines: diphenhydramine HCl (Benadryl)
	Anesthetics: benzocaine, lanolin
	Antibiotics: neomycin
	Preservatives: EDTA, ethylenediamine, thimerosal

an invaluable agent for enabling patients to identify potential nickel contactants.

Other physical clues to etiologic agents include involvement of axillary borders with clothing contact (often formaldehyde in permanent-press clothes is the sensitizer) or involvement of the dorsal foot from shoes (often from chromates or dyes). The use of hair dye containing paraphenylenediamine can result in ACD, which presents as an eruption along the hairline and severe facial edema.

MANAGEMENT

Acute. Initial treatment of contact dermatitis is aimed at drying the vesicular lesions and decreasing the pruritus by soaking with cool water or Burow's solution (1 packet Domeboro powder in 1 pint of cool water). For soaking eyelid lesions, 2% boric acid is the preferred solution. Compresses may be applied two to three times per day, for 20 minutes each application, for several days. Prolonged use of compresses may cause excessive drying of the skin and should be avoided. Cool compresses should not be performed on more than one quarter of the body surface at a time because of the risk of excessive heat loss through inflamed skin. An alternative method of drying widespread lesions is soaking in tepid colloidal oatmeal baths several times each day (Aveeno, one packet in tepid bath water). Following compresses, topical steroid cream mixed in a drying agent (such as triamcinolone cream 0.1%, 30 gm in milk of bismuth lotion or calamine lotion in quantity sufficient to make 120 cc) may be used. Widespread disease may be improved by bed rest, or immobilization of involved extremities.

After the oozing has subsided, topical corticosteroid preparations may be used two or three times per day. Ointments are generally the preferred vehicle in patients with unknown sensitivities, as these lack many of the potential sensitizers found in creams. Some choices of paraben-free creams include Lidex, Valisone, Aristocort, and Hytone. Potent topical steroids such as Lidex or Valisone may be used on moderate to severe dermatitis involving the extremities or trunk. Potent topical steroids should not be used on the face or genitals, as these areas are susceptible to the development of atrophy from use of fluorinated steroids. In addition, perioral dermatitis or rosacea-like dermatitis may develop if fluorinated steroids are used on the face. Mild to moderate facial dermatitis may be treated with hydrocortisone (1% to 2%) ointment or cream. A medium-potency ointment may be used, limiting its use to several days, in more severe cases. Dermatitis involving the eyelids is best treated with Decadron ophthalmic ointment for short periods.

Chronic. Topical steroids and emollients are the mainstays of therapy for chronic dermatitis. In addition to using the above named regimens of topical steroids, as for acute dermatitis, patients must concentrate on increasing the hydration of the skin. This can be accomplished by avoidance of hot water and use of mild soaps such as Dove, Eucerin, or Basis. To enhance absorption of emollients, patients should pat dry and apply a cream or lotion with the skin still slightly damp. Eucerin cream or lotion is suitable for very dry climates; patients in milder climatic zones may do well with less occlusive emollients such as Nutraderm (by Owen Laboratories) or Moisturel lotions. Topical treatment of chronic dermatitis may be enhanced by occluding the topical steroid applications with plastic wrap, but this should be carefully supervised: use for prolonged periods may cause cutaneous atrophy to develop, as well as possible systemic corticosteroid effects. Cotton gloves may be worn for occlusion of hand dermatitis, and white cotton socks for dermatitis of the feet.

ANTIBIOTICS

Weeping and crusted lesions encourage secondary bacterial infection and often require treatment with systemic antibiotics. Erythromycin and tetracycline are good broad-spectrum antibiotics that are inexpensive and well tolerated. Studies have shown that, even without obvious signs of infection, extensive dermatitis resolves more quickly with antibiotic treatment.

PRURITUS

Treatment of pruritus is a vital part of the therapy for contact dermatitis. In addition to the cool soaks previously discussed and avoidance of excessive dryness, patients should be advised to keep their fingernails clipped short and to resist scratching. These measures help to prevent additional damage to barrier function and the possible spread of infection. Several medications have been found to be useful for pruritus. The antihistamines hydroxyzine HCl (Atarax, 25 mg every eight hours) and diphenhydramine HCl (Benadryl, 25 or 50 mg PO every eight hours) have been found to have antipruritic effects. Doxepin hydrochloride (Sinequan, 10 mg PO every six hours, which can be increased to a total of 100 mg/day) is an antidepressant with both H_1- and H_2-receptor blocking activity that has been demonstrated as very effective.

SYSTEMIC STEROIDS

Patients with severe acute dermatitis may require systemic steroids. The initial dose is 40 to 60 mg of prednisone given in a single dose each morning, continued in a tapering dose over three weeks. Intramuscular steroids may be erratically absorbed or may cause atrophy within the injection site if not administered correctly. Systemic steroids must be used cautiously, because of their multitude of side effects. Weight and blood pressure measurements are advisable before prednisone is prescribed and at each follow-up visit. Patients with diabetes who must have prednisone should be followed carefully. Supplemental short-acting insulin may be needed for optimal control. Systemic steroids should generally be avoided in patients with chronic contact dermatitis because of the risk of exacerbation after withdrawal.

TAR, ULTRAVIOLET LIGHT, PUVA

Long-standing chronic dermatitis unresponsive to topical steroids alone may be treated with tar and ultraviolet-B light, or with oral psoralens and ultraviolet-A light (PUVA). Tar may also be added to steroid preparations (an effective combination is Ester gel, 60 gm and triamcinolone 0.1%, 60 gms in Nutraderm lotion in quantity sufficient to make 240 cc).

PATCH TESTING

Long-term management of patients with contact dermatitis may ultimately be defined by patch testing. A properly executed patch test may indicate whether the patient has developed delayed hypersensitivity to a specific antigen. Patch test kits with standardized contactant concentrations are available commercially. In these kits the proper concentration of each antigen has been determined to give a positive delayed hypersensitivity response with a low risk of an irritant reaction. If an industrial exposure is suspected that is not included in a standard patch test kit, the manufacturer must be contacted for information on the proper dilution of the chemical for patch testing. Petrolatum is the usual vehicle as it is nonirritating.

Once a list of possible sensitizers has been formed from the patient's history and the physical examination, the suspect allergens are placed on normal skin on the patient's back under occlusion. The most convenient method of occlusion is the Finn Chamber, which consists of an adhesive strip with ten small metal wells attached. The patches are removed and the results read 48 hours after application, and rechecked 24 hours later. Although simple to apply, patch tests are difficult to interpret and require an experienced eye. A positive test is indicated by a well-demarcated area of acute dermatitis and is graded from 1 to 4 according to the severity of the eruption.

There are many potential sources of error in the patch test, such as false-negative results caused by inappropriately applied patches or excessively low concentrations of the antigens. False-positive results may occur from irritant reactions produced by excessively high concentrations of the hapten or by increased skin irritability causing a decrease in the usual barrier function of normal skin. Furthermore, when the eruption is suspected to be a photocontact (i.e., an allergen that requires exposure to light before a delayed hypersensitivity response can occur), special patch testing (photograph testing) is required. Special patch test kits are also available for airborne contact dermatitis or vehicle contact dermatitis. Optimal patch testing is done after the patient has been cleared of the inflammatory dermatitis.

The relevance of individual patch results to the patient's dermatitis must ultimately be decided by the physician. To determine the agents responsible for the dermatitis, the physician may need to use clinical judgment from physical clues, as previously described, rather than categorically accepting patch test results.

PREVENTIVE MEASURES

Once it is decided that the patient has a specific contact dermatitis and the possible agents are identified, avoidance measures may be taken. Industrial exposure may require protective clothing. Hand exposure may be minimized with the use of vinyl gloves over cotton gloves (Dermal Gloves, Stanley Pulizer, Inc., New Orleans, LA). The cotton gloves help maceration. In addition to physical barriers such as gloves or long sleeves, the barrier function of the skin itself may be improved by specific preparations such as Acid Mantle Creme or Lotion. Photocontact reactions require careful use of sunscreens effective against UVA (containing oxybenzophenone), sun avoidance, and avoidance of the photosensitizer. In each case, the patient's life style must be closely examined and altered to avoid exposure to the offending contactant. A list of agents to avoid should be provided for each patient.

Clearly, successful treatment of contact dermatitis depends on avoidance of exposure and careful patient education.

REFERENCES

Emmett EA: Contact dermatitis. *In* Provost TT, Farmer ER (eds): Current Therapy in Dermatology, 1985–1986. C. V. Mosby Co, St. Louis, 1985, pp 26–29.

Fisher AA: Contact Dermatitis. Lea & Febiger, Philadelphia, 1975, pp 1–70.

Galen WK: Dermatitis. Primary Care 10:355–367, 1983.

Larsen WG, Maibach HI: Contact Dermatitis. *In* Moschella SL, Hurley HJ (eds): Dermatology, 2nd ed. W. B. Saunders Co, Philadelphia, 1985, pp. 289–322.

THE NERVOUS SYSTEM

H. ROYDEN JONES, JR.

1 · CURRENT PERSPECTIVES OF CEREBROVASCULAR DISEASE: AN OVERVIEW

H. Royden Jones, Jr.
LAHEY CLINIC MEDICAL CENTER

During the past 30 years the incidence of stroke from both ischemic and hemorrhagic causes has decreased dramatically. This has been attributed primarily to the highly successful control of hypertension and perhaps to a lesser degree to the prevention of rheumatic heart disease, with its consequent potential for cerebral emboli. Recently, the declining incidence of coronary artery disease may also be a factor. Despite these successes, cerebrovascular disease remains the third most common cause of death in Western societies, exceeded only by heart disease and cancer. Because of the brain's unique vulnerability to ischemia, prophylaxis of stroke is the cornerstone of ideal therapy.

The concepts of transient ischemic attack, residual ischemic neurologic dysfunction, and completed infarction have been well established for more than 30 years. However, these terms provide only the temporal profile of stroke. Unfortunately, these classifications were also used as a means for deciding on effective therapeutic approaches without precisely defining the underlying pathophysiologic mechanisms. Recent technologic advances have made more exact diagnosis possible. For example, because of the use of computed tomography, primary intracerebral hemorrhage is now recognized to be sometimes less severe than previously thought, and it may easily be confused with ischemic stroke. CT also provides an effective means of concomitantly excluding other diseases that may mimic a stroke, such as subdural hematoma, brain tumor, or abscess. Magnetic resonance imaging appears to have an added potential but will not be available outside the major medical centers for at least a few more years. Through the use of these and other techniques, a more objective view of various therapeutic options is now available.

The proper investigation of the asymptomatic carotid bruit is controversial. Noninvasive vascular laboratories have proliferated throughout the United States, and abnormalities observed in these studies have led to an increase in the number of "prophylactic" carotid endarterectomies. A subsequent chapter on the asymptomatic bruit (Sect. XII, Chap. 3) discusses the controversies surrounding proper use of these techniques as they apply to the individual patient.

In the hands of skillful neuroradiologists, particularly with digital arterial subtraction techniques, arteriography is now a much less hazardous procedure and permits more precise pathophysiologic definition of stroke than other radiographic studies. However, physicians should know the exact risks of the procedure in their own hospital before depending on arteriography as a major source of diagnostic information. If the risks of the procedure outweigh the benefits gained, it may be appropriate to refer the patient to a major center before arteriography is undertaken.

Carotid endarterectomy has become one of the most commonly performed surgical procedures in the U.S., with more than 80,000 procedures undertaken in 1983. The major question for physicians is whether the risks of having the procedure performed at their own hospital are fewer than when the disease has followed its natural course. A mortality rate of less than 1% may be achievable. However, in two studies the risk of operation appears to be far greater. Attending physicians must carefully consider their institution's rate of success before deciding whether this procedure can be recommended.

Anticoagulant agents have been the mainstay of therapy in acute vertebral basilar disease. Usually, patients with this condition have not undergone arteriography. As emphasized by Caplan, however, this part of the cerebral circulation should be examined with the same detail as is necessary for the patient with carotid system disease. It must be hoped that future therapeutic protocols will be based on more exact definitions of the anatomic site and underlying disease.

Diagnostic uncertainties still persist in a large percentage of patients in whom no specific cause for a stroke can be defined, i.e., embolic, thrombotic, lacunar, or hemorrhagic. Some uncommon factors are responsible, as outlined in Section XII, Chapter 7, and consideration of these possibilities may occasionally result in a diagnosis of a treatable condition. Unfortunately, in many patients a precise cause still cannot be established. In our own computerized data base for strokes, for example, no definitive cause of stroke has been determined in one third of patients. Many physicians believe that an unrecognized embolic mechanism may be present because of the abrupt onset of symptoms in 74% of patients in one series, and the finding of an embolus in 66% of patients in another series in whom angiography was performed within 48 hours of onset of stroke. To date, however, noninvasive cardiac studies, such as echocardiography, have failed to increase appreciably the percentage of recognized sources of emboli. New investigative methods may permit a more accurate diagnosis in a higher percentage of these patients and consequently lead to a more definitive therapeutic plan of management.

REFERENCES

Brott T, Thalinger K: The practice of carotid endarterectomy in a large metropolitan area. Stroke 15:950–955, 1984.

Caplan LR: Vertebrobasilar disease: time for a new strategy. Stroke 12:111–114, 1981.

Caplan LR: Are terms such as completed stroke or RIND of continued usefulness? Stroke 14:431–433, 1983.

Drury I, Whisnant JP, Garraway WM: Primary intracerebral hemorrhage: impact of CT on incidence. Neurology 34:653–657, 1984.

Easton JD, Sherman DG: Stroke and mortality rate in carotid endarterectomy: 228 consecutive operations. Stroke 8:565–568, 1977.

Eisenberg RL, Bank WO, Hedgcock MW: Neurologic complications of angiography for cerebrovascular disease. Neurology 30:895–897, 1980.

Jones HR Jr: Disease of the vertebral basilar system. Primary Care 6:733–743, 1979.

Jones HR, Millikan CH: Temporal profile (clinical course) of acute carotid system cerebral infarction. Stroke 7:64–71, 1976.

Lees RS, Kistler JP: Noninvasive diagnosis of extracranial cerebrovascular disease. Neurol Clin 2:667–675, 1984.

Pessin MS, Hinton RC, Davis KR, et al: Mechanisms of acute carotid stroke. Ann Neurol 6:245–252, 1979.

Whisnant JP: The decline of stroke. Stroke 15:160–168, 1984.

Whisnant JP, Sandok BA, Sundt TM Jr: Carotid endarterectomy for unilateral carotid system transient cerebral ischemia. Mayo Clin Proc 58:171–175, 1983.

Yatsu FM, Fields WS: Asymptomatic carotid bruit: stenosis or ulceration, a conservative approach. Arch Neurol 42:383–385, 1985.

2 · ISCHEMIC CEREBROVASCULAR DISEASE: CAROTID SYSTEM

David O. Wiebers
MAYO CLINIC AND MAYO FOUNDATION

DEFINITION AND DIAGNOSTIC CRITERIA

Focal neurologic deficits caused by ischemic cerebrovascular disease are classified by the temporal profile of the deficit. All these cerebrovascular episodes usually develop and evolve rapidly regardless of the total duration of symptoms. A transient ischemic attack (TIA) is defined as a temporary episode of focal ischemic neurologic dysfunction that completely resolves within 24 hours (usually within 15 minutes). When a focal ischemic deficit persists for longer than 24 hours but resolves within three weeks, the episode is termed a reversible ischemic neurologic deficit (RIND). Deficits lasting longer than three weeks are called cerebral infarctions (ischemic strokes). An exception to the usual rapid evolution of ischemic cerebrovascular events occurs in patients who have increasing neurologic deficit for up to 48 hours with infarction of the carotid system. These patients are classified as having progressing cerebral infarction.

PATHOPHYSIOLOGY

Any of a variety of pathophysiologic mechanisms may be responsible for focal ischemic neurologic dysfunction of any duration. These mechanisms can be categorized into four major groups progressing from proximal to distal in the vascular system as follows: cardiac disease, cervical vessel disease, cranial vessel disease, and hematologic disease. Cardiac disease may produce cerebral ischemic symptoms (1) by disturbances associated with pump failure producing generalized cerebral ischemia (syncope) or infarction (anoxic encephalopathy) and (2) by providing sources for distal emboli, including fragments from heart valves, intracardiac thrombi from local stagnation or endocardial alterations, and systemic venous thrombi shunted into the arterial circulation. Cervical vessel disease includes atherosclerosis (the most common disease process producing cerebral ischemia), carotid artery dissection, fibromuscular dysplasia, idiopathic regressing arteriopathy, and external compression or trauma to the cervical vessels. Cranial vessel disease includes noninfectious and infectious arteritides as well as lipohyalinosis secondary to hypertension. Atherosclerosis, although seen in cranial vessels, is much less common than in carotid arteries in the neck, except in diabetics and blacks. Abnormalities in blood cell constituents (i.e., polycythemia and sickle cell anemia) and plasma proteins (i.e., dysproteinemias) may result in hypercoagulable states with increased blood viscosity and stasis predisposing the patient to cerebral ischemia.

CLINICAL ASPECTS

In addition to knowing the temporal profile and possible underlying mechanisms for episodes of focal cerebral ischemia, the clinician must attempt to localize the area of dysfunction within the brain to facilitate optimal patient management. This is accomplished by relating clinical findings to the underlying anatomic cerebral structures and their blood supply.

The distinction between lesions involving the anterior circulation (internal carotid systems) and the posterior circulation (vertebrobasilar systems) is the most pertinent. The blood supply for the eyes and the major portion of the cerebral hemisphere comes from the internal carotid arteries, which take origin at or near the level of the thyroid cartilage in the neck. An ischemic lesion involving the ophthalmic arterial system produces ipsilateral visual loss, which may be transient (amaurosis fugax) or permanent (retinal infarction). Visual loss in amaurosis fugax may take the character of an ascending or descending dark shade or, less commonly, may progress from the periphery to the center. The two major terminal branches of the internal carotid artery are the anterior cerebral and the middle cerebral arteries. Ischemia in the distribution of the anterior cerebral artery usually causes contralateral weakness, apraxia, and sensory loss, primarily in the leg. There may also be intellectual dysfunction and behavioral alterations from frontal lobe involvement. Middle cerebral artery occlusion at its origin usually results in contralateral weakness and sensory loss, maximal in the face and arm. With dominant hemisphere lesions, dysphasia or aphasia may result. Nondominant hemisphere intellectual dysfunction may include construction apraxia, dressing apraxia, motor impersistence, and prominent neglect of the left body, particularly the left arm. Involvement of the optic pathways in either hemisphere may produce contralateral homonymous hemianopsia.

In summary, various combinations of monocular visual loss, hemiparesis, hemisensory deficit, apraxia, behavioral changes, aphasia or dysphasia, and homonymous hemianopsia suggest an internal carotid system (anterior circulation) lesion. Of these features, monocular visual loss, apraxia, and aphasia or dysphasia are seen only with anterior circulation problems, whereas the other features may be seen with either anterior or posterior circulation lesions.

MANAGEMENT

Whenever possible, management of patients with focal ischemic cerebrovascular symptoms is based on a precise definition of the underlying pathophysiologic mechanism and its appropriate treatment. Before the underlying mechanism can be defined, patients are managed according to the temporal profile of the focal deficit. Usually, therapy is commenced on the basis of the physician's clinical impression, while studies are performed to define the etiologic mechanism.

TRANSIENT ISCHEMIC ATTACKS

Approximately one third of patients with TIA have a stroke within five years of the first attack. More than 20% of these occur within one month of the initial attack and about 50% within one year. I recommend that all such patients be hospitalized and, if no contraindications exist (including clinical or CT scan evidence of intracranial hemorrhage), that heparin therapy by continuous infusions be started during the medical neurologic evaluation. The usual starting dose for heparin is 1000 units per hour, to be adjusted by monitoring the activated partial thromboplastin time (APTT) so that the APTT is approximately twice the baseline APTT After complete medical and neurologic examinations, certain diagnostic studies are usually performed (Table 1) to help identify the underlying pathophysiologic mechanism for the TIA symptoms. These examinations and studies help to identify many nonatherosclerotic vascular mechanisms for producing cerebral ischemia, including cardiac disease (valvular abnormalities, blood stagnation, paradoxical embolism), hypertension, hematologic disorders with hypercoagulable states, and arteritis. In addition, other lesions such as primary or metastatic brain tumor, arteriovenous malformation, intracranial aneurysm, and subdural hematoma must be considered since they may rarely cause TIA symptoms.

With these evaluations completed and the unusual causes of TIA-like symptoms taken into account, patients are considered for angiographic investigation provided the medical evaluation indicates that the risk of surgery is low. The operative morbidity of carotid endarterectomy may increase to 7% or 8% in patients with recent myocardial infarction, active unstable angina, or severe chronic obstructive pulmonary disease. Therefore, these patients are often treated medically. Noninvasive neurovascular studies such as ocular pneumoplethysmography (OPG) provide a safe, reliable means of detecting internal carotid system pressure-significant lesions (≥ 75% luminal area stenosis). Patients with underlying pressure-significant lesions of the internal carotid system are at higher risk of subsequent cerebral infarction, and these patients should undergo cerebral arteriography if they are in a low-risk surgical category. Patients with normal or equivocal findings on noninvasive studies may benefit from an intravenous digital subtraction angiogram (DSA) to help determine the nature of any underlying lesions in the carotid system without the risk of cerebral arteriography. If these studies all suggest no underlying pressure-significant carotid lesion, arteriography is not undertaken.

If arteriography is performed, it is important not only to examine the extracranial vasculature but also to assess the structure and dynamics of the intracranial circulation. Patients with TIA of the carotid system and pressure-significant ipsilateral carotid artery stenosis (more than 75% luminal area stenosis) with or without ulceration are usually advised to undergo endarterectomy, provided a surgeon capable of operating with a low morbidity and mortality risk is available.

Microneurosurgical techniques are also available that allow the anastomosing of branches of the extracranial arterial system (most often the superficial temporal artery) to branches of the intracranial circulation (most often branches of the middle cerebral artery). This procedure was thought to benefit patients with poor collateral circulation around an internal carotid artery occlusion, siphon stenosis, or stenosis or occlusion of the middle cerebral artery, especially if postural TIA symptoms were present, although a recent cooperative study (EC/IC Bypass Study Group) does not support this technique.

Patients who do not undergo operation are treated medically. For those with recent onset of TIA (two months or less), I suggest a three-month course of warfarin therapy unless there are contraindications. These latter include bleeding diatheses, previous sensitivity to warfarin therapy, severe hepatic or renal failure, propensity toward recurrent trauma such as falling down from unstable gait, significant alcoholism, and inability to follow instructions or receive adequate supervision for monitoring. Warfarin is also relatively contraindicated in pregnancy, particularly the first trimester. During the course of warfarin therapy, the dose is adjusted to maintain the prothrombin time (PT) at one and one-half to two times the control value. It is usually necessary to check the PT daily for the first five

Table 1. LABORATORY STUDIES IN PATIENTS WITH FOCAL CEREBRAL ISCHEMIC EVENTS

Routine	Selected Cases
Blood	
CBC	Antinuclear antibody
Platelet count	Cryoglobulins, immunoglobulins
Chemistry panel	Sickle cell screen
Serology	Blood cultures
Erythrocyte sedimentation rate	2D and M-mode echocardiogram
Cholesterol/triglycerides	Radionuclide cardiac scan
Activated partial thromboplastin time	EEG
Prothrombin time	Noninvasive neurovascular studies
Urinalysis	IV DSA
Chest x-ray	Cerebral arteriography (angiography)
Electrocardiogram	
Head CT scan	

to seven days of treatment and then after another four to seven days. Numerous exogenous and endogenous factors may affect the PT, including alcohol, vitamin K, concomitant liver and renal disease, and several other drugs metabolized by the liver. Side effects of warfarin other than hemorrhage are infrequent (alopecia, urticaria, GI upset, and a severe hypersensitivity reaction including hemorrhagic infarction and necrosis of the skin).

If patients treated medically are free of symptoms on warfarin over the first three months, I generally switch them to aspirin, 325 mg t.i.d., and dipyridamole, 75 mg t.i.d. or aspirin alone for the next nine months. Recent experimental evidence suggests that aspirin doses as low as 80 mg PO q day may be as effective as the more commonly used doses of 325 mg PO b.i.d. or t.i.d. Possible side effects include a slightly increased bleeding tendency with both drugs. Aspirin may cause GI irritation and bleeding, hypersensitivity, and (at higher doses) tinnitus and acid-base imbalances. Persantine may cause headache, dizziness, nausea, flushing, and hypersensitivity reactions. Patients with frequent ongoing TIA of several months' duration are given antiplatelet therapy unless there has been a recent change in the character of the TIA symptoms suggesting a new anatomic distribution of ischemia. In the latter situation, I advise a three-month trial of warfarin after the most recent TIA, followed by antiplatelet therapy.

REVERSIBLE ISCHEMIC NEUROLOGIC DEFICIT

Approximately 25% of patients with RIND have an ischemic stroke or RIND within five years of the initial event. This figure is approximately midway between the comparable figures for TIA (32%) and ischemic stroke (20%). Patients with RIND whose symptoms resolve within seven days have a probability of subsequent ischemic stroke or RIND analogous to that of patients with TIA and significantly greater than that of patients with RIND, whose symptoms resolve in eight to 21 days. The greatest difference in these groups occurs within the first year after the initial RIND.

Currently, no data define the results of treatment for patients with RIND. Since the pathogenesis of this syndrome probably differs little from that of either TIA or ischemic stroke, similar methods of evaluation and treatment are used. If a surgically correctable, pressure-significant atherosclerotic lesion is defined in the carotid system ipsilateral to symptoms, carotid endarterectomy or extracranial to intracranial bypass surgery is considered, particularly for patients whose symptoms resolve in the first week. In patients with atherosclerotic lesions that are not surgical or without identifiable underlying mechanisms for ischemia whose symptoms resolve within one week, anticoagulant therapy with warfarin is given for three months, followed by the use of antiplatelet agents over the next nine months, as indicated for TIA. In the remaining patients, I favor the use of antiplatelet agents alone.

CEREBRAL INFARCTION

Management of patients with cerebral infarction includes supportive care, prevention and treatment of secondary complications, treatment of the acute and chronic neurologic deficits, and prevention of subsequent cerebral infarction.

A computed tomography (CT) scan should be performed on all patients (preferably before and after contrast injection), to distinguish cerebral infarction from intracerebral hemorrhage and perhaps help confirm the clinical localization of the lesion. In addition, the scan may show underlying disease related to the infarction (e.g., arteriovenous malformation) or other lesions capable of producing similar symptoms (e.g., brain abscess, neoplasm, or subdural hematoma). Electroencephalography seldom contributes additional diagnostic information unless the CT scan is negative or the differential diagnosis includes other more diffuse nonischemic disorders, such as herpes simplex encephalitis. Many patients undergo noninvasive neurovascular studies to assess the integrity of the major extracranial vessels. These tests serve primarily to help recognize hemodynamically significant lesions of the carotid bifurcation area. Cerebral angiography is the most reliable method of identifying pathologic changes in the extracranial or intracranial vessels. Despite improvements in equipment and technique, the procedure carries a major morbidity risk of about 1% when performed in patients with ischemic cerebrovascular symptoms. Therefore, arteriography is used primarily in patients with minimal deficits in whom the information obtained may be helpful in planning surgical or medical treatment. In recent years, digital subtraction angiography has proved useful for defining the underlying stroke mechanism, primarily to facilitate medical treatment without the risk of arteriography. Even more recently, the nuclear magnetic resonance scan (magnetic resonance imaging scan) has been shown to be more sensitive for detecting cerebral infarction than CT. However, experience with this technique is still limited, and its cost is much greater and its availability much more limited than CT.

While efforts are under way to determine the mechanism of cerebral infarction, the patient is given the supportive care necessary to maintain general medical status. Particular attention is paid to monitoring fluid intake and output and serum and urine electrolytes, to ensure proper fluid balance. An indwelling catheter should not be used in patients who are awake, alert, and able to cooperate with a voluntary voiding program.

Bedridden patients have an increased risk of deep vein thrombosis and subsequent pulmonary embolism. Elastic stockings, passive physical therapy, and mini-dose heparin therapy (5000 units SQ every 12 hours) may help prevent deep vein thrombosis. Bronchopneumonia and urinary tract infections are frequent in patients with cerebral infarction. Vigorous tracheobronchial toilet and avoidance of unnecessary urinary catheterization are helpful preventive measures. Antibiotic therapy is used only for clinical infection and not prophylactically. Over the first 96 hours following a relatively large cerebral infarction, many patients may show progressive decrease in level of consciousness owing to cerebral edema. Although corticosteroids have been widely used to treat cerebral edema, they have little effect on the type of edema associated with cerebral infarction. Hyperosmolar agents such as glycerol (1 gm/kg PO every six hours) and mannitol (1 gm/kg IV in a 20% solution administered over a 30-minute period every two hours) may have some effect in reducing intracranial pressure. The stable patient who remains awake and alert receives no antiedema therapy.

Vasodilator therapy and other efforts to increase cerebral blood flow to the area of dysfunction have been ineffective, and attempts to reduce cerebral metabolism by induced hypothermia or barbiturate therapy, although possibly effective in experimental animals, have not yet been shown to be of practical benefit in human clinical situations.

Patients with seizures are treated with diazepam (10 to 20 mg IV at a rate of 5 mg/min). This is followed immediately by a loading dose of phenytoin (15 mg/kg IV at a rate of 50 mg/min in isotonic sodium chloride solution) with appropriate cardiorespiratory monitoring. Appropriate measures are instituted to treat any patient with superimposed metabolic encephalopathy.

A rehabilitation program designed to provide an environment of high motivation to help achieve maximal physical and psychologic functional capacity is tailored to meet the needs of each patient and family. Physiotherapy in the form of passive exercises is begun as soon as the deficit is stable, and active exercise and ambulation are attempted as soon as tolerated. Speech therapy to assist in language retraining and articulation is begun when the patient is awake and alert. Psychosocial therapy is started with the family at the time of hospitalization and begun with the patient as soon as feasible. Reactive depression can often be treated by encouraging verbalization of the patient's fears and anger. Psychotherapeutic agents and formal psychotherapy may be necessary in the exceptional patient.

The amount of rigor with which one approaches treatment to prevent subsequent cerebral infarction depends on several factors, including (1) the pathophysiologic mechanism responsible for the infarction; (2) the size, location, and character of the infarction (agents that alter blood coagulability are best avoided in the presence of larger hemorrhagic infarctions); (3) the degree of functional deficit; and (4) the potential benefits and risks of the therapy being considered.

The risk of intracranial hemorrhage is increased in patients taking anticoagulants after cerebral infarction. Because there is no evidence that anticoagulant therapy decreases the risk of subsequent cerebral infarction in the absence of a clearly identifiable responsive pathophysiologic mechanism (such as atrial fibrillation or valvular heart disease), this form of treatment is not generally advised. The effectiveness of antiplatelet agents such as aspirin and dipyridamole have not been clearly demonstrated. However, in patients without identifiable mechanisms for their symptoms or in patients with atherosclerotic disease who are not surgically treated, I often use antiplatelet therapy over a period of approximately one year.

Carotid endarterectomy is considered for patients with minimal residual neurologic deficit in clearly defined lesions. Endarterectomy is generally reserved for patients with pressure-significant stenotic lesions ipsilateral to carotid system symptoms, and is best delayed for seven to 14 days after infarction to help avoid hyperperfusion and intracranial hemorrhage into the infarcted area. Microneurosurgical extracranial to intracranial bypass procedures had previously been considered in some of these patients with various underlying pathophysiologies, as outlined earlier for TIA. However, a recent cooperative study does not support these procedures.

Correction of associated cerebrovascular risk factors may also help reduce the risk of subsequent cerebral infarction. Elevated blood pressure in patients with cerebral infarction is usually managed in the same manner as in patients without cerebral infarction. If the level of hypertension and cardiovascular status require rapid reduction in BP levels, this can be accomplished by a carefully monitored infusion of sodium nitroprusside (see Section XII, Chap. 10). If the level of hypertension and cardiovascular status allows gradual reduction in BP levels, this is preferable and can be done by the means most familiar to the physician. Treatment should also be instituted for diabetes mellitus, hyperlipidemia, gout, and obesity. The patient should eliminate smoking.

PROGRESSING INFARCTION

In approximately 20% of patients with infarction of the distribution of the carotid system, the neurologic deficit may progress over 24 to 48 hours. It is critical that these patients be monitored closely and that the clinician attempt to identify the underlying mechanism responsible for the progression. One must consider not only the possible ischemic mechanisms that may be responsible, but also other disorders with a similar clinical picture.

In some patients the neurologic deficit may progress as a result of widening of the marginal ischemic zone associated with cerebral infarction. This phenomenon is often attributed to a decrease in systemic BP because the vessels of the marginally ischemic area are maximally vasodilated and the blood flow is therefore largely dependent on systemic BP. In other patients, the infarction becomes hemorrhagic and there is a concomitant increase in deficit. Still others have deterioration because of cerebral edema associated with the area of cerebral infarction, as mentioned earlier. Many patients with a progressing infarction are believed to have propagation of the intra-arterial thrombus or subsequent additional embolization from a proximal source, with associated failure of collateral circulation and decrease in blood supply to the ischemic area. These patients often have sudden stepwise increases in neurologic deficits. Finally, some patients with a progressive neurologic course believed to be related to cerebral infarction have other types of intracranial pathologic processes causing their symptoms. Such processes include intracerebral hemorrhage, subdural hematoma, neoplasms, demyelinating disease, brain abscess, and encephalitis.

Diagnostic studies are performed to elucidate which of the above mechanisms is causing the patient's progression. This in turn dictates the proper treatment. Metabolic abnormalities and hypotension should be identified and corrected. CT scan should be performed early in the course of management. In patients with progression caused by evolving cerebral edema, anti-edema agents such as glycerol (1 to 2 gm/kg PO every six hours) or mannitol (1 to 2 gm/kg IV in a 20% solution administered over a 30-minute period every two hours). Dexamethasone (10 mg IV followed by 4 mg either IV or PO every six hours) may also be given concomitantly with one of the above agents, or alone.

If the intracranial process is still considered to be ischemic and the lesion is nonhemorrhagic on CT scan, heparin (1000 units per hour by constant IV infusion) should be considered. If instituted, treatment is usually continued for three to five days beyond the time when the clinical course has stabilized. For patients in whom the neurologic deficit continues to progress despite therapy, cerebral arteriography should be considered. A few patients in this group may be considered for emergency neurovascular surgical intervention.

REFERENCES

Dyken ML: Anticoagulant and platelet antiaggregating therapy in stroke and threatened stroke. Neurol Clin 1:223–242, 1983.

EC/IC Bypass Study Group: Failure of extracranial/intracranial arterial bypass to reduce the risk of ischemic stroke. Results of an international randomized trial. N Engl J Med 313:1191–1200, 1985.

Matsumoto N, Whisnant JP, Kurland LT, et al: Natural history of stroke in Rochester, Minnesota, 1955–1969: an extension of a previous study, 1945–1954. Stroke 4:20–29, 1973.

Sandok BA, Furlan AJ, Whisnant JP, et al: Guidelines for the management of transient ischemic attacks. Mayo Clin Proc 53:665–674, 1978.

Sundt TM Jr, Sandok BA, Houser OW: The selection of patients for intracranial and extracranial surgery for cerebrovascular occlusive disease. Clin Neurosurg 22:185–198, 1975.

Whisnant JP: Indications for medical and surgical therapy for ischemic stroke. Adv Neurol 16:133–144, 1977.

Wiebers DO, Whisnant JP, O'Fallon WM: Reversible ischemic neurologic deficit (RIND) in a community. Rochester, Minnesota, 1955–1974. Neurology 32:459–465, 1982.

3 · ASYMPTOMATIC CAROTID DISEASE

Donald J. Breslin
LAHEY CLINIC MEDICAL CENTER

No randomized clinical trial has yet studied the benefits of surgical versus medical management of patients with asymptomatic carotid disease. The risk of stroke in this group may not be any greater than the risk of surgery. Within the asymptomatic population, however, a subgroup may exist for whom a higher risk of stroke justifies carotid endarterectomy.

Occlusion of the internal carotid artery without signs or symptoms of cerebral ischemia is common, as shown by autopsy studies and clinical reports. In a nonrandomized series of patients observed over a mean period of about four years, Thompson and colleagues reported a 4.6% stroke rate in patients with asymptomatic carotid disease who underwent endarterectomy of the internal carotid artery, in contrast to a 17.4% stroke incidence in a nonoperated group. In this study, however, the population who underwent surgery may not have been comparable to the control group.

CAROTID BRUIT

The populations studied in various series are not comparable. Some studies report on patients with carotid bruit, and others evaluate patients with evidence of internal carotid disease as determined by noninvasive testing. In a few instances, patients with asymptomatic carotid disease demonstrated by arteriography have been evaluated.

Even experienced physicians often fail to identify a carotid bruit correctly, and the absence of bruit does not exclude the possibility of stenosis of the carotid artery. When angiographic findings were correlated with the presence or absence of carotid bruits in asymptomatic patients at the Cleveland Clinic, 65% of carotid arteries with bruits were associated with stenotic lesions. A cervical bruit in an asymptomatic patient indicates an increased risk of stroke. Only one third of such strokes, however, result from infarctions in areas of the brain that are supplied by the specific artery with the bruit. Although stroke may be preceded by one or more transient ischemic attacks (TIA) in a previously asymptomatic patient with cervical bruit, stroke may also take place without warning in this group.

The annual rate of stroke in asymptomatic patients with carotid bruit is much higher in the practices of individual surgeons than rates reported from community studies. Reported annual rates of stroke from Framingham, MA (1.7%) and Evans County, GA (2.3%) were appreciably lower than those noted by Cooperman and co-workers (3%) and Thompson and colleagues (4.3%).

NONINVASIVE TESTING

Attempts have been made to define a subgroup of asymptomatic patients with carotid bruits who are at particularly high risk of stroke. In a retrospective nonrandomized study of patients seen in a noninvasive laboratory and followed over a mean period of two years, the incidence of stroke was 2.9% when there was no evidence of decreased flow through the internal carotid artery, and 11.9% when the lesion seemed to be hemodynamically significant. Similar findings have been reported in prospective studies using noninvasive testing.

PROGRESSION OF CAROTID DISEASE

Javid and co-workers studied the natural history of atheroma of the carotid bifurcation with repeated arteriography over at least a 12-month period for an average of three years. All these patients initially had less than 60% stenosis of the internal carotid artery. Rapidly progressive stenosis (i.e., more than 25% change per year) was seen in 22% of the total group; in 40% no evidence of severe progression of stenosis was observed. In another series of patients evaluated by serial noninvasive studies, risk factors for progression were identified as cigarette smoking, diabetes mellitus, and age of less than 65 years.

DEATHS IN ASYMPTOMATIC DISEASE

The presence of an asymptomatic carotid bruit, particularly in an elderly person, is an indicator of generalized systemic atherosclerotic disease. Those with asymptomatic carotid bruit are reported to have an annual stroke rate of approximately 2%. However, the annual nonstroke death rate is approximately 4%, with cardiac disease as a major cause. Over an average period of 36 months after carotid endarterectomy, the mortality rate for patients with coronary disease was 21%. A high-risk group was identified in which the mortality rate for those with coronary disease in the same period was 66%, with a mean survival period of 18 months. Risk factors associated with deaths in this group included hypertension, overt coronary disease, and age greater than 65 years. Any decision regarding treatment of asymptomatic carotid disease must take into account the life expectancy of the patient.

PROPHYLACTIC CAROTID ENDARTERECTOMY

Should prophylactic carotid endarterectomy be performed in the patient with asymptomatic carotid disease who requires noncarotid surgery? In most studies that address this subject, the reports of the incidence of postoperative stroke in patients with carotid bruit do not indicate whether they had flow-reducing stenosis of the internal carotid artery. In three reported series, no perioperative strokes occurred in 160 patients with asymptomatic carotid bruit who underwent abdominal aortic or other peripheral vascular surgery without prophylactic carotid endarterectomy.

In another study, noninvasive testing was performed in patients with asymptomatic carotid bruits to determine whether there was stenosis of the internal carotid artery. These patients subsequently underwent operation for peripheral vascular disease or aortocoronary bypass without prophylactic carotid endarterectomy. No correlation was found between the incidence of perioperative stroke and the presence of stenotic lesions of the internal carotid artery as determined by noninvasive studies.

Routine prophylactic carotid endarterectomy is not advisable in asymptomatic patients with disease of the internal carotid artery who are to undergo surgery for coronary artery or peripheral vascular disease. Probably there is a relatively small subgroup of patients with flow-reducing internal carotid disease with poor collateral flow or with bilateral internal carotid disease in whom the risk of perioperative stroke is increased. Such patients may benefit from prophylactic carotid endarterectomy. At the Cleveland Clinic, 174 patients with asymptomatic carotid disease underwent prophylactic carotid endarterectomy either before aortocoronary bypass in a staged procedure or at the same time as aortocoronary bypass in a combined procedure. Patients who underwent staged carotid endarterectomy had a 1.5% rate of stroke, and those with combined coronary and carotid surgery had a 4.3% perioperative stroke rate. The group who underwent prophylactic carotid endarterectomy obviously had excellent results in terms of perioperative stroke, but these figures do not indicate whether definite benefits resulted from carotid surgery.

CONTRALATERAL CAROTID DISEASE AFTER ENDARTERECTOMY

Patients who have carotid endarterectomy for symptomatic carotid disease sometimes have asymptomatic disease in the contralateral carotid artery. The natural history of this condition has been studied by several investigators. Such patients have been observed over a period of two to 20 years, and during this time an appreciable number have undergone carotid endarterectomy because of episodes of transient cerebral ischemia or nonspecific symptoms referable to the central nervous system. No strokes occurred in 204 patients who did not have carotid endarterectomy of the contralateral artery and who remained asymptomatic. In another series, three strokes occurred in 67 patients who were observed for five years; two of these strokes occurred without a warning TIA. These findings agree with those in earlier series of patients, not all of whom had prior endarterectomy. Patients who have undergone carotid endarterectomy for symptomatic carotid stenosis and who have contralateral asymptomatic carotid stenosis appear to be at low risk of stroke if carotid endarterectomy is performed as soon as symptoms appear that suggest cerebral ischemia. A few remaining patients, however, have a stroke unheralded by previous warning symptoms.

ASYMPTOMATIC NONSTENOTIC INTERNAL CAROTID ULCERS

In one study, asymptomatic patients identified by arteriography as having small intimal ulcers of the carotid bifurcation were compared with those who had large ulcers. The latter had a high incidence of stroke. Arteriograms were not repeated, however, and therefore the number of patients in whom carotid stenosis developed in the intervening years is unknown. When a similar group was studied for a shorter period that averaged three years, no strokes were reported among patients with large ulcers. At present we must conclude that the natural history of these asymptomatic lesions is unknown.

COMPLICATIONS OF CAROTID ENDARTERECTOMY

The risk of stroke or death associated with carotid endarterectomy varies greatly among different institutions and different surgeons. Whenever carotid endarterectomy is being considered, the associated morbidity and mortality rates for this procedure should be monitored carefully. Endarterectomy for asymptomatic carotid disease was associated with a 1.2% incidence of stroke and no deaths as reported by Thompson and associates. On the other hand, in 16 hospitals in Cincinnati, Ohio, in 1980, the perioperative incidence of stroke was 7.9%, with a mortality rate of 3.1%. Reported perioperative complications for internal carotid endarterectomy vary from 1.5% to 21.1%.

INDICATIONS FOR ENDARTERECTOMY

After reviewing the natural history of asymptomatic carotid disease, Roederer and co-workers recommended carotid endarterectomy for those with symptoms of transient cerebral ischemia or progression of stenosis to more than 80%. Adequate determination includes consideration of several relevant factors. First, if the associated morbidity and mortality rates for carotid endarterectomy in the experience of the particular surgeon are not extremely low, all other considerations are negated. In patients with asymptomatic disease, the surgeon's rate of associated mortality and morbidity should be less than 3% and preferably from 1% to 2%. Second, the life expectancy of the patient must be considered and particularly the likelihood of death from coronary disease within one to two years. Patients who have overt coronary disease, are older than 65, or are hypertensive are at increased risk. In view of the current uncertainty with respect to benefits, aggressive treatment of asymptomatic carotid disease should not be considered when the anticipated life expectancy of the patient is brief.

Although the overall risk of stroke in patients with asymptomatic carotid disease appears to be low, a small subgroup of patients may exist in whom the benefit of carotid endarterectomy outweighs the risk. These patients should be identified among those with either varying stenosis of the internal carotid artery of more than 80% or progressive stenosis, or who cease to be asymptomatic and have TIAs.

The approach to patients with asymptomatic carotid disease must remain arbitrary until multicenter randomized controlled studies provide more data. At the Lahey Clinic our current practice is to follow such asymptomatic patients with noninvasive testing every six months and to instruct them carefully in the symptoms of transient cerebral ischemia. If appreciable progression of internal carotid stenosis is evidenced or if symptoms of cerebral ischemia develop, carotid endarterectomy is performed when there are no contraindications. Otherwise, patients are simply observed. The value of antiplatelet agents in the management of such asymptomatic patients remains unknown.

REFERENCES

Brott T, Thalinger K: The practice of carotid endarterectomy in a large metropolitan area. Stroke 15:950–955, 1984.

Busuttil RW, Baker JD, Davidson RK, et al: Carotid artery stenosis—hemodynamic significance and clinical course. JAMA 245:1438–1441, 1981.

Carney WI Jr, Stewart WB, DePinto DJ, et al: Carotid bruit as a risk factor in aortoiliac reconstruction. Surgery 81:567–570, 1977.

Chambers BR, Norris JW: The case against surgery for asymptomatic carotid stenosis. Stroke 15:964–967, 1984.

Cooperman M, Martin EW Jr, Evans WE: Significance of asymptomatic carotid bruits. Arch Surg 113:1339–1340, 1978.

David TE, Humphries AW, Young JR, et al: A correlation of neck bruits and arteriosclerotic carotid arteries. Arch Surg 107:729–731, 1973.

Evans WE, Cooperman M: The significance of asymptomatic unilateral carotid bruits in preoperative patients. Surgery 83:521–522, 1978.

Fields WS, Lemak NA: Joint study of extracranial arterial occlusion: X. Internal carotid artery occlusion. JAMA 235:2734–2738, 1976.

Hertzer NR, Loop FD, Taylor PC, et al: Staged and combined surgical approach to simultaneous carotid and coronary vascular disease. Surgery 83:803–811, 1978.

Heyman A, Wilkinson WE, Heyden S, et al: Risk of stroke in asymptomatic persons with cervical arterial bruits: a population study in Evans County, Georgia. N Engl J Med 302:838–841, 1980.

Humphries AW, Young JR, Santilli PH, et al: Asymptomatic significant carotid artery stenosis: a review of 182 instances. Surgery 80:695–698, 1976.

Javid H, Ostermiller WE Jr, Hengesh JW, et al: Natural history of carotid bifurcation atheroma. Surgery 67:80–86, 1970.

Javid H, Ostermiller WE Jr, Hengesh JW, et al: Carotid endarterectomy for asymptomatic patients. Arch Surg 102:389–391, 1971.

Johnson N, Burnham SJ, Flanigan DP, et al: Carotid endarterectomy: a follow-up study of the contralateral non-operated carotid artery. Ann Surg 188:748–752, 1978.

Kartchner MM, McRae LP: Noninvasive evaluation and management of the "asymptomatic" carotid bruit. Surgery 82:840–847, 1977.

Kroener JM, Dorn PL, Shoor PM, et al: Prognosis of asymptomatic ulcerating carotid lesions. Arch Surg 115:1387–1392, 1980.

Levin SM, Sondheimer FK, Levin JM: The contralateral diseased but asymptomatic carotid artery: to operate or not? An update. Am J Surg 140:203–205, 1980.

Martin MJ, Whisnant JP, Sayre GP: Occlusive vascular disease in the extracranial cerebal circulation. Arch Neurol 5:530–538, 1960.

Mohr JP: Asymptomatic carotid artery disease (editorial). Stroke 13:431–433, 1982.

Moore WS, Boren C, Malone JM, et al: Natural history of nonstenotic, asymptomatic ulcerative lesions of the carotid artery. Arch Surg 113:1352–1359, 1978.

Podore PC, DeWeese JA, May AG, et al: Asymptomatic contralateral carotid artery stenosis: a five-year follow-up study following carotid endarterectomy. Surgery 88:748–752, 1980.

Roederer GO, Langlois YE, Jager KA, et al: The natural history of carotid arterial disease in asymptomatic patients with cervical bruits. Stroke 15:605–613, 1984.

Thompson JE, Patman RD, Talkington CM: Asymptomatic carotid bruit: long-term outcome of patients having endarterectomy compared with unoperated controls. Ann Surg 188:308–316, 1978.

Treiman RL, Foran RF, Shore EH, et al: Carotid bruit: significance in patients undergoing an abdominal aortic operation. Arch Surg 106:803–805, 1973.

Turnipseed WD, Berkoff HA, Belzer FO: Postoperative stroke in cardiac and peripheral vascular disease. Ann Surg 192:365–368, 1980.

Wolf PA, Kannel WB, Sorlie P, et al: Asymptomatic carotid bruit and risk of stroke: the Framingham study. JAMA 245:1442–1445, 1981.

4 · ISCHEMIC CEREBROVASCULAR DISEASE: VERTEBROBASILAR SYSTEM

W. Neath Folger
MAYO CLINIC AND MAYO FOUNDATION

Ischemic disease in the vertebrobasilar (VB) system presents some unusual and challenging problems in diagnosis and management. The symptoms and signs are extremely variable, reflecting the complex and somewhat variable arterial network supplying structures with a wide variety of functions. The VB arterial system supplies all the structures in the posterior fossa (brain stem and cerebellum) plus a number of supratentorial structures (posterior thalamus, inferior and medial temporal lobes, and both occipital lobes). The symptoms and signs of disease in these structures can be predicted by knowing the function of each. The following may characteristically be present:

Group I	Group II
Hemiparesis/hemiplegia	Diplopia
Hemisensory impairment	Dysarthria
Homonymous hemianopsia	Dysphagia
	Vertigo and/or ataxia

Carefully chosen criteria are necessary for the diagnosis of lesions occurring in the VB system. Minimal criteria for a confident anatomic diagnosis of vertebral basilar distribution involvement include:

1. a combination of at least two segmental signs or symptoms represented in group II, or

2. bilateral involvement of the motor, sensory, or visual systems represented in group I (e.g., quadriparesis or cortical blindness), or

3. involvement of at least one system each from both group I and group II above (e.g., a segmental sign such as vertigo combined with an intersegmental sign such as hemiparesis).

Although vertigo is the most common single symptom, vertigo alone is not sufficient for the diagnosis since it is commonly due to a labyrinthine disturbance. Likewise, syncope and drop attacks are not included.

PATHOPHYSIOLOGY

Patients may be seen at various points in the spectrum of ischemia, i.e., with a transient ischemic attack (TIA) or minor to major infarction. Management may, in part, depend on the degree of ischemia, but should focus on identifying and treating the pathophysiologic mechanism responsible for the ischemia. Both a TIA and a completed infarct may share a common mechanism; dynamic processes may still be in effect after the initial attack, posing an ever-present risk to noninfarcted tissue.

Atherosclerosis is the most common underlying cause of ischemic stroke. As a relatively fixed condition, additional factors must be at work for symptoms to occur. For instance, a relatively well tolerated, hemodynamically significant lesion may cause focal symptoms only after a drop in systemic blood pressure or fall in cardiac output. Likewise the same lesion may ulcerate and the resulting platelet deposition and thrombogenesis may occlude the vessel or be a source of distal emboli.

The search for an etiology focuses on the following: heart, large vessels, small vessels, and blood constituents.

The heart may be (1) a source of embologenic material (e.g., infected and noninfected vegetations on heart valves, mural thrombi following myocardial infarction or associated with atrial enlargement and stagnation); or (2) a cause of impaired cardiac output (e.g., aortic stenosis, myocardial ischemia, arrhythmia).

Atherosclerosis is the most common disorder affecting medium- and large-sized vessels. Sites of prediction include the origin of both vertebral arteries and multiple intracranial sites, the latter relatively more important in the VB system than in the carotid system. Other important medium-to-large vessel diseases include arterial dissections (either spontaneous, associated with fibromuscular dysplasia or chiropractic manipulation) and temporal arteritis. In each instance, symptoms may occur on either a hemodynamic or thromboembolic basis.

Small and medium-sized vessels may be affected by noninflammatory diseases (e.g., hypertensive lipohyalinotic arteriopathy) and inflammatory disorders, both infectious (e.g., syphilis, fungal conditions) and those immunologically related (e.g., systemic lupus erythematosus, periarteritis nodosa, granulomatous arteritis, rheumatoid disease).

Finally, abnormalities of blood constituents may alter viscosity or increase coagulability, or both. Examples include polycythemia, leukemia, macroglobulinemia, sickle cell disease, thrombocytosis, thrombotic thrombocytopenia purpura, thrombosis associated with a circulating (lupus) anticoagulant, pregnancy, and exogenous estrogen use.

This is not an exhaustive list of etiologies underlying ischemic vascular disease, but each area should be considered during the history, physical examination, and laboratory studies.

An important clue to the etiology may be derived from knowledge of the portion of the VB system affected. Caplan has separated cases of posterior circulation ischemia into a number of clinically recognizable syndromes, each often having a common etiologic basis. He divides the VB vascular system into discrete anatomic regions; when characteristic signs and symptoms occur, coupled with the results of cerebral angiography, identification of the most likely affected subdivision becomes possible along with recognition of the most likely mechanism responsible (see Table 1). On the basis of this information, important management decisions can be made, such as whether to anticoagulate and if so for how long, whether to proceed with angiography, and so forth.

One must be alert to the possibility that the cause is not ischemic at all. Arteriovenous malformation, intracerebral hemorrhage, neoplasm, demyelinating disease and labyrinthine disorders may at times cause acute and nonprogressive symptoms. Neurologic symptoms from migraine with or without headache can create a real dilemma at times. Usually the characteristic, slow build-up of positive symptoms over 10 to 20 minutes is helpful, but sometimes an angiogram may be required.

CLINICAL ASPECTS

About 15% of ischemic strokes occur in the VB system. The search for a pathophysiologic mechanism begins with a detailed history and examination including the neurovascular exam (BP in both arms, cardiovascular exam, and auscultation for bruits). On the basis of this clinical data, an inference can sometimes be made as to the specific vessel involved, its relative size, and the most likely mechanism. For instance, basilar branch syndromes cause unilateral symptoms or signs confined to a well-defined area; the mechanism is frequently related to hypertension and usually self-limited (e.g., lacunar infarcts). Symptoms and signs of basilar artery stenosis or occlusion, on the other hand, are usually bilateral, involving structures primarily in the

Table 1. SYNDROMES OF VERTEBROBASILAR ISCHEMIA

Subdivision	Course	Etiology
Top of basilar	Unstable; ? recurrent	Embolic
Basilar artery occlusion	Unstable; ? progressive	Atherosclerosis and thrombosis
Basilar branch diseases and lacunes	Self-limited	Atherosclerosis of penetrating vessels, lipohyalinosis
Intracranial vertebral artery stenosis or occlusion	Usually self-limited	Atherosclerosis and thrombosis
Extracranial vertebral artery disease	Rare cause of infarction	Atherosclerosis, thrombosis, and distal embolism

basis pontis with bilateral long tract signs; here the course is frequently progressive over several days. The mechanism is usually thrombotic and related to large-vessel atherosclerosis. The top of the basilar artery syndrome may produce pupillary and eyelid abnormalities, bilateral visual field deficits, and changes in behavior and alertness. The fact that two vertebral arteries feed a vessel of larger size is unique in the human vascular system and is the reason this syndrome is usually due to emboli from a proximal arterial or cardiac source.

Historical details may also be very helpful in predicting the mechanism of stroke. Pain in the neck often suggests vertebral artery dissection but may also occur with occlusion. The relationship of transient symptoms to changes in posture may suggest a flow-restricting lesion.

In most cases arterial lesions cannot be predicted from a set of clinical details. This is, in part, related to the very great anatomic variation present in these vessels and the effect collateral channels may have. Occasionally, one or another vertebral artery may be hypoplastic and the clinical effect will depend on the vessel involved. Potential collateral channels are present in the vessels of deep cervical musculature (via the thyrocervical trunk and occipital arteries). The paired posterior communicating arteries linking the posterior cerebral arteries to the carotid system are very important. In 23% to 40% of patients this connection in the circle of Willis is not complete, however.

In summary, without knowledge of the arterial anatomy and pathology from a cerebral angiogram, the etiology and pathophysiologic mechanism will not be known in most cases.

MANAGEMENT

Patients with a recently acquired fixed neurologic deficit or TIA (less than two months) should be hospitalized for evaluation and initial stabilization (see Fig. 1). In patients with impaired consciousness or with severe deficit, general medical management alone is advised. This includes securing an airway and maintenance of hydration and nutrition (initially with IV fluids and later with a feeding tube). Very elevated arterial pressure should be judiciously lowered using a nitroprusside drip, but pressure should be allowed to stay in the high-normal range to prevent worsening ischemia in areas with impaired autoregulation. Mini-dose heparin, 5000 units SQ twice daily, is recommended to prevent phlebothrombosis.

Patients with minor deficits or with TIA remain at risk of further ischemic episodes. Following the history and examination, blood is drawn for routine and special studies as suggested from the history (Table 1 in Chapter 2). An IV line should be inserted at this time. A CT scan is then done to exclude a hemorrhagic lesion and other structural lesions that may simulate ischemic disease. There are many pathophysiologic mechanisms for stroke and it is unlikely that one treatment will apply to all. The clinical data may infer a mechanism that is self-limiting, e.g., a lateral medullary syndrome usually associated with vertebral artery thrombosis. In this case only short-term anticoagulation (five to seven days) may be necessary to prevent extension of the thrombus in the basilar artery. More commonly the mechanism will not be known and immediate anticoagulation with IV heparin is advised if there are no contraindications (e.g., uncontrolled hypertension or active bleeding). The risk associated with a continuous IV heparin infusion is minimal in this setting and may prevent further thromboembolic episodes during the evaluation phase. A reasonable starting dose is 1000 units per hour following an appropriate loading dose, e.g., 5000 units. Dose adjustments should be made as necessary to maintain a partial thromboplastin time at approximately twice the control value. Platelet counts are checked every other day to detect the thrombocytopenia and associated paradoxical thrombosis occasionally seen with heparin.

Patients with a fixed neurologic deficit should be carefully observed for signs of progression. This may best be done in a specialized monitoring unit by nurses

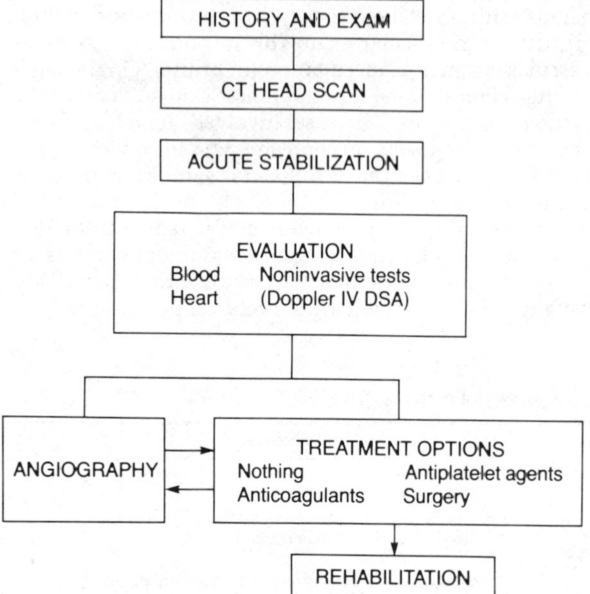

Figure 1. Evaluation of patients with vertebrobasilar ischemia.

accustomed to handling neurologic cases. Progression may be secondary to extension of the ischemia or to edema and the associated mass effect. When edema is suspected or shown to be present and responsible, antiedema measures should be instituted. Rapid but short-term control can be obtained if necessary using hyperventilation, maintaining the P_{CO_2} between 25 and 30 mm Hg. If herniation is not imminent, an osmotic agent may be given initially or may accompany hyperventilation. A 20% solution of mannitol (1.5 to 2.0 gm/kg) can be given over 30 to 60 minutes. Corticosteroids do not have a significant effect on edema secondary to ischemia, so plans should be made for surgical decompression if functional clinical recovery is possible. This is particularly relevant in patients with cerebellar infarction; as in patients with cerebellar hemorrhage, tonsillar herniation may threaten survival. Those with both lesions may have very satisfactory outcomes with exploration and debulking of the necrotic or hemorrhagic mass.

When progressing stroke is secondary to extension of the ischemia and anticoagulant levels are therapeutic, gentle elevation of BP can be attempted using vasopressors. Circulation in the ischemic bed may improve since the normal autoregulatory ability is paralyzed and flow becomes pressure dependent. Alternatively, flow may be increased simply by increasing blood volume. A technique of hypervolemic hemodilution has been reported to be useful in this situation. Here 250 cc of 5% albumen is infused every four hours to keep the hematocrit at approximately 33%. A central line should be inserted to monitor central venous pressure and observe for fluid overload.

Noninvasive laboratory techniques do not lend themselves easily to the VB system. Flow direction and velocity can be measured in the extracranial vertebral arteries; this is of doubtful value except in documenting a subclavian steal syndrome, which rarely causes significant permanent neurologic problems. A new transcranial technique is being developed in which a pulsed Doppler ultrasonic probe is directed through the foramen magnum, and from the signal analysis an estimate of vertebral and basilar flow is made. This technique may be useful in detecting stenosis or occlusion in these vessels.

Sophisticated cardiac studies (2D and M-mode echocardiography and radionuclide scans) are rarely helpful unless there is evidence of cardiac disease from the clinical data, chest x-ray, or electrocardiogram. IV digital subtraction angiography usually is not adequate to assess the intracranial VB vessels because of contrast dilution, superimposition of vessels, and misregistration artifact.

Unless the mechanism has been established at this point, further definition of a potential vascular lesion would require a conventional transfemoral cerebral angiogram. Knowledge of the vascular anatomy and pathology in each patient must be balanced against the associated risk of the study (1% risk for permanent or serious complications in the best centers). This may be accomplished by arterial digital subtraction techniques; the contrast load is lower and therefore is potentially less risky. Angiogaphy is recommended in patients who have

1. a progressing or unstable deficit.

2. failed the best available medical treatment.

3. a suspected hemodynamic mechanism where anticoagulant or antiplatelet therapy will be of little value.

4. an unusual mechanism suspected (e.g., arterial dissection or strokes in young patients).

In most uncomplicated TIA or minor stroke patients, cerebral angiography is not done initially. Treatment then is based not on a known but on a presumed thromboembolic mechanism. A three-month course of oral anticoagulant therapy with warfarin is recommended unless there are contraindications. These latter include severe renal or hepatic disease, bleeding diathesis, lack of adequate supervision or access to a laboratory capable of determining the prothrombin time (PT), an unreliable patient such as an alcoholic, or one with a gait disturbance that increases the risk of injury. Warfarin is adjusted to maintain the PT time at one and one-half to two times the control value. There is evidence that oral anticoagulation does reduce stroke risk used in this manner. At the three-month interval, a single daily 80-mg (children) aspirin is substituted and continued for at least the first year. In some circumstances, long-term anticoagulation is recommended when the identified arterial lesion suggests an unfavorable long-term prognosis (e.g., tight basilar stenosis or embolic source in the heart).

There is an increased risk of intracerebral hemorrhage in patients treated with oral anticoagulants. With careful monitoring and when these are used for less than one year, the risk appears to be small.

Nevertheless, when oral anticoagulants are contraindicated, antiplatelet treatment may be used. The evidence from available studies using 1000 to 1300 mg of aspirin in ischemic cerebrovascular disease are not convincing, but on the basis of newer laboratory studies, a single daily 80-mg (children) dose of aspirin may be more effective. At this dose there is inhibition of the proaggregant thromboxane A_2 in platelets, while there is little effect on the vessel wall generation of the antiaggregant prostacyclin. Also, at this dose there are few if any adverse side effects. Dipyridamole (Persantine), 75 mg three times a day, may be added as well, since it affects plate aggregation by a different mechanism from that of aspirin; however, there is little available evidence that it is effective in stroke reduction. The most common adverse side effects with dipyridamole are headaches and dizziness, which may require stopping the drug or reducing the dose.

Surgery is infrequently used in the management of VB disease. The diseased vessels are usually intracranial and have numerous small branches supplying vital brain stem structures. Revascularization procedures (e.g., extracranial-intracranial bypass) may be helpful, however, in patients with hemodynamic or flow-reducing lesions of the vertebral or basilar arteries. Such patients usually have well-defined and reproducible symptoms with changes in posture, or may have failed anticoagulant therapy. The recently published report on extracranial-intracranial bypass in the carotid system, however, casts significant doubt on the value of bypass procedures for any ischemic cerebrovascular disorder. Other surgical techniques such as vertebral endarterectomy or transluminal angioplasty are of doubtful use and have a significant risk.

CHRONIC (REHABILITATION) PHASE

For surviving patients with a deficit, psychologic support from the family and attending physician is very important. Physical and occupational therapy can help patient motivation and assist in gait retraining and in restoring activities of daily living. A speech therapist may be necessary and can sometimes help the patient learn techniques for swallowing.

Patients surviving an infarct in the VB distribution appear to have a better prognosis than those with carotid system infarctions, with respect to both survival and impairment.

REFERENCES

Caplan LR: Vertebrobasilar disease—time for a new strategy. Current Concepts Cerebrovasc Dis 15:11–16, 1980.

EC/IC Bypass Study Group: Failure of extracranial-intracranial arterial bypass to reduce the risk of ischemic stroke—results of an international randomized trial. N Engl J Med 313:1191–1200, 1985.

Kistler JP, Ropper AH, Heros RC: Therapy of ischemic cerebrovascular disease due to atherothrombosis. N Engl J Med 311:100–105, 1984.

Marshall J: A survey of occlusive disease of the vertebrobasilar arterial system. *In* Vinken PJ, Bruyn GW (eds): Handbook of Clinical Neurology, Vol 12. American Elsevier, New York, 1972, pp 1–12.

Sandok BA, Furlan AJ, Whisnant JP, et al: Guidelines for the management of transient ischemic attacks. Mayo Clin Proc 53:665–674, 1978.

Whisnant JP, Cartlidge NEF, Elveback LR: Carotid and vertebral basilar transient ischemic attacks: effect of anticoagulants, hypertension, and cardiac disorders on survival and stroke occurrence—a population study. Ann Neurol 3:107–115, 1978.

5 · *CARDIOEMBOLIC STROKE*

Anthony J. Furlan
CLEVELAND CLINIC FOUNDATION

The frequency of cardioembolic stroke has been reported to be as low as 8% in population studies and as high as 34% in referral center series. In the Harvard Stroke Registry, 20% of brain infarcts occurred in patients with an *identified* cardioembolic source (atrial fibrillation, valvular heart disease, recent myocardial infarction). Thus, emboli from cardiac sources are common causes of stroke, especially in individuals under 45 years of age. Although atherothrombotic stroke predominates in older age groups, there not infrequently is a coexistent cardiac source of embolism such as atrial fibrillation or mitral annulus calcification (MAC). In such older patients it may be impossible to identify the cause of stroke with certainty.

CLINICAL ASPECTS

Cardioembolic stroke should be considered in every patient who has sudden onset of a focal neurologic deficit that is maximal at or near onset and in whom there is a cardiac source. Other clues to cardioembolic stroke include

1. a patient under 45 years of age without atherosclerotic risk factors.

2. loss of consciousness or a seizure at the stroke onset.

3. rapid resolution of the neurologic deficit.

4. certain localized deficits such as Wernicke's aphasia, monoparesis, or isolated hemianopsia.

5. a history of stroke in a different vascular distribution or a history of systemic embolization.

Although strokes in multiple vascular territories always suggest a central embolic source, recurrent cardiac emboli may travel to the same vessel, usually to the middle cerebral artery. Embolic infarcts occur in a vertebrobasilar distribution about 15% of the time, and posterior cerebral artery occlusion is often embolic, either from the basilar artery or the heart. Embolization to the anterior cerebral artery is uncommon. It is sometimes stated that ocular ischemia is rarely caused by cardiac emboli, but amaurosis fugax or retinal infarction may be the only manifestation of cardiac embolization. Although cardiac emboli tend to be large and therefore produce severe strokes, a cardiac embolic source should also be considered in any patient with transient ischemic attacks (TIA) or minor stroke. Lastly, cardioembolic stroke may occasionally have a nonsudden onset. This possibly reflects fragmentation and distal embolization of the initial embolus, or thrombus formation in a vessel partially occluded by embolus.

LABORATORY INVESTIGATION

Computed Tomography. A brain CT scan may suggest embolic infarction if there are infarcts in multiple vascular territories. Deep basal ganglia infarcts or lacunar-type infarcts are rare with cardioembolism but can occur. The classic CT finding associated with embolic stroke is hemorrhagic infarction; 3% to 5% of embolic infarcts are hemorrhagic on an initial CT done within 48 hours of stroke onset. As many as 22% of large embolic infarcts that are initially nonhemorrhagic on CT undergo spontaneous hemorrhagic transformation within eight days of onset. Such transformation may or may not be correlated with clinical worsening (see below).

Cerebral Angiography. This may show occlusion or delayed perfusion of distal arterial branches. Occlusion of the origin of the middle cerebral artery is often embolic. Angiographic changes suggesting embolism are more frequent when the study is performed within 48 hours of stroke onset. Because of clot lysis, angiography is often normal when done beyond this period. Arterial branch occlusions cannot be visualized with intravenous digital subtraction angiography (IV-DSA). IV-DSA is a useful screening test for carotid artery atherosclerosis in patients with an otherwise typical profile of cardiac embolic infarction.

Cardiac Monitoring. Prolonged cardiac monitoring may reveal a variety of dysrhythmias in patients with brain infarction. Rarely, an unsuspected dysrhythmia predisposing to embolization (paroxysmal atrial fibrillation) is discovered in a patient with acute stroke and no history of cardiac disease. It may be difficult to determine if the findings on prolonged monitoring are the cause of the stroke or a secondary manifestation of brain infarction. Prolonged monitoring should be reserved for patients with unexplained stroke, especially younger individuals or patients with cardiac symptoms and signs.

Echocardiography. This should be done in young patients with unexplained stroke and in individuals with cardiac symptoms and signs. Echocardiography is not cost effective in older patients with brain infarction, although it can be done in selected cases. Most of the cardiac conditions that can produce embolic infarction are best visualized with two-dimensional echocardiography. The most frequent occult cardiac lesion detected on echocardiography in stroke patients is mitral valve prolapse. Unsuspected rheumatic mitral valve disease is only rarely discovered in a patient with unexplained stroke. MAC may be detected in older patients with brain infarction. Asymmetric septal hypertrophy is another common echocardiographic finding but should be viewed as coincidental in most patients with acute stroke. All these echocardiographic findings may be associated with dysrhythmia, such as atrial fibrillation, that should be submitted for prolonged electrocardiographic monitoring. Echocardiography is sometimes useful for visualizing mural or valvular thrombi or vegetations, but the false-negative rate is very high for these lesions.

Cardiac Catheterization. The need for cardiac catheterization in patients with cerebral infarction is usually determined by the cardiac/hemodynamic status. The role of catheterization in searching for occult sources of embolism is unclear. It should be considered in young patients with multiple unexplained brain infarctions. Certain conditions, such as patent foramen ovale with paradoxical embolism, are best visualized with heart catheterization. Sometimes mitral valve prolapse can be detected only with catheterization; whether such mild valvular lesions can produce cerebral embolism is uncertain.

SELECTED CARDIAC CONDITIONS CAUSING EMBOLIC STROKE

ATRIAL FIBRILLATION

Chronic atrial fibrillation not associated with valvular heart disease (NVAF) is the most common cardiac source of embolism. NVAF is frequently caused by ischemic heart disease but may be related to hyperthyroidism and other medical conditions. Epidemiologic studies indicate that NVAF increases the risk of stroke sixfold compared with controls. Patients with chronic atrial fibrillation associated with rheumatic valvular heart disease have a 17-fold increased risk of stroke. Paroxysmal atrial fibrillation can also cause embolic stroke. The risk of early embolism following cardioversion is about 2%.

About 15% of all ischemic strokes occur in patients with NVAF. One study found that about 14% of strokes occurred in the first year after onset of NVAF, with a 5% per year stroke rate thereafter. It is estimated that 75% of strokes in patients with NVAF are embolic infarcts. However, it may be difficult to distinguish an atherothrombotic infarct from an embolic infarct in patients with NVAF, since both types of stroke occur in older patients with numerous atherosclerotic risk factors.

RHEUMATIC HEART DISEASE

Clinical embolic events occur in about 20% of patients with rheumatic heart disease. Mitral stenosis with or without atrial fibrillation carries a 20% risk of embolization, and 50% of these events involve the brain. Aortic stenosis and insufficiency are infrequent sources of embolism.

ACUTE MYOCARDIAL INFARCTION

Mural thrombi are most common with large anterior wall myocardial infarctions. About 3% of patients with acute myocardial infarction have a clinical embolic event, and 85% of embolic strokes related to myocardial infarction occur within one month.

MITRAL VALVE PROLAPSE (MVP)

The prevalence of MVP in otherwise healthy young women ranges from 6% to 17%. Since its original recognition as a cause of stroke by Barnett and co-workers, several series of patients with stroke and associated MVP have been reported. Barnett estimates that 1% of cerebral infarcts per year are related to prolapsed mitral valve. However, the absolute risk of stroke in patients with prolapsed mitral valve is low, with an estimated incidence of one per 6000 patients per year.

MITRAL ANNULUS CALCIFICATION (MAC)

MAC is a frequent cause of apical systolic heart murmurs in the elderly. The average age at diagnosis is 65 years or older. DeBono and Warlow popularized the concept of MAC as a source of brain embolism. Another study, however, found that brain embolization from isolated MAC is rare and difficult to prove because of the frequent coexistence of atherosclerosis. Cardiac conditions, such as atrial fibrillation and mitral stenosis, which may increase the risk of embolism, are usually associated with MAC >5 mm thickness. In many patients with stroke, MAC may be better viewed as a marker of generalized calcific atherosclerotic disease than as an immediate embolic source.

PROSTHETIC HEART VALVES

In patients with prosthetic heart valves, more than 50% of clinical embolic events involve the brain. The best mechanical cloth-covered ball valves, disc valves, and tilting disc valves carry a similar risk of thromboembolic complications in anticoagulated patients. Mechanical aortic valve prostheses carry about a 2% risk per patient per year of embolism in anticoagulated patients. The risk is approximately 4% per year for anticoagulated patients with mechanical mitral prostheses. Tissue valves have been developed in an attempt to reduce the risk of embolism and the need for long-term anticoagulation. The embolic rates for biologic prostheses are comparable with the rates in anticoagulated patients with the best mechanical valves. Since most embolic complications associated with biologic prostheses appear to occur in the first three months after surgery, warfarin therapy is sometimes employed during this period. Antiplatelet agents are ineffective when used alone to prevent emboli in patients with prosthetic valves, but combinations of aspirin or dipyridamole with warfarin may further reduce the risk of embolism.

INFECTIOUS ENDOCARDITIS

Stroke is the most dreaded neurologic complication of bacterial endocarditis. The most common cerebrovascular complication is embolic cerebral infarction. Septic emboli may lodge anywhere in the brain, although they are most frequent in the middle cerebral artery territory. Cerebral emboli usually result in macroscopic infarction, which presents as the sudden onset of a focal neurologic deficit. Less commonly recognized are microscopic infarcts from multiple embolic occlusions of small intracerebral vessels. The presentation is that of a diffuse encephalopathy or fluctuating focal neurologic signs.

Neurologic complications may be the first manifestation of underlying endocarditis. In the Massachusetts General Hospital series, 16% of patients with endocarditis presented with a neurologic complication. More than 50% of patients with septic embolic brain infarction have no recognizable preceding peripheral embolic event.

The other major cerebrovascular complication of bacterial endocarditis is mycotic aneurysm, which occurs in about 5% of patients with endocarditis. Mycotic aneurysms develop as a result of septic embolization to the vasa vasorum of a major intracranial artery, with subsequent disruption of the adventitial and muscular arterial layers. The middle cerebral artery is the most frequent site of mycotic aneurysm formation, particularly on the distal branches at or beyond the sylvian fissure. This location distinguishes mycotic aneurysms from the more common berry aneurysms, which tend to occur proximally near the circle of Willis. Mycotic aneurysms are often unsuspected until they rupture, resulting in a catastrophic subarachnoid or intracerebral hemorrhage.

The management of mycotic aneurysms is controversial. Surgical treatment of accessible aneurysms is often successful but carries a significant risk. Mycotic aneurysms may resolve with intensive antibiotic treatment.

Other important cardiac sources of embolism include cardiomyopathy, paradoxical embolization related to atrial septal defect or patent foramen ovale, atrial myxomas, nonbacterial thrombotic endocarditis, and open heart surgery.

TREATMENT OF CARDIOGENIC EMBOLIC INFARCTION

ACUTE NONSEPTIC EMBOLIC INFARCTION

The risk of recurrent embolism must be weighed against that of brain hemorrhage in deciding on the timing and use of anticoagulant therapy after acute, nonseptic embolic brain infarction. Early recurrent brain embolism occurs in 10% to 13% of patients with embolic stroke from a variety of cardiac sources. Aggregate data suggest that early heparin therapy can reduce the rate of early recurrent brain embolism by as much as 67%. About 5% of nonseptic embolic infarcts are shown as hemorrhagic on CT performed within 48 hours of onset. As many as 22% of large embolic infarcts undergo spontaneous hemorrhagic transformation within eight days of onset. The Cerebral Embolism Study Group estimates that about 5% of unselected embolic stroke patients who are immediately anticoagulated will experience worsening associated with brain hemorrhage. In the one third of such patients with large embolic strokes, the incidence may reach 20%, which exceeds the risk of early recurrent embolism. The Study Group recommends immediate anticoagulation of small and moderate-sized nonseptic embolic infarcts, regardless of embolic source, if a CT performed after 24 hours from stroke onset does not show hemorrhage. In patients with large infarcts who are at special risk of spontaneous, late-onset hemorrhagic transformation, a delay of at least seven days before anticoagulation is initiated seems prudent. In patients who are receiving anticoagulants at the time of stroke onset, the Study Group recommends continuing anticoagulation in those with submassive infarcts who do not show hemorrhage on CT and in whom blood pressure is well controlled.

There is no standard way to administer anticoagulation therapy. Bolus doses of heparin, excessive anticoagulation, and elevated BP should be avoided. We typically begin heparin therapy by constant IV pump infusion at a rate of 1000 units/hour. Most patients require 300 to 500 units/kg/24 hr of heparin to maintain the activated partial thromboplastin time (APTT) at one and one-half to two times control. Occasionally the APTT remains "subtherapeutic" even with these doses of heparin. If this situation arises, the dose of heparin may be cautiously raised by increments of 50 to 100 units/hr, not to exceed a daily dose of 40,000 units. The APTT may also be supplemented with one of the new chromogenic or fluorogenic heparin assay systems. The APTT is best viewed as a guard against excessive anticoagulation; inter- and intrapatient APTT variabilities are high. I usually continue heparin for two or three days before initiating long-term warfarin therapy. Heparin therapy is discontinued when the PT is one and one-half to two times control. Others favor overlapping heparin and therapeutic warfarin therapy for five to seven days to ensure suppression of all vitamin K–dependent clotting factors. Lastly, I routinely check another CT before discharging the patient once therapeutic warfarin therapy is established, since hemorrhage into an infarction is often clinically silent.

SEPTIC EMBOLISM

Anticoagulation should still be regarded as contraindicated in patients with infectious endocarditis and septic embolism. However, in those with prosthetic valve endocarditis who are receiving warfarin, anticoagulation may be continued in the absence of systemic or brain embolism. Anticoagulation should also be considered in patients who experience multiple embolic events, but in this situation it is safest first to perform cerebral angiography to exclude a mycotic aneurysm.

LONG-TERM MANAGEMENT

There is ample evidence that long-term anticoagulation (with warfarin) decreases the risk of embolism in patients with mechanical prosthetic valves. The addition of dipyridamole or aspirin probably gives further protection without significantly increasing the risk of hemorrhagic complications. However, antiplatelet agents are relatively ineffective in preventing embolization when used alone in patients with prosthetic valves. Long-term anticoagulation is also an accepted form of therapy in patients with rheumatic mitral stenosis and atrial fibrillation. In patients with acute myocardial infarction, anticoagulation is sometimes used for a six-month period to allow organization of mural thrombus in patients who have embolized. Long-term anticoagulation is also recommended for patients with chronic atrial fibrillation who have suffered any embolic event. Patients with mitral valve prolapse who have embolized are usually first treated with antiplatelet agents, and then anticoagulation, should this fail. Prophylatic antiplatelet therapy should be considered in patients with chronic atrial fibrillation or other cardiac conditions that carry a significant stroke risk but in whom the dangers of long-term anticoagulation do not seem justified.

REFERENCES

Barnett HJM: Heart in ischemic stroke—a changing emphasis. Neurol Clin North Am 1:291–313, 1983.

Barnett HJM, Boughner DR, Taylor DW, et al: Further evidence relating mitral valve prolapse to cerebral ischemic events. N Engl J Med 302:139–144, 1980.

Cerebral Embolism Study Group: Immediate anticoagulation of embolic stroke: a randomized trial. Stroke 14:668–676, 1983.

Cerebral Embolism Study Group: Brain hemorrhage and management options. Stroke 15:779–789, 1984.

Come PC, Riley MF, Bivas NK: Roles of echocardiography and arrhythmia monitoring in the evaluation of patients with suspected systemic embolism. Ann Neurol 13:527–531, 1983.

DeBono DP, Warlow CP: Mitral-annulus calcification and cerebral or retinal ischaemia. Lancet 2:383–385, 1979.

Easton JD, Sherman DG: Management of cerebral embolism of cardiac origin. Stroke 11:433–442, 1980.

Furlan AJ, Breuer AC: Central nervous system complications of open heart surgery. Stroke 15:912–915, 1984.

Furlan AJ, Conomy JP: Stroke related to cardiac dysrhythmia and valvular heart disease. In Barnett HJM, Mohr JP, Stein B, et al (eds): Stroke. Churchill Livingstone, New York, 1985, pp 763–773.

Mohr JP, Caplan LR, Melski JW, et al: The Harvard Cooperative Stroke Registry: a prospective registry. Neurology 28:754–762, 1978.

Myers MG, Norris JW, Hachinski VC, et al: Cardiac sequelae of acute stroke. Stroke 13:838–842, 1982.

6 · LACUNAR INFARCTION

Robert T. Simkins
K. M. A. Welch
HENRY FORD HOSPITAL

Lacunar infarcts are small infarctions that involve the deeper subcortical regions of the cerebral hemispheres and brain stem. They represent the result of occlusion of penetrating branches of the larger cerebral arteries. After such an occlusion occurs, the necrotic tissue is ultimately phagocytized, leaving a small cavity, a lacune. The term lacune was first described in the medical literature in 1843 in a monograph by Durand-Fardel on softening of the brain.

The most common locations for lacunes, in descending order of frequency, are the putamen, caudate nucleus, thalamus, pons, internal capsule, and convolutional white matter. They are less easily seen in gray matter where the tissue tends to collapse. The smaller lacunes are usually asymptomatic unless strategically placed. Small, deep infarcts that vary in size from approximately 3 mm to 2.0 cm are frequently seen as part of larger cortical infarctions and are not categorized as lacunar infarcts.

INCIDENCE

Lacunes are responsible for clinically symptomatic strokes in approximately 19% of patients. They are also found in up to 10% of unselected autopsies.

PATHOGENESIS

RISK FACTORS

By far the most important risk factor is hypertension. The incidence in patients with lacunar infarction varies from 65% to 75%. Diabetes is present in 11% to 43% of patients with lacunar disease. Previous transient ischemic attacks (TIA) are seen in about 20% of patients, compared with an incidence of about 5% in embolic stroke and 50% in large artery atherosclerosis.

VASCULAR ANATOMY

Lenticulostriates. These vessels arise from the circle of Willis and main trunk of the anterior and middle cerebral arteries. They supply the putamen, caudate nucleus, and internal capsule. A medial group averages 100 to 200 μ in diameter, and a lateral group varies from 200 to 400 μ.

Thalamoperforates. These vessels arise from the posterior half of the circle of Willis and main trunks of the posterior cerebral arteries, and supply the midbrain and thalamus. They vary in diameter from 100 to 400 μ.

Paramedian Branches of Basilar Artery. These vessels range from 40 to 500 μ in diameter and mainly supply the pons.

Collectively, these vessels, known as "penetrators," have certain features in common. They are all less than 500 μ in diameter. They arise directly from much larger vessels and for the most part exhibit unbranching end-artery configuration without appreciable collateral flow. Because of this lack of collaterals, occlusion of one of these vessels results in a wedge-shaped infarct, the apex of which is at the point of occlusion. Most occlusions occur in the first half of the course of the penetrator, resulting in an infarct smaller in size than the total territory of supply. If the most proximal portion is occluded, the resulting infarct is larger and involves a greater proportion, or perhaps even the entire territory, of supply.

VASCULAR PATHOLOGY

Microatheroma. This is the most common cause of lacunar infarction, particularly when symptomatic. Tiny foci of atheromatous deposits involve the walls of the penetrating vessels. In the absence of hypertension, atheroma is usually confined to the extracranial internal carotid and basilar arteries and only occasionally involves other major cerebral arteries. However, in the presence of long-standing hypertension, these lesions advance faster and spread more distally to involve vessels as small as 100 to 400 μ.

Lipohyalinosis. This is the most frequent cause of small lacunes (0.2 to 3 mm), many of which may be clinically asymptomatic. The lumen of an artery (usually less than 200 μ in diameter) is occluded. The wall of the artery is thinned and reduced to connective tissue shreds. Similar characteristics are seen in fibrinoid necrosis associated with severely elevated levels of blood pressure.

Other Pathologic Processes that Produce Lacunar Lesions. Atherosclerosis of the wall of a major cerebral artery may affect the penetrating vessels at their origin. The frequency of this occurrence is unknown but it is probably less common than microatheroma or lipohyalinosis of penetrating arteries in the case of brain stem lacunes. The incidence of microembolization is unknown. Macroembolization to the middle cerebral artery stem, with infarction confined to the territory of one or more of the lenticulostriate arteries, commonly occurs with embolic strokes. These usually result in a large deep infarction and are not considered lacunes. Arteritis secondary to chronic meningitis resulting from neurosyphilis and granulomatous meningitis from any cause are other processes that produce lacunar lesions.

CLINICAL ASPECTS

COMMON MANIFESTATIONS

Twenty per cent of patients who experience lacunar infarctions have had previous TIAs. A gradual onset of neurologic signs occurs in 30% of patients (usually over a period of up to 36 hours), compared with 5% for major atheromatous or embolic strokes. Sudden onset occurs in only 40% of patients. The rate of development of physical signs does not appear to predict the severity of the eventual defect. The progression of deficit is usually preceded by intensification of initial deficits and only occasionally by spread into unaffected limbs.

SPECIFIC SYNDROMES

The following is a review of the lacunar syndromes with which the clinician is likely to be confronted in clinical practice. Rare syndromes and those whose "lacunar" identity has not been documented are not included. The syndrome of lacunar infarction is approached from the aspect of clinical presentation rather than location of the lesion. These syndromes may occur secondary to lesions in variable anatomic locations, and only by computed tomography (CT) can the actual location of the responsible lesion be identified. Others may occur in the absence of any confirmatory diagnostic test such as CT. The lacunar nature of these syndromes has been documented pathologically, and in such cases the diagnosis can usually be made with confidence by the characteristic presentation, even though results of such tests as CT scan may be negative. Magnetic resonance imaging is likely to increase the diagnostic yield of positive confirmatory results in patients with lacunar infarctions.

Pure Sensory Stroke. Pure sensory stroke is one of the most common lacunar syndromes. It usually manifests itself as an isolated numbness of the face, arm, and leg in the absence of weakness, visual loss, or aphasia. Only 10% of patients with recurrent TIAs go on to develop persistent numbness, which most frequently involves the face, arm, and leg, although all

three sites need not be involved. An associated sensory deficit may or may not involve all sensory modalities. The infarct lies in the posteroventral nucleus of the thalamus. Sensory TIAs may occasionally occur as a prodrome of posterior cerebral artery occlusion, and very rarely as a manifestation of internal carotid artery occlusion.

Pure Motor Hemiparesis. This is a pure motor stroke involving the face, arm, and leg on one side without associated sensory deficit, visual loss, or aphasia. It was the lacunar syndrome most often seen in one series. Some numbness may occur at the onset but no sensory deficit is found on examination. A TIA featuring pure motor hemiparesis may precede the stroke. The patient may awake with the stroke. The stroke may evolve gradually over a day or two or may even develop in a stepwise fashion over as long as six days. Brisk deep tendon reflexes develop early. The infarct may have various anatomic sites, having been reported to occur in the internal capsule, the lower basis pontis, or rarely the cerebral peduncle, medullary pyramid, or corona radiata.

Ataxic Hemiparesis. This syndrome presents as a pure motor lesion combined with cerebellar dysmetria in the affected limbs, assuming that enough residual motor strength is left to identify the cerebellar dysmetria. The leg is predominantly affected, with little involvement of the arm or face. Clinical findings include footdrop combined with cerebellar ataxia, increased deep tendon reflexes, and a Babinski sign. The infarct is usually in the upper basis pontis but may occur in the corona radiata or the posterior limb of the internal capsule.

Dysarthria–Clumsy Hand Syndrome. A lesion in the anterior portion or the genu of the internal capsule or the basis pontis may result in facial weakness, dysarthria, and dysphagia together with slight weakness and clumsiness of the hand, increased deep tendon reflexes, and a Babinski sign (a variant of ataxic hemiparesis). No sensory deficit is apparent.

Sensorimotor Stroke. The sensory and motor deficits are essentially the same as those seen in the more usual pure motor hemiparesis or pure sensory stroke. As in the more typical pure motor or sensory strokes, behavior abnormalities, aphasia, ophthalmoparesis, and visual field deficits are not observed. The lesion has usually been either a lacune involving the thalamus together with portions of the posterior limb of the internal capsule, or a large caudatoputaminal infarct. The former would require some aberrant blood supply to the internal capsule from the thalamoperforans artery. This relatively uncommon syndrome is seen more often as a result of hematoma, embolism, and atherosclerotic stenosis or occlusion of major extracranial vessels.

LABORATORY STUDIES

Initial evaluation of the patient with possible lacunar stroke is similar to that outlined in Section XII, Chapter 2 on carotid disease. However, some points deserve amplification.

ELECTROENCEPHALOGRAPHY

Results of electroencephalography (EEG) are usually negative in the patient with a lacunar infarction.

The absence of a specific abnormality thus lends support to the diagnosis of a lacune in contrast to a cortical (probably embolic) infarct, which should have focal EEG changes.

COMPUTED TOMOGRAPHY

Most lacunes smaller than 2 mm are not visualized on CT. Overall, the yield on scans obtained within the first two days tends to be low, but increases over time with the quality of the scanner. With respect to capsular infarctions, studies have shown 69% to 76% positivity on CT. One study revealed positive results in 29 of 30 patients with hemiparesis, although this high rate of positivity may have been an artifact of patient selection. In another study, sequential scans were performed over a seven-month period on patients thought to have had a capsular lacunar infarct. In 41 of 75 patients (55%), CT results were positive within the first ten days. By the end of one month, 48 of 75 patients (64%) scanned exhibited an appropriate area of infarction. This increased to 69% by seven months. Interestingly, in 13 of 25 patients with TIAs there were positive CT findings. The chance of detecting an infarct in the TIA group of patients was appreciably higher for those who had had multiple TIAs within the previous 24 hours.

MAGNETIC RESONANCE IMAGING

Magnetic resonance imaging may permit earlier observation of lacunar infarctions, will likely detect a higher percentage of lacunes compared with CT, and may be particularly useful for posterior fossa lacunes where the lack of signal from bone provides exceptional anatomic visualization. This technique may also identify the relative age of lacunes when multiple lacunes exist in patients who have had neurologic deficits disseminated in time. Magnetic resonance imaging thus promises to be a powerful tool for the study of lacunar lesions.

ANGIOGRAPHY

Conventional angiography does not have the technical capability to define adequately these small (40 to 500 μ in diameter), penetrating vessels. However, in the presence of giant lacunes, stenosis of the middle cerebral artery stem or of one of the larger lenticulostriate vessels may be demonstrated. In general, if there is strong clinical or CT support, or both, for a lacunar lesion, angiography is not performed.

TREATMENT

ANTICOAGULATION

No guidelines exist for this specific therapy in patients with lacunar disease. Although one might speculate that short-term use of anticoagulants is indicated in patients with microatheroma, perhaps with the potential for critical stenosis or distal emboli, it is not clinically possible to differentiate these patients from those with lipohyalinosis in whom anticoagulants would be potentially hazardous. Therefore, there are no established indications for the use of anticoagulants in patients with lacunar disease. At present, some physicians are prescribing aspirin or dipyridamole, although the efficacy of such treatment awaits a careful clinical trial.

ANTIHYPERTENSIVE THERAPY

Vigorous treatment of hypertension in the acute phase of stroke may precipitate more clinical deficits. Unless the BP level is excessively elevated, antihypertensive therapy is delayed until the stroke syndrome stabilizes (see Sect. XII, Chap. 10). After the acute phase of the stroke has stabilized, control of hypertension is usually attempted in the hope of preventing recurrent lacunes, although the efficacy of such therapy has not been established.

CONCLUSIONS

The early presentation of true lacunar syndromes can be extremely variable and of uncertain pathogenesis. When patients are seen during the acute stages of presentation, the clinician should be able to identify the type of lesion by careful examination. A more precise anatomic definition may be gained with imaging techniques, which also help exclude a hemorrhage. Rarely, cerebral arteriography may be utilized. A well-defined treatment protocol has yet to be developed.

REFERENCES

Buonanno FS, Kistler JP, DeWitt LD, et al: Proton (IH) nuclear magnetic resonance (NMR) imaging in stroke syndromes. Neurol Clin 1:243–262, 1983.

Damasio AD, Damasio H, Rizzo M, et al: Aphasia with nonhemorrhagic lesions in the basal ganglia and internal capsule. Arch Neurol 39:15–20, 1982.

Davis KR, Kistler JP, Buonanno FS: Clinical neuroimaging approaches to cerebrovascular diseases. Neurol Clin 2:655–665, 1984.

Donnan GA, Tress BM, Bladin PF: A prospective study of lacunar infarction using computerized tomography. Neurology 32:49–56, 1982.

Durand-Ferdel M: Traite du Ramollissement de Cerveau. Baillière, Paris, 1843.

Fisher CM: A lacunar stroke: the dysarthria–clumsy hand syndrome. Neurology 17:614–617, 1967.

Fisher CM: The arterial lesions underlying lacunes. Acta Neuropathol (Berl) 12:1–15, 1969.

Fisher CM: Bilateral occlusion of basilar artery branches. J Neurol Neurosurg Psychiatry 40:1182–1189, 1977.

Fisher CM: Ataxic hemiparesis. Arch Neurol 35:126–128, 1978.

Fisher CM: Thalamic pure sensory stroke: a pathologic study. Neurology 28:1141–1144, 1978.

Fisher CM: Capsular infarcts: the underlying vascular lesions. Arch Neurol 36:65–73, 1979.

Fisher CM: Lacunar strokes and infarcts: a review. Neurology 32:871–876, 1982.

Mohr JP: Lacunes. Stroke 13:3–10, 1982.

Mohr JP: Lacunes. Neurol Clin 1:201–221, 1983.

Mohr JP, Caplan LR, Melski JW, et al: The Harvard Cooperative Stroke Registry: a prospective registry. Neurology 28:754–762, 1978.

Rascol A, Clanet M, Manelfe C, et al: Pure motor hemiplegia: CT study of 30 cases. Stroke 13:11–17, 1982.

Ropper AH, Fisher CM, Kleinman GM: Pyramidal infarction in the medulla: cause of pure motor hemiplegia sparing the face. Neurology 29:91–95, 1979.

7 · UNCOMMON CAUSES OF STROKE

H. Royden Jones, Jr.
LAHEY CLINIC MEDICAL CENTER

Most patients who present with a stroke of acute onset are found to have a specific causative mechanism. This usually is related to emboli secondary to diseases of the carotid artery or heart, lacunar intracerebral vascular disease (in hypertensive patients), or a hemorrhagic lesion, either intracerebral or subarachnoid. However, careful evaluation sometimes fails to demonstrate any of these well-known mechanisms in a modest number of these patients. Because a patient who has sustained a stroke is at increased risk of having a recurrent event, the physician should search for other potential sources, including uncommon mechanisms, when none of the more common ones are evident. These causes are best categorized as uncommon cardiac emboli, other arterial lesions, drug-induced stroke, hematologic conditions, or infectious diseases. Specific clinical studies are available that will enable the physician to identify these factors and lead to proper management of the patient.

UNCOMMON CARDIAC LESIONS

Clinical history and examination usually suggest an obvious source for potential cardiac emboli: e.g., atrial fibrillation associated with either rheumatic heart disease or arteriosclerotic heart disease; recent or occasionally remote myocardial infarction with mural thrombi or latent aneurysm; an artificial heart valve; or bacterial endocarditis. Idiopathic myocardopathy predisposes patients to formation of clots with a potential for the development of cerebral emboli. Usually these patients have already presented with an episode of frank congestive heart failure. Except for patients with bacterial endocarditis, long-term therapy with anticoagulants is indicated to prevent further formation of emboli.

In patients under 50 years of age who present with stroke, about 25% may be found to have a previously unsuspected mitral valve prolapse, easily confirmed by echocardiography. Short-term administration of anticoagulants (three to six months) followed by antiplatelet agents is usually indicated. An atrial myxoma, another rare source of cerebral emboli diagnosed by echocardiography, may be removed surgically. Unfortunately, the routine use of echocardiography in patients who have sustained a cerebral infarct has failed to improve appreciably the diagnostic yield in a general group of patients who have had a stroke. However, echocardiography still merits consideration when one of the usual causes of stroke is not found, particularly in a patient under age 50. Marantic endocarditis is seen mainly in patients with underlying cancer and is usually of the mucin-secreting variety. These valvular deposits are too small even for two-dimensional echocardiography to define. However, such lesions produce cerebral emboli, and no specific therapy has proved of value even when the lesion is clinically suspected.

Paradoxical emboli through a probe patent foramen ovale (PPFO) or an occult atrial septal defect usually occurs in clinical situations, predisposing the patient to the development of venous stasis. Examples include use of birth control pills, appreciable obesity, underlying cancer, or patients who have had prolonged bed rest for an orthopedic or neurologic condition. Although a PPFO is found in 25% of the normal population, and 6% overall have a PPFO large enough to admit a pencil probe, high left-sided atrial pressure usually keeps this lesion functionally closed. In an acute event, however, increasing right-sided atrial pressure in a patient with occult venous thrombosis, associated with pulmonary embolus or Valsalva's maneuver, may permit a venous clot to enter the systemic circulation and produce paradoxical cerebral embolic infarction. Administration of anticoagulant agents and/or use of a Greenfield vena caval filter (Medi-Tech, Watertown, MA) are indicated.

UNCOMMON PRIMARY ARTERIAL LESIONS

In patients with hemiplegic migraine, symptoms usually evolve slowly and clear with onset of the headache. These symptoms include visual, sensory, language, and motor dysfunction with a characteristic march reminiscent of a focal seizure taking place over a matter of five to 20 minutes, rather than abruptly and totally as in patients with a transient ischemic attack (TIA) or stroke. It is uncommon for patients with migraine and focal neurologic deficits to have a permanent infarction. Propranolol (Inderal), 80 to 320 mg per day, is particularly effective in preventing these attacks in individuals in whom they may occur frequently. At times, a strong hereditary tendency may be seen.

Dissecting aneurysm of the carotid artery occurs spontaneously and is usually accompanied by Horner's syndrome and unilateral facial pain. The combination mimicks a cluster headache. In a similar way and particularly after trauma, which may be minimal, vertebral dissection may occur. A TIA or stroke may develop in some of these patients with either carotid or vertebral dissection. In general, short-term administration of anticoagulants prevent thrombi with subsequent potential for embolization from forming at the site of intimal tear. Surgery is not indicated because the vessel usually reconstitutes itself within three to six months.

Most patients with cerebral aneurysms have a history of subarachnoid hemorrhage. Occasionally, however, symptoms secondary to spasm or emboli arising from the aneurysm may be the presenting complaint. The clinician does not become aware of this lesion until cerebral angiography is performed. Treatment is surgical.

Most individuals with temporal granulomatous arteritis present with a classic pattern of headache. Occasionally, this lesion may also primarily affect the intracerebral arteries, presenting with a TIA or stroke. The erythrocyte sedimentation rate (ESR) should always be obtained in patients with TIA or stroke. Patients with temporal arteritis most often have ESR values between 60 and 120 mm/hr. When other conditions or lesions that cause such high values (e.g., bacterial endocarditis, atrial myxoma, or meningitis) are excluded, biopsy of the temporal artery may be indicated, since therapy with corticosteroid agents is curative in this disease.

DRUG-INDUCED STROKE

Drug-induced mechanisms are uncommon. Epidemiologic studies have indicated a slight increased potential for stroke in women who use oral hormonal contraceptives, particularly when they smoke. A variety of vascular lesions may be observed in these women, including an indeterminate arteriopathy; primary cerebral venous thrombosis; emboli, including paradoxical ones associated with deep venous thrombosis; and subarachnoid hemorrhage. Patients should not continue or ever resume taking birth control pills when an unexplained acute focal neurologic deficit is suggestive of a stroke or TIA, including those women who have hemiplegic migraine headaches.

An arteritis may develop in abusers of amphetamines, which may predispose them to the development of primary intracerebral hemorrhage. A few reports have also associated some of the proprietary anorectic medications, such as phenylpropanolamine, with a stroke. Heroin addicts using unsterile needles are predisposed to develop bacterial endocarditis and are at risk of stroke. Rarely, hypertensive crisis may be precipitated by the interaction of various foods, particularly wine and cheese, with the monoamine oxidase variety of antidepressants. This combination may lead to subarachnoid or intracerebral hemorrhage.

HEMATOLOGIC MECHANISMS

Various hematologic disorders may predispose patients to TIAs, stroke, or both. Polycythemia with a hematocrit level greater than 55%, with consequent increase of viscosity, usually results in a relative ischemia with slow blood flow. Phlebotomy is indicated when no other mechanism is found. Similarly, any form of anemia resulting in relative tissue oxygen ischemia may precipitate a focal cerebral lesion in an area already compromised perhaps by an intrinsic vascular lesion. Young blacks with sickle cell disease may sustain a cerebral infarct as part of a sickle cell crisis. Primary thrombocytosis may also lead to occlusion of small intracerebral arterioles due to aggregation of platelets, which occurs when the platelet count exceeds 500,000/mm^3, and particularly when it is more than 1,000,000/mm^3.

INFECTIOUS MECHANISMS

Primary infectious mechanisms leading to strokes are uncommon today. Historically, tertiary syphilis with a luetic arteritis was a common cause of recurrent cerebral infarction, and this infection still merits consideration. Although rare, fungal meningitis may develop into enough of an inflammatory response at the base of the brain to affect a branch of one of the arteries and lead to a focal cerebrovascular lesion. Evaluation of cerebrospinal fluid may provide the only indication of an infection as the cause. An unexplained pleocytosis should always be followed by studies to identify a luetic or fungal infection in the central nervous system. Blood cultures should also be obtained, as septic emboli may lead to a leukocytic response in the CSF. Rarely, in a patient with ophthalmic division herpes zoster, a secondary viral arteritis and stroke may develop in the carotid artery where it lies contiguous to the affected trigeminal nerve. No specific therapy is available. In populations still at risk of development of malarial infections, focal cerebral infarcts may occur during a falciparum malarial crisis, the so-called black water fever. Therapy for this condition is discussed in Section IV, "Infectious Diseases."

REFERENCES

Caplan LR, Hier DB, Banks G: Stroke and drug abuse. Stroke 17:9–14, 1982.

Come PC, Riley MF, Bivas NK: Roles of echocardiography and arrhythmia monitoring in the evaluation of patients with suspected systemic embolism. Ann Neurol 13:527–532, 1983.

Fisher M, Davidson RI, Marcus EM: Transient focal cerebral ischemia as a presenting manifestation of unruptured cerebral aneurysms. Ann Neurol 8:367–372, 1980.

Fisher CM, Ojemann RG, Roberson GH: Spontaneous dissection of cervico-cerebral arteries. Can J Neurol Sci 5:9–19, 1978.

Graus F, Rogers LR, Posner JB: Cerebrovascular complications in patients with cancer. Medicine 64:16–35, 1985.

Holmes MD, Brant-Zawadzki MM, Simon RP: Clinical features of meningovascular syphilis. Neurology 34:553–556, 1984.

Igarashi M, Gilmartin RC, Gerald B, et al: Cerebral arteritis and bacterial meningitis. Arch Neurol 41:531–540, 1984.

Jabaily J, Iland HJ, Laszlo J, et al: Neurologic manifestations of essential thrombocythemia. Ann Intern Med 99:513–518, 1983.

Jackson AC, Boughner DR, Barnett HJM: Mitral valve prolapse and cerebral ischemic events in young patients. Neurology 34:784–787, 1984.

Jones HR Jr, Caplan LR, Come PC, et al: Cerebral emboli of paradoxical origin. Ann Neurol 13:314–319, 1983.

Jones HR Jr, Siekert RG, Geraci JE: Neurologic manifestations of bacterial endocarditis. Ann Intern Med 71:21–28, 1969.

Kott HS: Stroke due to vasculitis. Primary Care 6:771–789, 1979.

Longstreth WT Jr, Swanson PD: Oral contraceptives and stroke. Stroke 15:747–750, 1984.

Millikan CH, Siekert RG, Whisnant JP: Intermittent carotid and vertebral-basilar insufficiency associated with polycythemia. Neurology 10:188–196, 1960.

Pruitt AA, Rubin RH, Karchmer AW, et al: Neurologic complications of bacterial endocarditis. Medicine 57:329–343, 1978.

Reshef E, Greenberg SB, Jankovic J: Herpes zoster ophthalmicus followed by contralateral hemiparesis: report of two cases and review of literature. J Neurol Neurosurg Psychiatry 48:122–127, 1985.

Sandok BA, von Estorff I, Giuliani ER: CNS embolism due to atrial myxoma: clinical features and diagnosis. Arch Neurol 37:485–488, 1980.

Thomas DJ, Marshall J, Russell RWR: Effect of haematocrit on cerebral blood-flow in man. Lancet 2:941–943, 1977.

Wood DH: Cerebrovascular complications of sickle cell anemia. Stroke 9:73–75, 1978.

8 · SUBARACHNOID HEMORRHAGE

Roger W. Countee
LAHEY CLINIC MEDICAL CENTER

DEFINITION AND DIAGNOSTIC CRITERIA

The subarachnoid space surrounds the brain, the spinal cord, and the cauda equina and freely communicates with the cerebral ventricles via the foramina of the fourth ventricle. All the large distributing arteries of these neural structures as well as the draining veins are contained in the subarachnoid space. Blood in the subarachnoid space may result from rupture of these vessels within the space itself or from primary intracerebral hemorrhage. Extension of primary intracerebral hemorrhage into the subarachnoid space may occur through the parenchymal surface or by rupture into the ventricular fluid, or both. Thus, the finding of blood within the subarachnoid space by lumbar puncture or computed tomography (CT) does not imply a specific anatomic site of origin.

Trauma, the most common cause of subarachnoid hemorrhage, is not within the scope of this chapter. Hemorrhagic infarct resulting from arterial occlusion may cause bloody cerebrospinal fluid but is discussed elsewhere. When primary intracerebral hemorrhage is excluded, ruptured intracranial aneurysm is the most common cause of nontraumatic (spontaneous) subarachnoid hemorrhage, accounting for an estimated 70% to 85% of cases. The remaining causes of subarachnoid hemorrhage are represented by a small heterogeneous group of disorders, including arteriovenous malformation, angioma, necrotizing lesions of the small and medium arteries, occlusion of the cerebral veins, intracranial neoplasm, infection, blood dyscrasias, and effects of "recreational" drugs; occasionally the etiologic factor is unknown.

Ruptured intracranial aneurysm, which accounts for 10% of all strokes, is the most common intracranial cause of sudden spontaneous death. The incidence and the associated mortality rate of aneurysmal subarachnoid hemorrhage have remained remarkably constant over the past 30 years in contrast to all other forms of cerebrovascular disease, which have continued to decline in incidence over the same period.

Despite major advances in radiographic diagnosis and surgical treatment of these lesions, only a small minority of persons with ruptured aneurysm survive long enough and are in adequate condition to undergo curative operation. This occurs in part because many persons do not see a physician when warning symptoms first arise. In addition, when these patients are seen by the physician the diagnosis of subarachnoid hemorrhage may remain unrecognized until a catastrophic hemorrhage occurs. Early and prompt identification and treatment of these lesions are therefore of paramount importance.

PREVALENCE AND NATURAL HISTORY

According to autopsy data, about 5% of the adult population in the United States harbor an intracranial berry aneurysm. Annually in the U.S., about 26,000 persons experience rupture of an aneurysm. Up to 60% of these individuals may have warning symptoms days to months in advance of a major hemorrhage. After rupture an estimated 20% of persons die before receiving medical attention. Within the next several days or weeks after rupture, an additional 30% to 35% die of hemorrhage or of complications of rebleeding or vasospasm (or both), with resultant cerebral ischemia. Of the remaining 45% to 50% of persons who do not undergo operation and survive 90 days after initial hemorrhage, about 20% have serious neurologic impairment. Those who do not undergo surgery and

survive the first six months and those with asymptomatic incidental aneurysm have a 3% likelihood of recurrent hemorrhage each year; the chance of death associated with each successive hemorrhage is 50%. Patients who are in good condition when they reach an experienced surgical team (about 30%) have an overall morbidity rate of 15%; the mortality rate for those who undergo operation is 5%. Life expectancy after successful surgery is normal.

PATHOGENESIS

The cerebral arteries at the base of the brain are the most common sites of aneurysm formation in the entire body. These lesions arise from defects in arterial walls where the vessels branch to form the circle of Willis. A congenital origin has often been suggested for these defects, although evidence to support this is weak. On the other hand, persons with certain congenital disorders, such as polycystic renal disease and coarctation of the aorta, or hereditary disorders of connective tissue, such as Marfan's syndrome and Ehlers-Danlos syndrome, are recognized to have a high incidence of berry aneurysm. The term berry is applied to describe the sessile appearance of the aneurysms as they dangle from the arterial tree in contrast to the fusiform dilatations seen less commonly with atherosclerotic ectasias of the cerebral arteries.

Acquired factors resulting in direct arterial injury, such as fibromuscular dysplasia, autoimmune necrotizing arteritis, and cranial trauma, are uncommon causes of intracranial aneurysm. Infection may occasionally cause mycotic aneurysm secondary to septic emboli from bacterial endocarditis. In populations with a high prevalence of abuse of parenterally administered drugs, mycotic aneurysm is reported to be as frequent as saccular aneurysm. Periarterial infection resulting from pyogenic meningitis or intracranial suppuration is a rare cause of intracranial aneurysm.

PATHOPHYSIOLOGY

Most berry aneurysms gradually expand over time and ultimately rupture. The severity of bleeding and the structures injured determine the clinical picture. Initial bleeding may occasionally be minor; a clot may precariously plug a small rent in the fundus of the aneurysm and thus temporarily prevent further bleeding. Because of the presence of fibrinolysin in CSF, however, lysis of clot occurs later, and subsequent hemorrhage, which is often massive, may recur. The incidence of rebleeding usually peaks within one to two weeks after initial hemorrhage. Extravasation of blood in the subarachnoid space provokes a reflex spasm in the arteries that also tends to arrest bleeding. This valuable protective reflex often leads to such severe arterial narrowing or spasm that cerebral ischemia and infarction may result. Spasm, which is prone to occur a few days to a week after initial hemorrhage, is a frequent cause of delayed neurologic deterioration.

A compressive mass lesion and a nonhemorrhagic stroke, occurring singly or in combination, are also important mechanisms of presentation of aneurysm. Recognition of these less common presentations may permit definitive therapy before potentially fatal rupture occurs. If the aneurysm is strategically located adjacent to pressure-sensitive neural structures, it may initially be evident as a compressive mass. A large aneurysm at the origin of the posterior communicating artery often compresses the contiguous oculomotor nerve, presenting as homolateral third-nerve paresis with diplopia. An aneurysm that arises at the origin of the ophthalmic artery commonly presents with disturbances in visual acuity and in visual fields caused by compression of the ipsilateral optic nerve or the adjacent optic chiasm, or both. Similarly, a large aneurysm of the supraclinoid segment of the internal carotid artery may compress the optic chiasm as well as the hypothalamus, and can mimic a typical suprasellar syndrome with bitemporal hemianopsia and pituitary dysfunction. If aneurysmal expansion is rapid, it often distends pain-sensitive structures, evoking localized head pain of variable severity.

Although most aneurysms are thin-walled, balloon-like sacs of turbulent blood, the walls of some may have areas of atherosclerotic plaque, laminated but friable thrombus, and aggregates of fibrin. This particulate matter may act as microembolic debris if discharged from the aneurysmal sac into the circulation of the parent artery, and thus transient embolic ischemic attacks or infarctions may be the first presentation of intracranial aneurysm. This presentation is now regarded as more common than previously recognized.

INFLUENTIAL FACTORS IN ANEURYSMAL EXPANSION AND RUPTURE

AGE OF PATIENT AND SIZE OF ANEURYSM

Most aneurysms are more commonly seen in older persons. Serial angiographic studies have demonstrated enlargement over intervals ranging from two weeks to ten years. The peak age for rupture is the fifth and sixth decades. Rupture of an aneurysm is rare in children but is the most common cause of subarachnoid hemorrhage in young adults, accounting for one half of fatal strokes in persons under the age of 45.

BLOOD PRESSURE

Although hypertension is believed to aggravate aneurysmal dilatation, its true importance is not clear. In some studies a considerably higher incidence of systolic and diastolic hypertension has been reported in patients with subarachnoid hemorrhage, especially in those under 45. Intracerebral hemorrhage is more common in hypertensive persons. Subarachnoid hemorrhage in normotensive persons is more commonly caused by aneurysm.

CIGARETTE SMOKING

Cigarette smoking has been demonstrated to be a notable risk factor, both singly and in combination with other risk factors for subarachnoid hemorrhage.

SEX

Up to age 40, men have a higher incidence of aneurysmal subarachnoid hemorrhage than women. In the 40s, sexual distribution appears to be equal, but after age 50 the prevalence in women increases over that in men. An association between pregnancy and subarachnoid hemorrhage has been suggested, but sufficient statistical evidence to support this is lacking. Of such aneurysms, however, 83% rupture during gestation (most occurring from the 26th to the 36th week), 4% rupture during labor, and 13% rupture post partum. The hemodynamic changes inherent in pregnancy are believed to be more important factors than hypertension or the stress of labor.

ORAL CONTRACEPTIVES

Orally administered contraceptive agents increase the risk of fatal subarachnoid hemorrhage, particularly in women who smoke cigarettes and are over 35.

PHYSICAL ACTIVITY

Although aneurysmal rupture may occur during extremes of physical exertion or emotional strain, twice as many ruptures take place during either sleep or normal daily activities.

"RECREATIONAL" DRUGS

Stroke and subarachnoid hemorrhage are frequent neurologic complications associated with the ingestion of amphetamines, particularly in large quantity. Phenylpropanolamine hydrochloride, which is similar to the amphetamines in chemical structure and action, is available without prescription in preparations for relief of colds and nasal decongestants. This is also the major anorectic ingredient in 36 of the 38 over-the-counter preparations for weight reduction. Subarachnoid hemorrhage, usually accompanied by marked hypertension, has been reported to occur within minutes of ingestion of excessive amounts of this drug.

Cocaine has also been reported to cause subarachnoid hemorrhage. Blood pressure is often normal in such individuals by the time they receive medical attention.

CLINICAL ASPECTS

Excruciating headache of sudden onset followed by nausea, vomiting, loss of consciousness, stiffness of the neck, and retinal hemorrhage (with or without such other symptoms as focal neurologic signs or third-nerve paresis) are the well-recognized hallmarks of ruptured aneurysm. Unfortunately, however, this clinical picture is apparent only after major aneurysmal hemorrhage when neurologic damage is often severe and the possibility of recovery is uncertain. Up to 60% of patients have warning symptoms of an impending rupture within days to months before the devastating hemorrhage. In these persons the clinical picture may be varied, symptoms may appear minor, and physical signs are often few. Warning symptoms may result from one or more of the three pathophysiologic consequences of aneurysm described previously, i.e., minor rupture, mass effect with compression, and transient cerebral or retinal ischemia.

Headache, the most common complaint, is frequently severe and abrupt in onset and sometimes follows vigorous exertion, including sexual intercourse. It is usually of variable location and characterized as notably "different," and is often described as worse than any headache experienced previously. Nausea with or without vomiting and nonspecific malaise are common. Pain may be restricted to the neck, shoulder(s), or back or may include all of these; only rarely is chest pain the major complaint. Episodes of sudden dizziness or confusion, transient loss of consciousness, seizures, sudden profuse perspiration, and palpitations may be prominent complaints that overshadow headache.

Physical findings depend on the location and severity of hemorrhage as well as the time elapsed between onset and presentation of the patient for medical evaluation. Unfortunately, many patients appear deceptively well when first seen, and physical signs are often subtle or absent. If the patient is seen within hours of onset of minor leakage, signs of meningism can usually be elicited; when signs are subtle, however, they may be misinterpreted as "only a sore neck." Although preretinal and subhyaloid hemorrhages are almost pathognomonic for aneurysmal hemorrhage, they are most commonly seen in patients with major hemorrhage who obviously are gravely ill. Fever is common. Incorrect diagnoses, which are frequent, include nonspecific viral illness, migraine, sinusitis, cervical sprain, arthritis, torticollis, and malingering. Antipyretics and analgesics containing aspirin are often prescribed, and the patient is dismissed. Many patients wander from one physician or emergency room to another until major aneurysmal hemorrhage makes the true diagnosis apparent.

DIAGNOSIS

The full-blown picture of subarachnoid hemorrhage consequent upon major aneurysmal rupture is easily recognized, but the other protean presentations, especially those seen in patients with minor warning leaks, often represent a major diagnostic challenge. Of paramount importance is a meticulous and detailed history-taking from the patient or family member or companion. Questions should focus on the characteristics of pain in the head or neck, particularly its prodrome, onset, and accompanying neurologic, visual, and systemic symptoms. Queries pertaining to known risk factors for aneurysmal rupture are imperative. In addition to a complete neurologic examination, a careful search must be conducted for signs of meningism and photophobia. The importance of serious attention to a suspicious headache cannot be overemphasized.

COMPUTED TOMOGRAPHY

When intracranial aneurysm or subarachnoid hemorrhage is strongly suspected, CT, lumbar puncture, or both are mandatory. When available, CT should be performed first. Subarachnoid blood is most likely to be demonstrated by CT performed within 48 hours after subarachnoid hemorrhage. Intracerebral and intraventricular hemorrhages as well as unsuspected arteriovenous malformations may also be shown by CT. Localized collections of subarachnoid blood occasionally help to identify the site of aneurysm. Large aneurysms (1.5 to 2.0 cm or larger) may be visualized after infusion of intravenous contrast material. Most ruptured aneurysms are smaller, however, and therefore not commonly seen on CT.

A CT scan performed 72 hours after subarachnoid hemorrhage demonstrates positive findings in only 25% of patients. Although diagnostic CT obviates the need for lumbar puncture, negative findings on CT do not exclude the possibility of subarachnoid hemorrhage or intracranial aneurysm, especially when CT is performed 48 hours or more after the ictus. Lumbar puncture should be performed when findings on CT are negative or when CT is unavailable.

CEREBROSPINAL FLUID

Diffusion of cerebral subarachnoid blood into the lumbar subarachnoid space takes about one hour. Therefore, lumbar puncture performed shortly after subarachnoid hemorrhage usually confirms the diagnosis by findings of uniformly bloody CSF and xanthochromic supernatant, although the latter may not be apparent for several hours. In traumatic lumbar puncture, blood in CSF results from the puncture itself. The finding of xanthochromia and a similar number of red cells in the first and last tubes of specimen at the initial spinal tap differentiates subarachnoid hemorrhage from traumatic puncture. Xanthochromia may be found, however, on a second spinal tap after an initial traumatic puncture. It may be necessary to obtain CSF by cisternal puncture to solve this dilemma. On rare occasions, if aneurysmal rupture is primarily into the parenchyma of the brain, CSF may initially be clear, or delayed xanthochromia without erythrocytes may be present. Red blood cells, elevated concentration of protein, and xanthochromia may persist in CSF for up to two weeks after initial subarachnoid hemorrhage. Arteriography of the four major cerebral vessels, which is necessary for definitive diagnosis or exclusion of intracranial aneurysms, must be performed before specific operative treatment.

MANAGEMENT

The most definitive treatment of cerebral aneurysm is intracranial surgical obliteration of the lesion with preservation of the parent artery. High rates of morbidity and mortality are associated with early operation, especially when the neurologic condition of the patient is poor or unstable and when vasospasm or increased intracranial pressure is evident. For this reason, surgery usually is electively deferred for seven to 14 days after recent subarachnoid hemorrhage. During this interval when the risk of rebleeding is highest, the mainstays of therapy are strict bed rest, a calm protected environment, sedatives and mild analgesics if necessary, stool softeners, and avoidance of rectally administered treatment. For control of hypertension, apotensive agents are cautiously used to avoid decreased cerebral perfusion and cerebral infarction. Patients should be given prophylactic phenytoin (Dilantin), 100 mg three times per day PO or IV after a loading dose of 1000 mg, or phenobarbital, 30 mg four times per day. Drugs that reduce coughing or vomiting should be given as needed.

Epsilon-aminocaproic acid (EACA) (Amicar) and tranexamic acid, agents that inhibit fibrinolysis, are used to forestall lysis of clot in the offending aneurysm and thus prevent rebleeding. Although one of these drugs usually is promptly administered, benefits remain controversial. Side effects include deep vein thrombosis, pulmonary embolus and communicating hydrocephalus. Usually EACA is given as a continuous IV infusion of 36 gm in 800 to 1000 ml of 5% dextrose solution every 24 hours. Increased intracranial pressure and cerebral edema are controlled by restricting fluid to 1500 to 2000 ml per 24 hours and dexamathasone, 4 to 10 mg every six hours. No uniformly effective treatment exists for cerebral vasospasm. When symptomatic vasospasm occurs, however, administration of human albumin (Albumisol) and transfusions of packed red cells are usually recommended to avoid hypotension and to increase the intravascular volume of fluids.

OUTLOOK

The primary physician must maintain a high level of suspicion to detect patients who harbor these potentially curable lesions. Early recognition of warning signs of minor aneurysmal leakage is of paramount importance. One must remember that the accompanying head pain may be atypical, associated only with mild meningism, and may mimic "just a stiff neck."

The public must be educated as to the common occurrence of intracranial aneurysm, its varied presentations, and its associated risk factors in a manner similar to the current dissemination of information on cancer and heart disease. The importance of serious attention to the acute headache of precipitous onset and to vague neurologic symptoms cannot be overemphasized. An occasional lumbar puncture or CT scan is preferable in terms of safety and cost effectiveness to failure in the prompt diagnosis of subarachnoid hemorrhage.

REFERENCES

Adams HP Jr, Jergenson DD, Kasell NF, et al: Pitfalls in the recognition of subarachnoid hemorrhage. JAMA 244:794–796, 1980.

Adams HP Jr, Kassell NF, Torner JC, et al: CT and clinical correlations in recent aneurysmal subarachnoid hemorrhage: a preliminary report of the Cooperative Aneurysm Study. Neurology 33:981–988, 1983.

Adams HP Jr, Sahs AL: Aneurysmal subarachnoid hemorrhage. Mod Concepts Cardiovasc Dis 50:49–54, 1981.

Drake CG: Management of cerebral aneurysm. Stroke 12:273–293, 1981.

Heros RC, Kistler JP: Intracranial arterial aneurysm—an update. Stroke 14:628–631, 1983.

King RB, Saba, MI: Forewarnings of major subarachnoid hemorrhage due to congenital berry aneurysm. NY State J Med 74:638–639, 1974.

Sacco RL, Wolf PA, Bharucha NE, et al: Subarachnoid and intracerebral hemorrhage: natural history, prognosis, and precursive factors in the Framingham study. Neurology 34:847–854, 1984.

9 · INTRACEREBRAL HEMORRHAGE

H. Royden Jones, Jr.
Edward C. Tarlov
LAHEY CLINIC MEDICAL CENTER

DEFINITION AND DIAGNOSTIC CRITERIA

Spontaneous intracranial hemorrhage is the underlying etiologic mechanism in approximately 10% of all strokes. Its two major categories are primary intracerebral hemorrhage and subarachnoid hemorrhage (Table

Table 1. INTRACRANIAL HEMORRHAGE

Type of Hemorrhage	Age Group at Which Commonly Seen	Pathologic and Clinical Findings
Intracerebral	Young adults	Arteriovenous malformation, bleeding into tumor, occurrence secondary to subarachnoid hemorrhage
	Middle age through elderly	Hypertension, use of anticoagulants, amyloid angiopathy
Subarachnoid	Young adults through middle age, occasionally elderly	Aneurysm, arteriovenous malformation, bleeding disorder less common, trauma, heat stroke

1). Intracerebral hemorrhage occurs five to six times more frequently than subarachnoid hemorrhage. Rarely a spontaneous intracerebral hemorrhage may be caused by a hematologic disorder or a primary tumor. However, the most important predisposing condition identified in 90% of patients with primary intracerebral hemorrhage is hypertension. Over the past 30 years the incidence of primary intracerebral hemorrhage has decreased more than twofold, which is similar to the experience with nonhemorrhagic stroke.

PATHOPHYSIOLOGY

The underlying associated pathologic changes of spontaneous intracerebral hemorrhage are fibrinoid necrosis and lipohyalinosis affecting the small penetrating arteries arising at the base of the brain. These are the lenticulostriate branches of the middle cerebral artery, the thalamoperforator branches of the posterior cerebral artery, and the paramedian and long circumferential branches of the basilar artery. Hemorrhage results when vessel walls are severely weakened by fibrinoid necrosis. Whether micromiliary aneurysms develop is not certain, but the primary predisposing pathophysiologic mechanism appears to be long-standing hypertension. The fact that most hemorrhages—subarachnoid and intracerebral—occur during waking hours, particularly during periods of physical exertion or emotional stress, suggests that a sudden increase in blood pressure is the precipitating event.

Spontaneous intracerebral hemorrhage does not occur commonly in normotensive patients. When it does occur, amyloid angiopathy is often found, particularly among patients in the seventh decade and older. The factors underlying this vasculopathy are not clear. Most of these hemorrhages take place in the cerebral hemispheres and are located mainly in the parietal and occipital lobes.

CLINICAL ASPECTS

Probably the single most important reason for the decreasing incidence of spontaneous intracerebral hemorrhage is increasingly careful evaluation and treatment of patients with elevated systolic or diastolic blood pressure. Early identification of hypertensive patients is an effective form of prophylaxis available to all physicians.

An important factor predisposing to primary intracerebral hemorrhage is the use of anticoagulant agents, which may increase the risk of such hemorrhage sixfold. Therefore, it behooves the physician to make a risk-benefit analysis and to be certain that the indications for the use of these medications are strong and that they are administered for as short a time as possible. Merely maintaining prothrombin time (PT) at a therapeutic level will not prevent bleeding, as many patients with primary intracerebral hemorrhage secondary to use of anticoagulants have had their PT within the therapeutic range of one and one-half to two times normal.

Emphasis on prophylaxis of primary intracerebral hemorrhage is important because, once hemorrhage occurs, therapy is often unsatisfactory. Before the advent of computed tomography (CT), small nonlethal hemorrhages were not identified and the prognosis for patients with primary intracerebral hemorrhage large enough to be recognized was poor. Acute mortality figures approached 80% to 90%. Now with CT scanning we can sometimes recognize small primary intracerebral hemorrhages, which tend to displace tissue planes without producing major destruction of brain. Thus, acute hospital mortality rates currently range between 25% and 50%. Certain clinical observations when the patient is first seen suggest a worse prognosis, including decreasing levels of consciousness, loss of pupillary reflexes, and evidence of intraventricular hemorrhage on CT. Patients with small lobar hemorrhage appear to have the best prognosis. However, some survivors, even those who are ambulatory at discharge, may not be able to return to an effective role in society.

The structures most likely to be damaged by primary intracerebral hemorrhage are the putamen in 55% of patients; the thalamus, the cerebellum, and the pons in 10% each; and the cerebral hemispheres (lobar) in 15%. Specific clinical findings that may suggest the presence of a lesion in these structures include gradual progressive hemiparesis with a putaminal lesion, the same finding associated with vertical gaze palsy with a thalamic lesion, and quadriparesis with a pontine lesion. Cerebellar hemorrhage is usually associated with rapid onset of nausea, vomiting, inability to sit or stand, or limb ataxia, gait ataxia, or both, and conjugate ipsilateral gaze palsy (Table 2). Lobar hemorrhages may mimic embolic stroke.

MANAGEMENT

All patients seen in a hospital in whom stroke is suspected should have an unenhanced CT scan to identify spontaneous intracerebral hemorrhage. Acute hemorrhage shows on CT as a white, high-density mass. The CT findings in this disease are not subtle. Ordinarily the patient is seen and scanned at the time of or soon after the ictus, and the white mass on CT is the rule. Following this, particularly if the patient is not hypertensive or the clinical findings are unusual, a contrast-enhanced CT scan may suggest an underlying arteriovenous malformation or neoplasm. However, in typical cases such a lesion is unlikely, and in most patients use of contrast is not helpful.

Because of the risk of transtentorial herniation in patients with elevated intracranial pressure, lumbar puncture may be hazardous and usually adds nothing to the diagnosis.

Table 2. NEUROLOGIC FINDINGS IN SYNDROMES OF INTRACEREBRAL HEMORRHAGE DUE TO HYPERTENSION

Type of Hemorrhage	Incidence (%)	Findings
Putaminal	55	Pupils usually equal until late stages (when ipsilateral pupil may dilate secondary to transtentorial herniation), contralateral hemiparesis
Thalamic	10	Eyes may be deviated downward or inward, pupils small, may have hemiparesis
Pontine	10	Small fixed pupils, quadriplegia, coma
Cerebellar*	10	Pupils equal, patient unable to sit or stand, may have mild ipsilateral facial weakness or corneal sensory loss, or eyes deviated laterally away from lesion
Lobar	15	Focal neurologic deficit with or without decreased consciousness

*Most important to recognize as surgical evacuation can be helpful.

In contrast to the importance of angiography in subarachnoid hemorrhage, cerebral angiography is not indicated in hypertensive patients in whom hemorrhage appears to arise in the region of the putamen, thalamus, pons, or cerebellum. Angiography is of importance when there is reason to suspect an arteriovenous malformation or an uncommon mechanism such as a ruptured mycotic aneurysm that may mimic a primary lobar hemorrhage.

The advent of magnetic resonance imaging (MRI) will have some bearing on diagnosis in these patients in the future. Chronic hematomas are probably shown better by magnetic resonance scanning than by CT. However, at this time acute clots appear to be demonstrated best by CT, and preliminary experiences suggest that CT will continue for the present to be the principal method of radiologic diagnosis of intracranial hemorrhage.

Supportive therapy is the mainstay of treatment for all patients with primary intracerebral hemorrhage. Control of hypertension and of elevated intracranial pressure are particularly important. Both subjects are discussed in Section XII, Chapters 10 and 12. Serum electrolyte levels should be monitored carefully and fluids restricted if necessary because of the possibility of inappropriate antidiuretic hormone secretion in patients with spontaneous intracerebral hemorrhage. Anticonvulsant agents probably should be considered in cerebral hemisphere (lobar) hemorrhage in which the likelihood of seizures seems high. In these patients, phenytoin (Dilantin) should be given, 1 gm the first day and 300 to 400 mg/day on subsequent days, to maintain a therapeutic level of 10 to 20 μ/ml.

SURGERY

For most hypertensive hemorrhages into the substance of the brain, surgical evacuation produces disappointing results. The reasons for this are many. The initial arterial force of the hemorrhage itself may already have produced a devastating and irreversible neurologic deficit. Moreover, the clot itself is semisolid material that requires open exposure to evacuate, and the common deep clots in the basal ganglia, thalamus, or pons usually cannot be exposed without worsening the effects of the hemorrhage. Many hemorrhages into the basal ganglia are either in, or so close to, the internal capsule that evacuation would certainly either lead to neurologic worsening or assure that a preoperative hemiparesis or hemiplegia remains complete. Once hypertensive hemorrhage has occurred, further bleeding is unlikely. This differs from the situation with ruptured intracranial aneurysm in which recurrence of bleeding is the major risk.

Lobar Hemorrhage. An occasional lobar hemorrhage may come so close to the surface that evacuation can be considered, particularly if an otherwise healthy patient is worsening. Although most patients with primary lobar hemorrhage should be managed medically, occasionally there may be a progressive clinical course despite medical therapy. In such a patient, surgical evacuation should be considered, particularly with non-dominant hemispheric lesions. Caution is advised, however, especially in the elderly in whom amyloid angiopathy may be the underlying pathologic mechanism. In patients with underlying amyloid angiopathy, surgery usually is not indicated because of the apparently increased risk of excessive bleeding at operation and possible recurrence of bleeding in the immediate postoperative period.

Putaminal Hemorrhage. Surgical removal of putaminal hemorrhage is rarely indicated in a patient with increasing focal neurologic deficit and concomitant decreasing levels of consciousness. This is true even if previous rigorous attempts have been made to treat signs of increasing intracranial pressure. To date, no well-defined set of indications for operation in patients with either thalamic or pontine hemorrhage has been formulated. Therefore, evacuation is likely to be disappointing in most hypertensive hemorrhages, and the procedure should not be carried out in most patients.

Cerebellar Hemorrhage. An exception to the above is cerebellar hemorrhage, in which surgery may be indicated. Physicians likely to see patients with stroke should be aware of this entity. The diagnosis can be made clinically, and in many patients measures can be undertaken that will be lifesaving. The typical patient has a history of hypertension, experiences sudden severe headache, and often collapses. After the ictus the patient is severely ataxic, unable to sit or stand. Nausea and vomiting may occur. A mild facial weakness may be noted on the side of the hemorrhage, along with inability to deviate the eyes conjugately to that side. Usually there is some depression of level of consciousness, but this may be slight in the early stages. As swelling and leakage of blood continue, brain stem compression with further change in level of consciousness will occur. In the early phases the plantar responses are flexor, but as brain stem compression increases they become extensor. The CT scan is diagnostic. Most cerebellar hemorrhages are in the hemisphere; the vermis is involved less frequently.

Surgery is indicated in cerebellar hemorrhage if the patient is in good general condition. Depression of level of consciousness and upgoing toes are signs of brain stem compression, and their presence is usually an indication for surgery. Patients without any depression of level of consciousness and with flexor plantar responses can usually be followed closely and may recover without operation. In between is a range of patients in whom the decision whether or not to operate requires careful surgical judgment. For those in deep coma, the overall prognosis even with surgery is poor.

Anticoagulant-Induced Hemorrhage. When primary intracerebral hemorrhage occurs in patients receiving warfarin (Coumadin) therapy, fresh-frozen plasma should be given immediately to reverse the anticoagulant effects. Administration of vitamin K_1 will maintain this reversal provided hepatic function is adequate. In the patient with thrombocytopenia, platelet transfusion should be given in an attempt to obtain a platelet count higher than $50,000/mm^3$, particularly if surgery is to be considered.

Intraventricular Hemorrhage. Intraventricular hemorrhage usually suggests a poor prognosis. It is believed to be associated with massive primary intracerebral hemorrhage and resulting rupture into the ventricles. The etiologic mehanisms resemble those found with primary intracerebral hemorrhage from other causes. Clot in the ventricle is usually a sign of massive bleeding and destruction of brain. The clot itself will liquefy and be absorbed more rapidly in the ventricle than in the brain itself. Occasionally blood is seen in the ventricles in patients without appreciable neurologic deficit, illustrating that this clot is not the cause of a major deficit. Drainage of clot in the ventricle is rarely indicated.

REFERENCES

Douglas MA, Haerer AF: Long-term prognosis of hypertensive intracerebral hemorrhage. Stroke 13:488–491, 1982.

Drury I, Whisnant JP, Garraway WM: Primary intracerebral hemorrhage: impact of CT on incidence. Neurology 34:653–657, 1984.

Furlan AJ, Whisnant JP, Elveback LR: The decreasing incidence of primary intracerebral hemorrhage: a population study. Ann Neurol 5:367–373, 1979.

Ojemann RG: Spontaneous brain hemorrhage: what treatment should we recommend? (editorial). Stroke 14:467, 1983.

Ojemann RG, Heros RC: Spontaneous brain hemorrhage. Stroke 14:468–475, 1983.

Ropper AH, King RB: Intracranial pressure monitoring in comatose patients with cerebral hemorrhage. Arch Neurol 41:725–728, 1984.

Scott WR, Miller BR: Intracerebral hemorrhage with rapid recovery. Arch Neurol 42:133–136, 1985.

10 · HYPERTENSION IN ACUTE STROKE AND HYPERTENSIVE ENCEPHALOPATHY

Donald J. Breslin
LAHEY CLINIC MEDICAL CENTER

The lowering of blood pressure in the patient with acute stroke is overshadowed by concern that such treatment will induce increased cerebral ischemia. This discussion does not duplicate the information presented in Section II, Chapter 4 on the use of various hypertensive agents, but rather indicates a perspective for their use in the presence of acute stroke.

CHRONIC HYPERTENSION AND THE CEREBRAL VASCULATURE

Chronically hypertensive individuals may experience an inability to maintain adequate cerebral perfusion because of their failure to compensate for rapid lowering of BP to levels that would be tolerated by persons without hypertension. Cerebral arterioles normally tend to maintain relatively constant cerebral blood flow over a range of mean BP from 60 to 160 mm Hg. This autoregulation, which is accomplished by constriction of arterioles as BP rises and by dilatation as it falls, is impaired in hypertensive individuals.

In the chronic treatment of hypertension in patients with known stable cerebrovascular disease, the lowering of BP does not present difficulties when it is carried out slowly. Strandgard and Paulson noted that BP can be lowered 25% in hypertensive patients in general before the limits of autoregulation are exceeded and that it can sometimes be lowered as much as 50% before symptoms of decreased blood flow occur. Rapid lowering of BP can be harmful, however, in patients with such conditions as acute cerebral infarction or hemorrhage, transient cerebral ischemia associated with disease of major extracranial arteries supplying the brain, or hypertensive encephalopathy. We do not have adequate control studies to demonstrate that antihypertensive agents decrease the associated rates of morbidity and mortality in such patients except for those with hypertensive encephalopathy.

Our approach to the treatment of patients with cerebral infarction is most cautious, but a more vigorous approach is taken in administering antihypertensive drugs to patients with subarachnoid or intracerebral hemorrhage. Prompt administration of antihypertensive agents for hypertensive encephalopathy usually results in reversal of the abnormal clinical state.

TRANSIENT ISCHEMIC ATTACKS

The rate of stroke in patients with hypertension and episodes of transient cerebral ischemia is decreased with chronic antihypertensive treatment. In the hypertensive patient who presents with a recent episode of transient cerebral ischemia, however, we usually avoid antihypertensive treatment until the status of the internal carotid system is clarified. Antihypertensive treatment is given when BP is greater than 200/110 mm Hg; otherwise, initial determination of possible severe stenosis of the extracranial internal carotid system is preferred. This is particularly important when angiography is planned; the contrast medium tends to lower BP, and hypotension should be avoided in the presence of severe stenosis of the extracranial internal carotid system.

ISCHEMIC INFARCTION

In areas of ischemia adjacent to a cerebral infarction, arterioles are dilated as a result of hypoxia, increased carbon dioxide tension, and increased accumulation of lactic acid. Blood flow in the marginally ischemic zone becomes dependent on levels of BP, modified by such factors as local cerebral edema. Rapid lowering of BP in the presence of acute cerebral infarction is potentially harmful, particularly in elderly persons or in those with multiple lacunar infarctions resulting from widespread cerebral arteriolar disease. My approach to lowering BP in these patients is much less aggressive than for those with intraparenchymal hemorrhage.

Elevated BP may often decrease spontaneously and gradually over a period of days after an acute cerebral infarction. Antihypertensive treatment is not usually given during the acute phases of cerebral infarction or for approximately three to four weeks after acute stroke. If BP consistently exceeds 200/110 mm Hg, however, antihypertensive therapy (orally administered if possible) is undertaken cautiously. The goal is BP of 160/100 to 110 mm Hg over the first two days after the acute event. Diastolic BP persistently higher than 140 mm Hg justifies treatment with an agent that has rapidly reversible effects, such as intravenously administered sodium nitroprusside (Nipride, Nitropress), which is often used in conjunction with IV furosemide (Lasix).

CEREBRAL HEMORRHAGE

Spontaneous intraparenchymal cerebral hemorrhage accounts for approximately 10% of all strokes, and hypertension is found in about one half of such patients. Approximately 50% are fatal. Although strong evidence suggests that chronic treatment of hypertension decreases the frequency of cerebral hemorrhage, it is unknown whether antihypertensive treatment lowers the associated mortality rate for acute cerebral hemorrhage. Nevertheless, our approach to lowering of BP is similar in these patients to that for subarachnoid hemorrhage.

Almost one fifth of patients who present with subarachnoid hemorrhage have systemic hypertension, and more than 40% have evidence of cerebral vasospasm. No correlation has been established between levels of BP and the degree of cerebral vasospasm in patients with subarachnoid hemorrhage. Mortality rates have been considerably greater in patients with higher BP, although rates of rebleeding cannot be correlated statistically with the presence or absence of hypertension.

When BP is higher than 200/100 mm Hg, we gradually lower it over one to two hours to 160/90 mm Hg, usually with IV sodium nitroprusside. Despite the theoretical disadvantages of increasing intracranial pressure caused by vasodilatation and resulting decreased vascular resistance, sodium nitroprusside remains useful in these patients. This agent has been shown to play no more than a minor role in cerebral hemodynamics in anesthetized patients. In the awake state, a 20% decrease in BP caused by administration of sodium nitroprusside can be accompanied by hyperventilation, hypocapnia, and decreased cerebral blood flow. The neurologic status of patients is monitored, and if it deteriorates the sodium nitroprusside is slowed or discontinued.

HYPERTENSIVE ENCEPHALOPATHY

Hypertensive encephalopathy results from the failure of cerebrovascular vasomotor control to respond to rising (usually severe) hypertension. Although hypertensive encephalopathy was originally attributed to exaggerated cerebral vasospasm, later concepts suggested that loss of the autoregulatory mechanism occurs, resulting in increased cerebral blood flow and cerebral edema. This is frequently accompanied by severe headache often associated with visual impairment, nausea, vomiting, lethargy, and confusion. Progression may take place to alterations of consciousness and finally coma, convulsions, and death. Focal neurologic signs, which may be transitory, are found. Retinal arteriolar spasm is present, usually with retinal hemorrhages, exudates, and papilledema. Impaired renal function is often noted. As mentioned previously, hypertensive encephalopathy is usually associated with severe hypertension (diastolic BP in adults of more than 130 mm Hg), but it may also be related to the rate of rise in BP as well as the level. Consequently, lower levels may produce the same syndrome if they are of recent onset.

Blood pressure must be lowered before the patient with hypertensive encephalopathy becomes stuporous or comatose, because when this stage has occurred the response to lowering is considerably decreased. Failure to respond to antihypertensive treatment requires prompt reevaluation of the diagnosis.

Modern techniques, such as computed tomography, have greatly simplified the exclusion of underlying brain tumor or hemorrhage. The history is also helpful because onset of hypertensive encephalopathy is slower than the usual sudden collapse after headache that is common in patients with subarachnoid or sometimes primary intracerebral hemorrhage. Uremic encephalopathy with associated extreme azotemia, usually accompanied by metabolic acidosis, must also be considered in evaluating these patients.

Prompt lowering of BP is important, but overzealous use of antihypertensive agents to the point of hypotension can be harmful. In a few rare instances, disastrous ischemic effects resulting from hypotension have been reported. This can occur, for example, when large boluses of diazoxide (Hyperstat) or intravenously administered vasodilators are given to a patient who is also receiving large amounts of a sympathetic beta-blocking agent.

My approach to this disorder is to treat hypertension with the initial goal of achieving a diastolic BP of 110 mm Hg within the first hour of treatment, and subsequently to lower BP further gradually over the next 24 hours to approximately 140 to 150/90 to 100 mm Hg. When the patient is capable of taking them, orally administered antihypertensive agents sometimes suffice to achieve these goals.

Antihypertensive agents given to patients with acute stroke are of striking benefit in hypertensive encephalopathy. Benefits are uncertain, however, in the other entities discussed. This is particularly true of acute cerebral infarction unless it is associated with myocardial infarction or congestive heart failure in which lowering of BP decreases demands on the heart.

REFERENCE

Strandgard S, Paulson OB: Cerebral autoregulation. Stroke 15:413–416, 1984.

11 · COMA AND CONFUSIONAL STATES

Maurice R. Hanson
CLEVELAND CLINIC FOUNDATION

Coma

Coma is one of the most serious circumstances in clinical medicine. In an age of advanced life support systems and organ transplantation, the subject of coma has taken on an urgency not envisioned in earlier years. Many comatose states are potentially reversible if prompt action is taken. This chapter outlines a step-by-step approach to the patient in coma, including initial management in the emergency room, neurologic work-up and history, ongoing therapeutic measures, differentiation of reversible from irreversible coma, and prognosis.

DEFINITION

Coma is an unarousable psychologic state in which the subject lies in repose with lids closed and is totally unresponsive. It is essentially the end point of a continuum from normal wakefulness through stupor, obtundation, and thence coma.

PATHOPHYSIOLOGY

Wakefulness and normal consciousness require proper functioning of the brain stem's reticular activating system (RAS), which is the core generator for arousal of both cerebral hemispheres. The RAS is a diffusely organized system localized in the midline regions of the pons, midbrain, and diencephalon, projecting to both hemispheres. From a strictly pathophysiologic standpoint, coma results from dysfunction in the RAS or the cerebral hemispheres bilaterally, or both. Generally speaking, a lesion of one hemisphere does not produce coma unless there is secondary involvement of the RAS, such as from herniation.

Three broad disease categories result in coma: (1) Cerebral hemispheric mass lesions that distort and compress the RAS are found in 15% to 20% of comatose patients. Examples include cerebral neoplasms, abscesses, hematomas, and infarctions. (2) Posterior fossa lesions directly involving the RAS either by intrinsic destruction (e.g., pontine infarction) or by extrinsic compression (e.g., cerebellar hemorrhage) cause coma in about 10% to 15% of cases. (3) Toxic-metabolic encephalopathy involving both hemispheres and the brain stem is by far the most common cause of coma. Toxic-metabolic disorders are due to substrate depletion (i.e., hypoglycemia, hypoxia); endogenous toxic disorders, such as hepatic, renal, adrenal, and pulmonary failure; or exogenous toxins, such as alcohol, drugs, and environmental poisons.

MANAGEMENT

The remainder of this discussion is directed toward the management of the comatose patient after entry into the emergency room. Since clinical evaluation is so deeply enmeshed in the management scheme, the history and physical techniques will be integrated into the decision analysis. Coma is one condition in which general therapeutic approaches often antedate discovery of the cause.

EMERGENCY MEASURES

Vital Functions. The first priority is to stabilize vital functions, and this requires a rapid team approach. A large-bore cannula is used to gain venous access. Prompt intubation may be required; otherwise, nasal oxygen at 5 ml per minute is administered after clearing of secretions and insertion of an oropharyngeal device to keep the upper airway patent. Hypotension is managed by prompt volume expansion with saline or colloidal solutions unless cardiac failure is apparent. While this is transpiring, blood is drawn for glucose and chemical and toxicologic analysis; an additional 25 ml is kept for further studies as needed. A sample for arterial blood gases is obtained. After the blood is drawn, a 50-ml ampule of 50% glucose is infused to treat presumptive hypoglycemia, since precious minutes may mean the difference between serious neurologic damage and recovery. Even if the cause of coma is later discovered to be nonketotic hyperglycemia, this additional glucose load is not likely to harm the patient. In the same line, 100 mg of thiamine hydrochloride is infused to prevent onset of Wernicke's disease, especially in a malnourished alcoholic patient with low thiamine reserves that may be consumed by the glucose infusion. A 0.4-mg infusion of naloxone is innocuous and will reverse an opiate-induced coma. Meanwhile, another member of the team inserts a nasogastric tube and aspirates the gastric contents, saving an aliquot for toxicologic analysis. An in-dwelling urinary catheter is inserted, and careful intake and output volumes are recorded.

CLINICAL EXAMINATION

Once these initial therapeutic maneuvers are completed and the vital functions stabilized, the clinician is free to find the cause of the coma. This begins with a rapid, focused physical examination. In order, the head, trunk, and extremities are inspected for evidence of trauma. In hypotensive patients in particular, the chest, abdomen, and extremities are scrutinized for evidence of compartmental volume accumulation that might reduce the intravascular volume, such as hemoperitoneum, hemothorax, pneumothorax, or extremity fractures. Once these concerns have been eliminated, attention is directed to the neurologic assessment, and objective findings are carefully recorded. Initially, the level of response to verbal and painful stimuli is noted. An adequate painful stimulus includes a gentle pinprick around the nasal mucosa, compression of the side of a pencil or pen against a nail, or firm Achilles' tendon pressure. Although many standardized scales are available, it is best simply to record the level of responsiveness to these various maneuvers.

Next, a few moments are spent carefully observing the dynamics of respiration. For example, regular hyperpnea and hyperventilation suggest either a midbrain compromise or metabolic acidosis. Periodic alternation between apnea and hyperpnea is indicative of bilateral cerebral dysfunction, whereas a totally chaotic and unpredictable respiratory pattern bespeaks a serious outcome, i.e., pontomedullary failure. The latter also indicates that the patient will soon require ventilatory support.

Attention is then focused on the pupils and their light reactions. The size of each pupil and its reactivity are carefully recorded and followed; it is most important to use a very bright light. Anisocoria, especially when attended by impaired light responses, is a sensitive indicator of pressure on the third cranial nerve from a supratentorial mass or structural brain stem disease. One rarely encounters a subtentorial lesion sufficient to result in coma that does not alter normal pupillary size and reactivity.

Next is an assessment of ocular movements. These are most easily tested by the so-called doll's-eye maneuver or oculocephalic reflexes. When the head is rapidly rotated to one side, such as the left, the eyes remain relatively stationary so that the right eye abducts and the left adducts. Slowly, both will refixate in the direction of the head movement. Observations are made of all movements and whether they are conjugate. If there is any evidence of trauma, these maneuvers are avoided for fear of aggravating an underlying potential cervical cord injury. A better stimulus to assess reflex ocular movements is the oculovestibular (OV) reflex, which is tested by caloric stimulation. The tympanic membrane is inspected for any evidence of bleeding or disruption, and patency of the external canal is established. The head of the bed is elevated 30 degrees, and 10 ml of ice water is slowly injected into either canal. The eyes are then observed for several minutes. In a state of depressed consciousness, the eyes will slowly deviate toward the irrigated canal, the fast phase of nystagmus having been abolished. If the brain stem is intact, they will move conjugately, although there may be a lag in the adducting eye (this should not be interpreted as abnormal unless it is persistent). The only clear abnormal result is complete failure of one or both eyes to move or a frank disruption of the ocular parallel axis. One should utilize up to 50 ml of ice water to be certain of this response. The findings can be recorded during the five-minute pause, after which the procedure is repeated on the opposite side. An intact OV reflex is further supportive evidence that the brain stem mechanisms are functioning. If the fast phase of eye movement is present, it also indicates a degree of wakefulness that may not have been suspected previously.

These three neuro-ophthalmologic signs, i.e., pupillary, oculocephalic, and oculovestibular reflexes, are among the most critical of bedside tests. If preserved, the signs suggest a metabolic etiology or hemispheric mass that has not yet violated brain stem integrity. If the latter is the case, precious time is still available to intercede and prevent irreversible brain death. If these reflexes are clearly aberrant, not only is brain stem integrity in jeopardy but also the prognosis for survival and functional recovery is in serious doubt. The exception is intoxication by certain drugs, such as opiates, glutethimide, antidepressants, and barbiturates.

The last important focus of the neurologic examination is motor response. Two observations are sought: unilateral localizing movements, and posturing to painful stimuli. In the face, the former is best assessed by pinprick around the nasal mucosa and observation of unilateral facial contractions. Otherwise, the most useful maneuver is to observe the patient for a few moments to see if there is asymmetry or unilateral lack of movement as well as any difference in withdrawal patterns to painful stimuli. Bilateral motor reflex responses to pain have a certain prognostic value. At a higher level is abduction of the arms, flexion of the elbows and wrists, and extension of the legs. A more serious response implying greater brain stem embarrassment is adduction of the arms, extension of the elbows and legs, and flexion of the wrists, i.e., the decerebrate posture.

HISTORY

Either concurrently with the assessment of physical signs or subsequently, a focused history should be obtained. The single most important information is the temporal course of events leading from intact mentation to coma. If the sequence is abrupt, the probable diagnosis is stroke or seizure. If there is a continuum and gradient, one should suspect an expanding mass or masses or toxic-metabolic disease. Other key historical points are presence or absence of headaches, focal weakness, prior medical history (insulin-dependent diabetes), access to drugs, and a history of depression and seizures. The patient should be thoroughly searched for relevant telephone numbers, ID bracelets or cards, medications, and so forth.

At this point, a reasonable differential diagnosis and localization can be entertained. The next step is to plan further tests and consultation preparatory to transfer to the intensive care unit.

RADIOLOGIC EVALUATION

If the signs and history suggest a mass lesion, neurosurgical consultation is requested and the patient is sent for an emergency computed tomography (CT) scan. If CT is not available, a less precise radiologic survey utilizing skull films, echoencephalography, and radionuclide scans will have to suffice. At the surgeon's discretion, emergency arteriography may be indicated. A member of the team should accompany the patient through the procedures, maintaining close attention to the critical physical findings and vital signs.

IMPENDING HERNIATION

If there is evidence of impending herniation at this point, urgent measures are undertaken medically to reduce intracranial pressure. Evidence may consist of a change in the respiratory pattern from Cheyne-Stokes respiration to central neurogenic hyperventilation, alteration in pupillary size or reactivity, or emergence of progression of unilateral signs. Procedures that achieve rapid reduction in intracranial pressure are combined with those producing a delayed reduction. Intubation

and hyperventilation will decrease the P_{CO_2}, resulting in cerebral vasoconstriction and reduction in intracranial pressure. Concurrently, 1 to 2/gm/kg of a 20% mannitol solution is infused over 20 to 30 minutes and repeated every six to 12 hours as indicated. Concurrently, 80 mg of furosemide is infused intravenously. Dexamethasone 20 mg IV is given, followed by 10 mg every four hours, although its effect will be delayed by several hours. Hyperthermia *increases* intracranial pressure and is controlled with cooling blankets. If the patient is having seizures, stabilization of vital signs should be ensured and hypoxia corrected. Then 5 mg of benzodiazepine is injected directly from the tubex over three to five minutes followed by a second dose in five minutes if seizures continue. Subsequently, phenytoin is infused to a total of 1 gm or about 15 mg/kg at a rate not to exceed 50 mg/min. During this time, one monitors electrocardiographic and blood pressure readings since the most likely complications will be hypotension and alteration of the QRS complex.

TRANSFER TO INTENSIVE CARE UNIT

Once the patient is stabilized and the need for emergency neurosurgical intervention has been excluded, the patient is transferred to the intensive care unit. By this time, results of several critical blood studies will be available and may modify treatment. General supportive measures are continued; the key process at this point is frequent assessment and recording of physical signs every 30 minutes. These include vital signs, level of consciousness, pupillary examination, oculocephalic maneuvers, and focal motor signs. At any point, increased intracranial pressure, hyperthermia, seizures, and so forth, may occur and are approached as noted above.

If these guidelines are followed, the cause of the coma will usually be evident within the first 12 hours. If it is still not clear, drug intoxication should be suspected and one must wait for toxicologic determinations. Frequently, when asked to assess patients in intensive care units, one notes absence of brain stem reflexes. A review of the medication list may reveal neuromuscular blocking agents. No judgments can be made in this setting since these agents produce apnea and abolish brain stem reflexes. Also, if the issues are not clear at this point and if there is any indication of an infectious process, a lumbar puncture is mandatory once a mass lesion has been excluded by CT or other studies. Additionally, a lumbar puncture is diagnostic in cases of subarachnoid hemorrhage.

PROGNOSIS

Prognostic aspects of coma may determine patient management and advice to families. In recent years, valuable data have been accumulated by many prospective studies, including those of Plum and Posner. The practical use of this information depends on the acceptance of brain death as the critical determinant.

With respect to nontraumatic coma, the most important determinants include age, duration and cause of coma, and status of brain stem reflexes. Not unexpectedly, advanced age and prolonged duration of coma denote a poorer outcome. The most decisive elements are brain stem reflexes. When drug intoxication is eliminated, 95% of patients with no brain stem reflexes six hours after onset will die. Stroke, anoxic-ischemic encephalopathy, and intracranial hemorrhage carry the poorest prognosis in comparison with metabolic encephalopathies. If coma of any cause persists for 72 hours in the absence of brain stem reflexes, and if drugs and hypothermia have been eliminated, it is reasonable to conclude that the chances of meaningful survival are nil.

Confusional States

The approach to confusional states is similar to that for comatose conditions except that the time frame is less urgent.

DEFINITION AND CLINICAL FINDINGS

Confusion in the neurologic context refers to an awake state in which the predominant deficit is disturbed concentration and attention. Delirium is often an important concomitant and generally implies acute or subacute change in mentation invariably accompanied by disorientation, incoherence of thought and speech, memory defects, and inattention. Visual hallucinations, delusions, fear, and agitation are common. Motor disturbances accompanying confusional states are frequent and take the form of spasms, multifocal myoclonus, tremor, and asterixis. Although the pupils are usually spared, certain delirious states may be accompanied by pupillary abnormalities that may be mistaken for structural lesions.

PATHOPHYSIOLOGY AND ETIOLOGY

Drugs are often involved. Glutethimide (Doriden) often produces poorly reactive and asymmetric pupils. Confusional states caused by anticholinergics may be accompanied by large, poorly reactive pupils, whereas narcotics produce small, pinpoint pupils. Confusional states can result from supratentorial lesions (especially when associated with increased intracranial pressure), or from lesions arising from certain cerebral regions, such as the temporal and parietal areas, or bilaterally. These stages are transient and shortly merge into coma. Prominent and progressive focal abnormalities should alert the clinician to the possibility of a mass lesion associated with confusion. Diffuse disorders of infectious causes such as viral, bacterial, or fungal meningoencephalitis are often attended by confusion and should be suspected when accompanied by fever, nuchal rigidity, and headache.

By far the most common causes of confusion are toxic-metabolic encephalopathies, and every confused or delirious patient should be screened promptly for systemic disturbances such as hypoglycemia, electrolyte imbalance, renal and hepatic dysfunction, and hyperglycemia. These unifactorial disturbances are usually recognized promptly. The most common and vexing problems arise in seriously ill patients with potential multifactorial abnormalities, especially in the elderly. All too often, clinicians fail to appreciate that apparently innocuous degrees of metabolic derangement and unimpressive doses of drugs can have a profound effect on the older, compromised brain. This is a direct reflection of altered metabolic processes and drug metabolism, combined with multiple systemic illnesses and failure of these patients to display the usual signs of somatic derangement, such as fever. Psychoactive drugs in seemingly small doses may result in significant confusion. Drugs not ordinarily considered to be intoxicants (e.g., digitalis, propranolol, quinidine, procainamide hydrochloride, and cimetidine) may lead to serious confusional states. Additionally, the elderly are high users of over-the-counter preparations containing agents such as antihistamines. The setting of the confusional change is often diagnostic, such as the postoperative state, or isolation.

MANAGEMENT

If after thorough investigation the clinical diagnosis is still in doubt, it is best to withhold all drugs possible and to monitor the outcome. It is wise to recall that some drugs have a very long half-life: e.g., phenobarbital, 96 hours; diazepam, 24 to 96 hours; morphine, 10 to 60 hours. There is also marked intersubject variation. Hence, sufficient time must elapse before one can be certain whether drugs were the cause of the confusion. This may take three or four days or longer.

Not infrequently, a confused patient recovers rapidly at home. This may be attributable to cessation of drugs or the natural resolution of the systemic illness. However, familiar surroundings and regular habits are of paramount importance for recovery. Once the patient is out of imminent danger, has been thoroughly evaluated, and has adequate home care, discharge may be advisable.

REFERENCES

Bates D, Caronna JJ, Cartlidge NEF, et al: A prospective study of nontraumatic coma. Ann Neurol 2:211–220, 1977.
Plum F, Posner JB: Diagnosis of Stupor and Coma, 3rd ed. F. A. Davis Co, Philadelphia, 1980, pp 1–73, 325–338, 345–361.
Sabin TD: Differential diagnosis of coma. N Engl J Med 290:1062–1064, 1974.
Satran R, Griggs RL: Metabolic encephalopathy. *In* Appel SH (ed): Current Neurology. John Wiley & Sons, New York, 1981, pp 231–254.
Tindall RSA: Evaluation and treatment of the comatose patient. *In* Rosenberg RN (ed): The Treatment of Neurological Diseases. SP Medical & Scientific Books, Jamaica, NY, 1979, pp 1–15.

12 · MANAGEMENT OF INCREASED INTRACRANIAL PRESSURE

Stephen R. Freidberg
LAHEY CLINIC MEDICAL CENTER

DEFINITION AND DIAGNOSTIC CRITERIA

The primary recognition and initial management of increased intracranial pressure are the province of the primary care or emergency physician, and the ultimate treatment usually falls to the neurosurgeon or neurologist. Uncontrolled and increasing intracranial pressure eventually lead to herniation of brain with its disastrous clinical sequelae of decreasing level of consciousness and coma. Apnea or change in breathing pattern, such as Cheyne-Stokes respiration, may be seen. Decorticate or decerebrate posturing, or both, and finally hemiplegia develop. An oculomotor nerve palsy with dilated pupils may occur. The patient who has recovered from herniation may be left with severe neurologic deficits, including dementia, diplopia, and hemiparesis. Therefore, increased intracranial pressure must be treated aggressively before the onset of herniation leading to neurologic deficit or death.

The normal level of intracranial pressure varies with the individual, depending on posture, hydration, and activity. Direct measurement of intracranial pressure in the normal person gives a reading below 15 torr, a level between 15 and 25 torr indicates need for treatment, and intracranial pressure of more than 25 torr is dangerously high. Within the skull are brain, cerebrospinal fluid, and blood in the vessels, mostly veins. The CSF provides the primary buffer for increasing intracranial pressure. As intracranial pressure is increased by an expanding mass, the CSF volume is reduced. A slowly expanding mass can enlarge without increasing intracranial pressure as long as an adequate amount of CSF is displaced. If the basal cisterns remain filled with CSF, increasing pressure in any one compartment is transmitted equally throughout the skull and spinal subarachnoid space. Herniation does not occur if only the intracranial pressure is elevated; this phenomenon is seen in pseudotumor cerebri. If, however, the CSF has been displaced and the cisterns are emptied, the subfalcine and tentorial incisurae and the foramen magnum contain brain tissue. Any change in pressure in one compartment can no longer be transmitted equally, and brain herniates.

The rate of growth of an intracranial mass is also a factor (Fig. 1). If an intracranial mass expands slowly, the buffering capacity of the brain may remain effective for several years. CSF is absorbed, intracranial blood volume is reduced, and (in the case of a very slowly growing meningioma) brain tissue is destroyed gradually by the tumor and removed by macrophages. Indeed, the mass can grow to considerable size with no change in intracranial pressure. However, when the capacity of the intracranial structures to buffer the enlarging mass is saturated, intracranial pressure rises precipitously. This is the cause of sudden deterioration in a patient who has clearly had an intracranial mass lesion for many years. On the other hand, if the mass grows rapidly, such as with an epidural hematoma, there is little time for the buffering effect to occur and intracranial pressure rises quickly.

PATHOPHYSIOLOGY

The first step in management of increased intracranial pressure is to ascertain its cause. In adults the brain lies within the rigid, compartmentalized skull. The tentorium separates the supratentorial portion from the infratentorial portion, the posterior fossa. The brain stem passes through the tentorial incisura and joins the spinal cord at the foramen magnum. Brain herniating through either of these relatively small holes can incarcerate and compress the brain stem, producing signs and symptoms of herniation, including very sudden death. The supratentorial compartment is further divided, right and left, by the falx. Subfalcine herniation produces a dramatic angiographic and computed tomographic (CT) appearance, but is rarely of clinical importance.

Increased intracranial pressure can be caused by various supratentorial and infratentorial lesions. A lesion may be within or outside the brain parenchyma and may have many pathologic causes. With a few exceptions, fast-growing and malignant tumors, such as glioma and metastatic tumors, produce considerable peritumor edema and therefore elevated intracranial pressure. More benign lesions such as meningioma, as a rule do not cause any appreciable edema. There are exceptions, however, and the clinical and radiologic diagnosis must be confirmed histologically. It is rare in a modern clinical setting that increased intracranial pressure caused by tumor is sufficient to result in

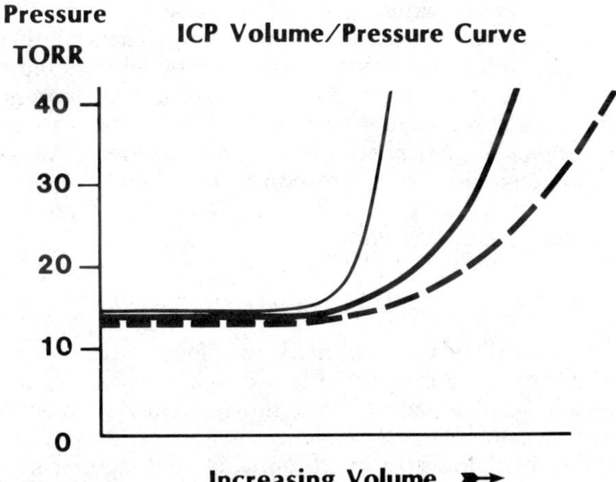

Figure 1. Volume/pressure curves showing rates of increase of intracranial pressure for a rapidly expanding mass lesion with little time for adaptation (*light solid line*), a mass lesion with a moderate rate of growth (*heavy solid line*), and a slowly expanding mass with considerable time for adaptation (*broken line*). As the volume of a mass enlarges, the intracranial pressure remains stable until the buffer capacity of the brain is exhausted. When the buffer capacity is exhausted, the pressure rises rapidly.

herniation before diagnosis. Tumors of the posterior fossa cause increased intracranial pressure not by reason of their size but because they block the fourth ventricle or aqueduct of Sylvius and cause hydrocephalus. Clinical deterioration in a patient with acutely decompensated hydrocephalus can be extremely rapid. Massive cerebral infarction associated with an occluded middle cerebral artery can result in brain swelling sufficient to cause herniation and death.

Increased intracranial pressure associated with trauma deserves special mention. Trauma is the most common cause of the increased intracranial pressure seen in emergency departments. The component of the clinical picture caused by direct contusion or laceration of brain with accompanying intrinsic edema must be differentiated from that component caused by an expanding subdural, epidural, or intraparenchymal hematoma mass. The hematoma is treated by surgical evacuation.

CLINICAL ASPECTS

In patients with increased intracranial pressure, clinical and etiologic diagnoses are both necessary because the urgency of treatment depends on the clinical findings, and the type of treatment is determined by the disease. The patient who walks into the physician's office with complaint of headache or focal neurologic symptoms and is found to have papilledema can usually be evaluated in a careful, expeditious fashion but without a sense of emergency. This is contrasted with the patient brought into the emergency room with reduced level of consciousness who may or may not have papilledema. In the latter patient the diagnostic evaluation must be performed immediately because delay in instituting treatment may have serious consequences. The etiology may or may not be obvious. Factors that direct the diagnostic and therapeutic approach are a history of major trauma, the presence of a diabetic or hypertensive condition, use of anticoagulant medications, use of drugs or alcohol, and whether the lapse into coma has been gradual or sudden. The Glasgow coma scale has become widely accepted as a standard by which a rapid and yet careful, quantifiable, and reproducible assessment of the patient's level of consciousness can be obtained. Numerical scores are given for eye opening, motor response, verbal response, and pupil reaction. This examination can easily be repeated periodically to establish a clinical trend.

MANAGEMENT

A CT scan is the primary diagnostic technique to establish the causes of the intracranial problem. It can usually be obtained in a few minutes and clearly demonstrates whether the patient has a mass lesion, i.e., tumor, hematoma, or hydrocephalus, that requires surgical treatment. CT also defines the involved intracranial compartment. If no mass lesion is present, diffuse swelling can be demonstrated by the loss of the basal cisterns and the pattern of sulci over the hemispheres. Normal CT findings in a stuporous patient suggest a metabolic cause probably not associated with increased intracranial pressure. For the patient with acute coma,

CT without intravenous administration of contrast agent should be performed initially to rule out fresh blood. If fresh clot, which appears very dense, is not found, IV contrast agent should be administered and the scan should be repeated. An acute brain infarction may not be obvious on an early CT scan.

Lumbar puncture should be avoided if increased intracranial pressure is suspected. Tapping the lumbar subarachnoid space in patients with increased intracranial pressure and cisterns filled with edematous brain tissue may lead to disastrous herniation through the tentorial incisura or the foramen magnum. If meningitis is suspected, CSF examination is essential but should be performed after a CT scan has ruled out a mass lesion, such as an abscess. If meningitis is suspected and an abscess is present on CT, a 22-gauge or smaller needle should be used for the lumbar tap, and the minimal amount of CSF should be removed for examination. Lumbar puncture can detect fresh bleeding but most often this diagnosis can also be obtained on CT. In patients with increased intracranial pressure, the danger of a spinal tap usually far outweights any useful information that may be obtained, except when the diagnosis is meningitis.

If a diagnosis of increased intracranial pressure is secondary to an intracranial mass lesion of tumor, hematoma, or hydrocephalus and the patient is not acutely ill, high doses of corticosteroid medication usually help to improve the clinical state while the patient is awaiting surgical treatment. Dexamethasone, 4 to 6 mg every four to six hours, is usually adequate, although doses up to 100 mg/day have been advocated.

For patients brought into the emergency department in a state of stupor, the approach is very different. Attention must initially be directed at urgent life-saving measures. If ventilation is not adequate, the patient must be intubated and hyperventilated. In the trauma victim the possibility of a cervical fracture must be kept in mind when attempting intubation. Impaired ventilation is detrimental to the brain in two ways. Lack of oxygen impairs neuronal function, especially in an already damaged brain in which tissue surrounding the lesion may have marginal supply of oxygen. Poor ventilation also increases arterial partial pressure of carbon dioxide (P_{CO_2}), the most potent dilator of cerebral blood vessels. This increases the volume of blood in the brain and noticeably increases the brain volume and elevates intracranial pressure. Optimally, the arterial partial pressure of oxygen (P_{O_2}) should be over 100 mm Hg and the P_{CO_2} should be around 30 mm Hg.

Concomitant with the management of ventilatory insufficiency, a search for associated injuries, especially hemorrhage, is essential. Hemorrhage may be external or may be internal from a lesion, such as a ruptured spleen or fractured femur. Shock and anemia are poorly tolerated by the injured brain. Clinical shock is not seen with an isolated brain injury unless the patient is experiencing terminal medullary failure. Shock implies an associated injury, usually with blood loss.

If the increased intracranial pressure is not acute and a mass lesion is diagnosed on CT, the patient can be given corticosteroid medication, and operation can be scheduled electively. If, on the other hand, a surgically treatable lesion is diagnosed in the acutely deteriorating patient, medical therapy can help stabilize intracranial pressure until the patient can be taken to the operating room. Intubation with hyperventilation is the most valuable procedure to be performed. If blood has been lost, it must be replaced. Mannitol, given as rapidly as possible in a dose of 1.5 gm/kg or 100 gm in a 20% solution, quickly reduces brain mass by osmotic diuresis. This may protect the brain for the time necessary to perform surgery. However, mannitol is not useful in the patient with a severely injured brain in which cerebral vasomotor autoregulation is impaired. Corticosteroid agents, even in massive doses, are frequently used in such a patient, but there is no convincing evidence that these are effective.

In a patient with increased intracranial pressure without a mass lesion or in whom increased intracranial pressure persists after operation, intracranial pressure should be monitored directly. This establishes a firm treatment goal. The methods for measuring intracranial pressure are varied. The simplest instrumentation involves a fluid line from the patient's brain to a standard pressure transducer found in all intensive care units. The calibration is uncomplicated and can be performed periodically. The line can begin as a catheter in a dilated ventricle or a bolt screwed into the skull and extending into the subarachnoid space. The intraventricular catheter has the advantage of permitting periodic withdrawal of CSF to reduce intracranial pressure. Fluid lines have the disadvantage of providing an avenue for the entrance of infection. A number of epidural devices have been marketed with electrical and fiberoptic lines from the skull. These have the advantages of safety and low risk of infection, but they are expensive and difficult to calibrate. Monitoring lines should be removed or changed within four to five days; the incidence of infection rises markedly after that time.

Monitoring allows the physician to respond to increases of intracranial pressure before the level becomes sufficiently high to cause herniation. Arterial P_{CO_2} can be reduced, ventricular fluid removed, and mannitol administered periodically. In the refractory patient, barbiturate coma can be induced in an attempt to reduce brain metabolism and intracranial pressure at the same time. In this situation, clinical evaluation of the patient is not possible. Physiologic measurements and laboratory data are used to guide continuing treatment until it is stopped at an appropriate time and the patient reevaluated. During the period of monitoring of intracranial pressure, repeat CT scans may demonstrate late development of an intracranial clot not present on earlier scans.

Increased intracranial pressure is a dangerous clinical condition associated with multiple causes. Careful diagnosis and treatment are necessary to preserve neurologic function and perhaps the patient's life.

REFERENCES

Jennett B, Teasdale G: Management of Head Injuries. F. A. Davis Co, Philadelphia, 1981.

Miller JD: Volume and pressure in the craniospinal axis. Clin Neurosurg 22:76–105, 1975.

Plum F, Posner JB: The Diagnosis of Stupor and Coma, 3rd ed. F. A. Davis Co, Philadelphia, 1980.

Teasdale G, Jennett B: Assessment of coma and impaired consciousness: a practical scale. Lancet 2:81–84, 1974.

13 · SEIZURE DISORDERS

A. David Rothner
CLEVELAND CLINIC FOUNDATION

DEFINITION

Epilepsy is the tendency to have recurrent seizures. A seizure, as defined by Hughlings Jackson, a 19th century neurologist, is "an occasional sudden, excessive, rapid, and local discharge of gray matter." Epilepsy is really a group of disorders with multiple etiologies. A seizure should be considered a symptom of central nervous system disease. Although there are many seizure types, all are due to excessive and paroxysmal neuronal discharge, and all result in a sudden disturbance of function. The episodes may be simple attacks of staring or altered consciousness, or frank tonic-clonic convulsive movements. The basic physiology of the seizure episode is beyond the scope of this discussion. However, its onset is traceable to an unstable cell membrane or its surrounding support cells. The stability of these cells can be affected by numerous factors, including pH, oxygen content, and serum levels of glucose, sodium, potassium, and calcium. Changes in these factors may lower the seizure threshold. The location of the abnormal focus of neurons determines the character of the seizure. A discharge arising from the right motor strip may result in tonic-clonic jerking of the extremities on the left. An occipital lobe focus on the left may cause visual disturbances in the right visual field.

Epilepsy consists of a group of disorders, the classification of which has undergone significant changes over the years. The International Classification of Epileptic Seizures was developed in 1969 and modified in 1981 (Table 1). The primary differentiation of the types of epilepsies depends on the localization of the epileptic focus. In partial seizures the epileptic focus is thought to arise in a focal area of cerebral cortex. In primarily generalized seizures, both hemispheres are affected simultaneously, presumably from a subcortical central focus. The most important types of partial seizures are the simple partial and the complex partial seizures. These have two things in common: they begin in a specific area of the brain and they may be associated with an underlying lesion. Any partial seizure may become secondarily generalized.

SIMPLE PARTIAL SEIZURE

During a simple partial seizure (focal seizure), consciousness is not affected. The clinical symptomatology is related to the affected area of cortex. A simple partial seizure may be either motor or sensory, and less frequently autonomic or psychic. A simple partial seizure with motor signs consists of recurrent contractions of muscles of one part of the body, such as the hand, arm, and face. There is no loss of consciousness. Each mus-

Table 1. INTERNATIONAL CLASSIFICATION OF EPILEPTIC SEIZURES

I. **Partial (Focal, Local) Seizures**
  A. Simple partial seizures (consciousness not impaired)
    1. With motor signs
    2. With sensory symptoms
    3. With autonomic symptoms or signs
    4. With psychic symptoms
  B. Complex partial seizures (temporal lobe or psychomotor seizures; consciousness impaired)
    1. Simple partial onset, followed by impairment of consciousness
      a. With simple partial features (A1–A4), followed by impaired consciousness
    2. With impairment of consciousness at onset
      a. With impairment of consciousness only
      b. With automatisms
  C. Partial seizures, evolving to secondarily generalized seizures (tonic-clonic, tonic, or clonic)
    1. Simple partial seizures (A), evolving to generalized seizures
    2. Complex partial seizures (B), evolving to generalized seizures
    3. Simple partial seizures, evolving to complex partial seizures, evolving to generalized seizures

II. **Generalized Seizures (Convulsive or Nonconvulsive)**
  A. Absence (petit mal) seizures
  B. Myoclonic seizures
  C. Clonic seizures
  D. Tonic seizures
  E. Tonic-clonic (grand mal) seizures
  F. Atonic seizures

III. **Unclassified Epileptic Seizures***

Modified from Dreifuss FE: Proposal for revised clinical and electroencephaolographic classification of epileptic seizures. Epilepsia 22:489, 1981.

*Data incomplete.

cular contraction is associated with a neuronal discharge of the contralateral motor cortex. This motor activity may remain confined and then cease. It may spread to other parts of the body (a jacksonian march) or it may spread to the other hemisphere and result in a secondarily generalized tonic-clonic seizure.

A simple partial sensory seizure consists of paresthesias in a single part of the body. It is associated with neuronal discharges from the contralateral sensory cortex. It may spread ipsilaterally or become secondarily generalized. Most partial seizures are brief, lasting approximately one to two minutes, and consciousness is retained.

COMPLEX PARTIAL SEIZURE

Complex partial seizures (temporal lobe or psychomotor seizures) are distinguished from simple partial seizures by an alteration in consciousness associated with the seizure. These complex partial seizures are often preceded by an aura, such as an abnormal or unpleasant sensation, a bad taste, a strange odor, or an unusual noise. Following the aura, patients may be able to seek a safe haven as they know the seizure is about to occur. Patients then have an altered consciousness (they usually do not fall), associated with abnormal movements called automatisms. These may consist of picking at their clothing, rubbing of a leg, lip-smacking, or swallowing. This semipurposeful behavior may last one or two minutes, followed by a period of confusion, drowsiness, and amnesia for the event. The complex partial seizure may also become secondarily generalized and result in a generalized tonic-clonic seizure.

GENERALIZED TONIC-CLONIC SEIZURE

The generalized tonic-clonic seizure (grand mal) simultaneously involves both hemispheres and usually lasts a matter of minutes. It is the most dramatic of all the generalized seizures. The patient immediately loses consciousness. This is followed by a sudden fall to the ground, the tonic phase of the seizure consisting of extension and stiffening of all the muscles of the body. The abdominal and chest muscles contract and an "epileptic cry" occurs. Cyanosis may occur secondary to inhibition of respiration. The jerking or clonic phase of the attack follows. It usually is bilaterally symmetric and intense initially and then slowly diminishes. Incontinence of urine and feces, as well as buccal-oral trauma, may occur during this attack. The attack is usually over in two to four minutes. Patients are generally unconscious afterwards and difficult to arouse. They then awaken but are confused and tired. There may be a severe headache and muscle pain after they recover from the attack.

Other forms of generalized seizures occur less frequently. These may be age-related or associated with other seizure types (mixed seizure disorder).

ABSENCE SEIZURE

Absence seizures, previously known as petit mal, consist of altered or impaired consciousness lasting 10 to 20 seconds. They usually occur in the school age child and only rarely in adult life. Patients stop what they are doing and stare blindly ahead or flutter the eyelids. There is usually no falling or incontinence. They usually recover consciousness immediately. The attacks occur 20 to 30 times a day and are quite responsive to medication. The electroencephalogram (EEG) shows a generalized 3 Hz spike and wave pattern. In two thirds or more the attacks disappear spontaneously as patients grow older, and in another third they may be replaced by or associated with generalized tonic-clonic seizures.

TONIC SEIZURE

Tonic seizures are more commonly seen in retarded individuals with mixed seizure disorders. The patient develops tonic muscular contraction affecting all extremities. He may arch his trunk, draw back his head, and fall to the ground. He may not lose consciousness during the attack. Tonic seizures frequently occur in neurologically impaired individuals. In atonic seizures, there is a diminution of muscle tone leading to falling without loss of consciousness. It is seen in a context similar to tonic seizures. Both conditions are associated with variably abnormal EEG findings and are difficult to control.

MYOCLONIC JERK

Myoclonic jerks, either singly or in combination, are sudden, brief, shocklike contractions involving one extremity or the entire body. They often occur early in the morning after awakening or as the patient is falling asleep. They may be associated with generalized tonic-clonic seizures. If they occur de novo in later adult life, they may be associated with a degenerative disorder.

INFANTILE SPASM

Infantile spasms usually occur in infancy and childhood. They consist of nodding of the head and then a jack-knifing of the entire body. They last for several seconds and may occur in clusters. The findings on EEG are chaotic or hypsarrhythmic in nature: the pattern consists of an abnormal combination of slow waves and multifocal spikes. This disorder can be associated with a wide variety of metabolic and congenital disorders. The prognosis is poor and there is often mental retardation.

STATUS EPILEPTICUS

Status epilepticus is a medical emergency consisting of a continuous seizure or multiple prolonged seizures without the patient regaining consciousness. It is most dramatically seen when generalized tonic-clonic seizures are involved. Status epilepticus may also involve focal seizures, complex partial seizures, and absence seizures. Generalized or tonic-clonic status epilepticus is a life-threatening condition necessitating emergency hospitalization and intensive care. This disorder may produce anoxia and severe neurologic deficits, and therefore must be treated quickly with intravenous medication and intensive support.

DIAGNOSIS

The history is the most important factor in determining the correct diagnosis and etiology. Both the patient and anyone who has observed an episode must be questioned. First, data should be obtained concerning the seizure itself and any precipitating factors. Important questions include: the types of seizures; their frequency and duration; the precipitating factors; the times of occurrence; the presence or absence of an aura; the type of ictal activity (focal, or generalized, tonic-clonic, or simple staring); and the condition during the postictal state, such as confusion and fatigue.

Second, the history-taking should determine whether the patient is prone to seizures. Relevant factors include any early childhood difficulties such as delay in development, any history of encephalopathic problems such as head injury, prolonged high fever, febrile seizures, or CNS infection. Further questioning should determine the presence or absence of seizures in close family members; whether the patient is taking any medication that could promote seizure activity; any medical disorder that may directly or indirectly affect the occurrence of seizures, such as diabetes, chronic lung disease, heart disease, allergy, or asthma; any emotional problems; and environmental conditions of employment.

The third part of the history-taking should determine whether the disorder is progressive or due to an intracranial lesion. Headaches, vomiting with or without nausea, lethargy, personality change, visual difficulties, focal weakness, cortical sensory loss, or intellectual deterioration suggest the need for immediate further evaluation. The affect of the patient throughout this history may also provide insight into associated problems such as anxiety, depression, or hostility. Throughout the history one should keep in mind other disorders that are paroxysmal in nature and may simulate epilepsy.

The general physical examination relates to all non-CNS organ systems, since these may indirectly influence the possibility of seizures.

The neurologic examination starts with the head: whether it is small (associated with CNS maldevelopment) or large (associated with hydrocephalus). Auscultation of the cranium and neck may reveal bruits indicating vascular disorders. The gait must be assessed for difficulties of balance or weakness. The cranial nerve examination should search for asymmetries. The fundi must be adequately visualized: any abnormality such as hemorrhage, papilledema, optic atrophy, or chorioretinal scarring is significant. An asymmetry of the cranial nerves should suggest a structural abnormality. Inability to move one or both of the eyes completely laterally may indicate a sixth nerve palsy, which is a nonspecific sign of increased intracranial pressure. Abnormalities of the lower cranial nerves, including ataxia or cerebellar dysfunction, may indicate a lesion of the posterior fossa. Strength and reflexes must be carefully noted along with the muscle tone. If asymmetry is apparent, a hemispheric abnormality should be suspected. Sensation testing is likewise important.

Before any laboratory tests are ordered, a differential diagnosis should be formulated since the extent of testing differs in a well individual with a single seizure as opposed to a patient with symptoms of a progressive neurologic disorder. The differential diagnosis should ask the following questions: (1) Does the patient have seizures or another paroxysmal disorder simulating seizures? (2) Is there an emotional problem causing hysterical seizures? (3) What is the type of seizure, partial or generalized? (4) At what age did seizures begin? (5) What other recent tests have been made, to avoid duplication? The mnemonic C-I-T-T-E-N-D-V-M-M may be useful (Table 2).

Electroencephalography. The EEG is extremely important in the diagnosis and treatment of epilepsy. However, it does not "make the diagnosis of epilepsy." Its value lies in assessing the type of seizure. At times it may determine the location of the discharge; at other times it may be useful in differentiating between hysterical and true seizures. A normal EEG does not rule out epilepsy, and an "epileptiform" EEG does not necessarily indicate a clinical seizure disorder. Most patients with epilepsy exhibit abnormal electrical discharges at some time. The more "active" the clinical seizure type, the more "active" the EEG is likely to be. The type of discharge may indicate the type of epilepsy. Infantile spasms often produce hypsarrhythmia, while atonic, akinetic, or myoclonic seizures are frequently associated with slow spike and wave patterns or multifocal spike-wave discharges. Petit mal seizures are

Table 2. DIFFERENTIAL DIAGNOSIS OF SEIZURE DISORDERS

C—Congenital malformation: porencephaly
I—Infection: acute, chronic, congenital
T—Trauma: subdural
T—Toxin: lead, alcohol
E—Endocrine: hypoglycemia
N—Neoplastic: primary or metastatic
D—Degenerative: Alzheimer's
V—Vascular: arteriovenous malformation
M—Metabolic: electrolytes, thiamine
M—Miscellaneous (autoimmune, neurocutaneous, genetic)

associated with three-per-second generalized spike and wave patterns; complex or partial seizures with spikes or sharp wave patterns limited to the temporal or frontotemporal region. Generalized tonic-clonic seizures may be associated with generalized spiking on the EEG. When the routine EEG is normal, activating techniques may be helpful and may elicit electrical abnormalities. Hyperventilation, sleep, and photic stimulation are among the most commonly used activation procedures. In some patients, nasopharyngeal electrodes or sphenoidal electrodes may show abnormality when routine scalp electrodes do not. Closed-circuit TV monitoring with continuous EEG is useful in evaluating patients for seizure surgery, those with spells of unknown etiology, those with hysterical seizures, and those with a hard-to-diagnose seizure disorder. Many normal children have minor abnormalities on the EEG that are nonspecific and are unrelated to epilepsy. Specific abnormalities, such as sharp waves, spikes, polyspike and waves, and focal slowing, may be related to seizures and require further evaluation.

Computed Tomography. The CT scan is a safe, rapid, and accurate method of evaluating the intracranial contents. In patients with epilepsy it may reveal a wide variety of etiologic conditions, including congenital malformations, hydrocephalus, intracranial infections, hemorrhages, neoplasms, degenerative disorders, and vascular disorders. CT is quite accurate and must be performed in any patient with focal seizures, focal or progressive neurologic symptoms or signs, or symptoms or signs of increased intracranial pressure. It is also useful in individuals who are dysmorphic and in whom a congenital anomaly of the brain is suspected.

Radionuclide Studies. These are infrequently used since CT appears to be more accurate. Cerebral arteriography and digital subtraction angiography are useful in delineating vascular abnormalities, but are not routinely used to diagnose epilepsy. However, if the patient is thought to have a vascular abnormality such as a carotid occlusion, aneurysm, or arteriovenous malformation, these tests can be quite useful.

Nuclear magnetic resonance imaging (NMR) is able to delineate some abnormalities not seen on CT. Its clinical applications are currently being investigated, but it has already proved useful in delineating the localized abnormalities in some patients with complex partial seizures.

Positron Emission Tomography (PET) uses signals from positron-emitting particles to create three-dimensional computer images, and measures cerebral blood flow and brain metabolism. This technique is not commonly in use but in the future may promote a better understanding of the etiology and pathogenesis of the seizures and of localized areas of abnormality.

The lumbar puncture is not routinely used to evaluate chronic seizure disorders.

Psychologic testing, both intellectual evaluation and projective tests, are useful in individuals with cognitive dysfunction or possible functional disease, either alone or associated with epilepsy. Such tests can help determine whether a neurodegenerative disorder is present or whether stressful circumstances are precipitating hysterical seizures.

MANAGEMENT

Effective treatment depends on selection of the appropriate drug in the appropriate amount for the specific seizure type. It also implies the removal of any seizure stimuli. Compliance with a therapeutic regimen depends on patient education. The patient should be followed with repeated histories, physical examinations, anticonvulsant blood determinations, and other laboratory tests as clinically indicated. If the clinical course changes, reevaluation is mandatory. A balance must be maintained between the therapeutic benefit and the potential side effects of the medications prescribed. One should try to use a single drug in the appropriate dosage to decrease the risk of side effects and increase the likelihood of seizure control. If seizures are not controlled with a single drug or if toxicity occurs, alternative treatments must be considered. If two drugs are used together, their side effects may be additive. Medication should never be discontinued abruptly, as this may precipitate status epilepticus. Special consideration should be given to medication for pregnant women or women of child-bearing age, since birth defects have occurred in infants of mothers taking anticonvulsant medication during pregnancy. When seizures seem to be refractory, consultation may be indicated, along with complete reevaluation and use of nonstandard anticonvulsant medications.

The major anticonvulsant drugs used today for epilepsy are listed in Table 3.

Phenobarbital. Phenobarbital was the first of the effective organic anticonvulsant drugs, introduced in 1912, replacing the more toxic bromides. It is particularly effective in tonic-clonic, simple partial, and complex partial seizures. It has long been established as a relatively nontoxic drug that can be used with little fear of serious side effects. In some children, phenobarbital paradoxically causes hyperactivity and behavioral disorders. In adults, drowsiness and sedation are significant problems. The usual adult daily dose is 90 to 180 mg per day. Since the drug has a long half-life (two to six days), it can be given once or twice daily. It may take two to three weeks of therapy to reach therapeutic levels. I utilize a low dosage initially and increase the dose weekly until either the seizures have ceased or

Table 3. COMMONLY USED ANTIEPILEPTIC DRUGS

	Adult Daily Dosage Range (mg)	Pediatric Daily Dosage Range (mg/kg)	Half-life Adults (hrs)	Half-life Children (hrs)	Time to Reach Steady State (days)	Therapeutic Serum Conc. (μg/ml)
Phenobarbital	90–180	3–7	45–125	35–75	14–21	15–40
Primidone	750–1500	10–25	5–15	5–12	4–7	5–12
Phenytoin	300–400	4–8	10–35	5–15	7–15	10–20
Carbamazepine	800–1400	20–40	12	12	5	8–12
Valproic acid	1500	15–60	8–12	8–12	5	60
Ethosuximide	750–1500	20–40	30–60	20–60	7–10	60–100

side effects have supervened. Blood levels should be determined two to three weeks after the dosage has been optimized, if toxicity occurs or if seizure control has not been achieved.

Primidone. Primidone (Mysoline), a congener of phenobarbital, was introduced in 1954. Some clinicians consider it useful for tonic-clonic seizures, simple partial seizures, and complex partial seizures. It should not be used in combination with phenobarbital as its side effects and therapeutic effects mimic those of phenobarbital, and it is metabolized to phenobarbital. The usual adult dosage is 750 to 1500 mg per day. It has a relatively short half-life, is quite soporific, and is usually administered t.i.d. or q.i.d. Blood levels of both primidone and phenobarbital should be monitored carefully in chronic therapy.

Phenytoin. Phenytoin was the first anticonvulsant to be discovered through planned and systemic screening in animals. It is structurally similar to phenobarbital. It is useful for tonic-clonic, complex partial, and simple partial seizures. If given in excess, it produces side effects, including dizziness, nystagmus, ataxia, and diplopia. It may also cause gingival hyperplasia, rash, and hirsutism. Serious toxic side effects involving the liver or bone marrow are rare. The usual half-life is 24 hours, and it can be given once or twice daily to adults. The usual dose is 300 to 400 mg per day. A therapeutic level is reached within 7 to 15 days.

Carbamazepine. Carbamazepine (Tegretol) is effective in simple partial, complex partial, or tonic-clonic seizures. It is related chemically to the tricyclic antidepressants. Common, but not serious, side effects include diplopia, dizziness, and drowsiness. It has been reported to cause serious life-threatening toxic effects, such as aplastic anemia and hepatotoxicity. It has a half-life of about 12 hours and is usually administered b.i.d. or t.i.d. The usual adult daily dosage is 800 to 1400 mg. Frequent monitoring of blood count and liver function is suggested. The therapeutic level is reached in about five days.

Valproate. Valproate as the acid or sodium salt has been used to treat epilepsy since 1963. It appears to be effective not only in generalized tonic-clonic and absence seizures, but in a variety of minor motor seizures. It seems to be less effective in simple partial and complex partial seizures. It elevates the levels of gamma-aminobutyric acid, a neuroinhibitory substance, in the brain. Its half-life is about eight to 12 hours and it must be taken b.i.d. or t.i.d. A steady-state level is reached within five days. Common side effects include gastrointestinal distress and tremor. It elevates the level of concomitantly administered phenobarbital. Therapy should be initiated at 10 mg/kg/day and increased slowly to a maximum of 60 mg/kg/day. The usual adult dose is 1500 mg per day. Minor elevations of hepatic enzymes are common. In rare instances, however, fatal hepatotoxicity can occur. About 60 deaths have been associated with this drug to date. Other abnormalities may include thrombocytopenia, bleeding abnormalities, and pancreatitis. It is contraindicated in women of childbearing age who have any potential for becoming pregnant. It carries significant risks of midline deformities, including cleft lip and palate and myelomeningocele.

Ethosuximide. Ethosuximide (Zarontin) is indicated for absence seizures. It is usually given t.i.d. and has a half-life of 30 to 60 hours. The usual dose is 750 to 1500 mg. The most common side effects are nausea, vomiting, and anorexia; serious side effects are rare. This drug is useful in absence or petit mal seizures, but does not control the frequently associated grand mal seizures.

Other Anticonvulsants. Other less frequently utilized anticonvulsants include diazepam, clonazepam, acetazolamide, and clorazepate. Other methods of treating epilepsy include the ketogenic diet, ACTH injections, psychotherapy and hypnosis, and surgery. Surgical removal of portions of the temporal lobe can sometimes eliminate or reduce the frequency of simple partial or complex partial seizures. The evaluation of such patients is complex and should be undertaken only in major medical centers specializing in this form of therapy.

FOLLOW-UP

When a patient has been free of seizures for two to five years, the need for continued therapy can be reevaluated. Risk factors that may preclude successful discontinuation of medication include an abnormal EEG, the frequent occurrence of seizures before control, the presence of a known structural lesion or neurologic disorder, mental retardation, onset of seizures before the age of 2 years, focal or complex partial seizures, and multiple seizure types. The decision to stop medication is difficult and must be individualized. Recurrence of seizures may involve loss of vocation and driver's license. If medication is withdrawn, it should be done slowly. I prefer to withdraw a single medication at a time over a period of three to six months.

SUPPORTIVE CARE

Because seizures disrupt and interfere with normal function, the patient with epilepsy is subject to a wide variety of social, psychiatric, vocational, and psychologic problems. Attitudes of friends, neighbors, and employers intensify the difficulties to be overcome. Control of seizures is the first step in treatment of the whole patient. A comprehensive program must also address itself to the other needs of the patient. Some physicians work directly with their patients toward rehabilitation; others find that referrals to agencies such as the Epilepsy Foundation of America or Bureau of Vocational Rehabilitation can be useful. Providing contacts with educational counselors, social service workers, and psychologic and psychiatric counseling should be part of the total treatment plan. The goal is to make the patient a fully functioning member of society.

REFERENCES

Booker HE: Phenobarbital: relation of plasma concentration to seizure control. *In* Woodbury DM, Penry JK, Pippenger CE (eds): Antiepileptic Drugs. Raven Press, New York, 1982.

Feldman RG: Borderline areas. *In* Browne TR, Feldman RG (eds): Epilepsy: Diagnosis and Management. Little, Brown & Co, Boston, 1983, pp 109–116.

Feldman RG, Ricks NL: Nonpharmacological and behavioral methods. *In* Ferriss GS (ed): Treatment of Epilepsy Today. Medical Economics Co, Oradell, NJ, 1978.

Fincham RW, Schottelius DD: Primidone: relation of plasma concentration to seizure control. *In* Woodbury DM, Penry JK, Pippenger CE (eds): Antiepileptic Drugs. Raven Press, New York, 1982.

Pippenger CE, Lesser RP: An overview of therapeutic drug monitoring principles. Cleve Clin Q 51:241–254, 1984.

Pippenger CE, Penry JK, Kutt H: Antiepileptic drugs: quantitative analysis and interpretation. Raven Press, New York, 1978.

Rothner AD: Evaluation of the child with seizures. Cleve Clin Q 51:267–272, 1984.

Wright GN (ed): Epilepsy Rehabilitation. Little, Brown & Co, Boston, 1975.

14 · SLEEP DISORDERS

Paul T. Gross
LAHEY CLINIC MEDICAL CENTER

DEFINITION AND DIAGNOSTIC CRITERIA

The two most common sleep-related problems seen by the clinician are excess daytime sleepiness (EDS) and insomnia. Less frequently, therapy is required for occurrences of abnormal events during sleep (parasomnias) and for disturbances of the circadian rhythm. In sleep disorders the diagnosis is usually made from the history or from the sleep log kept by the patient. When indicated, diagnosis can be confirmed and abnormalities quantified by the all-night sleep study, which records sleep events, and the multiple sleep latency test, which measures daytime sleepiness.

Many patients complain of EDS when they actually are experiencing weariness, fatigue, or depression. True EDS is marked by periods of involuntary sleep during the day or, at least, urges to sleep that are difficult to resist. EDS is usually due to insufficient sleep at night, impaired brain control of the sleep-wake cycle as in the narcolepsy syndrome, or severely disturbed nocturnal sleep as with sleep apnea or periodic movements in sleep (PMS).

NARCOLEPSY SYNDROME

Diagnosis of the narcolepsy syndrome is made on the basis of a history of associated symptoms, such as cataplexy, hypnagogic hallucinations, and sleep paralysis; demonstration of EDS and rapid eye movement (REM) sleep on a multiple sleep latency test; and absence of a significant sleep disturbance on an all-night sleep study. Excess daytime sleepiness without other symptoms of the narcoleptic syndrome and without disturbance of nocturnal sleep or a disorder of REM sleep is called idiopathic central nervous system hypersomnolence.

SLEEP APNEA

Sleep apnea can be central, resulting from lack of respiratory drive, or obstructive, occurring secondary to intermittent blockage of the upper airway. The diagnosis of obstructive sleep apnea should be considered when the history includes EDS and loud snoring. The diagnosis of PMS is often unsuspected clinically, although a history of restless legs syndrome or leg twitching may be obtained. Confirmation and quantification of sleep apnea and PMS are made with the all-night sleep study.

INSOMNIA

Insomnia involves the perception of insufficient sleep. Thus, the diagnosis depends as much on the patient's impression as on the inability to sleep for a certain period. Insomniacs commonly underestimate their sleep time. Causes of insomnia include transient situational factors, depression, and most commonly long-term behavioral maladaptation to sleep, which is termed chronic psychophysiologic insomnia.

PATHOPHYSIOLOGY

The narcolepsy syndrome is the result of impaired brain stem control of the sleep-wake cycle and REM sleep. It is usually idiopathic, sometimes familial, and rarely secondary to a known brain stem lesion. Obstructive sleep apnea is usually the result of a combination of factors that serve to obstruct the upper airway and diminish respiratory drive. Causes of obstruction include narrow oropharynx, macroglossia, a long soft palate, large uvula or tonsils, retrognathia, obesity, and sleeping in the supine position. Decreased respiratory drive appears also to be a factor, possibly secondary to brain stem dysfunction or use of alcohol. Nonobstructive apnea and hypopnea may result from brain stem or neuromuscular disorders or from morbid obesity. Chronic insomnia is a psychosomatic disorder whereby tension and anxiety impair sleep, poor sleep habits develop, and the pattern becomes self-perpetuating.

CLINICAL ASPECTS

The narcolepsy syndrome usually begins with sleepiness in the teenage years. Naps are brief and refreshing. Episodes of cataplexy, or sudden loss of muscle tone, are the second most common symptom of the narcoleptic syndrome and are precipitated by laughter, anger, or other sudden emotional change. Consequently, social withdrawal is common. Sleep paralysis and hypnagogic hallucinations occur in the transition period between waking and sleep, but are less common and generally less troublesome than narcoleptic sleep attacks and cataplexy.

The sleep disturbance in patients with obstructive sleep apnea and PMS is often unrecognized by the patient, who only experiences daytime sleepiness. A bed partner's observations are helpful. Not all patients with sleep apnea are obese, and obesity may become a moot point since weight loss is often not achieved. Most patients with sleep apnea are male.

Most adults need between seven and nine hours of sleep per night. After the age of 50 years, many persons have lighter sleep and a reduced total sleep time. If a person feels adequately rested and is alert during the day, reduced sleep time should not be a concern. Depression should be considered in any patient with insomnia, especially if early morning waking is also present.

MANAGEMENT

NARCOLEPSY

Most patients with narcolepsy find some relief by allowing themselves to take naps, and they should be encouraged to try to introduce naps into their daily schedules. However, this usually is not totally successful, and stimulant medications such as pemoline (Cylert) may be needed. Pemoline has an advantage over other stimulants in that it is not strictly controlled by the Drug Enforcement Administration. It is effective for six to 18 hours, depending on the individual. A good starting dose is a single 37.5-mg tablet one hour before the time of day when sleepiness begins. The dose is then titrated by 18.75 to 37.5 mg, either added to the starting dose or given approximately six hours later in the day. Most patients require about 75 mg daily and may need as much as 225 mg. Alternatives are methylphenidate (Ritalin), 5 to 60 mg daily in divided doses taken between meals, and dextroamphetamine (Dexedrine), 5 to 30 mg daily in divided doses. These medications last from four to six hours and longer if sustained release preparations are used. All stimulants may produce weight loss, mood change, paranoia, hypertension, and a feeling of "crashing" when the drug wears off. Tolerance may develop with these medications, and therefore drug-free intervals may be needed. Pemoline may produce chorea. Many patients respond well to pemoline plus a small dose of methylphenidate or dextroamphetamine on special occasions. Narcoleptic patients require individualized treatment programs as symptoms develop and change over time, and physicians should be flexible and allow patients to titrate their medications within agreed-upon limits. Patients, families, and employers should realize that no schedule of naps or medications will eliminate all the symptoms.

IDIOPATHIC CENTRAL NERVOUS SYSTEM HYPERSOMNOLENCE

This is a related sleep disorder characterized by EDS, impaired sleep control, and no REM sleep abnormality. It is treated with the same stimulants or with methysergide (Sansert), 2 to 4 mg three times per day.

CATAPLEXY, SLEEP PARALYSIS, AND HYPNAGOGIC HALLUCINATIONS

Specific therapy for these manifestations in the narcolepsy syndrome should not be given until enough time has been allotted to determine if treatment for EDS has eliminated the symptoms. Imipramine (Tofranil), 25 to 100 mg daily, may be added if needed.

SLEEP APNEA

Obstructive. Treatment of obstructive sleep apnea should also be tailored to the patient. When obesity seems to be a factor, weight loss is advised. Commonly the apneas are most frequent and prolonged when the patient is in the supine position. A change in sleep position can be accomplished by advising patients to pin a sock containing a tennis ball to the back of their night clothes, and to place blocks under the head of the bed or a wedge under the mattress. Alcohol and other respiratory suppressants should be avoided before bedtime, and respiratory stimulants such as protriptyline, 5 to 30 mg taken at bedtime, may be helpful. Tonsillectomy, palatopharyngoplasty (reconstruction of the posterior pharynx), and relief of nasal obstruction may be beneficial in selected patients. Continuous positive airway pressure can be used nocturnally at home and is a good alternative for the cooperative patient. Supplemental oxygen may be helpful in reducing nocturnal oxygen desaturation, although the patient must be monitored carefully to ensure that respiratory suppression is not occurring. Tracheostomy provides dramatic relief of obstructive sleep apnea and is the treatment of choice when apnea becomes life-threatening because of severe nocturnal hypoxemia, cardiac arrhythmia, or daytime sleepiness severe enough to result in a fall or an automobile accident.

Nonobstructive. Nonobstructive sleep apnea should be treated with a program for weight loss (when obesity is a factor); with respiratory stimulants, especially medroxyprogesterone (Provera), 10 to 20 mg three times a day, or acetazolamide (Diamox), 250 mg two to four times a day; and in extreme cases with mehanical respiratory aids such as a rocking bed, phrenic pacer, or ventilator.

Sleep apnea is a chronic condition and continued follow-up is needed. The patient with severe nocturnal oxygen desaturation or cardiac arrhythmia needs to be monitored after therapy to ensure that these parameters have improved. When EDS remains after therapy, a reevaluation is needed to determine if frequent interruptions of sleep are still present.

INSOMNIA

In treatment of insomnia the physician should first determine if the condition is transient or chronic. Transient insomnia due to self-limited events, such as a period of hospitalization or an episode of grief, can be treated with counseling and, if needed, hypnotic agents. The ideal hypnotic has a rapid onset, lasts as long as needed, and has no after-effects. If initiating sleep is the principal problem, diphenhydramine (Benadryl), 25 to 50 mg, or chloral hydrate, 500 to 1500 mg, is given at bedtime. For the patient who has difficulty maintaining sleep, the benzodiazepines are used. Flurazepam (Dalmane), 15 to 30 mg, is a common choice, but it has active metabolites that could result in sleepiness on the following day, especially in older patients. Triazolam (Halcion), 0.25 to 0.5 mg, and temazepan (Restoril), 15 to 30 mg, are newer medications that are less likely to have this effect.

For chronic insomnia not due to depression, a behavioral approach is emphasized. The goals are to permit sufficient sleep for rest and to prevent daytime sleepiness rather than to reach a specified number of hours of sleep. The patient is instructed to use the bed only for sleeping and not for reading and watching television, because long periods of wakefulness in bed reinforce the notion that it is all right to be awake in bed. The number of hours actually spent sleeping is calculated, and only that much time is allowed in bed. When most time in bed is spent sleeping, the time allotted can be increased gradually until daytime sleepiness ceases. Daytime naps should be eliminated.

Patients with chronic insomnia are encouraged not to use coffee, tea, soft drinks, and other products containing caffeine after noon and to avoid alcohol in the late evening. Although alcohol may induce sleep, it frequently results in disturbed sleep after several hours. Daily exercise may be used to improve sleep, but is best not performed in the evening when it may be stimulating. For some persons a snack at bedtime may help to overcome insomnia.

If sleep does not improve with this behavioral program, the physician should reconsider the possibility that anxiety or depression may be a major factor and seek appropriate therapy. Alternatively, some patients respond well if the program described is reinforced with administration of a hypnotic agent twice a week. This schedule provides needed sleep two nights of each week, does not result in drug dependency, and helps to remove anxiety on the other nights since some sleep in the near future is assured.

Delayed Sleep Phase Insomnia. This results from an inability to advance one's circadian rhythm to conform to society's schedule. The patient complains of sleep onset insomnia and morning sleepiness, but obtains sufficient sleep if allowed to sleep late. The appropriate treatment is to delay sleep progressively until an appropriate bedtime is achieved. Similarly, jet lag and work shift sleep disturbances improve more readily if sleep time is delayed rather than advanced. Hypnotic medications may be helpful in some patients when frequent readjustment of the circadian rhythm is needed.

PARASOMNIAS

Arousals from deep or slow wave sleep in the form of enuresis and night terrors (usually but not always in patients under the age of 10 years) and somnambulism are the most significant of the parasomnias. Their cause is unknown. The diagnosis can often be made from the history, the most common time of occurrences being about one hour after onset of sleep. When the history is uncertain or seizures are suspected, a sleep recording is helpful. Explanation and reassurance are usually sufficient treatment for night terrors and somnambulism. Enuresis or frequent episodes of night terror or somnambulism may respond to imipramine, 25 to 75 mg at bedtime, or diazepam (Valium), 5 to 10 mg at bedtime, which may reduce the time spent in slow wave sleep.

REFERENCES

Association of Sleep Disorders Centers and the Association for the Psychophysiological Study of Sleep: Diagnostic classification of sleep and arousal disorders. Sleep 2:1–154, 1979.

Guilleminault C, Tilkian A, Dement WC: The sleep apnea syndromes. Annu Rev Med 27:465–484, 1976.

Orr WC, Altshuler KZ, Stahl ML: Managing Sleep Complaints. Year Book Medical Publishers, Chicago, 1982.

Tobin MJ, Cohn MA, Sackner MA: Breathing abnormalities during sleep. Arch Intern Med 143:1221–1228, 1983.

van den Hoed J, Kraemer H, Guilleminault C, et al: Disorders of excessive daytime somnolence: polygraphic and clinical data for 100 patients. Sleep 4:23–37, 1981.

15 · DEMENTIA SYNDROME

E. Prather Palmer
LAHEY CLINIC MEDICAL CENTER

Prevalence of the dementia syndrome, which has been called "the silent epidemic" and "the disease of the century," is increasing rapidly in the Western world, especially in elderly persons. In the United States about 25 million persons (10% of the total population) are over 65 years of age. Approximately 5% of these have severe dementing illness and an additional 10% to 15% have mild to moderate dementia. Dementia may appreciably shorten life expectancy in the elderly and therefore is currently the fourth or fifth most common cause of death in the U.S.

As a result of the break-up of the nuclear family, society now bears the major expense of caring for persons with dementia. The annual cost of this care in the U.S., estimated to be approximately $25 million, is expected to double by about the year 2000. The worldwide implications of these costs will be experienced during the next few decades as life expectancy increases in third-world countries.

Recent advances in our understanding of neurobehavior, neuropsychology, and neurochemistry have resulted in an improved understanding of the dementia syndrome and its various causes.

DEFINITION AND DIAGNOSTIC CRITERIA

Dementia is a clinical term that describes a syndrome characterized by an acquired and progressive impairment of intellectual function. The condition must be differentiated from the mental retardation syndromes in which normal intellectual function fails to develop, and from the static dementia syndrome in which permanent damage to a large portion of the association cortex (usually as the result of trauma, stroke, or tumor) results in a circumscribed deficit that prohibits return to the pre-illness level of intellectual function. Dementia is not applicable to the normal changes in cognitive function and memory that occur with age (i.e., benign senescent forgetfulness).

The operational definition of the dementia syndrome provided by Cummings and Benson is useful. The *first* criterion is that the syndrome be persistent, thus excluding the confusional states (delirium) usually seen in patients with trauma or metabolic or toxic disorders. Confusional states, which are present for hours or days, involve clouding of consciousness, alteration in attention, loss of coherent thought, and fluctuation in clinical course. The dementia syndrome, on the other hand, does not typically fluctuate and is relentlessly progressive without notable remissions over a period of months or years.

The *second* criterion is that there be an impairment of intellectual function involving at least three of the following five spheres of mental activity: language, memory, visual spatial skills, and emotional and cognitive functions. Cognitive function refers to the ability to manipulate old knowledge to arrive at a new answer. Patients with the dementia syndrome frequently have difficulty in shifting from one task to another.

Although the terminal stages of dementia are similar in most patients, the initial clinical impairment may be variable and prominent in only one or two spheres of intellectual activity. Diagnosis is based on careful history-taking as well as a probing examination of mental status. The patient is usually a poor historian, and therefore family members, acquaintances, and even employers must be consulted for confirmation of deficits in any of the five spheres of mental activity.

DIFFERENTIAL DIAGNOSIS

The differential diagnosis of dementia syndrome is vast (Table 1) and the frequency with which certain syndromes are seen depends on patterns of referral. When proper screening procedures are used and patients with confusional states are eliminated, most cases of the dementia syndrome are found to result from Alzheimer's disease. Dementia is potentially reversible or treatable in less than 20% of patients, who must be identified by a search for causative mechanisms. Multi-infarct, communicating hydrocephalus, alcoholism, intracranial mass lesions, and depression (pseudodementia) are the most common potentially treatable causes. Other causative illnesses, such as thyroid or parathyroid dysfunction, general paresis, hepatic or renal disease, deficiency in vitamin B_{12} or folic acid, exposure to industrial toxins, Wilson's disease, drug toxicity, and other psychiatric disorders, are also potentially reversible.

When the diagnosis is not clear, neuropsychologic or psychiatric consultations or both may be helpful. Laboratory tests (Table 2) usually detect most treatable causes of dementia that are not suspected on clinical history and physical examination. Invasive procedures, such as angiography and brain biopsy, although rarely indicated, may occasionally provide diagnostic information with therapeutic potential.

ALZHEIMER'S DISEASE

Alzheimer's disease, the most common form of dementia, accounts for approximately one half of all cases. Its prevalence increases with each decade of life; however, some evidence suggests that the incidence may peak and decrease after the age of 80. Although a definite diagnosis can be made only at autopsy, Alzheimer's disease can be suspected strongly during life. Diagnosis is primarily made by exclusion using clinical and laboratory methods; no specific laboratory tests exist at present for the diagnosis of Alzheimer's disease. Brain biopsy is seldom justified. After a follow-up period of several months the clinical diagnosis is accurate in about 80% of patients. Pick's disease and other unclassified neurodegenerative disorders account for most of the remaining 20%.

Subtle differences in the clinical syndrome with respect to age of onset, behavior, genetic factors, results of pathologic studies, and even findings on physical examination have revived the former distinction between presenile (dementia of the Alzheimer's type) and postsenile (senile dementia of the Alzheimer's type) with an age of onset in the early 60s as the approximate line of division. Dementia of the Alzheimer's type, in contrast to senile dementia of the Alzheimer's type, is usually more rapidly progressive, is associated with a shorter life expectancy, has more genetic markers and a greater familial incidence, exhibits more widespread and severe pathologic and biochemical changes, displays more evidence of disturbances in language and

Table 2. LABORATORY TESTS THAT MAY BE USEFUL IN THE INITIAL EVALUATION OF DEMENTIA

Blood
  Complete blood count, erythrocyte sedimentation rate, serologic test for syphilis, thyroxine, blood chemistry profile (sequential multiple analyzer, 12–16), levels of vitamin B_{12} and folate, ammonia, copper, ceruloplasmins
Urine
  Urinalysis, drug screen
Electroencephalography
Radiography
  Chest film, CT or magnetic resonance scan of head
Lumbar puncture
  Protein concentration, serologic test for syphilis, cytologic studies

praxis, and has a higher incidence in left-handed individuals. There are no racial or sexual differences in incidence.

MULTI-INFARCT DEMENTIA

Multi-infarct dementia results from multiple cerebrovascular occlusions. It is less common than, and usually is readily distinguished clinically from, Alzheimer's disease. The decline in intellectual function results from multiple bilateral occlusions of arteries and arterioles as a result of either a distant embolic source or intrinsic arterial occlusive disease. The course is usually stepwise in progression as each new infarct causes worsening of the clinical condition. The infarcts may involve the sensorimotor cortex and deeper hemispheric structures as well as the association cortex. The change in intellectual function, unlike that in Alzheimer's disease, is usually associated with a pseudobulbar affect as well as disturbances in gait, sensorimotor functions, praxis, and attention. Personality change is often characterized by slowness of thought, apathy, inertia, and irritability.

Multi-infarct dementia has several recognized causes. Hypertension and diabetes are often associated with multiple large infarcts of the cortical vessels or lacunar infarcts of the arterioles in the area of the deep basal ganglia (i.e., lacunar state) or both. Involvement of the penetrating arteries from the surface of the brain may lead to loss of an appreciable portion of hemispheric white matter (Binswanger's disease), and malignant hypertension may disrupt the blood-brain barrier, leading to neuronal dysfunction. Inflammatory vasculopathies (e.g., systemic lupus erythematosus) and multiple cardiac emboli are less common causes of multi-infarct dementia.

PSEUDODEMENTIA

Pseudodementia, an apparent intellectual impairment associated with a psychiatric disorder, is usually applied to two groups of patients. The first and larger group consists of those depressed individuals with cognitive impairment that improves with treatment of the depression. Care must be taken, however, in the diagnosis of depressive pseudodementia in elderly persons. Some patients with Alzheimer's disease, aware of declining intellectual function, may initially present as depressed, but treatment of the depression does not restore cognitive function to its previous level. Drug therapy for depression in patients with early Alzheimer's disease may in fact worsen cognition.

Table 1. CAUSES OF PROGRESSIVE DEMENTIA

Cause	Approximate %
Dementia of Alzheimer's type (probable)	50
Multi-infarct	10
Combination Alzheimer's disease and multi-infarct	10
Alcoholism	5
Intracranial mass lesion	5
Drug toxicity	5
Pseudodementia of depression	3
Communicating hydrocephalus	2
Less common causes	10
Infectious disease (Jakob-Creutzfeldt, general paresis, progressive multifocal leukencephalopathy), degenerative disease (Pick's Disease, Huntington's chorea, parkinsonism, spinocerebellar disease, multiple sclerosis), metabolic (thyroid, Wilson's, liver, nutritional), trauma, other psychiatric illnesses	

The second group, which is more general, includes persons with apparent intellectual impairment secondary to psychiatric disturbances. Patients who make up this group are usually much younger than those with depressive pseudodementia. This syndrome is produced by several psychiatric diseases, including mania, schizophrenia, hysterical conversion reaction, and Ganser's syndrome. Ganser's syndrome is a peculiar, rare, and usually short-lived hysterical twilight state in which the patient may provide utterly incorrect and often absurd answers to questions although it is clear that the meaning of the questions has been understood. Such patients appear to be disoriented with respect to time and distance, but they are alert and not confused in the usual sense.

DRUG TOXICITY DEMENTIA

Most drugs taken in excess produce toxicity of the central nervous system. An idiosyncratic susceptibility to normal doses of medications, however, rather than excessive doses is responsible for most cases of drug toxicity dementia. This paradoxical effect is especially prominent in the aging brain—persons over age 65 constitute only 10% of the population but consume more than 25% of all prescription drugs.

Barbiturates, benzodiazepines, beta-blocking agents, neuroleptics, tricyclic antidepressants, monoamine oxidase inhibitors, anticholinergics, corticosteroids, reserpine, cimetidine (Tagamet), and digitalis are the drugs most often responsible. Phenytoin (Dilantin), baclofen (Lioresal), levodopa (Laradopa), methyldopa (Aldomet), clonidine (Catapres), orally administered hypoglycemic agents, and nonsteroidal anti-inflammatory agents are implicated only rarely. A meticulous history of medications should be taken in all patients with the dementia syndrome. Abuse of nonprescription drugs, except alcohol, is unusual in this age group, but the patterns of drug abuse are rapidly changing in the U.S. Inquiries on this subject should be made, especially in patients with early-onset dementia. Fortunately, the toxic effects of most drugs are usually reversed when they are discontinued.

COMMUNICATING HYDROCEPHALUS

Communicating hydrocephalus (normal pressure hydrocephalus) may cause a gradually progressive dementia syndrome. There may be history of subarachnoid hemorrhage, meningeal infection, or recurrent head trauma but the cause of the hydrocephalus often is unknown. Rarely, the cause may be thought to be decompensation in the patient with long-standing, often previously undiagnosed aqueductal stenosis.

Computed tomographic (CT) scan shows marked enlargement of the ventricular system, reduced or absent cortical sulcal markings, and attenuation of the periventricular white matter as a result of increased water content. The classic syndrome of a frontal lobe type of dementia with spastic ataxic gait, positive Babinski's signs, and urinary incontinence is seldom seen. The diagnosis is therefore dependent on a suggestive clinical picture, characteristic findings on CT scan, and cerebrospinal fluid pressure in the upper normal range (i.e., 160 to 220 mm H_2O).

An elevated protein concentration or white count in CSF suggests an active meningeal process. CSF shunts may improve intellectual and motor function in about one half of selected patients. Patients with a demonstrated probable cause of meningeal obstruction are most likely to show improvement. The complication rate associated with CSF shunts is appreciable in these patients, and such procedures should be recommended only after thorough evaluation.

PICK'S DISEASE

Pick's disease is an uncommon form of progressive dementia with clinical features similar to those of Alzheimer's disease. Patients with Pick's disease have severe atrophy of the frontal and temporal gyri, with relative preservation of the pre- and postcentral gyri and posterior portions of the superior temporal gyrus. Onset is usually earlier than in Alzheimer's disease and progression is more rapid, but these distinctions are not useful in clinical differentiation.

Consistent with the distribution of atrophy, patients with Pick's disease demonstrate severe progressive impairment of language and memory as well as frontal lobe behavioral disturbances. Visual spatial function is relatively preserved. Incontinence develops early and production of language may decline rapidly, often to the level of mutism. Signs of extrapyramidal and cortical motor dysfunction usually present late in the course of disease. The diagnosis may be suspected from the history, the examination, and the CT scan, which shows the typical distribution of atrophy. There is no treatment for Pick's disease.

MANAGEMENT

DRUG THERAPY

No satisfactory medical treatment exists for Alzheimer's disease or for the other neurodegenerative dementia syndromes. In all patients a thorough search for a treatable cause should be undertaken, as outlined previously. Medications that are not absolutely necessary should usually be discontinued, and substitutions should sometimes be made to eliminate potentially toxic agents.

Various agents have been used to treat Alzheimer's disease. Cholinergic precursors, cholinergic receptor agonists, cerebral vasodilators, CNS stimulants, vitamins, chelating agents, hyperbaric oxygen, amino acid precursors, and anabolic agents have been tried with little success.

Ergoloid mesylate preparations (Hydergine), 3 to 9 mg per day, have been used for more than 30 years in Alzheimer's disease. Some studies suggest that this drug produces a small but statistically significant improvement in behavior, at least in the short term. Formerly classified as a cerebral vasodilator, ergoloid mesylate is now considered to be a metabolic enhancer. The mechanism of improvement in Alzheimer's disease is unclear and many clinicians regard this drug as a placebo. No other drug therapy has proved better, however, and its side effects are minimal. The administration of ergoloid mesylates often reassures the patient's family that "something is being done," an important consideration in the course of the disease as family members learn to cope with the heavy burden that the diagnosis implies.

Medication used to treat the behavioral changes of

the demented patient should be kept to a minimum. As a general rule, drugs should be used only to treat specific medical illnesses. Most patients with dementia do not routinely require either major or minor tranquilizers. An acute decompensation may occur, however, when a demented patient is placed in unfamiliar surroundings, and sedation and antianxiety agents may be needed to control the resultant agitation and catastrophic reactions. Although high doses of medications may be required in an acute situation, constant attempts should be made to reduce and discontinue these agents as soon as possible. Paradoxically, continued use of an increasing number of tranquilizers, neuroleptics, and antidepressants produces a progressively more severe confusional state. Benzodiazepines are relatively contraindicated because of ineffectiveness, i.e., their tendency to accumulate in the body and cause increasing confusion and loss of memory. Diphenhydramine hydrochloride (Benadryl), 50 mg per day administered intramuscularly or orally as needed, is recommended as a mild sedative. Haloperidol (Haldol), 0.5 to 1 mg two to three times per day as needed, or thioridazine (Mellaril), 25 to 50 mg three to four times per day, may be necessary for more resistant problems.

Depression may be a factor early in the course of Alzheimer's disease. Tricyclic antidepressant drugs in relatively small doses may be useful, such as amitriptyline (Elavil) or imipramine hydrochloride (Tofranil), 30 to 100 mg per day. Tricyclic medication has an appreciable anticholinergic action, however, and thus may worsen confusion or loss of memory as the disease progresses. Patients should therefore be monitored and the drug discontinued as soon as side effects outweigh beneficial effects.

Shortening of the sleep time or alteration in the sleep-wake cycle is a common problem in demented patients. Use of hypnotic medication, at least on a regular basis, should be discouraged. During daylight hours the patient should be kept active and awake in an attempt to maintain a normal sleep-wake pattern. During the night a soft light or a radio tuned to quiet music may help to orient the patient who awakens.

GENERAL PRINCIPLES

Although there is no satisfactory medical treatment of dementia, optimal maintenance of the patient's abilities should always be attempted. The demented patient who is not stimulated and who is allowed to vegetate may deteriorate more quickly and ultimately present a more serious management problem. Maintenance of the patient's independence and personal dignity within the limits of safety should be a primary goal. In familiar surroundings with tolerant support and a structured program, the demented patient may function at a surprisingly satisfactory level for years. This is particularly true in the family setting where older remote memories, which are usually better preserved than recent memories, can be utilized by the patient. The learning of new material is hindered in these patients, but some learning may be accomplished with repetition in a structured setting. An active rehabilitation program is far better than a custodial one.

Demented patients commonly exhibit extreme emotional lability, agitation, and anger (catastrophic reaction) when confusing, constantly changing, or unfamiliar stimuli are encountered. This may occur when the patient is removed from familiar surroundings (e.g., on a vacation or trip, or to a hospital or nursing home) or is surrounded by unmanageable stimuli (e.g., a large party). To avoid this reaction a routine should be established that controls environmental stimuli and allows ample time for orientation and completion of a task. Instructions should be simple, and, if necessary, tasks should be subdivided into components that can be performed separately. Measures that maintain basic orientation, such as calendars, diaries, reality orientation, and memory aides, may be useful.

Demented patients are vulnerable to accidents and neglect of basic health measures because of disorientation, slowed reaction time, impaired judgment, forgetfulness, and distractibility. Safety and health topics should therefore be reviewed repeatedly by the physician and responsible family member or care giver. Such topics as driving, ability to call for emergency help, orientation outside the home, and personal hygiene must be evaluated frequently.

SUPPORT OF FAMILY MEMBERS AND OTHER CARE GIVERS

Family members and other care givers experience varying degrees of distress, depression, anxiety, and guilt. Early in the course of the illness, the extent of the dementing process is often denied by or not obvious to family members who are not in constant contact with the patient. This oversight can add greatly to the distress of the spouse or care giver.

A detailed and open discussion of dementia, especially as it relates to the patient, is necessary. Often the patient should be present at the outset of such a discussion to facilitate the initial confrontation between the care giver who must impose limits and the patient who may resist these restrictions. The discussion should focus (with or without the patient present) on cause, genetic implications, prognosis, course, and treatment or lack of treatment of the illness. Genetic transmissibility, a fear that is often unvoiced by family members, should be discussed. The physician should emphasize that Alzheimer's disease is progressive and untreatable, but that the patient may be helped in many ways. The unsuitability of "miracle cures" such as diets, hormones, and dubious medications should be emphasized so that the family will not waste limited resources and energy. Although most demented persons remain in the home, the family should be prepared for the possibility that the patient may have to be placed in a facility for long-term care if home care becomes impossible. As the disease progresses, assistance with and close monitoring of the patient's financial, business, and legal matters will eventually be required. Legal advice and power of attorney or guardianship are often necessary.

The care giver often benefits from the support and advice of others with similar difficulties, and the physician should encourage the care giver to contact local support groups, day care facilities, and informational meetings within the community. The Alzheimer's Disease and Related Disorders Association, Inc. (360 North Michigan Ave, Chicago, IL 60601), established in 1979, has proved active at the local and national levels. Referral to appropriate publications written for the lay person may also be helpful (e.g., Male and Rabins).

ROLE OF THE PHYSICIAN

The physician, who obviously plays an essential role in the care of the demented patient, sets an important example for family members and the caregiver by demonstrating an unwillingness to "give up" on the patient. Frequent initial follow-up visits (every three to four months) provide an opportunity for the care giver to express distress and to discuss difficulties in management. Such visits also permit the physician to evaluate the rate and progression of the illness and to ensure that the patient's general health and safety are being addressed. As the care giver becomes more familiar with the patient, follow-up visits may be required less frequently (every 12 months). Communication and cooperation with the family physician are also important.

Vigorous treatment of medical conditions is required to avoid deterioration and possible decompensation or catastrophic reactions. Hospitalization should be planned carefully and the patient should be returned to a familiar environment as soon as possible. Permission for a family member or care giver to remain with the patient in the hospital may be helpful. Because dementia is such an important and common illness, physicians should have knowledge not only of the illness itself but also of advances in the field, in order to answer questions and provide appropriate advice regarding care and treatment.

REFERENCES

Cummings JL, Benson DF: Dementia, A Clinical Approach. Butterworths, Stoneham, MA, 1983.

Eslinger PJ, Damasio AR, Benton AL, et al: Neuropsychologic detection of abnormal mental decline in older persons. JAMA 253:670–674, 1985.

Hershey LA, Miller DD: Adverse psychiatric drug reactions. Neurol Neurosurg Update Series 5:2–7, 1985.

Hollister LE, Yesavage J: Ergoloid mesylates for senile dementias: unanswered questions. Ann Intern Med 100:894–898, 1984.

Male NL, Rabins PV: The 36-hour Day: A Family Guide to Caring for Persons with Alzheimer's Disease, Related Dementing Illnesses, and Memory Loss in Later Life. Johns Hopkins University Press, Baltimore, 1981.

Mesulam M-M: Dementia: its definition, differential diagnosis, and subtypes (editorial). JAMA 253:2559–2561, 1985.

Wurtman RJ: Alzheimer's disease. Sci Am 252:62–74, 1985.

16 · PARKINSON'S DISEASE AND OTHER MOVEMENT DISORDERS

Stephen L. Wanger
LAHEY CLINIC MEDICAL CENTER

DEFINITION AND DIAGNOSTIC CRITERIA

Developments in the treatment of Parkinson's disease during the past 20 years have done much to dispel the myth of therapeutic nihilism from the discipline of neurology. Paradoxically, these advances have also led to increased uncertainty regarding both the pathophysiology and the management of patients with this disorder. The outlook for patients with Parkinson's disease has gone from hopeless to optimistic to questionable.

Parkinson's disease is a chronic neuronal degenerative disease of the central nervous system. It is one of the most common neurologic diseases found in the United States with an estimated prevalence of almost 1 million persons and an annual incidence of approximately 50,000 new cases. Tremor, rigidity, bradykinesia, and impairment of posture and balance are the cardinal features. Its course is insidiously but relentlessly progressive and it produces disability over a variable number of years.

PATHOPHYSIOLOGY

The fundamental anatomic defects in Parkinson's disease are loss of pigmented neurons in the substantia nigra and degeneration of the nigrostriatal dopaminergic tract. This pathway normally exerts an inhibitory influence on the corpus striatum and is counterbalanced by facilitative cholinergic impulses. In Parkinson's disease striatal dopamine is deficient, thus producing a relative cholinergic excess. This can be conceptualized as a seesaw, and therapeutic strategies have been conceived to subtract from the cholinergic end of the balance or to add to the dopaminergic end by either administering dopamine or substituting for it.

The recently identified neurotoxin methylphenyltetrahydropyridine (MPTP), a contaminant of synthetic heroin, induced an acute Parkinson-like state in some users, and selective degeneration of the substantia nigra was found on autopsy. Experiments with primates have reproduced these changes, creating the first true animal model of Parkinson's disease. A promising hypothesis holds that Parkinson's disease might be a consequence of subclinical nigral damage that occurred earlier in life, possibly caused by exposure to a toxin similar to MPTP, followed by the clinical symptoms from further degeneration in the substantia nigra and decline in striatal dopamine that occur with normal aging.

CLINICAL ASPECTS

The diagnosis of Parkinson's disease depends entirely on the history and neurologic examination; no diagnostic laboratory tests exist. The major features are those of motor dysfunction.

Tremor, resulting from the relatively rhythmic alternating contraction of agonist and antagonist muscle groups, is usually maximal when the limb is at rest and temporarily diminishes when movement of the involved limb is initiated, although it intensifies when other limbs are in use and is absent during sleep.

Rigidity, a form of hypertonicity that is present simultaneously and equally in agonists and antagonists, may assume a characteristic cogwheel quality because of superimposed tremor.

Bradykinesia produces exasperating slowness in initiating movements, and appreciable reduction in both spontaneous movements and automatic and auxiliary movements.

Impairment of postural and righting reflexes leads

to loss of balance either forward or backward and frequent falls, which cannot be prevented by the patient.

Serious problems in functional self-sufficiency result from these basic symptoms, which combine to produce decreased speed and amplitude of tasks that require repetitive movements and affect facial expressiveness, speech, writing, eating, dressing, rising from bed or chair, and turning in bed. Autonomic involvement may cause orthostatic hypotension, and prominent sialorrhea and seborrhea may embarrass the patient. Intellectual functioning may become impaired by a depressive reaction to the physical disability and also to some degree by a true dementing process.

Parkinson's disease is easily recognized when the symptoms and signs are fully developed, but the diagnosis may be difficult to establish in early stages of the disorder when subtle slowness of movement may be confused with normal senescence. Tremor at rest, often the first sign of the disease, must be differentiated from the action tremor of essential-familial tremor, which usually is benign. Serial examinations over many months may be necessary, and the development of impairment in walking and in the performance of daily activities may be a most important factor in establishing the diagnosis.

The clinical identification of secondary forms of parkinsonism may also be difficult. The basal ganglia syndrome produced by the use of neuroleptic drugs, especially the phenothiazines, and by reserpine, most frequently seen in older patients, cannot be distinguished clinically from idiopathic Parkinson's disease but it usually disappears within several months after the medication is discontinued. Instances of other symptomatic disease, such as after hypoxia, carbon monoxide poisoning, or chronic exposure to manganese, are infrequent. So-called "arteriosclerotic parkinsonism" combines features of the basal ganglia syndrome with signs of more widespread and less selective neurologic dysfunction; it occurs episodically, chiefly in hypertensive patients who have sustained multiple small strokes, producing a lacunar state. Parkinsonian features coexisting with other neurologic symptoms and signs in several other disorders are termed "multiple system atrophy" and include progressive supranuclear palsy, the Shy-Drager syndrome, striatonigral degeneration, and olivopontocerebellar degeneration. Postencephalitic parkinsonism, related to the pandemic Economo's encephalitis lethargica seen during the years 1918 to 1926, was a cause of disease of relatively early onset in the third or fourth decade of life. New cases are no longer encountered, but those of long duration can often be distinguished by the occurrence of prominent oculogyric crises, producing spasms of intense tonic conjugate deviation of the eyes.

MANAGEMENT

PLAN

The establishment of a diagnosis of Parkinson's disease marks the beginning of a long-term partnership between the physician and the patient and family. It is essential at the outset to discuss at great length the implications of this diagnosis. Emphasis should be focused on the many recent advances and the continuing active research in treatment, because many persons still visualize Parkinson's disease as a totally hopeless and rapidly disabling condition, and they interpret the diagnosis as signaling the end of useful life.

Degree of Disability. Determination of the degree of disability is of equal importance to the establishment of the diagnosis. This can be evaluated by rating the severity of the cardinal signs—rigidity, tremor, bradykinesia, postural stability, and impairment of gait—on a reproducible scale; by timing the performance of certain tasks, such as buttoning, tying shoes, writing a one-line sentence, or walking a measured distance; and by questioning the patient and family regarding activities of daily living at home and, if applicable, at work. Rating scales may be obtained from several drug companies or can easily be originated by the physician. Periodic repetition of such a scoring routine permits objective evaluation of the progress of the disease and the effectiveness of treatment.

Physical Activity. At all stages of the disease the patient must remain as physically and intellectually active as possible. For patients with mild tremor or slowness, this means reassurance that they may continue working and driving a car. As activities of daily living become limited, continuing independence must be encouraged. Active exercises, which do not require frequent postural corrections, must be performed in a daily routine. Consultation with a physical therapist may eventually become necessary to establish an exercise program to preserve mobility of the joints and coordinated functioning of the limbs, and to improve posture of the trunk and patterns of gait. Difficulty in rising from a seated position can be minimized by the use of chairs with arm rests and the installation of hand rails at toilet and bathtub. The tendency of patients to freeze upon initiating gait can be helped by teaching them to lift one foot as if about to step over an object, to bend the knee and lift the foot with each step, and to keep the shoulders back, thus transforming the automatic involuntary act of walking into a more conscious and voluntary one.

As the disease progresses, the frequency of office visits must increase and the physician must be available for telephone consultation whenever questions arise. The cornerstone of successful management remains close contact with patient and family.

DRUG THERAPY

Treatment with medications should be appropriate to the clinical situation. They need not be prescribed until real impairment of functional activity has developed. Many patients become uneasy when no medication is given, and it is necessary to explain that withholding early treatment will in no way foster more rapid progression of the disease but is, in fact, desirable to minimize long-term side effects.

Medications currently available for Parkinson's disease include anticholinergic and antihistamine drugs, amantadine (Symmetrel), levodopa alone or in combination with a peripheral decarboxylase inhibitor, and bromocriptine (Parlodel).

Anticholinergic Medications. These have the longest history of use based on empiric observations of the beneficial effects of atropine and scopolamine, and continuing with the synthesis of compounds that possess the ability to block acetylcholine receptors but produce fewer undesirable side effects than the naturally occurring belladonna alkaloids. Of the five compounds commercially available, my practice is limited to the use of two, trihexyphenidyl (Artane) and benztropine (Cogentin). Therapeutic effects are similar: they are most helpful for tremor, less so for rigidity, and least for bradykinesia. Although the benefits of these agents often seem to be minimal, an increase in all parkinsonian symptoms when they are withdrawn indicates how truly effective they are. A side effect is reduction of salivation, often helpful in controlling drooling, but dryness of the mouth may be unpleasant. Other peripheral side effects caused by parasympathetic blockade include constipation; decreased sweating, with resultant intolerance to heat; urinary retention, especially in men with prostatic enlargement; blurred vision from mydriasis; and impaired accommodation. The risk of development of narrow-angle glaucoma is also increased. Some degree of impairment of mental acuity, ranging from subtle difficulty in concentration and memory through more dramatic confusion and vivid hallucinations, is a common central side effect.

Antihistamines. Antihistamine preparations combine some degree of anticholinergic activity with a sedative effect, but most of the side effects of the anticholinergics, especially confusion and hallucinations, are minimized. Diphenhydramine (Benadryl) is the only antihistamine I prescribe for Parkinson's disease.

Amantadine. Developed in the late 1960s as a prophylactic drug against Asian influenza, amantadine was found by serendipity to improve all symptoms of Parkinson's disease. Its mechanism of action is not known, but it may combine elements of anticholinergic effect and dopaminergic action, especially enhancing the release of endogenous dopamine at the synapse. This may explain its rapid onset of benefit within a few days and its characteristic decline in effect after several months of use when endogenous stores of dopamine may have become depleted. The extent of initial response to amantadine alone may be a predictor of the degree of benefit to be expected when administration of levodopa is subsequently begun. The effect of amantadine is enhanced when given together with levodopa, and periods of withdrawal from amantadine also may enhance its subsequent effectiveness after reintroduction by permitting stores of dopamine to undergo partial replenishment. As with the anticholinergics, however, some temporary worsening of symptoms occurs with this program. Intrinsic side effects associated with amantadine are usually mild; these most prominently include edema of the ankles, mottled livedo reticularis of the legs, and an increased tendency toward orthostatic hypotension. Amantadine can enhance symptoms of confusion and cause vivid hallucinations, especially when used in combination with an anticholinergic drug.

Levodopa. Developed as a direct consequence of the discovery of deficiency of striatal dopamine, levodopa was pioneered during the 1960s by Cotzias and associates. Large doses of levodopa were found to be necessary to saturate the peripheral dopa decarboxylase enzymatic mechanism and enable even a small fraction of the medication to reach the brain, where it could be metabolized to dopamine. Dopamine itself does not cross the blood-brain barrier. Although tremor responds least well, all other symptoms of Parkinson's disease are improved to a much greater degree than with any previous medication. Levodopa has truly revolutionized the treatment of Parkinson's disease, and its dramatic success has stimulated continuing research into neurotransmitters in neurologic disease. However, its use is restricted by prominent peripheral adverse side effects, especially nausea and vomiting, which cannot be controlled reliably even by taking the drug with food. The optimal dose of levodopa should be determined and carefully titrated for each patient. Initial dosage is usually 0.5 to 1.0 gm daily, divided into two or three equal doses. This amount is increased gradually in small increments every three to seven days, as tolerated. Only in exceptional cases should patients receive more than 8 gm. Benefits of therapy may not be seen for as long as six months. Levodopa has been replaced by a compound that avoids these problems, and its use is now limited almost exclusively to a small number of patients who are doing well taking levodopa begun before the advent of peripheral decarboxylase inhibition.

Carbidopa-Levodopa (Sinemet). This agent is a combination of levodopa and a peripheral decarboxylase inhibitor. The extracerebral metabolism of levodopa is minimized by blocking most of the decarboxylase enzyme with an inhibitor that does not cross the blood-brain barrier. The ratio of inhibitor to levodopa is fixed at 1:4 and 1:10 in the available preparations. Peripheral side effects of nausea and vomiting are least likely to occur with the 1:4 combination, and largely obviate the need to take the drug with food, thus minimizing the competition for intestinal absorption. However, the drug is also more potent in the brain because of more complete peripheral inhibition at this ratio. Other side effects of combined central and peripheral mechanism include postural hypotension and cardiac arrhythmia. Central side effects are of the greatest importance and include psychiatric symptoms and abnormal involuntary movements. The sequence of psychiatric side effects usually begins with fragmentation of the sleep cycle and the appearance of vivid dreaming, which progresses to florid and usually visual hallucinations that are at least initially understood by the patient as not being real. A paranoid confusional state may develop eventually. Abnormal involuntary movements, which appear to be the most common side effect, are related to strength of dose and duration of treatment, and ultimately limit the dose in most patients. These movements may range from facial grimacing or posturing of the neck to prominent choreiform movements of individual limbs and to florid writhing of limbs and trunk. Such dyskinetic movements are not easily confused with any of the cardinal signs of Parkinson's disease, and may resemble more closely the relative dopaminergic excess and cholinergic deficiency seen with Huntington's chorea. Their exact mechanism is not well understood, but they may represent the inappropriate stimulation of dopamine receptors beyond their normal site of action, and they may herald the final phase of treatment of Parkinson's disease in which exogenous levodopa loses its effectiveness.

Bromocriptine. This is an ergot derivative that has been synthesized as a direct agonist of dopamine receptors in response to the emerging problem with long-term use of exogenous levodopa. When administered jointly with levodopa, bromocriptine potentiates all the side effects of levodopa with a heightened risk of behavioral abnormalities and dyskinetic movements, as well as nausea. These problems may be much less prominent when bromocriptine is taken alone without levodopa, especially in small doses. It has not been established clearly whether bromocriptine is a selective agonist of the D-2-receptors, specific for the nigrostriatal pathway and not for other dopaminergic receptors, which are not involved in Parkinson's disease.

SEQUENCE OF MEDICAL TREATMENT

The current use of medications for Parkinson's disease is based on the following five considerations:

Suppression of cholinergic activity is beneficial only as long as some dopaminergic activity persists. The continuing degeneration of pigmented neurons progressively reduces the supply of endogenous dopamine available to the nigrostriatal pathway.

Replenishment of dopamine by means of its precursor, levodopa, is an effective strategy only as long as nigral cells retain the ability to convert levodopa to dopamine and to release it into the synaptic cleft. This ability declines with progressive nigral neuronal degeneration, as the loss of dopa decarboxylase enzymes restricts the utilization of exogenous levodopa.

The success of levodopa administration also depends on the functional capacity of the postsynaptic dopaminergic receptors. Because of the phenomenon of denervation supersensitivity, these receptors appear to increase in number and density in response to a reduced amount of endogenous dopamine, acquiring the ability to react to lower concentrations of neurotransmitter. The very act of replacement of dopamine may reduce this enhanced sensitivity, decrease the number of postsynaptic receptor terminals, and thus undercut the effectiveness of treatment.

Loss of dopamine receptor function may be heralded by prominent abnormal involuntary movements, which accompany the therapeutic response at progressively increasing frequency, leading to both dose-related "wearing-off" of effect and the random occurrence of "on-off" loss of therapeutic benefit as the disease nears its end stages. Attempts to deal with such end-stage decline of therapeutic effectiveness include the temporary withdrawal of dopaminergic medication to try to reestablish supersensitivity of postsynaptic receptors, and the use of direct postsynaptic dopamine receptor agonists.

This inexorable sequence of decline may possibly be delayed by withholding initial levodopa therapy until the nondopaminergic medications have become ineffective. This remains controversial.

Initial Therapy. When (1) medication is to be started at an early stage of Parkinson's disease, (2) the patient is relatively compensated from a functional standpoint, and (3) no previous drugs for Parkinson's disease have been given, amantadine, 100 mg twice per day, is prescribed. In addition, when tremor is prominent, one of the anticholinergic medications is prescribed, either trihexyphenidyl, 2 mg, or benztropine, 0.5 mg, starting with one-half tablet per day and increasing at weekly increments of one-half tablet per day to a maintenance dose of one tablet three times per day. The patient or family should notify the physician of any problem or

side effect and the patient should be reexamined within one month. The dose of anticholinergic medication may be increased by use of trihexyphenidyl, 5 mg, or benztropine tablets, 1 or 2 mg, in divided doses three or four times per day, the maximal dose usually not to exceed trihexyphenidyl, 10 mg/day, or benztropine, 6 mg/day. Monthly follow-up visits are desirable until a maintenance dose is reached, after which the patient should be seen at definite intervals of two to three months or sooner if indicated by telephone reports of progressive disease or troublesome side effects.

Dopaminergic Therapy. The questions of when to begin more specific dopaminergic treatment and whether the patient is best served by starting replacement of dopamine or treatment with a receptor agonist have emerged as unanticipated dilemmas in the current management of Parkinson's disease. As knowledge and experience increase, the answers may become clearer. At present, my practice is to begin replacement of levodopa when the amantadine-anticholinergic combination therapy is no longer effective in controlling functional disability or can no longer be tolerated by the patient. Carbidopa-levodopa is begun at the 10/100 strength, one-half tablet per day, while other current medications are continued. At weekly intervals, the dose of carbidopa-levodopa is increased by one-half tablet per day at approximately four-hour intervals, taken on an empty stomach to facilitate intestinal absorption. If nausea or vomiting develops, medication should be taken with food. If gastrointestinal intolerance persists, the 25/100 tablet should be used instead of the 10/100. Most patients tolerate weekly increases to a maintenance schedule of 10/100, four tablets per day, by the end of two months, at which time administration of any anticholinergic medication should be tapered and eventually stopped during the third month while amantadine is continued. If tremor remains prominent, a small dose of anticholinergic drug may be continued. Should the tremor have features of a nonparkinsonian postural or action tremor, propranolol (Inderal) can be tried, but the potential for hypotension or bradycardia is increased by this combination of drugs.

Once carbidopa-levodopa has been established at a tolerable schedule, treatment should be continued at the smallest effective dose. The aim should never be for complete abolition of all symptoms and signs of parkinsonism but rather for maintenance of optimal functional ability with minimal side effects. Most patients achieve this goal with a total daily dose of levodopa of between 400 and 1250 mg in the 10/100 or 25/250 preparation.

Bromocriptine. The appearance of abnormal involuntary movements is the sign to decrease the dose of carbidopa-levodopa by one-half tablet decrements and to begin bromocriptine, one half of a 2.5-mg tablet per day, taken with food, increasing at the rate of one-half tablet per day each week, to a schedule of one tablet three times per day with meals by the sixth week of treatment. Periodic reassessment is again necessary during this titration phase and the patient will require much explanation and emotional support. Abnormal involuntary movements typically appear during the time of peak therapeutic effect of each dose of levodopa, and are often of more concern to the family than to the patient. When given the choice, patients almost unanimously prefer such nuisance dyskinetic movements to the more disabling symptoms of Parkinson's disease itself. It may be difficult to convince them of the importance of decreasing the dose of levodopa at this stage of treatment.

End-Stage Treatment. The most difficult and therapeutically frustrating stage of managing a patient with Parkinson's disease begins once abnormal involuntary movements become difficult to control after an average of about five years' treatment. Fluctuations in response to medication become prominent; dyskinesias may either accompany peak medication effect or may occur both before and after peak effect. Duration of benefit from each dose may become progressively shorter.

"Wearing-off" Effect. End-of-dose bradykinesia may appear after only two hours in contrast to previous durations of four or more hours, and nocturnal and morning bradykinesia may become prominent. At first, increasing the frequency of administration of carbidopa-levodopa to as often as every two hours, while not exceeding a daily total of 1500 mg of levodopa, may be effective. The dose of bromocriptine may be increased to a total of 15 to 20 mg/day. Amantadine may be administered for intervals of two to three months then withheld for a month and resumed in similar cycles. These therapeutic maneuvers are of variable success but rarely control the problem with consistency.

"On-off" Effect. This is an even more difficult problem to manage: a random and sudden loss of therapeutic benefit without regard to the time at which medication is taken. The patient may rapidly become immobile and "frozen," within minutes, totally unable to function for intervals of minutes to an hour or more, and then regain functional ability without the benefit of any intervening medication. The comparison with turning a switch off and on explains the term used for this phenomenon. The risk of falling is greatly increased at such times, and frequent falling may indicate "on-off" episodes.

Paranoid Psychosis. A further ominous sign is worsening of a chronic confusional state leading to a paranoid psychosis. Earlier in the course of treatment, such a development could represent simply the effect of polypharmacy and might respond to withdrawal of anticholinergics and amantadine, followed if necessary by a decrease in the total dose of levodopa. However, when it occurs at the stage of rapid clinical fluctuations, it is another indicator of probable failure of the dopaminergic response.

"Drug Holiday." An extreme strategy employed to try to deal with these manifestations of loss of dopaminergic response is the "drug holiday." This misleading term belies the drastic physical and emotional consequences of the abrupt withdrawal of all dopaminergic medication. The patient and family must be prepared for the predictable deterioration that will occur, even with continued administration of anticholinergics and amantadine, and the patient may well become helpless and confined to bed. The patient must be hospitalized and may require passive physical therapy and total nursing, nutritional and supportive care (including parenteral or nasogastric feeding), and precautions against possible aspiration and phlebitis during the period of five to seven days' withdrawal of levodopa and bromocriptine. To legitimize the need for hospitalization to third-party payers, the admitting diagnosis should be "severe toxic effects of drug therapy." Clearing of dyskinesias, some improvement in confusion and other psychiatric symptoms, and the reappearance of severe parkinsonian signs can be expected. Unless the "holiday" must be ended sooner because of severe medical complications, carbidopa-levodopa is reintroduced in small doses, as if never having been given before, with the goal of a maintenance dose at least one third lower than the prewithdrawal total. The theoretical rationale for this procedure is the reestablishment of supersensitivity of the dopaminergic receptors after a period free from the desensitizing feedback of dopaminergic stimulation. Increased sensitivity to bromocriptine would be expected by the same rationale.

The concept of periodic two-day drug holidays, at the patient's home under family supervision, has been developed to manage milder problems of fluctuation of therapeutic effect, dyskinesias, confusion, and hallucinations. Although less likely to produce the drastic clinical deterioration of a full seven-day "holiday," it also has less evident immediate benefits, and several cycles of such semiholidays may simply be equivalent to a partial reduction in the daily maintenance dose.

The problems of fluctuation and loss of therapeutic effect, and of behavioral and psychiatric abnormalities, remain at this time barriers to continuing effective drug treatment as the end stage of Parkinson's disease is reached after periods of five to 15 years of dopaminergic treatment in most patients.

Experimental Drugs. Current experimental approaches to this problem are aimed at prolonging the effectiveness of dopaminergic treatment and reducing side effects. Although not presently available for approved use for treating Parkinson's disease, pargyline (Eutonyl), a potent antihypertensive agent that is an inhibitor of monoamine oxidase-B, has been shown experimentally to block the neurotoxicity of MPTP in animals and may also increase the synaptic concentration of dopamine by inhibiting its metabolic degradation. Domperidone, a peripherally acting dopaminergic agonist, has been used experimentally to reduce the peripheral side effects of both levodopa and bromocriptine, and is especially effective in reducing the incidence and severity of nausea and vomiting. The use of low doses of bromocriptine or of other experimental postsynaptic dopamine receptor agonists as the sole dopaminergic therapy, without administration of any exogenous levodopa, is being investigated as a means of preventing the sequence of dyskinesias and failure of treatment.

Although the limitations of dopaminergic treatment are becoming increasingly obvious with added years of clinical experience, it is nevertheless true that therapeutic advances of the past 20 years have improved life expectancy and quality for patients with Parkinson's disease.

OTHER MOVEMENT DISORDERS

Disorders of movement can be classified as hypokinetic, with slowness and paucity of voluntary movements, and hyperkinetic, with excessive involuntary movements. Parkinson's disease is the preeminent example of the hypokinetic condition. Only those hyperkinetic disorders most likely to be encountered in office and emergency practice will be mentioned here.

ESSENTIAL TREMOR

Essential tremor, occurring with posture-holding and use of the affected limb, is often a familial condition and is characteristically reduced temporarily by ingestion of alcoholic beverages. While it usually is easily differentiated from resting tremor, which diminishes with intention, it may coexist in patients with Parkinson's disease. The medication of choice is the long-acting form of propranolol (Inderal LA), beginning at 80 mg once per day and increasing at weekly intervals until a satisfactory response is produced or a maximal dose of 320 mg/day is reached. If propranolol is contraindicated or cannot be tolerated, primidone (Mysoline), starting at one half of a 50-mg tablet per day and increasing weekly to a maximum of 500 mg/day, may be of benefit; drowsiness is a common side effect. Stereotaxic thalamic surgery, no longer advised for patients with Parkinson's disease, is rarely indicated to suppress disabling action tremor.

TARDIVE DYSKINESIA

Tardive dyskinesia, the most feared complication of long-term neuroleptic drug therapy, encompasses a variety of choreiform movements affecting the face, tongue, trunk, and limbs. The mechanism is thought to involve supersensitivity of the dopamine receptor resulting from chronic blockade by neuroleptics. No single medication is uniformly effective in treating tardive dyskinesias and the best treatment remains prevention. Phenothiazines and other dopamine antagonists should be reserved only for psychoses and prescribed in the smallest effective dose for the shortest possible time. If dyskinetic movements persist after neuroleptic withdrawal, therapeutic strategies are aimed at enhancing central cholinergic activity and reducing dopaminergic transmission. Medications currently recommended include lecithin, reserpine, and clonazepam (Klonopin), but optimal doses have not been established and response to treatment is variable.

CHRONIC DYSTONIAS

Spasmodic torticollis is the most common form of chronic dystonia; blepharospasm and writer's cramp are other familiar examples of focal dystonia. Trihexyphenidyl, gradually increased to the highest tolerated dose, is effective for some patients, and diazepam (Valium) and carbamazepine (Tegretol) may also be tried. Surgical procedures to denervate the affected muscles provide inconsistent relief.

ACUTE MOVEMENT DISORDERS

Acute movement disorders may require emergency treatment. *Acute dystonic reactions* to phenothiazines may seriously impair movements of the tongue, swallowing, and breathing and can produce acute torticollis and even opisthotonos. Diphenhydramine, 25 to 50 mg IV, or benztropine, 1 to 2 mg IM, usually relieves this condition promptly, and supportive measures for airway and hydration are generally not necessary. *Idiopathic paroxysmal choreoathetosis*, characterized by sudden and often violent choreoathetoid movements of the limbs and face that usually terminate within one minute but may recur many times a day, responds well to phenytoin (Dilantin). *Acute hemichorea* and *hemiballismus* can be produced by infarcts of the basal ganglia; improvement may occur within days after a hypertensive hemorrhage or within months after a nonhemorrhagic infarct, and treatment with reserpine or haloperidol (Haldol) may reduce persisting choreic movements.

REFERENCES

Fahn S: The extrapyramidal disorders. *In* Wyngaarden JB, Smith LH Jr (eds): Cecil Textbook of Medicine, 17th ed. W. B. Saunders Co, Philadelphia, 1985, pp 2068–2079.

Fahn S (ed): Management of Parkinson's disease at different stages of the illness. Clin Neuropharmacol 5(Suppl):S1–S43, 1982.

Janovic J (ed): Symposium on movement disorders. Neurol Clin 2:415–631, 1984.

Marsden CD, Fahn S (eds): Movement Disorders. Butterworth Scientific, London, 1982.

Wanger SL: The management of Parkinson's syndrome. Med Clin North Am 56:693–709, 1972.

Yahr MD: Extrapyramidal disorders. *In* Conn RB (ed): Current Diagnosis. W. B. Saunders Co, Philadelphia, 1985, pp 982–992.

17 · MULTIPLE SCLEROSIS

H. Stephen Kott
LAHEY CLINIC MEDICAL CENTER

DEFINITION AND DIAGNOSIS

Multiple sclerosis is probably the most common neurologic disease affecting young adults living in the northern latitudes of Europe and North America. The prevalence rate in these areas is 40 to 60 per 100,000 population. Pathologically, focal areas of demyelination appear in the white matter of the cerebrum, the brain stem, the cerebellum, and the spinal cord. These lesions, known as plaques, occur in greatest number during the first few years after onset of the disease. However, the frequency of their formation diminishes in subsequent years. The accumulation of the effects of the plaques eventually produces severe disability.

In the past the criteria for diagnosis of multiple sclerosis depended on clinical documentation of separate lesions appearing at different times. Thus, the diagnosis could not be confirmed on the basis of the initial symptoms or attack. In the patient with a gradually progressive paraparesis the possibility of multiple sclerosis was considered only if involvement of other areas of the central nervous system could be documented.

In recent years laboratory tests have been helpful in establishing the diagnosis at an earlier stage. Cerebrospinal fluid electrophoresis reveals more than one band in the IgG region in a majority of patients. Another test demonstrating increased CNS IgG synthesis is the comparison of IgG levels in serum and CSF, or the IgG index. Evoked potential testing may suggest scattered areas of abnormal conduction and thus support the diagnosis. Computed tomographic (CT) scanning may show low-density lesions in white matter, and acute plaques can be enhanced with injection of contrast media.

The advent of magnetic resonance imaging (MRI) has greatly facilitated the ability to make a diagnosis at an early stage. Plaques are often easily demonstrable with this technique. Even at the time of the first clinical episode, MRI may show several lesions in the white matter characteristic of demyelination.

PATHOPHYSIOLOGY

The etiology of multiple sclerosis remains a mystery, but considerable evidence is now available to suggest that alterations in the immune system are major factors. Genetic and environmental influences may be important pieces in the puzzle. Susceptibility is probably inherited and it is now thought that 60% to 70% of white patients with multiple sclerosis carry the HLA-DRw2 antigen. The risk of contracting multiple sclerosis is 15 to 25 times greater in a relative of a patient with the disease than in the general population.

Whatever the etiology, the primary process seems to be inflammatory. Initially, lymphocytes and macrophages responding to the unknown immunologic stimulus penetrate the blood-brain barrier and damage myelin while sparing axons. Oligodendroglia disappear from involved foci, but it is not clear whether demyelination occurs coincidentally with or secondary to the attack on these cells. Edema may be present, and the borders of the lesions are indistinct. Myelin is digested by microglia and macrophages. Astrocytes infiltrate the region, producing a glial scar. The plaques are areas of demyelination with variable degrees of scar formation. Helper T cells appear to predominate in the outer margin of the plaques, and suppressor T cells are decreased in the blood during many acute exacerbations of the disease.

Plaques are scattered widely throughout the white matter of the brain and the spinal cord but tend to be close to cerebrospinal pathways. Common areas of involvement include the cervical posterior columns, optic nerves, corpus callosum, periventricular white matter, cerebellum, brain stem, and pyramidal tracts.

The number and location of plaques determine the clinical signs and symptoms, and the length of intervals between appearances of new lesions determines the clinical course. Factors that govern the location and frequency of new lesions are completely unknown.

CLINICAL ASPECTS

Multiple sclerosis usually occurs in young adults 20 to 40 years of age. Onset in persons under 10 or over 50 years old accounts for only 2% to 5% of all cases. Exacerbation and remission are characteristic of the disease in the earlier years. Although the first attack tends to remit, subsequent episodes heal incompletely and contribute to progressive disability. When the disease begins in later years, the course is frequently that of progressive paraparesis.

An exacerbation often appears acutely but may progress for days or weeks. The duration of an attack may vary from three to 12 weeks. The disease may continue in a remitting form for many years but eventually advances in a stuttering or gradually progressive manner. Nevertheless, at least 50% of patients are able to work or manage a home for ten years after onset.

The overall survival rate at 25 years after onset is 50% or higher.

Symptoms and signs of multiple sclerosis depend on the number and location of plaques. Optic neuritis is one of the commonest early manifestations and occurs eventually in 25% to 40% of patients at some point in the course. Involvement of optic nerve, which may be subclinical, occurs in 80% to 90% of all patients eventually. Symptoms involve one eye at a time and include decrease in color vision, blurring, and complete blindness.

Sensory phenomena are an early manifestation and signify demyelination of the posterior column. The patient complains of paresthesia, dysesthesia, or Lhermitte's phenomenon. Examination may be negative or may reveal a decrease in two-point discrimination along with diminished vibration and position sense. A positive Romberg sign is common.

Lesions in the corticospinal pathways may result in stiffness or spasticity, a feeling of heaviness, and weakness. Severe disturbance in the motor system can produce an acute hemiplegia or paraplegia. Motor involvement of the bladder usually results in a hyperreflexic neurogenic bladder with urinary frequency and urgency. Presence of plaques in the sacral cord or chronic infection tends to produce a hypotonic bladder.

Diplopia and vertigo are frequent brain stem symptoms. Occasionally, trigeminal pain is noted. Nystagmus, third and sixth nerve palsies, internuclear ophthalmoplegia, and occasionally peripheral seventh nerve palsy may be seen on examination.

Cerebellar ataxia occurs in about 50% of all patients but is usually not an early sign. Symptoms include poor balance, intention tremor, dysarthria, and titubation. Cerebellar symptoms tend to be progressive and severely disabling.

Mental changes also occur in a large percentage of patients but are initially subtle. Mood changes are common and include depression and effects of frontal lobe disinhibition. Seizures appear in 2% to 4% of patients and dementia may be prominent in later years. CT scanning shows white matter atrophy with large ventricles in this late stage.

MANAGEMENT

GOALS AND NONPHARMACOLOGIC MEASURES

First Goal. When patients with multiple sclerosis first learn of the diagnosis, they often think of eventual confinement in a wheelchair. The first goal of management, therefore, is reassurance that the diagnosis is compatible with many years of productive life. Counseling of patient and spouse at this time is important and should include information about the symptoms and characteristics of an exacerbation. They should be told that symptoms of brief duration do not constitute an attack. Family planning should be discussed, and the importance of rest and minimizing stress mentioned. Activities that are personally fulfilling should be encouraged, and the importance of employment for as long as possible may be emphasized.

Later in the course of the disease, when physical disability, sexual dysfunction, and personality change may produce stresses within the family, formal counseling by a psychiatrist, psychologist, or primary physician is helpful. Introduction to a multiple sclerosis support group at this time may also assist the patient and family in coping with effects of the disease. Later the help of visiting nurses and home health aides may be valuable.

Second Goal. The second goal of therapy is to help the patient deal with exacerbations and to promote remission. Many attacks do not require pharmacologic treatment and remit spontaneously. An examination in the office often provides the opportunity for reassurance that the attack is mild and that aggressive intervention is not necessary. Telephone consultation with the physician during the exacerbation is also supportive. Employment can often be continued if symptoms are mild, but extra rest and the removal of some responsibilities should be advised. Even with more disturbing symptoms, pharmacotherapy can often be avoided, but two to three weeks of rest at home may help speed remission. Serious attacks manifested by paraplegia, hemiplegia, brain stem dysfunction, or encephalopathy require hospitalization.

Third Goal. The third goal of treatment is to delay and minimize disability. Physical therapy plays a definite role here but its limitations should be recognized. Exercises can improve muscle strength and help prevent shortening of tendons and spastic contractures. However, patients with multiple sclerosis have poor endurance, and when exercise is too vigorous or prolonged, increased weakness may appear.

At first the effects of ataxia can be offset by visual cueing and by widening the gait. As symptoms progress, a cane, a platform cane, Lofstrand crutches, and a walker may be required, in that order. Bracing may be helpful when footdrop is prominent. Braces of light metal or molded plastic are well tolerated, and their use improves endurance in walking and helps to prevent falls. Leg and knee braces may prevent buckling and damage to the knee from hyperextension. Compensation for dysfunction of the upper extremities can be obtained to some degree by specially designed pens and pencils, eating utensils, and cups.

Urinary incontinence can be a major problem. Pharmacotherapy may be effective, but in patients with a hypotonic bladder and urinary retention the technique of self-catheterization has been successful. Infection is the main complication. When self-catheterization is not possible, an indwelling Foley catheter or suprapubic diversion may be required. In some male patients, sphincterotomy and permanent condom catheter drainage is satisfactory.

Surgical Interventions. Occasionally, other surgical interventions such as tenotomy, rhizotomy, or cord tractotomy may be required to relieve spastic contractures and facilitate nursing care. When pressure sores fail to heal, skin grafting is sometimes attempted. Finally, thalamotomy may abolish severe intention tremor, but its use should be limited to special circumstances. Even when thalamotomy is successful, the extremity may not be useful because of weakness or proprioceptive loss. Also, the procedure adds another lesion near the pyramidal system that could produce pseudobulbar palsy.

DRUG THERAPY

Exacerbations

Exacerbations of multiple sclerosis have traditionally been treated with intramuscular or intravenous injections of adrenocorticotropic hormone (ACTH) or by oral administration of corticosteroid agents, such as prednisone or dexamethasone. High-dose IV pulse therapy with prednisolone has been advocated. The rationale is to reduce plaque edema, stabilize vascular membranes, and reduce inflammatory response. One study has demonstrated that corticosteroids decrease enhancement of plaques on CT scan.

Unfortunately, the effectiveness of short-term treatment with corticosteroids has had few controlled trials and is still being debated. Those who advocate the use of ACTH cite results of the National Cooperative Study published in 1970. Patients with acute exacerbations were hospitalized and treated with 80 units of ACTH gel IM for a week, followed by tapering over two more weeks. After six weeks 86% of treated patients had improved compared with 69% of controls. Later the two groups were identical, indicating that ACTH had no long-term beneficial effects. The study points out that most exacerbations improve spontaneously but that ACTH may hasten recovery.

When exacerbations require hospitalization, I give ACTH in a dose of 80 units IM for one week followed by gradual tapering over 10 to 14 days. This treatment is effective for acute severe weakness. ACTH also helps to relieve spasticity but the results are temporary. Clearly, for cerebellar symptoms, which do not remit spontaneously, ACTH and corticosteroid medications are of little value.

Side effects of this treatment have included stomach distress, weight gain and edema, hypokalemia, thrush, insomnia, hypomanic or manic behavior, depression, and (very rarely) steroid-induced psychosis and seizures. Peptic irritation can be prevented or controlled with a low-sodium bland diet and cimetidine (Tagamet), 300 mg four times a day. I have seen no instance of peptic ulceration or gastrointestinal bleeding with this regimen. If edema does appear, it can be controlled with diuretic medications, such as a combination of triamterene and hydrochlorothiazide (Dyazide or Moduretic).

Insomnia and hypomanic behavior occur with some frequency, but severe mania and steroid-induced psychosis have been extremely rare. I have not considered it necessary to prescribe lithium carbonate prophylactically. Flurazepam (Dalmane), 15 to 30 mg, is usually effective in inducing sleep, and occasionally a low dose of a benzodiazepine, such as chlordiazepoxide (Librium) or diazepam (Valium), is useful for daytime tranquilization.

To prevent hypokalemia, a high-potassium diet should be given and blood levels should be monitored every few days. If the serum level drops, potassium chloride elixir, 50 mEq/day by mouth, is usually sufficient to correct the situation. Intravenous doses are not required if blood levels are monitored appropriately.

Exacerbations that do not require hospitalization but produce appreciable decrease in vision, severe proprioceptive loss, mild weakness, and mild brain stem dysfunction may be treated with prednisone, 60 to 80 mg for one week and then tapered by 10 mg every three or four days. The patient should be seen in the office two or three times during this period so that results and side effects can be noted.

Preventive Measures

In the past few years, great interest has developed in immunosuppressive therapy for prevention of the progressive disability of multiple sclerosis. As early as the 1970s, azathioprine (Imuran) was believed by some to have a possible effect in decreasing the frequency of exacerbations and in delaying the appearance of disability.

Interest has now shifted to cyclophosphamide (Cytoxan). Hauser and colleagues in 1983 indicated that this drug produced stabilization for periods of up to one year in 80% of patients with progressive disease. Cyclophosphamide is given in doses of 400 to 500 mg/day IV until the white blood cell count drops below 4000 µL. Seven to ten days of treatment may be required. After treatment is stopped the WBC count is monitored daily until it reaches its low point and begins to rebound. When this occurs the patient is discharged from the hospital.

Short-term side effects of immunosuppressive therapy include alopecia, nausea and vomiting, fatigue, cystitis caused by chemical irritation, and infection, especially if the WBC count drops to very low levels. Possible long-term side effects include the risk of bladder cancer, leukemia, and infection with slow virus or other opportunistic agents. Short-term side effects have been rare with the program outlined, and so far none of the long-term possibilities have been reported. Nevertheless, at present this treatment should be reserved for patients with rapidly progressive disease or for those who may soon lose the ability to walk. In the future, monthly pulse therapy with cyclophosphamide may be the method of choice.

Currently, several other agents that act on the immune system are being studied. These include interferon, cyclosporine (Sandimmune), copolymer A, and monoclonal antibodies against helper T cells. Further investigation will be required to determine their effectiveness.

Palliative Agents

Patients with multiple sclerosis often experience disturbing symptoms that can be acute or chronic. Control of these problems may sometimes be possible with pharmacologic agents.

Pain. Some patients experience typical trigeminal neuralgic attacks. These episodes often subside spontaneously, but they may persist or recur sporadically over many years. Carbamazepine (Tegretol) usually controls pain when given in a dose of 200 to 400 mg three times a day. Side effects include dose-related nausea, dizziness, ataxia, and diplopia. Bone marrow suppression and hepatotoxicity are rare and do not usually occur after the third month of use. Until that time, however, complete blood count, platelet count, and serum glutamic-oxaloacetic transaminase (SGOT) should be monitored weekly.

Occasionally, paresthesias can be so disturbing as to require symptomatic treatment. Carbamazepine may be helpful, and also tricyclic agents such as amitriptyline, 10 to 25 mg twice a day or 25 to 75 mg at bedtime. Tricyclics should be used with great caution in patients who have hypotonic neurogenic bladder with residual urine, because these agents tend to produce urinary retention.

Fatigue. Most patients with multiple sclerosis complain of fatigue or poor endurance that limits functional performance. It is difficult to judge when such a subjective symptom requires treatment, but in some patients I have prescribed pemoline (Cylert) with good results. Pemoline is a CNS stimulant with a six- to 18-hour duration of action. It is given in doses of 37.5 mg once or twice a day and never later than early afternoon. Insomnia is the most frequent side effect, but other symptoms of CNS stimulation include anorexia, irritability, depression when the effects of the drug wear off, nausea, dizziness, and dyskinesia. Liver enzyme abnormalities may appear after several months of use.

Spasticity. The symptoms of spasticity vary from a feeling of stiffness and tightness to extensor and flexor spasms of the legs. Several agents may affect spasticity, such as anticonvulsants, phenothiazine derivatives, dantrolene (Dantrium), and glycine. The benzodiazepines and baclofen (Lioresal) are used most frequently. The main problem with all antispasticity agents is that they may reduce muscle tone that is useful in ambulation. Patients taking these drugs may experience enough decrease in muscle tone to produce falling.

Baclofen works by stimulating gamma-aminobutyric acid receptors at bicuculline-insensitive receptors and inhibiting calcium influx into presynaptic terminals. It may also decrease the release of excitatory neurotransmitters. The two actions produce a diminution of reflex activity. A low dose, such as 5 to 10 mg three times a day, may improve stiffness in ambulatory patients. The drug is most helpful, however, in later stages of the disease when spasms of the bladder and legs occur. At this time larger doses may be required, but more than 20 mg four times a day often produces side effects. Adverse reactions include nausea, vomiting, diarrhea, lethargy, weakness, hypotension, ataxia, confusion, dizziness, headache, insomnia, and behavioral changes.

Bladder Dysfunction. Urinary frequency and urgency incontinence can be distressing and socially embarrassing. These symptoms are most often due to a hyperreflexic neurogenic bladder, for which anticholinergic agents are helpful. Oxybutynin chloride (Ditropan), 5 mg two or three times a day, or propantheline bromide (Pro-Banthine), 15 to 30 mg three times a day, decreases cholinergic stimulation of the bladder and allows the patient three or four hours between voidings. Adverse effects are those of cholinergic blockage: blurred vision, dry mouth, constipation, drowsiness, dizziness, bradycardia, impotence, poor memory, toxic psychosis, and increase in intraocular pressure.

When the bladder is hyporeflexic and found to be infected, specific antibiotic therapy may convert the bladder to a hyperreflexic state. For an uninfected hypotonic bladder, bethanechol chloride (Urecholine) may be used in a dose of 25 mg/day, gradually increased to 25 mg four times a day. Its effectiveness should be determined by cystometry or by measuring the volume of residual urine. Symptoms of cholinergic stimulation, such as diaphoresis, abdominal cramping, and diarrhea, are the chief side effects.

In some patients, relaxation of the muscles of the bladder neck and urethra may improve emptying. This can be accomplished by diazepam, 5 mg three times a day; baclofen, 10 to 20 mg three times a day; or the alpha-adrenergic blocker phenoxybenzamine (Dibenzyline), 10 mg two or three times a day. Side effects of phenoxybenzamine are sympathetic blockage, such as postural hypotension, miosis, and ejaculatory dysfunction.

Intention Tremor. Cerebellar tremor is one of the most disabling symptoms of multiple sclerosis and when present may render a patient unable to eat, write, or dress. Pharmacotherapy has little to offer, but beta-blockers that cross the blood-brain barrier, such as propranolol (Inderal), should be tried. Doses ranging from 60 to 320 mg/day may dampen the tremor. Isoniazid (INH), because of its effect of stimulating gamma-aminobutyric acid receptors, has been advocated in large doses, such as 800 mg/day. In our experience this agent has not been useful.

REFERENCES

Adams RD, Victor M: Principles of Neurology, 2nd ed. McGraw-Hill Book Co, New York, 1981.

Antel JP (guest ed): Symposium on multiple sclerosis. Neurol Clin 1:571–782, 1983.

Hauser SL, Dawson DM, Lehrich JR, et al: Intensive immunosuppression in progressive multiple sclerosis: a randomized three-arm study of high-dose intravenous cyclophosphamide, plasma exchange, and ACTH. N Engl J Med 308:173–180, 1983.

McFarlin DE, McFarland HF: Multiple sclerosis. N Engl J Med 307:1183–1188, 1246–1251, 1982.

Rose AS, Kuzma JW, Kurtzke JF, et al: Cooperative study in the evaluation of therapy in multiple sclerosis: ACTH vs. placebo. Final report. Neurology 20(suppl):1–59, 1970.

18 · ACUTE SPINAL CORD DISORDERS

Robert P. Dinapoli
MAYO CLINIC AND MAYO FOUNDATION

The spinal cord is susceptible to a variety of pathologic processes. In this chapter we review the recognition and management of the most important nontraumatic disorders of the spinal cord and its extension, the cauda equina, which develop within hours or a few days. Although specific treatment is not currently available for some of the conditions, prompt recognition and appropriate management may help to reduce or prevent permanent neurologic impairment.

These disorders are recognized by a characteristic pattern of symptoms and signs indicating exclusive involvement of one or more portions of the spinal cord, nerve roots, cauda equina, meninges, or vertebral column. The etiologies include inflammation or infection, vascular disorders, neoplasms, skeletal disorders, toxic conditions, and physical agents.

RECOGNITION

HISTORY

Patients with spinal cord disease present with a combination of pain, bilateral limb weakness, bilateral sensory abnormalities, and variable bladder and bowel difficulties. Pain localized to the spine suggests periosteal or meningeal involvement. Radicular pain is more readily recognized and usually is intermittent, worse in recumbency when the spine lengthens, and aggravated by any activity that increases intraspinal pressure or stretches spinal nerves. Radicular pain may simulate a variety of intrathoracic and intra-abdominal conditions.

Weakness is usually bilateral and symmetric and often recognized by progressive interference with the patient's usual activities. Occasionally, subtle involvement is described as "heaviness" or "clumsiness." Sensory symptoms such as numbness, tingling, or deadness are easily recognized, and useful information can be obtained by the patient's localization of them. Autonomic symptoms such as hesitancy, urgency, and incontinence predominate in acute disorders, while constipation, fecal incontinence, and various sexual dysfunctions are more common in chronic disorders.

EXAMINATION

With a pertinent neurologic examination, it should be possible to ascertain the rostral-caudal level as well as the transverse extent of any lesion. A complete transverse spinal cord lesion produces paralysis, a sharply-defined sensory level to all modalities, and sphincter paralysis. Because of the phenomenon of spinal shock, the paralysis is initially flaccid with reduced or absent muscle stretch reflexes and absent Babinski signs. Several weeks later, the usual signs of spasticity appear. A partial section or hemisection of the spinal cord produces ipsilateral mono- or hemiparesis, ipsilateral loss of position and vibration sensations, and contralateral loss of pain and temperature sensations several dermatomes below the lesion. At the level of the lesion, segmental loss of motor, sensory, and reflex function also occurs, but this is difficult to demonstrate with thoracic lesions. Involvement of the ventral or anterior two thirds of the cord produces bilateral loss of pain and temperature, bilateral weakness, and sphincteric paralysis with preservation of touch, position, and vibration. Dorsal lesions cause impairment of position and vibration with ataxia of gait; similar findings, however, may also be produced by nerve root and peripheral nerve involvement. A central or intramedullary cord lesion results in bilateral loss of pain and temperature in affected segments; preserved touch, position and vibration; segmental weakness, atrophy, and reflex loss; and variable upper motor neuron weakness below the lesion. A cauda equina lesion produces radicular pains, flaccid weakness, loss of reflexes, dermatomal sensory loss, and late involvement of sphincters.

DIAGNOSTIC STUDIES

Standard roentgenograms may reveal bone erosion or destruction, abnormal calcification, and degenerative disc and vertebral changes. The spine should be visualized well above the level suspected clinically, because small or early lesions frequently produce signs at a lower level. Electromyography may reveal denervation in paraspinal as well as distal muscles from involvement of anterior horn cells or proximal nerve roots. Computed tomographic (CT) scanning of the spine can disclose changes in bone texture as well as encroachment on neural structures by bones, discs, and some tumors. Examination of cerebrospinal fluid is mandatory if infection or inflammation is suspected, but should only be done cautiously and as part of a myelogram with a neurosurgeon available if a mass lesion is a serious consideration. Myelography should be performed whenever a compressive or mass lesion is possible. It should be discussed with the radiologist and performed with specific possibilities in mind so that an optimal examination is done. If a subarachnoid block is detected, it may be necessary to visualize the upper level of the block as well. This is particularly important if the block appears epidural and in a patient who may have cancer. A lateral puncture at C1–2 is performed and additional dye injected so that the upper level of the block and the rest of the subarachnoid space can be examined for other lesions. An aortogram or spinal angiogram may be warranted in patients suspected of having various spinal cord vascular syndromes, particularly arteriovenous malformations.

MANAGEMENT

ACUTE CARE

Most patients with acute spinal cord disorders require hospitalization for further diagnostic tests, medical or surgical treatment, and initiation of a comprehensive physical therapy and rehabilitation program.

The goals of acute care are to relieve or control symptoms and signs and to preserve neurologic and general functions. Long-term goals are to prevent disease recurrence and to help the patient resume as normal a life as possible. The following categories of care should be carefully assessed in each patient on admission, and specific treatment strategies developed.

Skin. Skin breakdowns and subsequent ulcerations are much easier to prevent than treat. Bedding should be kept clean, dry, and smooth; patient's skin should be bathed and thoroughly dried each day. Patients should be turned every two hours, day and night, if unable to reposition themselves. Vulnerable areas such as over the sacrum, trochanters, ischia, and heels should be regularly inspected. Early areas of pressure are treated with massage, heat, and avoidance of further pressure. Minor skin infections are treated with povidone-iodine (Betadine) applications. Foam rubber over pressure points, specially lined boots, and specialized mattresses may be indicated in some cases.

Nutrition. Nutritional status and dietary intake should also be reviewed. Inadequate protein intake may contribute to skin breakdown. If the patient is on corticosteroids, antacids are given between meals and at bedtime. Cimetidine, 300 mg four times daily, or ranitidine, 150 mg twice daily, is used if the patient has preexisting peptic ulcer disease. A moderate low-sodium diet should be followed and electrolytes and glucose should be checked twice weekly.

Venous Complications. Patients immobilized with paraparesis or paraplegia are at risk for systemic venous thrombosis including pulmonary embolus. I use prophylactic anticoagulation with subcutaneous heparin, 5000 units every 12 hours, in most of these patients so long as they are confined to bed and inactive. Support hose are also applied and a regular program of passive limb exercise initiated.

Bladder. Some patients require intravenous fluids and accurate output measurements that necessitate an indwelling urinary catheter. As soon as feasible, however, each patient should be placed on a scheduled oral fluid intake, a schedule of voiding attempts, and intermittent catheterization. An intake of 2000 ml per day is given as 400 ml with each meal at 8:00 AM, 12:00 noon, and 6:00 PM and 200 ml at two-hour intervals in the morning, afternoon, and evening. Patients should attempt to void by straining or the Credé maneuver about every three hours during their waking hours. Intermittent catheterization is performed about every six hours after each voiding attempt, and residual urine volumes are measured. Since there is a direct correlation between the frequency of urinary tract infections and residual urine volumes, it is important to attempt to reduce the latter with an appropriate program. Infections can also be reduced by acidification of the urine. Fruit juices such as cranberry, apple, and grape can be added to the diet, but hippuric acid and mandelic acid are more effective means. Ascorbic acid (vitamin C) is widely used, but studies have not found it to be an effective urinary acidifier and it may contribute to the formation of kidney stones. Bacterial suppressant drugs such as methenamine mandelate (Mandelamine), 1 gm three times a day and at bedtime; methenamine hippurate (Hiprex), 1 gm twice a day, morning and evening; or trimethoprim-sulfamethoxazole (Septra, Bactrim), two tablets every 12 hours are also prescribed. Urinalyses and urine cultures are obtained periodically and whenever symptoms suggest infection.

Bowel. A high-fiber diet along with adequate fluid intake should be instituted along with other measures needed to reproduce the patient's natural schedule. Important additional measures include stool softeners such as docusate sodium (Colace); laxatives such as bisacodyl (Dulcolax) tablets, 5 mg; suppositories, 10 mg; enemas; and periodic rectal examination for impaction.

Spasticity, Spasms, Pain. Occasionally, patients with acute cord lesions have flexor or extensor spasms. These can be treated with baclofen (Lioresal), beginning with 5 mg three times daily. The dosage can be increased by 15 mg daily every three to five days until a response is obtained. Diazepam (Valium) can also be used but may produce troublesome drowsiness and occasionally depression; an initial dosage of 2 mg three times daily can be adjusted upward as needed. Pain can be a major symptom in cord compression of various types. Corticosteroids are often dramatically effective in some patients with mass lesions. I generally give dexamethasone orally in conventional dosage, 4 mg four times daily, or large doses, 24 mg four times daily, and rapidly taper the dose over 10 to 14 days.

Physical Therapy. Physical therapy should begin as soon as possible. Passive range-of-motion exercises for the limbs are performed several times each day. Active exercise, transfer techniques, and gait training should proceed as permitted by the patient's progress. Foot-drop is treated with a foot board or boot device, and on ambulation a molded ankle-foot orthosis or metal short leg brace can be used. A four-leg walker provides initial support and stability for patients with paraparesis; if sufficient improvement occurs, tripod or quad canes can be substituted.

GENERAL CARE

Patients and their families should be provided with instructional information concerning their disease. This is best initiated by discussion and later supplemented by written material, lectures, and conferences.

Follow-up visits for neurologic reevaluation and modification of treatment and rehabilitative regimens are extremely important. These also provide an opportunity to review the patient's and family's understanding of the problem, their degree of adjustment, and their need for psychosocial emotional support. In addition, compliance with various drug schedules and bladder, bowel, and skin techniques can be assessed. The patient's sexual function should also be reviewed and counseling provided for specific problems, including contraceptive options, if appropriate. Since many patients are permanently impaired, in some cases during their occupationally productive years, vocational rehabilitation should be reviewed when appropriate. Patient support groups and private and governmental agencies and services should also be investigated.

SPECIFIC DISORDERS

TRANSVERSE MYELITIS

Acute or subacute transverse myelitis or myelopathy refers to a group of disorders with rapid development of a horizontal intramedullary lesion. The etiologies are diverse and in many cases it is not possible to determine the specific disease.

The most common pathologic process is necrosis or inflammation in a number of segments in the thoracic spinal cord. It occurs in association with viral, exanthematous, respiratory, and nonspecific illnesses as well as after vaccinations. In a few cases, it may be the first episode of multiple sclerosis.

The clinical picture varies with the spinal cord level, the number of segments involved, and the extent of involvement of the spinal gray matter and ascending and descending spinal tracts. The usual features are those of a thoracic cord lesion with paraparesis or paraplegia, a sensory level and sphincter paralysis, developing over days, followed by stabilization and variable improvement. Some patients have spine or radicular pain mimicking a compressive lesion.

Management. Following emergency hospitalization, acute supportive care as detailed elsewhere should be instituted. Physical and laboratory evidence of systemic disease such as viral infection, collagen vascular disease, and malignancy should be sought. The most important consideration is whether a compressive lesion is present. X-rays of the spine should be obtained, and in most cases an iophendylate (Pantopaque) myelogram and spinal fluid analysis should be performed. Lymphocytic pleocytosis and a mild elevation of protein without block are common. Occasionally an intramedullary mass is demonstrated and there may be difficulty in establishing whether it is inflammatory or not.

Specific Treatment. Since most cases are due to inflammation and edema, it is reasonable to use corticosteroids once other more specific causes have been excluded. Unfortunately, there are no randomized trials of any forms of treatment.

I administer dexamethasone PO, in an an initial dose of 10 mg followed by 8 mg twice a day every twelve hours for the first seven to ten days of the illness. If there is further progression, I continue this dosage for an additional five to seven days, then tapering to 0 over the next 10 to 14 days. Prednisone, ACTH, and IV methylprednisolone have also been used. If the patient has a collagen vascular disease and is already on steroids, I simply increase the dosage.

MULTIPLE SCLEROSIS

This disorder is discussed in Section XII, Chapter 17.

VIRAL MYELITIS

A more diffuse, although frequently patchy and asymmetric involvement of the entire spinal cord is caused by several viruses. These may produce an acute or subacute syndrome with pain, flaccid weakness, and variable sensory signs.

The classic example is poliomyelitis, now a rarity owing to widespread vaccination. Enteroviruses, particularly echovirus 19 and coxsackievirus A-7, have been responsible for a milder clinical picture. Herpes zoster virus usually affects the sensory neurons in the dorsal root ganglia, but occasionally anterior horn cell involvement over several segments or a more diffuse myelitis develops. A similar myelitis has been associated with herpes simplex virus.

Management. These disorders are usually mild and can be managed with general supportive measures.

SPINAL MENINGOVASCULAR SYPHILIS

This is an uncommon form of tertiary neurosyphilis that produces an acute or subacute focal cord syndrome. There is an obliterative endarteritis with secondary occlusion and infarction producing a pachymeningitis, meningomyelitis, or myelomalacia, often in the distribution of the anterior spinal artery.

The clinical picture can be similar to that of transverse myelitis. CSF examination reveals an active infection with pleocytosis of 20 to 100 cells, elevated protein, elevated IgG, and positive reagin test or specific antibody test for *Treponema pallidum.*

Specific Treatment. Penicillin in large doses should be given provided the patient has no allergy to the drug. I follow the recommendations of the Communicable Disease Center and give aqueous procaine penicillin G, 600,000 units daily IM for 15 days or aqueous penicillin G, 12 million units daily IM for 10 days. With penicillin allergy, erythromycin or tetracycline is used. Follow-up, including CSF examination, should be performed every three to six months.

EPIDURAL CORD COMPRESSION

An acute spinal cord syndrome in cancer patients is usually due to invasion of the epidural space from an involved vertebra in carcinoma of the lung, breast, or prostate or from nearby lymph nodes in lymphoma. Occasionally, intramedullary metastases develop by hematogenous spread.

The neurologic deficit results from mechanical compression of neural structures by the tumor. With progression, secondary vascular compromise may also occur. There may be additional involvement by vertebral compression, pathologic fracture, or fracture dislocation.

The clinical presentation is stereotyped, with pain, initially local, then radicular, followed by sensory, motor, and sphincter dysfunction evolving over a variable period. Some patients experience a sudden catastrophic course, probably related to secondary infarction of the cord.

Management. Further evaluation is guided by the nature of the pain and the presence of neurologic abnormalities. Individuals with nonradicular back pain and a normal neurologic examination remain outpatients, but an immediate plain roentgenogram is taken of the entire spine. Patients with radicular pain are hospitalized as an emergency and plain films obtained. Approximately 85% of patients with epidural metastases have x-ray abnormalities including bony destruction or paraspinal mass. CT of the pelvis with bone windows may be useful in those who have sacral involvement.

If spine x-rays are abnormal, myelography is performed to determine the exact location and extent of the process. If a complete block is found, contrast material is also introduced at C1–2 in order to determine the upper level of the block as well as the presence of lesions at other levels. Contrast material may be left in the subarachnoid space for repeat fluoroscopy after treatment.

Specific Treatment. Patients with radiculopathy or myelopathy are given corticosteroids as soon as the diagnosis is suspected. Clinical experience and experimental studies indicate the presence of edema, which is responsive to steroid therapy. I use dexamethasone: an initial 10-mg IV bolus followed by 4 mg PO every six hours in patients with radiculopathy and larger doses up to 100-mg IV bolus initially, followed by 24 mg PO every six hours in patients with myelopathy. The dosage is tapered to 0 over the next 10 to 14 days of treatment.

In recent years, retrospective studies have indicated that the results of radiation therapy are comparable with those of surgical decompression and radiation. I recommend surgery for all patients who present with epidural cord compression of unknown cause, as well as for those who relapse during or after radiation therapy. Radiation therapy is recommended for all other cases; we usually give 3000 rads in 10 to 12 fractions over about two weeks.

I have found a multidisciplinary "Cancer Adaptation Team" approach particularly helpful in addressing the extensive physical, psychologic, and social needs of these patients and their families. The team consists of a phychiatrist and coordinating nurse as well as chaplain, dietician, occupational therapist, physical therapist, and social worker.

ACUTE EPIDURAL ABSCESS

Acute epidural abscess along with subdural empyema and intramedullary spinal cord abscess are rare, but treatable, infections producing acute spinal syndromes. They arise from localized skin infections, systemic infections, or recent nonpenetrating back trauma.

The infection is usually produced by *Staphylococcus aureus*, streptococci, and gram-negative bacilli forming a localized infection in the dorsal epidural space. Continuing infection produces an arteritis with secondary infarction or frank abscess formation in the spinal cord.

Patients complain of localized back pain followed quickly by radicular pain and limb weakness, and there are usually systemic signs of infection.

Management. The diagnosis must be established quickly if permanent sequelae are to be avoided. X-rays may suggest disc space or vertebral body infection but can be normal. Myelography with CSF examination usually shows a complete block with pleocytosis, elevated protein, and negative cultures.

Emergency laminectomy and drainage of the infection is performed, and definitive antibiotic coverage is determined by cultures and sensitivities.

SPINAL EPIDURAL HEMATOMA

Spinal epidural hematoma also produces an acute cord compression syndrome. The diagnosis should be suspected in patients receiving anticoagulant therapy or chemotherapy that has produced thrombocytopenia. It may be spontaneous or initiated by lumbar puncture. In either case, sudden localized back pain or cauda equina deficits are present.

Management. Patients with epidural hematoma require emergency myelography, which usually shows subarachnoid block; most patients require surgical decompression. Those with subdural hematoma secondary to spinal puncture may be treated conservatively and recover satisfactorily. Corticosteroids for presumed edema are also appropriate.

Spinal punctures should not be performed in patients on anticoagulants or who are thrombocytopenic from any cause. If absolutely necessary, vitamin K is given and a relatively normal prothrombin time is awaited. Thrombocytopenic patients are given fresh-frozen platelets just before the procedure.

PROTRUDED DISC AND CORD COMPRESSION

Although a protruded disc usually compresses a nerve root and presents as an acute radiculopathy, a myelopathy may occur with a central disc protrusion in either the cervical or thoracic region. Onset can be spontaneous but more often is related to a traumatic event or severe exertion. Severe and localized spine pain is followed by paraparesis, sensory loss, and sphincter dysfunction. Radicular pain may or may not be present.

Management. Patients undergo immediate evaluation in the hospital. Spine films are taken followed by myelography and usually posterior laminectomy and decompression.

SPINAL CORD INFARCTION

Infarction of the spinal cord can occur when the aorta, cervical, intercostal, lumbar, medullary, or spinal arteries are occluded by any process. The most common pattern is an anterior spinal artery syndrome with involvement of the anterior two thirds of the spinal cord at a thoracic level.

There are many causes, including dissecting aortic aneurysm, aortic bypass surgery, trauma, aortoiliac occlusion, collagen vascular disease with arteritis, sickle cell disease, systemic hypotension, and secondary compression from spinal cord tumor.

Management. Diagnosis requires careful clinical examination, including myelography, to exclude treatable causes. Many cases are painless, sudden, and catastrophic with little chance of recovery.

SPINAL CORD HEMORRHAGE

Subarachnoid hemorrhage may also produce an acute cord syndrome. The most common cause is an arteriovenous malformation, usually on the dorsal aspect of the thoracic cord. There is sudden pain, variable cord dysfunction, and later signs of meningeal irritation.

An intramedullary hemorrhage may also occur with vascular malformations or in patients with clotting defects. There is sudden paraplegia and other signs, with or without back pain.

Management. Both subarachnoid and intramedullary hemorrhage present difficulties in management. In subarachnoid hemorrhage, myelography is performed after stabilization. Some malformations are readily apparent; prone and supine films should be taken. Aortography with selective injection of appropriate segmental vessels is often needed. Depending on the anatomy of the malformation and the neurologic status, surgery is indicated in selected cases.

Intramedullary hemorrhage may produce a central cord syndrome with extensive damage over several segments. On myelography there is fusiform swelling of the cord, with or without block. The role of surgery is uncertain in these cases, which fortunately are rare.

RADIATION MYELOPATHY

Two forms of radiation effect on the spinal cord can present acutely. An "early" delayed reaction may occur weeks or a few months after incidental irradiation of a normal spinal cord. Usually the cervical region is affected in patients with head or neck radiotherapy. Tingling or other sensory symptoms down the spine and into the lower limbs are noted, often related to neck flexion and similar to so-called Lhermitte's phenomenon or syndrome. The condition is transient and benign, symptoms disappearing in weeks. It is presumably due to demyelination.

A late delayed reaction occurs in six to 18 months in patients who have usually received radiation for various intrathoracic malignancies. This usually presents as an incomplete hemicord syndrome with ipsilateral weakness and contralateral sensory loss. There is painless, progressive dysfunction over many months. The primary cause is thought to be vascular with degenerative and obliterative changes in blood vessels and occlusion, edema, demyelination, and coagulative necrosis.

Diagnosis requires that the spinal cord must have been included in the area irradiated, the main lesion must be within segments previously irradiated, and myelography and CSF examination must be performed to exclude other causes, such as cord compression from metastasis. In early cases the spinal cord may be slightly enlarged but subarachnoid block is rare. In late cases there may be localized atrophy in affected segments. An MRI of the spine may also be useful. Autopsy may be necessary to exclude other rare causes.

Management. Patients with the transient syndrome are simply reassured and require no other specific treatment. Management of patients with the progressive form is controversial. The course is generally more chronic, and time and repeated examinations can help establish a diagnosis.

Specific Treatment. There is no proven specific treatment for radiation myelopathy. I generally use corticosteroids, either dexamethasone or prednisone in conventional doses for two to six weeks.

CERVICAL SPONDYLOSIS WITH MYELOPATHY

Cervical spondylosis is a chronic degenerative disorder of the intervertebral discs and vertebral spine with compression of nerve roots and spinal cord. Occasionally it presents as an acute syndrome following a flexion-extension neck injury in a patient who may or may not have had previous symptoms.

Initially there is deterioration and bulging of intervertebral discs followed by fibrosis of ligaments, hypertropy of bone, and finally a series of bony ridges with narrowing of the intervertebral foramina and spinal canal. Mechanical compression may be associated with secondary vascular compromise; some patients present with a relatively pure anterior cord syndrome from occlusion of the anterior spinal artery.

Patients complain of a combination of nerve root and spinal cord symptoms and usually have a mixed picture with radiculopathy and myelopathy. Progression can be gradual or abrupt and stepwise.

Management. Most patients can be evaluated as outpatients with spine x-rays, electromyography, and eventually myelography. Differential diagnosis should include amyotrophic lateral sclerosis, spinal cord tumor, multiple sclerosis, and combined system degeneration.

In acute cases patients should be hospitalized for further observation, immobilization in a neck brace or collar, and additional evaluation. I usually treat patients who have mild to moderate radiculopathy conservatively with rest and gentle cervical traction. Those with significant or progressive myelopathy are considered for surgery, primarily to prevent further progression. Postoperatively, they usually require an additional period of rehabilitation, with an emphasis on gait training.

ELECTRICAL MYELOPATHY

Myelopathy due to the passage of lightning or high-voltage electric current is one of the most dramatic acute spinal cord syndromes. The risk is said to be greatest if the current passes longitudinally from head to foot, as frequently occurs with a direct lightning strike. Pathologically, there is edema, necrosis, hemorrhage, and vascular occlusion.

Respiratory and cardiac arrest is the primary risk to life. A variety of cord syndromes have been reported, including transient flaccid paraplegia, immediate and persistent paraplegia, and a delayed diffuse myelopathy with both anterior horn cell and long tract deficits.

Management. Patients may require cardiopulmonary resuscitation at the site of injury. In the hospital, general supportive measures as well as corticosteroids for possible edema are indicated. Many patients make a satisfactory recovery.

ACUTE TOXIC MYELOPATHY

Fortunately, spinal cord syndromes due to subarachnoid or intravascular administration of various agents are now rare. In the past, aortography utilizing sodium acetrizoate or other agents, spinal anesthesia, myelography with radioactive thorium dioxide, and intrathecal phenol, alcohol, and penicillin have all been associated with an acute myelopathic process or adhesive arachnoiditis.

Intrathecal methotrexate and cytosine arabinoside, as well as other agents, have been associated with an acute or a delayed myelopathy. Possible mechanisms include a direct toxicity of the drug or a metabolite, drug kinetic and distribution factors associated with leptomeningeal tumor, or toxicity of a diluent or preservative used with the drug. In addition, rare cases of a more diffuse encephalomyelopathy, coma, and death have been reported after accidental overdosage with some of these agents.

Management. Such complications are much easier to prevent than to treat. Intrathecal drugs should be administered only by experienced personnel, and the preparations of such agents should be rigorously controlled. Preservative-containing drugs or diluents should not be given intrathecally. Instead, a CSF substitute such as Elliott's B solution, Ringer's lactate, saline, or the patient's own spinal fluid should be used.

Specific Treatment. Any intrathecal injection should be immediately discontinued if the patient complains of symptoms during the procedure. Persistent minor symptoms can be observed. Corticosteroids may be considered for more serious reactions.

If it is determined that a dosage error has been made, an emergency regimen should be instituted. A repeat lumbar puncture should be performed and all CSF allowed to drain by gravity. A spinal washout is then performed as rapidly as possible, using the same needle or with a second needle placed in the cisterna magna, with Elliott's B or some other physiologic solution. If methotrexate has been given, leucovorin can be added to the solution or given intravenously. Corticosteroids and other supportive measures should also be instituted.

REFERENCES

Dinapoli RP, Cascino TL: Intraspinal neoplasms. *In* Spittell JA (ed): Clinical Medicine. Harper & Row, Philadelphia, 1984, pp 1–9.

Hahn AF, Feasly TE, Gilbert JJ: Paraparesis following intrathecal chemotherapy. Neurology 33:1032–1038, 1983.

Hogan EL, Dale AJD: Disorders of the spinal cord. *In* Spittell JA (ed): Clinical Medicine. Harper & Row, Philadelphia, 1984, pp 1–36.

Johnson RT: Current Therapy in Neurologic Disease. B.B. Decker, Philadelphia, 1985.

Ropper AH, Poskanzer DC: The prognosis of acute and subacute transverse myelopathy based on early signs and symptoms. Ann Neurol 4:51–59, 1978.

19 · *MOTOR NEURON DISEASE*

Hiroshi Mitsumoto
CLEVELAND CLINIC FOUNDATION

DEFINITION

In discussing motor neuron diseases (MND) in adults we must focus on amyotrophic lateral sclerosis (ALS), often called Lou Gehrig's disease by lay persons, which recently has received special public attention because of its devastating impact on suffering patients and their families. The condition of advanced ALS is often described as "living death." Despite vigorous research, the cause is still unknown, and thus no specific treatment is available. It should be remembered that we often use MND synonymously with ALS either when the clinical features in the early stages do not meet the strict criteria for the diagnosis of ALS or when the disease is somewhat atyical. The diagnosis of ALS should be made when (1) upper and lower motor neurons are affected in a widespread distribution (occasionally either upper or lower motor neuron involvement may predominate the clinical features in the early stages); (2) the course is progressive; and (3) no sensory, autonomic, ocular, or intellectual impairment is present.

PATHOPHYSIOLOGY

Neuronal degeneration develops in upper and lower motor neurons and results in a progressive diminution in number of these cells. Loss of lower motor neuron function is manifested by muscle fiber atrophy due to denervation, which is detected by clinical examination, electromyography (EMG), and muscle biopsy. Partial denervation in muscles may lead to reinnervation of once-denervated muscle fibers by remaining neurons, which is expressed by the presence of high-amplitude polyphasic motor unit potentials in the EMG, an increased fiber density in the single-fiber EMG (SFEMG), and muscle fiber type grouping on muscle biopsy. Some muscle fibers have unstable neuromuscular transmission, which may cause excessive fatigue in patients. The pathophysiology of the fasciculations and muscle cramps that frequently occur in ALS is not well understood. Spasticity, hyperreflexia, and extensor plantar responses are results of upper motor neuron involvement.

CLINICAL ASPECTS

Weakness, atrophy, fasciculations, and spasticity are the major clinical signs. Contractures may develop in muscles that are not sufficiently mobilized. Two thirds of the patients have both upper and lower motor neuron involvement, and 10% have mainly lower motor neuron disease. Twenty-five per cent of the patients have so-called bulbar ALS, or weakness restricted to muscles innervated by nonocular lower cranial nerves. The presence of spasticity or hyperreflexia, or both, in severely weak and atrophied muscles is unusual in conditions other than ALS.

The clinical features of ALS allow most physicians to reach the correct diagnosis with remarkable uniformity, particularly when the disease is well developed. However, in the early stages the clinical presentation may be confusing: motor paralysis can predominantly involve the upper or lower motor neurons for some time before the fully developed disease appears. Sometimes weakness starts on only one side. In a minority of patients, weakness and atrophy begin in the distribution of a main peripheral nerve. In such instances the diagnosis of ALS can be difficult, requiring further observation of the patient. Neck extensor muscle weakness, resulting in a so-called hangman posture, is not unusual in ALS. Dysarthria can be flaccid or spastic or, more commonly, a combined form, but forced crying and laughing are not very common. Dysphagia often begins with difficulty swallowing liquids. Drooling saliva is a bothersome complaint with dysphagia. Respiratory muscle weakness develops with increased frequency of sighing, exertional dyspnea, and preference for the semi-upright posture during sleep.

In advanced stages a weak cough, visible accessory respiratory muscle contraction, and paradoxical respiration ensue. Muscle spasms and cramps are very common complaints and often precede muscle weakness. The majority of patients do not complain of fasciculations, and fasciculations have never been reported to be the chief complaint in ALS. On rare occasions, however, muscle cramps and fasciculations become prominent. Almost always, the sensory system is spared in ALS. Dementia is not a component of ALS itself but may occur if Alzheimer's disease is also present. In 5% to 10% of patients with ALS, an autosomal dominant inheritance is found.

MANAGEMENT

GENERAL PLAN

The course of the illness is usually predictable. Facing a highly publicized, devastating disease, we must offer careful diagnostic evaluation to exclude all possible treatable conditions. Furthermore, we should focus on evaluating the degree of functional impairment in respiration, speech, and swallowing. Our long-term plan should provide comprehensive care with emotional and physical support. Maintaining a patient's personal independence and comfort in social activities is important to his or her well-being. Most of the care should be maintained at home with family support, visiting nurses, or other health care personnel.

NONPHARMACOLOGIC MEASURES

For loss of motor function, effective devices and equipment, including an electric wheelchair, should be acquired. Preventing falls is important. Lack of joint motion often precipitates painful disuse arthropathy. Range-of-motion exercises should be performed every day. The beneficial effect of active exercise on weakened muscles has not been established. Nevertheless, patients doing mild but active exercise appear to function better than those not doing exercises.

Speech Therapy. Careful evaluation with instruction in the use of residual function improves early dysarthria. We have found that teamwork with speech therapists who have an interest in ALS helps patients greatly. We have achieved temporary improvement of speech function following vocal cord Teflon injection or a palatal prosthesis. In advanced stages, use of an alphabet board, a computer, or other communicators should be tried. Inability to express oneself can be a major cause of depression, and early supportive care is extremely important.

Nutrition. In the early stages of dysphagia, blending already cooked food and changing food into a semiliquid form can be helpful. We have had only limited success with cricopharyngeal myotomy. Progressive weight loss, choking, and radiologic evidence of aspiration suggest the need for a feeding tube, but a nasopharyngeal tube should be avoided because of aspiration.

We prefer jejunostomy over gastrostomy because of the low frequency of regurgitation and reflux into the esophagus with jejunostomy. Again, this requires close teamwork with a designated general surgeon and a specially trained nutritionist.

Respiratory Failure. Patients should receive influenza and pneumonia vaccinations. I would not hesitate to give antibiotics, such as tetracycline HCl, 500 mg q.i.d. or erythromycin, 500 mg q.i.d., to empirically treat upper respiratory infections. Spirometry and maximum negative inspiratory force measurement (diaphragmatic strength) can provide objective data to monitor the patient's respiratory status. A blow bottle should be tried in the early stages, but with progressive respiratory failure IPPB with room air should be given.

Whether to use chronic respirator care or not is a major decision for the patient, but we can provide our own advice. Complete understanding by the patient and family of what will be involved is crucial to the success of long-term respirator care. Our respirator team evaluates the patient's respiratory function and discusses this in detail with the patient and family. It should be clearly understood that a major effort is generally required by the family and that management problems occur after chronic respirator care is started. Generally speaking, patients with ALS limited to the bulbar and respiratory muscles do better with chronic respirator care than do those who have generalized weakness.

DRUG THERAPY

Drug therapy is used for symptomatic relief. Tricyclic antidepressants, such as doxepin (Sinequan) or amitriptyline (Elavil), help to elevate the patient's mood and also help to diminish drooling by their anticholinergic effect. Usually a small dose of 10 or 25 mg at bedtime is used, with increasing dose increments if the patient can tolerate them. These medications are also effective for pseudobulbar symptoms. For spasticity we try baclofen (Lioresal), 10 mg t.i.d., occasionally increasing the dosage to 20 mg t.i.d.; alternatively, diazepam (Valium), 2 mg to 5 mg t.i.d. can be used to decrease spasticity, but drowsiness and fatigue are major side effects. Unfortunately, these drugs are not very helpful. Muscle cramps and pains are often quite bothersome; quinine sulfate, 5 grains before bedtime, may decrease nocturnal cramps. On rare occasions patients have rather profound fasciculations and cramps, which may respond to carbamazepine (Tegretol), 200 mg t.i.d. to q.i.d. Often patients complain of arthralgia and pain from contractures, for which appropriate analgesics may be prescribed. In cases of excessive drooling, atropine sulfate, 0.4 mg b.i.d. to t.i.d. can be tried, but decreased secretions in the bronchial tree may facilitate bronchial infection.

In recent years, experimental drugs such as antiviral agents, interferon, and gangliosides have been tried without beneficial effects. Plasmapheresis also has had no therapeutic effects. We have investigated thyrotropin-releasing hormone (TRH) but it had no beneficial effects.

PATIENT INFORMATION AND EDUCATION

Generally, the discussion of the diagnosis of ALS requires empathy and thoughtful consideration. Sometimes the diagnosis may be overwhelming to the patient. Some do not accept the diagnosis and actually deny it, but one should allow time for the patient to accept the diagnosis. Actually, the time spent in careful diagnostic and laboratory evaluation is sometimes helpful to patients. Literature and brochures about ALS from national organizations such as the National Institutes of Health, the ALS Association, and the Muscular Dystrophy Association are useful. When we discuss the prognosis we should emphasize the positive facts—that 10% of patients live more than 10 years and that a few live more than 20 years. One should have a firm belief that "incurable" is not synonymous with "nontreatable." Continuing discussion and emotional ventilation are quite supportive to the patient and the family. A group meeting composed of the patients and families can provide helpful communication and a positive attitude toward the disease.

At some point in the disease course, before significant dysphagia and respiratory distress begin, we must openly discuss with the patient and family the matters of tube feeding and chronic respirator care. If the patient decides not to be placed on a respirator, he or she might prepare a living will that states this decision. Without such a living will and/or a clear statement in the chart by the physician, signed by the patient (if able to sign), and witnessed by the family and a third party, the patient might receive full life-supportive care against his or her wishes in an emergency situation.

Dr. Hershel Goren, Cleveland Clinic Foundation, reviewed this manuscript and offered valuable advice.

REFERENCES

Brooke MH: A Clinician's View of Neuromuscular Diseases. The Williams & Wilkins Co, Baltimore, 1977.

Mitsumoto H, Munsat TL: Problem of nerve and muscle. *In* Kaye D, Rose LF (eds): Fundamentals of Internal Medicine. C.V. Mosby Co, St. Louis, 1983, pp 1169–1178.

Mulder DW (ed): The Diagnosis and Treatment of Amyotrophic Sclerosis. Houghton Mifflin Professional Publisher, Boston, 1979.

Mulder DW: Motor neuron disease. *In* Dyck et al (eds): Peripheral Neuropathy. W.B. Saunders Co, Philadelphia, 1984, pp 1525–1536.

Rowland LP: Human Motor Neuron Diseases. Raven Press, New York, 1982.

Sivak ED, Gipson WT, Hanson MR: Longterm management of respiratory failure in amyotrophic lateral sclerosis. Ann Neurol 12:18–23, 1982.

20 · PERIPHERAL NEUROPATHY

Kerry H. Levin
Asa J. Wilbourn
CLEVELAND CLINIC FOUNDATION

The peripheral nervous system includes, for motor fibers, the territory between the anterior horn cell and the neuromuscular junction, and for sensory fibers, the territory between the dorsal root ganglion cell and the terminal cutaneous receptor. However, by convention, only the portions of the nerve fibers that originate from the plexuses, or more distally, are designated peripheral nerves. There are a great many peripheral nerve disorders, each with its specific location for damage along the peripheral nerve axis, each with its specific pattern of involvement, and many with pathogenesis and potential treatment yet unknown. This chapter will concentrate on the most common and treatable peripheral nerve disorders, with greatest emphasis placed on their management.

DIAGNOSTIC CRITERIA

Peripheral nerve disorders of different etiology may appear similar on physical examination. The electromyogram (EMG) is helpful in defining the nature of peripheral nerve damage. Nerve conduction studies give information about the integrity of sensory and motor nerves, can often localize focal lesions, and can distinguish degeneration of axons from primary degeneration of the myelin sheath. The needle examination detects minimal motor axon degeneration and provides information about the chronicity of the process as well as its extent. With acute nerve lesions, although the clinical deficit is maximal at onset, the onset of EMG changes is delayed for varying periods of time. The conduction studies are maximally abnormal after the tenth day, while at least three weeks are required before the needle examination abnormalities are clearly defined.

The routine laboratory work-up is summarized in Table 1.

Peripheral nerve disorders can be distinguished based upon their pathology and their mechanisms of injury. From a clinical point of view, some distinction can also be made based on rapidity of onset and progression. Acute peripheral polyneuropathies, those developing over days to weeks, include the acute inflammatory polyradiculoneuropathies (Guillain-Barré syndrome), porphyric neuropathy, acute compressive neuropathies ("Saturday-night palsy," crossed-leg palsy), and neuropathies due to nerve trunk infarction

Table 1. BASIC WORK-UP OF PERIPHERAL NEUROPATHY

Blood tests	CBC
	Sedimentation rate
	Liver function tests
	BUN, creatinine
	Serum protein electrophoresis and immunoelectrophoresis
	Fasting serum glucose (consider tolerance test)
	Vitamin B_{12}
	Folate
	Thyroid function tests
Urine	Routine urinalysis
	24-hour urine collection for arsenic, lead, mercury, thallium
EMG	Nerve conduction studies and needle examination
In special cases	Selected tissue analysis for heavy metals (hair, nails)
	Porphyrin screen
	CSF analysis for cells, protein, glucose
	Spine and long bone radiographs (consider CT scan in cases of progressive localized nerve damage)

(mononeuropathy multiplex). Although most peripheral polyneuropathies secondary to chronic toxic (environmental) exposures occur subacutely (over weeks to months), certain metal exposures (gold, thallium, mercury, arsenic) and other massive acute exposures can produce neuropathy acutely. Other subacutely developing neuropathies include the metabolic neuropathies (uremia, vitamin deficiency, diabetes, hypervitaminosis B_6). Finally, chronic neuropathies that develop over years are, in general, genetically determined (Charcot-Marie-Tooth disease, Déjérine-Sottas disease, Friedreich's ataxia, Fabry's disease), although some acquired metabolic neuropathies tend to progress very slowly over years (amyloid neuropathy, diabetic peripheral neuropathy, vitamin B_{12} deficiency).

THE METABOLIC NEUROPATHIES

The metabolic neuropathies occur because of some change in the general metabolic homeostasis of the body: hormonal deficiency (hypothyroidism), vitamin or nutritional deficiency (B_{12}, thiamine), enzymatic deficiency (porphyria), or waste product excess (uremia). Although the precise mechanism of nerve injury is not known, it is thought that dysfunction occurs in the axon transport of cell body products to the periphery. From the resulting biochemical injuries, abnormal energy metabolism and disassembly of the axonal cytoskeleton occur, with more severe effects felt at the distal-most portions of peripheral nerves. This scenario gives rise to what is defined clinically and histopathologically as distal ("dying-back") axonopathy. While some metabolic neuropathies manifest themselves in a single way (distal axonopathy), other disorders (diabetes, uremia) are associated with multiple types of nerve pathology.

DIABETIC NEUROPATHIES

Diabetic neuropathies make up the majority of all acquired peripheral neuropathies in the United States. Diabetic neuropathies fall into several categories: generalized distal axonopathies (diabetic polyneuropathy), single or multiple mononeuropathies, and polyradiculopathies.

Diabetic Polyneuropathies. Clinically, these disorders may be primarily sensory, sensorimotor, or autonomic. There may be mild EMG evidence of the disorder at the clinical onset of diabetes, without specific neuropathic symptoms. Diabetic polyneuropathies often present as tingling numbness in the feet, later extending to the hands. These neuropathies may produce uncomfortable positive symptoms, such as burning or "pins and needles." On examination, the findings are typically rather minimal: reduced deep tendon reflexes, especially at the ankles, and blunted vibratory and pin sensation distally. These patients may develop a more severe sensorimotor neuropathy, in which all sensory modalities are affected and there is evidence of weakness and wasting in intrinsic muscles of the feet, and later, in the hands. A concurrent small-fiber, or autonomic, neuropathy may develop, most commonly manifesting as bowel and sexual dysfunction. Sweating, pupillary, and cardiovascular changes may also appear. It is uncommon for these diabetic "autonomic" neuropathies to occur in isolation, but sometimes they do so in young diabetics.

There is no known, definitely proven treatment for diabetic distal polyneuropathy, although there is mounting evidence that tight serum glucose control can prevent the onset and favorably modify the symptoms. The deleterious effect of prolonged elevated blood glucose levels on peripheral nerves is now well appreciated. Management goals include pain control and prevention of pressure damage to feet due to poor sensory feedback.

Anticonvulsants such as carbamazepine and phenytoin may relieve symptoms because of their ability to stabilize nerve membranes. Carbamazepine should be started slowly because of initial complaints of abdominal upset and dizziness. A beginning dose of 100 mg twice daily can be augmented weekly to as much as 1 gm per day, if well tolerated. Some clinicians use amytriptyline. This drug may have a twofold usefulness: as an analgesic and as an antidepressant. Dosage should begin slowly, at 50 mg once or twice daily, and can be increased on a biweekly basis to 150 to 200 mg daily. As steady-state blood levels are not reached for several weeks, at least a one-month trial is necessary before any benefit can be expected. Vitamin therapy has not been found useful. In our experience, most diabetic polyneuropathies eventually reach a stage of quiescence, during which the process becomes static and some symptoms may even subside.

Diabetic Mononeuropathies. These conditions include commonly occurring entrapments such as carpal tunnel syndrome, ulnar neuropathy at the elbow, radial neuropathy at the spiral groove, and peroneal neuropathy at the knee, all of which are discussed under entrapment neuropathies. They also include abrupt-onset, single or multiple mononeuropathies caused by nerve infarction.

Diabetic Polyradiculopathies. Finally, diabetes can cause multiple radiculopathies (diabetic polyradiculopathies). These most often affect the high lumbar or thoracic roots, resulting in diabetic amyotrophy and diabetic thoracic radiculopathy, respectively. Diabetic amyotrophy usually affects the elderly and presents as back and thigh pain, often accentuated nocturnally. It is accompanied by unilateral or bilateral weakness of the hip flexors and anteromedial thigh muscles, sometimes with wasting of the anterior thigh muscles. It can be mistaken for femoral mononeuropathy, but the EMG examination invariably demonstrates that the process is more widespread. Many patients with bilateral diabetic amyotrophy have a concurrent polyneuropathy and often appear chronically ill, with significant weight loss.

As with diabetic polyneuropathy, there is no specific treatment for the multiple mononeuropathies of diabetic origin. Although isolated entrapment neuropathies may require surgical intervention in nondiabetics, in diabetics an apparent entrapment neuropathy must initiate a search for the possible presence of an underlying polyneuropathy. Hence, during the EMG examination of diabetic patients it is critical to evaluate more than the nerve in question; study should be made of other nerves of the same extremity, nerves of the opposite extremity, and distal nerves of the leg to exclude a distal polyneuropathy. In our experience, what may at first have appeared as an isolated entrapment mononeuropathy may really be a focal manifestation of a generalized polyneuropathy or a nonlocalizable mononeuropathy due to infarct. In diabetics with a severe, localized entrapment neuropathy, however, even in the presence of a mild underlying generalized polyneuropathy, surgical intervention may be necessary.

When confronted with a diabetic patient with thoracic or lumbar polyradiculopathy, proper management requires definitive diagnosis. In relatively few patients will the EMG and clinical examination specify the diabetic nature of the abnormality. In all other cases, other causes must be excluded. Depending on the severity and tempo of the disorder, lumbosacral spine films, myelography, CT scan of the pelvis, and CSF analysis (including cytology) may be necessary to exclude more ominous, or treatable, diagnoses. In some cases the pain associated with diabetic amyotrophy may be controlled by phenytoin or carbamazepine.

OTHER METABOLIC NEUROPATHIES

Deficiencies in vitamins B_1, B_6, and B_{12}, pantothenic acid, and vitamin E can cause peripheral polyneuropathy. Deficiencies of vitamin B_1 and pantothenic acid are found in patients with poor nutritional status. Deficiencies of vitamins B_{12} and E occur primarily because of malfunction of their respective absorption mechanisms. Deficiencies in these vitamins cause widespread damage in the central as well as the peripheral nervous systems. The peripheral neuropathy of vitamins B_1 and B_6 appears to be primarily a smaller-fiber distal polyneuropathy, whereas vitamin B_{12} and E deficiencies lead to severe large-fiber sensory loss, characterized by proprioception and vibration loss, loss of deep tendon reflexes, and accompanying ataxia. Vitamin B_6 deficiency is almost always associated with concurrent use of isoniazid or hydralazine and can be prevented by prophylactic oral B_6 supplementation of 50 mg daily. Depending upon the severity of the polyneuropathy, remarkable improvement is possible with nutritional therapy and vitamin replacement. Recently it has been appreciated that excessive consumption of vitamin B_6 (currently popularized as a perimenstrual diuretic) can lead to a severe large-fiber sensory polyneuropathy. As little as several hundred mg per day over prolonged periods can lead to this disorder, which responds well to discontinuance of the supplement.

TOXIC NEUROPATHIES

Toxic polyneuropathies can be the result of industrial exposure, pharmaceutical toxicity, or criminal intent. Most occur subacutely, but at times they can present with alarming rapidity. Although most toxins produce distal axonal degeneration, manifested by distal extremity symptoms and signs, some may begin by demyelination and produce a chemical picture like that of Guillain-Barré syndrome (GBS). Unless specifically questioned about toxic or drug exposure, patients may not offer this critical diagnostic information. Most toxic neuropathies do not occur in isolation; signs of multiple organ system involvement are usually associated.

METALS

Those metals most commonly associated with nerve toxicity are arsenic, lead, mercury, thallium, gold, and platinum. Arsenic polyneuropathy is the most common type of metal neuropathy encountered. It usually presents as a slowly progressive symmetric sensory and, later, motor distal neuropathy. With single large-dose exposure, a rapidly progressive polyneuropathy, which can appear both clinically and electromyographically similar to GBS, can occur. Elemental mercury has been shown to produce both clinical and subclinical symmetric sensory and motor distal polyneuropathy. Gold and platinum have been used recently as therapeutic agents, producing multiple systemic toxic effects, one of which is peripheral neuropathy. Whereas gold can produce a relatively severe symmetric motor and sensory process, cisplatin tends to produce a more purely sensory abnormality; this has been corroborated by EMG studies. Gold has also been associated with a rapidly progressive polyneuropathy similar to GBS.

PHARMACEUTICALS

Most important among drugs that cause neuropathy are dapsone, disulfiram, hydralazine, isoniazid, nitrofurantoin, vincristine, and nitrous oxide. All these drugs produce a symmetric distal axonopathy involving sensory and motor fibers, although dapsone tends to produce more motor disability. Hydralazine and isoniazid appear to act by interference with vitamin B_6 (pyridoxine) metabolism. Although most of the polyneuropathies produced are mild, continued use of the drugs can produce devastating disability in some cases. Dentists can develop neuropathy from the long-term exposure to nitrous oxide, as can those who abuse this drug for euphoria. Fortunately, in general, discontinuance of the drug in question usually produces significant improvement over months to years.

INDUSTRIAL TOXINS

The most frequently incriminated toxins in this group include acrylamide (grouting materials), hexacarbons (solvents for lacquers and glues), and organophosphates (insecticides, petroleum additives, and plastics additives). Prominent sensory and motor signs may develop rapidly after exposure in the case of some toxins (organophosphates). Reversal of the damage occurs after discontinuance of exposure (although with hexacarbons, worsening can proceed for up to four months), and the degree of recovery depends upon the amount of neurogenic damage that was produced.

MONONEUROPATHY MULTIPLEX

Damage can occur to single large nerve trunks, usually owing to entrapment or compression (see further on), but involvement of multiple nerve trunks can also occur and is usually the manifestation of systemic disease. Disorders that may lead to multiple entrapment neuropathies include diabetes, rheumatoid arthritis, hypothyroidism, acromegaly, alcoholism/malnutrition, amyloidosis, renal failure, and gout. Other disorders can cause localized infarction or conduction block of major nerve trunks in a sporadic, asymmetric fashion. The clinical picture in these cases can be misconstrued as multiple entrapment neuropathies. Examples include vasculitides (polyarteritis nodosa, Churg-Strauss syndrome, sulfonamide and amphetamine drug reactions), inflammatory demyelinating polyneuropathies, acute idiopathic brachial neuritis/mononeuropathies, and infectious disorders such as leprosy and Lyme arthritis.

Although all the foregoing disorders can lead to multiple mononeuropathies, in common medical parlance "mononeuritis" multiplex suggests an inflammatory or vasculitic etiology, classically polyarteritis nodosa. In some cases these patients have clinically obvious systemic disease, but in others the neuropathy is the major clue. EMG examination can define the multifocal nature of the condition and can sometimes direct the clinician to a specific nerve or muscle for biopsy diagnosis. Although treatment depends upon the pathologic diagnosis and extent of organ system involvement, it usually begins with prednisone. Cytotoxic therapy, such as with cyclophosphamide, methotrexate, or nitrogen mustard, may be required.

ENTRAPMENT AND COMPRESSION NEUROPATHIES

In this section we will discuss only the most common entrapment syndromes. As mentioned earlier, although in most cases entrapments occur singly, and secondary to long-standing local trauma, they may be a manifestation of systemic disease.

MEDIAN NEUROPATHIES

Median neuropathy at the wrist, or carpal tunnel syndrome (CTS), is the most common entrapment mononeuropathy. Symptoms most frequently mentioned include intermittent hand and finger numbness (all five fingers in some patients), sometimes accompanied by a deep toothache-like forearm pain. Classically the symptoms are worst during activity that increases the pressure within the carpal tunnel: holding a newspaper, driving, typing, playing the piano. Patients often awaken at night with the symptoms and try to "shake out" the numbness in the hand. CTS is diagnosed much earlier now and often without any objective evidence of sensory or motor dysfunction. Nerve conduction studies, especially palmar sensory conductions in the hand, can identify almost all the entrapment neuropathies.

Mild to moderate CTS can be treated conservatively with cock-up wrist splints and, if necessary, local corticosteroid injections. More common systemic disorders should be excluded during the work-up. If the EMG shows significant axon loss, or if the symptoms and EMG findings progress despite conservative treatment, surgical section of the carpal retinaculum is necessary. This surgery is simple to perform and has a high cure rate.

ULNAR NEUROPATHIES

Ulnar entrapment neuropathies usually occur at the elbow, at one of two locations. At the ulnar groove (formed by the medial epicondyle and olecranon process), the nerve can undergo slowly progressive compression caused by remote fracture of the medial epicondyle (tardy ulnar palsy) or by displacement of the ulnar nerve from a congenitally shallow groove. At the cubital tunnel (just below the elbow, where the nerve pierces the fascial plane between the two heads of the flexor carpi ulnaris), the nerve can undergo chronic local trauma. These ulnar mononeuropathies usually present with sensory complaints in the ulnar hand distribution (medial half of the fourth and the entire fifth digit), sometimes accompanied by interosseous and hypothenar wasting.

Conservative therapy for ulnar neuropathies should always be considered initially, because surgery at the elbow is seldom curative and can sometimes lead to disabling causalgia or severe ulnar impairment. The best surgical indication remains the detection, on EMG examination, of progressive axon loss of ulnar nerve fibers that can be localized to a single point of entrapment.

Ulnar nerve lesions in the hand are often mistaken for ulnar neuropathies at the elbow. They commonly present with pure motor dysfunction and may involve the lateral ulnar innervated hand muscles while sparing the hypothenar ones. When sensory fibers are involved, ulnar cutaneous function over the dorsum of the hand is spared because that branch leaves the main trunk before entering the wrist. Which nerve structures are involved depends upon where in the wrist (Guyon's canal) or palm the compression occurs. These lesions are most frequently caused by local chronic trauma (hand drills, prolonged gripping of bicycle handles, volleyball playing) or tumors. Treatment of traumatic lesions involves either abstinence from the offending activity or protection of the hand.

THORACIC OUTLET SYNDROME

Entrapment of the neurovascular bundle at any of several points at the base of the neck has been called thoracic outlet syndrome (TOS). Once called scalenus anticus syndrome, this entity was frequently considered the source of brachialgia in the past before clinical entities such as CTS and cervical radiculopathy were described. Today TOS should be diagnosed with extreme caution. Although many patients complain of nonspecific numbness of the arm or hand, a falling-asleep sensation, or pain when using the arm or elevating it, few have angiographic or blood-flow criteria for vascular TOS, and only rare patients have clinical or electrodiagnostic evidence of the so-called true neurogenic TOS. Patients with true neurogenic TOS have sensory loss or symptoms in the C8–T1 distribution along with weakness and atrophy in muscles innervated by the lower trunk of the brachial plexus, most severely the abductor pollicis brevis. Surgery to relieve compression of a neurogenic TOS is not indicated unless there is electrodiagnostic evidence of lower trunk damage.

RADIAL NEUROPATHIES

Most radial nerve lesions not associated with fracture occur at the spiral groove of the humerus. Many are caused by acute compression of the nerve between the groove and a solid surface, such as a chair or edge of a bed ("Saturday-night palsy," "paralyse des amoureux—lovers' palsy"). Other traumatic causes include spiral fractures of the humerus and injection injuries. In radial nerve entrapment at the spiral groove there is weakness of wrist and finger extensors, totally sparing triceps strength and usually sparing brachioradialis strength. Typically, with compressive lesions function returns spontaneously, often after a relatively brief period, because the lesion is primarily demyelinating in nature (conduction blocks). In contrast, lesions associated with fractures and injections are usually axon-loss in type, and recovery is slow and often imperfect. Prognosis can be predicted based on EMG evidence of degree of axon loss performed at least one month after injury.

PERONEAL NEUROPATHIES

Almost all clinically important peroneal entrapments occur at the fibular head. This is especially common among chronic leg-crossers and bedridden patients who have lost weight and as a surgical complication of positioning and strapping onto the operating table. Although a few lesions are severe and never improve, most return to good function in two to 12 months. A foot drop brace may be helpful during this recovery period. The best treatment is protection of the nerve from additional trauma. Special precautionary care should be given any bedfast patient, using knee pads and proper positioning. Similar to radial lesions, peroneal mononeuropathies are usually caused by either axon loss or focal demyelination (producing conduction block). EMG can assist in defining the nature and hence the prognosis of the lesions.

ACUTE INFLAMMATORY DEMYELINATING POLYRADICULONEUROPATHY

Of the inflammatory neuropathies, the most common and most important is acute inflammatory demyelinating polyradiculoneuropathy, more commonly known as Guillain-Barré syndrome (GBS). This is a presumed autoimmune disorder, in which half of those affected have had a recent viral (CMV, EBV, influenza) infection, vaccination, or surgery. Others at risk for GBS include those with disorders of immune compromise: Hodgkin's disease, lupus erythematosus, or renal transplantation.

GBS is the most common cause of rapidly progressing weakness, and it is one of the few peripheral nerve emergencies. It is most important to recognize how subtly this condition can begin. Often the first symptoms are vague sensory complaints, such as distal paresthesias or a sense that something is crawling under the skin (formications). Symptoms of weakness begin with a sense of easy fatigability or lack of energy. To the physician many of these complaints may seem functional and are sometimes confused with hyperventilation.

These symptoms may smolder but may rapidly progess to severe weakness. On examination, the findings may be mild. Weakness may be predominantly proximal or distal and is sometimes more profound in the arms. Deep tendon reflexes are depressed or absent. Some patients develop cranial nerve involvement, with weakness of ocular, facial, or bulbar muscles.

The most worrisome developments include autonomic and respiratory dysfunction. Sympathetic and parasympathetic fluctuations lead to precipitous changes in blood pressure and heart rate. Arrhythmias may develop. Respiratory failure may develop slowly; many of these patients are young adults, with a large pulmonary reserve that will mask the progressive ventilatory impairment clinically until severe hypercapnia supervenes.

All patients with symptoms of recent onset should be admitted to an intensive care unit for careful monitoring of cardiovascular and respiratory function. Because blood gas abnormalities and deterioration of tidal volume are late findings, monitoring of forced vital capacity and negative inspiratory pressure is preferred and should be carried out every two to four hours. In most patients the condition stabilizes within two weeks, but careful monitoring may be necessary until improvement becomes apparent. During hospitalization, precautions should be taken against deep vein thrombosis, pulmonary embolism, and aspiration.

The diagnosis of GBS rests upon the clinical manifestations as well as the EMG evidence of demyelination along peripheral nerves. Cerebral spinal fluid (CSF) analysis classically shows elevation in protein without abnormal cell count. However, the CSF may remain normal for up to two weeks after onset of symptoms. GBS is a self-limited process, and 80% to 90% of patients have good or excellent recoveries.

Management. There is no specific treatment for GBS. Clinical trials with corticosteroids have failed to show statistically significant improvement in the time required for recovery. There is preliminary evidence that plasmapheresis may be of some help in shortening the disease course, when started within one week of clinical onset in severely affected patients. The foundation of treatment therefore remains careful monitoring and precautions during hospitalization, with rehabilitation and physical therapy during the posthospitalization recovery. Some patients develop recurrent bouts of demyelination with a chronic, slowly progressive course. Immunosuppressive drugs have been found to be helpful in these cases.

ANTICOAGULANT-RELATED PERIPHERAL NERVE COMPRESSION

Compartment syndromes from anticoagulant-associated hemorrhage are another type of peripheral nerve emergency. Examples include bleeding into the gluteal or posterior thigh compartment, leading to sciatic nerve infarction; and bleeding into forearm compartments, leading to median, ulnar, or radial nerve infarction. Infarction occurs secondary to compression of the nerve's blood supply from the rapid expansion of a hematoma in a closed space. Once neurologic symptoms develop, surgical decompression must be performed within four hours to preserve nerve function. Hemorrhage into the iliacus compartment, leading to acute, painful lumbar plexopathy or femoral neuropathy, can be treated with bed rest and correction of the bleeding diathesis. However, when a large psoas hematoma is found on CT scan of the pelvis, surgical decompression may be necessary. Suspicion of these compartment syndromes should be raised whenever an anticoagulated patient develops severe limb pain, swelling, and weakness, often associated wtih a drop in the hematocrit. CT scanning can confirm the clinical impression and guide surgical drainage. Persistence of the distal arterial pulses does not exclude a compartment syndrome, as the major arteries passing through the compartment maintain patency.

PERIPHERAL POLYNEUROPATHY ASSOCIATED WITH MALIGNANCY

These neuropathies can result from direct invasion of neoplastic cells into nervous tissue, remote humoral effects, and chemotherapeutic agents. Direct invasion of neoplastic cells into distal peripheral nerves is a rare cause of clinical neuropathy, but invasion into the meninges surrounding spinal nerves (i.e., the cauda equina) can cause devastating polyradiculopathies leading to paraplegia. Diagnosis can be made cytologically by analysis of cells collected by lumbar puncture. Intrathecal chemotherapy and sometimes local radiation therapy can arrest the process in some individuals.

Paraproteinemias associated with plasma cell dyscrasias, lymphomas, and leukemias have been associated with peripheral neuropathies; these paraproteins in the IgG and IgM classes have been found to bind with antigenic determinants on Schwann cells and axon membranes. Some patients have shown evidence of demyelinating neuropathy based on EMG; others have had clinical courses identical to that of GBS, perhaps because of an antecedent viral infection engendered by altered immune status. Several chemotherapeutic agents associated with polyneuropathy have been mentioned previously.

REFERENCES

American Association of Electromyography and Electrodiagnosis: Syllabus from Course B-1: Toxic Neuropathies, Seventh Annual Continuing Education Course, September 19, 1984, Kansas City, MO. Rochester, MN.

Brown WV, Greene DA: Diabetic neuropathy: Pathophysiology and management. *In* Asbury AK, Gilliatt RW (eds): Peripheral Nerve Disorders. Butterworths, London, 1984, pp 126–153.

Dawson DM, Hallett M, Millender LH: Entrapment Neuropathies. Little, Brown & Co, Boston, 1983.

Dyck PJ, Thomas PK, Lambert EH, et al: Peripheral Neuropathy. W.B. Saunders Co, Philadelphia, 1984.

Kimura J: Electrodiagnosis in Diseases of Nerve and Muscle: Principles and Practice. F.A. Davis Co, Philadelphia, 1983, pp 463–510.

Mubarak SJ, Hargens AR (eds): Compartment Syndromes and Volkmann's Contracture. W.B. Saunders Co, Philadelphia, 1981.

Pirart J: Diabetes mellitus and its degenerative complications: A prospective study of 4,400 cases observed between 1947 and 1973. Diabetes Care 1:168–188, 252–263, 1978.

21 · TREATMENT OF DISEASES AFFECTING NEUROMUSCULAR TRANSMISSION

Frank M. Howard, Jr.
MAYO CLINIC and MAYO FOUNDATION

Myasthenia Gravis

DEFINITIONS AND DIAGNOSTIC CRITERIA

Myasthenia gravis can cause weakness of any striated muscle, but it is the fluctuating degree of weakness that characterizes this illness.

CONGENITAL MYASTHENIA GRAVIS

The congenital form is rare and is suspected in patients who appear to have myasthenia gravis but do not have acetylcholine receptor antibodies (AChRab). Most patients have had a decremental response to 2-Hz stimulation. The onset is usually at birth, although the condition may not be recognized until later in life, and there is usually a family history of one or more similarly afflicted relatives. The patient does not respond to thymectomy, steroids, azathioprine, or plasma exchange, and minimal benefit is derived from anticholinesterase medication. The diagnosis requires a laboratory that can study muscle biopsy specimens. The specimens do not show immune complexes. Abnormalities identified include (1) defect in acetylcholine synthesis or storage, (2) deficiency of acetylcholinesterase at the junction, (3) prolonged open ion channel time, and (4) acetylcholine receptor deficiency.

AUTOIMMUNE MYASTHENIA GRAVIS

The vast majority of patients (>90%) have the autoimmune form of the disease, characterized by the presence of circulating AChRab. AChRab may be absent early during the course of the disease in patients with only ocular involvement or in those with disease in remission. The more severe the disease, the higher is the incidence of elevated antibodies. The most widely used assay determines *binding* antibodies. At my institution, the assay of human acetylcholine receptors is positive in 87% of patients with generalized disease, 63% with ocular myasthenia gravis, and 58% with disease in remission. Acetylcholine *blocking* antibodies are less often detected, but in 1% of patients these antibodies may be present when binding antibodies are not. The newest and most sensitive assay is for *modulating* antibodies, which requires cultured human skeletal muscle.

The antibody titer is not correlated with the severity of disease. Patients in remission, even for years, may have fairly high titers. If antibodies are not present, the possibility that myasthenia gravis is not the correct diagnosis should be considered.

False-positive test results are rare, but are seen when the patient has been treated with cobra venom or when the serum has been obtained during general anesthesia and muscle relaxants have been used. AChRab has been detected in patients with thymoma who show no clinical evidence of myasthenia gravis. These individuals may later experience overt myasthenia gravis. Antibodies are also found in patients with penicillamine-induced myasthenia gravis and have been noted in two patients with the Lambert-Eaton syndrome (see later).

ANTISTRIATIONAL ANTIBODIES

These antibodies are found in more than 90% of patients who have thymoma but may be present in 15% to 25% of those without it. Their presence is related to the age of the patient; antibodies are rarely found in young patients, and the frequency is increased in patients over 40 years of age. In addition, 25% of patients with a thymoma but without clinical evidence of myasthenia gravis may have antibodies. This figure of 25% may be artificially high because the symptoms of myasthenia may appear many years after a thymoma has been removed.

The presence of antistriational antibodies is an indication for computed tomography (CT) of the mediastinum. Unfortunately, CT has a notoriously high incidence of false-positive reports of thymoma.

TENSILON TESTING

Although this test is useful in suggesting the diagnosis, it may be misleading, since the increase in strength may result from an increased effort rather than from a pharmacologic effect. To avoid this, an initial intravenous injection of sterile saline is given. This injection is followed in 2 minutes by 0.2 ml (2 mg) of Tensilon (edrophonium chloride, 1.0 ml = 10 mg). If definite improvement occurs within 15 to 30 seconds after the second injection, the result is positive. If there is no improvement after a two-minute rest period, an additional 0.5 ml (5 mg) is injected and the strength again is tested. The increased strength usually lasts two to five minutes. False-negative results occur when the muscles are very weak and if too much Tensilon has been injected, resulting in a cholinergic block. For small children, 0.1 ml (1 mg) is used. I do not routinely premedicate my patients with atropine. I always exclude relatives during the test because of the potential side effects of nausea, palpitation, hypotension, and rarely syncope with a few clonic jerks and urinary incontinence. Resuscitation equipment should always be available.

ELECTROMYOGRAPHY AND NERVE CONDUCTION STUDIES

If the diagnosis of myasthenia gravis is suspected, regardless of the results of the Tensilon test, an electromyogram (EMG) should be ordered. A defect in neuromuscular transmission, manifested by a decline of more than 10% in the amplitude of the evoked muscle action potential to supramaximal stimulation of the nerve at slow rates of stimulation (2 to 3 Hz), is a positive result. If this defect is not present, a single-fiber needle electrode study is performed to check for increased jitter or blocking. This test is more sensitive than repetitive stimulation. If possible, patients should refrain from medication for 12 hours before these tests are given. Neither an EMG nor the single-fiber needle study is diagnostic. Myasthenia gravis is a clinical diagnosis.

In ocular myasthenia gravis, the Lancaster red-green test with Tensilon is very helpful in diagnosis.

PATHOPHYSIOLOGY

In normal neuromuscular transmission, a nerve impulse arriving in the terminal axon triggers the release of acetylcholine from the synaptic vesicles. Calcium has an important role in this incompletely understood release mechanism. The acetylcholine molecules diffuse across the primary synaptic cleft and bind to the acetylcholine receptors located on the crests of the postsynaptic muscle membrane. Each receptor has two receptor sites. Binding results in an opening of a central ion channel in the receptor. The ensuing ion exchange results in depolarization of the membrane and an end-plate potential. If a critical number of receptors are activated, the threshold is exceeded and the muscle contracts. The enzyme acetylcholinesterase in the synaptic cleft then lyses the acetylcholine molecule, terminating the reaction and allowing repolarization to occur.

Miniature end-plate potentials due to the random release of quanta of acetylcholine are reduced in amplitude in myasthenia gravis.

In autoimmune myasthenia gravis, the abnormality is a loss of receptor sites. As a result of the antibody-mediated autoimmune process, the postsynaptic membrane is destroyed. Some of the crests of the muscle folds are lost (the site of the receptors) and the primary synaptic cleft is widened. Immune complexes have been found on the postsynaptic membrane.

Experimental autoimmune myasthenia gravis may be produced in animals by the injection of purified receptor protein obtained from the electric eel or torpedo fish. The resulting disease is identical to human disease, differing only in a pronounced inflammatory response early during its course.

Myasthenia gravis can be induced in animals by passive transfer, using the serum or immunoglobulins from a human myasthenic patient or using monoclonal antibodies produced by a B-cell line from a myasthenic patient.

The thymus gland is abnormal in about 80% of patients with myasthenia gravis. About 15% have a thymoma and the remaining 65% have a hyperplastic gland with germinal follicles. There are also striated muscle fibers with acetylcholine receptors in the thymus. However, the role of the thymus in the development of myasthenia gravis is not known.

Young female patients under 40 years of age have an increased association of HLA-A1, HLA-B8, and HLA-DRw3 antigens. In male patients over 40 the association with HLA-A3, HLA-B7, and/or HLA-DRw2 has been reported. In patients with thymoma, no sex or HLA type predominates. From the clinical standpoint, HLA typing adds further expense and need not be obtained.

CLINICAL ASPECTS

The disease can begin at any age from birth to 90 or more years, and about one in 20,000 persons is afflicted. The incidence increases in women from puberty to 50 years of age and in men after the age of 50. The disease affects all races. In about 50% of patients, the initial symptoms are ptosis, diplopia, or both (Table 1). At some time during the disease, more than 90% of patients have these ocular symptoms.

In patients who present with ptosis and diplopia, in addition to weakness in other striated muscles, the disease is easily diagnosed. The three groups of patients

Table 1. INITIAL AND LATER SYMPTOMS REPORTED BY PATIENTS WITH ACQUIRED AUTOIMMUNE MYASTHENIA GRAVIS

Symptoms	Percentages*	
	With Initial Symptoms	*With Later Symptoms*
Ptosis and/or diplopia	54	94
Dysarthria	14	
Dysphagia	7	71
Facial weakness	6	
Difficulty with chewing	1	
Weakness of legs	10	
Weakness of arms	8	55
Weakness of neck	3	

*Many patients had more than one symptom.

whose diagnosis is most delayed are (1) adolescents whose main complaint is weakness of the extremities, (2) patients with largely ocular symptoms, and (3) older patients who present with bulbar symptoms of dysarthria and dysphagia. If no weakness is present on the regular examination, the extremities should be exercised (e.g., have the patient hold the arms or legs extended for at least two minutes). If the complaints are ocular, having the patient look up at a bright light for two minutes often produces ptosis and, less often, diplopia. In the third group, symptoms such as dysarthria and dysphagia are immediately apparent, and their abrupt appearance can lead to the erroneous diagnosis of a brain stem infarct.

Atrophy of muscles (in about 10% of patients) is most apparent in the muscles of mastication or of the neck, and needle electrode examination may reveal fibrillation potentials in these areas. Paretic nystagmoid jerks on lateral gaze should not be misinterpreted as internuclear ophthalmoplegia. The deep tendon reflexes are intact but may decrease in amplitude with repeated percussion. Although seldom mentioned, the sphincters may be affected, and the patient may complain of urinary and fecal incontinence. There are no objective sensory abnormalities, though patients may report peculiar sensations, most often a tightness around the mouth.

There are many problems in trying to separate the total population of patients into similar groups. In this regard the modified classification of Osserman and Genkins has been widely used: group I, ocular findings only (15% to 20%); group IIA, mild generalized disease (30%); group IIB, moderate generalized disease with bulbar symptoms (20%); group III, acute fulminating disease, rapid progression with severe bulbar involvement (10%); and group IV, late, severe disease, implying significant progression two years or more after onset (9%). Approximately one third of patients referred to my institution with a diagnosis of myasthenia gravis have a psychoneurotic illness.

Acute worsening, especially in the bulbar muscles, is referred to as crisis. Exacerbation due to infection or emotional upset or the failure to take pyridostigmine (Mestinon) is referred to as a myasthenic crisis. Increased weakness due to excessive anticholinesterase medication is a cholinergic crisis.

MANAGEMENT

After the initial symptoms appear, the disease may progress at a variable rate, although progression may be rapid. Generally, the disease reaches its maximum within two years, though infections and certain medications may produce an exacerbation in later years. Spontaneous remissions sometimes lasting for years do occur, most often within the first two years. The aim of treatment is to minimize disability and side effects. Treatment is designed to enhance neuromuscular transmission or alter the abnormal immune response.

GENERAL TREATMENT PHILOSOPHY

I almost always initiate treatment with anticholinesterase medication for one to three months. If patients cannot function without a significant handicap, I advise transsternal thymectomy unless they are older than 60 years. Above that age, the odds are great that the thymus is severely involuted and thymectomy is probably not beneficial, except for removal of a thymoma. Unless there are major medical contraindications, all patients with thymoma should undergo thymectomy, because the tumor is often invasive.

Older patients and those with a significant restriction after thymectomy are given prednisone. I try to avoid giving this agent to children. If prednisone fails, I use azathioprine and, very infrequently, cyclophosphamide. Plasma exchange is used in patients who have been on a respirator for more than 24 hours, in those with severe bulbar symptoms before thymectomy, or in those who have severe effects from steroids, in order to improve their condition until azathioprine can exert its effect while the dose of prednisone is being reduced. All patients undergoing plasma exchange should be given prednisone and/or azathioprine. All these forms of treatment have the potential for major side effects and death, and patients must agree to be reexamined and to undergo laboratory testing at appropriate intervals.

ANTICHOLINESTERASE MEDICATION

Anticholinesterases act by inhibiting the action of cholinesterase in the lysing of acetylcholine. Too much anticholinesterase will lead to a depolarization block, resulting in increasing weakness and a cholinergic crisis.

The most widely used anticholinesterase is pyridostigmine bromide (Mestinon, 60-mg tablets), with a duration of action of two to four hours. Treatment is started with a test dose of half a 60-mg tablet. If there are no side effects, the dose is increased to one tablet, given at approximately four-hour intervals. If the patient has trouble chewing or swallowing, the medication should be taken an hour before meals. The tablet can be crushed and placed in a teaspoonful of apple sauce for easier ingestion. Syrup of Mestinon (5 ml = 60 mg) is seldom required, except for young children. To avoid a cholinergic crisis, I never increase an individual dose by more than half a tablet (30 mg) at a time. There is very little benefit from using more than two tablets per dose. Some patients can take the medication when they notice weakness rather than on a fixed time schedule. In my opinion, the Tensilon test is widely overused to adjust the dosage of Mestinon.

I prescribe Mestinon Timespan (180 mg) to be taken only at bedtime to provide a sustained effect during the night. The rate of release is too unpredictable for this medication to be used during the day. For the rare patient who requires intramuscular medication, 2 mg of injectable Mestinon is equivalent to 60 mg by mouth. For intravenous use, 1.0 mg of prostigmine methylsulfate or 2 mg of Mestinon bromide can be taken.

Anticholinesterase medication should be kept in a tightly sealed container with an absorbent pad in the bottle. The shell of the Mestinon Timespan tablet may appear in the stool. There is little benefit in switching to other anticholinesterase medication, except for the very rare patient who gets a bromide rash, for whom ambenonium chloride (Mytelase) may be prescribed. To switch to Mytelase, begin with half a 10-mg tablet. Mestinon is excreted by the kidney, and patients with renal failure should be given only small doses.

Potential side effects of anticholinesterase medica-

**Table 2. UNWANTED EFFECTS OF
ANTICHOLINESTERASE MEDICATION
(CHOLINERGIC REACTIONS)**

Muscarinic Effects	Nicotinic Effects
On smooth muscle	On skeletal muscle
Epigastric discomfort	Fasciculations (twitching)
Abdominal cramps	Spasm
Anorexia	Weakness
Nausea	**CNS Effects**
Vomiting	Irritability
Diarrhea	Anxiety
Pupillary miosis	Insomnia
On glands	Unpleasant dreams
Increased salivation	Dysarthria
Cold, moist skin	Mental clouding
Increased lacrimation	Syncope
Increased bronchial secretion	Coma
	Convulsions

tion may be muscarinic or nicotinic (Table 2). The most ominous side effect is an increase in weakness one hour after the medication is taken, indicating overdose. With this complication, the patient must be carefully monitored and additional Mestinon withheld until the weakness subsides. Complications of the central nervous system rarely occur. The most troublesome complications usually are the muscarinic side effects on the gastrointestinal tract. In this situation, diphenoxylate (Lomotil) or atropine sulfate, gr. 1/150, may be helpful. For the patient bothered by fecal soiling, 15 mg of codeine sulfate can provide four carefree hours to enjoy athletic events, amusements, or long automobile trips. If bulbar signs are not a problem, the GI side effects are decreased when Mestinon is taken with a small snack.

In myasthenic patients, no drug is absolutely contraindicated if its use is essential. However, when any new medication is prescribed, patients should be carefully observed for signs of increasing weakness. Cephalosporin antibiotics, which have a blocking effect on the junction, belong in this category, erythromycin being the one most likely to cause problems. Local anesthetics and analgesics are safe to use. For severe pain, meperidine (Demerol) is the drug of choice. Antiarrhythmic drugs such as procainamide or quinidine, as well as calcium channel blockers, may increase the weakness. Sedatives, tranquilizers, and antidepressants can be used in low doses. Magnesium sulfate should be avoided if at all possible.

The vast majority (95%) of patients with myasthenia gravis need other treatment. I believe that before other potentially hazardous therapies are initiated, a defect in neuromuscular transmission, preferably an elevated titer of AChRab, should be demonstrated. The exception would be for patients with ocular myasthenia gravis who may not have AChRab and who generally respond well to relatively low doses of alternate-day prednisone. Mestinon is of very limited value for patients with ocular myasthenia gravis.

THYMECTOMY

Since there have never been any control studies, there is still controversy over the benefit of thymectomy and the extent and the timing of the operation. At present, no one knows how thymectomy causes improvement, except that it interferes with the immune system in some way.

Some institutions recommend immediate thymectomy at the time of diagnosis, but I prefer a brief trial of anticholinesterase therapy initially so that the patient and the family are aware of the limitations of this treatment and will more readily accept the gamble of an operation. Results at my institution have been remarkably consistent over the years, 40% of patients obtaining a prolonged remission, 40% being improved, and 20% being unchanged. Early surgery (within one year after diagnosis) results in a higher remission rate. There are no consistent guidelines for selection of the patient who is likely to be improved by thymectomy. I do not recommend thymectomy for patients with ocular myasthenia gravis or for those over 60 years old.

Thymectomy eliminates the possibility of a thymoma developing later, and even when patients are at a very early age has not led to an increased incidence of other diseases.

A conventional thymectomy is performed using a sternal-splitting incision. At a few institutions the thymus is removed through a transcervical approach. The mortality rate at my institution is much less than 1% and the average hospital stay is less than six days. Hospitalization is longer if there is postoperative respiratory difficulty. Patients with significant bulbar symptoms undergo plasmapheresis before surgery, which leads to an uncomplicated recovery.

The most important point in treatment during the immediate postoperative period is to withhold all anticholinesterase medication until there is a clear indication that the medication is required, usually not until 24 to 72 hours have passed. Rarely, patients do not require Mestinon after surgery. (This same rule of withholding Mestinon medication applies to all types of surgery on myasthenic patients.) The reason for the transient improvement in strength after surgery is unknown.

I believe that, if a thymoma is removed, the patient should have radiation therapy and be placed immediately on prednisone and azathioprine. Before the use of these agents, two thirds of patients who had thymoma died of myasthenia gravis within five years and only 10% went into remission. Fortunately, these distressing statistics have greatly improved.

STEROID THERAPY

Patients who fail to respond adequately to Mestinon and thymectomy, as well as older patients (over 60 years of age), should have a trial of alternate-day prednisone. My preference is to start with 60 mg of prednisone daily, in single oral dose in the morning for ten days, and then to change to an alternate-day schedule. It is safest to hospitalize patients for the first week of treatment because they can become weaker during this initial treatment phase. If there is no sign of improvement with therapy of 60 mg every other day for three months, the dose should be reduced gradually and discontinued. At times, patients may require from 10 to 20 mg on the day that they do not take the medication, but an effort should always be made to reach an alternate-day schedule in order to minimize side effects. Improvement may be noted in a few weeks or may take several months. After three months of therapy with 60 mg every other day, the dose should be gradually reduced by small increments (5 to 10 mg) every two weeks to a level of 30 mg every other day. After this, the dose should be reduced by 2.5 mg at a time. In most patients, there is a critical level between 20 and 25 mg every other day, and reduction below this level often leads to a recurrence of myasthenic symptoms. When this happens, the dose often has to be increased to 50 to 60 mg every other day. If a thymectomy has been performed, an attempt should be made eventually to discontinue the use of prednisone completely. In older patients or those who had a thymoma, I generally keep the dose at 20 to 25 mg every other day indefinitely. The use of azathioprine (discussed later) has led to some modification in this plan.

The hazards of prolonged prednisone therapy are well known. In my experience, the most common side effect is the accelerated formation of cataracts, although osteoporosis is common in older women.

Patients with ocular myasthenia gravis do not need to be hospitalized, and therapy is started with 30 mg of prednisone daily for ten days, after which it is changed to an every-other-day schedule for three months. This is followed by a 2.5-mg reduction in dose every two weeks. Relapses are common when the dose is reduced below 20 to 25 mg every other day. The ocular myasthenic patient, however, has a propensity for spontaneous remissions, so an effort should always be made to discontinue the use of prednisone eventually.

AZATHIOPRINE AND CYCLOPHOSPHAMIDE

Azathioprine has been used in Europe for many years, but only during the past five years has it had extensive use in the United States. The mode of action of this immunosuppressive drug is still not well understood, except that it decreases the titer of AChRab. In animals pretreated with azathioprine, experimental autoimmune myasthenia gravis cannot be induced.

In contrast to prednisone, azathioprine does not require the patient to be hospitalized because it does not cause any initial increase in weakness. I prescribe a dose of 2.5 mg per kg of body weight. Some physicians give an amount sufficient to decrease the leukocyte count to below 3000/mm^3. The treatment requires patience on the part of both physician and patient, because little benefit is noted for six months and maximal benefit may be delayed as long as one year. When the dose is decreased, the weakness usually returns.

The major side effects are bone marrow suppression, nausea, and liver toxicity. As in any immunosuppressed patient, infections also may occur. Toxic symptoms invariably disappear when the dose is discontinued or reduced. In experience with more than 50 patients at my institution, only three had to discontinue the drug because of nausea, vomiting, and pronounced elevation of the serum glutamic-oxaloacetic transaminase, alkaline phosphatase, and bilirubin levels. All these reactions occurred during the first week of therapy. A hemogram and liver function blood test should be repeated within four days after treatment has been started and then at monthly intervals. There have not been any reports of oncogenicity, except in patients who have undergone renal transplantation. Azathioprine should not be used in pregnant patients or in young females who may become pregnant. Despite these possible side effects, the drug probably is safer than long-term large-dose prednisone.

Azathioprine should be used in patients who receive plasma exchange, in those who have failed to respond to thymectomy and prednisone, and in those who require large doses of prednisone to control their symptoms. In several instances, patients have been able to discontinue prednisone completely.

Cyclophosphamide, more potent than azathioprine and with a higher risk of inducing malignancy, is rarely used but has been reported to be effective when all other modalities have failed.

Cyclosporin may prove useful, but there are only small series reported of its effects in myasthenic patients.

PLASMA EXCHANGE

After an initial wave of enthusiasm for and somewhat indiscriminate use of plasmapheresis, the indications have become more clear. Plasma exchange is effective in patients who have significant respiratory problems—either in crisis or before thymectomy. It is also beneficial in patients who require large doses of steroids, enabling steroids to be reduced at a more rapid rate.

At my institution, treatment involves three usually consecutive daily exchanges each of 3000 to 4500 ml. Our practice is to replace the plasma with human serum albumin. Because the beneficial effects are relatively brief, lasting a few days to several months, these patients should be placed on prednisone and azathioprine therapy; the prednisone covers the first six months after exchange, and azathioprine should be helpful after that.

Plasma exchange is a safe procedure if access can be obtained with needles placed in the peripheral veins. If a fistula or shunt is required, complications are common: infection, embolization, and bleeding. During the procedure, all anticholinesterase medication should be withheld.

Although plasmapheresis is an outpatient procedure at my institution, it generally is safer to hospitalize the individual.

INFORMATION AND EDUCATION

The results of treatment are best in patients with whom all aspects of their disease, including the various treatments, have been thoroughly discussed.

Myasthenic patients are invariably frightened by their illness and are very dependent on their physician for emotional support. They are also very perceptive and become upset by any indication of uncertainty on the part of the physician. Because many appear to be healthy, it is often necessary to provide the patient with a letter documenting their disability, to be shown to a school administrator or employer.

PERIODIC EXAMINATION

All myasthenic patients should be thoroughly examined at least every six months. This includes both neurologic and medical examinations and roentgenograms of the chest (posteroanterior and lateral views). Appropriate tests on a monthly basis are required for patients taking prednisone or azathioprine. At the six-month examination, patients on prednisone therapy should be checked for cataracts, and bone densitometry or roentgenography of the pelvis should be done to monitor for osteoporosis. At yearly intervals I obtain thyroid function tests, and in older patients I obtain vitamin B$_{12}$ and folate determinations. Myasthenic patients have a higher incidence of other autoimmune diseases. A test for antistriational antibodies also is done, and if positive, CT scans, tomograms, or both are obtained.

PREVENTIVE MEASURES

Because myasthenic symptoms worsen with infection, patients should receive pneumococcal vaccine and influenza immunizations. They should never stop prednisone therapy abruptly. In addition, common sense measures to reduce the possibility of upper respiratory infections should be stressed. Emotional upsets may also lead to increased weakness and should be treated with counseling and the careful use of tranquilizers or antidepressants.

Myasthenic women usually tolerate birth control medication. However, many have increased weakness at the time of menses and need more anticholinesterase medication. Thymectomy for these patients should be timed to avoid menses. During pregnancy, 40% to 60% of patients improve, usually during the second and third trimesters, and about one third get worse during the postpartum period. Delivery is accomplished vaginally. Their children should be closely monitored for transient neonatal myasthenia gravis, which occurs in about 15% of children born to myasthenic mothers. Involved infants have a weak cry, difficulty sucking, and sparse extremity movement and AChRab in their blood. In most instances the antibodies are transmitted through the placenta, and normal babies born to myasthenic mothers may have antibodies. It is believed that symptomatic children briefly produce their own antibodies, possibly because of a transient immunologic response. If symptoms are significant, small doses of Mestinon, either by injection or as syrup, should be given. The disease is self-limited and usually subsides after four days to several weeks. My colleagues and I have seen only one of these children develop myasthenia later in life.

MYASTHENIA CRISIS

Crisis, a life-threatening emergency, is characterized by increased bulbar symptoms and respiratory insufficiency. The first step is to secure an adequate airway and assisted ventilation if necessary. Because progression may be rapid, treatment should not be delayed. A Tensilon test should not be attempted, because the response to Tensilon cannot be accurately assessed in a patient with respiratory insufficiency. When adequate ventilation is assured, the remainder of the examination and further history can be completed. All anticholinesterase drugs should be stopped and plasma exchange done early.

Penicillamine-Induced Myasthenia Gravis

The coexistence of myasthenia gravis and rheumatoid arthritis occurs more frequently than can be explained by chance. Patients with rheumatoid arthritis, Wilson's disease, or scleroderma who are taking penicillamine have developed myasthenia gravis with clinical and electrophysiologic findings that are the same as in idiopathic myasthenia gravis. Other autoimmune diseases also have been induced by this drug. About 90% of patients have elevated titers of AChRab. The mechanism producing this syndrome is not known.

Weakness may appear within two days after penicillamine has been taken or not until several years of treatment. The eye muscles are most often involved but bulbar and extremity weakness does occur. In a few patients the weakness is severe. Results of Tensilon testing are often positive and patients are improved by anticholinesterase medication. Other treatment is seldom needed because the antibody titer progressively decreases with cessation of drug use, and in approximately 80% of patients the disease disappears in eight to 12 months. On occasion, thymectomy has been performed and a hyperplastic thymus removed. The very high remission rate is the principal difference between induced and idiopathic myasthenia gravis.

Myasthenic Syndrome Sometimes Associated With Small-Cell Carcinoma of the Lung

This disease (the Lambert-Eaton syndrome) causes weakness of the proximal muscles, but strength increases with the initial use of the extremities. In approximately two thirds of the patients the condition is a paraneoplastic syndrome occurring secondary to malignancy, usually small-cell carcinoma of the lung but at times other malignancies. The remaining one third have no associated malignancy but there is an autoimmune state.

PATHOLOGY

The defect in neuromuscular transmission, in contrast to that in myasthenia gravis, is presynaptic, with impaired release of acetylcholine from the terminal axon. The storage of acetylcholine and its reaction with the receptor protein on the postsynaptic muscle membrane are normal. There is evidence that calcium entry in the nerve terminal is impaired. This calcium entry triggers the release of acetylcholine. The autoimmune cause is based on an increased incidence of HLA-B8 and HLA-DRw3 antigens in these patients, as well as the ability to transfer the disease passively to mice, with a characteristic electrophysiologic response. There is a high prevalence of organ-specific autoantibodies in patients who do not have a malignancy.

CLINICAL ASPECTS

The disease is rare, less than one tenth as common as myasthenia gravis. In patients with cancer, the onset is in middle age or older. Some young patients have been reported but they had no associated malignancy. The initial complaints usually are referable to the proximal muscles. Infrequently, there may be bulbar weakness, diplopia, and ptosis, in contrast to the high frequency of these symptoms in myasthenia gravis. The prime finding on examination, suggesting the disease, is a pronounced reduction or absence of the reflexes in the face of a patient with only mild to moderate weakness, although in patients without malignancy the reflexes may be only slightly reduced or normal. If the proximal muscles are tested from rest, the weakness is evident. If, however, one tries to evaluate weakness in a contracted muscle, weakness may not be apparent. With sustained contraction (e.g., squeezing the examiner's fingers), an increase in grip may be noted. With repeated percussion, the amplitude of the deep tendon reflexes may increase. The patient is often bothered by dryness of the mouth, paresthesia without sensory loss, and impotence (males). These symptoms may not be spontaneously described and may require direct questioning. Some patients also have a fine intention tremor.

Diagnosis is most often made on the basis of nerve stimulation studies. Characteristically, a single supramaximal shock elicits a very low-amplitude muscle action potential. At 2-Hz stimulation, there is a further decline, but at high rates of stimulation (40 Hz) or after exercise, there is a pronounced facilitation.

If miniature end-plate potentials are studied on intercostal biopsy specimens, the amplitude is normal but the frequency is reduced.

In any patient with this syndrome, the possibility of cancer must be considered. Heavy smokers invariably have small-cell carcinoma of the lung, but even with careful examinations, bronchoscopy, and cytology, it may not be detected for as long as ten years. If the tumor is completely excised, the condition may disappear, only to recur when metastasis develops. It has rarely been seen in association with multiple sclerosis and collagen disease.

Acetylcholine receptor antibodies have rarely been found, and patients with these antibodies may have both the myasthenic syndrome and myasthenia gravis.

Weakness tends to progress slowly. When death occurs, it is caused by the malignancy and not by the myasthenic syndrome.

TREATMENT

If operable, any malignant lesion should be removed or treated with radiation or chemotherapy. Guanidine, which stimulates the release of acetylcholine, should not be used because of the high incidence of side effects, including aplastic anemia and renal failure. Anticholinesterase medication is of limited value. Many patients respond well to prednisone or azathioprine in the same doses used for myasthenia gravis. There is also a transitory improvement after plasma exchange. Recent reports have indicated that 3,4-diaminopyridine may be useful in combination with Mestinon, but the former drug is still classed as an experimental agent. Thymectomy is of no benefit.

FOLLOW-UP EXAMINATIONS

Patients should be seen at six-month intervals to be examined for malignancy, especially of the lung. In young nonsmokers, in whom the incidence of malignancy is low, yearly examinations are adequate, but all patients on steroid or azathioprine therapy require more frequent monitoring.

Botulism

The neurotoxins of *Clostridium botulinum* produce an illness characterized by descending paralysis and initial involvement of the bulbar muscles. The organism is ubiquitous but the spores do not cause illness, except possibly in infantile botulism. Generally, the illness arises from the ingestion of foods that contain preformed toxin. Home-canned vegetables, fermented fish, improperly processed meat, and honey have been incriminated. Rarely, botulism occurs with wound infection by the bacteria. Diagnosis is based on detection of the toxin in serum, feces, or suspected food or on cultures of the organism from the stool, wound, or food.

The disease results from the toxin fixing irreversibly to the neuromuscular junction and preventing the usual release of acetylcholine (by exocytosis) from the presynaptic terminal, probably by interference with the calcium-mediated release mechanism. Results of Tensilon testing may or may not be positive. There is a small muscle action potential elicited by supramaximal nerve stimulation. Repetitive nerve stimulation studies at low rates of stimulation (2 to 3 Hz) show a decrement, while facilitation is shown at high stimulation (30 to 40 Hz). These changes are usually not seen until there is clinical evidence of weakness of the extremity. For unknown reasons, the defect may be found in one extremity and not the other.

Clinically, three syndromes are recognized: food poisoning, infant botulism, and wound botulism.

FOOD POISONING

Symptoms appear between two and 36 hours after ingestion of toxin-contaminated food. Initially, there are usually gastrointestinal symptoms with nausea, vomiting, abdominal pain, and diarrhea. Dryness of the mouth and a sore throat are very common. Bulbar musculature is affected first with diplopia, ptosis, blurring of vision and difficulty focusing, dysphagia, dysarthria, and dizziness. Respiratory failure comes on rapidly and can occur on the first day of the illness. Later, peripheral weakness occurs.

On examination, the pupils may be fixed and dilated or normal. Ptosis and extraocular palsies, particularly bilateral sixth-nerve involvement, are found, and nystagmus may be present. The muscles of the face and the tongue are usually weak. Peripheral weakness is most often symmetric but not invariably so. The tendon reflexes are normal or hypoactive. The patient may complain of paresthesia but there is no objective sensory loss. Respiratory insufficiency is common and may last for months. The large majority of patients are awake, alert, and afebrile. Mortality rates of 10% to 20% are reported but patients who survive make a complete recovery. Death is caused by respiratory failure or intercurrent infection.

Early intubation and assisted respiration are the main component of treatment. If the disease is diagnosed early, gastric lavage and enemas are used to eliminate the toxin. The Centers for Disease Control (CDC) in Atlanta should be contacted as soon as the disease is suspected for its assistance in identifying the toxin and to obtain the trivalent antitoxin. This consists of A, B, and E antitoxin and is given intravenously every two to four hours, but specific instructions should be obtained from the CDC. The antitoxin is a horse serum preparation, and hypersensitivity reactions occur, including anaphylactic shock. The benefit from administering antitoxin has not been established, except for that from the E antitoxin. The major line of treatment remains in the respiratory intensive care unit, along with adequate nutritional support.

INFANT BOTULISM

In the past decade, it has been recognized that infants under 9 months of age can get botulism. In some, contaminated honey has been the vehicle of transmission. In others, the botulism organism may have remained in the gut, where it multiplied and produced the exotoxin. In these patients, antitoxin is not found in the serum but can be found in the stool, and botulism organisms can be cultured from the stool. The clinical picture is that of a floppy infant with flaccid weakness, constipation, lethargy, ptosis, and usually large, sluggish pupils, extremity weakness, a weak cry, impaired sucking, and poor head control. Respiratory failure with arrest may occur and is one of the causes of the sudden infant death syndrome. The endotoxin can be found in the stool for months after clinical recovery. Treatment is supportive, as previously outlined, and antitoxin and antibiotics in an attempt to eliminate the organism are seldom used. The mortality rate is about 2%.

WOUND BOTULISM

The clinical picture of wound botulism is the same as with the other varieties, except that the portal of entry is an infected wound. Wound botulism differs from food poisoning in that GI symptoms are not present and patients often have fever secondary to other bacterial infections. Treatment is the same as for food poisoning, except that antibiotics are used for the secondary infection.

PREVENTION

Proper preservation of canned foods, meat, and fish eliminates the toxin. Preserved foods should be heated to 90°C for 10 minutes or 80°C for 20 minutes before consumption, since this destroys the toxin.

Once the diagnosis has been suspected, it is important to ask patients about their recent diet and to examine any other persons who may have ingested similar food. Often the first person seen in an outbreak has received the largest amount of toxin and is likely to be the most seriously afflicted.

REFERENCES

Albers JW, Hodach RJ, Kimmel DW, et al: Penicillamine-associated myasthenia gravis. Neurology 30:1246–1249, 1980.
Engel AG: Myasthenia gravis and myasthenic syndromes. Ann Neurol 16:519–534, 1984.
Hughes JM, Blumenthal JR, Merson MH, et al: Clinical features of types A and B food-borne botulism. Ann Intern Med 95:442–445, 1981.
Lennon VA, Howard FM Jr: Serological diagnosis of myasthenia gravis. *In* Nakamura RM, O'Sullivan MB (eds): Clinical Laboratory Molecular Analyses: New Strategies in Autoimmunity Cancer and Virology. Grune & Stratton, New York, 1985.
Seybold ME, Lindstrom JM: Immunopathology of acetylcholine receptors in myasthenia gravis. Springer Semin Immunopathol 5:389–412, 1982.

22 · TREATMENT OF MYOPATHIES

Raymond G. Auger
MAYO CLINIC AND MAYO FOUNDATION

The term myopathy refers to a group of disorders that primarily involve muscle fibers. The clinical hallmarks are symmetric weakness (usually proximal), preserved reflexes (except in advanced forms of the disease), and intact sensation. Serum creatine kinase (CK) or serum creatine phosphokinase (CPK) levels are often elevated, particularly in inflammatory myopathies and rapidly progressive dystrophies. Motor and sensory nerve conduction studies are normal. Needle electrode examination may show small motor units with increased recruitment of units after a voluntary contraction (increased interference pattern). Clinicians often refer to this as a "myopathic pattern." The condition must be differentiated from anterior horn cell diseases, polyradiculopathies, polyneuropathies, and disorders of neuromuscular transmission.

LABORATORY EVALUATION

In addition to electromyographic and nerve conduction studies, other laboratory tests are frequently helpful in the evaluation of muscle disease. The CK or CPK determination is useful as a diagnostic aid and in following the course of treatment.

The sedimentation rate may be elevated in some cases of polymyositis but this is inconsistent. Again, however, some clinicians find this test useful to follow the course of treatment.

In patients suspected of having McArdle's syndrome or phosphofructokinase (PFK) deficiency, the ischemic exercise test performed by measuring serum lactate can be diagnostic. To confirm the metabolic defect, lactate concentrations are measured in blood samples obtained from an antecubital vein before and after ischemic exercise; the latter is achieved by applying a sphygmomanometer cuff around the upper arm inflated to a level above the systolic pressure. The patient exercises the forearm muscles by gripping forcefully 20 to 30 times in one minute. In normal individuals the serum lactate rises three- to fivefold, but in patients with McArdle's syndrome or PFK deficiency lactate levels do not change.

Endocrine studies that may be useful include determination of serum thyroxine, calcium metabolism including parathyroid hormone assay, serum cortisol determination, and (in selected instances) growth hormone assays.

MUSCLE BIOPSY

Once it has been determined that the condition is probably a myopathy, it may be necessary to perform a muscle biopsy to search for the underlying disease process, which in turn will determine whether specific treatment is possible. In addition to the hematoxylin and eosin and trichrome stains, histochemical staining techniques can be used to measure oxidative enzymes, enzymes associated with glycogen metabolism, and enzymes associated with lipid metabolism. In selected instances, electron microscopy may be an invaluable aid to diagnosis.

CLASSIFICATION

The classification shown in Table 1 is not a complete list of the myopathies; some of the rare forms for which no specific treatment is available have been omitted.

PRINCIPLES OF TREATMENT

The following principles of management apply to all myopathies:

1. Activity should be encouraged as much as possible, without precipitating undue fatigue; usually the aid of a skilled physical therapy team is essential.

2. Contractures should be prevented.

3. Orthopedic deformities should be avoided and treated with appropriate bracing or surgical procedures if necessary.

4. Complications of the disease such as decubiti, pulmonary infections, cardiac arrythmias, and aspiration should be recognized and promptly treated.

5. Obesity should be avoided. Many patients are likely to become obese because of inactivity.

6. Social issues should not be neglected. The school nurse and guidance counselor should be involved when children of school age are afflicted. Realistic goals should be set for the patient's future occupation.

7. For genetically determined illnesses, genetic counseling for the patient and other family members at risk is important.

Most states have branches of the Muscular Dystrophy Association that can provide financial assistance for medical diagnosis and treatment, not only for the dystrophies but also for other types of neuromuscular disease.

PHARMACOLOGIC TREATMENT

Some myopathies can be treated pharmacologically (see Table 1).

Polymyositis. Polymyositis may exist by itself or may coexist with a rash, in which case the term dermatomyositis is applied. The incidence of malignancy is increased in polymyositis. Earlier reports suggested a very high correlation, but more recent articles have indicated an overall incidence of about 8%, with a somewhat greater incidence in patients over 65 years of age. Polymyositis may also coexist with other collagen

diseases and may have more of a secondary role in the illness.

Steroids. Once the diagnosis has been confirmed by muscle biopsy, the initial treatment in adults consists of high-dose steroids, usually prednisone, 60 mg per day (15 mg four times a day). Therapy for females may be started at a smaller dose (about 40 mg per day) because they seem to be more likely to suffer toxic effects from steroids. At these doses, the CK level becomes normal in approximately six weeks and the dose can then be reduced gradually while the clinical status, as well as the CK level, is monitored. Generally, the prednisone dose can be reduced by 5 mg every two weeks. The maintenance dose is usually between 5 and 15 mg per day. Steroid therapy generally has to be continued indefinitely at a low level, but in some pa-

Table 1. CLASSIFICATION OF MYOPATHIES*

Inflammatory
  Polymyositis, dermatomyositis*

Hereditary
  Dystrophies
    Sex-linked recessive forms (Duchenne and Becker)
    Limb girdle dystrophy (some inherited in an autosomal recessive
      pattern; some inherited in an autosomal dominant pattern;
      some sporadic)
    Facioscapulohumeral dystrophy (usually autosomal dominant)
    Distal dystrophy
    Ocular and oculopharyngeal dystrophy (usually autosomal domi-
      nant)
    Scapuloperoneal atrophy (variable forms of inheritance)
  Myotonic disorders*
    Myotonic dystrophy
    Myotonic congenita
    Paramyotonia congenita (often associated with hyperkalemic peri-
      odic paralysis)
  Congenital nonprogressive myopathies (several histologic types)

Infections*
  Parasites (toxoplasmosis, trichinosis, cysticercosis)
  Viruses
  Bacterial infections (e.g., gas gangrene, septic myositis)

Toxic*
  Alcohol
  Chloroquine
  Clofibrate
  Steroids
  Long-term injections of pentazocine or meperidine

Metabolic
  Endocrine*
    Thyroid disease (hyperthyroidism or hypothyroidism)
    Hyperparathyroidism (primary or secondary)
    Cushing's syndrome
    Addison's disease
    Acromegaly and hypopituitarism
  Glycogen storage diseases
    Acid maltase deficiency (type II glycogenosis)
    Debranching enzyme deficiency (type III glycogenosis)
    Branching enzyme deficiency (type IV glycogenosis)
    Muscle phosphorylase deficiency (type V glycogenosis)
    Phosphofructokinase deficiency (type VII glycogenosis)
  Lipid storage diseases
  Mitochondrial myopathies
  Periodic paralysis*
    Hypokalemic
      Primary
      Secondary
        Hyperthyroidism
    Hyperkalemic
      Primary
      Secondary
    Normokalemic
  Myopathy associated with malignant hyperthermia*

*Condition that may benefit from pharmacologic treatment.

tients the dose may be decreased slowly after three years of treatment. In most patients treatment should be continued for at least five years before complete withdrawal can be achieved. If control is readily achieved, a switch to an alternate-day schedule can be made.

The usual side effects of steroids are to be expected, including weight gain, hirsutism, easy bruising, and the typical cushingoid appearance. Other more serious side effects to monitor include the development of cataracts, osteoporosis, avascular necrosis of the hip, diabetes, hypertension, decreased resistance to infection, and gastric ulcer. When higher doses are used, an antacid regimen is recommended.

Immunosuppressive Agents. In patients who are steroid resistant and do not respond to an adequate dose after three to four months, the addition of other immunosuppressive agents should be considered. Azathioprine, cyclophosphamide, and methotrexate have been used with some success. Patients must realize that these agents involve significant risks, and the decision to use them should be made only after consultation with a physician experienced in managing these agents.

Myotonic Disorders. In myotonia, there is a delayed relaxation of muscle following contraction. In myotonic dystrophy, the distribution of the weakness is often more pronounced distally in the early stages of the illness, although in the later stages proximal muscle weakness is usually prominent also. There are many other systemic manifestations including cataracts, diabetes, cardiac arrhythmias, frontal baldness, testicular atrophy, and other endocrine abnormalities. Patients with myotonia congenita have prominent myotonia without the associated muscle weakness or any of the other systemic manifestations.

Most patients with myotonia can tolerate it quite well without treatment, and many elect to do so. However, in some the myotonia may be sufficiently disabling to warrant therapy. In these, phenytoin may be helpful, 300 to 400 mg per day. Only rarely is it necessary to resort to procainamide.

Infections. Antihelmintic agents may be of benefit to treat some parasitic infestations. The most common parasitic infestation of muscle is trichinosis, caused by the ingestion of poorly cooked pork infested with *Trichinella spiralis*. The combination of periorbital edema, eosinophilia, myalgia, and a history of ingestion of raw or rare meat makes the diagnosis of trichinosis highly likely. Serologic tests are quite reliable and in most cases should be positive 17 days after infection. Muscle biopsy is not indicated in all infections but it provides a definitive diagnosis when larvae are recovered. Thiabendazole appears to be the drug of choice. If there is associated neurologic or myocardial involvement, corticosteroids should be administered in addition to thiabendazole. Antibiotics are required in pyogenic muscle infections.

Toxic Causes. Slow recovery may occur after removal of the offending agent.

Endocrine Causes. Correction of the underlying endocrine abnormalities often results in slow improvement. The most common endocrine myopathies are those related to hypo- or hyperthyroidism, and those associated with hypercortisolism, usually iatrogenic.

Glycogen Storage Diseases. Treatment of these conditions is usually unsatisfactory, but there have been recent reports of dietary manipulations, the idea being to provide an alternative fuel in order to bypass the metabolic block. This approach has been moderately successful in patients with carnitine palmityl transferase deficiency who are unable to metabolize long-chain fatty acids, and in patients with McArdle's disease. In the latter, a high protein diet may provide a remarkable improvement of endurance. It is speculated that a similar diet may be effective in PFK deficiency and possibly other glycolytic disorders.

Periodic Paralysis. This condition is characterized by recurrent attacks of flaccid paralysis. In most patients the respiratory and cranial muscles are not significantly affected. If the patient can be observed during an attack, the serum potassium level should be measured as soon as possible to determine whether it is increased, decreased, or normal. In the primary form of the illness (inherited as an autosomal dominant trait), the potassium level is normal between attacks, whereas it is either high or low in the secondary forms. In the primary form, in which the potassium level is normal between attacks, provocative testing in the hospital may be required to confirm the diagnosis if the attacks are infrequent. In the secondary forms, treatment is directed toward the underlying abnormality. Hyperthyroidism should be excluded in all patients with hypokalemic periodic paralysis, particularly if there is no family history.

Primary Hypokalemic Periodic Paralysis. In this form, patients have attacks of flaccid quadriplegia that may last several hours. The most important predisposing factors are prolonged rest after vigorous exercise, a heavy meal a few hours beforehand, anxiety or emotion, and cold. Patients with acute attacks are treated with 2.0 to 10.0 gm of potassium chloride orally. Preventive therapy consists of a low-sodium, low-carbohydrate diet, avoidance of exposure to cold and overexertion, and supplemental doses of potassium chloride.

Primary Hyperkalemic Periodic Paralysis. A typical attack develops when the patient is sitting in a chair after exercise. Most attacks are relatively short and largely subside within one to three hours. Patients with acute attacks can be treated with 2.0 gm of glucose per kg of body weight, and 15 to 20 units of regular insulin subcutaneously. In some patients, calcium gluconate, 0.5 to 2.0 gm IV, terminates the attacks. Prevention consists of frequent high-carbohydrate meals and avoidance of exposure to cold and overexertion.

Patients with the primary form of either hypokalemic or hyperkalemic periodic paralysis can be given acetazolamide, which seems to be effective in preventing recurrent attacks.

Malignant Hyperthermia. This potentially fatal syndrome, inherited in an autosomal dominant fashion, is caused by a hypermetabolic state involving skeletal muscle. The syndrome is usually associated with administration of halogenated inhalational anesthetic agents as well as with succinylcholine, and these agents should not be given to patients at risk. Typically, the increased muscle metabolism leads to elevated body temperature, muscle rigidity, and (in full-blown cases) rhabdomyolysis with myoglobinuria and possibly renal failure. The fatality rate is high for untreated patients.

The condition can be recognized in presymptomatic patients with a positive family history by in vitro study of the response of muscle to halothane and caffeine. In patients known to have the condition, alternative anesthetic agents can be used.

If the syndrome has developed, dantrolene is the primary specific therapeutic drug at present, 2.4 mg per kg IV. Other measures, including cooling, treatment of acidosis, and diuresis, should also be undertaken.

REFERENCES

Bohan A, Peter JB, Bowman RL, et al: A computer-assisted analysis of 153 patients with polymyositis and dermatomyositis. Medicine 56:255–286, 1977.

Currie S: Inflammatory myopathies. Part 1. Polymyositis and related disorders. *In* Walton JN (ed): Disorders of Voluntary Muscle, 4th ed. Churchill Livingstone, Edinburgh, 1981, pp 525–568.

Engel AG: Metabolic and endocrine myopathies. *In* Walton JN (ed): Disorders of Voluntary Muscle, 4th ed. Churchill Livingstone, Edinburgh, 1981, pp 664–711.

Layzer RB: McArdle's disease in the 1980s (editorial). N Engl J Med 312:370–371, 1985.

Mastaglia FL, Ojeda VJ: Inflammatory myopathies. Parts I and II. Ann Neurol 17:215–277, 317–323, 1985.

Munsat TL: Therapy of myotonia: a double-blind evaluation of diphenylhydantoin, procainamide, and placebo. Neurology 17:359–367, 1967.

Nelson TE, Flewellen EH: The malignant hyperthermia syndrome. N Engl J Med 309:416–418, 1983.

23 · COMMON EYE PROBLEMS IN INTERNAL MEDICINE

Monica L. Monica
Thom J. Zimmerman
OCHSNER CLINIC AND ALTON OCHSNER MEDICAL FOUNDATION

The eye acts as a "window" to the body and often reflects evidence of systemic disease. Certain eye findings may alert the physician to evaluate the patient for hypertension or diabetes. Therefore, it is important to be familiar with basic ocular problems.

We will discuss eye problems related to the anterior segment, containing the eyelids, conjunctiva, cornea, iris, sclera, and lens, and the posterior segment, consisting of the vitreous, retina, and optic nerve. The eye problems will be grouped into the appropriate divisions.

ANTERIOR SEGMENT OCULAR PROBLEMS

The red eye is the most common anterior segment eye problem and may be due to any of the following causes: (1) infection, (2) allergy, (3) trauma, (4) glaucoma, (5) tear film abnormalities, or (6) systemic diseases, such as collagen vascular or thyroid disease. The red eye is a cardinal sign of ocular inflammation.

INFECTION

Conjunctivitis is an inflammation of the mucous membranes lining the eyelids and covering the eye and is characterized by cellular infiltration and exudation. Bacterial conjunctivitis has an acute onset, involves all age groups, and produces a purulent to mucopurulent exudate with crusting and swelling of the eyelids. Viral or allergic types demonstrate a watery-to-stringy exudate. There is often evidence of a preauricular node in viral conjunctivitis. In those cases in which there is difficulty discriminating between bacterial and viral etiologies, a Gram stain, Giemsa stain, and conjunctival culture are helpful.

Epidemic keratoconjunctivitis (EKC) is a common viral infection caused by adenovirus type 8. Onset is abrupt, often unilateral at first, with involvement of the second eye within a week. The eye is red and watery and has a foreign body sensation. There is often a history of a preceding upper respiratory infection and evidence of adenopathy. On slit-lamp examination the conjunctiva has numerous follicles that are collections of lymphoid tissue. Vision is usually good unless there is corneal involvement.

Treatment of bacterial conjunctivitis differs from that of viral conjunctivitis. For bacterial conjunctivitis a broad-spectrum topical sulfonamide, such as sodium sulfacetamide, is used, since it is bacteriostatic against a wide range of microorganisms. The eye should not be patched with an eyepad because this will promote bacterial growth. Treatment of viral conjunctivitis is mainly supportive. The importance of good hygiene with frequent hand washing should be stressed to the patient, since EKC is contagious; cold compresses will minimize eyelid swelling; and topical decongestant eyedrops containing naphazoline hydrochloride will decrease conjunctival chemosis. Bacterial or viral conjunctivitis needs to be followed closely for signs of corneal involvement resulting from the infection.

A serious ocular infection causing a red eye is the bacterial corneal ulcer. There may be symptoms and signs of a bacterial conjunctivitis. The ulcer may occur in the visual axis, causing decreased vision, or near the periphery of the cornea, where it is obscured from recognition unless a slit-lamp microscope is used to examine the eye. The infection can be spread rapidly and lead to corneal perforation.

Prompt care by an ophthalmologist is necessary for the treatment of a bacterial corneal ulcer. Corneal scrapings and cultures aid in identifying the organism. Frequent instillation of broad-spectrum antibiotic eyedrops should be used in addition to supportive measures to reduce pain.

ALLERGY

Allergy can produce a conjunctivitis identical to that caused by viruses. The eye is red with conjunctival chemosis and vascular engorgement. A specific allergen such as pollen, dust, or animal hair may provoke the attack. Conjunctival scrapings show eosinophils. Allergic conjunctivitis can be differentiated from viral conjunctivitis by patient history and absence of preauricular adenopathy. The treatment for allergic conjunctivitis is mainly supportive.

Vernal conjunctivitis is a recurrent, bilateral inflammation of the conjunctiva occurring during the spring and summer in the northwestern hemisphere and during the fall and winter in the southern hemisphere. The principal symptoms are itching and burning, and most cases occur in patients between ages 5 and 20 years. There is a male predominance and often a history of atopic allergies. The disease lasts an average of four to ten years. Treatment is based on topical astringents, with careful "pulsing" of topical steroids. It is often difficult to wean patients from topical steroids. Recently, topical cromolyn sodium has been marketed for use in vernal conjunctivitis, since it prevents mast cell degranulation and release of histamine.

Another allegic cause of a red eye is contact with a specific allergen, such as medication or cosmetics. The skin around the eye becomes edematous. A unilateral distribution of the periocular edema suggests contact dermatitis, whereas bilateral involvement suggests airborne contact reaction. Allergic reaction to cosmetics affects primarily the area of distribution, usually the eyebrows and upper eyelids.

TRAUMA

Chemical Injuries. Chemical burns are urgent ocular emergencies. Common household agents capable of causing chemical burns include household ammonia, toilet bowl cleaners, drain cleaners, scouring compounds, bleaches, and disinfectants. Chemical burns may result from explosion of the mixture in a lead-acid storage battery upon recharging. In general, the alkalis are more damaging to the eye than the acids.

Among the three most common alkalis, calcium hydroxide (lime) most commonly causes superficial opacification of the cornea; sodium hydroxide (lye) induces opacification of the deep corneal layers; and ammonium hydroxide (ammonia) causes deep injury, with corneal edema and cataract formation. In alkali burns there is rapid penetration of the chemical through the cornea. Immediate irrigation with water or saline to flush the chemical from the eye is important to help to minimize the severity of the damage.

Corneal Abrasion. The most common traumatic cause of a red eye is the corneal abrasion. Characteristic symptoms are eye pain and tearing. The patient demonstrates blepharospasm (inability to keep the eyelids open). A drop of topical anesthetic with 0.5% proparacaine eliminates the blepharospasm and allows examination of the eye. A drop of fluorescein stains the abrasion. Under white light the abrasion stains a yellowgreen and under cobalt light, a bright green. One must look for a foreign body on the cornea or under the eyelid, and eversion of the upper eyelid often reveals a hidden foreign body. Foreign body removal is performed at the slit-lamp microscope using a special microsurgical instrument or a dull needle. In addition to topical antibiotics, a dilating eyedrop, such as 1% Cyclogyl, is placed in the eye to relieve ciliary spasm causing pain. A pressure patch is placed on the eye for 24 hours to promote corneal epithelium regeneration.

Ruptured Globe. The most serious traumatic injury is a ruptured globe. This may be caused by a missile, blunt trauma, or head injury. Diagnosis is made on examination of the anterior segment of the eye. There may be blood in the anterior chamber, a corneal laceration with prolapse of iris, or a scleral laceration with protrusion of retina. The intraocular pressure is low. The injury demands prompt ophthalmic surgery to repair the wound and reestablish the integrity of the eye. Prior to surgery, a Fox shield should be placed over the eye to protect it and intravenous antibiotics started to guard against infection.

GLAUCOMA

Most forms of glaucoma are "silent," and the patient is unaware that the intraocular pressure is elevated. However, an acute attack of angle-closure glaucoma produces a painful red eye. Angle-closure glaucoma results from inability of the aqueous to drain from the eye owing to anatomic blockage of the iris against the outflow area. The vision is blurred, with colored halos seen around lights. This phenomenon results from the intraocular pressure elevation producing corneal edema and the hazy cornea diffracting white light into its rainbow components. The pupil is mid-dilated owing to paralysis of the iris sphincter. Nausea and vomiting may accompany the attack.

On examination, there is swelling and vascular engorgement of the conjunctiva. The cornea demonstrates a dull reflex and appears hazy. The iris is bowed forward and may produce a shadow when a light from the side is directed across the eye. The pupil appears slightly dilated.

The medical treatment for angle-closure glaucoma is directed toward decreasing the intraocular pressure. This is accomplished by topical Timoptic 0.5% and oral hyperosmotic and carbonic anhydrase inhibitor agents. If the intraocular pressure remains elevated, mannitol 20% is administered intravenously in a dose of 1 to 2 gm/kg at a rate of 60 drops/minute. One must carefully titrate the dose because of drug-induced side effects on the renal and central nervous systems. After the intraocular pressure is reduced, a topical miotic is used to constrict the pupil and pull the iris away from the area of aqueous drainage. Later, an ophthalmic laser is used to create an opening for aqueous to flow between posterior and anterior portions of the iris.

TEAR FILM ABNORMALITIES

One of the most common causes of a red eye in the elderly is lacrimal insufficiency, or the dry eye. Patients with this condition may or may not demonstrate systemic disease. The dry eye is associated with systemic lupus erythematosus, pemphigoid, Sjögren's syndrome, erythema multiforme, scleroderma, periarteritis nodosa, and sarcoidosis.

Treatment of the dry eye involves tear replacement by means of artificial tears. In difficult cases, tear duct punctal occlusion is used to prevent any drainage of the tears. Moist chambers are placed around the eyes by means of plastic shields. Lubricating ointment is placed in the eyes at bedtime, and the eyes are even taped closed if there is lagophthalmos, or inability to close the eyes.

Interference with the normal lubrication and lysozyme function of the tears makes the dry eye susceptible to infection. Infections of the eyelid margin, namely blepharitis, can aggravate the tear deficiency and are treated aggressively with lid hygiene and topical antibiotics.

SYSTEMIC DISEASE

Scleritis is a painful, often bilateral cause of red eye seen in patients with connective tissue disease. The majority of patients are female, ranging in age from 40 to 60 years. The pain is so severe that it may awaken the patient from sleep. This condition is destructive and can cause perforation of the globe and loss of the eye. The inflammation localizes in the anterior or posterior portions of the sclera. It is thought to be due to activation of antigen-antibody complexes and complement that produce a vasculitis.

Treatment with topical steroid eyedrops every few hours helps to make the patient more comfortable. In order to suppress the inflammation, systemic nonsteroidal anti-inflammatory agents, such as indomethacin (Indocin), should be tried. To suppress inflammation until remission occurs, treatment should be started with 25 mg every day, increasing the dosage to 75 mg until the condition is controlled. If the disease is very destructive, 80 to 120 mg prednisolone per day can be given in divided doses and tapered to a maintenance dose of 15 mg per day. The patient may need to be on a maintenance dose for a few weeks, after which the drug is slowly withdrawn. If, upon withdrawal, the disease recurs, one should return to the initial high dose of systemic steroids and start to taper again. The intraocular pressure should be monitored, since glaucoma may occur. If glaucoma is developing, we place the patient on acetazolamide (Diamox), 500 mg twice a day.

Scleromalacia perforans is an actual necrosis of the sclera seen in long-standing polyarticular rheumatoid arthritis. The majority of patients are female. Large necrotic areas of sclera may require scleral grafting, since treatment with local and systemic steroids is often unsuccessful.

Thyroid disease can involve the eyes. Orbital Graves' disease is the most common cause of proptosis in adults. For a patient with thyroid ophthalmopathy, results of thyroid screening tests are often normal. On examination, the eyes show conjunctival injection over the extraocular muscles, lid retraction with appearance of a stare look, and symmetric proptosis between the two eyes. Visual loss may occur from optic nerve compression by the enlarged extraocular muscles.

Treatment is directed toward the associated problems in orbital Graves' disease, such as corneal drying from exposure. This is treated with lubricating ointment at bedtime, taping the eyes closed at bedtime, and using artificial tears frequently during the day. If corneal decompensation occurs, one should perform a lateral tarsorrhaphy to temporarily close the eye. With serious orbital congestion and optic nerve compression, high-dose systemic steroids, i.e., 120 mg daily, are started and slowly tapered. If there is progressive loss of vision due to optic nerve compression, a surgical orbital decompression procedure is performed.

POSTERIOR SEGMENT OCULAR PROBLEMS

The two principal retinopathy problems seen in the outpatient clinic population are caused by diabetes mellitus and hypertension. Ocular signs of these diseases are evident on direct opthalmoscopic examination.

DIABETES MELLITUS

Diabetes mellitus is the leading cause of blindness in the 45- to 75-year age group. There are approximately 2 to 5 million diabetic patients in the United States and an enormous number of undetected cases. Efforts are aimed at controlling blood glucose levels in the hope of arresting or preventing serious retinopathy. The incidence of diabetic retinopathy increases with the duration of the disease.

The earliest sign of diabetic retinopathy is venous dilatation. Eventually, chronic venous congestion produces tortuous, irregular vessels and structural changes, such as microaneurysms. These structures exhibit focal leakage of blood products due to a combination of factors, such as incompetent endothelium, pericyte degeneration, and thickened basement membrane. Hard exudates are the bright yellow starbursts seen around the microaneurysms that contain lipid. An early sign of retinal ischemia in diabetes is the appearance of the cotton-wool spot, or soft exudate. This represents an infarct in the neural retina. In addition, flame-shaped and dot-and-blot hemorrhages are scattered throughout the retina. With advanced retinal ischemia, new, friable blood vessels grow along the retinal surface and into the vitreous. The vessels may bleed, causing retinal and vitreous hemorrhages. Fibrosis and contraction of the vessel fronds pull on the retina, causing retinal detachment.

Photocoagulation is the mainstay of treatment for diabetic retinopathy. Laser is used to ablate areas of leakage or ischemia. Currently, an Early Treatment Diabetic Retinopathy Study (ETDRS) is being conducted to ascertain the effect of photocoagulation on milder forms of retinopathy. This innovative approach could mean earlier treatment with photocoagulation. The ETDRS is also trying to determine whether aspirin influences development of diabetic retinopathy. There is some evidence that diabetics with arthritis who take large doses of aspirin have less diabetic retinopathy.

HYPERTENSION

At least 15 million Americans suffer from hypertension, with its effects upon the heart, brain, kidney, and eyes. The eye changes involve the retina. The retinal vasculature shows arteriolar wall thickening and permeability changes. Sustained elevation of blood pressure produces necrosis of the vessel wall. Systemic hypertension may also produce branch retinal vein occlusion, with retinal hemorrhages and cotton-wool spots in the area of occlusion. Usually, hypertensive retinopathy does not seriously impair vision unless there is macular edema.

Retinal changes are graded from moderate arteriolar attenuation to retinal edema, hemorrhages, and soft exudates, which, if present, indicate a more serious state. When disc edema occurs, the patient is categorized as having malignant hypertension, and the prognosis for return of visual acuity is poor.

Obviously, treatment is aimed at controlling the hypertension. Photocoagulation for macular edema is controversial. Neovascularization may occur after branch vein occlusion and requires laser treatment.

It is important to remember that diabetic and hypertensive retinopathy is bilateral. If a patient demonstrates unilateral involvement of the diabetic retinopathy or if one eye appears to be worse, one should evaluate the patient for carotid occlusive disease. Unilateral total or partial carotid artery occlusion prevents or eliminates diabetic retinal manifestations so that there is a marked discrepancy between the two eyes.

Thus, certain ocular problems can alert the physician to look for evidence of systemic disease. We hope that this brief overview of common ocular problems will help the internist in patient evaluation and management.

REFERENCES

Ballantyne AJ, Michaelson IC: Textbook of the Fundus of the Eye. Livingstone, London, 1965, p 178–192.

Beigleman MN: Vernal conjunctivitis. University of Southern California Press, Los Angeles, 1950.

Cox J: Disodium cromoglycate (FPL 670) (Intal): A specific inhibitor of reagenic antigen-antibody mechanisms. Nature 216:1329, 1967.

Duke-Elder S, Leigh AG: System of ophthalmology. *In* Diseases of the Outer Eye, Vol 18. CV Mosby, St. Louis, 1965.

Grant WM: Toxicology of the Eye, 2nd ed. CC Thomas, Springfield, 1974, pp 88–101.

Hughes WF Jr: Alkali burns of the eye. I. Review of the literature and summary of present knowledge. Arch Ophthalmol 35:423, 1946.

Jawetz E, Thygeson P, Hanna L, et al: The etiology of epidemic keratoconjunctivitis. Am J Ophthalmol 43(Suppl):79, 1957.

Michaelson IC: Textbook of the Fundus of the Eye, 3rd ed. Livingstone, London, 1980, p 171–199.

Neumann E, Gutman MJ, Blumenkrantz J, et al: A review of 400 cases of vernal conjunctivitis. Am J Ophthalmol 47:166, 1959.

Watson DG, Hayreh SS: Scleritis and episcleritis. Br J Ophthalmol 60:163, 1976.

Watson P: Diseases of the sclera and episclera. *In* Duane T (ed): Clinical Ophthalmology. Vol. 4. Harper & Row, New York, 1983, pp 18–22.

Werner SC: Classification of the eye changes of Graves' disease. J Clin Endocrinol Metab 29:782, 1969.

Werner SC: The eye changes of Graves' disease. Overview. Mayo Clin Proc 47:969, 1972.

DISEASES OF THE JOINTS AND CONNECTIVE TISSUE

A. DEAN STEELE

1 · OSTEOARTHRITIS

*George L. Allen**
Robert J. Quinet†
**MAYO CLINIC AND MAYO FOUNDATION*
†OCHSNER CLINIC AND
ALTON OCHSNER MEDICAL FOUNDATION

DEFINITION AND PATHOPHYSIOLOGY

Osteoarthritis (OA, degenerative joint disease) is a noninflammatory disease that causes pain and deformity of joints and is characterized by deterioration and alteration of articular cartilage, surrounding ligaments, and underlying bone. Structural changes occur in the articular cartilage and new bone forms in the subchondral area and at the margins of the joints. Joint surface deterioration is progressive with aging. Osteoarthritis is of diverse causation and represents a final common pathway that is compounded by a failed repair mechanism. This repair, consisting of production of new cartilage and bone, seems to cause additional mechanical problems.

Osteoarthritis may exhibit a low-grade inflammation. Hydroxyapatite and calcium pyrophosphate dihydrate crystals have been demonstrated in synovial fluid and in the synovium of some osteoarthritic patients. These observations have aroused interest in abnormal mineral metabolism as a possible underlying cause of osteoarthritis and inflammation, as these crystals may evoke synovitis.

CLINICAL ASPECTS

Pain with motion or weight-bearing is the chief complaint, but pain at rest may occur with severe disease. Localized stiffness (gelling) may be present after periods of inactivity. Progressive disease is associated with limitation of motion, crepitus, and occasional localized tenderness. Symptoms are uncommon before the age of 40 unless there are associated preceding congenital, metabolic, or traumatic events. There are no systemic manifestations.

The joints most commonly involved by osteoarthritis include the distal interphalangeal joints, the proximal interphalangeal joints, the carpometacarpal and metacarpophalangeal joints of the thumb, the cervical and lumbar apophyseal joints, the hips, the knees, and the first metatarsophalangeal joint of the foot. The joints affected vary with sex, race, and associated occupational factors.

MANAGEMENT

Treatment of osteoarthritis has as its objective relieving pain and discomfort and minimizing disability. Effective treatment may delay progression of osteoarthritic changes and preserve joint function but will not reverse joint damage. Discomfort may be relieved even though pathologic changes continue to be present on roentgenograms and physical examination. Long-term goals are to restore function and reestablish individual independence. Hospitalization is rarely necessary except for operation.

NONPHARMACOLOGIC MEASURES

Certain general measures apply regardless of location of the joints involved. A program of management should be individually formulated, and the patient must understand the objectives of treatment. A successful program considers each joint involved, the nature and severity of symptoms, including occupational factors, and the effect of activities of daily living. All too frequently, treatment emphasis is on medication, which represents only one part of an overall program.

General measures include rest, the use of exercise and physical therapy, protection from trauma, proper positioning, and weight reduction. Surgery has a well-established role and is beneficial when part of a planned program.

Rest. The aching most patients experience is associated with overuse of the joint and is relieved by rest. Stiffness accompanies immobility and is usually greatest with the first few motions after a period of rest. Stiffness is significantly improved by a balanced program of rest and activity. Obviously, an osteoarthritic joint cannot tolerate as much stress as a normal one, and therefore, the pathologic process may accelerate if the joint is forced to perform beyond its limits. While in rare instances complete bed rest may be required, total joint immobilization is usually not necessary. When weight-bearing joints (knees, hips, lumbar spine) are involved, rest periods of up to an hour (several times daily) may be quite helpful. Dividing the day into periods of activity frequently proves useful. Periods of planned nonuse are usually sufficient for non-weight-bearing joints.

Spinal osteoarthritis usually responds to rest, heat, and salicylates. If the cervical spine is involved, immobilization with the use of a cervical collar may be helpful. A range-of-motion program combined with physical therapy (including traction) also is helpful but must be individualized.

Patients who have symptoms in the lumbar spine may find a firm mattress helpful. On occasion, severe muscle spasm may require the use of sedatives and muscle relaxants. Muscle relaxants should be avoided, particularly in elderly patients, because of side effects and habituating qualities.

Protection. If occupational factors are present, changes in the workplace may be necessary. Correction of abnormal forces acting upon the cartilage not only can decrease joint pain but also may slow developing osteoarthritic changes.

In some patients, body position and mechanics play an important role. The extra strain put on the knees, low back, and other weight-bearing joints by pronated feet, genu valgum or varum, and spinal curvature accelerates the rate of the pathologic process. Faulty posture can be helped by appropriate foot support, correction of lordotic changes within the lumbar spine, better support for large breasts, and reduction of a protuberant abdomen. A review of work habits and the role they play may be quite rewarding. Slouching while sitting or standing and prolonged bending over counters are examples of poor postural habits that may add to stiffness and muscle discomfort.

Diet. There is no evidence that diet plays a role in the pathogenesis of osteoarthritis. Although obesity may not be a factor in the pathogenesis of osteoarthritis, it may worsen symptoms in damaged weight-bearing joints and should be treated with appropriate weight reduction diets. Frequently patients who are obese become less active than normal, and this leads to additional weight gain, poor muscle tone, and decreased joint use. Behavioral reinforcement through diet clinics and group therapy is helpful.

Physical Therapy. Planned use of physical modalities such as heat and appropriate exercises is important to relieve pain and stiffness. Although these modalities are not curative, they are palliative. Control of pain permits patients to enjoy increased activity and to rest more comfortably. Heat can be effectively delivered by the use of bakers, hot packs, electric pads, and hot soaks. Contrast or paraffin baths are useful for hands and wrists. Diathermy and ultrasound are also helpful. Some patients receive benefit from moist or dry heat. In general, more expensive forms of heat delivery are no more effective than are simple measures. In a few patients, local heat increases symptoms and, therefore, should not be used. Patients should receive instruction to ensure that they are able to carry through individual treatment measures in their home environment. On occasion, massage may be necessary to relieve local muscle pain, but its effects are only temporary.

Exercise of the involved joint is important to decrease muscle spasm and prevent muscle atrophy. In patients with severe disease, only mild exercise can be tolerated. Beginning exercises should be provided in small amounts and then gradually increased. Emphasis should be on active rather than passive exercise. Isometric exercises are frequently helpful, particularly in treating weight-bearing joints such as the knees. Non-weight-bearing exercises may be important when there is lower extremity involvement.

Swimming is an excellent form of exercise because it does not restrict joint use and is not weight-bearing. Although walking rather than riding a stationary bicycle is frequently recommended, in some patients either or both may be stressful and should be avoided.

Some patients exercise their joints continuously in an attempt to avoid stiffness. Excessive exercise overloads involved joints and should be avoided. For each individual there is an important balance between rest and exercise that takes into consideration the degree of osteoarthritic changes, the joint involved, and the severity of symptoms.

Assistive Devices. Protection of a joint while it is being used is frequently helpful. Some patients with cervical pain are helped by the use of cervical collars. Lumbosacral corsets may give better spinal support, and various shoe orthoses give better foot support. Canes or crutches may be useful to take weight off a weight-bearing joint and redistribute it. Many patients are too proud to use such assistive devices, and although they realize their usefulness, are unwilling to compromise their attitude. Education will help reinforce the need for assistive devices, especially when combined with physical therapy training and information on use of local measures.

DRUG THERAPY

Increasingly, emphasis has been placed on drug management. Although relief of pain is important, the analgesic and anti-inflammatory qualities of available drugs have been overemphasized.

Aspirin remains the drug of choice. An adequate serum level of salicylates is 20 mg/dl, and it is usually obtained if the patient takes three to four aspirin tablets four times a day. Taking the tablets with meals is convenient and may avoid gastric intolerance. Taking aspirin crushed in yogurt, applesauce, or cottage cheese may be helpful in patients who have difficulty swallowing pills.

Although osteoarthritis is a degenerative process, an inflammatory component may be present to such a degree that simple analgesic medications are not totally adequate for control. However, in most instances, the use of anti-inflammatory medications and the local measures discussed above adequately control the patient's symptoms. In general, the use of other pain relievers, such as propoxyphene hydrochloride (Darvon), pentazocine (Talwin), and stronger analgesics should be avoided. Gastric distress can be decreased by the concomitant use of antacids. In some patients, liquid forms of salicylate, such as choline salicylate or choline magnesium trisalicylate, may be useful. Several forms of nonacetylated salicylates are helpful and are available in tablet form. These include magnesium trisalicylate (Trilisate), magnesium salicylate (Magan), and salsalate (Disalcid). Acetaminophen in doses of 650 mg every four to six hours may provide equivalent relief of pain in patients who cannot tolerate any form of salicylate.

In recent years, many nonsteroidal anti-inflammatory drugs (NSAID) have become available and are used instead of salicylates. Although there is no evidence that these medications are more advantageous than aspirin, they are frequently used to avoid gastric side effects, because of prejudice on the part of the patient or doctor, and to decrease the number of tablets taken per day. In older patients, toxic side effects must constantly be kept in mind and the dose somewhat decreased. In prescribing these medications, one should always consider the side effects and the possible interaction with other drugs. These NSAIDs and their dosages are briefly described in Table 1.

NSAIDs must be used cautiously in geriatric patients because of their effect on renal prostaglandins and blood flow. Gradually increasing the dose and careful monitoring of BUN and creatinine may decrease the risk of renal complications. They are to be avoided in chronic renal insufficiency and in situations associated with low renal perfusion.

Corticosteroid Therapy. The administration of systemic corticosteroids is rarely justified in the treatment of osteoarthritis. Well-known side effects associated with their prolonged use contraindicate their application in osteoarthritis. However, the local injection of corticosteroids into a joint has a definite place in management when combined with other local measures and medications. When corticosteroids are given intra-articularly, symptoms may be completely relieved in several days to weeks. In selected patients, relief is very gratifying. Sterile technique should always be followed to avoid infection.

Steroid preparations that have been most useful include methylprednisolone (Depo-medrol), triamcinolone hexacetonide (Aristospan), and betamethasone acetate (Celestone). Although symptomatic improvement may be of variable duration, relief of pain and stiffness may lead to overuse and, therefore, could be detrimen-

Table 1. NONSTEROIDAL ANTI-INFLAMMATORY DRUGS

	Trade Name	Recommended Daily Dose (mg)
Salicylates		
Aspirin	Ecotrin	325–500 mg/tabs, 2 q.i.d. (pc + hs)
Choline magnesium trisalicylate	Trilisate	500–750 mg, 2–3 tabs b.i.d. (pc)
Magnesium salicylate	Magan	545 mg, 2 tabs t.i.d. (pc)
Salicylsalicylic acid	Disalcid	500–750 mg, 2 b.i.d./t.i.d. (pc)
Diflunisal	Dolobid	250–500 mg, b.i.d. (pc)
Indole-related		
Indomethacin	Indocin	25–50 mg, t.i.d./q.i.d. (pc)
Sulindac	Clinoril	150–200 mg, b.i.d. (pc)
Tolmetin	Tolectin	200–400 mg, q.i.d. (pc)
Phenylpropionic acid		
Ibuprofen	Motrin, Rufen Advil	400–800 mg, t.i.d./q.i.d. (pc)
Naproxen	Naprosyn	250–500 mg, b.i.d. (pc)
Fenoprofen	Nalfon	300–600 mg, t.i.d./q.i.d. (pc)
Fenamates		
Meclofenamate	Meclomen	50–100 mg, t.i.d. (pc)
Oxicams		
Piroxicam	Feldene	20 mg, q.d. (pc)

tal. However, the relief of pain and stiffness may permit more effective use of physical therapy and appropriate balance of rest and exercise. Masking of pain may lead to serious overuse, particularly when injections are repeated in short intervals. A single joint should not be injected more than two or three times a year.

SPLINTING

Other local measures include splinting of selected joints, such as those in the thumb. Instruction in hand care helps to avoid hand or extremity overuse; it includes the use of mechanical devices for opening jars, lids, and cans and use of built-up handles. Problems with limitation of motion can be helped with such devices, which afford a greater degree of independence. A booklet illustrating these devices is obtainable upon request from the Arthritis Foundation for a nominal fee.

SURGERY

Probably the most significant advance in rehabilitation of osteoarthritis has come about through the use of total joint replacement. Remarkable strides have been made in the types of prosthetic joints available. When the degree of destructive change within a joint is such that joint replacement is recommended, overexpectation on the part of the patient should be avoided because the degree of individual patient success is variable. Joint replacements are most successful in the hip and knee.

Surgical measures (other than joint replacement) can be considered. For example, with unicompartmental narrowing (such as the medial compartment of the knee), an upper tibial osteotomy may be all that is necessary to change the weight relationship and relieve the symptoms. After an osteotomy, it may be years before another surgical procedure is required. In selected joints of the hands and fingers, an arthrodesis may be the best procedure. This is particularly true in conditions affecting the stability at the base of the thumb. Despite the advances in surgical replacement techniques, no good prosthetic joints have been developed for the distal interphalangeal joints of the hands, and fusion may be the best means of controlling pain and dysfunction.

In the foot, local measures to afford better arch support and to distribute weight-bearing should be used before operation is recommended. Pain and associated hypertrophic changes and deformity are common with disease at the first metatarsophalangeal joint (bunion joint). With disease at this joint, weight distribution frequently is shifted to the second and third metatarsal heads and results in associated hammer toes and metatarsalgia. Surgery may be helpful to relieve these symptoms. Surgery, in itself, is never a substitute for local measures of control to give better foot support. Many patients resist wearing the type of shoes necessary to obtain good foot support and do not like arch supports and orthotic appliances. Treatment is such an individual matter that it must be discussed with each patient, whose specific expectations must be kept in mind.

PATIENT INFORMATION AND EDUCATION

In the treatment of a specific joint, physical medicine measures include range of motion and muscle strengthening to avoid contractures and atrophy. It is an excellent educational experience for the patient to learn the importance of a daily program of range-of-motion and strengthening exercises, and use of local physical modalities. Reinforcing these techniques through periodic reassessment is important. It is surprising how many patients misunderstand directions that they have received. Frequently, it helps to give the patient a pamphlet to read. An excellent pamphlet on osteoarthritis is available at a modest cost through the Arthritis Foundation, 1314 Spring Street, N.W., Atlanta, Georgia 30309. In this way, a patient can review his or her problem without the pressure of having to ask questions and remembering all the information presented in an initial consultation.

PERIODIC EVALUATION

Unless a patient is taking medications that require follow-up blood studies, there are no specific routine laboratory studies required. Follow-up visits to assess progress are helpful to prevent misunderstanding of instructions and serve to reinforce the need to continue protective programs. They also help to ensure patient compliance.

PREVENTIVE MEASURES

When a patient continues to abuse his or her joints, it may be helpful to counsel family members. Instruction in a hand-care program helps when osteoarthritis is a result of hand abuse. To retard progression, it is useful to ask an occupational therapist to review activities of daily living and to suggest methods of joint protection.

SOCIOECONOMIC ASPECTS

Some patients may avoid recommended treatments because of financial concerns. This is particularly true in younger patients. For that reason, physicians should be aware of the disability provisions and refer to the Social Security Administration for advice. In some instances vocational rehabilitation is indicated, and help can be provided through local and state resources for both reeducation and counseling. Medications are normally not available through these sources. Medicare does not pay for drugs that can be self-administered, and it will not pay for special shoes unless they are part of a compound leg brace. In most states, Medicaid does help provide for these services. In addition, psychosocial problems may arise because of the threat to life style and imposition of loss of mobility, function, and independence. Depression and low self-esteem then occur and must be recognized and treated. A frank discussion between the physician and the patient usually helps to modify these factors.

REFERENCES

Blockshear JL, Napier JS, Davidman M, et al.: Renal complications of nonsteroidal anti-inflammatory drugs: identification and monitoring of those at risk. Semin Arthritis Rheum 14:163–175, 1985.

Brandt KD: Osteoarthritis: clinical patterns and pathology. In Kelley WN, Harris ED Jr, Ruddy S, et al (eds): Textbook of Rheumatology, 2nd ed. W.B. Saunders Co, Philadelphia, 1985, pp 1432–1448.

Ehrlich GE: Erosive inflammatory and primary generalized osteoarthritis. In Moskowitz RW, Howell DS, Goldberg VM, et al (eds): Osteoarthritis: Diagnosis and Management. W.B. Saunders Co, Philadelphia, 1984, pp 199–209.

Gerber LH, Hicks JE: Rehabilitation in the management of patients with osteoarthritis. In Moskowitz RW, Howell DS, Goldberg VM, et al (eds): Osteoarthritis: Diagnosis and Management. W.B. Saunders Co, Philadelphia, 1984, pp 287–315.

Sokoloff L: Current concepts of the pathogenesis of osteoarthritis. In Nelson CL, Dwyer AP (eds): The Aging Musculoskeletal System: Physiological and Pathological Problems. D.C. Heath & Co, Collamore Press, Lexington, MA, 1984, pp 113–120.

2 · RHEUMATOID ARTHRITIS

Ronald L. Kaye
PALO ALTO MEDICAL CLINIC

DEFINITION AND DIAGNOSTIC CRITERIA

Rheumatoid arthritis (RA) is a chronic systemic disease affecting not only joints and other connective tissues but various organs and the body as a whole. It is an inflammatory disease of unknown cause that is usually progressive, especially in terms of joint involvement. Various diagnostic criteria have been developed, the most commonly used of which are the American Rheumatism Association criteria, devised in 1958, which are listed below. In criteria numbers one through five, the joint signs or symptoms must be continuous for at least six weeks. A diagnosis of "classic" RA requires seven of the following criteria, "definite" RA five of the criteria, "probable" RA three of the criteria, and "possible" RA two of the criteria. In addition, 20 exclusions to the diagnosis are enumerated and include conditions that might mimic or be confused with RA, such as rheumatic fever or gouty arthritis. In drug studies and for most epidemiologic studies, usually only "classic" or "definite" RA patients are included. The criteria are:

1. Morning stiffness.
2. Pain on motion or tenderness in at least one joint.
3. Swelling in at least one joint.
4. Swelling of at least one other joint (within three months of criterion number three).
5. Symmetrical joint swelling (simultaneously).
6. Subcutaneous nodules.
7. X-ray changes typical of RA.
8. Positive agglutination test—demonstration of the "rheumatoid factor."
9. Poor mucin precipitate from synovial fluid.
10. Characteristic histologic changes in synovial membranes.
11. Characteristic histologic changes in nodules.

Because criteria numbers nine through 11 often are not present or testable, usually the diagnosis relies on criteria numbers one through eight.

ETIOLOGY

The etiology is unknown and appears to be multifactorial, including probable genetic, hormonal, and environmental relationships. Evidence for genetic influences is based on twin surveys, family aggregations, and the association of histocompatibility antigens HLA-Dw4 and DR4 with seropositive RA. Possible hormonal considerations reflect the facts that the disease is three times more prevalent in females than in males, the well-known phenomenon of disease remission in perhaps half of all women with rheumatoid arthritis during pregnancy, and the results of a few studies demonstrating some reduced incidence of RA in females on oral contraceptives. For years a possible infectious etiology has been sought, and despite present consideration that the immunologic phenomena seen are possibly "released" in a susceptible individual by an organism such as a virus, no definite agent has been conclusively identified. Environmental phenomena, both internal and extenal, such as physical and psychological stresses, have also been felt to play a part in aggravating the condition. Hence, current thought of etiology considers a genetically and hormonally predisposed individual who, given an inciting event such as a viral infection, in a matrix of possible emotional and/or physical stress, develops an autoimmune disease with immunologic and inflammatory characteristics.

PATHOPHYSIOLOGY

The earliest events in RA appear in the synovial lining with microvascular injury and proliferation of synovial lining cells. The synovium becomes grossly edematous and protrudes into the joint cavity in villous projections. There is proliferation of both synovial type A and B cells, and mononuclear cells aggregate into follicles in the subsynovial areas. These mononuclear cells are predominantly lymphocytes with some macrophages and plasma cells. It is felt that antibodies against an unknown antigen, perhaps altered IgG, are produced in the synovium, cartilage, and joint fluid. An immune complex results, which activates the complement sequence. An inflammatory process results as polymorphonuclear leukocytes (PMNs) are attracted by complement-released chemoactive factors. During the PMN phagocytosis of immune complexes, lysosomal enzymes, oxygen radicals, and arachidonic acid metabolites are released. The chemicals facilitate destruction of the nearby tissues such as cartilage and bone. This PMN phenomenon goes on concomitantly in the pannus and the proliferation of granulation tissue growing over and into the cartilage from the synovial lining. Overgrowth of fibrous connective tissue can lead to bony ankylosis.

CLINICAL ASPECTS

The *prevalence* of RA is approximately 1% or 2% in most Caucasian groups with a low prevalence of approximately 0.1% among African blacks and a high of around 6% in some North American Indians. The disease appears to be relatively "new," only described during the last few hundred years and present in some old masters' paintings during the same period.

The *sex incidence* reflects a female preponderance of approximately three to one. Individuals of any age can be affected, with a peak incidence of *onset* somewhere between the age of 35 and 45. The disease in children as many varieties, appearing often to be almost distinctly different from that which occurs in adults.

The *course* of the disease can vary from a mild articular illness of brief duration to a marked, progressive destructive process with systemic involvement. In adults, the onset is more commonly insidious than acute and more frequently polyarticular than monoarticular.

The majority of patients display a slowly progressive polyarthritis, some have an intermittent arthritis, and a relatively few demonstrate a self-limited disease. The mode of onset is not related to the subsequent course of the disease or prognosis.

JOINT MANIFESTATIONS

Articular manifestations are the symptoms and signs of inflammation and include pain, redness, heat, swelling, stiffness, and limitation of motion. Morning stiffness is characteristic of RA and usually lasts more than 30 minutes. Stiffness after inactivity, such as after sitting for a long period of time, is notable and usually is referred to as "gelling."

Any diarthrodial joint in the body can be involved. The small joints of the hands and feet are most often involved, while wrists and knees are also commonly involved. The disease may spread throughout the body with even temporomandibular ("jaw" pain) and cricoarytenoid (manifested as laryngitis) joint involvement.

Hand involvement characteristically is in the metacarpophalangeal joints, especially the second and third, and the proximal interphalangeal joints. Complications and deformities include ulnar deviation, swan-neck and boutonnière deformities, and rupture of extensor tendons. Pressure on the median nerve at the wrist may produce a carpal tunnel syndrome. Enlargement of the gastrocnemius-semimembranosus bursa (Baker's cyst) may rupture into the calf and mimic an acute thrombophlebitis. Anterior dislocation of the first cervical vertebra or subluxation of the odontoid process of the second cervical vertebra can lead to neurologic manifestations.

GENERAL AND EXTRA-ARTICULAR MANIFESTATIONS

It is not unusual for the patient with RA to have general systemic signs and symptoms, such as fatigue, weakness, and perhaps weight loss. Often, these general manifestations are the first to come and the last to go.

Extra-articular manifestations include those that are specific to the disease but occur outside the joint (e.g., rheumatoid nodules) and those that may occur from a variety of conditions (e.g., pleural effusion). Following is a list of some of the extra-articular manifestations seen in RA:

1. Systemic: general malaise, weakness, fever, weight loss.
2. Rheumatoid nodules.
3. Cardiac: pericarditis, granulomas, myocarditis, endocarditis, amyloidosis, arteritis.
4. Pulmonary: pleurisy, pleural effusion, pulmonary rheumatoid nodules, interstitial fibrosis, rheumatoid pneumoconiosis.
5. Ophthalmologic: keratoconjunctivitis sicca, episcleritis, scleritis, scheromalacia performans.
6. Blood vessel: vasculitis, Raynaud's phenomenon.
7. Hematologic: anemia, thrombocytosis, hyperviscosity syndrome.
8. Lymphatic: Felty's syndrome (RA, splenomegaly, and leukopenia), lymphadenopathy.

9. Neurologic: carpal tunnel syndrome, vasculitis with mononeuritis multiplex, distal sensory neuropathy.

LABORATORY FINDINGS

The erythrocyte sedimentation rate (ESR) is elevated in most patients and may parallel the disease activity. Rheumatoid factor (RF) is found in approximately three quarters of patients with this disease. It is also found in increasing incidence with age and is not specific for RA. Other common findings, nonspecific, include anemia, elevation of acute phase reactants such as C-reactive protein and alpha$_2$-globulin, and hypergammaglobulinemia. Antinuclear antibodies can be present in 25% to 50% of patients with RA at some time during the course of their disease. These usually are of the diffuse pattern by immunofluorescent straining. Synovial fluid analysis is helpful but not specific. Acetic acid added to rheumatoid joint fluid forms a loose mucin clot, reflecting depolymerization of hyaluronate. Hemolytic complement in the joint fluid is usually reduced. There is an increase in white blood cells in the synovial fluid, mostly mononuclear early in the disease, and later polymorphonuclear. Synovial biopsy may reveal characteristic abnormalities as outlined under "Pathophysiology."

RADIOLOGY

Characteristic findings are very helpful, but not diagnostic. Symmetrical involvement with a narrowed joint space, juxta-articular osteoporosis, and erosion of bone, especially the second and third metacarpophalangeal and proximal interphalangeal joints of the hands, are highly suggestive.

MANAGEMENT

PLAN, GOALS, AND THE RHEUMATOID ARTHRITIS HEALTH CARE TEAM

The main goals of management are (1) preservation of function of the involved joints and surrounding tissues; (2) suppression of the disease process; (3) relief of pain; and (4) maintenance of quality of life, including abilities to relate to other persons and to continue one's occupation.

Most treatment can be offered in the outpatient setting with the utilization of an appropriate health care team consisting of the primary physician, specialists such as rheumatologists, surgeons and podiatrists when necessary, physical and occupational therapists, and social workers. Hospitalization is rarely necessary except for surgery or treatment of extra-articular manifestations and complications such as cardiac or pulmonary involvement. Sometimes hospitalization may be desirable for observation of whether a patient will respond to a concentrated physical medicine program, for complete rest, and for initiation of drug therapy with assessment of its effects. In this era of cost-effectiveness and utilization concerns, this is rarely done.

Home health care for the home-bound is usually possible through visiting nurse and physical therapist associations. Surgery for RA is quite advanced and includes synovectomies, debridement, fusion, artificial joint replacement, and tendon repair. Indications for surgery include failure of drug treatment with progressive destruction of a joint and/or surrounding tissue, and the need for rehabilitative surgery to allow functional improvement.

Since RA is a systemic disease and has many manifestations, it is imperative in the care of the patient with RA that the physician focus not just on the joints but on all involved organ systems.

NONPHARMACOLOGIC MEASURES

Patients with RA will require both general body and local joint rest, good nutrition, patient education, sex counseling, psychological support, social services, and physical and occupational therapy.

Physical therapy modalities include heat therapy, massage, exercises, and appropriate assistive devices, such as canes, crutches and walkers. Joint protection, splinting, and functional rehabilitation, as well as preservation of energy in various activities, all contribute toward the goals of management outlined above. Consultation with physical and occupational therapists will provide detailed instruction to patients.

DRUG THERAPY

A stepwise approach to the treatment of rheumatoid arthritis extends from the least specific to more specific therapy as outlined in Figure 1. However, as one ascends the steps toward more specific drugs, there is usually also an increase in toxicity. An exception may be low-dose corticosteroids, compared with disease-modifying drugs. Some of the immunosuppressive drugs mentioned in Figure 1 are still considered experimental.

With very mild disease, such as that manifested chiefly by stiffness and with little pain or inflammation, the patient may require only rest, physical therapy, education, and perhaps a mild analgesic. With signs and symptoms of inflammation, especially with persistence, an anti-inflammatory drug is indicated. The agents of choice for initial therapy are the nonsteroidal anti-inflammatory drugs (NSAIDs). These include both salicylates and nonsalicylates. These drugs and other NSAIDs discussed below are classified and listed in Table 1.

Salicylates

Aspirin has always been the cornerstone of RA therapy because it works, is ubiquitous, and is inexpensive. In small doses it is analgesic; in sufficient larger doses it is also anti-inflammatory. The problem is that it may require the equivalent of 16 to 24 aspirin to be truly anti-inflammatory and at that dosage the toxicity may be great. However, some of the special coatings or delivery systems of some acetylated salicylates may make them better tolerated and less toxic, and so they provide an alternative to aspirin. Because of potential gastrointestinal upset, most physicians prescribe salicylates with food or milk or antacids; however, both approaches may decrease absorption. I usually start acetylated salicylates in a dose of 10 grains four times a day, usually with meals and at bedtime. If the patient does well and the disease appears under good control clinically, I do not administer more and do not obtain serum salicylate levels. If the patient does not do well and/or there are signs of active synovitis, I increase the dosage 10 grains at a time, giving the additional doses

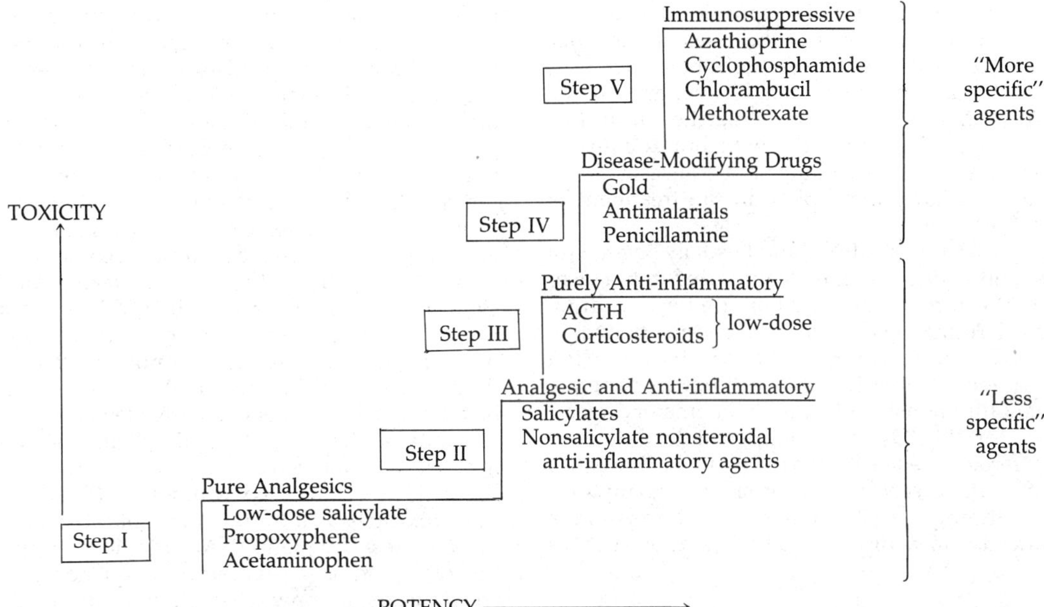

Figure 1. Stepwise approach to the drug treatment of rheumatoid arthritis.

at times when the patient has the most difficulty, for example, on arising, for morning stiffness. Salicylates are given in increasing amounts until (1) there is a clinically adequate effect or (2) there is toxicity or (3) a serum salicylate level of 20 to 25 mg/dl is achieved. Potential side effects include gastrointestinal bleeding, abnormal liver function, and tinnitus.

Because of toxicity at anti-inflammatory levels of some salicylates, many physicians utilize nonacetylated salicylates or nonsalicylate NSAIDs initially or after a trial of acetylated salicylate. These drugs are as efficacious as high-dose aspirin. They are more expensive, but in studies against aspirin, their advantages are less minor gastrointestinal upset, less microscopic bleeding, and less tinnitus.

Nonsalicylate NSAIDs

There has been a tremendous proliferation of nonsalicylate NSAIDs, listed in Table 1. Oraflex (benoxaprofen), Zomax (zomepirac), and Tandearil (oxyphenbutazone) were removed from use in recent years and are, consequently, not listed. With many NSAIDs available, the question is how does a physician determine which one is appropriate. Multi-drug trials in the same individual have demonstrated that some NSAIDs appear to be more consistently efficacious than others. Each drug, however, may have better or best efficacy in a given individual. Thus, one might have to try three to four different NSAIDs to find the one that is most effective. An NSAID should be given for approximately a month before concluding that it will not work and moving on to the next NSAID.

Side effects common to all the NSAIDs include allergic reactions, photosensitivity, edema, both minor and major gastrointestinal and renal toxicity, potential impaired hepatic function, and mild central nervous system effects and tinnitus.

There are significant differences in terms of special properties and side effects between the NSAIDs. It should be stressed that the following side effects are rare, but are mentioned to alert the clinician to these differences. All of the NSAIDs can be given either with or without food, except Clinoril and Nalfon. Clinoril must be taken with food to achieve a good blood level, whereas the absorption of Nalfon will be significantly lessened if taken with food. Tolectin can cause a false-positive test for proteinuria. Motrin can cause amblyopia, and aseptic meningitis has been described with its

Table 1. NONSTEROIDAL ANTI-INFLAMMATORY AGENTS FOR RHEUMATOID ARTHRITIS

Salicylates
Acetylated (acetylsalicylic acid)
  Aspirin 650–1300 mg q.i.d.
  Easprin 975 mg t.i.d., q.i.d.
  Ecotrin 500–1000 mg q.i.d.
  Zorprin 1600 mg b.i.d.
Nonacetylated
  Arthropan (choline salicylate) 650 mg q.i.d.
  Disalcid (salsalate) 500 mg b.i.d.
  Dolobid (diflunisal) 500 mg b.i.d., t.i.d.
  Trilisate (choline magnesium trisalicylate) 1500 mg b.i.d.

Nonsalicylates
Carboxylic Acid derivatives
  Acetic acid derivatives (indoles, indenes)
    Clinoril (sulindac) 200 mg b.i.d.
    Indocin (indomethacin) 25–50 mg t.i.d., q.i.d.
    Tolectin (tolmetin) 400 mg t.i.d., q.i.d.
  Proprionic acid derivatives
    Motrin, Rufen, Advil, Nuprin (ibuprofen) 300–600 mg q.i.d.
    Nalfon (fenoprofen) 300–600 t.i.d., q.i.d.
    Naprosyn (naproxen) 250–500 mg b.i.d.
    Anaprox (naproxen sodium) 275–550 mg b.i.d.
    Orudis (ketoprofen) 75–100 mg t.i.d.
  Fenamates
    Meclomen (meclofenamate sodium) 50–100 mg b.i.d., t.i.d., q.i.d.
Enolic Acid derivatives
  Oxicams
    Feldene (piroxicam) 20 mg single dose
  Pyrazolones
    Butazolidin (phenylbutazone) 100 mg t.i.d., q.i.d.

use in patients with systemic lupus erythematosus. Nalfon has accounted for half of the cases of nephrotic syndrome, 30% of the cases of acute tubular necrosis, and 28% of the cases of acute interstitial nephritis noted with NSAIDs. Meclomen can cause diarrhea in up to a third of patients. Chief concerns with Butazolidin are agranulocytosis and aplastic anemia; because of these, it is felt to have no present place in the treatment of rheumatoid arthritis.

Dosage with the NSAIDs should usually begin with a moderate dose and be gradually increased until reaching either (1) control of the condition, (2) toxicity, or (3) the maximal recommended dosage. As mentioned, it may be necessary to continue the NSAID for a full month to know whether it will or will not work before going to another nonsteroidal anti-inflammatory agent. Other uses for NSAIDs are to reduce the total amount of corticosteroid needed in a patient, to help wean a patient off corticosteroids, and for signs or symptoms that break through, such as morning stiffness in a patient already on a disease-modifying drug such as gold.

Disease-Modifying Agents

When the NSAIDs fail to control the disease and RA progresses, becomes destructive, and causes erosions of bone, one should consider the disease-modifying agents such as gold, antimalarials, or penicillamine. Usually one waits until at least six months of more conservative therapy is attempted.

Gold. Gold has been utilized in the treatment of RA for over 50 years. Gold salt–induced remissions in RA are excellent, and are seen in 50% or more of patients with active disease treated with gold during the first five years of the disease. Gold sodium thiomalate (Myochrysine) and aurothioglucose (Solganal) are given intramuscularly. Now there is also an oral gold compound, auranofin (Ridaura). The standard regimen of intramuscular gold consists of a 10-mg test injection followed in a week by a 25-mg injection. A week later 50 mg is injected, and 50 mg is injected weekly thereafter until 1 gm total is administered. If the patient improves earlier, then the gold salt injections are spaced farther apart. If there is a remission at the end of 1 gm total gold salt, then maintenance therapy is approximately 50 mg once a month. The usual dose of oral gold is 6 mg/day in divided doses. Because a second course of gold often is not as efficacious as the first, as long as gold therapy is effective it is continued indefinitely.

Side effects of gold commonly include pruritus, rashes, mouth ulcerations, and a metallic taste in the mouth. Injections must be stopped until mouth ulcerations or rashes clear, and after clearing, then a small dose may be instituted with caution to see if they will reappear. A nitritoid reaction with vasomotor flushing and weakness within minutes of an injection of gold salt occurs almost exclusively with the water-soluble Myochrysine, and substitution of fat-soluble Solganal will generally preclude further reactions. Serious complications include agranulocytosis, aplastic anemia, thrombocytopenia, pancytopenia, exfoliative dermatitis, nephrotic syndrome, obliterative bronchiolitis, and colitis. These complications require immediate cessation of the gold and treatment with corticosteroids. Because of these potential hazards, a complete blood count,

including a platelet count, and urinalysis should precede each gold injection. Thrombocytopenia less than 150,000 or proteinuria that persists contraindicates continued use in general. Some clinicians feel proteinuria over 1 gm or so is a contraindication; I do not continue gold if proteinuria of any degree does not clear when gold is withheld. Hematuria should alert one to proceed cautiously. Usually, hematuria does not occur without proteinuria in gold toxicity. Leukopenia may be difficult to assess, since it may be simply secondary to a virus, to other drugs the patient may be taking, or to Felty's syndrome. Leukopenia less than 3000 white cells/mm^3 requires one to temporarily discontinue gold. If the white blood count returns to normal, then a smaller dose of gold can be instituted as a test. If the white blood count again falls below this level, it is prudent to discontinue the gold. Periodic chemistry panels help monitor liver and renal function.

The new oral gold compound (Ridaura) has the same toxicities as intramuscular gold, but they are said to occur less frequently. An additional problem with the oral gold is a significant frequency of diarrhea, which leads to only a small percentage of patients having to discontinue the drug. Precautions are those stated for intramuscular gold.

Antimalarials. Antimalarials such as hydroxychloroquine (Plaquenil) and chloroquine (Aralen) can also induce remissions in RA. They also take up to six months of use for an adequate trial. The usual dosage is 200 to 400 mg of Plaquenil (hydroxychloroquine) per day and no more than 6 mg/kg/day. After a remission is apparent, one can reduce the dose from twice to once daily or even to every other day, judging by the patient's response. Gastrointestinal upsets may occur, but they are more uncommon than with NSAIDs and salicylates. Very rare side effects include a proximal neuromyopathy, interstitial keratitis, and an irreversible retinopathy. The ophthalmologic hazards have precluded its more widespread use. The retinopathy appears to be dose- and time-related, and the current guidelines of dosage relate to this. Usually, three or four years of therapy are required for retinopathy to appear. A baseline ophthalmologic examination to be sure there is no contraindication and for comparison later is highly recommended, and follow-up examinations are needed every six months as well as for any visual symptoms.

Penicillamine. Penicillamine (Cuprimine, Depen) can also induce remissions of RA. The remissions may also require six months of therapy. Because of potential toxicity, a "go low, go slow" program is advocated, starting with 125 mg/day with perhaps a doubling to 250 mg/day in three months as the usual initiation of therapy. Doses of up to 1000 mg are sometimes eventually administered. Failure at this dose dictates discontinuing the drug. Penicillamine must be taken on an empty stomach for appropriate absorption. This drug may chelate heavy metals (iron, zinc, copper), and so adjustments of compounds containing these elements must be made if taken concomitantly. Just as with gold, a CBC, urinalysis, and platelet count must be done frequently and periodically, and periodic chemistry panels, especially for serum creatinine and liver function, are important in monitoring for side effects.

Not only can this drug cause the same side effects as gold in the bone marrow and kidneys, but it can also cause diseases such as systemic lupus erythematosus, myasthenia gravis, pemphigus vulgaris, Goodpasture's syndrome, dermatomyositis, and polymyositis. Taste impairment is often an early concomitant and does not preclude the use of this drug. Often it takes a year for this toxicity to disappear. Rashes are not uncommon, both early and late in its administration. An early-onset rash often subsides and does not reappear, but one occurring late often precludes continued use. Because the side effects of penicillamine are so severe, it should be used only if other therapies fail.

Corticosteroids

Corticosteroids usually affect the signs and symptoms of RA, and if they do not have some effect on the disease, one must question the diagnosis! One tries to use the smallest dose of corticosteroid possible in a given patient, not only because of side effects, but also because the patient (or the disease) becomes so dependent on it that it is often difficult to discontinue or reduce the dosage. Doses of 5 to 7½ mg/day may be efficacious and 1-mg tablets may be obtained to keep the dose low and to reduce it by small decrements (for example, ½ or 1 mg). Toxicity of corticosteroids long term has precluded their more extensive use in RA, since the disease requires so many years of such therapy. Side effects, however, are usually very much dose-related, and low-dose corticosteroids, for example, under 5 to 7.5 mg/day, are enjoying a somewhat cautious resurgence. Although ideally one would like to give corticosteroids as alternate-day therapy, it is often not efficacious administered in this fashion. It may be given as a single daily AM dose. Corticosteroids may be necessary for extra-articular, often life-threatening complications of RA, such as pericarditis, vasculitis, and mononeuritis multiplex. They are also used judiciously and infrequently intra-articularly. ACTH and intramuscular corticosteroids may be very helpful as adjunctive therapy on occasion when a patient is not responding to NSAIDs, when one does not wish to utilize oral corticosteroids, or when other disease-modifying drugs are contraindicated.

The side effects of corticosteroids are well known and include moon facies, hirsutism, "buffalo hump," purple striae, glaucoma, posterior subcapsular cataracts, hypertension, peptic ulcer, renal stones, diabetes mellitus, hypercholesterolemia, personality changes and psychoses, osteoporosis and collapsed vertebrae, and aseptic necrosis of bone. With long-term steroid administration, vitamin D, 50,000 units twice per week, and 1500 mg of calcium daily should be given to mitigate osteoporosis. Although corticosteroids do not induce a remission of RA in the usual sense, review of original papers does show some decrease in bone erosion in patients receiving higher dose corticosteroids.

Other Drugs

Immunosuppressive drugs are used in patients with severe progressive RA when the drugs mentioned previously fail. They are also sometimes used for severe life-threatening conditions, such as vasculitis or mononeuritis multiplex, either when corticosteroids fail or in conjunction with them.

Azathioprine (Imuran) is the only one with current FDA approval for treatment of RA. The dose is 1.5 to 2.5 mg/kg/day by mouth. It is a purine analogue and is converted to 6-MP in vivo. 6-MP is metabolized by xanthine oxidase. If one gives a xanthine oxidase inhibitor, such as allopurinol, to the patient concomitantly, the 6-MP level will be increased with increased potential for toxicity. Hence, the dose of azathioprine should be reduced to one third or one fourth if given to a patient concomitantly taking allopurinol. Toxicity includes gastrointestinal disturbances, hepatic dysfunction, thrombocytopenia, leukopenia, increased susceptibility to infection due to bone marrow depression, and teratogenicity. Monitoring requires watching for signs of infection, periodic laboratory testing, and emphasis on birth control in patients of child-bearing age.

Methotrexate does not yet have FDA approval for treatment of RA, but along with its success in psoriatic arthritis and recent studies in RA, it is enjoying more widespread use. Dosage is interpolated from its use in psoriatic patients. By mouth it is given in a total dose of 5 to 30 mg once weekly in three divided doses every 12 hours, for example 5 mg every 12 hours × three doses at weekly intervals. Alternative administration includes 15 to 50 mg intravenously every week as a single dose. Toxicity includes gastrointestinal disturbances, stomatitis, bone marrow depression, megaloblastic anemia, hepatitis with or without cirrhosis, and teratogenicity. Monitoring includes those aspects mentioned under azathioprine. In addition, it should be noted that even periodic liver function tests and/or liver biopsies cannot always predict who will develop cirrhosis.

Other immunosuppressive drugs include *cyclophosphamide* (Cytoxan) and *chlorambucil* (Leukeran). These agents are not approved for RA, but may be helpful with unrelenting severe progressive RA not responding to the previously mentioned drugs, or in a patient with severe life-threatening complications, such as vasculitis. The dosage of cyclophosphamide is 1.5 to 2.5 mg/kg/day by mouth or as an intravenous bolus, 10 to 15 mg/kg at three to four week intervals. Chlorambucil is given by mouth in a dosage of 0.5 to 0.2 mg/kg/day. These drugs both can cause bone marrow depression and gastrointestinal disturbances, and teratogenicity. Cyclophosphamide can cause hemorrhagic cystitis and sterility, and has a fair incidence of alopecia. Careful laboratory monitoring is imperative. These drugs, as well as others that have been used as anticancer drugs, may cause tumors, some of which are malignant. Consequently, they should be used only when all other drugs fail and life-threatening complications are present in RA.

PERIODIC DISEASE EVALUATION

Assessments as to the outcome of management include (1) change in the duration of morning stiffness; (2) change in ability to do activities of daily living; (3) magnitude of pain; (4) objective changes in the redness, heat, swelling, and limitation of motion of joints; and (5) significant changes in the ESR and RF. X-ray changes are important, but require a much longer period of time for significant change.

PATIENT EDUCATION

Social services and psychologists/psychiatrists are very helpful to patients in their education and handling of the disease and in managing socioeconomic aspects of this condition.

The National Arthritis Foundation and its local chapters have readily available a myriad of pamphlets and booklets on various aspects of RA, including facts about the conditon, diet, surgery, and quackery. These sources, as well as self-help books and courses, should be an integral part of the management of the RA patient. Through such sessions there can be reinforcement of such concepts as compliance with drug regimens and physical therapy as well as the psychological support system necessary to sustain one through a chronic painful devastating disease process.

Utilizing all the elements mentioned in this chapter, the prognosis for most patients with the disease is, indeed, usually a good one.

REFERENCES

Allbeck P: Epidemiological investigations on rheumatoid arthritis in Stockholm. The use of different data sources. Scand J Rheumatol [Suppl] 55:10, 1984.

Carmichael J, Shankel SW: Effects of nonsteroidal anti-inflammatory drugs on prostaglandins and renal function. Am J Med 78:992–1000, 1985.

Harris ED Jr: Rheumatoid arthritis: the clinical spectrum. In Kelley WN, Harris ED, Ruddy S, et al (eds): Textbook of Rheumatology, 2nd ed. W.B. Saunders Co., Philadelphia, 1985, pp 915–950.

Katz WA: Rheumatic Diseases: Diagnosis and Management. J.B. Lippincott Co, Philadelphia, 1977.

Lightfoot RW Jr: Treatment of rheumatoid arthritis. In McCarty DJ (ed): Arthritis and Allied Conditions: A Textbook of Rheumatology, 10th ed. Lea & Febiger, Philadelphia, 1985, pp 668–676.

Ropes MW, Bennett GA, Cobb S, et al: Revision of diagnostic criteria for rheumatoid arthritis. Bull Rheum Dis 9:175–176, 1958.

3 · SCLERODERMA AND MIXED CONNECTIVE TISSUE SYNDROME

R. K. Winkelmann
MAYO CLINIC AND MAYO FOUNDATION

Scleroderma is a complex systemic disease that involves the production of increased amounts of collagen, vascular endarterial fibromucinosis, and inflammatory immunologic reactivity. These pathologic changes are expressed in various degrees in skin, gastrointestinal tract, lung, heart, and kidneys. Scleroderma may principally affect the vascular system of an organ or may be associated with sclerosis and atrophy of the organ parenchyma. Patients may show limited, slowly progressive disease or rapidly spreading diffuse scleroderma. Scleroderma syndromes include acrosclerosis, diffuse scleroderma, and gastrointestinal, pulmonary, myocardial, and renal scleroderma. The CREST syndrome is equivalent to acrosclerosis and represents calcinosis, Raynaud's phenomenon, esophageal disease, sclerodactyly, and telangiectasia.

Exposure to environmental chemicals such as polyvinyl chloride and other organochlorine compounds must be sought because they may be the cause of the disease (Table 1). Scleroderma may be associated with

Table 1. ETIOLOGY OF SCLERODERMA SYNDROMES

Genetic	Tumors
Progeria	Carcinoid
Werner's syndrome	Malignant
Phenylketonuria	Immunologic
Porphyria	Graft-vs.-host disease
Environmental	Lupus erythematosus
Vibration	Dermatomyositis
Pneumococcosis	Sjögren's syndrome
Polyvinyl chloride	Hashimoto's thyroiditis
Chlorinated hydrocarbons	Vasculitis

a neoplastic disease. Pseudoscleroderma syndromes such as scleromyxedema (papular mucinosis) with its unusual paraprotein may be recognized and treated successfully with alkylating agents. Finally, associated medical diseases that deposit mucin (myxedema) or cause fibrosis (diabetes mellitus) need to be recognized and treated before the scleroderma problem is approached.

The patient with scleroderma may present with varied degrees of organ involvement and function impairment. The stage of the disease may be identified by assessment of gastrointestinal motility and function, pulmonary structure and function, and renal and myocardial functions. A decrease in carbon monoxide diffusing capacity of the lung and a decrease in esophageal and small bowel motility can precede symptoms in these organs by many years (Table 2). No single assessment can establish the prognosis, but signs of a more unfavorable prognosis include extensive cutaneous sclerosis, rapid progression, multiple organ involvement, male sex, older patient age, elevated sedimentation rate, hypergammaglobulinemia, and stage III disease.

The skin biopsy will confirm the clinical diagnosis. Direct immunofluorescence of the skin biopsy may indicate the presence of other connective tissue diseases or immunoreactive diseases. Antinuclear antibody studies and serologic tests of connective tissue will show the degree of immunoreactivity. The use of special substrates will reveal antibodies in most patients with scleroderma. More specific antibodies are the nucleolar antibody, SCL-70 antibody, ribonucleoprotein antibody, and centromere antibody. The first two antibodies are related to systemic scleroderma, whereas the last two are related to mixed connective tissue disease and to acrosclerosis (CREST), respectively.

OVERLAP OR MIXED CONNECTIVE TISSUE SYNDROMES

Occasionally scleroderma develops manifestations of other connective tissue disease. The presence of myositis or lupus erythematosus may be indicated by

Table 2. STAGING OF SCLERODERMA

Stage I
Skin, esophagus, Raynaud's phenomenon
Stage II
Lung, gastrointestinal change in function
Symptoms
Stage III
Cardiovascular
Renal

edema and erythema of the hands and face. The renal lesion of scleroderma resembles that of lupus erythematosus and malignant hypertension. The esophageal dysmotility of scleroderma may be observed in lupus or myositis. The treatment program for these other connective tissue diseases is so different from that of usual scleroderma that identification of the pattern of other connective disease such as rheumatoid arthritis or lupus may change the emphasis of therapy.

The term "mixed connective tissue disease" is best reserved for an uncommitted or indeterminate connective tissue disease, which represents an early indeterminate stage of what later will be recognized as a typical connective tissue disease, usually scleroderma. The patient presents with arthralgia, edema of the hands, Raynaud's phenomenon, dysphagia, and, at times, pulmonary changes or myositis. The absence of renal disease in these patients also has been considered important. The process is similar to sclerodermatomyositis in that it responds to corticosteroids (40 to 80 mg/day), with loss of arthralgia and edema. The Raynaud's phenomenon often can be reversed with this treatment, and the esophageal and pulmonary changes also can improve.

In this indeterminate connective tissue disease syndrome, there is usually a high titer of antibody to ribonucleoprotein. Laboratory tests do not define disease but can confirm its presence. Direct immunofluorescence in a skin biopsy specimen may be positive and the pattern may be one of nuclear or basement membrane fluorescence, similar to that seen in lupus erythematosus. When features of lupus predominate, antimalarial therapy, such as hydroxychloroquine (200 mg/day), may be used to supplement corticosteroids.

STAGE I SCLERODERMA

Scleroderma may be defined as stage I when the sclerosis of the skin is limited to the acral areas of face and hands (acrosclerosis), associated with Raynaud's phenomenon. Chronic vascular sclerotic disease produces secondary telangiectasia and calcinosis. These findings, together with esophageal dysmotility and dysphagia, represent the syndrome usually shortened to the acronym CREST (see above). The prognosis for such patients is good, and renal disease is infrequent. The anticentromere antibody is present in most cases, and the antinuclear antibody titer is low. The diagnosis may be confirmed by skin biopsy, and direct immunofluorescence of the skin only rarely shows any immunoreactants.

A patient with stage I disease requires limited treatment only. Control of the environment and physical medicine are of great importance and may be the only treatment required. The temperature of the extremities may be increased by the use of heated gloves or socks, or more preferably, down slippers. Warm clothing needs to be worn at all times, and air conditioning should be avoided. Care of the skin requires daily lubrication and avoidance of tasks that involve sharp objects that may produce surface cuts or physical damage to the skin. If the sclerosis shows progression in the skin or in the viscera, additional drugs as suggested in stage II disease may be used.

Treatment of the vasospastic changes may be of greatest importance in this stage of the disease. All patients should be instructed to stop smoking. Active treatment includes drugs such as those listed in Table 3. Drugs that deplete or block the formation of catecholamines may be useful, but they produce side effects in the central nervous system or cardiovascular system. Alpha-adrenergic receptor blockers may be very helpful, but as the dose of drugs such as Dibenzyline or prazosin is increased, vascular side effects may appear. Synergism between the drugs may make it possible for the patient to tolerate one or two of the drugs given concurrently that cannot be tolerated at larger doses individually. For instance, a combination of reserpine and Dibenzyline can be used successfully. The combination of prazosin and reserpine or of prazosin and methyldopa may equally be useful in patients with severe Raynaud's phenomenon. The calcium channel–blocking agents nifedipine and verapamil are effective in controlling Raynaud's phenomenon. However, they are of limited value when the disease is severe. They should be useful adjunct forms of therapy to other agents that inhibit catecholamine formation or function. The agents listed in Table 3 provide a powerful armamentarium for the control of Raynaud's phenomenon in scleroderma. With physical therapy and environmental control, these drugs give good results in most patients.

STAGE II SCLERODERMA

The treatment of active, progressive scleroderma with extending sclerosis and involvement of the lungs and gastrointestinal tract requires penicillamine. D-Penicillamine increases the soluble collagen in the skin of patients with scleroderma by preventing intermolecular bridges during the maturation of collagen. Also, the turnover of insoluble collagen accelerates, although the drug does not modify the capacity of fibroblast to synthesize collagen. Many series have been published showing significant benefit in the manifestations of

Table 3. VASOACTIVE THERAPY FOR SCLERODERMA

Drug	Proprietary Name	Action	Starting Dose (mg/day)
Reserpine	——	Depletes catecholamine	0.1
Methyldopa	Aldomet	Blocks catecholamine formation	500–1000
Captopril	Capoten	Blocks angiotensin formation	75
Phenoxybenzamine	Dibenzyline	Blocks α-adrenergic receptors	20
Prazosin	Minipress	Blocks α-adrenergic receptors	15
Propranolol	Inderal	Blocks β-adrenergic receptors	160
Nifedipine	Procardia	Blocks calcium channel	30
Verapamil	Calan, Isoptin	Blocks calcium channel	240
Ketanserin	——	Blocks serotonin receptors	10

scleroderma of patients treated with this drug. In these early series, doses of 1 to 3 gm/day were used, which produced significant side effects that often overshadowed the benefits of treatment.

For the last decade, it has been recognized that 250 to 500 mg of D-penicillamine per day is adequate therapy for patients with scleroderma. It is important that D-penicillamine be given as early in the development of the scleroderma as possible in order to have an opportunity to prevent formation of significant sclerosis. Six to 12 months of therapy are required before any benefit can be observed. Recent reviews showed that treatment may remain beneficial when used for two to five years or more. A plan of treatment of two to four years probably is conservative.

Penicillamine should be used in the lowest effective dosage because it can produce multiple side effects: lupus and myositis, pemphigus, cholestasis, myasthenia syndrome, and vasculitis. Loss of taste, leukopenia, skin rash, and proteinuria are common side effects. The use of the drug should be stopped if untoward reactions develop. Monitoring the hematopoietic, renal, and hepatic systems at four- to eight-week intervals is required.

The occurrence of vasculitis, lupus erythematosus, dermatomyositis, pemphigus vulgaris, nephritis, and many other immunologic and immunoreactive syndromes after D-penicillamine therapy at the higher dosages has resulted in some reluctance to use the drug for the treatment of scleroderma. In many patients, the treatment of scleroderma using small doses for a long period is safe and effective.

Colchicine may be used at a dose of 5 to 10 mg/week for one to two years. Although some series have reported no benefit, Alarcon-Segovia has reported a series of 19 patients in which he found that 17 were improved. Housset used trimethylcolchicine in higher dosages because the gastrointestinal side effects were less than that with colchicine, and showed that nine of 22 patients with stage I disease and nine patients with stage II disease improved. The dose of colchicine is limited by the occurrence of gastrointestinal side effects. Leukopenia may occur, and hepatic function should be tested at monthly intervals.

GASTROINTESTINAL SCLERODERMA

The entire gastrointestinal tract may be involved with scleroderma, but the esophagus and small intestine are usually the major areas involved. Systemic scleroderma is difficult to diagnose if the esophagus is not involved. The loss of the smooth muscle of the gastrointestinal wall and its replacement by fibrosis produce an aperistaltic, dilated, and poorly functioning organ.

THE ESOPHAGUS

The smooth muscle in the lower two thirds of the esophagus is lost, and, with time, the esophagus becomes rigid, shortened, and dilated. Diaphragmatic hernia and loss of the gastroesophageal sphincter are common sequelae. Dysphagia is the first symptom and may precede serious disease by months or years. Pyrosis, pain, and gastric reflux may produce ulcers and sclerosis of the lower portion of the esophagus. Barrett's esophagus and carcinoma may subsequently occur.

Treatment of esophageal scleroderma must be symptomatic. Multiple small meals are practical. Elevation of the head of the bed on six-inch blocks is necessary. The routine use of antacids, particularly at bedtime, is required. The H_2-blocking agents, such as cimetidine and ranitidine, which suppress gastric acidity, may be used daily and at bedtime with very effective results. The dose of cimetidine should be 450 mg three times a day and of ranitidine 150 mg a day, until the symptoms are controlled, after which a maintenance dose of 450 mg or 150 mg, respectively, given at bedtime is appropriate.

Operations for diaphragmatic hernia have usually been unsuccessful. The fundoplication operation in which the stomach is wrapped around the lower end of the esophagus has produced relief of symptoms in some patients, particularly when the operation is done early enough so that chronic scarring does not occur. Scarring may produce esophageal stricture that may be relieved by repeated dilations or, if necessary, by surgery.

INTESTINAL SCLERODERMA

In one of every three patients with systemic scleroderma, the small bowel is involved. The loss of smooth muscle motility and the dilation and fibrosis of the small bowel may be accompanied by villous atrophy and loss of function. A major consequence of these changes is the slow transit time associated with intestinal stasis. Intermittent or persistent diarrhea may occur, which often has been attributed to bacterial overgrowth in the region of stasis in the intestine. A two- to four-week course of tetracycline (250 to 500 mg/day) or ampicillin (250 to 500 mg/day) will frequently control the diarrhea, supporting this view. Patients with malabsorption may be treated with low-residue diet, vitamins, and iron.

Progressive intestinal changes may produce intermittent atonic ileus (intestinal pseudo-obstruction) or pneumocystoides intestinalis. Small bowel infarction and ulceration may result from segmental mesenteric vascular infarction. All of these changes may be catastrophic and, in the past, have occasionally led to death. Nasogastric suction may reduce the obstruction, and total parenteral nutrition provides relief for these patients. The capacity to manage total parenteral nutrition in the patient's home has made it possible for patients to use this technique for years. After one to two years of total parenteral nutrition and therapy with penicillamine or prednisone (or both), oral feeding may be reinstituted in some patients. Scleroderma of the colon also may rarely produce obstruction, volvulus, or fecal impaction.

LIVER DISEASE AND SCLERODERMA

Primary biliary cirrhosis is associated with systemic scleroderma as a distinct syndrome. Ten per cent of patients with primary biliary cirrhosis have anticentromere antibody and should be examined for signs and progression to systemic scleroderma. Currently, penicillamine therapy is the treatment of choice in primary biliary cirrhosis associated with systemic scleroderma. Maintenance doses of as much as 1 gm/day have been given when primary biliary cirrhosis is present, but my experience indicates that low-dosage therapy is better tolerated.

PULMONARY SCLERODERMA

Pulmonary hypertension may be noted before visible fibrosis occurs in the lungs. Basal linear fibrosis is typical, but more extensive changes are not rare. Pulmonary hypertension is more common in the CREST variant. No specific treatment for these lesions exists, but in rare cases, alkylating agents, penicillamine, and prednisone have seemed to have some benefit. Pulmonary hygiene, respiratory exercises, and influenza and pneumococcal vaccines are necessary. The effects of long-term low-dose penicillamine on the development of pulmonary findings are not known. The use of low-dose antibiotics intermittently for intestinal scleroderma can have some benefit in controlling the secondary pulmonary infection.

STAGE III SCLERODERMA

CARDIOVASCULAR SCLERODERMA

Heart failure in systemic scleroderma may be due to primary cardiomyopathy or may be secondary to pulmonary hypertension, producing predominantly right-sided heart failure, or may be due to a combination of both events. Pericarditis has been treated with corticosteroids, without demonstrated benefit. Symptomatic treatment of these changes may include using digitalis, diuretics, and low-salt diet. There is no evidence that any of the agents used for primary systemic sclerosis has affected the myocardial tissue favorably.

RENAL SCLERODERMA

In chronic scleroderma, the kidney may manifest only mild proteinuria. Clearance tests and radioactive scans have shown early changes in cortical blood flow. The basic pathologic change is an intravascular fibromyxoid occlusion of the arteries, which can progress to a more acute fibrinoid degeneration, perhaps related to ischemia. The acute renal crisis in scleroderma may be recognized by an increase in blood pressure—sometimes to malignant levels—resulting in hypertensive retinopathy, elevated plasma renin activity, and progressive renal failure. This acute renal failure is life-threatening and may lead to death within one month or more. Such an episode occurs more frequently in winter, thus raising the question of a Raynaud-type temperature-related vasospastic onset. Most patients are females, approximately 50 years old, who have had their systemic scleroderma for two to three years. A rapid increase in generalized cutaneous sclerosis may precede the renal failure.

Until the past decade, the renal crisis of scleroderma has been uniformly fatal. The progressive development of malignant hypertension, renal failure, coma, and death was an inevitable progression. Reduction of the blood pressure to normotensive levels is now possible, using the much more effective antihypertensive agents such as minoxidil and beta-adrenergic blocking agents. If these agents are used early, they can control the hypertensive crisis in most patients. The elevated plasma renin level and its effect may be treated with captopril or enalapril—angiotensin-converting enzyme blocking agents—which prevent the formation of angiotensin II. The usual dose of captopril is 75 to 350 mg/day. Many, but not all, patients will respond to captopril, although occasionally severe side effects such as neutropenia and agranulocytosis are seen. Enalapril has been used successfully in a dose of 10 to 80 mg and seems to be free of these adverse effects.

However, renal failure may progress despite antihypertensive therapy, and renal dialysis may be necessary. Bilateral nephrectomy was the first successful treatment for the hypertensive renal crisis of scleroderma. Patients have been maintained on dialysis and have had renal function reestablished even as long as one year after the onset of renal failure from a renal crisis of systemic scleroderma. Patients have successfully received kidney transplants, but the occurrence and progression of scleroderma to involve the new kidney has been observed. Early recognition of renal changes offers an opportunity for plasma exchange to be added to the other measures in an effort to alter the course of events.

MUSCULOSKELETAL SYMPTOMS

Most patients with scleroderma have aches and pains in the joints, tendons, or muscles (or all three). The chronic fibrosis of muscles and tendons may cause daily discomfort. Nonsteroidal anti-inflammatory agents may be used regularly for relief. Degenerative bone changes secondary to fixation and sclerosis of digits or extremities can cause severe discomfort. Nonsteroidal anti-inflammatory agents may not be adequate to control this discomfort. Low-dose corticosteroids, such as 4 mg/day of triamcinolone orally, may produce pronounced relief for a patient with such chronic discomfort and severe disability.

Sclerodermatomyositis is one of the corticosteroid-responsive sclerodermoid states. Oral therapy with large doses of prednisone (40 to 80 mg/day according to body size) will bring remission in the signs and symptoms of myositis, Raynaud's phenomenon, and edematous sclerosis. Treatment for six to 12 months or more will be necessary. Physical therapy should be only passive until the serum enzyme levels become normal and symptoms have subsided. Later, active physical therapy can help resolve the edematous sclerosis and achieve rehabilitation.

CHRONIC SCLERODERMA

CALCIFICATION

One of the common side effects of chronic scleroderma is calcinosis cutis. The calcinosis occurs around the joints, usually in the hands. Small masses of calcium may work their way to the surface and form sterile abscesses before perforating and producing small ulcers. These ulcers are not infected until the skin surface has been opened. However, they may be mistaken for pyogenic infections because the aseptic necrosis may result in fever, pain, and pronounced swelling. Continuous saline compresses will reduce the pain, swelling, and discomfort until the calcium is extruded. The calcium mass may be excised or, more simply, adhesive tape may be placed over the mass, which will soften the skin and promote extrusion of the mass.

ULCERS

Vascular ulcers on the tips of the fingers accompany the vasospastic disease of scleroderma, and characteristic focal scars on the fingertips are a sign of long-standing disease. These painful ulcers must be treated by controlling the vasospasm, by maintaining a warm digit, and by thermal mittens.

Vascular ulcers and ulcers secondary to calcinosis occur elsewhere on the extensor extremities, particularly the lower legs. These ulcers are best treated by bed rest and sterile saline compresses. Small ulcers may be treated by the application of Castellani's paint or a similar dye or an antibiotic ointment, such as 1% neomycin cream. When a clean-based ulcer has been obtained, a stomal adhesive (Duoderm) may be placed over the ulcer and left for four to five days as a dressing that promotes healing.

GENERAL THERAPY MEASURES

SUPPORTIVE THERAPY

The environment of the patient with scleroderma should be warm and protected. Changes in temperature should be avoided, and the patient's moving from an air-conditioned room to a warm environment can cause Raynaud's phenomenon. The use of protective clothing and insulated underwear should be routine in winter. Warm mittens and socks should be used as necessary to maintain warmth. Down-filled outerwear is necessary, and a down-filled vest may be useful indoors. Down boots or slippers are important in day-to-day wear.

NUTRITION

Nutrition should include multiple meals that are attractive and nutritious and contain readily chewed and swallowed material. It is important to avoid a large bolus of food, and particularly materials such as bread, which can consolidate with saliva and form a mass that is difficult to swallow. High-protein supplements may be useful, except in patients with renal failure. Many patients find vitamin supplements helpful. Although such supplements are usually not required, they do no harm in commonly used doses.

PHYSICAL THERAPY

All patients should be instructed in physical therapy, particularly in the use of heat and massage. The source of heat is not important and may be warm compresses, warm baths, infrared lamp, or hot paraffin. Massage is very important and should be done twice a day to maintain mobility and reduce edema. Joint and muscle symptoms are relieved by this means, and other types of treatment may not be necessary. Lubrication of the skin is necessary, both before and after physical therapy.

SURGERY

Patients with scleroderma tolerate surgery (and pregnancy) in a similar fashion as most other patients. The wound healing is not delayed significantly, and while elective surgery should generally be postponed, emergency surgery can be performed safely. Most surgery performed for scleroderma is of a reconstructive nature. It is often possible to move the fixed and flexed fingers of a claw hand into a more useful position of function. Sometimes the anterior maxilla can be recon-

structed so that the protruding teeth can fit comfortably within the mouth.

GENERAL COMMENTS

Many patients with systemic scleroderma are frightened by their disease, by the information available, and by what they have been told. A positive, comforting approach by the physician is necessary to help most patients cope with the difficulties that this chronic disease presents. It cannot be too frequently repeated that the five- and ten-year survival rate of systemic scleroderma is high enough that the physician should reassure the individual patient and make every effort to support and treat the organs and tissues that are involved.

REFERENCES

Asboe-Hansen G: Treatment of generalized scleroderma with inhibitors of connective tissue formation. Acta Derm Venereol (Stockh) 55:461–465, 1975.
Jabłońska S (ed): Scleroderma and Pseudoscleroderma, 2nd ed. Polish Med Publishers, Warsaw, 1975.
Priollet P, Boudot N, Fiessinger JN, et al: Traitement de la sclérodermia systémique. Ann Dermatol Venereol 111:595–607, 1984.
Rodnan GP (ed): Progressive systemic sclerosis. Clin Rheum Dis 5:1–306, 1979.
Winkelmann RK, Kierland RR, Perry HO, et al: Management of scleroderma. Mayo Clin Proc 46:128–134, 1971.

4 · POLYARTERITIS NODOSA

Dennis Torretti
GEISINGER MEDICAL CENTER

DEFINITION AND DIAGNOSTIC CRITERIA

Polyarteritis nodosa (PAN) is a systemic necrotizing vasculitis characterized by inflammation and necrosis of small and medium-sized muscular arteries. In 1866, Kussmaul and Maier used the term periarteritis nodosa to define a systemic disorder with palpable nodules along the course of many medium-sized arteries.

Numerous classification schemes of the vasculitic disorders have evolved, but none remains completely satisfactory in clinical practice. Considerable difficulty may be encountered in distinguishing PAN from a hypersensitivity vasculitis. Although the latter process typically involves smaller blood vessels, larger vessels may occasionally be involved with clinical manifestations similar to PAN. Similarly, considerable overlap occurs between allergic granulomatosis and angiitis (Churg-Strauss syndrome) and PAN. Patients with allergic granulomatosis have a history of asthma or atopy, often severe, usually with eosinophilia associated with or preceding the manifestations of a necrotizing vasculitis. Involvement of the pulmonary arteries with eosinophilic infiltrates and granulomas in the vessel walls characterizes allergic granulomatosis. Nonetheless, the patterns of vascular damage and clinical manifestations may be very similar in these processes, and precise clinical categorization is not always possible.

PATHOPHYSIOLOGY

Available evidence suggests that immune-mediated mechanisms, primarily immune complex deposition in vessel walls, are the predominant effectors of arterial inflammation in PAN. Although many questions remain unanswered regarding this mechanism, it provides an adequate explanation for a number of clinical and laboratory observations.

In the early 1940s, Rich described a series of patients with polyarteritis that occurred following the administration of sulfonamides or hyperimmune serum and raised the question of hypersensitivity to foreign antigens as a mechanism of tissue damage. In the early 1970s, an important association between PAN and the hepatitis B virus was discovered. The demonstration of immunoglobulin, complement, and hepatitis B surface antigen in vessel walls, the presence of circulating immune complexes, and the demonstration of hepatitis B surface antigen in immune complexes of patients with PAN have given considerable support to the proposed immune complex mechanism of disease. However, immune complexes are not detected in all patients, and when present, do not correlate consistently with disease activity.

PAN has been described in association with other potential antigenic stimuli including allergic hyposensitization procedures, serous otitis media, trichinosis, hairy-cell leukemia, and drug abuse, particularly methamphetamines. The role of hepatitis B disease in the latter group remains uncertain.

CLINICAL ASPECTS

PAN occurs more frequently in males with a male:female ratio of approximately 2:1. It may affect patients at any age but is most common between 40 and 60 years of age.

The presentation of PAN is quite variable and often represents a diagnostic challenge to the clinician. The clinical course may be intermittent, chronic, gradually progressive, or acute and fulminant. The majority of patients experience systemic symptoms such as fever, fatigue, malaise, and weight loss, which may dominate the clinical picture for weeks to months prior to the appearance of localized organ system involvement.

Joints. Most patients experience diffuse or localized myalgias and arthralgias. A nondeforming inflammatory arthropathy may also occur. The arthropathy is usually asymmetric and may be intermittent, but a symmetric polyarthritis can also be seen.

Cutaneous Manifestations. Cutaneous manifestations may vary depending on the size of vessels involved. If small vessel involvement is present, patients may have petechial or palpable purpuric lesions. Ulcerative lesions may occur on the extremities or trunk. Livedo reticularis, vasospastic phenomenon, nodules, and digital ischemia, occasionally with gangrene, reflect involvement of larger vessels.

Peripheral Nerves. Involvement of peripheral nerves occurs in the majority of patients and may be the initial manifestation. The most common pattern of peripheral neuropathy is a mononeuritis multiplex characterized by the abrupt onset of pain and an emerging deficit in the distribution of the involved nerve over hours to days. Upper and lower extremities are affected with an equal frequency. Other patterns of neuropathy include patches of diminished sensation or paresthesias in the distribution of small cutaneous nerves and a distal sensory neuropathy. Recovery from the neuropathy is usually slow and may be incomplete.

Renal Disease. Renal disease occurs in 60% to 70% of patients and contributes significantly to morbidity and mortality. The most common abnormalities are proteinuria and changes in the urinary sediment such as microscopic hematuria and red blood cell casts. Histologic changes include a focal or diffuse glomerulonephritis or changes of a necrotizing vasculitis of the medium-sized arteries. Microaneurysm formation may occur, particularly in the arcuate and interlobular arteries. The development of accelerated, refractory hypertension in polyarteritis usually reflects a diffuse renal vasculitis with renal ischemia and secondary hyperreninemia and hyperaldosteronism.

Gastrointestinal Manifestations. Gastrointestinal manifestations usually occur as a result of ischemic injury to the bowel, gallbladder, liver, pancreas, or appendix. Abdominal pain is the most common symptom. Localized polyarteritis of the gallbladder and appendix may occur without evidence of a systemic vasculitis. Catastrophic gut involvement may present as severe gastrointestinal bleeding, bowel infarction, or a perforated viscus and requires surgical intervention.

Other Manifestations. Although common pathologically, cardiac involvement is not often clinically evident. Myocardial infarction, coronary artery microaneurysms, pericarditis, and arrhythmias are recognized features. Although occasionally patients with PAN may have pulmonary infiltrates, pulmonary involvement is uncommon and suggests an overlap syndrome or one of the granulomatous vasculitides.

Testicular pain, episcleritis, scleritis, and an ischemic retinopathy are additional features of the disease.

Laboratory studies are generally nonspecific. Diagnosis of PAN depends on a high index of suspicion, thorough history and physical examination, and tissue confirmation. Cutaneous lesions, when present, offer the most accessible site for biopsy. Information obtained from a skin biopsy has limited value, since only small vessels are being sampled. A full-thickness biopsy, including panniculus, should be obtained so that vessels of varying size can be assessed.

Biopsy of a sural nerve, when clinical or electrophysiologic evidence of a neuropathy is present, and muscle biopsy remain the most useful diagnostic procedures. Angiography of the renal, mesenteric, and celiac arteries should be considered if tissue confirmation is not readily obtained.

MANAGEMENT

THERAPEUTIC PLAN

Although the outlook for patients with untreated PAN is poor, there is marked variability in the course of the disease and its response to treatment. Some patients have limited, steroid-responsive disease whereas others exhibit a progressive, refractory course. The therapeutic plan must be individualized depending on the extent and severity of involvement. It must be aggressive initially, prior to the development of irreversible tissue damage, and adaptable to the changing clinical status of the patient. The goals of the therapeutic plan should include:

1. Rapid suppression of the inflammatory process with amelioration of systemic symptoms.

2. Prevention of end organ damage.

3. Facilitation of the healing process and recovery of end organ function.

4. Education of the patient and family.

5. Eradication of the disease process with maintenance of a sustained remission.

6. Avoidance, if possible, of adverse effects of therapy.

In the majority of patients, therapy is initiated in the hospital setting immediately following diagnosis. Some patients with major visceral involvement and changing clinical parameters require prolonged hospitalization to monitor the efficacy of initial therapy. Examples of such patients include those with gut involvement and increasing abdominal pain and those with renal involvement who manifest increasing blood pressure and diminishing renal function. Once the patient's status is stable, management can be continued in the outpatient setting. The recovery process is often long, requiring months. The use of home health care services may be of considerable benefit in the outpatient management of selected patients. Patients requiring daily care of lower extremity ulcerations and gangrenous digits or serial blood pressure measurements may have their hospital stay shortened with the use of such services. A home physical therapy program for the patient with an extensive neuropathy may also be of benefit.

NONPHARMACOLOGIC MEASURES

If an offending agent responsible for initiation of a vasculitic syndrome can be identified, the agent should be removed. Although this is not feasible in the majority of patients with PAN, patients who develop PAN during allergic hyposensitization treatment should have such treatments discontinued.

Plasmapheresis has been used as an adjunctive form of therapy in combination with cytotoxic agents in patients with rapidly progressive vasculitis. Improvement of the splenic component of reticuloendothelial cell function has been suggested following plasmapheresis and removal of circulating immune complexes. However, its use remains unproven and must be considered an experimental form of therapy.

DRUG THERAPY
Corticosteroids

Corticosteroid therapy has resulted in significant improvement of survival in patients with PAN. The cumulative five-year survival rate for patients treated with corticosteroids is approximately 50%, while in untreated patients the five-year survival is generally less than 15%. The inflammatory vascular changes are suppressed by corticosteroids, but proliferative changes may progress. Some patients with PAN respond favor-

ably to corticosteroid therapy and do not require more aggressive treatment. This subset of patients usually has milder and less extensive disease. In other patients, high-dose corticosteroids alone are insufficient to suppress disease activity. Although not rigorously proven in randomized trials, considerable evidence has been accumulated documenting the beneficial effects of immunosuppressive agents. The cumulative five-year survival of patients treated with corticosteroids and immunosuppressive agents is approximately 80%. Remissions induced by cyclophosphamide in patients with advanced disease refractory to corticosteroids have been well documented. Other immunosuppressive agents, most notably azathioprine, have also been used. Few data are available regarding comparative efficacy of the various immunosuppressive agents, but current clinical practice favors the use of cyclophosphamide in severe disease.

The major therapeutic question posed by each patient with PAN is whether corticosteroid therapy alone is sufficient or whether a cytotoxic agent should be added to their regimen. Visceral involvement, particularly gastrointestinal and renal, and the presence of microaneurysms on visceral angiography suggest a poor prognosis. More aggressive therapy with a cytotoxic agent should be considered in those circumstances. Patients who present with disease limited to the skin, joints, or muscle may respond favorably to corticosteroids alone. The effect on outcome of a neuropathy such as mononeuritis multiplex remains uncertain. Initial therapy with corticosteroids is appropriate, but as in all patients with this disease, serial assessment is necessary.

The initial prednisone dose is 60 to 80 mg daily in divided doses. When a favorable response has been obtained, consolidation into a single daily dose should be accomplished. Alternate-day corticosteroid therapy is not sufficiently effective when used as the only agent initially. The role of high-dose "pulse therapy" with intravenous methylprednisolone is uncertain. Corticosteroids should be continued at the starting dose for approximately one to two months, depending on the patient's response. Following improvement in clinical and laboratory parameters, gradual reduction in corticosteroid dose at approximately monthly intervals can be accomplished. When a daily dose of 20 mg is achieved, further reduction should be of a smaller magnitude. Decrements of 2 to 2.5 mg in the daily dose at one- to two-month intervals are appropriate. An attempt should be made to reduce the corticosteroid dose to the lowest possible amount sufficient to suppress the disease activity.

Adverse Effects. Prolonged therapy is often necessary and the risk of patients' developing complications of steroid therapy is considerable. Adverse effects of corticosteroids are familiar to physicians and include weight gain, cushingoid features, hypertension, glucose intolerance, cataracts, diminished resistance to infections, demineralization of bone, ischemic necrosis of bone, myopathy, gastric ulceration, and emotional lability. Rigorous caloric and salt restriction should be maintained. The prophylactic use of high doses of vitamin D (50,000 units three times weekly) and supplemental daily calcium (1000 mg of elemental calcium) may delay or prevent steroid-induced bone demineralization and its attendant problems such as compression fractures. The presence of hypercalciuria or a history of nephrolithiasis is a contraindication to the use of vitamin D and calcium.

Cyclophosphamide

Indications for treatment with cyclophosphamide are listed in Table 1. Cyclophosphamide should be initiated at a dose of 2 mg/kg/day. Frequent monitoring of the white blood cell count at two-week intervals is necessary initially. The daily dose of cyclophosphamide is titrated to maintain the white blood cell count above 4000/mm³. If the white blood cell count decreases to less than 4000/mm³, the drug is withheld until the count exceeds this level. The dose is then diminished by 25 mg and restarted. Continued gradual reductions in the dose of cyclophosphamide should be expected with chronic oral therapy.

Clinical response to cyclophosphamide may be dramatic with rapid reversal of progressive disease activity, improved control of refractory hypertension, and resolution of microaneurysms. The addition of cyclophosphamide to a patient's regimen may permit further reduction of the corticosteroid dose and a lower incidence of steroid-related adverse effects. The precise mechanism of action of low-dose oral daily cyclophosphamide in this setting is uncertain but may reflect a selective suppression of B cell function.

Adverse Effects. A major factor limiting the use of cyclophosphamide in PAN is its long-term irreversible toxicity. Toxic effects of this alkylating agent include dose-dependent myelosuppression, temporary hair loss, damage to germ cells, azoospermia that is often permanent, anovulation, and amenorrhea. An increased risk of serious opportunistic infections and herpes zoster accompanies long-term immunosuppressive therapy. Untoward effects on the urinary bladder remain a major drawback of chronic therapy. Painful hemorrhagic cystitis may occur while the drug is administered as a result of a direct irritative effect on the bladder by acrolein, a metabolite of cyclophosphamide. In addition, submucosal bladder fibrosis and telangiectasias may occur in 10% to 30% of patients. These problems can present months to years after the drug has been discontinued. Ingestion of large quantities of fluid to dilute the untoward chemical effect on the bladder is recommended. An increased risk of carcinoma of the bladder has been identified in patients receiving chronic oral cyclophosphamide. The absence of hemorrhagic cystitis does not preclude the development of bladder carcinoma.

In addition to bladder cancer, the late development of other malignancies in patients treated with cyclophosphamide poses a significant problem. Hematologic and lymphoreticular malignancies are most notable in

this regard with a 10- to 14-fold increase in incidence when compared with the general population. The mechanism of the development of malignancies in cytotoxic treated patients is uncertain. An effect on the immune surveillance system allowing mutant or transformed cells to persist that would otherwise have been destroyed is suspected.

The duration of therapy is variable, depending upon the individual patient response. Some patients require continued chronic therapy. In patients who achieve a complete remission, treatment can be gradually discontinued approximately 12 months after all evidence of disease activity has abated. If the patient is receiving both prednisone and an immunosuppressive agent, the prednisone should be tapered and discontinued first while the immunosuppressive agent is maintained at a stable dose.

Management of the complications of PAN is an integral part of treatment. Congestive heart failure and hypertension must be treated vigorously. Captopril may be effective in the treatment of refractory accelerated hypertension associated with renal vasculitis. Renal transplantation has been performed successfully in PAN. The role of antiplatelet agents is uncertain.

PATIENT INFORMATION AND EDUCATION

Successful treatment of the patient with PAN requires considerable cooperation between the patient and the physician over an extended period of time. If a patient is to comply with the treatment program, he must understand the serious nature of the disease process, the need for continued treatment and regular clinical and laboratory examinations, the rationale behind the therapy, and its potential complications. Realism coupled with optimism in the educational process helps to establish an atmosphere of trust, cooperation, and improved compliance.

The value of rest and principles of energy conservation deserve emphasis. Setting priorities, eliminating low priority activities, planning ahead, establishing rest periods, and resting before fatigue develops are useful strategies for the patient with PAN. Caloric and salt restriction while taking corticosteroids should be emphasized. The patient must be instructed not to stop or reduce his medication on his own, even if he is feeling well, and to report immediately any change in his status such as fevers, bleeding, abdominal pain, or hematuria.

PERIODIC EVALUATION

Serial assessment of disease activity and response to therapy is based primarily on clinical judgment with some assistance from the laboratory. Information regarding systemic symptoms such as fever, fatigue, myalgias, and arthralgias should be sought. Organ systems known to be affected must be evaluated for change and any new symptoms addressed that might reflect progressive disease or complications of therapy. Laboratory studies that may be helpful in assessing disease activity include the hemoglobin, white blood cell count, erythrocyte sedimentation rate, urinalysis, and renal function tests. Serial assessment of complement levels, cryoglobulins, and immune complex levels are not of sufficient value in the majority of patients to warrant routine testing. They may be of some utility in selected patients. An overall assessment of the patient's

---

Table 1. INDICATIONS FOR TREATMENT WITH CYCLOPHOSPHAMIDE IN PAN

Major visceral involvement
Microaneurysms on visceral angiography
Failure to respond to corticosteroid therapy after an adequate trial
Requirement of a high corticosteroid dose to suppress disease activity and the development of major complications of steroid therapy
Patients with an increased risk of major complications of high-dose corticosteroid therapy, e.g., the older female patient with involutional osteopenia and diabetes mellitus

current clinical status must be made by the physician and compared with the patient's former status. If consistent unfavorable trends are noted, modification of the drug regimen is appropriate. Changes in therapy based solely on a single laboratory parameter such as the erythrocyte sedimentation rate in the absence of clinical symptoms should be avoided.

Monitoring for potential toxicity is an integral part of the management plan. Blood pressure, weight, and blood glucose should be checked frequently. Patients receiving supplemental vitamin D and calcium to forestall steroid-induced osteopenia should have a 24-hour urine calcium measurement to avoid hypercalciuria and nephrolithiasis. Patients receiving cyclophosphamide must have their white blood cell count checked every two weeks initially and subsequently monthly.

Initial visits should be at two- to three-week intervals. Once the disease process is controlled and appears clinically stable, monthly visits are appropriate.

REFERENCES

Cohen RD, Conn DL, Ilstrup DM: Clinical features, prognosis, and response to treatment in polyarteritis. Mayo Clin Proc 55:146–155, 1980.

Cupps TR, Fauci AS: The Vasculitides. W.B. Saunders Co, Philadelphia, 1981.

Faucie AS, Katz P, Haynes BF, et al: Cyclophosphamide therapy of severe systemic necrotizing vasculitis. N Engl J Med 301:235–238, 1979.

Gocke DJ, Hsu K, Morgan C, et al: Association between polyarteritis and Australia antigen. Lancet 2:1149–1153, 1970.

Leib ES, Restivo C, Paulus HE: Immunosuppressive and corticosteroid therapy of polyarteritis nodosa. Am J Med 67:941–947, 1979.

5 · SYSTEMIC LUPUS ERYTHEMATOSUS

Randall S. Vollertsen
MAYO CLINIC AND MAYO FOUNDATION

DEFINITION AND DIAGNOSTIC CRITERIA

Systemic lupus erythematosus is a multisystemic disorder in which the cause is unknown and the severity varies. The American Rheumatism Association has established diagnostic criteria (Table 1). The prevalence approximates 0.05%, with predilection for women, blacks, and the young.

PATHOGENESIS

The pathogenesis seems to involve immunologic, genetic, hormonal, infectious, and environmental factors. Autoantibodies, immune complexes, tissue immune deposits, and an apparent deficiency of T-lymphocyte suppression with polyclonal B-cell activation are common abnormalities. Racial and familial predilection and an association with major histocompatibility complex (HLA) genotypes and complement deficiency suggest genetic involvement.

The predisposition of women and men with Klinefelter's syndrome indicates a permissive effect of estrogens. However, the variable sexual preponderance found in different murine models dictates caution in attributing lupus to a specific hormone. Concentrations of interferon and antiviral antibodies are increased, suggesting an infectious cause, but these findings may be nonspecific consequences of abnormal immune regulation. Worsening after exposure to ultraviolet light or certain drugs indicates a role for physical factors.

CLINICAL ASPECTS

Musculoskeletal. Myalgias, arthralgias, and arthritis are the most common manifestations. Involvement affects the small joints of the hands, the wrists, the knees, and, less frequently, the ankles, elbows, shoulders, hips, and feet. This pattern with associated morning stiffness mimics rheumatoid arthritis, but deformities are reversible and rarely do erosions or nodules occur. Aseptic necrosis and myositis are rare.

Cutaneous. An erythematous, maculopapular eruption predominantly in sun-exposed areas, which may assume a classic malar distribution, is frequent. Discoid lesions with hyperpigmented telangiectatic margins, hyperkeratotic plugging, and central scarring are less common in systemic disease. Photosensitivity occurs in one third of patients. Patchy alopecia is frequent.

Lupus profundus, cutaneous vasculitis, urticaria or bullae, livedo reticularis, and nail and pigmentary changes are uncommon.

General Systemic Symptoms. Fatigue, weight loss, and fever may be associated with active disease.

Renal Manifestations. Clinically significant renal involvement is manifested by hematuria, pyuria, casts, proteinuria, and renal insufficiency. Histologic examination may reveal mesangial, glomerular, interstitial, and tubular abnormalities.

Neurologic. Psychologic symptoms are common. Migraine headaches, seizures, and peripheral neuropathies including mononeuritis multiplex, meningoencephalitis, focal defects, transverse myelitis, or a movement disorder occur. Diffuse central involvement is manifested by disorientation, abnormal cognition, hallucinations, or coma. Vasculitis and thrombocytopenia are more common in those patients who have neuropsychiatric manifestations.

Ophthalmologic. The classic cytoid bodies are ischemic retinal exudates. Keratoconjunctivitis sicca, episcleritis, central retinal arterial occlusion, and vasculitis are unusual.

Hematologic. The mild anemia of chronic disease is frequent, but symptomatic autoimmune hemolysis is uncommon. Mild leukopenia, granulocytopenia, and lymphocytopenia are common. Leukocytosis is unusual; when it does occur, most often it signifies active disease or infection or is a consequence of glucocorticosteroid therapy.

Mild thrombocytopenia is common but only rarely becomes sufficiently severe to cause bleeding. The common "lupus anticoagulant" predisposes to thrombosis, not hemorrhage; it is associated with recurrent abortion, thrombocytopenia, and a false-positive serologic test for syphilis and is not specific for lupus. Characteristic increases in the partial thromboplastin and prothrombin times are not corrected with normal plasma. The lupus anticoagulant is an antibody directed against the phospholipid portion of the prothrombin activator. It may also inhibit prostacyclin and thereby favor thrombosis. Rare causes of hemorrhage are prothrombin deficiency,

Table 1. AMERICAN RHEUMATOLOGY ASSOCIATION 1982 REVISED CRITERIA FOR CLASSIFICATION OF SYSTEMIC LUPUS ERYTHEMATOSUS*

Criterion

1. Malar rash
    Fixed erythema, flat or raised, over malar eminences, tending to spare nasolabial folds
2. Discoid rash
    Erythematous, raised patches with adherent keratotic scaling and follicular plugging; atrophic scarring may occur in old lesions
3. Photosensitivity
    Skin rash as result of unusual reaction to sunlight (observed by physician or recounted by patient)
4. Oral ulcers
    Oral or nasopharyngeal ulceration, usually painless, observed by physician
5. Arthritis
    Nonerosive arthritis involving two or more peripheral joints, characterized by tenderness, swelling, or effusion
6. Serositis
    Pleurisy (convincing history of pleuritic pain or rub heard by physician or evidence of pleural effusion)
    Pericarditis (confirmed by ECG or rub or evidence of pericardial effusion)
7. Renal disorder
    Persistent proteinuria (>0.5 gm/day or $>3+$ if quantitation is not performed)
    Cellular casts (may be RBC, hemoglobin, granular, tubular, or mixed)
8. Neurologic disorder
    Seizures (in absence of offending drugs or known metabolic derangements, e.g., uremia, ketoacidosis, or electrolyte imbalance)
    Psychosis (in absence of offending drugs or known metabolic derangements, e.g., uremia, ketoacidosis, or electrolyte imbalance)
9. Hematologic disorder
    Hemolytic anemia with reticulocytosis
    Leukopenia ($<4000/mm^3$ on two or more occasions)
    Lymphopenia ($<1500/mm^3$ on two or more occasions)
    Thrombocytopenia ($<1500/mm^3$ in absence of offending drug therapy)
10. Immunologic disorder
    Positive LE-cell preparation
    Anti-n-DNA (antibody to native DNA in abnormal titer)
    Anti-Sm (presence of antibody to Sm nuclear antigen)
    False-positive serologic test result for syphilis known to be positive for at least 6 months and confirmed by *Treponema pallidum* immobilization or fluorescent treponemal antibody absorption test
11. Antinuclear antibody (ANA)
    Abnormal ANA titer by immunofluorescence or equivalent assay at any time and in absence of drugs known to be associated with "drug-induced lupus" syndrome

*The proposed classification is based on 11 criteria. For the purpose of identifying patients in clinical studies, a person shall be said to have systemic LE if any four or more of the 11 criteria are present, serially or simultaneously, during any interval of observation.

inhibitors of factors VII, IX, XI, XII, and XIII, and acquired von Willebrand's disease.

Pulmonary. Roentgenograms commonly show elevated diaphragms and basilar atelectasis, and pulmonary function tests show diminished carbon monoxide diffusion and lung volumes. None of these ordinarily causes symptoms. Pleuritis is very common and also can be asymptomatic. Less commonly, significant interstitial fibrosis causes cough and dyspnea. Acute "lupus pneumonitis," pulmonary hemorrhage, and pulmonary hypertension are rare.

Cardiovascular. Asymptomatic pericarditis is frequent; rarely it leads to tamponade. Heart failure or conduction disturbances due to myocarditis are unusual. Endocarditis with classic Libman-Sacks lesions is of doubtful clinical significance.

Mortality from premature coronary atherosclerosis in lupus patients who receive glucocorticosteroids may be increased. Vasculitis of the main coronary arteries is rare, as is congenital heart block in the offspring of mothers with lupus.

One fifth of lupus patients have Raynaud's phenomenon and one tenth have thrombophlebitis. The latter is common in those with the lupus anticoagulant. Arterial thrombosis is rare.

Hypertension may occur in association with renal disease, glucocorticosteroid therapy, or vasculitis.

Reticuloendothelial. Lymphadenopathy and minimal splenomegaly are common. Rarely, functional asplenia or a thymoma with myasthenia gravis is an associated finding.

Gastrointestinal. Mildly abnormal liver function is commonly associated with active disease and nonsteroidal anti-inflammatory therapy. Mild hepatomegaly may occur. "Lupoid hepatitis" refers to chronic active hepatitis in association with systemic features and antinuclear antibodies. Pancreatitis and malabsorption are rare.

Erosions of the oral or nasal mucosa are common. Dysphagia due to impaired peristalsis and abnormal sphincter pressure may be complicated by reflux esophagitis. Evidence of peritonitis is present in most patients at autopsy, but few complain of abdominal pain during life. Uncommonly, bowel erosions lead to hemorrhage. Colonic perforation due to vasculitis is frequently fatal. Angiography and paracentesis may help to differentiate between serositis and vasculitis, but sometimes the diagnosis rests upon clinical observation.

Menstrual Abnormalities and Pregnancy. Menstrual irregularity and increased fetal loss occur. Pregnancy and the postpartum period are associated with flare-ups, especially when active renal disease is present immediately prior to conception. Differentiation between an exacerbation of lupus nephritis and pre-eclampsia may be impossible. With appropriate planning and careful management, most patients can successfully deliver without undue risk to the infant or themselves.

Infections. Patients with systemic lupus erythematosus have a greater incidence of infection, and this is independent of renal disease and glucocorticosteroid therapy, which further predispose them to infection.

Drug-induced Systemic Lupus Erythematosus. An illness that is quite similar to systemic lupus erythematosus may occur after exposure to drugs. Hydralazine, procainamide, and isoniazid are recognized causes. Anticonvulsants, major tranquilizers, quinidine, penicillamine, antithyroid medications, and lithium carbonate also are suspect. Many other drugs, including oral contraceptives, have been reported to be associated but solid epidemiologic evidence is lacking. Serositis and anti-histone antibodies are more frequent in drug-induced than in idiopathic lupus, and neurologic and renal involvement are less frequent. Ordinarily, symptoms resolve after discontinuation of therapy. The presence of antinuclear antibodies without clinical symptoms does not necessarily contraindicate continuation of therapy.

Although oral contraceptives may not cause lupus, those containing estrogens often exacerbate the disease compared with those containing only progesterone.

ADDITIONAL LABORATORY STUDIES

Antinuclear antibodies (ANA) are a family of antibodies directed against components of the cell nuclei such as deoxyribonuclear protein, native deoxyribonucleic acid (n-DNA), denatured DNA, and extractable nuclear antigens (ENA) including the Sm antigen, histones, or the centromere. Different antibodies have relative specificity for different diseases but these additional clues may be of marginal benefit to the clinician. Two possible exceptions are the anti-n-DNA and anti-Sm, which are more common in systemic lupus than in other rheumatologic diseases. The anti-n-DNA titer may correlate with activity. The lupus erythematosis (LE) clot test, which measures antibody against deoxyribonuclear protein, has been supplanted by measurement of antinuclear antibodies. The erythrocyte sedimentation rate often correlates with activity in lupus, but the C-reactive protein is normal. Measurement of complement components helps to assess activity. A false-positive serologic test for syphilis, cryoglobulins, or rheumatoid factor may be present. The immune complex concentration and cellular immune function tests are neither widely available nor of established benefit in assessing the individual patient.

DIAGNOSIS

A carefully taken history and a thorough physical examination are paramount. Initial laboratory tests should include erythrocyte sedimentation rate, antinuclear antibody, hemoglobin, total and differential leukocyte counts, platelet count, measurement of renal and hepatic function, screening test for syphilis, urinalysis, chest roentgenogram, electrocardiogram, and appropriate bone roentgenograms. If the antinuclear antibody result is positive, measurement of anti-n-DNA and complement may quantitate severity.

If the patient is strongly suspected to have lupus but does not have antinuclear antibodies, the test may be repeated with a different substrate or anti-n-DNA or extractable nuclear antigen, or LE clot tests may be ordered. Such testing is necessary in few patients.

A more accurate assessment of renal function is provided by the creatinine clearance when the serum creatinine value is less than twice normal and by quantitation of urinary protein if qualitative proteinuria is present.

The role of renal biopsy is controversial. Biopsy may help determine other causes of renal disease and has some prognostic significance in lupus. If the result will not alter management, biopsy may be deferred. Renal biopsy may be warranted prior to instituting cytotoxic-immunosuppressive therapy because widespread glomerulosclerosis and a paucity of subendothelial deposits make improvement less likely. Examination of other tissues such as skin, muscle, or a sural nerve may confirm suspected vasculitis. Immunofluorescent examination of a skin biopsy specimen, the lupus band test, neither confirms the diagnosis nor affects the therapy.

The prothrombin and activated partial thromboplastin times are useful in detecting a coagulopathy, but additional testing is required to identify a specific abnormality. Psychometric testing, computed tomographic or magnetic resonance imaging, electroencephalography, electromyography, and cerebrospinal fluid examination can be helpful in defining neurologic involvement.

In evaluating a patient with lupus, one must remember that drug toxicity, a complicating infection, or another disease can mimic many of the manifestations.

PROGNOSIS

The prognosis may vary depending upon which outcome—progression of disease, renal failure, or survival—is analyzed. Increases in concentrations of anti-n-DNA and immune complexes and a decrease in complement concentrations may precede flares.

The clinical predictors of renal failure are young age, high creatinine value, and low complement value at diagnosis. When considered alone, the microscopic classification of glomerulopathy into mesangial, membranous, focal proliferative, or a diffuse proliferative lesion predicts survival, but when clinical parameters are concurrently considered, the microscopic classification predicts only renal function. Specifically, glomerulosclerosis or an index of chronicity (glomerulosclerosis, fibrinoid necrosis, interstitial fibrosis, tubular atrophy) is associated with renal deterioration, whereas subendothelial deposits are associated with preserved function.

The better survival of lupus patients in the past 40 years may be due to the detection of milder disease, use of glucocorticosteroids, and better supportive treatment. Hypertension, renal insufficiency, low hematocrit, proteinuria, and wide extension of disease all adversely affect survival. Those whose care is publicly funded also have increased mortality.

MANAGEMENT

Relief of symptoms, prevention and detection of complications, and prolongation of life are the therapeutic goals. Occasionally, hospitalization is necessary for those who are incapacitated by their symptoms.

NONPHARMACOLOGIC MEASURES

A well-balanced diet that maintains normal weight is warranted. Patients with hypertension or who receive glucocorticosteroids should be on a sodium-restricted diet. Home physical therapy, orthoses, gait aids, and assistive devices are helpful for musculoskeletal involvement. Those with photosensitivity should avoid the sun, wear protective clothing, and use sunscreens. New patients should be warned about possible adverse effects from sun exposure.

Patients must not use tobacco and should avoid taking alcohol and anti-inflammatory drugs simultaneously. Because of potential exacerbations, use of a method of contraception other than oral estrogens is prudent. Women with active disease should be advised to defer pregnancy.

In view of an increased susceptibility to infection, immunization against *Streptococcus pneumoniae* and influenza is indicated. Some authorities recommend avoiding use of live vaccines.

Perhaps all patients, and certainly those with hypertension or renal disease, must monitor their blood pressure. Avoidance of cold and trauma are indicated for patients who have Raynaud's phenomenon.

DRUG THERAPY

Nonsteroidal Anti-Inflammatory Drugs

These agents are useful for musculoskeletal and serosal symptoms. Aspirin is as efficacious as, probably is no more toxic than, and definitely is less expensive than newer drugs. Because these drugs may cause peptic ulceration, it is prudent to take them with food and possibly with an antacid. Patients with reflux esophagitis may do better with a drug that is given once or twice daily. Aspirin may cause audiovestibular symptoms. Less common are mild impairments of hepatic or renal function; these rarely require discontinuing therapy. Aseptic meningitis is a very rare complication that has been reported in association with the use of ibuprofen, tolmetin, and sulindac. Thrombocytopenia, a hemorrhagic diathesis, or anticoagulation therapy may contraindicate use of these drugs.

Antimalarials

These drugs are effective for cutaneous and musculoskeletal symptoms and fever and possibly for serositis. They may decrease the glucocorticosteroid requirement. They are additions to therapy with nonsteroidal and anti-inflammatory drugs, and a response to them is not evident for two to six months.

Hydroxychloroquine is preferred because it does not cause skin pigmentation and may have less retinal toxicity than chloroquine. One may begin with 200 mg daily; after a response, the dose may carefully be decreased by omitting one or more days each week as tolerated. However, exacerbations may not recur for several months after a decrease in dose. Accordingly, one should wait several months before the dose is further reduced.

Patients must know of possible retinal toxicity and the necessity for surveillance. With low-dosage hydroxychloroquine therapy and eye examinations twice yearly, significant impairment of vision is extremely rare. Preliminary and periodic eye examinations by an ophthalmologist who is familiar with antimalarial toxicity are mandatory. An examination every six months seems prudent, although quarterly evaluation is reasonable for patients at high risk—the elderly and those whose intake exceeds 300 gm. Patients who note reading difficulty, field disturbances, photophobia, blurred vision, or light flashing should be examined promptly. Corneal deposition of antimalarials does not require interruption of therapy. Prescriptions with limited refills ensure appropriate surveillance.

Other adverse effects include anorexia, nausea, diarrhea, abdominal cramps, cycloplegia, and rash. Rare complications include a myopathy, marrow aplasia, and hemolysis associated with glucose-6-phosphate dehydrogenase deficiency.

Glucocorticosteroids

The sparing topical application of a glucocorticosteroid ointment or cream of intermediate potency may resolve the rash. For the head and groin, a low-potency cream is indicated. Stubborn lesions may require more potent preparations. Because of complicating atrophy and telangiectasia, consultation with a dermatologist is indicated if therapy is necessary for more than several weeks. Systemic absorption of steroid also occurs.

Low to moderate systemic doses of glucocorticosteroids may be required for resistant skin, joint, or serosal symptoms or fever. Serious involvement of the renal, neurologic, or hematologic system calls for more aggressive therapy.

A one- to three-month trial of glucocorticosteroids is reasonable for significant proteinuria, an active urinary sediment, or renal insufficiency even if a biopsy shows focal proliferative or membranous lesions. If improvement follows, one can carefully decrease the dose while monitoring renal status. More prompt reduction is indicated for nonresponders.

Data supporting glucocorticosteroid efficacy for neurologic lupus is limited. Extremely large doses can result in decreased survival due to infection. Nonetheless, it is rational to proceed with a course of such therapy for acute manifestations such as seizures, focal lesions of the brain or peripheral nerves, organic brain syndromes, or a movement disorder. The response after several weeks will dictate dosage adjustment.

Even less clear is the indication in the event of psychological symptoms, especially because they may be a complication of the glucocorticosteroid. Active lupus elsewhere or other neurologic involvement strongly favors an organic cause. Increasing the steroid dose and carefully observing the response is rarely harmful.

Glucocorticosteroids are indicated for symptomatic hemolysis, usually when the hemoglobin value is less than 10.0 gm/dl and for thrombocytopenia when the platelet count is less than 50,000/μl. After control is achieved, reducing the dose or conversion to alternate-day therapy may be possible and can be guided by hematologic tests. A bleeding diathesis due to circulating anticoagulants may respond to treatment. A patient with the common lupus anticoagulant ordinarily requires no therapy; however, suppression of the lupus anticoagulant and maintenance of a normal activated partial thromboplastin time may allow successful pregnancy in a woman who previously has lost a fetus.

Progressive interstitial lung disease or pulmonary vasculitis may respond to high-dosage therapy. Chest roentgenograms and pulmonary function studies corroborate improvement. Conversion to an alternate-day regimen may be possible. In the absence of improvement after three months, the risks of continuing therapy may outweigh the benefits. Mild transient infiltrates and mild abnormalities of pulmonary function do not require glucocorticosteroids.

Active systemic vasculitis should be treated promptly, although periungual infarctions and minimal cutaneous involvement do not necessarily require treatment.

Prednisone is short-acting, inexpensive and available in a wide range of doses, allowing easy administration of moderate (0.25 mg/kg/day) to large (1.0 mg/kg/day) doses. Multiple daily doses increase efficacy and toxicity and alternate-day doses decrease them. Some manifestations decrease with alternate-day dosing, but others, such as arthralgias and arthritis, do not.

Decreasing the dose rapidly may precipitate flares with resultant need for a higher than average dose. In general, decrements should approximate 10% of the daily dosage. The initial interval of one or two weeks between decrements ordinarily has to be increased—perhaps to two to four weeks when dosages are below 40 mg/day and to four to eight weeks when below 10 mg/day. Consolidation of multiple daily doses and conversion to an alternate-day regimen are "decreases." Some patients require prolonged therapy but the vast majority of these require less than 10 mg daily.

Hypothalamic-pituitary-adrenal suppression requires extra glucocorticosteroids at times of stress such as general anesthesia, trauma, or infection, for up to 12 months after therapy. Obesity, fat redistribution, acne, hirsutism, stria, thin skin, easy bruising, delayed healing, and slight neutrophilia, lymphopenia and monocytopenia are common. Glucocorticosteroids may precipitate or worsen hypertension, diabetes, and glaucoma. Osteoporosis, menstrual irregularity, peptic ulceration, cataract formation, psychiatric disturbance, myopathy, or, rarely, intracranial hypertension or pancreatitis may ensue.

Glucocorticosteroids predispose to infection, a major cause of death in patients with lupus. If the clinical situation permits, one should obtain a tuberculin skin test prior to beginning therapy and prescribe appropriate prophylaxis if necessary. The possible acceleration of coronary atherosclerosis and consequent late mortality in patients with lupus who receive glucocorticosteroids are disturbing.

Recently, some authorities have experimented with "pulse" glucocorticosteroid therapy—administration of extraordinarily large doses, the equivalent of 1 to 1.5 gm of prednisone daily, parenterally for three successive days. The clinical benefit of such therapy is uncertain.

Cytotoxic-Immunosuppressive Drugs

The role of these drugs in systemic lupus erythematosus is controversial. When analyzed individually, randomized, controlled studies have not shown cytotoxic-immunosuppressive drugs to be efficacious in lupus. This may be due to insufficient numbers of properly stratified patients. Indeed, the pooled results from all such studies demonstrated that patients with nephritis did better with azathioprine or cyclophosphamide in addition to glucocorticosteroids than with glucocorticosteroids alone. Specifically, there was less renal

scarring, less end-stage renal disease, and lower mortality from kidney disease. These experimental results are most applicable to patients with more severe disease, since they were performed at tertiary care institutions. The findings were most dramatic in patients with diffuse proliferative glomerulonephritis.

Cytotoxic-immunosuppressive agents are carcinogenic. Their effect on overall survival remains to be determined because the aforenoted studies may not have been of sufficient duration to fully assess drug-induced mortality. Bone marrow suppression, infection, mucosal ulceration, interstitial cystitis, and potential teratogenesis warrant further caution.

In summary, cytotoxic-immunosuppressive drugs appear to be beneficial for severe lupus nephritis but are associated with significant complications and may adversely affect overall survival. For now, it is prudent to reserve these drugs for those patients with severe disease, particularly nephritis, who do not readily respond to tolerable doses of glucocorticosteroids. Such therapy should be directed by a physician who is experienced in using these drugs.

Other Drugs

Hypertension, seizures, and psychosis should be promptly treated. Although there seems to be no special risk for the development of drug-induced lupus in patients with idiopathic lupus, the coincidental occurrence of these disorders could lead to confusion. Because alternative medications are available, one may avoid hydralazine and perhaps phenytoin and phenothiazines. Patients who are reactive to a tuberculin skin test and will be receiving glucocorticosteroids or cytotoxic-immunosuppressive drugs may be given isoniazid and carefully observed.

Those who develop deep venous phlebitis can receive anticoagulants if carefully observed for thrombocytopenia or a hemorrhagic diathesis. Appropriate restriction of protein intake and phosphate binders are indicated for renal insufficiency; antacids or histamine(H_2^-)-blockers for esophagitis and peptic ulceration; and artificial tears for keratoconjunctivitis sicca.

Vasodilation with nifedipine, prazosin, or alpha-methyldopa may relieve Raynaud's phenomenon. If the symptoms are unabated or toxicity develops, therapy should be discontinued.

OTHER THERAPY

Renal failure may respond to hemodialysis, although infection, thrombosis of the fistula, and death may be more frequent for lupus patients than for others. Renal transplantation has been successful. Survival of the patient and the graft is comparable with the experience in other transplant recipients who do not have diabetes and recurrence of lupus in the allograft appears to be rare.

Progressive aseptic necrosis may require arthroplasty. Therapeutic thoracentesis, pericardiocentesis, or pericardiectomy are rarely required. Prompt laparotomy may be lifesaving if bowel perforation occurs. Splenectomy may reverse recalcitrant hemolytic anemia or thrombocytopenia. This should be limited to those who do not respond satisfactorily to tolerable doses of glucocorticosteroids. Thrombocytopenia may recur after apparently successful splenectomy.

EXPERIMENTAL THERAPY

In addition to pulse glucocorticosteroid therapy and cytotoxic-immunosuppressive drugs, investigators have tried other manipulations of the immune system. There are isolated reports of improvement after thoracic duct drainage, plasmapheresis, and leukopheresis. The only controlled study reported thus far demonstrated no benefit from plasmapheresis. An immune modulator, cyclosporin A, has yet to be tried systematically for lupus. Empiric opinion is that gold salts are of little help in lupus but the question has never been thoroughly studied. There are isolated reports of improvement in cases of cutaneous lupus produced by thalidomide and by sulfones.

Hormonal manipulation with anabolic steroids and tamoxifen has not shown definite clinical benefit, although it may increase the platelet count.

Bone marrow transplantation, antibodies directed against class II proteins encoded by the major histocompatibility complex, anti-idiotypic antibodies directed against anti-DNA antibodies, and dietary manipulation of prostaglandin precursors have produced improvement in murine models.

PERIODIC EVALUATION

Serious manifestations may require weekly reassessment, but for most patients a review every three to 12 months will suffice. In addition to a pertinent interview and physical examination, reassessment of the hemoglobin concentration, leukocyte count, platelet count, serum creatinine value or creatinine clearance, and urinalysis is indicated.

Measurements of the anti-n-DNA antibody and complement may be helpful but are unnecessary if the results do not correlate with the clinical course or affect therapy. Observation during the initial months of disease will help determine the usefulness of these tests.

PATIENT INFORMATION AND EDUCATION

A general overview of the disease with emphasis on the patient's own manifestations is helpful. Patients should also know about therapy, with emphasis on nonpharmacologic measures as well as drugs and their potential toxicity, and the need for appropriate tests to monitor for toxic side effects.

The Arthritis Foundation, the Lupus Foundation of America, the American Lupus Society, and local groups provide literature and support.

PATIENT COMPLIANCE

A good relationship between the patient and the physician and appropriate education are the foundations of good compliance. This is especially true in lupus because individual manifestations are variable and management is empiric.

PREVENTIVE MEASURES

Many patients worry about transmitting lupus to others. One may tell them that although there is a weak genetic predisposition, it is not likely that their children or other close relatives will develop lupus and that lupus is not known to be contagious.

SOCIOECONOMIC ASPECTS OF MANAGEMENT

Although most patients do well, a minority suffer devastating socioeconomic consequences. The ability to discuss disability issues frankly and to direct patients to appropriate social service agencies should be part of every physician's repertoire.

REFERENCES

Felson DT, Anderson J: Evidence for the superiority of immunosuppressive drugs and prednisone over prednisone alone in lupus nephritis. N Engl J Med 311:1528–1533, 1984.

Hughes GRV: Clinics in Rheumatic Diseases: Systemic Lupus Erythematosus, Vol 8. W.B. Saunders Co., Philadelphia, 1982.

Kelley WN, Harris ED, Ruddy S, et al: Textbook of Rheumatology, Vol 1, 2nd ed. W.B. Saunders Co., Philadelphia, 1985.

Schur PH: The Clinical Management of Systemic Lupus Erythematosus. Grune & Stratton, New York, 1983.

Steinberg AD: Systemic lupus erythematosus: insights from animal models. Ann Intern Med 100:714–727, 1984.

Vollertsen RS: The laboratory in rheumatology. Postgrad Med 76:155–162, 1984.

6 · SERONEGATIVE SPONDYLO-ARTHROPATHIES

Luis Fernandez-Herlihy
LAHEY CLINIC MEDICAL CENTER

DEFINITION AND DIAGNOSTIC CRITERIA

Seronegative spondyloarthropathies (SNSAs) are chronic inflammatory diseases of the spine and peripheral joints in which rheumatoid nodules and factors are not found. Examples are ankylosing spondylitis, psoriatic arthritis, Reiter's disease, the enteropathic arthritis of inflammatory bowel disease (chronic ulcerative colitis, Crohn's disease), and the arthritis that may occur in Whipple's or Behçet's disease or following intestinal bypass operations for morbid obesity. At least 50% of the patients with spondylitis of these diseases are carriers of HLA-B27.

Useful guidelines for diagnosis of SNSA are (1) pain, with or without swelling, of the peripheral joints without rheumatoid factors or nodules; (2) chronic back pain and stiffness, especially in the morning; (3) x-ray evidence of sacroiliitis or syndesmophytes; (4) evidence of psoriasis, inflammatory bowel disease, Reiter's disease, iritis, or uveitis; and (5) presence of HLA-B27. The occurrence of (1) or (2) together with one other criterion should raise a strong suspicion of SNSA.

This chapter will focus on ankylosing spondylitis, psoriatic arthritis, and enteropathic arthritis.

PATHOPHYSIOLOGY

The characteristic early lesion of ankylosing spondylitis is inflammation at the attachment of ligament to bone, the enthesis. Enthesopathy results in sacroiliitis and progressive ossification of spinal ligaments and can lead to the formation of thin syndesmophytes, fusion of the sacroiliac joints, and complete ankylosis of the spine. Similar changes are found in up to 40% of patients with psoriasis and 9% of patients with enteropathies. Enteropathic spondylitis resembles ankylosing spondylitis, but spinal ankylosis is rare. In psoriatic spondylitis, the syndesmophytes may be thick and asymmetric, and sacroiliitis is often absent or asymmetric.

Peripheral arthritis occurs in about 35% of patients with ankylosing spondylitis, in 5% to 7% of patients with psoriasis, and in 10% to 20% of patients with inflammatory bowel disease. This often consists of only a mild chronic synovitis, but some patients with psoriasis have marked resorption of the ends of phalanges that results in "pencil-in-cup" deformity or in shortening of the fingers and toes with extensive crippling of the hands and feet.

CLINICAL ASPECTS

ANKYLOSING SPONDYLITIS

Ankylosing spondylitis usually appears in the second or third decades of life. Formerly considered a disease primarily of men, the male to female ratio appears to be about 3:1, but in women the disease is often milder, ankylosis of the spine is rare, and the diagnosis is often missed. Back and neck pain and stiffness in the morning are common at the onset. There may be progressive limitation of motion of the spine until it is bent forward and immobile. Decrease in chest expansion (the chest circumference at mid-thorax should increase by at least 4 cm from full expiration to full inspiration) and limitation of motion of hips and shoulders are common in later stages. X-ray changes reflect the ligamentous and sacroiliac joint disease. There is sclerosis of both iliac and sacral sides of the sacroiliac joints and there may be eventual fusion of these joints. The ossification of the spinal ligaments results in radiographically visible syndesmophytes. Iritis or uveitis occurs in 25% and aortic regurgitation in up to 10% of patients. More than 90% of patients with ankylosing spondylitis are carriers of HLA-B27.

PSORIATIC ARTHRITIS

Psoriatic arthritis appears in several patterns: (1) asymmetric oligoarthritis affecting any joint, especially distal and proximal interphalangeal joints of the hands and feet; (2) symmetric arthritis affecting any joint; and (3) sacroiliitis with or without other features of ankylosing spondylitis or peripheral arthritis.

Onset occurs at any age and is generally independent of the extent and the activity of the rash. HLA-B27 is found in more than 50% of patients with psoriatic spondylitis and in about 23% of those with peripheral arthritis alone. X-ray changes in the peripheral joints are found almost exclusively in the interphalangeal joints and may appear as "pencil-in-cup" deformity. The symptoms of early psoriatic spondylitis and ankylosing spondylitis are similar. The x-ray appearance of the spine may also be similar, but in psoriasis the sacroiliac joint changes may be absent or asymmetric and the syndesmophytes are often thicker and asymmetric.

ENTEROPATHIC ARTHRITIS

Enteropathic arthritis appears as symmetric synovitis of the larger joints, such as ankles, knees, elbows, and wrists, or as backache with or without sacroiliitis and other features of ankylosing spondylitis. X-ray changes are uncommon in peripheral joints and in the spine are often limited to the sacroiliac joints. Peripheral arthritis is an indicator of active chronic ulcerative colitis or Crohn's disease, but spondylitis follows an independent course. The prevalence of HLA-B27 in patients with or without peripheral enteropathic arthritis is about the same as that of the general population but is found in 50% to 70% of those with enteropathic spondylitis.

Laboratory studies are not helpful in the diagnosis of SNSA. There may be an elevation of the erythrocyte sedimentation rate (ESR) and a mild anemia, but these tests are relatively unreliable as indicators of inflammation in these diseases.

MANAGEMENT

PLAN

Short-term and Long-term Goals. Short-term goals of treatment of SNSA are relief of pain and the achievement of more mobility. Long-term goals are prevention of joint damage and deformity and preservation or improvement of functional capacity and posture.

We cannot, at present, arrest progressive ankylosis in ankylosing spondylitis. The principal long-term goal is maintenance of an erect posture even if ankylosis occurs. This goal is usually attainable.

Psoriatic arthritis is not seriously disabling in most patients, and remissions can often be induced in peripheral arthritis with drug therapy.

Peripheral enteropathic arthritis implies active inflammatory bowel disease, and treatment should be directed at control of the enteritis.

The management of psoriatic and enteropathic spondylitis is the same as that of ankylosing spondylitis.

Indications for Hospitalization. Most patients with SNSA can be managed outside the hospital; exceptions are those who need surgery or whose inflammatory bowel disease is debilitating. Joint surgery is not often needed in SNSA; however, total joint replacement of the hip or knee is occasionally necessary in patients with ankylosing spondylitis.

NONPHARMACOLOGIC MEASURES

These are of the utmost importance in SNSA. Patients should be as active as they wish as long as pain is not aggravated and as long as they obtain adequate rest. The amount of rest depends on the amount of inflammation. An average rest program consists of ten hours of bed rest at night and one hour after the noon meal. This can be varied in proportion to the number of hot, swollen joints, the amount of generalized stiffness, nocturnal waking due to back pain, and elevation of the ESR. When pain results from joint damage rather than inflammation, rest limited to that joint is indicated. This can be accomplished by using lightweight splints, by reducing weight bearing, and by using a cane or crutches when necessary.

The application of heat or ice for 15 to 20 minutes two or three times each day provides symptomatic relief of joint pain. Patients are advised to use whichever is more comfortable. Ice has the advantage of reducing swelling; heat facilitates joint mobility.

An exercise program is of great importance. In ankylosing spondylitis, lifelong adherence to an exercise program can result in erect posture even if spinal ankylosis occurs. Exercises should be started as early as possible, before ankylosis occurs, and they should be performed every day. Our physical therapists instruct patients in the following program:

1. *Supine position*
   Inhale—Take a deep breath, spread ribs, raise chest, and swing arms overhead. Exhale—Slowly force air out through mouth and lower arms to sides of the body.
2. *Prone position*
   a. *Clasp hands on buttocks, pull shoulder blades together, and raise head and chest.*
   b. *Clasp hands behind head and raise elbows, head, and chest.*
   c. *With arms stretched out beyond head, raise opposite arm and leg. Alternate.*
   d. *With arms out at sides, circle arms five times, then rest.*
3. *Standing*
   Face corner of room and place hands on wall at shoulder level. Lean forward into corner bringing shoulder blades together. Keep chin in and heels on floor.

These exercises should be done a few times at first and gradually increased until each exercise is repeated ten times at least twice daily. The patient is warned to expect more myalgias at first, but these subside in time. Other exercises, such as walking, bicycling, and swimming, are also recommended.

Range-of-motion exercises for affected joints are prescribed for peripheral arthritis of SNSA and to maintain optimal muscle strength and prevent atrophy. Examples are quadriceps isometric exercises and progressive-resistance exercises for the knees. Exercises are performed more easily after a hot bath or local application of heat.

DRUG THERAPY

Selection of Drugs

Mild, early forms of SNSA may respond to non-pharmacologic measures alone, but most require the addition of analgesic and anti-inflammatory drugs.

Salicylates. Our preference is to begin treatment with enteric-coated (not buffered) aspirin. In mild disease, one 500-mg enteric-coated aspirin tablet (Maximum Strength Ecotrin) three times a day might suffice; in severe disease, a larger dose, such as 975 mg (one Easprin tablet) four times each day may be more effective. The use of enteric-coated aspirin in patients with delayed gastric emptying may result in acute and chronic salicylate toxicity.

Indomethacin and Corticosteroids. Some patients with SNSA have pain that is not relieved by salicylates. In these cases, especially if there is severe night pain, the use of indomethacin (Indocin) is often helpful. Doses range from 25 mg every eight hours to 50 mg every six hours. A useful formulation is sustained-release indomethacin (Indocin SR, 75 mg), which may be taken as a single bedtime dose or once every 12 hours. Corticosteroid treatment is reserved for those patients who have a severe inflammatory flare with intractable night pain, anemia, and a high ESR. In such cases, 10 to 20 mg of prednisone once daily, usually at bedtime, and gradually reduced to zero over a few weeks may be helpful. Oral corticosteroid agents should be avoided in psoriatic arthritis because stopping them can result in severe exacerbation of psoriasis. We encourage vigorous treatment of the psoriasis even though the rash and the arthritis follow independent courses.

Gold. The symptoms of psoriatic arthritis and spondylitis often respond to salicylates or indomethacin. When inflammation persists and there is peripheral joint damage despite adequate treatment with nonsteroidal anti-inflammatory drugs (NSAIDs), a course of gold injections may induce a remission. The procedure we recommend at the Lahey Clinic is the following:

Preparation: Aurothioglucose (Solganal), 50 mg/ml.
Method: Intramuscular (gluteal).
Dose: First week: 10 mg; second week: 25 mg; third week to 20th week: 50 mg/week. *Thereafter:* 50 mg IM every two weeks for six doses. *Then:* 50 mg IM every three weeks for six doses and, finally, every month for six doses or indefinitely.
On each visit: (a) Examine patient for rash and petechiae. (b) Ask about pruritus, rash, metallic taste, and diarrhea. (c) Check urine for red blood cells and albumin. (d) Check white blood count and differential and peripheral smear for platelets.
If patient has (a) pruritic rash, (b) petechiae, (c) leukopenia, (d) neutropenia, (e) reduced platelets on smear, (f) unexplained microhematuria, (g) unexplained albuminuria, (h) stomatitis, or (i) unexplained diarrhea, discontinue gold injections. There are numerous rare reactions to gold, some of which are very serious. The physician and the patient should be aware of these before embarking on a course of gold therapy.

The rash is most common and usually begins after about 400 mg of Solganal has been given. Eosinophilia is not unusual and has no serious implications; gold treatment may be continued.

Subjective improvement is not expected until at least 400 mg of Solganal has been given. If there is no significant improvement after 800 to 1000 mg of Solganal, stop gold treatment. Gold therapy is not known to be effective in psoriatic spondylitis or any other SNSA.

Methotrexate. Methotrexate, given once a week by mouth or by intramuscular injection, has been beneficial to some patients with psoriatic arthritis, but its use awaits the results of controlled studies of efficacy and safety.

Enteropathic arthritis and spondylitis respond quite well to NSAIDs, but these should be avoided when there is active bleeding. In such cases we use unacetylated salicylates, such as salsalate (Disalcid), 3 gm daily divided into two or three doses, or choline magnesium trisalicylate (Trilisate), 3 gm daily in one or two doses. The unacetylated salicylates do not inhibit platelet aggregation. However, the best treatment of enteropathic arthritis is control of the bowel disease.

Other Nonsteroidal Anti-Inflammatory Drugs. If salicylates cannot be used or are ineffective and indomethacin is not needed or desirable, other NSAIDs, such as ibuprofen (Motrin), tolmetin (Tolectin), or naproxen (Naprosyn), may be effective. All NSAIDs should be used with caution in the presence of active bleeding or chronic renal insufficiency.

PATIENT INFORMATION AND EDUCATION

The patient with SNSA must have a good understanding of the disease, its prognosis, and goals of management. Adequate time to discuss these fully with the patient is rewarded with compliance and optimal short- and long-term results. A frank and reassuring discussion about the genetic aspects of SNSA is helpful. The patient should be told that 6% to 14% of whites and 0% to 4% of blacks in the United States are carriers of HLA-B27, but only about 10% to 20% of these carriers have spondylitis. In addition, it is becoming apparent that the heredity of these diseases is multigenic and that environmental triggers for disease expression are multifactorial. Therefore, there is no good reason to interfere with the patient's normal family plans. Patients with enteropathic arthritis are taught to recognize that flares of peripheral arthritis usually indicate active enteritis even when there are no gastrointestinal symptoms.

PERIODIC EVALUATION

Patients with ankylosing spondylitis should be seen at least once each year to assess progression of disease and maintenance of an erect posture. This is best done by careful history, measurement of patient's height, chest expansion and spine mobility, follow-up x-ray films when necessary, and a review of the exercise program. More frequent visits may be necessary when the disease is more active. In some patients with peripheral arthritis, periodic hemoglobin and ESR determinations may be useful as measures of inflammation. Serial x-ray films of the affected joints at intervals of six to 12 months help to assess the progression of damage. The patient with ankylosing spondylitis should be asked to report eye symptoms that might indicate the presence of uveitis, which may require topical steroid treatment.

Early in the course of SNSA, the diagnosis may be difficult to confirm. Seronegative peripheral arthritis may occur months before inflammatory bowel disease or psoriasis appears. The symptoms of ankylosing spondylitis often precede the appearance of x-ray changes, and the presence of HLA-B27 alone is not diagnostic. This latent period may be frustrating to patient and physician, but the dilemma should be explained to the patient, his symptoms should be treated symptomatically with exercises and appropriate medications, and a schedule of visits should be established to look for diagnostic signs and to encourage the patient.

The majority of patients with SNSA, although faced with a chronic painful disease, do not often require hospitalization or joint surgery, and they are rarely seriously disabled. These patients and their physicians have good reason to embark optimistically on a structured management program.

REFERENCES

Ball J: Enthesopathy of rheumatoid and ankylosing spondylitis. Ann Rheum Dis 30:213–223, 1971.

Carette S, Graham D, Little H, et al: The natural disease course of ankylosing spondylitis. Arthritis Rheum 26:186–190, 1983.

Kammer GM, Soter NA, Gibson DJ, et al: Psoriatic arthritis: a clinical, immunologic and HLA study of 100 patients. Semin Arthritis Rheum 9:75–97, 1979.

Moll JMH, Haslock I, Macrae IF, et al: Associations between ankylosing spondylitis, psoriatic arthritis, Reiter's disease, the intestinal arthropathies, and Behcet's syndrome. Medicine 53:343–364, 1974.

Skinner M, Fernandez-Herlihy L: Entero-arthropathy: the coexistence of articular and gastrointestinal manifestations in systemic disease. Med Clin North Am 50:417–425, 1966.

7 · TENDINITIS AND BURSITIS

Jack Waxman
OCHSNER CLINIC AND ALTON OCHSNER MEDICAL FOUNDATION

DEFINITION AND DIAGNOSTIC CRITERIA

Inflammation adjacent to joints usually involves either the inserting tendon or the paratenon, that portion of the tendon attaching to muscle. Strictly speaking, such inflammation can be either tendinitis or peritendinitis, but for the purpose of this discussion, the single term *tendinitis* will be used. Such inflammatory processes often extend to the surrounding synovial tendon sheath and even to the fibrous tendon sheath surrounding all the structures. Bursae, synovial cell-lined cavities adjacent to joints and tendons, may also become inflamed and mimic tendon and joint symptoms. These periarticular sites become inflamed in rheumatoid arthritis and the seronegative spondyloarthropathies and are treated as part of the basic disease. However, they may require specific interventions as well, i.e., injection, incision, or excision. Gout and pseudogout may also occur in these structures, and occasionally sepsis develops and must be differentiated for proper therapy. Trauma usually results in a lower grade of inflammation, which tends to be repetitively aggravated by the partial, but inevitable, continued use of joints in the activities of daily life. These inflammatory processes may then become chronic, and it becomes difficult to separate the inciting cause from the continued mechanical insults to the structures in question. The prevalence of chronic tendinitis has increased with the sudden burgeoning interest in recent years of fitness via sports activities. Novice sportsmen and women initiating new physical activities in their 30s, 40s, and 50s, particularly jogging, have added to the legions of individuals with these chronic probems. New hobbies and activities also add regularly to the list of tendon and bursal disorders. For example, tendinitis has been documented in habitual video game players from joy-stick manipulation, and bursal sacs have been excised from the backs of break dancers.

PATHOPHYSIOLOGY

Elongating forces cause microtears in tendons when excessive force is applied or the forces are overly repetitious. Insufficient blood supply, loss of elasticity with age, and diabetes (which hastens both) may be contributing factors. Hormonal changes during pregnancy or at the menopause also favor tendinitis. Damaging, too, are compressive forces via external blows or internal spurs or continuous external pressures such as kneeling. These compressive forces usually affect bursae. The tendon is most vulnerable at its junction with bone or with muscle where partial or even complete tears tend to occur. Local pathologic processes include tenosynovial hypertrophy, tendon sheath adherence, calcium deposition, and a variable, chronic inflammatory infiltrate. Hydroxyapatite deposition is the most common crystalline deposit, but uric acid and calcium pyrophosphate dihydrate deposition may also occur. Minor trauma following such deposition may continue to shed such crystalline material into the periarticular structures, adding to the inflammatory process. Hydroxyapatite has been shown to undergo resorptive changes by surrounding inflammatory cells as well.

Hematogenous dissemination of organisms such as gonococci may deposit such organisms into tenosynovial regions such as the wrist, while direct inoculation of *Staphylococcus aureus* occurs in septic bursitis at the elbow and knee. Addicts inoculate this organism into wrist tendons while attempting to inject these veins. Bursae are significantly less reactive than a comparable joint when infected. In particular, leukocytosis is milder, with brisk elevations in only one half of the patients.

Responses to these inflammatory stimuli occur within hours after trauma, resulting in hematomas, soft tissue fluid accumulation, then organization with eventual resorption and scar tissue formation. Collagen repair occurs over six to eight weeks for restoration of proper tendon length and orientation, but adhesive restriction of sheath to the tendon may occur along with secondary atrophy of muscle from joint limitation. The worst sequel is a virtually frozen joint such as a "frozen shoulder." Repeated overuse prior to healing may result in eventual tendon rupture if sufficient retearing occurs prior to sufficient repair. This is especially true at the Achilles and rotator cuff and bicipital tendons, but in rheumatoid arthritis it may occur in dorsal wrist tendons at the fourth and fifth finger extensors.

The repair of small tendon defects is likely over a period of weeks to months but there is less success in larger tears. Unfortunately, present radiologic and physical examination techniques do not allow full definition of the healing process, making it difficult to determine when the patient can resume full activities. One often must proceed by trial and error to document the degree of healing response (see "Management"). Proper care, thus, will require a prompt, accurate diagnosis based predominantly on history and physical examination, and adequate follow-up will be required once a treatment plan is instituted.

CLINICAL ASPECTS

Pain, the predominant complaint, may be constant in severe cases but more often occurs during or after activities, even up to 24 to 48 hours later, and tends to radiate along superficial nerves distally for several inches. Examination reveals areas of localized tenderness, usually a small zone with or without local heat, redness, or nodule formation. Severe inflammation with bursal or tendon sheath swelling will require aspiration for crystal examination, Gram stain, and cell count. Culture will be essential to prove infection in such cases because white cell count, sugar, and lactate levels are not diagnostic in 50% of cases of septic bursitis. X-ray examination of the area usually documents a normal joint adjacent to a clinically abnormal tendon or bursa, assuring the physician that the inflammatory process is not related to a chronic intra-articular disease. However, acute joint disease processes usually appear normal on joint x-ray films and, therefore, are not excluded. In the periarticular space, amorphous calcium deposition helps document the chronicity of the tendon or bursal inflammatory reaction but is also present in far less than 50% of cases. Fine stippling should suggest calcium pyrophosphate dihydrate. However, the presence of calcification does not prove that an active, ongoing inflammatory process is occurring. Xeroradiographs are the preferred views to document such calcification, and other specially angled views may be required also, such as the "gunsight view" for calcification at the lateral epicondyle. CAT scanning or ultrasound examination may be useful in identifying fluid accumulations, particularly within bursae and especially in sites that tend to be relatively inaccessible to the palpating finger such as the posterior knee, the anterior hip, and at the shoulder.

The most important diagnostic technique remains reproduction of the patient's pain by palpation with resistive muscle maneuvers such as isometric contraction, which place tension on selective tendons and reproduce pain at the partially torn area. Impingement methods can also be used at the shoulder where compression of bursa and/or tendon against the overlying acromion occurs with abduction and more so with rotation in abduction. The technique of simultaneous palpation of symmetric tendons or bursae compares one side with the other and helps the patient and the examiner to identify small areas of tenderness that might otherwise be mistaken as normal palpatory sensitivity. The patient should be taught to palpate the sites himself to help judge the degree of healing or the recurrence of soreness when resuming various activities.

MANAGEMENT

After trauma, the inflammatory site should be immobilized to prevent bleeding and ice applied to minimize excess edema. Compression and elevation may be useful too, but venous constriction should be avoided. Anti-inflammatory medications are useful six to 12 hours later after the risk of bleeding is over, particularly if aspirin is the drug of choice, since even small doses may prolong the bleeding time excessively. Shorter-acting nonsteroidals (i.e., ibuprofen, meclofenamic acid) cause less platelet interference, and nonacetylated salicylates cause no platelet aggregation defects and may provide sufficient anti-inflammatory effect and pain control. Such medication effects are rarely clinically important except in patients with hemostatic defects. Severe inflammation may require steroid injection (between 10 and 40 mg of a long-acting preparation), which provides relief for seven to 14 days. Triamcinolone acetonide (or hexacetonide) is commonly utilized. When instilling such injections, the physician should carefully avoid the tendon itself to avoid weakening the structure and promoting rupture. It should be emphasized to the patient who takes pain medication (or is injected) that his pain relief does not indicate healing, and that premature use of the tendon may further weaken the partially torn site.

IMMOBILIZATION

The degree of tearing, which must be estimated based on the history and physical examination, will determine the length of time for immobilization. For tears of greater than 50%, the area should be immobilized for six to eight weeks. Lesser injuries may not require such strict immobilization, and avoidance of those sports or other activities that caused the initial injury will be sufficient. Splinting is useful in this phase of joint limitation and serves both as a reminder to the patient to restrict his activities as well as an actual physical barrier to prevent overstretching and retearing prior to full healing. The splint should be removed at least twice daily for a gentle stretching maneuver to prevent permanent stiffness and adhesions. Isometric exercises also help during this period to provide some continued muscle action and may gradually be increased to the point of pain. Exercise is particularly important for the shoulder and hip, where progressive stretching activities are essential as therapy advances.

After the several weeks required for the initial healing phase, a slower tendon remodeling takes place over a period of months, and the patient is gradually able to resume activities during this time regulated by recurrence of signs and symptoms of inflammation. If properly instructed initially, the patient is able to make this assessment by judging his pain and palpating his own wound. On follow-up visits the physician should establish the degree of inflammation by palpation, document any limitation of joint range of motion, and then treat accordingly with medication or progressive exercise.

PHYSICAL THERAPY

Tendon repair and stretching of contractures are aided by heat applications and gentle massage, which promote blood flow. Occasionally, the assistance of a physical therapist is needed, particularly for shoulder bursitis and tendinitis, which commonly lose the most motion. Certain patients, too, will be less willing to exert themselves in this somewhat painful process of stretching. Patients with hysterical or hypochondriacal personalities may require supplemental pretherapy pain medications to suppress even small pains and thus promote their cooperation. Therapists can use special techniques to help restore motion, including hot (hydrocolator) or ice packs, therapeutic massage, and even the application of transcutaneous nerve stimulators to block pain. Ultrasound as a source of deep heat has also been occasionally helpful in the management of tendinitis and bursitis.

FIBROSITIS OR SECONDARY FIBROMYALGIA

A particular patient subgroup is very prone to need the assistance of therapists. These patients have secondary fibrositis (also called "secondary fibromyalgia") and are anxious and often depressed. Their mood often compounds minor bursitic and arthritic complaints, and they have waxing and waning pain-spasm cycles and hyperirritable "tender" points or "trigger points," many of which overlie tendon origins or insertions. These sites are often the focal points of their multiple and virtually constant complaints. This patient group utilizes the most medication and therapeutic assistance to return to normal after even small injuries. Moreover, the de-

gree of tendon tearing will be difficult if not impossible to evaluate because pain complaints are so exaggerated. Small palpations tend to elicit startle responses with attempts at posturing and withdrawal, thus confusing the examiner unless he is aware of the patient's psychic state.

CHRONIC PAIN SYNDROMES

A small minority of patients with chronic tendon trauma will continue to have chronic pain syndromes during the long-term healing phase. This group constitutes about 10% of all patients seen. Included are those who have too rapidly returned to aggravating sports or work activities. Surgical repair may be necessary in this patient subgroup and in those with excessive deposits of calcium or bony spurring adjacent to tendon sites, which serve as repetitive foci of inflammation. Such surgical therapy should be delayed for many months (or even years) to allow slow healing, and care should be taken to exclude patients with fibromyalgia from this patient subgroup, since they characteristically do poorly with surgery. Other surgical candidates are those patients with major tendon tears seen early who are thought unlikely to heal with immobilization alone.

Traumatic bursitis is treated like tendinitis except that recurrent compressive forces are minimized instead of elongating ones. It must be recalled that these blows may inoculate crystals or bacteria into the bursa with an accelerated inflammatory response.

BURSAL GOUT

Acute bursal gout is treated like a joint attack of gout with high-dose anti-inflammatory medication early on, and tapering over days. Treatment includes ice packing, rest of the affected areas, and nonsteroidal medication, which replaces aspirin, which is contraindicated in gout because it causes shifts in serum uric acid. Renal function should be monitored carefully in those patients on nonsteroidals with concomitant diabetes, diuretic therapy, congestive failure, or renal impairment because progressive oliguric renal failure may occur within days of initiating therapy. Local steroid instillation into gouty bursae may be useful particularly when nonsteroidals need to be avoided, and intravenous colchicine is a good choice in the postoperative patient who is not eating.

SEPTIC BURSITIS

Septic bursae or tendons are usually identified by their heat or by skin discoloration, adjacent cellulitis or edema, and joint limitation of motion, but occasionally none of these signs are identified. In fact, a normal peripheral white count and sedimentation rate and good general status are common. Temperature elevation may be absent as well, and studies in the future will document whether succinic acid determination within bursal fluid and C-reactive protein determination in serum are more useful prognosticators of sepsis. If bursal fluid does reveal a high white count ($>$20,000/mm^3), sepsis should be presumed, but the absence of this finding should not delay therapy if sepsis is suspected clinically.

Repeated bursal aspiration and culture are presently the best methods for following cases of septic bursitis. Parenteral oxacillin is preferred, since most cases are staphylococcal. Intravenous therapies are continued until cultures are negative (usually within seven to 12 days). A course of oral cloxacillin or dicloxacillin is added for several days to prevent recurrence of infection. Some success has been documented with the initial use of 4 gm of cloxacillin per day orally, taken over two weeks. Such therapy needs careful monitoring of clinical signs and repeat aspiration and culture. Unusual organisms may occur in rare instances. Even *Mycobacterium marinum* has been documented and also *Sporothrix schenckii* in a few cases. Patients treated late (after two weeks of infection) are more resistant and will ordinarily require parenteral antibiotics.

LATE SEQUELAE AND FOLLOW-UP

Full resolution of septic prepatellar and/or olecranon bursal swelling and soreness requires 40 days on average. Occasionally late sequelae are noted, including the presence of chronic sinus tracts or sterile postinfectious bursitis. Surgical drainage is indicated in cases that do not demonstrate response to intravenous medication over 24 to 48 hours, although partial response with continued daily reaspiration over one to two weeks is adequate in the majority of cases. Since 85% of patients sustain localized infection in these sites via direct trauma with minor skin breakage, they must be educated to change their job routines in order to prevent recurrences. For example, tile workers and housemaids who do a lot of kneeling should be instructed to wear knee guards, which are also useful to diminish swelling and postinfectious bursitis by protecting against repeat trauma.

In summary, the physician's job is to assess the degree of inflammation, restriction of motion, weakness, and chronicity and then determine the most appropriate additional therapies. For example, for a patient with Achilles tendinitis, after treating the acute phase with rest and aspirin or a nonsteroidal, the physician may allow some running but only with better quality shoes (i.e., raised heels or orthotic inserts for overpronation). Ice application may be needed for minor bouts of recurrent inflammation. The patient should be taught proper strengthening and stretching exercises, and heat applications may be prescribed to speed healing in the subacute and chronic phases of therapy.

Tables 1 and 2 review the major clinical tendinitis and bursitis syndromes by site, diagnosis, causes, and

Table 1. TENDINITIS

Area	Diagnosis	Major Cause (but also consider)	Best Treatment Methods (beyond ASA/NSAID and less abuse)
Hand	Flexor tenosynovitis, ± trigger finger	Trauma .... RA, DM, Dupuytren's contracture	{Ice; massage; finger splint; steroid injection; excision
Wrist	Flexor tenosynovitis, ± carpal tunnel syndrome	Trauma .... RA, DM, pregnancy, amyloid, myxedema, ganglion tumors	{Ice; massage; wrist splint; steroid injection; excision
	Extensor tenosynovitis	RA, ... Gonorrhea, ... Sepsis (addict) .... Ganglion	{Rx of RA ± local steroid {Penicillin {Oxacillin {Rupture ± excision
	De Quervain's tenosynovitis	Trauma .... Pregnancy	{Molded thumb-wrist splint; steroid injection; excision
Elbow	Lateral epicondylitis ("tennis elbow")	Trauma .... radiohumeral synovitis, cervical root syndrome	{Ice → heat; elastic forearm or elbow support; steroid injection; wrist strengthening exercises (extension)
	Medial epicondylitis	Trauma	Ice → heat; steroid injection; wrist strengthening exercises (flexion)
Shoulder	Rotator cuff tendinitis	Trauma .... RA, PMR, AS	{Ice → heat; steroid injection; restretch-manipulation; surgery
	Bicipital tendinitis	Trauma	Ice → heat; steroid injection; restrengthen biceps (curls); surgery
Ankle-foot	Achilles tendinitis	Trauma .... AS, Reiter's syndrome	{Ice → heat, restretch (wall leans); restrengthen (toe risers); surgery
	Plantar fasciitis ("heel bursitis")	Trauma .... Reiter's syndrome	{Foam heel cusions or cups; steroid injection; toe curling exercises; arch support
	Posterior tibial tendinitis	Trauma	Elastic ankle support; foot adduction exercises
	Peroneal tendinitis	Löfgren's syndrome .... RA .... Trauma	{Ice; oral steroids {Rx of RA ± local steroid injection {Ice → heat; elastic ankle support; abduction exercises
Knee	Iliotibial tract tendinitis	Trauma	Ice → heat; resole shoe (outer); restretch
	Popliteal tendinitis	Trauma	Ice → heat; elastic knee brace
	Patellar tendinitis	Trauma	Ice → heat; patellar knee brace; quadriceps exercises; surgery

ASA = aspirin; NSAID = nonsteroidal anti-inflammatory drug; RA = rheumatoid arthritis; DM = diabetes mellitus; Rx = treatment; PMR = polymyalgia rheumatica; AS = ankylosing spondylitis.

Table 2. BURSITIS

Area	Diagnosis	Major Cause (but also consider)	Best Treatment Methods (beyond ASA/NSAID and less abuse)
Elbow	Olecranon bursitis	Trauma	{Ice → heat; cushioned sleeve
		Sepsis	{Oxacillin
		Gout	{Ice ± steroid injection; cushioned sleeve
		RA	{Cushioned sleeve ± local steroid and Rx of RA
Shoulder	Subacromial bursitis	Trauma	{Ice → heat; restretch-manipulate; steroid injection; surgery
		RA, PMR, AS	
Ankle/foot	Retrocalcaneal bursitis	Trauma	{Ice → heat; steroid injection
		Reiter's syndrome	
	Metatarsal bursitis (plantar 1–5)	Trauma	{Lower heels; spongy shoe inserts (or metatarsal bar)
		RA, Morton's neuroma	
	1st metatarsal bursitis (bunion)	Trauma	{Lower heels; broader-tipped shoe
		OA	{Rx of OA ± surgery; molded shoes
		RA	{Rx of RA ± surgery; molded shoes
		Gout	{Ice ± steroid injection
Knee	Anserine bursitis	Trauma	{Quadriceps and adductor knee exercises; elastic knee brace; cane (opposite hand); steroid injection; weight loss
		Medial knee OA	
	Gastrocnemius bursitis (Baker's cyst)	Trauma	{Steroid injection (knee or bursa); cane (opposite hand)
		RA, OA	
	Pre-patellar bursitis	Trauma	{Ice → heat; cushioned sleeve;
		Sepsis	{Oxacillin; drainage;
		Gout	{Ice → steroid injection; cushioned sleeve
Hip	Trochanteric bursitis	Trauma	{Steroid injection; restretch; weight loss; shoe insert for leg length correction; cane (opposite hand)
		L5 radiculopathy	{Corset; traction
	Iliopsoas bursitis	OA	{Steroid injection; cane (opposite hand); Rx of OA
		RA	{Steroid injection; cane (opposite hand); Rx of RA

NSAID = nonsteroidal anti-inflammatory drug; ASA = aspirin; PMR = polymyalgia rheumatica; AS = ankylosing spondylitis; RA = rheumatoid arthritis; Rx = treatment; OA = osteoarthritis.

best therapies. Anti-inflammatory medications and resting the involved area are standard treatment and are not listed individually.

REFERENCES

Brody DM: Running injuries. Clin Symp 32:1–36, 1980.

Clement DB, Taunton JE, Smart GW: Achilles tendinitis and peritendinitis. Am J Sports Med 12:179–184, 1984.

Ho G Jr, Tice AD: Comparison of nonseptic and septic bursitis. Arch Intern Med 139:1269–1273, 1979.

Hollingsworth GR, Ellis RM, Hattersley TS: Comparison of injection techniques for shoulder pain: results of a double-blind randomized study. Br Med J 2:87, 1983.

Steinbrucker O, Neustadt DH: Aspiration and Injection Therapy in Arthritis and Musculoskeletal Disorders. Harper & Row, Hagerstown, MD, 1972.

8 · FIBROSITIS

A. Dean Steele
SCOTT AND WHITE CLINIC

DEFINITION AND DIAGNOSTIC CRITERIA

Fibrositis is a nonarticular syndrome of musculoskeletal aches and pains that are diffuse in distribution and accompanied by tenderness to palpation in characteristic anatomic locations. The disorder is primary when no rheumatic or other diseases are present that could account for the patient's symptom complex. Fibrositic symptoms can be secondary to other rheumatic disorders such as rheumatoid arthritis or degenerative joint disease, but should be recognized as secondary in these instances.

PATHOPHYSIOLOGY

The mechanism of production of aches and pains is not known. Laboratory studies are uniformly normal or negative and serve primarily to help rule out other rheumatic diseases or illnesses that may cause the patient's symptom complex.

CLINICAL ASPECTS

The discomfort in the fibrositic is diffuse and difficult for the patient to describe in terms of its location. Most typically it involves the cervical and lumbar areas. It may shift from one location to another. The severity of the pain may show marked variation during the course of illness, and may range from a minimally symptomatic state to one of temporary functional disability. The symptoms are often worsened by exposure to cold and dampness. Morning stiffness is common.

Complaints of ease of fatigability and tiredness are frequent. Patients will often state that they feel as tired on arising in the morning as when they retire at night, in spite of a seemingly good night of sleep. Sleep disturbance is common in fibrositis, but this finding

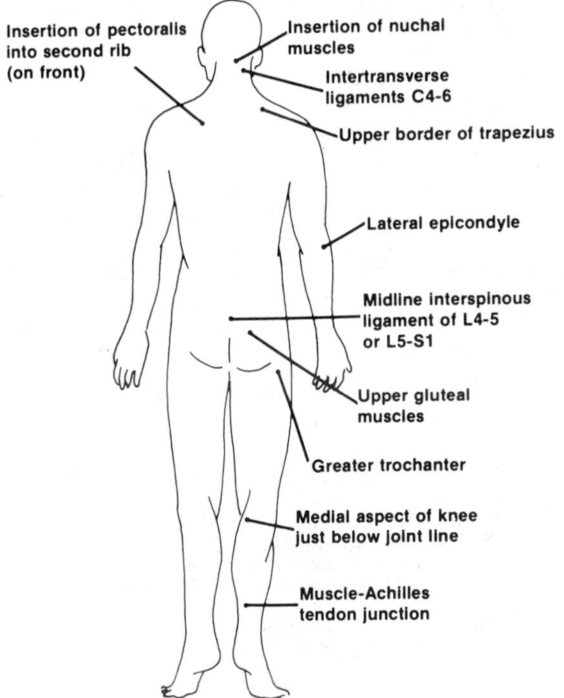

Figure 1. Characteristic sites of tenderness to palpation (bilateral) in fibrositic patients.

may not be recognized unless the physician specifically asks that patient about sleeping patterns. Patients with fibrositis have shown characteristic EEG changes during sleep indicating a disturbance in stage four, non-REM (rapid eye movement), sleep.

Psychological factors are associated with fibrositis, and study has shown that some fibrositic patients are psychologically disturbed when compared with control patients. The role of such disturbances in the pathogenesis of fibrositis remains to be determined.

Tender points on palpation exhibit remarkable consistency in location from patient to patient. Characteristic tender points are shown in Figure 1. While many of these sites are apt to be tender in normal persons, they are much more tender in fibrositic patients. Patients are frequently unaware that these sites are tender until they are palpated. While similar tender points may be demonstrable in normal patients, they are found much less frequently and require significantly greater pressure to elicit tenderness. An absolute requirement for a given number of tender points to make the diagnosis of fibrositis has not been defined, but the larger the number, the more likely the diagnosis.

Symptoms are characteristically worsened by cold, particularly damp cold. Conversely, symptoms tend to be improved by heat.

MANAGEMENT

PLAN

Treatment efforts are aimed at helping the patient understand what fibrositis is and is not, relieving discomfort, returning the patient to as normal a functional state as possible, and maintaining improvement of the patient's condition.

NONPHARMACOLOGIC MEASURES

The first step in any treatment program is education of the patient. While it is difficult to explain the fundamental nature of the fibrositic disorder, the patient must be reassured strongly that fibrositis does not represent a serious illness and is not a crippling disease. It should be stated that aches and pains do not lead to deterioration of muscles, tendons, or ligaments. The patient should be told that activity and exercise will not lead to damage of muscles in spite of any discomfort experienced. It should be pointed out that aside from the discomfort and distress, the syndrome is otherwise unharmful to the body. The pamphlet "Fibrositis" (published by the Arthritis Foundation and readily available from local chapters) provides excellent adjunctive information written specifically for the patient.

It is important for patients to understand that they must assume significant responsibility for much of their treatment, especially nonpharmacologic measures. Exercise programs are prescribed that typically might include walking, bicycling, or swimming. Programs must be significantly tailored to each patient in view of varying exercise tolerances. Periods of rest and exercise must be balanced, and it is appropriate to begin at low levels of activity with gradual increases as tolerated. Patients may be referred to a physical therapist or to patient education programs to learn muscle stretching and relaxation techniques. Application of heat, either wet or dry, may be prescribed one or more times a day depending on the severity of symptoms and the patient's response. Soaking in a hot tub of water (at home or at the local health club or spa) or use of hot towels covered by a heating pad, or the heating pad alone for periods of 10 to 20 minutes, two or three times a day, provides symptomatic relief. Applications of heat may be followed by gentle massage of symptomatic muscle sites.

DRUG THERAPY

Selection of Drugs. Aspirin and other nonsteroidal agents may be used in an effort to reduce pain, but these agents are usually of limited benefit. Aspirin may be given in doses of 650 to 775 mg, three or four times a day, while nonsteroidal anti-inflammatory drugs may be used in standard doses.

Tricyclic antidepressants are useful in patients with sleep disorders. Amitriptyline may be prescribed in a dose of 10 mg before retiring at night. The dose may be increased to 20 mg and occasionally to 50 to 75 mg depending on patient response. In some patients it is more helpful to give the dose one or two hours before retiring. Cyclobenzaprine is chemically a close relative of amitriptyline and may be useful in some patients. It may be prescribed in a dose of 10 mg at bedtime. Additionally another 5 to 10 mg may be given during the daytime.

Judicious injections of severely tender points, especially those in the upper or lower back with 1% lidocaine may occasionally afford symptomatic relief.

Adverse Effects. The common side effect from taking aspirin is gastrointestinal intolerance. Gastric erosion or ulceration may occur in some patients with associated minor or major episodes of bleeding. Decreased hearing and tinnitus may occur and are reversible with lowering doses or discontinuing use of aspirin. Gastrointestinal intolerance occurs in variable degrees with use of nonsteroidal anti-inflammatory drugs. In addition, these drugs may cause fluid retention, headache, or skin rash. Amitriptyline and cyclobenzaprine may cause excessive drowsiness, lethargy, and anticholinergic side effects such as dry mouth or urinary retention.

Interference with Concomitant Disease or Disorders. Salicylates should not be given to patients with active peptic ulcer disease or patients with asthma who are allergic to the drug. Nonsteroidal agents should be avoided or used with great caution in patients with severe congestive heart failure, cirrhosis with ascites, or significantly impaired renal function. Inhibition of prostaglandin synthesis in these patients may lead to further impairment of renal function and secondary worsening of the underlying conditions.

Amitriptyline and cyclobenzaprine must be used with caution or avoided in patients with problems of urinary retention or glaucoma.

Interference with Concomitant Drug Therapy. Aspirin will interfere with the use of oral anticoagulants, causing further prolongation of the prothrombin time, and it should not be given to patients taking these drugs. Amitriptyline and cyclobenzaprine should not be used in patients receiving monoamine oxidase inhibitors.

PATIENT INFORMATION AND EDUCATION

Patients should be informed of common side effects of medications that are prescribed (see earlier). When patients are given amitriptyline, it should be explained to them that the drug is being used to alleviate their sleep disorder. Similarly they should be told that cyclobenzaprine is being used as a muscle relaxant. At the same time it is appropriate to tell the patient that whereas amitriptyline is an antidepressant, it is not being prescribed for its antidepressant effect. Patients should be warned specifically to be careful with regard to operating motor vehicles or machinery if drowsiness presents a problem with use of tricyclic medications.

If gastrointestinal intolerance is a problem with regular aspirin, enteric-coated preparations may be used to avoid these side effects.

PERIODIC EVALUATION

The time and frequency of return visits will vary from patient to patient depending on the response or lack thereof to treatment efforts. Initial visits following the establishment of the basic treatment program are useful to reiterate educational information given to the patient and to reinforce specific instructions regarding the use of nonpharmacologic measures and medications.

PATIENT COMPLIANCE

It is appropriate to repeatedly question the patient to determine whether prescribed treatment programs are being followed. It is important to determine whether new situational problems at home or on the job have occurred that could have an adverse effect on the patient's course.

Practicing the art of medicine presents a significant opportunity and challenge in the fibrositic population. One must strive to convey a sense of caring and understanding and to provide continued encouragement and support.

PREVENTIVE MEASURES

Patients should be encouraged to look for stress factors that seem to aggravate their symptoms. When they can be identified either in the workplace or at home, appropriate measures should be taken to alleviate or eliminate such factors. Interpersonal problems with a spouse or other family members may require third-party counseling when the patient and other involved individuals cannot resolve their problems without assistance. If working conditions or requirements clearly aggravate underlying symptoms, it may be appropriate or necessary to consider a change in job.

REFERENCES

Ahles TA, Yunus MB, et al: Psychologic factors associated with primary fibromyalgia syndrome. Arthritis Rheum 27:1101–1106, 1984.
Bennett RM: Fibrositis; misnomer for a common rheumatic disorder. West J Med 134:405–413, 1981.
Moldofsky H, Scarisbrick P, England R, et al: Musculoskeletal symptoms and non-REM sleep disturbance in patients with "fibrositis syndrome" and healthy subjects. Psychosom Med 38:35–44, 1976.
Smythe HA: The "fibrositis" syndrome. In Kelley WN, Harris ED, Ruddy S, et al (eds): Textbook of Rheumatology. W.B. Saunders Co., Philadelphia, 1981, pp 488–493.

9 · CRYSTAL-INDUCED ARTHRITIS: CALCIUM PYROPHOSPHATE DEPOSITION DISEASE AND PSEUDOGOUT

William P. Beetham
LAHEY CLINIC MEDICAL CENTER

DEFINITION AND DIAGNOSTIC CRITERIA

Calcium pyrophosphate deposition disease can cause both acute inflammatory and chronic degenerative forms of arthritis. The diagnosis is confirmed by identification of calcium pyrophosphate dihydrate crystals in synovial fluid. Pseudogout is characterized by acute attacks of arthritis resembling gout that occur in patients with deposits of calcium pyrophosphate. Chondrocalcinosis is the term used to describe the radiologic appearance of calcification in joint cartilage and, although frequently associated with pseudogout, is not diagnostic of that condition. Gout, which is also a form of crystal-induced arthritis, is discussed in Chapter 8 of Section IX.

PATHOPHYSIOLOGY

The acute attack of arthritis represents an inflammatory host response to crystals of calcium pyrophosphate released from adjacent joint cartilage. These crystals are weakly positively birefringent when viewed under compensated polarized light microscopy. Calcium pyrophosphate deposition arthropathy can be classified as hereditary or idiopathic. The idiopathic type is seen more frequently. This type of arthropathy can also be associated with underlying disease or metabolic disorders, such as hyperparathyroidism, hemochromatosis, hypothyroidism, or neuropathic joint disease. The incidence of calcium pyrophosphate deposition and chondrocalcinosis increases with advancing age. Trauma predisposes to deposition of calcium pyrophosphate, and surgery can provoke acute symptoms.

CLINICAL ASPECTS

Calcium pyrophosphate deposition may not cause symptoms or it may be associated with a variety of clinical symptoms resembling other arthritic diseases. The acute pseudogout syndrome, which occurs in about 25% of symptomatic patients, is characterized by acute or subacute attacks of pain and swelling in involved joints lasting from one to two days to three or four weeks. It usually involves only one or two joints, thereby simulating gout. The knee is the most frequently involved joint, and the big toe is usually spared. The inflammation may begin in a single joint and spread to nearby joints, a pattern called cluster attack.

Less often, calcium pyrophosphate deposition arthropathy causes symmetric multiple joint involvement lasting several months and resembles rheumatoid arthritis.

A pseudo-osteoarthritic syndrome may occur causing chronic arthritis or chronic arthritis with superimposed acute episodes. This group accounts for two thirds of all symptomatic disease and resembles osteoarthritis although it has several differences. The knees are most often involved followed by wrists, metacarpophalangeal joints, hips, shoulders, intervertebral discs, elbows, and ankles. Although true osteoarthritis also involves the knees and hips, it would be unusual for osteoarthritis to involve wrists, metacarpophalangeal joints, elbows, and shoulders, which are often involved with calcium pyrophosphate deposition arthropathy. Occasionally, severe destruction of a joint and loss of cartilage resemble neuropathic or Charcot's joint, either with or without neurologic abnormalities.

Most joints with chondrocalcinosis are asymptomatic. However, recognition of articular calcification can be helpful in diagnosing symptomatic calcium pyrophosphate deposition arthropathy. Small calcifications in soft tissues and within articular cartilage can be overlooked easily on radiography. Articular calcification can be detected 90% of the time by frontal radiologic views of both knees and in almost all instances by a radiologic screen of knees, wrists, and the pelvis. Isolated patellofemoral or radiocarpal joint disease is a radiologic clue to underlying calcium pyrophosphate deposition disease.

The uric acid level, latex fixation test, and antinuclear antibody test are usually within normal limits, but the white blood cell count and sedimentation rate may be elevated if acute inflammation of the joint is present.

MANAGEMENT

OBJECTIVES AND THERAPEUTIC PLAN

The objectives of management are to relieve pain, prevent disability, and if possible stop progression of the degenerative process. Discomfort often can be relieved even though the degenerative changes in the joint persist. The great majority of patients can be treated as outpatients.

Aspiration of an acutely inflamed, painful joint is recommended whenever the diagnosis is uncertain to confirm the diagnosis by crystal analysis of joint fluid and to rule out infection by culture and white blood cell count of synovial fluid.

Acute attacks in large joints, such as the knee, ankle, or wrist, are often treated successfully by aspiration of synovial fluid and injection of a corticosteroid agent into the joint. Intra-articular injection can usually be performed easily as an outpatient procedure, but when the lower extremity is involved, it should be followed by limitation of weight-bearing activity until clinical improvement occurs. Intra-articular injection of the shoulder and hip is difficult and may require consultation with an orthopedic surgeon. Nonsteroidal anti-inflammatory drugs are often helpful in relieving acute attacks of pseudogout. However, the success of these drugs is variable. Steroid injections are frequently unnecessary, especially in mild attacks, since the response to oral medication is often satisfactory.

The treatment of milder, chronic symptoms is less specific, and techniques used to manage osteoarthritis can be applied to patients with this pattern of involvement. Hospitalization is usually unnecessary but is justified for persistent, disabling symptoms because it provides an opportunity for rest, physical therapy, emotional support, and reassessment of the drug therapeutic program. When the patient's symptoms are severe and the diagnosis is uncertain, hospitalization can also be helpful to rule out other underlying disease as well as to perform special studies, such as arthroscopy, tissue biopsy, or myelography, which can be difficult to obtain on an outpatient basis. Surgical intervention and total joint replacement may be necessary when severe degenerative changes and loss of joint cartilage are associated with pain and deposits of calcium pyrophosphate in weight-bearing joints such as the hip or knee.

NONPHARMACOLOGIC MEASURES

Physical therapy is useful in the management of calcium pyrophosphate disease involving the knee. Quadriceps muscle strengthening not only helps prevent muscle atrophy and joint instability but may also decrease further cartilage destruction caused by excessive wear on one side of the joint in the unstable knee. A properly fitted cane can help relieve pain involving joints of the lower extremity. The cane should be held in the hand opposite the symptomatic side. The patient is instructed to lean onto the cane away from the painful extremity to reduce weight bearing on the involved side.

A wrist splint can be useful in relieving pain in an inflamed wrist by reducing motion in the joint. Range-of-motion exercises for involved joints can prevent contractures and limitation of motion.

DRUG THERAPY

Nonsteroidal anti-inflammatory drugs are useful in the management of both acute and chronic forms of calcium pyrophosphate deposition disease. It may be necessary to try a number of different drugs before finding one with optimal efficacy.

In acute attacks of arthritis, large initial doses of medication are given and then reduced as the pain abates. Indomethacin (Indocin), 50 mg three times a day, or naproxen (Naprosyn), 500 mg twice a day, can be effective in acute pseudogout. These drugs are usually more effective if taken within several hours after the onset of acute symptoms. The medication should be continued for three to five days for a minor attack and for two to three weeks for a more severe episode. The dose can usually be reduced within one week as symptoms subside.

Chronic Arthritis. A wide variety of nonsteroidal anti-inflammatory drugs can be used to treat chronic calcium pyrophosphate deposition arthropathy. Long-acting drugs like piroxicam (Feldene), 20 mg once a day, sulindac (Clinoril), 200 mg, diflunisal (Dolobid), 500 mg, or naproxen, 375 mg twice a day, may be effective and improve compliance, since the patient has to take the drug only once or twice a day. If these drugs are not well tolerated, aspirin, 600 to 900 mg four times a day, ibuprofen (Motrin), 600 mg three or four times a day, tolmetin (Tolectin), 400 mg three times a day, meclofenamate (Meclomen), 50 to 100 mg three or four times a day, or fenoprofen calcium (Nalfon), 600 mg three times a day, may prove effective without serious side effects.

Adverse Effects. Adverse side effects common to all nonsteroidal anti-inflammatory drugs include rash, gastric intolerance and bleeding, aggravation of asthma and allergic rhinitis, and renal effects in patients with compromised renal function. Other reactions may be peculiar to certain drugs. Usually these medications are given after meals or with fluids to reduce irritation to the gastrointestinal tract.

Other Drugs. Simple analgesic drugs, such as codeine and propoxyphene, are usually of limited value. Narcotics should not be prescribed. Drugs with both analgesic and anti-inflammatory activity are especially effective. The prolonged use of phenylbutazone should be avoided because of the risk of blood dyscrasia. Oral steroids may suppress inflammation in acute pseudogout but usually are not necessary. Nonsteroidal anti-inflammatory drugs are usually preferable to colchicine.

Intra-articular Injection. Acutely inflamed joints are frequently relieved by aspiration of joint fluid and injection of a soluble corticosteroid agent. The anti-inflammatory effect usually occurs within 24 hours. The most common injectable corticosteroid agents used include hydrocortisone, prednisolone, dexamethasone, betamethasone, methylprednisolone, and triamcinolone. The duration of action may vary, but no corticosteroid agent has clearly been shown to be more effective than another. For small joints of the hands and feet, prednisolone suspension, 5 to 12.5 mg, or its equivalent is suggested. For medium-sized joints, such as the wrist, ankle, and elbow, 10 to 20 mg may be used; large joints, such as the knee, hip, and shoulder, require 20 to 50 mg of this agent.

PATIENT EDUCATION AND PREVENTIVE MEASURES

The physician should explain carefully the nature of the disease to the patient and, if appropriate, reassure the patient that the condition is not likely to cause crippling or deformity. A specific plan of therapy based on the site of involvement, severity of symptoms, occupational activities, and life style should be formulated for each patient. Medication is only one part of such a program. Modification of activity, control of weight, and physical therapy are especially useful in helping the patient adapt to chronic symptoms and disability. Reduction of weight is especially important in the obese patient with symptoms in weight-bearing joints. Anxiety and depression can often be controlled by relief of pain, reassurance, and the use of antidepressant medication or less often by tranquilizers.

Discomfort can frequently be relieved by an appropriate balance between rest and exercise. Patients with chronic degenerative joint disease are urged to live within their limitations. When weight-bearing joints are involved, rest periods can be helpful. Prolonged periods of weight-bearing activity should be avoided.

PERIODIC EVALUATION

Periodic evaluation is necessary for patients with chronic or recurrent symptoms to provide an opportunity to review the effectiveness of therapy and to detect adverse drug reactions. The patient should be encouraged to ask questions and should receive emotional support and encouragement.

REFERENCES

Arthritis Foundation: Calcium pyrophosphate deposition disease. *In* Rodnan GP, Schumacher HR, Zvaifler NJ (eds): Primer on the Rheumatic Diseases, 8th ed. Arthritis Foundation, Atlanta, 1983, pp 128–131.

Howell DS: Diseases due to the deposition of calcium pyrophosphate and hydroxyapatite. *In* Kelley WN, Harris ED Jr., Ruddy S, et al (eds): Textbook of Rheumatology, Vol 1, 2nd ed. W.B. Saunders Co., Philadelphia, 1985, pp 1398–1416.

Ryan LM, McCarty DJ: Calcium pyrophosphate crystal deposition disease; pseudogout; articular chondrocalcinosis. *In* McCarty DJ (ed): Arthritis and Allied Conditions: A Textbook of Rheumatology, 10th ed. Lea & Febiger, Philadelphia, 1985, pp 1515–1546.

10 · CERVICAL AND LUMBAR DISC DISEASE

Russell W. Hardy
Francis Boumphrey
CLEVELAND CLINIC FOUNDATION

SOCIOECONOMIC CONSIDERATIONS

Disease of the intervertebral discs is extremely common and has significant social and economic implications. Disc disease causes a tremendous national economic burden in medical expenses, lost work time, and compensation payments. It has been estimated that, in a recent year, well over 100,000 operations were performed for herniated lumbar discs alone. In addition to those patients requiring surgical intervention, literally millions of individuals have symptomatic disc disease treated nonoperatively (or not treated at all).

PATHOPHYSIOLOGY

Although the clinical manifestations of cervical and lumbar disc disease are different, the pathophysiology of disc disease is similar throughout the spine. At each level of the spinal column, the vertebral bodies are separated by a cartilaginous intervertebral disc, which acts as a cushion for the spinal column and also permits a certain amount of mobility between adjacent vertebrae. The disc consists of two parts, the central nucleus pulposus, and the more peripheral annulus fibrosus that encircles and supports the nucleus.

In youth the disc has a high water content, which diminishes with age. As the disc loses water, nuclear degeneration occurs, leading to loss of disc volume and elasticity and to fragmentation of the disc. Similar changes occur in the annulus, leading to splitting of the fibrotic elements and weakening of that structure. These changes occur at different rates in different individuals and may be accelerated by chronic and acute trauma.

As the disc degenerates, fragments of nuclear material may be extruded through defects in the annulus, leading to herniated cervical or lumbar discs. Such extrusions may be asymptomatic, or cause minor spinal or radicular pain that may subside spontaneously. On the other hand, if significant root, cord, or cauda equina compression occurs, severe pain or neurologic deficit may result, and aggressive treatment may be indicated.

In addition to acute or subacute herniation, symptoms may also arise from chronic degenerative changes in the spinal column. As degeneration occurs, reactive calcification develops at the disc margins, leading to osteophyte formation. Additional changes may occur in the synovial joints or ligamentous structures of the spine. These chronic degenerative changes may also give rise to symptoms if they cause neural compression.

Because of differences in clinical presentation, cervical and lumbar disc disease will be considered separately.

Cervical Disc Disease

There are seven cervical vertebrae, and six intervertebral discs (there are no discs between the occiput and C1 and between C1 and C2). Disc disease is most common in the midcervical spine, since this portion of the spine is most mobile and presumably subject to the greatest stress.

REGIONAL ANATOMY

The regional anatomy is seen in Figure 1. At each vertebral level, the nerve root leaves the spinal canal by

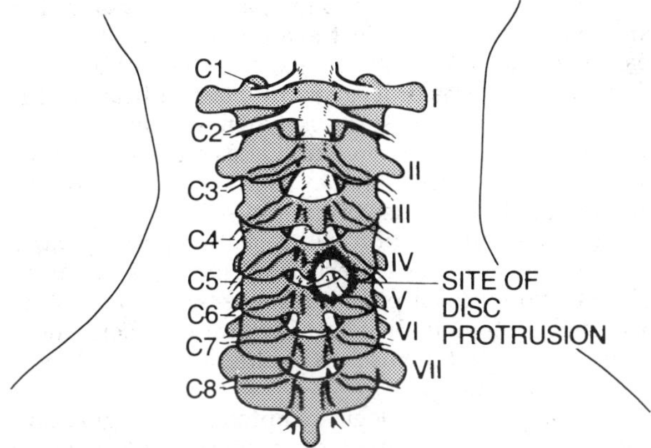

Figure 1. Diagram of the cervical spine, cord, and nerve roots. The root levels are shown in arabic and the vertebral levels in roman numerals. The location of a C4–5 lateral disc protrusion is shown. Normally a disc protrusion at C4–5 compresses the C5 root.

way of the neural foramen. The foramen is bounded anteriorly by the disc and vertebral body and posteriorly by the articular process. Because of the presence of the posterior spinal ligament, disc herniations most commonly occur laterally, compressing the root as it enters the bony confines of the neural foramen. It should be noted that although there are seven cervical vertebrae, there are eight cervical roots (Fig. 1). As the root enters the foramen, it crosses the disc corresponding numerically to the more superior vertebra. For this reason, a lateral herniated cervical disc typically compresses the root numbered one higher than the disc (for example, a C5 herniated disc compresses the C6 root).

CLINICAL ASPECTS

NEUROLOGIC SYNDROMES

The neurologic syndromes seen from root compression at each level are well defined and of considerable localizing significance. The cardinal presenting symptom is pain, beginning in the neck and radiating to the arm. There may be associated paresthesias in a radicular distribution. Physical examination may reveal sensory loss, motor weakness, or reflex changes. Compression of the C5 root may result in shoulder and upper arm pain, sensory loss over the deltoid, biceps and deltoid weakness, and loss of the biceps reflex. A C6 lesion will give shoulder pain with radiation along the outer arm to the thumb and first finger; sensory loss may occur in the thumb and first finger, and may be accompanied by biceps weakness and reduction in the biceps and brachioradialis reflex. Shoulder and lateral arm pain, with sensory loss in the index and middle fingers, together with triceps weakness and loss of that reflex may follow C7 root compression. Finally, C8 root compression may lead to medial forearm and hand pain, sensory loss in the fourth and fifth fingers, and intrinsic hand weakness. Not all of the above signs are seen with every lesion, and some variation is possible.

While the majority of cervical disc herniations occur laterally, some may be more central, causing pain of cord compression, either alone or in combination with signs of root compression. Such patients may complain of cervical pain as the first symptoms, but often neck pain is trivial or absent. The patient may notice paresthesias in the arms or legs, or complain of heaviness in the legs, spasms, or stiffness when walking; bladder symptoms may also be present. Occasionally, the symptoms of cord compression may even be overlooked until pointed out by a spouse or the physician.

Physical examination will reveal a spastic paraparesis or quadriparesis, including increased reflexes, clonus, and extensor plantar responses. A true sensory level is less commonly seen. Cervical disc herniations may also manifest themselves as anterior cord or Brown-Séquard syndromes.

Usually the neurologic symptoms begin gradually and develop over weeks or months. Unless major trauma has caused the ruptured disc, sudden profound neurologic deficit is quite rare.

The syndromes produced by acute disc herniations may also be seen in chronic degenerative disease. In these patients, compression is caused by osteophytes, or by a combination of osteophytes plus herniated disc material. Both radicular and cord symptoms may result. The radicular symptoms appear acutely and mimic disc herniation or they may present gradually as chronic arm pain. In some cases, multiple roots may be affected. Symptoms of cord compression appear over a period of months to years. In general, symptoms due to osteophytic compression appear more often in older patients, whereas acute herniated discs appear in younger individuals, but there are exceptions on both ends of the spectrum.

MANAGEMENT

The type of treatment employed will depend on the degree of pain, the nature and severity of neurologic symptoms, and the type of disease process that is suspected.

NONOPERATIVE MEASURES

For patients presenting with radicular symptoms and no evidence of cord compression, nonoperative treatment with traction and cervical immobilization is usually employed first (a possible exception may exist for individuals with a profound radicular motor deficit).

When arm pain and weakness are not too severe, this program may be carried out on an outpatient basis. Cervical immobilization is done with a soft cervical collar (worn at night and during the day). The collar should fit properly, and hold the head in a neutral position. Cervical traction can be done at home after the patient is instructed in its use. Generally we employ 15 pounds of weight initially, for 10 minutes twice a day, and increase the weight and duration as tolerated (up to 30 pounds several times a day). A common error is to use insufficient weight; frequently no improvement will be seen unless higher levels are reached.

Pain is controlled with appropriate non-narcotic or narcotic analgesics. If cervical muscle spasm is present, muscle relaxants may also be employed; I usually use diazepam, 5 mg t.i.d. or q.i.d., or methocarbamol, 1.0 gm q.i.d. Local heat may be useful in reducing spasm prior to traction. Nonsteroidal anti-inflammatory drugs may also be helpful as a short-term measure in some individuals (my own choices are phenylbutazone, 100 mg q.i.d., or indomethacin, 25 mg t.i.d., or q.i.d., for seven to ten days).

Non-operative measures may be continued for several weeks in patients with mild to moderate symptoms. When arm pain is severe, or a substantial motor deficit exists, we often hospitalize patients for traction and close neurologic observation. In this latter group, operative treatment may be necessary if improvement does not occur within a few days.

INDICATIONS FOR MYELOGRAM AND SURGERY

When patients do not respond to treatment, further diagnostic steps are indicated. In general, a cervical myelogram is the next logical step, although it is possible that myelography will someday be supplanted by magnetic resonance imaging (MRI). CT scanning following water-soluble contrast is used in many centers; however, we feel it offers no advantage over conventional myelography, and usually do not employ it in the diagnosis of herniated cervical discs. A myelogram is a prelude to an operation, and unless there is serious doubt about the diagnosis, should not be done prior to appropriate conservative treatment.

If the myelogram demonstrates a herniated disc or osteophytic compression, surgical treatment is indicated when nonoperative treatment has failed. Lateral cervical discs may be treated with either posterior or anterior operations, depending on the surgeon's preference and experience. A fusion may be employed as part of the anterior procedure, but is incidental to the primary goal of surgery, namely, nerve root decompression.

SPINAL CORD COMPRESSION

A different approach is used for patients with cord signs. In these individuals a myelogram is first carried out in order to confirm the diagnosis and determine the type and extent of cord compression.

In elderly patients with minimal symptoms and spondylotic compression, conservative treatment with a soft collar might suffice with operation reserved for patients who demonstrate neurologic progression. Most commonly, however, the symptoms are severe enough to warrant operation. In individuals with midline compression at one level, we prefer anterior operation. We employ an anterior operation for cases of two-level compression and some surgeons may use it at multiple levels. In general, however, we recommend a posterior decompressive laminectomy if more than two levels are involved, or if there is any doubt about the diagnosis. A decision regarding the operative approach also may hinge on whether diagnostic studies suggest anterior or posterior compression. For this reason, high quality myelographic films are essential; CT scanning may also be useful in localizing the compression. Preliminary work with MRI scanning of the cervical spine suggests these scanners may be highly useful in localizing the site of compression.

The results of cervical operations are variable, but the best results may be anticipated on individuals with symptoms of short duration. Postoperative results are less good in patients with severe, long-standing disease.

Lumbar Disc Disease

Lumbar disc disease commonly presents as an acute process (disc herniation), but also has a chronic form (lumbar spondylosis). These will be discussed separately because of significant differences in clinical presentation and management.

LUMBAR DISC HERNIATION

CLINICAL ASPECTS

Acute lumbar disc herniation usually occurs laterally, causing compression of nerve roots as they cross the disc space and leave the spinal canal. When root compression occurs, the cardinal symptom is pain radiating in a radicular distribution. Although back pain may often precede the development of sciatica, it is only rarely per se a symptom of disc herniation. In fact, the vast majority of patients with acute or chronic back pain alone do *not* have a demonstrable herniated disc.

Sciatica may also be accompanied by motor and sensory symptoms, such as weakness, paresthesias, or numbness.

There are substantial variations in the severity and duration of symptoms seen with acute herniated disc. Some individuals have severe, very disabling pain with accompanying neurologic signs and symptoms. Such acute attacks may subside or require early intervention. Other patients may have relapsing symptoms in which episodes of acute pain alternate with pain-free intervals. Still other patients may have constant pain, which is not severe and does not completely resolve.

Physical examination may reveal a variety of mechanical and neurologic findings. Inspection of the spine may disclose flattening of the normal lordotic curve, with a scoliosis toward or away from the affected side. There is often marked restriction of motion and local tenderness to percussion.

The most important sign of a herniated lumbar disc is an abnormal straight-leg raising test. Flexion of the hip with the leg extended will stretch the nerve root over the protruded disc, causing severe radiating leg pain. This test is positive in the vast majority of patients with ruptured discs, especially those with L4 and L5 protrusions. The rare herniated discs in the upper spine may cause pain on straight-leg extension rather than flexion. Finally, some patients with large disc herniations may have ipsilateral pain on raising the contralateral leg. This occurs because of contralateral movement of the root when the opposite leg is raised. The importance of the straight-leg raising test cannot be overemphasized. When positive, it is very suggestive of a ruptured disc and its absence should raise questions about the diagnosis.

Lumbar disc herniations most commonly occur at the L4 and L5 disc levels. It is important to realize that a ruptured disc at L4–5 usually compresses the L5 root, and one at L5–S1 usually compresses the S1 root (Fig. 2). The neurologic findings from S1 root compression include loss of ankle jerk, sensory loss on the lateral foot, and occasionally weakness of plantar flexion.

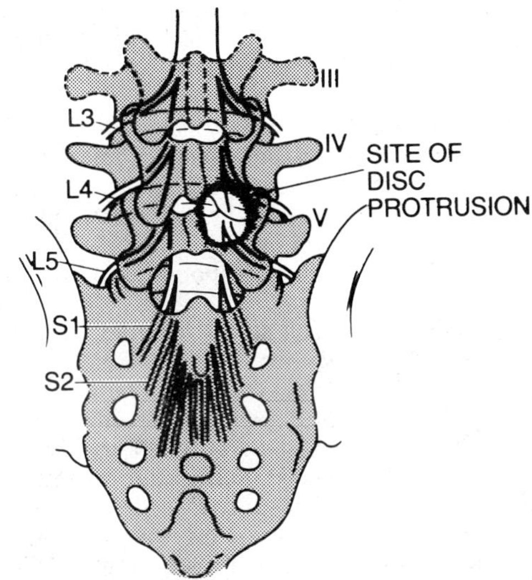

Figure 2. Diagram of the lower lumbar spine and nerve roots. A disc protrusion is shown at L4–5. Because of the relationship of the nerve root to the disc, an L4–5 disc herniation usually compresses the L5 root.

Weakness of toe or foot extension is seen with L5 root lesions. Sensory deficit is less characteristic but such patients may complain of pain radiating to the great toe.

Disc protrusions are relatively uncommon at L3, and rare at L2 or L1. Patients with upper lumbar lesions may have radiation of pain to the anterior leg, quadriceps weakness, or a reduced knee jerk. Rarely, patients with upper lumbar discs have back pain with little leg pain.

Midline disc protrusions are distinctly unusual. They may cause back pain alone, or unilateral symptoms, but they can also cause cauda equina compression with sphincter disturbance, bilateral leg pain, and motor and sensory abnormalities.

MANAGEMENT

Nonoperative Treatment

The treatment of herniated discs may be operative or nonoperative, depending on the duration and severity of symptoms, and the presence or absence of neurologic deficit.

Patients with the acute onset of severe sciatica should be treated with complete bed rest, with the patient either flat or in a semi-Fowler position. Appropriate narcotic or non-narcotic analgesics are used to control pain; muscle spasm, when present, may be controlled with diazepam (5 to 10 mg t.i.d.) or methocarbamol (1 gm q.i.d.). Nonsteroidal anti-inflammatory drugs may be useful in some individuals with moderately severe symptoms. The short-term use of oral corticosteroids has also been recommended, but I personally do not use them since they may obscure the normal recovery processes.

In general, patients with sciatica should be treated nonoperatively for seven to ten days before further steps are taken. Although some individuals advocate a longer period of conservative treatment, I believe that a patient who does not show some improvement in one to two weeks is unlikely to benefit from further bed rest.

Indications for Surgery

A patient with a cauda equina syndrome constitutes a surgical emergency, and should be treated aggressively from the outset. I also believe a patient with a complete or near-complete footdrop should be treated aggressively if he does not respond promptly to bed rest.

In general, diagnostic studies should be deferred pending a trial of bed rest. If the patient does not improve during the time indicated, neurodiagnostic studies should be the next step. A CT scan of the spine is a very accurate diagnostic test when positive. I also prefer to perform a myelogram in order to confirm the diagnosis and to help plan surgical tactics. Unless there is doubt about the diagnosis, a myelogram should not be done unless sugical treatment is contemplated.

The traditional treatment for patients who have not responded to nonoperative treatment is disc excision via laminectomy (so-called micro-discectomy is very similar to the traditional operation, and in my opinion has certain disadvantages over conventional surgery). In general, patients with herniated discs will respond well to laminectomy, which should have a high (80% to 90%) success rate and a low morbidity.

Chemonucleolysis. The introduction of chemonucleolysis (intradiscal injection of chymopapain) has led to controversy about the operative management of herniated discs. In general, chemonucleolysis has a somewhat lower success rate than open operation, although comparative statistics are difficult to obtain. The morbidity and mortality of the two procedures is similar.

The indications for surgery and chemonucleolysis are similar, and both should be reserved for patients with clear-cut, symptomatic herniated discs. Chemonucleolysis should not be used where there is doubt about the diagnosis, or where a complete myelographic block or cauda equina syndrome exists.

Preventive Measures

The management of patients with less severe forms of sciatica is somewhat different from those with acute, incapacitating pain. Some of these individuals will have chronic sciatica that is not completely incapacitating but never goes away. Such patients often benefit from a program of postural back exercises (swimming being an excellent alternative). In addition, simple measures such as a firm sleeping surface or a change in work habits may be helpful. Certain individuals may also obtain relief from the caudal epidural injections of local anesthetic and corticosteroids. If none of these measures is effective, further diagnostic tests and surgery may be required.

Another type of patient may present with acute attacks of pain that subside on bed rest but persistently recur. In these individuals, surgery may be required when the frequency of exacerbations becomes burdensome.

LUMBAR SPONDYLOSIS

As noted earlier, the end result of the degenerative process is spondylotic change in the lumbar spine. A number of changes occur, including disc protrusion, osteophyte formation, facet hypertrophy, thickening of the ligamentum flavum, and spondylotic spondylolisthesis. These processes may give rise to cauda equina or nerve root compression, particularly in patients with a narrow spinal canal. The end result is lumbar canal stenosis or its variant, the lateral recess syndrome.

LUMBAR CANAL STENOSIS

The cardinal symptom of lumbar canal stenosis is bilateral leg pain, produced by walking or standing, and relieved by sitting or lying down. This is called pseudoclaudication, and is distinguished from vascular claudication because it appears on standing as well as walking. The symptom is highly characteristic of lumbar canal stenosis, and indeed the diagnosis can almost be made from history alone. Some patients may also complain of postural paresthesias, and rare patients will have weakness in distal muscle groups. Sphincter disturbance is rare.

The condition should be distinguished from central disc protrusions, in which the pain is more constant and less postural. Tumors of the conus medullaris may produce bilateral pain, but this is also more constant and dysesthetic. Intradural, extramedullary spinal tumors cause pain that is more constant and may increase at night. Metastatic spinal tumors tend to cause more severe back pain and a more rapid course than lumbar canal stenosis.

When lumbar canal stenosis is suspected, plain spine films should be obtained to exclude obvious metastatic tumors or infection, and to determine if spondylolisthesis is present. CT scanning will document the degree of stenosis. I believe a myelogram should be done both to determine the extent of the stenosis and to exclude rare intraspinal tumors. When myelography is done, the study should extend to the conus medullaris (up to T10) in order to exclude lesions in this region.

Management. Except in rare individuals with very mild symptoms and poor general health, surgical decompression is the treatment of choice. Results of decompressive laminectomy are generally quite good.

LATERAL RECESS STENOSIS

Lateral recess stenosis is essentially unilateral lumbar canal stenosis. In this condition the nerve root is compressed by osteophytic changes as it traverses the lateral recess of the canal and enters the neural foramen. The patient complains of postural sciatica confined to one leg. Findings on physical examination may be minimal, and in particular the straight-leg raising test may be negative.

Plain films may be normal or show degenerative changes. Myelography (with water-soluble contrast agents) may show minimal evidence of root deviation or lack roof sleeve filling. CT scanning may be very helpful in demonstrating a narrow lateral recess.

Management. Hemi-laminectomy and foraminotomy is the treatment of choice; disc exploration should also be carried out, since a protruded disc may contribute to the patient's symptoms.

REFERENCES

Ciric I, Mikhael MA, Tarkington JA, et al: The lateral recess syndrome: a variant of spinal stenosis. J Neurosurg 53:433–443, 1980.

Ehni G: Extradural spinal cord and nerve root compression from benign lesions in the cervical area. *In* Youmans JR (ed): Neurological Surgery, Vol. 4. W.B. Saunders Co., Philadelphia, 1982, pp 2574–2612.

Hardy RW Jr (ed): Lumbar Disc Disease. Raven Press, New York, 1982.

Weinstein PR, Ehni G, Wilson CB: Lumbar Spondylosis. Yearbook Medical Publishers, Chicago, 1977.

Wilkinson M (ed): Cervical Spondylosis: Its Early Diagnosis and Treatment. W.B. Saunders Co., Philadelphia, 1971.

11 · REITER'S DISEASE

Andrea Dlesk
MARSHFIELD CLINIC

DEFINITION

Classic Reiter's disease or syndrome* is a triad of arthritis, conjunctivitis, and urethritis. In addition, patients frequently develop mucocutaneous lesions. The index case was described by Professor Hans Reiter. On August 21, 1916, Lieutentant N. developed abdominal pain and diarrhea lasting 48 hours. Seven days later urethritis and conjunctivitis developed. Eight days later he complained of polyarthralgias and polyarthritis involving knees, ankles, elbows, wrists, and interphalangeal joints. These persisted for three days. The patient did well for the next three weeks; then urethritis and uveitis recurred. Long-term follow-up of this patient is not available.

Several documented observations predate Reiter's description. In 1776 Stoll described urethritis, conjunctivitis, and arthritis following an episode of dysentery. In 1886 Sir Benjamin Brodie described the triad following venereal infection. And in 1916, the same year Reiter published his case report, Feisinger and LeRoy described their "conjunctivae-urethral-synovial" syndrome.

Reiter's disease is one of the so-called seronegative (i.e., rheumatoid factor–negative) spondyloarthropathies (SNSAs). These include idiopathic ankylosing spondylitis, the arthritis of inflammatory bowel disease, psoriatic arthritis, and "reactive arthritis" following various infectious diseases (discussed in Chapter 6). All of these share an association with HLA-B27 alloantigen.

DIAGNOSTIC CRITERIA

Diagnosis of Reiter's syndrome is difficult because it is a disease in time and space. The distinguishing urethritis, conjunctivitis, and arthritis do not necessarily occur simultaneously. Likewise, associated mucocutaneous lesions, i.e., keratoderma blennorrhagicum (psoriasiform hyperkeratotic lesions occurring primarily on palms and soles), circinate balanitis, iritis, conjunctivitis, and nail lesions (hyperkeratosis and onycholysis), do not always occur with other symptoms.

To deal with diagnostic difficulty, the American Rheumatism Association's Committee on Criteria for Reiter's Syndrome has developed a set of criteria for

---

*Since the cause is unknown, "syndrome" is felt by many to be a more accurate term than "disease."

definite disease. The committee found that an episode of peripheral arthritis of more than one month's duration occurring in association with urethritis and/or cervicitis was 84.3% sensitive and 98.2% specific for Reiter's during the initial episode. HLA-B27 was not included in this set of preliminary criteria.

ETIOLOGY

The cause of Reiter's syndrome is unknown. Two epidemics have been described. In the first, Paronen (1948) described 344 cases of Reiter's syndrome among 150,000 Finnish patients with *Shigella flexneri* dysentery. In the second, Noer (1966) described nine cases of Reiter's syndrome among 602 crew members with *Shigella* dysentery. Subsequently, Reiter's syndrome has been described following both enteric infection (*Salmonella*, *Yersinia*, and *Campylobacter*) and genitourinary infection (nongonococcal urethritis due to *Chlamydia* or *Ureaplasma*). Although these associations suggest an infectious cause, Reiter's syndrome can occur without antecedent enteric or genitourinary infection.

Genetics appear to play an important role in the development of Reiter's disease. Evidence for this is the fact that over 80% of Caucasian patients with Reiter's syndrome possess HLA-B27. The overall frequency of HLA-B27 in this population is only 6% to 8%. Among blacks, the association between HLA-B27 and Reiter's is less strong, although still significant. HLA-B27 is present in 40% to 60% of blacks with Reiter's syndrome and in less than 4% of the United States black population. It thus appears that given the appropriate genetic background, arthritis, conjunctivitis, and urethritis may occur de novo or following enteric or genitourinary infection with one of a number of microorganisms.

PATHOPHYSIOLOGY

The pathologic lesion responsible for many of the manifestations of Reiter's is an enthesopathy. Inflammation of entheses (the points of insertion of ligaments or tendons onto bone) is thought to be responsible for the arthritis, tendinitis, fasciitis, and spondylitis seen in Reiter's disease. Inflammation of entheses results in radiographic phenomena of peri-insertional osteopenia, new bone formation, and plantar spurs. The classic "sausage-shaped" digit seen in Reiter's is thought to result from inflammation of the synovium, entheses, and soft tissue around involved joints. In addition to entheses, patients with Reiter's develop inflammation of the anterior uveal tract and occasionally the heart muscle and/or cardiac conduction system.

CLINICAL ASPECTS

Reiter's patients tend to be young adult males—a highly mobile population that is easily lost to follow-up. The history of venereal infection may be suppressed. Many "silent" features exist: painless oral ulcerations may go unnoticed; cervicitis may easily be missed; urethritis in females may be dismissed as simply a bladder infection; circinate balanitis may go unnoticed; keratodermia blennorrhagicum may be mistaken for postular psoriasis; episodes of diarrhea may be forgotten. The patient may be misdiagnosed as seronegative rheumatoid arthritis or as one of the other seronegative spondyloarthropathies. Compounding all of the above is the lack of an absolute diagnostic test for Reiter's syndrome.

Reiter's disease occurs in an estimated 1% to 3% of patients following nongonococcal urethritis. Twenty per cent of HLA-B27–positive individuals will develop Reiter's syndrome following an episode of nonspecific urethritis. A similar incidence follows diarrheal illnesses that are due to *Salmonella*, *Shigella*, or *Yersinia* in B27-positive individuals.

Arthritis occurs in all patients with "complete Reiter's"* (urethritis, conjunctivitis, and arthritis). The arthritis is asymmetric and oligoarticular with large joints of the lower extremities most frequently affected. Acute, inflammatory monoarticular arthritis affecting primarily lower extremities occurs in 4% of patients. The spine is involved in 25% of patients, who usually complain of low back pain with predominant morning stiffness. The back pain typically improves with time and recurs following periods of immobility. With spinal involvement, physical examination reveals loss of lumbar lordosis and decreased range of motion.

Urethritis and/or cervicitis is the second most frequent clinical manifestation of Reiter's syndrome, occurring in close to 90% of patients. Eye disease including conjunctivitis, iritis, and iridocyclitis occurs in over half of Reiter's patients. Sixty per cent complain of heel pain. Fifty per cent have tendinitis, most often Achilles tendinitis. About half of affected males will develop balanitis. Skin and oral mucosa are involved in one quarter of patients; 15% complain of diarrhea.

Laboratory data in Reiter's syndrome are nonspecific and variable. The hallmark radiographic finding in Reiter's syndrome is sacroiliitis, initially manifested by subchondral sclerosis and finally fusion of sacroiliac joints. Juxta-articular osteopenia may be seen in actively inflamed joints. Periostitis involving the pelvis, metatarsals, tarsals, and phalangeal joints is common. Inflammatory spurs frequently occur at the insertion of the plantar fascia on the calcaneus. Spine disease is evidenced by the presence of asymmetric nonmarginal syndesmophytes, unlike the symmetric marginal syn-

---

*Patients with only one or two of the classic triad have been said to have "incomplete Reiter's."

desmophytosis that is seen in idiopathic ankylosing spondylitis.

MANAGEMENT

DRUG THERAPY

Nonsteroidal Anti-inflammatory Drugs. The arthritis of Reiter's is often difficult to treat. Nonsteroidal anti-inflammatory drugs (NSAIDs) are the mainstay of drug therapy. Patients with Reiter's syndrome seem to respond better to indomethacin (Indocin) or phenylbutazone (Butazolidin, Azolid) than to other NSAIDs. The reason for this is unknown.

Any of the NSAIDs may be used in the treatment of Reiter's syndrome. It is impossible to predict which will be most effective for a given patient. If the patient fails to respond to one class member of NSAID, he or she is less likely to respond to other members of that class. For this reason, I try to switch drug classes when therapy must be changed because of the patient's failure to respond. For example, if a patient has had an adequate therapeutic trial of ibuprofen (Motrin, Rufen, Advil), I prefer not to use other propionic acid derivatives next. Instead, I might pick meclofenamate (Meclomen), a fenamic acid. Patients are encouraged to continue NSAID therapy for at least two weeks before passing judgment on efficacy. The major classes of NSAIDs and representative doses are listed in Table 1.

NSAIDs share similar adverse side effects, largely due to inhibition of the enzyme cyclo-oxygenase with resultant prevention of prostaglandin synthesis. They include gastrointestinal disturbances, central nervous system toxicity, skin rashes, tinnitus, bone marrow suppression, edema, fluid retention, and hepatic dysfunction and renal toxicity. Of these, renal toxicity deserves special note. Its risk factors are age, extracellular volume depletion from any cause, congestive heart failure, sepsis, or concomitant use of any nephrotoxic drug. Patients with asthma, urticaria, nasal polyps, and aspirin sensitivity should avoid all NSAIDs because of potential hypersensitivity reactions. All NSAIDs interfere with platelet function to some extent, making them relatively contraindicated for patients on anticoagulant therapy. Also, NSAIDs may abrogate the antihypertensive effect of beta-blocking agents because of drug-induced salt and water retention.

Table 1. NONSTEROIDAL ANTI-INFLAMMATORY DRUG CLASSES AND DOSES FOR USE IN ADULTS WITH REITER'S

Class	Generic Name (Trade Name)	Dose	Schedule
Salicylates	Acetylsalicylic acid, aspirin (Bayer, Ecotrin, Ascriptin, many others)	325 mg	3–5 q.i.d.*
	Sodium Salicylate (Pabalate)	300 mg	3–5 q.i.d.
	Magnesium salicylate (Magan, Magsal)	500 mg	2–4 t.i.d.
	Choline magnesium trisalicylate (Trilisate)	500, 750 mg	2 b.i.d.
	Salicylsalicylic acid (Disalcid, Mono-gesic)	500, 750 mg	2 b.i.d.
	Diflunisal (Dolobid)	250, 500 mg	b.i.d.
Indoleacetic acids	Indomethacin (Indocin, Indocin SR)	25, 50, 75 mg	b.i.d.-q.i.d.
	Tolmetin (Tolectin)	200, 400 mg	t.i.d.
	Sulindac (Clinoril)	150, 200 mg	b.i.d.
Pyrazoles	Phenylbutazone (Butazolidin, Azolid)	100 mg	t.i.d.-q.i.d.
Propionic acids	Ibuprofen (Motrin, Rufen, Advil)	200, 400, 600 mg	b.i.d.-q.i.d.
	Fenoprofen (Nalfon)	200, 300, 600 mg	t.i.d.-q.i.d.
	Naproxen (Naprosyn)	250, 375, 500 mg	b.i.d.-t.i.d.
Fenamic acids	Meclofenamate (Meclomen)	50, 100 mg	t.i.d.
Oxicams	Piroxicam (Feldene)	10, 20 mg	q.d.

*Appropriate anti-inflammatory doses should be based on serum levels 10 to 14 days after initiation of therapy.

Because of potential toxicity, laboratory tests including complete blood counts, liver function tests (i.e., AST, ALT, LDH, and bilirubin), and renal function tests (i.e., creatinine) should be monitored at periodic intervals in all patients taking NSAIDs. Although specific guidelines do not exist, I recommend the following: In healthy young adults, repeat values four to six weeks after initiation of therapy and every six months to yearly thereafter. Among the elderly with underlying cardiac or renal disease, I would advise repeating tests of hepatic and renal function ten days to two weeks after starting therapy, again at six weeks, and every three to four months thereafter.

For initial NSAID therapy in Reiter's, I prefer indomethacin in doses of 25 mg t.i.d. to 50 mg q.i.d. depending upon patient weight. To improve patient compliance, one indomethacin slow release 75-mg tablet can be used twice daily. The most frequent adverse side effect of this drug is gastrointestinal (GI) disturbance. Three to 9% of patients will complain of nausea or dyspepsia. GI bleeding and peptic ulceration can occur. Active peptic ulcer disease is a contraindication to the use of indomethacin. Adverse GI side effects may be reduced by giving the medication after meals, with food, or with antacids.

For those patients in whom indomethacin fails to provide symptomatic relief, I usually try one of the other NSAIDs listed in Table 1. In general, I start with a relatively high dose for two weeks, then try to taper down according to the patient's symptoms. If other NSAIDs fail, phenylbutazone may be used in doses ranging from 100 mg t.i.d. to q.i.d. Long-term use of this drug is not advised because of potential marrow toxicity. I usually treat patients no longer than two to three weeks with this agent.

Antibiotic Therapy. Empiric use of antibiotic therapy in Reiter's is controversial. Most feel that antibiotics are not indicated. However, concomitant gonococcal disease, nonspecific urethritis, or enteric infection should be treated according to currently accepted protocol. Antibiotics are generally not recommended for the enteric pathogens associated wtih Reiter's unless there is another underlying chronic disease.

Corticosteroid Therapy. Systemic corticosteroid therapy is not indicated in the treatment of Reiter's syndrome. Local injection of corticosteroid preparations in one or two symptomatic joints is acceptable. I usually use triamcinolone hexacetonide (Aristospan) 20 mg/ml or betamethasone (Celestone Soluspan) 6 mg/ml mixed with 1% lidocaine (Xylocaine). For large joints such as the hip or knee, I use 1 ml of each. For smaller joints such as wrists or interphalangeal joints, I use 0.5 or 0.25 ml each, respectively. I do not like to inject joints more frequently than every two to three months to avoid potential weakening of periarticular supportive tissues or general immunosuppression of the patient. For refractory Achilles tendinitis, I occasionally use intralesional steroids. When using this treatment, patients should be advised of the potential for tendon rupture and/or immunosuppression following injection. Local tissue atrophy rarely occurs at the site of injection.

Cytotoxic Therapy. Patients with Reiter's syndrome occasionally develop an aggressive, deforming peripheral arthropathy with massive acro-osteolysis. These patients may be candidates for therapy with cytotoxic agents including methotrexate and azathioprine. Patients who require such aggressive therapy should be referred to a rheumatologist.

Conjunctivitis, urethritis, keratoderma blennorrhagicum, circinate balanitis, and mucosal ulcerations in general do not require specific therapy since they are usually self-limited. Inflammation of the anterior uveal tract (iritis, anterior uveitis) requires topical and occasionally systemic corticosteroid treatment following ophthalmology referral.

PHYSICAL THERAPY

In addition to NSAIDs, therapy for patients with Reiter's should include patient education and physical therapy. The same physical therapeutic modalities used for patients with idiopathic ankylosing spondylitis should be employed for Reiter's patients with spine involvement. Patients should be instructed in a home program of physical therapy including daily range-of-motion exercises. Principles of good posture should be emphasized. Patients should be discouraged from retiring to their reclining chairs. They should be advised to use a flat, firm mattress. The use of pillows, either under the head or under knees, is to be discouraged. This will help prevent deformities from occurring and/or progressing. Modified pushups should be done according to the physical therapist's instruction to maintain maximum chest expansion.

PATIENT EDUCATION

Unfortunately, Reiter's syndrome has been classified as one of the venereal diseases. Because of this, many patients feel guilty about this disease. Patients should be reassured that sexual promiscuity is not a sine qua non of their disease. They should be informed of the association of antecedent diarrheal illness, nonspecific urethritis, and genetically inherited HLA-B27 positivity with Reiter's syndrome.

Sexual promiscuity has been touted as a cause for exacerbation of Reiter's syndrome. This is not well documented in the literature and stating it as a fact is potentially harmful to patients. To allay such concerns, all patients should be given the American Rheumatism Association patient education pamphlet on Reiter's.

FOLLOW-UP

For patients with aggressive, active, highly inflammatory disease, I recommend follow-up visits every three to four weeks. This is done for three reasons: first, to change NSAID therapy if the patient is not responding to the present NSAID; second, to assess the need for cytotoxic therapy; and third, to assess the need for hospitalization for physical therapy, occupational therapy, patient education, rehabilitation psychology, and/or vocational rehabilitation. For patients with minimally active disease, I recommend a follow-up visit every six months to one year. This is done to assess interval disease activity, potential drug toxicity, and overall health maintenance.

PROGNOSIS

Reiter's syndrome was originally thought to be a self-limited disease. The illness was said to last six weeks, leaving patients symptom-free for the rest of their lives. Subsequent studies have disproved this. In an analysis of 131 patients with Reiter's, Fox et al. found 38% with some disease activity at a mean of 5.6 years. Thirty-four per cent had sustained disease, 16% had to change jobs, and 11% were unemployable. Thus, Reiter's syndrome may carry a significant risk of sustained morbidity.

REFERENCES

Calin A: Reiter's syndrome. *In* Calin A (ed): The Spondylarthropathies. Grune & Stratton, Orlando, FL, 1984, pp 119–150.

Calin A: Reiter's syndrome. *In* Kelley WM, Harris ED Jr, Ruddy S et al (eds): Textbook of Rheumatology. W.B. Saunders Co., Philadelphia, 1985, pp 1007–1031.

Fox R, Calin A, Guber RC, et al: The chronicity of symptoms and disability in Reiter's syndrome: an analysis of 131 consecutive patients. Ann Intern Med 91:190–193, 1979.

Fries JF: The reactive enthesopathies. Disease-a-Month 31:32–39, 1985.

Wilkens RF, Arnett FC, Bitter T, et al: Reiter's syndrome: Evaluation of preliminary criteria for definite disease. Bull Rheum Dis 32:31–34, 1982.

12 · GIANT CELL ARTERITIS AND POLYMYALGIA RHEUMATICA

Donald J. Dalessio
Gary W. Williams
SCRIPPS CLINIC AND RESEARCH FOUNDATION

DEFINITION AND DIAGNOSTIC CRITERIA

Giant cell arteritis (GCA) is an inflammatory disease of the branch arteries of the aortic arch. The cranial branches are most frequently involved. In addition, lesions may be seen in the major arteries of the upper and lower extremities. Patients are usually over the age of 50. The disease is also referred to as temporal arteritis, cranial arteritis, or granulomatous arteritis.

Polymyalgia rheumatica (PMR) does not have an official set of criteria for its diagnosis. It may represent a group of related disorders; however, it is generally recognized as a clinical syndrome characterized by the following:

1. Marked stiffness and pain in the muscles of the shoulder and pelvic girdles at night and especially in the morning. Improvement occurs throughout the day with activity.

2. Patients generally over age 50.

3. Absence of prominent symmetrical synovitis.

4. Negative latex fixation test for rheumatoid arthritis.

5. Elevation of the erythrocyte sedimentation rate (ESR) to >50 mm/hour (Westergren).

6. Prompt (usually within 48 hours) response to 15 mg/day of prednisone.

The cause of these two disease processes is unknown, and although they are often found together, their precise relationship is controversial. They may represent stages in a common inflammatory process, and the clinical picture may reflect certain host responses to an inciting agent.

PATHOPHYSIOLOGY

GIANT CELL ARTERITIS

In giant cell arteritis the involved arteries are grossly seen as tortuous, swollen, nodular vessels with or without pulsation, with cellulitis of contiguous tissue. Microscopic examination reveals a panarteritis. The typical section reveals hypertrophy of the intima, medial necrosis associated with formation of granulomatous tissue and the presence of foreign body giant cells, periarterial cellular infiltration, and thrombus formation. The presence of giant cells in the segment of artery removed may vary, and the reporting of giant cells is in part related to the diligence with which they are sought.

Senile changes in temporal arteries are not associated with giant cell reaction and should not be confused with the active phase of the disease. The residual changes of giant cell arteritis, which may persist for many years, are sufficiently different from the ordinary changes of senescence to enable one to distinguish between the senescent arteries and the arteries previously involved with the inflammatory reaction characteristic of the disease. Multiple cranial arteries as well as branches of the aorta other than cranial arteries may be involved, including branches to the extremities. We have recently observed two cases in which the patient presented with symptoms of upper extremity claudication as a primary manifestation of this disorder.

POLYMYALGIA RHEUMATICA

Pathologic changes are very limited in PMR and are generally not sought nor are they considered a part of the diagnostic work-up of such patients. As will be mentioned, there are mild degrees of hepatic inflammation that have been documented on biopsy. In addition, there is evidence of synovitis in many patients, which, although mild, may be associated with small effusions. In the group of patients we have studied, the WBC count in the synovial fluid is between 1000 and 2000 cells/mm³. Evidence of synovitis has also been documented by technetium scans. In spite of the prominent proximal muscle pain, muscle biopsies do not demonstrate inflammatory changes.

BIOPSY

Should the temporal artery be biopsied when a diagnosis of giant cell arteritis is suspected? In most cases, yes. In an emergency, for example, where vision is threatened, the biopsy can be done after corticosteroid therapy has been started. When consigning patients to long-term therapy with corticosteroids, however, we prefer to have a tissue diagnosis whenever possible. In patients with a diagnosis of polymyalgia rheumatica and in whom there is no clinical or historical evidence of GCA, we do not proceed to biopsy.

CLINICAL ASPECTS

The symptoms of the disease may be divided into the nonspecific complaints of a generalized systemic nature and specific complaints directly attributable to inflammation and distention of the temporal and other arteries.

Not all patients with giant cell arteritis have headache, but when present, the headache is of high intensity, of a deep aching quality, throbbing in nature, and persistent. In addition to the aching and throbbing there is often a burning component, unlike most other vascular headaches. The headache is slightly worse when the patient lies flat in bed and is diminished in intensity by the upright or half-upright position. It is somewhat reduced in intensity by digital pressure on the common carotid artery on the affected side and is made worse by stooping over. There is hyperalgesia of the scalp, and the distended arteries are extremely tender so that any pressure greatly increases the pain.

Some patients may suffer pain on mastication, and in some, it may be the initial symptom. Facial swelling and redness of the skin overlying the temporal arteries, with the addition of the burning component of pain, are usually noted after the onset of headache. Immediate relief from burning pain and headache may follow biopsy of the inflamed temporal artery, and it is assumed that this follows the interruption of the afferents for pain about the vessel.

Prior to the onset of the full-blown picture of giant cell arteritis, there is often pain in the teeth, ear, jaw, zygoma, nuchal region, and occiput. The distribution of these symptoms suggests primary involvement of other branches of the external carotid artery, notably the external and internal maxillary arteries.

Ocular Symptoms. The presenting complaint may be of ocular origin. It has become evident that more than one third of patients with cranial arteritis are threatened with partial or even complete loss of vision. Diplopia and photophobia have been noted; ophthalmoscopic evidence of occlusion of the central retinal artery has been apparent in some cases, and some cases with complete loss of vision have been reported.

Cerebral Symptoms. Some patients have presented signs suggestive of cerebral damage and encephalitis during the acute stage of the illness. Mental sluggishness, dizziness, vomiting, dysarthria, delirium, and even coma have been described.

Cases of giant cell arteritis with involvement of intracranial arteries may occur. In addition to the usual constitutional symptoms of weight loss, anorexia, low-grade fever, and headache, these patients also demonstrate lethargy, depression, and cranial nerve palsies. Major stroke may occur.

Other Symptoms. In every case there have been signs and symptoms that cannot be related plausibly to the sterile inflammation of the temporal arteries alone and that are more suggestive of systemic arteritis.

Prevalent symptoms and signs are weight loss, anorexia, general malaise, fever, sweating, and weakness. The weight loss may be profound and the patient emaciated. This is probably secondary to anorexia, which, while in certain cases is concomitant with the excruciating pain and headache, may antedate the onset of pain. Sweating is a common symptom.

Inconstant low-grade fever unassociated with shaking chills is recorded in 70% of the cases. The average temperature is 37.8° C, although recordings as high as 39.5° C have been made.

Table 1. PRESENTING SYMPTOMS IN 50 PATIENTS WITH GCA

Symptoms*	Patients (No.)	%
Headache	45	90
Jaw pain	20	40
Generalized aching, stiffness	19	38
Visual complaints	17	34
Cerebral symptoms	15	30
Tender, aching temporal arteries	12	24
Fatigue, malaise, insomnia	14	28
Neck and back pain	10	20

*Not mutually exclusive.

Other complaints of a nonspecific nature are weakness, lassitude, malaise and "grippy feelings," and fatigue (occasionally to the point of prostration) (Table 1).

MANAGEMENT

PLAN

Short-term and Long-term Goals. Giant cell arteritis can be considered a semiacute inflammatory disease that demands rapid treatment. On occasion, if vision is threatened, treatment should be considered a medical emergency. In the short term, the goal is to relieve the patient's complaints. Longer term goals are to suppress the disease sufficiently using the least amount of medication, presuming that the illness will eventually prove self-limited and will "burn out."

Indications for Hospitalization. Indications for hospitalization include rapid progression of complaints, especially if vision is threatened. Usually patients with giant cell arteritis are easily managed on an outpatient basis. The temporal artery biopsies are well suited to an outpatient surgical procedure. Long-term management will almost always be in the outpatient department.

NONPHARMACOLOGIC MEASURES

A graduated physical therapy program should be instituted for patients with polymyalgia rheumatica particularly emphasizing range of motion, exercise, heat, and hot packs. After the diagnosis has been made and corticosteroids begun, similar programs may be useful for patients with giant cell arteritis.

DRUG THERAPY

Selection of Drug. Corticosteroids should be used promptly in the therapy of giant cell arteritis and in PMR. They should be begun as soon as the diagnosis is made—if necessary, prior to a temporal artery biopsy. Corticosteroids control the progress of the arteritis, reduce symptoms, and prevent the development of ocular complications. Because blindness or defects in vision do not always correlate with the severity of the cranial arteritis, all patients should be treated promptly. In giant cell arteritis, treatment is usually initiated with 40 to 60 mg of prednisone daily. Thereafter, this dose may be rapidly tapered to a maintenance level, depending upon the relief of symptoms and the decline in the sedimentation rate toward normal. In PMR, prednisone may be started at a dose of 15 mg given as a single dose in the morning. The duration of therapy is uncertain. It may be necessary to continue corticosteroids for months or even years, although eventually it is possible to discontinue treatment in almost all patients.

Absence of response to prednisone within five to seven days is unusual and indicates a need for more comprehensive evaluation of the presenting complaints. In PMR the response is usually, but not invariably, within the first 24 to 72 hours.

Alternate-day corticosteroid therapy is not advisable in giant cell arteritis, at least initially, since systemic symptoms will not be controlled by the drug when used in this manner. It is advisable to use a single morning dose of prednisone to minimize the additional side effects associated with split-dose regimens, although the latter may be useful in the initial treatment program when the maximal effect of the drug is desired.

If treatment is stopped in less than two years, in about 20% of patients with GCA mild to moderate symptoms of PMR may become evident. Generally this does not constitute an indication to increase the prednisone levels unless there is significant elevation of the sedimentation rate. The sedimentation rate should be checked for several months after the cessation of therapy, and the physician should be aware of possible relapses at extended intervals. We have recently observed a relapse of the development of a vasculitic lesion in another patient previously treated for PMR for 18 months with, again, a two-year drug-free interval. These examples illustrate the continued risk of patients with this disease and point out the problems in considering the disease as "cured" in any individual patient.

In long-term treatment of PMR, it may be possible to manage the patient on a low maintenance steroid dose, in the range of 1 to 5 mg/day. If this is done, the clinician should be alert to the appearance of GCA despite the low-dose steroid therapy; involvement of the ophthalmic artery, producing blindness, is a particular concern in this situation.

It is known that other anti-inflammatory drugs, such as the nonsteroidals, are capable of lowering the sedimentation rate and relieving some of the constitutional symptoms of PMR. However, these agents do *not* protect patients from serious complictions, and we do not advocate their use in the initial management of PMR or GCA. They may have a role in the later therapy of patients when corticosteroids have been tapered to a low level and the patient experiences symptoms of a musculoskeletal nature associated with the steroid discontinuation. In all cases, the physician must be aware of the potential for relapse, and in this group of patients the use of the nonsteroidal anti-inflammatory agent may mask the sedimentation rate elevation accompanying a relapse of either GCA or PMR.

Finally, it is important to realize that in every series of patients there are those who in the process of tapering of corticosteroids eventually develop a polyarthritis and go on to classic rheumatoid arthritis. Such patients may or may not have positive latex fixation tests. We have observed several patients who have had biopsy-proven GCA go on to develop seropositive rheumatoid disease.

Complications of Treatment. The complications are those of treatment with corticosteroids. In a personal series of patients with GCA, about 40% developed a moonface-Cushingoid appearance; 15% had symptomatic vertebral compression fractures; and 10% had demonstrable proximal muscle weakness.

Some diabetic patients will note increased insulin requirements. The physician needs to be alert to rapid development of cataracts, exacerbation of peptic ulcers, avascular necrosis of bone, and reappearance of pulmonary infection, especially tuberculosis, which may occur in patients with GCA being treated with prednisone.

PATIENT INFORMATION AND EDUCATION

Patients should be advised regarding the proper use of corticosteroids as follows:

—Do not take more medication than prescribed.

—Missed dose: take as soon as remembered.

—Do not double dose.

—For oral dosage forms—take with food to minimize gastrointestinal irritation.

—Alcohol may enhance ulcerogenic effects of this medication.

Precautions and Concerns while Taking Corticosteroids

—Regular visits to physician to check progress during and following therapy

—Checking with physician before discontinuing medication; gradual dosage reduction may be necessary

—Possible need for sodium restriction and/or potassium supplementation during long-term therapy.

—Ophthalmologic examinations during long-term therapy

—Carrying medical identification card during long-term therapy

—Possible need to watch calories during long-term therapy

—Caution in receiving vaccinations, other immunizations, and skin tests

—Caution if any kind of surgery or emergency treatment is required

—Caution if serious infections or injuries occur

—Possible increased blood sugar levels (for diabetics)

—Risk of osteoporosis and the need for calcium supplementation (1000 to 1500 mg/day), and in women, consideration of estrogen therapy

—Possibility of blurring of vision during alterations in steroid dose due to changes in the water content of the lens

PERIODIC EVALUATION

Patients should be seen monthly with follow-up of the sedimentation rate at these visits. Patients should be checked for evidence of hypertension, excessive weight gain, cataract formation, and, if necessary, glucose intolerance. Evidence of proximal muscle weakness or developing synovitis should be sought.

PATIENT COMPLIANCE

Ordinarily patients with GCA and/or PMR will comply with the treatment regimen prescribed. Generally the response to corticosteroids in both conditions is brisk, rapid, and gratifying, enhancing the patient-physician relationship. Occasionally, the side effects of corticosteroids, especially those associated with weight gain and mental stimulation, may cause the patient to request a rapid reduction in dose or discontinuation. The use of antianxiety agents is helpful in the case of excessive mental stimulation; all patients should be cautioned regarding the potential for weight gain and the increase in appetite that they will experience. With such prior warning, weight gain can often be avoided: "Prednisone has no calories."

The patient needs to be carefully educated, however, regarding the chronic nature of the disease and the need for long-term and continuous reexamination, particularly while corticosteroids are being prescribed. During this phase, when corticosteroid side effects may be a problem, patient compliance may waver.

PREVENTIVE MEASURES

The cause of GCA/PMR is not understood; hence, risk factor modification and family counseling in this illness are of little value.

SOCIOECONOMIC ASPECTS OF MANAGEMENT

It is unusual for GCA/PMR to produce invalidism or prolonged disability. Referral to a chronic care facility based on this disease must be rare. The disease often appears in the elderly and may hasten early retirement in selected cases.

REFERENCES

Dalessio DJ: Cranial arteritis. *In* Dalessio DJ (ed): Wolff's Headache and Other Head Pain. Oxford University Press, New York, 1980, pp 220–232.

Hunder GG, Sheps SG, Allen GL, et al: Daily and alternate-day corticosteroid regimens in the treatment of giant-cell arteritis: comparison in a prospective study. Ann Intern Med 82:613–618, 1975.

Huston KA, Hunder GG, Lie JT, et al: Temporal arteritis: a 25 year epidemiologic, clinical and pathologic study. Ann Intern Med 88:162–167, 1978.

Liang GC, Simkin PA, Maunek M: Immunoglobulins in temporal arteritis: an immunofluorescent study. Ann Intern Med 81:19–24, 1974.

Nusinow SR, Federici AB, Zimmerman TS, et al: Increased von Willebrand factor antigen in the plasma of patients with vasculitis. Arthritis Rheum 27:1405–1410, 1984.

Wilkinson IM, Russell RW: Arteries of the head and neck in giant-cell arteritis. Arch Neurol 27:378–391, 1972.

13 · COMMON ORTHOPEDIC PROBLEMS IN INTERNAL MEDICINE

Wallace E. Lowry, Jr.
SCOTT AND WHITE CLINIC

This chapter discusses several common orthopedic problems resulting from trauma, which may be encountered by the "general internist," the family practitioner, and anyone working in the emergency room or weekend clinics.

The Contusion

DEFINITION

A contusion is an injury that does not break the skin, but does cause damage to the subcutaneous and/or muscle tissues. It occurs in association with all varieties of trauma.

CLINICAL ASPECTS

The presenting complaint is almost always pain in a specific place that corresponds to the area of trauma. Patients also may complain of localized numbness.

Physical exam may reveal localized ecchymosis, swelling, and tenderness to palpation. Most important, and critical to determining the prognosis, is examining the contiguous joints, and noting the neurologic and vascular status of the distal hand or foot. If there is nearly normal pain-free motion in the joints proximal and distal to the contusion, and if there is no deformity, then x-ray examination is not usually needed. Only when severe pain is present is an x-ray film really necessary. The vast majority of such contusions resolve uneventfully, and even if an occasional nondisplaced fracture is not diagnosed until a later time, nothing will have been lost relative to the ultimate outcome. What will have been avoided, however, are many unnecessary x-rays.

Neurologic and vascular status of the distal hand or foot must be critically examined. The absence of normal neurovascular function following a contusion may signal a true emergency. Vascular deficit usually requires immediate surgical repair. Neurologic deficits, while usually handled conservatively, signal a more severe injury and much more morbidity, and potential for disability. Either of these deficits should signal rapid referral to an orthopedic specialist.

If the joints are not involved, and these complications are not present, no real requirement for orthopedic referral exists, and these patients can be followed in the generalist's office as needed.

MANAGEMENT

The hallmark of treatment for the acute contusion is cooling the local area. This is best done by applying a simple ice pack. The cold will cause local vasoconstriction, which will decrease the blood supply of the area and thereby minimize the edema. Most individuals also perceive an analgesic effect from the cold therapy. Cold treatment is most effective during the first 48 hours post injury. Other points of treatment are elastic bandage wrapping of the local area, and strict instructions to the patient to maintain motion of the proximal and distal joints. These injuries can be quite painful, and a potent analgesic should be prescribed.

The Sprained Joint

DEFINITION

A sprain is a joint injury in which some ligamentous fibers are ruptured but there is no fracture or enough ligament damage to cause instability. Sprains occur with all varieties of trauma, but commonly involve much more morbidity because of the joint injury.

CLINICAL ASPECTS

In taking the history of the etiologic injury, it is most important to determine from what direction the trauma occurred. This can give one a valuable hint in trying to determine if any significant ligamentous injury has been sustained. Although ligamentous injuries may occur in the upper extremity joints, they are much more common in the knee and ankle.

Physical exam will show an obviously painful joint with swelling and possible discoloration. Particular efforts should be made to localize the area of maximum pain to one side, or one bony prominence of the joint. The direction of the traumatic agent provides the examining physician a clue to the location of fractures that might be present on the x-ray film. A critical exam of the involved joint under both medial and lateral stress (the orthopedic terms are varus and valgus) should be done and compared with the contralateral normal joint. If there appears to be instability of the injured joint compared with the normal one, confirmatory stress x-rays may be done. Sometimes this is not possible because the degree of pain causes involuntary splinting and muscle contraction. These involuntary reactions on the part of the patient may mask instability.

Even if the stress exam is normal, a significant joint injury should be x-rayed. Whereas a nondisplaced or minimally displaced fracture away from a joint is quite benign, similar intra-articular fractures have the potential for disaster. Every effort to make the definitive diagnosis should be made on the initial exam.

All these problems (intra-articular fracture, ligamentous instability, or inability to stress the joint due to pain) should be promptly referred for orthopedic specialty care.

MANAGEMENT

Appropriate initial care is to splint the injured joint with either a prefabricated commercial splint, a plaster splint, or a simple immobilization cast. In a lower extremity joint, the patient should be advised to either limit or eliminate weight-bearing, depending on the amount of pain. Aspiration of the hemarthrosis supposedly to relieve pain is mentioned only to be condemned. Although unusual, there is a danger that this can introduce infection into the joint and significantly increase the morbidity and long-term disability. If sufficient pain is present to seriously consider joint aspiration, an orthopedic specialist should be requested on an emergency basis. As with contusions, sprains are quite painful, and a potent analgesic should be prescribed. If prompt resolution of the joint sprain is not

clearly occurring within two to three weeks, these patients should also be referred.

Repetitive Stress Tenosynovitis

DEFINITION

When associated with repetitive stress, localized inflammatory symptoms occurring in specific synovial lined tendons and sheaths indicate "repetitive stress tenosynovitis." This syndrome is most common in the hands and wrists.

CLINICAL ASPECTS

The etiologic repetitive stress takes many forms. A poorly trained "weekend athlete" may vigorously take up racquetball. A housewife may become enthusiastic over her neglected flower beds and work long hours for several days planting bulbs and digging holes, or an assembly line worker may be required to perform a manual task several hundred times per day. A common denominator of all these is repetitive excursion of the tendons through their sheaths and surrounding tissues where this has not been the prior norm.

The tenosynovial swelling of the flexor tendons within the closed confines of the carpal tunnel actually causes diffuse pressure on the median nerve. Carpal tunnel syndrome may ensue with symptoms of pain, weakness, and/or numbness in the median nerve distribution. If the same pathophysiologic process occurs in the flexor tendon tenosynovium entering the tendon sheaths of the fingers, stenosing tenosynovitis (trigger finger) symptoms will occur. Tenosynovitis involving the extensor and abductor tendons of the thumb (DeQuervain's syndrome) is particularly common in industrial workers. Another common denominator is that some diminution of symptoms will occur with simply stopping the offending activity.

Physical exam frequently reveals only tenderness in the specific area involved. An exception is when the palpable triggering of stenosing tenosynovitis is present. X-ray examination usually is not indicated in patients with tenosynovitis. I attempt to limit x-ray evaluation to those cases where some acute trauma may be superimposed, where obvious coincidental degenerative joint disease is present, or in cases that have persisted two or three months in spite of treatment.

Few of these cases need surgical treatment and orthopedic referral can be restricted to those cases that either have some coincidental additional problem making the diagnosis difficult, or those that persist with symptoms for long periods of time.

MANAGEMENT

Treatment consists of resting the inflamed part, and careful use of nonsteroidal anti-inflammatory drugs (NSAID) such as indomethacin. To accomplish rest of the wrist, a splint is applied with instructions to the patient to remove it only for bathing. If it can be worn

22 to 23 hours per day, and if the patient will take the NSAID medication for two to three weeks, a high incidence of relief can be obtained. If needed, a depository steroid can be injected into the painful tendon sheath. In the industrial case where the repetitive stress results from the workman's job, counseling with him and his employer must be initiated by the physician about job reassignment. Without this, a high percentage of cases will quickly recur after the initial improvement with rest and NSAID medication.

Stress Fracture

Stress fractures occur in the bones of the lower extremity including the pelvis, femur, tibia, and most commonly in the metatarsals. Patients usually present with vague pain and are surprised to find they have a variety of fracture.

The history includes repetitive use of the legs for long periods of weight-bearing in situations to which the patient is not accustomed. A classic history is of spontaneous foot pain occurring in the military recruit after having to run unaccustomed distances. Fractures also occur in joggers, or various persons who walk or stand for long periods each day in their occupations. Frequently the patients are overweight.

Patients present with pain at the site of the fracture. The pain is much worse with weight-bearing and recedes with rest. If an x-ray film is made within the first few weeks of symptoms, it is usually normal. Sufficient diagnostic callus is commonly not present on a plain film for up to six weeks after the onset of symptoms. If a high degree of suspicion is present, an early diagnosis can be made with the use of a ^{99}technetium bone scan.

There is no real danger in these situations unless the stress fracture is where slight displacement might impair an adjacent joint. The unusual femoral neck fracture is just such a potential disaster and warrants prompt orthopedic referral. The common metatarsal stress fractures are quite benign and require only limitation of activity until the pain recedes. Ordinarily healing is progressing well when the diagnosis is entertained, and no other treatment than reassurance is indicated.

Extensor Tendinitis of the Elbow

The so-called tennis elbow syndrome is related to any chronic stress that involves repeated rotational stresses to the forearm. Participants in racket sports, dentists pulling teeth, and mechanics using screwdriver-type tools are only three of many groups that can develop this syndrome.

The basic pathophysiologic process is inflammation in the extensor muscle origins of the lateral humeral epicondyle. All gradations of inflammation from acute to chronic may be present. If acute, the prime symptom will be marked pain, localized to a point at or immediately distal to the lateral epicondyle. The pain will be worsened with wrist extension against resistance. In the chronic variety, symptoms will be more of aching and soreness. With these symptoms, the history can be expected to indict some specific physical activity that involves forearm rotational stresses.

X-ray evaluation may be deferred unless a specific injury has occurred or treatment has failed.

Orthopedic referral is not indicated for this problem unless there is a significant suiperimposed injury, or unless the syndrome does not respond to standard treatment after several months.

The hallmarks of treatment for this problem are NSAID medications, heat modalities, rest of the elbow and forearm, and depository steroid injections into the point of maximal tenderness when the inflammation is acute. Other secondary treatments sometimes used are electrical penetrating physical therapy modalities and circular forearm bands that restrict forearm muscle excursion. By using these varieties of conservative treatments persistently, I have found that only a small fraction of patients fail to improve significantly. Unfortunately, many of those not responding may have motives of secondary gain relative to their employment. Very few ever require surgery.

REFERENCES

American Society for Surgery of the Hand: Regional Review Course in Hand Surgery Syllabus, 1984, p 135.

Crenshaw AH: Campbell's Operative Orthopaedics, Vol. 1. C.V. Mosby Co, St. Louis, 1971, p 605.

Rockwood CA, Green DP: Fractures, Vol 2. J.B. Lippincott Co, Philadelphia, 1975, p 1483.

Salter RB: Textbook of Disorders and Injuries of the Musculoskeletal System. Williams & Wilkins Co, Baltimore, 1983, p 422.

Turek SL: Orthopaedics. J.B. Lippincott Co, Philadelphia, 1967, p 579.

PHYSICAL AND CHEMICAL INJURIES

ELEANOR T. HOBBS

1 · HEAT-RELATED ILLNESSES

Richard Y. McConnell
OCHSNER CLINIC AND
ALTON OCHSNER MEDICAL FOUNDATION

Normal body temperature is maintained through a number of compensatory mechanisms. Under conditions of high ambient temperature, high humidity, and low wind velocity, coupled with exercise and increased activity as blood goes from skeletal muscle to the hypothalamus, a reflex action is initiated with peripheral vasodilatation, sweating, and intense splanchnic vasoconstriction under control of the hypothalamus. If the individual cannot lose heat, the core temperature at rest rises 1.1°C per hour, and during moderate work the temperature rises at least 5°C per hour.

Who is at risk of heat illnesses? When are they at risk? What are the predisposing factors? What are the physiologic ways the body adapts to heat?

PREDISPOSING FACTORS

Predisposing factors are listed in Table 1 and include:

1. Ambient temperature—the higher the ambient temperature, the more heat the body gains.

2. Humidity—high levels of humidity interfere with the evaporation of sweat. At 75% or greater humidity, the ability to vaporize decreases significantly; at 90% or greater humidity, vaporization is negligible.

3. Wind velocity—at low wind velocity, the loss of heat through convection is minimal.

4. Inappropriate clothing—dark colors absorb heat from radiation. Heavy, impervious materials (e.g., plastic sweat suits) interfere with evaporation. Individuals should wear light-colored, lightweight, loose-fitting clothing.

5. Lack of acclimatization—the unacclimatized person who sweats to a maximum of 1500 ml per hour for one to two hours can theoretically dissipate 882 kcal per hour (590 cal/ml). However, evaporation may be only 80% efficient, since 20% of the sweat falls off the body and is unavailable. Therefore, a loss of 650 kcal per hour is more realistic.

PATHOPHYSIOLOGY

Ninety-seven per cent of heat loss occurs at the air/skin interphase. The necessary physiologic alterations include massive cutaneous vasodilatation, which lowers systemic vascular resistance. During rest, the skeletal muscle blood flow is 1 ml/100 gm/min, but during activity and heat dissipation it increases 20 to 40 times.

There is compensation for this shunting with intense increased splanchnic vascular resistance (hepatic blood flow decreases at least up to 50%) and increased cardiac output (up to 16 to 17 liters/min). Ultimately, the effective arterial volume decreases with increased heart rate and stroke volume (significant in unacclimatized individuals). Cutaneous vasodilatation may in-

Table 1. PREDISPOSING FACTORS TO HEAT-RELATED ILLNESSES

1. Ambient temperature
2. Humidity
3. Wind velocity
4. Inappropriate clothing
5. Lack of acclimatization
6. Physical conditioning—a well-conditioned individual is less likely to develop heat illness because he generates less endogenous heat with the same exercise or work
7. Obesity—the obese individual is usually less well conditioned and less well acclimatized
8. Age—extremes of age are more susceptible to heat illness; 80% of people who die from heat illness are over 55 years
9. Amount of exercise
10. Fluid and electrolyte status—individuals with decreased intake during exercise and work, dehydration, and hypokalemia are very prone to heat illness
11. Cardiovascular diseases
12. Acute febrile illnesses and acute infections
13. Previous heat stroke
14. Underlying diseases and debilitating illness, e.g., diabetes, thyrotoxicosis, Addison's disease, and alcoholism
15. Skin conditions that impair sweating—scleroderma, sweat gland necrosis (e.g., previous heat stroke), ectodermal dysplasia, miliaria, cystic fibrosis, burn damage with extensive scar tissue
16. Agitated states—overdose of sympathomimetics, hallucinogens, LSD, ethanol withdrawal, delirium tremens, barbiturate withdrawal, psychosis or psychotic-like behavior
17. Fatigue and loss of sleep
18. Drugs—barbiturates, atropine, antihistamines, anticholinergics, antiparkinsonian drugs, phenothiazines, salicylates
    a. Increased heat producers (LSD, PCP, thyroid, amphetamines, salicylates, cocaine, MAOs)
    b. Decreased blood volume (diuretics)
    c. Decreased thirst (haloperidol)
    d. Increased heat absorption (ethanol)
    e. Decreased sweating (antihistamines, anticholinergics, phenothiazine and beta-blockers, tricyclic antidepressants)

crease peripheral blood flow to 20% of total cardiac output. Occasionally, central venous pressure and stroke volume fall. During moderate work in severe heat, sweating and dehydration may decrease the plasma volume by 3% to 5%. Osmotically active intermediary products of glycolysis cause a net fluid shift into the cells. This may result in an additional 15% loss of plasma volume into the intercellular space and contribute to an acute mild hypernatremia and hyperosmolality. A loss of sodium and potassium in the sweat occurs, and urinary sodium increases secondary to increased aldosterone levels. Renal blood flow may decrease as much as 50% with a significant decrease in glomerular filtration rate. The increased metabolic rate produces more heat and a rise in core temperature.

SPECIFIC HEAT-RELATED DISORDERS

HEAT EDEMA

Heat edema is seen especially in the aged, and particularly in tropical and subtropical climates. It is believed to be caused by cutaneous vasodilatation and venostasis, which leads to vascular leak and accumulation of interstitial fluid in the hands and feet. Usually, there is no predisposing cardiac abnormality or other underlying illness. There is mild swelling in the hands and feet during the first few days of exposure to this new climate. Pitting edema, which rarely occurs, is thought to result from secondary aldosteronism that eventually subsides because of "escape" of the kidney.

Management

No specific treatment is necessary. Elevation may help, as will support stockings and cool compresses. Heat edema usually resolves spontaneously after several days; if not, it will certainly resolve when the individual leaves the hot environment. Diuretics are not recommended.

HEAT TETANY

Heat tetany occurs in normal individuals exposed to extremes of heat, who may be merely at rest. This results from respiratory alkalosis secondary to hyperventilation when they are exposed to short periods of intense heat stress. It manifests itself as carpopedal spasm with normal serum calcium levels.

Management

Treatment consists of reassurance and elimination of the heat stress.

PRICKLY HEAT (HEAT RASH, LICHEN TROPICUS, AND MILIARIA RUBRA)

This condition occurs more commonly in patients who are obese or who are wearing tight-fitting clothing. It usually occurs after two to three days of exposure to hot humid weather. A blockage of sweat pores occurs as a result of skin maceration and subsequent bacterial infection of the pores (staphylococcal). There is sweat duct rupture and the development of subcutaneous vesicles that rupture more deeply, producing a deeper obstruction. Clinically, there are glistening red vesicles on a red base limited to the areas covered by clothing (usually the arms and legs).

These areas are anhidrotic. The condition may progress to chronic dermatitis or anhidrotic heat exhaustion caused by sweat gland dysfunction.

Management

Treatment consists of chlorhexidine and the wearing of loose-fitting clothes. Patients should be advised not to expose themselves to heat until the vesicles resolve and normal sweating occurs. It may be necessary to treat with a penicillinase-resistant penicillin such as dicloxacillin, 250 to 500 mg four times a day for seven days.

ANHIDROTIC HEAT EXHAUSTION

This is a subacute disorder of temperature regulation secondary to sweat gland dysfunction. In over 80% of cases, this is preceded by prickly heat. Patients experience an inability to sweat owing to sweat gland ductal blockage; this usually occurs approximately three weeks after initial exposure to the hot humid environment. Patients demonstrate anhidrosis over the back, trunk, and limbs, usually with increased compensatory sweating over the face. They may complain of moderate fatigue with exertion and headache. Clinically, there may be tachycardia, temperature elevation, and potassium depletion. There is no nausea, vomiting, clinical dehydration, or muscle cramps.

Management

Treatment involves rest and avoidance of the hot humid environment until sweating occurs normally.

HEAT SYNCOPE

Heat syncope is a frequent occurrence. It is a rather benign disorder in the unacclimatized individual and is seen early during heat exposure. The condition is a result of increased sweating, loss of plasma volume, and cutaneous vasodilatation and may follow prolonged sitting or standing, or strenuous work. It may be related to venous pooling associated with prolonged standing. The patient experiences syncope but there is no nausea, vomiting, or cramps. Heat syncope is a diagnosis of exclusion.

Management

Treatment consists of rest and oral fluids for volume repletion. Patients should avoid prolonged sitting or standing in the hot environment.

HEAT CRAMPS

Heat cramps is an acute disorder of skeletal muscle characterized by brief, intermittent, paroxysmal, and excruciatingly painful cramps in skeletal muscles (usually the arms and legs) subjected to intense activity in the hot environment. The fingers are often affected initially. Heat cramps occur in healthy individuals who are well conditioned and acclimatized. The cramps develop after the activity during a latent period of one to two hours; the patient may be resting or taking a shower at the time. The cramps may occur in any muscle but tend to occur in those most heavily used. They rarely involve the abdominal wall. They may occur in athletes and heavy laborers who sweat profusely and replace their losses with a very hypotonic intake (usually water). The resulting hyponatremia in the muscle cell is believed to interfere with calcium-dependent relaxation processes.

Physical examination is unremarkable except for the muscle cramps. Patients are very uncomfortable and at times uncooperative. The serum sodium is rarely low but there is total body sodium depletion. Blood pressure and mental status are normal.

Management

Treatment includes rest in a cool place and replacement of fluid and electrolytes. Oral fluids such as diluted Gatorade or a solution prepared with ¼-teaspoon of table salt in 1 liter of water are suitable. Salt tablets are not recommended since they may produce gastrointestinal upset with nausea and vomiting. In severe cases, an intravenous solution of normal saline, 1000 ml over 1 to 1½ hours, may be better tolerated and more effective.

HEAT EXHAUSTION

Traditionally, there are two major types of heat exhaustion, but the clinical presentation is rarely exactly characteristic of one type or the other.

1. *Water Depletion Type (Hypertonic/Hypernatremic Dehydration).* These individuals cannot voluntarily replace their fluid losses. Examples include the debilitated, infirm, elderly individual in a hot nursing home or apartment; a baby left in a crib or a young child left in a poorly ventilated automobile parked in the summer sun; or a lost hiker or desert soldier unable to find water. The patient develops intense thirst, headache, vague malaise, fatigue, syncope, changes in mental status with anxiety, hyperventilation, and impaired judgment. This may progress to heat stroke. On physical examination, the patient demonstrates dehydration, mild hypotension with orthostatic blood pressure changes, mild to moderate hyperpyrexia, sweating, tachycardia, and increased respiratory rate. There usually is an elevated serum osmolality.

2. *Sodium Depletion Type.* This type of heat exhaustion may be seen early in the sports season in an athlete who is not well acclimatized or is in poor physical condition. This also may occur in a jogger, heavy laborer, soldier, or a member of a chain gang. There is massive sweating with fluid replacement. This condition may occur acutely or may develop over several days. Patients develop weakness, giddiness, lassitude, anorexia, nausea, vomiting, diarrhea, headache, fatigue, and muscle cramps. On physical examination, they do not appear to be dehydrated and they have a near-normal temperature. Very rarely, these patients may have developed water intoxication.

Management

Treatment for heat exhaustion should be individualized, based on examination and laboratory findings. Patients should rest in a cool environment with clothing removed. They should be fanned. Fluid and electrolytes should be replaced, preferably intravenously, because nausea is a common problem. Healthy young patients may require as much as 4 liters of 0.45 NaCl IV over six hours. The amount of fluid replacement should be based on clinical status, blood pressure, pulse, hematocrit, orthostatic BP changes, BUN, sodium, potassium, and serum osmolality. Be sure to watch for delayed rhabdomyolysis, particularly if there has been strenuous activity and exercise. Rhabdomyolysis produces muscle and soft tissue tenderness with swelling and myoglobinuria.

It may be very difficult to differentiate heat exhaustion from heat stroke. In the former, patients are often irritable and anxious with impaired judgment, but otherwise mental status is intact. Patients with heat exhaustion do not have seizures and coma. It is possible in heat exhaustion to have mild elevation of LDH, SGOT, SGPT, and CPK. Consider hospitalizing elderly symptomatic patients with predisposing factors to heat illness, or any individual whose symptoms do not clear completely within two to three hours of initiating treatment.

HEAT STROKE

Heat stroke is a total failure of normal thermoregulation in response to heat stress. Fortunately, heat stroke is very uncommon. It is a medical emergency because of the high mortality and morbidity associated with it. Mortality rates may be 20% to 60%. In patients who survive, there still may be a 50% to 70% residual disability depending on the underlying risk factors.

Heat stroke is characterized by exposure to heat, severely altered mental status, extreme hyperpyrexia (greater than 42°C), and (in approximately 50% of patients) anhidrosis. Traditionally, two types of heat stroke are described.

1. *Classic heat stroke* is seen mostly during prolonged heat waves and involves either the very young or the elderly. Elderly persons who have multiple medical problems or multiple drug therapies, who are socially or economically disadvantaged, who live in urban settings, and who are unable to care for themselves properly are most commonly involved. This type of heat stroke is very likely to present in the classic way with uniformly flushed skin and absence of sweating. Symptoms include malaise, weakness, anorexia, nausea, vomiting, muscle cramps, headache, confusion, and disorientation. Patients often present to the emergency department with fever, hypotension, and coma. The CNS manifestations are more severe than those associated with exertional-type heat stroke.

2. *Exertional-type heat stroke* usually occurs in previously healthy individuals such as athletes, military recruits, and construction workers. During strenuous activity, the patient's ability to rapidly dissipate body heat is overwhelmed by strenuous physical activity and heat production. This develops so acutely that the ability to sweat may still be maintained at the time of initial examination. The patient often presents to the emergency department after collapse or after manifesting bizarre behavior. Be aware that the core temperature may have already started dropping subsequent to treatment in the prehospital setting.

A typical case of exertional heat stroke is a healthy young athlete who starts with a subjective sense of physical deterioration and concentration lapse. The sweating rate may or may not decrease. Piloerection is common. Symptoms include chills, nausea, irritability, paresthesia of the hands and feet, ashen-gray coloring in the face, and an appearance of imminent collapse. This is followed by overt confusion, general collapse, and often seizures.

Electrolyte disturbances and rhabdomyolysis are common. In the second and third week of acclimatization and physical training, potassium depletion is significant secondary to increased aldosterone secretion. Hypokalemia impairs skeletal muscle perfusion, which results in increased anaerobic metabolism, lactic acid production, and failure to dissipate heat. This can be an important factor predisposing to exertional heat stroke and rhabdomyolysis.

Heat stroke affects all organ systems and may be insidious or sudden in onset. In heat stroke, hypoperfusion of vital organs, muscle breakdown, metabolic acidosis, and consumptive coagulopathy may occur. This leads to shock, brain damage, bleeding, acute renal failure, and cardiac arrhythmia.

Central Nervous System

The sine qua non of heat stroke is CNS dysfunction. The patient begins to lose the ability to function mentally at 38°C, with complete mental deterioration at 42° to 45° C (107° to 113° F). All the changes may be reversible; so it is very important to remember that resuscitation attempts should continue until a normal temperature is achieved. CNS dysfunction may include the entire spectrum of disturbance, including impaired consciousness, bizarre or psychotic behavior, hallucinations, confusion, seizures, coma, and focal neurologic deficits. The patient may have a positive Babinski sign, dystonia, muscle rigidity, nuchal rigidity, decorticate posturing, hemiplegia, flaccid muscles, incontinence, fixed and dilated pupils, and flat-line EEG. Ataxia and dysarthria are frequent and, when present, are often permanent. Seizures are very common. CNS pathology consists of neuronal necrosis, particularly in the cerebellum; diffuse petechial and gross hemorrhages; and cerebral edema.

Cardiovascular

Cardiovascular problems account for 80% of deaths in heat stroke. One of two states may be present.

1. A hyperdynamic state with increased cardiac output (up to 16 or 17 liters/min), increased heart rate, and decreased pulmonary and systemic vascular resistance, which correct with lowering of body core temperature.

2. A hypodynamic state with decreased cardiac output, increased heart rate, a variable increased pulmonary vascular resistance with pulmonary hypertension, and increased systemic vascular resistance. Myocardial and vascular necrosis may be present.

Arrhythmias occur most commonly during the cooling period and are a result of acidosis, hyper- or hypokalemia, hypoxia, and myocardial damage. A wide variety of EKG abnormalities may be seen.

Hepatic

Centrilobular hepatic degeneration and necrosis result from direct thermal injury (hepatothermolysis). Liver enzymes are frequently elevated with increased SGOT, SGPT, and bilirubin. An SGOT or SGPT greater than 1000 is a poor prognostic sign. The enzymes usually peak at 48 to 72 hours. Jaundice is rare and occurs at 48 hours. Alkaline phosphatase is normal.

There is decreased synthesis and thermal inactivation of clotting factors. A coagulation disorder appears in 60% of cases with abnormal prothrombin time (PT), partial thromboplastin time (PTT), and platelets. Liver damage is more common with exertional-type heat stroke. Disseminated intravascular coagulation (DIC) is rare and is a result of direct thermal trauma to the vascular endothelium with release of thromboplastic substances. DIC is more common with exertional-type heat stroke. Coagulopathy, therefore, is related to thrombocytopenia, hypoprothrombinemia, and hypofibrinogenemia.

Muscle damage may occur with rhabdomyolysis and myoglobinuria. In rhabdomyolysis, the muscle breakdown may result from direct thermal injury, mechanical trauma, muscular hyperactivity, or tissue ischemia. Severe hypokalemia contributes to decreased blood flow to the contracting skeletal muscle, resulting in ischemia. Rhabdomyolysis releases potassium from the damaged muscle cell, myoglobin, creatine, muscle enzymes (CPK, aldolase), and purines (metabolized to uric acid). Rhabdomyolysis produces muscle tenderness, swelling, stiffness, and CPK elevations. CPK is the best monitor of the severity of rhabdomyolysis.

Renal

Acute renal failure (acute tubular necrosis) occurs in 10% to 35% of patients with heat stroke, being more common with the exertional type. Hypovolemia leads to hypotension, renal ischemia, and increased aldosterone-renin-angiotensin activity. This, combined with direct thermal damage and blood viscosity, contributes to renal failure. Muscle damage with resultant rhabdomyolysis releases myoglobin. In the acid urine, myoglobin is converted to a very nephrotoxic compound, ferrihemate.

Gastrointestinal

Nausea and vomiting are universal. Diarrhea may be present. There is a risk of epistaxis and GI bleeding secondary to coagulopathy.

Chemistries

Potassium. Hypokalemia results in a decreased response to catecholamines; a decreased insulin release and decreased ability of skeletal muscle to synthesize glycogen; and muscle vasoconstriction leading to ischemia and rhabdomyolysis. *Hyperkalemia* results from muscle damage and renal failure.

Sodium. If hypernatremia is present, consider giving judicious amounts of free water.

Acid-base. Elevated lactate levels with lactic acidosis may be present with heat stroke. Normally, elevated lactate levels may be seen in marathon runners without heat stroke, but in classic heat stroke elevated levels correlate with a very poor prognosis.

Calcium. Hypocalcemia may be present secondary to soft tissue musculoskeletal damage and subsequent sequestration of calcium in the damaged muscle.

Management

Treatment must begin immediately!

1. It is absolutely necessary to protect the airway and maintain ventilation. Start supplemental oxygen at 4 to 6 liters/min. Consider intubation early for patients with seizures and coma. IV lines should be secured (peripheral and central), with consideration of a Swan-Ganz catheter and an arterial line if hypotension persists after cooling.

2. Administer IV fluids cautiously. Start with dextrose 5% in 0.45% NaCl. If hypotension persists after

initial fluid challenge and despite cooling, increased fluid administration with Ringer's lactate or normal saline is justified. Hypotension is usually due to high-output cardiac failure rather than severe dehydration.

3. Monitor the body core temperature continuously. This is best done with an electronic rectal thermister probe.

4. If alcoholism is a possible complicating risk factor, administer thiamine, 100 mg IV.

5. Patients with altered mental status should initially receive 50 ml of 50% dextrose IV (1 ml/kg in children).

6. Monitor the EKG continuously, because arrhythmias commonly occur during the cooling period.

7. Monitor urine output with a Foley catheter. Maintain urine output of 50 ml/hr in adults.

8. Carry out laboratory studies: complete blood count, electrolytes, urinalysis, BUN, creatinine, glucose, phosphorus, calcium, CPK (MM and MB fractions), SGOT, SGPT, LDH, bilirubin, alkaline phosphatase, PT, PTT, platelet count, fibrin degradation products, uric acid, lactate level.

9. Check arterial blood gases (corrected for temperature). If pH is less than 7.2, sodium bicarbonate should be administered (1 to 2 mEq/kg).

10. Administer antishivering drugs (remember that shivering will occur when the skin temperature drops to 28° C): diazepam (Valium), 5 to 10 mg IV push over several minutes; chlorpromazine (Thorazine), 25 to 50 mg IV push over several minutes. This is the second-line drug since, theoretically, chlorpromazine lowers the seizure threshold, is an alpha-blocker, and may worsen hypotension, and as a phenothiazine may impair heat dissipation.

11. If hypotension persists despite IV fluids and cooling, use vasopressors such as isoproterenol (Isuprel) (preferred), dopamine (beta doses), or dobutamine. Avoid norepinephrine (Levofed) because of severe peripheral vasoconstriction that will interfere with heat dissipation. Cardiac failure may be very difficult to manage owing to myocardial insufficiency and increased pulmonary vascular resistance, and may require invasive hemodynamic monitoring.

12. Consider calcium replacement—this is not necessary unless tetany, seizures, or arrhythmias are present with hypocalcemia.

13. Prevent pigment nephropathy if rhabdomyolysis and myoglobinuria are suspected. Add mannitol, 1 gm/kg and sodium bicarbonate, 100 mEq to 1 liter of 5% dextrose in water and give at 250 to 500 ml/hr. Furosemide (Lasix) may also be used to increase urinary output.

14. Administer steroids IV if cerebral edema is suspected.

15. Do not use dextran for fluid replacement, since it inhibits platelet aggregation.

16. To treat seizures (advance in sequence if they are uncontrolled), administer (a) diazepam (Valium), 5 to 10 mg IV push every five to ten minutes as necessary; (b) phenytoin (Dilantin), IV push 50 mg/min to a total of 18 mg/kg; (c) phenobarbital, 100 mg/min IV push to 20 mg/kg; or (d) general anesthesia with thiopental.

17. Give potassium: (a) hypokalemia, if present, is usually due to hyperventilation (respiratory alkalosis); if present in an acidotic state, administer IV potassium supplement with caution; (b) hyperkalemia may be present in exertional heat stroke as a result of rhabdomyolysis. Because of the high risk of renal failure secondary to rhabdomyolysis, dialysis is often required to control hyperkalemia.

18. Administer antipyretic agents (aspirin does not work and is contraindicated).

19. Do not use isopropyl alcohol for cooling because of possible percutaneous absorption.

20. Administer ranitidine (Zantac), 50 mg every 8 hours IV, to decrease the risk of GI bleeding.

21. Evaluate the coagulopathy present. Fresh whole blood, fresh-frozen plasma, platelets, and heparin may all be necessary.

22. *Rapid physical cooling is the mainstay of treatment.*

In the prehospital setting, the patient should be taken immediately to a cool environment and all clothing removed. Wet the skin and place ice in the more vascular areas such as the neck, axilla, lateral chest, inner thighs, and groin. Massage the muscles of the extremities to decrease vasoconstriction resulting from the skin-cooling process. The patient should be fanned.

At the hospital, one of several methods of more effective cooling must be used.

In the past, many hospitals used the ice bath method, in which the patient is totally immersed in ice water. The skin is rapidly cooled, but cutaneous vasoconstriction results and there is a significant decrease of heat conductance by a factor of 7 as the temperature of the skin approaches 28°C. Shivering occurs at this skin temperature, which subsequently raises heat production by as much as a factor of 7. Therefore, it is possible for a patient shivering in an ice bath not to be able to drop an elevated core temperature.

A variation of this method is not to immerse the patient in ice water but to cover him or her with wet towels covered with ice slush. Air currents in the room are stimulated with a fan, and the extremities are massaged in the hope of decreasing shivering and vasoconstriction. This method is common and more practical, particularly in view of other necessary interventions.

I prefer the evaporative method of cooling. The evaporation of 1 gm of water (1 ml) relieves 590 Cal (0.590 kcal) of heat. In contrast, melting of 1 gm of ice relieves only 8 Cal of heat. The evaporative cooling method consists of continually wetting the skin with warm water and generating a rapid air current of low relative humidity over the skin. The patient can be supported on a net, cot, or stretcher and should not be covered with towels or sheets. This method maximizes vaporization and minimizes patient discomfort, cutaneous vasoconstriction, and shivering. It also allows the medical personnel to examine the patient effectively and perform the necessary procedures and supportive care. It is estimated that this method relieves 31 kcal of heat per minute and provides a core temperature cooling rate of 0.31°C per minute, which is five times greater than passive cooling and three times greater than ice water baths.

Other methods have been used to lower core temperature. Unfortunately, there are no control studies available to evaluate these methods. I consider them less effective and less practical than the evaporative cooling method. These other methods include ice water gastric lavage, ice water enema and colonic lavage, peritoneal lavage with cold dialysate solution, extracorporeal bypass, cold IV infusion, and cold air inhalation.

The cooling process should be discontinued when the body core temperature reaches 39°C (102°F) in order to prevent hypothermia. The core temperature may continue to drop a few degrees, but beware of rebound elevation in 30 to 60 minutes or as late as three to six hours. The temperature will certainly remain labile with thermoregulatory instability for several weeks.

Poor Prognostic Signs

Coma lasting longer than ten hours is usually fatal. Coma lasting less than three to four hours has a good outcome.

In patients exhibiting temperatures greater than 42.2°C (108°F), the prognosis appears to be directly related to the degree and duration of hyperpyrexia.

Other poor diagnostic signs are severe hypotension, status epilepticus, SGOT and SGPT greater than 1000 units, coagulopathy, and conditions in which respiratory support is required.

PREVENTION

We have an obligation to teach patients how to prevent heat-related illnesses. To prevent exertional heat stroke, athletes in hot, humid weather should exercise in the early morning or late afternoon, and take a five-minute break at least every 30 minutes during training and competition. They should drink at least 500 ml of fluid 20 to 30 minutes before exercising. Replacement fluids should be cold (10° to 15°C) and hypotonic (less than 200 mOsm/L). During heavy exercise 6 to 10 oz should be taken every 15 minutes. Athletes and heavy workers need the proper physical conditioning, nutrition, hydration, rest, sleep, and training. Individuals should acclimatize slowly, spending at least five to seven days adjusting to the hot environment. Daily weights should be obtained during hot, humid weather and an individual who drops more than 3% of body weight in one day should not exercise actively until this is corrected. Proper clothing should include light-colored, loose-fitting, lightweight material.

Individuals at high risk of heat illness during heat waves should be advised to take precautions by providing air conditioning, fans, and hydration.

MEASUREMENT OF ENVIRONMENTAL HEAT STRESS

The ambient air temperature is only one of three aspects of environmental heat stress that should be accessed, the others being humidity, wind velocity, and radiant heat. The regular dry bulb thermometer that measures ambient temperatures is inadequate. The most useful method is the *wet bulb globe temperature (WBGT)*.

    WBGT = (0.7 Twb) + (0.2 Tg) + (0.1 Tdb)
    Twb =   temperature (wet bulb thermometer)
    Tg =   temperature (black globe thermometer)
    Tdb =   temperature (dry bulb thermometer)

This temperature index is very helpful in monitoring environmental conditions for athletes and those participating outdoors in hot, humid weather. An index of 60°F requires no particular precautions. A temperature reading of 70° to 75°F suggests postponement of sports practice; 80°F or above indicates that no sports participation should take place. Heavy work and vigorous exercise are very dangerous at a WBGT of 32°C (89.6°F).

REFERENCES

Bova CN: Heat Illness. *In* Greenberg MI, Roberts JR: Emergency Medicine: A Clinical Approach to Challenging Problems. F.A. Davis Co, Philadelphia, 1981, pp 197–217.
Callahan ML: Heat Illness. *In* Rosen P, Baker FJ, Braen GR, et al: Emergency Medicine, Concepts and Clinical Practice, Vol. 1. C.V. Mosby Co, St. Louis, 1983, pp 498–522.
Callahan ML: Hyperthermia. *In* Kravis TC, Warner CG (eds): Emergency Medicine, A Comprehensive Review. Aspen Systems Publication, Rockville, MD, 1983, pp 419–427.
Olson KB, Benowitz NL: Environmental and drug-induced hyperthermia. Emer Med Clin North Am 12:459–474, 1984.

2 · ILLNESSES CAUSED BY COLD

David J. Bechtel
LAHEY CLINIC MEDICAL CENTER

Hypothermia

DEFINITION

Hypothermia is defined as a core temperature below 35°C (95°F). Hypothermia occurs when production of heat by the body is unable to equal loss of heat. It may be a consequence of environmental stresses, or alterations in the body's normal mechanisms of thermal homeostasis, or a combination of both.

CLASSIFICATION AND PATHOPHYSIOLOGY

Patients presenting with hypothermia can be divided into three general groups: healthy patients with hypothermia secondary to exposure, healthy patients with hypothermia secondary to exposure in association with ingestion of drugs or alcohol, and patients with acute or chronic predisposing medical conditions. This grouping has major prognostic importance, which will be discussed later.

As the body cools, the metabolic activity of all organ systems decreases. Consumption of oxygen decreases 7% per degree centigrade, so that at 30°C (86°F), oxygen consumption is 50% of normal, and at 20°C (68°F) it is 10% of normal. Production of carbon dioxide is similarly decreased. This decreased metabolic activity is the physiologic basis for the observation that patients may be relatively protected from anoxic insult, which would cause major morbidity or mortality if it occurred at normal body temperature—the so-called metabolic icebox.

The body cools in three stages (Table 1).

Table 1. CLINICAL PRESENTATION OF HYPOTHERMIA*

Core Temperature (°C)	General	Percentage of Patients with			Neurologic Findings
		Blood Pressure <100 mm Hg†	*Heart Rate ≦60 beats/min†*	*Respiratory Rate ≦12 breaths/min†*	
37.6	Normal rectal temperature				
36	↑ Metabolic rate				
35	Maximum shivering; thermogenesis				Lethargic; confused; normal pupillary responses; normal reflexes likely
32	Temperature required for termination of cardiopulmonary resuscitation	18	20		Verbal response still likely; ↑ Muscle tone
	Fine tremor begins				Normal reflexes in 75% of patients
31	Atrial fibrillation in 50% of patients				
30	Basal metabolic rate in 50% of baseline	45		10	
	Shivering ceases				
	J wave in 80% of patients				
29					
28	Ventricular fibrillation increasingly possible		33		
27					
22	Maximum risk of ventricular fibrillation	56	72	50	Verbal response unlikely
20	Cardiac standstill; basal metabolic rate 10% of baseline				Purposeful response to noxious stimuli unlikely
18	Flat electroencephalography				
16	Lowest accidental hypothermia survival				↑ Muscle tone; sluggish or fixed pupils

*Adapted from Fischbeck KH, Simon RP: Ann Neurol 10:384–387, 1981.
†Percentage of patients at given temperature.
NOTE: Mild = 32° to 35°C.
       Moderate = 24° to 31.9°C.
       Severe = <24°C.

Stage 1—Mild. In the responsive or excitation stage, mild hypothermia is found: 32° to 35°C (89° to 95°F). In this stage the normal physiologic thermoregulatory responses are activated to maintain body temperature.

Stage 2—Moderate. In the slowing phase, moderate to severe hypothermia occurs: 24° to 31.9°C (75° to 89°F). Biochemical kinetics decrease, shivering ceases, and blood pressure, heart rate, and respiratory rate progressively fall.

Stage 3—Severe. The poikilothermic phase is characterized by severe hypothermia: less than 24°C (75°F). Below this temperature, heat loss occurs as if from an inanimate object. Indeed, the single differential diagnosis is death.

A broad spectrum of clinical findings and physiologic alterations in hypothermic patients exists. The mildly hypothermic patient may be only lethargic or confused, with essentially normal cardiorespiratory function. The deeply hypothermic patient may have puffy pale or cyanotic skin, be stiff with fixed pupils, have areflexia, and have imperceptible cardiorespiratory activity. These patients may appear to be dead. At a given body temperature, tremendous individual variations and findings may exist.

CLINICAL ASPECTS AND MANAGEMENT

In treating victims of hypothermia, the physician must be aware that patients who appear dead and without hope of resuscitation may recover to lead meaningful lives. Numerous cases have appeared in the medical literature and lay press reporting "miraculous" recoveries from circumstances seemingly as hopeless as 40 minutes of immersion in cold water, 3½ hours of cardiopulmonary resuscitation, and 70 minutes of asystolic arrest without cardiopulmonary resuscitation in severe hypothermia. Such patients may recover without long-term sequelae. Because of the protective effects of hyperthermia on critical organs, resuscitation should be attempted if any chance of recovery exists. The only irrefutable criterion for death is irreversibility after the body has been rewarmed—hence, "a patient is not dead until warm and dead."

ASSESSMENT

Hypothermia may be anticipated in the rescued mountaineer or the winter drowning victim but must also be looked for in a person who has experienced prolonged immersion or harsh environmental exposure of any season and also in confused or unconscious elderly persons. Specific information regarding the circumstances in which the patient was found, the duration of exposure, preexisting medical conditions, therapeutic ingestion of drugs or intoxication, changes in the level of consciousness, vital signs, and medical status during extrication and transport must be obtained. Although clinically inapparent at first, associated frostbite and trauma must be a consideration, and a cervical spinal injury must be ruled out in those with diving-related hypothermia.

Careful and gentle handling of the patient is important to avoid precipitation of ventricular fibrillation. Measures should be taken to prevent further heat loss or exposure, and frostbitten areas should be protected from trauma. Definitive efforts at rewarming should be carried out in the hospital with careful monitoring.

Except for mild hypothermia in an otherwise healthy individual, the diagnosis of hypothermia should convey a sense of critical medical need. Temperature must be taken with a thermometer that will record temperatures lower than 34.4°C. Deep (15 cm) rectal temperatures approximate core temperature and clinically are the most convenient to obtain. Monitoring of the esophageal and tympanic membranes may have some theoretical advantages, since these results closely indicate temperatures in the heart and brain stem, respectively.

VENTILATION AND RESUSCITATION

Oral or nasal intubation should be performed gently after preoxygenation with bag/mouth mask apparatus if protective airway reflexes are absent or respirations are depressed. Humidified oxygen warmed to 40° to 45°C should be administered by way of an endotracheal tube or by mask. The temptation to hyperventilate the patient should be resisted, as this may precipitate ventricular fibrillation.

When the patient is in cardiopulmonary arrest, compression of the chest and ventilation begin at one half the standard rate and are adjusted according to changes in the arterial blood gases. Efforts at resuscitation should not be terminted unless cardiac arrest persists despite rewarming the body to 32°C.

Volume depletion should be expected, and deficits of up to several liters may be present. The magnitude of the volume deficit may be unmasked as the patient's body is warmed and peripheral vasoconstriction is reversed. Uncorrected, the relative increasing volume deficit will perpetuate hypotension and poor tissue perfusion, leading to a condition known as rewarming shock. As a guideline, 1 L of 5% dextrose in normal saline solution is administered in the first hour of rewarming, with further replacement guided by monitoring of central venous pressure/Swan-Ganz data and blood pressure. For patients with hypothermia of moderate or severe degree, intravenous fluids should be warmed to 40° to 45°C. The 5% dextrose in normal saline solution is preferred over lactated Ringer's solution because lactate cannot be converted to bicarbonate by the hypothermic liver.

Inotropic agents are rarely indicated, as maximum peripheral vasoconstriction is usually present, and bradycardia and impaired myocardial contractility reverse with rewarming. Occasionally cardiac depression persists after rewarming, and the patient's condition will respond to administration of dopamine once adequate filling pressure is ensured.

MONITORING

Core temperature and cardiac rhythm should be monitored continuously. The urinary bladder should be catheterized and urine output measured carefully. Monitoring of central venous pressure or pulmonary artery pressure, or both, is helpful in guiding volume replacement. Nasogastric intubation is recommended because of decreased gastric motility and resulting distention.

LABORATORY STUDIES

Recommended studies include complete blood cell and platelet counts, glucose, electrolytes, hepatic and cardiac enzymes (serum glutamic-oxaloacetic transaminase, creatine phosphokinase), prothrombin time, partial thromboplastin time, blood urea nitrogen, creatinine, urinalysis, amylase, arterial blood gases, 12-lead electrocardiography, and stool guaiac. When occult sepsis is a consideration, blood cultures should be obtained.

A toxicology screen is ordered, and the level of ethanol is determined when the level of consciousness is inappropriate for the degree of hypothermia or when serum levels may have therapeutic consequences. Radiographs of the chest, cervical spine, and abdomen should be obtained as indicated. Tests to determine function of the thyroid gland and levels of cortisol may be performed if endocrine failure is suspected.

Tests for arterial blood gases and serum levels of potassium should be repeated at every few degrees centigrade of temperature increase. Rewarming reverses cold-induced vasoconstriction and permits reperfusion of peripheral tissues and "washout" of metabolic products, including large amounts of lactate from anaerobic metabolism and potassium from altered membrane permeability and rhabdomyolysis. Minor disturbances in electrolytes are usually corrected by rewarming, but severe hyperkalemia may require peritoneal dialysis or hemodialysis.

DRUG THERAPY

Drug therapy is relatively limited. Humidified oxygen warmed to 42° to 45°C should be administered by way of a face mask or endotracheal tube. Dextrose, 50 ml of a 50% solution, should be given to a patient with an altered mental state. Thiamine, 100 mg, should be given IV, especially in the alcoholic patient. Therapy with sodium bicarbonate should be restricted to in-hospital use and is guided by temperature-corrected determinations of arterial blood gases. Overcorrection of metabolic acidosis should be avoided.

ARRHYTHMIAS

Management of arrhythmias and conduction disturbances often requires the physician's forbearing restraint. Almost all arrhythmias, including asystole and ventricular fibrillation, revert spontaneously as the body is rewarmed. Although ventricular fibrillation is usually considered resistant to electric defibrillation when the temperature is below 25° to 30°C, a single attempt with 200 W/s should be made initially and repeated as the patient is rewarmed. The effects of antiarrhythmic agents are unpredictable at low temperature; at least one agent, procainamide, increases the incidence of ventricular fibrillation. Although bretylium tosylate (Bretylol) may be a useful antiarrhythmic medication for hypothermic animals, its use in the hypothermic human has not yet been established. If used, this drug should be administered IV as a 5 to 10 mg/kg bolus and repeated every 30 minutes to a total dose of 30 mg/kg.

INFECTION

The incidence of infection in severely hypothermic patients is as high as 40%. Rates of infection are high in elderly urban patients with underlying medical problems. Whether or not to begin antibiotics after cultures of blood, urine, and sputum have been obtained is a matter of clinical judgment based on the age and previous health of the patient.

HORMONE REPLACEMENT

Corticosteroid agents should be given only to treat patients with suspected adrenal insufficiency and before beginning thyroid replacement in patients with suspected hypothyroidism. When hypothyroidism is strongly suspected, thyroid replacement with triiodothyronine (Thyrolar), 50 to 100 µg IV every 12 hours until warm, is the therapy of choice, as it increases the thermogenesis within 24 hours compared with thyroxine, which takes between six and eight days to improve thermogenesis.

REWARMING

Considerable controversy surrounds the subject of rewarming. No controlled studies in humans are available that compare various rewarming techniques in moderately and severely hypothermic patients. However, treatment protocols have been derived from composite clinical experience. The choice of specific technique(s) depends on the degree of hypothermia and its acuteness, associated underlying diseases, and cardiovascular stability. Complications of rewarming include rewarming shock (mentioned previously) and core temperature afterdrop. Core temperature afterdrop occurs as warming induces vasodilatation of peripheral vascular beds, permitting the return of cool blood to the core compartment. This contributes to lowering the threshold for ventricular fibrillation. The three general methods of rewarming are passive external rewarming, active external rewarming, and active core rewarming.

Passive external rewarming consists of removing wet clothing, wrapping the patient in blankets, and placing him in a warm room with a temperature of 21°C or higher. This is the therapy of choice for patients with mild hypothermia (32°C) and cardiovascular stability, especially elderly persons whose onset of mild hypothermia was gradual. Rewarming rates vary from 0.5° to 2°C per hour, and this should be considered the minimum rate of adequate rewarming regardless of the method employed. To maintain an adequate rate of spontaneous rewarming, the patient must metabolically be capable of generating sufficient heat. If core temperature fails to rise by 0.55°C per hour, a more active method of rewarming should be instituted, as complications and mortality rates are related to the duration of hypothermia.

Active external rewarming is the application of heat to the external surface of the body by heating pads, water bottles, plumbed sarongs, or immersion in warm water. Initially, heat should be applied to the torso to rewarm the core structures before the periphery, thereby minimizing afterdrop and rewarming shock. The most effective method is to immerse a patient in a tub of water heated to 40° to 45°C, with the arms and legs outside the tub. The patient may be suspended by a sling to facilitate prompt removal from the tub, if necessary. When core temperature reaches 32°C, the patient is removed from the tub and is warmed passively. Active external rewarming is suitable for patients with hypothermia of moderate to severe degree (less than 32°C) and with cardiovascular stability, especially when they are otherwise healthy and acutely hypothermic from immersion. Rates of rewarming using the immersion technique are rapid and may be difficult to monitor. The patient must be watched closely for signs of clinical deterioration, which would dictate immediate removal from the water, stabilization, and use of an alternative method of rewarming.

Active core rewarming is the application of heat to any of the large internal body structures—the lung, peritoneum, blood (vessels), or stomach—thereby warming the core before the periphery. The method(s) used depend on medical urgency and availability. The simplest technique is to heat IV fluids to 45°C. Intubation and ventilation with humidified oxygen warmed to 46°C is an effective technique that can raise the core temperature up to 1.5°C per hour. Gastric lavage with warm fluid is less effective and may cause vomiting and aspiration.

Peritoneal dialysis has been shown to be a safe, effective, and readily available method of rewarming severely hypothermic patients. Two peritoneal catheters are placed, one in each lower quadrant of the abdomen. Isotonic dialysate is passed through a blood-warming coil and heated to 40° to 43°C before instillation. The fluid equilibrates in the peritoneum and then is either drained by gravity or suctioned through the second catheter. Flow rates of up to 10 L/hr are obtainable, raising body temperature by rates up to 10°C per hour. Dialysis should be discontinued as core temperature approaches 35°C. Previous abdominal operation is a relative contraindication to peritoneal dialysis, although passage of a catheter under direct visualization through a small incision is possible.

Peritoneal dialysis has many advantages. A rapid rate of core warming can be achieved regardless of cardiovascular status, abnormalities of electrolytes can be corrected, and toxic drugs can be removed. Furthermore, this method does not interfere with monitoring or cardiopulmonary resuscitation. Peritoneal dialysis is widely available and is not technically difficult to perform.

Mediastinal lavage, which has been advocated by some physicians, requires opening the chest and bathing the heart and mediastinum with a warm solution containing salt. Although this method warms the core first, less invasive techniques usually achieve the same result.

The most effective method of active core rewarming is through the *extracorporeal circulation* with either a hemodialysis unit or a heart-lung machine with inclusion of a heat exchanger. Hemodialysis requires the presence of adequate circulation, but with the use of the heart-lung machine, circulation can be maintained artificially. The rate of rewarming may approach 14°C per hour with these methods. Unfortunately, availability of these machines is limited, special skills are essential, the procedure is invasive, and full anticoagulation of the patient is required.

Recommendations for choosing an appropriate method of rewarming are summarized as follows.

For hypothermia of mild degree (greater than 32°C), passive rewarming is advised. When temperature rises at rates less than 0.55°C per hour, initiate active external rewarming or a simple method of active core rewarming.

For hypothermia of moderate to severe degree with cardiac stability, passive rewarming plus heated humidified oxygen and heated IV fluids should be tried. When the rate of rewarming is inadequate, consider active external rewarming with immersion of the torso or initiate an additional active core rewarming method, preferably peritoneal dialysis.

For hypothermia of moderate to severe degree with cardiovascular instability, rapid core rewarming with heated humidified oxygen, heated IV fluids, peritoneal dialysis, or extracorporeal circulation with hemodialysis or heart-lung machine and heat exchanger is suggested.

PROGNOSIS

The mortality rates range from 20% to 70%. The major determinant of survival is the presence of underlying disease. If appropriately managed, healthy patients have survival rates of greater than 80% even with severe hypothermia. Ingestion of drugs or alcohol does not usually affect survival adversely in an otherwise healthy individual unless the ingestion itself has created a serious problem. Both depth and duration of hypothermia influence survival. In drowning-related hypothermia, the water temperature is inversely related to survival rates: the colder the water, the better the prognosis.

Other Injuries Related to the Cold

Exposure to the cold may cause local injury to the extremities and body appendages that can result in loss of tissue and functional disability. Subfreezing temperatures are not required if the duration of exposure is prolonged, if extremities are wet, or if underlying vascular abnormalities are present. The two classes of injury are nonfreezing (chilblain and trench foot or immersion foot) and freezing (frostbite). The pathophysiologic common denominator is the intense vasoconstrictive response caused by cold.

Injury to civilians is almost always associated with inadequate protective clothing, fatigue, and unexpected injury, immersion, or immobilization. Alcohol is a predisposing factor in the majority of victims. Cigarette smoking increases risk because of nicotine-induced vasoconstriction. Because of differing vasomotor responses to cold, a racial predisposition to frostbite is apparent, blacks being six times more susceptible to frostbite than whites and Alaskan natives. The presence of atherosclerotic or vasospastic vascular disease increases susceptibility and the severity of injury to tissues. A previous episode of frostbite increases the vulnerability of that body part to recurrent cold injury. Acclimatization to cold weather increases resistance to cold injury by decreasing the vasospastic response and augmenting heat production.

CHILBLAIN

Chilblain is a type of nonfreezing injury that occurs with exposure to wet, windy weather that is sufficiently cool (less than 10°C) to cause the normal vasoconstrictive response. It is most commonly seen on the dorsa of the hands and feet, the cheeks, and the exposed legs of individuals, especially those predisposed to chilblain by such conditions as Raynaud's disease or collagen vascular disease. Chilblain is characterized by red to purple, warm, tender, and pruritic patches of the skin and edema. The affected area should be warmed in air, since immersion in warm water increases the itching and provides no additional benefit. The condition tends to recur with subsequent exposure to cold unless the part is protected with extreme care.

IMMERSION FOOT OR TRENCH FOOT

Immersion foot or trench foot results from prolonged (greater than 12 hours) exposure to cold and wetness at temperatures above freezing. Three stages have been described. During the vasospastic or ischemic phase, the foot is cold, swollen, and white or mottled with cyanotic patches. Pulses are decreased, and sensation is diminished or absent. The prolonged, intense vasoconstriction of this phase results in tissue hypoxia, cellular damage, and altered vascular permeability, which leads to formation of edema. After rewarming, a hyperemic stage, which may last from days to weeks, develops, with pain, bounding pulses (celer et altus), and warm, dry, hyperemic skin. During the recovery phase, the pulses return to normal but hypersensitivity to cold and pain on weight bearing may persist for years.

Treatment of patients with trench foot includes drying the foot, protecting it from further cold injury, and avoiding weight bearing. The foot should be rewarmed passively in a warm environment. Direct sources of heat, such as a stove or immersion in hot water, should be avoided, as these can cause additional thermal injury.

FROSTBITE

Frostbite occurs when tissue freezes. Two hypotheses have been suggested about the mechanism of injury to tissue in frostbite. One theory is that crystals of ice form within the cell, causing disruption of the cell. The other suggestion holds that crystallization occurs in the extracellular free water, leading to extracellular hypotonicity and cellular dehydration without rupture of the cell.

Before freezing occurs, cold-induced vasoconstriction results in decreased tissue perfusion and, together with cold-induced hyperviscosity, leads to intravascular sludging, thrombosis, increased vascular permeability, edema, and ischemia of tissues. As the tissues thaw, the severity of formation of edema, sludging, and thrombosis may increase. For this reason, heparin and dextran have been advocated in the treatment of patients with frostbite, although convincing clinical evidence to support their use in humans is unavailable.

Frostbite, like a burn, is classified by the degree of injury, which may not be apparent for days to weeks after presentation. First-degree frostbite causes erythema, swelling, and edema without formation of blisters. Edema occurs within three to four hours, peaks in 24 to 48 hours, and persists for one to two weeks. Second-degree frostbite results in erythema and edema, with formation of blisters and some loss of epidermal tissue. Third-degree frostbite refers to a full-thickness injury involving the dermis and subcutaneous tissues without loss of the body part. Blisters form along the margin of viable tissue. Fourth-degree frostbite results in complete necrosis (including bone) of the body part.

On initial presentation, it is helpful to use the clinical classification of frostnip, superficial frostbite, and deep frostbite. With frostnip, the skin is blanched and anesthetic. When the skin is rewarmed promptly, sensation returns, some erythema and edema are present, and no tissue is lost. In superficial frostbite, the skin appears waxy and white and is anesthetic, but remains soft and resilient when compressed. Thawing is painful and is followed by formation of blisters with subsequent slow healing. As a consequence of deep frostbite, the skin is hard, white, and noncompressible; after thawing, it remains cold and gray. Blisters form only along the line of demarcation between viable and nonviable tissue. Demarcation and sloughing of mummified tissue may take between two and three months.

MANAGEMENT

Rapid rewarming is the most important part of initial therapy, as it decreases the amount of tissue lost. The frozen part should be immersed in warm water (40° to 42°C, or 104° to 108°F) for 20 to 30 minutes. Thawing is usually accompanied by intense pain, often requiring narcotic analgesics. The thawed part should be handled carefully under sterile conditions, covered with dry sterile dressings, and restricted from use or weight bearing, or both. Blisters should be left intact. Administration of prophylactic antibiotics is not recommended, but prophylaxis with tetanus antitoxin is a requirement.

Subsequent management in the hospital includes debridement in a whirlpool bath and care of the wound. Surgical intervention should be deferred until unequivocal demarcation of nonviable tissue occurs; in some patients this may take as long as six to eight weeks.

Additional modalities that have been tried are anticoagulation with heparin, low-molecular-weight dextran (Rheomacrodex), reserpine, antiprostaglandin agents, thromboxane inhibitors, and sympathectomy. Although all have theoretical reasons to support their use, their clinical efficacy has not been proved.

When hypothermia and frostbite coexist, management of the hypothermia takes precedence, and thawing of a frozen part should be deferred until the circulatory status is stable and adequate core temperature is achieved. Late sequalae of frostbite include sensitivity to cold, paresthesias, pain, hyperhidrosis, and hyperkeratosis or ulceration.

PREVENTION

In many instances, cold injury can be prevented by proper planning and preparation for outdoor activities, choice of adequate clothing, and attention to basic safety. Ingestion of alcohol and drugs increases the risk of injury or exposure.

Attention should be directed not only to the management of the medical emergency but also to the underlyng social and behavioral problems that predispose to continuing susceptibility. The elderly, with their altered physiologic response to cold, are increasingly affected if limited resources require them to choose between food and a warm home. Medical education should be directed at increasing the awareness of this risk in the elderly, and social efforts should be made to provide adequate warmth and shelter.

REFERENCES

Danzl DF: Acidental hypothermia. *In* Rosen P, Baker FJ, Braen GR, et al (eds): Emergency Medicine: Concepts and Clinical Practice, Vol. 1. C.V. Mosby Co, St. Louis, 1983, pp 477–497.
Fischbeck KH, Simon RP: Neurological manifestations of accidental hypothermia. Ann Neurol 10:384–387, 1981.
Fitzgerald FT, Jessop C: Accidental hypothermia: a report of 22 cases and review of the literature. Adv Intern Med 27:128–150, 1982.
Gage AM, Gage AA: Frostbite. Compr Ther 7:25–30, 1981.
Miller JW, Danzl DF, Thomas DM: Urban accidental hypothermia: 135 cases. Ann Emerg Med 9:456–461, 1980.
Paton BC: Accidental hypothermia. Pharmacol Ther 22:331–377, 1983.
Reuler JB: Hypothermia: Pathophysiology, clinical settings and management. Ann Intern Med 89:519–527, 1978.
Shaw JF: Frostbite. *In* Rosen P (ed): Emergency Medicine: Concepts and Clinical Practice, Vol. 1. C.V. Mosby Co, St. Louis, 1983, pp 444–450.

3 · DISEASES DUE TO HYPOBARIC AND HYPERBARIC ENVIRONMENTS

Christopher J. Degnen
LAHEY CLINIC MEDICAL CENTER

A spectrum of medical problems can occur in individuals who have been subjected to either hypobaric (decreased ambient pressure) or hyperbaric (increased ambient pressure) environments. Exposure to a hypobaric environment, such as occurs in mountain climbing or flying in an unpressurized aircraft, causes one group of clinical syndromes; exposure to a hyperbaric environment, such as occurs in scuba diving, may cause different problems. Physicians need not reside in areas where these sports are popular to see the resulting medical problems. In view of air travel today, these conditions may present anywhere; in fact, air travel itself may be the final insult precipitating one of the problems.

Since recognition of the sometimes subtle clinical presentations is crucial to adequate treatment, diagnosis is emphasized. Treatment is relatively simple, but delay in its initiation may have disastrous consequences.

Altitude Sickness

DEFINITION AND DIAGNOSTIC CRITERIA

Ascent above 7000 feet is necessary before altitude illness develops. Four forms of this problem—acute mountain sickness, pulmonary edema, cerebral edema, and retinal hemorrhage—may occur singly or in combination.

Acute Mountain Sickness. Symptoms of acute mountain sickness include, in decreasing order of frequency, headache, insomnia, anorexia, nausea, and vomiting. A survey* of unacclimatized skiers visiting resorts at or

---

*Houston CS: Going Higher: The Story of Man and Altitude. Queen City Printers, Burlington, VT, 1983.

higher than 8000 feet revealed that about 25% of individuals experienced some symptoms of acute mountain sickness. The symptoms are usually self-limited and last 24 hours or less.

Pulmonary Edema. This usually occurs within 12 to 72 hours of rapid ascent to 9000 feet or higher. The initial symptoms are dyspnea and dry cough. When the climber continues to ascend, symptoms and signs progress to a wet productive cough (pink, frothy, or bloody sputum), rales, cyanosis, and progressive dyspnea. Results of chest radiography reveal the classic, fluffy perihilar infiltrates of pulmonary edema. When untreated, the edema may rapidly progress and lead to death.

Cerebral Edema. This is unusual at heights less than 12,000 feet. It causes confusion, ataxia, visual symptoms, dysarthria, hallucinations, coma, and ultimately death. It may be seen as a progression of acute mountain sickness, but onset may also be unheralded.

Retinal Hemorrhage. Involving the development of small, usually asymptomatic fundal flares, retinal hemorrhage rarely occurs at altitudes less than 17,000 feet. Most of these hemorrhages gradually resolve without sequelae even when the climber remains at altitude.

In addition to the four syndromes already described, a generalized edema detectable by a gain in weight or tightness of clothing may develop. Usually this edema produces only mild discomfort, but it can be a predictor of more serious problems if higher ascent is attempted. For some persons, prolonged stays at altitude can result in hemoconcentration and increased risk of development of thromboembolism. Subacute and chronic forms of mountain sickness are also apparent with prolonged headache, depression, and dyspnea occurring in persons residing at moderate elevations (8000 to 12,000 feet).

Of several factors predisposing to the development of altitude illness, speed of ascent appears to be the most important. Automobiles and tramways permit ascent within hours to heights such as the 13,796-foot Mauna Kea, Hawaii, and Pike's Peak, Colorado. For anyone planning more than a brief visit to such locations, a 24-hour acclimatization period at 9000 feet is recommended with a maximum ascent of 2000 feet per day.

PATHOPHYSIOLOGY

The barometric pressure at 9000 feet is about 540 mm Hg, in contrast to 760 mm Hg at sea level, and the partial pressure of oxygen in inspired air (PIO_2) is about 110 mm Hg, as opposed to 150 mm Hg at sea level. Without supplemental oxygen, mild hypoxia results. A mild tachypnea may compensate for this, often resulting in a mild hypocapnia. Alcohol and sedatives can inhibit this normal response, especially during sleep. Hypoxia causes pulmonary vasoconstriction with an initial increase in cardiac output. In susceptible individuals, a net increase in pulmonary vascular flow may result in pulmonary edema. Opposing effects are produced on cerebral blood flow; blood flow is decreased by hypocapnia and increased by hypoxia. This balance is tipped in favor of increased flow (and potential cerebral edema) by respiratory depression, which may occur during sleep, or worsening hypoxia, which occurs with continued ascent.

MANAGEMENT

The keystone of therapy for all forms of mountain sickness is to return the patient to a lower altitude as rapidly as possible. This alone usually causes symptoms to resolve totally or improve greatly.

Oxygen is the second mainstay of therapy and should be initiated before transport if possible. Furosemide (Lasix) is given for emergency treatment of pulmonary edema but rarely may result in hemoconcentration and complications secondary to increased viscosity. Morphine sulfate can also be administered, but only when ventilation is closely monitored and can be supported should the need arise. The further management of patients with high-altitude pulmonary edema and cerebral edema is the same at lower altitudes as the standard therapy for these problems.

Prophylaxis includes avoidance of the predisposing factors of rapid ascent, use of alcohol and sedatives, and a high level of physical activity at altitude for persons whose physical condition is not at optimal level. The occurrence and severity of acute mountain sickness are decreased by taking acetazolamide (Diamox), 250 mg three times daily, beginning one day before ascent and while at altitude. The mechanism of this is not completely understood, however. The thirst mechanism is suppressed at altitude, and the intake of fluids should be generous to promote adequate flow of urine. Women taking birth control pills should be cautioned that they are at an increased risk for the development of thromboembolism, especially with prolonged stays at altitude.

Barotrauma

MEDICAL PROBLEMS FROM SCUBA DIVING

When diving with pressurized gas, humans are exposed to a variety of potential hazards. Although patients are best treated by specialists trained in hyperbaric medicine, recognition of the symptoms and quick referral are critical steps for the general practitioner.

Air or artificial gaseous mixtures may be supplied to a diver by scuba equipment, pressure lines from the surface, or trapped air in an open chamber (e.g., in a submerged automobile). For each 33 feet of sea water a diver descends, the ambient pressure increases by 1 atmosphere (760 mm Hg). The two types of medical problems are those from barotrauma and those from decompression sickness (DCS).

PATHOPHYSIOLOGY AND CLINICAL ASPECTS

Barotrauma can occur as the result of gas expanding or contracting within a closed space. The air-containing body spaces—lungs, pleural cavity, sinuses, middle ear, and intestine—represent potential sites for problems to develop. Gases behave according to Boyle's law, which states that at a constant temperature, pressure times volume equals a constant ($PV = k$). Thus, a given volume of air at sea level (760 torr) occupies one half that space at 33 feet sea water, one third at 66 feet sea water, one fourth at 99 feet sea water, and so on.

Similarly, one unit volume at 33 feet sea water expands to two units at sea level, and one unit at 66 feet sea water expands to three units at sea level.

Barotrauma of descent is experienced to a certain degree by virtually all divers. Divers are taught to equilibrate pressure in the middle ear and sinuses on descent by performing a modified Valsalva maneuver against closed lips and nares. Inability to equilibrate may cause bleeding into the middle ear, rupture of the tympanic membrane, or bleeding in the sinus resulting from pressure gradients across these tissues. The symptoms of barotrauma of descent are referred to as "squeeze," and this term accurately describes what divers feel in their ears and sinuses when they are unable to equilibrate. The presence of an upper respiratory tract infection, allergies, or anatomic abnormalities may inhibit equilibration and temporarily or permanently preclude diving. Barotrauma of descent, although painful, is seldom life-threatening.

Conversely, barotrauma of ascent can be a serious or life-threatening event. Air inhaled under pressure at depth expands in the pulmonary cavities on ascent. When the volume of this expanding gas is restrained by holding the breath or by airway obstruction (e.g., by mucous plugs or bronchospasm), pulmonary barotrauma results. Alveolar rupture may occur into the pleural space, leading to pneumothorax; into the mediastinum, causing pneumomediastinum, subcutaneous emphysema, or both; or into the pulmonary veins, causing an arterial air embolism.

MANAGEMENT

Treatment of patients with hemorrhage in the middle ear, rupture of the tympanic membrane, or pain and bleeding in the sinuses from barotrauma includes administration of a systemic decongestant, such as pseudoephedrine hydrochloride, 30 to 60 mg every six hours; topically applied nasal decongestants; analgesics; and avoidance of diving until the symptoms have abated and the patient can easily equilibrate. Since the physical findings may mimic those of otitis media or sinusitis, antibiotics may also be prescribed. Patients with a ruptured tympanic membrane should be referred to an otolaryngologist for follow-up examination.

Arterial air embolism presents as a catastrophic event within seconds to minutes of surfacing from a dive. Presentation may include nausea, vomiting, confusion, central neurologic deficit (stroke), seizures, and coma. A diver with these symptoms or signs on or shortly after surfacing must be presumed to have an embolism and is placed in the Trendelenburg position with the head tilted downward 30° to prevent further air embolization. Pure oxygen is administered by face mask. Positive airway pressure should be avoided because it may cause additional gas to be forced into abnormal locations. Rapid transport to a recompression chamber for hyperbaric therapy is mandatory. (Call National Dive Alert Network [(919) 684–8111] for information.) In the treatment of pneumothorax, the usual indications for tube thoracostomy prevail. Persons with subcutaneous and mediastinal emphysema should be given 100% oxygen by face mask and supportive measures initiated.

Decompression Sickness (DCS)

PATHOPHYSIOLOGY AND CLINICAL ASPECTS

Whereas barotrauma represents the purely mechanical effects of contracting and expanding gas volumes, the increased solubility of nitrogen gas in body tissues under conditions of increased ambient pressure results in DCS, commonly known as the bends. The amount of nitrogen gas dissolved in body tissues during a dive is dependent on both duration and depth of the dive. During ascent, as ambient pressure decreases, the dissolved nitrogen gas comes out of solution and may form bubbles in various body tissues, leading to symptoms of DCS.

Divers are rigorously trained to adhere to the tables listing the maximal depth and duration of a dive or series of dives that can safely be made without the use of decompression stops. When these critical depth and duration levels are exceeded, divers are at risk for the development of DCS unless decompression stops are made during the return to the surface so that the nitrogen coming out of solution is released gradually. At depths of less than 30 feet, divers may spend unlimited time under water without danger of DCS developing. It should be emphasized, however, that fatal air embolism has occurred in as little as 7 feet of water.

Decompression sickness is divided into two categories based on clinical manifestations: type 1 DCS, often called "pain only bends," which includes symptoms referable to skin or joints; and type 2 DCS, which involves neurologic or respiratory systems, or both. Type 1 DCS commonly presents as pain in the joints, which in persons diving for sport most frequently affects the joints of the upper extremities, particularly the shoulder and elbow. Interestingly, caisson disease, the DCS seen in tunnel-construction workers, commonly affects the major joints in the lower extremity. Any recently injured joint, such as a sprained ankle or finger, may also be affected. The pain is described as steady and boring and is unaffected by movement or position. Results of physical examination and radiography of the joint are unrevealing.

Cutaneous DCS presents as pruritus or a burning sensation of the affected skin. The skin may be mottled or cyanotic, and blanches when pressure is applied. Edema or a peau d'orange texture may be present with lymphatic involvement.

The application of pressure to the area (e.g., with a blood pressure cuff) is a quick test to help establish DCS as the cause of pain in the joints. Relief of pain usually indicates that DCS was the cause. Complete relief of pain while the person is in a hyperbaric chamber is also diagnostic of DCS-caused pain in the joint. Cutaneous symptoms are usually self-limited but may augur more serious symptoms of DCS. Whether hyperbaric therapy should be instituted for decompression sickness affecting only the skin is controversial, and an expert in hyperbaric medicine should be consulted before making this decision. Persons with type 1 DCS involving one joint or multiple joints should be referred for treatment in a hyperbaric chamber. Hyperbaric therapy is diagnostic as well as therapeutic when the cause of the pain is in doubt.

Type 2 DCS can involve the lungs, central nervous system, or both. The pulmonary form, known as the chokes, presents with a substernal chest pain, cough, dyspnea, and other signs and symptoms of acutely increased pulmonary artery pressure. This type of sickness is thought to be caused by widespread obstruction of pulmonary blood flow by intravascular bubbles.

Decompression sickness involving the CNS most commonly affects the spinal cord. This seems to be a function of the anatomy of the epidural venous plexus where the normally slow blood flow is easily obstructed by formation of even minimal bubbles, resulting in venous stasis, edema, and further obstruction of flow. The white matter of the cord, especially the thoracic, upper lumbar, and lower cervical segments, is most commonly affected. An important early warning sign is unexplained back, abdominal, or girdle pain after a dive, which may precede the development of a neurologic deficit. Paresthesias of the leg, ataxia, and weakness are examples followed by urinary retention and paralysis.

A stroke syndrome may result when type 2 DCS involves the cerebral cortex, and it may be difficult to distinguish this form of DCS from pulmonary barotrauma with resultant air embolism. Knowledge of the depth and duration of the dive may help to distinguish the two causes because DCS is less likely to occur when standard dive tables are strictly followed. Additionally, cerebral air embolism usually produces an immediate maximal deficit when the diver surfaces whereas DCS often develops over minutes to hours. Fortunately, it is not critical for the practicing physician to determine the cause since both entities require expeditious referral of the patient to a hyperbaric facility for recompression therapy.

Air travel after diving can precipitate DCS even when the diver has adhered strictly to the standard dive tables. Commercial airline cabins are pressurized to the equivalent of 8000 feet, and such a decrease in ambient pressure from that of sea level enables more nitrogen to come out of solution and potentially cause bubble formation.

When any form of DCS is suspected, a complete dive profile, including duration and depth of all dives for the previous 72 hours, should be obtained. Symptoms and signs referred to earlier should be recorded, and a complete physical examination and neurologic evaluation carried out. When DCS is a possibility, consultation with a specialist should be obtained through the National Dive Alert Network.

MANAGEMENT

Immediate treatment of persons suspected of having type 2 DCS includes administration of 100% oxygen by face mask to speed the diffusion of inert nitrogen out of the body. When neurologic deficits are present, dexamethasone, 10 mg, should be administered intravenously. Hydration should be maintained by means of an isotonic solution. General supportive measures include cardiopulmonary and circulatory support as necessary.

Definitive therapy supervised by experienced personnel is accomplished by recompression in a hyperbaric chamber according to established schedules of treatment. Recompression by placing the patient under water is not recommended; it is fraught with hazard and precludes adequate medical supervision. The importance of recompression therapy cannot be overemphasized even when treatment or diagnosis has been long delayed or the hyperbaric chamber is many hours away. Hyperbaric therapy may result in improvement or resolution of neurologic deficits that have been present for many days or even a week.

Most medical problems related to diving could be prevented if persons who dive for sport had thorough knowledge of the physiology and hazards of diving and adhered strictly to the rules of safety. Physicians should not grant medical clearance for diving, which is required for certification, to persons with obstructive airway disease, seizure disorders, dangerous arrhythmias, unexplained syncopal episodes, or conditions impairing the ability to equilibrate pressures in the middle ear or sinuses.

REFERENCES

Bennett PB, Elliott DH (eds): The Physiology and Medicine of Diving and Compressed Air Work, 2nd ed. Williams & Wilkins Co., Baltimore, 1975.

Boettger ML: Scuba diving emergencies: pulmonary overpressure accidents and decompression sickness. Ann Emerg Med 12:563–567, 1983.

Heath D, Williams DR: Man at High Altitude: The Pathophysiology of Acclimatization and Adaptation. Churchill Livingstone, Edinburgh, 1977.

Sutton JR, Jones NL, Houston CS (eds): Hypoxia: Man at Altitude. Thieme-Stratton, New York, 1982.

4 · SNAKEBITES, SPIDER BITES, AND FIRE ANT STINGS

Charles N. Verheyden
Dennis J. Lynch
Raleigh R. White IV
SCOTT AND WHITE CLINIC

Snakebite

More than 100,000 people are bitten by poisonous snakes in the United States each year. Pit vipers from the family Viperidae (Crotalidae), including rattlesnakes, copperheads, and water moccasins, inflict most of these bites. The remainder are from the family Elapidae, which includes the coral snakes. Occasional bites are received from imported snakes.

The severity of an individual snakebite depends on the amount and site of envenomation and is influenced by several factors. *First,* the amount of venom present in the snake's venom sacs may be large or depleted by a previous strike. *Second*, the snake can inject venom through either or both fangs at will, using voluntary muscles. *Third*, the venom may be injected superficially into subcutaneous tissue or deeply into muscle or joint. The depth can vary with fang length (size of snake) or thickness of clothing worn at the time of the bite. *Fourth*, the components of the venom can vary greatly. Pit viper venom may contain as many as 20 different proteins. Those may vary within the same species and can even change in the same snake at different times. Coral snake venom is usually less complex. Identification of the snake is important since rattlesnake venom is usually more potent than that of other snakes endemic to the U.S.

CLINICAL ASPECTS

Snake venom can produce both local tissue damage and systemic reactions. Envenomation is graded according to the amount of local reaction, the number and extent of systemic symptoms and signs, and the presence or absence of laboratory abnormalities (Table 1). Systemic signs and symptoms include hypotension, nausea, vomiting, bradycardia, tachycardia, sweating, and weakness. Neurotoxic symptoms are more common in coral snake bites. Anemia and altered clotting studies are frequently observed. Pit viper venom usually produces an anticoagulation response when it affects the clotting mechanism, but infrequently it can be a coagulant. Components of a single venom can evoke both responses.

MANAGEMENT

Few areas in medicine are so controversial as the management of poisonous snakebite. Whether to perform surgery and if so, how much, or whether to administer antivenin are questions that stimulate vigorous debate. Some authors always, and others never, use each method. We advocate the balanced use of both modalities. The snakebite victim is treated initially like any patient who has sustained major trauma. Assessment of respiratory and circulatory status is followed by determination of the extent of envenomation, bite wound inspection, and, if possible, snake identification.

Medical

Intravenous fluids are started and electrocardiographic monitoring is established. Hemoglobin and hematocrit, prothrombin time (PT), plasma thromboplastin time (PTT), fibrinogen, fibrin split products, clotting time, and type and crossmatch are obtained as soon as possible. Snakebite wounds are tetanus-prone wounds and are treated with Td booster (0.5 ml). If the patient has not been previously immunized, tetanus immune globulin (TIG) is given according to the recommendations of the Committee on Trauma of the American College of Surgeons. Since bacteria can be carried to deep tissues, a broad-spectrum prophylactic antibiotic (cefazolin, 500 mg IV every eight hours in adults), is also given. Cultures are usually not helpful.

All victims of poisonous snakebite should be hospitalized, at least overnight, since the degree of envenomation may not be immediately apparent, depending on venom components and the type of first aid they may have received. Rattlesnake venom increases capillary permeability, resulting in loss of fluid volume, protein, and red cells into the interstitial space. Any hypotension, therefore, is managed with IV fluid replacement, and large volumes of Ringer's lactate may be required. Vasopressors should be used only secondarily.

Surgical

Examination of the bite wound includes a conservative excision of the fang marks, perhaps with a small extension of the incision, so that the underlying tissues can be evaluated. This small wound often permits egress of a large volume of edema fluid. More extensive surgical incision is employed if edema becomes severe, or if apparent necrosis of fat or muscle is extensive. If venom has been injected into a joint space, tendon sheath, or muscle compartment, this is opened and thoroughly irrigated. Fasciotomy through small skin incisions is frequently all that is required, and is done to relieve increasing pressure in fascial compartments. Debridement of hemorrhagic tissues should be extremely conservative at initial exploration. Skin wounds are left open at this time. Necrosis of skin and soft tissue and limitation of movement due to scarring and fibrosis have occasionally required digital amputations. Surgical treatment is directed at reducing or preventing long-term disability since the mortality rate is little affected. Death from snakebite is a rare event.

Antivenin

The use of antivenin is controversial but is indicated when moderate to severe envenomation causes systemic signs or symptoms. These include not only shock and clotting abnormalities, but also nausea, vomiting, paresthesias, fasciculations, weakness, sweating, chills, and edema extending beyond the local bite area. Antivenin (Wyeth) is available for both pit vipers (Crotalidae) and coral snakes (Elapidae). The directions for antivenin use are found on the package insert and should be followed precisely. A skin test is always applied before antivenin is used, but should not be done unless the decision has been made that antivenin is required in treatment. Three to five vials are usually given to initiate therapy, and subsequent amounts are given until symptoms or signs indicate improvement. The number of vials used often does not correlate with the size of the patient, since children may need more than adults. Antivenin is given in the intensive care unit, because adverse reactions to the drug itself are not uncommon, even if the skin test is negative. Serum sickness, caused by the horse serum antivenin, may also occur several weeks after treatment and can be bothersome.

Table 1. ENVENOMATION

Minimal
 Few systemic symptoms or signs
 Minimal abnormalities in laboratory values
Moderate
 Swelling beyond area of bite
 Some systemic symptoms and signs
 Abnormal laboratory values
Severe
 Marked local and systemic symptoms and signs
 Significant abnormalities in laboratory values

First Aid

First aid treatment of snakebite has been of great interest to campers, scouts, and other outdoorsmen for many years. The most effective treatment for snakebite victims is to get them to a hospital as quickly as possible. Incisions made by untrained persons have resulted in lacerated tendons, nerves, and arteries and have often been made unnecessarily. Cooling a bite wound may be of some theoretic benefit in reducing blood flow, but ice has led to instances of tissue necrosis in poorly vascularized limbs in older patients or to frostbite, even in younger patients. We do not advocate its use. Lymphatic tourniquets above and below the bite wound on an extremity are helpful until the patient reaches the hospital, but time should not be lost if they are not readily available. A bitten extremity should be immobilized to minimize systemic spread of venom.

Spider Bite

BLACK WIDOW SPIDER

Two species of spiders produce virtually all the clinically significant bites in the U.S. *Latrodectus mactans*, the black widow spider, is found in undisturbed woods or old buildings and is characterized by an orange-red, hourglass-shaped spot on the ventral surface of its black body.

CLINICAL ASPECTS

The black widow produces a neurotoxic venom that has its effect at synapses, leading to such symptoms and signs as pain, muscle rigidity, urinary retention, hyperactive reflexes, priapism, and nausea and vomiting. Mortality rates in the range of 5% have been reported.

MANAGEMENT

The bite of the black widow spider does not itself produce much pain and may go unnoticed until the onset of symptoms. Treatment consists of 10% calcium gluconate, 10 ml IV for pain, relief of which is diagnostic. *Latrodectus mactans* antivenin (Merck Sharp & Dohme) is then given IV. Usually one vial is all that is needed and may prevent some of the more serious problems if given early enough. The bite wound itself does not require any specific care other than cleansing of the area.

BROWN RECLUSE SPIDER

The brown recluse spider, *Loxosceles reclusa*, is also a reclusive creature, as its name implies. It can be found not only in basements, underneath rocks or bark, and in building cracks, but also in closets, old shoes, or pockets of clothing. A violin-shaped mark is found on the dorsal surface of the spider, leading to its nickname, "fiddle-back" spider.

CLINICAL ASPECTS

The venom contains enzymes that produce local tissue destruction. Systemic reactions are unusual, although more common in children. Deaths are rarely reported. Like that of the black widow, the bite of the brown recluse spider may not be noticed initially. A subsequent local stinging pruritus is the harbinger of a hemorrhagic blister, which causes considerable local pain. Ischemic changes are noted in the blistered area, with resultant necrosis and ulceration that are usually proportional to the amount of venom injected and the length of time since injection. These wounds often become chronic and relapsing, occasionally persisting for many months.

MANAGEMENT

Excision of the wound, usually after it delineates, and closure or skin grafting has been a standard form of treatment with satisfactory results. More recently, dapsone, a drug used in the treatment of leprosy and effective in skin diseases in which polymorphonuclear leukocytes play a role, has been used with invariable success (in brown recluse bites only, not black widow bites). Fifty to 100 mg PO is given twice daily for 14 days, often producing a dramatic response. A specific brown recluse antivenin has been produced, but is not commercially available and may not be as effective as dapsone if given more than 24 hours after the bite.

Fire Ant Stings

The fire ant, *Solenopsis invicta*, has become an increasing problem in the southern U.S. as it has continued to spread along the Gulf Coast. Its bites in large numbers have been known to kill dogs and newborn calves, and could theoretically produce the same result in small children. The ant bites and then stings, injecting an inoculum only one hundredth the volume of a honeybee sting. The bite is extremely painful and a local wheal rapidly forms. A small vesicle then develops and evolves into a sterile pustule. At this stage, secondary infection with a streptococcus is common, but may be prevented with proper cleansing and use of antibacterial cream or ointment. Systemic antibiotics are not usually required. The pustule soon crusts over and ultimately yields a punctate scar. Urticaria and angioedema occur in about 10% of patients, and antihistamines or epinephrine may be necessary. Once the initial episode has resolved, local wound care leads to rapid healing.

REFERENCES

Glass TG: Management of Poisonous Snakebite. Crumrine, San Antonio, 1976.

Hunt GR: Bites and stings of uncommon arthropods 1. Spiders. Postgrad Med 70:91–102, 1981.

Hunt GR: Bites and stings of uncommon arthropods 2. Reduviids, fire ants, puss caterpillars, and scorpions. Postgrad Med 70:107–114, 1981.

King LE Jr, Rees RS: Dapsone treatment of a brown recluse bite. JAMA 250:648, 1983.

Russell FE: Snake Venom Poisoning. J. B. Lippincott Co, Philadelphia, 1980.

5 · APPROACH TO THE POISONED PATIENT

Eleanor T. Hobbs
LAHEY CLINIC MEDICAL CENTER

Accidental or intentional poisoning is not usually seen by the internist in an outpatient setting. Most commonly, such patients are seen first in the emergency department where the diagnosis is made and therapy is instituted, and the emergency physician later consults the internist if inpatient therapy is needed. In many hospitals emergency physicians are the experts in toxicology, despite the fact that internists ultimately care for the most seriously poisoned patients. General internists should have a solid understanding of the correct approach to a poisoned patient and should know how to obtain detailed information about management of specific poisonings from reference books and a local poison control center. The *Physicians' Desk Reference* contains a listing of poison control centers in the United States.

DEFINITION AND DIAGNOSTIC CRITERIA

Most poisoned patients who require aggressive therapy present with acute toxic ingestion from a known substance. Others, however, may have more subtle multiple or nonspecific complaints owing to chronic toxic effects of prescribed or over-the-counter medications. A drug may have been improperly administered by the patient or family, or the consequences of altered metabolism or known side effects may have been cumulative. For example, salicylate poisoning may gradually develop in persons who chronically self-administer high doses of aspirin, and these patients present with life-threatening salicylism. The discussion that follows on the management of acute toxic ingestion also applies to patients with severe chronic poisoning.

CLINICAL ASPECTS

When a patient with a toxic ingestion is brought to a medical facility or a physician is notified by telephone of an ingestion, the first priorities are rapid evaluation and, if necessary, support of the cardiovascular and respiratory systems. Therapy must proceed concurrently with history-taking and a complete physical examination.

An accurate history coupled with the clinical presentation of the patient usually allows the physician to assess the potential severity of the ingestion, anticipate the clinical course, and take appropriate steps to prevent complications or treat them as they arise. With most oral ingestions the toxic symptoms, if they occur, begin within two to three hours after ingestion; large doses often show toxicity earlier. An ingestion is assumed to be potentially serious if the estimated dose is in the toxic range, if the patient presents with signs and symptoms of toxicity, or if the history is unobtainable

or cannot be verified. When in doubt, the physician should give treatment.

HISTORY

The history is of paramount importance but frequently difficult to obtain, and the physician may need to do detective work. Even if the patient is willing and able to give information, it may not be accurate, and attempts should always be made to verify the identity and amount of the drug ingested. Family and friends should be contacted; empty pill bottles should be examined; pharmacies should be called to obtain verification of dates and numbers of pills dispensed and information on any other recent prescriptions; and ambulance attendants or others who transported the patient should be questioned about the surroundings and condition of the patient when found. The important data regarding the ingestion are confirmation that an ingestion occurred, and determination of the substance or substances, route, dose, time, and subsequent clinical course. Any history of previous overdoses, psychiatric hospitalizations, suicide attempts, or recent losses or episodes of depression should also be obtained to aid in the psychiatric evaluation and in deciding the ultimate disposition of the patient.

PHYSICAL EXAMINATION

In examining a patient with an acute ingestion, the physician's attention should focus on vital signs, neurologic function, cardiopulmonary function, skin findings, abdominal findings, and excretory function. Vital signs, including temperature, must be obtained initially and followed at frequent intervals. Aspects of the neurologic examination that must be noted are level of consciousness, pupillary size and reactivity, extraocular movements (including presence of nystagmus), and presence or absence of gag reflex.

With the information obtained from this focused physical examination together with accumulated clinical experience or a reference guide (Table 1), the physician can frequently make a presumptive diagnosis as to the class of drug involved, even when no history is available.

LABORATORY EVALUATION

Patients with serious ingestions require laboratory testing, but those with minor ingestions usually do not. Between these extremes are a large number of cases that call for judgment by the physician. When in doubt as to the need for laboratory testing, the physician should request that samples of blood and urine be obtained early and held for subsequent analysis if the clinical course takes an unexpected turn.

Laboratory evaluation of the poisoned patient should include both routine and specific tests. In patients with a serious ingestion, routine tests include complete blood count, renal and hepatic function tests, urinalysis, possibly a coagulation profile, and measurements of serum electrolyte level, serum glucose level, and arterial blood gases. An electrocardiogram and chest radiograph should be obtained.

Specific tests are required to determine or confirm the presence and level of toxic substances in the blood, urine, or vomitus. Testing levels of particular substances is usually less expensive and more expeditious than

Table 1. SELECTED TOXIDROMES

Class of Drug	Vital Signs	Eye Findings	Central Nervous System	Skin	Other
Anticholinergics and atropinics (including tricyclic antidepressants)	Hyperthermia, tachycardia, hypertension	Mydriasis	Delirium/psychosis, seizures, coma	Dry, hot, flushed	Decreased bowel sounds, urinary retention
Barbiturates and sedative hypnotics	Hypothermia, hypotension, respiratory depression	Pupils variable, nystagmus	Lethargy, ataxia, stupor or coma	May have bullae	
Amphetamines and sympathomimetics (including cocaine)	Hyperthermia, tachycardia, hypertension	Mydriasis	Hyperactivity, tremors, delirium, hallucinations, psychosis or seizures	Diaphoretic	
Opiates and narcotics	Hypothermia, bradycardia, hypotension, respiratory depression	Pinpoint pupils	Euphoria to stupor and coma	May have needle marks	
Organophosphates and carbamates	Bradycardia or tachycardia, tachypnea	Miosis, lacrimation	Muscle fasciculations, weakness, confusion to lethargy and coma, seizures	Diaphoresis	Garlic odor, salivation, bronchorrhea, vomiting, stimulation of defecation and urination
Phenothiazines and haloperidol	Hypothermia or hyperthermia, tachycardia, postural hypotension	Miosis (most commonly)	Extrapyramidal reactions, lethargy to coma, seizures		
Phencyclidine	Hyperthermia, hypertension, tachycardia, respiratory depression	Nystagmus, pupils midposition or small	Decreased perception of pain, muscle rigidity, agitation, combativeness, ataxia, delusions, catatonia, euphoria, hyperreflexia, coma, seizures	Flushed, diaphoretic	Rhabdomyolysis with myoglobinuria, salivation, drooling, self-inflicted trauma
Salicylates	Hyperthermia, tachypnea, tachycardia		Tinnitus, vertigo, seizures, confusion, coma		Vomiting, GI bleeding

routine qualitative drug screens. Not only are such screens costly, but often four to six hours elapse before results are available, and for many patients the findings add nothing to the plan of management. A well-equipped laboratory in a hospital with a busy emergency department can usually provide immediate reports on a 24-hour basis for ethanol, salicylates, phenobarbital, phenytoin (Dilantin), theophylline, carboxyhemoglobin, iron and iron binding capacity, and acetaminophen. Levels of ethylene glycol and methanol are not as readily obtained but may be of critical importance in selected patients. When in doubt, specimens of blood, urine, and gastric contents should be obtained for a toxic screen. These can be refrigerated and held for about two hours rather than sent immediately to the laboratory, and if it later appears that the results of such tests may be helpful the specimens can be sent for processing. Situations in which a toxic screen may be advantageous include the presence of toxicity from a drug or toxin unknown, deviation of the clinical course from that expected for the alleged toxin, and the existence of medicolegal considerations.

MANAGEMENT

Treatment of the poisoned patient must proceed concurrently with history, physical examination, and laboratory tests. The four complementary components of therapy are resuscitation and stabilization, nonspecific therapy, specific therapy, and supportive care.

Resuscitative and stabilizing measures must be employed immediately in the patient with serious alterations in cardiorespiratory function. When the patient needs respiratory support or airway protection, nasotra-

cheal intubation is preferred to endotracheal intubation because a nasal airway in place facilitates passage of a large-bore orogastric tube for lavage. Hypotension in the setting of an overdose is most commonly due to vasodilation and venous pooling, and should initially be treated with a volume challenge of lactated Ringer's or normal saline solution, 300 ml over 30 minutes. Vasopressors should be used only when hypotension persists after adequate volume replacement. In unresponsive patients the initial treatment should include supplemental oxygen, glucose (50 ml of 50% solution), and naloxone (Narcan). Naloxone, a narcotic antagonist, is given intravenously, 0.4 to 0.8 mg every two to three minutes, until the patient awakens or an initial dose of 2 to 4 mg is reached; alternate parenteral routes are also effective. Large doses of naloxone, 2 to 5 mg, may be required to reverse the effects of some narcotics, such as propoxyphene. The duration of action of naloxone is one to four hours, considerably less than that of many narcotics. Thus, the patient must be observed continuously, and additional doses of naloxone given as necessary.

NONSPECIFIC THERAPY

Immediate resuscitative therapy should be followed by nonspecific measures to reduce absorption and enhance elimination. Although some toxins are absorbed through the skin or respiratory tract or received parenterally, most are ingested orally and absorbed in the stomach and small bowel.

Gastric Emptying. This is therefore critical. Although most drugs are well absorbed within two hours after ingestion, some medications that delay gastric emptying (anticholinergic agents) or form concretions in the stomach (salicylates, glutethimide, meprobamate) may show delayed absorption. The general rule should be to assume that absorption is not complete and to empty the stomach even when several hours have passed since ingestion.

Emesis. In the alert adult patient with an intact gag reflex, emesis may be induced by syrup of ipecac, 30 ml, followed by two to three cups of water. In 85% of patients emesis occurs within 20 minutes after a first dose of ipecac, and in another 10% of patients after a second dose. If emesis does not take place within 20 minutes after the second dose, gastric lavage should be initiated. Emesis should never be induced after ingestion of caustic substances nor after ingestion of substances containing highly volatile hydrocarbons, except in cases involving mixture with another highly toxic substance, in which the risk of aspiration of the hydrocarbon is less serious than the risk of toxicity from the other substance ingested.

Gastric Lavage. This is the method of choice for emptying the stomach in the obtunded patient or when syrup of ipecac has failed to produce emesis. When the patient has an intact gag reflex, gastric lavage can usually be performed rapidly and safely without endotracheal intubation. When the gag reflex is absent, endotracheal intubation (preferably nasotracheal) with a cuffed tube must precede lavage in order to avoid the danger of aspiration. A large-bore orogastric tube (36 F if available) is used to permit removal of fragments of pill. During lavage the patient should be positioned on the left side with the head slightly lower than the feet. The contents of the stomach should be removed as completely as possible before lavage is begun. Tap water or isotonic saline solution is instilled in 200- to 300-ml aliquots and allowed to drain. Lavage should continue until the effluent fluid is clear, which usually requires a volume of 3 to 4 L of water or solution. Gentle massage of the stomach during lavage may help to break up concretions of tablets that sometimes form.

Activated Charcoal. After emesis is induced or lavage is performed, a slurry of activated charcoal should be administered either orally or through an orogastric tube. Activated charcoal is an inert, fine, black, powdery material that almost irreversibly adsorbs drugs and chemicals in the gastrointestinal tract and prevents their absorption. The standard adult dose is 50 to 100 gm of charcoal mixed as a slurry with water or with a solution containing 30 gm of magnesium sulfate. When ipecac is used, 20 to 30 minutes must be allowed to elapse after the last emesis before the charcoal is given, otherwise the patient may vomit the slurry. Recently advocated is the use of "pulsed" charcoal with the dose repeated every few hours in an attempt to prevent reabsorption of drugs that have an enterohepatic circulation or are secreted into the stomach.

Cathartic Agents. The rationale for treatment of toxic ingestion with cathartic agents is that decreased intestinal transit time will result in less absorption of the toxin. Saline cathartics have not been proved of value but are nonetheless commonly accepted if bowel obstruction is not present and if diarrhea is not already occurring as a result of the ingestion. Magnesium sulfate or magnesium citrate, 250 mg/kg or a maximum of 30 gm, is given every one or two hours until charcoal is observed in the stool or until diarrhea occurs.

Enhancement of drug elimination once it has been absorbed is complicated. The method employed and the likelihood of success depend largely on the pharmacologic properties of the drug. Forced diuresis, dialysis, and hemoperfusion all present inherent risks to the patient and should be used only when a life-threatening ingestion has occurred and a major clinical benefit is anticipated.

Forced Diuresis. Forced diuresis by IV administration of fluids at a rate of 200 to 400 ml/hr in adults or 5 ml/kg/hr in children, with use of furosemide (Lasix) or mannitol, is indicated only in specific circumstances. Enhancement of renal excretion is difficult after ingestion of drugs that have a large volume of distribution (usually basic drugs that tend to enter fat) or are highly protein bound. Conversely, intoxication from agents with a small volume of distribution (usually acidic drugs) and little protein binding is more amenable to forced diuresis. The method is particularly effective in patients with intoxication from long-acting barbiturates, salicylates, and bromides. For some drugs the effectiveness of forced diuresis can be increased by "ion trapping," i.e., altering the pH level of the urine so that equilibrium favors the ionized form of the drug in the urine, inhibiting its reabsorption in the renal tubule. When the substance ingested is a weak acid, such as a salicylate agent, phenobarbital, or isoniazid, alkalinization of the urine to a pH level of 7.5 to 8.5 further enhances excretion during forced diuresis. This may be accomplished by initially adding 25 mEq of sodium bicarbonate and 75 mEq of sodium chloride to each liter of IV fluid of 5% dextrose in water, and thereafter adjusting the amount of added bicarbonate according to pH levels in urine and serum. The excretion of weak bases, such as amphetamines and phencyclidine, can be enhanced by acidification of the urine to a pH level of less than 5.5. This can be achieved by use of ascorbic acid in a dose of 1 gm PO every six hours or ammonium chloride in a dose of 4 gm PO every two hours, or by nasogastric tube in a 1% or 2% solution. Any type of forced diuresis requires careful monitoring of fluid balance, electrolyte level, and pH levels in serum and urine and is contraindicated in patients with congestive heart failure, renal failure, or shock.

Dialysis. Dialysis has a limited but important role in management of poisoning. Hemodialysis, which is far more effective than peritoneal dialysis, should be used when a drug with delayed high toxicity, such as methanol, ethylene glycol, or paraquat, has been ingested, and it is also effective for serious intoxication from lithium.

Hemodialysis should also be considered for life-threatening intoxications with dialyzable drugs (usually those with high water solubility and low protein binding) in the following situations: (1) when clinical deterioration has occurred despite intensive standard supportive therapy (specifically hypotension, thermoregulatory failure, or severe acid-base imbalance); or (2) when drug excretion is impaired because of liver, heart, or kidney failure. Standard dialysis is of no benefit in treating overdoses of highly lipid-soluble drugs, such as glutethimide, or highly protein-bound drugs, such as tricyclic antidepressants or phenothiazines.

Hemoperfusion. Hemoperfusion can greatly assist the removal of most drugs, including those not readily cleared by standard hemodialysis. Columns may contain various forms of adsorbent, coated carbon particles, such as acrylic hydrogel-coated granular carbon (Hemacol) or cellulose nitrate-coated granular carbon (Adsorba-300), or an Amberlite resin, such as Amberlite XAD-4 or Ambersorb XR-004. The Amberlite XAD-4 resin is particularly effective in removing highly lipid-soluble drugs, such as glutethimide. The clearance of tricyclic antidepressants, methaqualone, meprobamate, digoxin, parathion, and many other substances that have high toxicity can be enhanced considerably by hemoperfusion. Hemoperfusion across one of the commercially available columns can be performed with either an arteriovenous or a venovenous shunt, utilizing a blood pump. Efficient removal of the substance is facilitated by high flow rates of approximately 300 ml/min. Side effects of hemoperfusion include platelet depletion with an average reduction in platelet count of 30%, and mild hypocalcemia, hypoglycemia, and hypothermia, all of which can be managed clinically. When a hypotensive patient is receiving a vasopressor agent intravenously during hemoperfusion, the vasopressor should be administered distal to the hemoperfusion column, as it is readily adsorbed along with the offending toxin.

SPECIFIC THERAPY

Specific therapies are available for intoxication with particular drugs and toxins, and the effects are often dramatic and life-saving. Resuscitative and other nonspecific therapies must continue to be used concurrently with a specific therapy if it is available. Management of particular ingestions is not discussed in detail here, but Table 2 lists many of the important toxins for which a specific therapy is required. Further information should be sought for a toxicology reference source (see Table 1) or a local poison control center.

Immunotherapy. Immunotherapy using Fab fragments of antibodies directed against drug antigens, which bind the antigen and neutralize the drug's toxic effects, has been employed only for overdoses of di-

Table 2. SOME INTOXICANTS AND THEIR ANTIDOTES OR SPECIFIC THERAPIES

Poison	Antidote*
Acetaminophen	N-Acetylcysteine, initially 140 mg/kg PO in cola or grapefruit juice, then 70 mg/kg every 4 hr for 17 doses
Anticholinergics Anticholinesterases	Physostigmine, 2 mg IV for adults (for serious arrhythmias and seizures)
Organophosphates	Atropine, 1–4 mg IV (in children 0.05 mg/kg) every 10–15 min until atropinization is achieved, then pralidoxime, 1 gm IV (in children 25–50 mg/kg); may be repeated after 8 to 12 hr
Carbamates	Atropine, 1–4 mg IV (in children 0.05 mg/kg) every 10–15 min until atropinization is achieved
Bromides	Sodium or ammonium chloride, 6–12 gm/day PO with 4 L of fluid daily or forced diuresis IV with saline solution
Carbon monoxide	100% oxygen inhalation or administration of hyperbaric oxygen
Cyanide	Cyanide antidote package† Step 1: Inhalation of amyl nitrite for 15–20 sec/min alternating with oxygen Step 2: Sodium nitrate, 10 ml of 3% solution IV (in children 0.33 ml/kg) Step 3: Sodium thiosulfate, 50 ml of 25% solution IV (in children 1.65 ml/kg)
Fluoride and oxalate	Calcium gluconate, 10 ml of 10% solution IV, slow infusion, repeated as necessary
Heavy metals	
Arsenic	Dimercaprol, 3–5 mg/kg deep IM every 4 hr for 2 days, then every 6–12 hr for 2 days, then every 12–24 hr for 10 days
Copper	Dimercaprol as for arsenic or penicillamine, 25–50 mg/kg/day (maximal dose, 4 gm/day) PO in 4 divided doses for up to 5 days
Gold	Dimercaprol as for arsenic
Lead	Edetate, 50 to 75 mg/kg/day (maximal dose, 1 gm/day) in 3–6 divided doses either deep IM or slow IV infusion for up to 5 days; dimercaprol as for arsenic; penicillamine as for copper
Mercury	Dimercaprol as for arsenic, penicillamine as for copper
Iodine	3%–10% starch solution PO or lavage, or both
Iron	Deferoxamine, 90 mg/kg IM every 8 hr for 3 doses (maximal dose, 6 gm/day) or 1 gm IV every 4–6 hr at a rate not to exceed 15 mg/kg/hr
Isoniazid	Pyridoxine (vitamin B_6), 1 mg/gm isoniazid ingested, in divided doses given by slow IV push (5 mg/50 ml each bolus), can be repeated every 5–15 min until clinical improvement occurs
Methanol, ethylene glycol	Ethanol, 0.6 gm/kg initial IV loading dose, followed by infusion of 60–150 mg/kg/hr titrated to maintain a level of 100 mg/dl
Methemoglobinemia-producing agents	Methylene blue, 0.2 ml of 1% solution (2 mg/kg), slow IV infusion for 5 min; may be repeated once after 1 hr
Narcotics	Naloxone, 0.4–5.0 mg by IV push, repeated as necessary
Phenothiazines (dystonic reactions only)	Diphenhydramine, 0.5–1.0 mg/kg IM or IV, or benztropine 2 mg IM or IV
Warfarin	Vitamin K, 0.5–1.0 mg/kg IM or IV

*Generic and trade names of drugs: N-acetylcysteine (Mucomyst); physostigmine (Antilirium); pralidoxime (Protopam chloride); dimercaprol (BAL); deferoxamine (Desferal mesylate); isoniazid (INH); naloxone (Narcan); benztropine (Cogentin); warfarin (Coumadin).
†Eli Lilly and Co, Indianapolis, IN.

goxin, for which it has been successful. In the future, immunotherapy will play a larger role in treating overdoses.

Because specific therapy is available for only a limited number of toxins, supportive care is the mainstay of treatment for overdose in most patients. However, the most seriously ill patients require intensive care with a multidisciplinary approach under the guidance of a knowledgeable physician. The interventions required may include intubation and artificial ventilation; Foley catheterization and nasogastric intubation; central venous or pulmonary artery catheterization to assess volume status in the presence of hypotension; administration of vasopressors; cardiac monitoring and treatment of arrhythmias; careful management of IV fluid with frequent measurement of serum electrolyte level, serum pH level, and blood gases; management of hypothermia or hyperthermia; control of seizures; and the careful attention to skin changes and pulmonary function that is needed in the management of all comatose patients. After sufficient recovery from the physical effects of the ingestion, the circumstances of the event should be reviewed with the patient. If the overdose was deliberate, psychiatric consultation should be sought to determine the appropriate follow-up. In cases of accidental poisoning, the physician should attempt to educate the patient and family so that future episodes can be avoided.

REFERENCES

Arena JM: Poisoning: Toxicology, Symptoms, Treatments, 4th ed. Charles C Thomas, Springfield, IL, 1979.

Aronow R, Done AK: Phencyclidine overdose: an emerging concept of management. J Am Coll Emerg Phys 7:56–59, 1978.

Bayer MJ, Warner CG, Eie KF (eds): Poisonings and overdose. Topics Emerg Med 1:1–137, 1979.

Gilman AG, Goodman LS, Gilman A (eds): The Pharmacological Basis of Therapeutics, 6th ed. Macmillan, New York, 1980.

Gosselin RE, Smith RP, Hodge HC: Clinical Toxicology of Commercial Products, 5th ed. Williams & Wilkins Co, Baltimore, 1984.

Haddad LM, Winchester JF: Clinical Management of Poisoning and Drug Overdose. W. B. Saunders Co, Philadelphia, 1983.

Hanson W Jr (ed): Toxic Emergencies. Clinics in Emergency Medicine, Vol 5. Churchill Livingstone, New York, 1984.

Physicians' Desk Reference, 39th ed. Medical Economics, Oradell, NJ, 1985.

Rumack BH (ed): Poisindex Information System, microfiche. Micromedex, Englewood, CO, 1974 (revised quarterly).

Walker WE, Levy RC, Hanenson IB: Physostigmine—its use and abuse. J Am Coll Emerg Phys 5:436–439, 1976.

6 · ALCOHOLISM

Richard D. Hurt
MAYO CLINIC AND MAYO FOUNDATION

DEFINITION AND DIAGNOSTIC CRITERIA

The diagnosis of alcoholism is not difficult when the patient presents with advanced medical complications, yet many physicians are reluctant to make this diagnosis even in this setting. Because denial and defensiveness are hallmarks of this disease, the diagnosis of alcoholism in the earlier stages requires from the physician skill, knowledge, and a willingness to become involved. A first and major part of outpatient management of alcoholism is recognition of the disease in a patient who does not volunteer the cardinal symptoms and who may skillfully avoid giving accurate information about problems related to drinking. As in most other diseases, the diagnosis must first be suspected, then confirmed, before further intervention can take place. If the diagnosis is overlooked, the alcoholic patient may go on for many years before the next opportunity for intervention occurs. More than one visit may be required to establish the diagnosis, and the physician plays the dual role of diagnostician and interventionist. The patient's spouse, close family member, or significant other should be regarded as an important resource in this process, and permission to communicate with such individuals should be obtained from the patient at the earliest possible time.

The definition of alcoholism has been clarified in recent years and is clearly made in the *Diagnostic and Statistical Manual of Mental Disorders*, 3rd edition (DSM-III), published in 1980 by the American Psychiatric Association. The diagnosis is dependent on the presence of a pattern of pathologic alcohol use or impairment in social or occupational functioning due to its use, coupled either with central nervous system tolerance of the effects of alcohol or with withdrawal symptoms. Pathologic alcohol use may include a variety of patterns: daily use of alcohol, inability to cut down or stop drinking, repeated efforts to control or reduce drinking, alcoholic blackouts, or continued drinking despite a serious physical disorder related to alcohol. Impairment of social or occupational functioning due to alcohol use may include absence from work, loss of job, legal difficulties, violence while intoxicated, or problems in family or social relationships. According to the DSM-III criteria, tolerance and withdrawal symptoms are the factors distinguishing alcoholism from alcohol abuse, and one or the other must be present in order to establish the diagnosis of alcoholism.

Tolerance is a CNS phenomenon characterized by the ability of the alcoholic to consume increasingly larger amounts of alcohol without showing the signs of intoxication expected for a given blood alcohol concentration. Withdrawal symptoms may occur in the alcoholic when alcohol intake is reduced or stopped. Early withdrawal symptoms may include morning shakes and generalized malaise, both of which are relieved by drinking. The four classic withdrawal syndromes are (1) tremulousness, (2) seizures, (3) hallucinosis, and (4) delirium tremens. Just as for the severe medical illnesses associated with alcoholism, the diagnosis is easy when there is a full-blown withdrawal syndrome. If the physician fails to make the diagnosis until the disease has progressed to these stages, many patients may die or suffer irreversible damage that might have been avoided.

PATHOPHYSIOLOGY

The pathophysiology of the addiction process is poorly understood, but the recent findings of CNS receptors for a variety of substances suggests a CNS basis for alcohol dependence. Genetic factors also play a role, as indicated by the familial tendency toward alcoholism. Thus, some alcoholics may acquire the disease after repeated exposures over many years, whereas those who have a familial predisposition for its development may develop alcohol dependence very rapidly.

The precise mechanism for development of CNS tolerance is unknown. It appears early in the course of the disease and can develop to a degree that the alcoholic can function with blood alcohol concentrations that would severely impair or incapacitate the nonalcoholic. In the later stages of alcoholism, tolerance may fade so that doses of alcohol that earlier would have produced little effect will render the alcoholic intoxicated. Alcoholic blackouts are true amnestic episodes that occur during periods of heavy drinking. The individual continues to function during the drinking episode but later cannot recall the events that took place. Although an occasional nonalcoholic may have had a previous alcoholic blackout, multiple and recurrent blackouts are noted only in alcohol abusers or alcoholics.

Alcohol is a relatively simple compound that requires no digestion. Absorption begins in the stomach but is more rapid and complete in the small bowel. Once absorbed, alcohol is evenly distributed throughout the body water. The hepatic enzyme alcohol dehydrogenase is the major pathway for alcohol metabolism but is saturated at low blood alcohol concentrations. Thus, the clearance of alcohol becomes a linear function of time and cannot be accelerated. Alcohol dehydrogenase cannot be induced by long-term, high-volume alcohol use, and the rate of metabolism is roughly proportional to the individual's body weight.

In the alcoholic, the microsomal ethanol oxidizing system (MEOS), a second hepatic enzyme system, may be responsible for as much as 25% of the metabolism of alcohol. This system is induced by alcohol use and accounts for the metabolic tolerance observed in alcoholics. Acetaldehyde is produced by the metabolism of alcohol by both alcohol dehydrogenase and the MEOS. A small amount of ingested alcohol is excreted unchanged in expired air, sweat, and urine. The concentration of alcohol in expired air is closely correlated with blood alcohol concentration, so that properly administered breathalizer tests are an accurate reflection of blood alcohol concentration. The volume of distribution is smaller in women and elderly persons, so that lesser quantities of alcohol produce a greater than expected intoxicating effect in these individuals.

Alcohol readily crosses the placenta and may produce toxic fetal effects. The fetal alcohol syndrome is a relatively frequent cause of birth defects and is characterized by a triad of features in the affected child: (1) facial dysmorphology, (2) prenatal and postnatal growth deficiencies, and (3) CNS involvement, including mental retardation. The complete syndrome is probably limited to fetuses of women who drink large quantities of alcohol during pregnancy, but as little as one drink a day has been associated with lower-birth-weight infants. The current recommendation from the Surgeon General is that pregnant women should totally abstain.

Excessive alcohol consumption may have a direct toxic effect on a variety of tissues, even in the presence of a nutritionally adequate diet. Nevertheless, nutrition continues to be an important issue, and in many alcoholics 40% to 50% of the daily caloric intake may be provided by alcohol. When in the form of distilled spirits, the nutrient value of alcohol is limited to its calories (7.1 kcal/gm), since vitamins or other nutrients are absent. This has led to the term "empty calories" to describe alcohol's contribution to nutrition, although beer and wine do provide a certain amount of other nutrients. The weight of the evidence in recent years indicates that the toxic effect of alcohol is the primary mode of tissue injury, though the secondary effects of malnutrition, especially in the skid row alcoholic, may be important.

CLINICAL ASPECTS

In the overall assessment of an uncomplicated alcoholic in the outpatient setting, it should be remembered that alcoholics are usually defensive concerning their intake and frequently misrepresent and minimize the volume consumed. An attempt to quantify the alcohol intake of an alcoholic by history is of little use and often very misleading. Only when a patient admits to drinking a large volume of alcohol (one fifth of hard liquor per day or its equivalent in wine or beer) can the diagnosis of alcoholism be made solely on the basis of quantity consumed. The ability to drink this amount of alcohol on a daily basis requires CNS tolerance.

It is more important to try to obtain information reflecting problems that may have occurred in the patient's life as a result of alcohol intake. The question "How much do you drink?" may evoke defensive reactions even in patients who are nonalcoholic. What is really desirable is to determine how the patient uses alcohol and whether it has caused problems in his or her life. The following four questions can be asked during the medical history: (1) Do you drink? (2) Tell me how you use alcohol (i.e., how do you drink?) (3) Has drinking ever caused problems in your life? (medical, legal, social, etc.) (4) Has anyone been concerned about your drinking?

A convenient and nonthreatening time to ask these screening questions is to link them to inquiries about caffeine intake and smoking. The clinician should be alert not only to the answer given but also to the manner in which it is given. The alcoholic may become defensive, evasive, and uncomfortable and tend to minimize or rationalize. Such responses can provide a clue to an underlying alcohol problem and warrant a more detailed history (tolerance, blackouts, etc.) to establish the diagnosis. If the patient gives consent, early contact with the spouse may provide valuable information and set the stage for effective intervention.

Another screening test that has been popularized consists of the "CAGE" questions: (1) Have you felt the need to Cut down your drinking? (2) Have you ever felt Annoyed by criticism of your drinking? (3) Have you had Guilty feelings about drinking? (4) Do you ever take a morning Eye-opener? A positive answer to all four is well correlated with alcoholism.

Short questionnaires such as the Michigan Alcoholism Screening Test (MAST) and the Self-Administered Alcoholism Screening Test (SAAST) are being used more widely and can be easily administered in almost any medical setting. The SAAST is a 35-item, short-answer questionnaire that requires only a few minutes to complete. The grading system is uncomplicated and a high score is highly predictive of the presence of alcoholism.

The physical examination of the uncomplicated alcoholic is rarely revealing, but laboratory tests frequently reveal abnormalities that should alert the physician to the presence of alcoholism. Aside from the blood alcohol concentration, no laboratory test can be used by itself to establish the diagnosis of alcoholism. In fact, alcohol-related abnormalities shown by laboratory tests are useful primarily to focus attention on alcohol as a possible problem. Table 1 lists tests that are most often abnormally elevated in middle-class alcoholics admitted for treatment.

The gamma-glutamyl transpeptidase (GGT) is a hepatic microsomal enzyme that is elevated in a variety of hepatobiliary disorders. In alcoholics the abnormality is due to a combination of both microsomal enzyme induction and hepatic damage produced by alcohol. After the alcoholic stops drinking, the elevated GGT returns to normal over a period of several weeks, depending in part on the height of the initial abnormality. The GGT may also be useful in monitoring compliance with an abstinence program.

On the basis of studies, including liver biopsies, abnormality of serum aspartate aminotransferase (AST) in alcoholics reflects hepatocellular necrosis in the majority, and enzyme induction does not seem to play a role. It usually returns to normal after two weeks of abstinence.

The presence of macrocytosis without anemia in alcoholics has been well known for many years and is thought to be due to the direct toxic effect of alcohol on bone marrow. The same mechanism is presumed to be the cause of mean corpuscular hemoglobin (MCH) in these patients.

Fasting hyperglycemia is much more common than alcoholic hypoglycemia and may range from 110 to 160 mg/dl or higher. This mild hyperglycemia is thought to be due to alcohol's peripheral interference with the insulin-glucose interaction. Hypertriglyceridemia and uric acid elevations are in part a physiologic effect produced by the hepatic metabolism of alcohol, and rapidly decline with abstinence. The mechanism of hyperphosphatemia is unknown.

The determination of blood alcohol concentration for recognizing alcoholics is underutilized in clinical practice. It is more commonly applicable to an emergency room or hospital setting but can be useful in the outpatient practice. Blood alcohol concentration can provide objective information regarding alcohol use and give a good estimate of CNS tolerance. It may be the only test needed to establish the diagnosis of alcoholism. Blood alcohol concentration is commonly reported in

Table 2. BLOOD ALCOHOL CONCENTRATION AND THE USUAL EFFECT IN NONALCOHOLICS

Blood Alcohol Concentration (mg/dl)	CNS Effect
50	Mild release of inhibitions
100	Ataxia, dysarthria
150	Behavioral changes, (e.g., becoming argumentative, boisterous)
200	Periods of sleep
300	Stupor
400	Coma
500	Paralysis of respiratory center

three different units: gm%, mg/dl, and μg/ml. Medical facilities most often report in mg/dl.

Table 2 shows blood alcohol levels and the expected effects seen in nonalcoholics.

Alcohol acts as a CNS depressant, and as blood alcohol concentration increases this effect is intensified. "Passing out" occurs in the nonalcoholic at a blood alcohol concentration of approximately 200 mg/dl. Because of tolerance, the alcoholic may continue to function despite blood alcohol concentrations that would severely depress the CNS of the nonalcoholic.

If a person has a blood alcohol concentration of greater than 100 mg/dl at the time of a routine general examination, there is a high probability of his being alcoholic. A blood alcohol concentration greater than 150 mg/dl in the absence of signs of gross intoxication indicates CNS tolerance and is a major criterion for the diagnosis of alcoholism. If an individual can drink enough to achieve a blood alcohol concentration of 300 mg/dl, the probability of alcoholism is very high. Aside from the presence of significant CNS tolerance, the only way in which a blood alcohol concentration of 300 mg/dl can be reached is by rapid consumption of a large quantity of alcohol.

The individual's mental status should be documented at the time a blood alcohol concentration is drawn. It is particularly frustrating to see patients after an emergency room visit and find a significant blood alcohol concentration, but no comment in the emergency room record as to their state of intoxication at the time the blood was drawn. A simple statement as to the level of intoxication is all that is needed to make the blood alcohol concentration a highly valuable test.

In response to the question concerning whether alcohol has caused problems, patients occasionally relate a previous arrest for driving while intoxicated (DWI) or under the influence of alcohol (DUI). The legal limit of blood alcohol concentration allowed by most states for persons driving an automobile is 0.1 gm% (equal to 100 mg/dl). In many states, a lesser charge of driving while impaired can be brought if blood alcohol concentration is between 0.08 and 0.1 gm% (80 to 100 mg/dl). Patients who have been stopped and cited for DWI will sometimes know what their blood alcohol concentration was at the time (through breathalizer or blood alcohol tests). If the blood alcohol level was very high and the patient was not observed to be intoxicated, the physician's index of suspicion should be heightened.

MANAGEMENT

OVERCOMING THE INITIAL INERTIA

There is a reluctance on the part of many physicians to make the diagnosis of alcoholism, even when the

Table 1. LABORATORY TESTS THAT ARE FREQUENTLY ELEVATED IN MIDDLE-CLASS ALCOHOLICS

Laboratory Test	Frequency of Abnormal Elevations (%)
Mean corpuscular hemoglobin (MCH)	61
Gamma-glutamyl transpeptidase (GGT)	51–63
Serum aspartate aminotransferase (AST)	46–48
Fasting plasma glucose	36
Mean corpuscular volume (MCV)	18–25
Serum triglycerides	16–22
Serum alkaline phosphatase	16
Serum phosphate	10.4
Uric acid	10

signs and symptoms are obvious. The doctor often is misled by the alcoholic's denial and wants to believe that the patient can stop or modify the drinking behavior without outside help. Some believe that alcoholics are a hopeless cause and not amenable to treatment. Other physicians do not want to label their patient with a disease around which there is such a stigma, and with all the attendant problems that such labeling brings (increased health insurance rates, possible loss of job, and so forth). Even when the diagnosis is clear-cut, many physicians couch the dismissal diagnosis in terms that disguise the severity of the problem. As a result, few of the consequences of drinking are brought home to the patient, who may continue to skirt the issue successfully.

The denial of the alcoholic must be met firmly but with compassion and understanding. The doctor often has to rely on objective evidence (laboratory findings) to negate some of the denial, and the use of another source of information (spouse) is frequently the key. In accepting a plan that calls for alcoholics to modify or stop drinking without outside help, they must agree to more aggressive therapy if efforts to stop or control drinking fail. Alcoholics are no more a hopeless cause than are patients with other diseases that are prone to relapse and remission. The outlook for the alcoholic who undergoes inpatient treatment is quite good, with a success rate (defined as no drinking at two years after treatment) of around 50%. An additional 16% of alcoholics are abstinent at two years and will have had no more than two minor drinking episodes. Thus, with inpatient treatment, an overall success rate of approximately two thirds can be expected. Unfortunately, the attitude of most physicians is unduly influenced by the recidivist alcoholic. Alcoholics who relapse are sometimes viewed with a degree of disdain, while the diabetic who relapses or the heart patient who has recurrent congestive heart failure is usually treated with compassion.

MAINTAINING THE PHYSICIAN-PATIENT RELATIONSHIP

An important aspect of management of a patient with alcoholism is to establish sincere rapport in an open and honest manner, and to be firm without appearing moralistic or accusatory. The doctor can best maintain the physician-patient relationship by avoiding threats and demonstrating appropriate sensitivity. The alcoholic needs support as well as confrontation. The physician should understand that alcoholism is a disease and not simply a problem of willpower that can be made to recede by advising the patient to decrease the level of alcohol intake or stop drinking altogether. Unfortunately, many physicians view the patient's inability to comply with medical advice as evidence of a lack of willpower, and a strained or broken patient-physician relationship results. The influence of the physician's advice on the patient should not be underestimated. At the same time, it is clear that most alcoholics will not stop drinking because the doctor says it is bad for them or is causing harm. The physician should not expect compliance with such advice unless other measures are taken.

The physician has to be sensitive to the diagnostic clues at the time of the examination and be willing to intervene on behalf of the patient. Many physicians are somewhat uncomfortable in this role, but it is essential if they are to provide the best available assistance. In many areas of the United States, once an alcohol problem has been identified, consultation may be sought with an experienced alcoholism counselor who can then manage the rest of the intervention. The physician is in an excellent position to do this without consultation but, as with most other diseases, the decision to obtain consultation is an individual one.

THE SPOUSE AS A RESOURCE

A second key to management of the alcoholic is obtaining permission to discuss the problem with the patient's spouse, significant other, or close family member. An interview with the spouse, even by telephone, often elicits enough additional information to establish a firm diagnosis and allows for an open and honest discussion about treatment alternatives. It also helps to allay some of the suspiciousness on the part of the patient and guilt feelings on the part of the spouse. In addition, the physician gets a better feel for the family dynamics and how the patient's alcoholism has disrupted other aspects of the family's daily living. What sound like minor difficulties from the patient's point of view are often major problems threatening the family relationship. Another reason for contacting people close to the patient is to seek their help in exerting influence on the patient to seek treatment. In contrast to a commonly held notion, alcoholics do *not* have to admit there is a problem before help can be administered. They rarely seek treatment voluntarily, as evidenced by the observation that almost all alcoholics in treatment facilities were forced into treatment by one factor or another.

INTERVENTION AND TREATMENT

The initial goal of intervention is to enroll the patient for treatment. At the time of initial contact, the patient usually will not recognize that there is a problem, much less agree to treatment. If the initial visit is for a general examination, the intervention process can begin with gentle confrontation. Even if the diagnosis is obvious after the history and physical, I usually avoid the term alcoholism, using instead terms such as alcohol abuse or alcohol-related problems. I express concern about alcohol being a potential problem and arrange for the usual laboratory tests, including those listed in Table 1. At this point I also ask if the spouse will be available to accompany the patient when the test results are reviewed.

If the spouse is present at the time of the return visit, I assess further the possible presence of significant alcohol-related problems. Alcohol-related laboratory test abnormalities can be used to demonstrate further the seriousness of the problem. The stage is then set for intervention on the patient's behalf, and the term alcoholism may be introduced into the discussion. This is most effectively carried out with both the patient and spouse present, but can be accomplished with the patient alone. He or she should be told that the diagnosis is alcoholism and that treatment is needed. Most respond that treatment is not necessary, that "I can handle it on my own. I can take it or leave it. It really is not a problem." It should be pointed out that, as with most other diseases, treatment is necessary, and that fortunately effective treatment is available for alcoholism. Another response often given is "Let me try it on my own. I'm sure I can stop." Usually the patient has made previous attempts at "going on the wagon" and has failed. Thus, the physician can firmly reply that "You have tried it your way in the past and it has not worked out. Now we need to try handling your alcoholism in a different way."

If an impasse is reached and further pursuit is likely to jeopardize the physician-patient relationship, it is appropriate to pull back and attempt to arrange future treatment. A verbal contract can be made whereby the patient agrees to enter treatment if unable to control his or her drinking or totally abstain. Since loss of control is a major factor in separating alcoholics from social drinkers, some experts recommend that the patient drink no more than a small quantity (one or two drinks a day) over a long period (six months or longer). If the patient is unable to keep the intake at or below this quantity, this demonstrates loss of control and the need for treatment. A similar scenario can be designed to test the ability of the patient to abstain totally for a prolonged period (three to six months). Some caution has to be exercised when using this plan, as some alcoholics *can* abstain for prolonged periods. Despite this limitation, I personally prefer the latter approach, since it is easier for the spouse to monitor. The patient should be asked to agree to go into treatment if efforts to abstain fail. The patient is then asked what should be done if drinking resumes but he or she refuses to follow through with the verbal agreement to enter treatment. The alcoholic usually says that if the agreement is broken, treatment will be accepted without resistance. The issue should be pressed further by pointing out that a change in attitude will likely occur if drinking is resumed, and a refusal to follow through with the agreement is likely. The physician can then review the spouse's options, which are as follows: (1) say and do nothing further, (2) leave the patient, or (3) try to commit the patient to a treatment program. The alcoholic usually recognizes that the spouse is unlikely to say or do nothing, and usually does not want the spouse to leave. Thus, commitment may be the only alternative that is applicable. When asked which option should be pursued, the alcoholic usually reiterates that all this discussion is unnecessary because of the agreement to go into treatment if drinking resumes, but will acknowledge that, if necessary, commitment is the best alternative. The physician must be prepared to assist in further intervention efforts, as the need will almost surely arise. The commitment laws for inebriates differ from state to state, and to undertake a commitment is usually not an easy task for either the spouse or physician. In most instances, the threat of commitment is the tool that can be used to show the alcoholic how serious the situation is and the lengths to which the loved ones are willing to go to seek help.

Whether or not the patient goes into treatment, the spouse should be referred to Al-Anon. Al-A-Teen is a similar resource available to the children of alcoholics. The purpose of both groups is to help the spouse and children deal with their own feelings and teach them to be able to detach themselves emotionally from the alcoholic's problems while continuing to demonstrate their love for the alcoholic.

Occasionally the physician receives a phone call from a concerned spouse about a patient who has recently been seen or is coming in for an examination. The spouse expresses concern about the patient's alcohol use but invariably asks that the phone call be kept secret. Although generally receptive to such calls, I tell the spouse of the need to be open and honest about the problem. The spouse should be told that the problem cannot be fully discussed without the patient's consent, but she or he can be encouraged to accompany the patient on the next visit so that the situation can be reviewed in the open. The spouse is a highly accurate source and rarely if ever provides information that leads to a false diagnosis of alcoholism.

An occasional patient agrees to go into treatment at the initial intervention. Under such circumstances, the physician should be prepared to help in the long-term follow-up, not only to check any medical abnormalities that may be present but to help in monitoring the patient's sobriety. The physician is often in the best position to do this, especially if good rapport has developed. Recovering alcoholics are generally very grateful, and as the recovery process proceeds, any hard feelings that may have resulted from the diagnosis and intervention fade and are replaced with genuine appreciation.

Much has been written concerning outpatient treatment for alcoholism and its relative cost in comparison to inpatient treatment, but we emphasize the need for inpatient treatment for most alcoholics, with few exceptions. Some individuals who have more insight and a greater degree of initial acceptance of their problem may be managed as outpatients, although inpatient therapy would be acceptable as well. Patients with more severe medical problems related to alcoholism and those with high potential for a withdrawal syndrome should be hospitalized in an inpatient treatment program so that detoxification can occur safely. Those who have had a previous withdrawal syndrome and those who have had a very high-volume, long-term intake are more likely to have withdrawal symptoms once they become abstinent, and are best treated as inpatients. The treatment program designed around a medical model includes detoxification, therapy for withdrawal symptoms, educational sessions, group therapy support, individual therapy, and evaluation and treatment of other medical illnesses. A variety of treatment facilities are available in most locations, and the physician should be aware of the availability of such resources to which referrals can be made and of the type of treatment offered.

Alcoholics Anonymous (AA) is sometimes successful as a primary treatment modality, but is most useful for after-care of a patient who has gone through a treatment program. AA is a highly worthwhile organization of daily assistance to millions of alcoholics in the U.S. Another source of support is the after-care that can be administered through local mental health centers. At such centers, health professionals trained in chemical dependence can help alcoholic patients through difficult times by various types of counseling. Mental health centers often offer outpatient programs for alcoholics who do not require inpatient treatment.

There has been great interest in studies showing that some alcoholics can return to "controlled drinking." Most of these studies are limited by a relatively short follow-up period. Widespread experience shows that there is a very high risk of returning to alcoholic drinking, regardless of how long a period of abstinence precedes the attempt to return to social drinking. At present, abstinence seems to be the best and perhaps the only realistic goal of alcoholism treatment.

DRUG THERAPY

Any type of mood-altering drug should be used with great caution in the alcoholic patient, and except during closely monitored detoxification, should be avoided altogether. Oral chlordiazepoxide (Librium) has proved very effective for detoxification. It has cross-tolerance to the CNS effects of alcohol and has a sufficiently long half-life to allow for a smooth withdrawal. Since CNS tolerance in the alcoholic may be marked, large doses of chlordiazepoxide are often required. For mild to moderate withdrawal symptoms, an initial dosage of 25 to 50 mg every two to four hours may be needed to control the symptoms, followed by 25 to 50 mg every four hours p.r.n. For more severe withdrawal symptoms, 25 to 100 mg every one to two hours may be needed to gain control of the symptoms, followed by 25 to 100 mg every two to four hours p.r.n. to keep control of the symptoms. Some latitude is necessary in the use of chlordiazepoxide; if allowed, nurses in attendance usually respond by closely observing the patients during withdrawal. The dose can be tapered by approximately 20% per day, and most patients can be off the medication within four to five days. The support of the milieu of a treatment unit is also important to help minimize the effects of withdrawal. Nursing and counseling staff in treatment units are particularly adept at helping the patient through difficult withdrawal symptoms.

Disulfiram (Antabuse) is a useful adjunct in the treatment of the alcoholic patient. Its major limitation is the need for self-administration, and the physician should be aware that simply giving a prescription to the patient and expecting abstinence to result is beyond the capabilities of this sometimes useful drug. The dose recommended is 250 mg per day. There is no need for a loading dose, and it is not necessary to test for a disulfiram-alcohol reaction by administering a dose of alcohol after a patient has been on the drug. Disulfiram blocks aldehyde dehydrogenase, and high levels of acetaldehyde are produced when alcohol is ingested. The severity of the reaction depends on the dose of alcohol and the resultant blood alcohol concentration. A blood alcohol concentration as low as 5 to 10 mg/dl produces a mild reaction characterized by flushing, cutaneous warmth, nausea, and palpitations. As blood alcohol concentration increases, more severe flushing with vasodilatation occurs along with nausea, vomiting, headache, dizziness, palpitations, tachycardia, and other reactions that are beyond the scope of this chapter. Clinicians should be aware that solutions containing alcohol, such as cough medicines, mouthwash, and aftershave lotions, may produce minor reactions. Disulfiram can be given under controlled circumstances, such as by the patient's spouse, at the site of employment, or at a treatment unit. This ensures that the agent is being taken and it overcomes the limitation of self-administration. Although rare individuals can drink a small amount of alcohol while taking disulfiram without

having a significant reaction, such patients have a more severe reaction if taking higher doses (500 mg/day) of disulfiram. Because of the cardiovascular effects of the disulfiram-alcohol reaction, significant coronary artery disease is a relative contraindication to the use of this drug. Follow-up hepatic biochemical tests (AST, alkaline phosphatase, bilirubin) should be obtained six months after institution of therapy because of the possibility of disulfiram-related mild hepatic dysfunction.

Daily disulfiram allows the alcoholic to make the decision only once a day whether or not to drink, rather than having to face that issue on several different occasions throughout the day. Many alcoholics find this very comforting and look upon disulfiram as an insurance policy that allows them to use their emotional energy in other more productive ways.

ALCOHOL-DRUG INTERACTIONS

In alcoholics the interactions of alcohol and other drugs can be very important for both diagnosis and management. These interactions can be divided into four categories: (1) the additive or antagonistic effect of coadministration of alcohol and a drug, (2) metabolic cross-tolerance, (3) CNS cross-tolerance, and (4) drugs that cause intolerance to alcohol.

The ingestion of alcohol plus minor tranquilizers, hypnotics, or sedatives may produce an additive sedative effect. The dose of alcohol and the other drug plus the degree of CNS tolerance determines the extent of the sedative effect. There does not appear to be an additive effect when alcohol and narcotic analgesics are used concurrently. The effects of stimulant ingestion are somewhat antagonized by alcohol ingestion.

The metabolic competition between alcohol and drugs that are predominantly metabolized by hepatic enzymes from the smooth endoplasmic reticulum causes significant alterations of drug metabolism in alcoholics taking anticoagulants (warfarin), oral hypoglycemic agents (tolbutamide), and anticonvulsants (phenytoin and barbiturates). The abstaining alcoholic metabolizes these drugs at a faster rate than a comparable nonalcoholic, thus reducing the clinical effect. However, if the alcoholic is drinking, the hepatic enzyme receptors are occupied by alcohol and the rate of metabolism of these drugs is less, enhancing their clinical effect. The alcoholic patient who requires one of these drugs but continues to drink is difficult to manage, and serious complications may result.

The CNS cross-tolerance presents similar problems but can also be useful in establishing the diagnosis of alcoholism. Because of the degree of CNS tolerance that may be present in the alcoholic, major tranquilizers, sedatives, or hypnotics may have little effect. The unintoxicated alcoholic undergoing anesthesia may require much larger doses of the short-acting barbiturate used for the induction of anesthesia, as well as the gaseous anesthetic agent, compared with a nonalcoholic of the same age, sex, and size. The alert anesthesiologist will question this at the time and ask about the patient's alcohol and drug history. In the acutely intoxicated alcoholic, the dose of the inducing agent and anesthetic agent may be closer to the expected dose or actually may be less than predicted.

The CNS cross-tolerance with minor tranquilizers and sedatives leads some alcoholics to use such drugs, especially in instances where drinking would be noticed and considered unacceptable (e.g., at work). Alcoholics are frequently found to be codependent on such drugs, which is the major reason why these drugs should not be administered to them except in an inpatient withdrawal regimen. Too often drugs such as diazepam (Valium) and chlordiazepoxide are prescribed to alcoholic patients under the false assumption that pathologic drinking has been the result of an anxiety state. In fact, these commonly prescribed minor tranquilizers tend to alter mood in such a way as to pose a risk that dependence will be transferred from alcohol to the prescribed drug, or that the patient will return to alcohol use while continuing to use the drug.

Some drugs may interfere with the metabolism of alcohol or its metabolic products. Metronidazole is well known to interfere with aldehyde dehydrogenase, producing a disulfiram-like reaction in a small but significant percentage of patients who take the drug and drink alcohol. Before patients are started on metronidazole, they should be cautioned about this potential reaction and advised to abstain from alcohol during treatment. A milder form of the same reaction may be observed in patients taking tolbutamide or chlorpropamide.

MANAGEMENT OF WITHDRAWAL SYNDROMES

Detoxification of the alcoholic patient should be under monitored conditions, and the management of withdrawal syndromes usually requires administration of a minor tranquilizer. There are basically four types of alcoholic withdrawal syndromes: (1) tremulousness, (2) alcoholic hallucinosis, (3) alcoholic withdrawal seizures, and (4) delirium tremens. The tremulousness syndrome is characterized by a coarse tremor that primarily involves the hands but can involve the head, neck, and lower extremities. It may occur any time within the first 24 hours after withdrawal has begun. The patient does not necessarily have to stop drinking altogether before the tremulousness begins. I have observed an alcoholic patient with a blood alcohol concentration of over 200 mg/dl who was having such severe shakes that he could not hold a half-filled cup of coffee without spilling it. Other manifestations of this syndrome include nausea, vomiting, headache, irritability, insomnia, and a craving for alcohol. The syndrome usually leads to use of alcohol at times of day when the tremulousness is worse, such as in the morning. Some alcoholics may take a minor tranquilizer or sedative to prevent these withdrawal symptoms, thus creating a codependency.

Alcoholic hallucinosis by itself is an uncommon withdrawal syndrome. It is characterized by hallucinations but these arise in the absence of a disordered sensorium, memory disturbance, confusion, or disorientation.

Alcoholic withdrawal seizures usually occur within the first three days after cessation of alcohol. The seizures are grand mal in type and usually single. An alcoholic who has had a previous withdrawal seizure is at a greater risk of developing another upon discontinuing alcohol. Prophylactic phenytoin can be administered to alcoholics being detoxified in whom there is a history of previous withdrawal seizures. There is no need for long-term anticonvulsant therapy in patients who have experienced an alcoholic withdrawal seizure, unless they have idiopathic epilepsy. Thus, in the alcoholic who has undergone a fairly typical alcohol withdrawal seizure, a normal electroencephalogram will obviate the need for continued anticonvulsant therapy.

Delirium tremens, the most severe alcoholic withdrawal syndrome, is fairly easily recognized. Physicians who have trained in inner city or V.A. hospitals may have a distorted view of alcoholism because of the frequent observation of delirium tremens. The syndrome is characterized by disorientation, hallucinations, tremor, hyperexcitability, tachycardia, and hyperpyrexia. The condition remains potentially fatal, requiring hospitalization with monitoring and adequate fluid and electrolyte replacement. The agitation and hyperexcitability can usually be controlled by large amounts of chlordiazepoxide PO, as outlined previously. If parenteral sedation is needed, IM chlordiazepoxide or diazepam can be used, but the absorption is erratic and the IV route is preferred. More commonly, haloperidol (Haldol) is preferable, 3 to 5 mg IM every four to six hours until adequate sedation is achieved. The dose of any of these drugs should be titrated to control symptoms, remembering that large doses may be required because of CNS tolerance.

SUMMARY

The prevalence of alcoholism in the U.S. is not known, but most sources estimate that it afflicts over 10,000,000 Americans and accounts for over 4% of all the nation's health expenditure. Despite the prevalence of alcoholism and the frequency with which alcoholics are seen in medical care facilities, the diagnosis is infrequently made. To establish the diagnosis, the physician needs not only an understanding of the diagnostic criteria but also skills in patient management.

REFERENCES

Ewing JA: Detecting alcoholism: the CAGE questionnaire. JAMA 252:1905–1907, 1984.
Hurt RD, Morse RM, Swenson WM: Diagnosis of alcoholism with a Self-Administered Alcoholism Screening Test. Mayo Clin Proc 55:365–370, 1980.
Lieber CS: Metabolism and metabolic effects of alcohol. Med Clin North Am 68:3–31, 1984.
Mills JL, Graubard BI, Harley EE, et al.: Maternal alcohol consumption and birth weight. JAMA 252:1875–1879, 1984.
Morse RM, Hurt RD: Screening for alcoholism. JAMA 242:2688–2690, 1979.

7 · DRUG ABUSE AND WITHDRAWAL

Gregory B. Collins
CLEVELAND CLINIC FOUNDATION

The phenomenon of drug abuse can present a frustrating and puzzling challenge to the primary care physician. The physician may perceive clear-cut evidence of drug-induced medical complications, trauma, or psychosocial consequences, but all too often these findings are met with denial and resistance by the patient. The patient's attitude and behavior are made more problematic at times by concealment of drug history, noncompliance, or even hostility. These drug-related behaviors place formidable obstacles in the path of the treating physician and challenge even the most experienced clinicians. However, the primary care physician often plays a pivotal role in the course of the illness. He or she is in a unique position to help, but can also worsen the problem through benign neglect or mismanagement. To be effective, the physician must clearly understand the phenomenon of drug abuse and appreciate his or her front-line role in treatment. Effective physician intervention involves the art and science of medical practice by combining common-sense psychotherapy and physical restoration. Intervention with the drug-involved person concerns four major areas: diagnosis, confrontation, detoxification, and follow-up. In many instances, competent intervention in these four areas means the difference between life and death for the patient.

Diagnosis of any medical condition, including drug abuse, is predicated on understanding and recognizing the disorder. However, there is something elusive and problematic about defining drug abuse. Is use always abuse? When does "prudent, recreational" use become "abuse?" At what point does abuse become dependency, and is dependency the same as addiction? It is easy for the treating physician to be caught up in these issues, especially if the involved patient wishes to impress the physician that his use is occasional, recreational, or medically necessary. If the drug use has created any problem serious enough to come to the attention of a physician, the problem is probably serious. As a general rule, minor problems of occasional misuse do not come to the attention of a physician. It is best to maintain a high index of suspicion, assuming that a serious problem is present, in the hope that additional information will clarify the diagnostic picture.

All the drugs of abuse afford the user a measure of temporary chemical pleasure. These drugs, regardless of their class or pharmacologic effect, produce a type of chemical experience perceived by the user as positive. Although the initial use of these substances may be experimental or even medically necessary, the user soon learns that they afford a chemical pleasurable experience and soon begins to take them for their own sake. This process may happen fully outside the user's conscious awareness, but the net effect is the same: the drugs induce their own taking. "Use" progresses to "abuse" and to "loss of control." In my view, the "loss of control" phenomenon is critical for the physician's assessment. Generally, patients deny any loss of control. They feel they are in complete volitional control of their actions, including drug taking or avoidance. Although the drug use itself may be heavy and frequent, this fact may seem only dimly apparent to the users, who seem instead preoccupied with reasons and excuses for drug use. These reasons may be situational, medical, or psychologic, but they convince users of the reasonableness of continued heavy involvement with mood-altering drugs. Thus, the "loss of control" is apparent to everyone but the users themselves. It is the "loss of control" that marks the phenomenon as a self-perpet-

uating disease process called chemical dependency or drug addiction. Bearing in mind that substance "abusers" possibly have an addiction or "sick compulsion" may help you as the physician to understand better the abusers' behavior, relapses, mood swings, and physical complications.

PATHOPHYSIOLOGY AND CHEMICAL DEPENDENCY

Addictions can be regarded as having both psychologic and physical components, but their pathophysiology has not yet been entirely elucidated. For now, the only practical way to diagnose addictions is to observe their consequences or symptoms. Usually, these symptoms are reflected in the deterioration of marital, occupational, emotional, spiritual, legal, financial, or physical well-being. If the drug use repeatedly causes problems in one or more of these areas, the diagnosis of chemical dependency or addiction can be made even though the patient may believe that he or she can stop using drugs.

Current thinking favors the view that chemical dependency is a result of complex genetic, environmental, psychologic, physical, and social factors. Because of these complexities, most professionals pay little attention to how the chemically dependent person came to be addicted. Looking for underlying problems or causes before stable abstinence has been achieved is generally fruitless and may be detrimental. It is better to direct treatment at completely eliminating the use of psychoactive substances, while recognizing that the patient is suffering from a sick compulsion to return to active drug use. Chemical dependency is a "great masquerader," disguising itself as a medical or psychiatric complaint. Patients rarely seek treatment for drug problems. Usually they are in the physician's office for one or more drug-related disorders such as seizures, systemic or local infections, accidents, trauma, burns, or hepatitis. The presenting complaint also may be psychiatric with the appearance of anxiety, depression, personality disorder, or paranoid ideation. The spouse or other family member may also be symptomatic because of the patient's drug abuse. The role of the physician is to *see through* the symptoms and diagnose the chemical problem. If alcohol, drugs, or both have anything to do with the problem, the chemical abuse should be investigated further.

Problems often arise because physicians tend to recognize only late-stage physical complications and withdrawal symptoms as indicative of drug addiction. They should, however, cultivate the skill of diagnosing substance dependency at a much earlier point in this progressive disability, when manifestations are subtle. The earliest symptoms are generally adverse effects on marriage and job, which often antedate by many years any detectable physical consequences. It is therefore a good idea to ask "did this problem have anything to do with your drug use?" or "were you using a drug when the problem occurred?"

DIAGNOSIS

Diagnosis of drug dependence is usually made on the basis of information obtained from the medical history, physical examination, psychologic assessment, laboratory tests, and reports of concerned others. For the medical history, ask about recent drug use including alcohol, analgesics, sedatives, tranquilizers, cocaine, marijuana, and any others. Has there been a pattern of increasing the dosage or frequency of these drugs? Has the patient received treatment from numerous doctors or hospitals? Is he unwilling to reveal the names or places of the previous treatment? Does he have a vague physical problem such as "back pain" without radiologic changes, or conversely, does he report an exotic chronic disease such as acute intermittent porphyria, which causes intermittent bouts of pain? Is there any deception or significant omission in the medical or psychiatric history? Does the patient acknowledge an earlier drug problem or previous drug treatment? Are other risk factors present such as easy access to drugs (in the case of health care professionals) or peer pressure (e.g., in sports or entertainment figures)? Has he been arrested for driving while intoxicated? Have there been any drug-related arrests? Is there a history of drug-involved marital discord or job trouble? Have there been any drug-related trauma, violence, explosion, or burns? Has there been a history of any drug withdrawal symptoms such as sweating, nausea, vomiting, or seizures?

The physical examination should be fairly comprehensive, since chronic drug misuse can adversely affect virtually any organ system. Are there complications of chronic drug administration such as needle marks, scars, ulcerations, cellulitis, or necrotic areas of skin? Does the patient have "no veins," making it difficult to obtain blood for laboratory sampling? Look for evidence of aseptic necrosis of large muscle masses, often with scarring and fibrosis. Muscles may take on a boardlike consistency. Look for elevated blood pressure, decreased or increased pulse rate. Pupillary constriction may be present (opiates) or pupils may be dilated (stimulants, or sedative withdrawal). Check for jaundice of the skin and icteric sclerae as well as heart murmurs (possible subacute bacterial endocarditis with valvular vegetations) or blood cells in the urine. Examine the liver for tenderness or enlargement. Check the nose for inflammation of the nasal mucosa, perforation of the nasal septum, or any residual white powdery substance (cocaine) in a "doughnut shape" around the nares. Listen for coarsened voice or chronic bronchitis from cocaine freebasing or chronic marijuana smoking.

PSYCHOLOGIC MANIFESTATIONS

Psychologic manifestations may include a recent drug-related personality change of any type. There may be evidence of intoxication: staggering gait, slurred speech, "nodding off," "not making sense," or forgetting. Clothing and personal effects may reveal an interest in drugs or the drug culture. Check for the presence of medications or drugs, as well as administering paraphernalia including syringes, needles, cellophane "bags," paper wrappers, freebasing pipe, volatile ether, or sodium bicarbonate. Look for razor blades, tiny spoons, and drug-related insignias on belts, shirts, rings, and so forth. Anxiety and nervousness may be present with anger, irritability, and impatience. Agitation or even assaultiveness may require emergency precautions. The patient may be confused or disoriented and may have evidence of hallucinosis or paranoid delusions. Conversely, behavior may be dull, apathetic, and listless. Drug-seeking may be in evidence.

LABORATORY STUDIES

Laboratory tests may help to confirm the presence of drugs or establish evidence of organ damage. Negative laboratory studies, however, do not rule out a significant drug problem. A toxicology screen for drugs of abuse is warranted in any suspicious circumstance. A supervised urine collection is best for this purpose. Blood studies may indicate elevated SGOT, lactate dehydrogenase, and bilirubin. Hepatitis antigens may be present. A TB skin test is advisable. The electrocardiogram may reflect arrhythmias (cocaine), and a posteroanterior and left lateral chest x-ray may show infectious granulomas, diffuse fibrosis, tuberculosis, or pneumonia.

Outside confirmation from concerned others such as the spouse or persons close to the patient is always helpful. In this regard, physicians must be very discreet in their enquiries so as not to reveal "privileged information" or jeopardize the patient's reputation. Generally, eliciting information from the family is the best way to proceed. If they reveal serious concerns because of drug use, the physician can support these concerns and assist the family to motivate the patient to accept help.

MANAGEMENT

For the physician, surely the most anxiety-producing aspect of drug abuse treatment is the initial confrontation of the patient. The prospect of confronting an evasive, resistant, denying addict is distressing for any physician. Experience has shown that there are basic steps in effective confrontation: (1) confrontation: mutual recognition of worsening progression, (2) self-diagnosis, and (3) the offer of hope through treatment.

MUTUAL RECOGNITION OF WORSENING PROGRESSION

Set aside an hour to interview the patient with the spouse present. If both are denying, bring in the patient's parents or mature children. Start by obtaining a good drug history. State your concern about the possibility that the presenting medical complaint is related to a drug problem and indicate that you would like to discuss this in more detail. Start with the patient's first drug use and develop a chronologic history of drug involvement to the present time. In the patient's early years, look for drug-related problems in high school, college, or military service. Look for drug-related effects on the marriage, such as complaints from the spouse, arguing and fighting, physical abuse, or drug-related separation or divorce. Get a good marital history, listing all marriages and significant relationships and the reasons for break-ups, separations, or divorces.

Obtain a good occupational history and ask about absenteeism from work, arriving late, leaving early, declining job performance, warnings on the job, or loss of job. Inquire about lost time at work related to health problems such as hospitalizations, injuries, auto accidents, or surgery. Ask about arrests and convictions, and ascertain whether these offenses were related to drug ingestion or use. Inquire about financial concerns.

Is the spouse complaining that bills are unpaid and money is going for drugs or "drug life style?" Is the patient behind on his medical account, and is this because of drugs? Have his wages been garnisheed? Has the patient ever had psychiatric difficulty involving alcohol or drugs in any way? Did he use any psychotropic drugs, and if so, what type, for how long, how many, and from whom? Is there a dual dependency, e.g., on psychotropic drugs as well as alcohol? Remember that most drug-dependent persons obtain their medications from physicians, so that the patient's assurance that "I only take drugs prescribed by a doctor" does not eliminate the possibility of medication misuse or dependency.

Focus on the pattern of drinking and drug use in the last year or two. Generally, a worsening progression is evident in the form of deterioration of functioning or health, or more and more frequent episodes of intoxication. Ask about the extent and severity of drug hunger, craving, and withdrawal symptoms.

SELF-DIAGNOSIS

Drug abuse and drug dependency are stigmatized diagnoses, and all the patient's defenses are usually geared to avoid having the physician apply those labels. Thus, whenever possible, it is helpful to allow the patient the dignity of self-diagnosis. This step can be made easier with the help of prepared questionnaires such as those available from Alcoholics Anonymous or Narcotics Anonymous, or such as the Michigan Alcoholism Screening Test (MAST). When taking these tests with you, patients will perceive that their patterns and problems are those of a drug-dependent person. Often it is helpful to ask the hypothetical question, "If I asked you if you had a drug problem, what would you say?" This clearly gives patients a chance for self-diagnosis and introduces the concept of a "drug problem" in a nonjudgmental way. After a careful history has been taken and spouses have reported their concerns, and when laboratory tests are clear-cut, patients generally admit to having a drug problem or "developing one."

The term "denial" is usually taken to mean the patients' refusal to admit to any problem with drugs. More often, however, they refuse to acknowledge loss of control over drugs, thus denying any need for help. This aspect of denial often takes the form of promises to "cut down" or "do better" and assertions that they want to "go it alone." However, since they have been struggling alone for years without much success, there is little reason to suspect that they will do better now without outside help. You should express specifically your concern that the situation is getting worse as time passes. Emphasize the need for immediate treatment if a worsening picture is to be avoided.

OFFERING HOPE THROUGH TREATMENT

Emphasize that the downward spiral can be interrupted and that the patient and the family do not have to continue to suffer. State that patients invariably do better in specialized programs in hospitals and in self-help groups such as Alcoholics Anonymous and Narcotics Anonymous. Know the treatment facilities in your area and recommend appropriate ones to the patient. Inpatient admission, especially in a specialized rehabilitation program, will greatly improve the outcome.

Outpatient treatment is less protective and should be used only for stable, well-motivated, detoxified patients in no medical danger. Modern comprehensive treatment centers for chemical dependency are available in many parts of the United States and have relatively high success rates (50% and more in some centers). Be optimistic, hopeful, and firm. Often the best first step in the treatment process is hospitalization for a thorough physical and psychiatric evaluation, as well as for detoxification.

DETOXIFICATION

Having patients in a hospital setting puts the physician at a decided advantage in the treatment of chemical dependency. I tend to favor a "restrictive/protective" policy with respect to hospitalized chemical dependents. I do not allow visitors other than immediate family or self-help group representatives and I allow no off-ward privileges. A comprehensive physical examination and laboratory studies are essential elements of the detoxification process. Physicians should make it absolutely clear to patients that evidence of any withdrawal symptom or drug-related medical complication is de facto evidence of drug dependency or addiction. They should also emphasize that the detoxification phase is merely the first step in a comprehensive treatment approach, which may include additional inpatient rehabilitation, outpatient after-care, self-help group attendance, and even toxicology checks. Unless patients are willing to commit themselves to such a comprehensive and long-term programmatic structure, the outlook remains poor, and I generally will not accept a patient for "detoxification only" without this commitment. On the other hand, some patients are too toxic or impaired to formulate rationally a sound decision in the direction of total treatment commitment and cooperation. I try to give such patients the benefit of the doubt, allowing time for detoxification, in the hope that I can persuade them to accept a comprehensive treatment approach.

Pharmacologically, the detoxification phase can be managed with a few general guidelines.

Ascertain as carefully as possible from the patient the exact type and amount of drug being used. Use every information source, including toxicology screens and family members, to obtain good data in this regard. Patients are often unreliable reporters of the type and amount of drug use. Some exaggerate in order to obtain more detoxification medications, and others minimize their use out of shame or embarrassment. In the end, the physician must exercise clinical judgment in evaluating this information.

It is also helpful to know that withdrawal reactions vary widely in severity. This reality has been borne out in animal experimentations, as it has been shown that animals can be selectively bred to have severe or mild withdrawal reactions. Clinically, this is apparent in that some individuals report a history of severe, disabling withdrawal reactions, whereas others report only mild reactions. Thus, the patient's own past history of withdrawal is likely to be the best indicator of the likely severity of the present withdrawal problem. The patient may also be able to supply information as to how previous withdrawals were managed (or mismanaged).

Try to avoid using the patient's "favorite" drug for detoxification, but use a drug from the same chemical family. Addicts have a strong psychologic attachment to their "drug of choice" and it is much easier to accomplish a successful detoxification program if, at the outset, a substitute but related drug is used. If no substitute drug is available, however, the patient's own drug of choice can be employed. In general, avoid nonaddictive psychoactive drugs such as major tranquilizers or antidepressants during the detoxification phase. These drugs do not substitute well for addictive drugs, and may actually lower seizure thresholds and produce toxic side effects and undesirable reactions.

Barbiturates. For barbiturates, I prefer an initial challenge dose of 200 mg of pentobarbital (Nembutal) to see if the person is "tolerant." If the patient becomes sleepy or ataxic or shows nystagmus, tolerance is mild and a modest dosage schedule is indicated, such as 100 to 200 mg of pentobarbital PO q.i.d. If no effect is seen two hours after the initial 200-mg challenge dose, a stronger regimen may be required, such as 300 to 400 mg PO q.i.d.

Amphetamines and Cocaine. For these there is no acceptable substitute medication for detoxification purposes. Withdrawal reactions generally consist of depression, irritability, and drug-seeking behavior. Psychologic supportive measures are best in a closed environment with adequate nursing supervision.

Marijuana. Marijuana is a dependency-producing drug that creates a moderately strong desire for repetitive use in the susceptible individual. There is no substitute drug for detoxification purposes. Isolation from the drug is the treatment of choice, again with supportive psychologic measures. Marijuana is fat soluble and the numerous metabolites are only slowly excreted from the body; thus, urine toxicologies for marijuana may remain positive for five to six weeks in heavy users.

Opiates. Opiates and related narcotic analgesics are generally best managed on an inpatient basis with a methadone detoxification regimen. Start-up dosages vary widely, depending on the amount, frequency, and quality of the user's medication. For "psychologic" dependence, at low dose, as with modest amounts of physician-prescribed low-potency pain medicines, I prefer 5 mg of methadone PO q.i.d. (20 mg daily total). For "street addicts" with variable access to poor-quality drugs, 10 mg PO q.i.d. (40 mg daily total) of methadone often suffices. For addicts with better-quality analgesics taken over a moderately long period such as three to six months, 10 to 15 mg PO q.i.d. (40 to 60 mg daily total) may be required. For the most chemically addicted patients, i.e., those who have been using high-quality narcotic analgesics in large amounts for long periods, 20 to 25 mg PO q.i.d. (80 to 100 mg daily total) or more of methadone may be required. These are admittedly rough guidelines, but they are offered in the hope that they may help the clinician arrive at an approximate starting dosage.

Benzodiazepine and Other Tranquilizers. Withdrawal from benzodiazepine is usually mild, but chlordiazepoxide, 25 to 50 mg PO t.i.d., generally reduces irritability and improves patient cooperation.

Other sedatives and tranquilizers such as glutethimide (Doriden) and meprobamate (Equanil, Miltown), when discontinued after heavy chronic use, can produce violent withdrawal reactions, including seizures. I tend to prefer sodium pentobarbital (Nembutal), 100 to 400 mg PO q.i.d., as a replacement drug for glutethimide, and chlordiazepoxide (Librium), 25 to 75 mg PO q.i.d., for meprobamate replacement.

Initiation of Detoxification

In general, great care must be exercised in establishing the initial detoxification dosage. After they receive the first dose, patients must be observed carefully for the next two to six hours to determine if the medication is adequate to "hold" them, i.e., to replace their usual drug, but also to determine that it is not excessively high, producing somnolence, lethargy, intoxication, or even respiratory suppression. One can be a little more generous with the "safe" drugs such as benzodiazepines, but one should be more cautious with those that have the capability to suppress respiration, such as barbiturates or opiates. Concern about the possibility of respiratory suppression is the reason for "test doses" and divided dosage schedules so that patients do not receive large quantities of drug at any one time. It should also be remembered that most of these drugs are metabolized in the liver and excreted by the kidney. Thus, liver disease, often present in addicts, may impair the conjugation and excretion of these drugs and their metabolites, and cause a corresponding accumulation of drug in the blood stream. Lethargy and somnolence usually indicate this phenomenon, which calls for discontinuation or sharp curtailment of the detoxification drug.

Continued Detoxification

Once the comfortable start-up dosage is established, one can generally proceed to reduce the amount of detoxification drug by approximately 10% per day. Periodic toxicology checks are advisable during the detoxification period to see if the patient is obtaining any additional medication surreptitiously. Generally, I try to keep the patient medicated to a level of mild irritability and tremor. Violent withdrawal reactions including nausea, vomiting, abdominal spasms, or seizures are to be avoided. These symptoms generally indicate that more detoxification medicine is needed. Usually the first sign of undermedication is irritability, anger, noncooperation, and a desire to leave the hospital. It is remarkable how many discharges "against medical advice" can be avoided by prompt supplements to medication.

Whenever possible, I try to administer detoxification medicines in elixir form in orange juice. Dosages are never discussed with patients, although symptoms and reactions to the medications are scrutinized closely and discussed freely. Insomnia is often present during the first few days of detoxification, and for this reason I occasionally allow a sedative to be administered at bedtime. In milder cases, I prefer 500 to 1000 mg of chloral hydrate (Noctec), and in severe cases, 100 to 200 mg of sodium pentobarbital. I generally allow this for only one to three days and then discontinue it. In the vast majority of cases, no bedtime sedatives are given.

Nursing Care

There is much to be said for good nursing care during the detoxification process. Verbal and emotional reassurance, patience, and encouragement help patients endure difficult and uncomfortable days and nights. Heating pads, hot baths, and relaxation therapies presented in a calm and dignified milieu do much to relieve tension and anxiety. If complaints of localized pain emerge as detoxification progresses, dosage reduction can be slowed, or acetaminophen can be allowed for minor discomforts. Most patients addicted to analgesics experience recurrences of localized pain as withdrawal progresses. Interestingly, this pain is generally experienced in the region that was originally painful, triggering the dependence on narcotics, perhaps years earlier. Pain is once again "felt" in that area even though the "painful" organ or limb may be normal, or may have been removed.

Supportive Therapy

Since many addicts are malnourished, aggressive nutritional support is advised, generally with vitamin supplementation. I prefer to encourage multivitamin preparations with additional vitamin C and thiamine. The usual goal of detoxification is to rid patients of all psychoactive substances. I generally try to get them to be free of all psychoactive medications for a period, such as 90 days. If, at the end of that time, it appears that nonaddictive psychiatric medications are indicated, I may cautiously initiate such treatment. I tend to prefer lithium, 150 to 300 mg t.i.d., for marked mood instability, and imipramine (Tofranil), 25 to 50 mg t.i.d., for cases of disabling depression. However, it should be emphasized that most mood lability and dysphoria in addicts is a nonspecific form of "drug hunger" that subsides spontaneously, but slowly, over a period of time. Reassurance and the avoidance of pharmacotherapy is the treatment of choice in most of these circumstances.

FOLLOW-UP

During hospitalization, the patient and physician must lay the groundwork for a long-term follow-up program and other specialized treatments. It must be decided whether an inpatient chemical dependency "rehabilitation" unit might be beneficial. I recommend these units in a large majority of cases; they generally provide an intense inpatient educational-motivational experience, overcoming denial and resistance in a supportive milieu. Most individuals require an inpatient stay of 28 days or so. If they have been through one or more of these recently, it may not be beneficial to repeat the experience if it appears that they are adequately motivated and insightful.

Urine Monitoring. The physician should try to mobilize additional long-term treatment supports, including outpatient specialized addiction counseling, preferably in a program where urine monitoring is the rule. Urine monitoring is an indispensable tool in dealing with drug-involved patients. I recommend frequent, randomized urine checks for a minimum of one to two years for most such patients. Most of these checks are obtained randomly, approximately once a week.

Self-Help Groups. Addiction self-help groups should also be a mandatory part of the recovery program. Such groups, including Alcoholics Anonymous, Narcotics Anonymous, Cocaine Anonymous, and others affiliated with treatment centers, provide frequent, powerful, therapeutic reinforcement for recovering patients. As a rule, patients must go to these self-help groups to maintain sobriety, and your task as a physician should be to endorse these organizations strongly and facilitate patients' participation. Avoid offering treatment alternatives to the self-help groups. Many physicians who are successful with chemical dependents will not even see them unless they are willing to be involved in the self-help groups. Knowledgeable physicians develop familiarity with local groups and cultivate friendships within them. Patients should become involved with the self-help groups while in the hospital. They should call the local representatives, who will visit them in the hospital or shortly after discharge.

After-Care. As the treatment physician, your role in after-care is to ask about abstinence and participation in the other treatment modalities. Continued sobriety usually hinges on regular and frequent attendance at self-help groups and professional counseling. Try to continue a physician-patient relationship after the detoxification phase. Insist that patients bring all requests for medication and other medical consultations to you *first* for your opinion. I generally prohibit the taking of any medicine other than acetaminophen without my expressed approval. Periodically check "needle addicts" for physical evidence of injection: examine the entire body surface carefully. Maintain contact with the toxicology laboratory to ascertain results of urine checks. If patients become lax in participation in any of these modalities, insist on reactivation. After detoxification, avoid the use of psychoactive drugs, especially sedatives, analgesics, and minor tranquilizers. These medications, even when taken under the supervision of a well-meaning physician, are poorly tolerated by such patients; they carry significant risk of reinducing medication dependency. I also strongly recommend to medication-dependent patients that they abstain from drinking alcohol. In many such patients, drinking escalates rapidly to full-blown alcoholism, and in others drinking leads to relapse of drug abuse. I regard alcohol as another mood-altering drug and insist on rigorous abstinence from it.

Maintain close contact with both patient and spouse for at least one to two years. In my view, the patient is never "cured"; "once an addict, always an addict." Follow-up visits may be scheduled to conform to a pattern of weekly, then bi-weekly, then monthly office visits, generally with the spouse attending or at least telephoned to ascertain compliance. As solid drug-free stability is achieved, visits can be spread out to quarterly or even yearly intervals. Give recovering patients respect and praise for maintaining an abstinence program and for participating in the treatment modalities. They have to sacrifice much in time, energy, and expense to conquer this potentially fatal illness. Understanding, praise, and firm support for "sticking to the treatment program" are the physician's most valuable psychotherapeutic tools.

REFERENCES

Collins GB, Janesz J, Byerly-Thrope J, et al: The Cleveland Clinic Alcohol Rehabilitation Program: a treatment outcome study preliminary report. Cleve Clin Q 52:245–251, 1985.
Selzer ML: The Michigan Alcoholism Screening Test: the quest for a new diagnostic instrument. Am J Psychiatry 12:1653–1658, 1971.

<h1>INDEX</h1>

Note: Page numbers in *italics* refer to illustrations. Page numbers followed by (t) refer to tables.

Abscess, acute epidural, 698
cutaneous, due to hyperimmunoglobulin E recurrent infection syndrome, 615
intra-abdominal, fever due to, 4(t)
of brain, 230–231
perianal, 433
putrid, of lung, 182–183
Accutane, for psoriasis, 624
Acetaminophen, for herpes zoster, 635
for pain, 7, 7(t)
nephropathy due to, 508
poisoning due to, 788(t)
Acetohexamide, dosing of, 546(t)
Acetylcholine receptor antibody, in myasthenia gravis, 707
Acetylcysteine, 15
N-Acetylcysteine, for poisoning, 788(t)
Acetylsalicylic acid. See *Aspirin.*
Achalasia, as precancerous condition, 388(t), 389
management of, 378
Achilles tendinitis, 749(t)
Achlorhydria, delayed gastric emptying due to, 381(t)
Acid, accidental ingestion of, 381
Acid maltase, disorder of, 561(t)
Acid-base balance, clinical derangements of, 574–577
disturbances of, 573–577
primary, 574(t)
in chronic renal failure, 491
in heat stroke, 772
in respiratory failure, 167–168
Acidosis, dyspnea and, 212
in tumor lysis syndrome, 367
metabolic, causes of, 575(t)
definition of, 575–576
in acute renal failure, 488
in chronic renal failure, 495
respiratory, causes of, 575(t)
definition of, 575
vomiting due to, 23(t)
Acne vulgaris, management of, 630–633
pathogenesis of, 630
Acquired immune deficiency syndrome, hemophilia and, 320
in homosexual males, 287(t), 288
Pneumocystis carinii pneumonia and, 261–262
Acrodermatitis enteropathica, 584
Acromegaly, clinical aspects of, 442–443
definition of, 442
management of, 443–444
Acrosclerosis, 730
Actifed, 16
Actinomycin D, emetic classification of, 369(t)
for soft tissue sarcoma, 362
Acyclovir, for herpes zoster, 635
in herpesvirus type II vaginitis, 479

Acyclovir (*Continued*)
in herpetic infection, 282–283
in outpatient therapy, 223
Addiction, definition of, 796
Addison's disease, surgery and, 58
vomiting due to, 23(t)
Adenocarcinoma, papillary
of thyroid gland, 453
pulmonary, sexual ratio in, 344
Adenoma, Hürthle cell, 452–453
macrofollicular, 452–453
Adenomectomy, transphenoidal, 445
Adenovirus, acute encephalitis due to, 234
common cold due to, 183(t), 184
exanthems due to, 255
pneumonia due to, 187
Adolescent(s), blood pressure levels of, 43, 43(t)
medical history of, 41
musculoskeletal screening examination for, 43, 43(t)
office visit and, 40
parental role and, 41
physician attitude toward, 40–41
screening tests for, 41–43, 42, 43(t)
sports physical for, 43
Adrenal gland, adenoma of, 463
carcinoma of, 463
in multiple endocrine neoplasia, 469, 469(t)
insufficiency of, 460–461
in pluriglandular autoimmune syndrome, 471, 471(t)
surgery and, 58
Adrenergic agonists. See *Beta-adrenergic agonist.*
Adrenocorticotropic hormone, deficiency of, 438–439, 460
unrecognized, 440
for multiple sclerosis, 693
Adrenocorticotropic hormone syndrome, ectopic, 463
Adult(s), healthy, medical care of, 60–63
vaccination in, 277–281
Aerobic point system, 71
Aerosols, for asthma, 166
for respiratory failure, 169
Affective disorder, bipolar
in chronic renal failure, 497
lithium toxicity in, 508
Aganglionosis, constipation in, 12(t)
Aging. See also *Elderly.*
chronic disease incidence and, 46
clinical implications of, 44–45
of U.S. population, 44–45, 44
socioeconomic impact of, 47
Agnogenic myeloid metaplasia, definition of, 336
management of, 336–337
Agoraphobia, 20

AIDS. See *Acquired immune deficiency syndrome.*
Albumin, synthesis of, in hepatic cirrhosis, 425
Albuterol, for chronic obstructive pulmonary disease, 158–159
Alcohol, abuse of. See also *Alcoholism.*
in healthy adult, 63
blood, concentration of, 791
-drug interactions, 794–795
sleep disorders and, 19
Alcoholics Anonymous, 793
Alcoholism, blood alcohol concentrations and, 791(t)
clinical aspects of, 790–791
definition of, 789
impotence and, 468
laboratory tests in, 791(t)
management of, 791–795
pancreatitis due to, 428–430, 428(t)
pathophysiology of, 789–790
screening tests for, 790
Aldosterone, deficiency of, 460–461
Alka II, neutralizing capacity of, 393(t)
Alkaline, accidental ingestion of, 381
Alkaline phosphatase, serum, in alcoholism, 791(t)
Alkalis, eye trauma due to, 718
Alkalosis, metabolic, causes of, 576(t)
definition of, 576
management of, 576–577
respiratory, causes of, 575(t)
definition of, 575
Allergen(s), antibody testing for, 609–611
food, 603–607
diagnostic diet for, 605(t)
immunotherapy for, 611–613
Allergen-specific IgE antibody test, in asthma, 163
Allergy, asthma and, 163
bronchopulmonary aspergillosis and, 166
conjunctivitis due to, 717–718
definition of, 601
to foods, 603–607
diagnosis of, 604(t)
to insect sting, 607–609
to insulin, 541
Allopurinol, acute tubulointerstitial nephritis due to, 509, 509(t)
fever due to, 4(t)
for gout, 568
for hyperuricemia, 566
for urate nephropathy, 509
in polycythemia rubra vera, 307
in renal impairment, 525
Alpha gene, in thalassemias, 304, 304(t)
Alpha-adrenergic agonists, in renal impairment, 524